Current Medical Diagnosis & Treatment 1991

Edited By

Steven A. Schroeder, MD
President, Robert Wood Johnson Foundation
Princeton, New Jersey
Clinical Professor of Medicine
University of Medicine & Dentistry of New Jersey
Robert Wood Johnson Medical School
Piscataway, New Jersey

Marcus A. Krupp, MD
Clinical Professor of Medicine Emeritus
Stanford University School of Medicine, Stanford
Director (Emeritus) of Research Institute
Palo Alto Medical Foundation, Palo Alto

Lawrence M. Tierney, Jr., MD
Professor of Medicine
University of California, San Francisco
Assistant Chief of Medical Services
Veterans Administration Medical Center, San Francisco

Stephen J. McPhee, MD
Associate Professor of Medicine
Division of General Internal Medicine
University of California, San Francisco

with Associate Authors

Appleton & Lange
Norwalk, Connecticut/San Mateo, California

0-8385-1430-8

91 92 93 94 95 / 10 9 8 7 6 5 4 3 2 1

Prentice-Hall International (UK) Limited, *London*
Prentice-Hall of Australia, Pty. Limited, *Sydney*
Prentice-Hall Canada, Inc. *Toronto*
Prentice-Hall Hispanoamericana, S.A., *Mexico*
Prentice-Hall of India Private Limited, *New Delhi*
Prentice-Hall of Japan, Inc., *Tokyo*
Simon & Schuster Asia Pte. Ltd., *Singapore*
Editora Prentice-Hall do Brasil Ltda., *Rio de Janeiro*
Prentice-Hall, Englewood Cliffs, *New Jersey*

ISBN: 0-8385-1430-8
ISSN: 0092-8682

Production Editor: Christine Langan
Cover: Steve Byrum

PRINTED IN THE UNITED STATES OF AMERICA

Table of Contents

Appendix 1191

Index 1207

From inability to let alone; from too much zeal for the new and contempt for what is old; from putting knowledge before wisdom, and science before art and cleverness before common sense; from treating patients as cases; and from making the cure of the disease more grievous than the endurance of the same, Good Lord, deliver us.

—*Sir Robert Hutchison*

Preface

Current Medical Diagnosis & Treatment 1991 is the 30th annual volume of a general medical text designed as a single-source reference for practitioners in both hospital and ambulatory settings. CMDT covers all internal medicine fields plus important topics outside internal medicine, emphasizing the practical features of diagnosis and patient management. Appropriate biochemical and pathophysiologic background information is provided as necessary to facilitate understanding of concepts.

OUTSTANDING FEATURES

- Reissued annually in January to incorporate current advances.
- All aspects of internal medicine plus gynecology/obstetrics, dermatology, ophthalmology, otolaryngology, psychiatry, neurology, and other topics of concern to the primary care physician and to all specialists who provide generalist care.
- Consistent, readable format, permitting efficient use in various practice settings.
- More than 1000 diseases and disorders.
- Only book of its kind to include an annual update on AIDS.
- Quick reference index to common presenting problems on inside front cover.
- Emphasis on prevention and cost-consciousness, reflecting the realities of modern medical practice.
- Brevity, conciseness, and easy accessibility of key information.
- Inexpensively priced.

INTENDED AUDIENCE

House officers and medical students will find the concise, up-to-date descriptions of diagnostic and therapeutic procedures, with citations to the current literature, of daily usefulness in the immediate management of patients.

Internists, family physicians, and other specialists who provide generalist care will find CMDT useful as a ready reference and refresher text.

Physicians in other specialties, surgeons, and dentists will find the book useful as a basic treatise on internal medicine.

Nurses and other health practitioners will find that the concise format and broad scope of the book facilitate their understanding of diagnostic principles and therapeutic procedures.

ORGANIZATION

CMDT is developed chiefly by organ system. Chapter 1 presents general information on patient care, including health maintenance and disease prevention, test selection and interpretation, and management of pain and other common symptoms. Chapter 2 addresses special problems of the elderly patient. Chapter 3 discusses medical management of cancer. Chapters 4—21 describe diseases and disorders and their treatment. Chapter 22 sets forth the basic concepts of nutrition in modern medical practice. Chapters 23—31 cover infectious diseases and antimicrobial therapy. Chapters 32—34 cover special topics: physical agents, poisoning, and medical genetics. The Appendix provides data on commonly used laboratory tests and diagnostic imaging techniques.

NEW TO THIS EDITION

- Drug information and bibliographies updated through May, 1990.
- Greatly revised and reorganized chapters on Infectious Diseases, including an up-to-date, expanded chapter on AIDS and information on AIDS in other relevant chapters.
- An update on antibiotics.
- Totally new chapter on Medical Genetics.
- Substantially revised chapter on the Heart and Great Vessels.
- Major changes and additions to the chapter on Arthritis and Musculoskeletal Disorders, Introduction to Infectious Diseases, Bacterial and Chlamydial Infections, and Poisoning—including a late comment on Chemical Warfare Agents added in October 1990.

ACKNOWLEDGEMENTS

We wish to thank our associate authors for participating once again in the annual updating of this important book. Many students and physicians have contributed useful suggestions to this and previous editions, and we are grateful. We continue to welcome comments and recommendations for future editions.

Steven A. Schroeder, MD
Marcus A. Krupp, MD
Lawrence M. Tierney, Jr., MD
Stephen J. McPhee, MD

San Francisco, California
November, 1990

Authors

Michael J. Aminoff, MD, FRCP
Professor of Neurology, University of California, San Francisco
Nervous System

Robert B. Baron, MD
Associate Professor of Clinical Medicine and Director of Primary Care, Internal Medicine Residency Program, University of California, San Francisco
Nutrition

James J. Brophy, MD
Associate Clinical Professor of Psychiatry, University of California School of Medicine, San Diego
Psychiatric Disorders

Carlos A. Camargo, MD
Associate Clinical Professor of Medicine, Stanford University School of Medicine, Stanford, California
Endocrine Disorders

Henry F. Chambers, MD
Associate Professor of Medicine, Division of Infectious Diseases, University of California, San Francisco, and San Francisco General Hospital
Infectious Diseases: Bacterial & Chlamydial

Richard Cohen, MD, MPH
Associate Clinical Professor, Division of Occupational Medicine, University of California, San Francisco
Disorders Due to Physical Agents

John M. Erskine, MD
Associate Clinical Professor of Surgery, University of California, San Francisco; and Associate in Surgery, Stanford University School of Medicine, Stanford, California
Blood Vessels & Lymphatics

Lawrence Z. Feigenbaum, MD
Clinical Professor of Medicine, University of California, San Francisco; and Associate Chief of Medicine, Mount Zion Medical Center of the University of California, San Francisco
Geriatric Medicine & the Elderly Patient

Armando E. Giuliano, MD
Professor of Surgery, University of California, Los Angeles
Breast

Robert S. Goldsmith, MD, MPH, DTM&H
Professor of Tropical Medicine and Epidemiology, University of California, San Francisco
Infectious Diseases: Protozoal; Infectious Diseases: Helminthic

Sadja Greenwood, MD, MPH
Assistant Clinical Professor of Obstetrics, Gynecology, and Reproductive Sciences, University of California, San Francisco
Gynecology & Obstetrics

Moses Grossman, MD
Professor of Pediatrics, University of California, San Francisco; and Chief of Pediatrics, San Francisco General Hospital
Infectious Diseases: Viral & Rickettsial; Infectious Diseases: Bacterial & Chlamydial

Carlyn Halde, PhD
Professor of Microbiology and Immunology and Professor of Dermatology, University of California, San Francisco
Infectious Diseases: Mycotic

David B. Hellman, MD
Mary Betty Stevens Associate Professor of Medicine, Deputy Directory of Department of Medicine, and Clinical Director of Division of Molecular and Clinical Rheumatology, The Johns Hopkins Hospital, Baltimore.
Arthritis & Musculoskeletal Disorders

Harry Hollander, MD
Associate Professor of Clinical Medicine and Director, AIDS Clinic, University of California, San Francisco
AIDS & Related Conditions; Infectious Diseases: Mycotic

Robert K. Jackler, MD
Assistant Clinical Professor of Otolaryngology, University of California, San Francisco
Ear, Nose, & Throat

Richard A. Jacobs, MD, PhD
Associate Clinical Professor of Medicine and Co-director, Outpatient Infectious Disease Service, University of California, San Francisco
Introduction to Infectious Diseases; Infectious Diseases: Spirochetal; Anti-infective Chemotherapeutic & Antibiotic Agents

Ernest Jawetz, MD, PhD
Professor of Microbiology and Medicine Emeritus, University of California, San Francisco
Infections of the Urinary Tract; Infectious Diseases: Viral & Rickettsial; Infectious Diseases: Bacterial & Chlamydial; Anti-infective Chemotherapeutic & Antibiotic Agents

Michael J. Kaplan, MD
Assistant Professor, Department of Otolaryngology-Head and Neck Surgery, University of California, San Francisco; and Chief, Otolaryngology-Head and Neck Surgery, San Francisco Veterans Administration Medical Center
Ear, Nose, & Throat

John H. Karam, MD
Professor of Medicine, Director of Diabetes Clinic, and Chief of Clinical Endocrinology, University of California, San Francisco
Diabetes Mellitus, Hypoglycemia, & Lipoprotein Disorders

Mitchell H. Katz, MD
Clinical Instructor of Medicine, Department of General Internal Medicine, University of California, San Francisco
AIDS & Related Conditions

C. Michael Knauer, MD
Chief of Division of Gastroenterology, Santa Clara Valley Medical Center, San Jose, California; and Clinical Professor of Medicine, Stanford University School of Medicine, Stanford, California
Alimentary Tract & Liver

Marcus A. Krupp, MD
Clinical Professor of Medicine Emeritus, Stanford University School of Medicine, Stanford, California; and Director Emeritus of Research Institute, Palo Alto Medical Foundation, Palo Alto, California
Fluid & Electrolyte Disorders; Genitourinary Tract; Normal Laboratory Values

Joseph LaDou, MD
Clinical Professor of Medicine and Chief, Division of Occupational and Environmental Medicine, University of California, San Francisco
Disorders Due to Physical Agents

Charles A. Linker, MD
Associate Clinical Professor of Medicine, University of California, San Francisco
Blood

Alan J. Margolis, MD
Professor of Obstetrics, Gynecology, and Reproductive Sciences Emeritus, University of California, San Francisco
Gynecology & Obstetrics

Barry M. Massie, MD
Professor of Medicine, University of California, San Francisco; Associate Staff Member, Cardiovascular Research Institute; and Chief, Hypertension Unit, and Director, Coronary Care Unit, San Francisco Veterans Administration Medical Center
Heart & Great Vessels

Richard B. Odom, MD
Clinical Professor of Dermatology, University of California, San Francisco
Skin & Appendages

Stephen J. McPhee, MD
Associate Professor of Medicine, Division of General Internal Medicine, University of California, San Francisco
General Approach to the Patient; Health Maintenance & Disease Prevention; Principles of Diagnostic Test Selection & Use; & Common Symptoms

Richard B. Odom, MD
Clinical Professor of Dermatology, University of California, San Francisco
Skin & Appendages

Kent R. Olson, MD
Assistant Clinical Professor of Medicine and Adjunct Lecturer in Pharmacy, University of California, San Francisco; and Medical Director of the San Francisco Bay Area Regional Poison Control Center
Poisoning

Reed E. Pyeritz, MD, PhD
Professor of Medicine and Pediatrics, Johns Hopkins University School of Medicine; Clinical Director, Center for Medical Genetics, Johns Hopkins Hospital, Baltimore
Medical Genetics

Rees B. Rees, Jr., MD
Clinical Professor of Dermatology Emeritus, University of California, San Francisco
Skin & Appendages

Paul Riordan-Eva, FRCS, FCOphth
Registrar in Ophthalmology, Moorfields Eye Hospital, London
Eye

Sydney E. Salmon, MD
Regents' Professor of Internal Medicine (Hematology and Oncology), University of Arizona College of Medicine, Tucson, Arizona; and Director of Arizona Cancer Center, Tucson
Malignant Disorders

Steven A. Schroeder, MD
President, Robert Wood Johnson Foundation, Princeton, New Jersey; Clinical Professor of Medicine, University of Medicine & Dentistry of New Jersey, Robert Wood Johnson Medical School, Piscataway, New Jersey
General Approach to the Patient; Health Maintenance & Disease Prevention; Principles of Diagnostic Test Selection & Use; & Common Symptoms

Martin A. Shearn, MD
Clinical Professor of Medicine Emeritus, University of California, San Francisco
Arthritis & Musculoskeletal Disorders

Sol Silverman, Jr., DDS
Professor of Oral Medicine and Chairman of the Division, University of California, San Francisco
Diseases of the Mouth

Maurice Sokolow, MD
Professor of Medicine Emeritus and Senior Staff Member, Cardiovascular Research Institute, University of California, San Francisco
Heart & Great Vessels

John L. Stauffer, MD
Associate Professor of Medicine, College of Medicine, The Pennsylvania State University; and Attending Physician, The Milton S. Hershey Medical Center, Hershey, Pennsylvania
Pulmonary Diseases

Daniel P. Stites, MD
Professor and Vice Chairman of the Laboratory Medicine Department and Director of the Immunology Laboratory, University of California, San Francisco
Allergic & Immunologic Disorders

Abba Terr, MD
Clinical Professor of Medicine, Stanford University School of Medicine, Stanford, California
Allergic & Immunologic Disorders

Lawrence M. Tierney, Jr., MD
Professor of Medicine, University of California, San Francisco; and Assistant Chief of Medical Services, San Francisco Veterans Administration Medical Center
Blood Vessels & Lymphatics; Infectious Diseases: Viral & Rickettsial

Daniel G. Vaughan, MD
Clinical Professor of Ophthalmology, University of California, San Francisco; and Member, Francis I. Proctor Foundation for Research in Ophthalmology, San Francisco
Eye

Susan D. Wall, MD
Associate Professor of Radiology, University of California, San Francisco; and Assistant Chief of Radiology, San Francisco Veterans Administration Medical Center
Selected Imaging Procedures: Descriptions, Indications, & Costs

General Approach to the Patient; Health Maintenance & Disease Prevention; Principles of Diagnostic Test Selection & Use; & Common Symptoms

1

Steven A. Schroeder, MD, & Stephen J. McPhee, MD

GENERAL APPROACH TO THE PATIENT

Arriving at a correct diagnosis and ensuring the best treatment and outcome for every patient are the ultimate missions of medical care. This book is a reservoir—replenished annually—of instructions and guidelines for medical practitioners. The successful practitioner, however, is more than a receptacle for facts that make up the body of knowledge called medicine. Success in diagnosis and treatment can only be achieved by considering all of the complex personal, familial, and economic circumstances of our patients and their families and by establishing and maintaining a supportive and open relationship with every patient.

The approach to diagnosis begins with the history and pertinent physical examination. If diagnostic procedures are indicated, they must be based on principles of diagnostic test selection, which in turn depend on principles of test characteristics (sensitivity and specificity), disease incidence and prevalence, the potential risk to the patient, and the cost:benefit profile of the test determined by reference to the indications for it. Appropriate treatment involves more than merely deciding what drug, operation, or other treatment is called for. Successful treatment—particularly management of patients with chronic illnesses—must be tailored to the circumstances of the individual patient and reinforced by a well-established doctor-patient relationship. For many illnesses, treatment depends on fundamental behavioral changes—including alterations in diet, exercise, smoking, and drinking—that may be difficult even for motivated patients. Compliance with prescribed drug regimens is a problem in every practice, with up to 50% of patients failing to achieve full compliance and a third never taking their medicines at all. Patient compliance is improved when strong and trusting doctor-patient relationships have been established.

Fundamental ethical principles must also undergird a successful approach to diagnosis and treatment: honesty, beneficence, justice, avoidance of conflict of interest, and the pledge to do no harm. Increasingly, Western medicine has involved patients in important decisions about medical care, including how far to proceed with treatment of patients who have terminal illnesses.

Finally, the physician's role does not end with diagnosis and the prescribing of a treatment regimen. The importance of the physician in helping patients and their families bear the burden of serious illness and death cannot be overemphasized. "To cure sometimes, to relieve often, and to comfort always" is a French saying as apt today as it was 5 centuries ago—as is Francis Peabody's admonition: "The secret of the care of the patient is in caring for the patient."

Green LW: How physicians can improve patients' participation and maintenance in self-care. West J Med 1987; 147:346.

Jonsen AR, Siegler M, Winslade WJ: *Clinical Ethics: A Practical Approach to Ethical Decisions in Clinical Medicine.* Macmillan, 1982.

HEALTH MAINTENANCE & DISEASE PREVENTION

Preventing disease is more important than treating it. Preventive medicine is categorized as primary, secondary, or tertiary. Examples in the case of cancer are giving up or not starting smoking, thereby reducing the incidence of lung carcinoma (primary prevention); routine periodic surveillance by cervical Papanicolaou smear (secondary prevention); and mastectomy to remove localized breast cancer (tertiary prevention). Primary prevention is by far the most effective and economical of all methods of disease control.

Table 1–1 lists the 5 leading causes of death in the USA, along with important risk factors linked to these causes. Physicians can have a major role in reducing almost all of these risk factors, thereby improving their patients' health.

Health maintenance and disease prevention usually begin with the office or clinic encounter. Table 1–2 lists recent recommendations for the periodic health examination as developed by the US Preventive Services Task Force. These recommendations include a variety of maneuvers: inquiring about and counseling for various risk factors, performing parts of the physical examination, and selecting laboratory and radiologic tests and procedures. The recommendations of the Task Force are stratified by age group, reflecting the different epidemiologic risks appropriate for each group. Based on a critical review of available evidence, the recommendations emphasize counseling activities and are more conservative about routine use of such procedures as periodic sigmoidoscopy than were earlier guidelines from groups such as the

Table 1–1. The 5 leading causes of death in the USA and associated modifiable risk factors.[1]

Cause of Death	Risk Factors
1. Cardiovascular disease	Tobacco use
	Elevated serum cholesterol
	High blood pressure
	Obesity
	Diabetes mellitus
	Sedentary life-style
2. Cancer	Tobacco use
	Improper diet
	Alcohol
	Occupational and environmental exposures
3. Cerebrovascular disease	High blood pressure
	Tobacco use
	Elevated serum cholesterol
4. Accidental injuries	Safety belt noncompliance
	Cycle helmet noncompliance
	Alcohol and substance abuse
	Reckless driving
	Occupational hazards
	Guns in the home
	Stress and fatigue
5. Chronic lung disease	Tobacco use
	Occupational and environmental exposures

[1] Adapted from National Center for Health Statistics/U.S. Department of Health and Human Services: *Health United States: 1986.* DHHS Pub. No. (PHS) 87–1232, 1987.

American Cancer Society. Cost considerations may limit the application of some of these (eg, mammography), depending on the setting and the circumstances.

Report of the US Preventive Services Task Force: Guide to Clinical Preventive Services. Williams & Wilkins, 1989. (Summary of extensive Task Force deliberations on the evidence for efficacy of prevention strategies.)

INFECTIOUS DISEASES

The impressive 20th century accomplishments in immunization and antibiotic therapy notwithstanding, much of the decline in the incidence and fatality rates of infectious diseases is attributable to improved social conditions and public health measures—especially improved sanitation, better nutrition, and greater prosperity.

Immunization remains the best means of preventing many infectious diseases, including tetanus, diphtheria, poliomyelitis, measles, mumps, rubella, hepatitis B, yellow fever, influenza, and pneumococcal pneumonia. Recommended immunization schedules for children and adults are set forth in Table 23–4. Persons traveling to countries where infections are endemic should take special precautions, as described in Chapter 23.

Skin testing for tuberculosis and then treating selected skin-positive patients with prophylactic isoniazid reduces the risk of reactivation tuberculosis. Treatment is recommended for high-risk reactors regardless of age. These patients include recent tuberculin converters, postgastrectomy patients, persons taking immunosuppressive drugs, patients with silicosis, and patients who test positive for infection with HIV. For tuberculin-positive patients without these risk factors, treatment with isoniazid is recommended only for those under the age of 35 in order to minimize the risk of drug-induced hepatitis. It now appears that prophylaxis for only 6 months (300 mg daily) is as effective as 12 months. BCG vaccine should be reserved for use in selected cases, such as protection of health workers in areas where tuberculosis is endemic.

AIDS is now the major infectious disease problem in the Western world. Until a vaccine or cure is found, prevention will be the major weapon against this disease. Since sexual contact is the usual mode of transmission, prevention must rely on safe sexual practices. These include abstinence, prudent selection of partners, avoidance of promiscuity, the use of condoms, and the limiting or avoidance of anal sex except with partners known to be uninfected (see Chapter 24). Increasingly, cases of HIV infection are transmitted among users of intravenous narcotics and crack cocaine. In some instances, sexual transmission occurs, as with drug addicts who support their habit by prostitution. In other cases, infection occurs by transmission

Table 1–2. Prevention surveillance in office practice. (Modified from: 1989 Report of the US Preventive Services Task Force: Guide to Clinical Preventive Services.)

I. Patients Ages 13–18

Leading causes of death:
- Motor vehicle crashes
- Homicide
- Suicide
- Injuries (non-motor vehicle)
- Heart disease

Schedule: One visit is required for immunizations. Because of lack of data and differing patient risk profiles, the scheduling of additional visits and the frequency of the individual preventive services listed in this table are left to clinical discretion (except as otherwise indicated below).

Remain alert for:
- Depressive symptoms
- Suicide risk factors: Depression, alcohol or other drug abuse, serious medical illnesses, or recent bereavement.
- Abnormal bereavement
- Tooth decay, malalignment, gingivitis
- Signs of child abuse and neglect

SCREENING

History
- Dietary intake
- Physical activity
- Tobacco/alcohol/drug use
- Sexual practices

Physical exam
- Height and weight
- Blood pressure

HIGH-RISK GROUPS
- Complete skin exam: Persons with increased recreational or occupational exposure to sunlight, a family or personal history of skin cancer, or clinical evidence of precursor lesions (eg, dysplastic nevi, certain congenital nevi).
- Clinical testicular exam: Males with a history of cryptorchidism, orchiopexy, or testicular atrophy.

Laboratory and diagnostic procedures

HIGH-RISK GROUPS
- Rubella antibodies: Females of childbearing age lacking evidence of immunity.
- VDRL: Persons who engage in sex with multiple partners, prostitutes, or contacts of persons with active syphilis.
- Chlamydial testing: Persons who attend clinics for sexually transmitted diseases; attend other high-risk health care facilities (eg, adolescent and family planning clinics); or have other risk factors for chlamydial infection (eg, multiple sex partners or a sexual partner with multiple sexual contacts).
- Gonorrhea culture: Persons with multiple sexual partners or a sexual partner with multiple contacts, sexual contact of persons with culture-proved gonorrhea, or persons with a history of repeated episodes of gonorrhea.
- Counseling and testing for HIV: Persons seeking treatment for sexually transmitted diseases; homosexual and bisexual men; past or present intravenous drug users; persons with a history of prostitution or multiple sexual partners; women whose past or present sexual partners were HIV-infected, bisexual, or intravenous drug users; persons with long-term residence or birth in an area with high prevalence of HIV infections; or persons with a history of transfusion between 1978 and 1985.
- Tuberculin skin test (PPD): Household contacts of persons with tuberculosis or others at risk for close exposure to infection; recent immigrants or refugees from countries in which tuberculosis is common (eg, Asia, Africa, Central and South America, Pacific Islands); migrant workers; residents of correctional institutions or homeless shelters; or persons with certain underlying medical disorders.
- Hearing: Persons exposed regularly to excessive noise in recreational or other settings.

COUNSELING

Diet and exercise
- Fat (especially saturated fat), cholesterol, sodium, iron (for females), calcium (for females)
- Caloric balance
- Selection of exercise program

Substance use
- Tobacco: cessation/primary prevention
- Alcohol and other drugs:
  - Driving/other dangerous activities while under the influence
  - Treatment for abuse

HIGH-RISK GROUPS
- Sharing/using unsterilized needles and syringes (intravenous drug users)

Sexual practices
- Sexual development and behavior (counseling often best performed early in adolescence and with the involvement of the parents)
- Sexually transmitted diseases: partner selection, condoms
- Unintended pregnancy and contraceptive options

Injury prevention
- Safety belts
- Safety helmets
- Violent behavior (for males)
- Firearms (for males)
- Smoke detector

Table 1–2 (cont'd). Prevention surveillance in office practice.

I. Patients Ages 13–18 (cont'd)

Dental health: Regular tooth brushing, flossing, dental visits
Other primary preventive measures
  HIGH-RISK GROUPS
    Discussion of hemoglobin testing: Persons of Caribbean, Latin American, Asian, Mediterranean, or African descent.
    Skin protection from ultraviolet light: Persons with increased exposure to sunlight.
IMMUNIZATION AND CHEMOPROPHYLAXIS
  Tetanus-diphtheria (Td) booster once between ages 14 and 16
    HIGH-RISK GROUPS
      Fluoride supplements: Persons living in areas with inadequate water fluoridation (< 0.7 ppm).

II. Patients Ages 19–39

Leading causes of death: Same as for ages 13–18.
Schedule: Periodic visit every 1–3 years.
Remain alert for:
  Depressive symptoms
  Suicide risk factors: Recent divorce, separation, unemployment, depression, alcohol or other drug abuse, serious medical illnesses, living alone, or recent bereavement.
  Abnormal bereavement
  Malignant skin lesions
  Tooth decay, gingivitis
  Signs of physical abuse
SCREENING
  History and physical exam: Same as for ages 13–18.
    HIGH-RISK GROUPS
      Complete oral cavity exam: Persons with exposure to tobacco or excessive amounts of alcohol, or those with suspicious symptoms or lesions detected through self-examination.
      Palpation for thyroid nodules: Persons with a history of upper-body irradiation.
      Clinical breast exam: Women aged 35 and older with a family history of premenopausally diagnosed breast cancer in a first-degree relative.
      Clinical testicular exam: Men with a history of cryptorchidism, orchiopexy, or testicular atrophy.
      Complete skin exam: Persons with family or personal history of skin cancer, increased occupational or recreational exposure to sunlight, or clinical evidence of precursor lesions (eg, dysplastic nevi, certain congenital nevi).
  Laboratory and diagnostic procedures
    Nonfasting total blood cholesterol
    Papanicolaou smear (every 1–3 years)
    HIGH-RISK GROUPS
      Fasting plasma glucose: The markedly obese, persons with a family history of diabetes, or women with a history of gestational diabetes.
      Rubella antibodies: Women lacking evidence of immunity.
      VDRL: Prostitutes, persons who engage in sex with multiple partners, or contacts of persons with active syphilis.
      Urinalysis for bacteriuria: Persons with diabetes.
      Chlamydial testing: Persons who attend clinics for sexually transmitted diseases, attend other high-risk health care facilities (eg, adolescent and family planning clinics), or have other risk factors for chlamydial infection (eg, multiple sexual partners or a sexual partner with multiple sexual contacts, age less than 20).
      Gonorrhea culture: Prostitutes, persons with multiple sexual partners or a sexual partner with multiple contacts, sexual contacts of persons with culture-proved gonorrhea, or persons with a history of repeated episodes of gonorrhea.
      Counseling and testing for HIV: Persons seeking treatment for sexually transmitted diseases; homosexual and bisexual men; past or present intravenous drug users; persons with a history of prostitution or multiple sexual partners; women whose past or present sexual partners were HIV-infected, bisexual, or intravenous drug users; persons with long-term residence or birth in an area with high prevalence of HIV infection; or persons with a history of transfusion between 1978 and 1985.
      Hearing: Persons exposed regularly to excessive noise.
      Tuberculin skin test (PPD): Household contacts of persons with tuberculosis or others at risk for close exposure to infection (eg, staff of tuberculosis clinics, shelters for the homeless, nursing homes, substance abuse treatment facilities, dialysis units, correctional institutions); recent immigrants or refugees from countries in which tuberculosis is common; migrant workers; residents of nursing homes, correctional institutions, or homeless shelters; or persons with certain underlying medical disorders (eg, HIV infection).
      Electrocardiogram: Persons who would endanger public safety were they to experience sudden cardiac events (eg, commercial airline pilots).
      Mammogram: Women aged 35 and older with a family history of premenopausally diagnosed breast cancer in a first-degree relative.
      Colonoscopy: Persons with a family history of familial polyposis coli or cancer family syndrome.
COUNSELING
  Diet and exercise: Same as for ages 13–18.
  Substance use:
    Tobacco: cessation/primary prevention
    Alcohol and other drugs:
      Limiting alcohol consumption

Table 1–2 (cont'd). Prevention surveillance in office practice.

II. Patients Ages 19–39 (cont'd)

Driving/other dangerous activities while under the influence
Treatment for abuse
HIGH-RISK GROUPS: Same as for ages 13–18.
Sexual practices
Sexually transmitted diseases: partner selection, condoms, anal intercourse
Unintended pregnancy and contraceptive options
Injury prevention
Safety belts
Safety helmets
Violent behavior (for young males)
Firearms (for young males)
Smoke detector
Smoking near bedding or upholstery
HIGH-RISK GROUPS
Back-conditioning exercises: Persons at increased risk for low back injury because of past history, body configuration, or type of activities.
Prevention of childhood injuries: Persons with children in the home or automobile.
Falls in the elderly: Persons with older adults in the home.
Dental health: Regular tooth brushing, flossing, dental visits.
Other primary preventive measures
HIGH-RISK GROUPS: Same as for ages 13–18.

IMMUNIZATIONS
Tetanus-diphtheria (Td) booster (every 10 years)
HIGH-RISK GROUPS
Hepatitis B vaccine: Homosexually active men, intravenous drug users, recipients of some blood products, or persons in health-related jobs with frequent exposure to blood or blood products.
Pneumococcal vaccine: Persons with medical conditions that increase the risk of pneumococcal infection (eg, chronic cardiac or pulmonary disease, sickle cell disease, nephrotic syndrome, Hodgkin's disease, asplenia, diabetes mellitus, alcoholism, cirrhosis, multiple myeloma, renal disease, or conditions associated with immunosuppression).
Influenza vaccine (annually): Residents of chronic care facilities or persons suffering from chronic cardiopulmonary disorders, metabolic diseases (including diabetes mellitus), hemoglobinopathies, immunosuppression, or renal dysfunction.
Measles-mumps-rubella vaccine: Persons born after 1956 who lack evidence of immunity to measles (receipt of live vaccine on or after first birthday, laboratory evidence of immunity, or a history of physician-diagnosed measles).

III. Patients Ages 40–64

Leading causes of death:
Heart disease
Lung cancer
Cerebrovascular disease
Breast cancer
Colorectal cancer
Obstructive lung disease
Schedule: Periodic visit every 1–3 years.
Remain alert for:
Depressive symptoms
Suicide risk factors: Recent divorce, separation, unemployment, depression, alcohol or other drug abuse, serious medical illnesses, living alone, or recent bereavement.
Abnormal bereavement
Signs of physical abuse or neglect
Malignant skin lesions
Peripheral arterial disease: Persons over age 50, smokers, or persons with diabetes mellitus.
Tooth decay, gingivitis, loose teeth

SCREENING
History: Same as for ages 13–18.
Physical exam
Height and weight
Blood pressure
Clinical breast exam (annually for women)

HIGH-RISK GROUPS
Complete skin exam: Persons with a family or personal history of skin cancer, increased occupational or recreational exposure to sunlight, or clinical evidence of precursor lesions (eg, dysplastic nevi, certain congenital nevi).
Complete oral cavity exam: Persons with exposure to tobacco or excessive amounts of alcohol, or those with suspicious symptoms or lesions detected through self-examination.
Palpation for thyroid nodules: Persons with a history of upper-body irradiation.
Laboratory/diagnostic procedures
Nonfasting total blood cholesterol

Table 1–2 (cont'd). Prevention surveillance in office practice.

III. Patients Ages 40–64 (cont'd)

Papanicolaou smear (every 1–3 years for women)
Mammogram (every 1–2 years for women beginning at age 50)

HIGH-RISK GROUPS

Fasting plasma glucose: The markedly obese, persons with a family history of diabetes, or women with a history of gestational diabetes.

VDRL: Prostitutes, persons who engage in sex with multiple partners, or contacts of persons with active syphilis.

Urinalysis for bacteriuria: Persons with diabetes.

Chlamydial testing: Persons who attend clinics for sexually transmitted diseases, attend other high-risk health care facilities (eg, adolescent and family planning clinics), or have other risk factors for chlamydial infection (eg, multiple sexual partners or a sexual partner with multiple sexual contacts).

Gonorrhea culture: Prostitutes, persons with multiple sexual partners or a sexual partner with multiple contacts, sexual contacts of persons with culture-proved gonorrhea, or persons with a history of repeated episodes of gonorrhea.

Counseling and testing for HIV: Persons seeking treatment for sexually transmitted diseases; homosexual and bisexual men; past or present intravenous drug users; persons with a history of prostitution or multiple sexual partners; women whose past or present sexual partners were HIV-infected, bisexual, or intravenous drug users; persons with long-term residence or birth in an area with high prevalence of HIV infection; or persons with a history of transfusion between 1978 and 1985.

Tuberculin skin test (PPD): Household contacts of persons with tuberculosis or others at risk for close exposure to infection (eg, staff of tuberculosis clinics, shelters for the homeless, nursing homes, substance abuse treatment facilities, dialysis units, correctional institutions); recent immigrants or refugees from countries in which tuberculosis is common (eg, Asia, Africa, Central and South America, Pacific Islands); migrant workers; residents of nursing homes, correctional institutions, or homeless shelters; or persons with certain underlying medical disorders (eg, HIV infection).

Hearing: Persons exposed regularly to excessive noise.

Electrocardiogram: Men with 2 or more cardiac risk factors (high blood cholesterol, hypertension, cigarette smoking, diabetes mellitus, family history of coronary artery disease); men who would endanger public safety were they to experience sudden cardiac events (eg, commercial airline pilots); or sedentary or high-risk males planning to begin a vigorous exercise program.

Fecal occult blood/sigmoidoscopy: Persons aged 50 and older who have first-degree relatives with colorectal cancer; a personal history of endometrial, ovarian, or breast cancer; or a previous diagnosis of inflammatory bowel disease, adenomatous polyps, or colorectal cancer.

Fecal occult blood/colonoscopy: Persons with a family history of familial polyposis coli or cancer family syndrome.

Bone mineral content: Perimenopausal women at increased risk for osteoporosis (eg, Caucasian race, bilateral oophorectomy before menopause, slender build) and for whom estrogen replacement therapy would otherwise not be recommended.

COUNSELING

Diet and exercise
Fat (especially saturated fat), cholesterol, complex carbohydrates, fiber, sodium, calcium (for women)
Caloric balance
Selection of exercise program
Substance use: Same as for ages 19–39.
Sexual practices
Sexually transmitted diseases: partner selection, condoms, anal intercourse
Unintended pregnancy and contraceptive options
Injury prevention
Safety belts
Safety helmets
Smoke detector
Smoking near bedding or upholstery
HIGH-RISK GROUPS: Same as for ages 19–39.
Dental health: Regular tooth brushing, flossing, dental visits
Other primary preventive measures
HIGH-RISK GROUPS

Skin protection from ultraviolet light: Persons with increased exposure to sunlight.

Discussion of aspirin therapy: Men who have risk factors for myocardial infarction (eg, high blood cholesterol, smoking, diabetes mellitus, family history of early-onset coronary artery disease) and who lack a history of gastrointestinal or other bleeding problems, and other risk factors for bleeding or cerebral hemorrhage.

Discussion of estrogen replacement therapy: Perimenopausal women at increased risk for osteoporosis (eg, Caucasian, low bone mineral content, bilateral oophorectomy before menopause or early menopause, slender build) and who are without known contraindications (eg, history of undiagnosed vaginal bleeding, active liver disease, thromboembolic disorders, hormone-dependent cancer).

IMMUNIZATIONS

Tetanus-diphtheria (Td) booster (every 10 years)
HIGH-RISK GROUPS

Hepatitis B vaccine: Homosexually active men, intravenous drug users, recipients of some blood products, or persons in health-related jobs with frequent exposure to blood or blood products.

Pneumococcal influenza vaccine: Persons with medical conditions that increase the risk of pneumococcal infection (eg, chronic cardiac or pulmonary disease, sickle cell disease, nephrotic syndrome, Hodgkin's disease, asplenia, diabetes mellitus, alcoholism, cirrhosis, multiple myeloma, renal disease, or conditions associated with immunosuppression).

Influenza vaccine: Residents of chronic care facilities and persons suffering from chronic cardiopulmonary disorders, metabolic diseases (including diabetes mellitus), hemoglobinopathies, immunosuppression, or renal dysfunction.

Table 1-2 (cont'd). Prevention surveillance in office practice.

IV. Patients Ages 65 and Over

Leading causes of death:
> Heart disease
> Cerebrovascular disease
> Obstructive lung disease
> Pneumonia/influenza
> Lung cancer
> Colorectal cancer

Schedule: Periodic visit every year.

Remain alert for:
> Depressive symptoms
> Suicide risk factors: Recent divorce, separation, unemployment, depression, alcohol or other drug abuse, serious medical illnesses, living alone, or recent bereavement.
> Abnormal bereavement
> Changes in cognitive function
> Medications that increase risk of falls
> Signs of physical abuse or neglect
> Malignant skin lesions
> Peripheral arterial disease
> Tooth decay, gingivitis, loose teeth

SCREENING

History
> Prior symptoms of transient ischemic attack
> Dietary intake
> Physical activity
> Tobacco/alcohol/drug use
> Functional status at home

Physical exam
> Height and weight
> Blood pressure
> Visual acuity
> Hearing and hearing aids
> Clinical breast exam (annually for women until age 75, unless pathology detected)

HIGH-RISK GROUPS
> Complete skin exam: Persons with a family or personal history of skin cancer or clinical evidence of precursor lesions (eg, dysplastic nevi, certain congenital nevi), or those with increased occupational or recreational exposure to sunlight.
> Complete oral cavity exam: Persons with exposure to tobacco or excessive amounts of alcohol, or those with suspicious symptoms or lesions detected through self-examination.
> Palpation for thyroid nodules: Persons with a history of upper-body irradiation.

Laboratory/diagnostic procedures
> Nonfasting total blood cholesterol
> Dipstick urinalysis
> Mammogram (every 1–2 years for women until age 75, unless pathology detected)
> Thyroid function tests (for women)

HIGH-RISK GROUPS
> Fasting plasma glucose: The markedly obese, persons with a family history of diabetes, or women with a history of gestational diabetes.
> Tuberculin skin test (PPD): Household members of persons with tuberculosis or others at risk for close exposure to infection (eg, staff or tuberculosis clinics, shelters for the homeless, nursing homes, substance abuse treatment facilities, dialysis units, correctional institutions); recent immigrants or refugees from countries in which tuberculosis is common (eg, Asia, Africa, Central and South America, Pacific Islands); migrant workers; residents of nursing homes, correctional institutions, or homeless shelters; or persons with certain underlying medical disorders (eg, HIV infection).
> Electrocardiogram: Men with 2 or more cardiac risk factors (high blood cholesterol, hypertension, cigarette smoking, diabetes mellitus, family history of coronary artery disease); men who would endanger public safety were they to experience sudden cardiac events (eg, commercial airline pilots); or sedentary or high-risk males planning to begin a vigorous exercise program.
> Papanicolaou smear (every 1–3 years): Women who have not had previous documented screening in which smears have been consistently negative.
> Fecal occult blood/sigmoidoscopy: Persons who have first-degree relatives with colorectal cancer; a personal history of endometrial, ovarian, or breast cancer; or a previous diagnosis of inflammatory bowel disease, adenomatous polyps, or colorectal cancer.
> Fecal occult blood/colonoscopy: Persons with a family history of familial polyposis coli or cancer family syndrome.

COUNSELING

Diet and exercise: Same as for ages 40–64.
Substance use: Same as for ages 19–39.
Injury prevention
> Prevention of falls
> Safety belts
> Safety helmets
> Smoke detector
> Smoking near bedding or upholstery
> Hot water heater temperature

Table 1–2 (cont'd). Prevention surveillance in office practice.

IV. Patients Ages 65 and Over (cont'd)

HIGH-RISK GROUPS
   Prevention of childhood injuries: Persons with children in the home or automobile.
Dental health: Regular dental visits, tooth brushing, flossing
Other primary preventive measures: Glaucoma testing by eye specialist
   HIGH-RISK GROUPS
   Discussion of estrogen replacement therapy: Women at increased risk for osteoporosis (eg, Caucasian, low bone mineral content,
      bilateral oopherectomy before menopause or early menopause, slender build) and who are without known contraindications (eg,
      history of undiagnosed vaginal bleeding, active liver disease, thromboembolic disorders, hormone-dependent cancer).
   Discussion of aspirin therapy: Men who have risk factors for myocardial infarction (eg, high blood cholesterol, smoking, diabetes
      mellitus, family history of early-onset CAD) and who lack a history of gastrointestinal or other bleeding problems, or other risk
      factors for bleeding or cerebral hemorrhage.
   Skin protection from ultraviolet light: Persons with increased exposure to sunlight.

IMMUNIZATIONS
   Tetanus-diphtheria (Td) booster (every 10 years)
   Influenza vaccine (annually)
   HIGH-RISK GROUPS
   Hepatitis B vaccine: Homosexually active men, intravenous drug users, recipients of some blood products, or persons in health-
      related jobs with frequent exposure to blood or blood products.

of infected blood. In these instances, prevention is best achieved by abstaining from intravenous drug use; failing that, secondary preventive maneuvers include avoidance of shared needles or using clean or sterilized needles and syringes. Antibody testing for infection with HIV is now widely available and highly sensitive and specific. However, in patients with no risk factors, a positive test is still likely to be falsely positive. Furthermore, serum conversion after infection can take as long as 6 months, and perhaps even longer, so false-negatives can also occur. Although indications for testing are controversial, most clinicians now favor elective testing for those at high risk. Detection of asymptomatic persons with HIV infection is important for preventive strategies and allows these persons to consider the newer treatments that may extend life in HIV-infected patients (see Chapter 24).

Centers for Disease Control: General recommendations on immunization. Ann Intern Med 1989;111:133. (Published also in 2 parts in JAMA 1989;262:22, 187.)
Rhame FS, Maki DG: The case for wider use of testing for HIV infection. New Engl J Med 1989;320:1248.

CARDIOVASCULAR & CEREBROVASCULAR DISEASES

Impressive declines in age-specific mortality rates from heart disease and stroke have been achieved in all age groups in North America during the past 2 decades. The chief reason for this favorable trend appears to be a modification of risk factors, especially cigarette smoking, hypercholesterolemia, and hypertension.

Cigarette Smoking

Cigarette smoking remains the most important cause of preventable morbidity and early demise in developed countries. Smokers die 5–8 years earlier than nonsmokers; have twice the risk of fatal heart disease, 10 times the risk of lung cancer and several times the risk of cancers of the mouth, throat, esophagus, pancreas, kidney, bladder, and cervix; and have a 2- to 3-fold greater incidence of peptic ulcers—which heal less well than in nonsmokers—and about a 2- to 4-fold greater risk of fractures of the hip, wrist, and vertebrae. Olfaction and taste are impaired in smokers, and facial wrinkles are increased. Smoking cessation lessens the risk of death or myocardial infarction in both men and women with coronary artery disease, slows the rate of progression of carotid atherosclerosis, and is associated with reversal of chronic bronchitis.

The children of patients who smoke have lower birth weights, more frequent respiratory infections, less efficient pulmonary function, and a higher incidence of chronic ear infections than children of nonsmokers and are more likely to become smokers themselves. In addition, passive smoking by adults has been shown to increase the risk of cervical cancer and probably of lung cancer and to promote endothelial damage and platelet aggregation.

There has recently been an encouraging national trend away from smoking. In 1987, fewer than 27% of United States adults were smokers—the lowest percentage ever recorded. Smoking was slightly more common in men than in women (29.5% versus 23.8%) and slightly higher in blacks than in whites. One-fourth of United States adults are former smokers.

The clinician should adopt a 4-step smoking cessation strategy: (1) Ask the patient about smoking and interest in quitting. (2) Motivate the patient to stop smoking. (3) Set a date to stop entirely. (4) Follow up to find out what happens. A recent survey showed that only 44% of smokers who had seen a physician in the previous year had been advised to quit. Table

Table 1–3. Some immediate consequences of smoking cessation.[1]

1. Improve ability to breathe.
2. Regain sense of smell.
3. Regain sense of taste.
4. Save money.
5. Require less sleep.
6. Increase energy.
7. Fresh breath.
8. Odor-free environment.
9. No ashtrays to empty.
10. No burn holes.
11. Cut risk of death by fire 50%.
12. Alleviate tobacco stains on teeth, fingers.
13. Decrease risks of passive smoking for family and coworkers.
14. More employable.
15. Better insurance risk and cheaper insurance premiums.
16. Improve lung cleansing through ability to cough and improved ciliary activity.
17. Improve coronary and peripheral circulation.
18. Decrease heart rate.
19. Reduce blood carbon monoxide levels.
20. Reduce perspiration.
21. Improve exercise tolerance.
22. Improve ability to perform physical work.
23. Lower grocery bills.
24. Extra time.
25. Decrease social pressure.

[1] Reproduced, with permission from Green HL, Goldberg RJ, Ockene JK: Cigarette smoking: The physician's role in cessation and maintenance. *J Gen Intern Med* 1988;**3**:75.

Table 1–4. The physician's role in smoking cessation.[1]

I. For the individual
1. Identify the smoker.
2. Present health consequences of smoking.
3. Present health benefits of cessation.
4. Assess and develop the desire to modify smoking behavior.
5. Develop and formalize a patient-centered plan for change.
6. Utilize pharmacologic adjuncts as appropriate.
7. Establish a quit day.
8. Arrange for follow-up.
9. Implement maintenance strategies.
10. Continue surveillance for relapse prevention and plan modifications as needed.

II. For society
1. Set a personal example.
2. Become involved in the legislative process.
3. Be an advisor to industry.
4. Work through public health and school health programs to prevent smoking initiation.
5. Work with voluntary agencies: American Heart Association, American Cancer Society, American Lung Association, etc.
6. Work toward a smoke-free society.

[1] Reproduced, with permission, from Green HL, Goldberg RJ, Ockene JK: Cigarette smoking: The physician's role in cessation and maintenance. *J Gen Intern Med* 1988;**3**:75.

1–3 lists immediate benefits from smoking cessation that the physician can call to the attention of smokers.

Pharmacologic aids may be useful in selected cases. Nicotine gum may be useful for some patients—particularly those who are in the process of quitting and are concerned about weight gain—but it is expensive and maintains the addiction to nicotine. Clonidine patches may help, but this is controversial.

Clinicians should avoid appearing to disapprove of patients who are unable to stop smoking. Concerned exhortation, family or social pressures, or the opportunity presented by intercurrent illness may eventually enable even the most addicted chronic smoker to give up the habit or at least to cut back. Even under the most pessimistic assumptions, such counseling is more cost-effective than treating hypertension or hypercholesterolemia. The physician's role in smoking cessation is summarized in Table 1–4.

Cohen SJ et al: Encouraging primary care physicians to help smokers quit: A randomized trial. Ann Intern Med 1989;110:648. (Labeling the medical records of smokers or offering nicotine gum increased the success rate of smoking cessation by 2- to 6-fold in one county teaching hospital.)

Cummings SR, Rubin SM, Oster G: The cost-effectiveness of counseling smokers to quit. JAMA 1989;261:75.

Cummings SR et al: Training physicians in counseling about smoking cessation: A randomized trial of the "quit for life" program. Ann Intern Med 1989;110:640. (Physicians trained in how to help smokers quit then spend more time helping patients quit.)

Franks P, Harp J, Bell B: Randomized, controlled trial of clonidine for smoking cessation in a primary care setting. JAMA 1989;262:3011. (Ineffective compared with placebo.)

Stokes J, Rigotti N: The health consequences of cigarette smoking and the internist's role in smoking cessation. Adv Intern Med 1988;33:431.

Hypercholesterolemia

Lowering elevated LDL cholesterol concentrations reduces the risk from coronary heart disease. The data in Table 1–5 can be used as a guide to lowering blood cholesterol. Calculated gain in life expectancy from modest decreases in blood cholesterol is low, especially in patients without other risk factors such as cigarette smoking and hypertension.

Specific methods of therapy, which include diet, weight reduction, exercise, and drugs, are discussed in Chapter 21.

Baron RB: Management of hypercholesterolemia: A primary care perspective. West J Med 1989;150:562.

Cleeman JJ: Report of the National Cholesterol Education Program expert panel on detection, evaluation, and treatment of high blood cholesterol in adults. Arch Intern Med 1988;148:36. (Most up-to-date, definitive reference.)

National Heart, Lung, and Blood Institute Workshop: Recommendations regarding public screening for measuring blood cholesterol. Arch Intern Med 1989;149:2650.

Hypertension

Over 60 million adults in the USA have hyperten-

Table 1–5. National Cholesterol Education Program guidelines for classification and treatment of elevated total and LDL cholesterol.[1]

I. Initial classification and recommended follow-up based on total cholesterol

Classification (mg/dL)

<200	Desirable blood cholesterol
200–239	Borderline to high blood cholesterol
≥240	High blood cholesterol

Recommended follow-up

Total cholesterol <200 mg/dL	Repeat within 5 years
Total cholesterol 200–239 mg/dL	
Without definite CHD or 2 other CHD risk factors (one of which can be male sex)	Dietary information and recheck annually
With definite CHD or 2 other CHD risk factors (one of which can be male sex)	Lipoprotein analysis; further action based on LDL cholesterol level

II. Classification and treatment decisions based on LDL cholesterol (fasting)

Classification (mg/dL)

LDL cholesterol

$$= \text{Total cholesterol} - (\text{HDL cholesterol}) - \left(\frac{\text{Triglycerides}}{5}\right)$$

<130	Desirable LDL cholesterol
130–159	Borderline to high-risk LDL cholesterol
≥160	High-risk LDL cholesterol

Treatment decisions	Initial Level mg/dL	Minimal Goal mg/dL
Dietary treatment		
Without CHD or 2 other risk factors[2]	≥160	<160[3]
With CHD or 2 other risk factors[2]	≥130	<130[4]
Drug treatment		
Without CHD or 2 other risk factors[2]	≥190	<160
With CHD or 2 other risk factors[2]	≥160	<130

[1] CHD = coronary heart disease; LDL = low-density lipoprotein.
[2] Patients have a lower initiation level and goal if they are at high risk because they already have definite CHD, or because they have any 2 of the following risk factors: male sex, family history of premature CHD, cigarette smoking, hypertension, low high-density lipoprotein (HDL) cholesterol, diabetes mellitus, definite cerebrovascular or peripheral vascular disease, or severe obesity.
[3] Roughly equivalent to total cholesterol level of <240 mg/dL.
[4] As goals for monitoring dietary treatment.

sion. In every adult age group, higher values of systolic and diastolic blood pressure carry greater risks of stroke and congestive heart failure. Even so, clinicians must be able to apply specific blood pressure criteria as a means of deciding at what levels treatment should be considered in individual cases. Table 1–6 presents a classification of hypertension based on blood pressures that was developed in 1988. Sixty-five percent of hypertensive patients in the United States are now adequately controlled, compared with only 16% in 1972 (see Chapter 8).

Joint National Committee: The 1988 Report of the Joint National Committee on detection, evaluation, and treatment of high blood pressure. Arch Intern Med 1988; 148:1023. (Most up-to-date, definitive reference.)

CANCER

Primary Prevention

Cigarette smoking is the most important preventable cause of cancer. Primary prevention of skin cancer consists of restricting exposure to ultraviolet light by wearing appropriate clothing and use of sunscreens. In the past 2 decades, there has been a 3-fold increase in the incidence of squamous cell carcinoma and a 4-fold increase in melanoma in the United States. Prevention of occupationally induced cancers involves minimizing exposure to carcinogenic substances such as asbestos, ionizing radiation, and benzene compounds.

Table 1–6. Classification of blood pressure.[1]

	Category[2]
Diastolic blood pressure (DBP) (mm Hg)	
<85	Normal blood pressure
85–89	High normal blood pressure
90–104	Mild hypertension
105–114	Moderate hypertension
≥115	Severe hypertension
Systolic blood pressure (SBP [mm Hg] when DBP <90 mm Hg)	
<140	Normal blood pressure
140–159	Borderline isolated systolic hypertension
≥160	Isolated systolic hypertension

[1] In individuals aged 18 years or older, based on the average of 2 or more readings on 2 or more occasions.
[2] A classification of borderline isolated systolic hypertension (SBP 140–159 mm Hg) or isolated systolic hypertension (SBP ≥160 mm Hg) takes precedence over a classification of high normal blood pressure (DBP 85–89 mm Hg) when both occur in the same individual. High normal blood pressure (DBP 85–89 mm Hg) takes precedence over a classification of normal blood pressure (SBP <140 mm Hg) when both occur in the same person.

Secondary Prevention

Generally accepted techniques exist for secondary prevention of cancers of the breast, colon, and cervix through cancer screening procedures (Table 1–7). Note that Table 1–7, derived from the American Cancer Society guidelines, differs in many instances from the recommendations of the US Preventive Services Task Force (Table 1–2), which takes a more conservative view of the efficacy of cancer screening maneuvers. In their own medical practices, the authors tend to follow the more conservative guidelines of the Task Force Recommendations. Screening for other cancers in normal asymptomatic or even high-risk segments of the population is not recommended.

Table 1–7. Screening for cancer: American Cancer Society (1988) guidelines for the early detection of cancer in people without symptoms.

Test or Procedure	Sex	Age	Frequency
Sigmoidoscopy	M&F	Over 50	Every 3–5 years after 2 negative examinations 1 year apart.
Stool test for occult blood	M&F	Over 50	Every year.
Digital rectal examination	M&F	Over 40	Every year.
Papanicolaou test	F	Women who are or have been sexually active or have reached 18 years.	Annually until at least 3 consecutive satisfactory normal examinations, then less often at discretion of physician.
Pelvic examination	F	20–40	Every 3 years.
		Over 40	Every year
Endometrial tissue sample	F	At menopause; women at high risk.[1]	At menopause.
Breast self-examination	F	Over 20	Every month
Breast physical examination	F	20–40	Every 3 years.
		Over 40	Every year.
Mammography	F	35–39	One baseline examination
		40–49	Every 1 or 2 years
		Over 50	Every year
Chest x-ray			Not recommended.
Sputum cytologic examination			Not recommended.
Health counseling and cancer checkup[2]	M&F	Over 20	Every 3 years.
		Over 40	Every year.

[1] History of infertility, obesity, failure of ovulation, abnormal uterine bleeding, or estrogen therapy.
[2] To include examination for cancers of the thyroid, testicles, prostate, ovaries, lymph nodes, oral region, and skin.

ACCIDENTS & VIOLENCE

Accidents remain the most important cause of loss of potential years of life before age 65, followed by cancer, heart disease, and suicide and homicide. Despite incontrovertible evidence that seat belt use protects against serious injury and death in motor vehicle accidents, fewer than 30% of all adults use seat belts routinely. It is estimated that fewer than 20% of bicycle and motorcycle riders use safety helmets, a simple protective device that can greatly reduce the risk of head and brain injuries following an accident. As part of routine medical care, physicians should try to educate their patients about seat belts, drinking and driving, and the risks of having guns in the home. Males aged 16–35 are at especially high risk for serious injury and death from accidents and violence, with blacks at especially high risk of dying violent deaths.

Thompson RS, Rivara FP, Thompson DC: A case-control study of the effectiveness of bicycle safety helmets. N Engl J Med 1989;320:1361.

SUBSTANCE ABUSE
(See also Chapter 19)

Substance abuse—including alcohol and illicit drugs—is a major public health problem in the United States and is estimated to be a factor in more than half of highway fatality accidents. Alcohol abuse effects both adolescents and adults. Approximately two-thirds of high school seniors are regular users of alcohol, and the lifetime prevalence of alcoholism is estimated to be between 12% and 16%. Underdiagnosis of alcoholism is substantial, both because of patient denial and lack of physician alertness to historical and physical clues of the condition. Although about 10% of all adults seen in medical practices are problem drinkers, that fact is seldom recognized. The CAGE test (see Table 1–8) is a simple screening test that is both sensitive and specific. Alternatively, asking the 2 questions: "Have you ever had a drinking problem?" and "When did you have your last drink?"—

Table 1–8. CAGE screening test for alcoholism.[1]

Have you ever felt the need to	**Cut down** on drinking?
Have you ever felt	**Annoyed** by criticism of your drinking?
Have you ever felt	**Guilty** about your drinking?
Have you ever taken a morning	**Eye opener?**

INTERPRETATION: Two "yes" answers are considered a positive screen. One "yes" answer should raise a suspicion of alcohol abuse.

[1] Modified from Mayfield D et al: The CAGE questionnaire: Validation of a new alcoholism screening instrument. Am J Psychiatry 1974:131;1121.

positive if in the past 24 hours—yields a 91% sensitivity for alcoholism but is obviously less specific than the CAGE test. Treatment of alcoholism and its complications is discussed in Chapter 19.

A 1988 survey showed that 28 million Americans had used illicit drugs during the preceding year, a 33% decline from 1985. Of these 28 million, nearly 3 million were current users of cocaine. Many of these drug users were employed, and many used drugs during pregnancy. As with alcohol abuse, the recognition of drug abuse presents special problems and requires that the physician actively consider the diagnosis. Treatment issues are discussed in Chapter 19.

Cyr MG, Wartman SA: The effectiveness of routine screening questions in the detection of alcoholism. JAMA 1988;259:51.

Johnson B, Clark W: Alcoholism: A challenging physician-encounter. J Gen Intern Med 1989;4:445. (A good working discussion of how to approach the diagnosis of alcoholism in the office setting, including a description of doctor-patient dynamics in the alcoholic patient.)

Linn LS, Yager J: Factors associated with physician recognition and treatment of alcoholism. West J Med 1989;150:468.

Mason JO: From the Assistant Secretary of Health. JAMA 1990;262:494. (Review of current state of affairs in prevention.)

PRINCIPLES OF DIAGNOSTIC TEST SELECTION & USE

USES OF LABORATORY TESTS

Laboratory Tests Have Many Uses

A. Screening Tests: Screening tests are used to identify asymptomatic persons with risk factors for disease. Early detection and treatment of occult disease may reduce disease morbidity and mortality, and identification of risk factors may allow early intervention to prevent disease occurrence or sequelae. Screening tests also allow clinicians to reassure patients found free of disease or without risk factors and to provide genetic counseling in familial conditions. Optimal screening tests meet the criteria listed in Table 1–9.

B. Diagnostic Tests: Diagnostic tests are used to help establish or exclude the presence of disease in symptomatic persons. Some tests assist in early diagnosis after onset of symptoms and signs; others assist in differential diagnosis of various possible diseases. Still others help determine the stage or activity of disease.

C. Tests Used in Management of Patients: Tests used in patient management enable the clinician

Table 1–9. Criteria for use of screening procedures.

Characteristics of disease
1. Sufficiently common to justify the effort to detect it.
2. Sufficient morbidity and mortality if untreated.
3. Effective treatment available and acceptable to alter its natural history.
4. Presymptomatic period during which detection and treatment may occur.
5. Detection and treatment during presymptomatic period yields better results than when treatment occurs during symptomatic period.

Characteristics of test
1. Acceptable to patients.
2. Sensitive enough to detect disease in presymptomatic individuals (few false-negatives).
3. Specific enough to exclude disease in normal individuals (few false-positives).
4. Low cost.
5. Safety.

Characteristics of population
1. Sufficiently high prevalence of disease.
2. Accessible.
3. Likely to be compliant with subsequently recommended diagnostic tests and treatment.

to (1) evaluate objectively and quantitatively the severity of disease and to estimate its prognosis, (2) monitor the course of disease (progression, stability, or resolution), (3) assist in selecting and adjusting therapy to avoid toxicity and ensure adequacy of treatment, (4) monitor the response of disease to treatment, and (5) detect disease recurrence.

Definitions & Attributes of Tests

Test **sensitivity** is a measure of the probability that a test result will be *positive* if the disease being investigated is *present*. A test with positive (abnormal) results in all patients with a given disease would have perfect (100%) sensitivity (ie, no false-negative results). A perfectly sensitive test can exclude ("rule out") a possible diagnosis if the result is negative (normal).

Test **specificity** is a measure of the probability that a test result will be *negative* if the disease being investigated is *not present*. A test with negative (normal) results in all patients without a given disease would have perfect (100%) specificity (ie, no false-positive results). A perfectly specific test can confirm ("rule in") a possible diagnosis if the result is positive (abnormal).

For example, serum creatine kinase measurement is a fairly sensitive test for ischemic necrosis of the myocardium. The finding of a normal serum creatine kinase during the 24–48 hours after onset of chest pain helps to exclude the diagnosis of acute myocardial infarction. However, the serum creatine kinase is not a very specific test, because several other factors (surgery, intramuscular injections, seizures, muscle trauma, etc) can cause an abnormal result.

By contrast, the finding of new Q waves on the ECG is quite specific and helps to confirm the diagnosis of acute myocardial infarction. However, this finding is not very sensitive, since acute myocardial infarction can occur also in the absence of detectable Q waves.

Virtually none of the laboratory tests used in clinical medicine have perfect sensitivity or specificity. A **false-positive result** occurs when a test result is positive (abnormal) even though the patient is disease-free. The false-positive rate for a test is the complement to its specificity (1 − specificity). A **false-negative result** occurs when a test result is negative (normal) even though the patient has the disease. The false-negative rate for a test is the complement to its sensitivity (1 − sensitivity).

Most tests are capable of giving both false-positive and false-negative results. False-negative results are of most concern in situations when missing a diagnosis would be very costly; false-positive results are troublesome in their potential to cause both unnecessary worry and to require further diagnostic evaluation.

Tests are also described in terms of their predictive value. The **positive predictive value** of a test is the probability that the patient has the disease if the test result is positive; the **negative predictive value** of a test is the probability that the patient is free of the disease if the test result is negative. The positive predictive value is related to the sensitivity of the test and the negative predictive value to its specificity (Fig 1–1). The **false-alarm rate** of a test is the complement to its positive predictive value (1 − PPV). The **false-reassurance rate** is the complement to its negative predictive value (1 − NPV).

Problems in Selecting Tests & Interpreting Test Results

Most clinicians have little trouble with the concepts of sensitivity and specificity and use them intuitively all the time. However, clinicians commonly have more difficulty understanding the concept of predictive value and the import of **Bayes' theorem,** ie, that the predictive values (positive and negative) of a test relate not only to the characteristics of the test but also to the population being tested (prevalence of disease). Often, for example, a new diagnostic test is reported to have very high sensitivity and specificity because it has been evaluated on a population of very sick persons. Later, as the same test is applied to a different population (of less ill or even asymp-

	Disease	
	Present	Absent
Positive (abnormal)	a	b
Negative (normal)	c	d

Test result

Definitions

$$\text{Sensitivity} = \frac{a}{a + c} \times 100\%$$
$$= \frac{\text{Number of persons with disease with positive tests}}{\text{Total number of persons with disease}}$$

$$\text{Specificity} = \frac{d}{b + d} \times 100\%$$
$$= \frac{\text{Number of persons without disease with negative tests}}{\text{Total number of persons without disease}}$$

$$\text{Positive predictive value} = \frac{a}{a + b} \times 100\%$$
$$= \text{Probability of disease if test positive}$$

$$\text{Negative predictive value} = \frac{d}{c + d} \times 100\%$$
$$= \text{Probability of no disease if test negative}$$

$$\text{False-negative rate} = \frac{c}{a + c} \times 100\%$$

$$\text{False-positive rate} = \frac{b}{b + d} \times 100\%$$

$$\text{False alarm rate} = \frac{b}{a + b} \times 100\%$$

$$\text{False reassurance rate} = \frac{c}{c + d} \times 100\%$$

Figure 1–1. Potential relationships between disease and test results.

tomatic individuals), the test appears to have considerably less favorable characteristics.

Indeed, Bayes' theorem means that clinicians must take into account not only the inherent uncertainty of the tests but also the (known or estimated) probability that the disease is present. For example, to exclude a disease with confidence, the clinician needs to order a very sensitive test (one with few false-negative results), whereas to confirm a diagnosis with confidence requires a very specific test (one with few false-positive results). In choosing between a sensitive test to exclude or a specific test to confirm a diagnosis, the clinician must first estimate whether the diagnosis in question is either unlikely or probable. Table 1–10 presents several such rules of thumb in use of laboratory tests.

The mistake clinicians most commonly make is to conclude that a disease is present when it is not, based on a positive test result. To help prevent this mistake, the clinician should roughly estimate the **pretest likelihood** of the disease being present before ordering the test. When the pretest likelihood is high, a positive (abnormal) result helps to confirm the diagnosis but an unexpectedly negative (normal) result does not help to rule out the diagnosis. When the pretest likelihood is low, a negative (normal) result helps to exclude the diagnosis but an unexpectedly positive (abnormal) result is not particularly helpful for confirmation. Tests are most likely to be useful

when the diagnosis is truly uncertain (pretest likelihood about 50%). Laboratory tests add little when the diagnosis is either extremely unlikely or almost certain.

Finally, clinicians often have trouble understanding that the definition of *normal* is often somewhat arbitrary. Most quantitative laboratory tests yield results that conform roughly to the Gaussian bell-shaped curve; the curve for healthy individuals usually overlaps that for diseased persons (Fig 1–2). When this occurs, the laboratory must assign a **cut-off point** to separate normal (negative) test results from abnormal (positive) results. As shown in Fig 1–2, the choice of the cut-off point determines the sensitivity and specificity of the test.

For most tests, normal results are defined as the range of values within 2 standard errors of the mean for healthy individuals, or the range of values within

Table 1–10. Rules of thumb in use of laboratory tests.

1. Before ordering a test, roughly estimate the likelihood that the disease is present. Interpret the test result with this likelihood in mind.
2. When a disease is highly unlikely, a positive test result will usually be a false-positive result.
3. When a disease is highly probable, a negative test result will usually be a false-negative result.
4. Ruling out a disease requires a negative result of a test with high sensitivity (few false-negatives). Make use of the value of a negative test result.
5. Ruling in a disease requires a positive result of a test with high specificity (few false-positives). Make use of the value of a positive test result.
6. Ask yourself if the test result will alter your diagnosis or management. If not, do not order the test.
7. To minimize the risk of false-positive results, limit the use of screening tests to those individuals who have risk factors or other findings increasing the likelihood for disease.
8. Limit screening or testing for uncommon diseases to situations in which the following apply:
   a. The disease is important to find (or not to miss).
   b. The disease is readily treatable.
   c. The test has high sensitivity and specificity.
   d. There is a practical means of separating true positives from false positives.
9. When evaluating claims regarding new diagnostic tests, ask yourself:
   a. How sensitive is the test among presymptomatic or minimally symptomatic individuals?
   b. How often are test results falsely positive in individuals with other diseases presenting with similar symptoms and signs—especially closely related diseases?

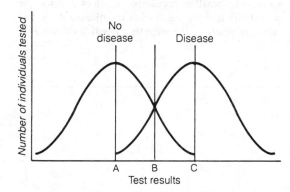

Figure 1–2. Hypothetical distribution of test results for healthy and diseased individuals (eg, serum uric acid values in men without and with gouty arthritis). Because no test unfailingly distinguishes between healthy and ill persons, the distribution of test results overlaps as shown. Defining the "cut-off point" between "normal" and "abnormal" (or "negative" and "positive") test results determines the relationship between test sensitivity and specificity. For example, if *A* is chosen as the cut-off point and all patients with values to the right of *A* are said to have "abnormal" or "positive" results, the test will have 100% sensitivity but low specificity. This would be an appropriate cut-off point if the test were being used to screen for or to exclude a disease. However, if *C* is chosen as the cut-off point and all patients with values to the right of *C* are said to have "abnormal" results, the test will have 100% specificity but low sensitivity. This would be an appropriate cut-off point if the test were being used to confirm a suspected diagnosis. For most tests, the cut-off point is usually at point *B*, somewhere between points *A* and *C*. Exactly where to fix point *B* depends on why the test is usually performed and the relative importance of false-positive and false-negative results. (Modified from Griner PF et al: Selection and interpretation of diagnostic tests and procedures: Principles and applications. Ann Intern Med 1981;84[4, Part 2]:453.)

which 95% of the healthy population falls. Therefore, by definition, 5% of healthy individuals have values either above or below this normal range. This means that the clinician performing 12 diagnostic tests on an apparently healthy person has a 46% chance of finding one abnormal test result; for 20 tests, a 64% chance of one abnormal result; and for 25 tests, a 72% chance of one abnormal result!

Normal or reference values vary with the method employed, the laboratory, and conditions of collection and preservation of specimens. The normal values established by individual laboratories should be clearly expressed to ensure proper interpretation.

Inaccurate collection of a 24-hour urine specimen, variations in concentration of the randomly collected urine specimen, hemolysis in a blood sample, addition of an inappropriate anticoagulant, and contaminated glassware or other apparatus are examples of causes of erroneous results.

Other common errors in use of laboratory tests are listed in Table 1–11.

When laboratory tests are used properly and efficiently, their results should assist in diagnosis, establish prognosis, guide therapy, lead to a better understanding of the disease process, and benefit the patient.

Griner PF, Mayewski RJ, Mushlin AI, Greenland P: Selection and interpretation of diagnostic tests and procedures: principles and applications. Ann Intern Med 1981;84(4, Part 2):453–600.

Table 1–11. Common errors in use of laboratory tests.[1]

1. Unnecessary test duplication (redundancy).
2. Overuse of emergent ("stat") tests.
3. Confusion between available tests.
4. Ordering without regard to previous results.
5. "Shotgun" approach.
6. Inappropriate use of screening tests.
7. Failure to distinguish patient benefit from clinical interest.
8. Failure to review test results.
9. Omission of indicated tests.
10. Too-frequent repetition of monitoring tests.
11. Failure to make a tentative clinical diagnosis and then decide on the most efficient and inexpensive tests to confirm or exclude it.
12. Failure to confirm with a more specific test a diagnosis based on the result of a very sensitive test.
13. Failure to appreciate the clinical import of a positive (abnormal) test result.
14. Failure to consider the potential significance of an incidental unexpected but highly suggestive test result.
15. Failure to weigh the consequences of missing or making a diagnosis based on a single test result.
16. Failure to consider pretest likelihood that a certain disease is present, leading to fruitless pursuit of nonexistent disease based on an isolated nonspecific test result.
17. Failure to assign the clinical evaluation (history and physical examination) sufficient importance relative to the laboratory test results.

[1] Modified from Johns RJ, Fortuin NJ, Wheeler PS: The collection and evaluation of clinical information. Chapter 1.2 in: *The Principles and Practice of Medicine,* 2nd ed. Harvey AM et al (editors). Appleton & Lange, 1988.

Johns RJ, Fortuin NJ, Wheeler PS: The collection and evaluation of clinical information. Chapter 1.2, pp 4–20, in: The Principles and Practice of Medicine, 22nd ed. Appleton & Lange, 1988.

Kassirer JP: Our stubborn quest for diagnostic certainty: A cause of excessive testing. N Engl J Med 1989; 320:1489.

Patterson RE, Horowitz SF: Importance of epidemiology and biostatistics in deciding clinical strategies for using diagnostic tests: A simplified approach using examples from coronary artery disease. J Am Coll Cardiol 1989;13:1653.

Sox HC: Probability theory in the use of diagnostic tests: An introduction to critical study of the literature. Ann Intern Med 1986;104:60.

Sox HC et al: Sensitivities and specificities of diagnostic tests. In: Medical Decision Making. Butterworth, 1988.

COMMON SYMPTOMS

PAIN*

Approach to the Patient

Pain is the most common symptom causing patients to seek medical attention. It can provide the clinician with important diagnostic information. Because pain is highly subjective, the patient's description may be difficult to interpret. Information about the timing, nature, location, severity, and radiation is crucial for proper treatment; the same is true for aggravating or alleviating factors.

Many emotional and cultural factors influence the perception of pain. The primary cause (eg, trauma, infection), pathogenesis (eg, inflammation, ischemia), and contributory factors (eg, recent changes in life situation, symbolic attributes of pain) must all be sought.

Administration of a systemic analgesic is the usual method of pain management, but many other nonpharmacologic methods are useful. Examples include graded physical activity, simple reassurance, support groups, and biofeedback training. For severe chronic nerve pain, such as occurs in metastatic cancer or neuropathic conditions, therapies such as nerve block, radiation, and even rhizotomy may be useful in selected patients.

1. DRUGS FOR SEVERE PAIN

Narcotics are indicated for severe pain that cannot be relieved with less effective agents. Examples include the pain of severe trauma, myocardial infarc-

* Management of chronic pain is discussed in Chapter 19.

tion, ureteral stone, and postoperative pain. Table 1–12 lists narcotic analgesics with some of their characteristics.

These drugs have pharmacologic similarities to opium. They are employed principally for the control of severe pain, but they also act to suppress cough and gastrointestinal motility. All can produce **physical dependence,** but to varying degrees and after varying periods of use. The risk of addiction or habituation should not prevent their appropriate use, especially in the management of terminal illness.

A common error in management of pain from cancer is to prescribe insufficient doses "prn" rather than adequate doses around-the-clock at staged intervals. In such cases, the major goal of management should be patient comfort.

The effects of all narcotics are reversed by naloxone. Continued narcotic use produces tolerance, so that increasing doses are needed to produce the same analgesic effect.

Contraindications

The narcotic drugs are relatively contraindicated in some acute illnesses. In acute abdomen, for example, the pattern of pain may provide important diagnostic clues. However, some analgesia may be necessary in order to perform an adequate physical examination for diagnostic purposes. In acute head injuries, these drugs interfere with clinical interpretation of neurologic changes.

Adverse Effects

The drugs in this category have the potential adverse effects listed below. Patients with hypothyroidism, adrenal insufficiency, hypopituitarism, acute intermittent porphyria, reduced blood volume, and severe debility are particularly apt to suffer adverse effects from the addicting analgesics.

(1) Opioid narcotics should be given with great caution to patients with pulmonary insufficiency, because of dose-dependent respiratory depression.

(2) Central nervous system effects include sedation, euphoria, nausea, and vomiting. Antidepressants, antihistamines, phenothiazines, hypnotics, and alcohol can potentiate these effects.

(3) Cardiovascular effects include hypotension. This is less common than hypoventilation, however.

(4) Gastrointestinal effects are chiefly decreased bowel motility and consequent constipation.

(5) Genitourinary effects include bladder spasm and urinary retention.

(6) Enhanced sensitivity to the drugs occurs in patients with hepatic impairment; biliary spasm may cause severe biliary colic.

(7) Allergic manifestations also occur, but rarely.

Frequently Used Narcotic Analgesics

A. Morphine sulfate, 8–15 mg subcutaneously or intramuscularly in adults, is the most effective drug for control of severe pain. The effects last 4–5

Table 1–12. Useful narcotic analgesics.[1]

	Approximate Equivalent Dose (mg)	Oral:Parenteral Potency Ratio	Duration of Analgesia (hours)	Maximum Efficacy	Addiction/Abuse Liability
Morphine	10	Low	4–5	High	High
Hydromorphone (Dilaudid)	1.5	Low	4–5	High	High
Oxymorphone (Numorphan)	1.5	Low	3–4	High	High
Methadone (Dolophine)	10	High	4–6	High	High
Meperidine (Demerol)	60–100	Low	2–4	High	High
Codeine	30–60[2]	High	3–4	Low	Medium
Oxycodone[3] (Percodan)	4.5[2]	Medium	3–4	Moderate	Medium
Hydrocodone[4] (Vicodin, others)	5[2]	Medium	3–5	Moderate	Medium

[1] Modified and reproduced, with permission, from Katzung BG (editor): *Basic & Clinical Pharmacology,* 4th ed. Appleton & Lange, 1989.
[2] Analgesic efficacy at this dose not equivalent to 10 mg of morphine. See text for explanation.
[3] Available only in tablets containing aspirin 325 mg (Percodan) or acetaminophen 325 mg (Percocet).
[4] In tablets or capsules with acetaminophen 500 mg (Vicodin) or aspirin.

hours. In acute myocardial infarction or in acute pulmonary edema due to left ventricular failure, 2–6 mg may be injected slowly intravenously in 5 mL of saline solution. Long-acting, sustained-release oral morphine preparations (MS Contin, Roxanol SR) are available and allow less frequent dosing. For severe, refractory pain, morphine solution may be given in a continuous intravenous drip. Dosage will depend on the previous 24-hour narcotics requirement.

B. Morphine congeners give effects equivalent to 10 mg of morphine sulfate but have no specific advantages—eg, hydromorphone or oxymorphone, 2–4 mg of either orally every 4 hours, or 1–3 mg of either subcutaneously every 4 hours.

C. Meperidine (Demerol), 50–150 mg orally or intramuscularly every 3–4 hours, provides analgesia similar to that achieved with morphine. Its indications and side effects are similar to those of morphine.

D. Methadone, 10 mg orally every 6–8 hours, is most often used for treatment of addiction based on its long duration of action. Its side effects are similar to those of morphine, but tolerance and physical dependence are slower to develop.

E. Codeine (sulfate or phosphate), 15–60 mg orally or subcutaneously every 4–6 hours, is somewhat less effective than morphine but also less habit-forming. It is often given together with aspirin or acetaminophen for enhanced analgesic effect. Codeine is a powerful cough suppressant in a dose of 15–30 mg orally every 4 hours, but is constipating.

F. Oxycodone and hydrocodone are given orally and prescribed with another analgesic. The dosage is 5 mg every 4–6 hours in tablets that contain aspirin (Percodan) or acetaminophen 325 mg (Percocet) or 500 mg (Vicodin).

2. DRUGS FOR MODERATE OR MILD PAIN

Most people can manage their minor aches and pains with OTC analgesics available at drugstores and food stores, which now stock ibuprofen in the 200-mg dosage. Drugs such as codeine, oxycodone, and pentazocine, listed above as "addictive narcotics," are sometimes used for moderate pain, but salicylates or acetaminophen in higher doses or the highly visible class of NSAIDs (which also include salicylates) are often better for this purpose. (See Table 1–13.)

The activity—both anti-inflammatory and analgesic—of aspirin and other NSAIDs is mediated through inhibition of the biosynthesis of prostaglandins. All of these drugs to varying degrees inhibit platelet aggregation and may cause gastric irritation (the risk of associated upper gastrointestinal bleeding is about one and one-half times normal), kidney damage (including acute renal failure, decreased glomerular filtration, nephrotic syndrome, and type IV renal tubular

acidosis), bone marrow suppression, rashes, anorexia, and nausea. Their principal advantage over aspirin is the longer duration of action—permitting less frequent dosing and better compliance—and the decreased frequency of gastrointestinal side effects. For most patients, however, aspirin remains the preferred (and much less expensive) drug—though the risk of gastrointestinal bleeding is higher with aspirin than with the other NSAIDs. All NSAIDs are analgesic, antipyretic, and anti-inflammatory in dose-dependent fashion. However, they may activate quiescent inflammatory bowel disease. Their principal uses are in the control of moderate pain of various musculoskeletal disorders, menstrual cramps, and other—mainly self-limited—conditions, including moderate postoperative discomfort. Suicide attempts with overdoses of the other NSAIDs are less serious and less often successful than attempts with aspirin.

Table 1–13 lists the most commonly used NSAIDs along with dosages and pertinent comments. The most widely used agents for these purposes are aspirin and acetaminophen.

Aspirin is the drug of first choice for management of mild to moderate pain and is an effective antipyretic and anti-inflammatory agent. Analgesia is achieved with much lower doses and blood levels than are needed for anti-inflammatory action. Aspirin is available in many forms for oral administration in a single 325-mg unit dose, as well as smaller (eg, 60 mg) and larger (eg, 500 mg) doses. The usual dose is 2 tablets (650 mg) every 4 hours as needed, taken with fluid. Gastrointestinal irritation can be reduced by ingestion with food or with an antacid. Enteric-coated aspirin, which is more expensive (Ecotrin; many others), can be used to avoid gastric irritation, but absorption is delayed.

The main untoward effect of aspirin—especially in large doses or when taken chronically—is gastric irritation and microscopic blood loss from the gut. Rarely, there may be massive gastrointestinal hemorrhage, most commonly in heavy drinkers or patients with a history of peptic ulcer disease. Gastrointestinal symptoms do not correlate with the amount of blood lost.

Aspirin allergy occurs infrequently and may be manifested as rhinorrhea, nasal polyps, asthma, and—very rarely—anaphylaxis. The incidence is less than 0.1%. Aspirin in high doses may produce a vitamin K-responsive prolongation of the prothrombin time.

Because of a possible association with Reye's syndrome, salicylates are best avoided by children and teenagers with febrile viral illnesses such as influenza and chickenpox.

Acetaminophen in the same dosage as aspirin (650 mg orally every 4 hours) has comparable analgesic and antipyretic effects but lacks the anti-inflammatory property of aspirin. It is useful for people who cannot tolerate aspirin, for those with bleeding disorders, and for those at risk for Reye's syndrome. In very

Table 1–13. Useful nonsteroidal anti-inflammatory drugs.

Generic Name	Proprietary Name	Dosage Range	Costs for 30 Days' Treatment[1]	Comments[2]
Aspirin		325–625 mg 2–4 times daily	$1.40	Available also in enteric-coated form that is more expensive and less well absorbed.
Ibuprofen	Advil (OTC), Motrin, etc	200–600 mg 3–4 times daily	$9.00	Now available without prescription; relatively well tolerated.
Naproxen	Anaprox, Naprosyn	250–500 mg twice daily	$75.00	
Piroxicam	Feldene	20 mg daily	$186.00	Single dosage convenient; may have higher rate of gastrointestinal bleeding.
Sulindac	Clinoril	150–200 mg twice daily	$100.00	May have higher rate of gastrointestinal bleeding, less nephrotoxic potential.
Tolmetin	Tolectin	200–600 mg 4 times daily	$44.00	
Fenoprofen	Nalfon	300–600 mg 3–4 times daily	$43.00	
Indomethacin	Indameth, Indocin, etc.	25–50 mg 2–4 times daily	$3.00	Higher incidence of dose-related toxic effects, especially gastrointestinal and bone marrow effects.
Meclofenamate sodium	Meclomen	100 mg 2–4 times daily	$29.00	Diarrhea relatively more common.
Diclofenac	Voltaren	50 mg 2 or 3 times daily	$68.00	May impose higher risk of aplastic anemia.
Acetaminophen	Tylenol	325–500 mg	$3.50	Not an NSAID because it lacks anti-inflammatory effects. Equivalent to aspirin as analgesic and antipyretic agent.

[1] Cost to pharmacist for 30 days' treatment based on lowest usual dosage (generic, when possible). When estimating daily costs for medications, dosage frequency should be taken into account.
[2] The adverse effects of headache, tinnitus, dizziness, confusion, rashes, anorexia, nausea, vomiting, gastrointestinal bleeding, diarrhea, nephrotoxicity, visual disturbances, etc, can occur with any of the drugs that have been available for shorter periods. Tolerance and efficacy are subject to great individual variations among patients.

large doses (eg, > 4 g/d chronically, > 7 g/d acutely), acetaminophen can be hepatotoxic, manifested by appreciable hepatic necrosis with very high serum transaminase levels, often in the thousands. Toxicity may occur at considerably lower doses in the chronic alcoholic.

See Chapter 33 for further details on salicylate and acetaminophen overdosage.

Brigden ML, Barnett JB: A practical approach to improving pain control in cancer patients. West J Med 1987; 146:580. (Explicit dosing guidelines.)
Foley KM: The treatment of cancer pain. N Engl J Med 1985;313:84.
Perlman SL: Modern techniques of pain management. West J Med 1988;148:54.
Whelton A et al: Renal effects of ibuprofen, piroxicam, and sulindac in patients with asymptomatic renal failure. Ann Intern Med 1990;112:568. (Even a brief course of ibuprofen can quickly result in acute renal failure in patients with asymptomatic, mild chronic renal failure.)

FEVER & HYPERTHERMIA

The average normal oral body temperature is 36.7 °C (range 36–37.4 °C), or 98 °F (range 96.8–99.3 °F). These ranges include 2 standard deviations and thus encompass 95% of a normal population, measured in mid-morning. The normal rectal or vaginal temperature is 0.5 °C (1 °F) higher than the oral temperature, and the normal axillary temperature is correspondingly lower. Rectal temperature is more reliable than oral temperature, particularly in the case of patients who are mouth-breathers or who are tachypneic.

The normal diurnal temperature variation may be as much as 1 °C, being lowest in the early morning and highest in the late afternoon. There is a slight sustained temperature rise following ovulation during the menstrual cycle and in the first trimester of pregnancy.

Fever is a regulated rise to a new "set point" of body temperature. When proper stimuli act on appropriate monocyte-macrophages, these cells elaborate interleukin-1, which causes elevation of the set point through effects in the hypothalamus. The elevation may result from either increased heat production (eg, shivering) or decreased heat loss (eg, peripheral vasoconstriction). Body temperature in interleukin-1 induced fever seldom exceeds 41.1°C unless there is structural damage in the hypothalamus.

Hyperthermia—not mediated by interleukin-1—occurs when body metabolic heat production or environmental heat load exceeds normal heat loss capacity or when there is impaired heat loss; heat stroke is an example. Body temperature may rise to alarming levels (> 41.1 °C [106 °F]) capable of producing irreversible brain damage; no diurnal variation is observed.

Neuroleptic malignant syndrome is a rare and potentially lethal idiosyncratic reaction to major tranquilizers, particularly haloperidol and fluphenazine. The syndrome, which may be a variant of malignant hyperthermia, consists of hyperthermia of anesthesia, muscular rigidity, autonomic dysfunction, and altered consciousness occurring after therapeutic doses of the medication; it is not dose- or duration-related. Some benefit has been reported from the use of amantadine, bromocriptine, and dantrolene.

Effect of Elevated Body Temperature

While fever as a symptom should generally be regarded with appropriate concern, in some circumstances it may play a beneficial role. However, markedly elevated body temperature may result in profound metabolic disturbances. High temperature during the first trimester of pregnancy may cause birth defects, such as anencephaly. Fever may increase insulin requirements and also alter the metabolism and disposition of drugs used for the treatment of the diverse diseases associated with fever.

The body temperature may provide important information about the presence of illness, particularly infections, and about changes in the clinical status of the patient. The fever pattern, however, is of rather limited use for specific diagnosis. Furthermore, the degree of temperature elevation does not necessarily correspond to the severity of the illness. In general, the febrile response tends to be greater in children than in adults; in elderly persons and neonates, the febrile response is less marked or absent, even in the face of bacteremia.

Diagnostic Considerations

The outline below illustrates the wide variety of clinical disorders that may cause fever. Most febrile illnesses are due to common infections, are short-lived, and are relatively easy to diagnose. In certain instances, however, the origin of the fever may remain obscure ("fever of undetermined origin," FUO) after lengthy diagnostic examination. The term FUO has traditionally been reserved for cases of fever of over 38.3 °C (101 °F) for three weeks in patients whose diagnosis is not apparent after 1 week or more of studies.

At least 90% of FUO cases are due to infection, neoplasm, or immune disorder. In 5–10% of cases, the diagnosis is never established. In view of recent advances in diagnostic technology, this distribution may change as certain diseases are diagnosed earlier. In recent years, HIV infection has been commonly encountered as a cause of FUO.

Though empiric use of antibiotics is warranted while awaiting culture results in seriously ill patients (eg, patients with severe neutropenia), such a practice is generally not valuable as a diagnostic test in cases of FUO.

Important Causes of Fever & Hyperthermia (With Examples)

A. Infections: Bacterial, viral, chlamydial, mycobacterial, fungal, spirochetal, rickettsial, parasitic.

B. Autoimmune Diseases: Systemic lupus erythematosus, polyarteritis nodosa, rheumatic fever, giant cell arteritis, Still's disease; less prominent in dermatomyositis, adult rheumatoid arthritis.

C. Central Nervous System Disease: Cerebral hemorrhage, head injuries, brain and spinal cord tumors, degenerative central nervous system disease (eg, multiple sclerosis), spinal cord injuries. (This category represents interference with the thermal regulatory process rather than true "fever.")

D. Malignant Neoplastic Disease: Primary neoplasms (eg, of lung, liver, pancreas, and kidney), tumors metastatic to the liver.

E. Hematologic Disease: Lymphomas, leukemias, hemolytic anemias, hemorrhage (gastrointestinal tract or soft tissue).

F. Cardiovascular Disease: Myocardial infarction, pulmonary embolism.

G. Gastrointestinal Disease: Inflammatory bowel disease, liver abscess.

H. Endocrine Disease: Hyperthyroidism, pheochromocytoma may raise temperature because of altered thermoregulation.

I. Diseases Due to Chemical Agents: Drug reactions (including serum sickness), neuroleptic malignant syndrome, malignant hyperthermia of anesthesia.

J. Miscellaneous Diseases: Sarcoidosis, familial Mediterranean fever.

K. Factitious, or "false," fever.

Treatment

Most fever is well tolerated. When the temperature is greater than 40 °C (104 °F), particularly if prolonged, symptomatic treatment may be required. *Temperature over 41 °C (105.8 °F) is a medical emergency.* (See Heat Stroke, Chapter 32.)

A. Measures for Removal of Heat: Alcohol sponges, cold sponges, ice bags, ice-water enemas, and ice baths will lower body temperature and provide physical comfort for patients who complain of feeling *hot.*

B. Antipyretic Drugs: In most instances, antipyretic therapy by itself is not needed except for reasons of comfort or in patients with fragile hemodynamic status. Aspirin or acetaminophen, 0.3–0.6 g every

4 hours as needed, is quite effective in reducing fever. If given, these drugs are best administered continuously rather than as needed, since "prn" dosing results in periodic chills and sweats due to varying levels of drug.

C. Fluid Replacement: Oral or parenteral fluids must be administered to compensate for increased insensible fluid and electrolyte losses as well as those from perspiration.

Brusch JL, Weinstein L: Fever of unknown origin. Med Clin North Am 1988;72:1247.

Dinarello CA, Cannon JG, Wolff SM: New concepts on the pathogenesis of fever. Rev Infect Dis 1988;10:48.

McGowan JE et al: Fever in hospitalized patients: With special reference of the medical service. Am J Med 1987;82:580.

Rosenberg MR, Green M: Neuroleptic malignant syndrome: Review of response to therapy. Arch Intern Med 1989;149:1927. (Literature review that supports use of dantrolene or bromocriptine.)

WEIGHT LOSS

Marked unexplained weight loss is often an indication of serious physical or psychologic illness. Significant weight loss may be due to a wide variety of disease processes of any organ system as well as to psychiatric disorders. It should be distinguished from voluntary weight loss and from the mild, gradual weight loss that occurs in some elderly persons. When the patient complains of weight loss but appears to be adequately nourished, inquiry should be made about exact weight changes (with approximate dates) and about changes in clothing size. Family members may provide confirmation of weight loss, as may old documents such as driver's licenses.

Once it has been established that the patient has marked weight loss, further laboratory and radiologic investigation may be indicated, such as chest x-ray, complete blood count, serum chemistries, urinalysis, and upper gastrointestinal series radiograph. Involuntary weight loss is rarely due to "occult disease." Almost all physical causes are clinically evident during the initial evaluation of the patient. Marked weight loss can sometimes occur in the absence of serious physical illness. Psychiatric consultation should be considered when there is evidence of depression, anorexia nervosa, or other psychologic problems (see Chapter 22).

Marton KI, Sox HC Jr, Krupp JR: Involuntary weight loss: Diagnostic and prognostic significance. Ann Intern Med 1981;95:568. (Best article on diagnostic approach to weight loss.)

FATIGUE

Fatigue is one of the most common symptoms confronting the office practitioner. Its prevalence may be as high as 25%, with higher rates in women than men. The symptoms of fatigue may be less well defined and explained by patients than symptoms associated with specific functions, such as fever or dyspnea. Fatigue or lassitude and the closely related complaints of weakness, tiredness, and lethargy are most often readily explained by common factors such as overexertion, poor physical conditioning, inadequate rest, obesity, undernutrition, stress, and emotional problems. Taking a history of the patient's daily living and working habits may obviate the need for extensive and unproductive diagnostic studies.

Important diseases that can cause fatigue include endocrine disorders such as hyperthyroidism and hypothyroidism, cardiac disease (congestive heart failure), infections (endocarditis, hepatitis), respiratory disorders (COPD), anemia, the arthritides and related disorders, cancer, alcoholism, drug side effects such as from sedatives and beta-blockers, and psychologic conditions such as depression and somatization disorder.

Chronic Fatigue Syndrome

A syndrome of chronic fatigue has received much recent attention. It is poorly defined and consists of chronic or recurrent fatigue and various combinations of other symptoms such as sore throat, lymph node tenderness, headache, and myalgias. Laboratory tests are not generally useful in uncovering previously undetected conditions or in determining the cause of fatigue. This syndrome does not appear to be related to chronic infection with Epstein-Barr virus (see Chapter 25) or to Lyme disease (see Chapter 27). Although testing for infection with EBV is commonly performed, studies have shown that the antibody to EBV is not helpful in evaluation of patients with chronic fatigue.

A variety of treatments have been tried for the syndrome of chronic fatigue. The antiviral drug acyclovir does not appear to improve symptoms. In all cases, patients should be encouraged to exercise and engage in life's activities to the extent possible and to be reassured that full recovery is eventually possible in most cases.

Holmes GP et al: Chronic fatigue syndrome: A working case definition. Ann Intern Med 1988;108:387.

Koo D: Chronic fatigue syndrome: A critical appraisal of the role of Epstein-Barr virus. West J. Med 1989; 150:590.

Kroenke K, Mangelsdorff D: Common symptoms in ambulatory care: Incidence, evaluation, therapy, and outcome. Am J Med 1989;86:262.

Manu P, Matthews DA, Lane TJ: The mental health of patients with a chief complaint of chronic fatigue: A prospective evaluation and follow-up. Arch Intern Med 1988;148:2213.

Swartz MN: The chronic fatigue syndrome: One entity or many? N Engl J Med 1988;319:1726.

Geriatric Medicine & the Elderly Patient

2

Lawrence Z. Feigenbaum, MD

The biologic changes associated with aging are influenced by hereditary and environmental factors. A distinction should be made between physiologic aging—the normal wear and tear that occurs with the passage of time—and pathologic phenomena occurring in old people that are the result of disease or adverse features of the individual's life-style. The long-term effects of disuse and physical deconditioning are other factors that should logically be distinguished from the physiologic aging process.

Aging ordinarily occurs gradually throughout life, but quite unevenly from individual to individual; some persons age more rapidly than others. Specific chronologic age criteria for designating older individuals as a group are unavoidably arbitrary and may be harmful. The terms "elderly" and "senior citizen" are better defined in terms of functional status rather than by chronologic age, though for purposes of administrative convenience, age 65, age 75, etc, are often used. Some writers now subclassify the elderly into the "young-old" (ages 65–74) and the most rapidly growing group, the "old-old" (over 80 or 85).

Some of the consequences of aging that determine the nature and degree of functional impairment are listed below:

(1) Decreased function of one or more organ systems. Table 2–1 lists changes that occur as a result of "normal" aging.

(2) Decreased stress tolerance. A major characteristic of aging is a diminution or slowing of homeostatic mechanisms required to meet stress. Thus, accidental hypothermia and heat stroke are more common in the elderly, and mortality rates associated with burns, trauma, and disease increase significantly with age.

(3) Increased psychologic stress due to personal losses, eg, loss of physical vigor, deaths of friends and family members, retirement, reduced income, loss of sense of identity and self-worth.

(4) Impaired immunity, eg, greater susceptibility to infection, neoplastic disease.

(5) Increased susceptibility to disease, often to multiple diseases.

(6) Altered pharmacokinetics, eg, adverse drug reactions.

(7) Decreased physical conditioning, eg, loss of muscle tone and shorter endurance.

It is important to recognize that there is immense variation in these changes within the elderly population and from organ system to organ system. Stereotypic concepts of hopelessness or progressive physical and mental deterioration must be avoided, since most older patients do enjoy good health and respond well to proper medical care.

An awareness of special problems of the elderly, a willingness to listen, careful assessment of the medical, psychologic, and socioeconomic problems and their impact on functional capacity, avoidance of overmedication, a realistic and understanding attitude in dealing with older patients, and a knowledge of community support services can help the elderly function independently and actively as long as possible.

HISTORY TAKING WITH ELDERLY PATIENTS

It must not be assumed that an older patient is unable to provide a reliable medical history. At the initial interview, the examiner should note any impairment of hearing or speech, mood disturbance, or apparent difficulty with thought processes, any of which may interfere with the history-taking process. If the patient is unable to comprehend or communicate, data should be sought from family and friends. If the patient has a hearing aid, be sure that it is used and is working properly. The elderly patient, just as any other patient, should be interviewed in an unhurried, reassuring manner in quiet, pleasant surroundings. It is important to note any differences between the patient's chief complaint and that of the family; both need to be attended to. The history should include pertinent information about daily living activities, presence or absence of stairs or elevator, availability of family and friends, and socioeconomic circumstances. A home visit may provide a very different perception from what is gained from the history regarding the patient's ability to cope, eg, a refrigerator and cupboards with little or no staples, rotting food, burned pots, major disarray.

Drug History

It is essential to review *all* drugs the patient has

Table 2–1. Physiologic changes frequently associated with aging.

Organ or System	Age-Related Change
Skin	Decrease in subcutaneous fat; atrophy of sweat glands; wrinkling and dryness; seborrheic keratoses.
Eyes	Presbyopia with marked decrease in accommodation; lens opacification and discoloration; decrease in pupil size; increase in drusen.
Ears	Decrease in hearing high frequencies; increase in sensitivity to loud noise.
Nose	Decrease in sense of smell.
Respiratory system	Decrease in bronchial ciliary activity; less lung elasticity; decrease in maximal breathing capacity; decrease in maximal oxygen uptake; decrease in sensitivity of cough reflex.
Cardiovascular system	Decrease in elasticity and compliance of arteries; sclerotic changes in aorta and valves; decrease in cardiac output and heart rate response to stress; decrease in baroreceptor response.
Gastrointestinal system	Decrease in salivary flow; decreased sense of taste; lower gastric acidity; decrease in absorption of calcium; decrease in colonic motility.
Genitourinary system	Atrophy and drying of vaginal mucous membrane; slower sexual response; enlargement of prostate; decrease in number of glomeruli; decrease in renal blood flow; decrease in maximal urine osmolality.
Nervous system	Decrease in size and weight of brain; slower psychomotor performance; decrease in "righting" reflexes; fewer nighttime hours of stage 4 and rapid eye movement (REM) sleep.
Musculoskeletal system	Decrease in bone mass; decrease in lean body mass; articular cartilage loss on weight-bearing joints.
Endocrine system	Glucose intolerance; increase in ADH response; decrease in estrogen secretion; decrease in aldosterone and renin response to upright posture and sodium restriction.
Immunologic system	Absent thymic hormone secretion; decrease in T cell function; increase in autoantibodies.
General	Decrease in total body water; decrease in lean body mass; increase in percentage of total body fat; decrease in height and weight; graying of hair.

been taking. Have the patient or family bring in both prescription and over-the-counter drugs. Review them one by one by name, inquiring about the reason for taking the drug, its dosage and frequency of administration, and any adverse side effects the patient may attribute to the drug. Repeat this important exercise as often as necessary to make certain the patient's drug intake is both rational and minimal.

Dietary History

Many elderly patients have limited nutritional intake. It is important to inquire about the diet, asking specifically about adequacy of income, problems with shopping or preparing meals, eating habits, impaired senses of taste and smell, difficulties with dentures, or unusual dietary habits.

Incontinence History

Close to 50% of women and 25% of men over age 80 residing in the community have some urinary incontinence, but only 10–30% of primary care physicians are aware of the extent of the problem. Many patients are too embarrassed to mention this distressing symptom, which can have serious psychologic and social impact and increase the risk of institutionalization; for these reasons, it is very important to ask about incontinence.

Psychiatric History

Depression and anxiety resulting from severe psychologic stress or organic disease are common in the elderly. (The highest incidence of suicide in the USA is in white men over age 75.) Depression is a treatable condition that may be overlooked unless one is alert to its possibility. Depression can easily be mistaken for early dementia, since decreased attention span, loss of sense of humor, irritability, and poor performance on mental status testing may occur in both conditions. Decrease in appetite, change in sleep patterns, and constipation are common in the well elderly but may also be signs of depression. Ask openly about suicidal thoughts and crying spells and any past history of mental illness. Psychiatric illness in old people can often be successfully treated, and psychiatric consultation should be recommended without hesitation if the history arouses concern about the patient's emotional status.

Do not avoid questions about sexual feelings or problems, since elderly patients may welcome an opportunity to discuss such matters. Many elderly people worry that it is abnormal for them to still have sexual feelings. Impotence or unreliable erections may be a significant problem for elderly men, and dryness of the vagina with a history of dyspareunia for elderly women.

Be aware of the possibility of drug abuse and alcoholism; they are more common in the elderly than is generally recognized.

A careful history is essential in any elderly patient who has recently demonstrated confusion. To assume that confusion is a manifestation of dementia without having inquired into factors such as other illnesses, new medications, or increased doses of drugs that may produce delirium may overlook an easily correctable and serious condition. To make matters worse, if delirium is overlooked and assumed to be dementia with behavioral abnormalities, tranquilizers or psychotropic agents may be prescribed (especially in the nursing home or hospital) that may then further aggravate the delirium.

PHYSICAL EXAMINATION

A complete physical examination, including pelvic examination in women and rectal examination in both sexes, is essential. Note abnormalities of gait and steadiness on standing. Observing the patient getting up from a chair is an excellent method of identifying persons at risk for falls. Examine the patient completely undressed (with gown) so that the skin can be carefully inspected. Check for postural blood pressure changes. Test and record hearing and vision in all elderly patients. Remove excess cerumen from the external auditory canals, look for cataracts, test ability to read, and check visual fields. Note redness or tenderness over the temporal artery. Look to see if dentures fit well, and inspect the oral cavity carefully with dentures removed, remembering that malignant lesions of the mouth are more often red than white. In auscultating the chest, bear in mind that the presence of an S_4 in an elderly patient does not imply clinically significant cardiac disease. The systolic murmur of aortic sclerosis is a common finding and may be difficult to differentiate from aortic stenosis.

Do not overlook the breast examination, since older women are more likely to have breast cancer and less likely to do breast self-examination. Be sure to check for fecal impaction in inactive patients and those with fecal or urinary incontinence. In patients with urinary incontinence—especially in men—check for a distended bladder, since that may be the only finding in urinary retention. Check muscle strength and range of motion of joints, and observe for neurologic deficit. Diminished or absent vibratory sense in the lower extremities may be found in elderly patients with no evidence of neurologic disease. Careful questionnaire of the feet, including how well the shoes

are fitted, is important in the patient with gait disturbance. If the patient uses a cane, be sure it is the correct length (ie, equal to the distance from the wrist crease to the ground) and has a good grip. If the patient is chair-bound or bed-bound, great care must be taken to examine the skin for reddening or evidence of early ulceration over pressure points.

MENTAL STATUS EXAMINATION

Some form of cognitive testing is desirable with all elderly patients. Remember that patients with mild degrees of dementia may mask intellectual impairment by a cheerful and cooperative manner. If the patient appears mentally competent, the physician should explain that a mental status evaluation is part of every complete examination, so that the patient will not feel singled out and insulted. An examination that tests only orientation as to person, place, and time is not sufficient to detect mild or moderate intellectual impairment. Many practical mental status tests are available such as the Jacobs Cognitive Capacity Screening Examination (see Jacobs J et al: Ann Intern Med 1977;86:40), the Short Portable Mental Status Questionnaire, and the Mini-Mental Status Examination of Folstein and provide a numerical score that can be of great value as a baseline test and can be completed in 5–10 minutes. Table 2–2 lists the specific components of mental status that each of these tests includes. Descriptions of these rather similar tests can be found in the Kane reference at the end of this chapter. In lieu of one of these formal tests, simply asking the patient to draw a clock with the hands at a set time (eg, 10 minutes before 2) can be very informative regarding cognitive status, visuospatial deficits, ability to comprehend and execute instructions in logical sequence, and presence or absence of perseveration. However, no single question or task can establish or rule out cognitive impairment.

Table 2–2. Components of the mental status examination.

	CCSE[1] (Jacobs)	MMS[2] (Folstein)	SPMSQ[3] (Pfeiffer)
Orientation	+	+	+
Attention	+	+	+
Calculation	+	+	+
Recall	+	+	0
Language	0	+	0
Abstractions	+	0	0
Remote memory	0	0	+
Reading: follows written command	0	+	0
Visuospatial	0	+	0

[1] Cognitive Capacity Screening Examination.
[2] Mini-Mental Status Examination.
[3] Short Portable Mental Status Examination.

EVALUATION OF FUNCTIONAL CAPACITY IN THE ELDERLY

Simply taking a history, performing a physical examination, and listing medical diagnoses are not sufficient for elderly patients, particularly those who are frail and at high risk, for institutional care. A clear description of the patient's degree of fitness or functional incapacity based on both medical and psychosocial problems is essential. Appropriate management of the elderly requires focusing on what the patient can and cannot do. The disability is not the same as the disease. Before nursing home placement is recommended, a thorough multidisciplinary geriatric functional assessment should be done in most instances. In addition to the physician, the assessment team may also include the following

(1) A social worker, who assesses the ability of the family, friends, and community agencies to provide those supports that will allow the patient to remain in his or her home. Financial and family problems are often elucidated by the social worker.

(2) An occupational therapist, who assesses the patient's ability to perform the activities of daily living, which are those activities needed for personal self-care. The Katz Index of Activities of Daily Living (ADL) is a commonly used instrument (Katz S et al: JAMA 1963;185:94), as are the Barthel Index and OARS: Physical ADL. These tests classify patients according to their functional independence or dependence in the following areas: bathing, dressing, feeding, transferring, using the toilet, and continence. For those patients who are less incapacitated, testing of more complex functions requiring both physical and cognitive ability should be done. These instrumental activities of daily living (IADL) are those personal activities that are more complex than ADLs and include writing, cooking, shopping, using the telephone, and managing money and medications. See Table 2–3 for a complete list of ADLs and IADLs and instruments used for assessing the patient's mastery of them. Assessment of these functions and careful consideration of what steps can be taken to help the patient become more independent are often the most important contributions the health team can make in improving the patient's quality of life and preventing or delaying institutionalization.

(3) A neuropsychologist, for more thorough testing for organicity and localization of deficits as well as evidence of affective or psychotic disorders.

(4) A psychiatrist or clinical psychologist, who may help differentiate depression (''pseudodementia'') from dementia as well as organic from psychogenic symptoms.

Other consultants may be required, most frequently a physiatrist, neurologist, speech pathologist, urologist, gynecologist, dentist, or nutritionist.

A home visit is of great value in assessing the patient's ability to function in his or her own environ-

Table 2–3. Tests of physical functioning.

Activities of Daily Living (ADL)
Ambulation
Bathing
Feeding
Toileting
Dressing
Transfer from bed
Transfer from toilet
Bowel and bladder control
Communication
Tests include: Katz Index of ADL
     Barthel Index
     OARS: Physical ADL
     Rapid Disability Rating Scale

Instrumental Activities of Daily Living (IADL)
Shopping
Cooking
Cleaning
Laundry
Using the telephone
Managing money
Writing
Reading
Taking medications
Climbing stairs
Walking outdoors
Using public transportation
Tests include: OARS:[1] IADL
     PACE II:[2] IADL
     PGC:[3] IADL

[1] Older Americans Research and Service Center Instrument.
[2] Patient Appraisal Care Evaluation.
[3] Philadelphia Geriatric Center.

ment. Practical advice can be given to the patient or family on how to decrease risks of accidents in the home. These may include installation of handrails, grab bars, better lighting, and smoke alarms as well as elimination of slippery throw rugs or long and loose extension cords.

About 25% of patients on waiting lists for nursing home care can remain in their homes if a multidisciplinary functional assessment is carried out and appropriate recommendations implemented.

LABORATORY EXAMINATIONS & IMAGING

Standard normal laboratory values are essentially the same for the elderly as for younger adults. (There is, for example, no ''anemia of old age.'') An elevated sedimentation rate should arouse a suspicion of polymyalgia rheumatica, cranial arteritis, infection, or cancer. The fasting blood glucose is not significantly altered by age, but the 2- and 3-hour postprandial blood glucose may be higher than normal. Hemoglobin A_{1c} is useful in managing the elderly diabetic; however, one must keep in mind that there may be a slight increase in levels in nondiabetic elderly patients. Serum creatinine is not a good index of renal sufficiency in the elderly, since creatinine levels may be low because of the decrease in lean body mass. The age-corrected creatinine clearance can be derived from the following Cockcroft-Gault equation and should be used as a used as a guide for dosage of ototoxic and nephrotoxic antibiotics: (For women, multiply the result by 0.85.)

$$\text{Creatinine clearance} = \frac{(140 - \text{Age}) \times \text{Body wt (kg)}}{72 \times \text{Serum creatinine}}$$

Since "apathetic" hyperthyroidism is commoner in the aged, thyroid function tests (including plasma TSH measurement) may be indicated.

In the confused elderly patient, the following may be of diagnostic value: urinalysis, chemistry panel, thyroid function tests, serum vitamin B_{12} and red cell folate levels (if there is an associated macrocytic anemia), and CT scan. These tests should be done in most cases when there are signs of early dementia of relatively short duration (months up to 1 or even 2 years). After that time, they should be ordered only upon specific indications.

CT scan is not in itself diagnostic of Alzheimer's disease but is useful in ruling out subdural hematoma, hydrocephalus, cerebral thrombosis or hemorrhage, and multiinfarct dementia, all of which may mimic dementia of the Alzheimer type. Keep in mind that a CT scan "consistent with Alzheimer's" is not diagnostic and may be found in normally cognitive elderly patients and thus should not keep the physician from doing other tests to rule out "treatable dementias."

MRI demonstrates cerebral ischemic lesions often not seen on CT scans. However, the demented patient is unlikely to be able to hold still long enough for a satisfactory MRI.

SPECIAL CLINICAL CONSIDERATIONS

The following clinical characteristics of the elderly differ from those of the young or middle-aged and must be kept in mind when evaluating and treating elderly patients:

(1) Multiple diseases frequent.

(2) Atypical presentations of disease.

(3) Frequent adverse drug reactions.

(4) More disability and dependence.

(5) Proper treatment and management must be based on functional assessment. "The disease is not the disability."

(6) Serious consequences from relatively minor insults.

(7) High frequency of associated social and psychologic problems.

(8) Higher mortality rates.

Diseases more common in the elderly are listed in Table 2–4. A number of medical problems do not usually present as clear-cut organ-specific diag-

Table 2–4. Diseases more common with aging.

Atherosclerotic cardiovascular and cerebrovascular diseases with resultant myocardial infarction, strokes, multi-infarct dementia, and abdominal aneurysms (see Chapters 8, 9, and 18).
Senile dementia of the Alzheimer type (see text).
Polymyalgia rheumatica (see Chapter 15).
Type II diabetes mellitus and nonketotic hyperglycemic coma (see Chapter 21).
Cancer—especially of the colon, prostate, lung, breast, and skin (see Chapter 3).
Decubitus ulcers.
Tuberculosis (see Chapter 7).
Macular degeneration.
Cataracts (see Chapter 5).
Deafness.
Constipation (see Chapter 11).
Osteoarthritis, spinal stenosis, osteoporosis, hip fracture, and Paget's disease (see Chapters 15 and 20).
Parkinson's disease (see Chapter 18).
Depression and suicide (the latter is most common in elderly white men) (see Chapter 19).
Chronic obstructive pulmonary disease.
Benign prostatic hypertrophy (see Chapter 17).
Diverticulitis (see Chapter 11).
Herpes zoster (see Chapters 4 and 25).
Systemic hypothermia (see Chapter 32).

noses. These problems are most common in the frail elderly, especially those over 80 years of age, and are often referred to as the "five *I*'s."

THE FRAIL ELDERLY & THE FIVE *I*'S

Frail elderly patients are subject to certain problems that are referred to as the "five *I*'s" of geriatrics: (1) intellectual impairment, (2) immobility, (3) instability, (4) incontinence, and (5) iatrogenic drug reactions.

INTELLECTUAL IMPAIRMENT (Dementia)

Dementia is defined as an acquired persistent and progressive impairment of intellectual function with compromise in at least 3 of the following spheres of mental activity: language, memory, visuospatial skills, emotional behavior or personality, and cognition (calculation, abstraction, judgment, etc). It is probably the most feared condition among the aging population. It is important to reassure elderly patients who may have some degree of benign forgetfulness that senile dementia is not inevitable. Clinically significant intellectual impairment affects an estimated 5–10% of people over age 65 and only 20% of people over age 80, though recent estimates are as high as 47% for people over 85. At least 60–70% of cases of senile dementia are of the Alzheimer type, and 15–20% are vascular dementias, usually called multi-infarct dementias. These include (1) multiple cortical infarcts, (2) Binswanger's disease (subcortical arteriosclerotic encephalopathy), and (3) lacunar infarcts. Another 15–20% of patients show evidence of both Alzheimer's disease and vascular dementia.

Clinical Features

Early manifestations of dementia include decrease in attention span, impaired powers of concentration, some personality change, and forgetfulness. These changes will often be noted by the family during periods of physical or emotional stress. Many patients with dementia maintain their social graces even in the face of significant cognitive impairment; thus, a clinical impression without mental status testing may miss the diagnosis. As the disease progresses, there is loss of computational ability, word-finding problems, difficulty with ordinary activities such as dressing, cooking, and balancing the checkbook, then severe memory loss and, ultimately, complete disorientation and social withdrawal. Senile dementia of the Alzheimer type has an insidious onset and is steadily progressive. Multi-infarct dementia is more common in men, associated with hypertension with or without a history of transient ischemic attacks or strokes, and is more likely to progress in a series of recognizably distinct steps. The modified Hachinski Ischemia score (see Table 2–5) is commonly used in making the clinical diagnosis, with a score of 4 or more considered diagnostic of multi-infarct dementia. Its progression may be slowed by antihypertensive therapy. Multi-infarct dementia is probably overdiagnosed, since many elderly Alzheimer patients also have coexistent hypertension.

Diagnosis

Diagnosis is based on the history and the physical, laboratory, and mental status examinations. CT scanning usually should be done as part of a complete diagnostic workup of dementia, even though it is not diagnostic of Alzheimer's disease, since it is very useful in ruling out structural brain disorders, such as hematomas, tumors, hemorrhage, hydrocephalus, and infarction. The scan may show minimal or no cerebral atrophy or ventricular enlargement in patients with severe dementia; conversely, these abnormalities may be incidental findings of no clinical significance in the normal elderly. At present, magnetic resonance imaging (MRI) offers no advantage except perhaps in head injury. MRI may be impractical for the demented patient who is restless, since the test requires that the patient lie still for a relatively long period.

The significance of the rather frequent diagnosis of Binswanger's disease (subcortical arteriosclerotic encephalopathy) by CT scan or MRI remains to be elucidated, since these findings (periventricular white matter hypodensity) may be found in normal as well as in demented patients.

Normal-pressure hydrocephalus should be considered in the demented patient who also has a gait disturbance and urinary incontinence. Surgical procedures for cerebrospinal diversion may be helpful, but it is difficult to predict which patients will show clinical improvement. A short duration of symptoms with early gait disturbance and a specific cause correlate best with surgical benefit. Regrettably, demented patients are seldom helped by surgery.

Creutzfeldt-Jakob disease is characterized by a rapidly progressive course of dementia, behavioral changes, myoclonus, and rigidity, with periodic triphasic waves on the EEG. This disease has no specific treatment and is uniformly fatal, usually within 1–2 years.

There is no single diagnostic test specific for dementia. It is essential to rule out other conditions (see Differential Diagnosis, below) that may mimic dementia.

A very small percentage of patients prove to have a condition whose treatment reverses or improves the dementia. Although this is relatively rare, it is a significant "therapeutic" success for both patient and family to avoid unnecessary institutionalization.

Differential Diagnosis

One of the most important tasks of the physician dealing with older people is to distinguish between delirium (see Table 2–6) and dementia and to rule out other treatable causes of confusional states that may mimic dementia. These treatable causes are uncommon, however. Delirium in the hospitalized elderly patient is easily missed and may be mistaken for dementia. It has multiple causes, the commonest of which are severe illness, abnormal (either high or low) serum sodium levels, fever, psychoactive drugs, and azotemia. The following common causes of confusional states may be missed if not specifically looked for.

A. Drugs: A wide variety of agents may cause

Table 2–5. Factors suggesting multi-infarct dementia: modified Hachinski Ischemia Score.[1]

Characteristic	Point Score[2]
Abrupt onset	2
Stepwise deterioration	1
Somatic complaints	1
Emotional incontinence	1
History or presence of hypertension	1
History of strokes	2
Focal neurologic symptoms	2
Focal neurologic signs	2

[1] Rosen et al: *Ann Neurol* 1988;**7**:486.
[2] The score is derived by adding up the points assigned to characteristics that apply. A score of 4 or more is considered diagnostic of multi-infarct dementia.

Table 2–6. Definition of delirium (*DSM-III*).

Clouded sense of consciousness
1. Awareness of environment
2. Sudden shifts
3. "Lucid" periods

Perceptual disturbances
Sensory misperceptions or misinterpretations
Illusions
Hallucinations (visual)

Disordered thought
Mild: Acceleration or slowing of thought
Severe: Total disorganization

Disorientation and memory impairment often not assessed
because of inattention, incoherence

confusion in the elderly. The most common are sedatives, hypnotics, neuroleptics, antidepressants, anticholinergics, antihypertensives, chronic salicylate use, and nonsteroidal anti-inflammatory drugs. If, as sometimes happens, the patient is receiving the same drug under different brand names, there is an increased likelihood of drug-induced confusion.

Chronic alcoholism can occur in the elderly. It is the third most common cause of mental disorder (after dementia and anxiety and phobic disorders) in elderly men but is frequently undiagnosed.

B. Depression: (See Psychiatric History, above; and Management of Depression, below. See also Chapter 19.) Depression of significant degree probably occurs in 10–15% of community-dwelling elderly but is often overlooked. It may mimic dementia ("pseudodementia") or may be superimposed on mild dementia. Differentiation may be difficult and may warrant a therapeutic trial of antidepressant drugs or psychiatric consultation. The depressed patient is more likely to complain of difficulty in answering mental status questions, whereas the demented patient usually is oblivious to the incorrect answers except in the early stages of the disease.

C. Other Psychiatric Problems: Confusion may result from the anxiety and disorienting effect of being in a hospital or other unfamiliar surroundings. Severe anxiety over normal forgetfulness or psychotic behavior may be misdiagnosed as dementia. Sleep deprivation may result in confusion.

D. Sensory Loss: Hearing loss not only leads to social isolation but results in inappropriate answers that may be misinterpreted as evidence of dementia. Behavior resulting from abnormalities of perception in patients with lesions of the nondominant parietal lobe may be mistaken for dementia.

E. Metabolic Disturbances: Hyponatremia is a common cause of confusional state in hospitalized elderly people because of the age-related increase in antidiuretic hormone (ADH) responsiveness to stress (eg, hypovolemia, morphine, trauma) and the syndrome of inappropriate antidiuretic hormone (SIADH) secretion, many of whose causes are common in the elderly (eg, tuberculosis, carcinoma of the lung and prostate, head injury, brain tumor). Other metabolic derangements such as liver failure, renal failure, and cardiopulmonary failure can also cause metabolic confusional states. Confusion due to hypercalcemia is particularly apt to occur in bone disorders that are more often seen in elderly patients (eg, Paget's disease, multiple myeloma, metastatic carcinoma).

F. Endocrine Abnormalities: Hypothyroidism and rarely hyperparathyroidism (even in the absence of hypercalcemia) may cause confusion and be interpreted as senile dementia.

G. Nutritional Deficiencies: Cognitive impairment can be produced by folate, niacin, riboflavin, and thiamine deficiencies. Many factors including poor appetite, loss of taste and smell, poorly fitting dentures, and difficulty in shopping for and preparing meals as well as alcoholism increase the likelihood of nutritional problems.

H. Trauma: Subdural hematoma must always be considered as a possible cause of confusion. Falls with head injury may be forgotten or not reported by the patient and unknown to the family.

I. Brain Tumor: Metastatic lesions and gliomas are the most common brain tumors in old people, but in published reports they are rare as a cause of dementia.

J. Infections: Acute infection in the elderly may cause confusion. Suspect acute infection (eg, pneumonia, pyelonephritis) when an older patient without fever or neurologic deficit suddenly becomes confused. Chronic infections of lung, bone, kidneys, skin (associated with pressure sores), and the central nervous system (including AIDS) may also present as dementia. Central nervous system syphilis is now a very rare cause of dementia.

K. Cardiovascular or Cerebrovascular Accidents: Acute myocardial infarction, acute congestive heart failure, or pulmonary embolism may present as an acute confusional state. Strokes that result in fluent or receptive aphasias are often mistaken for dementia.

Treatment

A. General Measures: The important first step in management of a "demented" elderly patient is the search for treatable factors contributing to the confusional state (see above). Patients with these treatable conditions should receive appropriate treatment, which at times may result in dramatic improvement. However, the patient and family should be advised that treatment seldom results in full recovery.

There is no specific pharmacologic treatment for the memory and cognitive deficits of dementia. This does not mean that the physician has no role in treating the patient and family.

1. Discontinue nonessential medications, particularly sedatives and hypnotics.

2. Provide for the patient's comfort and safety. Whenever possible, allow patients to remain in their own living quarters to minimize confusion and disorientation. Remember that the patient who becomes confused for the first time during a hospital stay is likely to recover at home. The adverse consequences of isolation must be balanced against the normal desire for an appropriate degree of privacy.

3. Provide adequate nutrition and hydration.

4. Treat coexisting medical problems such as heart failure, anemia, and infections. Improvement in these conditions may result in striking amelioration of behavioral and functional disturbances.

5. Remember that no drug treatment has consistently been shown to alter the course of dementia.

6. Help the patient's family cope with this devastating condition. Urge the family to read The Thirty-Six-Hour Day, by Mace and Rabins (Johns Hopkins University Press, 1981). Support groups such as the Alzheimer's Disease and Related Disorders Association (ADRDA) often are of great value to the family and help to anticipate problems.

7. Ethical decisions about such issues as life support, treatment of acute conditions in a severely demented patient, tube feeding, etc, should be anticipated and, when appropriate, discussed with the patient or family.

B. Management of Depression: The elderly patient with early dementia deserves evaluation for possible depression. Since early dementia and depression may be indistinguishable, a cautious therapeutic trial of antidepressant medication may be required.

There is no ideal antidepressant drug. All of the tricyclic antidepressants seem about equally effective, but there are significant differences in side effects (see Chapter 19) that must be considered. Initial dosage should be low, and drug increases should be made slowly to avoid serious side effects; in addition, tricyclics in low doses (eg, doxepin, 10–20 mg daily; desipramine, 25–75 mg daily) may be effective in the elderly. Careful follow-up supervision is required in order to anticipate and minimize anticholinergic side effects, orthostatic hypotension, sedating effects, confusion, bizarre mental symptoms, cardiovascular complications, and drug overdose with suicidal intent. Provide the patient and family with all of the necessary information and warnings, so that adverse drug reactions are not assumed to be due to the aging process.

Experience in the elderly with the tetracyclic agents and other new antidepressants has been limited. The monoamine oxidase inhibitors, used cautiously, are sometimes of benefit when other antidepressants are ineffective. Monoamine oxidase inhibitors should not be used in combination with the cyclic compounds. Electroconvulsive therapy has been successfully used and is usually well tolerated by elderly patients who remain severely depressed despite drug treatment.

IMMOBILITY
(Chair- or Bed-Bound)

The main causes of immobility in the elderly are weakness, stiffness, pain, imbalance, and psychologic problems. Weakness may result from disuse of muscles, malnutrition, electrolyte disturbances, anemia, neurologic disorders, or myopathies. The commonest cause of stiffness in the elderly is osteoarthritis, but rheumatoid arthritis, gout, and pseudogout also occur in this age group. Polymyalgia rheumatica should not be overlooked in the elderly patient with pain and stiffness, particularly of the pelvic and shoulder girdle, and with associated systemic symptoms (see Chapter 15).

Pain, whether from bone (eg, osteoporosis, osteomalacia, Paget's disease, metastatic bone cancer, trauma), joints (eg, osteoarthritis, rheumatoid arthritis, gout), or muscle (eg, polymyalgia rheumatica, intermittent claudication), may immobilize the patient. Foot problems are common and include plantar warts, ulceration, bunions, corns, and ingrown toenails. Poorly fitting shoes are a frequent cause of these disorders.

Imbalance and fear of falling are major causes of immobilization. Imbalance may result from general debility, neurologic causes (eg, stroke; loss of postural reflexes; peripheral neuropathy due to diabetes, alcohol, or malnutrition; vestibulocerebellar abnormalities), anxiety, or drugs or may occur following prolonged bed rest (see Instability, below).

Psychologic conditions such as severe anxiety, depression, or catatonia may produce or contribute to immobilization.

Iatrogenic factors, particularly excessive bed rest and drugs (eg, haloperidol), may immobilize the patient.

Treatment
A. General Measures: Treatment should be directed toward correction of malnutrition, anemia, and electrolyte disturbances that may be responsible for the patient's immobilized status. Installing handrails, lowering the bed, and providing chairs of proper height with arms and rubber skid guards may allow the patient to be safely mobile in the home. A properly fitted cane or walker may be necessary for getting the patient out for walks. (These aids should not be encouraged if the patient can manage without them.) Podiatric care, including proper footwear, is often essential.

In treating arthritis in the elderly, it must be remembered that nonsteroidal anti-inflammatory drugs, especially indomethacin, may cause central nervous system side effects with resultant confusion or even hallucinations. Aspirin remains a useful and inexpensive drug, although chronic use can lead to salicylism. Enteric-coated aspirin may be used for patients with upper gastrointestinal problems.

The hazards of bed rest must be recognized and avoided. Prevention is the best means of dealing with the serious and sometimes life-threatening complications of immobilization. Appropriate active exercises, no matter how limited the patient's capacity, should be encouraged on a regular basis when the patient is chair- or bed-bound.

B. Management of Specific Complications:

1. Pressure sores (decubitus ulcers)– Pressure sores are a serious complication of immobility and usually are associated with prolonged and expensive hospitalization, complications (eg, sepsis and osteomyelitis), and high mortality rates. Prevention requires frequent and careful observation of the skin, particularly over pressure points. Keep the skin clean and dry. The multiplicity of topical therapies underlines the fact that no single one is clearly more effective than others. Surgical debridement may be required for severely undermined lesions. A special mattress (eg, foam-rubber egg-crate) or air-fluidized bed or water bed may be required for the very debilitated patient. If the patient is chair-bound, the skin over the coccyx and ischial tuberosities must be inspected daily. Correction of malnutrition and anemia is essential (see Chapter 4).

2. Muscle weakness and wasting and osteoporosis– Graded exercises and early ambulation are effective even in very old and frail patients.

3. Contractures– These may be avoided by early institution of range-of-motion exercises. Getting the immobile patient out of bed and into the chair is not enough; unless leg exercises are done regularly, 90-degree knee contractures may result.

4. Venous thrombosis– (See Chapter 9.) Frequent ankle flexion while in bed, elastic stockings, correction of dehydration, and early ambulation are important.

5. Incontinence– Spurious urinary incontinence is a common problem in immobilized elderly patients who cannot get to the bathroom if the bedpan or urinal is not made easily available. Such functional incontinence must be avoided because of its devastating psychologic effect as well as the potential for skin maceration, bedsores, and secondary skin infections. The patient should be toileted frequently, preferably in the bathroom or on a bedside commode rather than a bedpan. Avoid restraints and side rails whenever possible. (See Urinary Incontinence, below.)

INSTABILITY
(Physical Instability, Falls, Unstable Gait)

Falls are a major problem for elderly people, especially women. Thirty percent of people over the age of 65 in the community fall each year; and one out of 4 of those who fall have serious injuries, including 6% who have fractures. Falls are a contributing factor in 40% of admissions to nursing homes. Resultant hip problems and fear of falls are major causes of loss of independence.

Causes of Falls

It is often difficult to tell from the history what caused a fall. The patient who is uncertain about what happened will often say, "I must have tripped."

Causes of falls in the elderly are often classified as intrinsic (host) or extrinsic (environmental). General physiologic impairments associated with aging that may increase the risk of falling include reduced vision, general debility and excessive bed rest, impaired "righting" reflexes, and increased body sway when the patient assumes the upright posture. The older and the more debilitated or demented the patient, the more likely it is that a fall will occur. A history of falls in the last 2 years is a strong predictor of further falls. Some specific factors that cause old people to fall are the following:

A. Environmental: The home environment (especially the bathroom) often poses hazards, particularly for a patient with poor vision, weakness, confusion, or problems of mobility. These consist of slippery floors or loose or worn carpeting, loose appliance and telephone cords, poor lighting, steep stairs, and absence of handrails in halls and bathrooms and on stairways. All of these are an even greater hazard if the patient wears loose-fitting slippers, walks in stocking feet, or uses appliances, such as walkers or canes, improperly. Accidental falls are probably more common than those associated with specific disease, but most falls are multifactorial.

B. "Drop Attacks": These occur without warning and without loss of consciousness, possibly as a result of sudden loss of antigravity reflexes. The patient usually falls backward. Pressure on the soles of the feet is one stimulus that often helps the patient to get up again.

C. Loss of Consciousness, Syncope, Vertigo: (See Chapters 6 and 18.) Such episodes may be due to cerebrovascular or cardiovascular disease (eg, arrhythmias, acute myocardial or pulmonary infarction, aortic stenosis, postural hypotension). Leading questions should be avoided, since many patients will say they are "dizzy" if asked.

D. Abnormalities of Balance and Gait: These may be due to strokes or other neurologic diseases involving the pyramidal, extrapyramidal, or cerebellar areas. Patients with Parkinson's disease may fall because of their spasticity as well as their abnormal center of gravity with festinating gait.

E. Alcohol: Excessive alcohol consumption is often overlooked as a cause of falls in old people. Falls occurring while the patient is intoxicated may be forgotten or denied, and a resulting subdural hematoma may be overlooked.

F. Drugs: Any drug that causes postural hypotension (eg, neuroleptics, antihypertensives, antidepressants), arrhythmias (eg, antidepressants), dizziness or vertigo, rigidity (eg, neuroleptics), excessive sedation, or confusion can affect balance and result in falls. Sedatives and hypnotics should be avoided whenever possible.

G. Genitourinary Factors: Urgency (especially at night), straining, and micturition syncope may be unrecognized factors in falls in elderly people.

H. Vision: Poor vision is an important risk factor for falls.

Complications of Falls

Fear of falling again is a major factor in the elderly person's loss of confidence and independence. The most common fractures resulting from falls are of the wrist, hip, and vertebrae. These are more likely to occur in thin white women. There is a high mortality rate (approximately 20% in 1 year) in elderly women with hip fractures, particularly if they were debilitated prior to the time of the fracture.

Subdural hematoma is a treatable but easily overlooked complication of falls that must be considered in any elderly patient presenting with new neurologic signs, including confusion.

Dehydration, electrolyte imbalance, and hypothermia may all occur and endanger the patient's life following a fall.

Prevention & Management

The risk of falling and consequent injury, disability, and potential institutionalization can be reduced by modifying those factors predisposing to falls. A home visit is often helpful to identify and correct environmental factors. Cataract surgery or correction of refractive errors may improve vision. Leg muscles usually can be strengthened by graded exercises. Instructing patients to change position slowly (from lying to sitting, from sitting to standing) may prevent lightheadedness and falls.

Teaching the patient how to get up after a fall if alone can have an important effect on the patient's confidence. Lightweight radio call systems are available that patients can wear to obtain help when out of reach of a telephone.

Prevention or retardation of bone loss started in the perimenopausal period is very important in reducing the risk of fractures in old age.

Medication use, especially sedatives and hypnotics, should be reduced or avoided whenever possible.

Discourage excessive bed rest.

URINARY INCONTINENCE

Loss of bladder control has a major psychologic and social impact and can seriously worsen the patient's life-style. Too often the patient is simply labeled "incontinent of urine" with no attempt to discern the type, to determine if it is transient or chronic, or to institute proper treatment.

Every patient or caregiver should keep an incontinence chart recording "accidents," estimating volumes as large or small, recording the presence or absence of a sense of urgency or discomfort, and relating the episodes to taking of medications (eg, diuretics, anticholinergics). Keeping such a chart helps a diagnosis, treatment, and follow-up.

Simple urodynamic testing can be done in the office to help differentiate the various types of incontinence:

(1) Stress pad test: Hold a pad at the urethral outlet and have the patient strain or cough while standing with a full bladder. This reveals stress incontinence.

(2) Check postvoiding residual by catheterizing the patient. This will show the presence or absence of urinary retention.

(3) Leave the catheter in the bladder, attach a 50-mL syringe, and instill 50-mL increments of sterile water at room temperature until the patient feels an urge to void. This demonstrates the bladder capacity. Uninhibited bladder contractions can be noted by fluctuation in water level (syringe should be held 15 cm above the symphysis pubis); be sure to avoid false-positive "contractions" by being certain that the patient is not straining or coughing, which will also produce fluctuations.

Classification

It is important to differentiate between transient and chronic incontinence (see Table 2-7).

A. Spurious (Functional) Incontinence: Inability of the patient to get to the toilet without a long delay is probably the most common cause of incontinence in a hospitalized patient. Do not assume the patient will need nursing home care if urinary incontinence occurs for the first time in the hospital, since the problem may disappear at home. The delay in toileting may be related to an inaccessible call light, restraints, side rails, immobility, communication problems, or debility. Medications (eg, hypnotics, sedatives, diuretics) are apt to aggravate the problem.

B. Medication-Induced Incontinence: Diuret-

Table 2-7. Types of urinary incontinence.

Transient
Spurious
Immobility
Side rails
Restraints
Inaccessible call light
Language problem
Medication
Diuretics
Sedatives and hypnotics
Anticholinergic drugs producing retention and overflow
Urinary tract infection
Chronic
Detrusor instability
Overflow incontinence
Stress incontinence
Urge incontinence

ics, particularly if taken at night, as well as sedatives or hypnotics may cause nocturnal incontinence. Anticholinergic drugs may cause urinary retention and overflow incontinence, especially in males.

C. Acute Urinary Tract Infection: Severe cystitis may cause frequency, urgency, and at times incontinence in the elderly.

D. Fecal Impaction: Fecal impaction in immobilized elderly patients is a common cause of urinary incontinence. This should be considered when the patient has both fecal leakage and urinary incontinence of short duration. The mechanism may be local irritative factors, change in urethrovesical angle, or other neurogenic stimuli. Whatever the cause, this is an easily treatable type of urinary incontinence.

E. Detrusor Instability (Spastic or Uninhibited Bladder): Detrusor instability is the commonest cause of chronic incontinence in patients with senile dementia of the Alzheimer type. Bladder volume is small, and uninhibited detrusor contractions result in urinary incontinence. This may also occur with bladder stones or tumor.

F. Overflow Incontinence: This may occur in elderly men with benign prostatic hypertrophy and partial bladder outlet obstruction. In addition, large neuropathic bladder as seen in diabetes and tabes dorsalis may result in overflow incontinence. Drugs with anticholinergic effects (eg, atropine, antidepressants, antipsychotics, antihistamines) may cause urinary retention and, secondarily, overflow incontinence.

G. Stress Incontinence: This is a common problem in postmenopausal women and may be due to estrogen deficiency, urethral and vaginal atrophy, or pelvic floor relaxation. If the latter is severe, it may result in persistent incontinence.

H. Psychogenic Incontinence: Incontinence may be associated with severe depression. It may also be an attention-getting device in neurotic or psychotic patients.

Treatment

Proper diagnosis is essential, since many disorders associated with urinary incontinence are treatable.

A. Spurious Incontinence: It is essential that the bed-bound or chair-bound patient be encouraged to toilet frequently. A bedside commode is often preferable to a bedpan or enclosed toilet at a distance from the bed. Restriction of fluids, especially coffee and tea in the evening, may help.

B. Medication-Induced Incontinence: The first step in treatment is to review all medications that may be inducing incontinence. Stop or decrease dosage whenever possible. To prevent nocturnal incontinence, avoid administration of diuretics at night, if possible. Avoid heavy sedation. Keep in mind that many drugs, especially psychotropics, have anticholinergic effects and may produce urinary retention and overflow incontinence (see below).

C. Urinary Tract Infection: Infection is less often a cause than a consequence of incontinence, but in either case it should be treated.

D. Fecal Impaction: The impaction must be broken up digitally or dislodged with a sigmoidoscope. Recurrence should be avoided by regular toileting; by increasing the amounts of fluids, fiber, and stewed fruit in the diet; and by using mild laxatives (eg, milk of magnesia, 15–30 mL at bedtime or as necessary), bowel softeners (eg, docusate (Colace)), and bulk-forming agents (eg, psyllium hydrophilic mucilloid (Metamucil), 15 g in a glass of water or fruit juice 2 or 3 times daily). Frequent oil retention enemas or rectal suppositories (glycerin, bisacodyl (Dulcolax)) may be necessary. It is equally important to increase the patient's physical activity if possible.

E. Detrusor Instability: The general measures noted for treatment of spurious incontinence are important here also. Anticholinergic drugs (eg, oxybutynin (Ditropan), 5 mg 2 or 3 times daily, or flavoxate, 100–200 mg 3 times daily), have been used and may help; however, they are likely to produce serious side effects in elderly people. Imipramine, 25 mg at bedtime, may be helpful but should be used cautiously. Calcium channel blockers (eg, nifedipine, 10–20 mg twice daily) may decrease incontinence in some patients. If senile vaginitis is also present, estrogen therapy (conjugated estrogens, 0.3–0.625 mg daily) may help.

F. Overflow Incontinence: Obstructive benign prostatic hypertrophy should be corrected surgically. Discontinue or decrease the dosage of anticholinergic drugs. Encourage frequent toileting. Bethanechol chloride, 5 mg cautiously 2 or 3 times daily, may be helpful. Prazosin, 1 mg twice daily, may be tried with extreme caution because of concern for syncope.

G. Stress Incontinence and Pelvic Floor Relaxation: Give estrogen as ethinyl estradiol, 0.02–0.05 mg orally every other day. For pelvic floor relaxation, exercises to strengthen the pelvic floor musculature should be tried. Cystocele and severe pelvic floor relaxation may require surgery. A pessary may be of help if the patient is a poor surgical risk or refuses surgery. If all else fails, a cautious trial of an α-adrenergic agonist to increase sphincter contraction may be attempted (eg, phenylpropanolamine, 25–50 mg twice daily).

H. Psychogenic Incontinence: If incontinence is associated with depression and no other treatable causes are found, a trial of antidepressants (eg, imipramine, 25 mg/d) may be helpful. If related to "acting out" by the "difficult" patient, giving the patient an opportunity to ventilate may help, or psychiatric consultation may be indicated.

General Comments

Diagnose the type of incontinence first. Stress incontinence and incontinence associated with bladder infection usually have a characteristic history. A distended bladder found on physical examination suggests urinary retention or obstruction and overflow incontinence. Detrusor instability is the usual cause of incontinence in the demented patient.

Avoid catheterization if possible, since it imposes a risk of urinary tract infection. If essential, a condom catheter may be used in men intermittently with proper hygienic care. Absorbent underpants may simplify management.

Frequent toileting is often the single most important feature of treatment.

Sedatives, hypnotics and diuretics should be discontinued whenever possible.

"IATROGENIC" DRUG REACTIONS

Older patients are 2 or 3 times more likely than young to middle-aged adults to have adverse drug reactions, for a number of reasons. Changes in absorption, even with achlorhydria, are usually not of clinical significance, but drug clearance is often markedly reduced. This is due to a decrease in renal plasma flow and glomerular filtration rate as well as reduced hepatic clearance. The latter is due to a decrease in activity of the drug-metabolizing microsomal enzymes as well as an overall decrease in blood flow to the liver with aging. The volume of distribution of drugs also is affected, since the elderly have a decrease in total body water and a relative increase in body fat. Thus, water-soluble drugs become more concentrated, and fat-soluble drugs have longer half-lives. In addition, serum albumin levels decrease, so that there is some decrease in protein binding of some drugs (eg, warfarin, phenytoin), leaving more free (active) drug available.

In addition, the older patient with multiple chronic conditions is likely to be receiving many drugs. Thus, adverse drug reactions and dosage errors are more likely to occur, especially if the patient has visual, hearing, or memory deficits.

Precautions in Administering Drugs

To avoid drug toxicity in the elderly, the following should be kept in mind:

A. Drug Selection and Administration:

1. Use drug therapy only when the benefit clearly outweighs the risk.

2. Start with less than the usual adult dosage, and increase the dosage slowly.

3. Keep the dosage schedule as simple as possible.

4. Keep the number of tablets or capsules to a minimum, but try to avoid combination drugs. Combinations may be used only after the benefit of and tolerance to each drug, given separately in the same dose as in the combination preparation, have been established.

5. Have the patient or a family member bring in all medications at frequent intervals for reinforcing instructions regarding reasons for drug use, dosage, frequency of administration, and possible adverse effects.

6. Serum drug levels may be necessary for monitoring certain potentially toxic drugs with narrow therapeutic indices such as digoxin, quinidine, aminoglycosides, lithium, and other psychotropic drugs.

7. As long as the special problems of drug therapy in the elderly are kept in mind, the physician should not withhold essential drugs from older patients.

8. Instruct the pharmacist not to use safety cap containers unless the patient is confused or at high risk for suicide or is living with small grandchildren, since it may be difficult or impossible for the patient to open them.

B. Over-the-Counter Drugs: Adverse drug reactions may result from taking over-the-counter drugs or drugs prescribed for others in the household in addition to those prescribed for the patient. Have the patient or a family member bring in for review all over-the-counter drugs as well as prescription drugs the patient may be taking. Most cold pills contain antihistamines that can produce drowsiness or confusion as well as anticholinergic side effects (eg, dryness of mouth, blurring of vision, confusion, urinary hesitancy or retention).

C. Sedative-Hypnotics: Remember that the effects of sedative-hypnotics persist much longer in the elderly and may produce confusional states. Avoid this class of drugs whenever possible. Even the shorter-acting benzodiazepines may have adverse effects.

D. Antibiotics: Serum creatinine is not a good index of renal function in old people. An age-corrected creatinine clearance determination should be used to calculate drug doses of ototoxic and nephrotoxic antibiotics. (See Laboratory Examinations & Imaging, above.)

E. Cardiac Drugs: Both digitalis and quinidine have prolonged half-lives in older patients and have narrow therapeutic windows, so toxicity is common at the usual dosages.

F. Cimetidine: Cimetidine lowers hepatic blood flow, which reduces drug metabolism and thus results in a higher incidence of toxicity of drugs metabolized mainly in the liver (eg, propranolol). In addition, cimetidine itself often produces confusion in the elderly.

G. Antidepressants and Antipsychotics: Antidepressants and antipsychotics are very likely to produce anticholinergic side effects in old people (eg, confusion, urinary retention, constipation, dry mouth). A period of cautious drug withdrawal should be attempted before assuming that such symptoms are age-related or due to other diseases.

H. Avoid Overtreatment: Drugs are not necessarily indicated in some common clinical situations:

1. Asymptomatic bacteriuria—Antibiotics need

not be given unless associated with obstructive uropathy, other anatomic abnormalities, or stones.

2. Ankle edema–Often due to venous insufficiency; diuretics are usually not indicated unless edema is associated with heart failure.

3. Sleep pattern changes–Avoid prescribing hypnotics until nonpharmacologic interventions have been tried.

SUMMARY

Special Considerations in Treating the Elderly

A. Encourage Hopeful Attitude: Remember that 80% of patients over age 80 function well and relatively independently in the community and should not be assumed to be demented, helpless, or hopeless. Remember also that the average 75-year-old man can expect to live to age 84 and the average 85-year-old woman to age 92.

B. Provide Prompt Medical Care: Impaired homeostasis or even mild changes in physical status in the frail elderly dictate *prompt* medical attention.

C. Attend to Psychosocial Problems: Early attention to social and psychologic problems may be critical factors in the patient's ability to remain independent.

D. Geriatric Assessment: The frail elderly patient facing institutionalization may benefit significantly (as may the family also) by referral for geriatric assessment. Assessment may prevent unnecessary nursing home placement and help families and patients cope with difficult problems by "case management," ie, coordination of available community health and social services.

E. Encourage Home Care: Every attempt should be made to allow the patient to stay at home. Some community resources that may be of value include the following: Home Health Care, Day Health Care, Respite Beds (families who care for elderly relatives at home often require periods of relief from that burden if they are to be able to continue to keep the patient at home), Meals on Wheels, Home Health Aides, Transportation Services for the Disabled, and Visiting Nurses. Daily telephone contact, emergency radio systems, and communal and sheltered living arrangements all have obvious advantages in overall management of old people needing care and attention. Keep in mind the burden that maintaining the patient at home may impose on the family's primary caregiver. This person will need a great deal of support.

F. Monitor Drug Therapy: Allow enough time for the patient to respond to treatment before switching to different medications or other forms of treatment.

G. Advance Directives: Once having established a comfortable relationship with the elderly patient, one should obtain explicit information about the patient's wishes regarding life support systems in case the patient should be unable to communicate those wishes when very ill. Executing a durable power of attorney for health care when still well may help avoid future conflicts, confusion, and potential legal problems.

H. Assess Feasibility of Surgery: Age alone should never be the sole criterion for deciding whether a surgical procedure should be done. Survival following surgery in the elderly has increased dramatically in recent years. Premorbid health status and the patient's wishes are far more important than age in making this decision.

I. Assist the Family: If the patient has dementia or other complex medical and psychosocial problems, the family often needs the physician's support even more than the patient.

Identification of the "High-Risk" Elderly

The following patients are at greater risk of rapid deterioration and institutionalization than others and should be monitored more closely;

(1) Those over age 80.

(2) Those who live alone.

(3) Those who are bereaved or depressed.

(4) Those who are intellectually impaired.

(5) Those who have fallen several times.

(6) Those with incontinence.

(7) Those who have not coped well in the past.

General Instructions to the Elderly Patient

The elderly patient should be given some general practical instructions for maintaining health, dignity, and independence. The following is a partial list of subjects that can be introduced as the occasion arises:

A. Outside Interests: Maintain an active interest in others and the outside world.

B. Nutrition: Eat nourishing food with adequate protein, fruit, vegetables, and fiber content. Avoid excess calories and salt intake. This sometimes requires smaller and more frequent meals.

C. Exercise: Exercise briskly by walking outside of the house at least 3–4 times weekly if possible. A patient who is unable to walk should be taught how to do muscle and movement exercises in a chair or in bed at least 4 times daily, accepting the use of a cane or walker when necessary.

D. Fluids: Drink 3–4 glasses of water daily to avoid dehydration.

E. Skin Hygiene: Devote proper attention to the skin, with adequate hygiene, but avoid overdrying of the skin by too frequent bathing.

F. Eyeglasses: Make sure eyeglasses are properly fitted and checked periodically.

G. Foot Care: Make sure that shoes are properly fitted and that feet are examined periodically.

H. Hearing Aid: Accept the use of a hearing aid when needed, and talk to a physician for advice in obtaining one. They are less visible now and, even if noticed, are evidence that the wearer is interested in communicating. Much less expensive assistive listening devices (''ALD'') to amplify sound may be found in radio or electronic stores.

I. Dentures: Obtain dental services as needed, including being sure dentures fit properly.

J. Unnecessary Drugs: Avoid all types of nonessential medicines, especially sleeping pills and tranquilizers. Remember that with age, it is normal for sleep patterns and sleep requirements to change.

K. Misuse of Alcohol: Avoid intemperate use of alcoholic beverages.

L. Physical Safety: Take appropriate measures to prevent home accidents and injuries. Install handrails, provide adequate lighting, resurface or replace slippery floors, and keep loose appliance and telephone cords off the floor. Night lighting in the bedroom and bathroom is very useful. Avoid hypothermia by means of adequate clothing, heating, and physical activity. Care is needed in preventing burns (eg, when using hot water or electric heating pads).

M. Medical Care: Seek prompt medical attention and openly discuss symptoms of dreaded diseases such as cancer or dementia. The physician should be contacted even when symptoms are equivocal. Let your physician know what your wishes are in all medical decisions, but particularly what you do or do not want done when you are terminally ill and perhaps unable to communicate.

N. Sexuality: It is not abnormal to have sexual thoughts and desires as we age. Feel free to discuss any sexual problems with your physician.

O. Natural Limitations: Recognize the natural limitations imposed by aging, but be certain that medical and other problems are given proper consideration and are not ascribed to ''old age'' without suitable diagnostic evaluation.

REFERENCES

Alman RM et al: Pressure sores among hospitalized patients. Ann Intern Med 1986;105:337.

Beers M et al: Psychoactive medication use in intermediate-care facility residents. JAMA 1988;260:3016.

Eslinger PJ et al: Neuropsychologic detection of abnormal mental decline in older persons. JAMA 1985; 253:670.

Ettinger B: A practical guide to preventing osteoporosis. West J Med 1988;149:691. (An excellent review that can be used to instruct women on the value of preventing osteoporosis.)

Evans D et al: Prevalence of Alzheimer's disease in a community population of older persons. JAMA 1986; 262:2551.

Francis J et al: A prospective study of delirium in hospitalized elderly. JAMA 1990;263:1097.

Gurland BJ et al: The assessment of cognitive function in the elderly. Clin Geriatr Med 1987;3:530. (Practical review, including specific tests available.)

Hall FM, Davis MA, Baran DT: Bone mineral screening for osteoporosis. N Engl J Med 1987;316:212.

Health and Public Policy Committee, American College of Physicians: Financing long-term care. Ann Intern Med 1988;108:279.

Heikoff LE: Practical management of demented elderly. West J Med 1986;145:397. (Practical aspects of management.)

Kane R, Kane R: Lexington Books, 1981.

Kelsey J, Hoffman S: Risk factors for hip fracture. (Editorial.) N Engl J Med 1987;316:404.

Kroenke K, Corrie GD: Urinary incontinence. West J Med 1987;146:623.

Larson EB, Bruce RA: Exercise and aging. Ann Intern Med 1986;105:783. (Brief good review of benefits of exercise with aging—especially regarding cardiovascular effects and muscle strengthening.)

Larson EB at al: Adverse drug reactions with global cognitive impairment in elderly persons. Ann Intern Med 1987;107:169.

Larson EB et al: Diagnostic tests in the evaluation of dementia: A prospective study of 200 elderly outpatients. Ann Intern Med 1986;146:1917.

Lipschitz DA et al: Cancer in the elderly: Basic science and clinical aspects. Ann Intern Med 1985;102:218.

Lipsitz LA: Orthostatic hypotension in the elderly. N Engl J Med 198321:658.

Mahler ME, Cummings JL, Tomiyasu U: Atypical dementia syndrome in an elderly man. J Am Geriatr Soc 1987;35:1116.

McIntosh JL: Suicide among the elderly: Levels and trends. Am J Orthopsychiatry 1985;55:288.

Morley JE et al: Nutrition in the elderly: UCLA conference. Ann Intern Med 1988;109:890.

Morley JE et al: UCLA geriatric grand rounds: Osteoporosis. J Am Geriatr Soc 1988;36:845. (Type 1 and type 2 osteoporosis, pathophysiology and treatment.)

Ouslander J et al: Simple versus multichannel cystometry in the evaluation of bladder function in an incontinent geriatric population. J Urol 1988;140:1482.

Palmore E, Nowlin J, Wang M: Predictors of function among the old-old: A 10-year follow-up. J Gerontol 1985;40:244.

Rango N: The nursing home resident with dementia: Clinical care, ethics and policy implications. Ann Intern Med 1985;102:835.

Resnick NM: Initial evaluation of the incontinent patient. J Am Geriatr Soc 1990;38:311.

Resnick NM, Greenspan SL: ''Senile'' osteoporosis reconsidered. JAMA 1989;261:1025. (Excellent critique of literature on type 2 osteoporosis.)

Salzman C: Geriatric psychopharmacology. Annu Rev Med 1985;36:217.

Schneider E, Reed JD Jr: Life extension. N Engl J Med 1985;312:1159.

Solomon D: National-Institutes-of-Health Consensus Development Conference Statement: Geriatric assessment methods for clinical decision-making. J Am Geriatr Soc 1988;36:342.

Solomon DH et al: UCLA Conference: New issues in geriatric care. Ann Intern Med 1988;108:718.

Terry RD, Katzman R: Senile dementia of the Alzheimer type. Ann Neurol 1983;14:497.

Tinetti ME, Speechley M: Prevention of falls among the elderly. N Engl J Med 1989;320:1055. (Excellent review of causes, evaluation, and prevention of falls.)

Wein AS: Pharmacologic treatment of incontinence. J Am Geriatr Soc 1990;38:317.

Wrenn K: Fecal impaction. N Engl J Med 1989;321:658.

3

Malignant Disorders

Sydney E. Salmon, MD

"Cancer" is a general term that denotes a complex series of proliferative disorders of cells associated with mutation in DNA sequences leading to amplification or increased expression of "oncogenes" or deletion of "tumor suppressor genes"—or both processes. Oncogenes are usually normal cellular genes and encode the sequences for cellular growth factor receptors, growth factors, or elements of the proliferative machinery of the cancer cell. Tumor suppressor genes encode for regulatory proteins that normally suppress cellular proliferation. The consequence of these and other mutations, which are usually due to environmental causes, is the disease process called cancer.

Cancer is associated with tumor growth, invasion, and metastasis of the transformed cells. General classes of environmental carcinogens include chemical carcinogens, oncogenic viruses, and physical causes such as environmental radiation. There are also apparent linkages to hereditary predisposition for some specific forms of cancer (eg, retinoblastoma). The single most important recognized carcinogen is tobacco, and tobacco-related cancers account for one-third of all fatal forms of cancer. Non-Hodgkin's lymphoma is now increasing in incidence in relation to HIV and the AIDS epidemic and other environmental carcinomas. Cancer is the second most common cause of death in the USA. Aside from nonmelanomatous skin cancers, there are over 1 million new cases of cancer in the USA every year and over 500,000 deaths. Table 3–1 summarizes current incidence figures for some of the major forms of cancer as well as for all sites combined.

While cancer prevention is an eventual goal, for most sites additional scientific information will be needed before effective prevention can be achieved. Early diagnosis of cancer involving some sites can be enhanced with standardized screening approaches (eg, Papanicolaou smears, routine mammography) and can increase the cure rate. For most sites, stage at presentation is related to curability, with the highest cure rates reported when the tumor is small and there is no evidence of metastasis. However, for some tumor sites (eg, lung cancer), distant metastasis occurs even from small tumors before they can be detected. More sensitive detection methods are needed for many forms of cancer (eg, ovary, pancreas, kidney). Standardized staging for tumor burden at the time of diagnosis (eg, using the TNM system) is extremely valuable for determining prognosis and making decisions about treatment for individual patients.

The major features of this chapter are the clinical aspects of cancer, including (1) syndromes that may be important in diagnosis and management, (2) diagnosis and treatment of emergency complications, (3) the role of surgery and radiotherapy in primary treatment, (4) chemotherapy for advanced disease, and (5) adjuvant chemotherapy for micrometastases. Specific cancers are discussed in the appropriate organ system chapters.

THE PARANEOPLASTIC SYNDROMES

The clinical manifestations of cancer are usually due to pressure effects of local tumor growth; to infiltration or metastatic deposition of tumor cells in a variety of organs in the body; or to certain systemic symptoms. General problems observed in many patients with advanced or widespread metastatic cancer include anorexia, malaise, weight loss, and sometimes fever. These characteristics must be considered when evaluating a patient with an undiagnosed illness. Except in the case of functioning tumors such as those of the endocrine glands, systemic symptoms of cancer usually are not specific, often consisting of weakness, anorexia, and weight loss. The term paraneoplastic refers to features of disease considered to be due to the remote effects of a cancer that cannot be attributed either to a cancer's direct invasive or metastatic properties and are often considered to be due to aberrant hormonal or metabolic effects not observed in a cancer's normal tissue equivalent. In the paraneoplastic syndromes, clinical findings may resemble those of primary endocrine, metabolic, hematologic, or neuromuscular disorders. At present, the mechanisms for such remote effects can be classed in 3 groups: (1) effects initiated by a tumor product (eg, carcinoid syndrome), (2) effects of destruction of normal tissues by tumor (eg, hypercalcemia with osteolytic skeletal metastases), and (3) effects due to unknown mechanisms (eg, osteoarthropathy with bronchogenic carcinoma). In paraneoplastic syndromes associated with ectopic hormone production, tumor tissue itself se-

Table 3–1. Incidence of the 10 most common cancers in the USA in males and females (all races).

Rank	Males	Rate[1]	Females	Rate[1]
1	Prostate	88	Breast	103
2	Lung	83	Colorectal	44
3	Colorectal	62	Lung	36
4	Leukemia	13	Endometrium	22
5	Bladder	29	Ovary	13
6	Lymphoma	18	Lymphoma	13
7	Oropharyngeal	16	Melanoma	9
8	Stomach	12	Cervix	8
9	Kidney	11	Bladder	8
10	Pancreas	11	Leukemia	7
	All sites	343	All sites	264

[1] Rates are per 100,000 in 1985–1986 and rounded to the nearest whole number and age-adjusted to the 1970 United States standard population. Both Hodgkin's disease and non-Hodgkin's lymphoma are included under lymphoma. Data from National Cancer Institute's SEER Program.

cretes the hormone that produces the syndrome. Ectopic hormones secreted by neoplasms are often prohormones of higher molecular weight than those secreted by the more differentiated normal endocrine cell. Such ectopic hormone production by cancer cells is believed to result from activation of genes in the malignant cells that are suppressed in the normal tissue equivalent and in most somatic cells. Autocrine growth factors secreted by neoplastic cells may also result in paraneoplastic syndromes. Small cell lung cancer is the one type of cancer most likely to be associated with paraneoplastic syndromes.

The paraneoplastic syndromes are of considerable clinical importance for the following reasons:

(1) They sometimes accompany relatively limited neoplastic growth and may provide the clinician with an early clue to the presence of certain types of cancer.

(2) The metabolic or toxic effects of the syndrome may constitute a more urgent hazard to the patient's life than the underlying cancer (eg, hypercalcemia, hyponatremia).

(3) Effective treatment of the tumor should be accompanied by resolution of the paraneoplastic syndrome, and, conversely, recurrence of the cancer may be heralded by return of the systemic symptoms. In some instances, rapid response to cytotoxic chemotherapy may briefly increase the severity of the paraneoplastic syndrome in association with tumor lysis (eg, hyponatremia with inappropriate antidiuretic hormone excretion). In some instances the identical symptom complex (eg, hypercalcemia) may be induced by entirely different mechanisms. A single syndrome such as hypercalcemia may be due to any one of a variety of humoral factors, such as secretion of parathyroid hormone precursors or homologs, an

osteoclast-activating factor (lymphotoxin), transforming growth factor alpha, or prostaglandins. Effective antitumor treatment usually results in return of serum calcium to normal.

Common paraneoplastic syndromes and endocrine secretions associated with functional cancers are summarized in Table 3–2.

Daughaday WH et al: Synthesis and secretion of insulinlike growth factor II by a leiomyosarcoma with associated hypoglycemia. N Engl J Med 1988;319:1434.

List AF et al: The syndrome of inappropriate secretion of antidiuretic hormone (SIADH) in small cell lung cancer. J Clin Oncol 1986;4:1191.

MANAGEMENT OF EMERGENCIES & COMPLICATIONS OF MALIGNANT DISEASE*

Cancer is a chronic disease, but acute emergency complications may occur as a consequence of local (spinal cord compression, superior vena cava syndrome, malignant effusions, etc) or generalized systemic effects (hypercalcemia, opportunistic infections, disseminated intravascular coagulation, hyperuricemia, etc).

SPINAL CORD COMPRESSION

Spinal cord compression by tumor mass is manifested by back pain, progressive weakness and sensory changes in the lower extremities, and blockage of contrast material as shown by myelography. It occurs as a complication of lymphoma or multiple myeloma or of metastatic solid tumor. Back pain at the level of the lesion occurs in over 80% of cases and may be aggravated by lying down, weight bearing, sneezing, or coughing; it usually precedes the development of neurologic symptoms or signs. Since involvement is usually epidural, a mixture of nerve root and spinal cord symptoms often develops.

The initial findings of impending cord compression may be quite subtle, and there should be a high index of suspicion when cancer patients develop back pain or weakness of the lower extremities. Prompt diagnosis and therapy are essential, since paralysis is irreversible once it develops; patients who are treated promptly may have complete return of function and, depending on tumor sensitivity to specific treatment, may respond favorably to subsequent anticancer therapy. Once a severe neurologic defect develops, it is

* Superior vena cava syndrome in discussed in Chapter 9.

Table 3–2. Paraneoplastic syndromes and certain endocrine secretions associated with cancer.

Hormone Excess or Syndrome	Broncho-genic Carci-noma	Breast Carci-noma	Renal Carci-noma	Adrenal Carci-noma	Hepa-toma	Multiple Myeloma	Lym-phoma	Thy-moma	Prostatic Carci-noma	Pan-creatic Carci-noma	Chorio-carci-noma	Sarcoma
Hypercalcemia	++	++++	++	++	+	++++	+	+	++	+	+	+
Cushing's syn-drome	+++		+	+++				++	+	++		
Inappropriate ADH se-cretion	+++						+			+		
Hypoglycemia				+	++		+					+++
Gonadotropins	+				+						++++	
Thyrotropin											+++	
Polycythemia			+++	+	++							
Erythroid apla-sia								++				
Fever			+++		++		+++	++		+		+
Neuro-myopathy	++	+						++	+	+		
Derma-tomyositis	++	+								+		
Coagulopathy	+	++			+	+			+++	+++		
Thrombophle-bitis			+							+	+++	
Humoral im-mune defi-cits						+++	+++	+++				

usually irreversible. Therefore, early diagnosis is essential.

While bone radiographs may show evidence of vertebral metastases, they are not a substitute for myelography. Magnetic resonance imaging (MRI) offers an excellent noninvasive alternative to the myelogram and provides sagittal images of the entire spinal cord and vertebral canal. When the symptoms or neurologic examination are at all suggestive, an emergency CT, myelogram or MRI scan should be performed. If a block is demonstrated on myelography, additional contrast is injected above the lesions to exclude the possibility of multiple lesions.

Emergency treatment. Radiation therapy to the involved area of the block and 2 adjacent vertebrae above and below represents the treatment of choice. High doses of glucocorticoids are usually administered on an emergency basis as soon as the diagnosis is established and often continued through the majority or all of the course of radiation therapy. The addition of chemotherapy is occasionally of use in treating lymphomas. Emergency surgery is indicated if there is doubt about the cause of the block.

Wilson JKV, Masaryk TJ: Neurologic emergencies in the cancer patient. Semin Oncol 1989;16:490.

MALIGNANT EFFUSIONS

The development of effusions in the pleural, pericardial, and peritoneal spaces presents diagnostic and therapeutic problems in patients with advanced neoplasms. Direct involvement of the serous surface with tumor appears to be the most frequent initiating factor in such cases. Benign processes such as congestive heart failure, pulmonary embolus, trauma, and infection (eg, tuberculosis) may be confused with malignant effusion. Bloody effusions are usually due to cancer but occasionally are due to pulmonary embolism or trauma. Chylous effusions may be associated with thoracic duct obstruction or may result from mediastinal lymph node enlargement in lymphoma. Cytologic or cell block establishes that the effusion is neoplastic in origin before local therapy is used to prevent recurrence. Pericardial effusions are best aspirated under fluoroscopy.

The management of effusions should be appropriate to the severity of involvement. Diuretics are often tried as an initial treatment for small to moderate-sized effusions and administered as an adjunct to local drainage with large effusions and to minimize the possibility of pulmonary edema that may occasionally occur after thoracentesis. Effusions due to lung, ovarian, and breast carcinoma often require more than simple drainage. Drainage of a large pleural effusion can be accomplished rapidly with a closed system using a disposable phlebotomy set connected to a vacuum phlebotomy bottle. Ultrasonography facilitates localization and removal of small or loculated effusions. For recurrent effusions, closed water-seal drainage with a chest tube for 3–4 days is an effective way to seal off the pleural space. Posttap radiographs are always indicated after thoracentesis to assess the results and exclude pneumothorax.

Recurrent effusions that do not respond to repeated taps or a chest tube may often be controlled by "chemosclerosis," which consists of instillation of tetracycline, bleomycin, quinacrine, or mechlorethamine. These agents are normally admixed with a small amount of lidocaine (to help control the pain associated with the local inflammation induced). The alkylating agent thiotepa and the antibiotic bleomycin appear to be preferable for suppression of malignant ascites, since they produce less local pain and discomfort in the peritoneum than do other agents.

The procedure is as follows: Most of the pleural, ascitic, or pericardial fluid is withdrawn. While a free flow of fluid is still present, a parenteral formulation of tetracycline (500 mg), mechlorethamine (20–30 mg), thiotepa (30 mg), or bleomycin (60 units) —admixed with a small amount of lidocaine (eg, 5 mL)—is instilled into the cavity. The solution should be freshly mixed at the time of injection. After the drug is injected and the needle withdrawn, the patient is placed in a variety of positions in order to distribute the drug throughout the cavity. Attendance to careful positioning is particularly important for pleurodesis. On the following day, the remaining fluid is withdrawn. Inasmuch as at least half of the instilled drug is absorbed systemically from the cavity, use of alkylating agents is not advised for patients who already have significant pancytopenia or bone marrow depression due to chemotherapy. In such cases, bleomycin, quinacrine, or tetracycline is indicated. Quinacrine is usually administered in a dose of 200 mg/d for 5 days, with daily drainage of residual fluid. Two or more daily doses of tetracycline are also frequently required.

Nausea and vomiting commonly follow the instillation of mechlorethamine but can often be controlled with prophylactic administration of an antiemetic agent prior to the procedure and at intervals afterward. Pleural pain and fever may occur after intracavitary administration of alkylating agents, tetracycline, or quinacrine but are more common with the latter compounds. Orders for narcotic analgesic administration should be written to cover at least the first 24 hours after pleurodesis. Bleomycin instillation may cause fever but generally is unassociated with significant toxicity. Effusions can also act as "sanctuaries" in which viable tumor stem cells are protected from systemic chemotherapy. Though the pleural or other potential space may be effectively sealed with such treatment, recurrent effusion is occasionally a problem.

Hausheer FH, Yarboro JW: Diagnosis and treatment of malignant pleural effusion. Semin Oncol 1985;12:54.

HYPERCALCEMIA

Hypercalcemia secondary to cancer is a fairly common medical emergency, particularly in lung and breast carcinoma and multiple myeloma but also with a variety of other cancers. Bone metastasis is not an essential feature of the syndrome. Various endocrine causes of hypercalcemia of cancer are discussed above under paraneoplastic syndromes. Typical findings in addition to elevated serum calcium are anorexia, nausea and vomiting, constipation, polyuria, muscular weakness and hyporeflexia, confusion, psychosis, tremor, and lethargy; some patients are asymptomatic. Electrocardiography often shows a shortening of the QT interval. When the serum calcium rises above 12 mg/dL, sudden death due to cardiac arrhythmia or asystole may occur. The presence of hypercalcemia does not invariably indicate a dismal prognosis, especially in breast or prostate cancer.

In the absence of signs or symptoms of hypercalcemia, a laboratory finding of elevated serum calcium should be retested immediately to exclude the possibility of error.

Emergency treatment consists of (1) intravenous fluids, 3–4 L daily (starting with saline); (2) intravenous administration of a potent diuretic (such as furosemide) once saline infusion has been initiated and the volume status normalized; (3) the diphosphonate, etidronate disodium (Didronel), 7.5 mg/kg/d orally; (4) calcitonin; and (5) prednisone, 60–80 mg/d orally for 4–5 days, followed by tapering. For refractory cases, mithramycin (Mithracin), 25 mg/kg, is given intravenously every other day for 2–4 doses. Although mithramycin therapy is often effective, the drug has significant toxicities, including potential hemorrhagic diathesis and myelosuppression after frequent repeated dosing.

Once the acute episode has been treated, chemotherapy may be considered. In breast cancer, hypercalcemia may appear as a "flare" after initiation of estrogen or antiestrogen therapy; the patient will often achieve excellent tumor remission with continued therapy. If chronic hypercalcemia persists–even if only to a moderate degree–the patient should be treated with small doses of prednisone, etidronate disodium, or Neutra-Phos, 3–4 g/d, and encouraged to maintain a high fluid intake. In most instances, if the cancer responds to chemotherapy, hypercalcemia subsides.

Insogna KL, Broadus AE: Hypercalcemia of malignancy. Annu Rev Med 1987;38:241.

Ringenberg QS, Ritch PS: Efficacy of oral administration of etidronate disodium in maintaining normal serum calcium levels in previously hypercalcemia cancer patients. Clin Ther 1987;9:318.

HYPERURICEMIA & ACUTE URATE NEPHROPATHY

Hyperuricemia is most often a complication of treatment for hematologic neoplasms such as leukemia, lymphoma, and myeloma, but it may occur with any form of cancer undergoing destruction and release of nucleic acid constituents. Less commonly, certain rapidly proliferating neoplasms with a high nucleic acid turnover (eg, acute leukemia) may present with hyperuricemia even in the absence of prior chemotherapy. If the patient is also receiving a thiazide diuretic, the problem may be compounded by decreased urate excretion. Initial follow-up of patients receiving cancer chemotherapy should include measurements of serum uric acid and creatinine. Rapid elevation of the serum uric acid concentration usually does not produce gouty arthritis in these patients but does present the danger of acute urate nephropathy. In this form of acute renal failure, uric acid crystallizes in the distal tubules, the collecting ducts, and the renal parenchyma. The danger of uric acid nephropathy is present when the serum urate concentration is above 15 mg/dL.

Prophylactic therapy consists of giving allopurinol, 100 mg orally 3 times daily, starting 1 day before initiation of chemotherapy. Allopurinol inhibits xanthine oxidase and prevents conversion of the highly soluble hypoxanthine and xanthine to the relatively insoluble uric acid. Patients who are to receive the purine antagonists mercaptopurine or azathioprine for cancer chemotherapy should be given only 25–35% of the calculated dose if they are also receiving allopurinol, inasmuch as the latter drug potentiates both the effects and toxicity of these drugs.

Emergency therapy for established severe hyperuricemia consists of (1) hydration with 2–4 L of fluid per day; (2) alkalinization of the urine with 6–8 g of sodium bicarbonate per day (to enhance urate solubility); (3) allopurinol, 200 mg 4 times daily orally; and (4) in severe cases, with serum urate levels above 25–30 mg/dL, emergency hemodialysis.

Since patients who suffer from this complication are often entering a stage of complete remission of the neoplasm, the prognosis is good if renal damage can be prevented.

BACTERIAL SEPSIS IN CANCER PATIENTS

Many patients with disseminated neoplasms have increased susceptibility to infection. In some instances, this results from impaired host defense mechanisms (eg, acute leukemia, Hodgkin's disease, multiple myeloma, chronic lymphocytic leukemia); in others, it results from the myelosuppressive and immunosuppressive effects of cancer chemotherapy or a combination of these factors. The bacterial organisms accounting for the majority of infections in cancer patients include Enterobacteriaceae *(Klebsiella-Enterobacter-Serratia-Escherichia coli)*, *Staphylococcus*, *Streptococcus*, *Corynebacterium*, *Pseudomonas*, *Clostridium*, *Mycobacterium*, and *Legionella* species. In patients with acute leukemia and in those with granulocytopenia (<600 granulocytes per microliter), infection is a medical emergency. Although fever alone does not prove the presence of infection, in these patients as well as in patients with multiple myeloma or chronic lymphocytic leukemia, it is highly suggestive. While infections in patients with myeloma or chronic leukemia are often due to sensitive organisms, patients with pancytopenia are less fortunate, as resistant gram-negative organisms are commonly responsible. Appropriate cultures (eg, blood, sputum, urine, cerebrospinal fluid) should always be obtained before starting therapy; however, one should not wait for results of these studies before initiating bactericidal antibiotic therapy. Gram-stained smears may show a predominant organism in sputum, urine, or cerebrospinal fluid.

Emergency Treatment

In the absence of granulocytopenia and in nonleukemic patients, the combination of a third-generation cephalosporin with an aminoglycoside (tobramycin or gentamicin) has proved useful for many patients with acute bacteremia. Whenever possible, empirically prescribed antibiotics should be directed against expected bacteria and susceptibilities until culture results are available. In the current era of intensive chemotherapy of acute leukemia, *Pseudomonas* bacteremia is the most frequent life-threatening infection in granulocytopenic patients. Until recently, empiric therapy generally consisted of 1- or 3-drug combinations including an aminoglycoside and an antipseudomonal penicillin, with resolution of fever and bacteremia in about 70% of patients. Current results using initial monotherapy with ceftazidime appear to yield similar results. In cases selected on the basis of culture results or clinical suspicion, either vancomycin or amphotericin B may be added to ceftazidime. *Pneumocystis carinii* is an important pathogen in patients with advanced Hodgkin's disease with T cell deficiency as well as in patients with epidemic Kaposi's sarcoma or Burkitt's lymphoma associated with AIDS. Trimethoprim-sulfamethoxazole, pentamidine, dapsone, and trimetrexate are all of use in such patients.

The recombinant bone marrow growth factors granulocyte colony-stimulating factor (GCSF) and granulocyte-macrophage colony-stimulating factor (GMCSF) have proved effective in reducing the duration of neutropenia and the frequency and severity of infection after myelosuppressive chemotherapy, and these agents will soon be licensed for this indication by the FDA. GMCSF has also been used to stimulate bone marrow stem cell production in both the circulating and bone marrow cell populations collected for autologous bone marrow transplantation. Administration after autologous or allogeneic transplantation reduces the toxicity of this procedure.

Gabrilove JL et al: Effect of granulocyte colony-stimulating factor on neutropenia and associated morbidity due to chemotherapy for transitional-cell carcinoma of the urothelium. N Engl J Med 1988;318:1414.

Herrmann F et al: Hematopoietic responses in patients with advanced malignancy treated with recombinant human granulocyte-macrophage colony-stimulating factor. J Clin Oncol 1989;7:159.

Lazarus HM et al: Infectious emergencies in oncology patients. Semin Oncol 1989;16:543.

Morstyn G et al: Effect of granulocyte colony stimulating factor on neutropenia induced by cytotoxic chemotherapy. Lancet 1988;1:667.

Pizzo PA et al: A randomized trial comparing ceftazidime alone with combination antibiotic therapy in cancer patients with fever and neutropenia. N Engl J Med 1986;315:552.

CARCINOID SYNDROME

Although tumors of argentaffin cells are rare, they secrete a variety of vasoactive materials, including serotonin, histamine, catecholamines, prostaglandins, and vasoactive peptides. Carcinoid tumors usually arise from the ileum, stomach, or bronchi and tend to metastasize early; in most patients with small intestinal carcinoid tumors, development of the syndrome usually requires hepatic metastases. Related syndromes occur in patients with pancreatic tumors secreting vasointestinal peptides. Such patients frequently have severe watery diarrhea (pancreatic cholera).

The manifestations of carcinoid syndrome include facial flushing, edema of the head and neck (especially with bronchial carcinoid), abdominal cramps and diarrhea, bronchospasm, cardiac lesions (pulmonary or tricuspid stenosis or insufficiency), telangiectases, and increased urinary 5-hydroxyindoleacetic acid (5-HIAA). Patients with symptomatic intestinal carcinoids usually excrete more than 25 mg of 5-HIAA per day in the urine. Ideally, all drugs should be withheld for several days prior to the urine collection.

Emergency therapy for patients with symptomatic bronchial carcinoids consists of giving prednisone, 15–30 mg orally daily. With intestinal carcinoids, abdominal cramps and diarrhea can often be managed with diphenoxylate with atropine (Lomotil), alone or in combination with an antiserotonin agent such as methysergide maleate.

The H$_1$ histamine receptor antagonist cyprohepta-dine, the H$_2$ receptor blocker cimetidine, and phenothiazines may prove useful. A new synthetic peptide somatostatin agonist, octreotide acetate (Sandostatin), is the most effective agent for reducing symptoms due to carcinoid syndrome in association with significant reduction in levels of 5-HIAA. Octreotide is effective also in the symptomatic treatment of vasointestinal peptide-secreting pancreatic tumors (vipomas) and markedly reduces the watery diarrhea syndrome with such neoplasms.

Chemotherapy with interferon alfa-2, doxorubicin plus cyclophosphamide, and fluorouracil or streptozocin is used for advanced-stage carcinoid patients.

Maton PN et al: Effect of a long-acting somatostatin analogue (SMS 201–995) in a patient with pancreatic cholera. N Engl J Med 1985;312:17.

Moertel CG: Treatment of the carcinoid tumor and the malignant carcinoid syndrome. J Clin Oncol 1983;1:727.

PRIMARY CANCER TREATMENT: THE ROLE OF SURGERY & RADIATION THERAPY

Most human cancers present initially as localized tumor nodules and cause local symptoms. Depending on the type of cancer, initial therapy may be directed locally in the form either of surgery or radiation therapy. This is the treatment of choice for a variety of potentially curable cancers, including most gastrointestinal and genitourinary cancers, central nervous system tumors, and cancers arising from the breast, thyroid, or skin as well as most sarcomas.

In other circumstances, surgery may be used for palliation of noncurable cases or for reconstruction and rehabilitation.

Surgery initially has both diagnostic and therapeutic effectiveness, since it permits pathologic staging of the extent of local and regional invasion as well as an opportunity for removal of the primary neoplasm. CT scanning and MRI play an increasing role in noninvasive tumor staging. However, it usually remains necessary for the surgeon to accurately identify those patients who can be potentially cured by local treatment alone.

For some specific sites, complete surgical removal of the tumor can be disfiguring, disabling, or unachievable. Under those circumstances, primary local treatment with ionizing radiation therapy may prove to be the treatment of choice. In other instances, surgery and radiation therapy are used in sequence.

Radiation therapy is usually delivered as brachytherapy or teletherapy. In brachytherapy, the radiation source is placed close to the tumor. This intracavitary approach is used for many gynecologic or oral neoplasms. In teletherapy, supervoltage radiotherapy is usually delivered with a linear accelerator, as this instrument permits more precise beam localization and avoids the complication of skin radiation toxicity. Various beam-modifying wedges, rotational techniques, and other specific approaches are used to increase the radiation dosage to the tumor bed while minimizing toxicity to adjacent normal tissues.

Well-oxygenated tumors are more radiosensitive than hypoxic tumors. Hypoxic tumors are often bulky, implying a potential synergistic role of surgical debulking prior to radiotherapy. Radiation therapy is normally delivered in a fractionated fashion, this method appearing to have radiobiologic superiority by permitting time for recovery of normal host tissues (but not the tumor) from sublethal damage during the period of treatment. Various normal tissues (particularly the skin, mucosal surfaces, spinal cord, bone marrow, and lymphoid system) can exhibit early or late toxicity from radiation therapy and limit radiation dosage. Fractionated radiation doses are usually administered for 5 days per week until the desired total dose has been delivered, usually over the course of 4–6 weeks.

For most tumor types, there is a sigmoid curve of increasing rate of control of the local tumor with increasing radiation dose. Radiosensitive tumors usually exhibit radiosensitivity over the dose range of 3500–5000 cGy.

Radiation therapy can play a special role in curative treatment of tumors of the larynx (permitting cure without loss of the voice), carcinoma of the uterine cervix, and early-stage breast cancer, Hodgkin's disease, and seminoma of the testis.

Increasingly, the primary local therapy of cancer is integrated with systemic therapy, an approach that has proved to be superior for apparently localized tumor types with a high propensity for early metastatic spread and for which anticancer drugs are available. Locoregional hyperthermia (40–42 °C) is a form of nonionizing irradiation that is of value as an adjunct to ionizing irradiation for some tumor sites. Hyperthermia's greatest use to date has been in relatively bulky hypovascular tumors with some degree of hypoxia.

SYSTEMIC CANCER THERAPY

Use of cytotoxic drugs, hormones, antihormones, and biologicals has become a highly specialized and increasingly effective means of treating cancer, and therapy is usually administered by a medical oncologist. Selection of specific drugs or protocols for various types of cancer has traditionally been based on results of prior clinical trials; however, many patients have drug-resistant tumors. Molecular mechanisms of drug resistance are now the subject of intense study. In many instances, specific drug resistance results from an amplification in the number of gene copies for an enzyme associated with drug resistance. A more general form of "multidrug resistance" to natural product anticancer drugs has also been described in association with expression of a 170,000-MW glycoprotein on the surface of tumor cells. This glycoprotein is an energy-dependent transport pump that facilitates drug efflux from tumor cells. Acquired multidrug resistance in multiple myeloma and lymphoma has been reversed clinically with addition of the calcium channel blocker verapamil to the chemotherapy regimen.

Cancer chemotherapy is usually curative in advanced stages of choriocarcinoma in women; in Burkitt's lymphoma and testicular tumors; and in some cases of acute leukemia, embryonal rhabdomyosarcoma, Hodgkin's disease, and diffuse large cell lymphoma. When combined with initial surgery—and in some instances with irradiation—chemotherapy also increases the cure rate in Wilms' tumor and may increase the rate of long-term control of breast cancer, colon cancer, and rectal cancer as well as of osteogenic sarcomas. Combination chemotherapy provides significant palliation of symptoms along with prolongation of survival in children with acute leukemia, Ewing's sarcoma, and retinoblastoma and in adults with Hodgkin's disease, non-Hodgkin lymphomas, mycosis fungoides, multiple myeloma, macroglobulinemia, and breast, ovary, prostate, and small-cell lung carcinoma. The results of currently available treatments are largely unsuccessful in squamous cancer of the lung as well as in metastatic melanoma and in adenocarcinomas of the colon, gallbladder, or pancreas.

While most anticancer drugs are used systemically, there are selected indications for local or regional administration (eg, intravesical therapy, intraperitoneal therapy, hepatic artery infusion).

A summary of the types of cancer responsive to chemotherapy and the current treatment of choice is offered in Table 3–3. In some instances (eg, Hodgkin's disease), optimal therapy may require a combination of therapeutic resources, eg, radiation therapy plus chemotherapy rather than chemotherapy alone. All patients with stage I or II Hodgkin's disease should receive radiation therapy. Table 3–4 outlines the currently used dosage schedules and the toxicities of the cancer chemotherapeutic agents. The dosage schedules given are for single-agent therapy. Combination therapy, as now used in advanced Hodgkin's disease, testicular tumors, and certain other neoplasms, often requires reductions of the dosages shown–otherwise, the combined toxicity would be prohibitive. Such combination therapy should be attempted only by oncologic specialists who have adequate supportive services available.

Table 3–3. Treatment choices for cancers responsive to systemic agents.

Diagnosis	Current Treatment of Choice	Other Valuable Agents
Acute lymphocytic leukemia	Induction: vincristine plus prednisone. Remission maintenance: mercaptopurine, methotrexate, and cyclophosphamide in various combinations.	Asparaginase, daunorubicin, VM-26,[1] carmustine, doxorubicin, cytarabine, allopurinol,[2] craniospinal radiotherapy.
Acute myelocytic and myelomonocytic leukemia	Combination chemotherapy: cytarabine and daunorubicin.	Vincristine, mitoxantrone, methotrexate, mercaptopurine, allopurinol,[2] azacitidine,[1] AMSA, prednisone, doxorubicin.
Chronic myelocytic leukemia	Busulfan or alfa-interferon.	Vincristine, mercaptopurine, hydroxyurea, melphalan, cytarabine, allopurinol.[2]
Chronic lymphocytic leukemia	Chlorambucil and prednisone (if indicated) or fludarabine[1]	Vincristine, androgens,[2] allopurinol,[2] doxorubicin.
Hairy cell leukemia	Interferon.	Deoxycoformycin[1] (pentostatin), chloroadenosine.
Hodgkin's disease (stages III and IV)	Combination chemotherapy: mechlorethamine, vincristine, procarbazine, prednisone ("MOPP").	Doxorubicin, bleomycin, vinblastine, dacarbazine ("ABVD"); lomustine, VM-26,[1] interferon, methotrexate.
Non-Hodgkin's lymphomas	Combination chemotherapy: cyclophosphamide, doxorubicin, vincristine, prednisone.	Bleomycin, lomustine, carmustine, methotrexate, cytarabine, VM-26,[1] AMSA, mitoxantrone, interferon.
Multiple myeloma	Combination chemotherapy: melphalan, cyclophosphamide, doxorubicin, vincristine, carmustine.	Prednisone or dexamethasone, interferon, androgens.[2]
Macroglobulinemia	Chlorambucil.	Melphalan, interferon.
Polycythemia vera	Busulfan, chlorambucil, or cyclophosphamide; radiophosphorus P 32.	
Carcinoma of lung	Etoposide plus cisplatin.	Quinacrine,[2] mitomycin, vincristine, vinblastine, doxorubicin, cyclophosphamide, fluorouracil.
"Head and neck" carcinomas	Cisplatin and fluorouracil.	Hydroxyurea, doxorubicin, vinblastine, methotrexate, bleomycin.
Carcinoma of uterus	Progestins or tamoxifen.	Cisplatin, fluorouracil, doxorubicin.
Carcinoma of ovary	Cyclophosphamide and cisplatin or carboplatin.	Doxorubicin, melphalan, fluorouracil, vincristine, hexamethylmelamine, taxol[2]
Carcinoma of cervix	Mitomycin, bleomycin, vincristine, and cisplatin.	Lomustine, cyclophosphamide, doxorubicin, methotrexate.
Breast carcinoma	(1) Combination chemotherapy or tamoxifen (see text). (2) Combination chemotherapy; hormonal manipulation for late recurrence (see text).	Cyclophosphamide, doxorubicin, vincristine, methotrexate, fluorouracil, mitomycin, vinblastine, mitoxantrone,[1] quinacrine,[2] prednisone,[2] megestrol, androgens, aminoglutethimide, and hydrocortisone.
Choriocarcinoma (trophoblastic neoplasms)	Methotrexate, alone or in combination with vincristine, dactinomycin, and cyclophosphamide.	Vinblastine, cisplatin, mercaptopurine, chlorambucil, doxorubicin.
Carcinoma of testis	Combination chemotherapy: cisplatin, vinblastine, bleomycin or etoposide plus cisplatin.	Methotrexate, dactinomycin, mithramycin, doxorubicin, ifosfamide, mesna.[2]
Carcinoma of prostate	Estrogens or leuprolide plus flutamide.	Cisplatin, estramustine, fluorouracil, progestins, aminoglutethimide, suramin[1]
Wilms' tumor (children)	Vincristine plus dactinomycin after surgery and radiotherapy.	Methotrexate, cyclophosphamide, doxorubicin.
Neuroblastoma	Cyclophosphamide, doxorubicin, and vincristine.	Dactinomycin, daunorubicin, cisplatin.
Carcinoma of thyroid	Radioiodine (^{131}I), doxorubicin.	Bleomycin, fluorouracil, melphalan, cisplatin.
Carcinoma of adrenal	Mitotane.	Doxorubicin, suramin[1]
Carcinoma of stomach or pancreas	Fluorouracil plus doxorubicin and mitomycin.	Hydroxyurea, lomustine.
Carcinoma of colon	Fluorouracil plus levamisole (adjuvant) or with leucovorin.	Mitomycin, carmustine, cisplatin.
Carcinoid	Interferon or doxorubicin plus cyclophosphamide.	Octreotide,[2] methysergide,[2] streptozocin.

Table 3–3 (cont'd) Treatment choices for cancers responsive to systemic agents.

Diagnosis	Current Treatment of Choice	Other Valuable Agents
Insulinoma	Interferon, streptozocin.	Doxorubicin, fluorouracil, mitomycin.
Osteogenic sarcoma	Doxorubicin, or methotrexate with citrovorum rescue initiated after surgery.	Cyclophosphamide, dacarbazine.
Miscellaneous sarcomas	Doxorubicin plus dacarbazine.	Ifosfamide, methotrexate, dactinomycin, vincristine, vinblastine.
Melanoma	Dacarbazine, interferon.	Lomustine, cisplatin, mitomycin, vinblastine, interferon, taxol[1]
Kaposi's sarcoma	High-dose interferon	Vinblastine, vincristine, etoposide, doxorubicin

Note: Interferon is now available as recombinant interferon alfa-2a: Roferon-A (Roche, alfa-2a); Itron A (Schering, alfa-2b).
[1] Investigational agent. Treatment available through qualified investigators and centers authorized by National Cancer Institute and Cooperative Oncology Groups.
[2] Supportive agent, not oncolytic.

Hormonal therapy also plays an important role in cancer management. Hormonal therapy or ablation is important in palliation of breast and prostatic carcinoma, while added progestins are useful in suppression of endometrial carcinoma. Studies have shown that women with metastatic breast cancer who show objective improvement with hormonal therapy have tumors that contain cytoplasmic estrogen and progesterone receptors. Patients whose tumors lack these receptor proteins are unresponsive to hormonal management but frequently respond to cytotoxic chemotherapy. Antiestrogens (eg, tamoxifen) and aromatase inhibitors (such as aminoglutethimide) that block peripheral conversion of adrenal androgens into estrogens have substantial additive effects to oophorectomy in premenopausal women whose tumors are estrogen or progesterone receptor-positive. Thus, estrogen and progesterone receptor status should be assessed on all breast cancers at the time of mastectomy and on biopsy material (if available) from patients who manifest metastatic breast cancer. Androgen receptors remain difficult to measure in prostate cancer. In addition to estrogens, new hormonal approaches are also appearing in prostate cancer. These include the use of analogues of gonadotropin-releasing hormone agonists (eg, leuprolide) and of aromatase inhibitors (eg, aminoglutethimide) and antiandrogens (eg, flutamide). The use of leuprolide plus flutamide can be considered as an alternative to orchiectomy but also induces impotence. Recombinant interferon alfa-2 has marked antitumor effects in hairy cell leukemia and chronic myelogenous leukemia, moderate effects in lymphomas, the epidemic form of Kaposi's sarcoma (AIDS-associated), and multiple myeloma. Interferon alfa-2 also has some utility in metastatic melanoma, hypernephroma, and carcinoid syndrome. The use of interferon together with other methods of treatment will increase significantly in the coming years. For example, the addition of interferon to systemic chemotherapy for multiple myeloma appears to significantly increase the degree of cytoreduction attained as compared to chemotherapy alone. Another cytokine, interleukin-2 (IL-2), when administered alone or in combination with lymphocyte-activated killer (LAK) cells or tumor-infiltrating lymphocytes (TIL), exhibits marked antitumor activity in a minority of patients with melanoma or renal cancer and has received regulatory approval in European countries. IL-2 remains investigational in the USA.

Dalton WS et al: Drug resistance in multiple myeloma and non-Hodgkin's lymphoma: Detection of P-glycoprotein and potential circumvention by addition of verapamil to chemotherapy. J Clin Oncol 1989;7:415.

MECHANISMS OF ACTION OF CANCER CHEMOTHERAPEUTIC AGENTS

Although the emphasis in this chapter is on the empirical applications of cancer chemotherapy, the cytokinetics and mechanisms of drug action should be discussed briefly. At the clinical level of detectability of tumors, growth characteristics vary considerably between tumors of different histologic appearance or tissue of origin. The key cells in a cancer are the clonogenic **tumor stem cells,** which make up less than 1% of cancer cells but provide for population renewal and serve as the seeds of metastasis. Another useful concept is that of the "growth fraction"–the percentage of tumor cells that are proliferating at any given time. The leukemias, certain lymphomas, and genital tract tumors have relatively high growth fractions and are quite susceptible to treatment with drugs that have specific toxicity for proliferating cells. These drugs include cytarabine, mercaptopurine, thioguanine, methotrexate, fluorouracil, azacytidine, vincristine, vinblastine, bleomycin, and certain steroid hormones. These drugs are therefore classed as **cell cycle specific (CCS)** agents, and their utility has proved to be greatest in tumors with high growth fractions such as those mentioned above. The sequential 4 phases of the cell cycle are G_1 (period of RNA and protein synthesis), S phase (period of DNA syn-

Table 3–4. Single-agent dosage and toxicity of anticancer drugs.

Chemotherapeutic Agent	Usual Adult Dosage	Acute Toxicity	Delayed Toxicity
Alkylating agents			
Mechlorethamine (nitrogen mustard, HN2, Mustargen)	0.4 mg/kg IV in single or divided doses.	Nausea and vomiting	Moderate depression of blood count. Excessive doses produce severe bone marrow depression with leukopenia, thrombocytopenia, and bleeding. Alopecia and hemorrhagic cystitis occur with cyclophosphamide, while busulfan occasionally causes pigmentation and other usual toxicities (see below). Acute leukemia may develop in 5–10% of patients receiving prolonged therapy with melphalan or chlorambucil.
Chlorambucil (Leukeran)	0.1–0.2 mg/kg/d orally; 6–12 mg/d.	None	
Cyclophosphamide	3.5–5 mg/kg/d orally for 10 days; 1 g/m^2 IV as single dose every 3–4 weeks.	Nausea and vomiting	
Melphalan (Alkeran)	0.25 mg/kg/d orally for 4 days every 6 weeks.	None	
Thiotepa	0.2 mg/kg IV for 5 days.	None	
Busulfan (Myleran)	2–8 mg/d orally; 150–250 mg/course.	None	
Carmustine (BCNU, bischloroethylnitrosourea)	200 mg/m^2 IV every 6 weeks.	Nausea and vomiting	Leukopenia and thrombocytopenia. Rarely hepatitis. Acute leukemia has been observed to occur in some patients receiving semustine.
Lomustine (CCNU) or semustine (methyl-CCNU)	130 mg/m^2 orally every 6 weeks.	Nausea and vomiting	
Procarbazine (N-methyl-hydrazine, Matulane)	50–300 mg/d orally.	Nausea and vomiting	Bone marrow depression, mental depression, monoamine oxidase inhibition.
Decarbazine (dimethyl triazeno imidazole carboxamide, DTIC)	250 mg/m^2/d for 5 days every 3 weeks.	Anorexia, nausea, vomiting	Bone marrow depression.
Cisplatin (Platinol)	50–100 mg/m^2 IV every 3 weeks.	Nausea and vomiting	Nephrotoxicity, mild otic and bone marrow toxicity, neurotoxicity.
Carboplatin (Paraplatin)	360 mg/m^2 IV every 3 weeks.	Nausea and vomiting, myelosuppression	Anemia.
Structural analogues or antimetabolites			
Methotrexate (amethopterin, MTX)	2.5–5 mg/d orally; 15 mg intrathecally weekly or every other week for 4 doses. 20–25 mg IM twice weekly is well tolerated and may be preferable.	None	Oral and gastrointestinal tract ulceration, bone and marrow depression, leukopenia, thrombocytopenia.
Mercaptopurine (Purinethol, 6-MP)	2.5 mg/kg/d orally.	None	Usually well tolerated. Larger dosages may cause bone marrow depression.
Thioguanine (6-TG)	2 mg/kg/d orally.	None	Usually well tolerated. Larger dosages may cause bone marrow depression.
Fluorouracil (5-FU)	15/mg/kg/d IV for 3–5 days, or 15 mg/kg weekly for at least 6 weeks.	None	Nausea, oral and gastrointestinal ulceration, bone marrow depression.
Cytarabine (Ara-C, Cytosar)	100 mg/m^2/d for 5–10 days given by continuous IV infusion, or in divided doses subcut or IV every 8 hours.	None	Nausea and vomiting, bone marrow depression, megaloblastosis, leukopenia, thrombocytopenia.
Hormonal agents			
Androgens			
Testosterone propionate	100 mg IM 3 times weekly.	None	Fluid retention, masculinization. There is a 10% incidence of cholestatic jaundice with fluoxymesterone.
Fluoxymesterone (Halotestin)	20–40 mg/d orally.	None	
Antiandrogen Flutamide (Eulexin)	500 mg/d orally.	None	None.
Estrogens			
Diethylstilbestrol	1–5 mg 3 times a day orally.	Occasional nausea and vomiting	Fluid retention, feminization, uterine bleeding.
Ethinyl estradiol (Estinyl)	3 mg/d orally.	None	
Antiestrogen Tamoxifen (Nolvadex)	20 mg/d orally.	None	None.

Table 3–4 (cont'd). Single-agent dosage and toxicity of anticancer drugs.

Chemotherapeutic Agent	Usual Adult Dosage	Acute Toxicity	Delayed Toxicity
Progestins Hydroxyprogesterone ca-proate (Delalutin)	1 g IM twice weekly.	None	Occasional fluid retention.
Medroxyprogesterone (Provera)	100–200 mg/d orally; 200–600 mg orally twice weekly.	None	
Megestrol acetate (Megace)	40 mg 4 times a day orally.	None	
Adrenocorticosteroids Prednisone	20–100 mg/d orally or, when effective, 50–100 mg every other day orally as single dose.	None	Fluid retention, hypertension, diabetes, increased susceptibility to infection, "moon facies," osteoporosis.
Aromatase inhibitors Aminoglutethimide	500 mg/d orally, along with hydrocortisone, 40 mg/d.	Initial drowsiness	Transient skin rash, which usually subsides with continued therapy.
Gonadotropin-releasing hormone inhibitors Leuprolide	1 mg/d subcutaneously.	Usually none	Usually none.
Biologic response modifiers Interferon alfa-2 (recombinant) (Roferon-A, Intron A)	3–5 million IU subcutaneously daily or 3 times weekly.	Fever, chills, anorexia	Fatigue, weight loss, confusion.
Natural products and miscellaneous agents Vinblastine (Velban)	0.1–0.2 mg/kg IV weekly.	Nausea and vomiting	Alopecia, loss of reflexes, bone marrow depression.
Vincristine (Oncovin)	1.5 mg/m^2 IV (maximum: 2 mg weekly).	None	Areflexia, muscle weakness, peripheral neuritis, paralytic ileus, alopecia (below).
Dactinomycin (actinomycin D, Cosmegen)	0.04 mg/kg IV weekly.	Nausea and vomiting	Stomatitis, gastrointestinal tract upset, alopecia, bone marrow depression.
Daunorubicin (daunomycin, rubidomycin)	30–60 mg/m^2 daily IV for 3 days, or 30–60 mg/m^2 IV weekly.	Nausea, fever, red urine (not hematuria)	Cardiotoxicity, bone marrow depression, alopecia.
Doxorubicin (Adriamycin)	60 mg/m^2 IV every 3 weeks to a maximum total dose of 550 mg/m^2.	Nausea, red urine (not hematuria)	Cardiotoxicity, alopecia, bone marrow depression, stomatitis.
Etoposide (Vepesid, VP-16)	100 mg/m^2 IV daily for 5 days every 3 weeks.	Nausea and vomiting; occasionally, hypotension	Myelosuppression.
Mithramycin (Mithracin)	25–50 μg/kg IV every other day for up to 8 doses.	Nausea and vomiting	Thrombocytopenia, hepatotoxicity.
Mitomycin (Mutamycin)	20 mg/m^2 every 6 weeks.	Nausea	Thrombocytopenia, leukopenia.
Mitoxantrone (Novantrone)	12 mg/m^2 daily IV for 3 days along with cytarabine every 4–6 weeks.	None	Leukopenia, thrombocytopenia.
Bleomycin (Blenoxane)	Up to 15 units/m^2 twice weekly to a total dose of 200 units/m^2.	Allergic reactions, fever, hypotension	Fever, dermatitis, pulmonary fibrosis.
Hydroxyurea (Hydrea)	300 mg/m^2 orally for 5 days.	Nausea and vomiting	Bone marrow depression.
Mitotane (o,p-DDD, Lysodren)	6–12 g/d orally.	Nausea and vomiting	Dermatitis, diarrhea, mental depression, muscle tremors.
Supportive agents Allopurinol (Zyloprim)	300–800 mg/d orally for prevention or relief of hyperuricemia.	None	Usually none. Enhances effects and toxicity of mercaptopurine when used in combination.
Quinacrine (Atabrine)	100–200 mg/d by intracavitary injection for 6 days.	Local pain and fever	None

thesis), G_2 (period of assembly of the mitotic spindle apparatus), and M (mitosis). Cytarabine is an excellent example of a drug with selective toxicity during just the S phase of the cell cycle, and its current use is virtually limited to the management of acute leukemia, in which it has had a major beneficial effect.

A second major group of drugs are classed as **cell cycle nonspecific (CCNS)** agents. Most of these drugs act by complexing with cellular DNA and are capable of doing this whether cells are proliferating or not. Examples are the alkylating agents (eg, mechlorethamine, cyclophosphamide, melphalan, carmustine), other chemical agents (cisplatin), and antibiotics such as dactinomycin, doxorubicin, and mitomycin. Such drugs are useful in the treatment of a variety of so-called "solid tumors," which generally have low growth fractions at the clinical phase of disease; but they are also quite useful in high growth fraction tumors. Tumor kinetics are far from static, however, and our strategy in cancer chemotherapy is now undergoing radical revision to exploit our expanding knowledge of cytokinetics, pharmacokinetics, selective cell line sensitivity, etc. Use of continuous infusion pumps and special routes of administration have also been important. The intraperitoneal route has been explored as a means of delivering high local concentrations of specific agents to the peritoneal space while minimizing systemic toxicity. Autologous bone marrow infusion has also been studied experimentally as a means of limiting bone marrow toxicity with high-dose therapy.

Drugs that have had the greatest value in humans are those that produce a fractional kill of at least 5–6 logs (100,000-fold to 1 million-fold reduction in tumor cell number) in animal tumor systems. Because patients with human tumors present with 10^{10}–10^{12} tumor cells, use of effective combination chemotherapy should be given serious consideration after a major reduction in the body burden of tumor is first accomplished with surgery or irradiation. Additionally, cytotoxic anticancer drugs have steep dose-response curves. Accordingly, dose intensity and high dose chemotherapy are important concepts, and—for many tumor sites—increasing response and survival are related to increased dose intensity. The development of bone marrow growth factors should further enhance the use of myelosuppressive chemotherapy by permitting increased dose intensity of myelosuppressive drugs. A new strategy that has already been proved effective in Hodgkin's disease is the use of alternating non-cross-resistant combinations of drugs (eg, "MOPP-ABVD") for induction of remission. A theoretic scheme of strategies in cancer chemotherapy is shown in Fig 3–1. Mechanisms of action of biologicals such as the interferons remain unclear, but they appear to be suppressive agents and may act analogously to hormones, or in some instances in concert with the host's immune system (eg, with interleukin-2).

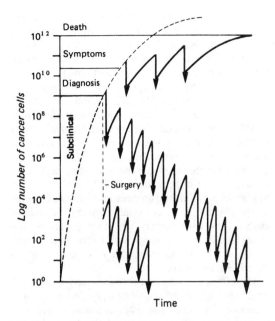

Figure 3–1. Relationship of tumor cell number to time of diagnosis, symptoms, treatment, and survival. Three alternative approaches to drug treatment are shown for comparison with the course of tumor growth when no treatment is given (dotted line). In the protocol diagrammed at top, treatment (indicated by the arrows) is given infrequently, and the result is manifested as prolongation of survival but with recurrence of symptoms between courses of treatment and eventual death of the patient. The combination chemotherapy treatment diagrammed in the middle section is begun earlier and is more intensive. Tumor cell kill exceeds regrowth; drug resistance does not develop; and "cure" results. In this example, treatment has been continued long after all clinical evidence of cancer has disappeared (1–3 years). This approach has been established as effective in the treatment of childhood acute leukemia, testicular cancers, and Hodgkin's disease. The recent introduction of the concept of "alternating non-cross-resistant" combination chemotherapy may further enhance this approach. In the treatment diagrammed near the bottom of the graph, early surgery has been employed to remove the primary tumor, and intensive adjuvant chemotherapy has been administered long enough (up to 1 year) to eradicate the remaining 10^3 tumor stem cells that comprise the remaining occult micrometastases. This approach is now widely applied and appears effective in the treatment of breast cancer, rectal cancer, osteosarcoma, and Wilms' tumor.

ADJUVANT CHEMOTHERAPY FOR MICROMETASTASES

One of the most important roles of cancer chemotherapy is undoubtedly as an "adjuvant" (to eradicate or suppress minimal residual disease) after "primary field" treatment with surgery or irradiation. Failures with primary field therapy are due principally to occult micrometastases of tumor stem cells outside the primary field. These distant micrometastases are usually present in patients with one or more positive lymph nodes at the time of surgery (eg, in breast cancer) and in patients with tumors having a known propensity for early hematogenous spread (eg, osteogenic sarcoma, Wilms' tumor). The risk of recurrent or metastatic disease in such patients can be extremely high (>80%). Only systemic therapy can adequately attack micrometastases. Chemotherapeutic regimens that induce regression of advanced cancer may have curative potential (at the right dosage and schedule) when combined with surgery for high-risk "early" cancer. Studies in experimental animals have shown that chemotherapy can eradicate small numbers of residual cancer cells after surgery. In other instances, micrometastases may be suppressed although not eradicated–such is the case when antiestrogen therapy is used in breast cancer.

The efficacy of adjuvant chemotherapy is also well established in pediatric neoplasms, eg, Wilms' tumor, rhabdomyosarcoma, and osteosarcoma, where substantial improvement in survival has been obtained with adjuvant therapy. Recent studies have shown significant prolongation of survival in both pre- and postmenopausal women with stage II breast cancer who received adjuvant chemotherapy. In breast cancer, women with positive or negative lymph nodes at breast cancer surgery have had prolonged disease-free survival from combination chemotherapy (stages I and II breast cancer). Several useful combination chemotherapy regimens for adjuvant therapy for breast cancer are "CMF" (cyclophosphamide-methotrexate-fluorouracil), alone or with the addition of vincristine and prednisone (CMFVP), and "D/C" (doxorubicin-cyclophosphamide), alone or with the addition of fluorouracil. There is clear evidence of a dose-response effect of adjuvant cytotoxic chemotherapy, and low-dose protocols are generally ineffective. For premenopausal women, chemotherapy is indicated, as is the antiestrogen tamoxifen for postmenopausal women; the latter is most effective if hormone receptors are present. The main challenge in women with stage I (node-negative) breast cancer is to identify prognostic factors to determine which patients in this group definitely require treatment with chemotherapy. In osteogenic sarcoma, doxorubicin alone and in combination with other drugs has proved useful as an adjuvant. Survival is clearly improved in patients with rectal cancer when they receive postoperative radiotherapy and the combination of fluorouracil plus semustine or mitomycin.

Adjuvant chemotherapy with fluorouracil plus levamisole is now indicated also in Dukes C colorectal cancer. Adjuvant therapy remains investigational and unproved for a number of common tumors, including non-small-cell lung cancer and pancreatic cancer. Adjuvant therapy is probably not indicated in early Hodgkin's disease or testicular carcinoma, since the cure rates with chemotherapy for these diseases when advanced and recurrent are high.

Eilber F et al: Adjuvant chemotherapy for osteosarcoma: Randomized prospective trial. J Clin Oncol 1987;5:21.

Fisher B et al: A randomized clinical trial evaluating sequential methotrexate and fluorouracil in the treatment of patients with node-negative breast cancer who have estrogen receptor-negative tumors. N Engl J Med 1989;320:473.

Salmon SE (editor): *Adjuvant Therapy of Cancer VI*. Saunders, 1990.

TOXICITY & DOSE MODIFICATION OF CHEMOTHERAPEUTIC AGENTS

A number of cancer chemotherapeutic agents have cytotoxic effects on rapidly proliferating normal cells in bone marrow, mucosa, and skin. Still other drugs such as the *Vinca* alkaloids produce neuropathy, and the hormones often have psychic effects. Acute and chronic toxicities of the various drugs are summarized in Table 3–4. Appropriate dose modification usually minimizes these side effects, so that therapy can be continued with relative safety.

Bone Marrow Toxicity

Depression of bone marrow is usually the most significant limiting toxicity in cancer chemotherapy. While autologous bone marrow transplantation can often reduce the myelosuppressive toxicity of high-dose chemotherapy, it is not yet clear that this will prove to be a generally useful strategy. Growth factors that stimulate myeloid proliferation (eg, granulocyte colony-stimulating factor [GCSF] and granulocyte-macrophage stimulating factor [GMCSF]) or erythroid proliferation (erythropoietin) are currently in clinical trial. These factors have the potential for markedly reducing the duration and severity of granulocytopenia or anemia after cytotoxic chemotherapy.

Commonly used short-acting drugs that affect bone marrow are the oral alkylating agents (eg, cyclophosphamide, melphalan, chlorambucil), procarbazine, mercaptopurine, methotrexate, vinblastine, fluorouracil, dactinomycin, and doxorubicin. In general, it is preferable to use alkylating agents in intensive "pulse" courses every 3–4 weeks rather than to administer in continuous daily schedules. This allows for complete hematologic (and immunologic) recovery between courses rather than leaving the patient continuously suppressed with a cytotoxic agent. This approach reduces side effects but does not reduce therapeutic efficacy. The standard dosage schedules that produce tumor responses with these agents often do induce some bone marrow depression. In such instances, if the drug is not discontinued or its dosage reduced, severe bone marrow aplasia may result in pancytopenia, bleeding, or infection. Simple guidelines to therapy can usually prevent severe marrow depression.

White blood counts (and differential counts), hematocrit or hemoglobin, and platelet counts should be obtained frequently. With long-term chemotherapy, counts should be obtained initially at weekly intervals; the frequency of counts may be reduced only after the patient's sensitivity to the drug can be well predicted (eg, 3–4 months) and cumulative toxicity excluded.

In patients with normal blood counts as well as normal liver and kidney function, drugs should usually be started at their full dosage and tapered if need be, rather than starting at a lower dose and escalating the dose to hematologic tolerance. When the dose is escalated, toxicity often cannot be adequately anticipated, especially if it is cumulative, and marrow depression is often more severe.

Drug dosage can usually be tapered on a fixed schedule as a function of the peripheral white blood count or platelet count (or both). In this fashion, smooth titration control of drug administration can usually be attained for oral alkylating agents or antimetabolites. A scheme for dose modifications is shown in Table 3–5. These modifications assume that the blood counts are checked shortly before the next course of chemotherapy is to be administered. Alternatively, the interval between drug courses can be lengthened, thereby permitting more complete hematologic recovery and repetition of full-dose chemotherapy.

Drugs with delayed hematologic toxicities do not always fit into such a simple scheme, and in general they should be administered by specialists familiar with the specific toxicities. Drugs requiring special precautions with respect to toxicity include doxorubicin, mitomycin, busulfan, cytarabine, bleomycin, mithramycin, carmustine, lomustine, semustine, and daunorubicin.

Chemotherapy-Induced Nausea & Vomiting

A number of cytotoxic anticancer drugs induce nausea and vomiting as side effects. In general, these symptoms are thought to originate in the central nervous system rather than peripherally. Parenteral administration of single agents such as doxorubicin, etoposide, or cyclophosphamide frequently is associated with mild to moderate nausea and vomiting, whereas parenteral administration of nitrosoureas, dacarbazine, and particularly cisplatin usually causes severe symptoms, which can limit patient acceptance of chemotherapy. Combination chemotherapy with agents including those listed above can also cause severe symptoms. Antiemetics clearly reduce and often eliminate nausea and vomiting associated with drugs such as cisplatin. Metoclopramide (Reglan) is a particularly useful agent, especially when administered parenterally at a dosage of 1 mg/kg, both 30 minutes before and again 30 minutes after the administration of chemotherapy. Extrapyramidal signs may be induced with this drug but frequently can be suppressed with diphenhydramine. Dexamethasone has antiemetic effects when administered at a dosage of 10 mg at similar intervals. Both of these agents are significantly more potent than conventional agents such as prochlorperazine, diphenhydramine, and thiethylperazine. Combinations of antiemetics (eg, metoclopramide along with dexamethasone and other agents) are often more effective than maximal doses of any one agent for blocking cisplatin-induced vomiting. Inclusion of diazepam in such combinations is often useful for its sedating effect. Cannabinoids such as tetrahydrocannabinol (Marinol) are also effective in some patients but generally cause more undesirable side effects. A patient receiving potent antiemetics along with chemotherapy on an outpatient basis must be escorted to and from the clinic, since the antiemetics often induce marked sedation and transient impairment of balance and reflexes.

Plezia PM et al: Immediate termination of intractable vomiting induced by cisplatin combination chemotherapy using an intensive five-drug antiemetic regiment. Cancer Treat Rep 1984;68:1493.

Gastrointestinal & Skin Toxicity

Since antimetabolites such as methotrexate and fluorouracil act only on rapidly proliferating cells, they damage the cells of mucosal surfaces such as the gastrointestinal tract. Methotrexate has similar effects on the skin. These toxicities are at times more significant than those that have occurred in the bone marrow, and they should be looked for routinely when these agents are used.

Erythema of the buccal mucosa is an early sign of mucosal toxicity. If therapy is continued beyond this point, oral ulceration will develop. In general, it is wise to discontinue therapy at the time of appearance of early oral ulceration. This finding usually heralds the appearance of similar but potentially more serious ulceration at other sites lower in the gastrointestinal tract. Therapy can usually be reinstituted when the oral ulcer heals (1 week to 10 days). The dose of drug used may need to be modified downward at this point, with titration to an acceptable level of effect on the mucosa.

Table 3–5. A common scheme for dose modification of cancer chemotherapeutic agents.

Granulocyte Count (/μL)	Platelet Count (/μL)	Suggested Drug Dosage (% of full dose)
>3000	>100,000	100%
2000–3000	75,000–100,000	50%
<2000	<50,000	0%

Miscellaneous Drug-Specific Toxicities

The toxicities of individual drugs have been summarized in Table 3–4; however, several of these warrant additional mention, since they occur with frequently administered agents, and special measures are often indicated.

A. Hemorrhagic Cystitis Induced by Cyclophosphamide or Ifosfamide: Metabolic products of cyclophosphamide that retain cytotoxic activity are excreted into the urine. Some patients appear to metabolize more of the drug to these active excretory products; if their urine is concentrated, severe bladder damage may result. In general, it is wise to advise patients receiving cyclophosphamide to maintain a large fluid intake. Early symptoms include dysuria and frequency despite the absence of bacteriuria. Such symptoms develop in about 20% of patients who receive the drug. Should microscopic hematuria develop, it is advisable to stop the drug temporarily or switch to a different alkylating agent, to increase fluid intake, and to administer a urinary analgesic such as phenazopyridine. With severe cystitis, large segments of bladder mucosa may be shed and the patient may have prolonged gross hematuria. Such patients should be observed for signs of urinary obstruction and may require cystoscopy for removal of obstructing blood clots. The cyclophosphamide analogue ifosfamide, which was recently approved by the FDA, can cause severe hemorrhagic cystitis when used alone. However, when its use is followed with a series of doses of the neutralizing agent mesna, bladder toxicity can be prevented. Mesna can also be used for patients who develop cystitis with cyclophosphamide.

B. Vincristine-Induced Neuropathy: Neuropathy is a toxic side effect that is peculiar to the *Vinca* alkaloid drugs, especially vincristine. The peripheral neuropathy can be sensory, motor, autonomic, or a combination of these effects. In its mildest form, it consists of paresthesias ("pins and needles") of the fingers and toes. Occasional patients develop acute jaw or throat pain after vincristine therapy. This may be a form of trigeminal neuralgia. With continued vincristine therapy, the paresthesias extend to the proximal interphalangeal joints, hyporeflexia appears in the lower extremities, and significant weakness develops in the quadriceps muscle group. At this point, it is wise to discontinue vincristine therapy until the neuropathy has subsided. A useful means of judging whether peripheral motor neuropathy is significant enough to warrant stopping treatment is to have the patient attempt to do deep knee bends or get up out of a chair without using the arm muscles.

Constipation is the most common symptom of autonomic neuropathy associated with vincristine therapy. Patients receiving vincristine should be started on stool softeners and mild cathartics when therapy is begun; otherwise, severe impaction may result in association with an atonic bowel.

More serious autonomic involvement can lead to acute intestinal obstruction with signs indistinguishable from those of an acute abdomen. Bladder neuropathies are uncommon but may be severe. These 2 complications are absolute contraindications to continued vincristine therapy.

C. Methotrexate Toxicity and "Citrovorum Rescue": In addition to standard uses of methotrexate for chemotherapy, this drug has some use in a very high dosage that would lead to fatal bone marrow toxicity if it were given without an antidote. The bone marrow toxicity of methotrexate can be prevented by early administration of citrovorum factor (folinic acid, leucovorin). If an overdose of methotrexate is administered accidentally, folinic acid therapy should be initiated as soon as possible, preferably within 1 hour. Intravenous infusion should be employed for large overdosages, inasmuch as it is generally advisable to give citrovorum factor repeatedly. Up to 75 mg should be given in the first 12 hours, followed by 12 mg intramuscularly every 4 hours for at least 6 doses.

Intentional high-dosage methotrexate therapy with citrovorum rescue should only be considered for osteosarcoma patients with good renal function.

Vigorous hydration and bicarbonate loading also appear to be important in preventing crystallization of high-dose methotrexate in the renal tubular epithelium. Daily monitoring of the serum creatinine is mandatory because methotrexate metabolism is slowed by renal insufficiency, and high-dosage methotrexate can itself cause renal injury. When high-dose methotrexate is used, folinic acid therapy should probably be started within 4 hours of the methotrexate dose and continued for 3 days (or longer if the creatinine level rises).

D. Busulfan Toxicity: The alkylating agent busulfan, frequently used for treatment of chronic myelogenous leukemia, has curious delayed toxicities including (1) increased skin pigmentation, (2) a wasting syndrome similar to that seen in adrenal insufficiency, and (3) progressive pulmonary fibrosis. Patients who develop either of the latter 2 problems should be switched to a different drug (eg, melphalan) when further therapy is needed. The pigmentary changes are innocuous and will usually regress slowly after treatment is discontinued.

E. Bleomycin Toxicity: This antibiotic has found increasing application in cancer chemotherapy in view of activity in squamous cell carcinomas, Hodgkin's disease, non-Hodgkin's lymphomas, and testicular tumors. Bleomycin produces edema of the interphalangeal joints and hardening of the palmar and plantar skin as well as sometimes also inducing an anaphylactic or serum sickness-like reaction or a serious or fatal pulmonary fibrotic reaction (seen especially in elderly patients receiving a total dose of over 300 units). If nonproductive cough, dyspnea, and pulmonary infiltrates develop, the drug is discontinued, and high-dose corticosteroids are instituted as well as empiric antibiotics pending cultures. Fever alone or with chills is an occasional complication of bleomycin treatment and is not an absolute contraindication to continued treatment. The fever may be avoided by prednisone administration at the time of injection. Moreover, fever alone is not predictive of pulmonary toxicity. About 1% of patients (especially those with lymphoma) may have a severe or even fatal hypotensive reaction after the initial dose of bleomycin. In order to identify such patients, it is wise to administer a test dose of 5 units of bleomycin first with adequate monitoring and emergency facilities available should they be needed. Patients exhibiting a hypotensive reaction should not receive further bleomycin therapy.

F. Doxorubicin-Induced Cardiomyopathy: The anthracycline antibiotics doxorubicin and daunomycin both have delayed cardiac toxicity. The problem is greater with doxorubicin because it has a major role in the treatment of acute leukemia, sarcomas, breast cancer, lymphomas, and certain other solid tumors. Studies of left ventricular function and endomyocardial biopsies indicate that some changes in cardiac dynamics occur in most patients by the time they have received 300 mg/m^2. The *mu*ltiple-*ga*ted ("MUGA") radionuclide cardiac scan appears to be the most useful noninvasive test for assessing toxicity. Doxorubicin should not be used in elderly patients with significant intrinsic cardiac disease, and in general, patients should not receive a total dose in excess of 550 mg/m^2. Patients who have had prior chest or mediastinal radiotherapy may develop doxorubicin heart disease at lower total doses. The appearance of a high resting pulse may herald the appearance of overt cardiac toxicity. Unfortunately, toxicity may be irreversible and frequently fatal at dosage levels above 550 mg/m^2. At lower doses (eg, 350 mg/m^2), the symptoms and signs of cardiac failure generally respond well to digitalis, diuretics, and cessation of doxorubicin therapy. Recent evidence suggests that cardiac toxicity can be correlated with high peak plasma levels obtained with intermittent high-dose bolus therapy (eg, every 3–4 weeks). Use of weekly injections or low-dose continuous infusion schedules appears to delay the occurrence of cardiac toxicity. Current laboratory studies suggest that cardiac toxicity may be due to a mechanism involving the formation of intracellular free radicals in cardiac muscle.

G. Cisplatin Nephrotoxicity and Neurotoxicity: Cisplatin is effective in testicular, bladder, and ovarian cancer as well as in several other types of tumor. Nausea and vomiting are common, but nephrotoxicity and neurotoxicity are more serious. Ototoxicity is a potentially serious neurotoxicity with cisplatin and can result in deafness. Vigorous hydration plus mannitol diuresis may substantially reduce nephrotoxicity. The neurotoxicity of this drug is delayed and

is more common after a total dose of 300 mg/m^2 has been administered. The neurotoxicity is usually manifested as a peripheral neuropathy of mixed sensorimotor type and may be associated with painful paresthesias. The neuropathy may be secondary to hypomagnesemia, which can be induced by cisplatin. Therefore, the serum magnesium should be measured if neuropathy develops, and treatment with parenteral magnesium sulfate should be tried. These supportive measures do not appear to reduce the therapeutic effectiveness of cisplatin. The second-generation platinum analogue carboplatin is now available and has been shown to be as effective as cisplatin in ovarian cancer. Carboplatin is nonnephrotoxic and does not often cause severe nausea or vomiting but does induce myelosuppression. A recent report suggests that an ACTH analogue may be useful in preventing cisplatin neurotoxicity.

H. Interferon Toxicities: While alfa-2 interferon is generally well tolerated in the standard doses listed in Table 3–4, it has increasing toxicity with increasing doses and is more toxic in elderly patients. Fever and chills are initial side effects but are infrequent after continued treatment. However, anorexia, fatigue, and weight loss can have cumulative effects, often representing dose-limiting toxicities, and can be severe. In some patients, central nervous system symptoms develop and usually are manifested as confusion or somnolence. Reduction in peripheral blood counts can develop, but this abnormality is usually not clinically important. These interferon-induced side effects can sometimes be confused with the symptoms of progressive cancer. Fortunately, the side effects usually clear within 1 week after cessation of interferon therapy.

EVALUATION OF TUMOR RESPONSE

Inasmuch as cancer chemotherapy can induce clinical improvement, significant toxicity, or both, it is extremely important to critically assess the beneficial effects of treatment in patients with advanced cancer to determine that the net effect is favorable. The most valuable signs to follow during therapy include the following:

(1) Tumor size: Shrinkage in tumor size can be demonstrated on physical examination, chest film or other x-ray, sonography, or radionuclide scanning procedure such as bone scanning (breast, lung, prostate cancer). CT scanning has assumed a significant role in evaluating tumor size and location for a wide variety of tumors and sites. Magnetic resonance imaging (MRI) appears to be the best noninvasive means of evaluating posterior fossa brain tumors and spinal cord tumors and spinal cord compression, but CT scanning is also useful. Sonography and MRI have special utility in pelvic neoplasms.

(2) Marker substances: Significant decrease in

the quantity of a tumor product or marker substance reflects a reduced amount of tumor in the body. Examples of such markers include paraproteins in multiple myeloma and macroglobulinemia, chorionic gonadotropin in choriocarcinoma and testicular tumors, prostatic acid phosphatase and prostate-specific antigen in prostatic cancer, urinary steroids in adrenal carcinoma and paraneoplastic Cushing's syndrome, and 5-hydroxyindoleacetic acid in carcinoid syndrome. Tumor-secreted fetal antigens are becoming of increasing importance. These include alpha$_1$-fetoprotein in hepatoma, in teratoembryonal carcinoma, and in occasional cases of gastric carcinoma; ovarian tumor antigen (CA 125) in ovarian cancer; and carcinoembryonic antigen in carcinomas of the colon, lungs, and pancreas. Monoclonal antibodies are now used for measurement of a number of the tumor markers and offer the potential of delineating a number of additional markers for diagnostic purposes.

(3) General well-being and performance status: A valuable sign of clinical improvement is the general well-being of the patient. Although this finding is a combination of subjective and objective factors and may be partly a placebo effect, it nonetheless serves as a sign of clinical improvement in assessing some of the objective observations listed above. Factors included in the assessment of general well-being are improved appetite and weight gain and increased "performance status" (eg, ambulatory versus bedridden). Evaluation of factors such as activity status enables the physician to judge whether the net effect of chemotherapy is worthwhile palliation.

REFERENCES

Berger NA (guest editor): Oncologic emergencies. Semin Oncol 1989;16:461.

Brenner DE: Intraperitoneal chemotherapy: A review. J Clin Oncol 1986;4:1135.

Chan HSL et al: Immunohistochemical detection of P-glycoprotein: Prognostic correlation in soft tissue sarcoma of childhood. J Clin Oncol 1990;8:689.

DeVita VT Jr, Hellman S, Rosenberg SA (editors): Principles and Practice of Oncology, 3rd ed. Lippincott, 1989.

Fisher B et al: A randomized clinical trial evaluating tamoxifen in the treatment of patients with node-negative breast cancer who have estrogen receptor-positive tumors. N Engl J Med 1989;320:479.

Golumb HM et al: Alpha-2 interferon therapy of hairy cell leukemia: A multicenter study. J Clin Oncol 1986;4:900.

Greene MH et al: Melphalan may be a more potent leukemogen than cyclophosphamide. Ann Intern Med 1986; 105:360.

Henderson IC et al: Effects of adjuvant tamoxifen and of cytotoxic therapy on mortality in early breast cancer: An overview of 61 randomized trials among 28,896 women. N Engl J Med 1988;319:1681.

Hryniuck W: Average relative dose intensity and the impact on design of clinical trials. Semin Oncol 1987;14:65.

Kraut EH, Bouronele BA, Grever MR: Pentostatin in the treatment of advanced hairy cell leukemia. J Clin Oncol 1989;7:168.

Leichman L et al: Preoperative chemotherapy for carcinoma of the esophagus: A potentially curative approach. J Clin Oncol 1984;2:75.

Link MP et al: The effect of adjuvant chemotherapy on relapse-free survival in osteosarcoma of the extremity. N Engl J Med 1986;314:1600.

Longo D et al: Twenty years of MOPP therapy for Hodgkin's disease. J Clin Oncol 1986;4:1295.

Mansour EG et al: Efficacy of adjuvant chemotherapy in high-risk node-negative breast cancer: An intergroup study. N Engl J Med 1989;320:485.

Marty M et al: Comparison of the 5-hydroxytryptamine$_3$ (serotonin) antagonist ondansetron with high dose metoclopramide in the control of cisplatin-induced emesis. N Engl J Med 1990;322:816.

Patchell RA et al: A randomized trial of surgery in the treatment of single metastasis to the brain. N Engl J Med 1990;322:494.

Perry MC et al: Chemotherapy with or without radiation therapy in limited small cell carcinoma of the lung. N Engl J Med 1987;316:912.

Rosen ST et al: Radioimmunodetection and radioimmunotherapy of cutaneous T cell lymphomas using a ^{131}I-labeled monoclonal antibody. J Clin Oncol 1987;5:562.

Rosenberg SA: The low grade non-Hodgkin's lymphomas: Challenges and opportunities. J Clin Oncol 1985;3:299.

Salmon SE: Adjuvant Therapy of Cancer V. Grune & Stratton, 1987.

Salmon SE, Sartorelli AC: Cancer chemotherapy. Chap 56 in: Basic & Clinical Pharmacology. 4th ed. Katzung BG (editor). Appleton & Lange, 1989.

Salmon SE et al: Prediction of doxorubicin resistance in vitro in myeloma, lymphoma, and breast cancer by P-glycoprotein staining. J Natl Cancer Inst 1989;81:696.

Sigurdsson H et al: Indicators of prognosis in node-negative breast cancer. N Engl J Med 1990;322:1045.

Steis RG et al: Resistance to recombinant interferon alfa-2a in hairy-cell leukemia associated with neutralizing anti-interferon antibodies. N Engl J Med 1988;318:1409.

Tandon AK et al: Cathepsin D and prognosis in breast cancer. N Engl J Med 1990;322:297.

Vander Hoop RG et al: Prevention of cisplatin neurotoxicity with an ACTH analog in patients with ovarian cancer. N Engl J Med 1990;322:89.

Yandell DW et al: Oncogenic point mutations in the human retinoblastoma gene: Their application to genetic counselling. N Engl J Med 1989;321:1689.

Yeager AM et al: Autologous bone marrow transplantation in patients with acute nonlymphocytic leukemia, using ex vivo marrow treatment with 4-hydroperoxycyclophosphamide. N Engl J Med 1986;315:141.

Young RC et al: Adjuvant therapy in stage I and II epithelial ovarian cancer. N Engl J Med 1990;322:1021.

Skin & Appendages

4

Richard B. Odom, MD, & Rees B. Rees, Jr., MD

Diagnosis of Skin Disorders

Important components of the diagnosis of skin disorders include taking a thorough history, assessing the role of systemic disorders, inquiring about systemic and topical medications, questioning about recent or unusual exposure to physical factors and chemical agents in the home and work environments, and examining the entire skin and mucous membrane surfaces in good (preferably natural) light.

Planning Topical Treatment

Many topical agents are available for the treatment of dermatologic disorders. In general, it is better to be thoroughly familiar with a few drugs and treatment methods than to attempt to use a great many. Dry skins usually require lubricating or softening agents; moist or oily skins, greaseless drying agents.

Treatment is begun with mild, simple remedies. In general, acute, inflamed lesions are best treated with soothing, nonirritating agents; chronic, thickened lesions with stimulating or keratolytic agents. When appropriate, apply a small amount of drug to a small area and observe for several hours for skin sensitivity.

Instruct the patient carefully on how to apply medications. When in doubt about the proper method of treatment, *undertreat* rather than overtreat.

General Rules Governing Choice of Topical Treatment of Various Stages of Dermatoses

Note: The choice of treatment will vary with the individual case, depending upon the characteristics of the dermatosis, the extent of the lesions, the general character of the patient's skin, previous medications and drug allergies, environment, and other factors.

A. Acute Lesions: (Recent onset; red, burning, swollen, itching, stinging, blistering, or oozing lesions.) Use wet preparations, such as soaks, for lesions localized to extremities; cool, wet dressings or compresses for localized lesions of the head, neck, trunk, or extremities; or baths for generalized lesions (see below under Pruritus). Lotions or powders may be used in intertriginous areas (axillas, groin, between toes, beneath breasts).

B. Subacute Lesions: (Intermediate duration; subsiding lesions or lesions that are less inflamed in appearance.) Use wet preparations as outlined above,

lotions, or both. Emulsions and water-soluble creams may also be used for soothing and drying effects and to deliver medication.

C. Chronic Lesions: (Longer duration; quiescent, thickened, crusted, fissured, scaly lesions.) Use wet preparations or compresses for crusted lesions and emulsions, hydrophilic ointments, pastes (high powder content), water-soluble (vanishing) creams, or greasy ointments, especially for thickened, scaly lesions. Special medications can be incorporated in these preparations.

Prevention of Complications

A. Pyoderma: Infected, inflamed, or denuded areas of skin are receptive environments for pyogenic organisms introduced by scratching, rubbing, or squeezing of skin lesions. Patients should be instructed to wash their hands frequently and to avoid manipulation of infected areas. Medications should be kept in closed containers. Crusts (scabs) should be removed by repeated soaks or compresses. If an infection occurs in a hairy portion of the body, cleanse or shave the area gently to avoid irritation.

B. Local or Systemic Spread of Infection: Almost any skin infection may spread by extension or through vascular or lymphatic channels. In most cases, this complication is a much greater threat to the patient's health and life than the primary skin infection. A most striking and serious example is the extension of staphylococcal infections of the face to the cavernous sinuses. Lymphangitis, lymphadenitis, septicemia, and glomerulonephritis may occur as sequelae to primary skin infection. For these reasons, it is important to institute vigorous local and systemic measures for the control of skin infections, and systemic antibiotics for potentially serious infections or those associated with systemic reactions.

C. Overtreatment Dermatitis: This may be avoided if the physician and the patient are aware that undertreatment is preferable to overtreatment and if the patient is warned to avoid overenthusiastic application of topical remedies (either too much or too long). Injudicious use of topical corticosteroids in large amounts or over prolonged periods, especially with occlusive plastic wrapping, can result in significant systemic absorption of steroids. Fluorinated topical corticosteroids may induce acnelike processes on the face (steroid rosacea) and atrophic striae in body folds and may induce acute adrenocortical insufficiency and aseptic bone necrosis.

D. Exfoliative Dermatitis: This complication cannot always be anticipated or avoided, but it may be minimized if a careful history of drug sensitivity is obtained before institution of drug therapy. In allergic individuals, it is important to apply a small amount of topical medication in order to determine hypersensitivity. Drugs that may be required for systemic use (eg, sulfonamides or antihistamines) should preferably not be used in topical preparations. Sodium sulfacetamide, silver sulfadiazine, erythromycin, clindamycin, and mupirocin appear to be safe for topical use. Neomycin in particular has high sensitizing potential.

E. Cosmetic Disfigurement: Disfigurement due to skin disorders may be avoided by early, careful treatment of skin lesions and by appropriate dermatologic operative techniques. Self-manipulation of skin lesions, especially on the face and exposed skin areas, should be avoided.

PRURITUS
(Itching)

Pruritus is a disagreeable sensation that provokes a desire to scratch. It is a primary sensory impulse carried on unmyelinated C fibers in the spinothalamic tract. It is modulated by central factors, including cortical ones. Not all cases of pruritus are mediated by histamine, although several mediators—bradykinin, neurotensin, secretin, and substance P—release histamine.

Although most cases of generalized pruritus can be attributed to dry skin—whether naturally occurring and precipitated or aggravated by climatic conditions or arising from disease states—there are many other causes: scabies, dermatitis herpetiformis, atopic dermatitis, pruritus vulvae et ani, miliaria, insect bites, pediculosis, contact dermatitis, drug reactions, urticaria, urticarial eruptions of pregnancy, psoriasis, lichen planus, lichen simplex chronicus, exfoliative dermatitis, folliculitis, sunburn, bullous pemphigoid, and fiberglass dermatitis.

Perhaps the commonest cause of pruritus associated with systemic disease at present is uremia in conjunction with hemodialysis. Both this condition and the pruritus of obstructive biliary disease may be helped by irradiation with ultraviolet B. Endocrine disorders, psychiatric disturbances, lymphoma, leukemia and other internal malignant disorders, iron deficiency anemia, and certain neurologic disorders may also be manifested by pruritus.

Burning or itching involving the face, scalp, and genitalia may be manifestations of primary depression and treatable with antidepressant heterocyclic drugs such as amitriptyline, imipramine, doxepin, and others.

Treatment

A. General Measures: External irritants (eg, rough clothing, occupational contactants) should be avoided. Soaps and detergents should not be used by persons with dry or irritated skin. Baths containing a small amount of bath oil may be used. Nails should be kept trimmed and clean (see below).

B. Specific Measures: Remove or treat specific causes whenever possible.

C. Local Measures:

1. Corticosteroids–Representative topical corticosteroid creams, lotions, ointments, gels, and sprays are presented in the following list:

Lowest potency: Hydrocortisone, desonide, and alclometasone dipropionate. Best for chronic use and for the face.

Mid potency: Flurandrenolide, fluocinolone, triamcinolone, hydrocortisone valerate, and hydrocortisone butyrate.

Higher potency: Desoximetasone, amcinonide, halcinonide, and fluocinonide.

Highest potency: Betamethasone, clobetasol, and diflorasone. These should be used for brief periods only, on limited areas, and not on the face or genitalia or in body folds.

2. Petrolatum–If the skin is too dry, wet it, as in a bath (to hydrate the keratin), and then apply petrolatum to the wet skin to trap the moisture.

3. Drying agents–If the skin is too moist, drying agents may afford relief, eg, wet dressings, soaks, shake lotions (eg, starch or calamine lotions), and powders (especially if the process is acute).

4. Tub baths–Generalized pruritus may often be effectively controlled by lukewarm baths, 15 minutes 2–3 times daily. Elderly patients with dry skin should bathe as infrequently as possible, because soaps and overbathing further aggravate xerosis. After bathing, the skin should be blotted (not rubbed) dry. Useful bath formulations are as follows: (1) Colloidal oatmeal baths, regular and oilated—especially beneficial for pruritic, sensitive, and dry skin. (2) Tar bath: 50–100 mL of coal tar solution USP dissolved in 1 tubful (50 gallons) of warm water. (Watch for sensitivity.) (3) Bath oils: 5–25 mL in 1 tubful (50 gallons) of warm water (eg, Alpha-Keri, DOB, Domol Lubath). Bubble baths should be avoided. Oils, creams, lotions, and ointments are preferably applied to hydrated skin immediately after the shower or bath.

5. Five percent lactic acid in petrolatum or a lotion vehicle may relieve the pruritus and the appearance of dry skin and ichthyosis. A 12% lactate lotion is useful (Lac-Hydrin).

6. Lotions that contain 0.5% each of camphor, menthol, and phenol (Sarna) are effective for mild pruritic dermatoses.

7. Pramoxine hydrochloride, 1% (Prax) cream or lotion, or pramoxine hydrochloride, 1%, with 0.5% menthol (Pramagel), as a surface anesthetic is an effective antipruritic agent. Hydrocortisone, 1% or

2.5%, may be incorporated for its anti-inflammatory effect (Pramosone cream, lotion, or ointment).

D. Potentiation of Topical Corticosteroid Creams: By covering selected lesions of psoriasis, lichen planus, and localized eczemas each night, first with the corticosteroid, then with a thin light plastic pliable film (eg, Saran Wrap), an appreciable amount of the medicament may be systemically absorbed. Complications include miliaria, striae, pyoderma, local skin atrophy, malodor, fungal infections, urticarial erythema, and, rarely, adrenocortical suppression when extensive areas of body surface are occluded.

E. Systemic Antipruritic Drugs:

1. Antihistaminic and "antiserotonin" drugs–In general, H_1 blockers are the agents of choice for pruritus, because H_2 receptors are not involved in itching. Hydroxyzine and doxepin are useful, as are all other agents that act as antihistamines. Cyproheptadine or chlorpheniramine may be useful when sedation is to be avoided. The newer nonsedating antihistamines—specifically terfenadine and astemizole—may be beneficial and appear to be well tolerated (see Chapter 1).

2. Diazepam may provide useful sedation in agitated or distracted patients.

3. Corticotropin or the corticosteroids–(See Chapter 20.) The role of corticosteroids in controlling the endogenous mediators of inflammation is not known. Histamine, kinins, lysosomal enzymes, and prostaglandins have been examined, but experimental clarification of modes of action is lacking. The antimitotic effects of corticosteroids on human skin may account for some benefit in psoriasis and in other diseases associated with increased cell turnover.

4. Psychotropic drugs–The analgesic and antihistaminic properties of some antidepressants, such as doxepin and imipramine (see Chapter 19), may alleviate intractable pruritus, since pain and pruritus share the same central nervous system pathways.

Prognosis

Elimination of external factors and irritating agents is often successful in giving complete relief from pruritus. Pruritus accompanying specific skin disease will subside when the disease is controlled. Idiopathic pruritus and that accompanying serious internal disease may not respond to any type of therapy.

Denman ST: A review of pruritus. J Am Acad Dermatol 1986;14:375.
Gupta M et al: Psychotropic drugs in dermatology: A review and guidelines for use. J Am Acad Dermatol 1986; 14:633.

ANOGENITAL PRURITUS

Essentials of Diagnosis

- Itching, chiefly nocturnal, of the anogenital area.
- Examination is highly variable, ranging from no skin reactions to excoriations and inflammation of any degree, including lichenification.

General Considerations

Most cases have no obvious cause, but multiple specific causes have been identified. Anogenital pruritus may have the same causes as intertrigo, lichen simplex chronicus, or seborrheic or contact dermatitis (from soaps, colognes, douches, contraceptives) or may be due to irritating secretions, as in diarrhea, leukorrhea, or trichomoniasis, or local disease (candidiasis, dermatophytosis, erythrasma). Diabetes mellitus must be ruled out. Psoriasis or seborrheic dermatitis may be present. Uncleanliness may be at fault. It has been postulated that fecal bacterial endopeptidases play a causative role in pruritus ani.

Many gynecologic patients experience pruritus vulvae. In women, pruritus ani by itself is rare, and pruritus vulvae does not usually involve the anal area, although anal itching will usually spread to the vulva. In men, pruritus of the scrotum is less common than pruritus ani. When all possible known causes have been ruled out, the condition is diagnosed as idiopathic or essential pruritus—by no means rare.

Proctosigmoidoscopic examination is seldom helpful. Oxyuriasis (pinworm) is rarely a cause in adults. Psychologic abnormalities are usually not evident. Lichen sclerosus et atrophicus may at times be the cause, but gross pathologic changes are evident in this disorder. Erythrasma is easily diagnosed by demonstration of coral-red fluorescence with Wood's light; it is easily cured with erythromycin, orally and topically.

Clinical Findings

A. Symptoms and Signs: The only symptom is itching, which is chiefly nocturnal. Physical findings are usually not present, but there may be erythema, fissuring, maceration, lichenification, excoriations, or changes suggestive of candidiasis or tinea.

B. Laboratory Findings: Urinalysis and blood glucose determination may lead to a diagnosis of diabetes mellitus. Microscopic examination or culture of tissue scrapings may reveal yeasts, fungi, or parasites. Stool examination may show intestinal parasites.

Differential Diagnosis

The etiologic differential diagnosis consists of *Candida* infection, parasitosis, local irritation from contact with drugs and irritants, and other primary skin disorders of the genital area such as psoriasis, seborrhea, intertrigo, or lichen sclerosus et atrophicus.

Prevention

Instruct the patient in proper anogenital hygiene after treating systemic or local conditions.

Treatment
(See also Pruritus.)

A. General Measures: Avoid "hot" (spicy) foods, and drugs that can irritate the anal mucosa. Treat constipation if present, preferably with high-fiber management (psyllium [Metamucil; many others]). Instruct the patient to use very soft or moistened tissue or cotton after a bowel movement and to clean the perianal area thoroughly. Women should use similar precautions after urinating. Anal douching is the best cleansing method for all types of pruritus ani. Instruct the patient regarding the harmful and pruritus-inducing effects of scratching.

B. Local Measures: Prax cream or lotion or Pramosone, 1% or 2.5% cream, lotion, or ointment, is helpful in managing pruritus in the anogenital area. Hydrocortisone or iodochlorhydroxyquin-hydrocortisone creams are quite useful. Potent fluorinated topical corticosteroids may lead to atrophy and striae if used for more than a few days. Sitz baths twice daily using silver nitrate, 1:10,000–1:200; potassium permanganate, 1:10,000; or aluminum subacetate solution, 1:20, are of value if the area is acutely inflamed and oozing. Underclothing should be changed daily. Affected areas may be painted with Castellani's solution. Balneol Perianal Cleansing Lotion or Tucks premoistened pads, ointment, or cream (all Tucks preparations contain witch hazel) may be very useful for pruritus ani.

Prognosis

Although usually benign, anogenital pruritus may be persistent and recurrent.

Jillson OF: Pruritus ani: Disputing the passage. Cutis 1984;33:537.

COMMON DERMATOSES

CONTACT DERMATITIS
(Dermatitis Venenata)

Essentials of Diagnosis
- Erythema and edema, often followed by vesicles and bullae in area of contact with suspected agent.
- Later, weeping, crusting, or secondary infection.
- Often a history of previous reaction to suspected contactant.
- Patch test with agent usually positive in the allergic form.

General Considerations

Contact dermatitis is an acute or chronic dermatitis that results from direct skin contact with chemicals or allergens. Lesions are most often on exposed parts. Four-fifths of such disturbances are due to excessive exposure to or additive effects of primary or universal irritants (eg, soaps, detergents, organic solvents). Others are due to actual contact allergy. The most common allergies to dermatologic agents include antimicrobials (especially neomycin), topical antihistamines, anesthetics, and preservatives, eg, parabens.

Clinical Findings

A. Symptoms and Signs: Itching, burning, and stinging are often extremely severe, distributed on exposed parts or in bizarre asymmetric patterns. The lesions consist of erythematous macules, papules, and vesicles. The affected area is often hot and swollen, with exudation, crusting, and commonly secondary infection. The pattern of the eruption may be diagnostic (eg, typical linear streaked vesicles on the extremities and erythema and swelling of the genitalia in poison oak or ivy dermatitis). The location will often suggest the cause: Scalp involvement suggests hair tints, lacquer, shampoos, or tonics; face involvement, creams, cosmetics, soaps, shaving materials; neck involvement, jewelry, fingernail polish, etc.

B. Laboratory Findings: The patch test may be useful but has limitations. In the event of a positive reaction, the clinical relevance of the chemical agent and the dermatitis must be determined. Photopatch tests (exposing the traditional patch test site to ultraviolet light after 24 hours) may be necessary in the case of suspected photosensitivity contact dermatitis.

Differential Diagnosis

Asymmetric distribution and a history of contact help distinguish contact dermatitis from other skin lesions. The commonest causes are poison oak and ivy, rubber antioxidants and accelerators, nickel and chromium salts, paraphenylenediamine, formalin, ethylenediamine, turpentine, benzocaine, and neomycin. Differentiation may be difficult if the area of involvement is consistent with that seen in other types of skin disorders such as scabies, dermatophytid, atopic dermatitis, dyshidrotic eczema, and other eczemas.

Prevention

Soaps and detergents are avoided, and cosmetics are either unscented or not used. Protective gloves may be used; in such cases, a cotton glove liner must be added. Protective (barrier) creams are almost useless.

Prompt and thorough removal of irritants by prolonged washing or by removal with solvents or other chemical agents may be effective if done very shortly after exposure.

Injection or ingestion of Rhus antigen is of limited practical clinical value for the prevention of *Rhus (Toxicodendron)* dermatitis.

Treatment

A. General Measures: For acute severe cases, one may give prednisone, 40–60 mg/d orally for 10 days. Triamcinolone acetonide (Kenalog-40), 40 mg once intragluteally, may be used instead. (See Chapter 20.) An age-old remedy for itching disorders is repeated exposure to hot water, as in a shower, without soap; this treatment may have the effect of prolonging and aggravating the underlying disorder (eg, atopic or nummular dermatitis).

B. Local Measures: Treat the stage and type of dermatitis (see above).

1. Acute weeping dermatitis–It is unwise to scrub lesions with soap and water. Apply solutions. Calamine or starch shake lotions may be indicated instead of wet dressings or in intervals between wet dressings, especially for involvement of intertriginous areas or when oozing is not marked. Lesions on the extremities may be bandaged with wet dressings. Potent topical corticosteroids, in ointment or cream form, may help suppress acute contact dermatitis and relieve itching. A soothing formulation is 0.1% triamcinolone acetonide in Sarna (0.5% in camphor, 0.5% menthol, 0.5% phenol) lotion. Frequent continued use may induce tachyphylaxis (acute tolerance).

2. Subacute dermatitis (subsiding)–Shake lotions or antipruritic-steroid lotions are used.

3. Chronic dermatitis (dry and lichenified)– Treat with hydrophilic, greasy ointments or creams. Tars, often combined with moderate-strength corticosteroid (eg, 0.1% triamcinolone), are useful.

Prognosis

Contact dermatitis is self-limited if reexposure is prevented. Spontaneous desensitization may occur. Increasing sensitivity to industrial irritants may necessitate a change of occupation.

Adams RM, Fisher AA: Contact allergen alternatives: 1986. J Am Acad Dermatol 1986;14:951.

Fisher AA: *Contact Dermatitis,* 3rd ed. Lea & Febiger, 1986.

ATOPIC DERMATITIS (Eczema)

Essentials of Diagnosis

- Pruritic, exudative, or lichenified eruption on face, neck, upper trunk, wrists, and hands and in the folds of knees and elbows.
- Personal or family history of allergic manifestations (eg, asthma, allergic rhinitis, eczema).
- Tendency to recur, with remission from adolescence to age 20.

General Considerations

Diagnostic criteria for atopic dermatitis must include pruritus, typical morphology and distribution (flexural lichenification in adults; facial and extensor involvement in infancy), and a tendency toward chronic or chronically relapsing dermatitis. In addition, there should be 2 or more of the following features: (1) personal or family history of atopic disease (asthma, allergic rhinitis, atopic dermatitis), (2) immediate skin test reactivity, (3) white dermographism or delayed blanch to cholinergic agents, and (4) anterior or posterior subcapsular cataracts; plus 4 or more of the following features: (a) xerosis-ichthyosis-hyperlinear palms, (b) pityriasis alba, (c) keratosis pilaris, (d) facial pallor with infraorbital darkening, (e) Dennie-Morgan infraorbital fold, (f) elevated serum IgE, (g) keratoconus, (h) tendency toward nonspecific hand dermatitis, and (i) tendency toward repeated cutaneous infections.

Clinical Findings

A. Symptoms and Signs: Itching may be extremely severe and prolonged, leading often to emotional disturbances, which have been erroneously interpreted by some as being causative. The distribution of the lesions is characteristic, with involvement of the face, neck, and upper trunk ("monk's cowl"). The bends of the elbows and knees are involved. An abortive form may involve the hands alone (in which case the history of atopy is all-important). In infants, the eruption usually begins on the cheeks and is often vesicular and exudative. In children (and later) it is dry, leathery, and lichenified, although intraepidermal vesicles are occasionally present histologically. Adults generally have dry, leathery, hyperpigmented or hypopigmented lesions in typical distribution.

The role of food allergy in atopic dermatitis is debatable. Several studies have implicated eggs, cow's milk, and peanuts in flare-ups of dermatitis, especially in younger children.

B. Laboratory Findings: Laboratory findings in general, including scratch and intradermal tests, are disappointing. Eosinophilia and increased serum IgE levels may be present.

Differential Diagnosis

Atopic dermatitis must be distinguished from seborrheic dermatitis (frequent scalp and face involvement, greasy and scaly lesions, and quick response to therapy), contact dermatitis (especially that due to weeds), and lichen simplex chronicus (flat, more circumscribed, less extensive lesions).

Treatment

A. General Measures: Systemic corticosteroids are indicated only in extensive and more severe cases. Oral prednisone dosages should be high enough to suppress the dermatitis quickly, usually starting with 60 mg daily. The dosage is then reduced over a period of 2–5 weeks. Triamcinolone acetonide suspension, 20–40 mg intramuscularly every 4–6 weeks (or less often), may exert control. In mild cases, topical corticosteroid therapy may be adequate. The antihistamines may be used to aid in the relief of severe pruritus. Hydroxyzine or doxepin may be useful, but the dosage must be increased gradually to avoid drowsiness. Warm temperate climates and exposure to ultraviolet rays are helpful for atopic dermatitis, reducing the need for topical corticosteroids. There is increased IgE binding to *Staphylococcus aureus*. Interaction of staphylococcal antigen and specific antistaphylococcal antibodies may induce mast cell release, causing itching and aggravation of the dermatitis. Painful fissures, crusts, or pustules indicate staphylococcal infection clinically. Therefore, antibiotics given systemically, such as erythromycin or dicloxacillin, may be helpful in management.

Eczema herpeticum, a generalized herpes simplex infection superimposed on atopic dermatitis or other extensive eczematous processes, is usually treated successfully with intravenous acyclovir in a dose of 1500 mg/m^2/d, administered over a 1-hour period 3 times a day. Nephrotoxicity is minimized by giving adequate fluids. Phlebitis may be a problem at the infusion site. Oral acyclovir, 400 mg 5 times daily, may be substituted in milder cases.

B. Specific Measures: Avoidance of temperature changes and stress may help to minimize abnormal cutaneous vascular and sweat responses.

The dry skin of atopic patients should be hydrated with hydrophilic creams and lotions.

Attempts at desensitization to various allergens by graded injections are disappointing and may cause exacerbations. Environmental irritants and allergens (wool, feather pillows) should be sought for and eliminated.

Treatment of emotional disturbances is of little practical value in management of the dermatitis.

C. Local Treatment: Soapless detergents are not advisable. Corticosteroids in lotion, cream, or ointment form have almost completely supplanted all other topical medications because of greater efficacy. They should be applied sparingly twice daily.

Treatment is dictated by the stage of the dermatitis:

1. Acute weeping lesions–Use saline, bicarbonate, or aluminum subacetate solution as soothing or astringent soaks, baths, or wet dressings for 30 minutes 3 or 4 times daily. Calamine or starch shake lotions may be employed at night or when wet dressings are not desirable. Lesions on extremities, particularly, may be bandaged for protection at night. Apply steroid lotions or creams for this stage.

2. Subacute or subsiding lesions may be treated with lotions, which may incorporate mild antipruritic or mild stimulating agents. Creams or ointments containing a steroid or mild tar should also be used.

3. Chronic, dry, lichenified lesions are best treated with ointments, creams, and pastes containing lubricating, keratolytic, antipruritic, and mild kerato-

plastic agents as indicated. Topical corticosteroids and tars are the most popular agents in chronic eczema. **Tachyphylaxis** may be overcome by applying a potent corticosteroid twice daily for 2 days, alternating with 2 days of less potent steroid preparations, coal tar products, or emollients. Coal tar is available as 2–5% ointment, creams, and pastes. The least irritating soaps are Alpha-Keri, Basis, Neutrogena, Purpose, and Emulave. The skin may be cleansed with lipid-free lotions, Cetaphil, Aquanil, and SFC.

Prognosis

The disease runs a chronic course, often with a tendency to disappear and recur. Poor prognostic factors for eventual complete remission in atopic dermatitis include onset early in childhood, early generalized disease, and asthma. Only 40–60% of these patients have lasting remissions.

Dahl MV: *Staphylococcus aureus* and atopic dermatitis. Arch Dermatol 1983;119:840.

Hanifin JM: Atopic dermatitis. J Am Acad Dermatol 1982;6:1.

Hannuksela M et al: Ultraviolet light therapy in atopic dermatitis. Acta Derm Venereol (Stockh) 1986;114 (Suppl):137.

Rystedt I: Long term follow-up in atopic dermatitis. Acta Derm Venereol (Stockh) 1985;114:117.

LICHEN SIMPLEX CHRONICUS (Circumscribed Neurodermatitis)

Essentials of Diagnosis

- Chronic itching associated with pigmented lichenified skin lesions.
- Exaggerated skin lines overlying a thickened, well-circumscribed scaly plaque.
- Predilection for nape of neck, wrists, external surfaces of forearms, inner thighs, genitalia, popliteal and antecubital areas.

General Considerations

A traditional explanation for lichen simplex chronicus (circumscribed neurodermatitis) is that it represents a self-perpetuating scratch-itch cycle. Hypertrophic nerve fibers have been found in lichenified, thickened lesions of long standing. Definite personality patterns seem to be associated with the disorder, including inability to be aggressive. In some instances, the disease may be a well-compensated equivalent of a psychosis.

Clinical Findings

Intermittent itching incites the patient to manipulate the lesions. Itching may be so intense as to interfere with sleep. Dry, leathery, hypertrophic, lichenified plaques appear on the neck, wrist, perineum, thigh, or almost anywhere. The patches are well-localized and rectangular, with sharp borders, and are thickened and pigmented. The lines of the skin are exaggerated and divide the lesion into rectangular plaques.

Differential Diagnosis

This disorder may be confused with plaquelike lesions such as psoriasis, lichen planus, seborrheic dermatitis, and nummular dermatitis.

Treatment

The area should be protected and the patient encouraged to avoid stressful and emotionally charged situations if possible. Topical corticosteroids give relief. The injection of dilute triamcinolone acetonide suspension into the lesions may occasionally be curative. Application of triamcinolone acetonide 0.1%, fluocinolone 0.025%, betamethasone valerate 0.1%, or fluocinonide 0.05% cream nightly with occlusive plastic wrap (eg, Saran Wrap) covering may be helpful. Betamethasone dipropionate 0.05% and clobetasol propionate 0.05% are effective creams and ointments without occlusion when applied twice daily. Stimulants (caffeine, etc) should be avoided. The mechanism of the itch-scratch cycle should be explained to the patient in hope of breaking the pattern.

Prognosis

The disease tends to remit during treatment but may recur, or another site may develop.

Arnold HL Jr: Paroxysmal pruritus: Its clinical characterization and a hypothesis of its pathogenesis. J Am Acad Dermatol 1984;11:322.

DERMATITIS MEDICAMENTOSA
(Drug Eruption)

Essentials of Diagnosis

- Usually, abrupt onset of widespread, symmetric erythematous eruption. May mimic any inflammatory skin condition. Constitutional symptoms (malaise, arthralgia, headache, and fever) may be present.

General Considerations

As is well recognized, only a minority of cutaneous drug reactions result from allergy. True allergic drug reactions involve prior exposure, an "incubation" period, reactions to doses far below the therapeutic range, manifestations different from the usual pharmacologic effects of the drug, involvement of only a small portion of the population at risk, restriction to a limited number of syndromes (anaphylactic and anaphylactoid, urticarial, vasculitic, etc), and reproducibility. Such factors as overdose, toxic side effects, neoplastic disease, superinfection, drug interaction, impaired degradation or excretion, conditions mimicking allergic reactions (eg, Jarisch-Herxheimer reaction), ampicillin reactions with infectious mononu-

cleosis, Stevens-Johnson syndrome, intolerance with low doses, and idiosyncrasy may be operative.

Rashes are among the most common adverse reactions to drugs and occur in 2–3% of hospitalized patients. Amoxicillin, trimethoprim-sulfamethoxazole, and ampicillin or penicillin are the commonest causes. Toxic epidermal necrolysis and Stevens-Johnson syndrome are most commonly produced by sulfonamides. Phenolphthalein, pyrazolone derivatives, and barbiturates are the major causes of fixed drug eruptions.

Clinical Findings

A. Symptoms and Signs: The onset is usually abrupt, with bright erythema and often severe itching, but may be delayed (penicillin, serum). Fever and other constitutional symptoms may be present. The skin reaction usually occurs in symmetric distribution. In a given situation, the physician may suspect one specific drug (or one of several) and must therefore inquire specifically whether it has been used or not.

1. Toxic erythema–This is the commonest skin reaction to drugs and causes many patterns of erythema; it is often more pronounced on the trunk than on the extremities. In previously exposed patients, the rash may start in 2–3 days. In the first course of treatment, the eruption often appears about the ninth day. Fever may be present. Common offenders include antibiotics (especially ampicillin), sulfonamides and related compounds (including thiazide diuretics, furosemide, and sulfonylurea hypoglycemics), barbiturates, phenylbutazone, and aminosalicylic acid.

2. Erythema multiforme–In this disorder, target-like lesions are noted mainly on the extensor aspects of the limbs. Bullae may occur. The commonest offenders are the sulfonamides, barbiturates, phenylbutazone, sulindac, and fenoprofen.

Inflammatory cutaneous nodules are usually limited to the extensor aspects of the legs and may be accompanied by fever, arthralgias, and pain.

3. Erythema nodosum–Oral contraceptives.

4. Allergic vasculitis– Inflammatory changes most severe around veins and venules. Lesions may present as urticaria, hemorrhagic papules ("palpable purpura"), vesicles, bullae, or necrotic ulcers. Common offenders include sulfonamides, phenylbutazone, indomethacin, phenytoin, and ibuprofen.

5. Purpura–(Results from thrombocytopenia, by damaging blood vessel or by affecting blood coagulation.) Itchy, brownish, petechial macular rash on dependent areas. Common offenders include thiazides, sulfonamides, phenylbutazone, sulfonylureas, barbiturates, quinine, and sulindac.

6. Eczema–Rare epidermal reaction similar to contact dermatitis in patients previously sensitized by external exposure who are given the same or a related substance systemically. The commonest offenders include penicillin, neomycin, phenothiazines, and local anesthetics.

7. Exfoliative dermatitis and erythroderma–(Entire skin surface is red and scaly.) Common offenders include allopurinol, sulfonamides, phenylbutazone, aminosalicylic acid, isoniazid, gold, carbamazepine.

8. Photosensitivity–(An exaggerated response to ultraviolet light.) Affects the exposed skin of the face, neck, and backs of the hands, and also, in women, the lower legs. On occasion, the ultraviolet emission from fluorescent lighting may be sufficient. Common offenders are sulfonamides and sulfonamide-related compounds (thiazide diuretics, furosemide, sulfonylurea hypoglycemics), tetracyclines (especially demeclocycline), phenothiazines, nalidixic acid, sulindac, amiodarone, piroxicam, and indomethacin.

9. Drug-related lupus erythematosus–May present with a photosensitive rash accompanied by fever, polyarthritis, myalgia, and serositis. Less severe than systemic lupus erythematosus, and recovery often follows drug withdrawal. Common offenders are hydralazine, isoniazid, procainamide, and phenytoin, as well as many other drugs.

10. Lichenoid and lichen planus-like eruptions–The lesions appear as pruritic, erythematous to violaceous polygonal papules that coalesce or expand to form plaques. Amiphenazole, benzthiazides, bismuth, carbamazepine, chlordiazepoxide, chloroquine, chlorpropamide, dapsone, ethambutol, furosemide, gold salts, hydroxychloroquine, levamisole, quinacrine, meprobamate, methyldopa, aminosalicylic acid, paraphenylenediamine salts, penicillamine, phenothiazines, pindolol, propranolol, quinidine, quinine, streptomycin, sulfonylureas, tetracyclines, thiazides, triprolidine.

11. Fixed eruptions–Demarcated, round, erythematous plaques that recur at the same site when the drug is repeated. Pigmentation remains after healing. Fixed drug eruptions have been described with numerous drugs, including antimicrobials, analgesics, barbiturates, cardiovascular drugs, heavy metals, antiparasitics, antihistamines, phenolphthalein, ibuprofen, and naproxen.

12. Toxic epidermal necrolysis–(Rare.) Large sheets of erythema develop, followed by separation, which looks like scalded skin. In adults, the eruption has occurred after administration of practically all classes of drugs, particularly barbiturates, phenytoin, sulfonamides, and nonsteroidal anti-inflammatory drugs.

13. Urticaria–(Rare in chronic form.) The penicillins, nonsteroidal anti-inflammatory drugs, sulfonamides, opiates, and salicylates may be responsible.

14. Pruritus–Itchy skin without rash may be due to a wide variety of drug reactions. Pruritus ani may be due to overgrowth of *Candida* after systemic antibiotic treatment. Contraceptive pills, phenothiazines,

and rifampin cause pruritus by producing cholestatic jaundice.

15. Hair loss–Predictable side effect of cytotoxic agents and oral contraceptives. Diffuse hair loss also occurs unpredictably with a wide variety of other drugs, including anticoagulants, antithyroid drugs, newer antimicrobials, cholesterol-lowering agents, heavy metals, corticosteroids, androgens, nonsteroidal anti-inflammatory drugs, retinoids (isotretinoin, etretinate), and nadolol.

16. Pigmentation–Drugs can cause many types of pigmentary disturbances.

a. Flat hyperpigmented areas on the forehead and cheeks (chloasma or melasma) are the most common pigmentary disorder associated with drug ingestion. Improvement is slow despite stopping the drug. Oral contraceptives are the usual cause.

b. Blue-gray discoloration on light-exposed areas may occur with chlorpromazine and related phenothiazines.

c. Generalized brown or blue-gray pigmentation may occur with heavy metals (silver, gold, bismuth, and arsenic). Arsenic is no longer used as a therapeutic agent.

d. Generalized yellow color is usually due to quinacrine (Atabrine).

e. Blue-black patches on the shins, pigmentation of the nails and palate, and depigmentation of the hair may be due to chloroquine or minocycline.

f. Slate gray color is observed with amiodarone.

17. Psoriasiform eruptions–Amodiaquine, chloroquine, debrisoquin, lithium, oxprenolol, pindolol, propranolol, quinacrine, sulfonamides.

18. Pityriasis rosea-like eruptions–Arsenic trioxide, barbiturates, bismuth, clonidine, gold salts, methopromazine, metoprolol, metronidazole, tripelennamine.

19. Seborrheic dermatitis-like eruptions–Arsenic, cimetidine, gold salts, methyldopa.

20. Bullous eruptions–Aspirin, barbiturates, bromides, chlorpromazine, warfarin, phenytoin, sulfonamides and related compounds, and promethazine.

B. Laboratory Findings: The complete blood count may show leukopenia, eosinophilia, agranulocytosis, or evidence of aplastic anemia. Patch tests performed with the suspect drug, although not routinely useful, may detect an offending drug when contact sensitivity is also present.

Direct immunofluorescence studies may help distinguish drug eruptions from other skin conditions in patients with a histologic pattern of lichenoid dermatitis, vasculitis, perivascular lymphocytic infiltrate, nonspecific inflammation, and mild dermatitis. Common drugs that may be associated with such changes include nonsteroidal anti-inflammatory drugs and antibiotics, as well as triamterene, trimethoprim-sulfamethoxazole, and quinidine.

Differential Diagnosis

Distinguish from other eruptions, usually by history and subsidence after drug withdrawal, although fading may be slow.

Complications

Blood dyscrasias, anaphylaxis, laryngeal edema, photosensitivity, and hepatic, renal, ocular, central nervous system, and other complications may occur with dermatitis medicamentosa.

Prevention

People who have had dermatitis medicamentosa should avoid analogues of known chemical "allergens" as well as known offenders. The physician should pay careful attention to a history of drug reaction.

Treatment

A. General Measures: Treat systemic manifestations as they arise (eg, anemia, icterus, purpura). Antihistamines may be of value in urticarial and angioneurotic reactions, but epinephrine, 1:1000, 0.5–1 mL intravenously or subcutaneously, should be used as an emergency measure. Corticosteroids may be used as for acute contact dermatitis in severe cases. Dialysis may speed drug elimination.

B. Local Measures: Treat the varieties and stages of dermatitis according to the major dermatitis simulated. Watch for sensitivity. Extensive blistering eruptions resulting in erosions and superficial ulcerations demand hospitalization and nursing care as for burn patients.

Prognosis

Drug rash usually disappears upon withdrawal of the drug and proper treatment. If systemic involvement is severe, the outcome may be fatal.

Bigby M, Stern R: Cutaneous reactions to nonsteroidal antiinflammatory drugs: A review. J Am Acad Dermatol 1985;12:866.

Bigby M et al: Drug-induced cutaneous reactions. JAMA 1986;256:3358.

Kauppinen K, Stubb S: Drug eruptions: Causative agents and clinical types. Acta Derm Venereol (Stockh) 1984;64:320.

Millikan LE: Cutaneous adverse drug reactions. Curr Concepts Skin Disorders (Spring) 1984;5:5.

Westly ED, Wechsler HL: Toxic epidermal necrolysis. Arch Dermatol 1984;120:721.

Wintroub BU, Stern R: Cutaneous drug reactions: Pathogenesis and clinical classification. J Am Acad Dermatol 1985;13:167.

PHOTODERMATITIS
(Dermatitis Actinica, Erythema Solare [Sunburn], Polymorphous Light Sensitivity, Contact Photodermatitis)

Essentials of Diagnosis

- Painful erythema, edema, and vesiculation on sun-exposed surfaces.
- Fever, gastrointestinal symptoms, malaise, or prostration may occur.
- Proteinuria, casts, and hematuria may occur.

General Considerations

Photodermatitis is an acute or chronic inflammatory skin reaction due to overexposure or hypersensitivity to sunlight or other sources of actinic rays, photosensitization of the skin by certain drugs, or idiosyncrasy to actinic light as seen in some constitutional disorders including the porphyrias and many hereditary disorders (phenylketonuria, xeroderma pigmentosum, and others). Contact photosensitivity may occur with perfumes, antiseptics, and other chemicals.

Clinical Findings

A. Symptoms and Signs: The acute inflammatory skin reaction is accompanied by pain, fever, gastrointestinal symptoms, malaise, and even prostration. Signs include erythema, edema, and possibly vesiculation and oozing on exposed surfaces. Exfoliation and pigmentary changes often result.

B. Laboratory Findings: Uncommonly, proteinuria, casts, hematuria, and hemoconcentration may be present. Look for porphyrins in urine and stool and protoporphyrins in blood when burning, stinging, vesicles, or bullae develop in sun-exposed skin. Elaborate testing for photosensitivity may be performed by experts.

Differential Diagnosis

Photodermatitis must be differentiated from contact dermatitis that may develop from one of the many substances in suntan lotions and oils. Sensitivity to actinic rays may also be part of a more serious condition such as porphyria cutanea tarda, erythropoietic protoporphyria, lupus erythematosus, or pellagra. Phenothiazines, sulfones, chlorothiazides, griseofulvin, oral antidiabetic agents, nonsteroidal anti-inflammatory agents, and antibiotics may photosensitize the skin. Polymorphous light eruption appears to be an idiopathic photodermatosis that affects both sexes equally.

Polymorphous light eruption is chronic in nature but shows diminishing sunlight sensitivity over the long term. Transitory periods of spontaneous remission do occur, and the risk of developing systemic lupus erythematosus and possibly other autoimmune disorders is negligible. The action spectrum often lies in both long (320–400 nm) and short (below 320 nm) ultraviolet wavelengths. Contact photodermatitis may be caused by halogenated salicylanilides (weak antiseptics in soaps, creams, etc).

Complications

Delayed cumulative effects in fair-skinned people include keratoses and epitheliomas. Some individuals become chronic light-reactors even when they apparently are no longer exposed to photosensitizing or phototoxic drugs.

Prevention

Persons with very fair, sensitive skins should avoid prolonged exposure to strong sun or ultraviolet radiation. Preliminary conditioning by graded exposure and protective clothing is advisable.

Protective sunscreening agents (eg, those containing PABA and oxy- or dioxybenzone) may be applied before exposure, although PABA itself may cause photosensitivity dermatitis. There are several PABA-free sunscreens of great efficacy.

Photoplex Broad Spectrum Sunscreen Lotion not only provides protection for UVB radiation but also offers absorbent protection from UVA rays and may be beneficial for the patient experiencing photosensitivity activated by UVA.

Sunscreens with an SPF (sun protective factor) of at least 15 should be used. Estimates indicate that if fair children were to use such a sunscreen regularly it might reduce the lifetime incidence of skin cancer by 75%.

Treatment

A. General Measures: Aspirin may have some specific value for fever and pain. Corticosteroids, both systemically and topically, may be required for severe reactions. Beta-carotene (Solatene), 60 mg/d orally, is effective treatment for erythropoietic protoporphyria. Beta-carotene, 90–300 mg/d orally, may be tried in adults with photosensitive eczema, polymorphous light eruptions, or solar urticaria, although double-blind studies have not been done because of unavoidable skin staining. Chloroquine, 125 mg orally twice weekly for 3–9 months, is effective in treating porphyria cutanea tarda. Patients must be followed clinically and ophthalmologically and with laboratory uroporphyrin determinations. This is not suitable if the patient has hepatitis or cirrhosis. Phlebotomy, letting 500 mL of blood every 2 weeks, is an alternative mode of therapy but is often complicated by anemia, other hematologic disorders, hypoproteinemia, or vasomotor dysfunction. Liver toxins, including alcohol, should be interdicted.

Triamcinolone acetonide suspension, 40 mg, may be given deep in the gluteal muscle once yearly for flare-ups of polymorphous light eruption.

Trioxsalen (Trisoralen), 25–30 mg orally, followed by sunlight exposure 2 hours later, may control polymorphous light eruption. Treatment may be given for 4 days each month if needed. Initial flare-ups may occur.

B. Local Measures: Treat as for any acute dermatitis. First use cooling and soothing wet dressings with saline, bicarbonate, or aluminum subacetate solutions and follow with calamine or starch lotions. Greases must be avoided because of the occlusive effect.

For maximum protection, sunscreens with a sun protective factor (SPF) of 15 or greater should be used. These aid in delaying sun damage and aging of fair skin and in the management of photodermatoses. Photoplex in particular may be helpful for a variety of photosensitive dermatoses. Unfortunately, contact or photoallergy may be caused by sunscreens themselves, in which case sunshades containing titanium dioxide, zinc oxide, or talc may be used instead.

Prognosis

Dermatitis actinica is usually benign and self-limiting unless the burn is severe or when it occurs as an associated finding in a more serious disorder.

Frain-Bell W (guest editor): Photodermatoses. Semin Dermatol 1982;1:153. (Entire issue.)

Jansen CT, Karvonen J: Polymorphous light eruption: A seven-year follow-up evaluation of 114 patients. Arch Dermatol 1984;120:862.

Stern RS, Weinstein MC, Baker SG: Risk reduction for nonmelanoma skin cancer with childhood sunscreen use. Arch Dermatol 1986;122:537.

ERYTHEMA NODOSUM

Essentials of Diagnosis

- Painful red nodules without ulceration on anterior aspects of legs.
- Slow regression over several weeks to resemble contusions.
- Some cases associated with infection or drug sensitivity. Women are predominantly affected.

General Considerations

Erythema nodosum is a symptom complex characterized by tender, erythematous nodules that appear most commonly on the extensor surfaces of the legs. It usually lasts about 6 weeks and may recur. The disease may be associated with various infections (streptococcosis, primary coccidioidomycosis, other deep fungal infections, primary tuberculosis, hepatitis B, or syphilis) or may be due to drug sensitivity (penicillin, progestins). It may accompany leukemia, sarcoidosis, rheumatic fever, and ulcerative colitis. Infections with unusual organisms such as *Pasteurella (Yersinia) pseudotuberculosis* and *Yersinia enterocolitica* may be responsible. Erythema nodosum may be associated with pregnancy.

Keep in mind the possibility of a hepatitis B virus when seeing a patient with erythema nodosum or erythema multiforme or even chronic urticaria if there is accompanying hepatomegaly.

Clinical Findings

A. Symptoms and Signs: The swellings are exquisitely tender and are usually preceded by fever, malaise, and arthralgia. They occur most often located on the anterior surfaces of the legs below the knees but may occur (rarely) on the arms, trunk, and face. The lesions, 1–10 cm in diameter, are at first pink to red; with regression, all the various hues seen in a contusion can be observed. The nodules occasionally become fluctuant, but they do not suppurate.

B. Laboratory Findings: The histologic finding of septal panniculitis is characteristic of erythema nodosum. Otherwise, the findings are those of the associated illness.

Differential Diagnosis

Erythema induratum is seen on the posterior surfaces of the legs and shows ulceration. Nodular vasculitis is usually on the calves and is associated with phlebitis. Erythema multiforme occurs in generalized distribution. In the late stages, erythema nodosum must be distinguished from simple bruises and contusions.

Treatment

A. General Measures: One first identifies and treats the underlying cause, eg, systemic infection and exogenous toxins. Saturated solution of potassium iodide, 5–15 drops 3 times daily, may result in prompt involution in many cases. Side effects of potassium iodide include salivation, swelling of salivary glands, and headache. Complete bed rest may be advisable. Focal infections should be treated, although this does not appear to influence the course of the disease. Systemic therapy directed against the lesions themselves may include corticosteroid therapy (see Chapter 20) unless contraindicated by associated infection; and salicylates are helpful for several days during the acute painful stage.

B. Local Treatment: This is usually not necessary. Hot or cold compresses may help.

Prognosis

The lesions usually disappear after about 6 weeks, but they may recur.

Horio T et al: Potassium iodide in the treatment of erythema nodosum and nodular vasculitis. Arch Dermatol 1981;117:29.

Maggiore G, Grifeo S, Marzani MD: Erythema nodosum and hepatitis B virus (HBV) infection. (Letter.) J Am Acad Dermatol 1983;9:602.

ERYTHEMA MULTIFORME

Essentials of Diagnosis

- Sudden onset of symmetric erythematous skin lesions with history of recurrence.
- May be macular, papular, urticarial, bullous, or purpuric.
- "Target" lesions with clear centers and concentric erythematous rings or "iris" lesions may be noted.
- Mostly on extensor surfaces; may be on palms, soles, or mucous membranes.
- Herpes simplex, systemic infection or disease, and drug reactions may be associated.

General Considerations

Erythema multiforme is an acute inflammatory, polymorphic skin disease due to multiple causes or of undetermined origin. Approximately 80% of cases of erythema multiforme follow outbreaks of herpes simplex. Of the remaining 20%, half have been associated with administration of a sulfonamide drug and half with miscellaneous causes—drug, viral, fungal, and bacterial. The most serious cases (Stevens-Johnson syndrome, or erythema multiforme major) by far have followed sulfonamide exposure, with possible renal damage and death. Those associated with herpes simplex were not serious.

Mycoplasma pneumoniae may be causative in the more severe cases (erythema multiforme major).

Clinical Findings

A. Symptoms and Signs: Erythema multiforme is characterized by fixed erythematous papules and wheals, some of which evolve into blisters or target lesions. It has rather characteristic histologic features. Stevens-Johnson syndrome and some cases of toxic epidermal necrolysis are major forms of erythema multiforme. Mucous membrane ulcerations are frequent. The tracheobronchial mucosa may be involved in severe cases (Stevens-Johnson variant), causing bronchitis and atelectasis. Chronic low-grade stomatitis may be an erythema multiforme variant.

Erythema multiforme-like eruptions may follow topical contact with medications, including ophthalmologic and intravaginal agents. Such topicals include balsam of Peru, chloramphenicol, econazole, ethylenediamine, furazolidone, mafenide acetate, neomycin, nifuroxime, promethazine, scopolamine, sulfonamides, and vitamin E.

B. Laboratory Findings: The characteristic epidermal change is necrosis. There is a prominent perivascular lymphocytic infiltrate in the upper dermis. Edema of the papillary dermis, leading to the formation of a subepidermal blister, is characteristic of bullous lesions. Direct immunofluorescence may show vascular deposits of IgM and C3.

Differential Diagnosis

Secondary syphilis, urticaria, drug eruptions, and toxic epidermal necrolysis must be ruled out. The bullous variety of erythema multiforme is more severe and should be differentiated from dermatitis herpetiformis, pemphigus, pemphigoid, and bullous drug eruptions. In erythema multiforme there is usually some constitutional reaction, including fever.

Complications

Visceral lesions are a complication (eg, pneumonitis, myocarditis, nephritis).

Treatment

A. General Measures: When fever is present, the patient should be at bed rest and good nursing care should be provided. Erythema multiforme major (Stevens-Johnson syndrome) may resemble toxic epidermal necrolysis, with extensive denudation of skin, and is best treated in a burn unit.

B. Specific Measures: Eliminate causative factors such as chronic systemic infections, focal infections, and sensitizing drugs. Corticosteroids may be tried in more severe cases, although their use is controversial. Oral acyclovir, 200 mg 5 times daily or 800 mg twice daily for 5 days, is effective in preventing recurrent herpes-associated erythema multiforme. Antibacterial preparations are used for secondary infection.

C. Local Measures: Treat the stage and type of dermatitis (see above). For acute lesions, employ simple wet dressings and soaks of soothing lotions. Zinc sulfate solution, 0.01–0.025%, may be used as a mouth rinse several times daily. Subacute lesions require soothing lotions.

Prognosis

The illness usually lasts 2–6 weeks and may recur. Stevens-Johnson syndrome, in which visceral involvement may occur, may be serious or even fatal. The prognosis depends in part on that of the primary disease.

Fisher AA: Erythema multiforme-like eruptions due to topical medications. (Part 2.) Cutis 1986;37:158.
Lemak MA, Duvic M, Ben SF: Oral acyclovir for the prevention of herpes-associated erythema multiforme. J Am Acad Dermatol 1986;15:50.
Schosser RH: The erythema multiforme spectrum: Diagnosis and treatment. Curr Concepts Skin Dis (Summer) 1985;6:6.

ERYTHEMA CHRONICUM MIGRANS
(See also Chapter 27.)

Erythema chronicum migrans is a unique cutaneous eruption that characterizes stage 1 of Lyme disease. Three to days (median: 7 days) after a tick bite, there is gradual expansion of redness around the papule representing the bite site. The advancing border is usually slightly raised, warm, red to bluish-red, and free of any scale. Centrally, the site of the bite may clear, leaving only a rim of peripheral erythema, or it may become indurated, vesicular, or necrotic. The annular erythema usually grows to a median diameter of 15 cm (range: 3–68 cm). It is accompanied by a burning sensation in half of patients; rarely, it is pruritic or painful. Twenty-five to 50 percent of patients will develop multiple secondary annular lesions similar in appearance to the primary lesion but without indurated centers and generally of smaller size.

Without treatment, erythema chronicum migrans and the secondary lesions fade in a median of 28 days, though some may be present for months. Ten percent of untreated patients experience recurrences over the ensuing months.

Berger BW, Johnson RC: Clinical and microbiologic findings in six patients with erythema migrans of Lyme disease. J Am Acad Dermatol 1989;21:1188.
Steere AC: Lyme disease. N Engl J Med 1989;321:586.

EXFOLIATIVE DERMATITIS
(Exfoliative Erythroderma)

Essentials of Diagnosis

- Scaling and erythema over large area of body.
- Itching, malaise, fever, weight loss.
- Primary disease or exposure to toxic agent (contact, oral, parenteral) may be evident.

General Considerations

As a causative factor, a preexisting dermatosis may be found in approximately 40% of cases, including psoriasis, atopic dermatitis, contact dermatitis, pityriasis rubra pilaris, and seborrheic dermatitis. Reactions to external and internal drugs account for perhaps one-fourth of cases and cancer for 10%. Causation of the remainder is undeterminable.

Clinical Findings

A. Symptoms and Signs: Symptoms may include itching, weakness, malaise, fever, and weight loss. Exfoliation may be generalized or universal and sometimes includes loss of hair and nails. Generalized lymphadenopathy may be due to lymphoma or leukemia or may be part of the clinical picture of the skin disease (dermatopathic lymphadenitis). There may be mucosal sloughs.

B. Laboratory Findings: Blood and bone marrow studies and lymph node biopsies may show evidence of lymphoma or leukemia. There may be pathologic serum electrophoresis, elevated erythrocyte sedimentation rate, eosinophilia, elevated serum IgE, elevated white blood count, anemia, and peripheral blood lymphocytosis. A complete blood count is indicated in all patients with this problem, and skin biopsy is mandatory and may show changes of a specific inflammatory dermatitis or cutaneous T cell lymphoma or leukemia.

Differential Diagnosis

It is often impossible to identify the cause of exfoliative dermatitis early in the course of the disease, so careful follow-up is necessary. Similar eruptions include psoriasis, lichen planus, severe seborrheic dermatitis, and dermatitis medicamentosa, which may themselves develop into exfoliative dermatitis.

Complications

Septicemia, debility (protein loss), dehydration, pneumonia, high-output cardiac failure, masking of fever, hypermetabolism, thermoregulatory disorders, and anemia may develop in patients with generalized inflammatory erythroderma.

Treatment

A. General Measures: If the erythroderma becomes chronic and is not manageable in an outpatient setting, hospitalize the patient at bed rest. Keep the room at a warm, constant temperature and avoid drafts.

B. Specific Measures: Stop all drugs, if possible. Systemic corticosteroids may provide spectacular improvement in severe or fulminant exfoliative dermatitis, but long-term therapy should be avoided if possible (see Chapter 20). For recalcitrant cases of psoriatic erythroderma and pityriasis rubra pilaris, either isotretinoin, etretinate, or methotrexate—or isotretinoin and methotrexate in combination—may be indicated. Erythroderma secondary to lymphoma or leukemia requires specific topical or systemic chemotherapy combined with radiation therapy. Suitable antibiotic drugs should be given when there is evidence of bacterial infection; pyoderma is a common complication of exfoliative dermatitis.

C. Local Measures: Observe careful skin hygiene and avoid irritating local applications. Treat skin as for acute extensive dermatitis first with midpotency topical steroids under wet dressings or plastic suit occlusion and soothing baths; and later with soothing oily steroid lotions and ointments. Topical anti-infective drugs may be used when necessary.

Prognosis

Most patients recover completely or improve greatly over time. Deaths have been reported but are rare unless there is underlying cancer. A minority will suffer from undiminished erythroderma for indefinite periods of time.

Hasan T, Jansen CT: Erythroderma: A follow-up of fifty cases. J Am Acad Dermatol 1983;8:836.

URTICARIA & ANGIOEDEMA

Essentials of Diagnosis

- Eruptions of evanescent wheals or hives.
- Itching is usually intense but may on rare occasions be absent.

- Special forms of urticaria have special features (hereditary angioedema, dermographism, cholinergic urticaria, solar urticaria, or cold urticaria).
- Most incidents are acute and self-limited over a period of 1–2 weeks.
- Chronic urticaria may defy the best efforts of the clinician to find and eliminate the cause.

General Considerations

Urticaria can result from many different stimuli. The pathogenetic mechanism may be either immunologic or nonimmunologic. The most common immunologic mechanism is the type I hypersensitivity state mediated by IgE. Another immunologic mechanism involves the activation of the complement cascade, which produces anaphylatoxins. These in turn can release histamine. Whether the pathogenesis is allergic or nonallergic, modulating factors affect mast cells and basophils to release mediators capable of producing urticarial lesions. These mediators include histamine, serotonin, kinins, leukotrienes, prostaglandins, acetylcholine, degradation products of fibrin, and anaphylatoxins that increase vascular permeability, producing wheals.

Clinical Findings

A. Symptoms and Signs: Itching is the classic presenting symptom but (paradoxically) may be absent in rare cases. Lesions are acute, with pseudopods and intense swelling. The morphology of the lesions may vary over a period of minutes to hours. There may be involvement of the lips, tongue, eyelids, larynx, palms, soles, and genitalia. Papular urticaria resulting from insect bites may persist for long periods and may occasionally be mistaken for lymphoma or leukemia cutis on the basis of histologic findings. A central punctum can usually be seen as with flea or gnat bites. Streaked urticarial lesions may be seen in acute allergic plant dermatitis, eg, poison ivy, oak, or sumac.

In familial angioedema, there is generally a positive family history, and the urticarial lesions may be massive. Death may occur from laryngeal obstruction.

Contact urticaria may be caused by a host of substances varying from chemicals to foods to medications on a nonimmunologic basis, or it may be due to allergy.

B. Laboratory Findings: Laboratory studies are not likely to be helpful in the evaluation of chronic urticaria unless there are suggestive findings in the history and physical examination. When urticarial lesions persist indefinitely, biopsy is necessary to rule out vasculitis, and it may be desirable to determine the erythrocyte sedimentation rate, quantitative immunoglobulins, cryoglobulins, cryofibrinogens, antinuclear antibodies, total hemolytic complement, and circulating immune complexes. Hepatitis B is one factor that may cause persisting lesions.

Differential Diagnosis

Distinguish from contact dermatitis and from dermographism.

Treatment

A. General Measures: Look for and eliminate the cause if possible. The chief nonallergic causes are drugs, eg, atropine, pilocarpine, morphine, codeine; arthropod bites, eg, insect bites and bee stings (although the latter may cause anaphylaxis as well as angioedema); physical factors such as heat, cold, sunlight, injury, and pressure; and, presumably, neurogenic factors such as tension states and cholinergic urticaria induced by physical exercise, excitement, hot showers, etc.

Allergic causes may include penicillin reactions, inhalants such as feathers and animal danders, ingestion of shellfish or strawberries, injections of sera and vaccines as well as penicillin, external contactants including various chemicals and cosmetics, and infections such as viral hepatitis.

A few patients with chronic urticaria may respond to a salicylate—and tartrazine-free diet. Although salicylates are ubiquitous in nature, drugs and food are the most obvious sources.

B. Systemic Treatment: Treatment includes antihistamines orally. Hydroxyzine, 10 mg twice daily to 25 mg 3 times daily, may be very useful. Cyproheptadine, 4 mg 4 times daily, may work where hydroxyzine fails and is especially useful for cold urticaria.

Doxepin, a tricyclic antidepressant, 25–50 mg 3 times daily, appears to be effective in some cases of chronic urticaria. It is given orally.

Enthusiasm for antihistamines has lessened. Clinicians no longer claim 95% symptomatic relief; 35% may be closer to the mark. Terfenadine (Seldane), a nonsedating antihistamine, has been reported to be effective in chronic idiopathic urticaria. The dosage is 60 mg twice daily. The drug is considerably more expensive than other antihistamines. Its use is not recommended during pregnancy and lactation. Another nonsedating antihistamine—astemizole—has been reported to be effective in a majority of patients with seasonal allergic rhinitis and chronic idiopathic urticaria. The recommended dosage is 30 mg on the first day, 20 mg on the second day, and 10 mg daily thereafter.

It may be necessary to give a course of oral prednisone in a dose of 40 mg/d for 10 days. Epinephrine 1:1000, 0.3–1 mL given subcutaneously sequentially, may be useful. Sus-Phrine (epinephrine suspension), 0.1–0.3 mL, may be injected subcutaneously for more prolonged action.

For hereditary angioedema, methyltestosterone buccal tablets, 10 mg once or twice daily, may reduce the episodes. Danazol is effective for hereditary angioedema but is expensive. Stanozolol is a cheaper anabolic agent and is effective. Lyophilized, partially purified C1-inhibitor concentrate, in 5% dextrose, given intravenously in 10–45 minutes, may be lifesaving during an acute attack.

There is a continuing search for effective treatment for chronic idiopathic urticaria. The combined use of H_1 and H_2 receptor blockers, such as chlorpheniramine and cimetidine or ranitidine, has given inconsistent results. Agents are needed to counteract the kinins, the slow-reacting substance of anaphylaxis leukotrienes, the prostaglandins, the components of complement, and the potent factor that activates platelets.

C. Local Treatment: Starch baths twice daily or Aveeno baths may be very useful. One cupful of finely refined cornstarch or a packet of Aveeno may be used in a comfortably warm bath. Alternatively, one may use a lotion containing 0.5% camphor, 0.5% menthol, and 0.5% phenol (Sarna) topically or in addition to the bathing.

Solar urticaria is treated by graded exposure to sunlight or with cyproheptadine, 4 mg 4 times daily.

Prognosis

Acute urticaria usually lasts only a few days. The chronic form may persist for years.

Goldsobel AB et al: Efficacy of doxepin in the treatment of chronic idiopathic urticaria. J Allergy Clin Immunol 1986;78:867.

Kailasam V, Mathews KP: Controlled clinical assessment of astemizole in the treatment of chronic idiopathic urticaria and angioedema. J Am Acad Dermatol 1987; 16:797.

Shelley WB: Commentary: Antihistamines and the treatment of urticaria. Arch Dermatol 1983;119:442.

Winton GB, Lewis CW: Contact urticaria. Int J Dermatol 1982;21:573.

PEMPHIGUS

Essentials of Diagnosis

- Relapsing crops of bullae appearing on normal skin.
- Often preceded by mucous membrane bullae, erosions, and ulcerations.
- Superficial detachment of the skin after pressure or trauma variably present (Nikolsky's sign).
- Acantholysis on biopsy.
- Immunofluorescence studies are confirmatory.

General Considerations

Pemphigus is an uncommon intraepidermal blistering disease occurring on skin and mucous membranes. The cause is unknown, and the condition, if untreated, is usually fatal within 2 months to 5 years. The bullae appear spontaneously and are relatively asymptomatic, but the lesions become extensive and the complications of the disease lead to great toxicity and debility. There is a surprising lack of pathologic findings; no primary lesions are found in internal organs at biopsy. The disease occurs almost exclusively in middle-aged or older adults and in all races and ethnic groups. Studies have demonstrated the presence of circulating autoantibodies to intercellular substances. Drug-induced autoimmune pemphigus from penicillamine and captopril has been reported. The pathogenetic role of IgG antibodies has been proved by passive transfer of antibodies to neonatal mice, reproducing the disease. There is an association with HLA-A10 antigen. Pemphigus may present with atypical features, and repeated reevaluation of clinical findings and changes shown by immunofluorescence and histopathologic studies may be necessary.

There are 2 forms of pemphigus: **pemphigus vulgaris** and its variant, **pemphigus vegetans;** and **pemphigus foliaceus** and its variant, **pemphigus erythematosus.** Both forms may occur at any age. The vulgaris form begins in the mouth in over 50% of cases. The foliaceus form, particularly, may be associated with other autoimmune diseases or may be drug-induced, eg, by exposure to penicillamine.

Clinical Findings

A. Symptoms and Signs: Pemphigus is characterized by an insidious onset of flaccid bullae in crops or waves. The lesions often appear first on the oral mucous membranes, and these rapidly become erosive. Toxemia and a ''mousy'' odor may occur soon. Rubbing the thumb laterally on the surface of uninvolved skin may cause easy separation of the epidermis **(Nikolsky's sign).**

B. Laboratory Findings: On a smear taken from the base of a bulla and stained with Giemsa's stain **(Tzanck test),** one may see an almost unique histologic picture of disruption of the epidermal intercellular connections called **acantholysis.** There may be leukocytosis and eosinophilia. As the disease progresses, low serum protein levels may be found, as well as serum electrolyte changes. The sedimentation rate may be elevated, and anemia may be present. Intercellular antibody may be detected by the indirect immunofluorescent test on the patient's serum. In some patients, the antibody titer correlates with disease activity and may be clinically useful.

Microscopically, acantholysis is the hallmark of pemphigus, but in some patients, there may be eosinophilic spongiosis initially. Immunoelectron microscopy shows deposits of IgG intercellularly in the epidermis. These IgG antibodies may have titers corresponding with disease activity. C3 and other immunoglobulins and complement components may be present on occasion. Acantholysis can develop in a culture of normal human skin tissue when pemphigus serum is added.

Differential Diagnosis

Acantholysis is not seen in other bullous eruptions such as erythema multiforme, drug eruptions, contact dermatitis, or bullous impetigo or in the less common dermatitis herpetiformis and pemphigoid. All of these diseases have gross clinical characteristics and different immunofluorescence test results that distinguish them from pemphigus. Transient acantholytic dermatosis (harmless) may be a source of confusion.

Complications

Secondary infection commonly occurs, often causing extreme morbidity. Disturbances of electrolyte balance, malnutrition, and septicemia may lead to a fatal outcome.

Treatment

A. General Measures: Hospitalize the patient at bed rest and provide antibiotics and intravenous feedings as indicated. Anesthetic troches used before eating ease painful oral lesions.

B. Specific Measures: High dosages of prednisone, 180–360 mg/d for 6–10 weeks, may be lifesaving in pemphigus when given in time. Intermediate dosages, between 40 mg every other day and 120 mg daily, should be avoided. After initial control is achieved, azathioprine, 100 mg/d, is given concurrently with prednisone, which is gradually reduced to 40 mg/d for the first week, 30 mg/d for the second week, and 25 mg/d for the third week. Thereafter, 40 mg is given every other day, as a single morning dose, together with 100 mg/d orally of azathioprine, for years if necessary. This regimen reduces the incidence of death due to therapy. Gold sodium thiomalate, given as for rheumatoid arthritis, is said to be effective following initial prednisone. Many investigators feel that by initiating and carefully monitoring treatment with concomitant use of methotrexate, azathioprine, gold, and corticosteroids, it is possible to reduce the dosage of steroids gradually with fewer of the hazards of long-term steroid therapy. Dapsone, 100 mg daily or less, controls some cases of pemphigus.

C. Local Measures: Skin and mucous membrane lesions should be treated as for vesicular, bullous, and ulcerative lesions due to any cause. Complicating infection requires appropriate systemic and local antibiotic therapy.

Prognosis

Infection is the most frequent cause of death, usually from *Staphylococcus aureus* septicemia. Signs and symptoms are often masked by high-dose corticosteroids, suggesting caution in their use. One-half of all deaths are not related to the complications of therapy.

Anhalt GJ, Patel H, Diaz LA: Mechanisms of immunologic injury: Pemphigus and bullous pemphigoid. Arch Dermatol 1983;119:711.

Bean SF, Fritz KA, Jordon RE: Bullous dermatoses: Pemphigus. J Am Acad Dermatol 1984;11:1151.

Lever WF, Schaumberg-Lever G: Treatment of pemphigus vulgaris. Arch Dermatol 1983;120:44.

Tuffanelli DL et al: Pemphigus, (Medical Staff Conference,

University of California, San Francisco.) West J Med 1983;138:699.

OTHER BLISTERING DISEASES

There is a wide variety of other skin disorders characterized by formation of bullae, or blisters. These include bullous pemphigoid, cicatricial pemphigoid, dermatitis herpetiformis, herpes gestationis, and other less common bullous disorders.

Bullous Pemphigoid

Bullous pemphigoid is relatively benign, usually remitting in 5 or 6 years, with a course characterized by exacerbations and remissions. Oral lesions are present in about one-third of affected persons. The disease may occur in various forms, including localized, vesicular, vegetating, erythematous, erythrodermic, and nodular. There is no statistical association with internal malignant disease. The subepidermal bullae that characterize pemphigoid may closely resemble those of dermatitis herpetiformis.

With immunoelectron microscopy, deposits of IgG and C3 are found in the lamina lucida of the basement membrane. Circulating basement membrane antibodies can be found in the sera of patients in about 70% of cases. With direct immunofluorescence, IgG and C3 are commonly found, but other immunoglobulins and complement components may be found.

Corticosteroids are the treatment of choice. Some authorities add methotrexate, azathioprine, or cyclophosphamide. In a few cases, sulfapyridine or dapsone may be adequate.

Cicatricial Pemphigoid

Cicatricial pemphigoid occurs most commonly in the mouth. The eyes are the second most common site. The nasal mucosa, larynx, pharynx, genitalia, anus, and esophagus may be involved. Desquamative gingivitis is a common presenting sign. The skin is involved in about one-third of cases. The **Brunsting-Perry variant** involves only the skin of the head and neck, sparing the mucous membranes. A subepidermal blister is seen microscopically. With immunologic techniques, C3, IgG, and other immunoglobulins and complement components are seen at the basement membrane zone.

The differential diagnosis includes acquired epidermolysis bullosa, but in that disorder clinical lesions of trauma-induced bullae are seen over the joints of the hands, feet, elbows, and knees as well as atrophic scars, milia, and nail dystrophy.

Dapsone, alone or with prednisone, may be tried initially, but prednisone in combination with azathioprine or cyclophosphamide may be necessary.

Dermatitis Herpetiformis

Dermatitis herpetiformis occurs most commonly on the scalp, the sacral area, elbows, and knees. The clinical lesions are tense, very pruritic vesicles. Excoriations and hyperpigmentation or hypopigmentation may be seen.

There are 3 different forms of the disease, each having a different pattern of immunoreactants in the lamina lucida and the sub-lamina densa zone. The commonest form has a granular pattern and a high prevalence of HLA-B8/Dw3 immunogens. This form is associated with a gluten-sensitive enteropathy and slowly responds to a gluten-free diet. The other 2 forms each have different linear patterns of IgA deposits localized in the lamina lucida or below the lamina densa. The pathophysiology of these 2 types differs from that of the first type. Sulfapyridine or dapsone is the drug of choice. Dapsone may cause profound methemoglobinemia in persons with glucose-6-phosphate dehydrogenase deficiency.

Serologic studies for IgA-class antiendomysial antibodies, when positive, are specific in 70% of cases of dermatitis herpetiformis.

Herpes Gestationis

Herpes gestationis occurs in about one in 50,000–60,000 pregnancies. The bullae often appear first in periumbilical distribution, and there may be erythematous papules and plaques, vesicles, and large bullae. It usually begins in the fifth or sixth month of pregnancy or the onset may be delayed to the postpartum period. The disease is self-limited, but it may recur in subsequent pregnancies. Use of estrogens or progesterone or the onset of menses may trigger flareups. The risks to mother and fetus appear to be less significant than was formerly thought. Blisters are subepidermal, with eosinophils present. Direct immunofluorescence shows C3 at the basement membrane zone in most cases. IgG is found less often. Herpes gestationis factor is an avid complement-fixing IgG antibody found in the serum but rarely in the basement membrane zone.

Corticosteroids are the treatment of choice and are sometimes effective when used topically only.

Accetta P et al: Anti-endomysial antibodies: A serologic marker of dermatitis herpetiformis. Arch Dermatol 1986;122:459.

Bean SF, Fritz KA, Jordon RE: Bullous pemphigoid. J Am Acad Dermatol 1984;11:1152.

Bean SF, Fritz KA, Jordon RE: Cicatricial pemphigoid. J Am Acad Dermatol 1984;11:1153.

Bean SF, Fritz KA, Jordon RE: Herpes gestationis. J Am Acad Dermatol 1984;11:1154.

Beutner EH, Chorzelski TP, Jablonska S: Immunofluorescence tests: Clinical significance of sera and skin in bullous diseases. Int J Dermatol 1985;24:405.

LICHEN PLANUS

Essentials of Diagnosis
- Pruritic, violaceous, flat-topped papules with fine white streaks and symmetric distribution.
- Commonly seen along linear scratch mark (Koebner phenomenon). Anterior wrists, sacral region, penis, legs, mucous membranes.
- Usually occurs in an otherwise healthy but emotionally tense person. Histopathology is diagnostic.

General Considerations
Lichen planus is an inflammatory pruritic disease of the skin and mucous membranes, characterized by distinctive papules with a predilection for the flexor surfaces and trunk. It may be an "allergic" reaction pattern, particularly following exposure to dyes, color film developers, and gold. The 3 cardinal findings are typical skin lesions, histopathologic features of band-like infiltration of lymphocytes, histiocytes, and melanophages in the dermis, and fluorescence with clumps of IgM subepidermally. Links have been seen with bullous pemphigoid, alopecia areata, vitiligo, chronic ulcerative colitis, hypogammaglobulinemia, and graft-versus-host reactions. Drugs associated with lichen planus include gold, demeclocycline, streptomycin, tetracycline, arsenic, iodides, chloroquine, quinacrine, quinidine, and paraphenylenediamine. Antimony, phenothiazine, aminosalicylic acid, chlorothiazide, hydrochlorothiazide, and amiphenazole have also been incriminated.

Clinical Findings
Itching is mild to severe. The lesions are violaceous, flat-topped, angulated papules, discrete or in clusters, on the flexor surfaces of the wrists and on the penis, lips, tongue, and buccal and vaginal mucous membranes. Mucosal lichen planus has been reported in the genital and anorectal areas, the gastrointestinal tract, the bladder, the larynx, and the conjunctiva. The papules may become bullous or ulcerated. The disease may be generalized. Mucous membrane lesions have a lacy white network overlying them that is often confused with leukoplakia. Papules are 1–4 mm in diameter, with white streaks on the surface (Wickham's striae).

A special form of lichen planus is the erosive variety. On palms and soles, it can be disabling. It is a major problem in the mouth, since squamous cell carcinoma may develop. The disease must be distinguished from systemic lupus erythematosus, both clinically and by laboratory findings.

Differential Diagnosis
Distinguish from similar lesions produced by quinacrine or bismuth sensitivity and other papular lesions such as psoriasis, lichen simplex chronicus, and syphiloderm. Lichen planus on the mucous membranes must be differentiated from leukoplakia. Certain photodeveloping or duplicating solutions may produce eruptions that mimic lichen planus.

Treatment
A. General Measures: Patients with lichen planus are sometimes tense and nervous, and episodes of dermatitis may be temporally related to emotional crises. Measures should be directed at relieving anxiety, and judicious use of sedatives or hydroxyzine may be helpful. Corticosteroids (see Chapter 20) may be required in severe cases.

Psoralens plus long-wave ultraviolet light (PUVA) is effective for most cases of lichen planus, and maintenance therapy apparently is not required.

Isotretinoin (Accutane) and etretinate (Tegison) by mouth appear effective for oral and cutaneous lichen planus, though this is not a listed indication for these drugs, and precautions must be observed.

After testing for the presence of glucose-6-phosphate dehydrogenase, treat erosive lichen planus with dapsone, 50 mg/d; this may be given over a period of many weeks, if necessary, with appropriate clinical and laboratory monitoring. Metronidazole, 250 mg 3 times daily, may help both mucous membrane and cutaneous lichen planus.

B. Local Measures: Use lotions containing tar. Intralesional injection of triamcinolone acetonide is useful for localized forms. Corticosteroid cream or ointment may be used nightly under thin pliable plastic film. Betamethasone dipropionate or clobetasol propionate creams or ointments applied twice daily are helpful.

Application of tretinoin cream (retinoic acid; vitamin A acid), 0.05%, to mucosal lichen planus, followed by a corticosteroid ointment, may be helpful. For disabling hypertrophic lichen planus of the soles, tretinoin cream applied and covered with thin, pliable polyethylene film nightly is said to be effective.

Prognosis
Lichen planus is a benign disease, but it may persist for months or years and may be recurrent. Oral lesions tend to be especially persistent, and neoplastic degeneration has been described. The oral retinoids appear to induce remissions and facilitate healing of erosive lesions in some patients.

Falk DK, Latour DL, King LE Jr: Dapsone in the treatment of erosive lichen planus. J Am Acad Dermatol 1985;12:567.

Fox B, Odom R: Papulosquamous diseases: A review. J Am Acad Dermatol 1985;12:597.

Gonzalez E, Momtaz TK, Freedman S: Bilateral comparison of generalized lichen planus treated with psoralens and ultraviolet A. J Am Acad Dermatol 1984;10:958.

Woo TY: Systemic isotretinoin treatment of oral and cutaneous lichen planus. Cutis 1985;35:385.

PSORIASIS

Essentials of Diagnosis

- Silvery scales on bright red plaques, usually on the knees, elbows, and scalp.
- Stippled nails.
- Mild itching unless psoriasis is eruptive or occurs in body folds.
- Possible associated psoriatic arthritis. Specific histopathologic features.

General Considerations

Psoriasis is a common benign, acute or chronic inflammatory skin disease that is based upon genetic predisposition. A genetic error in the epidermal mitotic control system has been postulated. For the relationship of psoriasis to histocompatibility (HLA) antigens, see Chapter 14. The decreased responsiveness of the cAMP system in psoriatic epidermis to prostaglandin E_1 suggests that altered response of the epidermis to prostaglandins may be one of the factors in the pathophysiology of psoriasis. Polyamines, proteases, and the leukotrienes have been proposed as mediators in psoriasis. Injury or irritation of psoriatic skin tends to provoke lesions of psoriasis in the site (Koebner's phenomenon). Psoriasis occasionally is eruptive, particularly in periods of stress or after streptococcal pharyngitis. Grave, life-threatening forms may occur. There is some evidence that immunologic factors may play a part in the pathogenesis of psoriasis, but this is inadequately confirmed. Extensive erythrodermic psoriasis with abrupt onset may accompany AIDS.

Clinical Findings

There are usually no symptoms. Eruptive psoriasis may itch, and psoriasis in body folds itches severely ("inverse psoriasis"). The lesions are dull red, sharply outlined plaques covered with silvery scales. The elbows, knees, and scalp are the most common sites. Nail involvement may resemble onychomycosis. Fine stippling ("pitting") in the nails is highly suggestive of psoriasis. There may be associated arthritis that resembles the rheumatoid variety but with a negative latex fixation test (see Chapter 15).

Differential Diagnosis

Differentiate in the scalp from seborrheic dermatitis; in body folds from intertrigo and candidiasis; and in the nails from onychomycosis. Many features of Reiter's syndrome mimic psoriasis.

Treatment

A. General Measures: Desert climates seem to exert a favorable effect. Severe psoriasis calls for treatment in the hospital or a day-care center with the Goeckerman regimen or PUVA.

Corticotropin or corticosteroids may be necessary to give relief in fulminating cases. Parenteral corticosteroids should not be used except in the most severe cases, because of the possibility of changing plaques to pustular lesions. Methotrexate is available for severe psoriasis. Guidelines published by the American Academy of Dermatology must be followed.

Reassurance is important, since these patients are apt to be discouraged by the difficulties of treatment. An attempt should be made to relieve anxieties.

B. Local Measures:

1. Acute psoriasis–Avoid irritating or stimulating drugs. Begin with a bland ointment containing 10% solution of coal tar. As the lesions become less acute, the tar should be incorporated into lotions and hydrophilic ointments. Betamethasone dipropionate (Diprolene ointment), clobetasol propionate (Temovate), and diflorasone diacetate (Psorcon), rubbed into the skin once or twice daily so that 60 g lasts 2 weeks, are sometimes highly effective in treating resistant psoriasis and other dermatoses; adrenal function remains relatively unaffected. It is best to restrict the ointment to 2–3 weeks' daily use and then switch to a less potent corticosteroid or pulse 2 or 3 times daily with the potent corticosteroid and apply either a less potent agent or plain ointment with 5% coal tar solution on the remaining days.

2. Subacute psoriasis–Give warm baths daily, scrubbing the lesions thoroughly with a brush, soap, and water. Solar or ultraviolet irradiations may be applied in gradually increasing doses.

3. Chronic psoriasis–The Goeckerman regimen in psoriasis day-care centers is highly effective and cost-effective and has high patient compliance. With treatment for 6 days a week for 6 or 7 hours daily, a remission rate of 90% clearing of the skin occurs in an average of 18 days. Long remissions may occur. Intensive exposure to 2–5% crude coal tar in petrolatum to which 2.5% polysorbate 80 is added, coupled with exposure to ultraviolet light in the B range (UVB in the 290- to 320-nm wavelength range), with the addition of 2% or 5% salicylic acid to the tar ointment for thick plaques, are the essentials of the treatment; mild corticosteroid creams are added, plus a 10% solution of coal tar USP in an oil base for the scalp. The Mayo Clinic Goeckerman treatment is the standard with which other forms of psoriasis treatment must be compared.

Estar gel, psoriGel, Aquatar, and Fototar are elegant substitutes for crude coal tar. Anthralin ointment 0.1% may be helpful for thickened plaques. It tends to be irritating, however, and it discolors white or gray hair. It should not be used near the eyes. Short-contact anthralin therapy (SCAT)—anthralin 1% applied for 15–30 minutes—is an effective and safe method of treatment.

Exposure to sunlamps or black light lamps, without systemic or topical therapy, may benefit chronic psoriasis.

PUVA (psoralen plus ultraviolet-A, ie, ultraviolet light in the 320- to 400-nm wavelength range; same as black light) tends to be a long-term form of treatment, as maintenance therapy is usually required. The ultraviolet dose is cumulative, and the relapse rate is about 63% in 1–6 months. The total safe dose is unknown, and the incidence of skin cancer is 9 times the normal incidence, with a reversal of the usual basal cell to squamous cell carcinoma ratio. Epidermal dystrophy by light microscopy is seen in 50% of patients treated with PUVA, and there is rapid aging of the skin. Cataracts are a potential threat, and there may be immunologic changes.

The simple application twice daily of commercial tar plus topical corticosteroids may be helpful.

For recalcitrant scalp lesions, one may rub in nightly, a cream or ointment containing 0.5% anthralin, followed at once by Neutrogena T/Derm oil. This treatment stains pillowcases and may irritate the eyes.

Etretinate (aromatic retinoid), 0.3–1 mg/kg/d, appears to be the first choice in the treatment of severe pustular psoriasis. It is also useful for psoriatic erythroderma, psoriasis vulgaris, and psoriatic arthritis. Liver enzymes and serum lipids must be checked periodically. The drug has a prolonged half-life. An ominous finding is that of diffuse idiopathic skeletal hyperostosis (DISH syndrome) from long-term, high-dose therapy (eg, 4 mg/kg/d orally for many months).

Acitretin (etretin), an analogue of etretinate, has a much shorter half-life, and it is hoped that this compound will soon be available in the United States.

Prognosis

The course tends to be chronic and unpredictable, and the disease may be refractory to treatment.

Johnson TM et al: AIDS exacerbates psoriasis. N Engl J Med 1985;313:1415.
Lowe NJ, Lazarus V, Matt L: Systemic retinoid therapy for psoriasis. J Am Acad Dermatol 1988;19:186. Muller SA,
Perry HO: The Goeckerman treatment in psoriasis: Six decades of experience at the Mayo Clinic. Cutis 1984;34:265.
Roenigk HH Jr, Maibach HI (editors): *Psoriasis.* Marcel Dekker, 1985.
Roenigk HH Jr et al: Methotrexate in psoriasis: Revised guidelines. J Am Acad Dermatol 1988;19:145.

PITYRIASIS ROSEA

Essentials of Diagnosis

- Oval, fawn-colored, scaly eruption following cleavage lines of trunk.
- Herald patch commonly precedes eruption by 1–2 weeks. Occasional pruritus.

General Considerations

This is a common, mild, acute inflammatory disease which is 50% more common in females. Young adults are principally affected, mostly in the spring or fall.

Concurrent household cases have been reported, and recurrences may take place over a period of years. The cause is unknown, but it is speculated that a picornavirus may be causative.

Clinical Findings

Occasionally, there is severe itching. The lesions consist of oval, fawn-colored macules 4–5 mm in diameter following cleavage lines on the trunk. Exfoliation of the lesions causes a crinkly scale that begins in the center. The proximal portions of the extremities are involved. An initial lesion ("herald patch") usually precedes the later efflorescence by 1–2 weeks. Attacks usually last 4–8 weeks.

Differential Diagnosis

Differentiate from secondary syphilis, especially when lesions are numerous or smaller than usual. Tinea corporis, seborrheic dermatitis, tinea versicolor, viral exanthems, and drug eruptions may simulate pityriasis rosea. Treatment

Acute irritated lesions (uncommon) should be treated as for acute dermatitis with wet dressings or steroid lotions or creams applied twice daily. Pruritic lesions also are relieved by steroid creams or ointments. Ultraviolet light is helpful.

Prognosis

Pityriasis rosea is usually an acute self-limiting illness that disappears in about 6 weeks.

Arndt KA et al: Treatment of pityriasis rosea with UV radiation. Arch Dermatol 1983;119:381.
Chuang T-Y et al: Pityriasis rosea in Rochester, Minnesota, 1969 to 1978: A 10-year epidemiologic study. J Am Acad Dermatol 1982;7:80.

SEBORRHEIC DERMATITIS & DANDRUFF

Essentials of Diagnosis

- Dry scales or dry yellowish dandruff with or without underlying erythema.
- Scalp, central face, presternal, interscapular areas, umbilicus, and body folds.

General Considerations

Seborrheic dermatitis is an acute or chronic papulosquamous dermatitis. It is based upon a genetic predisposition mediated by an interplay of such factors as hormones, nutrition, infection, and emotional stress. The possibility exists that *Pityrosporum orbiculare (Malassezia furfur)* or *Pityrosporum ovale* plays a central role in the pathogenesis of seborrheic dermatitis. Dandruff per se is merely an intensification of the physiologic process of desquamation. Induction or aggravation of seborrheic dermatitis has been described from overgrowth of *P ovale (Malassezia ovalis)* in AIDS patients, with clinical response to application of 2% ketoconazole cream.

It is difficult to distinguish between seborrheic dermatitis, simple dandruff, and scalp psoriasis on clinical or histologic grounds. The etiology and pathogenesis of seborrheic dermatitis and dandruff are poorly understood. Numerous disparate agents are useful in controlling dandruff, including selenium sulfide, zinc pyrithione, and antifungals (against yeasts) such as nystatin and the imidazoles. There is a reawakening of interest in *Pityrosporum* yeasts as possible agents of seborrheic dermatitis, but opinion is divided about whether imidazoles help these conditions because of their antifungal activity or because they have a nonspecific cytostatic effect.

Clinical Findings

Pruritus may be present but is an inconstant finding. The scalp, face, chest, back, umbilicus, and body folds may be oily or dry, with dry scales or oily yellowish scurf. Eyelid margins (seborrheic blepharitis) may be involved in the process. Erythema, fissuring, and secondary infection may be present. Patients with Parkinson's disease frequently develop moderately severe seborrheic dermatitis.

Differential Diagnosis

Distinguish from other skin diseases of the same areas such as intertrigo and fungal infections; and from psoriasis (location).

Treatment

A. General Measures: Treat aggravating systemic factors such as infections, Parkinson's disease, and emotional stress.

B. Local Measures:

1. Acute, subacute, or chronic eczematous lesions–Treat as for dermatitis or eczema. Corticosteroid creams, lotions, or solution may be used in all stages. Potent fluorinated corticosteroids used regularly on the face may produce steroid rosacea. Therefore, nonfluorinated steroids are recommended for the face and intertriginous areas.

P ovale folliculitis of the scalp, previously resistant to treatment, responds to a brief course of ketoconazole by mouth (200 mg/d for 1 week).

Two percent ketoconazole cream appears to benefit most patients with seborrheic dermatitis and may prevent use of topical steroids, especially on the face and eyelids.

2. Seborrhea of the scalp–Use one of the following: (1) Selsun (selenium sulfide) suspension or Exsel once a week as a shampoo. Fostex cream (containing soapless cleansers, wetting agents, sulfur, and salicylic acid) or Sebulex may be used as a weekly shampoo for oily seborrhea. The patient should be instructed to shampoo vigorously once and then shampoo again, leaving the shampoo on for 5–10 minutes to loosen the scales. (2) Neutrogena T/Gel shampoo,

Sebutone, Ionil-T, and DHS Tar, containing tar, may succeed where others fail. (3) Shampoos and soaps containing zinc pyrithione may be helpful. (4) Betamethasone valerate (Valisone), fluocinonide (Lidex), betamethasone dipropionate (Diprosone), and clobetasol propionate (Temovate) solution and lotion are excellent.

An alcoholic solution of aluminum chloride plus an antibiotic topical lotion rubbed in once or twice daily, may work where other measures fail.

Newer antifungal lotions (miconazole, clotrimazole, econazole) may help.

3. Seborrhea of nonhairy areas–Mild stimulating coal tar lotion, mild sulfur-salicylic acid ointment, or 3–5% sulfur in hydrophilic ointment may be used. (The addition of 1% salicylic acid to these preparations aids in removing scales.) Low-potency steroid creams—ie, 1% or 2.5% hydrocortisone, desonide, hydrocortisone valerate or butyrate, or alclometasone dipropionate—are highly effective.

4. Seborrhea of intertriginous areas–Avoid greasy ointments. Apply low-potency steroid lotions or creams twice daily for 5–7 days and then once or twice weekly for maintenance as necessary.

5. Involvement of eyelid margins ("marginal blepharitis") usually responds to rubbing in of undiluted Johnson's Baby Shampoo.

Prognosis

The tendency is to lifelong recurrences. Individual outbreaks may last weeks, months, or years.

Editorial: Scales in the balance: Dandruff reconsidered. Lancet 1985;2:703.

Ford GP et al: The response of seborrheic dermatitis to ketoconazole. Br J Dermatol 1984;111:603.

Skinner RB et al: Double-blind treatment of seborrheic dermatitis with 2% ketoconazole cream. J Am Acad Dermatol 1985;12:852.

Skinner RB et al: Seborrheic dermatitis and acquired immunodeficiency syndrome. (Correspondence.) J Am Acad Dermatol 1986;14:147.

ACNE VULGARIS

Essentials of Diagnosis

- Pimples (papules or pustules) over the face, back, and shoulders occurring at puberty.
- Open and closed comedones. Cyst formation, slow resolution, scarring.
- The most common of all skin conditions.

General Considerations

Acne vulgaris is a common inflammatory disease of unknown cause that is apparently activated by androgens in those who are genetically predisposed. It may occur from puberty through the period of sex hormone activity. Eunuchs are spared. Similar involvement may occur in identical twins.

The disease is more common and more severe in males. Contrary to popular belief, it does not always clear spontaneously when maturity is reached. If untreated, it may persist into the fourth, fifth, or even sixth decade of life. The skin lesions follow sebaceous overactivity, plugging of the infundibulum of the follicles, retention of sebum, overgrowth of the acne bacillus *(Propionibacterium acnes)* in incarcerated sebum, irritation by accumulated fatty acids, and foreign body reaction to extrafollicular sebum. The role of antibiotics in controlling acne is not clearly understood, but they may work because of their antianabolic effect on the sebaceous gland or antibacterial or anti-inflammatory properties. (Topical occlusive or systemic corticosteroids may produce acne.)

When a resistant case of acne is encountered in a woman, hyperandrogenism may be suspected. Look for hirsutism, irregular menses, or other signs of virilism. Dexamethasone, 0.5 mg nightly, may help.

Clinical Findings

There may be mild soreness, pain, or itching; inflammatory papules, pustules, ectatic pores, acne cysts, and scarring. The lesions occur mainly over the face, neck, upper chest, back, and shoulders. Comedones are common.

Self-consciousness and embarrassment may be the most disturbing symptoms.

Differential Diagnosis

Distinguish from acneiform lesions caused by bromides, iodides, steroids, and contact with chlorinated naphthalenes and diphenyls.

Complications

Cyst formation, severe scarring, and psychic trauma.

Treatment

A. General Measures:

1. Education of the patient–It should be explained that treatment is essential not only to produce an acceptable cosmetic result while the condition is active but also to prevent permanent scarring.

2. Diet–Specific dietary factors are less important than formerly thought in causing acne.

3. Avoid exposure to oils and greases.

4. Aggravating or complicating emotional disturbances must be taken into consideration and treated appropriately.

B. Systemic Treatment:

1. Antibiotics–Tetracycline, 500–1000 mg daily; erythromycin, 500–1000 mg daily; minocycline, 100–200 mg daily. Tetracycline may discolor growing teeth.

Blood counts, blood chemistries, and urinalyses give essentially normal findings in persons on long-term low-dose tetracycline or erythromycin therapy for acne. Gram-negative folliculitis developing from acne during broad-spectrum antibiotic therapy will respond to oral isotretinoin *(caution)*. Chloramphenicol should not be used. A number of commercial topical antibiotic lotions are available. The most effective are erythromycin and clindamycin, in hydroalcoholic or other special vehicles. Clindamycin phosphate should be used topically instead of the hydrochloride. Erythromycin with benzoyl peroxide (Benzamycin) topical gel is an effective combination product.

2. Isotretinoin (Accutane; 13-*cis*-retinoic acid), a vitamin A analogue, is approved for treatment of severe cystic acne in the USA. A dosage of 0.5–1 mg/kg/d for 4–5 months is usually adequate for severe cystic acne. The drug is *absolutely contraindicated during pregnancy* because of teratogenicity; serum pregnancy tests should be obtained prior to starting the drug in a female, and therapeutic abortion should be considered if the patient becomes pregnant during therapy. Side effects occur in most patients, usually related to dry skin and mucous membranes (dry lips, nosebleed, and dry eyes). If headache occurs, pseudotumor cerebri must be ruled out. At the higher dosage level, about 25% of patients will develop hypertriglyceridemia, 15% hypercholesterolemia, and 5% a lowering of high-density lipoproteins. Miscellaneous adverse reactions, usually not seen with doses of 0.5 mg/kg/d, include musculoskeletal or bowel symptoms, rash, thinning of hair, exuberant granulation tissue in lesions, and bony hyperostosis (seen only with very high doses). No serious liver or hematologic disturbances have been reported.

Isotretinoin, in contrast to its prototype, vitamin A (retinol), is not stored in the liver, and few significant laboratory abnormalities have been reported. At doses of 1 mg/kg/d or less in teenage patients, even elevations of serum triglycerides have rarely been high enough to be of concern. Elevations of liver enzymes and triglycerides return to normal once the drug is stopped.

C. Local Measures: Desquam-X wash or Benzac W wash may be used. Avoid greasy cleansing creams and other cosmetics. Shampoo the scalp 1–2 times a week. Extract blackheads with a comedo extractor. Incise and drain fluctuant cystic lesions with a small sharp scalpel.

1. Keratoplastic and keratolytic agents–A sulfur-zinc acne lotion may be applied locally to the skin at bedtime and washed off in the morning. Tretinoin (Retin-A) cream or gel is recommended for comedo acne, but it may be irritating, in which case a lower concentration may be necessary.

2. Commercial preparations for acne include Fostex cream and cake; Acne-Dome cleanser, cream, and lotion; Benzac W gel and wash; Desquam-X gel and wash; Benzagel, Persa-Gel, Clear By Design; and Xerac BP. All of these gels contain benzoyl peroxide. Benzoyl peroxide products are available in concentrations of 2.5%, 5%, and 10%.

3. Dermabrasion–Cosmetic improvement may be achieved by abrasion of inactive acne lesions, particularly flat, superficial scars. The skin is first frozen and anesthetized with ethyl chloride or Freon and then carefully abraded with fine sandpaper, special motor-driven abrasive brushes, or diamond fraises. The technique is not without untoward effects, since hyperpigmentation, hypopigmentation, grooving, and scarring have been known to occur. Dark-skinned individuals do poorly.

4. Irradiation–Simple exposure to sunlight in graded doses is often beneficial. Ultraviolet irradiation may be used as an adjunct to other treatment measures. Use suberythema doses in graded intervals up to the point of mild erythema and scaling.

5. Intralesional triamcinolone acetonide suspension, 3 mg/mL, is helpful for acutely inflamed acne cysts.

6. Topical antibiotics–If dryness occurs with benzoyl peroxide-containing agents or topical antibiotics in hydroalcoholic vehicles, 2% erythromycin ointment (Akne-mycin) is an alternative.

Prognosis

Untreated acne vulgaris often remits spontaneously, but the condition may persist throughout adulthood and may lead to severe scarring. The disease is chronic and tends to recur in spite of treatment. Remissions following systemic treatment with isotretinoin tend to be lasting.

Dicken CH: Retinoids: A review. J Am Acad Dermatol 1984;11:541.
Lesher JL et al: An evaluation of a 2% erythromycin ointment in the topical therapy of acne vulgaris. J Am Acad Dermatol 1985;12:526.
Nader S et al: Acne and hyperandrogenism: Impact of lowering androgen levels with glucocorticoid treatment. J Am Acad Dermatol 1984;11:256.
Shalita AR et al: Isotretinoin revisited. (Symposium.) Cutis 1988;42(Suppl 6A):1. [Entire issue.]
Strauss JS et al: Isotretinoin therapy for acne: Results of a multicenter dose-response study. J Am Acad Dermatol 1984;10:490.

ROSACEA

Essentials of Diagnosis

- A chronic facial disorder of middle-aged and older people.
- There is a large vascular component (erythema and telangiectasis).
- An acneiform component (papules, pustules, and seborrhea) may also be present.
- There is a glandular aspect accompanied by hyperplasia of the soft tissue of the nose (rhinophyma).

General Considerations

Aside from obvious genetic overtones, no single factor adequately explains the pathogenesis of this disorder. Emotional disturbances, chronic alcoholism, a seborrheic diathesis, and a dysfunction of the gastrointestinal tract may be significant associated factors. A statistically significant incidence of migraine headaches accompanying rosacea has been reported.

A variant of rosacea is so-called **demodex acne (demodicidosis),** in which large numbers of the mite *Demodex folliculorum* are found in pores. These may be demonstrated under the microscope when squeezings from pores are examined in glycerin on a microscope slide.

Potent topical steroids can change trivial dermatoses of the face into recognizable entities called **perioral dermatitis** and **steroid rosacea.** These occur predominantly in young women and may be confused with acne rosacea. It yields to 1% hydrocortisone cream topically, plus tetracycline orally.

Clinical Findings

These are described above. The entire face may have a rosy hue. One sees few or no comedones. Inflammatory papules are prominent, and there may be pustules. Associated seborrhea may be found. The patient often complains of burning or stinging with episodes of flushing.

Differential Diagnosis

Distinguish from acne, bromoderma, iododerma, other acneiform eruptions, and demodicidosis, as described above. The rosy hue of rosacea generally will pinpoint the diagnosis.

Treatment

A. General Measures: Tetracycline, 250 or 500 mg orally daily on an empty stomach, when used in conjunction with the topical treatment described below, may be very effective.

Isotretinoin (13-*cis*-retinoic acid; Accutane) may succeed where other measures fail. A dosage of 0.5–1 mg/kg/d orally for 12–28 weeks is recommended.

Metronidazole, 250 mg twice daily for 3 weeks, may be worth trying for rosacea. Side effects appear to be minimal. Though it may have a disulfiram-like effect when the patient uses alcohol.

B. Local Measures: Hydrocortisone cream 0.5–1%, desonide cream 0.05%, hydrocortisone valerate (Westcort) 0.1%, hydrocortisone butyrate (Locoid), or alclometasone dipropionate 0.05% (Aclovate), used morning and night, along with tetracycline orally, is a very effective regimen. Topical antibiotics in special vehicles may be helpful (see Acne Vulgaris). Benzoyl peroxide, 5–10% in an acetone gel, apparently will clear erythema, papules, pustules, and nodules but not telangiectasia of rosacea. Five to 8 weeks of treatment are needed for significant response. About one person in 6 or 7 experiences irritation, burning edema, and erythema from the applications. Metronidazole, 0.75% gel (MetroGel) applied twice daily, is frequently effective.

Prognosis

Rosacea tends to be a stubborn and persistent process. With the regimens described above, it can usually be controlled adequately. Complicating rhinophyma may require surgical correction.

Bleicher PA, Charles JH, Sober AJ: Topical metronidazole therapy for rosacea. Arch Dermatol 1987;123:609.

Plewig G, Nikolowski J, Wolff HH: Action of isotretinoin in acne rosacea and gram-negative folliculitis. J Am Acad Dermatol 1982;6:766.

INTERTRIGO

Intertrigo is caused by the macerating effect of heat, moisture, and friction. It is especially likely to occur in obese persons and in humid climates. Poor hygiene is an important etiologic factor. There is often a history of seborrheic dermatitis. The symptoms are itching, stinging, and burning. The body folds develop fissures, erythema, and sodden epidermis, with superficial denudation. Urine and blood examination may reveal diabetes mellitus, and the skin examination may reveal candidiasis. A direct smear may show abundant cocci. "Inverse psoriasis," tinea cruris, erythrasma, and candidiasis must be ruled out.

Maintain hygiene in the area and apply talc powder. If there is evidence of colonization of yeasts or bacteria, apply a topical antifungal or antibacterial solution, lotion, or powder. Recurrences are common.

MILIARIA
(Heat Rash)

Essentials of Diagnosis

- Burning, itching, superficial aggregated small vesicles, papules, or pustules on covered areas of the skin.
- Hot, moist climate.
- May have fever and even heat prostration.

General Considerations

Miliaria is an acute dermatitis that occurs most commonly on the upper extremities, trunk, and intertriginous areas. A hot, moist environment is the most frequent cause, but individual susceptibility is important, and obese persons are most often affected. Bedridden febrile patients are also susceptible. Plugging of the ostia of sweat ducts occurs, with consequent ballooning and ultimate rupture of the sweat duct, producing an irritating, stinging reaction. Increase in numbers of resident aerobes, notably cocci, apparently plays a role.

Clinical Findings

The usual symptoms are burning and itching. In severe cases, fever, heat prostration, and even death may result. The lesions consist of small, superficial, reddened thin-walled, discrete but closely aggregated vesicles, papules, vesicopapules, or pustules. The reaction occurs most commonly on covered areas of the skin.

Differential Diagnosis

Miliaria is to be distinguished from similar skin manifestations occurring in drug rash and folliculitis.

Prevention

Provide favorable working conditions when possible, ie, controlled temperature, ventilation, and humidity. Avoid overbathing and the use of strong, irritating soaps. Graded exposure to sunlight or ultraviolet light may benefit persons who will later be subjected to a hot, moist atmosphere. Susceptible persons should avoid exposure to hot, humid environments.

Treatment

Triamcinolone acetonide, 0.1% in Sarna lotion, should be applied 2–4 times daily. Alternative measures that have been employed with varying success are drying shake lotions and antipruritic powders or other dusting powders. Treat secondary infections (superficial pyoderma) with erythromycin or cloxacillin, 250 mg 4 times daily by mouth. Tannic acid, 10% in 70% alcohol, applied locally twice daily, serves to toughen the skin. Anticholinergic drugs given by mouth may be very helpful in severe cases, eg, glycopyrrolate, 1 mg twice daily.

Prognosis

Miliaria is usually a mild disorder, but death may occur with the severe forms (tropical anhidrosis and asthenia) as a result of interference with the heat-regulating mechanism. The process of the severe form may also be irreversible to some extent, requiring permanent removal of the individual from the humid or hot climate.

CALLOSITIES & CORNS OF FEET OR TOES

Callosities and corns are caused by pressure and friction due to faulty weight bearing, orthopedic deformities, improperly fitting shoes, or neuropathies such as occur in diabetes mellitus. Some persons are hereditarily predisposed to excessive and abnormal callus formation. It is crucial to provide optimal foot care for diabetics and those with insensitive extremities.

Tenderness on pressure and "after-pain" are the only symptoms. The hyperkeratotic well-localized overgrowths always occur at pressure points. On paring, a glassy core is found (which differentiates these disorders from plantar warts, which have multiple capillary bleeding points when cut). A soft corn often occurs laterally on the proximal portion of the fourth toe as a result of pressure against the bony structure of the interphalangeal joint of the fifth toe.

Treatment consists of correcting mechanical abnormalities that cause friction and pressure. Shoes must be properly fitted and orthopedic deformities corrected. Callosities may be removed by careful paring of the callus after a warm water soak or with keratolytic agents, eg, Keralyt gel, which contains 6% salicylic acid. Apply locally to the callus every night and cover with a polyethylene plastic film (Saran Wrap); remove in the morning. Repeat until the corn or callus is removed.

Extensive and severe palmar and plantar hyperkeratosis can be treated successfully by applying equal parts of propylene glycol and water nightly and covering with thin polyethylene plastic film (Baggies), or by soaking in 3% acetic acid solution.

A metatarsal leather bar, 1.25 cm (1/2 inch) wide and 0.65 cm (1/4 inch) high, may be placed on the outside of the shoe just behind the weight-bearing surface of the sole.

Women who tend to form calluses and corns should not wear confining footgear and high-heeled shoes.

Gibbs RC, Boxer MC: Abnormal biomechanics of feet and their cause of hyperkeratoses. J Am Acad Dermatol 1982;6:1061.

CHRONIC DISCOID LUPUS ERYTHEMATOSUS (Chronic Cutaneous Lupus Erythematosus)

Essentials of Diagnosis

- Red, asymptomatic, localized plaques, usually on the face, often in butterfly distribution.
- Scaling, follicular plugging, atrophy, and telangiectasia of involved areas.
- Histology distinctive.
- May be photosensitive.

General Considerations

This type of lupus erythematosus is a superficial, localized discoid inflammation of the skin occurring most frequently in areas exposed to solar or ultraviolet irradiation. The cause is not known. The systemic type is discussed in Chapter 15.

Clinical Findings

A. Symptoms and Signs: There are usually no symptoms. The lesions consist of dusky red, well-localized, single or multiple plaques, 5–20 mm in diameter, usually on the face and often in a "butterfly pattern" over the nose and cheeks. The scalp, external ears, and oral mucous membranes may be involved. There is atrophy, telangiectasia, and follicular plugging. The lesion is usually covered by dry, horny, adherent scales.

Complete medical evaluation should be made to rule out systemic lupus erythematosus.

B. Laboratory Findings: There are usually no significant routine laboratory findings in the chronic discoid type. If there is leukopenia or proteinuria, with or without casts, one must suspect the systemic form of the disease. Histologic changes are distinctive. The antinuclear antibody test is perhaps best for ruling out systemic lupus erythematosus. A direct immunofluorescence microscopy test reveals basement membrane antibody. "Uninvolved" skin adjacent to a lesion tends to be negative to direct immunofluorescence testing in discoid lupus erythematosus but positive in the systemic form of the disease.

One may also obtain a complete blood count, sedimentation rate, urinalysis, anti-ds DNA, and serum complement determinations.

In patients with marked photosensitivity and negative antinuclear antibody tests, tests of other cellular—and organ—tissues may be required.

Differential Diagnosis

The scales are dry and "tacklike" and can thus be distinguished from those of seborrheic dermatitis and psoriasis. Differentiate also from the sclerosing type of basal cell epithelioma and, by absence of nodules and ulceration, from lupus vulgaris.

Complications

Lesions may be widespread, resulting in dyspigmentation and scarring.

Treatment

A. General Measures: Provide protection from sunlight in photosensitive patients. *Caution:* Do not use any form of radiation therapy. Avoid using drugs that are potentially photosensitizing, eg, thiazides, piroxicam.

B. Local Infiltration: Triamcinolone acetonide suspension, 2.5–10 mg/mL, may be injected into the lesions once a week or once a month. This should be tried before internal treatment (see above).

C. Corticosteroids: Corticosteroid creams applied each night and covered with airtight, thin, pliable plastic film may be useful. Clobetasol propionate (Temovate) cream or ointment applied twice daily without occlusion should be attempted before systemic therapy.

D. Medical Treatment: *Caution:* The following drugs may cause serious eye changes. If the medication is continued, ophthalmologic examination should be done every 3 months. Chloroquine, 250 mg/d, or hydroxychloroquine, no more than 400 mg/d, is unlikely to cause retinopathy or other eye damage.

Wherever possible, chronic discoid lupus erythematosus should be considered a cosmetic defect only and treated topically or with camouflaging agents.

1. Chloroquine phosphate, 0.25 g daily for 1 week, then 0.25 g twice weekly. Watch for signs of toxicity.

2. Hydroxychloroquine sulfate, 0.2–0.4 g orally daily and 0.2 g daily for several weeks, may occasionally be effective when chloroquine is not tolerated.

3. Quinacrine (Atabrine), 100 mg daily, may be the safest of the antimalarials, since eye damage has not been reported. It colors the skin yellow.

E. Dapsone: Dapsone, 50 mg/d orally, may be helpful.

F. Isotretinoin: In a limited open study, isotretinoin, 80 mg/d, was effective in returning the skin and laboratory findings to normal in chronic or subacute cutaneous lupus erythematosus. Because of teratogenicity, the drug cannot be used if there is any possibility of pregnancy.

Prognosis

The disease is persistent but not life-endangering, unless it turns into the systemic variety.

McCormack LS, Elgart ML, Turner MLC: Annular subacute cutaneous lupus erythematosus responsive to dapsone. J Am Acad Dermatol 1984;11:397.

Newton RC et al: Mechanism-oriented assessment of isotretinoin in chronic or subacute cutaneous lupus erythematosus. Arch Dermatol 1986;122:170.

Olansky AJ: Antimalarials and ophthalmologic safety. J Am Acad Dermatol 1982;6:19.

VIRAL INFECTIONS OF THE SKIN

HERPES SIMPLEX
(Cold or Fever Sore)

Essentials of Diagnosis

- Recurrent small grouped vesicles on an erythematous base, especially around oral and genital areas. May follow minor infections, trauma, stress, or sun exposure. Regional lymph nodes may be swollen and tender.
- Tzanck smear is positive for large multinucleated epithelial giant cells surrounded by acantholytic balloon cells.

General Considerations

Although approximately 90% of the population acquire herpes simplex infection before the age of 4 or 5 years based on antibody studies, it is generally type 1 infection, following which the virus may remain in some form in the regional ganglia for life. No present means of treatment can eliminate the hidden foci of infection. The disease may manifest itself as severe gingivostomatitis in small children, or the initial infection may be subclinical. Thereafter, the subject may have recurrent attacks, provoked by fever, a viral infection, fatigue, menstruation, and other triggering factors such as sun and wind. Herpes simplex virus type 1 and the AIDS virus are the most important causes of fatal sporadic encephalitis in the USA.

The incidence of genital herpes, most commonly caused by HSV-2, in the USA in patients treated in private clinics increased about 10-fold from 1966 to 1981.

In addition to mucocutaneous lesions, the virus may cause encephalitis, with a high morbidity and fatality rate, ophthalmitis, and a virulent infection in neonates.

Herpes simplex virus antibodies are found in 85% of young adults in lower economic classes.

Clinical Findings

A. Symptoms and Signs: The principal symptoms are burning and stinging. Neuralgia may precede and accompany attacks. The lesions consist of small, grouped vesicles which can occur anywhere but which most often occur on the lips, mouth, and genitals. Regional lymph nodes may be swollen and tender.

B. Laboratory Findings: Lesions clinically diagnosed as chancroid, syphilis, pyoderma, or trauma have been found to be herpes simplex virus infections on culture. Viral culture, although not completely sensitive, is most helpful in confirming the clinical diagnosis and for showing viral shedding in asymptomatic patients. Other methods rely on detection of viral particles by electron microscopy, detection of viral antigen by immunologic methods (immunoperoxidase or immunofluorescence), or demonstration of multinucleated cells or intranuclear inclusion cells. The latter (Tzanck test) is the least sensitive but is readily available and easy to perform.

Complications

Complications include pyoderma, eczema herpeticum, whitlow, esophagitis, transplacental fetal infection, keratitis, and a severe encephalitis.

Treatment

For persistent or severe, recurrent herpes:

A. General Measures: Eliminate precipitating factors (sunburn) when possible.

Acyclovir is effective systemically (intravenously or orally) and is practically nontoxic. With episodes of primary genital herpes simplex, the period of viral shedding, pain, crusting, and other symptoms can be shortened and healing can be hastened by giving acyclovir, 200 mg orally 5 times daily—or 800 mg twice daily—for 10 days. Acyclovir is effective in preventing subsequent genital recurrences if suppressive dosages of 200 mg 3 times daily are maintained. If recurrences are infrequent (every 3–6 months), episodic treatment employing 200 mg orally 5 times daily or 800 mg twice daily is effective if initiated at the first sign or symptom of recurrence. Long-term acyclovir therapy appears to be effective and safe. Intravenous acyclovir is nephrotoxic and is reserved for patients with severe and life-threatening infections.

Recurrences and symptoms may be reduced by giving L-lysine by mouth for several months. Two grams daily are needed.

B. Local Measures: Apply a moistened styptic pencil several times daily to abort lesions. Zinc sulfate solution, 0.025–0.05%, may be used as a warm compress, 10 minutes twice daily. Or one may apply epinephrine, 1:100 solution, frequently. Applied topically, toluidine blue has an anesthetic effect and appears to hasten drying of vesicles.

If there is associated cellulitis and lymphadenitis, apply cool compresses. Treat stomatitis with water and milk of magnesia mouthwashes.

There is no really safe and effective systemic approach to cure recurrent herpes simplex infections of the skin. It is strongly urged that topical use of 5% acyclovir ointment (Zovirax) be limited to the restricted indications for which it has been approved, namely, initial herpes genitalis and mucocutaneous herpes simplex infections in immunocompromised patients, because of promotion of resistant strains of the virus and the possible mutagenicity of the drug.

Prognosis

Aside from the dread complications described above, recurrent attacks last 1–2 weeks. Many patients with genital herpes are essentially free of frequently recurring episodes several years after onset.

Becker TM, Blount JH, Guinan ME: Genital herpes infections in private practice in the United States, 1966 to 1981. JAMA 1985;253:1601.

Bierman SM: A retrospective study of 375 patients with genital herpes simplex infections seen between 1973 and 1980. Cutis 1983;31:548.

Guinan ME: Oral acyclovir for treatment and suppression of genital herpes simplex virus infection: A review. JAMA 1986;255:1747.

HERPES ZOSTER
(Shingles)

Essentials of Diagnosis

- Pain along course of a nerve followed by painful grouped vesicular lesions.
- Involvement is unilateral.
- Lesions are usually on face and trunk.

- Swelling of regional lymph nodes (inconstant).
- Tzanck smear is positive.

General Considerations

Herpes zoster is an acute vesicular eruption due to a virus that is morphologically identical with the virus of varicella. It usually occurs in adults. With rare exceptions, one attack of zoster confers lifelong immunity. In immunocompromised patients, generalized, life-threatening dissemination (varicella) may occur.

Zoster is the response to the varicella-zoster virus of a partially immune person. In patients at risk for HIV infection, development of zoster may be one sign that precedes marked depression of cellular immunity associated with AIDS or ARC.

Clinical Findings

Pain usually precedes the eruption by 48 hours or more and may persist and actually increase in intensity after the lesions have disappeared. The lesions consist of grouped, tense, deep-seated vesicles distributed unilaterally along the neural pathways of the trunk. The commonest distributions are on the trunk or face. Regional lymph glands may be tender and swollen.

It used to be felt that herpes zoster appearing in an older adult was a sign of occult malignant neoplastic disease. This suspicion has not been verified by controlled studies.

Differential Diagnosis

Since poison oak and poison ivy dermatitis may be produced unilaterally and in a streak by a single brush with the plant, it must be differentiated at times from herpes zoster. Differentiate also from similar lesions of herpes simplex, which is usually less painful. The pain of preeruptive herpes zoster may lead the clinician to diagnose migraine, myocardial infarction, acute abdomen, herniated nucleus pulposus, etc, depending on the dermatome.

Complications

Persistent neuralgia, anesthesia of the affected area following healing, facial or other nerve paralysis, and encephalitis may occur.

Treatment

A. General Measures: Attacks of shingles in the normal host can be ameliorated by acyclovir. Both intravenous and high-dose (800 mg 5 times daily for 7 days) oral acyclovir have been reported to accelerate rash healing and reduce acute pain, but no study has yet shown an effect on postherpetic neuralgia. Aspirin with or without codeine phosphate, 30 mg, usually controls pain. A single intragluteal injection of 40 mg of triamcinolone acetonide suspension may give prompt relief. Prednisone, 60 mg orally for 10 days, may be the treatment of choice for patients over age 50–60 years. Steroid therapy may decrease the incidence of postherpetic neuralgia. Ophthalmologic consultation should be considered, especially if the tip of the nose is involved, to avoid serious ocular complications. Hospitalization may be necessary in serious cases. Zoster has developed despite normal varicella-zoster antibody levels, indicating that cell-mediated immunity is more important in preventing zoster than are circulating antibodies. (See Chapters 23, 25, and 31.)

The supply of varicella-zoster immune globulin is limited, and its use is restricted to susceptible children under 15 years of age who have underlying immunosuppression or immunodeficiency diseases and have had intimate exposure to chickenpox; the globulin must be given within 72 hours after exposure. It is not effective in established zoster. Zoster immune plasma is ineffective in established zoster.

The goal of herpes zoster therapy for immunocompromised patients is prevention of possibly life-threatening viral spread. Both intravenous acyclovir and vidarabine will prevent progression in this patient population. The advantages of using intravenous acyclovir for herpes zoster, especially in the immunocompromised patient, probably outweigh the disadvantages. Adverse effects include decreased renal function from crystallization, and nausea, vomiting, and abdominal pain. One may give acyclovir sodium, 7.5 mg/kg of ideal body weight, 3 times daily for 7 days. Acyclovir alone has not been shown to prevent post-herpetic neuralgia.

B. Local Measures: Calamine or starch shake lotions are often of value. Apply lotion liberally and cover with a layer of cotton. Do not use greases.

C. Postzoster Neuralgia: Severe initial pain—or age over 50–60 years—tends to increase the likelihood of postherpetic neuralgia. Infiltration of skin with triamcinolone acetonide and lidocaine has been disappointing. High doses of systemic corticosteroids and oral acyclovir, 400–800 mg 5 times daily, early in the disease may reduce the incidence of postherpetic neuralgia. Topical capsaicin (Zostrix) appears to help about 3 out of 4 patients with neuralgia. Chronic post-herpetic neuralgia is usually not relieved by regional blocks (stellate ganglion, epidural, local infiltration, or peripheral nerve) with bupivacaine hydrochloride, with or without corticosteroids added to the injections. Amitriptyline, 25 mg orally 3 times daily, and perphenazine, 4 mg orally 3 times daily, or fluphenazine, 1 mg 4 times daily, has also been suggested. Doxepin, 25–50 mg 3 times daily, has also been reported to be helpful. Somnolence may occur with either type of drug.

Prognosis

The eruption persists 2–3 weeks and does not recur. Motor involvement in 2–3% may lead to temporary palsy. No age group is exempt from the possibility of post-zoster neuralgia persisting for a year or more, but the likelihood is greater in the 60- to 69-year

age group. (20%) and in those over 70 (30%). Ocular involvement may lead to blindness.

Balfour HH Jr: Acyclovir therapy for herpes zoster: Advantages and adverse effects. JAMA 1986;255:387.

Bernstein JE et al: Treatment of chronic postherpetic neuralgia with topical capsaicin: A preliminary study. J Am Acad Dermatol 1987;17:93.

Keczkes K, Basheer AM: Do corticosteroids prevent postherpetic neuralgia? Br J Dermatol 1980;102:551.

Riopelle JM, Naraghi M, Grush KP: Chronic neuralgia incidence following local anesthetic therapy for herpes zoster. Arch Dermatol 1984;120:747.

Wood MJ, Geddes AM: Antiviral therapy. Lancet 1987;2:1189.

WARTS

Essentials of Diagnosis

- Warty elevation anywhere on skin or mucous membranes, usually no larger than 0.5 cm in diameter.
- Prolonged incubation period (average 2–18 months). Spontaneous "cures" are frequent (50%), but warts are often unresponsive to any form of treatment.
- "Recurrences" (new lesions) are frequent.

General Considerations

Nearly a million visits to physicians for warts took place in 1981, nearly triple the incidence for genital herpes. Over 40 different subtypes of human papilloma viruses have been identified by serologic typing of viral proteins, molecular hybridization of viral DNA, and monoclonal antibody assays, using immunoperoxidase staining. About 25% of abnormal Papanicolaou smears are associated with the presence of human papilloma viruses, and 80% of cases of carcinoma of the cervix have similar associations, indicating that wart viruses may be more important than herpes simplex virus.

Six human papilloma virus types are associated with malignant neoplasms: types 5, 8, and 14 with squamous cell carcinomas occurring in the rare **epidermodysplasia verruciformis;** and types 6, 16, and 18 with uterine cervical carcinomas. Type 6 has also been implicated in giant condylomas of Buschke-Lowenstein and type 16 with bowenoid papulosis.

Cervical warts may be transmitted to the newborn via passage through the infected birth canal. Colposcopy with application of 3% acetic acid to suspicious lesions on the cervix may detect premalignant flat warts. A number of children with laryngeal papillomas (types 11 and 6) treated with x-rays have developed squamous cell carcinoma of the larynx.

Clinical Findings

There are usually no symptoms. Tenderness on pressure occurs with plantar warts: itching occurs with anogenital warts. Occasionally a wart will produce mechanical obstruction (eg, nostril, ear canal, urethra).

Warts vary widely in shape, size, and appearance. Flat warts are most evident under oblique illumination. Subungual warts may be dry, fissured, and hyperkeratotic and may resemble hangnails or other nonspecific changes. Plantar warts resemble plantar corns or calluses.

Prevention

Avoid contact with warts. A person with flat warts should be admonished not to scratch the areas. Using an electric shaver will in occasional cases prevent the spread of warts in razor scratches. Anogenital warts may be transmitted sexually.

Treatment

A. Removal: Remove the warts whenever possible by one of the following means:

1. Surgical excision– Inject a small amount of local anesthetic into the base and then remove the wart with a dermal curet or scissors or by shaving off at the base of the wart with a scalpel. Trichloroacetic acid or Monsel's solution on a tightly wound cotton-tipped applicator may be painted on the wound, or electrocautery may be applied.

2. Liquid nitrogen applied for a few seconds may be used every 2 weeks for a period of 3 months if necessary.

3. Keratolytic agents–Any of the following may be used for treatment or removal of common warts or plantar warts: Occlusal, Occlusal-HP, Trans-Ver-Sal, Duofilm, Duoplant, and Viranol.

4. Anogenital warts are best treated by painting them weekly with 25% podophyllum resin in compound tincture of benzoin if they are moist and occluded by apposing skin surfaces. Dry genital warts are best treated with applications of liquid nitrogen. Intralesional recombinant interferon alfa-2a is more effective than placebo in clearing a single condyloma, but plantar warts do not respond.

5. Plantar Warts may be treated by applying a 40% salicylic acid plaster after paring. The plaster may be left on for 5–6 days, then removed, pared down, and reapplied. Although with this method it may take weeks to months to eradicate the wart, it is safe and effective with almost no side effects.

Application of cantharidin (Cantharone, Cantharone Plus) is also effective in managing plantar warts. It is applied to the wart after it is pared, allowed to dry, and covered by tape. The area may be sensitive or slightly painful for 2 or 3 days. It should be debrided in 10–14 days and the treatment repeated.

Bleomycin diluted to 0.1% with physiologic saline may be injected under warts, not exceeding 0.1 mL per puncture; with multiple punctures, it has been shown to have a high cure rate for plantar and common warts. It may cause loss of nails and symptoms similar to those of Raynaud's syndrome when used for periungual warts.

B. Immunotherapy: Dinitrochlorobenzene (DNCB) is useful for resistant warts. Initially, 400 μg of freshly prepared dinitrochlorobenzene is applied as a sensitizing dose to 2 or 3 sites on the forearm. Then the warts are painted with an Eppendorf pipette with precisely 20 μL of dinitrochlorobenzene at 2-week intervals until they recede. DNCB gives positive results with the Ames test.

Persistent conservative application of topical irritants may cure warts by nonspecific boosting of wart antibodies. Specific wart antibodies (especially IgG) have been found in the serum of individuals with regressing warts.

C. Laser Therapy: The carbon dioxide laser is particularly effective for treating recurrent warts, plantar warts, and condylomata acuminata. The wart tissue is vaporized under magnified vision in a bloodless procedure without damage to surrounding areas. The plume of vaporization has been shown to contain wart virus particles.

D. Retinoids: Tretinoin (Retina-A) cream or gel applied topically twice daily may be effective for facial or beard area warts. Extensive warts have been reported to disappear when etretinate was given by mouth for a month. This drug is now available for use in the USA. Oral isotretinoin may cure some warts (see Acne Vulgaris).

Prognosis

There is a striking tendency to the development of new lesions. Warts may disappear spontaneously or may be unresponsive to treatment.

Bailin PL: Lasers in dermatology: 1983. (Editorial.) Cleve Clin Q 1983;50:53.

Bender ME: Papillomavirus infection of the urogenital tract: Implications for the dermatologist. Curr Concepts Skin Disorders (Spring) 1985;6:16.

Donagin WG, Millikan LE: Dinitrochlorobenzene immunotherapy for verrucae resistant to standard treatment modalities. J Am Acad Dermatol 1982;6:40.

Jablonska S, Orth G (editors): Warts/human papilloma viruses. Clin Dermatol 1985;3:No. 4. (Entire issue.)

Mackie RM: Extensive warts treated with etretinate. Br J Dermatol 1982;107(Suppl 22):97.

Rees RB: The treatment of warts. Clin Dermatol 1985;3:179.

Vance JC et al: Intralesional recombinant alpha-2 interferon for the treatment of patients with condyloma acuminatum or verruca plantaris. Arch Dermatol 1986;122:272.

MOLLUSCUM CONTAGIOSUM

Molluscum contagiosum is characterized by single or multiple rounded, dome-shaped, waxy papules 2–5 mm in diameter that are umbilicated and contain a caseous plug. Lesions at first are firm, solid, and flesh-colored but upon reaching maturity become softened, whitish, or pearly gray and may suppurate. The principal sites of involvement are the face, hands, and lower abdomen and genitals, but the papules are commonly found on other parts of the skin and at times are widely distributed.

The lesions are probably spread by autoinoculation. In sexually active individuals, they may be confined to such genital areas as the penis, pubis, and inner thighs. Molluscum contagiosum is one of the common viral infections seen in patients with AIDS. These individuals tend to develop extensive lesions over the face and neck as well as the genital area.

The diagnosis is easily established in most instances because of the distinctive central umbilication of the dome-shaped lesion. The best treatment is by curettage or applications of liquid nitrogen as for warts. Other forms of treatment include light electrosurgery with a fine needle and applications of cantharidin. Lesions tend to resolve spontaneously, and it has been estimated that individual lesions persist for about 2 months.

Brown ST, Nalley JF, Kraus SJ: Molluscum contagiosum. Sex Transm Dis 1981;8:227.

BACTERIAL INFECTIONS OF THE SKIN

IMPETIGO

Impetigo is a contagious and autoinoculable infection of the skin caused by staphylococci or streptococci or both. Two forms are recognized: (1) a vesiculopustular type with thick golden-crusted lesions caused by group A β-hemolytic *Streptococcus* or coagulase-positive *Staphylococcus aureus* and (2) a bullous type generally associated with phage group II *S aureus*.

Itching is the only symptom. The lesions consist of macules, vesicles, bullae, pustules, and honey-colored gummy crusts (streptococcal) that when removed leave denuded red areas. The face and other exposed parts are most often involved.

Ecthyma is a deeper form of impetigo caused by streptococci, with ulceration and scarring. It occurs frequently on the legs and other covered areas, often as a complication of debility and local cutaneous trauma.

Impetigo neonatorum is a highly contagious, potentially serious form of staphylococcal impetigo occurring in infants. It requires prompt systemic treatment and protection of other infants (isolation, exclusion from the nursery of personnel with pyoderma, etc).

The lesions are bullous and massive and accompanied by systemic toxicity. Death may occur.

Impetigo must be distinguished from other vesicular and pustular lesions such as herpes simplex, varicella, and contact dermatitis (dermatitis venenata). A Gram stain and a Tzanck smear may be useful in differentiating the organisms.

Treatment is as for folliculitis. Some question has been raised about the efficacy of topical antibiotics. Two percent topical mupirocin (Bactroban) is as effective as systemic erythromycin and cloxacillin in primary and secondary skin infections. If there is fever or toxicity or any concern over the possibility of a nephritogenic strain of *Streptococcus* being causative, systemic antibiotics should be given. Either erythromycin or dicloxacillin, 1 g daily, is usually effective, or one may use cephalexin, 50 mg/kg/24 h. For furunculosis in the family setting or in a live-in group of people, a course of rifampin, 600 mg daily, may be necessary.

Coskey RJ, Coskey LA: Diagnosis and treatment of impetigo. J Am Acad Dermatol 1987;17:62.
Feingold DS, Wagner RF Jr: Antibacterial therapy. J Am Acad Dermatol 1986;14:535.

FOLLICULITIS
(Including Sycosis Vulgaris, [Barber's Itch], Pseudofolliculitis)

Essentials of Diagnosis
- Itching and burning in hairy areas.
- Pustules in the hair follicles.
- In sycosis, inflammation of surrounding skin area.

General Considerations
Folliculitis is caused by staphylococcal infection of a hair follicle. When the lesion is deep-seated, chronic, and recalcitrant, it is called sycosis. Sycosis is usually propagated by the autoinoculation and trauma of shaving. The upper lip is particularly susceptible to involvement in men who suffer with chronic nasal discharge from sinusitis or hay fever.

Bockhart's impetigo is a staphylococcal infection that produces painful, tense, superficial globular pustules at the follicular orifices. It is a form of folliculitis.

Gram-negative folliculitis, which may develop from antibiotic-treated acne, may be best treated with isotretinoin given orally, although this is not a listed indication for the drug. A range of gram-negative organisms has been implicated as the cause. An absolute contraindication to use of isotretinoin is pregnancy.

"Hot tub folliculitis," caused by *Pseudomonas aeruginosa*, is characterized by pruritic follicular, maculopapular, vesicular, or pustular lesions occurring within 1–4 days after bathing in hot tub, whirlpool, or public swimming pool. Rarely, systemic infections may result.

Pseudofolliculitis is caused by ingrowing hairs in the beard area and on the nape. It may be treated by growing a beard or by using chemical depilatories or the PFB (pseudofolliculitis barbae) shaving system, American Safety Razor Co., Staunton, VA 24401.

Clinical Findings

The symptoms are slight burning and itching, and pain on manipulation of the hair. The lesions consist of pustules of the hair follicles. In sycosis, the surrounding skin becomes involved also and so resembles eczema, with redness and crusting.

Differential Diagnosis

Differentiate from acne vulgaris or pustular miliaria and infections of the skin such as impetigo or fungal infections.

Complications

Abscess formation is the major complication.

Prevention

Correct any precipitating or aggravating factors: systemic (eg, diabetes mellitus) or local causes (eg, irritations of a mechanical or chemical nature, discharges).

Treatment

A. Specific Measures: Systemic antibiotics may be tried if the skin infection is resistant to local treatment, if it is extensive or severe and accompanied by a febrile reaction, if it is complicated, or if it involves the so-called danger areas (upper lip, nose, and eyes) associated with the rare complication cavernous sinus thrombosis.

Topical 2% mupirocin (Bactroban) is extremely effective in achieving clinical cure, bringing about improvement in primary and secondary skin infections, and eliminating infecting organisms. It should be applied 3 times daily and protected by dressings; soaks should be applied during the day.

Penicillin and sulfonamides should not be used topically.

B. Local Measures: Cleanse the area gently with chlorhexidine (Hibiclens) and apply saline or aluminum subacetate soaks or compresses to the involved area for 15 minutes twice daily. When skin is softened, gently open the larger pustules and trim away necrotic tissue.

Anhydrous ethyl alcohol containing 6.25% aluminum chloride (Xerac AC), applied to lesions and environs and followed by an antibiotic ointment (see above), may be very helpful. It is especially useful for chronic folliculitis of the buttocks.

Prognosis

Folliculitis is often stubborn and persistent, lasting for months and even years.

James WD, Leyden JJ: Treatment of gram-negative folliculitis with isotretinoin: Positive clinical and microbiologic response. J Am Acad Dermatol 1985;12:319.

FURUNCULOSIS (BOILS) & CARBUNCLES

Essentials of Diagnosis

- Extremely painful inflammatory swelling of a hair follicle that forms an abscess.
- Primary predisposing debilitating disease sometimes present.
- Coagulase-positive *Staphylococcus aureus* is the causative organism.

General Considerations

A furuncle (boil) is a deep-seated infection (abscess) involving the entire hair follicle and adjacent subcutaneous tissue. The most common sites of occurrence are the hairy parts exposed to irritation and friction, pressure, or moisture or to the plugging action of petroleum products. Because the lesions are autoinoculable, they are often multiple. Thorough investigation usually fails to uncover a predisposing cause, although an occasional patient may have unsuspected diabetes mellitus.

A carbuncle consists of several furuncles developing in adjoining hair follicles and coalescing to form a conglomerate, deeply situated mass with multiple drainage points.

Clinical Findings

A. Symptoms and Signs: Pain and tenderness may be prominent, and more severe with carbuncles than with furuncles. The follicular abscess is either rounded or conical. It gradually enlarges, becomes fluctuant, and then softens and opens spontaneously after a few days to 1–2 weeks to discharge a core of necrotic tissue and pus. The inflammation occasionally subsides before necrosis occurs.

Infection of the soft tissue around the nails (paronychia) is usually due to staphylococci when it is acute. This is a variant of furuncle. Other organisms may be involved, including herpes simplex (herpetic whitlow).

B. Laboratory Findings: There may be slight leukocytosis.

Differential Diagnosis

Furuncle is to be distinguished from deep mycotic infections such as sporotrichosis and blastomycosis; from other bacterial infections such as anthrax and tularemia; and from acne cysts and infected epidermoid or pilar cysts.

Complications

Serious and sometimes fatal cavernous sinus thrombosis may occur as a complication of a manipulated furuncle on the central portion of the upper lip or near the nasolabial folds. Perinephric abscess, osteomyelitis, and even endocarditis may also occur from manipulation of any furuncle.

Treatment

A. Specific Measures: Systemic anti-infective agents are indicated (chosen on the basis of cultures and sensitivity tests if possible). Sodium cloxacillin or erythromycin, 1 g daily in divided doses by mouth for 10 days, is usually effective. Cephalexin is an effective alternative drug. Ciprofloxacin is effective against strains of staphylococci resistant to other antibiotics.

Recurrent furunculosis may be effectively treated with a combination of dicloxacillin, 250–500 mg 4 times daily, and rifampin, 300 mg twice daily. Family members and intimate contacts may need evaluation for staphylococcal carrier state and perhaps concomitant treatment. Applications of topical 2% mupirocin (Bactroban) to the nares, axillas, and anogenital areas 3 times daily for 5–7 days, eliminates the staphylococcal carrier state.

Strains of pathogenic staphylococci may carry a plasmid, or episome, causing resistance to antibiotics such as erythromycin.

B. Local Measures: Immobilize the part and avoid overmanipulation of inflamed areas. Use moist heat to help larger lesions "localize." Use surgical incision and debridement *after* the lesions are "mature." Do not incise deeply. Apply anti-infective ointment and bandage the area loosely during drainage. It is not necessary to incise and drain an acute staphylococcal paronychia. Inserting a flat metal spatula or sharpened hardwood stick into the nail fold where it adjoins the nail will release pus from a mature lesion.

Prognosis

Recurrent crops may harass the patient for months or years. Carbunculosis is more severe and more hazardous than furunculosis.

An alcoholic aluminum chloride solution (see above) may be very useful in controlling repeated attacks of furuncles.

Gorbach SL (guest editor): Antibacterial therapy update: 1985: Skin and soft tissue infections. Cutis 1985;36(No. 5A):1. [Special issue.]

ERYSIPELAS

Essentials of Diagnosis

- Edematous, spreading, circumscribed, hot, erythematous area, with or without vesicle or bulla formation.
- Pain, chills, fever, and systemic toxicity may be striking.
- Leukocytosis.

General Considerations

Erysipelas is an acute inflammation of the skin and subcutaneous tissue caused by infection with β-hemolytic streptococci. It occurs classically on the cheek.

Clinical Findings

A. Symptoms and Signs: The symptoms are pain, malaise, chills, and moderate fever. A bright red spot appears first, very often near a fissure at the angle of the nose. This spreads to form a tense, sharply demarcated, glistening, smooth, hot area. The margin characteristically makes noticeable advances from day to day. The patch is somewhat edematous and can be pitted slightly with the finger. Vesicles or bullae occasionally develop on the surface. The patch does not usually become pustular or gangrenous and heals without scar formation. The disease may complicate any break in the skin that provides a portal of entry for the organism.

B. Laboratory Findings: Leukocytosis and increased sedimentation rate almost invariably occur.

Differential Diagnosis

Cellulitis has a less definite margin and involvement of deeper tissues; erysipeloid is a benign bacillary infection producing redness of the skin of the fingers or the backs of the hands in fishermen and meat handlers.

Complications

Unless erysipelas is promptly treated, death may result from extension of the process and systemic toxicity, particularly in the very young and in the aged.

Treatment

Place the patient at bed rest with the head of the bed elevated, apply hot packs, and give aspirin for pain and fever. Penicillin is specific for β-hemolytic streptococcal infections. Erythromycin is a good alternative in penicillin-allergic patients.

Prognosis

Erysipelas formerly was a life-threatening infection, it can now usually be quickly controlled with systemic penicillin or erythromycin therapy.

CELLULITIS

Cellulitis, a diffuse spreading infection of the skin, must be differentiated from erysipelas (a superficial form of cellulitis) because the 2 conditions are quite similar. Cellulitis involves deeper tissues and may be due to one of several organisms, usually gram-positive cocci, though gram-negative rods such as *E coli* may also be responsible. The lesion is hot and red but has a more diffuse border than does erysipelas. Cellulitis usually occurs after a break in the skin. Recurrent attacks may sometimes affect lymphatic vessels, producing a permanent swelling called "solid edema."

The response to systemic anti-infective measures (penicillin or broad-spectrum antibiotics) is usually prompt and satisfactory.

ERYSIPELOID

Erysipelothrix insidiosa infection must be differentiated from erysipelas and cellulitis. It is usually a benign infection commonly seen in fishermen and meat handlers and characterized by purplish erythema of the skin, most often of a finger or the back of the hand, which gradually extends over a period of several days. Systemic involvement occurs rarely; endocarditis may occur.

Penicillin is usually promptly curative. Broad-spectrum antibiotics may be used instead if the patient appears toxic and the diagnosis is uncertain.

DECUBITUS ULCERS
(Bedsores, Pressure Sores)

Bedsores (pressure sores) are a special type of ulcer caused by impaired blood supply and tissue nutrition due to prolonged pressure over bony or cartilaginous prominences. The skin overlying the sacrum and hips is most commonly involved, but bedsores may also be seen over the occiput, ears, elbows, heels, and ankles. They occur most readily in aged, paralyzed, debilitated, and unconscious patients. Low-grade infection may occur.

Good nursing care and nutrition and maintenance of skin hygiene are important preventive measures. The skin and the bed linens should be kept clean and dry. Bedfast, paralyzed, moribund, or listless patients who are candidates for the development of decubiti must be turned *frequently* (at least every hour) and must be examined at pressure points for the appearance of small areas of redness and tenderness. Water-filled mattresses, rubber pillows, alternating pressure mattresses, and thick papillated foam pads are useful in prevention and in the treatment of lesions.

Early lesions should also be treated with topical antibiotic powders and adhesive absorbent bandage (Gelfoam). Established lesions require surgical consultation and care. A spongy foam pad placed under the patient may work best in some cases. It may be laundered often. A continuous dressing of 1% iodochlorhydroxyquin (Vioform) in Lassar's paste may be effective.

Deep infections are usually present in pressure sores, often requiring systemic antibiotics.

Parish LC, Witkowski JA, Crissey JT: *The Decubitus Ulcer.* Masson, 1983.
Sugarman B: Infection and pressure sores. Arch Phys Med Rehabil 1985;66:177.

FUNGAL INFECTIONS OF THE SKIN

Mycotic infections are traditionally divided into 2 principal groups: superficial and deep. In this chapter we will discuss only the superficial infections: tinea capitis, tinea corporis, and tinea cruris; dermatophytosis of the feet and dermatophytid of the hands; tinea unguium (onychomycosis, or fungal infection of the nails); and tinea versicolor. Candidiasis belongs in an intermediate group but will be considered here as well as with the deep mycoses.

The diagnosis of fungal infections of the skin is usually based on the location and characteristics of the lesions and on the following laboratory examinations: (1) Direct demonstration of fungi in 10% potassium hydroxide preparations of scrapings from suspected lesions. (2) Cultures of organisms. Dermatophytes responsive to griseofulvin are easily detectable, with color change from yellow to red on dermatophyte test medium (DTM); or one may use a microculture slide that produces color change and allows for direct microscopic identification. (3) Examination with Wood's light (an ultraviolet light with a special filter), which causes hairs to fluoresce a brilliant green when they are infected by *Microsporum* organisms. The lamp is also invaluable in following the progress of treatment. *Trichophyton*-infected hairs do not fluoresce. (4) Histologic sections stained with periodic acid-Schiff (Hotchkiss-McManus) technique. Fungal elements stain red and are easily found.

Serologic tests are of no value in the diagnosis of superficial fungal infections.

Delayed sensitivity to intradermal trichophytin appears to be a correlate of immunity, whereas immediate trichophytin reactivity is associated with chronic tinea infections.

Principles of Treatment

Treat acute active fungal infections initially as for any acute dermatitis. It may be necessary to treat the associated dermatitis before applying specific topical fungistatic medication.

Ketoconazole is now approved for treatment of candidiasis, chronic mucocutaneous candidiasis, oral thrush, candiduria, coccidioidomycosis, histoplasmosis, chromoblastomycosis, and paracoccidioidomycosis. It is also indicated for the treatment of patients with severe recalcitrant cutaneous dermatophyte infections who have not responded to topical therapy or oral griseofulvin or who are unable to take griseofulvin. Chief concerns are abnormal levels of liver enzymes, gynecomastia, nausea, and urticaria.

One person in 10,000–15,000 may have liver damage. It is critical to warn patients to stop the drug at the first onset of nausea, indigestion, dark urine, clay-colored stools, or jaundice. Of those who developed jaundice, 82% did so within 11–168 days of treatment (average, 49 days). Liver function tests rapidly return to normal when the drug is stopped. Tests may be done every 2–4 weeks, though clinical signs and symptoms are more reliable. Gynecomastia can be avoided by giving the total dose once daily. It is best to avoid giving more than 200 mg/d (one tablet) if possible.

General Measures & Prevention

Keep the skin dry, since moist skin favors the growth of fungi. A cool climate is preferred. Reduce exercise and activities to prevent excessive perspiration. Dry the skin carefully after bathing or after perspiring heavily. Loose-fitting underwear is advisable. Socks and other clothing should be changed often. Sandals or open-toed shoes should be worn. Skin secretions should be controlled with talc or other drying powders or with drying soaks. Sedatives may be effective in reducing skin secretions in tense, nervous people. Graded daily sunbaths or quartz lamp exposure may be helpful.

Duarte PA et al: Fatal hepatitis associated with ketoconazole therapy. Arch Intern Med 1984;144:1069.
Rippon JW: A new era in antimycotic agents. (Editorial.) Arch Dermatol 1986;122:399.

TINEA CAPITIS
(Ringworm of Scalp)

Essentials of Diagnosis

- Round, gray, scaly "bald" patches on the scalp. Usually in prepubertal children.
- Occasionally fluorescent under Wood's lamp.
- Microscopic examination or culture identifies the fungus.

General Considerations

This persistent, contagious, and sometimes epidemic infection occurs almost exclusively in children and disappears spontaneously at puberty. Two general species (*Microsporum* and *Trichophyton*) cause ringworm infections of the scalp. *Microsporum* accounts for a small percentage of the infections, and hairs infected with this genus fluoresce brilliantly under Wood's light. *Trichophyton tonsurans* is the most common cause of tinea capitis in the USA today. *Trichophyton* species account for some of the very resistant infections, which may persist into adulthood.

Clinical Findings

A. Symptoms and Signs: There are usually no symptoms with noninflammatory tinea capitis, although there may be slight itching. The lesions are round, gray, scaly, apparently bald patches on the scalp. (The hairs are broken off, and the patches are not actually bald.) "Black-dot" ringworm caused primarily by *T tonsurans* presents as multiple areas of alopecia studded with black dots representing infected hairs broken off at or below the surface of the scalp. At times, scalp ringworm presents as a localized spot accompanied by pronounced swelling and develops into boggy and indurated areas exuding pus known as kerion celsi. Regional lymphadenopathy is frequently associated.

B. Laboratory Findings: Microscopic or culture demonstration of the organisms in the hairs may be necessary.

Differential Diagnosis

Differentiate from other diseases of scalp hair such as pediculosis capitis, pyoderma, alopecia areata, and trichotillomania (voluntary pulling out of one's own hair).

Prevention

Exchange of headgear must be avoided, and infected individuals or household pets must be vigorously treated and scrupulously reexamined for determination of cure. The scalp should be washed after haircuts.

Complications

Kerion (a nodular, exudative pustule), possibly followed by scarring, is the only complication. It responds dramatically to saturated solution of potassium iodide orally and prednisone, 1 mg/kg daily for 10–14 days.

Treatment

Microcrystalline griseofulvin, 0.125–0.25 g/d for children weighing 3–50 lb, 0.2–0.5 g/d for children weighing 50–90 lb, and 0.5–1 g/d for children and adolescents over 90 lb and for adults, may be given by mouth for 8 weeks or more. The drug is best taken with the midday meal. Selenium sulfide shampoo is recommended to reduce spore shedding.

Prognosis

Tinea capitis may be very persistent but usually clears spontaneously by puberty, except for infections caused by certain resistant organisms such as *T tonsurans*. Kerion responds promptly to saturated solution of potassium iodide by mouth or short-term prednisone therapy.

Rudolph AH: The diagnosis and treatment of tinea capitis due to *Trichophyton tonsurans*. Int J Dermatol 1985;24:426.

TINEA CORPORIS OR TINEA CIRCINATA (Body Ringworm)

Essentials of Diagnosis

- Pruritic, ringed, scaling, centrally clearing lesions; small vesicles in a peripherally advancing border.
- On exposed skin surfaces.
- History of exposure to infected domestic animal.
- Laboratory examination by microscope or culture confirms diagnosis.

General Considerations

The lesions are often on exposed areas of the body such as the face and arms. A history of exposure to an infected cat may be obtained. All species of dermatophytes may cause this disease, but some are more common than others.

Clinical Findings

A. Symptoms and Signs: Itching is usually intense; this distinguishes the disease from other ringed lesions. Rings, erythema, or vesicles with central clearing are grouped in clusters and distributed asymmetrically, usually on an exposed surface.

B. Laboratory Findings: Hyphae can be demonstrated by removing scale or the cap of a vesicle and examining it microscopically in a drop of 10% potassium hydroxide. The diagnosis may be confirmed by culture.

Material can be obtained for culture on Sabouraud's medium by thoroughly rubbing a cotton swab over the lesion and then rotating the swab while thoroughly rubbing it on the medium; this technique is just as accurate as scraping the lesions with a scalpel or curet.

Differential Diagnosis

Itching distinguishes tinea corporis from other skin lesions with annular configuration, such as the annular lesions of psoriasis, syphilis, erythema multiforme, and pityriasis rosea.

Complications

Complications include extension of the disease to the scalp hair or nails (in which case it becomes much more difficult to cure), overtreatment dermatitis, pyoderma, and dermatophytid.

Prevention

Avoid contact with infected household pets and exchange of clothing without adequate laundering.

Treatment

A. Specific Measures: Griseofulvin (microcrystalline), 0.5 g orally daily for children and 1 g orally daily for adults. Ketoconazole (Nizoral) is also indicated for the treatment of patients with severe recalcitrant cutaneous dermatophyte infections starting at doses of 200 mg/d.

B. Local Measures: Compound undecylenic acid ointment may be used in less chronic and nonthickened lesions. The following applied topically are effective against dermatophyte infections other than those of the nails: tolnaftate, 1% solution or cream; haloprogin, 1% solution or cream; miconazole, 2% cream; clotrimazole, 1% liquid, cream, or lotion; ketoconazole, 2% cream; econazole, 1% cream; sulconazole, 1% cream; oxiconazole, 1% cream; ciclopirox, 1% cream; and naftifine hydrochloride, 1% cream. Betamethasone dipropionate with clotrimazole (Lotrisone) applied twice daily for 3–5 days is beneficial for acutely inflamed tinea lesions. After the inflammation subsides, switch to a topical antifungal without a steroid component.

Prognosis

Body ringworm usually responds promptly to griseofulvin by mouth or to conservative topical therapy.

Head ES, Henry J, MacDonald EM: The cotton swab technic for the culture of dermatophyte infections: Its efficacy and merit. J Am Acad Dermatol 1984;11:797.

TINEA CRURIS (Jock Itch)

Essentials of Diagnosis

- Marked itching in intertriginous areas.
- Peripherally spreading, sharply demarcated, centrally clearing erythematous macular lesions, with or without vesicle formation.
- May have associated tinea infection of feet.
- Laboratory examination with microscope or culture confirms diagnosis.

General Considerations

Tinea cruris lesions are confined to the groin and gluteal cleft and are as a rule more indolent than those of tinea corporis and tinea circinata. The disease often occurs in athletes as well as in persons who are obese or who perspire a great deal. Any of the dermatophytes may cause tinea cruris, and it may be transmitted to the groin from active dermatophytosis of the foot. Intractable pruritus ani may occasionally be caused by a tinea infection.

Clinical Findings

A. Symptoms and Signs: Itching is usually more severe than that which occurs in seborrheic dermatitis or intertrigo. Inverse psoriasis, however, may itch even more than tinea cruris. The lesions consist of erythematous macules with sharp margins, cleared centers, and active, spreading peripheries in intertriginous areas. There may be vesicle formation at the borders, and satellite vesicular lesions are sometimes present. Follicular pustules are sometimes encountered.

B. Laboratory Findings: Hyphae can be demonstrated microscopically in 10% potassium hydroxide preparations. The organism may be cultured readily.

Differential Diagnosis

Differentiate from other lesions involving the intertriginous areas, such as candidiasis, tinea versicolor, seborrheic dermatitis, intertrigo, psoriasis of body folds ("inverse psoriasis"), and erythrasma.

Treatment

A. General Measures: Drying powder should be dusted into the involved area 2–3 times a day, especially when perspiration is excessive. Keep the area clean and dry but avoid overbathing. Prevent intertrigo or chafing by avoiding overtreatment, which predisposes a further infection and complications. Underwear should be loose-fitting. Rough-textured clothing should be avoided.

B. Specific Measures: Griseofulvin is indicated for severe cases. Give 1 g orally daily for 1–2 weeks.

C. Local Measures: Treat the stage of dermatosis. Secondarily infected or inflamed lesions are best treated with soothing and drying solutions, with the patient at bed rest. Use wet compresses of potassium permanganate, 1:10,000 (or 1:20 aluminum acetate solution), or, in case of anogenital infection, sitz baths.

Fungistatic preparations. Any of the following may be used: (1) Tolnaftate (Tinactin) solution or cream. (2) Haloprogin (Halotex), 1% cream or solution. (3) Miconazole, 2% cream. (4) Clotrimazole, 1% liquid or cream. (5) Ketoconazole, 2% cream. (6) Econazole, 1% cream. (7) Sulconazole, 1% cream. (8) Oxiconazole, 1% cream. (9) Ciclopirox, 1% cream. (10) Naftifine hydrochloride, 1% cream (fungicidal).

Initial control of symptoms of tinea cruris and tinea corporis can be achieved with use of an antifungal-corticosteroid combination (clotrimazole plus betamethasone dipropionate [Lotrisone cream]). After 2 weeks' use, results with clotrimazole alone are as good as with the combination.

Prognosis

Tinea cruris usually responds promptly to topical or systemic treatment.

Katz HI et al: SCH 370 (clotrimazole-betamethasone dipropionate) cream in patients with tinea cruris or tinea corporis. Cutis 1984;34:183.

TINEA MANUUM & TINEA PEDIS (Dermatophytosis, Tinea of Palms & Soles, "Athlete's Foot")

Essentials of Diagnosis

- Itching, burning, and stinging of interdigital webs, palms, and soles. Deep vesicles in acute stage.
- Exfoliation, fissuring, and maceration in subacute or chronic stages.
- Skin scrapings examined microscopically or by culture may reveal fungus.

General Considerations

Tinea of the feet is an extremely common acute or chronic dermatosis. It is possible that some causative organisms are present on the feet of most adults at all times. Certain individuals appear to be more susceptible than others. Most infections are caused by *Trichophyton* and *Epidermophyton* species.

Clinical Findings

A. Symptoms and Signs: The presenting symptom is usually itching. However, there may be burning, stinging, and other sensations, or frank pain from secondary infection with complicating cellulitis, lymphangitis, and lymphadenitis. Tinea pedis often appears as a fissuring of the toe webs, perhaps with denudation and sodden maceration. Toe web "tinea" may not be tinea at all but rather an intertrigo that may be called "athlete's foot." It may respond better to 30% aqueous aluminum chloride or to carbolfuchsin paint or a keratolytic agent (Keralyt gel) than to antifungal agents. However, there may also be grouped vesicles distributed anywhere on the soles or the palms, a generalized exfoliation of the skin of the soles, or destructive nail involvement in the form of discoloration and hypertrophy of the nail substance with pithy changes. Acute reddened, weeping vesicular lesions are seen on the skin in the acute stages.

B. Laboratory Findings: The dermatophytosis complex includes white maceration and soggy interdigital scaling, with itching and malodor. Anatomically occluded tinea pedis is invaded by coryneform bacteria and *Brevibacterium* species. Combined topical antifungal and antibacterial therapy are needed. Hyphae can often be demonstrated microscopically in skin scales treated with 10% potassium hydroxide. Culture with Sabouraud's medium is simple and often informative but does not always demonstrate pathogenic fungi.

Differential Diagnosis

Differentiate from other skin conditions involving the same areas such as interdigital intertrigo, candidiasis, gram-negative toe web infection, psoriasis, contact dermatitis (from shoes, powders, nail polish), dyshidrosis, atopic eczema, and scabies.

Prevention

The essential factor in prevention is personal hygiene. Rubber or wooden sandals should be used in community showers and bathing places. Careful drying between the toes after showering is recommended. Socks should be changed frequently. Apply dusting and drying powders as necessary.

Treatment

A. Specific Measures: Griseofulvin has been disappointing in the treatment of dermatophytosis of the feet and should be used only for severe cases or those that are recalcitrant to topical therapy.

Ketoconazole, 200 mg daily by mouth, is an effective agent for griseofulvin-resistant dermatophytosis, although relapse may occur after discontinuing therapy. The drug is well tolerated; hepatotoxicity has been reported from its use.

Itraconazole, a new oral antifungal medication not yet approved by the FDA, appears to be effective for relief of clinical aspects of recalcitrant dermatophyte infections.

B. Local Measures: *Caution:* Do not overtreat.

1. Acute stage (lasts 1–10 days)—Give aluminum subacetate solution soaks for 20 minutes 2–3 times daily. If secondary infection is present, use soaks of 1:10,000 potassium permanganate. If secondary infection is severe or complicated, treat as described on p 115.

2. Chronic stage—Use any of the following: (1) Sulfur-salicylic acid ointment or cream. (2) Whitfield's ointment, one-fourth to one-half strength. (3) Compound undecylenic acid ointment twice daily. (4) Alcoholic Whitfield's solution. (5) Carbolfuchsin solution (Castellani's paint). (6) Tolnaftate (Tinactin) solution or cream. (7) Haloprogin, 1% cream or solution. (8) Miconazole, 2% cream. (9) Clotrimazole (Lotrimin or Mycelex), 1% cream or lotion. (10) Ketoconazole cream (Nizoral), 2%. (11) Sulconazole, 1% cream. (12) Oxiconazole, 1% cream. (13) Naftifine hydrochloride (Naftin), 1% cream. (14) Ciclopirox, 1% cream.

C. Mechanical Measures: Carefully remove or debride dead or thickened tissues after soaks or baths.

Prognosis

Tinea of the hands and feet usually responds well to treatment, but recurrences are common in strongly predisposed persons.

Hanifin JM, Tofte SJ: Itraconazole therapy for recalcitrant dermatophyte infections. J Am Acad Dermatol 1988;18:1077. Robertson MH et al: Ketoconazole in griseofulvin-resistant dermatophytosis. J Am Acad Dermatol 1982;6:224. Roth RR, James WD: Microbiology of the skin: Resident flora, ecology, infection. J Am Acad Dermatol 1989;20:367.

DERMATOPHYTID
(Allergy or Sensitivity to Fungi)

Essentials of Diagnosis

- Pruritic, grouped vesicular lesions involving the sides and flexor aspects of the fingers and the palms.

- Fungal infection elsewhere on body, usually the feet. Trichophytin skin test positive.
- No fungus demonstrable in lesions.

General Considerations

Dermatophytid is a sensitivity reaction to an active focus of dermatophytosis elsewhere on the body, usually the feet. Fungi are present in the primary lesions but are not present in the lesions of dermatophytid. The hands are most often affected, but dermatophytid may occur on other areas also.

Clinical Findings

A. Symptoms and Signs: Itching is the only symptom. The lesions consist of grouped vesicles, often involving the thenar and hypothenar eminences. Lesions are round, up to 15 mm in diameter, and may be present on the side and flexor aspects of the fingers. Lesions occasionally involve the backs of the hands or may even be generalized.

B. Laboratory Findings: The trichophytin skin test is positive, but it may also be positive with other disorders. A negative trichophytin test rules out dermatophytid. Repeated negative microscopic examination of material taken from the lesions is necessary before the diagnosis of dermatophytid can be established. Culture from the primary site tends to reveal *Trichophyton mentagrophytes* organisms rather than *Trichophyton rubrum*. There appears to be selective anergy in patients with chronic *T rubrum* infections.

Differential Diagnosis

Differentiate from all diseases causing vesicular eruptions of the hands, especially contact dermatitis, dyshidrosis, and localized forms of atopic dermatitis.

Prevention

Treat fungal infections early and adequately, and prevent recurrences.

Treatment

General measures are as outlined on p 53. The lesions should be treated according to type of dermatitis. The primary focus should be treated with griseofulvin or by local measures as described for dermatophytosis (see above). A single injection of triamcinolone acetonide suspension, 40 mg intragluteally, may suppress the eruption until the causative focus is controlled.

Prognosis

Dermatophytid may occur in an explosive series of episodes, and recurrences are not uncommon; however, it clears with adequate treatment of the primary infection elsewhere on the body.

TINEA UNGUIUM & CANDIDAL ONYCHOMYCOSIS

Essentials of Diagnosis

- Lusterless, brittle, hypertrophic, friable nails.
- Fungus demonstrated in nail section or nail dust by microscope or culture.

General Considerations

Tinea unguium is a destructive *Trichophyton* infection of one or more (but rarely all) fingernails or toenails. The species most commonly found are *Trichophyton mentagrophytes* and *Trichophyton rubrum*. *Candida albicans* causes candidal onychomycosis. "Saprophytic" fungi may cause onychomycosis.

Clinical Findings

A. Symptoms and Signs: There are usually no symptoms. The nails are lusterless, brittle, and hypertrophic, and the substance of the nail is friable and even pithy. Irregular segments of the diseased nail may be broken.

B. Laboratory Findings: Laboratory diagnosis is mandatory. Portions of the nail should be cleared with 10% potassium hydroxide and examined under the microscope for branching hyphae or collections of spores. Fungi may also be cultured, using Sabouraud's medium. Periodic acid-Schiff stain of a histologic section will also demonstrate the fungus readily.

Differential Diagnosis

Distinguish from nail disorders due to psoriasis, lichen planus, candidiasis, and trauma.

Treatment

A. General Measures: See p 53.

B. Specific Measures: Onychomycosis is an unlisted indication for ketoconazole. Griseofulvin ultramicrosize, 1000 mg/d, is about as effective as ketoconazole, 200 mg/d. Increasing ketoconazole to 400 mg/d will substantially increase the cure rate of onychomycosis, but the side effects of ketoconazole (liver abnormalities, effects on the adrenal cortex, and antiandrogenic activity) must be taken into account.

C. Local Measures: Sandpaper or file the nails daily (down to nail bed if necessary). Ciclopirox (Loprox) is a topical fungicidal cream that contains a pyridone-ethanolamine salt and seems to penetrate nails better than other topical agents. To date, no topical agent has been very effective.

Prognosis

Cure is difficult, even with microcrystalline griseofulvin by mouth in a dose of 1–2 g daily for months, or with ketoconazole, miconazole, or clotrimazole topically. Even when the nails clear after months of treatment, recurrences can be expected shortly after discontinuance of systemic therapy.

Scher RK: Differential diagnosis and treatment of onychomycosis. Curr Concepts Skin Dis 1985;6:4.

Zaias N, Drachman D: A method for the determination of drug effectiveness in onychomycosis: Trials with ketoconazole and griseofulvin ultramicrosize. J Am Acad Dermatol 1983;9:912.

TINEA VERSICOLOR (Pityriasis Versicolor)

Essentials of Diagnosis

- Pale macules that will not tan.
- Velvety, chamois-colored macules that scale with scraping.
- Trunk distribution the most frequent site.
- Fungus observed on microscopic examination of scales.

General Considerations

Tinea versicolor is a mild, superficial *Pityrosporum orbiculare (Malassezia furfur)* infection of the skin (usually of the trunk). The eruption is called to the patient's attention by the fact that the involved areas will not tan, and the resulting pseudoachromia may be mistaken for vitiligo. A hyperpigmented form is not uncommon. The disease is not particularly contagious and is apt to occur more frequently in those who wear heavy clothing and who perspire a great deal. Epidemics may occur in athletes.

Pityrosporum folliculitis is common. Stubborn scalp folliculitis may occur.

Clinical Findings

A. Symptoms and Signs: There may be mild itching. The lesions are velvety, chamois-colored macules that vary from 4 to 5 mm in diameter to large confluent areas. Scales may be readily obtained by scraping the area. Lesions may appear on the trunk, upper arms, neck, face, and groin.

B. Laboratory Findings: Large, blunt hyphae and thick-walled budding spores ("spaghetti and meatballs") may be seen under the low-power objective when skin scales have been cleared in 10% potassium hydroxide. *P orbiculare* and *P ovale* are difficult to culture.

Differential Diagnosis

Distinguish from vitiligo on basis of appearance. Differentiate also from seborrheic dermatitis of the same areas.

Treatment & Prognosis

Encourage good skin hygiene. Topical treatments include Selsun suspension or Exsel lotion (both contain selenium sulfide), which may be applied daily and left on for 5 minutes; or one may use equal parts of propylene glycol and water topically, diluting with water if there is irritation. Other choices are

3% salicylic acid in rubbing alcohol and Tinver lotion (contains sodium thiosulfate). Relapses are common.

Sulfur-salicylic acid soap or shampoo (Sebulex) used on a continuing basis may be effective.

Ketoconazole, 200 mg daily orally for 1 week or a 400 mg as a single oral dose, apparently results in cure of 90% of cases.

Newer imidazole creams, solutions, and lotions are quite effective for localized areas.

Badck O, Faergemann J, Hornqvist R: *Pityrosporum* folliculitis: A common disease of the young and middle-aged. J Am Acad Dermatol 1985;12:56.

Savin RC: Systemic ketoconazole in tinea versicolor: A double-blind evaluation and 1-year follow-up. J Am Acad Dermatol 1984;10:824.

MUCOCUTANEOUS CANDIDIASIS

Essentials of Diagnosis

- Severe pruritus of vulva, anus, or body folds.
- Superficial denuded, beefy-red areas with or without satellite vesicopustules.
- Whitish curdlike concretions on the oral and vaginal mucous membranes.
- Fungus on microscopic examination of scales or curd.

General Considerations

Mucocutaneous candidiasis is a superficial fungal infection that may involve almost any cutaneous or mucous surface of the body. It is particularly likely to occur in diabetics, during pregnancy, and in obese persons who perspire freely. Antibiotics and oral contraceptive agents may be contributory. When the patient presents with chronic mucocutaneous candidiasis, baseline and yearly follow-up tests will screen for development of endocrinopathy. Oral candidiasis may be the first sign of HIV infection. Esophageal candidiasis can be detected by endoscopy in all patients with AIDS and oral candidiasis.

Clinical Findings

A. Symptoms and Signs: Itching may be intense. Burning sensations are sometimes reported, particularly around the vulva and anus. The lesions consist of superficially denuded, beefy-red areas in the depths of the body folds such as in the groin and the intergluteal cleft, beneath the breasts, at the angles of the mouth, and in the umbilicus. The peripheries of these denuded lesions are superficially undermined, and there may be satellite vesicopustules. Whitish, curdlike concretions may be present on the surface of the lesions (particularly in the oral and vaginal mucous membranes). Paronychia and interdigital erosions may occur.

B. Laboratory Findings: Clusters of budding cells and short hyphae can be seen under the high-power lens when skin scales or curdlike lesions have been cleared in 10% potassium hydroxide. The organism may be isolated on Sabouraud's medium. In the more severe forms of mucocutaneous candidiasis, there may be negative skin tests to all common antigens including *Candida,* as well as inability to be sensitized to dinitrochlorobenzene.

Tests for diabetes include glycosylated hemoglobin (hemoglobin A_{1c}) and fasting and 2-hour postprandial glucose; for thyroid function, TSH, T_4, resin T_3 uptake, thyroglobulin, and microsomal antibody tests; for parathyroid function, calcium, phosphorus, and alkaline phosphatase tests; for adrenal function, electrolyte, blood glucose, and adrenal antibody tests and ACTH and cortisol levels.

Differential Diagnosis

Differentiate from intertrigo, seborrheic dermatitis, tinea cruris, "inverse psoriasis," and erythrasma involving the same areas.

Complications

In the debilitated or immunosuppressed patient, candidiasis may spread from the skin or mucous membranes to the bladder, lungs, and other internal organs.

Treatment

A. General Measures: Treat associated diabetes, obesity, or hyperhidrosis. Keep the parts dry and exposed to air as much as possible. If possible, discontinue systemic antibiotics; if not, give nystatin by mouth concomitantly in a dose of 1.5 million units 3 times daily. Ketoconazole, 200 mg daily by mouth, will eradicate lesions with minimal side effects except for rare instances of liver damage. Liver function must be monitored. Recurrences follow discontinuance of therapy.

B. Local Measures:

1. Nails and skin–Apply 1% ciclopirox cream, nystatin cream, 100,000 units/g, or miconazole, ketoconazole, or clotrimazole cream or lotion, 3–4 times daily. Gentian violet, 1%, or carbolfuchsin paint (Castellani's paint) may be applied 1–2 times weekly as an alternative.

2. Vulva, anal mucous membranes–For vaginal candidiasis, use miconazole cream (Monistat 7), one applicatorful vaginally at bedtime for 7 days; or clotrimazole (Gyne-Lotrimin, Mycelex-G), one suppository vaginally per day for 7 days; or terconazole vaginal cream (Terazol 7) or suppositories (Terazol 3); or nystatin, one tablet (100,000 units) vaginally twice daily for 7 days. Gentian violet or carbolfuchsin (see above) can also be used. Clotrimazole troches have proved effective in controlling chronic oral candidiasis. Ketoconazole, 200 mg daily for 10 days, is quite effective for chronic, recurrent, or recalcitrant vulvovaginal candidiasis.

Prognosis

Cutaneous candidiasis may be intractable and prolonged, particularly in children, in whom the disturbance may take the form of a granuloma.

Jorizzo JL: Chronic mucocutaneous candidiasis: An update. Arch Dermatol 1982;18:963.

Tkach JR, Rinaldi MG: Severe hepatitis associated with ketoconazole therapy for chronic mucocutaneous candidiasis. Cutis 1982;29:482.

PARASITIC INFESTATIONS OF THE SKIN

SCABIES

Essentials of Diagnosis

- Nocturnal itching.
- Pruritic vesicles and pustules in "runs" or "galleries," especially on the sides of the fingers and the heels of the palms.
- Mites, ova, and brown dots of feces visible microscopically.

General Considerations

Scabies is a common dermatitis caused by infestation with *Sarcoptes scabiei*. An entire family may be affected. The infestation usually spares the head and neck (although even these areas may be involved in infants). The mite is barely visible with the naked eye as a white dot. Scabies is usually acquired by sleeping with an infested individual or by other close contact. This infestation is on the increase worldwide.

Clinical Findings

A. Symptoms and Signs: Itching occurs almost exclusively at night. The lesions consist of more or less generalized excoriations with small pruritic vesicles, pustules, and "runs" or "galleries" on the sides of the fingers and the heels of the palms. The run or gallery appears as a short irregular mark (perhaps 2–3 mm long), as if made by a sharp pencil. Characteristic lesions may occur on the nipples in females and as pruritic papules on the scrotum or penis in males. Pruritic papules may be seen over the buttocks. Pyoderma is often the presenting sign.

B. Laboratory Findings: The adult female mite may be demonstrated by probing the fresh end of a run or gallery with a pointed scalpel. The mite tends to cling to the tip of the blade. One may shave off the entire run or gallery (or in the scrotum, a papule) and demonstrate the female mite, her ova, and small brown dots of feces. A sharp bone or dermal curet yields an excellent specimen. The diagnosis should be confirmed by microscopic demonstration of the organism, ova, or feces in a mounted specimen in glycerin, mineral oil, or immersion oil. The diagnosis can be confirmed in most cases with the burrow ink test. Apply ink to the burrow and then do a superficial shave biopsy by sawing off the burrow with a No. 15 blade, painlessly and bloodlessly. The mite, ova, and feces can be seen under the light microscope.

Differential Diagnosis

Distinguish from the various forms of pediculosis and from other causes of pruritus.

Treatment & Prognosis

Unless the lesions are complicated by severe secondary pyoderma, treatment consists primarily of disinfestation. If secondary pyoderma is present, it should be treated with systemic and topical antibiotics.

Disinfestation with lindane (gamma benzene hexachloride), 1% in cream or lotion base, applied from the neck down overnight, is a popular treatment. A warning has been issued by the FDA regarding potential neurotoxicity, and any use in infants and pregnant women, as well as overuse in adults, is discouraged. Bedding and clothing should be laundered or cleaned. This preparation can be used before secondary infection is controlled. Permethrin 5% dermal cream (Eli-Mite) is highly effective and safe in the management of scabies. Treatment consists of a single application. The drug has been used safely in infants aged 2 months to 5 years. An alternative drug is crotamiton (Eurax) cream or lotion, which may be applied in the same way as lindane (gamma benzene hexachloride). The old-fashioned medication consisting of 5% or 6% sulfur in petrolatum may still be used, applying it nightly from the collarbones down, for 3 nights, but one must be prepared to treat irritant dermatitis. Benzyl benzoate may be compounded as a lotion or emulsion in strengths from 20% to 35% and used as generalized (from collarbones down) applications overnight for 2 treatments 1 week apart. The NF XIV formula is 275 mL benzyl benzoate (containing 5 g of triethanolamine and 20 g of oleic acid) in water to make 1000 mL. It is cosmetically acceptable, clean, and not overly irritating. Persistent pruritic postscabietic papules may be painted with undiluted crude coal tar or Estargel.

Unless treatment is aimed at all infected persons in a family or institutionalized group, reinfestations will probably occur.

Resistant forms requiring multiple forms of treatment are appearing.

Davies JH et al: Lindane poisonings. Arch Dermatol 1983;119:142.

Felman YM, Nikitas JA: Scabies. Cutis 1984;33:266.

Orkin M, Maibach HI (editors): *Cutaneous Infestations and Insect Bites*. Marcel Dekker, 1985.

PEDICULOSIS

Essentials of Diagnosis
- Pruritus with excoriation.
- Nits on hair shafts; lice on skin or clothes.
- Occasionally, sky-blue macules (maculae ceruleae) on the inner thighs or lower abdomen in pubic louse infestation.

General Considerations
Pediculosis is a parasitic infestation of the skin of the scalp, trunk, or pubic areas. It usually occurs among people who live in overcrowded dwellings with inadequate hygiene facilities, although pubic lice may be acquired by anyone sitting on an infested toilet seat—and, more commonly, by sexual transmission. There are 3 different varieties: (1) pediculosis pubis, caused by *Pthirus pubis* (pubic louse, "crabs"); (2) pediculosis corporis, by *Pediculus humanus* var *corporis* (body louse); and (3) pediculosis capitis, by *Pediculus humanus* var *capitis* (head louse).

Head and body lice are similar in appearance and are 3–4 mm long. Head louse infestations may be transmitted by shared use of hats or combs. The body louse can seldom be found on the body, because the insect comes onto the skin only to feed and must be looked for in the seams of the underclothing.

Trench fever, relapsing fever, and typhus may be transmitted by the body louse, but this would be an extremely rare event in the USA.

Clinical Findings
Itching may be very intense in body louse infestations, and scratching may result in deep excoriations over the affected area. The clinical appearance is of gross excoriation. Pyoderma may be present and may be the presenting sign in any of these infestations. Head lice can be found on the scalp or may be manifested as small nits resembling pussy-willow buds on the scalp hairs close to the skin. They are easiest to see above the ears and at the nape of the neck. Body lice may deposit visible nits on the vellus hair of the body. Pubic louse infestations are occasionally generalized, particularly in a hairy individual; the lice may even be found on the eyelashes and in the scalp.

Differential Diagnosis
Distinguish head louse infestation from seborrheic dermatitis, body louse infestation from scabies, and pubic louse infestation from anogenital pruritus and eczema.

Treatment
For all types of pediculosis, lindane lotion (Kwell, Scabene) is used extensively. A thin layer is applied to the infested and adjacent hairy areas. It is removed after 12 hours by thorough washing. Remaining nits may be removed with a fine-toothed comb or forceps. Sexual contacts should be treated. Permethrin (Nix), 1% cream rinse, is a topical pediculocide and ovicide for the treatment of head lice and eggs. It is applied to the scalp and hair and left on for 10 minutes before being rinsed off with water. Synergized pyrethrins (A-200 Pyrinate, Pyrinyl, Rid) are over-the-counter products that are applied undiluted until the infested areas are entirely wet. After 10 minutes, the areas are washed thoroughly with warm water and soap and then dried. Nits may be treated as indicated above. For involvement of eyelashes, petrolatum is applied thickly twice daily for 8 days, and remaining nits are then plucked off. There is controversy about whether lice and the acarus of scabies can develop resistance to lindane.

Malathion lotion, 0.5% (Prioderm), compared with A-200 Pyrinate shampoo, R&C shampoo, Rid, Kwell shampoo (lindane), and A-200 Pyrinate liquid, is the only product for pediculosis capitis that shows excellent ovicidal activity. Hatching of eggs following treatment with the other agents leads to recurrence of the infestation.

Prognosis
Pediculosis responds to topical treatment.

Meinking TL et al: Comparative efficacy of treatments for pediculosis capitis infestations. Arch Dermatol 1986;122:267.
Parish LC, Witkowoski JA, Kucirka SA: Lindane resistance and pediculosis capitis. Int J Trop Dermatol 1983; 22:572.

SKIN LESIONS DUE TO OTHER ARTHROPODS

Essentials of Diagnosis
- Localized rash with pruritus.
- Furuncle-like lesions containing live arthropods.
- Tender erythematous patches that migrate ("larva migrans").
- Generalized urticaria or erythema multiforme.

General Considerations
Some arthropods (eg, most pest mosquitoes and biting flies) are readily detected as they bite. Many others are not, eg, because they are too small, because there is no immediate reaction, or because they bite during sleep. Reactions may be delayed for many hours; many severe reactions are allergic. Patients are most apt to consult a physician when the lesions are multiple and pruritus is intense. Severe attacks may be accompanied by insomnia, restlessness, fever, and faintness or even collapse. Rashes may sometimes cover the body.

Many persons will react severely only to their earliest contacts with an arthropod, thus presenting pruritic lesions when traveling, moving into new quarters, etc. Body lice, fleas, bedbugs, and local mosquitoes should be borne in mind. Spiders are often incorrectly believed to be the source of bites; they rarely attack humans, although the brown spider *(Loxosceles laeta, Loxosceles reclusa)* may cause severe necrotic reactions and death due to intravascular hemolysis, and the black widow spider *(Latrodectus mactans)* may cause severe systemic symptoms and death.

In addition to arthropod bites, the most common lesions are venomous stings (wasps, hornets, bees, ants, scorpions) or bites (centipedes), dermatitis due to vesicating Furuncle-like lesions due to fly maggots or sand fleas in the skin, and a linear creeping eruption due to a migrating larva.

Clinical Findings

The diagnosis may be difficult when the patient has not noticed the initial attack but suffers a delayed reaction. Individual bites are frequently in clusters and tend to occur either on exposed parts (eg, midges and gnats) or under clothing, especially around the waist or at flexures (eg, small mites or insects in bedding or clothing). The reaction is often delayed for 1–24 hours or more. Pruritus is almost always present and may be all but intolerable once the patient starts to scratch. Secondary infection, sometimes with serious consequences, may follow scratching. Allergic manifestations, including urticarial wheals, are common. Papules may become vesicular. The diagnosis is aided by searching for exposure to arthropods and by considering the patient's occupation and recent activities. The principal arthropods are as follows:

(1) Bedbugs: In crevices of beds or furniture; bites tend to occur in lines or clusters. Papular urticaria is a characteristic lesion of bedbug bites. It is thought that *Cimex lectularius* (bedbug) may play a significant role in the transmission of hepatitis B. The closely related kissing bug has been reported with increasing frequency as attacking humans.

(2) Fleas: Fleas are bloodsucking ectoparasites that feed on dogs, cats, humans, and other species. Flea saliva produces papular urticaria in sensitized individuals. *Ctenocephalides felis* and *Ctenocephalides canis* are the most common species found on cats and dogs, and both species attack humans. The human flea, *Pulex irritans,* is not commonly recognized by veterinarians as a pet animal problem.

To break the life cycle of the flea, one must treat the home, pets, and outside environment, using quick-kill insecticides, residual insecticides, and a growth regulator. Obviously, this is a repetitive job for the exterminator. Home foggers and flea collars are not adequate. Birds and fish are especially sensitive and must be protected during disinfestation.

(3) Ticks: Usually picked up by brushing against low vegetation. Larval ticks may attack in large numbers and cause much distress; in Africa and India they have been confused with chiggers. Ascending paralysis may occasionally be traced to a tick bite, and removal of the embedded tick is essential. Ticks may transmit Rocky Mountain spotted fever, Lyme disease, and relapsing fever.

(4) Chiggers or red bugs are larvae of trombiculid mites. A few species confined to particular countries and usually to restricted and locally recognized habitats (eg, berry patches, woodland edges, lawns, brush turkey mounds in Australia, poultry farms) attack humans, often around the waist, on the ankles, or in flexures, raising intensely itching erythematous papules after a delay of many hours. The red chiggers may sometimes be seen in the center of papules that have not yet been scratched. Chiggers are the commonest cause of distressing multiple lesions associated with arthropods.

(5) Bird mites: Larger than chiggers, infesting chicken houses, pigeon lofts, or nests of birds in eaves. Bites are multiple anywhere on the body, although poultry handlers are most often attacked on the hands and forearms. Room air conditioning units may suck in bird mites and infest the inhabitants of the room. Rodent mites from mice or rats may cause similar effects.

The diagnosis of bird mites, rodent mites, or carpet mites may readily be overlooked and the patient treated for other dermatoses or for psychogenic dermatosis. Intractable "acarophobia" (delusions of parasitosis) may result from early neglect or misdiagnosis.

(6) Mites in stored products: These are white and almost invisible and infest products such as copra ("copra itch"), vanilla pods ("vanillism"), sugar, straw, cottonseeds, and cereals. Persons who handle these products may be attacked, especially on the hands and forearms and sometimes on the feet. Infested bedding may occasionally lead to generalized dermatitis.

(7) Caterpillars of moths with urticating hairs: The hairs are blown from cocoons or carried by emergent moths, causing severe and often seasonally recurrent outbreaks after mass emergence, eg, in some southern states of the USA.

(8) Tungiasis is due to the burrowing flea known as *Tunga penetrans* (also known as chigoe, jigger; not the same as chigger), found in Africa, the West Indies, and South America. The female burrows under the skin, sucks blood, swells to 0.5 cm, and then ejects her eggs onto the ground. Ulceration, lymphangitis, gangrene, and septicemia may result, possibly with fatality. Ethyl chloride spray will kill the insect when applied to the lesion, and disinfestation may be accomplished with insecticide applied to the terrain.

Differential Diagnosis

Arthropods should be considered in the differential diagnosis of skin lesions showing any of the above symptoms.

Prevention

Arthropod infestations are best prevented by avoidance of contaminated areas, personal cleanliness, and disinfection of clothing, bedclothes, and furniture as indicated. Lice, chiggers, red bugs, and mites can be killed by lindane (gamma benzene hexachloride; Gammexane, Kwell, Scabene) applied to the head and clothing. (It is not necessary to remove clothing.) Benzyl benzoate and dimethylphthalate are excellent acaricides; clothing should be impregnated by spray or by dipping in a soapy emulsion.

Treatment

Caution: Avoid local overtreatment.

Living arthropods should be removed carefully with tweezers after application of alcohol. Preserve in alcohol for identification. (*Caution:* In endemic Rocky Mountain spotted fever areas, do not remove ticks with the bare fingers, because infection may occur.) Children in particular should be prevented from scratching.

Apply corticosteroid lotions or creams. Crotamiton (Eurax) cream or lotion may be used; it is a miticide as well as an antipruritic. Calamine lotion or a cool wet dressing is always appropriate. Antibiotic creams, lotions, or powders may be applied if secondary infection is suspected.

Localized persistent lesions may be treated with intralesional corticosteroids. Avoid exercise and excessive warmth. Codeine may be given for pain. Creams containing local anesthetics are not very effective and may be sensitizing.

Stings produced by many arthropods may be alleviated by applying papain powder (Adolph's Meat Tenderizer) mixed with water, or Xerac AC.

Extracts (expensive) from venom sacs of bees, wasps, yellow jackets, and hornets are now available for immunotherapy of patients at risk for anaphylaxis. Approximately 5% of patients fail to respond.

Chipps BE et al: Diagnosis and treatment of anaphylactic reactions to Hymenoptera stings in children. J Pediatr 1980;97:177.

Crissey JT: Bedbugs: An old problem with a new dimension. Int J Dermatol 1981;20:411.

Medleau L, Miller WH Jr: Flea infestation and its control. Int J Dermatol 1983;22:378.

Pien FD, Grekin JL: Common ectoparasites. West J Med 1983;139:382.

TUMORS OF THE SKIN

Excessive exposure of fair skin to sun radiation is a cancer risk of major degree. Inculcation of new attitudes about sunbathing and development of measures to counteract the adverse effects of sun damage are important public health objectives. Sunlight on sandy complexions can induce actinic (solar) keratoses, nevi, basal and squamous cell carcinoma, and melanoma. The best protection is shelter, but protective clothing, avoidance of direct sun exposure during the 5 peak hours of the day, and the assiduous use of commercially available chemical sunscreens or sunshades are helpful.

A number of highly effective sunscreens are available. Fair-complexioned persons should not use a sunscreen with a rating less than SPF 15 (sun protective factor 15). For those who are sensitive to PABA (*p*-aminobenzoic acid), Neutrogena PABA-free sunscreen SPF 15, Solbar SPF 15 PABA-free cream, TI-Screen SPF 15, or PreSun 29 may be used. SolBar PF (PABA-free) cream with an SPF rating of 50 is available. Photoplex Broad Spectrum Sunscreen Lotion affords protection against UVA and UVB light exposure and may be helpful in managing photosensitivity disorders.

The sunshades include those containing opaque materials such as titanium dioxide or zinc oxide.

Classification

The following classification is admittedly oversimplified; almost any tumor arising from embryonal tissues in the various stages of their development can be found in the skin.

A. Benign: Seborrheic keratoses, considered by some to be nevoid, consist of benign overgrowths of epithelium that have a pigmented velvety or warty surface. They are relatively common, especially in the elderly, both on exposed and covered parts, and are commonly mistaken for melanomas or other types of cutaneous neoplasms. Skin tags frequently develop on the eyelids, around the neck, and in the axillae and groins.

Keratoacanthomas are rapidly growing tumors resembling squamous cell carcinomas.

B. Nevi: Any of the following (except freckles) may be excised if there are suspicious features.

1. Junctional nevi, which consist of clear nevus cells and usually some melanin, have nevus cells on both sides of the epidermal junction. They are possible forerunners of malignant melanoma, although most melanomas arise de novo. If a nevus grows rapidly, develops color changes, darkens, or bleeds, the possibility of melanomatous degeneration should be considered.

2. Compound nevi, composed of junctional elements as well as clear nevus cells in the dermis, also may develop into malignant melanoma.

3. Dermal nevi are almost always benign, and almost everyone has at least a few of these lesions. They usually appear in childhood and tend to undergo spontaneous fibrosis in old age. Pigmented nevi that are present at birth show a greater tendency toward the development of melanoma than those developing in later years and should be excised wherever possible.

This is especially true of bathing trunk nevi, which should be excised in decrements if possible.

4. Dysplastic nevi range from 6 to 12 mm in diameter. They may be pebbly, papular, nodular, or plaquelike. They may be tan to dark brown, perhaps with a pink component, and may have an inflamed appearance. They may occur anywhere on the body but are usually on unexposed areas. An individual may have more than 100 lesions—instead of about 25, as is the case with common melanocytic nevi (''moles''). They usually appear in adolescence, may continue developing throughout life (ordinary moles tend to disappear with aging), and may be familial, in which case the rate of development of malignant melanoma may be much higher than in sporadic cases. Patients with dysplastic nevi have an overall lifetime risk for malignant melanoma of between 5 and 10%, with the rate approaching 100% in familial cases—especially if there is a history of malignant melanoma in close relatives. Several lesions should be biopsied and the rest followed carefully.

5. Blue nevi are benign, although in some instances they behave in an invasive manner requiring multiple excisions. These lesions in the pristine state are small, slightly elevated, and blue-black.

6. Epithelial nevi include several types of verrucous epithelial overgrowths, usually in linear distribution. Microscopically, cells found normally in the epidermis are present. Such lesions rarely degenerate into squamous or basal cell carcinomas. The nevus sebaceus of Jadassohn, which occurs commonly in the scalp, is composed of a number of embryonal elements and is considered to be particularly likely to give rise to carcinomas.

7. Freckles, which in the juvenile form are called ephelides and in the adult delayed form are called lentigines, consist of excess amounts of melanin in the melanocytes in the basal layer of the epidermis. Juvenile freckles tend to disappear with time, whereas lentigines come on in later life and are more persistent.

C. Premalignant: Actinic or solar keratoses are flesh-colored and feel like little patches of sandpaper when the finger is pulled over them. When they degenerate, they become squamous cell carcinomas. They occur on exposed parts of the body in persons of fair complexion. Nonactinic keratoses may be provoked by exposure to arsenic systemically or occupational irritants such as tars. In keratoses, the cells are atypical and similar to those seen in squamous cell epitheliomas, but these changes are well contained by an intact dermoepidermal junction. Application of liquid nitrogen is a rapid and effective method of eradication. The lesions are frozen for a few seconds with a cotton-tipped applicator that has been dipped in liquid nitrogen or with a spraying unit containing liquid nitrogen. The lesions disappear in a few days. They may be excised or removed superficially with a scalpel followed by cautery or fulguration. An alter-native treatment is the use of 1–5% fluorouracil in propylene glycol or in a cream base. This agent may be rubbed into the lesions morning and night until they become briskly sore (usually 1–3 weeks); the treatment should then be continued for several days longer and then stopped. The eyes and the mouth should be avoided. Any lesions that persist may then be excised for histologic examination.

D. Malignant:

1. Squamous cell carcinoma usually occurs on exposed parts in fair-skinned individuals who sunburn easily and tan poorly. They may arise out of actinic or solar keratoses. They tend to develop slowly in the course of a few months. These lesions appear as small red, conical, hard nodules that quickly ulcerate. Squamous cell carcinomas of the lip, oral cavity, tongue, and genitalia are serious cancers and deserve special care and management. Metastases may occur early, although they are said to be less likely with squamous cell carcinoma arising out of actinic keratoses than in those that arise de novo. Keratoacanthomas are benign growths that resemble squamous cell carcinoma but which for all practical purposes should be treated as though they were skin cancers. The preferred treatment of squamous cell carcinoma is excision. Electrodesiccation and curettage and x-ray radiation may be used instead, and Mohs' fresh tissue microscopically controlled excision, where available, is excellent treatment also.

2. Basal cell carcinoma occurs mostly on exposed parts. These lesions grow slowly, attaining a size of 1–2 cm in diameter only after a year's growth. There is a waxy appearance, with telangiectatic vessels easily visible. Metastases almost never occur. Neglected lesions may ulcerate and produce great destruction, ultimately invading vital structures. It is important to widely excise basal cell carcinomas where possible. Excision and suturing may be used, or one may carve out the entire growth (called a ''shave biopsy'' by some physicians), following which the base of the wound is treated with curettage and electrodesiccation. If the growth is in areas such as the inner canthus of the eye or the nasolabial fold, where pockets of extension may occur, fresh tissue microscopically controlled excision may be done (modified Mohs' technique). X-ray therapy and cryosurgery are alternative methods of treatment.

3. Bowen's disease (intraepidermal squamous cell carcinoma) is relatively uncommon, occurs on cutaneous surfaces and mucous membranes, and resembles a plaque of psoriasis. The course is relatively benign, but malignant progression may occur, and it is best to excise the lesion widely if possible.

4. Paget's disease, considered by some to be a manifestation of apocrine sweat gland carcinoma, may occur around the nipple, resembling chronic eczema, or may involve apocrine areas such as the genitalia (extramammary Paget's disease). There seems to be less likelihood of an underlying sweat gland carcinoma if the lesions are on the vulva than if they are on the nipple or perianal area.

5. Malignant melanoma–Malignant melanoma is the leading cause of death from skin disease. It is estimated that 27,300 cases of melanoma occurred in the USA in 1988, causing melanoma to be ranked as the ninth most common cancer, with nearly 6000 deaths. Five-year survival rates, related to thickness in millimeters, are as follows: < 0.76 mm, 99%; 0.76–1.49 mm, 95%; 1.5–2.49 mm, 84%; 2.5–3.99 mm, 70%; and > 4 mm, 44%. With lymph node involvement, the 5-year survival rate is 30%; and with distant metastases, it is less than 10%. Deaths from malignant melanoma are increasing at a faster rate than death from any other malignant neoplastic disease except lung cancer. Melanomas cause most of the deaths from skin cancer. The mean age of those dying from melanomas is less than that of those dying from other skin cancers. There is a trend toward a younger age incidence each year. Primary malignant melanomas may be classified into 6 clinicohistologic types, including lentigo maligna melanoma; superficial spreading malignant melanoma (the most common type, occurring in two-thirds of individuals developing melanoma); nodular malignant melanoma; acral-lentiginous melanomas; malignant melanomas on mucous membranes; and miscellaneous forms such as those arising from blue nevi and congenital and giant nevocytic nevi.

True melanomas vary from macules to nodules, with a surprising play of colors from flesh tints to pitch black and a frequent admixture of white, blue, purple, and red. The border tends to be irregular, and growth may be rapid.

Treatment of melanoma consists of wide excision, with lymph node dissection varying with the depth and location of the lesions and the background of the surgeon. Deaths from melanoma are increasing at a rate of 2% per year for females and 3% for males. Depth of invasion is the single most important prognostic factor (according to Breslow; see Balch reference, below).

6. Kaposi's sarcoma–Until recently in the USA, this rare malignant skin lesion was seen mostly in elderly white men, had a chronic clinical course, and was rarely fatal. Kaposi's sarcoma occurs endemically in an often aggressive form in young black men of equatorial Africa, but it is rare in American blacks. Within the past few years, epidemic clusters of Kaposi's sarcoma, predominantly in homosexual men, have been found in various large cities of the USA. Disseminated Kaposi's sarcoma in the homosexual population occurs as one feature of AIDS. The HIV retrovirus is the cause of AIDS. Fever, adenopathy, and gastrointestinal complaints associated with red, purple, or dark plaques or nodules on cutaneous or mucosal surfaces should alert the clinician to the possibility of the disease.

Management of AIDS-associated Kaposi's sarcoma consists of observation and supportive care for slowly progressive disease; cryotherapy, vinblastine, 0.1–0.5 mg/mL, and α_1-interferon intralesionally, for cosmetically objectionable lesions; radiation therapy for accessible and space-occupying lesions; laser surgery for certain intraoral and pharyngeal lesions; and, for progressive disease, intravenous chemotherapy.

Successful treatment and remission of Kaposi's sarcoma unfortunately do not affect patient survival.

Balch CM: Measuring melanomas: A tribute to Alexander Breslow. J Am Acad Dermatol 1981;5:96.

Brooks NA: Curettage and shave excision: A tissue-sparing technic for primary cutaneous carcinoma worthy of inclusion in graduate training programs. J Am Acad Dermatol 1984;10:279.

Dixon SL: Dysplastic nevus syndrome: A clinical review. Curr Concepts Skin Disorders (Spring) 1985;6:5.

Friedman RJ, Rigel DS, Kopf AW: Early detection of malignant melanoma: The role of physician examination and self-examination of the skin. CA (May-June) 1985; 35:130.

Koh HK, Lew RA, Prout MN: Screening for melanoma/skin cancer: Theoretic and practical considerations. J Am Acad Dermatol 1989;20:159.

Lane HC, Fauci AS: Immunologic reconstitution in the acquired immunodeficiency syndrome. Ann Intern Med 1985;103:714.

Silverberg E, Lubera JA: Cancer statistics, 1988. CA 1988;38:5.

Volberding P et al: Vinblastine therapy for Kaposi's sarcoma in the acquired immunodeficiency syndrome. Ann Intern Med 1985;103:335.

MISCELLANEOUS SKIN, HAIR, & NAIL DISORDERS*

PIGMENTARY DISORDERS

Melanin is formed in the melanocytes in the basal layer of the epidermis. Its precursor, the amino acid tyrosine, is slowly converted to dihydroxyphenylalanine (dopa) by tyrosinase, and there are many further chemical steps to the ultimate formation of melanin. This system may be affected by external influences such as exposure to sun, heat, trauma, ionizing radiation, heavy metals, and changes in oxygen potential. These influences may result in hyperpigmentation, hypopigmentation, or both. Local trauma may destroy melanocytes temporarily or permanently, causing hypopigmentation, sometimes with surrounding hyperpigmentation as in eczema and dermatitis. Hypermelanosis appears to be associated with increased plasma immunoreactive β-MSH (melanocyte-stimulating

---

* Hirsutism is discussed in Chapter 20.

hormone from the pituitary) only in Addison's disease. Melatonin, a pineal hormone, regulates pigment dispersion and aggregation.

Other pigmentary disorders include those resulting from exposure to exogenous pigments such as carotenemia, argyria, deposition of other metals, and tattooing. Other endogenous pigmentary disorders are attributable to metabolic substances, including hemosiderin (iron), in purpuric processes and in hemochromatosis; mercaptans, homogentisic acid (ochronosis), bile pigments, and carotenes.

Classification

Pigmentary disorders may be classified as primary or secondary and as hyperpigmentary or hypopigmentary.

A. Primary Pigmentary Disorders: These are nevoid or congenital and include pigmented nevi, Mongolian spots, and incontinentia pigmenti, vitiligo, albinism, and piebaldism. In vitiligo, pigment cells (melanocytes) are destroyed. The greater the pigment loss, the fewer the number of melanocytes. At the borders of lesions, the melanocytes are often large and have long dendritic processes, and they resemble pigment cells in tissue cultures that are blocked in the G phase of the cell cycle. Loss of pigment surrounding nevi, and in melanomas, may represent immune responses. Vitiligo, found in approximately 1% of the population, may be associated with hyperthyroidism and hypothyroidism, pernicious anemia, diabetes mellitus, addisonism, and carcinoma of the stomach. Albinism, partial or total, occurs as a genetically determined recessive trait. Piebaldism, a localized hypomelanosis, is an autosomal dominant trait.

B. Secondary Pigmentary Disorders: Hyper- or hypopigmentation may occur following overexposure to sunlight or heat or as a result of excoriation or direct physical injury. Hyperpigmentation occurs in arsenical melanosis or in association with Addison's disease (due to lack of the inhibitory influence of hydrocortisone on the production of MSH by the pituitary gland). Several disorders of clinical importance are as follows:

1. Melasma—This occurs as patterned hyperpigmentation of the face. The localized pigmentation of chloasma may be a direct effect of certain steroid hormones, estrogens, and progesterones in predisposed clones of melanocytes. It occurs not only during pregnancy but also in 30–50% of women taking oral contraceptives.

2. Berloque hyperpigmentation can be provoked by phototoxicity from essential oils in perfumes, and these should be excluded wherever possible.

3. Leukoderma, or secondary depigmentation, may complicate atopic dermatitis, lichen planus, psoriasis, alopecia areata, lichen simplex chronicus, and such systemic conditions as myxedema, thyrotoxicosis, syphilis, and toxemias. It may follow local skin trauma of various sorts or may complicate dermatitis due to exposure to gold or arsenic. Antioxidants in rubber goods, such as monobenzyl ether of hydroquinone, cause leukoderma from the wearing of gauntlet gloves, rubber pads in brassieres, etc. This is most likely to occur in blacks.

4. Ephelides (juvenile freckles) and lentigines (senile freckles)—The number of functioning melanocytes decreases by about 10% per decade. The loss is often blotchy, particularly in areas of solar degeneration. Compensatory hypertrophy of some melanocytes gives rise to lentigines.

5. Drugs—Pigmentation may be produced by chloroquine, chlorpromazine, minocycline, and amiodarone.

Differential Diagnosis

One must distinguish true lack of pigment from pseudoachromia, such as occurs in tinea versicolor, pityriasis simplex, and seborrheic dermatitis. It may be difficult to differentiate true vitiligo from leukoderma and even from partial albinism.

Complications

Solar keratoses and epitheliomas are more likely to develop in persons with vitiligo and albinism. Vitiligo tends to cause pruritus in anogenital folds. There may be severe emotional trauma in extensive vitiligo and other types of hypo- and hyperpigmentations, particularly when they occur in naturally dark-skinned persons.

Treatment & Prognosis

There is no increase of pigment in partial or total albinism; return of pigment is rare in vitiligo; in leukoderma, repigmentation may occur spontaneously. Therapy of vitiligo is long and tedious. Cosmetics such as Covermark and Dermablend are highly effective for concealing disfiguring patches. The patient must be strongly motivated. If less than 20% of the skin is involved (most cases), topical methoxsalen, 0.1% in ethanol and propylene glycol or in Acid Mantle cream or Unibase, is used, with cautious exposure to long-wavelength ultraviolet light (UVA), followed by thorough washing and application of an SPF 15 sunscreen. With 20–25% involvement, oral methoxsalen, 0.6 mg/kg 2 hours before UVA exposure, is best. Severe phototoxic response may occur with topical or oral psoralens plus UVA. For more than 50% skin involvement, the use of 20% monobenzone cream to totally depigment the skin has been reported.

Potent topical corticosteroids have been advocated for the treatment of vitiligo. Betamethasone dipropionate ointment may be rubbed thoroughly into the moistened skin once daily for 10 days, followed by 10 days' rest, then repetition, over a period of time. Caution must be exercised, especially on the face and on thin skin, to avoid pseudoatrophy and other changes.

Localized ephelides and lentigines may be destroyed by careful application of a saturated solution of liquid phenol on a tightly wound cotton applicator, or by brief application of liquid nitrogen. Chloasma and other forms of hyperpigmentation may be treated by protecting the skin from the sun and with cosmetics such as Covermark, Dermablend, or Maxafil. Cosmetics containing perfumes should not be used.

Bleaching preparations generally contain hydroquinone or its derivatives. This is not without hazard, and it is best to start with the weakest preparation offered by the manufacturer. The use of this kind of bleach may result in unexpected hypopigmentation, hyperpigmentation, or even ochronosis and pigmented milia, particularly with prolonged use.

Treatment of other pigmentary disorders should be directed toward avoidance of the causative agent if possible (as in carotenemia) or treatment of the underlying disorder. Melasma, ephelides, and postinflammatory hyperpigmentation may be treated with 3–4% hydroquinone solution or cream and a sunscreen with an SPF of 15. Tretinoin cream, 0.05%, may be added. The superficial melasma responds well, but if there is predominantly dermal deposition of pigment, the prognosis is poor. Senile lentigines are resistant to topicals but respond to liquid nitrogen application.

Alpha-hydroxy acids may be useful in treating seborrheic keratoses, "age spots," and actinic keratoses and in modifying wrinkles. One such preparation is Lac-Hydrin cream, which contains 12% ammonium lactate.

Fisher AA: Hydroquinone uses and abnormal reactions. Cutis 1983;31:240.
Kenney JA Jr, Grimes P: How we treat vitiligo. Cutis 1983;32:347.
Vanscott EJ, Yu RJ: Alpha hydroxy acids: Procedures for use in clinical practice. Cutis 1989;43:222.

BALDNESS
(Alopecia)

Baldness Due to Scarring

Cicatricial baldness may occur following chemical or physical trauma, lichen planopilaris, severe bacterial or fungal infections, severe herpes zoster, chronic discoid lupus erythematosus, scleroderma, and excessive ionizing radiation. The specific cause is often suggested by the history, the distribution of hair loss, and the appearance of the skin, as in lupus erythematosus and other infections. Biopsy may be necessary to differentiate lupus from the others.

Scarring alopecias are irreversible and permanent. There is no treatment, except for surgical hair transplants.

Baldness Not Due to Scarring

Alopecia areata (patchy baldness) is a form of temporary, noncicatricial baldness that may progress to alopecia totalis (complete scalp hair loss) or alopecia universalis (generalized total hair loss).

Nonscarring alopecia may occur in association with various **systemic diseases** such as systemic lupus erythematosus, cachexia, lymphomas, uncontrolled diabetes, severe thyroid or pituitary hypofunction, and dermatomyositis. The only treatment necessary is prompt and adequate control of the underlying disorder, in which case hair loss may be reversible.

Male pattern baldness, the most common form of alopecia, is of genetic predetermination. The earliest changes occur at the anterior portions of the calvarium on either side of the "widow's peak." Associated seborrhea may be evident as excessive oiliness and erythema of the scalp, with scaling. Premature loss of hair in a young adult male may create some anxiety. The extent of hair loss is variable and unpredictable. Extensive studies with minoxidil applied topically have shown good results in the treatment of androgenetic (male pattern) alopecia. The commercial product, Rogaine, is a solution containing 2 mg/mL of minoxidil. The best results are achieved in patients under 50 years of age and in those with recent onset (< 5 years) and smaller diameters of alopecia. Seborrhea may be treated as described on p 115.

Hair loss or thinning of the hair in women results from the same cause as common baldness in men (androgenetic alopecia). Treatment is aimed at antagonizing the follicular effects of androgens. Cyproterone acetate is the only widely available antiandrogen in Europe; it is not available in the USA. Spironolactone, a synthetic steroidal aldosterone antagonist, has been used successfully for the treatment of diffuse hair loss in women (androgenetic alopecia) in a dose of 25 mg daily by mouth. This is not a listed indication for the drug, which has been shown to be a tumorigen in long-term toxicity studies in rats. Oral corticosteroids have been recommended to suppress adrenal androgen production; give prednisolone, 2.5–7.5 mg/d plus oral antiandrogens. There are no well-documented studies to prove the efficacy of these approaches. Topical estrogens are of occasional value. Minoxidil (Rogaine) is also indicated for women with androgenetic alopecia.

Women who complain of thin hair but show little evidence of alopecia need follow-up, because 20% of the scalp hair can be lost before the clinician can perceive it.

Telogen effluvium may be the cause of temporary hair loss in some women. A transitory increase occurs in the number of hairs in the telogen (resting) phase of the hair growth cycle. This may occur spontaneously, may appear at the termination of pregnancy, may be precipitated by "crash dieting" or malnutrition, or may be provoked by hormonal contraceptives, especially the monophasic contraceptives. Whatever the cause, telogen effluvium usually has a latent period of 2–4 months. the prognosis is generally good. If an abnormally high proportion of telogen hairs is present before taking the contraceptive, lasting improvement in hair growth may be expected. In one study, the only cause of telogen effluvium was found to be iron deficiency, and the hair counts bore a clear relationship to serum iron levels.

Alopecia areata is of unknown cause. Histopathologically, there are numerous small anagen hairs and a lymphocytic infiltrate. The bare patches may be perfectly smooth, or a few hairs may remain. Severe forms may be treated by systemic corticosteroid therapy, although systemic therapy is rarely justified unless the disease is of serious emotional or economic significance. Alopecia areata is occasionally associated with Hashimoto's thyroiditis, pernicious anemia, Addison's disease, vitiligo, several of the connective tissue autoimmune diseases, and atopy.

Anthralin, 0.5% ointment applied daily, may provoke hair growth *(caution)*. Intralesional corticosteroids are frequently effective. Triamcinolone acetonide, in a concentration of 5 mg/mL, is injected in aliquots of 0.1 mL at approximately 1- to 2-cm intervals, not exceeding a total dose of 50 mg per month for adults. Alopecia areata is usually self-limiting, with complete regrowth of hair, but some mild cases are permanent and the extensive forms are usually permanent, as are the totalis and universalis types. Both topical dinitrochlorobenzene (DNCB) and an experimental topical allergen, squaric acid dibutyl ester, have been used to treat persistent alopecia areata. The principle is to sensitize the skin, then intermittently apply weaker concentrations to produce and maintain a slight dermatitis. Hair regrowth in 3–6 months in some patients has been reported to be remarkable. Long-term safety and efficacy have not been established.

New contact allergens are being sought to replace DNCB for the treatment of alopecia areata because of the positive Ames test, which has shown that the substance is carcinogenic in laboratory animals. Squaric acid dibutyl ester and diphencyprone apparently are as effective as DNCB.

Minoxidil, a peripheral vasodilator given orally for hypertension, causes hypertrichosis in 80% of users. As Rogaine, it is available for topical application in male pattern baldness and alopecia areata.

Cataracts may complicate extensive alopecia areata.

In **trichotillomania** (the pulling out of one's own hair), the patches of hair loss was irregular, and growing hairs are always present, since they cannot be pulled out until they are long enough.

Drug-induced alopecia is becoming increasingly important. Such drugs include thallium, excessive and prolonged use of vitamin A, retinoids, antimitotic agents, anticoagulants, clofibrate (rarely), antithyroid drugs, oral contraceptives, trimethadione, allopuri-

nol, propranolol, indomethacin, amphetamines, salicylates, gentamicin, and levodopa.

Bergfeld WF, Redmond GP: Androgenetic alopecia. Dermatol Clin 1987;5:491.
Nelson DA, Spielvogel RL: Alopecia areata: A review. Int J Dermatol 1985;24:26.
Stern RS: Topical minoxidil: A survey of use and complications. Arch Dermatol 1987;123:62.

KELOIDS & HYPERTROPHIC SCARS

Keloids are tumors consisting of actively growing fibrous tissue and occur as a result of trauma or irritation in predisposed persons, especially those of dark-skinned races. The trauma may be relatively trivial, such as an acne lesion. Keloids behave as neoplasms, although they are not malignant. Spontaneous digitations may project from the central growth, and the tumors may become large and disfiguring. There may be itching and burning sensations with both types of tumor.

Hypertrophic scars, usually seen following surgery or accidental trauma, tend to be raised, red, and indurated. After a few months or longer, they lose their redness and become soft and flat. Removal should not be attempted until all induration has subsided.

Intralesional injection of a corticosteroid suspension is effective against hypertrophic scars. The treatment of keloids is less satisfactory; surgical excision, x-ray therapy, and freezing with liquid nitrogen are used, as well as injection of corticosteroid suspensions into the lesions. They tend to involute in older age groups.

Keloids can be removed with carbon dioxide laser excision. Ring block anesthesia is accomplished with 1% lidocaine with epinephrine 1:200,000. The bulk of keloidal tissue is removed, using the focused mode to perform a shave excision. The base of the wound is palpated to remove residual areas of firmness, and the base is injected with triamcinolone acetonide suspension, 40 mg/mL. The wound is allowed to heal by granulation.

Wheeland RG, Bailin PL: Dermatologic application of the argon and carbon dioxide lasers. Curr Concepts Skin Disorders (Summer) 1984;5:5.

NAIL DISORDERS
(See also Candidal Onychomycosis, above.)

Nail changes are generally not diagnostic of a specific systemic or cutaneous disease. All of the nail manifestations of systemic disorders may be seen also in the absence of any systemic illness.

Nail dystrophies cannot usually be related to changes in thyroid function, hypovitaminosis, nutritional disturbances, or generalized allergic reactions.

Classification

Nail disorders may be classified as (1) local, (2) congenital or genetic, and (3) those associated with systemic or generalized skin diseases.

A. Local Nail Disorders:

1. Onycholysis (distal separation of the nail plate from the nail bed, usually of the fingers) is caused by excessive exposure to water, soaps, detergents, alkalies, and industrial keratolytic agents. Candidal infection of the nail folds and subungual area, nail hardeners, and demeclocycline may cause onycholysis. Hyper- and hypothyroidism may also be a cause.

2. Distortion of the nail occurs as a result of chronic inflammation of the nail matrix underlying the eponychial fold.

3. Discoloration and pithy changes, accompanied by a musty odor, are seen in ringworm infection.

4. Grooving and other changes may be caused by warts, nevi, synovial cysts, etc, impinging on the nail matrix.

5. Allergic reactions (to formaldehyde and resins in undercoats and polishes) involving the nail bed or matrix formerly caused hemorrhagic streaking of the nails, accumulation of keratin under the free margins of the nails, and great tenderness of the nail beds.

6. Beau's lines (transverse furrows) may be due to faulty manicuring and acute systemic illness.

7. Onychogryphosis, usually involving the nails of the great toes, is characterized by grossly distorted, hypertrophic, and misshapen nails. The disorder may respond to correction of chronic edema associated with stasis dermatitis, stasis ulcers, and other conditions of the lower extremities that are adversely affected by gravitational factors.

B. Congenital and Genetic Nail Disorders:

1. A longitudinal single nail groove may occur as a result of a genetic or traumatic defect in the nail matrix underlying the eponychial fold.

2. Nail atrophy may be congenital.

3. Clubbed fingers may be congenital.

C. Nail Changes Associated With Systemic or Generalized Skin Diseases:

1. Beau's lines (transverse furrows) may follow any serious systemic illness.

2. Atrophy of the nails may be related to trauma or vascular or neurologic disease.

3. Clubbed fingers may be due to the prolonged hypoxemia associated with cardiopulmonary disorders.

4. Spoon nails may be seen in anemic patients.

5. Stippling or pitting of the nails is seen in psoriasis.

6. Nail changes may be seen also with alopecia areata, lichen planus, and keratosis follicularis.

7. Nail hyperpigmentation may be caused by zidovudine, doxorubicin, cyclophosphamide, methotrexate, bleomycin, dacarbazine, daunorubicin, fluorouracil, hydroxyurea, melphalan, mechlorethamine, and nitrosoureas.

Differential Diagnosis

It is important to distinguish congenital and genetic disorders from those caused by trauma and environmental disorders. Nail changes due to dermatophyte fungi may be difficult to differentiate from onychia due to *Candida* infections. Direct microscopic examination of a specimen cleared with 10% potassium hydroxide, or culture on Sabouraud's medium, may be diagnostic. Onychomycosis may be closely similar to the changes seen in psoriasis and lichen planus, in which case careful observation of more characteristic lesions elsewhere on the body is essential to the diagnosis of the nail disorders. Suspect cancer (eg, Bowen's disease or squamous cell carcinoma) with any persistent solitary subungual or periungual lesion.

Complications

Secondary bacterial infection occasionally occurs in onychodystrophies and leads to considerable pain and disability and possibly more serious consequences if circulation or innervation is impaired. Toenail changes may lead to an ingrown nail, in turn often complicated by bacterial infection and occasionally by exuberant granulation tissue. Poor manicuring and poorly fitting shoes may contribute to this complication. Cellulitis may result.

Treatment & Prognosis

Treatment consists usually of careful debridement and manicuring and, above all, reduction of exposure to irritants (soaps, detergents, alkali, bleaches, solvents, etc). Antifungal measures may be used in the case of onychomycosis and candidal onychia; antibacterial measures may be used for bacterial complications. Congenital or genetic nail disorders are usually uncorrectable. Longitudinal grooving due to temporary lesions of the matrix, such as warts, synovial cysts, and other impingements, may be cured by removal of the offending lesion. Intradermal triamcinolone acetonide suspension, 2.5 mg/mL, may be injected in the area of the nail matrix at intervals of 2–4 weeks for the successful management of various types of nail dystrophies (psoriasis, lichen planus, onycholysis, longitudinal splitting, grooving from synovial cysts, and others).

If it is necessary to remove nails for any reason (eg, fungal nails or severe psoriasis), one may apply urea 40%, anhydrous lanolin 20%, white wax 5%, white petrolatum 25%, and silica gel type H. The nail folds are painted with compound tincture of benzoin and then covered with cloth adhesive tape. Apply the urea ointment generously to the nail surface, and cover with plastic film and then adhesive tape. Avoid water. Leave the ointment on for 5–10 days; then lift off the nail plate. Medication can then be applied that is appropriate for the condition being treated.

South DA, Farber EM: Urea ointment in the nonsurgical avulsion of nail dystrophies. Cutis 1980;25:609.

Stone OJ: Resolution of onychogryphosis. Cutis 1984; 34:480.

REFERENCES

Arnold HL Jr, Odom RB, James WD: *Andrews' Diseases of the Skin*, 8th ed. Saunders, 1990.

Braverman IM: *Skin Signs of Systemic Disease*, 2nd ed. Saunders, 1981.

Burgdorf WHC et al: *Dermatopathology*. Springer-Verlag, 1984.

Ely H, Thiers BH (editors): Dermatologic therapy II. (Symposium.) Dermatol Clin 1989;7:1. (Entire issue.)

Fitzpatrick TB et al: *Dermatology in General Medicine*, 3rd ed. McGraw-Hill, 1987.

Lever WF, Schaumberg-Lever G: *Histopathology of the Skin*, 6th ed. Lippincott, 1983.

Moschella SL, Hurley HJ: *Dermatology*, 2nd ed. 2 vols. Saunders, 1985.

Pinkus H, Mehregan AH: *A Guide to Dermatohistopathology*, 3rd ed. Appleton-Century-Crofts, 1981.

Sande MA, Volberding PA: *The Medical Management of AIDS*. Saunders, 1988.

Shelley WP, Shelley ED: *Advanced Dermatologic Therapy*. Saunders, 1987.

Taylor JS et al: Environmental reactions to chemical, physical, and biologic agents. J Am Acad Dermatol 1984; 11(5–Part 2):1007.

5

Eye

Paul Riordan-Eva, FRCS, FCOphth, & Daniel G. Vaughan, MD

SYMPTOMS OF OCULAR DISEASE

Redness

Redness is the most frequently encountered symptom of ocular disorders. It is due to hyperemia of the conjunctival, episcleral, or ciliary vessels; erythema of the eyelids; or subconjunctival hemorrhage. The major differential diagnoses are conjunctivitis, corneal disorders, acute glaucoma, and acute uveitis (Table 5–1).

Ocular Discomfort

Ocular pain may be caused by trauma (chemical, mechanical, or physical), infection, inflammation, or sudden increase in intraocular pressure.

Foreign body sensation is most commonly due to corneal or conjunctival foreign bodies. Other causes are disturbances of the corneal epithelium and rubbing of eyelashes against the cornea (trichiasis).

Photophobia is commonly due to corneal inflammation, aphakia, iritis, or albinism. A less common cause is fever associated with viral infections.

Itching is characteristically associated with allergic eye disease.

Scratching and burning due to dryness of the eyes are common complaints of older people but may occur at any age. Deficiency of tear film components may be due to dry environment, local ocular disease, systemic disorders, or drugs (eg, atropine-like agents).

Watering is usually due to inadequate tear drainage through obstruction of the lacrimal drainage system or malposition of the lower lid. Reflex tearing occurs with any disturbance of the corneal epithelium and thus may occur paradoxically with dryness of the eye.

"Eyestrain" & Headache

Eyestrain is a common complaint that usually means discomfort associated with prolonged reading or close work. Significant refractive error, presbyopia, inadequate illumination, and phoria (usually exophoria with poor convergence) should be ruled out. Headache is only occasionally due to ocular disorders, but these same conditions should be considered, as well as corneal inflammation, iritis, and acute glaucoma. Headache with scalp tenderness is a major feature of giant cell arteritis, which should always be considered in older patients.

Conjunctival Discharge

Purulent discharge usually indicates bacterial infection of the conjunctiva, cornea, or lacrimal sac. Viral conjunctivitis or keratitis produces watery discharge. Allergic conjunctivitis usually causes tearing and ropy discharge associated with itching.

Visual Loss

The most important causes of blurred vision are refractive error, cataract, macular degeneration, diabetic retinopathy, vitreous hemorrhage, retinal detachment involving the macula, central retinal vein occlusion, central retinal artery occlusion, corneal opacities, and optic nerve disorders. Amblyopia, due to failure of development of visual processing mechanisms, is an important cause of treatable visual loss in children. Strabismus, refractive error, and media opacity are the major causes. Any child with poor vision should be referred for ophthalmic assessment as soon as possible.

Monocular field loss indicates disease of the retina or optic nerve. Important causes are retinal detachment, chronic glaucoma, branch retinal artery or vein occlusion, optic neuritis, and anterior ischemic optic neuropathy. (All these conditions may of course produce bilateral visual field loss.) Lesions of the optic chiasm due to pituitary tumors characteristically produce bitemporal field loss. Retrochiasmal lesions cause contralateral homonymous field defects. The more posterior the lesion in the visual pathway, the more congruous (similar in size, shape, and location) are the defects in the 2 eyes. Cerebrovascular disease and tumors are responsible for most lesions of the retrochiasmal visual pathways.

Visual Impairment & Blindness

An individual may be considered to be visually impaired if the best corrected distant visual acuity in the better eye is 20/80 or less or if visual fields are significantly restricted. Legal blindness (partial) in the USA is defined for practical purposes as visual acuity for distant vision of 20/200 or less in the better eye with best correction or widest diameter of the visual field subtending an angle of less than 20 de-

Table 5–1. The inflamed eye: differential diagnosis of common causes.

	Acute Conjunctivitis	Acute Uveitis	Acute Glaucoma[1]	Corneal Trauma or Infection
Incidence	Extremely common	Common	Uncommon	Common
Discharge	Moderate to copious	None	None	Watery or purulent
Vision	No effect on vision	Often blurred	Markedly blurred	Usually blurred
Pain	Mild	Moderate	Severe	Moderate to severe
Conjunctival injection	Diffuse; more toward fornices	Mainly circumcorneal	Diffuse	Diffuse
Cornea	Clear	Usually clear	Steamy	Clarity change related to cause
Pupil size	Normal	Small	Moderately dilated and fixed	Normal
Pupillary light response	Normal	Poor	None	Normal
Intraocular pressure	Normal	Commonly low but may be elevated	Elevated	Normal
Smear	Causative organisms	No organisms	No organisms	Organisms found only in corneal ulcers due to infection

[1] Angle-closure glaucoma.

grees. There are approximately 500,000 legally blind people in the USA; about half are over the age of 65. The leading causes of blindness are glaucoma, diabetic retinopathy, and age-related macular degeneration.

WHO estimates that at least 28 million of the world's population have vision of 10/200 or less, and millions more have loss of sight sufficient to interfere with normal living. The most frequent causes of preventable blindness worldwide are trachoma, leprosy, onchocerciasis, and xerophthalmia.

Diplopia & Strabismus

Double vision results from extraocular muscle imbalance. This may be caused by disturbance of third, fourth, or sixth cranial nerve function by head injury, vascular disturbance, intracranial tumors, or intraorbital lesions; direct involvement of muscle as in dysthyroid eye disease; or entrapment as a result of orbital blowout fracture.

In children, suppression of the abnormal image eliminates double vision but at the risk of amblyopia. Childhood strabismus thus usually presents as a misalignment of the eyes noticed by the parents or other relatives, or poor vision. The underlying cause is usually not a structural lesion—refractive error, abnormal relationships between accommodation and convergence, and more subtle abnormalities of ocular motor coordination are much more common—but neurologic lesions must always be appropriately excluded. Any child said to have strabismus after the age of 3 months should be referred as soon as possible for ophthalmic assessment.

"Spots Before the Eyes" & "Flashing Lights"

Spots before the eyes (floaters) are usually caused by vitreous opacities that have no significance. However, they may also be caused by posterior vitreous detachment, vitreous hemorrhage, or posterior

uveitis. Sudden onset of floaters, particularly when associated with flashing lights (photopsiae), necessitates dilated fundal examination to exclude a retinal tear or detachment.

OCULAR EXAMINATION

Visual Acuity

Corrected distant visual acuity should be tested for each eye in turn, using a standardized chart such as the Snellen chart. If appropriate refractive correction is not available, a pinhole will overcome most refractive errors. The Snellen chart is annotated according to the distance at which each line can be read by a normal individual. Visual acuity is expressed as a fraction—the test distance over the figure assigned to the lowest line the patient can read. If the patient is unable to read the top line of the chart, acuity is recorded as counting fingers, hand movements, perception of light, or no perception of light. Distant acuity is usually measured at 20 feet. A corrected acuity of less than 20/30 is abnormal.

If assessment of distant visual acuity is not possible, near acuity should be tested with a reduced Snellen chart or standardized reading test types. The patient must be wearing an appropriate reading correction.

Visual Fields

Confrontation field testing is extremely valuable for assessment of field defects. Use of a red target enhances the detection of neurologic field defects. Amsler charts are the easiest method of detecting central field abnormalities due to macular disease.

Pupils

The pupils should be examined for absolute and relative size and reactions to both light and accommodation. A large, poorly reacting pupil may be due to third nerve palsy, iris damage caused by acute glaucoma, or pharmacologic mydriasis. A small, poorly reacting pupil may be due to Horner's syndrome, inflammatory adhesions between iris and lens (posterior synechiae), or Argyll Robertson pupils of neurosyphilis. Physiologic anisocoria is a common cause of unequal pupils that react normally.

A relative afferent pupillary defect, in which the pupillary light reaction is of reduced intensity when light is shined into the affected eye compared to when light is shined into the normal eye, is an important objective sign that usually indicates optic nerve disease. It is most easily detected with the "swinging light test," in which the pupillary light reactions are compared as a bright light is moved from one eye to the other. It is only necessary to observe the pupillary reactions of one eye to detect the presence of a relative afferent pupillary defect.

Extraocular Movements

Examination of extraocular movements begins with the detection of any manifest deviation. (Manifest deviation is any deviation present when both eyes are open. Latent deviation is any additional deviation that then becomes apparent when one eye is covered.) This can be quickly achieved by comparing the relative positions of the corneal light reflexes. More accurate assessment requires a cover test in which the deviated eye moves to take up fixation when the other eye is occluded. This correctional movement is in a direction opposite to that of the original manifest deviation. (This movement may not occur if the deviated eye is poorly sighted.)

Recently acquired unilateral third, fourth, and sixth nerve palsies produce restricted movement in one eye only. (In long-standing lesions, changes may also occur in movements of the contralateral eye.) The false outer image of the resulting diplopia arises from the affected eye. Horizontal diplopia indicates dysfunction of horizontally acting muscles (medial and lateral recti), and vertical diplopia indicates dysfunction of vertically acting muscles (superior and inferior recti and the obliques), The direction of gaze in which image separation is greatest indicates the direction of action of the underacting muscle.

Minor degrees of nystagmus at the extremes of gaze are normal. Other forms of physiologic nystagmus include optokinetic nystagmus and those induced by rotation or caloric stimulation. Exaggerated gaze-evoked nystagmus may be due to drugs or posterior fossa disease. Nystagmus in the primary position is always abnormal. Certain acquired forms specifically localize lesions within the nervous system. Congenital nystagmus may be a benign isolated anomaly or due to poor vision.

Proptosis (Exophthalmos)

Proptosis may be suspected by observing widening of the palpebral aperture, with exposure of sclera both superiorly and inferiorly. (Eyelid retraction generally causes exposure only superiorly.) By viewing the patient from above, while the patient is asked to look down and the upper lids are lifted by the examiner, a further estimate of the degree of proptosis can be made. Exophthalmometry should be performed for objective assessment. In nonaxial proptosis, there is also horizontal or vertical displacement of the globe, indicating the presence of a mass lesion outside the extraocular muscle cone.

The most frequent cause of proptosis in adults is dysthyroid eye disease. Other causes of (usually unilateral) proptosis include cellulitis, tumors, and pseudotumor of the orbit.

Ptosis

Neurologic causes of ptosis include third nerve palsy and Horner's syndrome, which are differentiated by pupil size. Local causes include congenital and acquired disorders of the levator muscle complex and tumors and infections of the eyelid. Myasthenia should always be considered.

Anterior Segment Examination

Although slit lamp examination is recommended for accurate documentation of anterior segment abnormalities, examination with a flashlight and loupe usually provides sufficient information for initial diagnosis. Patterns of redness indicate the site of the underlying problem. Conjunctivitis produces redness that extends diffusely across the globe and the inner surface of the lids. Keratitis, intraocular inflammation, and acute glaucoma produce predominantly circumcorneal injection. Episcleritis and scleritis cause localized or diffuse deep injection, which in the case of scleritis is associated with blue discoloration.

Focal lesions of the cornea due to infection or trauma can be differentiated from the diffuse corneal haze of acute glaucoma and from the cloudiness of the anterior chamber and perhaps hypopyon (accumulation of white cells within the anterior chamber) of iritis. Instillation of fluorescein and examination with a blue light aids in detection of corneal epithelial defects. Palpation of the globe will reveal the stony hardness of acute glaucoma.

Direct Ophthalmoscopy

Direct ophthalmoscopy is principally used for examining the retina, but much other useful information can also be gained. Assessment of the red reflex and clarity of fundal details indicates the degree of media opacity. Abnormalities may then be localized to the cornea, lens, or vitreous by variations of focus of the ophthalmoscope and use of parallax.

The optic disk should be examined for disk swelling and the size of the optic cup in relation to the disk. Macular lesions causing poor central vision are usually apparent. The retinal vessels are examined for caliber and wall changes. Retinal hemorrhages, exudates, and cotton-wool spots should be noted.

Dilation of the pupil aids direct ophthalmoscopy but should be done with caution in patients with shallow anterior chambers (see below).

OPHTHALMOLOGIC REFERRALS

Sudden loss of vision is a serious symptom requiring urgent or emergency ophthalmologic consultation. The most important causes of painless sudden visual loss are vitreous hemorrhage, retinal detachment, exudative age-related macular degeneration, retinal vein occlusions, retinal artery occlusions, and anterior ischemic optic neuropathy. Painful sudden visual loss may be due to acute anterior uveitis, acute glaucoma, corneal ulcer, or optic neuritis. Other ophthalmologic emergencies include orbital cellulitis, gonococcal keratoconjunctivitis, and major ocular trauma.

Any patient developing gradual loss of vision should be referred for ophthalmologic assessment. Important causes include cataract, atrophic age-related macular degeneration, chronic glaucoma, chronic uveitis, and intraorbital and intracranial tumors.

Patients with diabetes mellitus must undergo regular fundus examination through dilated pupils. Myopic patients should be warned of the increased risk of retinal detachment and made aware of the importance of reporting relevant symptoms. Close relatives of patients with chronic glaucoma should be encouraged to undergo annual glaucoma screening once they have reached adulthood.

REFRACTIVE ERRORS

Refractive errors are the most common cause of blurred vision. In **emmetropia,** objects at infinity are seen clearly with the unaccommodated eye. Objects nearer than infinity are seen with the aid of accommodation, which increases the refractive power of the lens. In **hyperopia,** objects at infinity are not seen clearly unless accommodation is used, and near objects may not be seen because accommodative capacity is finite. Hyperopia is corrected with plus (convex) lenses. In **myopia,** the unaccommodated eye brings to a focus images of objects closer than infinity, the distance of such objects from the patient becoming shorter and shorter with increasing myopia. (Thus, the high myope is able to focus on very near objects without glasses.) However, objects beyond this distance cannot be seen without the aid of corrective (minus, concave) lenses. In **astigmatism,** the refractive error in the horizontal and vertical axes differs. **Presbyopia** is the natural loss of accommodative capacity with age. Emmetropes usually notice inability to focus on objects at a normal reading distance at about age 40. Hyperopes experience symptoms at an earlier age. Presbyopia is corrected with plus lenses for near work.

Use of a pinhole will overcome most refractive errors and thus allows their exclusion as a cause of visual loss. Transient refractive errors occur in diabetes—often when diabetic control is erratic—and may be the presenting feature. Autoinoculation of scopolamine from seasickness patches or atropine from vials for parenteral use leads to pupillary dilatation and loss of accommodation.

DISORDERS OF THE LIDS & LACRIMAL APPARATUS

Hordeolum

Hordeolum is a common staphylococcal abscess that is characterized by a localized red, swollen, acutely tender area on the upper or lower lid. Internal hordeolum is a meibomian gland abscess that points onto the conjunctival surface of the lid; external hordeolum or sty (infection of the glands of Moll or Zeis) is smaller and on the margin. The chief symptom is pain of an intensity directly related to the amount of swelling.

Warm compresses are helpful. Incision is indicated if resolution does not begin within 48 hours. An antibiotic instilled into the conjunctival sac every 3 hours may be beneficial during the acute stage. Internal hordeolum may lead to generalized cellulitis of the lid.

Chalazion

Chalazion is a common granulomatous inflammation of a meibomian gland that may follow an internal hordeolum. It is characterized by a hard, nontender swelling on the upper or lower lid. The conjunctiva in the region of the chalazion is red and elevated. If the chalazion is large enough to impress the cornea, vision will be distorted.

Excision is done by an ophthalmologist.

Tumors

Verrucae and papillomas of the skin of the lids can often be excised by the general physician if they do not involve the lid margin; otherwise, surgery should be performed by an ophthalmologist so as to avoid permanent notching of the lid. Cancer—including basal cell carcinoma, squamous cell carcinoma, meibomian gland carcinoma, and malignant melanoma—should be ruled out by microscopic examination of the excised material.

Blepharitis

Blepharitis is a common chronic bilateral inflammation of the lid margins. It may be ulcerative (*Staphylococcus aureus*) or nonulcerative (seborrheic). Both types are commonly present. Seborrhea of the scalp, brows, and frequently the ears is almost always associated with seborrheic blepharitis.

Symptoms are irritation, burning, and itching. The eyes are "red-rimmed," and scales or "granulations" can be seen clinging to the lashes. In the staphylococcal type, the scales are dry, the lid margins are red and ulcerated, and the lashes tend to fall out; in the seborrheic type, the scales are greasy, ulceration is absent, and the margins are less red. In the more common mixed, type, both dry and greasy scales are present and the lid margins are red and may be ulcerated.

Cleanliness of the scalp, eyebrows, and lid margins is essential to effective local therapy. Scales must be removed from the lids daily with a damp cotton applicator.

An antistaphylococcal antibiotic or sulfonamide eye ointment is applied daily to the lid margins with a cotton-tipped applicator. The treatment of both types is similar except that in severe staphylococcal blepharitis, antibiotic sensitivity studies may be required.

Entropion & Ectropion

Entropion (inward turning of usually the lower lid) occurs occasionally in older people as a result of degeneration of the lid fascia, or may follow extensive scarring of the conjunctiva and tarsus. Surgery is indicated if the lashes rub on the cornea.

Ectropion (outward turning of the lower lid) is fairly common in elderly people. Surgery is indicated if ectropion causes excessive tearing, exposure keratitis, or a cosmetic problem.

Dacryocystitis

Dacryocystitis is infection of the lacrimal sac due to obstruction of the nasolacrimal system. It may be acute or chronic and occurs most often in infants and in persons over 40. It is usually unilateral.

In acute dacryocystitis, the usual infectious organisms are *S aureus* and β-hemolytic streptococci; in chronic dacryocystitis, *Streptococcus pneumoniae* (rarely, *Candida albicans*). Mixed infections do not occur.

Acute dacryocystitis is characterized by pain, swelling, tenderness, and redness in the tear sac area; purulent material may be expressed. In chronic dacryocystitis, tearing and discharge are the principal signs. Mucus or pus may be expressed from the tear sac.

Acute dacryocystitis responds well to systemic antibiotic therapy, but recurrences are common if the obstruction is not surgically removed. The chronic form may be kept latent by using antibiotic drugs, but relief of the obstruction is the only cure.

CONJUNCTIVITIS

Conjunctivitis is the most common eye disease. It may be acute or chronic. Most cases are due to bacterial (including chlamydial) or viral infection. Other causes include keratoconjunctivitis sicca, allergy, and chemical irritants. The mode of transmission of infectious conjunctivitis is usually direct contact via fingers, towels, handkerchiefs, etc, to the fellow eye or to other persons.

Conjunctivitis must be differentiated from acute uveitis, acute glaucoma, and corneal disorders (Table 5–1).

Bacterial Conjunctivitis

The organisms found most commonly in bacterial conjunctivitis are *S pneumoniae, S aureus, Haemophilus aegyptius,* and *Moraxella lacunata.* All may produce a copious purulent discharge. There is no blurring of vision and only mild discomfort. In severe cases, examination of stained conjunctival scrapings and culture studies are recommended.

The disease is usually self-limited, lasting about 10–14 days if untreated. A sulfonamide (eg, sulfacetamide, 10% ophthalmic solution or ointment) instilled locally 3 times daily will usually clear the infection in 2–3 days. Topical antibiotics are usually to be avoided for minimal infections and limited to those unlikely to be used systemically.

Gonococcal Conjunctivitis

Gonococcal conjunctivitis, usually acquired through contact with infected genital secretions, is manifested by a copious purulent discharge. It is an ophthalmologic emergency because corneal involvement may rapidly lead to perforation. The diagnosis should be confirmed by stained smear and culture of the discharge. Treatment is primarily with intravenous antibiotics—aqueous penicillin, or cefotaxime if penicillin resistance is likely. Topical treatment should include frequent saline lavage. Topical antibiotics may also be used.

Ullman S, Roussel TJ, Forster RK: Gonococcal keratoconjunctivitis. Surv Ophthalmol 1987;32:199.

Chlamydial Keratoconjunctivitis

A. Trachoma: Trachoma is a major cause of blindness worldwide. Recurrent episodes of infection occur in childhood. Manifested by redness, itching, tearing, and slight discharge, the clinical picture consists of bilateral follicular conjunctivitis, epithelial keratitis, and corneal vascularization (pannus). Visual loss occurs from early adulthood. Cicatrization of the tarsal conjunctiva produces entropion and trichiasis, leading to central corneal scarring.

The specific diagnosis can be made in Giemsa-stained conjunctival scrapings. Treatment should be started on the basis of clinical findings without waiting for laboratory confirmation. Oral tetracycline or erythromycin is given in full doses for 3–5 weeks. Local treatment is not necessary. *Caution:* Tetracyclines are contraindicated during pregnancy and in young children. Surgical treatment includes correction of eyelid deformities and corneal transplantation.

B. Inclusion Conjunctivitis: The agent of inclusion conjunctivitis is a common cause of genital tract disease in adults. The eye is usually involved following accidental contact with genital secretions, and adult inclusion conjunctivitis thus occurs most frequently in sexually active young adults. The disease starts with acute redness, discharge, and irritation. The eye findings consist of follicular conjunctivitis with mild keratitis. A nontender preauricular lymph node can often be palpated. Healing leaves no sequelae. Cytologic examination of conjunctival scrapings shows a picture similar to that of trachoma. Treatment is with oral tetracycline or erythromycin for 2–3 weeks. Before treatment, all cases should be appropriately assessed for genital tract infection so that management can be adjusted accordingly.

Viral Conjunctivitis

One of the most common causes of viral conjunctivitis is adenovirus type 3. Conjunctivitis due to this agent is usually associated with pharyngitis, fever, malaise, and preauricular adenopathy (pharyngoconjunctival fever). Locally, the palpebral conjunctiva is red, and there is a copious watery discharge and scanty exudate. Children are more often affected than adults, and contaminated swimming pools are sometimes the source of infection. Epidemic keratoconjunctivitis (EKC) is caused by adenovirus types 8 and 19. There is no specific treatment for viral conjunctivitis, though local sulfonamide therapy may prevent secondary bacterial infection. The disease usually lasts at least 2 weeks.

Keratoconjunctivitis Sicca

This is a common disorder, particularly in elderly women. A wide range of conditions predispose to or are characterized by dry eyes. Hypofunction of the lacrimal glands, causing loss of the aqueous component of tears, may be due to aging, hereditary disorders, systemic disease (eg, rheumatoid arthritis and other autoimmune disorders), or systemic and topical drugs. Excessive evaporation of tears may be due to environmental factors (eg, a hot, dry, or windy climate) or abnormalities of the lipid component of the tear film, as in blepharitis. Mucin deficiency may be due to malnutrition, infection, burns, or drugs.

The patient complains of dryness, redness, or a scratchy feeling of the eyes. In severe cases there is persistent marked discomfort, with photophobia, difficulty in moving the eyelids, and often excessive mucus secretion. In many cases, gross examination reveals no abnormality, but on slit lamp examination there are subtle abnormalities of tear film stability and reduced volume of the tear film meniscus along the lower lid. In more severe cases, damaged corneal and conjunctival cells stain with 1% rose bengal. (Rose bengal staining should be avoided in severe

cases because of the intense pain it may cause.) In the most severe cases there is marked conjunctival injection, loss of the normal conjunctival and corneal luster, epithelial keratitis that may progress to frank ulceration, and mucous strands. Schirmer's test, which measures the rate of production of the aqueous component of tears by the amount of wetting of filter paper strips during a 5-minute period, may be helpful when the diagnosis is in doubt, but false-positive and false-negative results are frequent.

Treatment depends upon the cause. In most early cases, the corneal and conjunctival epithelial changes are reversible. Aqueous deficiency can be treated by replacement of the aqueous component of tears with various types of artificial tears. Mucin deficiency can be partially compensated for by the use of ophthalmic vehicles of high molecular weight—eg, water-soluble polymers—or by use of the patient's own serum as local eye drops. Serum used for this purpose must be kept refrigerated at all times. If the mucus is tenacious, mucolytic agents (eg, acetylcysteine, 20%) may provide some relief. Blepharitis should be treated appropriately (see above).

Allergic Conjunctivitis

Hay fever conjunctivitis is a common disorder that is usually chronic and recurrent but benign. It causes bilateral tearing, itching, redness, and a minimal stringy discharge. It is the usual cause of the alarming sudden painless chemosis seen in children. Topical vasoconstrictors and antihistamines are usually effective, but short-term local corticosteroid therapy may be· necessary for severe episodes.

Vernal conjunctivitis is a potentially very disabling form of allergic eye disease, particularly in atopic individuals. There is often seasonal variation. The conjunctivitis is characterized by "cobblestone" papillae on the upper tarsal conjunctiva. Corneal involvement, including refractory ulceration, is frequent during acute exacerbations. The mainstay of treatment is topical corticosteroids, but steroid-induced cataracts and glaucoma are major problems. Sodium cromoglycate drops are generally effective in reducing the severity and frequency of episodes but they must be used as prophylaxis rather than for treatment of acute symptoms.

Vaughan D: Conjunctiva. Chap 5, pp 74–103, in: *General Ophthalmology*, 12th ed. Vaughan D, Asbury T, Tabbara KF (editors). Appleton & Lange, 1989.

PINGUECULA & PTERYGIUM

Pinguecula is a yellow elevated nodule on either side of the cornea (more commonly on the nasal side) in the area of the palpebral fissure. It is common in persons over age 35.

Pterygium is a fleshy, triangular encroachment of

the conjunctiva onto the nasal side of the cornea and is usually associated with constant exposure to wind, sun, sand, and dust. Pterygium may be either unilateral or bilateral. There may be a genetic predisposition, but no hereditary pattern has been described. Pterygium is fairly common in the southwestern USA.

Histologically, pinguecula and pterygium show similar features of which the most important is elastoid degeneration of the conjunctival substantia propria.

Pingueculae rarely grow, but inflammation (pingueculitis) may occur. No treatment is indicated.

Excision of a pterygium is indicated if the growth threatens to interfere with vision by approaching the visual axis. Recurrences are frequent and often more aggressive than the primary lesion. Various forms of treatment are available to reduce the frequency of recurrence.

CORNEAL ULCER

Corneal ulcers are most commonly due to infection, which may involve bacteria, viruses, fungi, or amebas. Noninfectious causes—all of which may be complicated by infection—include neurotrophic keratitis (resulting from loss of corneal sensation), exposure keratitis (due to inadequate eyelid closure), severe dry eyes, severe allergic eye disease, and various inflammatory disorders, that may be purely ocular or part of a systemic vasculitis. These noninfectious conditions will not be discussed further.

Delayed or ineffective treatment of corneal infection may lead to devastating consequences through intraocular infection or corneal scarring. Prompt effective treatment is essential, and for that reason patients must be referred immediately to an ophthalmologist.

Patients present with pain, photophobia, tearing, and reduced vision. The eye is red, with predominantly circumcorneal injection, and there may be purulent or watery discharge. The corneal appearance varies according to the organisms involved, of which the major types will be discussed.

Bacterial Keratitis

Bacterial keratitis tends to pursue an aggressive course. Precipitating factors include corneal trauma—usually caused by a foreign body—and contact lens wear, especially soft contact lenses worn continuously for extended periods. The pathogens most commonly isolated are *Pseudomonas aeruginosa,* pneumococcus, *Moraxella* sp, and staphylococci. The cornea is hazy, with a central ulcer and adjacent stromal abscess. Sterile hypopyon is often present. The ulcer should be scraped to recover material for Gram's stain and culture prior to starting treatment with frequent application of topical antibiotics. Subconjunctival antibiotics may also be used. The choice of antibiotics is usually empirical initially but is subsequently altered according to culture results and response to treatment.

Herpes Simplex Keratitis

Herpes simplex keratitis is an important cause of ocular morbidity, particularly in adults of working age. The ability of the virus to colonize the trigeminal ganglion leads to recurrences that may be precipitated by specifically identifiable forms of stress such as fever and excessive exposure to sunlight.

The dendritic (branching) ulcer is the most characteristic manifestation of epithelial keratitis due to the herpes simplex virus. More extensive (''geographic'') ulcers may also occur, particularly if topical corticosteroids have been used. These ulcers are most easily seen after instillation of sterile fluorescein and examination with a blue light. Epithelial disease in itself does not lead to corneal scarring. It responds well to simple debridement and patching. More rapid healing can be achieved by the addition of topical antivirals such as acyclovir (Zovirax), trifluridine (Viroptic), and idoxuridine (Herplex, Stoxil). Topical corticosteroids must not be used.

Stromal herpes simplex keratitis produces increasingly severe corneal opacity and irregularity with each recurrence. Topical corticosteroids are frequently used in combination with topical antivirals to control stromal disease, but steroid dependence is a common consequence. Corticosteroids may also enhance viral replication, which is most likely to be a problem if there is coexisting epithelial disease. Whether topical antivirals alone are sufficient to fully control stromal disease has yet to be demonstrated. How epithelial and stromal disease are related and what factors influence development of the latter and its frequency of recurrence are as yet unclear. *Caution:* For patients with known or possible herpetic disease, topical corticosteroids should be prescribed only under strict ophthalmologic supervision.

Fungal Keratitis

Fungal keratitis tends to occur after corneal injury involving plant material or in an agricultural setting and in immunocompromised patients. There is often an indolent course. The cornea characteristically has multiple stromal abscesses with relatively little epithelial loss. Intraocular infection is common. Corneal scrapings must be cultured on media suitable for fungi whenever the history or corneal appearance is suggestive of fungal disease.

Acanthamoeba Keratitis

Acanthamoeba has recently become a more commonly recognized cause of suppurative keratitis in contact lens wearers, particularly those who use homemade saline solutions. Severe pain is a characteristic feature. Culture requires specialized media. Treatment is severely hampered by the organism's ability to encyst within the corneal stroma.

Jones DB: *Acanthamoeba:* The ultimate opportunist? (Editorial.) Am J Ophthalmol 1986;102:527.

Smith RE, MacRae SM: Contact lenses: Convenience and complications. (Editorial.) N Engl J Med 1989;321:824.

ORBITAL CELLULITIS

Orbital cellulitis is manifested by an abrupt onset of fever, proptosis, restriction of extraocular movements, and swelling and redness of the lids, usually in a child. Infection of the paranasal sinuses is the usual underlying cause. Immediate treatment with intravenous antibiotics is necessary to prevent optic nerve damage and spread of infection to the cavernous sinuses—manifested as increased restriction of extraocular movements, impaired visual acuity, diminished pupillary reflexes, and papilledema, all of which may be bilateral—meninges, and brain. The response to antibiotics is usually excellent, but abscess formation may necessitate surgical drainage.

ACUTE (ANGLE-CLOSURE) GLAUCOMA

Primary acute angle-closure glaucoma can occur only with closure of a preexisting narrow anterior chamber angle, as is found in elderly persons (owing to physiologic enlargement of the lens), hyperopes, and Asians. About 1% of people over age 35 have narrow anterior chamber angles, but many of these never develop acute glaucoma; thus, the condition is uncommon. Angle closure is associated with pupillary dilatation and thus might occur with sitting in a darkened movie theater, at times of stress (owing to increased circulating epinephrine), and with pharmacologic mydriasis for ophthalmoscopic examination or incidentally with systemic anticholinergic medications such as atropine (eg, preoperative medication). Dilation of the pupil should be undertaken with caution if the anterior chamber is shallow (readily determined by oblique illumination of the anterior segment of the eye). A short-acting mydriatic such as tropicamide should be used and the patient warned to report immediately if ocular discomfort or redness develops. Angle closure is probably more likely to occur if pilocarpine is used to overcome pupillary dilation than if the pupil is allowed to constrict naturally.

Acute angle-closure glaucoma may also occur secondary to long-standing anterior uveitis or dislocation of the lens. Symptoms are the same as in primary acute angle-closure glaucoma, but differentiation is important because of differences in management.

Patients with acute glaucoma usually seek treatment immediately because of extreme pain and blurred vision, though there are subacute cases in which presentation is delayed. The blurred vision is characteristically associated with halos around lights. Nausea and even abdominal pain may occur, and for this reason acute glaucoma must be remembered in the differential diagnosis of abdominal pain and vomiting in elderly patients. The eye is red, the cornea steamy, and the pupil moderately dilated and nonreactive to light. Tonometry (or palpation of the globe) reveals elevated intraocular pressure.

Acute glaucoma must be differentiated from conjunctivitis, acute uveitis, and corneal disorders (Table 5–1).

Untreated acute glaucoma results in severe and permanent visual loss within 2–5 days after onset of symptoms. In primary acute angle-closure glaucoma, laser peripheral iridectomy will usually result in permanent cure. Intraocular pressure must be lowered preoperatively by intravenous and oral acetazolamide, supplemented by osmotic diuretics if necessary, and topical pilocarpine (4%), which also treats the underlying angle closure. Available osmotic agents are intravenous urea and mannitol and oral glycerol, the usual dosage of all 3 being 1.5 g/kg. The fellow eye should be dealt with by prophylactic iridectomy.

In secondary acute angle-closure glaucoma, systemic acetazolamide is also used, with or without osmotic agents, to control intraocular pressure. Further treatment is determined by the underlying pathogenesis.

OPEN-ANGLE GLAUCOMA

Essentials of Diagnosis
- Insidious onset in older age groups.
- No symptoms in early stages.
- Gradual loss of peripheral vision over a period of years, resulting in tunnel vision.
- Persistent elevation of intraocular pressure associated with pathologic cupping of the optic disks.
- "Halos around lights" are not present unless the intraocular tension is markedly elevated.

General Considerations
In open-angle glaucoma, the intraocular pressure is consistently elevated. Over a period of months or years, this results in optic atrophy with loss of vision varying from slight constriction of the upper nasal peripheral fields to complete blindness.

The cause of the decreased rate of aqueous outflow in open-angle glaucoma has not been clearly established. The disease is bilateral and is genetically determined, multifactorial, with no clear inheritance pattern. Glaucoma occurs at an earlier age and more frequently in blacks and may result in more severe optic nerve damage.

In the USA, it is estimated that 1–2% of people over 40 have glaucoma; about 25% of these cases are undetected. About 90% of all cases of glaucoma are of the open-angle type.

Clinical Findings

Patients with open-angle glaucoma have no symptoms initially. On examination, there may be slight cupping of the optic disk. Changes in the retinal nerve fiber layer may be observed as an earlier finding in some patients. The visual fields gradually constrict, but central vision remains good until late in the disease.

Tonometry, ophthalmoscopic visualization of the optic nerve, and central visual field testing are the 3 prime tests for the diagnosis and continued evaluation of glaucoma. The normal intraocular pressure is about 10–21 mm Hg. Except in acute glaucoma, however, the diagnosis is never made on the basis of one tonometric measurement, since various factors can influence the pressure (eg, diurnal variation). Transient elevations of intraocular pressure do not constitute glaucoma (for the same reason that periodic or intermittent elevations of blood pressure do not constitute hypertensive disease). Field testing may prove unreliable in some patients.

Prevention

All persons over age 20 should have tonometric and ophthalmoscopic examinations every 3–5 years. The examination may be performed by a general physician, internist, or ophthalmologist. It is important, however, that ophthalmologic assessment be carried out before treatment is started. If there is a family history of glaucoma, annual examination is indicated.

Treatment

Timolol, a β-adrenergic blocking agent, is an effective antiglaucoma agent in a dosage of 1 drop of 0.25% or 0.5% solution every 12 hours. It should not be used in patients with reactive airway disease or heart failure. Betaxolol (Betoptic) 0.5% and levobunol (Betazan) 0.5%—β_1-receptor selective blocking agents—may be safer in patients with reactive airway disease. Epinephrine eye drops, 0.5–1%, or the prodrug dipivefrin (Propine) 0.1%, is often used instead of or in combination with β-adrenergic blocking agents. Pilocarpine, which has been the standard drug for a century, is still very useful and may be employed along with timolol and epinephrine. Carbonic anhydrase inhibitors (eg, acetazolamide) have been used less commonly since the advent of timolol. When local eye drops are ineffective, laser trabeculoplasty is an effective method of reducing intraocular pressure. Surgical trabeculectomy is necessary for patients whose intraocular pressure remains elevated despite medical and laser therapy and may be used as primary treatment in some individuals.

Prognosis

Untreated chronic glaucoma that begins at age 40– 45 will probably cause complete blindness by age 60–65. Early diagnosis and treatment will preserve useful vision throughout life in most cases.

Hitchings RA: Screening for glaucoma. (Editorial.) Br Med J 1986;292:505.
Quigley HA: Better methods in glaucoma diagnosis. (Editorial.) Arch Ophthalmol 1985;103:186.

UVEITIS

Uveitis means inflammation of the uveal tract, which is formed by the iris (iritis), ciliary body (cyclitis), and choroid (choroiditis). Inflammatory eye disease may, however, also originate primarily in the retina (retinitis) or retinal blood vessels (retinal vasculitis).

Intraocular inflammation is classified as anterior uveitis, posterior uveitis, or panuveitis according to whether inflammatory signs are predominantly present in the anterior or posterior segment of the eye or equally distributed between the two. Uveitis may also be categorized as acute or chronic and granulomatous or nongranulomatous.

Clinical Findings

Anterior uveitis is characterized by inflammatory cells and flare within the aqueous. Cells may also be seen on the corneal endothelium as keratic precipitates (KPs). In granulomatous uveitis, these are large "mutton-fat" KPs, and iris nodules may be seen. In nongranulomatous uveitis, the KPs are smaller and iris nodules are not seen. Occasionally, granulomatous uveitis may initially masquerade as nongranulomatous disease. In severe nongranulomatous anterior uveitis, there may be hypopyon and fibrin within the anterior chamber. In virtually all forms of anterior uveitis, the pupil is small, and with the development of posterior synechiae, it also becomes irregular.

Nongranulomatous anterior uveitis tends to present acutely with unilateral pain, redness, photophobia, and visual loss. Granulomatous anterior uveitis is more likely to present less acutely with blurred vision in a mildly inflamed eye.

In posterior uveitis, there are cells in the vitreous. Inflammatory lesions may be present in the retina or choroid. Fresh lesions are yellow, with indistinct margins, whereas older lesions have more definite margins and are commonly pigmented. Retinal vessel sheathing may occur adjacent to such lesions or more diffusely. In severe cases, vitreous opacity precludes visualization of retinal details.

Posterior uveitis tends to present with gradual visual loss in a relatively quiet eye. Bilateral involvement is common. Visual loss may be due to vitreous haze and opacities, inflammatory lesions involving the macula, macular edema, retinal vein occlusion, or, rarely, associated optic neuropathy.

Etiology

The systemic disorders associated with acute nongranulomatous anterior uveitis are the HLA-B27-related conditions sacroiliitis, ankylosing spondylitis, Reiter's syndrome, psoriasis, ulcerative colitis, and Crohn's disease. Behcset's syndrome produces both anterior uveitis with recurrent hypopyon and posterior uveitis with marked retinal vascular changes. A chronic nongranulomatous anterior uveitis occurs in children with juvenile rheumatoid arthritis, and without periodic screening it may remain undetected. Both herpes simplex and herpes zoster infections may cause nongranulomatous anterior uveitis.

Diseases producing granulomatous anterior uveitis also tend to be causes of posterior uveitis. These include sarcoidosis, which is commonly bilateral; tuberculosis; syphilis; toxoplasmosis; Vogt-Koyanagi-Harada syndrome; and sympathetic ophthalmia. Syphilis produces a characteristic "salt and pepper" fundus, often with surprisingly little visual loss unless there is also primary syphilitic optic atrophy. In congenital toxoplasmosis, there is usually evidence of previous episodes of retinochoroiditis. Leprosy does not affect the posterior segment.

Autoimmune retinal vasculitis and pars planitis (intermediate uveitis) are idiopathic conditions that produce posterior uveitis.

Retinal detachment, intraocular tumors, central nervous system lymphoma, and multiple sclerosis may all masquerade as uveitis.

Evaluation & Treatment

Besides the history and physical examination, investigations may include erythrocyte sedimentation rate, VDRL and FTA-ABS tests, and chest x-ray. PPD skin test and x-rays of sacroiliac joints may also be indicated; serum angiotensin-converting enzyme and serologic tests for toxoplasmosis are of limited use.

Anterior uveitis will usually respond to topical corticosteroids. Occasionally, periocular steroid injections or even systemic steroids may be required. Dilation of the pupil is important to relieve discomfort and prevent posterior synechiae.

Posterior uveitis more commonly requires systemic corticosteroid therapy and occasionally systemic immunosuppression with azathioprine or cyclosporine. Pupillary dilation is not usually necessary.

In all cases if an infective cause is identified, specific chemotherapy may be indicated. In general, the prognosis for anterior uveitis, particularly the nongranulomatous type, is better than that for posterior uveitis.

Management of patients with uveitis must remain primarily in the hands of an ophthalmologist, but the cooperation of other physicians is essential for determining causes and in assisting in the administration of antimicrobials, high-dose systemic corticosteroids, and systemic immunosuppressants.

Henderly DE et al: Changing patterns of uveitis. Am J Ophthalmol 1987;103:131.

Smith RE, Nozik RM: *Uveitis: A Clinical Approach to Diagnosis and Management,* 2nd ed. Williams & Wilkins, 1988.

CATARACT

Essentials of Diagnosis

- Blurred vision, progressive over months or years.
- No pain or redness.
- Lens opacities (may be grossly visible).

General Considerations

A cataract is a lens opacity. Cataracts are usually bilateral. They may be congenital (owing to intrauterine infections such as rubella and cytomegalovirus, inborn errors of metabolism such as galactosemia, or as yet unidentified hereditary factors); traumatic; or secondary to systemic disease (diabetes, myotonic dystrophy, atopic dermatitis), systemic corticosteroid treatment, or uveitis. Senile cataract is by far the most common type; most persons over age 60 have some degree of lens opacity.

Clinical Findings

Even in its early stages, a cataract can be seen through a dilated pupil with an ophthalmoscope, a slit lamp, or an ordinary hand illuminator. As the cataract matures, the retina will become increasingly more difficult to visualize, until finally the fundus reflection is absent. At this point, the pupil is white and the cataract is mature.

The degree of visual loss corresponds to the density of the cataract.

Treatment

Functional visual impairment is the prime criterion for surgery. The cataract is usually removed by one of the techniques in which the delicate posterior lens capsule remains (extracapsular).

Over recent years, it has become routine practice to implant an intraocular lens at the time of surgery. This dispenses with the need for heavy cataract glasses or contact lenses. With modern techniques and improved intraocular lenses, the success rate is high. Intraocular lens implants are generally not suitable for patients with uveitis-associated cataract or those with significant diabetic retinopathy.

Prognosis

If surgery is indicated, lens extraction improves visual acuity in 95% of cases. The remainder either have preexisting retinal damage or develop postoperative complications such as glaucoma, hemorrhage, retinal detachment, or infection.

RETINAL DETACHMENT

Essentials of Diagnosis

- Blurred vision in one eye becoming progressively worse. ("A curtain came down over my eye.")
- No pain or redness.
- Detachment seen by ophthalmoscopy.

General Considerations

Detachment of the retina is usually spontaneous but may be secondary to trauma. Spontaneous detachment occurs most frequently in persons over 50 years of age. Aphakia and myopia are the 2 most common predisposing causes.

Clinical Findings

As soon as the retina is torn, fluid vitreous is able to pass through the tear and lodge behind the sensory retina. This, combined with vitreous traction and the pull of gravity, results in progressive detachment. The superior temporal area is the most common site of detachment. The area of detachment rapidly increases, causing corresponding progressive visual loss. Central vision remains intact until the macula becomes detached.

On ophthalmoscopic examination, the retina is seen hanging in the vitreous like a gray cloud. One or more retinal tears, usually crescent-shaped and red or orange, are usually present and can be seen by an experienced examiner.

Treatment

All cases of retinal detachment should be referred immediately to an ophthalmologist. During transportation, the patient's head should be positioned so that the detached portion of the retina will fall back with the aid of gravity.

Treatment is aimed at closing retinal breaks so as to facilitate reattachment of the retina. Cryotherapy is applied to the sclera in the region of the tear, and an indentation is made in the sclera with a silicone sponge or buckle. Certain cases require drainage of subretinal fluid. Occasionally, removal of vitreous and internal tamponade of the retina with air, expansile gases, or even silicone oil is necessary. (The presence of an expansile gas within the eye is a contraindication to air travel. Such gases may last for a number of weeks from the time of surgery.)

Certain types of uncomplicated retinal detachment are now being treated by the technique of pneumatic retinopexy. The retina is made to reattach by injection of expansile gas into the vitreous cavity, a procedure that can be performed under local anesthesia as an office procedure, followed by careful positioning of the head. Once the retina is reattached, the retinal tear can be sealed by photocoagulation or cryotherapy. The last stage is the same as is used to seal retinal tears without associated detachment as prophylaxis against detachment.

Prognosis

About 80% of uncomplicated cases can be cured with one operation; an additional 15% will need repeated operations; and the remainder never reattach. The prognosis is worse if the macula is detached or if the detachment is of long duration. Without treatment, retinal detachment often becomes total within 6 months. Spontaneous detachments are ultimately bilateral in 2–25% of cases.

Chignell AH: *Retinal Detachment Surgery,* 2nd ed. Springer-Verlag, 1988.
Tornambe PE, Hilton GF: The Retinal Detachment Study Group: Pneumatic retinopexy: A multicentre randomized controlled clinical trial comparing pneumatic retinopexy with scleral buckling. Ophthalmology 1989;96:772.

VITREOUS HEMORRHAGE

Patients with vitreous hemorrhage complain of sudden visual loss, sudden onset of floaters that may progressively increase in severity, or, occasionally, "bleeding within the eye." Visual acuity ranges from 20/20 to light perception only. The eye is not inflamed, and the clue to diagnosis is the inability to see fundal details clearly despite the presence of a clear lens. Causes of vitreous hemorrhage include diabetic retinopathy, retinal tears (with or without retinal detachment), retinal vein occlusions, exudative age-related macular degeneration, blood dyscrasias, and trauma. In all cases, examination by an ophthalmologist is essential. Retinal tears and detachments necessitate urgent treatment (see above).

O'Malley C: Vitreous. Chap 10, pp 154–164, in: *General Ophthalmology,* 12th ed. Vaughan D, Asbury T, Tabbara KF (editors). Appleton & Lange, 1989.

AGE-RELATED MACULAR DEGENERATION

Age-related macular degeneration is the leading cause of permanent visual loss in the elderly. The exact cause is unknown, but the incidence increases with each decade over age 50 (to almost 30% by age 75). Other associations besides age include race (usually white), sex (slight female predominance), family history, and a history of cigarette smoking.

Age-related macular degeneration includes a broad spectrum of clinical and pathologic findings that can be classified into 2 groups: atrophic ("dry") and exudative ("wet"). Although both types are progressive and usually bilateral, they differ in manifestations, prognosis, and management.

Atrophic degeneration is characterized by gradually progressive bilateral visual loss of moderate severity due to atrophy and degeneration of the outer retina, retinal pigment epithelium, Bruch's membrane, and choriocapillaris. In exudative degeneration, visual loss is of more rapid onset and greater severity, and the 2 eyes are usually affected sequentially over a period of a few years. The exudative form accounts for about 90% of all cases of legal blindness due to this disorder. Impairment of the barrier function of Bruch's membrane (between the retinal pigment epithelium and the choriocapillaris) allows serous fluid or blood to leak into the retina to produce elevation of the retinal pigment epithelium from Bruch's membrane (retinal pigment epithelial detachment) or separation of the neurosensory retina from the retinal pigment epithelium (serous retinal detachment). These changes may resolve spontaneously, with variable visual outcome, but are often associated with neovascularization arising from the choroidal vessels and extending between the retinal pigment epithelium and Bruch's membrane (subretinal neovascular membrane). This membrane produces permanent progressive visual loss.

Sudden visual loss in patients with exudative age-related macular degeneration occurs at the time of pigment epithelial or sensory retinal detachment or hemorrhage from a subretinal neovascular membrane. All these changes may occur in previously undiagnosed patients, in patients known to have atrophic changes, and in the other eye of patients with exudative disease. Laser photocoagulation of subretinal neovascular membranes may delay the onset of permanent visual loss but only when the membrane is far enough away from the fovea to permit such treatment. Elderly patients developing sudden visual loss due to macular disease—particularly paracentral distortion or scotoma with preservation of central acuity—should be referred urgently to an ophthalmologist for assessment.

There is no specific treatment for atrophic age-related macular degeneration, but—as with the exudative form—patients often benefit from carefully prescribed low vision aids. It is important to reassure all patients that the disorder results in loss of central vision only. Peripheral fields and hence navigational vision are always maintained, though these may become impaired by cataract formation for which surgery may well be helpful.

Bressler NM, Bressler SB, Fine SL: Age-related macular degeneration. Surv Ophthalmol 1988;32:375.

CENTRAL & BRANCH RETINAL VEIN OCCLUSIONS

The severity of visual loss in central retinal vein occlusion is variable. Younger patients may present with near-normal acuity. Older patients present with acuities ranging from 20/40 to hand movements only. The visual impairment is commonly first noticed upon waking in the morning. Ophthalmoscopic signs include disk swelling, venous dilatation and tortuosity, retinal hemorrhages, and cotton-wool spots.

In those with initially good acuity (20/60 or better), the visual prognosis is good. In those with poor initial acuity (20/200 or worse), extensive hemorrhages and multiple cotton-wool spots indicate widespread retinal ischemia, which can be confirmed by demonstrating extensive areas of capillary closure on fluorescein angiography. These eyes are at high risk of developing neovascular (rubeotic) glaucoma, typically within 3 months after venous occlusion, and should be considered for prophylactic laser panretinal photocoagulation. The visual prognosis in these cases is poor.

Branch retinal vein occlusions may present in a variety of ways. Sudden loss of vision may occur at the time of occlusion if the fovea is involved or some time afterward from vitreous hemorrhage due to retinal new vessels. More gradual visual loss may occur with development of macular edema or exudate. In a significant proportion, the occlusion is noted incidentally in patients with glaucoma, systemic hypertension, diabetes mellitus, or uveitis.

In acute branch retinal vein occlusion there are signs similar to those of central retinal vein occlusion but affecting only the retina drained by the obstructed vein. There is no specific treatment, but if retinal neovascularization develops, the area of retina affected by the initial occlusion should be laser-photocoagulated. Macular edema may also respond to laser treatment.

All patients with retinal vein occlusion should be referred urgently to an ophthalmologist for confirmation of the diagnosis and further management. It is important to look for glaucoma, systemic hypertension, diabetes mellitus, and hyperlipidemia. Hyperviscosity syndromes and other hematologic abnormalities are only rarely associated with retinal vein occlusions but may worsen their prognosis. Branch retinal vein occlusion is an important feature of Behçet's syndrome.

CENTRAL & BRANCH RETINAL ARTERY OCCLUSIONS

Central retinal artery occlusion presents as sudden profound visual loss. Visual acuity is reduced to counting fingers or worse, and visual field is commonly restricted to an island of vision in the temporal field. Ophthalmoscopy reveals pallid swelling of the retina, most obvious in the posterior segment, with a cherry-red spot at the fovea. The retinal arteries are attenuated, and "box-car" segmentation of blood in the veins may be seen. Occasionally, emboli are seen in the central retinal artery or its branches. The retinal swelling subsides over a period of 4–6 weeks, leaving a relatively normal retinal appearance but a pale optic disk and attenuated arterioles.

The patient should be referred as an emergency

to an ophthalmologist. If seen within a few hours after onset, emergency treatment—including laying the patient flat, ocular massage, high concentrations of inhaled oxygen, intravenous acetazolamide, and anterior chamber paracentesis—may influence the visual outcome.

The main management problem is identifying any treatable underlying disorder. Giant cell arteritis must be excluded in all older patients, especially because of the risk—highest in the first few days—of involvement of the other eye. If giant cell arteritis is diagnosed, either on the basis of associated symptoms (especially headache or polymyalgia), clinical signs, or a high erythrocyte sedimentation rate, high-dose systemic corticosteroids must be started immediately. Carotid and cardiac sources of emboli must be identified and appropriate treatment given to reduce the risk of stroke. Risk factors for atherosclerosis, including systemic hypertension, diabetes mellitus, hyperlipidemia, and smoking should be identified and managed appropriately.

Branch retinal artery occlusion may also present with sudden loss of vision if the fovea is involved, but more commonly sudden loss of visual field is the presenting complaint. Fundal signs of retinal swelling and adjacent cotton-wool spots are limited to the area of retina supplied by the occluded vessel. Embolic causes are proportionately more common than in central retinal artery occlusion. Migraine, oral contraceptives, and vasculitis must also be considered. Patients with branch retinal artery occlusions should be referred urgently to an ophthalmologist.

AMAUROSIS FUGAX

Amaurosis fugax ("fleeting blindness") is characteristically caused by retinal emboli from ipsilateral carotid disease. The visual loss is usually described as a curtain passing vertically across the visual field with complete monocular visual loss lasting a few minutes and a similar curtain effect as the episode passes. These patients should be investigated to ascertain their suitability for carotid endarterectomy or medical treatment (with aspirin or other antiplatelet drugs) to reduce the risk of stroke. Emboli from cardiac sources may also be responsible. Early ophthalmologic consultation is advisable to ratify the diagnosis.

Similar obscurations of vision may occur with poor ocular perfusion due to severe occlusive carotid disease. More transient obscurations (lasting only a few seconds to 1 minute) affecting both eyes occur in patients with raised intracranial pressure.

Callow AD et al: Carotid endarterectomy: What is its current status? Am J Med 1988;85:835.

RETINAL DISORDERS ASSOCIATED WITH SYSTEMIC DISEASES

Many systemic diseases are associated with retinal manifestations. These include diabetes mellitus, essential hypertension, preeclampsia-eclampsia of pregnancy, blood dyscrasias, and AIDS. The retinal changes caused by these disorders can be easily observed with the aid of the ophthalmoscope.

Diabetic Retinopathy

Diabetic retinopathy is the leading cause of new blindness among US adults aged 20–65. It is broadly classified as proliferative and nonproliferative.

Nonproliferative retinopathy is characterized by dilatation of veins, microaneurysms, retinal hemorrhages, retinal edema, and hard exudates. A major subgroup are those patients in which visual loss develops owing to edema, ischemia, or exudates at the macula (diabetic maculopathy). This is the most common cause of legal blindness in maturity-onset diabetes.

Proliferative retinopathy is characterized by neovascularization, arising either from the optic disk or the major vascular arcades. Vitreous hemorrhage is a common sequela. Proliferation into the vitreous of blood vessels, with their associated fibrous component, leads to tractional retinal detachment. Without treatment, the visual prognosis with proliferative retinopathy is generally much worse than that with nonproliferative retinopathy. Severe proliferative retinopathy is often complicated by maculopathy.

Nonproliferative retinopathy is present at the time of diagnosis in a significant number of maturity-onset diabetics and may be the presenting feature. Treatment is focused on optimizing control of blood glucose and any associated systemic hypertension. Regular assessment of visual acuity and fundal examination are essential for the detection of macular changes. As soon as there is a decline in acuity or the fovea is seen to be threatened by exudates, the patient should be referred to an ophthalmologist. Laser photocoagulation is helpful in treating macular exudates. Maculopathy due to ischemia or edema is assessed by fluorescein angiography. Laser treatment may be helpful.

It is essential that proliferative retinopathy be recognized early and treated by panretinal laser photocoagulation to prevent blindness. Unfortunately, the presence of neovascularization is all too often diagnosed only at the time of vitreous hemorrhage. In some patients, a "preproliferative" retinopathy—characterized as nonproliferative retinopathy complicated by multiple cotton-wool spots and gross venous abnormalities—may be identified. Whether panretinal laser photocoagulation should be undertaken at this time is currently under investigation. Fluorescein angiography is helpful in determining the degree of retinal ischemia in these patients and deciding whether neovascularization is indeed present when clinical findings are equivocal.

Surgical treatment (vitrectomy) is being used increasingly in the treatment of severe proliferative retinopathy, either to remove vitreous hemorrhage or to deal with retinal detachments involving the macula.

Patients with diabetes mellitus should have at least yearly ophthalmoscopic examination through dilated pupils. Examination by an ophthalmologist is usually advisable in juvenile-onset diabetes of more than 5 years' duration; at the time of diagnosis in maturity-onset diabetes; if ocular symptoms develop; or if there are suspicious findings of retinopathy, especially neovascularization or macular exudates. Failure to diagnose diabetic retinopathy by ophthalmoscopic examination is common, particularly if the pupils are not dilated. Many clinicians believe that the severity of diabetic retinopathy can be lessened by careful control of blood glucose levels. It is probable that good diabetic control is most important in preventing the development of retinopathy rather than influencing its subsequent course.

Klein R: Recent developments in the understanding and management of diabetic retinopathy. Med Clin North Am 1988;72:1415.

Hypertensive Retinopathy

One method of classifying hypertensive retinopathy (modified after Keith and Wagener) is shown in Table 5–2.

Preeclampsia-eclampsia is manifested in the retina as rapidly progressive hypertensive retinopathy, and extensive permanent retinal damage may occur if the pregnancy is not terminated. Occasionally, the choroidal circulation is mainly affected, leading to infarction of the retinal pigment epithelium.

Blood Dyscrasias

In blood dyscrasias characterized by thrombocytopenia and severe anemia, various types of hemorrhages are present in both the retina and choroid and may lead to visual loss. If the underlying dyscrasia is successfully treated and macular hemorrhages have not occurred, it is possible to regain normal vision.

Proliferative retinopathy (sickle cell retinopathy) is particularly common in hemoglobin SC disease but may also occur with other hemoglobin S variants. Severe visual loss is rare, and retinal photocoagulation, although it reverses the retinal abnormalities, does not affect the long-term outcome in terms of visual acuity or frequency of vitreous hemorrhage.

AIDS

Cotton-wool spots, retinal hemorrhages, and microaneurysms are the most common ophthalmic abnormalities in AIDS patients. (Cotton-wool spots are also seen in patients with AIDS-related complex [ARC].) These microvascular changes have no prognostic significance. They may arise from direct retinal infection by HIV or from deposition of circulating immune complexes.

Cytomegalovirus retinopathy occurs in many AIDS patients. It is characterized by progressively enlarging yellowish-white patches of retinal opacification, which are accompanied by retinal hemorrhages; they usually begin adjacent to the major retinal vascular arcades. Patients are often asymptomatic until there is involvement of the fovea or optic nerve or until retinal detachment develops.

Ganciclovir has been shown to be useful in the management of cytomegalovirus retinopathy in patients with AIDS. Unfortunately, progression of the disease is common even when maintenance therapy is used. Ganciclovir must be administered intravenously and commonly causes bone marrow suppression.

Other opportunistic ophthalmic infections occurring in AIDS patients include herpes simplex retinitis, toxoplasmic and candidal chorioretinitis, and herpes zoster ophthalmicus. Kaposi's sarcoma of the conjunctiva and orbital lymphoma may also be seen. Central nervous system involvement by primary HIV infection, opportunistic infections, and intracranial neoplasms may produce a variety of neuro-ophthalmologic abnormalities.

Jabs DA et al: Ocular manifestations of acquired immune deficiency syndrome. Ophthalmology 1989;96:1092.
Kreiger AE, Holland GN: Ocular involvement in AIDS. Eye 1988;2:496.

Table 5–2. A classification of hypertensive retinopathy. (Modified after Keith and Wagener.)

Stage	Ophthalmoscopic Appearance	Clinical Classification
I	Minimal narrowing or sclerosis of arterioles.	"Essential" hypertension (chronic, benign, "arteriosclerotic").
II	Thickening and dulling of vessel reflection (copper wire appearance). Localized and generalized narrowing of arterioles. Changes at arteriovenous crossings (A-V nicking). Scattered tiny round or flame-shaped hemorrhages. Vascular occlusion may be present.	
III	Sclerotic changes may not be marked. "Angiospastic retinopathy": localized arteriolar spasm, hemorrhages, exudates, "cotton-wool patches," retinal edema.	Malignant hypertensive retinopathy.
IV	Same as III, plus optic disk swelling.	

ANTERIOR ISCHEMIC OPTIC NEUROPATHY

Anterior ischemic optic neuropathy—due to occlusion of the posterior ciliary arteries that supply the anterior portion of the optic disk—produces sudden visual loss, usually with an altitudinal field defect, and optic disk swelling. In older patients, it is often caused by giant cell arteritis, which is treated with high-dose systemic corticosteroids. In all other patients, systemic hypertension, arteriosclerosis, systemic lupus erythematosus, and polyarteritis nodosa should be considered. Urgent ophthalmologic consultation should be arranged. There is a significant risk of subsequent involvement of the fellow eye.

Hayreh SS: Anterior ischaemic optic neuropathy: Differentiation of arteritis from non-arteritis type and its management. Eye 1990;4:25.
Mehler MF, Rabinowich L: The clinical neuro-ophthalmologic spectrum of temporal arteritis. Am J Med 1988;85:839.

OPTIC NEURITIS

Optic neuritis is characterized by unilateral loss of vision which usually develops suddenly and may increase during the following few days. At its worst, the level of vision may vary from 20/30 to no perception of light. Visual acuity often then improves within 2–3 weeks and may return to normal. Commonly there is pain in the region of the eye, particularly on eye movements. Field loss is usually a central scotoma, but a wide range of monocular field defects are possible. There is marked loss of color vision and a relative afferent pupillary defect. The optic disk may be swollen, with occasional flame-shaped peripapillary hemorrhages. (In retrobulbar optic neuritis, the optic disk is normal.) In all forms of optic neuritis, optic atrophy subsequently develops if there has been destruction of sufficient optic nerve fibers.

Demyelination, particularly that due to multiple sclerosis, is a frequent cause of optic neuritis. Optic neuritis may also occur in association with viral infections, including measles, mumps, influenza, and those caused by the varicella-zoster virus and by spread of inflammation from meninges, orbital tissues, or paranasal sinuses.

All patients with "idiopathic" optic neuritis should be assessed for symptoms and signs of previously undiagnosed episodes of demyelination. Cerebrospinal fluid oligoclonal bands and evoked potentials may also be helpful in establishing a diagnosis of multiple sclerosis. Magnetic resonance imaging will reveal multiple white matter lesions in the brains of many patients with truly isolated optic neuritis. However, this does not establish a diagnosis of multiple sclerosis—a diagnosis that should be deferred until develop-

ment of further clinical evidence, which will indeed occur in the majority of such patients.

Systemic steroids may accelerate the rate of recovery in optic neuritis due to demyelination and in idiopathic cases. A favorable influence on the eventual visual outcome has not yet been proved, though a major study is currently being undertaken. Whether systemic steroids are to be used in an individual patient should be determined by the degree of visual loss, the state of the other eye, and the patient's visual requirements. Optic neuritis due to herpes zoster necessitates systemic steroid treatment. All patients with optic neuritis should be referred urgently for neuro-ophthalmologic assessment.

Francis DA et al: A reassessment of the risk of multiple sclerosis developing in patients with optic neuritis after extended follow-up. J Neurol Neurosurg Psychiatry 1987;50:758.
Rizzo JF, Lessell S: Risk of developing multiple sclerosis after uncomplicated optic neuritis: A long-term prospective study. Neurology 1988;38:185.

OPTIC DISK SWELLING

Optic disk swelling may result from intraocular disease, orbital and optic nerve lesions, systemic hypertension (grade IV retinopathy), or raised intracranial pressure. Intraocular causes include central retinal vein occlusion, posterior uveitis, and posterior scleritis. Optic nerve lesions causing disk swelling include optic neuritis, anterior ischemic optic neuropathy; optic disk drusen (pseudopapilledema); optic nerve sheath meningioma; and optic nerve infiltration by sarcoidosis, leukemia, or lymphoma. Any orbital lesion causing optic nerve compression may produce disk swelling.

Papilledema (optic disk swelling due to raised intracranial pressure) is usually bilateral and produces enlargement of the blind spot without loss of acuity. Optic neuritis causes visual loss, usually with a central scotoma; loss of color vision; and a relative afferent pupillary defect. Anterior ischemic optic neuropathy is usually associated with an altitudinal field defect.

Optic disk drusen are a major source of confusion. Recognizing their presence may avoid much needless investigation. Optic disk drusen should be considered when disk swelling is not associated with any visual disturbance or symptoms of raised intracranial pressure. Exposed optic disk drusen may be obvious clinically or can be demonstrated by their autofluorescence. Buried or exposed drusen are best detected by CT scanning. Other family members may be similarly affected.

OCULAR MOTOR PALSIES

In complete third nerve paralysis, there is complete ptosis and the eye is divergent and slightly depressed.

Extraocular movements are restricted in all directions except laterally (preserved lateral rectus function). Intact fourth nerve (superior oblique) function is detected by the presence of inward rotation on attempted depression of the eye.

Pupillary involvement (dilated pupil that does not react to accommodation or to light shined in either eye) is an important sign differentiating "surgical" from "medical" causes of isolated third nerve palsy. (Compressive lesions of the third nerve, such as aneurysm of the posterior communicating artery and uncal herniation due to a supratentorial mass lesion, characteristically have pupillary involvement.) It is crucial that patients presenting with isolated third nerve palsy with pupillary involvement be assumed to have a posterior communicating artery aneurysm until this has been excluded by cerebral arteriography—and thus they should be referred immediately for neuro-ophthalmologic assessment. Medical causes of isolated third nerve palsy include diabetes, systemic hypertension, syphilis, and giant cell arteritis.

Fourth nerve paralysis causes upward deviation of the eye with failure of depression on adduction. There is vertical diplopia that becomes most apparent on attempted reading and descending stairs. Many cases of isolated fourth nerve palsy are due to decompensation of a congenital lesion. Trauma is a major cause of acquired—particularly bilateral—fourth nerve palsy, but cerebral neoplasms and medical causes such as in third nerve palsies should also be considered.

Sixth nerve paralysis causes convergent squint in the primary position with failure of abduction of the affected eye, producing horizontal diplopia that increases on gaze to the affected side. It is an important sign of raised intracranial pressure, particularly in children. Sixth nerve palsy may also be due to trauma, neoplasms, brain stem lesions, or medical causes (see above).

Any patient presenting with an isolated ocular motor palsy must be investigated to exclude an intracranial or intraorbital mass lesion. In all patients with isolated ocular motor nerve palsies presumed to be due to medical causes, such investigations should be repeated if recovery has not begun within 3 months.

Ocular motor nerve palsies occurring in association with other neurologic signs may be due to lesions in the brain stem, around the cavernous sinus, or in the orbit. Lesions around the cavernous sinus involve the upper divisions of the trigeminal nerve, the ocular motor nerves, and occasionally the optic chiasm. Orbital apex lesions involve the optic nerve and the ocular motor nerves.

Myasthenia and dysthyroid eye disease must always be considered in the differential diagnosis of disordered extraocular movements.

OCULAR TRAUMA

Conjunctival & Corneal Foreign Bodies

If a patient complains of "something in my eye" and gives a consistent history, a foreign body is usually present on the cornea or under the upper lid even though it may not be readily visible. Visual acuity should be tested before treatment is instituted, as a basis for comparison in the event of complications.

After a local anesthetic is instilled, the eye is examined with the aid of a hand flashlight, using oblique illumination, and loupe. Corneal foreign bodies may be made more apparent by the instillation of sterile fluorescein. They are then removed with a sterile wet cotton-tipped applicator. Antibiotic ointment should be instilled. It is not necessary to patch the eye, but the patient must be examined 24 hours later for secondary infection of the crater. If a corneal foreign body cannot be removed in this manner, the patient should be referred to an ophthalmologist.

Steel foreign bodies usually leave a diffuse rust ring. This requires excision of the affected tissue and is best done under local anesthesia using a slit lamp. *Caution:* Anesthetic drops should not be given to the patient for self-administration.

If there is no infection, a layer of corneal epithelial cells will line the crater within 24 hours. It should be emphasized that the intact corneal epithelium forms an effective barrier to infection, but once it is disturbed it becomes extremely susceptible to infection. Early infection is manifested by a white necrotic area around the crater and a small amount of gray exudate. These patients should be referred immediately to an ophthalmologist, since untreated corneal infection may lead to severe corneal ulceration, panophthalmitis, and loss of the eye.

In the case of a foreign body under the upper lid, a local anesthetic is instilled and the lid is everted by grasping the lashes gently and exerting pressure on the mid portion of the outer surface of the upper lid with an applicator. If a foreign body is present, it can easily be removed by passing a wet sterile cotton-tipped applicator across the conjunctival surface.

Intraocular Foreign Body

Intraocular foreign body requires emergency treatment by an ophthalmologist. Patients giving a history of "something hitting the eye"—particularly if it happens while hammering on metal or using grinding equipment—must be carefully assessed for the possibility of an intraocular foreign body, especially when no corneal foreign body is seen, a corneal or scleral wound is apparent, or there is marked visual loss or media opacity. Such patients must be treated as for corneal laceration (see below) and referred without delay to an ophthalmologist.

Corneal Abrasions

A patient with a corneal abrasion complains of severe pain and photophobia. There is often a history of trauma to the eye, commonly involving a fingernail or piece of paper. Visual acuity is recorded, and the cornea and conjunctiva are examined with a light and loupe to rule out a foreign body. If an abrasion is suspected but cannot be seen, sterile fluorescein is instilled into the conjunctival sac: the area of corneal abrasion will stain a deeper green than the surrounding cornea.

Treatment includes antibiotic ointment and application of a bandage with firm pressure to prevent movement of the lid. The patient should rest at home, keeping the fellow eye closed, and should be observed the following day to be certain the cornea has healed. Recurrent corneal erosion may follow corneal abrasions.

Contusions

Contusion injuries of the eye and surrounding structures may cause ecchymosis ("black eye"), subconjunctival hemorrhage, edema or rupture of the cornea, hemorrhage into the anterior chamber (hyphema), rupture of the root of the iris (iridodialysis), paralysis of the pupillary sphincter, paralysis of the muscles of accommodation, cataract, subluxation or luxation of the lens, vitreous hemorrhage, retinal hemorrhage and edema (most common in the macular area), detachment of the retina, rupture of the choroid, fracture of the orbital floor ("blowout fracture"), or optic nerve injury. Many of these injuries are immediately obvious; others may not become apparent for days or weeks. Patients with moderate to severe contusions should be seen by an ophthalmologist.

Any injury severe enough to cause hyphema involves the danger of secondary hemorrhage, which may cause intractable glaucoma with permanent visual loss. Any patient with traumatic hyphema should be advised to rest quietly until complete resolution has occurred. Daily ophthalmologic assessment is essential. Aspirin and related drugs increase the risk of secondary hemorrhage and must be avoided.

Affeldt JC et al: Microbial endophthalmitis resulting from ocular trauma. Ophthalmology 1987;94:407.
Schein OD et al: The spectrum and burden of ocular injury. Ophthalmology 1988;95:300.

Lacerations

A. Lids: If the lid margin is lacerated, the patient should be referred for specialized care, since permanent notching may result. Lacerations of the lower eyelid near the inner canthus often sever the lower canaliculus. Lid lacerations not involving the margin may be sutured just like any other skin laceration.

B. Conjunctiva: In superficial lacerations of the conjunctiva, sutures are not necessary. In order to prevent infection, sulfonamides or other antibiotics are instilled into the eye until the laceration is healed.

C. Cornea or Sclera: Patients with suspected corneal or scleral lacerations must be seen by an ophthalmologist as soon as possible. Manipulation is kept to a minimum, since pressure may result in extrusion of the intraocular contents. The eye is bandaged lightly and covered with a metal shield that rests on the orbital bones above and below. The patient should be instructed not to squeeze the eye shut and to remain as quiet as possible. The eye is routinely studied radiographically to exclude the presence of foreign bodies.

Ultraviolet Keratitis (Actinic Keratitis)

Ultraviolet burns of the cornea are usually caused by use of a sunlamp without eye protection, exposure to a welding arc, or exposure to the sun when skiing ("snow blindness"). There are no immediate symptoms, but about 6–12 hours later the patient complains of agonizing pain and severe photophobia. Slit lamp examination after instillation of sterile fluorescein shows diffuse punctate staining of both corneas.

Treatment consists of binocular patching and instillation of cycloplegic agents. All patients recover within 24–48 hours without complications. Local anesthetics should not be prescribed.

Chemical Conjunctivitis & Keratitis

Chemical burns are treated by irrigation of the eyes with saline solution or plain water as soon as possible after exposure. Neutralization of an acid with an alkali or vice versa generates heat and may cause further damage. Alkali injuries are more serious and require prolonged irrigation, since alkalies are not precipitated by the proteins of the eye as are acids. It is important to remove any retained particulate matter such as is typically present in injuries involving cement and building plaster. This may require double eversion of the upper lid. The pupil should be dilated with 0.2% scopolamine or 2% atropine to relieve discomfort and prophylactic topical antibiotics should be started. In moderate to severe injuries, intensive topical corticosteroids and topical and systemic vitamin C are also necessary. Complications include mucus deficiency, scarring of the cornea and conjunctiva, symblepharon, tear duct obstruction, and secondary infection.

Morgan SJ: Chemical burns of the eye: Causes and management. Br J Ophthalmol 1987;71:854.

PRINCIPLES OF TREATMENT OF OCULAR INFECTIONS

Before one can determine the drug of choice, the causative organisms must be identified, but in most instances empirical treatment, based on clinical experience, is used in the first instance. In the treatment of conjunctivitis and for prophylaxis against ocular infection, it is preferable to use a drug that is not given systemically. Of the available local antibacterial agents, the sulfonamides are effective and inexpensive. Two reliable sulfonamides for ophthalmic use are sulfisoxazole and sodium sulfacetamide. The sulfonamides have the added advantages of low allergenicity and effectiveness against the chlamydial group of organisms. They are available in ointment or solution form. Combined bacitracin-polymyxin ointment is often used prophylactically after corneal foreign body removal for the protection it affords against both gram-positive and gram-negative organisms.

Among the most effective broad-spectrum antibiotics for ophthalmic use are gentamicin, tobramycin, and neomycin. These drugs have some effect against gram-negative as well as gram-positive organisms but are generally not effective against the pneumococcus. Allergic reactions to neomycin are common. Other antibiotics frequently used are erythromycin, the tetracyclines, and the cephalosporins.

Method of Administration

Most ocular anti-infective drugs are administered locally. Ointments have greater therapeutic effectiveness than solutions, since contact can be maintained longer. However, they do cause blurring of vision; if this must be avoided, solutions should be used.

Systemic administration is required for all intraocular infections, orbital cellulitis, dacryocystitis, gonococcal keratoconjunctivitis, inclusion conjunctivitis, and severe external infection that does not respond to local treatment.

TECHNIQUES USED IN THE TREATMENT OF OCULAR DISORDERS

Instilling Medications

The patient is placed in a chair with head tilted back, both eyes open, and looking up. The lower lid is retracted slightly, and 2 drops of liquid are instilled into the lower cul-de-sac. The patient looks down while finger contact is maintained, so that the eyes are not squeezed shut. Ointments are instilled in the same general manner.

For self-medication, the same techniques are used except that medications are usually better instilled with the patient lying down.

Eye Bandage

Most eye bandages should be applied firmly enough to hold the lid securely against the cornea. An ordinary patch consisting of gauze-covered cotton is usually sufficient. Tape is applied from the cheek to the forehead.

PRECAUTIONS IN MANAGEMENT OF OCULAR DISORDERS

Use of Local Anesthetics

Unsupervised self-administration of local anesthetics is dangerous because the patient may further injure an anesthetized eye without knowing it. The drug may also prevent the normal healing process.

Pupillary Dilation

Dilating the pupil can very occasionally precipitate an acute glaucoma attack if the patient has a narrow anterior chamber angle. Dilation of the pupil should still be undertaken, but with caution if the anterior chamber is obviously shallow (readily determined by oblique illumination of the anterior segment of the eye). A short-acting mydriatic such as tropicamide should be used and the patient warned to report immediately if ocular discomfort or redness develops. Angle closure is probably more likely to occur if pilocarpine is used to overcome pupillary dilatation than if the pupil is allowed to constrict naturally.

Local Corticosteroid Therapy

Repeated use of local corticosteroids presents several hazards: herpes simplex (dendritic) keratitis, fungal infection, open-angle glaucoma, and cataract formation. Furthermore, perforation of the cornea may occur when the corticosteroids are used for herpes simplex keratitis.

Contaminated Eye Medications

Ophthalmic solutions are prepared with the same degree of care as fluids intended for intravenous administration, but once bottles are opened there is always a risk of contamination, particularly with solutions of tetracaine, proparacaine, and fluorescein. The most dangerous is fluorescein, as this solution is frequently contaminated with P aeruginosa, an organism that can rapidly destroy the eye. Sterile fluorescein filter paper strips are now available and are recommended for use in place of fluorescein solutions.

Whether in plastic or glass containers, eye solutions should not remain in use for long periods after the bottle is opened. Two weeks after opening is a reasonable maximal time to use a solution before discarding. Any solution should of course be checked for signs of bacterial contamination prior to use.

If the eye has been injured accidentally or by surgical trauma, it is of the greatest importance to use freshly opened bottles of sterile medications or single-use eyedropper units.

Toxic & Hypersensitivity Reactions to Topical Therapy

Patients receiving long-term topical therapy may develop local toxic or hypersensitivity reactions to the active agent or preservatives, especially if there

Table 5–3. Adverse ocular effects of systemic drugs.

Drug	Possible Side Effects
Respiratory agents	
Oxygen	Retinopathy of prematurity.
Cardiovascular system drugs	
Digitalis	Disturbances of color vision, blurring of vision, scotomas.
Quinidine	Toxic amblyopia.
Thiazides (Diuril, etc)	Xanthopsia (yellow vision), myopia.
Carbonic anhydrase inhibitors (acetazolamide)	Ocular hypotony, transient myopia.
Amiodarone	Corneal deposits.
Oxyprenolol	Photophobia, ocular irritation.
Gastrointestinal drugs	
Anticholinergic agents	Risk of angle-closure glaucoma due to mydriasis. Blurring of vision due to cycloplegia (occasional).
Central nervous system drugs	
Barbiturates	Extraocular muscle palsies with diplopia, ptosis, cortical blindness.
Chloral hydrate	Diplopia, ptosis, miosis.
Phenothiazines	Toxic amblyopia, deposits of pigment in conjunctiva, cornea, lens, and retina. Oculogyric crises.
Amphetamines	Widening of palpebral fissure. Dilatation of pupil, paralysis of ciliary muscle with loss of accommodation.
Monoamine oxidase inhibitors	Nystagmus, extraocular muscle palsies, amblyopia (toxic).
Tricyclic agents	Dilatation of pupil (risk of angle-closure glaucoma), cycloplegia.
Phenytoin	Nystagmus, diplopia, ptosis, slight blurring of vision (rare).
Neostigmine	Nystagmus, miosis.
Morphine	Miosis.
Haloperidol	Capsular cataract.
Lithium carbonate	Exophthalmos, oculogyric crisis.
Diazepam	Nystagmus, allergic conjunctivitis.
Hormones	
Corticosteroids	Cataract (posterior subcapsular), local immunologic suppression causing susceptibility to viral (herpesvirus hominis), bacterial, and fungal infections; steroid-induced glaucoma.
Female sex hormones	Retinal artery thrombosis, retinal vein thrombosis, papilledema, ocular palsies with diplopia, nystagmus, optic neuritis and atrophy, retinal vasculitis, scotomas, migraine, mydriasis and cycloplegia, and macular edema.
Antibiotics	
Chloramphenicol	Optic neuritis and atrophy and aplastic anemia. Toxic amblyopia (rare).
Streptomycin	Toxic amblyopia (rare).
Tetracycline	Pseudotumor cerebri, transient myopia.
Antimalarial agents	
Eg, chloroquine	Macular changes, central scotomas, pigmentary degeneration of the retina, chloroquine keratopathy, ocular palsies, ptosis, ERG depression.
Amebicides	
Iodochlorhydroxyquin	Optic atrophy.
Chemotherapeutic agents	
Sulfonamides	Stevens-Johnson syndrome. Toxic amblyopia (rare).
Ethambutol	Toxic amblyopia, optic neuritis and atrophy.
Isoniazid	Toxic amblyopia, optic neuritis and atrophy.
Aminosalicylic acid	Toxic amblyopia.
Heavy metals	
Gold salts	Deposits in the cornea and conjunctiva.
Lead compounds	Toxic amblyopia, papilledema, ocular palsies.
Chelating agents	
Penicillamine	Ocular pemphigoid, optic neuritis, ocular myasthenia.
Oral hypoglycemic agents	
Chlorpropamide	Transient change in refractive error, toxic amblyopia, diplopia.
Vitamins	
Vitamin A	Papilledema, retinal hemorrhages, loss of eyebrows and eyelashes, nystagmus, diplopia, blurring of vision.
Vitamin D	Band-shaped keratopathy.
Antirheumatic agents	
Salicylates	Toxic amblyopia, cortical blindness (rare).
Indomethacin	Corneal deposits, toxic amblyopia, diplopia, retinal changes.
Phenylbutazone	Toxic amblyopia, retinal hemorrhages.

is inadequate tear secretion. Preservatives in contact lens cleaning solutions may produce similar problems. Burning and soreness are exacerbated by drop instillation or contact lens insertion; occasionally, fibrosis and scarring of the conjunctiva and cornea may occur.

An antibiotic instilled into the eye can sensitize the patient to that drug and cause a hypersensitivity reaction upon subsequent systemic administration.

Systemic Effects of Ocular Drugs

The systemic absorption of certain topical drugs (through the conjunctival vessels and lacrimal drainage system) must be considered when there is a systemic medical contraindication to the use of the drug. Ophthalmic solutions of the beta-blocker timolol (Timoptic) may worsen patients with cardiac failure or asthma. Atropine ointment should be prescribed for children rather than the drops, since absorption of the 1% topical solution may be toxic. Phenylephrine

eye drops can precipitate hypertensive crises and angina. Also to be considered are adverse interactions between systemically administered and ocular drugs. Using only 1 or 2 drops at a time and a few minutes of nasolacrimal occlusion or eyelid closure ensure maximum efficacy and decrease systemic side effects of topical agents.

ADVERSE OCULAR EFFECTS OF SYSTEMIC DRUGS

Systemically administered drugs produce a wide variety of adverse effects on the visual system. Table 5–3 lists the major examples.

Fraunfelder FT, Mayer SM: Ocular and systemic side effects of drugs. Pages 407–410 in: *General Ophthalmology,* 12th ed. Vaughan D, Asbury T, Tabbara KF (editors). Appleton & Lange, 1989.

REFERENCES

Ellis PP: Commonly used eye medications. Chap 26, pp 399–411, in: *General Ophthalmology,* 12th ed. Vaughan D, Asbury T, Tabbara KF (editors). Appleton & Lange, 1989. Vaughan D, Asbury T, Tabbara KF

(editors): *General Ophthalmology,* 12th ed. Appleton & Lange, 1989.
Zun LS: Acute visual loss. Emerg Med Clin North Am 1988;6:57.

6

Ear, Nose, & Throat

Robert K. Jackler, MD, & Michael J. Kaplan, MD

DISEASES OF THE EAR

HEARING LOSS

Classification

A. Conductive Hearing Loss: Conductive hearing loss results from dysfunction of the external or middle ear. There are 4 mechanisms, each resulting in impairment of the passage of sound vibrations to the inner ear: (1) obstruction (eg, cerumen impaction), (2) mass loading (eg, middle ear effusion), (3) stiffness effect (eg, otosclerosis), and (4) discontinuity (eg, ossicular disruption). Conductive hearing loss is generally correctable with medical or surgical therapy—or in some cases both.

B. Sensory Hearing Loss: Sensory hearing loss results from deterioration of the cochlea, usually due to loss of hair cells from the organ of Corti. Among the many common causes are noise trauma, ototoxicity, and aging (presbycusis). Sensory hearing loss is not correctable with medical or surgical therapy but often may be prevented or stabilized.

C. Neural Hearing Loss: Neural hearing loss occurs with lesions involving the eighth nerve, auditory nuclei, ascending tracts, or auditory cortex. It is the least common clinically recognized cause of hearing loss. Examples include acoustic neuroma, multiple sclerosis, and cerebrovascular disease.

Epidemiology of Hearing Loss

A. Children: Conductive losses in children are very common, especially before age 6. Most are due to middle ear effusion resulting from immaturity of the auditory tube (eustachian tube). Significant conductive losses during this critical period of speech and language acquisition are especially deleterious. Uncorrected hearing loss during this time may lead to a lasting deficit in communication skills.

Sensorineural loss in children may be congenital (eg, familial, teratogenic) or acquired (eg, meningitis, viral infection). Profound congenital deafness is usually not recognized by parents until age 12–18 months. For this reason, careful screening of high-risk infants is indicated in order to implement auditory rehabilita-

tion at the earliest possible time. Some criteria for high risk include prematurity, congenital malformation involving the head and neck region or urinary tract, hyperbilirubinemia, meningitis, exposure to teratogens, and a familial history of deafness.

B. Adults: Conductive losses in adults are most commonly due to cerumen impaction or transient auditory tube dysfunction associated with upper respiratory tract infection. Persistent conductive losses usually result from chronic ear infection, trauma, or otosclerosis.

Sensorineural losses in adults are common. A gradually progressive, predominantly high-frequency loss with advancing age is typical though not invariable. Other than aging effects, common causes of sensorineural loss include excessive noise exposure, head trauma, and systemic diseases such as diabetes mellitus.

Evaluation of Hearing (Audiology)

In a quiet room, the hearing level may be estimated by having the patient repeat aloud words presented in a soft whisper, a normal spoken voice, or a shout. Tuning forks are useful in differentiating conductive from sensorineural losses. A 512-Hz tuning fork is employed, since frequencies below this level elicit a tactile response. In the **Weber test,** the tuning fork is placed on the forehead or front teeth. In conductive losses, the sound appears louder in the poorer-hearing ear, whereas in sensorineural losses it radiates to the better side. In the **Rinne test,** the tuning fork is placed alternately on the mastoid bone and in front of the ear canal. In conductive losses, bone conduction exceeds air conduction; in sensorineural losses, the opposite is true.

Formal audiometric studies are performed by an audiologist in a soundproofed room. Pure-tone thresholds in decibels (dB) are obtained over the range of 250–8000 Hz (the main speech frequencies are between 500 and 3000 Hz) for both air and bone conduction. Conductive losses create a gap between the air and bone thresholds, whereas in sensorineural losses both air and bone conduction are equally diminished. The threshold of normal hearing is from 0 to 20 dB, which corresponds to the loudness of a soft whisper. Mild hearing loss is indicated by a threshold of 20–40 dB (soft spoken voice), moderate loss by a threshold of 40–60 dB (normal spoken voice), severe loss by a threshold of 60–80 dB (loud spoken voice), and profound loss by a threshold of 80 dB (shout). The clarity of hearing is often impaired in sensorineural hearing loss. This is evaluated by speech discrimination testing, which is reported as percentage correct (90–100% is normal). The site of the lesion responsible for sensorineural loss—whether it lies in the cochlea or in the central auditory system—may be determined with auditory brain stem-evoked responses.

Katz J: *Handbook of Clinical Audiology,* 3rd ed. Williams & Wilkins, 1985. (A comprehensive textbook on the diagnosis and rehabilitation of hearing disorders.)

Hearing Rehabilitation

Patients with hearing loss not correctable by medical therapy may benefit from hearing amplification. Contemporary hearing aids are comparatively free of distortion and have been miniaturized to the point where they often may be contained entirely within the ear canal. To optimize the benefit, a hearing aid must be carefully selected to conform to the nature of the hearing loss. Digitally programmable hearing aids are now becoming available that promise substantial improvements in speech intelligibility, especially under difficult listening circumstances.

Aside from hearing aids, many assistive devices are available to improve comprehension in individual and group settings, to help with hearing television and radio programs, and for telephone communication. In individuals with profound sensory deafness, the cochlear implant—an electronic device that is surgically implanted to stimulate the auditory nerve—offers socially beneficial auditory rehabilitation to most adults with acquired deafness.

Hecox KE, Punch JL: The impact of digital technology on the selection and fitting of hearing aids. Am J Otol 1988;9 (Suppl):77.
Nadol JB Jr, Eddington DK: Treatment of sensorineural hearing loss by cochlear implantation. Annu Rev Med 1988;39:491.
Rupp RR, Vaughn GR, Lightfoot RK: Nontraditional "aids" to hearing: Assistive listening devices. Geriatrics 1984;39:55.

DISEASES OF THE AURICLE

Disorders of the external ear are for the most part dermatologic. Skin cancers due to actinic exposure are common and may be treated with standard techniques. Traumatic auricular hematoma must be recognized and drained to prevent significant cosmetic deformity (cauliflower ear) resulting from dissolution of supporting cartilage. Similarly, cellulitis of the auricle must be treated promptly to prevent development of perichondritis and its resultant deformity.

Relapsing polychondritis is a systemic disorder often associated with recurrent, frequently bilateral, painful episodes of auricular erythema and edema. Treatment with corticosteroids may help forestall cartilage dissolution. Respiratory compromise may occur as a result of progressive involvement of the tracheobronchial tree. Chondritis and perichondritis may be differentiated from auricular cellulitis by sparing of involvement of the lobule, which does not contain cartilage.

DISEASES OF THE EAR CANAL

1. CERUMEN IMPACTION

Cerumen is a protective secretion produced by the outer portion of the ear canal. In most individuals, the ear canal is self-cleansing. Recommended hygiene consists of cleaning the external opening with a washcloth over the index finger without entering the canal itself. In most cases, cerumen impaction is self-induced through ill-advised attempts at cleaning the ear. It may be relieved with detergent ear drops (eg, 3% hydrogen peroxide; 6.5% carbamide peroxide [Debrox]), mechanical removal, suction, or irrigation. Irrigation is performed with water at body temperature to avoid a vestibular caloric response. The stream should be directed at the ear canal wall adjacent to the cerumen plug. Irrigation should be performed only when the tympanic membrane is known to be intact.

2. FOREIGN BODIES

Foreign bodies in the ear canal are more frequent in children than in adults. Firm materials may be removed with a loop or a hook, taking care not to displace the object medially toward the tympanic membrane. Aqueous irrigation should not be performed for organic foreign bodies (eg, beans, insects), because water may cause them to swell. Living insects are best immobilized before removal by filling the ear canal with lidocaine.

3. EXTERNAL OTITIS

External otitis, commonly known as swimmer's ear, presents with otalgia, frequently accompanied by pruritus and purulent discharge. There is often a history of recent water exposure or mechanical trauma (eg, scratching, cotton applicators). External otitis is usually caused by gram-negative rods (eg, *Pseudomonas, Proteus*) or fungi (eg, *Aspergillus*), which grow in the presence of excessive moisture.

Examination reveals erythema and edema of the ear canal skin, often with a purulent exudate. Manipulation of the auricle often elicits pain. Because the lateral surface of the tympanic membrane is ear canal skin, it is often erythematous. However, in contrast to acute otitis media, it moves normally with pneumatic otoscopy. When the canal skin is very edematous, it may be impossible to visualize the tympanic membrane. Fundamental to the treatment of external otitis is protection of the ear from additional moisture and avoidance of further mechanical injury by scratching. Otic drops containing a mixture of aminoglycoside antibiotic and anti-inflammatory corticosteroid in an acid vehicle are generally very effective (eg, Cortisporin Otic). Purulent debris filling the ear canal should be gently removed to permit entry of the topical medication. Drops should be used abundantly (5 or more drops), since too much is harmless and too little will fail to penetrate the depths of the canal. When substantial edema of the canal wall prevents entry of drops into the ear canal, a wick is placed to facilitate entry of the medication.

4. MALIGNANT EXTERNAL OTITIS

Persistent external otitis in the diabetic or immunocompromised patient may evolve into osteomyelitis of the skull base, often called malignant external otitis. Usually caused by *Pseudomonas aeruginosa*, osteomyelitis begins in the floor of the ear canal and may extend into the middle fossa floor, the clivus, and even the contralateral skull base. The patient usually presents with persistent foul aural discharge, granulations in the ear canal, deep otalgia, and progressive cranial nerve palsies involving nerves VI, VII, IX, X, XI, or XII. Diagnosis is confirmed by the demonstration of osseous erosion on CT and radionuclide scanning.

Treatment is chiefly medical, requiring prolonged antipseudomonal antibiotic administration, often for several months. Although intravenous therapy is often required, selected patients may be managed with the oral agent ciprofloxacin (500–1000 mg orally twice daily), which has proved effective against many of the causative *Pseudomonas* strains. To avoid relapse, antibiotic therapy should be continued, even in the asymptomatic patient, until gallium scanning indicates a marked reduction in the inflammatory process. Surgical debridement of infected bone is reserved for cases of deterioration despite medical therapy.

Bell DN: Otitis externa: A common, often self-inflicted condition. Postgrad Med (Sept) 1985;78:101.

Joachims HZ, Danino J, Raz R: Malignant external otitis: Treatment with fluoroquinolones. Am J Otolaryngol 1988;9:102. (Success with ciprofloxacin in 4 cases.)

Rubin J, Yu VL: Malignant external otitis: Insights into pathogenesis, clinical manifestations, diagnosis, and therapy. Am J Med 1988;85:391.

5. EXOSTOSES & OSTEOMAS

Bony overgrowths of the ear canal are a frequent incidental finding and occasionally have clinical significance. Clinically, they present as skin-covered mounds in the medial ear canal obscuring the tympanic membrane to a variable degree. Solitary osteomas are of no significance as long as they do not cause obstruction or infection. Multiple exostoses, which are generally acquired from repeated exposure to cold water, often progress and require surgical removal.

6. NEOPLASIA

The most common neoplasm of the ear canal is squamous cell carcinoma. Clinically, this tumor may simulate persistent external otitis. When an apparent otitis externa does not resolve on therapy, early biopsy is warranted. This disease carries a very high 5-year mortality rate and must be treated with wide surgical resection and radiation therapy. Adenomatous tumors, originating from the ceruminous glands, generally follow a more indolent course.

Arriaga M et al: Squamous cell carcinoma of the external auditory meatus (canal). Otolaryngol Head Neck Surg 1989;101:330.

DISEASES OF THE AUDITORY (EUSTACHIAN) TUBE

1. AUDITORY TUBE DYSFUNCTION

The tube that connects the middle ear to the nasopharynx—the auditory tube, or eustachian tube—provides ventilation and drainage for the middle ear cleft. It is normally closed, opening only during the act of swallowing or yawning. When auditory tube function is compromised, air trapped within the middle ear becomes absorbed and negative pressure results. The most common causes of auditory tube dysfunction are diseases associated with edema of the tubal lining, such as viral upper respiratory tract infections and allergy. The patient usually reports a sense of fullness in the ear and mild to moderate impairment of hearing. When the tube is only partially blocked, swallowing or yawning may elicit a popping or crackling sound. Examination reveals retraction of the tympanic membrane and decreased mobility on pneumatic otoscopy. Following a viral illness, this disorder is usually transient, lasting days to weeks. Treatment with systemic and intranasal decongestants combined with autoinflation by forced exhalation against closed nostrils may hasten relief. Air travel, rapid altitudinal change, and underwater diving should be avoided. Autoinflation should not be recommended to patients with active intranasal infection, since this maneuver may precipitate middle ear infection. Allergic patients may also benefit from desensitization or intranasal corticosteroids.

Bluestone CD, Doyle WJ: Anatomy and physiology of eustachian tube and middle ear related to otitis media. J Allergy Clin Immunol 1988;81:997.

2. SEROUS OTITIS MEDIA

When the auditory tube remains blocked for a prolonged period, the resultant negative pressure will result in transudation of fluid. This condition, known as serous otitis media, is especially common in children because their auditory tubes are narrower and more horizontal in orientation than adults. It is less common in adults, in whom it usually follows an upper respiratory tract infection or barotrauma. In an adult with persistent unilateral serous otitis media, nasopharyngeal carcinoma must be excluded. The tympanic membrane in serous otitis media is dull and hypomobile, occasionally accompanied by air bubbles in the middle ear and conductive hearing loss. The treatment of serous otitis media is similar to that for auditory tube dysfunction. When medication fails to bring relief after several months, a ventilating tube placed through the tympanic membrane may restore hearing and alleviate the sense of aural fullness. Recent evidence suggests that adenoidectomy modifies the underlying pathology of serous otitis media in young children and constitutes effective therapy regardless of whether the adenoids are of normal size or enlarged.

Gates GA et al: Chronic secretory otitis media: Effects of surgical management. Ann Otol Rhinol Laryngol 1989; 98(Suppl 138):2. (Entire issue.) (Most favorable results with adenoidectomy and concomitant myringotomy.)
Paradise JL: Management of secretory otitis media: State of the art. Adv Otorhinolaryngol 1988;40:99.

3. BAROTRAUMA

Individuals with auditory tube dysfunction due either to congenital narrowness or to acquired mucosal edema may be unable to equalize the barometric stress exerted on the middle ear by air travel, rapid altitudinal change, or underwater diving. The problem is generally most acute during airplane descent, since the negative middle ear pressure tends to collapse and lock the auditory tube. Several measures are useful to enhance auditory tube function and avoid otic barotrauma. The patient should be advised to swallow, yawn, and autoinflate frequently during descent. Systemic decongestants (eg, pseudoephedrine, 30–60 mg) should be taken several hours before anticipated arrival time so that they will be maximally effective during descent. Topical decongestants such as 1% phenylephrine nasal spray should be administered 1 hour before arrival. It is important that the susceptible individual not sleep during the descent phase, since one may awaken with severe pain and markedly negative pressure from a collapsed auditory tube. Infants are especially prone to barotrauma and should be given a bottle to suck during descent.

The treatment of acute negative middle ear pressure that persists on the ground is with decongestants and attempts at autoinflation. Myringotomy provides immediate relief and is appropriate in the setting of severe otalgia and hearing loss. Repeated episodes of barotrauma in persons who must fly frequently may be alleviated by insertion of ventilating tubes.

DISEASES OF THE MIDDLE EAR

1. ACUTE OTITIS MEDIA

Acute otitis media is a bacterial infection of the mucosally lined air-containing spaces of the temporal bone. Purulent material forms not only within the middle ear cleft but also within the mastoid air cells and petrous apex when they are pneumatized. Acute otitis media is usually precipitated by a viral upper respiratory tract infection that causes auditory tube edema. This results in accumulation of fluid and mucus, which becomes secondarily infected by bacteria. The most common pathogens both in adults and in children are *Streptococcus pneumoniae, Haemophilus influenzae,* and *Streptococcus pyogenes.* In newborn infants, gram-negative enteric bacilli predominate.

Acute otitis media is most common in infants and children, though it may occur at any age. The patient presents with otalgia, aural pressure, decreased hearing, and often fever. The typical physical findings are erythema and decreased mobility of the tympanic membrane. Occasionally, bullae will be seen on the tympanic membrane. Although it is commonly taught that this represents infection with *Mycoplasma pneumoniae,* most cases involve more common pathogens.

Rarely, when middle ear empyema is severe, the tympanic membrane can be seen to bulge outward. In such cases, tympanic membrane rupture is imminent. Rupture is accompanied by a sudden decrease in pain, followed by the onset of otorrhea. With appropriate therapy, spontaneous healing of the tympanic membrane occurs in most cases. When perforation persists, chronic otitis media frequently evolves. Mastoid tenderness often accompanies acute otitis media and is due to the presence of pus within the mastoid air cells. At this stage, this does not indicate suppurative (surgical) mastoiditis.

The treatment of acute otitis media is specific antibi-

otic therapy, often combined with nasal decongestants. Surgical drainage of the middle ear (myringotomy) is reserved for patients with severe otalgia
or when complications of otitis (eg, mastoiditis,
meningitis) have occurred.

Tympanocentesis for bacterial (aerobic and anaerobic) and fungal culture may be performed by any
experienced physician. A 20-gauge spinal needle bent
90 degrees to the hub of a 3-mL syringe should be
inserted atraumatically through the inferior portion
of the tympanic membrane. Interposition of a pliable
connecting tube between the needle and syringe permits an assistant to aspirate without inducing movement of the needle. Tympanocentesis is useful for
otitis media in immunocompromised patients; in neonates, in whom gram-negative organisms are common; and in cases of persistent infection despite multiple courses of antibiotics.

The first-choice antibiotic treatment is either amoxicillin (20–40 mg/kg/d) or erythromycin (50 mg/
kg/d) plus sulfonamide (150 mg/kg/d). Alternatives
useful in resistant cases are cefaclor (20–40 mg/kg/
d) or amoxicillin-clavulanate (20–40 mg/kg/d) combinations.

Recurrent acute otitis media may be managed with
long-term antibiotic prophylaxis. Single daily doses
of sulfamethoxazole (500 mg) or amoxicillin (250
or 500 mg) are given over a period of 1–3 months.
Failure of this regimen to control infection is an indication for insertion of ventilating tubes. In children
with recurrent nasopharyngitis and nasal obstruction,
adenoidectomy may be a useful adjunct to tympanos-
tomy tubes.

Bluestone CD: Management of otitis media in infants and
children: Current role of old and new antimicrobial
agents. Pediatr Infect Dis J 1988;7(Suppl 11):S129.
Fireman P: Otitis media and its relationship to allergy.
Pediatr Clin North Am 1988;35:1075.
Heald MM et al: Pressure equalization tubes in treatment
of otitis media: National Survey of Otolaryngologists.
Otolaryngol Head Neck Surg 1990;102:334.
Leonetti JP, Stankiewicz JA: Antimicrobial prophylaxis for
recurrent otitis media. Otolaryngol Head Neck Surg
1988;99:81. (Includes a review of the literature through
1988.)
Lim DJ (editor): Recent advances in otitis media. Ann Otol
Rhinol Laryngol 1989;98(Suppl 139):1.

2. CHRONIC OTITIS MEDIA & CHOLESTEATOMA

Chronic infection of the middle ear and mastoid
generally develops as a consequence of recurrent acute
otitis media, although it may follow other diseases
and trauma. Perforation of the tympanic membrane
is usually present. This may be accompanied by mucosal changes such as polypoid degeneration and granulation tissue and osseous changes such as osteitis
and sclerosis. The bacteriology of chronic otitis media
differs from that of acute otitis media. Common organisms include *P aeruginosa*, *Proteus* sp, *Staphylococcus aureus,* and mixed anaerobic infections. The clinical hallmark of chronic otitis media is purulent aural
discharge. Drainage may be continuous or intermittent, with increased severity during upper respiratory
tract infection or following water exposure. Pain is
uncommon except during acute exacerbations. Conductive hearing loss results from destruction of the
tympanic membrane and ossicular chain. The medical
treatment of chronic otitis media includes regular removal of infected debris, use of earplugs to protect
against water exposure, and topical antibiotic drops
for exacerbations. Ciprofloxacin, a new antipseudomonal agent, may help to dry a chronically discharging ear when given in a dosage of 500 mg orally
twice a day for several weeks.

The definitive management of chronic otitis media
is surgical in most cases. Tympanic membrane repair
may be accomplished with temporalis muscle fascia
or with homograft middle ear structures. Successful
reconstruction of the tympanic membrane may be
achieved in about 90% of cases, often with elimination
of infection and significant improvement in hearing.
When the mastoid air cells are involved by irreversible
infection, they should be exenterated through mastoidectomy.

Cholesteatoma is a special variety of chronic otitis
media. The most common cause is prolonged auditory
tube dysfunction, with resultant chronic negative middle ear pressure that draws inward the upper flaccid
portion of the tympanic membrane. This creates a
squamous epithelium-lined sac, which—when its
neck becomes obstructed—fills with desquamated
keratin and becomes chronically infected. Cholestea-
tomas typically erode bone, with early penetration
of the mastoid and destruction of the ossicular chain.
Over time, they may erode the inner ear or facial
nerve and on rare occasions may spread intracranially.
Physical examination reveals an epitympanic retraction pocket or marginal tympanic membrane perforation that exudes keratin debris. The treatment of cholesteatoma is surgical marsupialization of the sac or
its complete removal. This often requires creation
of a "mastoid bowl" in which the ear canal and
mastoid are joined into a large common cavity that
must be periodically cleaned.

Scularati N, Bluestone CD: Pathogenesis of cholesteatoma.
Otolaryngol Clin North Am 1989;22:859.
Sheehy JL: Acquired cholesteatoma in adults. Otolaryngol
Clin North Am 1989;22:967.

3. COMPLICATIONS OF OTITIS MEDIA

Mastoiditis

Acute suppurative mastoiditis usually evolves following several weeks of inadequately treated acute

otitis media. It is characterized by postauricular pain and erythema accompanied by a spiking fever. Radiography reveals coalescence of the mastoid air cells due to destruction of their bony septa. Initial treatment consists of intravenous antibiotics and myringotomy for culture and drainage. Failure of medical therapy indicates the need for surgical drainage (mastoidectomy).

Rubin JS, Wei WI: Acute mastoiditis: A review of 34 patients. Laryngoscope 1985;95:963. (Contemporary diagnosis and management.)

Petrous Apicitis

The medial portion of the petrous bone between the inner ear and clivus may become a site of persistent infection when the drainage of its pneumatic cell tracts becomes blocked. This may cause foul discharge, deep ear and retro-orbital pain, and sixth nerve palsy (Gradenigo's syndrome). Treatment is with prolonged antibiotic therapy and surgical drainage via petrous apicectomy.

Otogenic Skull Base Osteomyelitis

Infections originating in the external or middle ear may result in osteomyelitis of the skull base, usually due to *P aeruginosa*. The diagnosis and management of this disease are discussed in the section on external otitis.

Beneke JE: Management of osteomyelitis of the skull base. Laryngoscope 1989;99:1220.

Facial Paralysis

Facial palsy may be associated with either acute or chronic otitis media. In the acute setting, it results from inflammation of the nerve in its middle ear segment, perhaps mediated through bacterially secreted neurotoxins. Treatment consists of myringotomy for drainage and culture, followed by intravenous antibiotics. The use of corticosteroids is controversial. The prognosis is excellent, with complete recovery in the vast majority of cases.

Facial palsy associated with chronic otitis media usually evolves slowly due to chronic pressure on the nerve in the middle ear or mastoid by cholesteatoma. Treatment requires surgical correction of the underlying disease. The prognosis is less favorable than for facial palsy associated with acute otitis media.

Olsen KD: Facial nerve paralysis. 2. ''All that palsies is not Bell's.'' Postgrad Med (July) 1984;76:95.

Sigmoid Sinus Thrombosis

Trapped infection within the mastoid air cells adjacent to the sigmoid sinus may cause septic thrombophlebitis. This is heralded by signs of systemic sepsis (spiking fevers, chills), at times accompanied by signs of increased intracranial pressure (headache, lethargy, nausea and vomiting, papilledema). If not recognized early, it may lead to widespread septic embolization and death. Treatment is with intravenous antibiotics, surgical drainage, and—when emboli are suspected—ligation of the internal jugular vein in the neck.

Southwick FS, Richardson EP Jr, Swartz MN: Septic thrombosis of the dural venous sinuses. Medicine 1986;65:82.

Central Nervous System Infection

Otogenic meningitis is by far the most common intracranial complication of ear infection. In the setting of acute suppurative otitis media, it arises from hematogenous spread of bacteria, most commonly *H influenzae* and *S pneumoniae*. In chronic otitis media, it results either from passage of infections along preformed pathways such as the petrosquamous suture line or from direct extension of disease through the dural plates of the petrous pyramid.

Epidural abscesses arise from direct extension of disease in the setting of chronic infection. They are usually asymptomatic but may present with deep local pain, headache, and low-grade fever. They are often discovered as an incidental finding at surgery. Intraparenchymal brain abscesses may arise in the temporal lobe or cerebellum. They most commonly evolve from retrograde thrombophlebitis adjacent to an epidural abscess. The predominant causative organisms are *S aureus*, *S pyogenes*, and *S pneumoniae*. Rupture into the subarachnoid space results in catastrophic meningitis and often rapid death.

Friedman EM et al: Central nervous system complications associated with acute otitis media in children. Laryngoscope 1990;100:149.

4. OTOSCLEROSIS

Otosclerosis is a progressive disease with a marked familial tendency that affects bone surrounding the inner ear. Lesions involving the footplate of the stapes result in increased impedance to the passage of sound through the ossicular chain, producing conductive hearing loss. This may be corrected through surgical replacement of the stapes with a prosthesis (stapedectomy). When otosclerotic lesions impinge on the cochlea, permanent sensory hearing loss occurs. Some evidence suggests that this level of hearing loss may be stabilized by treatment with oral sodium fluoride over prolonged periods of time (Florical—8.3 mg sodium fluoride and 364 mg calcium carbonate—2 tablets orally each morning). Fluorides have minimal adverse effects other than occasional mild gastric irritation, which may be eliminated by ingesting the drug with meals.

Bretlau P et al: Otospongiosis and sodium fluoride: A blind experimental and clinical evaluation of the effect of sodium fluoride treatment in patients with otospongiosis. Ann Otol Rhinol Laryngol 1985;94:103. (Less hearing deterioration in the fluoride-treated group.)

5. TRAUMA TO THE MIDDLE EAR

Tympanic membrane perforation may result from impact injury or explosive acoustic trauma. Spontaneous healing occurs in the great majority of cases. Persistent perforation may result from secondary infection brought on by exposure to water. Patients should be advised to wear earplugs while swimming or bathing during the healing period. Hemorrhage behind an intact tympanic membrane (hemotympanum) may follow blunt trauma or extreme barotrauma. Spontaneous resolution over several weeks is the usual course. When a conductive hearing loss greater than 30 dB persists for more than 3 months following trauma, disruption of the ossicular chain should be suspected. Middle ear exploration with reconstruction of the ossicular chain, combined with repair of the tympanic membrane when required, will usually restore hearing.

6. MIDDLE EAR NEOPLASIA

Primary middle ear tumors are rare. Glomus tumors arise either in the middle ear (glomus tympanicum) or in the jugular bulb with upward erosion into the hypotympanum (glomus jugulare). They present clinically with pulsatile tinnitus and hearing loss. A vascular mass may be visible behind an intact tympanic membrane. Large glomus jugulare tumors are often associated with multiple cranial neuropathies, especially involving nerves VII, IX, X, XI, and XII. Treatment may require surgery, radiotherapy, or both.

EARACHE

External otitis and acute otitis media are both painful conditions. In external otitis, there is often a recent history of swimming, Q-tip use, or physical trauma, while in acute otitis media there is usually an antecedent or concurrent upper respiratory infection. The physical findings also differ. In external otitis, the ear canal skin is erythematous, while in acute otitis media this generally occurs only if the tympanic membrane has ruptured, spilling purulent material into the ear canal. Also, in external otitis the tympanic membrane may be erythematous, but it retains its mobility owing to the normal aeration of the middle ear cavity. Acute severe pain out of proportion to the physical findings may be due to herpes zoster oticus, especially when vesicles appear in the ear

canal or concha. Chronic otitis media is usually not painful except during acute exacerbations. Persistent pain and discharge from the ear suggest osteomyelitis of the skull base or cancer.

The sensory innervation of the ear is derived from the trigeminal, facial, glossopharyngeal, vagal, and upper cervical nerves. Because of this rich innervation, referred otalgia is quite frequent. Temporomandibular joint dysfunction is a common cause of ear pain. It is often made worse by chewing or psychogenic grinding of the teeth (bruxism) and may be associated with dental malocclusion. Management includes soft diet, local heat to the masticatory muscles, massage, analgesics, and dental referral. Repeated episodes of severe lancinating otalgia may occur in glossopharyngeal neuralgia. Treatment with carbamazepine often confers substantial symptomatic relief. Infections and neoplasia that involve the oropharynx, hypopharynx, and larynx frequently cause otalgia. Persistent earache demands specialty referral to exclude cancer of the upper aerodigestive tract.

DISEASES OF THE INNER EAR

1. SENSORY HEARING LOSS

Diseases of the cochlea result in sensory hearing loss, a condition that is usually irreversible. Most cochlear diseases result in bilateral symmetric hearing loss. The presence of unilateral or asymmetric sensorineural hearing loss suggests a lesion proximal to the cochlea. Lesions affecting the eighth nerve and central auditory system are discussed in the section on neural hearing loss. The primary goals in the management of sensory hearing loss are prevention of further losses and functional improvement with amplification and auditory rehabilitation.

Presbycusis

Presbycusis is the progressive, predominantly high-frequency symmetric hearing loss of advancing age. It is difficult to separate the various etiologic factors (eg, noise trauma) that may contribute to presbycusis, but genetic predisposition appears to play a role. Most patients notice a loss of speech discrimination that is especially pronounced in noisy environments. About 25% of people between the ages of 65 and 75 years and almost 50% of those over 75 experience hearing difficulties.

Gates GA et al: Presbycusis. Otolaryngol Head Neck Surg 1989;100:266.

Noise Trauma

Noise trauma is the second most common cause of sensory hearing loss. Sounds exceeding 85 dB are potentially injurious to the cochlea, especially with prolonged exposures. The loss typically begins in the high frequencies (especially 4000 Hz) and progresses to involve the speech frequencies with continuing exposure. Among the more common sources of injurious noise are industrial machinery, weapons, and excessively loud music. In recent years, monitoring of noise levels in the workplace by regulatory agencies has led to preventive programs that have reduced the frequency of occupational losses. Individuals of all ages, especially those with existing hearing losses, should wear earplugs when exposed to moderately loud noises and specially designed earmuffs when exposed to explosive noises such as gunfire.

Riko K, Alberti PW: Hearing protectors: A review of recent observations. J Occup Med 1983;25:523.
Sataloff RT, Sataloff J: Occupational Hearing Loss. Marcel Dekker, 1987.

Physical Trauma

Head trauma has effects on the inner ear similar to those of severe acoustic trauma. Some degree of sensory hearing loss may occur following simple concussion and is frequent after skull fracture.

Ototoxicity

Ototoxic substances may affect both the auditory and vestibular systems. The most common ototoxic medications are salicylates, aminoglycosides, loop diuretics, and several antineoplastic agents, notably cisplatin. The latter 3 categories may cause irreversible hearing loss even when administered in therapeutic doses. When using these medications, it is important to identify high-risk patients such as those with preexisting hearing losses or renal insufficiency. Patients simultaneously receiving multiple ototoxic agents are at particular risk owing to ototoxic synergy. Useful measures to reduce the risk of ototoxic injury include serial audiometry and monitoring of serum peak and trough levels and substitution of equivalent nonototoxic drugs whenever possible.

Brummett RE, Morrison RB: The incidence of aminoglycoside antibiotic-induced hearing loss. Arch Otol Head Neck Surg 1990;116:406.
Meyerhoff WL: Audiologic threshold monitoring of patients receiving ototoxic drugs. Ann Otol Radiol Laryngol 1989;98:950.

Sudden Sensory Hearing Loss

Sudden loss of hearing in one ear may occur at any age but is more common in the elderly. It most probably is the result of sudden vascular occlusion of the internal auditory artery or of a viral inner ear infection. Prognosis is mixed, with many patients suffering permanent deafness in the involved ear while others have complete recovery. Oral corticosteroids are felt by many to improve the odds of recovery.

A common regimen is prednisone, 80 mg/d, followed by a tapering dose over a 10-day period.

Cole RR, Jahrsdoerfer RA: Sudden hearing loss: An update. Am J Otol 1988;9:211.

Other Causes of Sensory Hearing Loss

There are numerous less common causes of sensory hearing loss. Metabolic derangements (eg, diabetes, hypothyroidism, hyperlipidemia, and renal failure), infections (eg, measles, mumps, syphilis), autoimmune disorders (eg, polyarteritis, lupus erythematosus), physical factors (eg, radiation therapy) and hereditary syndromes are some of the chief examples. Identification of metabolic, infectious, or autoimmune sensory hearing losses is especially important, as these may occasionally be reversible with medical therapy. Meniere's syndrome and labyrinthitis are discussed in the section on vestibular disorders.

Rybak LP: Treatable sensorineural hearing loss. Am J Otol 1985;6:482.
Wackym PA, Linthicum FH Jr: Diabetes mellitus and hearing loss: Clinical and histopathologic relationships. Am J Otol 1986;7:176.

2. TINNITUS

Tinnitus is the perception of abnormal ear or head noises. Persistent tinnitus usually indicates the presence of sensory hearing loss. Intermittent periods of mild, high-pitched tinnitus lasting for several minutes are common in normal-hearing persons. When severe and persistent, tinnitus may interfere with sleep and the ability to concentrate, resulting in considerable psychologic distress.

The most important treatment of tinnitus is avoidance of exposure to excessive noise, ototoxic agents, and other factors that may cause cochlear damage. Masking the tinnitus with music or through amplification of normal sounds with a hearing aid may also bring some relief. Although pharmacologic treatment with antiarrhythmic drugs has been advocated, recent evidence suggests no benefit with available oral regimens. Among the numerous drugs that have been used in attempts to suppress tinnitus, oral antidepressants (eg, nortriptyline) have proved to be the most efficacious.

Pulsatile tinnitus should be distinguished from tonal tinnitus. Pulsations most often result from conductive hearing loss, which renders transmitted carotid pulsations more apparent. However, it may also indicate a vascular abnormality such as glomus tumor, carotid vaso-occlusive disease, arteriovenous malformation, or aneurysm. CT scan and vascular studies are often necessary to establish a definitive diagnosis.

Mattox DE, Richtsmeier WJ: Tinnitus: The initial evaluation. Otolaryngol Head Neck Surg 1987;96:172. (History, physical examination, and current audiologic and radiographic evaluation of this symptom.)

Sullivan MD et al: Treatment of depressed tinnitus patients with nortriptyline. Ann Otol Rhinol Laryngol 1989; 98:867.

3. VERTIGO
(Table 6–1)

Vertigo is the cardinal symptom of vestibular disease. It is either a sensation of motion when there is no motion or an exaggerated sense of motion in response to a given bodily movement. Thus, vertigo is not just "spinning" but may present, for example, as a sense of tumbling, of falling forward or backward, or of the ground rolling beneath one's feet ("earthquake-like"). It should be distinguished from imbalance, light-headedness, and syncope, all of which are usually nonvestibular in origin. The vertigo that results from peripheral vestibulopathy is usually of sudden onset, may be so severe that the patient is unable to walk or stand, and is frequently accompanied by nausea and vomiting. Tinnitus and hearing loss may be associated and provide strong support for a peripheral origin.

A minimal physical examination of the patient with vertigo includes the Romberg test, an evaluation of gait, and observation for the presence of nystagmus. Nystagmus is usually horizontal with a rotatory component; the fast phase usually beats away from the diseased side. Visual fixation tends to inhibit nystagmus except in very acute peripheral lesions or with central nervous system disease. The Nylen-Baaraany maneuvers are intended to induce positioning nystagmus but are of limited use when the patient is able to visually fixate. This objection may be overcome either by placing +2-diopter lenses (Fresnel glasses) over the eyes or by making observations in the dark by means of electronystagmographic recording. The Fukuda test, in which the patient marches in place with eyes closed, is useful for detecting subtle defects. A positive response is observed when the patient ro-

tates, usually toward the side of the disease labyrinth. Vertigo arising from central lesions tends to develop gradually and then become progressively more severe and debilitating. Nystagmus is not always present but can occur in any direction and may be dissociated in the 2 eyes. The associated nystagmus is often nonfatigable, vertical rather than horizontal in orientation, without latency, and unsuppressed by visual fixation. Electronystagmography is useful in documenting these characteristics. The evaluation of central audiovestibular dysfunction usually requires imaging of the brain with CT scans or, particularly, MRI.

Episodic vertigo can occur in patients with diplopia from external ophthalmoplegia and is maximal when the patient looks in the direction where the separation of images is greatest. Cerebral lesions involving the temporal cortex may also produce vertigo, which is sometimes the initial symptom of a seizure. Finally, vertigo may be a feature of a number of system disorders and can occur as a side effect of certain anticonvulsant, antibiotic, hypnotic, analgesic, and tranquilizing drugs or of alcohol.

Laboratory investigations such as audiologic evaluation, caloric stimulation, electronystagmography, CT scan, and brain stem auditory evoked potential studies are indicated in patients with persistent vertigo or when central nervous system disease is suspected. These studies will help to distinguish between central and peripheral lesions and to identify causes requiring specific therapy. Electronystagmography consists of objective recording of the nystagmus induced by head and body movements, gaze, and caloric stimulation. It is helpful in quantifying the degree of vestibular hypofunction and may help with the differentiation between peripheral and central lesions. Computer-driven rotatory chairs and posturography platforms offer improved diagnostic abilities but are not widely available.

Vertigo Syndromes Due to Peripheral Lesions

A. Endolymphatic Hydrops (Meniere's Syndrome): Meniere's syndrome results from distention of the endolymphatic compartment of the inner ear.

Table 6–1. Common vestibular disorders: Differential diagnosis based on classic presentations.

Duration of Typical Vertiginous Episodes	Auditory Symptoms Present	Auditory Symptoms Absent
Seconds	Perilymphatic fistula	Positioning vertigo (cupulolithiasis), vertebrobasilar insufficiency, cervical vertigo
Hours	Endolymphatic hydrops (Meniere's syndrome), syphilis	Recurrent vestibulopathy, vestibular migraine
Days	Labyrinthitis, labyrinthine concussion	Vestibular neuronitis
Months	Acoustic neuroma, ototoxicity	Multiple sclerosis, cerebellar degeneration

The primary lesion appears to be in the endolymphatic sac, which is thought to be responsible for endolymph filtration and excretion. Although a precise cause of hydrops cannot be established in most cases, 2 known causes are syphilis and head trauma. The classic syndrome consists of episodic vertigo, usually lasting 1–8 hours; low-frequency sensorineural hearing loss, often fluctuating; tinnitus, usually low-tone and "blowing" in quality, and a sensation of aural pressure. Symptoms wax and wane as the endolymphatic pressure rises and falls. Caloric testing commonly reveals loss or impairment of thermally induced nystagmus on the involved side.

Specific treatment is intended to lower endolymphatic pressure. A low-salt diet (< 2 g sodium daily), at times supplemented by diuretics, adequately controls symptoms in the great majority of patients. A typical diuretic regimen is hydrochlorothiazide, 50–100 mg daily. In those who have failed medical therapy and remain disabled by their vertigo, surgical decompression of the endolymphatic sac may bring relief.

Episodic vertigo resembling that of Meniere's syndrome but without accompanying auditory symptoms is known as recurrent vestibulopathy. The pathogenic mechanism of this symptom complex is unknown in most cases, though a few patients suffer from a variant of migraine whereas others go on to develop the classic syndrome of endolymphatic hydrops.

B. Labyrinthitis: Patients with labyrinthitis suffer from continuous, usually severe vertigo lasting several days to a week, accompanied by hearing loss and tinnitus. During a recovery period that lasts for several weeks, rapid head movements may bring on transient vertigo. Hearing may return to normal or remain permanently impaired in the involved ear. The cause of labyrinthitis is unknown, although it frequently follows an upper respiratory tract infection. For this reason, it is generally known as "viral" or "infectious" labyrinthitis.

C. Vestibular Neuronitis: In vestibular neuronitis, a paroxysmal, usually single attack of vertigo occurs without accompanying impairment of auditory function and may persist for several days to weeks before clearing. Examination reveals nystagmus and absent responses to caloric stimulation on one or both sides. The cause of the disorder is unclear. Viral mononeuritis has been suggested as the cause. Treatment is symptomatic.

D. Traumatic Vertigo: The most common cause of vertigo following head injury is labyrinthine concussion. Symptoms generally diminish within several days but may linger for a month or more. Basilar skull fractures that traverse the inner ear usually result in severe vertigo lasting several days to a week and deafness in the involved ear. Chronic posttraumatic vertigo may result from cupulolithiasis. This occurs when traumatically detached statoconia (otoconia) settle on the ampulla of the posterior semicircular canal

and cause an excessive degree of cupular deflection in response to head motion. Clinically, this presents as episodic positioning vertigo. A less common source of posttraumatic vertigo is disruption of the oval or round window with leakage of perilymph into the middle ear. Perilymphatic fistulization may follow physical or barometric trauma or may result from erosion of the inner ear by cholesteatoma or neoplasm. Symptomatic fistulas are usually associated with both vertigo and hearing loss. Surgical repair may be necessary.

E. Positioning Vertigo: This form of vertigo is usually peripheral in origin, though it occasionally occurs with central lesions. Transient vertigo following changes in head position is a frequent complaint. The term "positioning vertigo" is more accurate than "positional vertigo" because it is provoked by changes in head position rather than by the maintenance of a particular posture. Use of the term "benign positional vertigo" is discouraged except for cases known to be unassociated with central nervous system disorders. True positional vertigo suggests either vertebrobasilar insufficiency or dysfunction of the cervical spine.

The typical symptoms of positioning vertigo occur in clusters that persist for several days. Typically with peripheral lesions, there is a latency period of several seconds following a head movement before symptoms develop, and they subside within 10–60 seconds. Constant repetition of the positional change leads to habituation. In central lesions, there is no latent period, fatigability, or habituation of the sign and symptoms.

F. Acoustic Neuromas: These tumors, which are schwannomas of the vestibular nerve, typically are associated with chronic vestibular symptoms in the form of unsteadiness and imbalance. Less commonly, they are manifested by repeated episodes of true vertigo. Unilateral hearing loss with relatively poor speech discrimination and tinnitus is common.

Vertigo Syndromes Due to Central Lesions

Central nervous system causes of vertigo include brain stem vascular disease, arteriovenous malformations, tumor of the brain stem and cerebellum, multiple sclerosis, and vertebrobasilar migraine. Vertigo of central origin often becomes unremitting and disabling. There are commonly other signs of brain stem dysfunction (eg, cranial nerve palsies; motor, sensory, or cerebellar deficits in the limbs) or of increased intracranial pressure. Auditory function is generally spared. The underlying cause should be treated.

Management of the Patient With Vertigo

Unfortunately, few specific treatments for labyrinthine disorders have been designed to reverse a known pathogenic mechanism. Examples include low-salt diet and diuretics in Meniere's disease, antibiotic treatment of infectious diseases, and surgical repair of perilymphatic fistulas.

Symptomatic treatment is useful in the vertiginous patient to lessen the abnormal sensation and to alleviate vegetative symptoms such as nausea and vomiting. The most common drug classes employed are the antihistamines, anticholinergics, and sedative-hypnotics. Ample evidence exists that vestibular suppressant medications adversely affect the process of central compensation following acute vestibular disease. For this reason, these drugs should be used only for brief periods. Generally, they are best administered to patients with prominent vegetative symptoms and are best tapered and halted when symptoms are resolved, usually within 1–2 weeks.

In acute severe vertigo, diazepam, 2.5–5 mg intravenously, may abate an attack. Relief from nausea and vomiting usually requires antiemetic delivered intramuscularly or by rectal suppository (eg, prochlorperazine, 10 mg intramuscularly, or 25 mg rectally every 6 hours). Less severe vertigo may often be successfully alleviated with antihistamines such as meclizine, 25 mg, or cyclizine or dimenhydrinate, 25–50 mg, orally every 6 hours. Scopolamine, administered in low dosage transdermally (0.5 mg/d), has proved beneficial to many patients with recurrent vertigo, although side effects (dry mouth, blurred vision, urinary obstruction) often limit its utility. Sometimes employing one-half or even one-fourth of a patch may allow therapeutic effect without the usual adverse consequences. A combination of drugs sometimes helps when the response to one drug is disappointing.

Bed rest may reduce the severity of acute vertigo. In chronic or recurrent vertigo, one of the most important therapies is exercise. Physical activity substantially enhances the central nervous system's ability to compensate for labyrinthine dysfunction and should be encouraged once nausea and vomiting have resolved. In general, the patient should be instructed to repeatedly perform maneuvers that provoke vertigo—up to the point of nausea or fatigue—in an effort to habituate them.

Surgical remedies are reserved for those who remain substantially disabled despite a prolonged and varied trial of medical therapy and exercises. Selective section of the vestibular portion of the eighth nerve brings relief of vertigo in over 90% of such patients. Surgical removal of the semicircular canals (labyrinthectomy) is also highly effective but is appropriate only for patients with little or no hearing in the involved ear.

Bagger-Sjoback D: Surgical treatment of vertigo. Acta Otolaryngol 1988;Suppl 455:86.

Baloh RW: The dizzy patient: Symptomatic treatment of vertigo. Postgrad Med (May) 1983;73:317.

Baloh RW, Furman JMR: Modern vestibular function testing. West J Med 1989;150:59. (A comprehensive review that includes advanced diagnostic techniques.)

Dix MR, Hood JD: Vertigo. Wiley, 1984.

Mohr DN: The syndrome of paroxysmal positional vertigo: A review. West J Med 1986;145:645.

Peppard SB: Effect of drug therapy on compensation from vestibular injury. Laryngoscope 1986;96:878.

Pyykko I et al: Pharmacological treatment of vertigo. Acta Otolaryngol 1988;Suppl 445:77.

Slater R: Vertigo: How serious are recurrent and single attacks? Postgrad Med (Oct) 1988;84:58.

Thomsen J: Defining valid approaches to therapy for Meniere's disease. Ear Nose Throat J (Sept) 1986;65:10.

DISEASES OF THE CENTRAL AUDITORY & VESTIBULAR SYSTEMS (Table 6–1)

Lesions of the eighth cranial nerve and central audiovestibular pathways produce neural hearing loss and vertigo. One characteristic of neural hearing loss is deterioration of speech discrimination out of proportion to the decrease in pure tone thresholds. Another is auditory adaptation, wherein a steady tone appears to the listener to decay and eventually disappear. Auditory evoked responses are useful in distinguishing cochlear from neural losses and may give insight into the site of lesion within the central pathways.

Vertigo arising from central lesions tends to be more chronic and debilitating than that seen in labyrinthine disease. The associated nystagmus is often nonfatigable, vertical rather than horizontal in orientation, without latency, and unsuppressed by visual fixation. Electronystagmography is useful in documenting these characteristics. The evaluation of central audiovestibular dysfunction usually requires imaging of the brain with CT scans or MRI. The paramagnetic contrast agent gadolinium-DTPA, when used with MRI scanning, substantially improves diagnostic sensitivity in the detection of central audiovestibular lesions.

Kumar A, Dobben GD: Central auditory and vestibular pathology. Otolaryngol Clin North Am 1988;21:377. (Review of imaging modalities in diagnosis of central audiovestibular diseases.)

1. ACOUSTIC NEUROMA

Tumors of the cerebellopontine angle, most notably acoustic neuroma, cause central audiovestibular symptoms. Acoustic neuromas are among the most common intracranial neoplasms. These schwannomas generally arise from the vestibular division of the eighth nerve. When small, they may occasionally be excised, with preservation of hearing. Large tumors can also be safely removed in most cases, but cranial nerve palsies—especially facial paralysis and deafness—are common sequelae.

Barrs DM, Olsson JE: The audiologic evaluation of cerebellopontine angle tumor suspects: A review of tumor and nontumor suspects. Otolaryngol Head Neck Surg 1987;96:523. (Reviews the diagnostic efficacy of both classic hearing tests and evoked responses in the diagnosis of acoustic neuroma.)

Shelton C et al: Hearing preservation after acoustic tumor removal: Long term results. Laryngoscope 1990; 1000:115.

2. VASCULAR COMPROMISE

Vertebrobasilar insufficiency is a common cause of vertigo in the elderly. It is often triggered by changes in posture or extension of the neck. Empirical treatment is with vasodilators and exercise.

Migraine may cause vertiginous attacks. The diagnosis is obvious when vertigo accompanies a typical headache pattern, but this is not always the case. In patients with a history of both migraine headaches and recurrent vertigo, a therapeutic trial of β-adrenergic blocking drugs and ergots is reasonable.

Vascular loops that impinge upon the brain stem root entry zone of cranial nerves have been shown to cause dysfunction. Widely recognized examples are hemifacial spasm and tic douloureux. It has been suggested that hearing loss, tinnitus, and disabling positioning vertigo may result from such a loop abutting the eighth nerve.

Ausman JI et al: Vertebrobasilar insufficiency: A review. Arch Neurol 1985;42:803.

3. MULTIPLE SCLEROSIS

Most patients with multiple sclerosis suffer from episodic vertigo and chronic imbalance. Hearing loss in this disease is most commonly unilateral and of rapid onset. Spontaneous recovery may occur.

Grenman R: Involvement of the audiovestibular system in multiple sclerosis: An otoneurologic and audiologic study. Acta Otolaryngol [Suppl] (Stockh) 1985;420:1.

DISEASES OF THE NOSE & PARANASAL SINUSES

INFECTIONS OF THE NOSE & PARANASAL SINUSES

1. VIRAL RHINITIS (Common Cold)

The nonspecific symptoms of the ubiquitous common cold are present in the early phases of many diseases that affect the upper aerodigestive tract. Because there are numerous serologic types of rhinoviruses, adenoviruses, and other viruses, patients remain susceptible throughout life. Headache, nasal congestion, watery rhinorrhea, sneezing, and a scratchy throat accompanied by general malaise are typical in viral infections. Nasal examination usually shows reddened, edematous mucosa and a watery discharge. The presence of purulent nasal discharge suggests bacterial infection.

There is no proved specific treatment for a cold, but supportive measures such as decongestants (pseudoephedrine, 30 mg every 4 hours, or 120 mg twice daily) may provide some relief of rhinorrhea and nasal obstruction. Nasal sprays such as oxymetazolone or phenylephrine are rapidly effective. They should not be used for more than a few days at a time, since chronic use leads to a rebound congestion that is often worse than the original symptoms. This chronic nasal stuffiness is known as rhinitis medicamentosa. Treatment requires complete cessation of the sprays. This triggers a period of severe nasal congestion that usually lasts 1–2 weeks. Topical intranasal corticosteroids (flunisolide [Nasalide]), 2 sprays in each nostril twice daily) or a short tapering course of oral prednisone may help during the process of withdrawal.

Other than transient middle ear effusion, complications of viral rhinitis are unusual. Secondary bacterial infection may occur and is suggested by a change in color of the rhinorrhea from clear and watery to mucoid and yellow or green. The most common pathogens are the same as those responsible for acute otitis media. Nasal cultures may help guide treatment.

2. ACUTE SINUSITIS

Acute sinus infections are uncommon compared to viral rhinitis. Because sinusitis usually has followed an acute respiratory infection and because media advertisements often use the term ''sinusitis'' when ''rhinitis'' would be more accurate, it is understandable that patients and physicians alike sometimes confuse these entities. In addition to the symptoms of rhinitis, the diagnosis of sinusitis requires clinical signs and symptoms that indicate involvement of the affected sinus or sinuses such as pain and tenderness over the involved sinus.

Sinusitis occurs when an undrained collection of pus accumulates in a sinus. Diseases that swell the nasal mucous membrane, such as viral or allergic rhinitis, are usually the underlying cause. Edematous mucosa causes obstruction of a sinus drainage tract, resulting in the accumulation of mucous secretion in the sinus cavity that becomes secondarily infected by bacteria. The typical pathogens of bacterial sinusitis are the same as those that cause acute otitis media: *S pneumoniae*, other streptococci, *H influenzae*, and, less commonly, *S aureus* and *Branhamella catarrhalis*.

Clinical Findings

A. Symptoms and Signs: Because the maxillary sinus is the largest of the paranasal sinuses and its ostium into the nose is superiorly placed, thereby failing to take advantage of gravity, it is the most commonly affected sinus. Pain and pressure over the cheek are the usual symptoms. Pain may refer to the upper incisor and canine teeth via branches of the trigeminal nerve, which traverse the floor of the sinus. It is not uncommon for maxillary sinusitis to result from dental infection, and teeth that are tender should be carefully examined for signs of abscess.

Acute ethmoiditis in adults is usually accompanied by maxillary sinusitis. In such cases, the symptoms of maxillary sinusitis generally predominate. Ethmoidal infection presents with pain and pressure over the high lateral wall of the nose that may radiate to the orbit. In children, however, because the maxillary sinus is poorly developed, isolated ethmoiditis is not rare. It usually presents as periorbital cellulitis, with the most common pathogen being *H influenzae*.

Sphenoid sinusitis is usually seen in the setting of pansinusitis. The patient may complain of a headache "in the middle of the head" and often points to the vertex. Sixth nerve palsy may occur as the abducens nerve courses just lateral to the sinus.

Acute frontal sinusitis usually causes pain and tenderness of the forehead. This is most easily elicited by palpation of the orbital roof just below the medial end of the eyebrow. Palpation here is more accurate than percussion of the supraorbital area or forehead.

B. Imaging: Although it is often possible to make the diagnosis of sinusitis on clinical grounds alone, radiologic confirmation allows a more definitive diagnosis and is an objective monitor of the course of infection. Transillumination may aid in diagnosis, but variations in soft tissue thickness and technique often make interpretation difficult. The authors have not found it particularly helpful in practice. The standard set of sinus films and the sinus best seen in each view are Caldwell (frontal), Waters (maxillary), lateral (sphenoid), and submentovertical (ethmoid). Opacification without bone destruction is a typical feature of sinusitis. An air-fluid level may be seen if the films are taken with the patient upright rather than supine. The frontal sinus may occasionally appear normal even in the face of clinically compelling evidence of sinusitis.

Treatment

In uncomplicated sinusitis with mild symptoms, outpatient management is usually successful. Oral decongestants, nasal decongestant sprays, and oral antibiotics are recommended. If purulent discharge is seen in the nose, it should be cultured. Maxillary sinus puncture and aspiration frequently provides a sample for culture. This is especially important when there is reason to suspect that the pathogen may not be typical, such as in nosocomial sinusitis in an intensive care unit. Interestingly, the bacterial spectrum seen in sinusitis in AIDS is similar to that in more common settings; but aspiration for cytology may lead to a diagnosis of lymphoma, a not uncommon finding in apparent "sinusitis" in AIDS patients. Because amoxicillin has better sinus penetration than ampicillin, it is an appropriate first choice. Alternatives are discussed in the section on acute otitis media. Antibiotic treatment for sinusitis should be continued for 2 weeks, with longer courses sometimes required to prevent relapses.

Failure of sinusitis to resolve after an adequate course of oral antibiotics may necessitate hospital admission for intravenous antibiotics and possible surgical drainage. Frontal sinusitis that does not promptly respond to outpatient care should be managed aggressively, because the posterior sinus wall is adjacent to the dura and because undertreated infection may lead to intracranial extension. If intravenous antibiotics fail to ameliorate symptoms, a frontal sinus trephine may be necessary to drain and irrigate the sinus. Persistent maxillary empyema may be cultured and relieved with a needle inserted through the lateral wall of the nose or anterior wall of the antrum through the gingivobuccal sulcus.

Complications

Local complications of sinusitis include osteomyelitis and mucocele. Mucoceles, a consequence of long-standing ductal obstruction, are more common in the supraorbital ethmoids and frontal sinuses and may become secondarily infected. They appear radiologically as a smoothly expanded sinus filled with homogeneous soft tissue density. Treatment is surgical, requiring either drainage of the mucocele intranasally or its complete excision with fat ablation of the sinus cavity.

Osteomyelitis requires prolonged antibiotics as well as removal of necrotic bone. The frontal sinus is most commonly affected, with bone involvement suggested by a tender puffy swelling of the forehead. Following treatment, secondary cosmetic reconstructive procedures may be necessary.

Intracranial complications of sinusitis occur either through hematogenous spread, as in cavernous sinus thrombosis and meningitis, or by direct extension, as in epidural and intraparenchymal brain abscesses. Fortunately, they are rare today. Cavernous sinus thrombosis is heralded by ophthalmoplegia, chemosis, and visual loss. Frontal epidural abscess is usually quiescent. It may be detected on CT scan, a study recommended in all cases of atypical or complicated sinusitis.

It should always be kept in mind that paranasal sinus cancer is in the differential diagnosis of sinusitis. The presence of bone destruction radiologically, cranial neuropathies (especially V2), persistent pain, epistaxis, or a prolonged clinical course should raise the suspicion of possible cancer.

Berg O, Carenfelt C, Kronvall G: Bacteriology of maxillary sinusitis in relation to character of inflammation and prior treatment. Scand J Infect Dis 1988;20:511. (*S pneumoniae* predominates. In treatment failures, *H influenzae* predominates, with 11% of these β-lactamase-producing. Pathogens are not found in nonpurulent sinusitis.)

Jousimies-Somer HR, Savolainen S, Ylikoski JS: Bacteriological findings of acute maxillary sinusitis in young adults. J Clin Microbiol 1988;26:1919. (76% of cultures are positive, with *H influenzae* and *S pneumoniae* predominating. Only 2 of 168 H influenzae strains produced β-lactamase.)

Linden BE, Aguilar EA, Allen SJ: Sinusitis in the nasotracheally intubated patient. Arch Otolaryngol Head Neck Surg 1988;114:860.

Maniglia AJ et al: Intracranial abscesses secondary to nasal, sinus, and orbital infections in adults and children. Arch Otol Head Neck Surg 1989;115:1424.

Som PM et al: Sinonasal tumors and inflammatory tissues: Differentiation with MR imaging. Radiology 1988;167:803.

Stool SE: Diagnosis and treatment of sinusitis. Am Fam Physician (Dec) 1985;32:101.

Wald ER: Sinusitis in children. Pediatr Infect Dis J 1988;7(11 Suppl):S150.

3. NASAL VESTIBULITIS

Inflammation at the nasal vestibule commonly results from folliculitis of the hairs that line this orifice. Systemic antibiotics effective against *S aureus* (such as nafcillin) are indicated. Topical mupirocin (applied 2–3 times daily) is a new antibiotic that appears to be a helpful addition. If recurrent, it is possible that the addition of rifampin (10 mg/kg orally twice daily for the last 4 days of treatment) may eliminate the S aureus carrier state. If a furuncle exists, it should be incised and drained, preferably intranasally. Adequate treatment of these infections is important to prevent retrograde spread of infection through valveless veins into the cavernous sinus and intracranial contents.

Villiger JW et al: A comparison of the new topical antibiotic mupirocin (''Bactroban'') with oral antibiotics in the treatment of skin infections in general practice. Curr Med Res Opin 1986;10:339.

4. RHINOCEREBRAL MUCORMYCOSIS

Although mucormycosis is rare, any physician seeing patients in a primary care setting must be aware of its presenting signs and symptoms. The fungus (*Mucor, Absidia, Rhizopus*) spreads rapidly through vascular channels and may be lethal if not detected early. Patients with mucormycosis almost invariably have an underlying disease, often diabetes mellitus or uremia. The initial symptoms may be similar to those of bacterial sinusitis, although facial pain is often more severe. Examination of the nasal mucosa is likely to show black, necrotic eschar adherent to the inferior turbinate. Cranial neuropathies and black necrotic skin overlying the ethmoid sinuses are advanced signs. Diagnosis requires biopsy, which reveals broad nonseptate hyphae within tissues.

Mucormycosis represents a medical and surgical emergency. Once recognized, prompt wide surgical debridement and amphotericin B by intravenous infusion are indicated. Close management of the underlying disease is also of great importance. Even with early diagnosis and immediate appropriate intervention, the prognosis is guarded. In diabetics, the mortality rate is about 20%; in patients with renal failure, the mortality rate is over 50%.

Goering P, Berlinger NT, Weisdorf DJ: Aggressive combined modality treatment of progressive sinonasal fungal infections in immunocompromised patients. Am J Med 1988;85:619.

Parfrey NA: Improved diagnosis and prognosis of mucormycosis: A clinicopathologic study of 33 cases. Medicine 1986;65:113.

ALLERGIC RHINITIS

The symptoms of ''hay fever'' are similar to those of viral rhinitis but are usually more persistent and show seasonal variation. Nasal symptoms are often accompanied by eye irritation, which causes pruritus, erythema, and excessive tearing. Numerous allergens may cause these symptoms: pollens are most common in the spring, grasses in the summer, and ragweed in the fall. Dust and household mites may produce year-round symptoms.

On physical examination, the mucosa of the turbinates is usually pale or violaceous because of venous engorgement—in contrast to the erythema of viral rhinitis. Nasal polyps, which are yellowish boggy masses of hypertrophic mucosa, may be seen.

Treatment is symptomatic in most cases. Oral decongestants alone are usually helpful, although antihistamines more specifically counteract allergic mechanisms. Numerous over-the-counter preparations are available. Nasal corticosteroid sprays such as beclomethasone and flunisolide (Nasalide), are remarkably effective if used appropriately. These sprays should be administered as 2 activations into each nostril twice daily for 1 month. Compliance is poor unless patients know that improvement usually does not begin until 1–2 weeks after starting therapy. Intranasal steroids are especially helpful in shrinking nasal polyps, often eliminating the need for surgery. Intranasal cromolyn (Nasalcrom) may be useful, especially when administered before expected contact with an offending allergen.

Maintaining an allergen-free environment by covering pillows and mattresses with plastic covers, substituting synthetic materials (foam mattress, acrylics) for animal products (wool, horsehair), and removing dust-collecting household fixtures (carpets, drapes, bedspreads, wicker) is worth the attempt to help more troubled patients. Air purifiers and dust filters (such as Bionair models) may also aid in maintaining an allergen-free environment. When symptoms are extremely bothersome, a search for offending allergens may prove helpful. This can either be done by skin testing or by serum RAST testing. Desensitization by gradually increasing subdermal exposure to identified allergens may be tried in selected patients, with variable results.

Becker GD, Radford ER: An otolaryngologic approach to the allergic patient. Ear Nose Throat J 1988;67:10. (Discusses diagnostic and therapeutic advances in allergic rhinitis.)

Broide D, Schatz M, Zeigler R: Current status of pharmacotherapy in the treatment of rhinitis. Ear Nose Throat J 1986;65:222.

Norman PS: Allergic rhinitis. J Allergy Clin Immunol 1985;75:531.

Osguthorpe JD: Current developments in diagnosis and treatment of otolaryngology. Ear Nose Throat J 1990;69:6. (Basic articles dealing with allergy.)

OLFACTORY DYSFUNCTION

The physiology of olfaction is less well understood than that of the other special senses. Odorous molecules must traverse the nasal vault to reach the cribriform area and become soluble in the mucus overlying the exposed dendrites of receptor cells. Anatomic lack of access to the receptor cells of the first cranial nerve is the most common cause of olfactory dysfunction (hyposmia or anosmia). Polyps, septal deformities, and nasal tumors may all contribute to this inability of air to reach the area of the cribriform plate high in the nose where these receptors are located. Transient olfactory dysfunction often accompanies the common cold, nasal allergies, and perennial rhinitis. About 20% of impaired olfactory function is idiopathic, although it often follows a viral illness. Some have suggested administering large doses of vitamin A and zinc to such patients, although little evidence supports their use. Central nervous system neoplasms, especially those that involve the olfactory groove or temporal lobe, may affect olfaction. Head trauma accounts for less then 5% of cases of hyposmia. Absent, diminished, or distorted smell or taste has been reported in a wide variety of endocrine, nutritional, and nervous disorders. A great many medications have also been implicated.

Evaluation of olfactory dysfunction should include a thorough history of systemic illnesses and medication use as well as a physical examination focusing on the nose and nervous system. Most clinical offices are not set up to test olfaction, but such feats may at times be worthwhile if only to assess whether a patient possesses any sense of smell at all. Odor threshold should be tested in increasing concentrations. For example, use n-butyl alcohol (1-butanolol) in concentrations up to 4% in deionized water. Serial 3:1 dilutions in 12 steps produce an initial test of 46 ppb (v/v) and the maximum of 3055 ppm (at 4%). Odor identification can be tested using standardized choices (see references). In permanent hyposmia, counseling should be offered about seasoning foods with spices (eg, pepper) that stimulate the trigeminal as well as olfactory chemoreceptors and safety issues such as the use of smoke alarms and electric rather than gas home appliances.

Cain WS: Testing olfaction in a clinical setting. Ear Nose Throat J 1989;68:316. (This issue is devoted to taste and smell disorders.)

Davidson TM et al: Evaluation and treatment of smell dysfunction. West J Med 1987;146:434.

Frank ME, Jafek BW, Scott AE: Assessment and management of taste and smell disorders. Ear Nose Throat J 1989;68:352.

Frank ME, Rabin MD: Chemosensory neuroanatomy and physiology. Ear Nose Throat J 1989;68:291.

Leopold DA: Physiology of olfaction. Pages 527–545 in: Otolaryngology: Head and Neck Surgery. Cummings CW, Frederickson J (editors). Mosby, 1986. (An indepth overview of current knowledge in olfactory function.)

Leopold DA et al: Aging of the upper airway and the senses of taste and smell. Otolaryngol Head Neck Surg 1989;100:288.

Scott AE: Clinical characteristics of taste and smell disorders. Ear Nose Throat J 1989;68:297.

Wright HN: Characterization of olfactory dysfunction. Arch Otolaryngol Head Neck Surg 1987;113:163. (Describes qualitative analysis of available tests for olfactory disorders.)

EPISTAXIS

Bleeding from Kiesselbach's plexus, a vascular plexus on the anterior nasal septum, is by far the most common type of epistaxis encountered. Predisposing factors include nasal trauma (nose picking, foreign bodies, forceful nose blowing), rhinitis, drying of the nasal mucosa from low humidity, and deviation of the nasal septum. Most cases of anterior epistaxis may be successfully treated by direct pressure on the bleeding site. The nasal alae should be firmly compressed for at least 10 minutes. Venous pressure is reduced in the sitting position, and leaning forward lessens the swallowing of blood. Nasal decongestant sprays, which act as vasoconstrictors, may also be helpful. When the bleeding does not readily subside, the nose should be examined, using good illumination and suction, in an attempt to locate the bleeding site.

Topical 4% cocaine applied either as a spray or on a cotton strip serves both as an anesthetic and as a vasoconstricting agent. When visible, the bleeding site may be cauterized with silver nitrate, diathermy, or electrocautery. A supplemental patch of Surgicel or Gelfoam may be helpful.

Occasionally, a site of bleeding may be inaccessible to direct control, or attempts at direct control may be unsuccessful. In such cases, nasal packing is necessary. A properly placed anterior pack requires several feet of half-inch iodoform packing lubricated with bacitracin or petroleum ointment. The packing is carefully and systematically placed along the floor and then the vault of the nose. If the equipment necessary to place a pack is not available, various manufactured nasal balloons may serve as either a temporizing or definitive solution.

About 5% of nasal bleeding originates in the posterior nasal cavity. This requires placement of a pack to occlude the choana before placement of a pack anteriorly. Because this is uncomfortable for the patient and because it requires oxygen supplementation to prevent hypoxia, hospitalization for several days is indicated. Narcotic analgesics are needed to reduce the considerable discomfort and elevated blood pressure caused by a posterior pack. Immediate ligation of the nasal arterial supply (internal maxillary artery and ethmoid arteries) is a reasonable alternative to posterior nasal packing. This surgery is certainly necessary when packing fails to control life-threatening hemorrhage. On rare occasions, selective arterial embolization or ligation of the external carotid artery may be necessary.

After control of epistaxis, the patient is advised to avoid vigorous exercise for several days. Avoidance of hot or spicy foods and tobacco is also advisable, as they may cause vasodilation. Avoiding nasal trauma is an obvious necessity and may require trimming children's nails. Lubrication with petroleum jelly or bacitracin ointment and increasing home humidity may be useful ancillary measures.

It is important in all patients with epistaxis, especially if recurrent, to consider underlying causes of the bleeding. A check of the PT, PTT, and platelet count may be indicated. Similarly, once the acute episode has passed, careful examination of the nose and paranasal sinuses to rule out neoplasia is wise.

Erwin SA: Epistaxis: How to control the persistent nosebleed. Postgrad Med (Sept)/1987;82:59. (Emphasizes the first requirement—of looking for [and how to do so] a specific bleeding site.)

Jackson KR, Jackson RT: Factors associated with active, refractory epistaxis. Arch Otolaryngol Head Neck Surg 1988;114:862. (Hypertension, alcohol, and aspirin were common.)

John DG et al: Who should treat epistaxis? J Laryngol Otol 1987;101:139. (Practical approach to triage.)

Perretta LJ, Denslow BL, Brown CG: Emergency evaluation and management of epistaxis. Emerg Med Clin North Am 1987;5:265.

NASAL TRAUMA

The nasal pyramid is the most frequently fractured bone in the body. Fracture is suggested by crepitance or palpably mobile bony segments. Epistaxis and pain are common, as are soft tissue hematomas ("black eye"). It is important to make certain that there is no palpable step-off of the infraorbital rim, which would indicate the presence of a zygomatic complex fracture. Radiologic confirmation may at times be helpful but is not necessary in uncomplicated nasal fractures.

Treatment is aimed at maintaining long-term nasal airway patency and nasal aesthetics. Closed reduction, using topical 4% cocaine and locally injected 1% lidocaine, should be attempted within 1 week of injury. In the presence of marked nasal swelling, it is best to wait several days for the edema to subside before undertaking reduction. Persistent functional or cosmetic defects may be repaired by delayed reconstructive nasal surgery.

Intranasal examination should be performed in all cases to rule out septal hematoma, which appears as a widening of the anterior septum, visible just posterior to the columella. The septal cartilage receives its only nutrition from its closely adherent mucoperichondrium. An untreated subperichondrial hematoma will result in loss of the nasal cartilage with resultant saddlenose deformity. Undrained septal hematomas may become infected, with S aureus the predominant organism. Treatment consists of incision and drainage via an intranasal septal mucosal incision. It is important to be sure that both sides of the septal cartilage are adequately drained. A small Penrose drain sutured in place is helpful. Antibiotics should be given and the drained fluid sent for culture.

Colton JJ, Beekhuis GJ: Management of nasal fractures. Otolaryngol Clin North Am 1986;19:73.

TUMORS & GRANULOMATOUS DISEASE

1. BENIGN NASAL TUMORS

Nasal Polyps

Nasal polyps are pale, edematous, mucosally covered masses commonly seen in patients with allergic rhinitis. They may result in chronic nasal obstruction and a diminished sense of smell. In patients with nasal polyps and a history of asthma, aspirin should be avoided, as it may precipitate a severe episode of bronchospasm. The presence of polyps in children should alert the physician to the possibility of cystic fibrosis.

Medical treatment with topical nasal steroid sprays (such as beclomethasone) is usually successful for small polyps. A short course of oral corticosteroids (eg, prednisone) may also be of benefit. When medical management is unsuccessful, polyps should be removed surgically. In healthy persons, this is a minor outpatient procedure. When frequent recurrence is likely or when surgery itself is associated with increased risk (such as in asthmatics), a more complete procedure, such as ethmoidectomy, may be advisable initially. In recurrent polyposis, it may be necessary to remove polyps from the ethmoid, sphenoid, and maxillary sinuses to provide longer-lasting relief. This may be done intranasally, endoscopically, via an anterior transantral route through the gingivolabial sulcus (Caldwell-Luc), or through an external skin incision depending on the extent of disease.

Perkins JA, Bladeslee DB, Andrade P: Nasal polyps: A manifestation of allergy? Otolaryngol Head Neck Surg 1989;101:641.

Levine HL: Functional endoscopic sinus surgery: Evaluation, surgery, and follow-up of 250 patients. Laryngoscope 1990;100:79. (High success rate in properly selected patients. Serious potential complications.)

Inverted Papilloma

Inverted papillomas are benign tumors that usually arise from the lateral wall of the nose. They present with unilateral nasal obstruction and occasionally hemorrhage. Because squamous cell carcinomas are seen in 5–10% of inverted papillomas, complete excision is necessary. Lateral rhinotomy and medial maxillectomy, with all tissue carefully processed for the pathology laboratory, is usually the procedure of choice.

Juvenile Angiofibroma

These highly vascular tumors arise in the nasopharynx, typically in adolescent males. Initially, they cause nasal obstruction and hemorrhage. Any adolescent male with recurrent epistaxis should be checked to be sure he is not harboring an angiofibroma. Though benign, these tumors expand locally from the nasopharynx to involve the nasal cavity, the sphenoid and other paranasal sinuses, the clivus, and the intracranial structures.

2. MALIGNANT NASAL TUMORS

Unfortunately, malignant tumors of the nose, nasopharynx, and paranasal sinuses tend to remain asymptomatic until late in their course. In general, the prognosis is poor. Early symptoms are nonspecific, mimicking those of rhinitis or sinusitis. Unilateral nasal obstruction and discharge are common, with pain and recurrent hemorrhage often clues to the diagnosis of cancer. Any patient with unilateral or persistent nasal symptoms should be thoroughly evaluated. A high index of suspicion remains a key to the earlier diagnosis of these tumors. Patients often present with advanced symptoms such as proptosis, expansion of a cheek, or ill-fitting maxillary dentures. Malar hypesthesia, due to involvement of the infraorbital nerve, is common in maxillary sinus tumors. Biopsy is necessary for definitive diagnosis, and MRI or CT scan will usually delineate the extent of disease.

Squamous cell carcinoma is the most common cancer seen in this anatomic region. It is especially common in the nasopharynx, where it obstructs the auditory tube and results in serous otitis media. Nasopharyngeal carcinoma (poorly differentiated squamous cell carcinoma, nonkeratinizing squamous cell carcinoma, or lymphoepithelioma) is usually associated with elevated IgA viral capsid antigen to Epstein-Barr virus. It is particularly common in patients of southern Chinese descent but is seen in all populations. Any adult with persistent serous otitis media, especially when unilateral, requires careful evaluation of the nasopharynx. Adenocarcinoma, mucosal melanomas, sarcomas, and non-Hodgkin's lymphomas are less commonly encountered neoplasms of this area.

Treatment depends on the tumor type and the extent of disease. Nasopharyngeal carcinoma may be treated, with considerable success, by radiotherapy alone. Other squamous cell carcinomas are best treated—when resectable—with a combination of surgery and irradiation. Numerous protocols investigating the role of chemotherapy are under evaluation.

Johns ME, Kaplan MJ: Advances in the management of paranasal sinus tumors. Page 53 in: Head and Neck Oncology. Wolf GT (editor). Martinus Nijhoff, 1984. (A detailed overview of evaluation, histology, and treatment recommendations.)

3. WEGENER'S GRANULOMATOSIS, POLYMORPHIC RETICULOSIS, SARCOIDOSIS

The nose and paranasal sinuses are involved in over 90% of cases of Wegener's granulomatosis. It is often not realized that involvement at these sites is more common than involvement of lungs or kidneys. Examination shows bloodstained crusts and friable mucosa. Biopsy classically shows necrotizing granulomas and vasculitis, but in practice the differential diagnosis may be more difficult. Sarcoidosis also commonly presents in the paranasal sinuses and is clinically similar. Biopsy shows nonnecrotic granulomas. Polymorphic reticulosis (midline malignant reticulosis, idiopathic midline destructive disease, lethal midline granuloma), as the multitude of apt descriptive terms suggest, is not well understood. In contrast to Wegener's granulomatosis, involvement is limited to the mid face, and there may be extensive bone destruction. Its progression in time to a T cell lymphoma is being described with increasing frequency, and recent studies suggest clonal T cell proliferation. Histologically, there is a dense infiltrate of mature lymphocytes, histiocytes, and immunoblasts. Even with appropriate immunohistochemical stains, differentiation from lymphoma may be difficult.

Unlike Wegener's granulomatosis, which is treated with drugs such as steroids and cyclophosphamide, polymorphic reticulosis is usually best managed by local irradiation and sustained vigilance for the development of lymphoma.

Fauci AS et al: Wegener's granulomatosis: Prospective clinical and therapeutic experience with 85 patients for 21 years. Ann Intern Med 1983;98:76. (A classic review.)
Maeda H et al: Malignant lymphomas and related conditions involving nasal cavity and paranasal sinuses: A clinicopathologic study of forty-two cases with emphasis on prognostic factors. Eur J Surg Oncol 1988;14:9.
O'Connor JC, Robinson RA: Review of diseases presenting as "midline granuloma": Clinical implications for the appropriate workup of patients with midline granuloma syndrome with emphasis on recent diagnostic advances in lymphoid neoplasms that present as midline destructive lesions. Acta Otolaryngol Suppl 1988;439:1.

DISEASES OF THE ORAL CAVITY & PHARYNX*

LEUKOPLAKIA & ERYTHROPLAKIA

Leukoplakia is any white mucosal lesion that cannot be removed by simply rubbing the surface. It may consist of simple hyperkeratosis resulting from chronic irritation (eg, dentures, chronic alcohol exposure, chewing tobacco) or may represent histologic dysplasia. In about 2–6% of cases, leukoplakia represents early squamous cell carcinoma. Erythroplakia is similar except that there is an erythematous component to it. About 90% of erythroplakia is early squamous cell carcinoma. Any leukoplakic area that enlarges or contains an erythematous component should be managed by incisional biopsy or scraping for cytologic examination.

A systematic and thorough intraoral examination, including the lateral tongue, the floor of the mouth, the gingiva, the buccal region, the palate, and the tonsillar fossa, should be part of any general physical examination, especially in patients over the age of 45 who smoke or drink immoderately. Numerous benign lesions may mimic carcinoma, including necrotizing sialometaplasia, pseudoepitheliomatous hyperplasia, median rhomboid glossitis, oral epithelial

residues, and the juxtaoral organ of Chievitz. The threshold for specialty referral should be low.

PHARYNGITIS & TONSILLITIS

As common as sore throats are, one would think the most appropriate management would be a matter of agreement among all physicians. However, the issues are deceptively complex. Controversy exists over when to culture an inflamed throat and how long to treat confirmed group A β-hemolytic streptococcal pharyngitis (GABHS)—and with what. Numerous well-conceived and well-controlled studies in the past few years as well as the recent availability of rapid laboratory tests for detection of streptococci (eliminating the delay caused by culturing) appear to make a rational approach possible.

The clinical features suggestive of GABHS include fever, anterior cervical adenopathy, and a pharyngotonsillar exudate. A leftward shift and elevated white blood count are also suggestive. Marked lymphadenopathy and a shaggy white-purple tonsillar exudate, often extending into the nasopharynx, suggest mononucleosis, especially if present in a young adult. Hepatosplenomegaly and a positive heterophil agglutination test or elevated anti-EBV titer of course are corroborative. It should be kept in mind that about one-third of patients with mononucleosis have secondary streptococcal tonsillitis. Diphtheria (extremely rare today) presents with high fever in an ill patient with a gray tonsillar pseudomembrane; it should be distinguished from the more common acute necrotizing ulcerative gingivitis (Vincent's angina) and herpangina discussed earlier.

The most common non-GABHS entity in the differential diagnosis of "sore throat" is of course viral infection. Rhinorrhea would suggest a virus, but in practice the most reasonable assumption is that it is not possible to distinguish viral upper respiratory infection from GABHS on clinical grounds alone.

The authors recommend culturing every patient and withholding treatment until a positive identification of GABHS can be made. This may be by culture in 24–48 hours or may be "rapid" (Centor, 1986). Delay in treating GABHS does not appear to increase intrafamilial spread, nor does immediate initiation of antibiotics significantly reduce morbidity due to pharyngitis (fever, malaise, odynophagia). Antibiotics have no impact on culture-negative pharyngitis.

Thirty years ago, a single injection of benzathine penicillin or procaine penicillin was standard antibiotic treatment. Penicillin remains effective even though the injections are painful; if compliance is an issue, it may be the best choice. Oral treatment, however, is also effective. The controversy over choice of preparation revolves around reducing the already low (10–20%) incidence of treatment failures (positive culture after treatment despite symptomatic

* Stomatitis is discussed in Chapter 11.

resolution) and recurrences. A review of recent controlled studies suggests that penicillin V potassium (250 mg orally 3 times daily for 10 days, not once or twice daily) or cefuroxime axetil (125 mg orally twice daily for 10 days in children, 250 mg orally twice daily for 10 days in adults) are both effective. A full 10-day antibiotic course (not less) is necessary. Cefadroxil (30 mg/kg once daily) also appears effective, as are several other cephalosporins in their usual dose schedules.

Adequate antibiotic treatment usually avoids the streptococcal complications of scarlet fever, glomerulonephritis, rheumatic myocarditis, and local abscess formation. About 10% of the time, studies have shown that repeat cultures show persistent presence of group A streptococci.

Antibiotic choices for treatment failures are also somewhat controversial. Perhaps surprisingly, penicillin-tolerant strains are not necessarily isolated more frequently in failed children than in those treated successfully with penicillin. The reasons for failure appear to be complex, and a second course of treatment with the same drug is therefore not necessarily unreasonable. Alternatives to penicillin include cefuroxime and certain other cephalosporins, dicloxacillin (which is β-lactamase-resistant), and amoxicillin with clavulanate. In penicillin-allergic patients, the usual alternatives should be used, such as erythromycin and—acknowledging the risk of crossover—cephalosporins.

Ancillary treatment of pharyngitis includes appropriate analgesics and anti-inflammatory agents, such as aspirin or acetaminophen. Some patients find that salt water gargling is soothing. In severe cases, anesthetic gargles and lozenges (eg, benzocaine) may provide additional symptomatic relief. Occasionally, odynophagia is so intense that hospitalization for intravenous hydration and antibiotics is warranted.

Centor RM, Meier FA, Dalton HP: Throat cultures and rapid tests for diagnosis of group A streptococcal pharyngitis. Ann Intern Med 1986;105:892. (Compares sensitivity and specificity of new rapid tests for streptococci with throat culture results.)

Gooch WM 3rd et al: Cefuroxime axetil and penicillin V compared in the treatment of group A beta-hemolytic streptococcal pharyngitis. Clin Ther 1987;9:670. (Both are effective, cefuroxime perhaps a bit more so.)

Hedges JR, Lowe RA: Approach to acute pharyngitis. Emerg Med Clin North Am 1987;5:335. (Includes considerations such as immunocompromise, gonococcal exposure.) Hedges JR, Lowe RA: Streptococcal pharyngitis in the emergency department: Analysis of therapeutic strategies. Am J Emerg Med 1986;4:107. (Cost-benefit analysis supporting immediate penicillin when the likelihood of a positive throat culture is high. Selective use of throat cultures is recommended. We disagree with this approach but include this reference for balance. It is possible that newer rapid tests for GABHS refute to some extent the rationale for the approach this article suggests.)

Middleton DB, Damico F, Merenstein JH: Standardized symptomatic treatment versus penicillin as initial therapy for streptococcal pharyngitis. J Pediatr 1988;113:1089. (Supports the statement that immediate initiation of penicillin is unwarranted.)

Pichichero ME et al: A multicenter, randomized, single-blind evaluation of cefuroxime axetil and phenoxymethyl penicillin in the treatment of streptococcal pharyngitis. Clin Pediatr 1987;26:453. (Both are effective, cefuroxime perhaps slightly more so.)

PERITONSILLAR ABSCESS & CELLULITIS

When infection penetrates the tonsillar capsule and involves the surrounding tissues, peritonsillar cellulitis results. Peritonsillar abscess and cellulitis present with severe sore throat, odynophagia, trismus, medial deviation of the soft palate and peritonsillar fold, and a "hot potato" voice. Following therapy, peritonsillar cellulitis usually either resolves over several days or evolves into peritonsillar abscess. The existence of an abscess may be confirmed by aspirating pus from the peritonsillar fold just superior and medial to the upper pole of the tonsil. A No. 19 or No. 21 needle should be passed no deeper than 1 cm, because the internal carotid artery passes posterior and deep to the tonsillar fossa. There is controversy about the best way to treat peritonsillar abscesses. Some incise and drain the area and continue with parenteral antibiotics, whereas others aspirate only and follow as an outpatient. At times it is appropriate to consider immediate tonsillectomy (quinsy tonsillectomy) both to drain the abscess and to avoid recurrence. Both approaches are rational and have support in the literature. Whichever approach is taken, one must be sure the abscess is adequately drained, since complications such as extension to the retropharyngeal, deep neck, and posterior mediastinal spaces are possible. Pus may also be aspirated into the lungs, resulting in pneumonia. While there is controversy about whether a single abscess is sufficient indication for tonsillectomy, most would agree that patients with recurrent abscesses should have their tonsils removed.

Ophir D et al: Peritonsillar abscess: A prospective evaluation of outpatient management by needle aspiration. Arch Otolaryngol Head Neck Surg 1988;114:661.

Stringer SP, Schaefer SD, Close LG: A randomized trial for outpatient management of peritonsillar abscess. Arch Otolaryngol Head Neck Surg 1988;114:296.

(These 2 randomized studies suggest that needle aspiration on an outpatient basis is a viable alternative to incision and drainage in uncomplicated peritonsillar abscesses.)

TONSILLECTOMY

Despite the frequency with which tonsillectomy is performed, the indications for the procedure remain controversial. Most would agree that airway obstruction causing sleep apnea or cor pulmonale is an absolute indication for tonsillectomy. Similarly, persistent marked tonsillar asymmetry should prompt an excisional biopsy to rule out lymphoma. Relative indications include recurrent streptococcal tonsillitis, causing considerable loss of time from school or work, recurrent peritonsillar abscess, and chronic tonsillitis.

Tonsillectomy is not an entirely benign procedure. Postoperative bleeding occurs in 2–8% of cases and on rare occasions can lead to laryngospasm and airway obstruction. Pain may be considerable, especially in the adult. The pros and cons of the procedure need to be discussed with each prospective patient. Although reports in the 1970s suggested an association of tonsillectomy with Hodgkin's disease, careful review of this literature reveals no causative association whatever.

Kornblut AD (editor): The tonsils and adenoids. Otolaryngol Clin North Am 1987;20:207. (Entire issue.) (A good starting point for further reading about immunology, controversies, misconceptions, and management.)

DEEP NECK INFECTIONS

Deep neck abscesses are emergencies because they may rapidly compromise the airway. They may also spread to the mediastinum or cause septicemia. Most commonly, they originate from odontogenic infections. Other causes include suppurative lymphadenitis, direct spread of pharyngeal infection, penetrating trauma, pharyngoesophageal foreign bodies, and intravenous injection of the internal jugular vein, especially in drug abusers. Fundamentals of treatment include securing the airway, intravenous antibiotics, and incision and drainage. The airway may be secured either by intubation or tracheostomy. Tracheostomy is preferable in the patients with substantial pharyngeal edema, since attempts at intubation may precipitate acute airway obstruction. CT scan may be helpful in defining the extent of the abscess. Bleeding in association with a deep neck abscess suggests the possibility of carotid artery or internal jugular vein involvement and requires prompt neck exploration both for drainage of pus and for vascular ligation.

Ludwig's angina is the most commonly encountered neck space infection. It is a cellulitis of the sublingual and submaxillary spaces, often arising from infection of the tooth roots that extend below the mylohyoid line of the mandible. Clinically, there is edema and erythema of the upper neck under the chin and often of the floor of the mouth. The tongue may be displaced upward and backward by the posterior spread of cellulitis. This may lead to occlusion of the airway and necessitate tracheostomy. Hospitalization and intravenous antibiotics effective against streptococci and staphylococci (such as nafcillin, 4–6 g/d intravenously in divided doses, until cultures and sensitivities become available) are necessary. Dental consultation is advisable. External drainage via bilateral submental incisions is required immediately if the airway is threatened and when medical therapy has not reversed the process.

Stiernberg CM: Deep-neck space infections. Arch Otolaryngol Head Neck Surg 1986;112:1274.

DISEASES OF THE SALIVARY GLANDS

The salivary glands are divided into the 2 large parotid glands, 2 submandibular glands, several sublingual glands, and 600–1000 minor salivary glands located throughout the upper aerodigestive tract.

ACUTE INFLAMMATORY SALIVARY GLAND DISORDERS

1. SIALADENITIS

Acute bacterial sialadenitis in the adult most commonly affects either the parotid or submandibular gland. It typically presents with acute swelling of the gland, increased pain and swelling with meals, and tenderness and erythema of the duct opening. Pus often can be massaged from the duct. Sialadenitis often occurs in the setting of dehydration, either postsurgical or associated with chronic illness. The pathogenesis is ductal obstruction, often by an inspissated mucous plug, followed by salivary stasis and secondary infection. The most common organism recovered from purulent draining saliva is S aureus. Treatment consists of intravenous antibiotics such as nafcillin and measures to increase salivary flow, including hydration, warm compresses, sialagogues (eg, lemon drops), and massage of the gland. Failure of the process to resolve on this regimen suggests abscess formation, ductal stricture, stone, or tumor causing obstruction. Ultrasound or CT scan may be helpful in establishing the diagnosis. Sialography is best avoided in acute cases.

Children are also subject to acute bacterial sialadenitis, and at times this is a recurrent problem. There need be no underlying pathologic process. Treatment is similar to that outlined for adults, though outpatient management is worth a try. Usually even recurrent sialadenitis of childhood resolves. Epidemic viral parotitis, better known as mumps, is uncommon today because of immunizations.

2. SIALOLITHIASIS

Calculus formation is more common in Wharton's duct (draining the submandibular glands) than in Stensen's duct (draining the parotid glands). Clinically, a patient may note postprandial pain and local swelling, often with a history of recurrent acute sialadenitis. Stones in Wharton's duct are usually large and radiopaque, whereas those in Stensen's duct are usually radiolucent and smaller. Those very close to the orifice of Wharton's duct may be palpated manually in the anterior floor of the mouth and removed intraorally by dilating or incising the distal duct. The duct proximal to the stone must be temporarily clamped (using, for instance, a single throw of a suture) to keep manipulation of the stone from pushing it back toward the submandibular gland. Those more than 1.5–2 cm from the duct are too close to the lingual nerve to be removed safely in this manner. Similarly, dilation of Stensen's duct, located on the buccal surface opposite the second maxillary molar, may relieve distal stricture or allow a small stone to pass. The location of the facial nerve makes intraoral retrieval of more proximal parotid stones unsafe.

Repeated episodes of sialadenitis invariably lead to stricture and chronic infection. If the obstruction cannot be safely removed or dilated, excision of the gland parenchyma is necessary.

CHRONIC INFLAMMATORY & INFILTRATIVE DISORDERS OF THE SALIVARY GLANDS

Numerous infiltrative disorders may cause unilateral or bilateral parotid gland enlargement (see Chapter 15). Sjogren's disease and sarcoidosis are examples of lymphoepithelial and granulomatous diseases that may affect the salivary glands. Metabolic disorders including alcoholism, diabetes mellitus, vitamin deficiencies, and certain thyroid disorders may also cause diffuse enlargement. Several drugs have been associated with parotid enlargement, including thioureas, iodine, and drugs with cholinergic effects (eg, phenothiazines), which stimulate flow and cause more viscous saliva.

SALIVARY GLAND TUMORS

Approximately 80% of salivary gland tumors occur in the parotid gland. In adults, about 80% of these are benign. In the submandibular triangle, it is sometimes difficult to distinguish a primary submandibular gland tumor from a metastatic submandibular space node. Only 50–60% of primary submandibular tumors are benign. Tumors of the minor salivary glands are most likely to be malignant, with adenoid cystic carcinoma predominating.

In children, the likelihood of salivary gland cancer is considerably greater than in the adult. Watchful waiting is not recommended management of a parotid mass in a child. Mucoepidermoid carcinoma is the most common salivary gland cancer in children.

Most parotid tumors present as an asymptomatic mass in the superficial part of the gland. Their presence may have been noted by the patient for months or years. Facial nerve involvement correlates strongly with malignancy. Tumors may extend deep to the plane of the facial nerve or may originate in the parapharyngeal space. In such cases, medial deviation of the soft palate is visible on intraoral examination. MRI and CT scans have largely replaced sialography in defining the extent of tumor.

Although the accuracy of fine-needle aspiration is improving, superficial parotidectomy with facial nerve dissection is required for both diagnosis and treatment of most primary tumors. Similarly, submandibular gland masses generally require excision of the gland. In benign and small low-grade malignant tumors, no additional treatment is needed. Postoperative irradiation is required for larger and high-grade cancers.

Johns ME, Kaplan MJ: Malignant neoplasms (of the salivary glands). Page 1035 in: *Otolaryngology: Head and Neck Surgery.* Cummings CW, Frederickson J (editors). Mosby, 1986. (Review of significant prognostic factors and treatment recommendations based on them.)

DISEASES OF THE LARYNX

HOARSENESS & STRIDOR

The primary symptoms of laryngeal disease are hoarseness and stridor. Hoarseness is caused by an abnormal flow of air past the vocal cords. The voice is "breathy" when too much air passes incompletely apposed vocal cords, as in unilateral vocal cord paralysis. The voice is harsh when turbulence is created by irregularity of the vocal cords, as in laryngitis or a mass lesion. Stridor, a high-pitched sound, is produced by lesions that narrow the airway. Airway impairment above the vocal cords produces predominantly inspiratory stridor. Lesions below the vocal cord level produce either expiratory or mixed stridor.

CONGENITAL LESIONS OF THE LARYNX

Although many congenital laryngeal lesions are strongly suggested by their clinical presentations, laryngoscopy and bronchoscopy are recommended investigative procedures for all pediatric patients with stridor. This is important both to ensure the diagnosis and because multiple abnormalities may be present.

By far the most common cause of congenital stridor is laryngomalacia, which is caused by an immature omega-shaped epiglottis that prolapses into the airway during inspiration. It resolves with time, usually within the first 18 months of life, and requires no additional treatment.

Stridor in an infant with a cutaneous hemangioma suggests the presence of a subglottic hemangioma. These tumors often involute in time without treatment but may require laser excision or tracheostomy if critical airway obstruction occurs. Other causes of congenital stridor include laryngeal webs, subglottic stenosis, and vocal cord paralysis.

INFECTIONS OF THE LARYNX

1. CROUP
(Laryngotracheobronchitis)

Croup is a viral infection of the subglottic region and tracheobronchial tree. It presents with inspiratory and expiratory stridor accompanied by a barking cough. The child with croup often has had a preceding upper respiratory infection. An anteroposterior soft tissue radiograph of the neck may show a narrowed subglottic airway (pencil sign), but this is not needed to make the diagnosis. Treatment is with cool humidity in a mist tent and hydration. Dexamethasone (0.6–1 mg/kg intramuscularly or intravenously) has been shown to shorten hospitalization and may avoid the need for intubation in moderately severe cases. Adequate ventilatory status is best ensured by using a pulse oximeter to monitor oxyhemoglobin saturation continuously. In severe cases, endotracheal intubation to safeguard the airway is necessary, usually for about 48 hours. Nebulized racemic epinephrine appears to be less effective than dexamethasone.

It should be kept in mind that an aspirated foreign body may mimic the symptoms of croup.

Differentiation of croup and epiglottitis is shown in Table 6–2.

2. EPIGLOTTITIS
(Supraglottitis)

Epiglottitis is an infection involving the supraglottic region of the larynx. In children, it is usually caused by *H influenzae* type B. Fever, odynophagia, dysphagia, and inspiratory stridor are prominent. In severe cases, the child may be quite agitated, leaning forward, drooling, and have little stridor owing to severe airway compromise. In a patient suspected of having epiglottitis, no attempt should be made to view the epiglottis, as doing so may precipitate acute obstruction. The child should be kept with its parents, given humidified oxygen, and transported to the operating room for direct laryngoscopy and intubation once an appropriate team has been assembled. This team should be prepared if necessary to perform rigid bronchoscopy (to establish an airway) and tracheotomy, though this is infrequently required today. After the airway is controlled, blood cultures may be obtained and are usually positive. Treatment includes hydration and intravenous antibiotics effective against *H influenzae*. Because of the potential life-threatening nature of epiglottitis and the increasing prevalence of b-lactamase-producing bacteria, reliance solely on ampicillin is unwise. In many centers, cefuroxime has replaced the previous standard of ampicillin plus chloramphenicol (until sensitivities are available). The addition of dexamethasone (0.6—1 mg/kg intravenously) and, to a lesser extent, racemic epinephrine may more rapidly resolve airway edema, usually allowing extubation at 48 hours.

Epiglottitis in adults should be suspected when odynophagia seems out of proportion to pharyngeal findings. It may be viral or bacterial in origin. Unlike the case of children, indirect laryngoscopy is generally safe and may demonstrate the swollen, erythematous epiglottis. Initial treatment is hospitalization for intravenous antibiotics, steroids, and observation of the airway. When adult epiglottitis is recognized early, it is usually possible to avoid intubation. In such cases, it would seem prudent to monitor oxyhemoglobin saturation with continuous pulse oximetry.

Deeb ZE, Yenson AC, DeFries HO: Acute epiglottitis in the adult. Laryngoscope 1985;95:289. (Rapid progres-

Table 6–2. Croup (laryngotracheobronchitis) and epiglottitis: Differential diagnosis

	Croup	Epiglottitis
Age	6 months to 3 years	3–6 years
Stridor	Inspiratory and expiratory	Inspiratory only
Pace	Days, then bark	Hours
Agent	Viral (often)	*H influenzae* type B (parainfluenzae)
Site	Subglottis	Supraglottis

sion of symptoms [< 8 hours' duration] or drooling requires intubation; otherwise, monitoring the airway for 24 hours in an ICU is sufficient.)

Mauro RD, Poole SR, Lockhart CH: Differentiation of epiglottitis from laryngotracheitis in the child with stridor. Am J Dis Child 1988;142:679.

MayoSmith MF et al: Acute epiglottitis in adults. An eight-year experience in the state of Rhode Island. N Engl J Med 1986;314:1133. (In contrast to the Shapiro article (below), emphasizes that epiglottitis in adults can be fulminant. Twenty-three percent grew *H influenzae,* and 7% died. This retrospective study is biased toward severe cases, however, in that, eg, records from medical examiners were included and less fulminant cases may not have been diagnosed and recorded as epiglottitis.)

Shapiro J, Eavey RD, Baker AS: Adult supraglottitis: A prospective analysis. JAMA 1988;259:563. (Emphasizes that the non-*H influenzae* variety can, if recognized early, follow a more benign course than epiglottitis in children.)

Vernon DD, Sarnaik AP: Acute epiglottitis in children: A conservative approach to diagnosis and management. Crit Care Med 1986;14:23. (Good review emphasizing a well-organized approach and the success of nasotracheal intubation.)

Wolf M et al: Conservative management of adult epiglottitis. Laryngoscope 1990;100:183. (Management without intubation. Ampicillin was associated with 27% abscess rate. In 1991, other antibiotics would be first choice. See text.)

3. LARYNGEAL PAPILLOMAS

Papillomas, thought to be caused by human papovavirus, are common lesions of the larynx in both children and adults. Patients present with hoarseness that progresses to stridor over weeks to months. Repeated laser excisions are often needed to control the disease. Tracheostomy should be avoided, as this may lead to seeding of papillomas in the tracheobronchial tree, a potentially lethal complication.

4. VIRAL LARYNGITIS

Viral laryngitis is probably the most common cause of hoarseness, which may persist for a week or so after other symptoms of upper respiratory infection have cleared. The patient should be warned to avoid vigorous use of the voice (singing, shouting) while laryngitis is present, since this may foster the formation of vocal nodules.

TUMORS OF THE LARYNX

1. BENIGN TUMORS OF THE LARYNX

Vocal cord nodules are smooth, paired lesions that form at the junction of the anterior one-third and posterior two-thirds of the vocal cords. They are a common cause of hoarseness resulting from vocal abuse. In adults, they are referred to as ''singer's nodules''; in children, ''screamer's nodules.'' Treatment requires modification of voice habits, and referral to a speech therapist is indicated. Recalcitrant nodules may require surgical excision.

Polypoid changes in the vocal cords may result from vocal abuse, smoking, or chemical industrial irritants or may be seen in hypothyroidism. Attention to the underlying problem may resolve the polypoid changes. Inhaled steroid spray (eg, beclomethasone) may hasten resolution. At times, removal of the hyperplastic vocal cord mucosa may be indicated.

A common but often unrecognized cause of hoarseness is contact ulcers on the vocal processes of the arytenoid cartilages secondary to esophageal reflux. Treatment of the underlying reflux with antacids or histamine H_2-receptor antagonists and elevation of the head of the bed is often curative. Intubation granulomas may also be seen posteriorly between the vocal processes.

2. LARYNGEAL LEUKOPLAKIA

Leukoplakia is a frequent cause of hoarseness, most commonly arising in smokers. Direct laryngoscopy with biopsy is advised. Histologic examination usually demonstrates mild, moderate, or severe dysplasia. Cessation of smoking may reverse dysplastic changes. A certain percentage of patients—estimated to be less than 5% of those with mild dysplasia and about 35–60% of those with severe dysplasia—will subsequently develop squamous cell carcinoma. In some cases, invasive squamous cell carcinoma is present in initial biopsy.

3. SQUAMOUS CELL CARCINOMA OF THE LARYNX

Squamous cell carcinoma is the most common cancer seen in the larynx. It occurs predominantly in heavy smokers, with alcohol an apparent cocarcinogen. It is most common between ages 50 and 70. Hoarseness is the usual presenting symptom. Any patient with hoarseness that has persisted beyond 2 weeks must be evaluated by indirect laryngoscopy. Odynophagia, hemoptysis, weight loss, referred otalgia, vocal cord immobility, and cervical adenopathy suggest more advanced disease.

Early squamous cell carcinoma is best treated with radiation, with cure rates in excess of 85–95%. Conservation surgery or total laryngectomy is necessary for radiation failures and for more advanced disease. Today, the use of tracheoesophageal valves following total laryngectomy restores useful speech for most laryngectomy patients.

VOCAL CORD PARALYSIS

Most cases of vocal cord paralysis result from lesions of the recurrent laryngeal nerve. In the adult, unilateral vocal cord paralysis generally presents as hoarseness with a breathy character. The most common cause is thyroid surgery. In left vocal cord paralysis, it is important to eliminate a mediastinal or pulmonary apical lesion (Pancoast's tumor) as the causative factor. Involvement of the vagus nerve by tumors involving the jugular foramen may cause vocal cord paralysis that is usually accompanied by additional cranial neuropathies (IX, XI). When no cause can be found, function may return spontaneously within 1 year. Hoarseness secondary to unilateral vocal cord paralysis may be improved by injecting Teflon into the paralyzed cord.

Bilateral vocal cord paralysis usually causes stridor. If sudden in onset, the stridor will be inspiratory and expiratory, causing sufficient airway compromise to warrant emergency cricothyrotomy. If insidious in onset, it may (curiously) be asymptomatic at rest. The voice may be quite good, as the cords are apposed in the midline. Thyroid surgery, neck trauma, and tumor invasion from anaplastic thyroid or esophageal carcinoma are among the more common causes. Immobility of the vocal cords may also result from cricoarytenoid arthritis, as seen in advanced rheumatoid arthritis. When airway obstruction is severe, tracheostomy is indicated. Various procedures, which open the glottis by lateralizing a vocal cord, have been used in order to remove the tracheostomy. A less powerful, breathy voice often accompanies these procedures.

TRACHEOSTOMY & CRICOTHYROTOMY

There are 2 primary indications for tracheostomy: airway obstruction at or above the level of the larynx and respiratory failure requiring prolonged mechanical ventilation. In an acute emergency, cricothyrotomy secures an airway more rapidly than tracheostomy, with fewer potential immediate complications such as pneumothorax and hemorrhage. In order to reduce the chance of subglottic stenosis, cricothyrotomy should be converted to tracheostomy as soon as the patient is stable.

The most common indication for elective tracheostomy is the need for prolonged mechanical ventilation. There is no firm rule about how many days a patient must be intubated before conversion to tracheostomy should be advised. The incidence of serious complications such as subglottic stenosis increases with extended endotracheal intubation. As soon as it is apparent that the patient will require protracted ventilatory support, tracheostomy should replace the endotracheal tube. Less frequent indications for tracheostomy are life-threatening aspiration pneumonia, the need to improve pulmonary toilet to correct problems related to insufficient clearing of tracheobronchial secretions, and sleep apnea.

Posttracheostomy care requires humidified air to prevent secretions from crusting and occluding the inner cannula of the tracheostomy tube. The tracheostomy tube should be cleaned several times daily. The most frequent early complication of tracheostomy is dislodgment of the tracheostomy tube. Surgical creation of an inferiorly based tracheal flap sutured to the inferior neck skin may make reinsertion of a dislodged tube easier. It should be recalled that the act of swallowing requires elevation of the larynx, which is prevented by tracheostomy. Therefore, frequent tracheal and bronchial suctioning is often required to clear the aspirated saliva as well as the increased tracheobronchial secretions. Care of the skin around the stoma is important to prevent maceration and secondary infection.

Astrachan DI, Kirchner JC, Goodwin WJ Jr: Prolonged intubation vs. tracheotomy: Complications, practical and psychological considerations. Laryngoscope 1988; 98: 1165. (Tracheotomy is far superior: fewer complications, ability to speak, comfort, ease of care.)

Berlauk JF: Prolonged endotracheal intubation vs tracheostomy. Crit Care Med 1986;14:742.

DeCarle B: Tracheostomy care. Nursing Times (Oct 2) 1985;81:50. (If a tracheotomy care protocol is unavailable at your institution, this article represents one reasonable approach.)

Kuriloff DB et al: Laryngotracheal injury following cricothyroidotomy. Laryngoscope 1989;99:125. (Cricothyrotomy should be used only in a true emergency and should be replaced with conventional tracheostomy as soon as convenient.)

Nash M: Swallowing problems in the tracheotomized patient. Otolaryngol Clin North Am 1988;21:701. (Some common misunderstandings of the effect of tracheostomy on swallowing and aspiration.)

FOREIGN BODIES IN THE UPPER AERODIGESTIVE TRACT

FOREIGN BODIES OF THE TRACHEA & BRONCHI

Aspiration of foreign bodies is not rare in young children. Tracheal foreign bodies produce immediate symptoms of obstruction and choking, while bronchial foreign bodies often have an initial asymptomatic period generally lasting a few hours. Following this, symptoms of obstruction and inflammation appear, ie, wheezing and coughing that may mimic asthma.

Plain chest radiographs may reveal a radiopaque foreign body, such as a coin. Detection of radiolucent foreign bodies may be aided by inspiration-expiration films that demonstrate air trapping distal to the obstructed segment. Atelectasis and pneumonia may occur later.

Tracheal and bronchial foreign bodies should be removed under general anesthesia by a skilled endoscopist working with an experienced anesthesiologist.

ESOPHAGEAL FOREIGN BODIES

Foreign bodies in the esophagus generally produce immediate symptoms of gagging and coughing. Dysphagia is often nearly complete. Patients can often point to the exact level of the obstruction. Indirect laryngoscopy often shows pooling of saliva at the esophageal inlet. Plain films may detect radiopaque foreign bodies such as chicken bones. Coins tend to align in the coronal plane in the esophagus and sagittally in the trachea. If a foreign body is suspected but not certainly known to be present, barium swallow may help make the diagnosis.

Although some have suggested that a Foley catheter may be used to remove an esophageal foreign body, this method risks displacing it into the larynx with resultant air obstruction. Endoscopic removal under general anesthesia is safer.

DISEASES PRESENTING AS NECK MASSES

The differential diagnosis of neck masses is heavily dependent on the location in the neck, the age of the patient, and the presence of associated disease processes. Rapid growth and tenderness suggest an inflammatory process, while firm, painless, and slowly enlarging masses are often neoplastic. In children, most neck masses are benign, arising due to congenital problems (eg, branchial cleft cysts, lymphangioma, hemangioma) or infection. The most common pediatric tumors involving the neck are neuroblastoma and rhabdomyosarcoma. In adults, the incidence of cancer is much greater. Among neoplasms, squamous cell carcinomas arising in the upper aerodigestive tract predominate. Persistent neck masses, especially when enlarging, deserve attention. Most important are a comprehensive otolaryngologic examination and histologic evaluation of the lesion, often via fine-needle biopsy.

CONGENITAL LESIONS PRESENTING AS NECK MASSES

1. HEAD & NECK HEMANGIOMA

Hemangiomas are common on the face and neck, with most appearing at birth or by age 1. Intervention should be delayed, as most hemangiomas will involute over the first few years of life. In those persisting beyond the age of 5 years, conventional surgical excision or photocoagulation with an argon laser should be considered. Intervention is mandatory in the rare cases where hemangioma interferes with swallowing or breathing.

2. HEAD & NECK LYMPHANGIOMA

Lymphangiomas, also known as cystic hygromas, present at birth in two-thirds of cases and by age 2 in 90%. They are palpable as a lobulated soft and transilluminable mass involving the subcutaneous and deep tissues of the neck. When large, they may compress the esophagus or trachea, causing dysphagia or stridor. Fine-needle aspiration yields a mucoid yellow fluid. Unlike hemangiomas, lymphangiomas do not regress. Meticulous dissection is required for complete excision with preservation of cranial nerves and important vascular structures.

3. BRANCHIAL CLEFT CYSTS

Branchial cleft cysts usually present as a soft cystic mass along the anterior border of the sternocleidomastoid muscle. These lesions are usually recognized in the second or third decades of life, often when they suddenly swell or become infected. To prevent recurrent infection and possible carcinoma, they should be completely excised, along with their fistulous tracts.

First branchial cleft cysts present high in the neck, sometimes just below the ear. A fistulous connection with the floor of the external auditory canal may be present. Second cleft cysts, which are far more common, may communicate with the tonsillar fossa. Third cleft cysts, which may communicate with the piriform sinus, are rare.

4. THYROGLOSSAL DUCT CYST

Thyroglossal duct cysts are remnants occurring along the embryologic course of the thyroid's descent from the tuberculum impar of the tongue base to its usual position in the low neck. Although they may occur at any age, they are commonest before age 20. They present as a midline neck mass, often just below the hyoid bone, that moves with swallowing. Surgical excision is recommended to prevent recurrent infection. This requires removal of the entire fistulous tract along with the middle portion of the hyoid bone.

INFECTIOUS & INFLAMMATORY NECK MASSES

1. REACTIVE CERVICAL LYMPHADENOPATHY

The normal cervical lymphatic chain is not palpable. Infections involving the pharynx, salivary glands, and scalp usually cause tender enlargement of neck nodes. In children with frequent upper respiratory tract infections, it is common to palpate small, soft, and mobile nodes in the neck. Reactive nodes are especially prominent in infectious mononucleosis. Except for the occasional node that suppurates and requires incision and drainage, treatment is directed against the underlying infection. Enlarged lymph nodes that persist beyond several months, are firm in consistency, or show steady growth should be examined histologically.

2. NECK INFECTIONS WITH ATYPICAL MYCOBACTERIA (Scrofula)

Granulomatous neck masses are not uncommon. The differential diagnosis includes cat-scratch disease (probably more common than realized), sarcoidosis, and, especially in children, mycobacterial adenitis. Atypical mycobacterial adenitis (scrofula) usually presents as persistent adenopathy and can become fixed to the skin and drain externally. Although fine-needle aspiration may suggest a granulomatous origin, demonstration of mycobacteria by acid-fast staining (of material taken by fine-needle aspiration or open excisional biopsy) or culture is necessary to confirm this diagnosis. Treatment of scrofula is most successful with total excision of the involved nodes and appropriate antituberculous antibiotics for at least 9 months. The antibiotics used will depend on sensitivity studies but are likely to include isoniazid, rifampin, and, for at least the first two months, ethambutol in standard doses (see Table 7–12). When total excision might pose formidable surgical risks (eg, facial nerve proximity), a trial of needle aspiration or incision and drainage (along with antituberculosis medication) is worthwhile.

Alessi DP, Dudley JP: Atypical mycobacteria-induced cervical adenitis: Treatment by needle aspiration. Arch Otolaryngol Head Neck Surg 1988;114:664. (Aspiration when injury to the facial nerve is possible is an acceptable alternative to excision.)

Castro DJ et al: Cervical mycobacterial lymphadenitis: Medical vs surgical management. Arch Otolaryngol 1985;111:816. (Surgery in addition to long-term antituberculosis drugs.)

Cheung WL, Siu KF, Ng A: Tuberculosis cervical abscess: Comparing the results of total excision against simple incision and drainage. Br J Surg 1988;75:563. (Total excision cured 94%, versus 77% for incision and drainage.)

Shikhani AF et al: Mycobacterial cervical lymphadenitis. Ear Nose Throat J 1989;68:662. (Describes 2 typical presentations with cervical involvement.)

TUMOR METASTASES

In older adults, 80% of firm, persistent, and enlarging neck masses are metastatic in origin. The great majority of these arise from squamous cell carcinoma of the upper aerodigestive tract. A complete head and neck examination may reveal the tumor of origin, but examination under anesthesia with direct laryngoscopy, esophagoscopy, and bronchoscopy is usually required to fully evaluate the tumor and exclude second primaries.

The initial evaluation of most persistent neck masses is fine-needle aspiration. It is important not to perform open biopsy on a neck mass when squamous cell carcinoma is in the differential diagnosis unless the surgeon is prepared to proceed immediately with a definitive procedure. There is an increased risk of recurrence and decreased survival when premature biopsy is performed.

Other than thyroid carcinoma, non-squamous cell metastases to the neck are infrequent. While tumors not involving the head and neck seldom metastasize to the middle or upper neck, the supraclavicular region is quite often involved by lung and breast tumors. Infradiaphragmatic tumors, with the exception of renal carcinoma, rarely metastasize to the neck.

LYMPHOMA

About 10% of lymphomas present in the head and neck. Multiple rubbery nodes, especially in the young adult, are suggestive of this disease. A thorough physical examination may demonstrate other sites of nodal or organ involvement. Needle aspiration may be diagnostic, but open biopsy is often required.

OTOLARYNGOLOGIC
MANIFESTATIONS OF AIDS
(See also Chapter 24.)

ORAL CAVITY & PHARYNX

Severe gingivitis and stomatitis are frequent presenting symptoms in AIDS patients. Candidiasis is common and may require prolonged ketoconazole or clotrimazole for control, with topical nystatin less effective. Giant intraoral ulcers have been seen in some patients. Hairy leukoplakia occurring on the lateral border of the tongue is often an early finding. It may develop quickly and appears as slightly raised leukoplakic areas with a corrugated or "hairy" surface. Histologically, parakeratosis and koilocytes are seen with little or no underlying inflammation. Among HIV-positive patients with oral lesions, hairy leukoplakia was seen in 19% in one study. Although clinical response following administration of azidothymidine, zidovudine, or acyclovir has been reported, the success of treatment or even the need for treatment is under active investigation. The greater significance of the appearance of hairy leukoplakia among seropositive patients is that it may correlate positively with subsequent more ominous manifestations of AIDS.

Kaposi's sarcoma is most common on the hard palate but may be seen anywhere in the oral cavity and pharynx. It usually appears as a raised violaceous lesion beneath an intact mucosa, although it may be ulcerated, erythematous, and bleeding. Radiation therapy may control the tumor. A brisk mucositis can be expected following radiation therapy.

In addition to Kaposi's sarcoma, an increased incidence of non-Hodgkin's lymphoma is seen in AIDS. An increase in squamous cell carcinoma is also seen in the homosexual population, perhaps related to AIDS.

THE NECK

Persistent generalized lymphadenopathy is extremely common in HIV infection. In this setting, a tender or growing node may represent secondary infection, lymphoma, or other tumor. Fine-needle aspiration for culture and cytology is the best initial diagnostic step. Open biopsy will be needed if granulomatous disease or lymphoma is suspected.

PARANASAL SINUSES

Sinusitis is common in AIDS, and the causative organisms are diverse. Early sinus irrigation, with aspirates sent for cytologic examination as well as fungal, viral, *Legionella,* and aerobic and anaerobic cultures is warranted. Initial antibiotic coverage should be based on the aspirate smear.

EAR

Given the common neurologic manifestations in AIDS, it is not surprising that there is a higher incidence of sensorineural hearing loss and auditory brain stem response abnormalities in AIDS patients than in the general population. Kaposi's sarcoma of the auricle is not uncommon. Seborrheic dermatitis, more common in AIDS, may be more difficult to treat in the external auditory canal.

Ficarra G et al: Oral hairy leukoplakia among HIV-positive intravenous drug abusers: A clinicopathologic and ultrastructural study. Oral Surg Oral Med Oral Pathol 1988;65:421.

Greenspan D et al: Relation of oral hairy leukoplakia to infection with the human immunodeficiency virus and the risk of developing AIDS. J Infect Dis 1987;155:475.

Schidt M et al: Clinical and histologic spectrum of oral hairy leukoplakia. Oral Surg Oral Med Oral Pathol 1987;64:716. (The development of hairy leukoplakia appears to represent a marked increased risk of developing AIDS.)

Marcusen DC, Sooy CD: Otolaryngologic and head and neck manifestations of acquired immunodeficiency syndrome (AIDS). Laryngoscope 1985;95:401.

REFERENCES

Alberti PW, Ruben RJ (editors): *Otologic Medicine and Surgery.* Churchill Livingstone, 1988. (A comprehensive and current reference source.)

Cummings CW, Frederickson J: *Otolaryngology—Head and Neck Surgery.* Mosby, 1986. (A comprehensive text in 4 volumes.)

Gates GA: *Current Therapy in Otolaryngology Head and Neck Surgery.* Mosby, 1986. (Useful for rapid review of treatment.)

Sande MA, Volberding PA: *The Medical Management of AIDS.* Saunders, 1988.

Pulmonary Diseases

7

John L. Stauffer, MD

DIAGNOSTIC METHODS

SYMPTOMS OF PULMONARY DISEASES

Dyspnea is the sensation of breathlessness that is excessive for any given level of physical activity. The severity of dyspnea can be graded by the patient but can only be inferred by the physician on the basis of signs of respiratory distress. Nevertheless, the physician should record the level of activity that induces dyspnea, to serve as a basis for assessing the results of therapy. Dyspnea of pulmonary origin may be due to disorders of the airway, lung parenchyma, pleura, respiratory muscles, or chest wall. Extrapulmonary disorders causing dyspnea include heart disease, shock, anemia, hypermetabolic states, and anxiety. **Paroxysmal nocturnal dyspnea** (inappropriate breathlessness at night) and orthopnea (dyspnea on recumbency) usually are caused by left ventricular failure but may also be observed in asthma, aspiration, and chronic obstructive pulmonary disease.

Platypnea, the opposite of orthopnea, is dyspnea in the upright position relieved by recumbency. This rare symptom is usually caused by right-to-left intracardiac or pulmonary vascular shunting of venous blood.

Persistent cough should always be considered abnormal. The cough reflex may be triggered by stimulation of receptors located in the tracheobronchial tree, the upper airway, and in other sites such as the sinuses, auditory canal, pleura, pericardium, esophagus, stomach, and diaphragm. Cough may also be caused by drugs (angiotensin converting enzyme inhibitors), cardiac disease, occupational agents, and psychogenic factors. Thus, the differential diagnosis of cough is considerable. Chronic, persistent cough is often caused by cigarette smoking, asthma, or chronic obstructive pulmonary disease. However, the physician may encounter patients with this complaint in whom the history, physical examination, chest x-ray, and pulmonary function tests do not suggest a specific cause. In such cases, the cough is usually found to be caused by postnasal drip, occult asthma, gastroesophageal reflux, bronchitis, or bronchiectasis. Complications of severe cough include worsening of bronchospasm, vomiting, rib fractures, urinary incontinence, and, occasionally, syncope.

Stridor is a crowing sound during breathing caused by turbulent airflow through a narrowed upper airway. Inspiratory stridor suggests extrathoracic variable airway obstruction, while expiratory stridor indicates intrathoracic variable airway obstruction. Inspiratory and expiratory stridor occurring together suggest fixed obstruction anywhere in the upper airway. Snoring is an inspiratory sound due to vibration in the pharynx during sleep.

Wheezes are continuous musical or whistling noises caused by turbulent airflow through narrowed intrathoracic airways. Most, but not all, complaints of wheezing are due to asthma. Wheezing may be accompanied by a sensation of chest tightness, a nonspecific feeling of labored breathing that implies bronchoconstriction.

Hemoptysis—the expectoration of blood or blood-tinged sputum—is often the first indication of serious bronchopulmonary disease; the history distinguishes it from hematemesis and from nasopharyngeal bleeding. The duration of symptoms, the appearance of the expectorated blood, and accompanying symptoms help narrow the differential diagnosis. Bright red, frothy blood implies a bronchopulmonary origin of bleeding. Patients are rarely able to accurately localize the site of bronchopulmonary bleeding. Though bronchitis and bronchiectasis are more common causes of hemoptysis, carcinoma must always be excluded. Massive hemoptysis, defined arbitrarily as the coughing up of more than 200–600 mL of blood in 24 hours, is often caused by bronchiectasis, tuberculosis (particularly from a Rasmussen aneurysm in cavitary disease), mycetomas, and other chronic suppurative parenchymal diseases.

Burki NK et al: Dyspnea: Mechanism, evaluation, and treatment. Am Rev Respir Dis 1988;138:1040.

Irwin RS, Curley FJ, French CL: Chronic cough. The spectrum and frequency of causes, key components of the diagnostic evaluation, and outcome of specific therapy. Am Rev Respir Dis 1990;141:640. (Can be effectively treated in nearly all cases after identification of specific cause.)

SIGNS OF PULMONARY DISEASES

Tachypnea may be defined arbitrarily as a respiratory rate greater than 25/min; a sudden onset or persistence of tachypnea is particularly alarming. **Hyperpnea** is rapid, deep breathing. **Hyperventilation** is an increase in the amount of air entering the alveoli, causing hypocapnia.

The thorax is normally symmetric, and both sides expand equally on inspiration. Asymmetry at rest is observed in scoliosis, chest wall deformity, severe fibrothorax, and conditions with unilateral loss of lung volume. Symmetrically reduced chest expansion during deep inspiration is seen in such conditions as neuromuscular disease, emphysema, and ankylosis of the spine. Asymmetric chest expansion during inspiration suggests unilateral airway obstruction, pleural or pulmonary fibrosis, or splinting due to chest pain. Expansion of the chest but collapse of the abdomen on inspiration indicates weakness or paralysis of the diaphragm. If the chest collapses and the abdomen rises on inspiration, airway obstruction or a flail deformity of the chest wall may be present.

The arterial blood pressure normally falls about 5 mm Hg on inspiration. **Paradoxic pulse,** an exaggeration of the normal response, is defined as a fall in systolic arterial blood pressure of 10 mm Hg or more on inspiration. This occurs in severe asthma or emphysema, upper airway obstruction, pulmonary embolism, pericardial constriction or tamponade, and restrictive cardiomyopathy.

Cyanosis is a bluish discoloration of skin or mucous membranes caused by increased amounts of unsaturated hemoglobin in the blood. Anemia may preclude detection of cyanosis in a hypoxemic patient. **Central cyanosis,** which is usually caused by hypoxemia from respiratory failure or a right-to-left intracardiac or intrapulmonary shunt, is apparent on inspection of the oral mucous membranes; **peripheral cyanosis** is more likely due to nonrespiratory causes such as reduced cardiac output and vasoconstriction.

Digital clubbing is present when the anteroposterior thickness of the index finger at the base of the fingernail exceeds the thickness of the distal interphalangeal joint. Nail bed sponginess, rounding of the nail plate, and flattening of the angle between the nail plate and proximal nail skin fold are helpful clues to clubbing. Symmetric clubbing occurs in lung cancer, bronchiectasis, lung abscess, pulmonary arteriovenous malformation, idiopathic pulmonary fibrosis, and cystic fibrosis. It is rarely seen in chronic obstructive pulmonary disease and asthma. Nonpulmonary causes of symmetric clubbing include cyanotic congenital heart disease, infective endocarditis, cirrhosis, and inflammatory bowel disease. Clubbing may be familial and is especially common in blacks.

Hyperresonance to percussion occurs in diseases accompanied by hyperinflation (asthma, emphysema) and in pneumothorax. **Dullness** to percussion is observed in thickening of the chest wall or pleura, pleural effusion, atelectasis, parenchymal infiltration or consolidation, elevation of the diaphragm, or displacement of abdominal contents into the thorax.

Vesicular breath sounds are normal soft, low-pitched sounds heard at the periphery of the lung. The finding of harsh **bronchial (tracheal) breath sounds** in areas where vesicular sounds are normally heard implies consolidation, compression, or infiltration of the lung with a patent bronchus. **Bronchovesicular breath sounds** are intermediate in tone quality between vesicular and bronchial sounds. Diminished breath sounds imply inspiratory obstruction to airflow in large airways, pleural disease (especially effusion), or pneumothorax.

Adventitious sounds are abnormal sounds on auscultation and may be classified as continuous **(wheezes, rhonchi)** or discontinuous **(crackles or rales).** Wheezes result from bronchospasm, bronchial or bronchiolar mucosal edema, or airway obstruction by mucus, tumors, or foreign bodies. Rhonchi are often caused by sputum in large airways and frequently clear after cough. Crackles are probably generated by the snapping open of small airways during inspiration. Fine crackles are heard in interstitial diseases and in early pneumonia or congestive heart failure. Coarse crackles are heard late in the course of pulmonary edema or pneumonia.

Tactile (vocal) fremitus denotes palpable voice vibrations on the chest wall. This is a normal finding. Localized reduction in fremitus occurs in pleural effusion, pneumothorax, or thickening of the chest wall. Increased fremitus suggests lung consolidation. **Rhonchal fremitus** means palpable coarse vibrations on the chest wall in patients with loud rhonchi.

Bronchophony refers to increased intensity and clarity of the spoken word during auscultation; it is heard over areas of consolidation or lung compression. **Whispered pectoriloquy** is an extreme form of bronchophony in which softly spoken words are readily heard by auscultation. **Egophony** refers to auscultation of an ''a'' sound when the patient speaks an ''e'' sound. It is demonstrated over compressed lung above a pleural effusion, and in consolidation.

DIAGNOSTIC TESTS: PULMONARY FUNCTION TESTS, PULMONARY EXERCISE STRESS TESTING, & BRONCHOSCOPY

Pulmonary Function Tests

Pulmonary function tests objectively measure the ability of the respiratory system to perform gas exchange by assessing its ventilation, diffusion, and mechanical properties. Indications for pulmonary function testing include the following:

(1) Evaluation of the type and degree of pulmonary dysfunction.

Table 7–1. Definitions of selected pulmonary function tests.

Tests	Definition
Tests derived from spirometry	
Forced vital capacity	The volume of gas that can be forcefully expelled from the lungs after maximal inspiration.
Forced expiratory volume in 1 second (FEV_1)	The volume of gas expelled in the first second of the FVC maneuver.
Forced expiratory flow from 25% to 75% of the forced vital capacity (FEF_{25-75})	The maximal midexpiratory airflow rate.
Peak expiratory flow rate (PEFR)	The maximal airflow rate achieved in the FVC maneuver.
Maximum voluntary ventilation (MVV)	The maximum volume of gas that can be breathed in 1 minute (usually measured for 15 seconds and multiplied by 4).
Lung volumes	
Slow vital capacity (SVC)	The volume of gas that can be slowly exhaled after maximal inspiration.
Total lung capacity (TLC)	The volume of gas in the lungs after a maximal inspiration.
Functional residual capacity (FRC)	The volume of gas in the lungs at the end of a normal tidal expiration.
Expiratory reserve volume (ERV)	The volume of gas representing the difference between functional residual capacity and residual volume.
Residual volume (RV)	The volume of gas remaining in the lungs after maximal expiration.

(2) Evaluation of dyspnea, cough, and other symptoms.

(3) Early detection of lung dysfunction.

(4) Surveillance in occupational settings.

(5) Follow-up of response to therapy.

(6) Preoperative evaluation.

(7) Disability assessment.

Relative contraindications to pulmonary function testing include severe acute asthma or respiratory distress, chest pain aggravated by testing, pneumothorax, brisk hemoptysis, and active tuberculosis. Most of the tests depend on the efforts of the patient; some patients may be too ill to make an optimal effort. Pulmonary function tests derived from **spirometry** (the measurement of airflow rates and forced vital capacity) and measurement of lung volumes are defined in Table 7–1.

Spirometry and measurement of lung volumes allow determination of the presence and severity of *obstructive* and *restrictive* pulmonary dysfunction. The hallmark of obstructive pulmonary dysfunction is reduction in airflow rates. Causes include asthma, chronic bronchitis, emphysema, small airway dysfunction, bronchiolitis, bronchiectasis, cystic fibrosis, and upper airway obstruction. Restrictive pulmonary dysfunction is characterized by reduction in lung volumes. Pulmonary infiltrates, lung resection, pleural diseases, chest wall disorders, reduced diaphragm movement, and neuromuscular disease may be responsible. Pulmonary function alterations in obstructive and restrictive disorders are summarized in Table 7–2. The changes in airflow rates and lung volumes in the restrictive category vary according to the specific cause of the disorder.

Obstructive dysfunction is graded according to the reduction in the ratio of forced expiratory volume in 1 second (FEV_1) to forced vital capacity (FVC). Restrictive dysfunction is graded by reduction in the FVC or total lung capacity (Table 7–3), comparing observed with predicted values. Predicted values are derived from studies of normals and in general vary with gender, age, and height. Spirometry provides a **spirogram** that displays time (*x*-axis) versus expired volume (*y*-axis) and an expiratory **flow-volume curve** (first derivative of the spirogram) that plots expiratory volume (*x*-axis) versus expiratory airflow rate (positive *y*-axis) (Fig 7–1). The **flow-volume loop** (Fig

Table 7–2. Results of pulmonary function tests in obstructive and restrictive pulmonary dysfunction.[1]

Tests	Obstructive[2]	Restrictive[2]
Spirometry		
FVC (liters)	N or ↓	↓
FEV_1 (liters)	↓	N or ↓
FEV_1/FVC (%)	↓	N or ↑
FEF_{25-75} (L/s)	↓	N or ↓
PEFR (L/s)	↓	N or ↑
MVV (L/min)	↓	N or ↓
Lung volumes		
SVC (liters)	N or ↓	↓
TLC (liters)	N or ↑	↓
FRC (liters)	↑	N or ↓
ERV (liters)	N or ↓	N or ↓
RV (liters)	↑	N, ↓, or ↑
RV/TLC ratio	↑	N or ↑

[1] See Table 7–1 for definitions of tests.
[2] N = normal; ↓ = less than predicted; ↑ = greater than predicted.

Table 7–3. Interpretation of pulmonary function tests.[1]

Obstructive dysfunction	FEV₁/FVC ratio
None	≥ 0.70
"Mild"	$0.61 - 0.69$
"Moderate"	$0.45 - 0.60$
"Severe"	< 0.45
Restrictive Dysfunction	**FVC observed/ FVC predicted ratio[2]**
None	≥ 0.81
"Mild"	$0.66 - 0.80$
"Moderate"	$0.51 - 0.65$
"Severe"	≤ 0.50

[1] Guidelines from Kanner RE, Morris AH (editors): *Clinical Pulmonary Function Testing.* Intermountain Thoracic Society, 1975.
[2] If lung volume measurements are available, this ratio is superseded by the TLC observed/TLC predicted ratio.

7–2) combines the expiratory and inspiratory flow-volume curves and is especially helpful for determining intrathoracic and extrathoracic airway dynamics and the site of airway obstruction.

Spirometry (cost approximately $30.00–50.00) is adequate for evaluation of most patients with suspected respiratory disease. If airflow obstruction is evident, spirometry is repeated 10–20 minutes after an inhaled bronchodilator is administered. Measurements of lung volumes and diffusing capacity are useful in selected patients, but these tests double the cost of pulmonary function testing and should not be ordered routinely.

Measurement of the single-breath diffusing capacity for carbon monoxide ($D_L CO$), which reflects the ability of the lung to transfer gas across the alveolar/capillary interface, is particularly helpful in evaluation of patients with diffuse infiltrative lung disease or emphysema. A diffusing capacity less than 80% of predicted value, after correction for the blood hemoglobin level,* suggests the presence of a diffusion defect. Reporting the ratio of measured diffusing capacity to alveolar volume (D_L) is helpful, because the diffusion capacity may be decreased by reduction in lung volume (lung resection, some alveolar filling precesses). In patients with emphysema, the diffusing capacity is characteristically low, the alveolar volume normal or increased, and the $D_L CO/V_A$ ratio is low. In patients with diffuse infiltrative lung disease, both the diffusing capacity and the alveolar volume are characteristically reduced, and the $D_L CO/V_A$ ratio is normal or near normal.

In patients with AIDS, $D_L CO$ is a highly sensitive screening test for the presence of pulmonary disease, especially *Pneumocystis carinii* pneumonia, but it lacks specificity. A normal $D_L CO$ in an AIDS patient is strong evidence against an AIDS-related pulmonary infection. An abnormal result indicates the need for

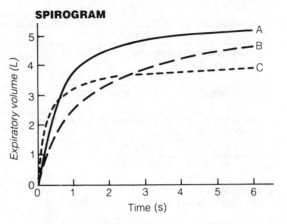

SPIROGRAM

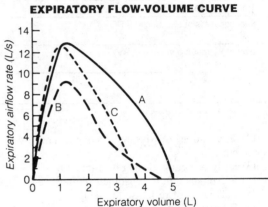

EXPIRATORY FLOW-VOLUME CURVE

Figure 7–1. Representative spirograms (upper panel) and expiratory flow-volume curves (lower panel) for normal *(A)*, obstructive *(B)*, and restrictive *(C)* patterns.

further diagnostic evaluation. Routine measurement of $D_L CO$ and other pulmonary function tests in AIDS patients with pulmonary disease is not advised.

Arterial blood gas analysis is fundamental to the modern practice of pulmonary medicine (see Chapter 16). An arterial blood gas profile (charges range from $35.00 to $75.00) is indicated whenever a clinically important acid-base disturbance or hypoxemia is suspected. **Oximetry** provides an inexpensive, noninvasive alternative means of monitoring oxyhemoglobin saturation with oxygen. Pulse oximeters are accurate and portable and monitor heart rate as well as saturation. It is important to recognize that all oximeters monitor oxygen saturation and not oxygen tension. Noninvasive oximetry has the added advantage of being safer than arterial puncture for health care providers in an era of concern about exposure to HIV virus through accidental needle sticks. Table 7–4 displays the normal relationship between oxyhemoglobin saturation and partial pressure of oxygen in blood; Table 7–5 displays the effect of altitude on arterial P_{O_2}.

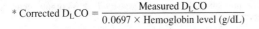

* Corrected $D_L CO = \dfrac{\text{Measured } D_L CO}{0.0697 \times \text{Hemoglobin level (g/dL)}}$

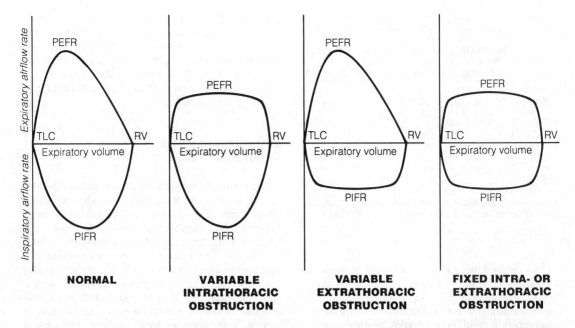

Figure 7–2. Maximal expiratory and inspiratory flow-volume curves are combined to form the flow-volume loop. Representative normal and abnormal patterns are illustrated. TLC equals total lung capacity; RV equals residual volume; PEFR equals peak expiratory airflow rate; PIFR equals peak inspiratory airflow rate.

Table 7–4. Relationship of oxyhemoglobin saturation and partial pressure of oxygen in blood.[1,2]

Saturation (%)	Partial Pressure (mm Hg)[3]
50	27
55	29
60	31
65	34
70	37
75	40
80	45
85	50
90	58
91	60
92	63
93	66
94	69
95	74
96	81
97	92
98	111
99	159
99.9	500

[1] Modified and reproduced, with permission, from Severinghaus JW: Values for a standard blood oxygen dissociation curve: Man. Page 204 in: *Respiration and Circulation.* Altman PC, Dittmer DS (editors): Federation of American Societies for Experimental Biology, 1971.
[2] This relationship assumes a normal position of the oxyhemoglobin dissociation curve.
[3] Rounded to the nearest whole number.

Gardner RM: Standardization of spirometry: A summary of recommendations from the American Thoracic Society. The 1987 update. Ann Intern Med 1988;108:217. (Standards for spirometry, including both hospital and office systems.)

Zibrak JD, O'Donnell CR, Morton K: Indications for pulmonary function testing. Ann Intern Med 1990;112:763.

Pulmonary Exercise Stress Testing

Pulmonary exercise testing is usually performed to evaluate patients with unexplained exertional dyspnea. A bicycle ergometer or treadmill is used. Minute ventilation, expired oxygen and carbon dioxide tension, heart rate, blood pressure, and respiratory rate are monitored. The exercise protocol is determined by the indications for the test and the ability of the patient to exercise. Complications are rare. The cost for a full exercise study (without arterial catheterization) is approximately $200.00.

Weber KT et al: Concepts and applications of cardiopulmonary exercise testing. Chest 1988;93:843.

Bronchoscopy

Flexible **fiberoptic bronchoscopy** is an essential tool in the diagnosis and management of many pulmonary diseases. Bronchoscopy is of value for diagnosis

Table 7-5. The effect of altitude on P_{O_2} in normals.

Altitude (feet)	Barometric Pressure (mm Hg)	Atmospheric[1] P_{O_1} (mm Hg)	Tracheal[2] P_{O_2} (mm Hg)	Arterial[3] P_{O_2} (mm Hg)
Sea level	760	159	149	99
2,000	707	148	138	88
4,000	656	137	127	77
6,000	609	127	118	68
8,000	564	118	108	58
10,000	523	109	100	50
15,000	428	90	80	30

[1] Dry gas.
[2] Saturated with water vapor.
[3] Actual values at altitude will be higher, depending on the degree of adaptation (ventilatory response to hypoxia).

and staging of bronchogenic carcinoma, evaluation of hemoptysis, biopsy of diffuse lung infiltrates, diagnosis of opportunistic pulmonary infections, facilitation of bronchoalveolar lavage, and removal of retained secretions and foreign bodies from the airway. The procedure is contraindicated in patients with severe bronchospasm. A bleeding diathesis is a contraindication to biopsy and brushing. Complications include hemoptysis, fever, and a transient reduction in P_{O_2} (< 10 mm Hg). The rate of major complications is less than 2%, and deaths are rare. Hospitalization for fiberoptic bronchoscopy is not necessary in most cases. The total cost of the procedure ranges from $500.00 to over $1000.00, depending on the need for fluoroscopy, processing of specimens in the laboratory, hospital outpatient stay charges, and other variables.

Rigid bronchoscopy is performed infrequently but is valuable in selected situations. These include massive bleeding, extraction of large obstructing objects (foreign bodies, blood clots, tumor masses, broncholiths), biopsy of tracheal or main stem bronchus tumors and bronchial carcinoids, facilitation of ventilation during bronchoscopy, and facilitation of laser therapy.

DEVELOPMENTAL DISORDERS

PULMONARY AGENESIS, APLASIA, & HYPOPLASIA

The development of the lungs is complex, so that the potential for developmental anomalies is considerable. Bilateral arrested lung development is usually incompatible with extrauterine life. An entire lung is more commonly affected by agenesis, aplasia, or hypoplasia than is a single lobe, and the condition is usually asymptomatic. Most patients with arrested development of a lung have associated anomalies in other organs. Isolated agenesis, aplasia, or hypoplasia is usually detected on routine chest x-ray, which shows volume loss and absence of aerated lung in the affected hemithorax.

BRONCHOPULMONARY SEQUESTRATION

The term bronchopulmonary sequestration denotes an area of nonfunctioning lung tissue that is discontinuous with the remainder of the lung and derives its blood supply from the systemic circulation, usually a branch of the descending aorta. **Intralobar** sequestrations share the same visceral pleural envelope with surrounding lung tissue and drain into the pulmonary venous system. The less common **extralobar** sequestration has its own visceral pleura and drains into systemic veins. Bronchopulmonary sequestration is located in the posterior basal segment of the lower lobes, more often on the left side than on the right. If no communication exists between the bronchial tree and the sequestration, the latter appears on x-ray as a soft tissue mass or infiltrate. If such communication exists, x-ray demonstrates a cystic, air-containing structure with or without air-fluid levels.

Bronchopulmonary sequestration is usually asymptomatic until pneumonia occurs and leads to infection of the sequestration; chronic infection follows.

Once sequestration becomes symptomatic, it should be resected. The aberrant systemic vessel supplying the sequestration is identified by preoperative aortography, so that the possibility of bleeding from an unrecognized anomalous artery is reduced. MRI has been proposed as a noninvasive method to diagnose intralobar pulmonary sequestration. Asymptomatic sequestration requires no treatment.

BRONCHOGENIC CYSTS

Bronchogenic cysts are thin-walled cystic structures lined with bronchial epithelium and filled with mucus. They arise when a portion of the bronchial tree becomes detached during organogenesis. Bronchogenic cysts are recognized on chest x-ray as round, sharply circumscribed structures containing fluid, air, or both. They usually are located near the trachea or main bronchi. CT scanning and MRI are useful in diagnosis.

Patients with bronchogenic cysts are usually asymptomatic. The major clinical significance of bronchogenic cysts lies in their presentation as pulmonary nodules in patients at risk for more serious disorders. Surgical excision is often necessary, because these cysts mimic lung cancer or produce symptoms resulting from bleeding, infection, compression of adjacent structures, or rupture into the trachea, lung, esophagus, or pleural space.

PULMONARY ARTERIOVENOUS MALFORMATIONS

Pulmonary arteriovenous malformation is a direct communication between a pulmonary artery and a pulmonary vein, producing a right-to-left shunt. They are multiple in as many as a third of cases and may be associated with hereditary hemorrhagic telangiectasias (Osler-Weber-Rendu disease). Pulmonary arteriovenous malformations are often asymptomatic, but they may cause hemoptysis or dyspnea. Potential physical findings include cyanosis, clubbing, and a continuous murmur heard over the malformation. **Platypnea** and **orthodeoxia** (hypoxemia aggravated by upright posture and improved by recumbency) have been observed. Laboratory studies reveal hypoxemia and often erythrocytosis. The severity of the shunt may vary as blood flow through the malformation is altered by changes in body position or lung volume. Complications include paradoxic systemic emboli, brain abscess, and hemothorax.

Arteriovenous malformations appear radiographically as sharply circumscribed round or lobulated densities within the lung parenchyma. Dilated vessels ("feeder" vessels) connecting the arteriovenous malformation to the hilum may be visible. Changes in size of the lesion induced by alterations in intrathoracic pressure (Valsalva and Müller maneuvers) during fluoroscopy suggest the diagnosis. Perfusion lung scanning and contrast echocardiography are useful as screening procedures. CT scanning with bolus contrast injection and rapid sequence imaging is an accurate method of diagnosis. CT scan may reveal the feeder vessels if they are not visible on the conventional chest x-ray. There is little experience to date with MRI in the diagnosis of pulmonary arteriovenous malformations. Pulmonary angiography, the imaging procedure of choice, is necessary to confirm the diagnosis and to rule out the presence of additional malformations. Arteriovenous malformation must be considered in the differential diagnosis of pulmonary nodules, because failure to do so may lead to excessive bleeding after transthoracic needle aspiration or transbronchial biopsy. Single symptomatic arteriovenous malformations should be resected; multiple arteriovenous malformations that are unresectable may be treated with therapeutic embolization.

Burke CM et al: Pulmonary arteriovenous malformations: A critical update. Am Rev Respir Dis 1986;134:334.

DISORDERS OF THE AIRWAYS

Diseases of the airways have diverse causes but share certain pathophysiologic and clinical features. Limitation of airflow is characteristic and results from intraluminal airway obstruction, thickening of airway walls, or the loss of distending support by interstitial tissues necessary to maintain patency of the airways. Hypersecretion of mucus, airway irritability, and gas exchange abnormalities result in cough, sputum production, wheezing, and dyspnea.

ASTHMA

Essentials of Diagnosis
- Episodic or chronic wheezing, dyspnea, cough, and feeling of tightness in the chest.
- Prolonged expiration and diffuse wheezing on physical examination.
- Limitation of airflow on pulmonary function testing, or positive bronchoprovocation challenge test.
- Complete or partial reversibility of obstructive dysfunction after bronchodilator therapy.

General Considerations
Asthma is defined as a "disease characterized by an increased responsiveness of the trachea and bronchi to various stimuli, and manifested by widespread narrowing of the airways that changes in severity either spontaneously or as a result of treatment" (American Thoracic Society). Asthma is characterized by such pathologic changes as hypertrophy of bronchial smooth muscle, mucosal edema and hyperemia, thickening of epithelial basement membrane, hypertrophy of mucous glands, acute inflammation, and plugging of airways by thick, viscid mucus. These changes result in obstruction of airways of all calibers.

The pathogenesis of asthma is poorly understood. It has recently been popular to consider asthma primarily as an inflammatory disease of airways, but this concept is now being challenged. The pivotal role of allergic mechanisms in asthma is gaining more attention. Multiple complex mechanisms probably are involved in reversible airflow obstruction. Mast cells, neutrophils, eosinophils, and platelets are important in various phases of bronchoconstriction. Putative chemical mediators of asthma include histamine, leukotrienes, prostaglandins and thromboxanes, bradykinin, neutrophil and eosinophil chemotactic factors, and platelet-activating factor. Complex neural factors also influence bronchoconstriction and mucus secretion. The interaction between airway inflammation and numerous neuropeptides in the airways, including vasoactive intestinal peptide and substance P, is gaining increasing attention.

Asthma is common in adults and even more common in children. Men and women are equally affected. About 3% of the population has asthma. Clinicians have sometimes found it useful to distinguish "extrinsic" from "intrinsic" asthma (Table 7–6), though recent work challenges the concept that there is a pathogenetic difference between the two.

Exercise-induced asthma occurs mainly in patients with a known diagnosis of asthma. Attacks occur 5–10 minutes after the patient starts to exercise and may be related to heat loss or water loss from the bronchial surface. **Triad asthma,** a combination of intrinsic asthma, aspirin sensitivity, and nasal polyposis, occurs in fewer than 10% of asthma patients. Bronchoconstriction in this condition is due to the effects on arachidonic acid metabolism of aspirin and other compounds, including indomethacin, ibuprofen, and tartrazine dyes. **Occupational asthma** may be triggered by various agents found in the workplace and occurs a few weeks to many years after initial exposure to an offending agent. Nocturnal cough may be the only symptom. **Cardiac asthma** represents bronchospasm precipitated by congestive heart failure. **Asthmatic bronchitis** denotes chronic bronchitis with features of bronchospasm that quickly responds to bronchodilator therapy. **Drug-induced asthma** is caused by many commonly used agents (Table 7–20).

Clinical Findings

A. Symptoms and Signs: Asthma is characterized by episodic wheezing, feelings of tightness in the chest, dyspnea, and cough. Cough may be the sole presenting complaint ("cough-variant asthma"). The frequency of asthma attacks is highly variable. Some patients may have very infrequent, brief attacks of asthma; others may suffer nearly continuous symptoms. Asthma is often worse at night. Nocturnal asthma is usually most severe around 4 AM, when circadian variations in bronchomotor tone and bronchial reactivity and the occurrence of late asthmatic responses to aeroallergens inhaled in the evening result in bronchoconstriction. Attacks occur spontaneously or result from various "trigger factors," including nonspecific irritants (dusts, odors, cold air, sulfur dioxide fumes), emotional stress, infection, exertion, exposure to aeroallergens, aspiration, and abrupt changes in weather. An immediate symptomatic response to an aeroallergen is often followed by a late asthmatic response 3–8 hours later. Aspirin, nonsteroidal anti-inflammatory drugs, sulfites added to foods and certain medications, and other drugs (Table 7–20) can trigger attacks of asthma.

Physical findings vary with the severity of the attack. A mild attack may produce only slight tachycardia and tachypnea, with prolonged expiration and mild diffuse wheezing. More severe attacks are associated with use of accessory muscles of respiration, distant breath sounds, loud wheezing, hyperresonance, and intercostal retraction. Ominous signs in severe asthma include fatigue, pulsus paradoxus (> 20 mm Hg), diaphoresis, inaudible breath sounds with diminished wheezing, inability to maintain recumbency, and cyanosis.

B. Laboratory Findings: The total white blood cell count may be slightly increased during an acute attack, and eosinophilia is common. Expectorated sputum is viscid on gross examination; microscopic findings include mucus casts of small airways (Curschmann's spirals), eosinophils, and elongated rhomboid crystals derived from eosinophil cytoplasm (Charcot-Leyden crystals). Pulmonary function tests reveal abnormalities typical of obstructive dysfunction, and partial reversibility (improvement in FVC or FEV_1 of at least 15% or improvement in FEF_{25-75} of at least 25%) is often demonstrated after an inhaled bronchodilator is administered. It is important to emphasize that the absence of improvement in the pulmonary function test after bronchodilator does not constitute proof of irreversible airflow obstruction. Arterial blood gas measurements in asthma (Table 7–7) may be normal during a mild attack, but respiratory alkalosis and mild hypoxemia are usu-

Table 7–6. Features distinguishing extrinsic from intrinsic asthma.

	Extrinsic	**Intrinsic**
Etiology	Mainly atopy	Complex
Antigen-related	Yes	No
IgE-mediated	Yes	No
Eczema, hay fever	Common	Uncommon
Family history	Usually positive	Often negative
Hypersensitivity skin tests	Often positive	Usually negative
Typical attack	Acute, mild	Often severe
Results of treatment	Effective	Variable
Environmental control	Useful	Not useful
Desensitization	Occasionally helpful	Not helpful
Relief between attacks	Complete	Often incomplete
Prognosis	Usually good	Less favorable

Table 7–7. Arterial blood gas measurements in asthma.

Severity of Attack	pH[1]	P_{CO_2}[1]	P_{O_2}[1]
Mild	N	N	N
Moderate	↑	↓	↓
Severe	N	N	↓ ↓
Very severe	↓	↑	↓ ↓ ↓

[1] N = normal; ↑ = increased; ↓ = reduced.

ally observed. In more severe cases, respiratory alkalosis disappears when respiratory muscle fatigue prevents hyperventilation. This is a poor prognostic sign that usually indicates the need for mechanical ventilation.

C. Imaging: Routine chest radiographs in adults and children with uncomplicated attacks reveal only hyperinflation; they are unnecessary in acute asthma unless pneumothorax, pneumonia, or another disorder mimicking asthma (see below) is suspected. Bronchial wall thickening and absence of vascular shadows in the periphery of the lung are sometimes observed.

D. Special Examinations: Skin testing for allergens that trigger attacks is most useful in young patients with extrinsic asthma. **Bronchial provocation testing** with methacholine or histamine is helpful in confirming asthma when the diagnosis is uncertain. This test is highly sensitive in the detection of bronchial hyperresponsiveness, the hallmark of asthma. It is not, however, entirely specific for asthma. Serum immunoglobulin E (IgE) levels are elevated in most cases of extrinsic asthma but are not specific. Serum-specific IgE antibody against a specific allergen can be measured with the radioallergosorbent (RAST) test, but this test is expensive and less sensitive than intradermal skin testing.

Differential Diagnosis

Wheezing occurs not only in bronchial asthma but also in chronic obstructive pulmonary disease (COPD), left ventricular failure, pulmonary embolism, and bronchogenic carcinoma. Stridor in upper airway obstruction or in vocal cord dysfunction may simulate wheezing. Asthma must be distinguished from functional disorders of the larynx. Foreign body aspiration may also present with features suggesting bronchial asthma. Reversible bronchial obstruction with eosinophilia occurs in infestations with parasitic infection (particularly *Strongyloides*), bronchopulmonary aspergillosis, and Churg-Strauss syndrome.

Complications

Complications of asthma include exhaustion, dehydration, airway infection, cor pulmonale, and tussive syncope. Pneumothorax is a rare complication. Acute respiratory failure with hypoxemia and hypercapnia occurs in severe disease. In most western countries, there has been over the last decade a gradual increase in the asthma mortality rate, despite advances in understanding the pathogenesis of this disorder and the availability of new pharmacologic agents. The explanation for this increased death rate is not clear. The death rate from asthma in the United States is approximately 0.4 cases per 100,000 population per year.

Prevention

Asthma is often preventable if environmental and occupational agents and other "trigger factors"

known to provoke asthma attacks can be identified and eliminated. Early treatment of chest infections, recognition and effective management of nasal and paranasal disorders, discontinuance of cigarette smoking, and a sympathetic attitude on the part of the physician are essential aspects of preventive care. Patient compliance with prescribed medication is essential to prevent flare-ups of asthma.

Treatment

A. Ambulatory Patients With Asthma: Most patients require bronchodilator therapy to control symptoms. Patients with infrequent attacks may use, on an "as needed" basis, inhaled sympathomimetic bronchodilator drugs. These include albuterol, metaproterenol, bitolterol, pirbuterol, terbutaline, isoetharine, and isoproterenol. All activate beta-agonist receptors on smooth muscle cells in the respiratory tract, thereby stimulating the intracellular enzyme adenylate cyclase. This increases production of cAMP, resulting in relaxation of bronchial smooth muscle (bronchodilatation). Inhaled sympathomimetics have replaced oral theophylline as the treatment of choice for bronchial asthma. Metered-dose inhaler (MDI) devices are the most convenient and practical way of administering these drugs. Anti-inflammatory drugs (inhaled corticosteroids and cromolyn) are considered by some authorities to be first-line therapy because of their ability to prevent attacks of asthma. Oral sympathomimetics should, in general, be avoided because of cardiac and neuromuscular side effects, but they may be useful in patients unable to use inhalers. Continuous treatment with theophylline derivatives is not recommended for infrequent, mild attacks of asthma; however, a long-acting theophylline compound taken at bedtime may be helpful for patients with nocturnal asthma. An extended-release albuterol tablet may accomplish the same purpose. Exercise-induced asthma may be avoided by treatment with inhaled bronchodilators or cromolyn sodium before exercise.

Patients with more frequent or more severe attacks of asthma require maintenance bronchodilator therapy with inhaled sympathomimetics, oral theophylline drugs, or both; most clinicians favor regular use of inhaled sympathomimetics both to prevent and to treat asthma. Table 7–8 summarizes drugs used in the treatment of asthma and COPD.

1. Inhaled sympathomimetics–Albuterol, bitolterol, and terbutaline are relatively long-acting and may be administered every 4–6 hours for stable asthma to maintain bronchodilatation; and metaproterenol, a shorter-acting agent, is given every 4 hours for this purpose. One or 2 inhalations are usually sufficient. For acute severe asthma, up to 4 inhalations of any of these agents, administered as often as every 3 hours, may be required.

The metered-dose inhaler is the preferred means of delivery of sympathomimetic and corticosteroid

Table 7–8. Selected drugs for obstructive airway diseases.[1]

Drug	Formulation	Usual Adult Dosage (stable patient)	Comments
Bronchodilators Sympathomimetics Albuterol (Proventil, Ventolin)[3]	Metered-dose inhaler (90 μg/ puff; 200 puffs/inhaler)	1–4 puffs every 4–6 hours[2]	Preferred formulation in most cases. Clinically similar to metaproterenol but slightly longer duration of action.
	Powder for inhalation (200-μg/ capsule)	200–400 μg every 4–6 hours	New formulation; limited experience.
	Nebulized solution (0.5%)	0.5 mL plus 2.5 mL normal saline every 4–6 hours[2]	Administer with powered nebulizer or, rarely, by IPPB.
	Syrup (2 mg/5 mL)	1–2 tsp orally every 6–8 hours	
	Tablets (2 mg, 4 mg)	2–4 mg orally every 6–8 hours	An extended-release 4-mg tablet is available for use every 12 hours.
Metaproterenol (Alupent, Metaprel)	Metered-dose inhaler (0.65 mg/puff; 300 puffs/inhaler)	1–4 puffs every 3–4 hours (or more frequently)[2]	Preferred formulation in most cases.
	Nebulized solution (5%)	0.3 mL plus 2.5 mL normal saline every 3–4 hours[2]	Administer with powered nebulizer or, rarely, by IPPB. Also available as unit dose vial.
	Syrup (10 mg/5 mL	2 tsp orally every 6–8 hours	
	Tablets (10 mg, 20 mg)	20 mg orally every 6–8 hours	
Bitolterol (Tornalate)[3]	Metered-dose inhaler (0.37 mg/puff; 300 puffs/inhaler)	2–3 puffs every 4–6 hours[2]	Longest duration of action.
Pirbuterol (Maxair)[3]	Metered-dose inhaler (200 μg/ puff; 300 puffs/inhaler)	2 puffs every 4–6 hours[2]	New formulation; limited experience.
Terbutaline (Brethaire)[3]	Metered-dose inhaler (0.2 mg/ puff; 300 puffs/inhaler)	2–3 puffs every 4–6 hours[2]	
(Brethine, Bricanyl)	Tablets (2.5 mg, 5 mg)	2.5–5 mg orally 3 times daily	Tremor, nervousness, palpitations common. Oral formulation therefore not recommended.
	Subcutaneous injection (1 mg/ mL)	0.25 mg subcutaneously; may be repeated once in 30 minutes	Slow onset of action (30 minutes). Not limited to β_2-adrenergic stimulation.
Isoetharine (Bronkometer)	Metered-dose inhaler (340 μg/ puff; 200 puffs/10-mL inhaler)	1–4 puffs every 3–4 hours[2]	
(Bronkosol)	Nebulized solution (1%)	0.5 mL plus 1.5 mL normal saline every 3–4 hours[2]	Administer with powered nebulizer or, rarely, by IPPB.
Isoproterenol (Isuprel and others)	Metered-dose inhaler (131 μg/ puff; 200 puffs/10 mL)	1–3 puffs every 2–4 hours	
	Nebulized solution (0.5%; 1% also available)	0.5 mL of 0.5% solution plus 1.5 mL normal saline every 2–4 hours	Administer with powered nebulizer or, rarely, by IPPB.
Epinephrine (many brands)	Metered dose inhaler (0.2 mg/ puff)	1–2 puffs every 2–4 hours	Available without prescription. β_1 and α stimulation limit usefulness.
	Subcutaneous injection (0.1%, 1:1000)	0.3–0.5 mL subcutaneously; may be repeated once in 30 minutes	Use with caution in older patients or those with tachycardia, hypertension, or arrhythmia. No more effective than inhaled β_2 agonist.
Anticholinergics Ipratropium bromide (Atrovent)	Metered dose inhaler (18 μg/ puff; 200 puffs/inhaler)	2–4 puffs every 6 hours	More potent than sympathomimetics in COPD. Minimal side effects.
Atropine sulfate	Nebulized solution (1 mg/mL)	0.025 mg/kg by inhalation every 6 hours; volume diluted to 2.5 mL with normal saline	Administer with powered nebulizer. Side effects common. Contraindicated in narrow-angle glaucoma or prostatic hypertrophy. Outpatient use is now practically obsolete because of availability of ipratropium bromide.

[1] Only those drugs and their formulations available in the United States are listed.
[2] More frequent dosing for acute or severe episodes of bronchoconstriction is acceptable.
[3] Preferential effect is on β_2-adrenergic receptors.

Table 7–8 (*cont'd*). Selected drugs for obstructive airway diseases.

Drug	Formulation	Usual Adult Dosage	Comments
Theophyllines Theophylline, oral (many brands)	Sustained-release tablets and bead-filled capsules	200 mg orally every 12 hours initially; thereafter, 200–600 mg orally every 8–12 hours	Maintenance dose is guided by serum theophylline level. Therapeutic level 10–20 µg/mL. Absorption varies with brand. Formulations are also available for administration every 24 hours.
Aminophylline	Intravenous	Loading dose is 5.6 mg/kg over 30 minutes for a person not using oral theophylline; maintenance dose is 0.7 mg/kg/h by constant infusion pump, lower if patient has liver disease, heart failure, or erythromycin or cimetidine therapy	Calculate dose on lean body mass. Monitor serum theophylline level.
Antimediators Cromolyn sodium (Intal)	Metered-dose inhaler (800 µg/puff; 200 puffs/14.2-g cannister)	2 puffs 4 times daily	Clinical response may require 2–4 weeks of treatment. Useful only for prophylaxis; younger patients with extrinsic asthma are more likely to benefit. To prevent bronchospasm, cromolyn may be used 15–30 minutes before exercise or exposure to cold air or allergens.
	Nebulized solution (20 mg/2-mL ampule)	20 mg 4 times daily by powered nebulizer	
	Powder for inhalation (20 mg/capsule)	20 mg 4 times daily by turboinhaler (Spinhaler)	Cough and airway irritation common with powder
Corticosteroids Prednisone (many names)	Tablets (2.5, 5, 10, 20, 50 mg)	Acute bronchospasm: 10–40 mg every 8 hours to 60 mg every 24 hours Chronic bronchospasm: 5–40 mg daily to every other day	
Methylprednisolone sodium succinate (several brands)	Intravenous injection (40, 125, 500 mg, and larger vials)	0.5–1 mg/kg every 6 hours	Clinical response may be delayed for several hours.
Hydrocortisone sodium succinate (several brands)	Intravenous injection (vials of 100, 250, 500, and 1000 mg)	4 mg/kg every 6 hours	Clinical response may be delayed for several hours.
Beclomethasone dipropionate (Beclovent, Vanceril)	Metered-dose inhaler (42 µg/puff; 200 puffs/inhaler)	2–4 puffs every 6–12 hours	Rinse mouth with water after use to prevent oral candidiasis; use 30 seconds after inhaled sympathomimetic to control cough and airway irritation. Spacer devices also helpful to prevent oral candidiasis.
Triamcinolone acetonide (Azmacort)	Metered-dose inhaler with spacer (100 µg/puff; 240 puffs/inhaler)	2–4 puffs every 6–8 hours	Cough and wheezing after inhalation are reported to be less than after inhalation of beclomethasone.
Flunisolide (AeroBid)	Metered-dose inhaler (250 µg/puff; 100 puffs/inhaler)	2–4 puffs ever 12 hours	Dosing frequency of twice daily offers an advantage.

aerosol drugs. Unfortunately, a single inhaler may cost the patient as much as $15.00–20.00. Various extension devices (''spacers'') may be attached to the inhaler to facilitate use and enhance aerosol deposition in the lung. Hand-bulb nebulizers have no practical advantage. Compressed air or oxygen may be used to nebulize certain sympathomimetic drug solutions and cromolyn solution. Jet nebulizers are expensive and inconvenient and have not been demonstrated to be more effective than metered-dose inhalers. Their use should be reserved for patients who are unable to use the metered dose inhalers effectively. Liquid solutions of different medications (eg, a sympathomimetic drug and cromolyn) may be mixed together in the nebulizer unit. IPPB is expensive and rarely indicated to deliver inhaled drugs.

2. Oral theophylline–The mechanism of action of theophylline in producing bronchodilatation is unknown. Airway smooth muscle cell adenosine receptor antagonism is the most popular of several proposed mechanisms. Phosphodiesterase inhibition is minimal at therapeutic dosage ranges. Theophyllines are now considered second-line agents for prevention and treatment of asthma. Long-acting oral theophylline preparations allow infrequent dosing. The usual starting dose for adults is 400–1000 mg/d in 2 divided doses. Serum theophylline levels should be measured 3–5 days after therapy is started and 4–5 hours after administration of a sustained-release formulation. Therapeutic levels of theophylline are 10–20 mg/mL; higher concentrations are associated with gastrointestinal, cardiac, and central nervous system side effects. Therapeutic benefits are commonly seen with levels between 5 and 10 μg/mL. Mild hypercalcemia may also occur. Short-acting theophylline derivatives such as aminophylline and oxtriphylline require dosing every 6 hours and are rarely (if ever) indicated. Drug interactions with theophylline are common. Decreases in theophylline clearance accompany the use of cimetidine, erythromycin and other macrolide antibiotics, quinolone antibiotics, and oral contraceptives. Increases in theophylline clearance are caused by rifampin, phenytoin, and barbiturates.

3. Cromolyn sodium–Inhaled cromolyn sodium is particularly useful in preventing exercise-induced asthma and attacks of extrinsic asthma but is ineffective in acute exacerbations of asthma. Cromolyn is sometimes effective in reducing the amount of corticosteroids needed by patients with severe asthma. The precise mechanism of action of cromolyn sodium is unknown. It probably stabilizes mast cell membranes, preventing mediator release, and inhibits reflux of calcium ions into mast cells, blocking bronchoconstriction. Cromolyn displays no anti-inflammatory or intrinsic bronchodilator activity. Unlike sympathomimetics, cromolyn inhibits late phase allergen-induced bronchospasm. Aerosol (2 puffs, 1 mg each), powder (20 mg per capsule), and nebulizer solution (20 mg/2 mL) formulations are available and should be used 4 times daily or 10–15 minutes before exercise. Toxicity is minimal.

4. Anticholinergics–Ipratropium bromide and atropine antagonize acetylcholine and prevent increases in intracellular levels of cyclic guanosine monophosphate, a substance that constricts bronchial smooth muscle. Ipratropium bromide, an atropine derivative, is a second-line drug for asthma. It may benefit selected ambulatory patients with asthma, such as older patients, those with nonallergic asthma, and those whose symptoms are poorly controlled by sympathomimetics alone. This drug is less effective than sympathomimetics in counteracting bronchospasm from specific stimuli. Combination therapy with inhaled ipratropium bromide and an inhaled sympathomimetic may benefit a few asthma patients. The

dose of ipratropium is 2–4 inhalations by metered-dose inhaler every 6 hours. Systemic toxicity is minimal. The availability of ipratropium bromide has rendered inhaled atropine for outpatient treatment of asthma practically obsolete.

5. Corticosteroids–Corticosteroids are effective in asthma because they suppress both acute and chronic airway inflammation. Their complex actions include attenuation of the release of and response to mediators of inflammation. These drugs may also potentiate the action of β_2-adrenergic agents.

Corticosteroid therapy is used only when other measures fail to relieve symptoms. Prednisone or prednisolone is preferred; the dosage is 40–60 mg/d orally to start, tapered in increments of 5–10 mg every 2–3 days over 1–3 weeks. Early treatment of severe asthma attacks with adequate doses of corticosteroids usually relieves symptoms and prevents hospitalization. Chronic maintenance therapy with corticosteroids is rarely necessary and is associated with many adverse effects. Repeated efforts should be made to eliminate daily corticosteroids or reduce the dose to the minimal amount necessary to control symptoms. Treatment every other day is preferred to daily treatment for corticosteroid-dependent patients.

Some patients will experience repeated severe exacerbations of asthma if corticosteroids are tapered too quickly. Inhaled corticosteroids are helpful for many such patients and may eliminate the need for oral corticosteroids or permit a substantial reduction in their dosage. They are best started when patients are stable or adequately controlled with other antiasthma medications. Many clinicians favor inhaled corticosteroids over theophyllines as second-line therapy for asthma. Choices include beclomethasone, beginning with 2 inhalations (84 μg) 2–4 times daily and progressing, if necessary, to 6 inhalations 4 times daily; flunisolide, beginning with 2 inhalations (500 μg) every 12 hours and progressing to 4 inhalations every 12 hours; or triamcinolone, beginning with 2 inhalations (200 μg) 4 times daily and progressing to 4 inhalations 4 times daily. Use of spacer devices for inhalation and mouth rinsing after dosing help prevent oral candidiasis. If inhalation provokes cough and wheezing, prescribe these drugs 20 minutes after inhalation of a sympathomimetic agent. Too rapid transfer from systemic to inhaled corticosteroids may precipitate adrenal insufficiency.

6. Antimicrobial drugs–The routine use of antibiotic therapy for acute or chronic asthma is not warranted. In a few cases, bacterial tracheobronchitis may occur simultaneously with an attack of asthma or may follow an attack, indicating the need for sputum Gram stain and treatment with the appropriate antibiotic. Empirical antibiotic therapy, which saves the additional cost of sputum Gram stain, is a reasonable alternative approach. Amoxicillin (500 mg orally every 8 hours for 7–10 days), tetracycline (250–500 mg 4 times daily by mouth for 7–10 days), and trimethoprim-sulfamethoxazole (160/800 mg orally every 12 hours for 7–10 days) are reasonable alternative choices for empirical therapy.

7. Hyposensitization–Desensitization therapy is indicated for patients with extrinsic asthma who fail to respond to conventional therapy and who have documented specific reactivity to allergens that have consistently induced asthma attacks. Overall, only a few adult patients with bronchial asthma are likely to benefit from hyposensitization.

8. Avoiding drugs that worsen symptoms– Beta-blocking drugs may worsen bronchospasm and should be avoided in patients with asthma. Angiotensin converting enzyme inhibitors may aggravate cough in patients with bronchial hyperresponsiveness.

B. Patients With Acute, Severe Asthma: Patients with acute, severe asthma are often exhausted, irritable, and apprehensive. Dehydration and toxic effects resulting from overuse of medications are common. Objective measurement of airflow is important in patients with acute asthma because the intensity of wheezing on auscultation is an unreliable indicator of the extent of airflow limitation; however, in severe cases, patients may be unable to cooperate. The peak expiratory flow rate (PEFR), the preferred index of airflow in an emergency setting, is measured initially to provide a baseline and then obtained at successive intervals during treatment. A PEFR under 100 L/min indicates severe airway obstruction.

All patients with acute, severe asthma should receive supplemental oxygen, 1–3 L/min by nasal cannula. Monitoring with oximetry is desirable. An inhaled sympathomimetic drug such as metaproterenol (0.3 mL of 5% solution) or albuterol (0.5 mL of 0.5% solution) may be tried, diluted in 2.5 mL sterile normal saline, using a powered nebulizer. A metered-dose inhaler is satisfactory if the patient is able to inspire deeply. If the patient fails to respond within 30 minutes, the dose may be repeated. Inhaled sympathomimetic therapy is superior to intravenous aminophylline in improving airflow. Subcutaneous epinephrine (0.3 mL of 1:1000 dilution) or terbutaline (0.25 mg) is an alternative form of sympathomimetic therapy, indicated only in patients unable to use aerosolized drugs.

Patients with severe, acute asthma who fail to respond to oxygen and sympathomimetic therapy are often given intravenous aminophylline, although data supporting the efficacy of this approach are lacking. Simultaneous administration of intravenous aminophylline and sympathomimetic may increase toxicity. If aminophylline is used at all, treatment is guided by serum theophylline levels. If the patient has not been receiving oral theophylline compounds, a loading dose of 5–6 mg/kg of aminophylline is administered intravenously over 30 minutes; the loading dose is eliminated or reduced if these agents are already part of the patient's ongoing regimen. Maintenance doses of aminophylline, 0.6 mg/kg/h intravenously,

are given if the patient is a nonsmoking, otherwise healthy adult. The dose is reduced substantially in patients with congestive heart failure, liver disease, or concurrent use of erythromycin, quinolone antibiotics, or cimetidine. A higher maintenance dose of aminophylline, 0.8 mg/kg/h, is recommended for young adult cigarette smokers because of increased clearance rates of the drug.

Corticosteroids are administered intravenously if the patient fails to respond to sympathomimetic therapy. Hydrocortisone (4 mg/kg) or methylprednisolone (1–2 mg/kg) is given initially and every 6 hours thereafter. A lag period of 4–6 hours before improvement occurs is common. Larger doses have no proved benefit. Inhaled corticosteroids have no proved role in acute, severe asthma and may worsen bronchospasm. Inhaled cromolyn is also not useful in severe acute asthma. The role of inhalation of ipratropium bromide aerosol in acute severe asthma is controversial. Further studies are needed before it can be concluded that this drug should be routinely added to sympathomimetic therapy.

The patient should be admitted to the hospital if any of the following are noted: failure to respond to the above regimen, a persistently low PEFR, respiratory acidosis, electrocardiographic abnormalities, pneumothorax or pneumomediastinum, respiratory fatigue, suspected airway infection, and a history of status asthmaticus or previous intubation for asthma.

Status asthmaticus is severe, prolonged asthma refractory to conventional modes of therapy. Management is similar to that for acute, severe asthma; it consists of controlled-flow oxygen therapy, corticosteroids, inhaled sympathomimetics, and antibiotics for presumed or proved airway infection; intravenous aminophylline may add marginally to the regimen. Intravenous fluids are given as needed to maintain a state of normal hydration; overhydration has no benefit and may be deleterious. Treatment in an intensive care unit with careful monitoring of arterial blood gases and continuous oximetry is necessary. The role of ipratropium bromide has not been established.

Most patients with status asthmaticus improve with this regimen; however, some develop progressive respiratory acidemia and require tracheal intubation and mechanical ventilation. The decision to intubate is a complex one and is better based on the general appearance of the patient (fatigue, respiratory distress, apprehension) than on any single laboratory finding. Status asthmaticus not controlled after intubation and mechanical ventilation requires highly aggressive therapy, eg, sedation with morphine or diazepam, paralysis with pancuronium, general anesthesia with a bronchodilating anesthetic agent, such as halothane, or segmental bronchial lavage to remove plugs of mucus. Fortunately, these extreme measures are rarely necessary.

Prognosis

The outlook for patients with bronchial asthma is excellent despite the small recent increase in the death rate. Attention to general health measures and use of pharmacologic agents permit control of symptoms in nearly all cases. The outlook is better for patients with extrinsic asthma who develop asthma early in life. Pneumococcal and yearly influenzal immunization should be part of every patient's regimen. A rigorous medical regimen may reduce hospitalization rates for patients with frequent exacerbations of asthma.

Drugs for asthma. Med Lett Drugs Ther (Jan 30) 1987;29:11.

Fitzgerald JM, Hargreave FE: The assessment and management of acute life-threatening asthma. Chest 1989; 95:888. (A succinct review of the emergency room management of acute, severe asthma.)

Holland WW (editor): International workshop on etiology of asthma. (Symposium.) Chest 1987;91(Suppl):65S. (Brief articles on etiologic and epidemiologic aspects of asthma.)

Mayo PH, Richman J, Harris HW: Results of a program to reduce admissions for adult asthma. Ann Intern Med 1990;112:864.

Petty TL et al: Cromolyn sodium is effective in adult chronic asthmatics. Am Rev Respir Dis 1989;139:694.

Rossing TH: Methylxanthines in 1989. Ann Intern Med 1989;110:502.

Sertl K, Clark T, Kaliner M (editors): Corticosteroids: Their biologic mechanisms and application to the treatment of asthma. (Symposium.) Am Rev Respir Dis 1990; 141(Suppl):1S. [Entire issue.]

CHRONIC OBSTRUCTIVE PULMONARY DISEASE (COPD)

Essentials of Diagnosis

- History of cigarette smoking (most cases).
- Chronic cough and sputum production (in chronic bronchitis) and dyspnea (in emphysema).
- Rhonchi, decreased intensity of breath sounds, and prolonged expiration on physical examination.
- Airflow limitation on pulmonary function testing.

General Considerations

The term chronic obstructive pulmonary disease (COPD) identifies patients with emphysema (type A COPD) or chronic bronchitis (type B COPD). Although emphysema and chronic bronchitis must be diagnosed and treated as specific diseases, most patients with COPD have features of both conditions. About 10 million Americans are affected. As a group, the chronic obstructive lung diseases, including COPD and asthma, represent the fifth leading cause of death in the United States. The death rate from COPD is increasing, especially among elderly men.

Chronic bronchitis is characterized by excessive secretion of bronchial mucus and is manifested by productive cough for 3 months or more in at least 2 consecutive years in the absence of any other disease that might account for this symptom. **Emphysema** denotes abnormal, permanent enlargement of air spaces distal to the terminal bronchiole, with destruction of their walls and without obvious fibrosis (American Thoracic Society). Cigarette smoking is clearly the most important cause of COPD, even though only 10–15% of smokers develop COPD. Air pollution, airway infection, familial factors, and allergy have also been implicated in chronic bronchitis, and hereditary factors (deficiency of α_1-antitrypsin) have been implicated in emphysema. Atopy and the tendency for bronchoconstriction to develop in response to nonspecific airway stimuli may be important risks for COPD. The pathogenesis of emphysema may be excessive lysis of elastin and other structural proteins in the lung matrix by elastase and other proteases derived from lung neutrophils, macrophages, and mononuclear cells.

Clinical Findings

A. Symptoms and Signs: The clinical, roentgenographic, and laboratory findings in chronic bronchitis and emphysema are summarized in Table 7–9.

Patients with COPD characteristically present in the fifth or sixth decade of life complaining of excessive cough, sputum production, and shortness of breath that have often been present for 10 years or more. Productive cough usually occurs in the morning. Dyspnea is noted initially only on extreme exertion, but as the condition progresses, it becomes more severe and occurs with mild activity. In severe disease, dyspnea occurs at rest. Frequent exacerbations of illness are common and result in absence from work and eventual disability. Pneumonia, pulmonary hypertension, cor pulmonale, and chronic respiratory failure characterize the late stage of COPD. Death usually occurs during an exacerbation of illness in association with acute respiratory failure. Hemoptysis occurs occasionally, often following the use of aspirin, presumably because of its antiplatelet action. Bronchitis alone may explain this finding, but occult lung cancer should always be considered in the differential diagnosis.

Clinical findings may be completely absent early in the course of COPD. Diminished breath sounds and prolonged expiration may be detectable during exacerbations of the disease. The physical findings presented in Table 7–9 become apparent as the disease progresses.

B. Laboratory Findings: Secondary polycythemia may be found in advanced COPD as a result of hypoxemia. During exacerbations of illness, examination of the sputum may reveal *Streptococcus pneumoniae* or *Haemophilus influenzae,* though these may be present in the carrier state between episodes of

Table 7–9. Emphysema versus chronic bronchitis: Clinical, roentgenographic, and laboratory findings.[1]

	Emphysema (Type A COPD)	Chronic Bronchitis (Type B COPD)
History		
Onset of symptoms	After age 50.	After age 35.
Dyspnea	Progressive, constant, severe.	Intermittent, mild to moderate.
Cough	Absent or mild.	Persistent, severe.
Sputum production	Absent or mild.	Copious.
Sputum appearance	Clear, mucoid.	Mucopurulent or purulent.
Other features	Weight loss.[2]	Airway infections, right heart failure, obesity.
Physical examination		
Body habitus	Thin, wasted.[2]	Stocky, obese.
Central cyanosis	Absent.	Present.[2]
Plethora	Absent.	Present.
Accessory respiratory muscles	Hypertrophied.	Unremarkable.
Anteroposterior chest diameter	Increased.	Normal.
Percussion note	Hyperresonant.	Normal.
Auscultation	Diminished breath sounds.	Wheezes, rhonchi.
Chest x-ray		
Bullae, blebs	Present.	Absent.
Overall appearance	Decreased markings in periphery.	Increased markings ("dirty lungs").
Hyperinflation	Present.	Absent.
Heart size	Normal or small, vertical.	Large, horizontal.
Hemidiaphragms	Low, flat.	Normal, rounded.
Laboratory studies		
Hematocrit	Normal.	Increased.
ECG	Normal.	Right axis deviation, right ventricular hypertrophy, "p" pulmonale.[2]
Hypoxemia	Absent, mild.	Moderate, severe.
Hypercapnia	Absent.	Moderate, severe.
Respiratory acidosis	Absent.	Present.
Total lung capacity	Increased.	Normal.
Static lung compliance	Increased.	Normal.
Diffusing capacity	Decreased.	Normal.

[1] As noted in the text, most patients with COPD have features of both emphysema and chronic bronchitis.
[2] In advanced disease.

deterioration. The ECG may show sinus tachycardia, and in advanced disease, chronic pulmonary hypertension may produce electrocardiographic abnormalities typical of cor pulmonale. Supraventricular arrhythmias (multifocal atrial tachycardia, atrial flutter, and atrial fibrillation) and ventricular irritability also occur.

Arterial blood gas measurements characteristically show no abnormalities early in COPD; indeed, they are unnecessary unless hypoxia or hypercapnia is suspected. Hypoxemia occurs in advanced disease, particularly when chronic bronchitis predominates. Compensated respiratory acidosis occurs in patients with chronic respiratory failure, particularly in chronic bronchitis, with worsening of acidemia during acute exacerbations.

Spirometry provides objective information about pulmonary function and assesses the results of therapy. Pulmonary function tests early in the course of COPD reveal only evidence of dysfunction in small airways (abnormal closing volume, reduced midexpiratory flow rate). Reduction in forced expiratory volume in 1 second (FEV_1) and in the ratio of forced expiratory volume to forced vital capacity (FEV_1:FVC) occurs later. In severe disease, the forced vital capacity is markedly reduced. Lung volume measurements reveal increase in the total lung capacity (TLC), marked increase in the residual volume (RV), and elevation of the RV/TLC ratio, indicative of air trapping, particularly in emphysema.

C. Imaging: When emphysema is the main clinical feature, hyperinflation is apparent. Parenchymal bullae or subpleural blebs are pathognomonic of emphysema. Radiographs of patients with chronic bronchitis may show only nonspecific peribronchial and perivascular markings. Pulmonary hypertension becomes evident as enlargement of pulmonary arteries in advanced disease. Doppler echocardiography is an effective way to estimate pulmonary artery pressure if pulmonary hypertension is suspected. Thoracic CT scanning may detect emphysema not apparent on the chest x-ray, but it is very costly and therefore rarely indicated for this purpose.

Differential Diagnosis

Clinical, roentgenographic, and laboratory findings usually enable the clinician to distinguish COPD from other obstructive pulmonary disorders such as bronchial asthma, bronchiectasis, cystic fibrosis, bronchopulmonary aspergillosis, and central airway obstruction. Bronchiectasis is distinguished from COPD by features such as recurrent pneumonia and hemoptysis, 3-layered sputum, digital clubbing, and radiographic abnormalities. Cystic fibrosis occurs in children and younger adults. Rarely, mechanical obstruction of the central airways simulates COPD. Flow-volume curves may help separate patients with central airway obstruction from those with diffuse intrathoracic airway obstruction characteristic of COPD.

Complications

Acute bronchitis, pneumonia, pulmonary embolization, and concomitant left ventricular failure may worsen otherwise stable COPD. Pulmonary hypertension, cor pulmonale, and chronic respiratory failure are common in advanced COPD. Spontaneous pneumothorax occurs in a small fraction of patients with emphysema. Hemoptysis may result from chronic bronchitis or may signal bronchogenic carcinoma.

Prevention

COPD is largely preventable. Many believe that early recognition of small airways dysfunction in patients who smoke, combined with appropriate treatment and cessation of smoking, may prevent relentless progression of the disease. Early treatment of airway infections and vaccination against influenza and pneumococcal disease may also be of benefit but have no effect on the progression of the disease.

Treatment

Management of COPD includes discontinuance of cigarette smoking, education of the patient about his or her disease, relief of bronchospasm, aerosol therapy, chest physiotherapy, treatment of complications such as airway infections and heart failure, use of supplemental oxygen, and other measures designed to promote rehabilitation.

A. Ambulatory Patients: The general health maintenance measures for patients with bronchial asthma are also important for patients with COPD. Goals in the treatment of COPD include control of symptoms, improvement in ability to carry out daily activities, reduction in the need for hospitalization, and rehabilitation. Controlling the frequency and severity of respiratory infections and acute exacerbations of COPD is also important.

A trial of bronchodilator drugs is warranted in all patients with symptomatic COPD. Inhaled ipratropium bromide or sympathomimetic drugs are the mainstay of this therapy; long-acting theophylline compounds may be of some added value. Although theophylline has value as a bronchodilator in COPD patients with partial reversibility of airflow limitation, its principal value in COPD may relate to improving respiratory muscle performance. The response to bronchodilator therapy is assessed with spirometry. Patients with asthmatic bronchitis and those with partially reversible airflow obstruction, frequent acute exacerbations of disease, or wheezing may benefit the most from bronchodilator therapy. The routine use of maintenance bronchodilator drugs in all patients with COPD is controversial. These drugs probably have little value in patients with pure emphysema. If a clinical trial of bronchodilators over several months demonstrates no objective (spirometric) or symptomatic improvement, they may be discontinued; however, this is not often the case.

Ipratropium bromide is superior to sympathomimetic aerosols in achieving bronchodilation in patients with moderate to severe COPD. In combination with other bronchodilators, it enhances and prolongs bronchodilation. Side effects are minimal, and effects on sputum production and viscosity are negligible. Two to 4 inhalations every 6 hours is recommended.

Corticosteroids are prescribed in the same fashion as in asthma. Candidates for a trial of corticosteroid therapy include patients with asthmatic bronchitis and those with frequent exacerbations or disabling symptoms who fail to respond to conventional therapy with sympathomimetics and theophylline; eosinophils in peripheral blood or sputum may also predict a response. Corticosteroids should be discontinued after 2–4 weeks if there is no objective (spirometric) improvement. Inhaled corticosteroids may be of value for corticosteroid-responsive patients, particularly those requiring less than 20 mg of prednisone (or equivalent) daily. Inhaled corticosteroids may permit discontinuance of systemic therapy. Cromolyn has no role in treatment of chronic bronchitis or emphysema; a trial in those with chronic asthmatic bronchitis may be warranted.

Bronchial hygiene decreases production of bronchopulmonary secretions and enhances their mobilization and clearance. Smoking cessation, avoiding airway irritants and allergens, controlling airway infection with broad-spectrum oral antimicrobials and preventing pulmonary aspiration may reduce the production of mucus. If airway infection is suspected, amoxicillin (500 mg every 8 hours), ampicillin or tetracycline (250–500 mg 4 times daily), or trimethoprim-sulfamethoxazole (160/800 mg every 12 hours) may be given orally for 7–10 days. Although routine antibiotic therapy for exacerbations of COPD is controversial, one recent study shows that COPD patients with increasing dyspnea and purulent sputum are particularly likely to benefit from antibiotics. Nicotine chewing gum (2-mg pieces chewed slowly over 30 minutes) is an effective aid to smoking cessation for patients highly motivated to stop smoking.

Increased mobilization of secretions may be accomplished through the use of adequate systemic hydration, effective cough training methods, and postural drainage, sometimes with chest percussion or vibration. One effective method of coughing up retained secretions is to have the patient lean forward and "huff" repeatedly, interspersed with relaxed breaths. Forceful paroxysms of cough should be discouraged. Inhalation of bland water aerosols is sometimes helpful. Postural drainage and chest percussion should be used only in selected patients with excessive amounts of retained secretions that cannot be cleared by coughing and other methods; these measures are of no benefit in pure emphysema. Expectorant-mucolytic therapy has generally been regarded as unhelpful in patients with chronic bronchitis, though a recent multicenter study showed some symptomatic benefit from iodinated glycerol (60 mg orally 4 times daily).

Cough suppressants and sedatives should be avoided as routine measures.

Graded aerobic physical exercise programs (eg, walking 20 minutes 3 times weekly, or bicycling) are helpful to prevent deterioration of physical condition and to improve the patient's ability to carry out daily activities. Pursed-lip breathing to slow the rate of breathing and abdominal breathing exercises to relieve fatigue of accessory muscles of respiration may reduce dyspnea in some patients. Training of inspiratory muscles by inspiring against progressively larger resistive loads improves exercise tolerance in some but not all patients.

Severe dyspnea in spite of optimal medical management may respond to a trial of an opiate drug (eg, hydrocodone, 5 mg orally 4 times daily). Constipation is a common side effect. Sedative-hypnotic drugs (eg, diazepam, 5 mg 3 times daily) are controversial in intractable dyspnea but may benefit very anxious patients. Bilateral carotid body resection is unacceptable because of the severe hypoxemia that ensues. Intermittent negative-pressure (cuirass) ventilation and transnasal positive pressure ventilation at home to rest the respiratory muscles are promising new approaches to improve respiratory muscle function and reduce dyspnea in patients with severe COPD. The routine use of intermittent positive-pressure breathing (IPPB) for stable ambulatory COPD patients has been proved to confer no benefits and is very expensive.

Home oxygen therapy is prescribed for selected patients with COPD or other severe lung diseases who have significant hypoxemia. Requirements for Medicare coverage for a patient's home use of oxygen and oxygen equipment are listed in Table 7–10. Arterial blood gas measurements, not ear or pulse oximetry, should be used to guide initial oxygen therapy. Oxygen may be prescribed for continuous use, only at night, or with exercise. Cardiovascular disorders without hypoxemia are not indications for this expensive therapy. Hypoxemic patients with pulmonary hypertension, chronic cor pulmonale, erythrocytosis, impaired cognitive function, exercise intolerance, nocturnal restlessness, or morning headache are particularly likely to benefit from home oxygen therapy.

Home oxygen may be supplied by liquid oxygen cylinders, gas tanks, or oxygen concentrators. Most patients benefit from having both stationary and portable systems. Oxygen by nasal prongs must be given at least 15 hours a day unless therapy is intended only for exercise or sleep. For most patients, a flow rate of 1–3 L/min achieves a Pa_{O_2} greater than 55 mm Hg. The monthly cost of home oxygen therapy ranges from $200.00 to $400.00 or more, being higher for liquid oxygen systems. Medicare covers approximately 80% of home oxygen expenses. **Transtracheal oxygen** is an alternative method of delivery. Reservoir nasal cannulas or "pendants" and demand oxygen delivery systems are also available to conserve oxygen.

Table 7–10. Home oxygen therapy: Requirements for Medicare coverage.[1]

Group I
1. $Pa_{O_2} \leq 55$ mm Hg, or $Sa_{O_2} \leq 88\%$, taken at rest, breathing room air, while awake.
2. During sleep (prescription for nocturnal oxygen use only):
   a. $Pa_{O_2} \leq 55$ mm Hg, or $Sa_{O_2} \leq 88\%$, whose awake, resting, room air $Pa_{O_2} \geq$ is 56 mm Hg or $Sa_{O_2} \geq 89\%$,

   or

   b. Decrease in $Pa_{O_2} > 10$ mm Hg or decrease in $Sa_{O_2} > 5\%$ associated with symptoms or signs reasonably attributed to hypoxemia (eg, impaired cognitive processes, nocturnal restlessness, insomnia).
3. During exercise (prescription for oxygen use only during exercise):
   a. $Pa_{O_2} \leq 55$ mm Hg, or $Sa_{O_2} \leq 88\%$ taken during exercise for a patient whose awake, resting, room air Pa_{O_2} is ≥ 56 mm Hg or $Sa_{O_2} \geq 89\%$,

   and

   b. There is evidence that the use of supplemental oxygen during exercise improves the hypoxemia that was demonstrated during exercise while breathing room air.

Group II:
$Pa_{O_2} = 56$–59 mm Hg or $Sa_{O_2} = 89\%$ *if* there is evidence of:
1. Dependent edema suggesting congestive heart failure.
2. P pulmonale on ECG (P wave > 3 mm in standard leads II, III, or AVF).
3. Hematocrit > 56%.

[1] Health Care Financing Administration, 1989.

Human α_1-proteinase inhibitor is available for replacement therapy of emphysema due to congenital deficiency of α_1-antitrypsin. The efficacy of this new agent is unknown, and it is very expensive. Lung transplantation for end-stage COPD is currently being evaluated in several centers.

B. Hospitalized Patients: Hospitalization is indicated for acute worsening of COPD that fails to respond to measures for ambulatory patients. Patients with acute respiratory failure or complications such as cor pulmonale and pneumothorax should also be hospitalized.

Management of the hospitalized patient with an **exacerbation of COPD** uses a comprehensive approach similar to that for patients hospitalized with asthma. Therapeutic options include supplemental oxygen, ipratropium bromide, inhaled sympathomimetics, and intravenous aminophylline, as well as broad-spectrum antibiotics, corticosteroids, and, in selected cases, chest physiotherapy. Oxygen therapy should not be withheld for fear of worsening respiratory acidemia; hypoxemia is more detrimental than hypercapnia. Cor pulmonale is treated with salt restriction and diuretics in addition to aggressive management of the underlying COPD. Cardiac arrhythmias are managed with antiarrhythmic drugs as indicated but usually respond to aggressive treatment of COPD itself. Verapamil (240–480 mg/d in divided doses every 8 hours, or 0.075 mg/kg given intravenously at a rate of 1–2 mg/min) is especially effective in multifocal atrial tachycardia. If progressive respiratory failure ensues, tracheal intubation and mechanical ventilation are necessary.

Prognosis

The outlook for patients with clinically significant COPD is poor. The median survival time of patients with severe COPD ($FEV_1 \leq 1$ L) is about 4 years. The degree of pulmonary dysfunction (as measured by FEV_1) at the time the patient is first seen is probably the most important predictor of survival. Comprehensive care programs and cessation of smoking apparently reduce the rate of decline of pulmonary function, but therapy with bronchodilators and other approaches probably has little, if any, impact on the natural course of COPD. Survival time varies widely and cannot be easily predicted. The prognosis is better in the chronic asthmatic form of COPD (chronic asthmatic bronchitis) than in the emphysematous form.

American Thoracic Society: Standards for the diagnosis and care of patients with chronic obstructive pulmonary disease (COPD) and asthma. Am Rev Respir Dis 1987; 136:225.

Anthonisen NR et al: Antibiotic therapy in exacerbations of chronic obstructive pulmonary disease. Ann Intern Med 1987;106:196. (Significant benefit from broad-spectrum antibiotics in exacerbation of COPD.)

Derenne JP, Fleury B, Pariente R: Acute respiratory failure of chronic obstructive pulmonary disease. Am Rev Respir Dis 1989;138:1006. (A state-of-the-art review of this subject, including mechanisms, diagnosis, and therapy.)

Eliasson O et al: Corticosteroids in COPD: A clinical trial and reassessment of the literature. Chest 1986;89:484.

Murciano D et al: A randomized, controlled trial of theophylline in patients with severe chronic obstructive pulmonary disease. N Engl J Med 1989;320:1521. (Improvements attributed to enhanced respiratory muscle performance.)

Petty TL: The national mucolytic study: Results of a randomized, double-blind, placebo-controlled study of iodinated glycerol in chronic obstructive bronchitis. Chest 1990; 97:75. (Some symptoms improved by prolonged treatment.)

Snider GL: Chronic obstructive pulmonary disease: A definition and implications of structural determinants of airflow obstruction for epidemiology. Am Rev Respir Dis 1989; 140(Suppl):S3.

Speizer FE (editor): The rise in chronic obstructive pulmonary disease mortality. (Symposium.) Am Rev Respir Dis 1989;140(Suppl):S1. [Entire issue.]

CYSTIC FIBROSIS
(See also Chapter 34.)

Essentials of Diagnosis

- Chronic obstructive pulmonary disease in childhood and early adulthood.
- Chronic *Pseudomonas aeruginosa* or *Staphylococcus aureus* bronchitis.
- Positive family history of cystic fibrosis.
- Sweat chloride concentration above 80 meq/L in adults (> 60 meq/L under age 20) on 2 occasions.
- Idiopathic obstructive azoospermia in males.

General Considerations

Cystic fibrosis is a generalized autosomal recessive disorder of the exocrine glands. Deletion of a single phenylalanine residue from a 1480-amino-acid protein coded by the cystic fibrosis gene, resulting from a mutation of the long arm of chromosome 7 (band q31), accounts for the large majority of cases of cystic fibrosis. Almost all exocrine glands are affected by secretion of an abnormal mucus that obstructs glands and ducts in various organs. Obstruction results in dilation of the secretory glands and eventual damage to exocrine tissue. Pulmonary manifestations, which occur in all patients who survive infancy, include acute and chronic bronchitis, bronchiectasis, pneumonia, atelectasis, and peribronchial and parenchymal scarring. Pneumothorax and mild hemoptysis are common. Cor pulmonale occurs in advanced cases and signifies a poor prognosis.

Cystic fibrosis is the most common fatal hereditary disorder of Caucasians in the USA and is the most common cause of chronic lung disease in children and young adults. About half of children with cystic fibrosis live beyond age 20. About one-third of the 25,000 cystic fibrosis patients in the USA are adults.

Clinical Findings

A. Symptoms and Signs: The diagnosis should be suspected in a young adult presenting with a history of chronic lung disease. Cough, exercise intolerance, and recurrent pneumonia are typical. Steatorrhea is common. Digital clubbing, increased anteroposterior chest diameter, hyperresonance to percussion, and basilar crackles are noted on physical examination. Nasal polyps occur in as many as 15% of patients with cystic fibrosis. Biliary cirrhosis and gallstones are common.

B. Laboratory Findings: Arterial blood gas studies reveal hypoxemia. Pulmonary function studies show reduction in forced vital capacity, airflow rates, and total lung capacity. Air trapping (high ratio of residual volume to total lung capacity) and reduction in pulmonary diffusing capacity are common. A mixed obstructive and restrictive pattern of dysfunction characterizes advanced disease.

C. Imaging: Common radiographic abnormalities include peribronchial thickening, obstructive emphysema, bronchiectasis, atelectasis, and cysts. MRI may detect hilar adenopathy, but this is usually not evident on conventional radiographs.

D. Special Examinations: The pilocarpine iontophoresis "sweat test" reveals elevated sodium and chloride levels (> 60 meq/L) in the sweat of patients with cystic fibrosis. Values higher than 80 meq/L are diagnostic. Two separate tests on consecutive days are required for accurate diagnosis.

Treatment

Early recognition and comprehensive, multidisciplinary therapy lengthen survival time and ameliorate symptoms. Treatment of the psychosocial aspects is of paramount importance in young people; genetic and occupational counseling is also critical. Antibiotics are used to treat active airway infections based on results of culture and susceptibility testing of sputum. *S aureus* and a mucoid variant of *P aeruginosa* are commonly present. *Haemophilus influenzae* and *Pseudomonas cepacia*—the latter a highly drug-resistant organism—are occasionally isolated. The use of aerosolized antibiotics (gentamicin and others) for prophylaxis or treatment of lower respiratory tract infections in patients with cystic fibrosis is controversial. Although some studies demonstrate reduced exacerbations in patients chronically infected with *P aeruginosa,* there is concern about the emergence of drug-resistant organisms, equipment contamination with *P cepacia,* and side effects such as bronchospasm.

Inhaled bland aerosols, chest physiotherapy, and inhaled bronchodilators are used to promote clearance of inspissated airway secretions. Cough suppressants should be avoided. Chronic use of mucolytic agents such as acetylcysteine is of no proved benefit and is potentially harmful. Yearly influenza vaccination is advised. Daily postural drainage and chest percussion are very helpful for patients with copious sputum production. Children with cystic fibrosis who were treated with alternate-day prednisone (2 mg/kg) demonstrated improved height, weight, and pulmonary function and reduced hospitalization needs compared to controls in one study. The routine use of corticosteroids in adults with cystic fibrosis cannot be recommended in the absence of controlled clinical trials.

Prognosis

The longevity of patients with cystic fibrosis is increasing, and the median survival age is now 25 years. Few patients survive beyond 35 years. Death occurs from pulmonary complications, eg, pneumonia, pneumothorax, or hemoptysis, or as a result of terminal chronic respiratory failure and cor pulmonale.

Fick RB, Jr, Stillwell PC: Controversies in the management of pulmonary disease due to cystic fibrosis. Chest 1989;95:1319.

UPPER AIRWAY OBSTRUCTION

Acute upper airway obstruction may cause life-threatening asphyxia and must be relieved promptly. Acute upper airway obstruction due to foreign body aspiration is discussed below. Other causes of acute upper airway obstruction include laryngospasm, trauma to the larynx and pharynx, laryngeal edema from airway burns, and various inflammatory conditions (Ludwig's angina, peritonsillar and retropharyngeal abscess, acute epiglottitis, and acute allergic laryngitis).

Chronic obstruction of the upper airway may be caused by carcinoma of the pharynx or larynx, laryngeal or subglottic stenosis, laryngeal granulomas or webs, or bilateral vocal cord paralysis. Laryngeal or subglottic stenosis may become evident weeks or months following a period of translaryngeal endotracheal intubation. Inspiratory stridor, intercostal retractions on inspiration, and a palpable inspiratory thrill over the throat are characteristic findings. Flow-volume curves may reveal evidence of fixed airway obstruction or variable extrathoracic obstruction. Plain films (soft tissue views of the neck) may demonstrate supra- and infraglottic narrowing, and CT scanning and MRI may be useful to image lesions in the pharynx and larynx. Fiberoptic endoscopy is helpful in diagnosis of upper airway obstruction, but caution is necessary because this procedure may exacerbate upper airway edema, leading to critical airway narrowing.

Occasionally, a functional disorder of the larynx may mimic bronchial asthma. This condition, variously called "episodic laryngeal dyskinesis," "factitious asthma," and "emotional laryngeal wheezing," may be distinguished from true asthma by the finding of variable extrathoracic airway obstruction on the flow-volume loop (Fig 7–2), a normal alveolar-arterial oxygen tension gradient, laryngoscopic evidence of adduction of the vocal cords on both inspiration and expiration, and lack of response to bronchodilator therapy. Fluoroscopy may also be helpful in diagnosis. Pulmonary function testing is normal immediately after the attack resolves. Treatment consists of speech therapy and psychotherapy. Bronchodilator drugs are of no benefit.

LOWER AIRWAY OBSTRUCTION

Tracheal obstruction may be intrathoracic (below the suprasternal notch) or extrathoracic. Fixed tracheal obstruction may be caused by acquired or congenital tracheal stenosis, primary and secondary tracheal neoplasms, compression by extrinsic diseases (tumors of the lung, thymus, or thyroid; lymphadenopathy; congenital vascular rings; aneurysms, etc), foreign body aspiration, tracheal granulomas and papillomas, and tracheal trauma.

Acquired **tracheal stenosis** is usually secondary to tracheostomy or endotracheal intubation. Dyspnea, cough, and inability to clear pulmonary secretions occur weeks to months after tracheal decannulation or extubation. Stridor implies severe stenosis. Physical findings may be absent until tracheal diameter is reduced 50% or more, when wheezing, a palpable tracheal thrill, and harsh breath sounds may be detected. The diagnosis is usually confirmed by plain films, conventional tomography of the trachea when plain films are not adequate, CT scan, and characteristic findings of the fixed airway obstruction on the flow-volume loop (Fig 7–2). Complications include recurring pulmonary infection and life-threatening respiratory failure. Management is directed toward ensuring adequate ventilation and oxygenation and avoiding manipulative procedures that may increase edema of the tracheal mucosa. Surgical reconstruction or laser photoresection is required in severe cases.

Bronchial obstruction is caused by retained pulmonary secretions, aspiration, primary lung cancer, compression by extrinsic masses, and (rarely) tumors metastatic to the airway. Clinical and radiographic findings vary depending on the location of the obstruction and the degree of airway narrowing. Symptoms include dyspnea, cough, wheezing, and if infection is present, fever and chills. A history of recurrent pneumonia in the same lobe or segment or slow resolution (> 3 months) of pneumonia on successive x-rays suggests the possibility of bronchial obstruction and the need for bronchoscopy. Complete obstruction of a main stem bronchus may be obvious on physical examination (asymmetric chest expansion, mediastinal shift, absence of breath sounds on the affected side, and dullness to percussion), but partial obstruction is often difficult to detect. Prolonged expiration and localized wheezing may be the only clues. Alterations of the flow-volume loop may be helpful in diagnosis. Segmental or subsegmental bronchial obstruction may produce no abnormalities on physical examination.

Roentgenographic findings range from **atelectasis** (lung collapse) to air trapping. The latter may be caused by unidirectional expiratory obstruction. Expiratory films are particularly useful to show air trapping. CT scanning may demonstrate the nature and the exact location of obstruction of the central bronchi. MRI may be superior to CT for delineating the extent of the underlying disease in the hilum, but it is usually reserved for cases in which CT findings are equivocal. Bronchoscopy is helpful, particularly if tumor or foreign body aspiration is suspected. The finding of tubular breath sounds on physical examination or an air bronchogram on chest radiography in an area of atelectasis rules out complete airway obstruction. Bronchoscopy is unlikely to be of benefit in this situation.

Right middle lobe syndrome is recurrent or persistent atelectasis of the right middle lobe, probably related to inadequate collateral ventilation. Fiberoptic bronchoscopy is necessary to rule out obstructing tumor or foreign body.

ALLERGIC BRONCHOPULMONARY ASPERGILLOSIS

Allergic bronchopulmonary aspergillosis is a pulmonary hypersensitivity disorder that is being recognized with increasing frequency in the USA. It is caused by allergy to antigens of *Aspergillus* species and usually occurs in atopic asthmatic individuals who are 20–40 years of age. Primary criteria for the diagnosis of allergic bronchopulmonary aspergillosis include a clinical history of asthma, peripheral eosinophilia, immediate skin reactivity to *Aspergillus* antigen, precipitating antibodies to *Aspergillus* antigen, elevated serum IgE levels, pulmonary infiltrates (transient or fixed), and central bronchiectasis. If the first 6 of these 7 primary criteria are present, the diagnosis is almost certain. Secondary diagnostic criteria include identification of *Aspergillus* in sputum, a history of brown-flecked sputum, and late skin reactivity to *Aspergillus* antigen. Corticosteroids are the treatment of choice, and the response is usually excellent. Prednisone (0.5 mg/kg/d) is given as a single morning dose for several weeks before a transition is made to alternate-day dosing. Several months of prednisone therapy may be required. Inhaled corticosteroids and cromolyn sodium are not currently recommended. Bronchodilators (Table 7–8) are also helpful. Complications include hemoptysis, severe bronchiectasis, and pulmonary fibrosis.

BRONCHIECTASIS

Bronchiectasis is a congenital or acquired disorder of the large bronchi characterized by permanent, abnormal dilatation and destruction of bronchial walls. It is caused by recurrent inflammation or infection of the airways and is primarily a disorder of childhood and young adulthood, with most cases being recognized during the first 2 decades of life. Cystic fibrosis causes about half of all cases of bronchiectasis. Other causes include lung infection (tuberculosis, fungal infections, lung abscess, pneumonia), abnormal lung defense mechanisms (humoral immunodeficiency, α_1-antitrypsin deficiency with cigarette smoking, mucociliary clearance disorders, rheumatic diseases), and localized airway obstruction (foreign body, tumor, mucoid impaction). Acquired primary bronchiectasis is now uncommon in the USA because of improved control of bronchopulmonary infections.

Symptoms of bronchiectasis include chronic cough, production of copious amounts of purulent sputum, hemoptysis, and recurrent pneumonia. Weight loss, anemia, and other systemic manifestations are common. Physical findings are nonspecific, but persistent crackles at the lung bases are common. Clubbing is infrequent. Foul-smelling, purulent sputum that separates into 3 layers in a cup is characteristic. Obstructive pulmonary dysfunction with hypoxemia is seen in moderate or severe disease. Roentgenographic abnormalities include crowded bronchial markings related to peribronchial fibrosis and small cystic spaces at the base of the lungs. Thin-section (1.5-mm) CT scanning may detect moderate to severe cases. Bronchography is usually not performed unless surgery is planned.

Treatment consists of antibiotics (selected on the basis of sputum smears and cultures), chest physiotherapy with postural drainage and chest percussion, and inhaled bronchodilators. Empiric oral antibiotic therapy for 10–14 days with amoxicillin (500 mg every 8 hours), ampicillin or tetracycline (250–500 mg 4 times daily), or trimethoprim-sulfamethoxazole (160/800 mg every 12 hours) is reasonable therapy in an acute exacerbation if a specific bacterial pathogen cannot be isolated. Alternating cycles of 2 or 3 of these antibiotics, given orally for 2–4 weeks, is sometimes employed in patients with copious, purulent sputum. The role of aerosolized antibiotics has not been established. Bronchoscopy is sometimes necessary to evaluate hemoptysis, remove retained secretions and rule out obstructing airway lesions. Surgical resection is reserved for a few patients with localized bronchiectasis who fail to respond to conservative management. Surgery is also indicated for massive hemoptysis. Complications of bronchiectasis include cor pulmonale, amyloidosis, and secondary visceral abscesses at distant sites, eg, brain.

Barker AF, Bardana EJ Jr: Bronchiectasis: Update of an orphan disease. Am Rev Respir Dis 1988;137:969.

IMMOTILE CILIA SYNDROME
(Primary Ciliary Dyskinesia)

Immotile cilia syndrome is an autosomal recessive disorder characterized by ultrastructural defects in the microtubular apparatus of both ciliated epithelial cells and spermatozoa, resulting in abnormal mucociliary clearance, reduced fertility in women, and male infertility. Cough productive of copious mucopurulent sputum, sinusitis, and otitis occur in almost all patients. Situs inversus is present in half of cases (Kartagener's syndrome). Nasal stuffiness, rhinorrhea, and childhood nasal polyposis are common. Bronchiectasis and signs of COPD occur in severe disease. Clubbing occurs occasionally. Chest radiography reveals features of chronic bronchitis and bronchiectasis. Paranasal sinus films reveal sinusitis. Definitive diagnosis requires biopsy of nasal or tracheal mucosa with electron microscopic examination of the ultrastructure of the cilia.

Treatment consists of maintenance of bronchial hygiene through coughing and chest physiotherapy and antibiotics (selected on the basis of sputum smears and cultures) for acute airway infections. Bronchodilator drugs and mucolytic agents are not effective.

Surgical resection may be considered if severe saccular bronchiectasis is present.

BRONCHOCENTRIC GRANULOMATOSIS & MUCOID IMPACTION SYNDROME

Bronchocentric granulomatosis is a rare chronic idiopathic disorder in which bronchi and bronchioles are destroyed and replaced by granulomas. Symptoms include fever, cough, chest pain, anorexia, malaise, and hemoptysis of short duration. In patients with bronchocentric granulomatosis and chronic asthma, the condition resembles allergic bronchopulmonary aspergillosis; eosinophilia is common. Chest radiography reveals air space consolidation, atelectasis, masses, abnormal bronchial shadows, and, occasionally, linear or reticulonodular infiltrates. Unilateral and upper lung zone distribution of these abnormalities is characteristic. The diagnosis of bronchocentric granulomatosis is confirmed by lung resection, which is also therapeutic if the condition is localized.

Mucoid impaction syndrome is characterized by obstruction of large, proximal bronchi by plugs of inspissated mucus. This syndrome has clinical features similar to those of bronchocentric granulomatosis, eosinophilic pneumonia, and allergic bronchopulmonary aspergillosis, but the cause of this condition and its relationship to hypersensitivity to fungal antigens are not clear. Most patients with mucoid impaction syndrome have symptoms of chronic bronchitis or asthma. Expectoration of large, rubbery plugs of mucus suggests the diagnosis. Radiographs show densities shaped like branching central airways in the upper lung; atelectasis or consolidation is a common associated feature. Mucolytic therapy (inhaled acetylcysteine, 10% solution, 5 mL 4 times daily by nebulizer) may be tried if bland aerosols fail to relieve mucus plugging. Pretreatment with bronchodilators is recommended, since acetylcysteine may provoke bronchospasm. Corticosteroids are not helpful.

BRONCHIOLITIS

Bronchiolitis is an acute, common, often severe respiratory illness of infants and young children under 2 years of age caused by respiratory syncytial virus, other viruses (occasionally), and *Mycoplasma pneumoniae*. The child presents with combined bronchospasm and pneumonia. Bronchiolitis in children is usually a self-limited entity. In some cases—particularly following infection with adenovirus, influenza, or measles viruses—obstruction of bronchioles by granulation and fibrous tissue may follow (**bronchiolitis obliterans**). The consequences of this condition include dyspnea, obstructive lung disease, atelectasis, bronchiectasis, and unilateral hyperlucent lung (see below).

An acute infectious bronchiolitis has not been recognized as a distinct entity in adults. However, bronchiolitis obliterans does occur. Once classified as a type of chronic interstitial pneumonia, bronchiolitis obliterans has been recently reclassified. Five clinical types have been described by Epler et al: (1985): (1) toxic fume bronchiolitis obliterans, (2) postinfectious bronchiolitis obliterans, (3) bronchiolitis obliterans associated with connective tissue disease and organ transplantation, (4) bronchiolitis obliterans associated with localized lung lesions, and (5) idiopathic bronchiolitis obliterans with organizing pneumonia.

Cough and dyspnea are common symptoms in each of these types. Toxic fume bronchiolitis obliterans follows 1–3 weeks after exposure to oxides of nitrogen, phosgene, and other noxious gases. The chest x-ray shows diffuse nonspecific alveolar or ''ground-glass'' densities. Postinfectious bronchiolitis obliterans is a late response to *Mycoplasma* or viral lung infection in adults and has a highly variable radiographic appearance.

Unilateral hyperlucent lung (Swyer-James syndrome; MacLeod syndrome) is a result of unilateral postinfectious bronchiolitis obliterans in infancy or early childhood. Unilateral hyperlucency is related to oligemia and obliteration of bronchioles and small bronchi on the affected side. Reduction in volume of the affected lung on inspiration, air trapping on expiration, a small hilum, and diversion of blood flow to the opposite lung are noted on chest x-ray. No treatment is available.

Bronchiolitis obliterans may occur in association with rheumatoid arthritis, polymyositis, and dermatomyositis. Penicillamine therapy has been implicated as a possible cause of bronchiolitis obliterans in patients with rheumatoid arthritis. Bronchiolitis obliterans is a common complication of heart-lung transplantation and a rare complication of allogeneic bone marrow transplantation, the latter occurring in the setting of chronic graft-versus-host disease.

It is important to recognize **bronchiolitis obliterans with organizing pneumonia (BOOP).** This idiopathic disorder affects men and women equally. Most patients are between the ages of 50 and 70. Dry cough, dyspnea, and a flulike illness, ranging in duration from a few days to several months, are typical. Fever and weight loss are common. Physical examination demonstrates crackles in most patients, and wheezing is present in about a third. Clubbing is uncommon. Pulmonary function studies demonstrate restrictive dysfunction and hypoxemia. The chest x-ray typically shows patchy, bilateral, ground glass or alveolar infiltrates. Solitary pneumonialike infiltrates and a diffuse interstitial pattern have also recently been described.

BOOP is usually a difficult diagnosis to make on clinical grounds alone. The presence of fever and weight loss, abrupt onset of symptoms (often with an upper respiratory tract infection), a relatively short duration of symptoms, the absence of clubbing, and the presence of alveolar infiltrates help the clinician distinguish this entity from idiopathic pulmonary fibrosis. However, open lung biopsy may be necessary. Buds of loose connective tissue and inflammatory cells fill alveoli and distal bronchioles. Corticosteroid therapy is effective in two-thirds of cases, often abruptly. Relapses are common if corticosteroid therapy is stopped before 6 months.

Respiratory bronchiolitis is a disorder of small airways in young cigarette smokers. Clinically and radiographically, this disorder resembles idiopathic pulmonary fibrosis. Cough, dyspnea, and crackles on chest auscultation are typical. However, the reduction in lung compliance seen in idiopathic pulmonary fibrosis is not found in this disorder. The condition may be recognized only on open lung biopsy, which demonstrates characteristic metaplasia of terminal and respiratory bronchioles and filling of respiratory and terminal bronchioles, alveolar ducts, and alveoli by pigmented alveolar macrophages.

Diffuse panbronchiolitis is an idiopathic disorder of respiratory bronchioles that is frequently diagnosed in Japan. The condition appears to be extremely rare in the United States. Men are affected about twice as often as women and are most often between ages 20 and 80. About two-thirds of patients are nonsmokers. The large majority have a history of chronic pansinusitis. Marked dyspnea, cough, and sputum production are cardinal features. Crackles and rhonchi are noted on physical examination. Pulmonary function tests reveal obstructive abnormalities. The chest x-ray shows a distinct pattern of diffuse small nodular shadows and hyperinflation. Open lung biopsy is necessary for diagnosis. This demonstrates thickening of the walls of respiratory bronchioles and extension of a chronic inflammatory cell infiltrate into peribronchiolar tissues. Airway infection, often by *P aeruginosa,* and features of bronchiectasis are common in advanced stages. Treatment is supportive, including smoking cessation, bronchodilators, and trials of antibiotics and corticosteroids. The prognosis is poor, and a rapidly progressive downhill course is typical.

Kindt GC, et al: Bronchiolitis in adults: a reversible cause of airway obstruction associated with airway neutrophils and neutrophil products. Am Rev Respir Dis 1989; 140:483.

BRONCHOLITHIASIS

In broncholithiasis, a calcified mass (broncholith) lies in the lumen of a bronchus or a cavity derived from a bronchus. Broncholiths are usually calcified hilar lymph nodes that have migrated through the wall of a bronchus into the lumen of the airway.

Tuberculosis and histoplasmosis are the most common causes. Broncholiths may be expectorated or retained in the airway, in which case they cause hemoptysis, atelectasis, and postobstructive pneumonia.

Broncholithiasis should be suspected in any patient with hilar calcification who complains of worsening cough or hemoptysis. Late complications include bronchoesophageal or aortotracheal fistula, erosion into the pleura, and bronchiectasis. The diagnosis is confirmed by examination of expectorated material or by disappearance of a calcified hilar or intracavitary density on serial chest x-rays. CT scanning is also helpful in diagnosis. Management includes observation, appropriate treatment of central airway obstruction or hemoptysis, bronchoscopic removal of the broncholith, and surgery (lung resection, debridement, or fistula repair) as required. Successful laser treatment has been reported.

PLEUROPULMONARY INFECTIONS

ACUTE TRACHEOBRONCHITIS

Acute tracheobronchitis is a poorly defined but common clinical condition caused by acute inflammation of the trachea and bronchi. This syndrome is usually attributed to infectious agents, though it may be difficult to distinguish from inflammation of the tracheobronchial tree by nonspecific irritants such as dust and smoke. Infectious agents causing acute tracheobronchitis in older children and adults include influenza A and B viruses, parainfluenza viruses, respiratory syncytial virus, adenovirus, rhinovirus, and others. Acute infectious tracheobronchitis often presents with cough (initially nonproductive but later productive of mucopurulent sputum) and substernal discomfort worsened by coughing. Symptoms of upper respiratory tract infection often precede and overlap the manifestations of tracheobronchitis.

Physical findings are minimal or absent. Rhonchi, which may disappear after productive cough, and wheezing may be evident. Signs of pulmonary consolidation are absent. The chest x-ray is normal.

Fever is usually minimal or absent except in cases of influenza. Chest x-ray examination should be reserved for those patients in whom influenza is suspected, those with underlying chronic obstructive pulmonary disease, and those with physical findings suggestive of pneumonia.

Treatment is symptomatic, aimed at controlling cough, chest discomfort, and fever. An inhaled bronchodilator, such as metaproterenol or albuterol, 2 puffs every 4 hours, may be tried if chest tightness or wheezing is present. Sputum Gram stain or culture is generally not indicated. Empiric antibiotic therapy is generally reserved for patients with underlying chronic obstructive pulmonary disease or those with persistent cough productive of purulent sputum, which suggests possible secondary bacterial infection with *S pneumoniae* or *H influenzae*. In this situation, amoxicillin (500 mg every 8 hours); ampicillin, erythromycin, or tetracycline (each in a dose of 250–500 mg 4 times daily); or trimethoprim-sulfamethoxazole (160/800 mg every 12 hours) may be given orally for 7–10 days.

PNEUMONIA

Pneumonia continues to be a major health problem despite the availability of potent antimicrobial drugs. Microorganisms gain access to the lower respiratory tract in 1 of 3 ways, of which aspiration of oropharyngeal secretions and associated bacterial flora occurs most commonly. Viruses, *Mycoplasma,* and other infectious organisms that cause pneumonia also reach the lungs through inhalation of infected aerosols. Pneumonia also occurs when lung parenchyma is infected as a result of hematogenous dissemination. Characteristics of pneumonia caused by specific agents and appropriate antimicrobial therapy are presented in Table 7–11.

Chlamydia pneumoniae (TWAR strain) and *Moraxella (Branhamella) catarrhalis* are both being increasingly recognized as important causes of pneumonia in adults. Infection with *C pneumoniae* is treated with tetracycline (500 mg orally 4 times daily for 14 days), the latter with amoxicillin-clavulanic acid (250–500 mg orally every 8 hours for 10–14 days).

Approach to the Immunocompetent Patient With Possible Pneumonia

A chest radiograph is included in the initial evaluation of a patient with symptoms and signs suggestive of pneumonia. The pattern of the infiltrate is not pathognomonic of a specific cause of pneumonia.

The attempt to establish a specific causative diagnosis should begin with a Gram-stained smear of expectorated sputum, which often reveals the predominant organism. An adequate sputum specimen demonstrates at least 25 polymorphonuclear leukocytes and fewer than 10 squamous epithelial cells per low-power field.

Sputum induction should be performed if the patient cannot produce an adequate sputum specimen by spontaneous cough. Direct instruction by the physician is often all that is necessary. Merely leaving a sputum container at the patient's bedside is futile. The mouth should be rinsed with water initially. The patient is instructed to take several deep breaths and then inhale deeply before coughing vigorously. Simultaneous chest clapping over the lower lobes posteriorly

Table 7–11. Characteristics of selected pneumonias.

Organism	Clinical Setting	Gram-Stained Smears of Sputum	Chest Radiograph[1]	Laboratory Studies	Complications	Antimicrobial Therapy[2]
Streptococcus pneumoniae (pneumococcus)	Chronic cardiopulmonary disease; follows upper respiratory tract infection.	Gram-positive diplococci.	Lobar consolidation.	Gram-stained smear of sputum; culture of blood, pleural fluid.	Bacteremia, meningitis, endocarditis, pericarditis, empyema.	Preferred: Penicillin G (or V, oral) Alternative: Erythromycin, cephalosporin.
Haemophilus influenzae	Chronic cardiopulmonary disease; follows upper respiratory tract infection.	Pleomorphic gram-negative coccobacilli.	Lobar consolidation.	Culture of sputum, blood, pleural fluid.	Empyema, endocarditis.	Preferred: Ampicillin (or amoxicillin). Cefotaxime or ceftriaxone for severe infections. Alternative: Cefuroxime, trimethoprim-sulfamethoxazole, tetracyline.
Staphylococcus aureus	Influenza epidemics; nosocomial.	Plump gram-positive cocci in clumps.	Patchy infiltrates.	Culture of sputum, blood, pleural fluid.	Empyema, cavitation.	Preferred: Nafcillin.[3] Alternative: A cephalosporin, vancomycin, clindamycin, ciprofloxacin, amoxicillin–clavulanic acid, ticarcillin-clavulanic acid.
Klebsiella pneumoniae	Alcohol abuse, diabetes mellitus; nosocomial.	Plump gram-negative encapsulated rods.	Lobar consolidation.	Culture of sputum, blood, pleural fluid.	Cavitation, empyema.	Preferred: A cephalosporin; for severe infection, a cephalosporin plus gentamicin, tobramycin, or amikacin. Alternative: Mezlocillin or piperacillin, amoxicillin-clavulanic acid, ticarcillin-clavulanic acid, imipenem, aztreonam.
Escherichia coli	Nosocomial; rarely community-acquired.	Gram-negative rods.	Patchy infiltrates, pleural effusion.	Culture of sputum, blood, pleural fluid.	Empyema.	Preferred: Aminoglycoside or a cephalosporin. Alternative: Ampicillin, carbenicillin, mezlocillin, ticarcillin, piperacillin, ciprofloxacin, ticarcillin-clavulanic acid, imipenem.
Pseudomonas aeruginosa	Nosocomial; cystic fibrosis.	Gram-negative rods.	Patchy infiltrates, cavitation.	Culture of sputum, blood.	Cavitation.	Preferred: Aminoglycoside plus anti-*Pseudomonas* penicillin. Alternative: Aminoglycoside plus ceftazidime, imipenem, or aztreonam; ciprofloxacin.
Anaerobes	Aspiration, periodontitis.	Mixed flora.	Patchy infiltrates in dependent lung zones.	Culture of pleural fluid or material obtained by transtracheal or transthoracic aspiration.	Necrotizing pneumonia, abscess, empyema.	Preferred: Penicillin G. Alternative: Clindamycin, chloramphenicol; metronidazole with penicillin.
Mycoplasma pneumoniae	Young adults; summer and fall.	PMNs and monocytes; no bacterial pathogens.	Extensive patchy infiltrates.	Complement fixation titer.[4] Cold agglutinin serum titers are not helpful as they lack sensitivity and specificity.	Skin rashes , bullous myringitis; hemolytic anemia.	Preferred: Erythromycin. Alternative: Tetracycline.
Legionella species	Summer and fall; exposure to contaminated construction site, water source, air conditioner; community-acquired or nosocomial.	Few PMNs; no bacteria.	Patchy or lobar consolidation.	Direct immunofluorescent examination of sputum or tissue; immunofluorescent antibody titer,[4] culture of sputum or tissue.[5]	Empyema, cavitation, endocarditis, pericarditis.	Preferred: Erythromycin, with or without rifampin. Alternative: Trimethoprim–sulfamethoxazole.

[1] See p 307 regarding the lack of specificity of x-ray findings.
[2] Antimicrobial sensitivities should guide therapy when available.
[3] Methicillin-resistant *S aureus* nfections are treated with vancomycin.
[4] Four-fold rise in titer is diagnostic.
[5] Selective media are required.

may assist the cough. Complementary techniques include chest percussion or vibration, inhalation of bland aerosols of water from a face mask or ultrasonic nebulizer, inhalation of sympathomimetic bronchodilators, intermittent positive-pressure breathing (IPPB), and combinations of these approaches.

In examining expectorated sputum, one must discriminate between lower respiratory tract pathogens and organisms that colonize the pharynx. For example, the presence of gram-negative bacteria and fungi such as *Candida albicans* and *Aspergillus* species on a smear of expectorated sputum may represent pharyngeal colonization and not lower respiratory tract infection.

The absence of a definitive bacterial organism on sputum Gram stain in a patient with pneumonia raises the possibility of lung infection by viruses, *Mycoplasma pneumoniae*, *Chlamydia*, *Legionella* sp, anaerobic organisms, and fungal or mycobacterial organisms. Cultures of sputum representative of lower respiratory tract secretions (ie, devoid of epithelial cells) should be obtained. Results of sputum cultures may be misleading because of contamination with flora of the upper respiratory tract; cultures are most helpful when correlated with Gram-stained smears. It is important to emphasize that *the diagnosis of pneumonia cannot be based solely on the results of culture of expectorated sputum.* In patients appearing especially ill, blood cultures should also be obtained before antimicrobial therapy is started; if cultures are positive, the causative organism has been definitively identified.

Thoracentesis should be performed in most cases of suspected bacterial pneumonia if a significant pleural effusion is present. Gram-stained smears and cultures of pleural fluid may reveal the causative organism. Pleural fluid with characteristics diagnostic of empyema (see Table 7–6) represents an indication for tube thoracostomy in most cases.

Antimicrobial therapy should be started after initial diagnostic studies have been performed. Empiric antibiotic therapy is initiated in most cases, because the clinical presentation and initial sputum Gram stain do not commonly indicate infection caused by a specific infectious agent. If the physician judges that the specific infecting organism must be identified with precision before antibiotic therapy is started, an invasive procedure such as transtracheal aspiration, fiberoptic bronchoscopy with bronchoalveolar lavage or protected brushing, or transthoracic needle aspiration must be performed. Such procedures are rarely necessary in patients with uncomplicated community-acquired pneumonia.

Empiric Treatment of Community-Acquired Pneumonia

Erythromycin is the drug of choice for *empiric* treatment of community-acquired atypical pneumonia in the young or middle-aged adult; the usual dose is 250–500 mg orally 4 times daily for 10–14 days. In contrast, if typical pneumonia is suspected in this setting and a Gram stain of sputum is consistent with pneumococcal infection, penicillin G or V is the drug of choice. The usual dose of penicillin G or V for pneumococcal pneumonia in an adult is 250 mg orally 4 times daily for 1 week. Cefuroxime is favored for empirical therapy of community-acquired typical pneumonia if the patient is elderly or has underlying COPD, chronic alcoholism, or a history of recent influenza. In such patients, hospitalization is usually necessary, and cefuroxime is given in doses of 0.75–1.5 g intravenously every 8 hours for 5–10 days, with adjustments as necessary for impaired renal function. If ambulatory treatment is considered acceptable, cefuroxime axetil is given in doses of 250–500 mg orally every 12 hours for 10–14 days. In patients with COPD, chronic heart disease, or alcoholism who are elderly or who have limited pulmonary reserve, empiric therapy for nonspecific community-acquired pneumonia often consists of both erythromycin and cefuroxime.

Invasive procedures may be justified in immunodeficient patients or patients who fail to respond to conventional therapy. The benefits of invasive methods to pinpoint a specific organism causing pneumonia must be weighed against their risks and costs. Knowledge of indigenous hospital flora and their antimicrobial sensitivities is vital in selecting empiric therapy for nosocomial pneumonia; therapy is modified when antimicrobial sensitivities become known or if the patient fails to respond.

Prevention

Polyvalent pneumococcal vaccine (containing capsular polysaccharide antigens of 23 strains of *S pneumoniae*) has the potential to prevent or lessen the severity of 85–90% of pneumococcal infections in immunocompetent patients (see Chapter 23). Although specific indications for routine vaccination remain controversial, the vaccine's potential value and proved safety have led the Centers for Disease Control to recommend vaccination of the following classes of adults:

(1) Those with chronic illnesses (eg, chronic cardiovascular and pulmonary diseases) that lead to increased morbidity from respiratory infections.

(2) Those with underlying illnesses associated with an increased risk of pneumococcal disease (eg, asplenia or splenic dysfunction, Hodgkin's disease, multiple myeloma, cirrhosis, alcoholism, renal failure, cerebrospinal fluid leaks, sickle cell anemia, symptomatic or asymptomatic HIV infection, and conditions associated with immunosuppression).

(3) Those aged 65 years and older in general good health.

Local discomfort at the injection site occurs in about 50% of those immunized. Systemic reactions (fever, malaise) are rare in those vaccinated for the first time but are common in those who are revaccinated. Pneumococcal vaccine should therefore be administered only once to each individual.

Annual vaccination against influenza is recommended for those at risk. Guidelines are updated yearly by the Centers for Disease Control (Influenza Branch, 7–112, Centers for Disease Control, Atlanta, GA, 30333; [404] 639–3311).

Douglas RG., Jr: Prophylaxis and treatment of influenza. N Engl J Med 1990;322:443.

Faling LJ: Advances in preventing nosocomial pneumonia. (Part 2.) Am Rev Respir Dis 1988:137:256.

Fedson DS: Influenza and pneumococcal immunization strategies for physicians. Chest 1987;91:436.

1. ACUTE BACTERIAL PNEUMONIA

Essentials of Diagnosis

- Fever, chills, pleuritic chest pain, cough, purulent sputum.
- Evidence of consolidation on examination of the chest.
- Leukocytosis with leftward shift; leukopenia in some.
- Patchy or lobar infiltrates on chest x-ray.
- Diagnostic sputum Gram smear or culture of blood or pleural fluid.

General Considerations

Information about the cause of acute bacterial pneumonia is incomplete because of the difficulty encountered in isolating the responsible organisms. Sputum cultures may fail to reveal the bacterial pathogen while demonstrating other organisms that have merely colonized the upper respiratory tract. Blood cultures and cultures of pleural fluid are positive in a minority of patients. Most studies of community-acquired acute bacterial pneumonia identify *S pneumoniae* (pneumococcus) as the causative organism in about two-thirds of cases; *H influenzae*, *S aureus*, enteric gram-negative rods, and anaerobes account for most of the remainder.

The bacterial pathogens of nosocomial acute bacterial pneumonia differ from those of the community-acquired variety. Hospitalized patients commonly develop oropharyngeal colonization with enteric gram-negative rods, particularly *P aeruginosa*, and *S aureus*, which are usually responsible for lower respiratory tract infections in these patients. *S pneumoniae* is an infrequent cause of nosocomial pneumonia.

In HIV-infected patients, the frequency of pneumococcal pneumonia is much higher than in the general population. Multiple defects in the systemic immune system and abnormal pulmonary defense mechanisms are presumably responsible for this increased risk.

Bacteremia and multilobar involvement are more commonly seen in HIV-infected patients with bacterial pneumonia than in immunologically normal patients.

Clinical Findings

A. Symptoms and Signs: Acute bacterial pneumonia is manifested by the abrupt onset of fever, chills, cough productive of purulent sputum, and pleuritic chest pain. Physical examination reveals a toxic-appearing, febrile patient with tachypnea and tachycardia. Evidence of consolidation may be present. In elderly patients, however, acute pneumonia may be heralded only by an alteration in mental status or an apparent worsening of underlying disease such as chronic obstructive pulmonary disease or congestive heart failure.

B. Laboratory Findings: An initial pair of blood cultures is necessary. Hematologic evaluation reveals leukocytosis with a shift to the left or sometimes leukopenia. Sputum is purulent or mucopurulent. Gram-stained smears of sputum reveal neutrophils and (usually) a single predominant organism.

Bronchoscopy may be helpful in evaluating patients with suspected nosocomial pneumonia, particularly in critical care settings. Insertion of a protected brush catheter through the fiberoptic bronchoscope permits a highly accurate (> 90%) diagnosis of nosocomial pneumonia, using a cutoff level of 10^3 bacteria colony-forming units/mL. Such accuracy cannot be achieved with clinical and radiographic assessment alone. Bronchoalveolar lavage with microscopic identification of a high percentage of intracellular bacteria is another useful tool. However, the physician must decide in each case whether the risks and expense of bronchoscopy with brushing or lavage, accompanied by the delays in obtaining a final culture and sensitivity report, are acceptable when compared with the results of empiric antibiotic therapy.

C. Imaging: Chest radiography shows lobar or segmental ("patchy") infiltrates. Ipsilateral pleural effusion may be present, particularly in *S aureus* or *Streptococcus pyogenes* pneumonia. Cavitation also suggests *S aureus* or *S pyogenes* infection. A downward bulging of the right minor fissure may occur in right upper lobe pneumonia caused by *Klebsiella pneumoniae*, but this finding is neither sensitive nor specific.

Treatment

The patient who is otherwise healthy and free of respiratory distress or complications of pneumonia may be managed as an outpatient with oral antibiotics (Table 7–11) and appropriate supportive care. A follow-up evaluation and chest x-ray within 1 week are advised. However, many patients with acute bacterial pneumonia should be hospitalized (1–4 days is usually adequate).

Neutropenia, involvement of more than one lobe,

and poor host resistance (eg, alcoholism, diabetes mellitus, malnutrition) suggest the possibility of a poor response to therapy and indicate the need for hospitalization. Bed rest, supplemental oxygen if hypoxemia is present, and antibiotics (Table 7–11) are the cornerstones of therapy. Respiratory and chest physical therapy are helpful in patients with specific problems such as bronchoconstriction and retained lung secretions but should not be routinely ordered.

The choice of antimicrobial drugs. Med Lett Drugs Ther 1990;32:41.
Fagon JY et al: Nosocomial pneumonia in patients receiving continuous mechanical ventilation: Prospective analysis of 52 episodes with use of a protected specimen brush and quantitative culture techniques. Am Rev Respir Dis 1989;139:877.
Faling LJ: New advances in diagnosing nosocomial pneumonia in intubated patients. (Part 1.) Am Rev Respir Dis 1988;137:253.
Nolan PE, Bass JB: New drugs for treating lung infection. Chest 1988;94:1076.

2. ATYPICAL PNEUMONIA

The clinical picture in atypical pneumonia is dominated by constitutional symptoms such as fever, malaise, and headache rather than by respiratory symptoms, though a nonproductive cough is usually present. Unfortunately, overlap of these symptoms with similar ones in bacterial processes precludes their use in establishing a diagnosis. Physical findings of consolidation are absent. Leukocytosis, if present, is mild. Gram-stained smears of sputum (if obtainable) reveal neutrophils or mononuclear cells but no predominant bacterial pathogens. Chest radiographs reveal patchy nonlobar infiltrates that are more extensive than might be predicted from the clinical presentation. Pleural effusions are very uncommon.

The most common cause of atypical pneumonia is *Mycoplasma pneumoniae*. Other less common causative agents include *Legionella* sp, *Chlamydia psittaci* (psittacosis), *C pneumoniae*, *Coxiella burnetii* (Q fever), adenovirus, and, in endemic areas, *Coccidioides immitis* and *Histoplasma capsulatum*. Viral pneumonia produces a similar clinical picture; influenza (types A and B) adenoviruses are the most common causes.

Antibiotic regimens are as follows: mycoplasmal pneumonia (erythromycin, 500 mg orally 4 times daily for 2 weeks); *Legionella* pneumonia (erythromycin, 1 g intravenously every 6 hours for 2 weeks); psittacosis or Q fever (tetracycline, 500 mg orally 4 times daily for 2–3 weeks).

Amantadine is 65–80% effective in prevention of symptomatic influenza A infection during outbreaks. If given during the first 1–2 days of illness, it also shortens the duration of symptoms of influenza A

infection. Adults should receive 100 mg of amantadine twice daily for 10 days. The dose is reduced in those over age 65, in children, and in patients with a seizure disorder or renal impairment. Treatment guidelines are available from the Influenza Branch, 7–112, Centers for Disease Control, Atlanta, GA 30333.

Finegold SM: Legionnaires' disease: Still with us. N Engl J Med 1988;318:571.
Grayston JT: Chlamydia pneumoniae, strain TWAR. Chest 1989;95:664.
Mansel JK et al: Mycoplasma pneumoniae pneumonia. Chest 1989;95:639.

3. ANAEROBIC PNEUMONIA & LUNG ABSCESS

Essentials of Diagnosis
- Predisposition to aspiration.
- Poor dental hygiene.
- Fever, weight loss, malaise.
- Foul-smelling sputum (fewer than half of patients).
- Infiltrate in dependent lung zone, with single or multiple areas of cavitation or pleural effusion.

General Considerations
Aspiration of small amounts of oropharyngeal secretions occurs during sleep in normal individuals and rarely causes disease. Sequelae of aspiration of larger amounts oo material include nocturnal asthma, bronchiectasis, chemical pneumonitis, mechanical obstruction of airways by particulate matter, and pleuropulmonary infection. Individuals predisposed to disease induced by aspiration include those with depressed levels of consciousness due to drug or alcohol use, seizures, general anesthesia, or central nervous system disease; those with impaired deglutition due to esophageal disease or neurologic disorders; and those with tracheal or nasogastric tubes, which disrupt the mechanical defenses of the airways.

Periodontal disease, which increases the number of anaerobic bacteria in aspirated material, is associated with a greater likelihood of anaerobic pleuropulmonary infection. Aspiration of infected oropharyngeal contents initially leads to pneumonia in dependent lung zones, such as the posterior segments of the upper lobes and superior and basilar segments of the lower lobes. Body position at the time of aspiration determines which lung zones are dependent. The onset of symptoms is insidious. By the time the patient seeks medical attention, necrotizing pneumonia, lung abscess, or empyema may be apparent.

About two-thirds of patients with necrotizing pneumonia, lung abscess, and empyema are found to be infected with multiple species of anaerobic bacteria only. Most of the remainder are infected with both anaerobic and aerobic bacteria. *Bacteroides melanino-genicus,* anaerobic streptococci, and *Fusobacterium nucleatum* are commonly isolated anaerobic bacteria.

Clinical Findings

A. Symptoms and Signs: Patients with anaerobic pleuropulmonary infection usually present with constitutional symptoms such as fever, weight loss, and malaise. Cough with expectoration of foul-smelling purulent sputum suggests anaerobic infection, though the absence of productive cough does not rule out such an infection. Dental hygiene is poor, but patients are rarely edentulous; if the patient is edentulous, an obstructing bronchial lesion is commonly present.

B. Laboratory Findings: Expectorated sputum is inappropriate for culture of anaerobic organisms because of contaminating mouth flora. Representative material for culture can be obtained only by transtracheal or transthoracic aspiration, thoracentesis, or bronchoscopy with a protected brush. Transthoracic or transtracheal aspiration is rarely indicated, because anaerobic pleuropulmonary infections respond well to penicillin or clindamycin.

C. Imaging: The different types of anaerobic pleuropulmonary infection are distinguished on the basis of their radiographic appearance. **Lung abscess** appears as a thick-walled solitary cavity surrounded by consolidation. An air-fluid level is usually present. Other causes of cavitary lung disease (tuberculosis, mycosis, cancer, infarction, Wegener's granulomatosis) should be excluded. **Necrotizing pneumonia** is distinguished by multiple areas of cavitation within an area of consolidation. **Empyema** is characterized by the presence of pleural fluid and may accompany either of the other 2 radiographic findings. Ultrasonography is of value in locating fluid and may also reveal pleural loculations.

Treatment

Penicillin G (1–2 million units intravenously every 4 hours) is the usual treatment for anaerobic pleuropulmonary infections. Penicillin V (0.5–1 g orally every 6 hours) may be used after improvement with intravenous penicillin G has occurred. Clindamycin (600 mg intravenously every 8 hours until improvement, then 300 mg orally every 6 hours) is regarded by most authorities as an acceptable alternative to penicillin for treatment of anaerobic pleuropulmonary infections. One study suggests that it is more effective than penicillin for treatment of community-acquired putrid lung abscess. Antibiotics should be given until the chest x-ray stabilizes. The treatment of anaerobic pleuropulmonary disease requires adequate drainage. Tube thoracostomy is required for the treatment of empyema, but open pleural drainage is often necessary because of the propensity of these infections to produce loculations in the pleural space.

Bartlett JG: Anaerobic bacterial infections of the lung. Chest 1987;91:901.

Styrt B, Gorbach SL: Recent developments in the understanding of the pathogenesis and treatment of anaerobic infections. (Two parts.) N Engl J Med 1989;321:240, 298.

PULMONARY INFILTRATES IN THE COMPROMISED HOST

Pneumonia in immunocompromised patients may be caused by bacterial, mycobacterial, fungal, protozoal, helminthic, or viral pathogens, but not all pulmonary infiltrates in compromised hosts are due to infection. Noninfectious processes such as pulmonary edema, drug reaction, pulmonary infarction, underlying malignant disease, and radiation pneumonitis may mimic infection. Although almost any pathogen can cause pneumonia in a compromised host, 2 clinical tools help the clinician narrow the differential diagnosis. The first of these is knowledge of the underlying immunologic defect: specific types of immunologic defects predispose to particular infections; eg, defects in humoral immunity predispose mainly to bacterial infections against which antibodies play an important role, whereas defects in cellular immunity predispose to infections with viruses, fungi, mycobacteria, and protozoa. Chest radiography is also helpful in clarifying the differential diagnosis. Diffuse infiltrates are usually seen with *Pneumocystis carinii* or viral pneumonias. Bacterial and fungal infections are typically associated with more localized infiltrates.

The time course of infection also provides clues to the etiology of pneumonia in immunocompromised patients. A fulminant pneumonia is probably caused by bacterial infection, whereas an insidious pneumonia is more apt to be caused by viral, fungal, protozoal, or mycobacterial infection. Pneumonia occurring within 2–4 weeks after organ transplantation is most likely to be bacterial, whereas several months or more after transplantation, infection caused by *P carinii*, viruses (CMV, others), and fungi (*Aspergillus*, others) is more likely.

Diagnostic procedures should include blood cultures and examination and culture of sputum and pleural fluid, if present. Examination of expectorated sputum for bacteria, fungi, mycobacteria, *Legionella,* and *P carinii* is important and may preclude the need for an expensive, invasive diagnostic procedure. An adequate sputum sample is frequently difficult to obtain. Sputum induction then becomes necessary. Repeated efforts to obtain sputum should be made.

Frequently, routine evaluation fails to identify the causative organism. The clinician must then either begin empirical antimicrobial therapy or proceed to invasive procedures such as bronchoscopy, transthoracic aspiration, or open lung biopsy. **Bronchoalveolar lavage** using the flexible fiberoptic bronchoscope is a safe and effective method for obtaining representative pulmonary secretions for microbiologic studies. It involves less risk of bleeding than transbronchial brushing and transbronchial biopsy. Lavage is especially suitable for the diagnosis of *P carinii* pneumonia in patients with AIDS (see Chapters 24 and 28), the yield approaching 90%. Examination of expectorated sputum for *P carinii* is a less expensive and noninvasive alternative to bronchoalveolar lavage, but yields average only about 60% even in centers experienced with this technique. Selection of the approach to management must be based on the severity of the pulmonary infection, the underlying disease, the risks of empiric therapy, and local expertise and experience with the diagnostic procedures. Open lung biopsy is considered the "gold standard" for diagnosis of pulmonary infiltrates in the compromised host, but choice of this procedure should be tempered by the realization that the information obtained rarely affects the ultimate outcome. Moreover, a specific diagnosis is obtained in only about two-thirds of cases in which this test is performed. Therefore, empiric treatment is generally preferred, especially when the risk-benefit ratio of lung biopsy is high.

Lipscomb MF: Lung defenses against opportunistic infections. Chest 1989;96:1393.

Murray JF, Mills J: Pulmonary infectious complications of human immunodeficiency virus infection. Am Rev Respir Dis 1990;141:1356.

Rankin JA: Role of bronchoalveolar lavage in the diagnosis of pneumonia. Chest 1989;95(Suppl):187S.

Smith CB: Cytomegalovirus pneumonia: State of the art. Chest 1989;95(Suppl):182S.

PULMONARY TUBERCULOSIS

Essentials of Diagnosis

- Fatigue, weight loss, fever, night sweats.
- Productive cough. Pulmonary infiltrates on chest radiograph.
- Positive tuberculin skin test reaction (most cases).
- Acid-fast bacilli on smear of sputum.
- Sputum culture positive for *Mycobacterium tuberculosis*.

General Considerations

Infection with *M tuberculosis* begins when aerosolized droplets containing viable organisms are inhaled by a person susceptible to the disease. When they reach the lungs, the organisms are ingested by macrophages and either die or persist and multiply. Widespread lymphatic and hematogenous dissemination of organisms occurs before development of an effective immune response when mycobacteria throughout the body are walled off by granulomatous inflammation. This type of infection, called **primary tuberculosis,** is usually asymptomatic. Uncommonly, the immune response is inadequate, and progressive primary tuberculosis develops, accompanied by both pulmonary and constitutional symptoms. Hematogenous dissemination from the primary focus throughout the lungs ("miliary" tuberculosis), to the pleural space (tuberculous pleural effusion), or to extrapulmonary sites (meninges, bone) is a rare complication of primary tuberculosis. Dormant but viable organisms persist for years, and reactivation of disease in any of these sites ("pulmonary" focus, "Simon" focus) may occur if the host's defense mechanisms become impaired. Most cases of tuberculosis in adults are due to reactivation of disease (postprimary or reactivation tuberculosis) and not to recent infection. As the number of reported cases decreases, however, the percentage of patients with atypical presentations—particularly elderly patients, patients with late stage HIV infection, and those in nursing homes—has increased.

Persons infected with the human immunodeficiency virus (HIV), with or without AIDS, are at increased risk of developing tuberculosis. HIV infection has emerged as the most important risk factor for the development of tuberculosis. Tuberculosis is also common in the homeless and in refugees from Asia and Central America.

Clinical Findings

A. Symptoms and Signs: The patient with reactivated tuberculosis typically presents with constitutional symptoms of fatigue, weight loss, anorexia, low-grade fever, and night sweats. Pulmonary symptoms include cough, which is initially dry but later productive of purulent sputum and (sometimes) blood. Occasionally, there may be no symptoms. On physical examination, patients often appear chronically ill and exhibit evidence of weight loss. Examination of the chest may reveal findings such as posttussive apical rales or may be normal.

B. Laboratory Findings: A high index of suspicion is critical to the diagnosis of tuberculosis. Definitive diagnosis depends on recovery of *M tuberculosis* from cultures. Diagnosis therefore starts with collection of an early morning sputum specimen for stain and culture. Drug susceptibility testing is ordered whenever there is a suspicion of drug resistance. Induction of sputum may be helpful in patients who cannot voluntarily produce good specimens. Multiple sputum specimens are often required to identify acid-fast bacilli. Demonstration of acid-fast bacilli on sputum smear does not confirm a diagnosis of tuberculosis, since saprophytic nontuberculous mycobacteria may colonize the airways or cause pulmonary disease. False-positive sputum cultures of *M tuberculosis* are, however, very rare.

If attempts to obtain sputum are unsuccessful, gastric washings may be useful, although they are suitable only for culture and not for stained smear, because nontuberculous mycobacteria may be present in the stomach in the absence of tuberculous infection. Fiberoptic bronchoscopy with bronchial washings may also lead to diagnosis in patients who are unable to produce adequate amounts of sputum or in those who are still thought to have tuberculosis despite negative results on sputum smears.

Cultures require 6–8 weeks for final interpretation. A radiometric culture system (Bactec) may allow detection of mycobacterial growth in as little as several days.

In patients with pleural effusions caused by *M tuberculosis,* needle biopsy of the pleura reveals granulomas in a high percentage of patients, though pleural fluid culture is usually not revealing.

C. Imaging: Because primary tuberculosis is usually asymptomatic, a chest x-ray is infrequently obtained. Radiographic abnormalities are particularly likely to occur in children and include small homogeneous infiltrates (usually in the upper lobe), hilar and paratracheal lymph node enlargement, and segmental atelectasis. Pleural effusion may be present, especially in adults, sometimes as the sole radiographic abnormality. Ghon (calcified primary focus) and Ranke (calcified primary focus and calcified hilar lymph node) complexes are detected as residual evidence of healed primary tuberculosis in a minority of patients.

Postprimary or reactivation tuberculosis is associated with various radiographic manifestations, including fibrocavitary apical disease, nodules, and pneumonic infiltrates. The usual location is in the apical or posterior segments of the upper lobes or in the superior segments of the lower lobes; as many as 30% of patients may present with radiographic evidence of disease in other locations, however. This is especially true in elderly patients, in whom lower lobe infiltrates with or without pleural effusion are encountered with increasing frequency. Lower lung zone tuberculosis, which may occur with endobronchial tuberculosis, may masquerade as pneumonia or lung cancer. In HIV-infected patients who develop pulmonary tuberculosis, the radiographic features of tuberculosis may vary with the stage of HIV disease. In patients with "early" HIV infection, the radiographic features of tuberculosis resemble those in patients without HIV infection. In contrast, atypical radiographic features predominate in patients with "late" stage HIV infection (AIDS). These patients often display lower lung zone, diffuse, or miliary infiltrates and enlargement of hilar and mediastinal lymph nodes.

D. Special Examinations: The **tuberculin skin test** (5 tuberculin units of purified protein derivative (PPD) intradermally) identifies individuals who have been infected at some time with *M tuberculosis* but does not distinguish between current disease and past infection. The transverse width (in millimeters) of the induration at the skin test site should be recorded after 48–72 hours. Patients with a high likelihood of infection with *M tuberculosis,* eg, those who are known contacts of an individual with active disease or those with findings consistent with tuberculosis on chest x-ray, should be considered to have "significant" tuberculin skin test results if induration is 5 mm or more. Patients with a lower likelihood of tuberculous infection or those with a high likelihood of infection with atypical mycobacteria should be considered to have significant results on tuberculin skin testing if induration is 10 mm or more. The criterion for a significant skin test reaction in patients with HIV infection or those with defects in cellular immunity is 5 mm of induration. In the early (asymptomatic) stage of HIV infection, cutaneous reactivity to tuberculin is intact. Patients with AIDS are usually anergic. HIV-seropositive patients should be monitored very closely with tuberculin skin tests.

Both false-positive and false-negative tuberculin reactions occur. False-positive reactions are due to infection with nontuberculous mycobacteria. False-negative reactions occur in patients with malnutrition, immunologic defects, renal failure, overwhelming tuberculosis, or old age.

"Boosting" of the skin test reaction by serial testing may cause a false impression of conversion, as dormant mycobacterial sensitivity is restored by the antigenic challenge of the initial skin test.

Vaccination with BCG has a variable effect on the tuberculin skin test reaction. A history of BCG vaccination should not alter the interpretation of the tuberculin skin test. A significant skin test reaction in a person vaccinated with BCG should be regarded as evidence of infection with *M tuberculosis.*

Treatment

All possible or proved cases of tuberculosis should be reported to local and state public health departments.

A. Hospitalization: Hospitalization for initial therapy of tuberculosis is not necessary in most patients, though it should be considered if a patient is incapable of self-care or is likely to expose susceptible individuals to the risk of tuberculosis. Monthly follow-up of compliant outpatients is recommended, including sputum smear and culture until conversion occurs. A private room with appropriate ventilation and instruction in the importance of covering the mouth while coughing are sufficient infection control measures for hospitalized patients receiving effective chemotherapy.

B. Drug Therapy: (Table 7–12.) (See also Chapter 31.) Standard therapy for pulmonary infection due to fully susceptible *M tuberculosis* in compliant adults and children over the age of 12 consists of isoniazid, rifampin, and pyrazinamide daily for 2 months, followed by isoniazid and rifampin for 4 more months. If isoniazid resistance is suspected, ethambutol should be added for the first 2 months or until drug susceptibility studies are available.

Table 7–12. First-line antituberculous drugs.[1]

	Dosage[2] Daily	Dosage[2] Twice Weekly	Most Common Side Effects	Tests for Side Effects	Drug Interactions	Remarks
Isoniazid (INH)	Adults: 5 mg/kg PO or IM Maximum 300 mg Children: 10–20 mg/kg PO or IM Maximum 300 mg	Adults: 15 mg/kg Maximum 900 mg Children: 20–40 mg/kg Maximum 900 mg	Peripheral neuritis, hepatitis, hypersensitivity.	SGOT (AST)/SGPT (ALT)	Phenytoin (synergistic); disulfiram.	Bactericidal to both extracellular and intracellular organisms. Pyridoxine, 10 mg orally as prophylaxis for neuritis; 50–100 mg as treatment.
Rifampin	Adults: 10 mg/kg PO Maximum 600 mg Children: 10–20 mg/kg PO Maximum 600 mg	Adults: 10 mg/kg Maximum 600 mg Children: 10–20 mg/kg Maximum 600 mg	Hepatitis, febrile reaction, purpura (rare).	SGOT (AST)/SGPT (ALT)	Rifampin inhibits the effect of oral contraceptives, quinidine, corticosteroids, coumarin anticoagulants, methadone, digoxin, oral hypoglycemics; PAS may interfere with absorption of rifampin.	Bactericidal to all populations of organisms. Colors urine and other body secretions orange. Discoloring of contact lenses.
Pyrazinamide	Adults: 15–30 mg/kg PO Maximum 2 g Children: 15–30 mg/kg PO Maximum 2 g	Adults: 50–70 mg/kg Children: 50–70 mg/kg	Hyperuricemia, hepatotoxicity.	Uric acid, SGOT (AST)/SGPT (ALT).	· · ·	Bactericidal to intracellular organisms. Combination with an aminoglycoside is bactericidal.
Ethambutol	Adults: 15–25 mg/kg PO Maximum 2.5 g Children: 15–25 mg/kg PO Maximum 2.5 g	Adults: 50 mg/kg Children: 50 mg/kg	Optic neuritis (reversible with discontinuance of drug; rare at 15 mg/kg), rash.	Red-green color discrimination and visual acuity (difficult to test in children under 3 years of age).	· · ·	Bacteriostatic to both intracellular and extracellular organisms. Mainly used to inhibit development of resistant mutants. Use with caution in renal disease or when ophthalmologic testing is not feasible.
Streptomycin	Adults: 15 mg/kg IM[3] Maximum 1 g Children: 20–40 mg/kg IM Maximum 1 g	Adults: 25–30 mg/kg IM Children: 25–30 mg/kg IM	Eighth nerve damage, nephrotoxicity.	Vestibular function (audiograms); blood urea nitrogen and creatinine.	Neuromuscular blocking agents may be potentiated and cause prolonged paralysis.	Bactericidal to extracellular organisms. Use with caution in older patients or those with renal disease.

[1] Modified and reproduced, with permission, from Bailey WC et al: Treatment of tuberculosis and other mycobacterial diseases. *Am Rev Respir Dis* 1983:**127**:790.
[2] Recommendations of American Thoracic Society: *Am Rev Respir Dis* 1986:**134**:355.
[3] In patients > 60 years of age, the daily streptomycin dose is 10 mg/kg with a maximum of 750 mg.

Twice-weekly administration of isoniazid and rifampin is acceptable for the last 4 months of the 6-month regimen, with dosage modification as in Table 7–12. A 9-month regimen of daily isoniazid and rifampin, supplemented as above with ethambutol when isoniazid resistance is suspected, is an alternative, but recent data suggest that the 6-month regimen is preferable. Treatment regimens of less than 6 months are unacceptable because of higher relapse rates. In patients with AIDS or HIV infection, drug-sensitive tuberculosis is treated with isoniazid, rifampin, and either ethambutol or pyrazinamide for 2 months, followed by isoniazid and rifampin for at least 7 more months. The total duration of treatment is 9 months *plus* at least 6 months after sputum culture conversion. Patients who are expected to be noncompliant with treatment programs should have supervised administration of medications, including confinement if necessary. A single recent study suggests that adult patients with smear-negative, culture-positive pulmonary tuberculosis can be effectively treated with a regimen of isoniazid, 300 mg, and rifampin, 600 mg, daily for 1 month, followed by isoniazid, 900 mg, and rifampin, 600 mg, twice weekly for 5 months. Drug side effects are common with this regimen (Dutt et al, 1990).

Resistance of *M tuberculosis* to isoniazid and streptomycin is common in certain geographic regions of the world and in Asians and Hispanics. Resistance to rifampin or ethambutol is less common. Until drug susceptibility tests are available, treatment must consist of at least 2 and preferably 3 drugs (bactericidal if possible) to which the patient has not been exposed. If isoniazid resistance is confirmed, rifampin and ethambutol are given for 12 months. The possibility of drug resistance must also be considered when re-treatment of tuberculosis is necessary. Re-treatment requires at least 2 drugs (bactericidal if possible) to which the patient has not been exposed and against which microbial resistance has not been demonstrated.

The physician will occasionally encounter patients with clinical and radiographic abnormalities consistent with tuberculosis, positive tuberculin reactions, and negative bacteriologic findings. In these patients, the bacillary population is presumed to be lower than in cases where sputum smears or cultures are positive. Recent evidence suggests the value of treatment of smear—and culture-negative pulmonary tuberculosis. A 4-month regimen of isoniazid and rifampin has been found to be effective (Dutt et al, 1989).

Extrapulmonary tuberculosis due to fully susceptible *M tuberculosis* should be treated with a 9-month daily regimen of isoniazid (300 mg orally) and rifampin (600 mg orally). Twice weekly therapy with 900 mg of isoniazid and 600 mg of rifampin for the last 8 months of this regimen appears to be acceptable. A recent study suggests that a 4-drug, largely twice-weekly, 6-month regimen for extrapulmonary tuberculosis is also effective (Cohn et al, 1990). Treatment of skeletal tuberculosis is enhanced by early drainage and debridement of necrotic bone.

Consultation with experts in the treatment of tuberculosis is advised, since therapeutic errors by inexperienced physicians are commonly observed. The reader is referred to recent guidelines on the treatment of tuberculosis (American Thoracic Society).

Adults should have measurements of serum bilirubin, hepatic enzymes, urea nitrogen, and creatinine and a complete blood count, including platelets, before starting chemotherapy for tuberculosis. Visual acuity tests are recommended before initiation of ethambutol, and serum uric acid should be measured before starting pyrazinamide. The patient beginning therapy should be cautioned to watch for symptoms of drug toxicity (Table 7–12). Routine monitoring of laboratory tests for evidence of toxicity is not recommended, but monthly questioning for symptoms of drug toxicity is advised. Appropriate laboratory tests are mandatory if signs or symptoms of toxicity develop.

C. Chemoprophylaxis: Patients infected with *M tuberculosis* but without active disease harbor small numbers of organisms. Isoniazid prophylaxis (300 mg/d for adults and 10–14 mg/kg/d—up to 300 mg/d—for children) for 12 months in such patients may reduce the expected incidence of reactivated tuberculosis by 93%. Six months of isoniazid therapy may offer equal protection and improved patient compliance. Rifampin rather than isoniazid should be given for chemoprophylaxis if the patient has had contact with someone known to have isoniazid-resistant organisms.

The following groups of individuals, regardless of age, should be offered isoniazid prophylaxis if they have significant tuberculin skin test results:

(1) Household members and other close contacts of individuals with potentially infectious tuberculosis. Children should be treated even if their skin test results are nonsignificant, and such tests should be repeated after 3 months of isoniazid therapy. Isoniazid should be continued for a total of 12 months if the skin test reaction becomes significant.

(2) Newly infected persons (conversion of skin test reaction from nonsignificant to significant within 2 years).

(3) Persons with a history of untreated or inadequately treated tuberculosis.

(4) Individuals with positive skin test reactions and chest x-ray abnormalities consistent with tuberculosis but without bacteriologic consistent with tuberculosis but without bacteriologic evidence of active disease. A course of 12 months of chemoprophylactic therapy is offered in this circumstance.

(5) Individuals with previous or current positive skin test reactions and underlying conditions that increase the risk of reactivated tuberculosis, including silicosis, diabetes mellitus, prolonged corticosteroid therapy, immunosuppressive therapy, end-stage renal

disease, chronic malnutrition due to any cause, hematologic and reticuloendothelial cancers, and AIDS or positive tests for antibodies to HIV.

(6) Individuals with positive skin test reactions who are under 35 years of age and who have none of the risk factors discussed above.

The major risk of isoniazid prophylaxis is drug-induced hepatitis, the incidence of which increases with age. Isoniazid should be discontinued if a patient develops clinical evidence of hepatitis during therapy. Failure to discontinue the drug may result in progressive and possibly fatal hepatic necrosis. The routine monitoring of biochemical tests of liver function periodically during isoniazid prophylaxis is recommended for persons 35 and older. Elevations of transaminase up to 3 times normal without symptoms do not constitute an indication to stop therapy.

D. Vaccine: A number of live tuberculosis vaccines are available and are known collectively as BCG after the original strain of bacterium used in the vaccine (bacillus Calmette-Guearin). BCG vaccination should be considered only if isoniazid chemoprophylaxis cannot be used. Current recommendations are that BCG vaccination be considered for tuberculin-negative persons, especially children, who are repeatedly exposed to individuals with untreated or ineffectively treated tuberculosis. Vaccination should be considered for communities or groups in which a high rate of new infections occurs despite aggressive treatment and surveillance programs.

Prognosis

Almost all properly treated patients with tuberculosis are cured. Relapse rates are less than 5% with current regimens. The only important cause of treatment failure is noncompliance.

American Thoracic Society: Treatment of tuberculosis and tuberculosis infection in adults and children. Am Rev Respir Dis 1986;134:355.

Centers for Disease Control: Diagnosis and management of mycobacterial infection and disease in persons with human immunodeficiency virus infection. Ann Intern Med 1987;106:254.

Cohn DL et al: A 62-dose, 6-month therapy for pulmonary and extrapulmonary tuberculosis. Ann Intern Med 1990;112:407.

Drugs for tuberculosis. Med Lett Drugs Ther 1988;30:43. (This statement summarizes modern treatment of tuberculosis.)

Dutt AK, Moers D, Stead WW: Smear-negative and culture-negative pulmonary tuberculosis: Four-month short-course chemotherapy. Am Rev Respir Dis 1989;139:867.

Dutt AK, Moers D, Stead WW: Smear-negative, culture-positive pulmonary tuberculosis: Six-month chemotherapy with isoniazid and rifampin. Am Rev Respir Dis 1990;141:1232.

Murray JF: The white plague: Down and out, or up and coming? Am Rev Respir Dis 1989;140:1788.

DISEASE CAUSED BY NONTUBERCULOUS MYCOBACTERIA

Mycobacteria other than *M tuberculosis* ("atypical" mycobacteria) are ubiquitous in nature. Only *Mycobacterium kansasii* and *Mycobacterium avium-intracellulare* complex are important causes of pulmonary disease in humans, which is clinically indistinguishable from *M tuberculosis*. The diagnosis rests on recovery of the pathogen from cultures. Infections with *M avium-intracellulare* are being seen with increasing frequency in patients with AIDS, in whom the disease is likely to be disseminated.

Sputum cultures positive for atypical mycobacteria do not in themselves prove the presence of atypical tuberculosis, because atypical bacteria may exist as saprophytes in the airways or as environmental contaminants. Sputum cultures are meaningful if the following criteria are met: (1) The patient has clinical and radiographic evidence of disease compatible with a diagnosis of pulmonary tuberculosis; and (2) multiple colonies are present on more than one culture. A positive result on culture of material obtained from tissue biopsies or pleural fluid is also diagnostic.

Disease caused by *M kansasii* responds well to drug therapy. Recent data suggest that a regimen of rifampin, isoniazid, and ethambutol for 12 months, with streptomycin added for the first 3 months, is sufficient.

In contrast, *M avium-intracellulare* is resistant in vitro to most antituberculosis drugs. Most nonimmunocompromised patients with lung infection caused by *M avium-intracellulare* are middle-aged or older men with underlying chronic lung disease. Traditional chemotherapeutic regimens have taken an aggressive approach using 5 or 6 drugs, but these have been associated with drug-induced side effects and patient noncompliance. An alternative regimen uses isoniazid, ethambutol, and rifampin for 18–24 months, plus streptomycin during the first 2–3 months. Medical treatment is initially successful in about two-thirds of cases, but relapses after treatment are common. Long-term benefit is demonstrated in about half of all patients treated medically. Those who do not respond favorably generally have active but stable disease. Surgical resection is an alternative for the patient with progressive disease that responds poorly to chemotherapy. The overall success with surgical therapy is favorable. Dissemination of *M avium-intracellulare* infection is rare in immunocompetent patients. In contrast, in patients with AIDS, *M avium-intracellulare* infections are systemic and tend to occur late in the course. The prognosis is dismal in such cases (see Chapter 24). Treatment of *M avium-intracellulare* infections in patients with AIDS is controversial. The drug regimens used for immunocompetent patients are not applicable to those with AIDS. Multiple combinations of drugs such as isoniazid, ethambutol, rifampin, clofazimine, cycloserine, amikacin, ciprofloxacin, pyrazinamide, and ansamycin have been tried, but clinical improvement and survival benefit have not been demonstrated.

Murray JF, Mills J: Pulmonary infectious complications of human immunodeficiency virus infection. Am Rev Respir Dis 1990;141:1356.

Prince DS et al: Infection with *Mycobacterium avium complex* in patients without predisposing conditions. N Engl J Med 1989;321:863. (Infection may occur in patients without the usual predisposing factors, particularly elderly women.)

NEOPLASTIC & RELATED DISEASES

BRONCHOGENIC CARCINOMA

Essentials of Diagnosis

- Cough, dyspnea, hemoptysis, anorexia, or weight loss in most patients.
- Variable findings on physical examination depending on stage of disease.
- Enlarging mass, infiltrate, atelectasis, cavitation, or pleural effusion on chest x-ray in most patients.
- Cytologic or histologic findings diagnostic of (primary) lung cancer in sputum, pleural fluid, or tissue.

General Considerations

About 157,000 new cases of lung cancer are expected in the USA in 1991. Lung cancer accounts for 34% of cancer deaths in men and 21% of cancer deaths in women, and its incidence in women is rising rapidly. Most cases present between the ages of 50 and 70. Fewer than 5% of lung cancer patients are under 40 years of age. Cigarette smoking is the most important cause of lung cancer in both men and women in the USA. Ionizing radiation (indoor radon gas, therapeutic radiation, atomic bomb blasts), asbestos, heavy metals (nickel, chromium), and industrial carcinogens (chloromethyl ether) are established but less potent pulmonary carcinogens. Lung scars, air pollution, and genetic factors are also implicated, but the data supporting these associations are not conclusive. Chronic obstructive pulmonary disease may represent a risk factor for lung cancer even after controlling for cigarette smoking. Primary lung cancer in nonsmokers is uncommon.

More than 20 benign and malignant primary neoplasms of the lung have been identified and classified histologically. Ninety percent of malignant cancers belong to one of the 4 major cell types of bronchogenic carcinoma, a term denoting primary malignant tumors of the airway epithelium. **Squamous cell carcinoma** and **adenocarcinoma** are the most common types of bronchogenic carcinoma and account for about 30–35% of primary tumors each. **Small cell carcinoma** and **large cell carcinoma** account for about 20–25% and 15%, respectively. Other malignant epithelial tumors of the lung include adenosquamous carcinoma, carcinoid tumor, bronchial gland carcinomas, and a few rare tumors.

Squamous cell carcinoma of the lung tends to originate in the central bronchi as an intraluminal growth and is thus more amenable to early detection through cytologic examination of sputum than are the other types of carcinoma. Squamous cell carcinoma tends to metastasize to regional lymph nodes. About 10% of squamous cell carcinomas cavitate. Small-cell carcinoma also occurs centrally and tends to narrow bronchi by extrinsic compression; widespread metastases are common. Adenocarcinoma and large-cell carcinoma resemble each other in their clinical behavior. These tumors usually appear in the periphery of the lung and therefore are not amenable to early detection through examination of sputum. They typically metastasize to distant organs. **Bronchioloalveolar cell carcinoma,** a subtype of adenocarcinoma, is a low-grade carcinoma that represents about 2% of cases of bronchogenic carcinoma and presents as single or multiple pulmonary nodules or an alveolar infiltrate.

Clinical Findings

The clinical features of lung cancer depend on the primary cancer itself, its metastases, systemic effects of the cancer, and any coexisting paraneoplastic syndromes.

A. Symptoms and Signs: Only 10–25% of patients are asymptomatic at the time of diagnosis of lung cancer. Symptomatic lung cancer is generally advanced and often not resectable. Initial symptoms include nonspecific complaints such as cough, weight loss, dyspnea, chest pain, and hemoptysis that are associated with other disorders. Any change in the pattern of cough, blood-streaked sputum, anorexia with weight loss, and hoarseness are symptoms that point to a diagnosis of bronchogenic carcinoma in the appropriate clinical setting.

Physical findings vary and may be totally absent. Central tumors that obstruct segmental, lobar, or main stem bronchi may cause atelectasis and postobstructive pneumonitis with typical physical findings. Peripheral tumors may cause no abnormalities on physical examination. Extension of the tumor to the pleural surface may cause pleural effusion. In one large series, lymphadenopathy, hepatomegaly, and clubbing were noted in about 20% of patients with lung cancer. Superior vena cava syndrome. **Horner's syndrome** (miosis, ptosis, enophthalmos, and loss of sweating on the affected side), **Pancoast's syndrome** (neurovascular complications of superior pulmonary sulcus tumor), recurrent laryngeal nerve palsy with hoarseness, phrenic nerve palsy with hemidiaphragm paralysis, and skin metastases are each seen in fewer than 5% of cases.

Paraneoplastic syndromes (extrapulmonary organ dysfunction not related to space-occupying metastases) occur in 15–20% of lung cancer patients (see Chapter 3). A number of tumor secretory products have been associated with lung cancer. The manifestations of paraneoplastic syndromes may precede, coincide with, or follow the diagnosis of lung cancer. Recognition of paraneoplastic syndromes in lung cancer is important, because treatment of the associated symptoms may improve the patient's well-being even though the primary tumor itself is not curable; occasionally, resection of the tumor is followed by immediate resolution of the paraneoplastic syndrome. Table 7–13 lists important paraneoplastic syndromes associated with lung cancer.

B. Laboratory Findings: All patients with suspected lung cancer should receive a complete blood count, liver function tests, and measurement of serum electrolytes and calcium in addition to a chest radio-

graph. Definitive diagnosis requires cytologic or histologic evidence of cancer.

Cytologic examination of sputum permits definitive diagnosis of lung cancer in many cases, especially in centrally located tumors. This test is inexpensive and highly specific; unfortunately, the sensitivity is low and influenced by a number of variables. However, a definitive diagnosis of lung cancer by sputum cytologic examination may spare the patient from having to submit to bronchoscopy or another invasive procedure. Examination of pleural fluid reveals cytologic findings positive for cancer in 40–50% of patients with malignant pleural effusion from lung cancer. Closed pleural biopsy (Cope or Abrams needle) yields a histologic diagnosis of cancer in about 55% of patients. Biopsy and cytologic study of pleural fluid combined establish a diagnosis of cancer in about 80% of patients with malignant pleural effusion.

Tissue for histologic confirmation of lung cancer may be obtained by various techniques, including bronchoscopy, percutaneous needle aspirate, mediastinoscopy, lymph node biopsy, or biopsy of other metastatic sites (eg, skin), and thoracotomy. Biopsy of mediastinal lymph nodes reveals cancer in about a third of lung cancer patients. Fine-needle aspiration of supraclavicular or cervical lymph nodes is useful if these nodes are enlarged on palpation. Thoracotomy is occasionally necessary to diagnose lung cancer when simpler cytologic and histologic evaluations are negative.

C. Imaging: Chest radiography demonstrates abnormal findings in nearly all patients with lung cancer. Comparison of old and current chest radiographs enables calculation of the (volume) doubling time. A doubling time of less than 30 days or more than 500 days makes the diagnosis of primary lung cancer unlikely.

Radiographic abnormalities in primary lung cancer are not specific. Common abnormalities are hilar masses or enlargement, peripheral masses, atelectasis, infiltrates, cavitation, and pleural effusions. Multiple masses, consolidation, and chest wall involvement are unusual. Squamous cell and small-cell carcinomas commonly produce a hilar mass and mediastinal widening. Cavitation suggests squamous cell carcinoma and is exceedingly rare in small-cell carcinoma. Small peripheral masses usually are adenocarcinomas.

CT scanning, MRI, and ultrasound are useful imaging methods in selected patients with suspected or proved lung cancer. All depend upon initial detection of a suspicious lesion on the plain chest x-ray. CT scanning is particularly useful for evaluation of the lung parenchyma and pleura. MRI excels in evaluation of the hilum and mediastinum, but experience is less extensive than with CT scanning at this time. Conventional tomography has some value in imaging the hila, central airways, and pulmonary nodules, but it has been rendered almost obsolete by CT scanning and MRI.

Table 7–13. Paraneoplastic syndromes in lung cancer.

Classification	Syndrome	Common Histologic Type of Cancer
Endocrine and metabolic	Cushing's syndrome	Small-cell
	Inappropriate secretion of antidiuretic hormone (SIADH)	Small-cell
	Hypercalcemia	Squamous cell
	Gynecomastia	Large-cell
Connective tissue and osseous	Clubbing and hypertrophic pulmonary osteoarthropathy	Squamous cell, adenocarcinoma, large-cell
Neuromuscular	Peripheral neuropathy (sensory, sensorimotor)	Small-cell
	Subacute cerebellar degeneration	Small-cell
	Myasthenia (Eaton-Lambert syndrome)	Small-cell
	Dermatomyositis	All
Cardiovascular	Thrombophlebitis Nonbacterial verrucous (marantic) endocarditis	Adenocarcinoma
Hematologic	Anemia Disseminated intravascular coagulation Eosinophilia Thrombocytosis	All
Cutaneous	Acanthosis nigricans Erythema gyratum repens	All

D. Special Examinations: Early detection of lung cancer in an asymptomatic stage is feasible with cytologic examination of sputum and chest radiography. Small-cell carcinoma, however, is nearly always metastatic when first detected. Routine screening for lung cancer with chest radiography or cytologic studies of sputum is not recommended because the mortality rate from lung cancer is not appreciably reduced by early detection.

Staging of lung cancer utilizes the TNM international staging system for lung carcinoma, in which T describes the primary tumor, N the nodal involvement, and M any distant metastases (Mountain, 1987). Small-cell carcinoma is staged as "limited" (tumor confined to one hemithorax and hilar, mediastinal, and supraclavicular nodes) or "extensive" (spread to more distant sites). CT scan of the lungs, mediastinum, and upper abdomen (liver, adrenal glands, and periaortic lymph nodes) is usually helpful in staging lung cancer. In a patient with known lung cancer, the finding of mediastinal lymph nodes larger than 2 cm in diameter on CT scan is strong evidence of mediastinal spread of the tumor; however, occasional false-positive results occur with this technique. Nodes smaller than 1 cm have a low probability of tumor involvement. At least 85% of lung cancer patients with negative results on mediastinal CT scans have no evidence of mediastinal lymphadenopathy at the time of surgery.

History, physical examination, and simple laboratory studies (complete blood count, including differential white blood count, liver function tests, bone alkaline phosphatase, and serum calcium) are usually sufficient to detect metastases to distant sites such as liver, brain, bone, heart, abdomen, and skin. Routine radionuclide scans to detect occult distant metastases are not recommended. Radionuclide bone scanning for asymptomatic skeletal metastases is more sensitive than plain x-rays of the skeleton, but it lacks specificity. Patients with skeletal complaints should have bone x-rays. If these are negative, a radionuclide bone scan should be ordered. Those with abnormal central nervous system findings should have a CT scan or MRI of the brain. The latter is preferred for infratentorial lesions.

Surgical exploration of the mediastinum from the suprasternal or parasternal approach should be strongly considered before thoracotomy if radiographic studies suggest significant mediastinal lymphadenopathy or direct extension of the lung cancer into the mediastinum. This approach reduces the number of thoracotomies that do not permit curative lung resection.

Complications

A. Superior Vena Cava Syndrome: See Chapter 9.

B. Phrenic Nerve Palsy: Tumor destruction of the phrenic nerve, which courses through the mediastinum to innervate the hemidiaphragm, occurs in about 1% of patients with lung cancer and results in hemidiaphragmatic paralysis.

C. Recurrent Laryngeal Nerve Palsy: Recurrent laryngeal nerve palsy due to destruction of the recurrent laryngeal nerve by tumor causes paralysis of the muscles of the larynx, resulting in hoarseness. This palsy almost always occurs on the left side and is seen in fewer than 3% of patients with lung cancer.

Treatment

The main treatment options in lung cancer include surgery, chemotherapy, and radiation therapy. Laser photocoagulation has been performed on obstructing central tumors to relieve dyspnea and control hemoptysis.

Surgery remains the treatment of choice for patients with non-small-cell carcinoma. Unfortunately, only about 25% of patients with lung cancer are appropriate candidates for surgery, and many of these are found to have unresectable disease at the time of thoracotomy. Contraindications to surgery include extrathoracic metastases; tumor involving the trachea, carina, or proximal main stem bronchi (< 2 cm from the carina); malignant pleural effusion; recurrent laryngeal nerve or phrenic nerve palsy; superior vena cava syndrome; tumor involving the esophagus or pericardium; spread to contralateral mediastinal lymph nodes; poor general health; and extensive involvement of the chest wall. Patients with lung cancer often have severe obstructive pulmonary dysfunction. Those whose FEV_1 is less than 2 L, those whose FVC is less than 70% of predicted, and those whose maximum voluntary ventilation is less than 50% of predicted will tolerate lung resection poorly. Elderly patients with severe COPD are especially likely to be functionally inoperable.

In patients with non-small-cell carcinoma, adjuvant therapy (chemotherapy, radiation therapy, or both given in the postoperative period) has in general yielded disappointing results. Single agent chemotherapy given postoperatively is of no value. In patients with stage II and stage III adenocarcinoma and large-cell carcinoma, chemotherapy with a combination of 3 drugs for completely resected tumors apparently increases disease-free survival. In patients with incompletely resected non-small-cell carcinoma, postoperative radiation therapy is frequently administered, and recent data suggest that the disease-free survival is further extended when postoperative radiation therapy is used with multidrug chemotherapy. Studies are currently under way to determine whether neoadjuvant therapy (combination chemotherapy given prior to surgical resection) improves resectability and survival in patients with non-small-cell carcinoma.

Combination chemotherapy (see Chapter 3) is the treatment of choice for small-cell carcinoma and results in considerable improvement in median survival.

Occasionally, posttreatment surgical debulking of primary lesions is carried out. Prophylactic cranial radiation is performed in patients with small-cell carcinoma who have responded to chemotherapy. Single-agent chemotherapy has no proved value. Although tumor regression in non-small-cell carcinoma is possible with combination chemotherapy, median survival time is not prolonged.

External beam radiation therapy is often used to palliate symptoms of lung cancer such as cough, hemoptysis, pain due to bone metastases, and dyspnea from bronchial or tracheal obstruction. It is also employed to treat bronchial obstruction (atelectasis, pneumonia). Radiation therapy is only about 20% successful for treatment of bronchial obstruction by lung cancer; laser therapy is superior when the obstructing lesion is in a main stem bronchus. Radiation therapy is also useful to treat superior vena cava syndrome resulting from non-small-cell carcinoma. Superior vena cava syndrome from small cell carcinoma may be treated with chemotherapy or radiation therapy. Symptomatic brain metastases are treated with radiation therapy and corticosteroids. Selected patients with unresectable lung cancer also receive external beam radiation to the primary tumor site. In patients with limited-stage small-cell carcinoma, this improves complete response rates and survival when compared to chemotherapy alone. However, in non-small-cell lung cancer, survival is not improved. Intraluminal radiation ("brachytherapy") is a new approach to relief of symptoms of recurrent endobronchial lung cancer.

Prognosis

The overall 5-year survival rate for lung cancer is 10–15%. Determinants of survival include the stage of disease at the time of presentation, the patient's general health, age, histologic type of tumor, tumor growth rate, and type of therapy. Overall, the 5-year survival rate after "curative" resection of squamous cell carcinoma is 35–40%, compared with 25% for adenocarcinoma and large-cell carcinoma. Patients with small-cell carcinoma rarely live for 5 years after the diagnosis is made.

Batra P et al: Evaluation of intrathoracic extent of lung cancer by plain chest radiography, computed tomography, and magnetic resonance imaging. Am Rev Respir Dis 1988;137:1456.

Ginsberg RJ, Joss RA, Feld R (editors): Fifth World Conference on Lung Cancer. Chest 1989;96(Suppl):1S [Entire issue.] (Update on epidemiology, biology, pathology, and therapy.)

Iannuzzi MC, Scoggin CH: Small cell lung cancer. Am Rev Respir Dis 1986;134:593. (Review of clinical and basic science aspects).

Matthay RA et al: Lung cancer 1987: Epidemiology, etiology, diagnosis, staging, and treatment. Am Rev Respir Dis 1987;136:1040.

Mountain CF: The new international staging system for lung cancer. Surg Clin North Am 1987;67:925.

SOLITARY PULMONARY NODULE

A solitary pulmonary nodule is a round or oval, sharply circumscribed pulmonary lesion (up to 5 cm in diameter; larger lesions are termed "masses") surrounded by normal lung tissue. Central cavitation, calcification, or surrounding ("satellite") lesions may occur. Although mass population screening for lung cancer by chest x-ray is not advised, the finding of a solitary pulmonary nodule on chest x-ray in an individual patient is important. About 25% of cases of bronchogenic carcinoma present as solitary pulmonary nodule, and the 5-year survival rate for bronchogenic carcinoma that is detected in this form approaches 50%, which is considerably higher than the 10–15% 5-year survival rate of lung cancer overall.

In large surgical series, about 60% of solitary pulmonary nodules are benign lesions and 40% are malignant. Infectious granulomas account for most benign lesions, whereas primary lung cancer accounts for more than three-quarters of all malignant solitary pulmonary nodules. Solitary pulmonary nodules occasionally represent metastases from another primary tumor. Determining whether the lesion is likely to be benign or malignant preoperatively is more important than establishing its precise cause.

A lesion is almost certainly benign if the volume doubling time is less than 30 days or more than 500 days or if the lesion is calcified (central, "clustered," or laminated calcium pattern). Factors favoring a benign diagnosis are young age, absence of symptoms, small size (< 2 cm in diameter), smooth margins on tomography, and presence of satellite lesions, but none of these criteria are foolproof. Malignant solitary pulmonary nodules are occasionally symptomatic, tend to occur in patients over 45 years of age, are usually larger than 2 cm, often have indistinct margins, and are rarely calcified. Typical features of solitary pulmonary metastases include smooth or lobulated margins, peripheral location, location in the lower lobe, and absence of satellite lesions.

Skin tests and serologic studies for fungal infection are generally not helpful. Cytologic examination of sputum should be considered for evaluation of a large centrally located pulmonary nodule; a positive result might preclude the need for bronchoscopy or needle biopsy. However, sputum cytology is rarely diagnostic of malignancy in small or peripheral pulmonary nodules. Radiographic studies and *comparisons with old chest radiographs* are of utmost importance. Conventional tomograms and CT scan are particularly useful approaches. Thin section (1.5–5 mm) CT scanning is the preferred method for detection of calcification within the nodule. Investigations for primary cancer elsewhere in the body are not indicated unless abnormal symptoms, signs, and results of simple laboratory studies suggest an extrapulmonary cancer. Routine percutaneous needle aspiration of all solitary pulmonary nodules is not advised; it seldom changes subsequent therapy, and false negatives are common.

Treatment

As a general rule, all solitary pulmonary nodules in patients over age 35 should be considered potentially malignant and should be resected unless calcification typical of benign lesions or stability on radiography for 2 years is documented. Prospective evaluation ("watchful waiting") is generally not appropriate if calcification is not present or if stability cannot be documented. However, strong indications of a benign diagnosis or contraindications to surgery may justify a conservative approach. Otherwise, exploratory thoracotomy is advised as soon as possible after a solitary pulmonary nodule is detected. Decision analysis suggests that the average life expectancy of patients with solitary pulmonary nodules is similar, whether immediate surgery, biopsy, or observation is chosen as the initial approach (Cummings et al, 1986). However, such an outcome has not been established by prospective clinical trials. Having the informed patient participate in the decision-making process is important.

Cummings SR, Lillington GA, Richard RJ: Managing solitary pulmonary nodules: The choice of strategy is a close call. Am Rev Respir Dis 1986;134:453.

SECONDARY LUNG CANCER

Secondary lung cancers represent metastases from extrapulmonary malignant neoplasms that spread to the lungs through vascular or lymphatic channels or by direct extension. Metastases to the lung usually occur via the pulmonary artery and typically present as multiple masses on chest radiography. Almost any cancer can metastasize to the lung. **Lymphangitic carcinoma** denotes diffuse involvement of the pulmonary lymphatic network by secondary lung cancer, probably a result of extension of tumor from lung capillaries to the lymphatics. **Tumor embolism** from extrapulmonary cancer (renal cell carcinoma, hepatoma, choriocarcinoma) is an uncommon way that tumor is spread to the lungs. Endobronchial metastases occur in fewer than 5% of patients dying of nonpulmonary cancer; most metastases are intraparenchymal. Carcinoma of the kidney, breast, colon, and cervix and malignant melanoma are the tumors most likely to cause endobronchial metastases. Secondary lung cancer also presents as malignant pleural effusion.

Clinical Findings

A. Symptoms and Signs: Symptoms are uncommon but include cough, hemoptysis, and in advanced cases, dyspnea. Symptoms are usually referable to the site of the primary tumor.

B. Laboratory Findings: The diagnosis of secondary lung cancer is usually established by identifying the primary tumor. Cytologic examination of sputum is not often helpful. If history and physical examination fail to reveal the site of the primary tumor, an expensive radiographic and endoscopic search for the primary lesion is ill-advised. Appropriate studies should be ordered if there is a suspicion of any primary cancer, such as breast, thyroid, testis, or prostate, for which specific treatment is available. In most cases, attention is better focused on the lung, where tissue samples obtained at aspiration bronchoscopy, needle or thoracotomy establish the histologic diagnosis and suggest the most likely primary. Occasionally, cytologic studies of pleural fluid or pleural biopsy reveal the diagnosis. If a solitary lung lesion is detected in a patient with known extrapulmonary cancer, primary lung cancer is the most likely diagnosis. Patients with sarcoma or melanoma are exceptions to this rule. Only about 3% of all solitary pulmonary nodules represent solitary metastases, and about a third of these are metastases from rectosigmoid tumors.

C. Imaging: Chest radiographs usually show multiple spherical densities with sharp margins. Solitary metastases are observed in fewer than 25% of cases of secondary lung cancer. The size of metastatic lesions varies from a few millimeters (miliary densities) to large masses. The lesions are usually bilateral, peripheral, and more common in lower lung zones. Cavitation suggests primary squamous cell tumor; calcification suggests osteosarcoma. Conventional chest radiography is less sensitive than CT scan in detecting pulmonary metastases. Whole lung conventional tomography for determining the extent of pulmonary metastases has been rendered almost obsolete by CT scanning. The radiographic differential diagnosis of multiple pulmonary nodules includes pulmonary arteriovenous malformation, pulmonary abscesses, granulomatous infection, sarcoidosis, rheumatoid nodules, and Wegener's granulomatosis.

Treatment

Surgical resection of a *solitary* pulmonary nodule is often prudent in the patient with known current or previous extrapulmonary cancer. A solitary pulmonary nodule in such a patient is more often primary lung cancer than a single metastasis.

Once the diagnosis of secondary lung cancer has been established (usually by percutaneous needle biopsy or transbronchial biopsy), management consists of treatment of the primary neoplasm and any pulmonary complications. Local resection of one or more pulmonary metastases via thoracotomy or median sternotomy is feasible in a few carefully selected patients with various sarcomas and carcinomas (breast, testis, colon, kidney, and head and neck). Surgical resection should be considered only if the primary tumor is under control, if the patient is a good surgical risk, if all of the metastatic tumor can be resected, if nonsurgical approaches are not available, and if there are no metastases elsewhere in the body. The overall 5-year survival rate in secondary lung cancer treated surgically is 20–35%. Surgery is not advised if the primary lesion is a melanoma, if metastases are synchronous, if pneumonectomy is required, or if there is pleural involvement.

MESOTHELIOMA

Mesotheliomas are primary tumors arising from the surface lining of the pleura (80% of cases) or peritoneum (20% of cases). About three-fourths of pleural mesotheliomas are diffuse (usually malignant) tumors, and the remaining one-fourth are localized (usually benign). Men outnumber women by a 3:1 ratio. Numerous studies have confirmed the association of **malignant pleural mesothelioma** with exposure to asbestos (particularly the crocidolite form). About 7% of asbestos workers are affected. The physician should inquire about asbestos exposure through mining, milling, manufacturing, shipyard work, insulation, brake linings, building construction and demolition, roofing materials, and a variety of asbestos products (pipe, textiles, paint, tile, gaskets, panels). Although cigarette smoking increases the risk of bronchogenic carcinoma in asbestos workers and aggravates asbestosis, there is no association between smoking and mesothelioma.

The mean age at onset of symptoms of malignant pleural mesothelioma is about 60 years. The latent period between exposure and onset of symptoms ranges from 20 to 40 years. Symptoms include the insidious onset of shortness of breath, nonpleuritic chest pain, and weight loss. Physical findings include dullness to percussion, diminished breath sounds, and finger clubbing. Radiographic abnormalities consist of nodular, irregular, unilateral pleural thickening and varying degrees of unilateral pleural effusion. CT scan helps demonstrate the extent of pleural involvement.

Pleural fluid is exudative and often hemorrhagic. Open pleural biopsy is usually necessary to obtain an adequate specimen for histologic diagnosis; even then, distinction from benign inflammatory conditions and from metastatic adenocarcinoma may be difficult.

Malignant pleural mesothelioma progresses rapidly as the tumor spreads quickly along the pleural surface to involve the pericardium, mediastinum, and contralateral pleura. The tumor may eventually extend beyond the thorax to involve abdominal lymph nodes and organs. Progressive pain and dyspnea are characteristic. Median survival time from onset of symptoms is 8–14 months, and about 75% of patients are dead within 1 year of diagnosis. Treatment with surgery, radiotherapy, chemotherapy, and a combination of methods has been attempted but is generally unsuccessful.

Pisani RJ, Colby TV, Williams DE: Malignant mesothelioma of the pleura. Mayo Clin Proc 1988;63:1234.

BENIGN TUMORS OF THE LUNG

Benign neoplasms of the lung typically present as asymptomatic solitary pulmonary nodules detected on routine chest radiography. They account for about 2% of all solitary pulmonary nodules.

Hamartoma is the most common benign lung tumor. Fibromas, lipomas, leiomyomas, hemangiomas, and papillomas account for most of the remainder. The clustered ("popcorn") pattern of calcification on chest x-ray or tomograms is a helpful diagnostic clue to hamartoma.

The medical history, physical examination, and radiographic studies do not permit reliable differentiation of malignant and benign lung tumors. Percutaneous needle biopsy, guided by fluoroscopy or CT scanning and using a needle large enough (18- to 20-gauge) to obtain a core of tissue, is occasionally successful in establishing a *specific* benign diagnosis. However, because of the suspicion of bronchogenic carcinoma, most patients will require thoracotomy for definitive diagnosis. Patients who are poor operative risks may be followed with serial chest films for progression. Even if cancer is present, short periods of observation do not appreciably affect the prognosis.

Gabrail NY, Zara BY: Pulmonary hamartoma syndrome. Chest 1990;97:962.
Wang KP, Kelly SJ, Britt JE: Percutaneous needle aspiration biopsy of chest lesions: New instrument and new technique. Chest 1988;93:993.

BRONCHIAL CARCINOID TUMORS

Carcinoid and bronchial gland tumors are sometimes termed **bronchial adenomas,** but this classification is a misnomer, because it implies that the lesions are benign, when in fact carcinoid tumors and bronchial gland carcinomas are low-grade malignant neoplasms.

Carcinoid tumors are about 6 times more common than bronchial gland carcinomas, and most of them occur as pedunculated or sessile growths in central bronchi. Men and women are equally affected. Most patients are under 60 years of age. Common symptoms of bronchial carcinoid tumors are hemoptysis, cough, wheezing, and recurrent pneumonia. Peripherally located bronchial carcinoid tumors are rare and present as asymptomatic solitary pulmonary nodules. Carcinoid syndrome (flushing, diarrhea, wheezing, hypotension, etc) is rare. Most carcinoid tumors are diagnosed at the time of fiberoptic bronchoscopy, the characteristic finding being a pink or purplish tumor protruding into the lumen of main stem, lobar, or segmental bronchi. Bronchoscopic biopsy is occasionally complicated by significant bleeding, because these lesions have a well-vascularized stroma. CT scanning is helpful to localize the lesion and to follow its growth over time.

Bronchial carcinoid tumors grow slowly and rarely metastasize. Complications involve bleeding and airway obstruction rather than invasion by tumor and metastases. Surgical excision is necessary in some cases, and the prognosis is generally favorable. Most bronchial carcinoid tumors are resistant to radiation and chemotherapy.

Rozenman J et al: Bronchial adenoma. Chest 1987;92:145. (Clinical and radiographic features, management, and prognosis.)

MEDIASTINAL MASSES

Various developmental, neoplastic, infectious, traumatic, and cardiovascular disorders may cause masses that appear in the mediastinum on chest x-ray (Table 7–14). A useful convention arbitrarily divides the mediastinum into 3 compartments—anterior, middle, and posterior—in order to classify mediastinal masses and assist in differential diagnosis. Specific mediastinal masses have a predilection for one or more of these compartments; most mediastinal masses are located in the anterior or middle compartment.

Symptoms and signs of mediastinal masses are nonspecific and are usually caused by the effects of the mass on surrounding structures. Insidious onset of retrosternal chest pain, dysphagia, or dyspnea is often an important clue to the presence of a mediastinal mass. In about half of cases, symptoms are absent, and the mass is detected on routine chest x-ray. Physical findings vary depending upon the nature and location of the mass.

CT scan is helpful in management; additional radiographic studies of benefit include barium swallow if esophageal disease is suspected, Doppler sonography or venography of brachiocephalic veins and the superior vena cava, and arteriography. MRI is complementary to CT scanning and is often advised when the results of CT scan are equivocal. Advantages of MRI include distinction between vessels and masses, no need for contrast media, and better delineation of hilar structures. MRI also allows imaging in multiple planes, whereas CT permits only axial imaging. Tissue diagnosis is necessary if a neoplastic disorder is suspected. Treatment and prognosis depend on the underlying cause of the mediastinal mass.

Gamsu G, Sostman D: Magnetic resonance imaging of the thorax. Am Rev Respir Dis 1989;139:254. (State-of-the-art review describing the advantages and limitations of MRI of the thorax in comparison with CT scanning.)

INTERSTITIAL LUNG DISEASES

Interstitial lung diseases comprise a heterogeneous group of disorders that have in common the features of inflammation and fibrosis of the interalveolar septum, which represent a nonspecific reaction of the lung to injury of diverse cause. Some 130 disease entities share the manifestations of interstitial lung disease (Table 7–15). In the majority of patients, no specific cause can be identified. In the remainder, drugs and a variety of inorganic and organic dusts are the predominant causes of the interstitial disease.

The pathogenesis of interstitial lung disease of unknown etiology is believed to be lung injury that leads to inflammation of the interalveolar septum (alveolitis). Persistent alveolitis may lead to eventual irreversible interstitial fibrosis.

Interstitial lung diseases share common clinical, physiologic, and radiographic features. Dyspnea and dry cough of insidious onset are the usual presenting symptoms. Chest examination is notable for fine inspiratory crackles at the bases of the lung. Digital clubbing is common. Pulmonary function testing reveals a restrictive ventilatory defect and a decreased diffusing capacity for carbon monoxide. Hypoxemia, especially with exercise, is common. Diffuse ground-glass, nodular, reticular, or reticulonodular infiltrates that may progress to "honeycomb lung" are noted on chest x-ray. Infrequently, the chest x-ray is normal when lung biopsy demonstrates interstitial lung disease.

The history, physical examination, chest x-ray, and laboratory studies may provide evidence of a specific cause of interstitial lung disease. Sputum is usually minimal or nonexistent. Induced sputum is likely to yield useful diagnostic information only if pulmonary infection or malignancy is suspected.

Techniques to evaluate the progression of alveolitis have been devised in an attempt to identify patients suitable for anti-inflammatory therapy. These techniques include lung biopsy, bronchoalveolar lavage, and Ga 67 lung scanning.

Transbronchial biopsy using a fiberoptic bronchoscope is easily performed and is associated with a low morbidity rate, but the tissue specimens obtained are small, and sampling errors may result. Open lung biopsy produces large specimens but has a higher rate of complications. Transbronchial biopsies and washings may be adequate to permit the diagnosis of diseases such as sarcoidosis, histiocytosis X, *Pneu-*

Table 7–14. Radiographic and clinical features of selected mediastinal masses.

Mass	Radiographic Features	Clinical Features
Anterior compartment		
Thymoma	Smooth or lobulated, round or oval homogeneous density; calcified rim in some cases.	One-fourth to one-half of patients have myasthenia gravis; otherwise, usually asymptomatic. Local symptoms suggest cancer (50% of thymomas).
Teratomas and dermoid cysts	Same as thymoma; teeth, bone may be present.	Asymptomatic young adults; expectoration of cyst contents may occur. Surgical excision advised because of potential for malignancy.
Thyroid masses	Smooth, lobulated, homogeneous densities; move with swallowing on fluoroscopy; calcification common.	Usually asymptomatic; thyroid gland often palpably enlarged; thyrotoxicosis and carcinoma uncommon.
Parathryoid masses	Smooth, lobulated; rare cause of anterior mediastinal masses.	Typical features of hyperparathyroidism; local effects rare.
Middle compartment		
Lymph node enlargement	Common cause of mediastinal masses; single or multiple lobulated masses; variable size; unilateral or bilateral.	Symptoms are those of underlying diseases, including bronchogenic carcinoma, lymphoma and leukemia, sarcoidosis, granulomatous infections.
Bronchogenic cysts	Oval or round, sharp margins; near carina or main bronchi.	Asymptomatic young adults; expectoration of contents, secondary infection may occur; surgery often warranted.
Pleuropericardial cysts	Round or oval, smooth margins; most at cardiophrenic angle; more common on right side; fluid contents move with change in position.	Asymptomatic.
Carcinoma of trachea	Paratracheal or intratracheal density.	Rare; cough, hemoptysis, stridor.
Foramen of Morgagni hernia	Abdominal contents in thorax; round or oval mass; usually on right side of pericardium.	Usually asymptomatic.
Enlarged pulmonary arteries	Smooth structures; usually bilateral and contiguous with hili; CT scan or angiography may be necessary for clarification.	Clinical evidence of pulmonary hypertension; rarely, pulmonic stenosis or aneurysm.
Dilatation of superior vena cava	Right-sided smooth-walled density; azygos vein usually dilated as well; size changes with change in intrapleural pressure.	Findings of right-sided heart disease or constrictive pericardial disease.
Dilatation of azygos or hemiazygos veins	Round or oval smooth-walled density at right tracheobronchial angle; Valsalva and Müller maneuvers help distinguish from azygos lymph node.	Symptoms depend on underlying cause.
Aneurysm of aorta or innominate artery	Variable saccular or fusiform masses adjacent to aorta or innominate artery; calcification common; angiography or CT scan required for clarification.	Symptoms vary depending on cause, location, and size.
Posterior compartment		
Neurogenic tumors	Round or oval homogeneous densities with sharp margins; paravertebral location; usually unilateral.	Usually asymptomatic; occasional pain and dyspnea; surgical excision usually required.
Meningocele	Single or multiple; slightly more common on right side; sharp margins.	Usually middle-aged adults; often associated with neurofibromatosis.
Esophageal tumors	Usually not visible on plain chest x-ray; barium swallow required.	Dysphagia; pain under sternum; bleeding.
Esophageal hiatus hernia	Retrocardiac location slightly to the right of midline; air and fluid contents; confirmation by barium swallow.	Dysphagia; postprandial pain on bending over or lying down.
Foramen of Bochdalek hernia	Round or oval; more common on left side; barium studies of gut and excretory urogram may be helpful.	Usually detected in children; strangulation of hernia contents may occur.
Thoracic spine diseases	Bone tumors produce round, paravertebral soft tissue masses; occasional destruction of vertebra; tomograms and CT scan helpful.	Variable; back pain common.
Extramedullary hematopoiesis	Smooth, lobulated, multiple masses; homogeneous densities; unilateral or bilateral; paravertebral location.	Usually asymptomatic; patients have chronic hemolytic anemia, usually with splenomegaly and other features of extramedullary hematopoiesis.

Table 7–15. Interstitial lung diseases.[1]

Known Cause	Unknown Cause
Inorganic dusts	Cryptogenic fibrosing
Silica	alveolitis
Silicates (including	Sarcoidosis
asbestos)	Histiocytosis X
Aluminum	Rheumatic disease-
Antimony	associated
Carbon	Goodpasture's syndrome
Beryllium	Idiopathic pulmonary
Hard metal dusts	hemosiderosis
Organic dusts	Wegener's granulomatosis
(hypersensitivity	Lymphomatoid
pneumonitis)	granulomatosis
Gases, fumes, vapors	Churg-Strauss syndrome
Chlorine	Angioimmunoblastic
Sulfur dioxide	lymphadenopathy
Mercury	Inherited diseases
Drugs	Tuberous sclerosis
Antineoplastic agents	Neurofibromatosis
Antibiotics	Pulmonary veno-occlusive
Sulfonamides	disease
Penicillins	Ankylosing spondylitis
Nitrofurantoin	Amyloidosis
Drugs inducing lupus	Chronic eosinophilic
erythematosus	pneumonia
Sulfonylureas	Pulmonary
Gold	lymphangiomyomatosis
Phenytoin	Whipple's disease
Penicillamine	Alveolar proteinosis
Amiodarone	Inflammatory bowel disease-
Poisons	associated
Paraquat	
Radiation	
Infections	
Disseminated	
mycobacterial or fungal	
infections	
Viral pneumonia	
Pneumocystis carinii	
pneumonia	
Residue of active infection	
of any type	
Pulmonary edema	
Lymphangitic carcinoma	

[1] Modified and reproduced, with permission, from Crystal RG et al: Interstitial lung disease: Current concepts of pathogenesis, staging, and therapy. *Am J Med* 1981;**70**:542.

mocystis carinii pneumonia, miliary tuberculosis, pulmonary alveolar proteinosis, and lymphangitic carcinomatosis. On the other hand, patients who are rapidly deteriorating may be best served by definitive open lung biopsy rather than potentially nondiagnostic transbronchial biopsy. The choice between transbronchial biopsy and open lung biopsy depends on the following factors: (1) the probable diagnosis, (2) the patient's condition, (3) the operator's expertise in these biopsy procedures, (4) the risks of empiric therapy, and (5) the risk of biopsy procedures. It is probably reasonable to begin with transbronchial biopsy in most patients because of the low rate of complications associated with this procedure. If no specific diagnosis can be reached and the patient is a good

candidate for surgery, open lung biopsy may then be performed.

Bronchoalveolar lavage is useful in the diagnosis of *P carinii* pneumonia and in selected patients with lung infection from other organisms (mycobacteria, fungi, cytomegalovirus, and *Legionella* species). It is occasionally employed for specific diagnosis of lung cancer, pulmonary alveolar proteinosis, histiocytosis X, beryllium-induced lung disease, amiodarone-induced pneumonitis, or pulmonary hemorrhage in thrombocytopenic patients. In ongoing studies, a very high percentage of T lymphocytes in bronchoalveolar lavage fluid suggests sarcoidosis or hypersensitivity pneumonitis; a predominance of neutrophils, eosinophils, and macrophages suggests idiopathic pulmonary fibrosis. Expertise in evaluation of lavage fluid is not widely available, limiting the application of serial bronchoalveolar lavage. Lung scanning with Ga 67 is nonspecific and has no proved value in diagnosis or management of patients with interstitial lung disease.

Known causes of interstitial lung disease are dealt with in their specific sections. The important idiopathic forms are discussed below.

Deremee RA: Diffuse interstitial pulmonary disease from the perspective of the clinician. Chest 1987;92:1068. (An algorithmic approach to the definitive diagnosis of diffuse interstitial lung disease.)

Reynolds HY: Bronchoalveolar lavage. Am Rev Respir Dis 1987;135:250.

Sibille Y, Reynolds HY: Macrophages and polymorphonuclear neutrophils in lung defense and injury. Am Rev Respir Dis 1990;141:471.

Smith CM, Moser KM: Management for interstitial lung disease: State of the art. Chest 1989;95:676.

CRYPTOGENIC FIBROSING ALVEOLITIS (Idiopathic Pulmonary Fibrosis)

Cryptogenic fibrosing alveolitis is the most common diagnosis among patients presenting with interstitial lung disease. Patients usually present in the sixth or seventh decade. The disease is more common in men than in women. A familial form of the disease (autosomal dominant trait with variable penetrance) has been described. Serologic tests for antinuclear antibody and rheumatoid factor are frequently positive (20–40% of cases). Symptoms, physical findings, and results on pulmonary function tests are typical of those of interstitial lung disease and are described above. Chest x-ray abnormalities are highly variable. Lower lung zone interstitial infiltrates of a reticular pattern are typical when the patient is first seen. High-resolution CT scan best demonstrates the extent of lung parenchymal fibrosis. Circulating immune complexes have been detected in patients with this disorder. However, the diagnosis is usually based on the clinical presentation and exclusion of other specific diagnoses, usually by means of bronchoalveolar lavage or lung biopsy. Histologic examination of lung tissue reveals a combination of cellular infiltration and fibrosis of the alveolar septum. Desquamated mononuclear cells, mainly macrophages, may be observed within alveoli; it is likely that fibrosis is preceded by other histologic stages (desquamative interstitial pneumonitis, usual interstitial pneumonitis) in many of these patients. Open lung biopsy for the diagnosis of cryptogenic fibrosing alveolitis is helpful to exclude other specific causes of interstitial lung disease. Its routine use for this purpose is controversial.

High doses of oral corticosteroids (eg, prednisone, 40–80 mg daily) are the usual treatment. Cytotoxic drugs such as cyclophosphamide and azathioprine have also been used. Controlled clinical trials have not demonstrated any beneficial effect of therapy, but clinical experience with these drugs suggests that about 20% of patients will improve. The response to corticosteroids is better in patients with more inflammation and less fibrosis noted on lung biopsy. Relentless progression of the disease with eventual respiratory insufficiency is the rule, and the average survival time is about 4 years. Lung transplantation for highly selected patients with end-stage pulmonary fibrosis has been reported. It is important to distinguish cryptogenic fibrosing alveolitis from bronchiolitis obliterans organizing pneumonia (BOOP) because of the excellent response of the latter disorder to corticosteroid therapy.

Burkhardt A: Alveolitis and collapse in the pathogenesis of pulmonary fibrosis. Am Rev Respir Dis 1989;140:513.
Raghu G: Idiopathic pulmonary fibrosis: A rational clinical approach. Chest 1987;92:148.

SARCOIDOSIS

Sarcoidosis is a systemic disease of unknown cause characterized by granulomatous inflammation that affects the lung in about 90% of patients. The incidence is highest in North American blacks and northern European whites; among blacks, women are more frequently affected than men. Onset of disease is usually in the third or fourth decade.

Patients may present with malaise, fever, and dyspnea of insidious onset. Alternatively, sarcoidosis may present with symptoms referable to the skin, eyes, peripheral nerves, liver, or heart. Some patients are asymptomatic and come to medical attention after abnormal findings on routine chest radiographs. Physical findings in the chest are typical of those associated with interstitial lung involvement, if the parenchyma is involved. Other findings may include skin rashes, erythema nodosum, parotid gland enlargement, hepatosplenomegaly, and lymphadenopathy.

Laboratory tests may show leukopenia, eosinophilia, an elevated erythrocyte sedimentation rate, and hypercalcemia (about 10% of patients) or hypercalciuria. Angiotensin-converting enzyme (ACE) levels may be elevated with active sarcoidosis, but this finding is neither sensitive nor specific enough to have diagnostic significance. ACE is derived from the cell membrane of epithelioid cells of the sarcoid granuloma. Its synthesis is controlled by T lymphocytes. Physiologic testing may reveal evidence of airflow obstruction, but decreased lung volumes and diffusing capacity are more common signs. Skin test anergy is present in 70%.

Radiographic findings are variable and include bilateral hilar adenopathy alone (stage I), hilar adenopathy and parenchymal involvement (stage II), or parenchymal involvement alone (stage III). Parenchymal involvement is usually manifested radiographically by diffuse reticular infiltrates, but focal infiltrates, acinar shadows, nodules, and, rarely, cavitation may be seen. Pleural effusion is noted in fewer than 10% of patients.

The diagnosis of sarcoidosis generally requires histologic demonstration of noncaseating granulomas in biopsies from a patient with other typical associated manifestations. Other granulomatous diseases must be ruled out. If indicated, biopsy of easily accessible sites, eg, palpable lymph nodes, skin lesions, or salivary glands, is likely to provide positive findings. Transbronchial lung biopsy has a high yield of positive findings, especially in patients with radiographic evidence of parenchymal involvement. Most clinicians would agree that tissue biopsy is not necessary when stage I radiographic findings are detected in a clinical situation that strongly favors the diagnosis of sarcoidosis (eg, a young black female with erythema nodosum). Biopsy is essential whenever clinical and radiographic findings suggest the possibility of an alternative diagnosis such as lymphoma. Bronchoalveolar lavage is useful in following the activity of sarcoidosis in selected patients but does not provide a specific diagnosis.

Indications for treatment with corticosteroids include constitutional symptoms, hypercalcemia, iritis, arthritis, central nervous system involvement, granulomatous hepatitis, cutaneous lesions, and symptomatic pulmonary lesions. ACE serum levels usually fall with clinical improvement. About 20% of patients with lung involvement suffer irreversible lung impairment. The outlook is best for patients with hilar adenopathy alone; radiographic involvement of the lung parenchyma is associated with a worse prognosis. Death due to pulmonary insufficiency occurs in about 5% of patients.

Thomas PD, Hunninghake GW: Current concepts of the pathogenesis of sarcoidosis. Am Rev Respir Dis 1987; 135:747.

HISTIOCYTOSIS X

Histiocytosis X is a generic term embracing 3 clinical syndromes that share a common histologic characteristic and are defined by age at onset, clinical course, and organ involvement. Letterer-Siwe disease is a rapidly fatal disseminated disorder occurring in children. Hand-Schuller-Christian disease is a slowly progressive disorder occurring in children and adolescents that involves bone and the posterior pituitary and may be disseminated. Pulmonary histiocytosis X **(pulmonary Langerhans cell granulomatosis, or eosinophilic granuloma)** is characterized by bronchiolitis and small-vessel vasculitis that progresses to fibrosis and destruction of alveolar walls; bone and posterior pituitary are uncommonly involved. Most patients present in the third or fourth decade. Nearly all are cigarette smokers. Symptoms may be absent or may include cough, dyspnea, chest pain, fever, and weight loss. Blood eosinophilia is not observed. Spontaneous pneumothorax occurs in about 10% of patients and may be bilateral. Chest x-ray is characterized by finely nodular interstitial infiltrates mostly in the upper lung zones. A honeycomb pattern may evolve. Physiologic testing may reveal a restrictive defect, obstructive defect with hyperinflation, or a combination of these patterns.

The diagnosis is confirmed by the demonstration of characteristic pentalaminar structures ("X bodies") within histiocytosis×cells (mononuclear phagocytes, ie, alveolar macrophages, similar to Langerhans cells in normal skin). These "X bodies" may be demonstrated by electron microscopic study of fluid obtained by bronchoalveolar lavage, thereby avoiding lung biopsy. The disease spontaneously stabilizes or improves in about half of patients and progresses to permanent loss of lung function in the other half. Corticosteroids are the usual form of therapy, although their efficacy has not been established.

INTERSTITIAL LUNG INVOLVEMENT IN OTHER DISEASES

Interstitial lung disease that clinically resembles cryptogenic fibrosing alveolitis has been described in a variety of rheumatic diseases. It also occurs with chronic active hepatitis, inflammatory bowel disease, biliary cirrhosis, autoimmune thrombocytopenia, and hemolytic anemia. Although other manifestations of these diseases usually dominate the clinical picture, interstitial lung disease may be symptomatic and progress to respiratory insufficiency, in which case treatment with anti-inflammatory drugs similar to those used in cryptogenic fibrosing alveolitis should be started. Nonspecific interstitial pneumonitis characterized by diffuse alveolar damage but lacking evidence of infection has been reported to account for one-third of all episodes of clinical pneumonitis in patients with AIDS.

Tazelaar HD, et al: Interstitial lung disease in polymyositis and dermatomyositis: Clinical features and prognosis as correlated with histologic findings. Am Rev Respir Dis 1990;141:727.

White DA, Matthay RA: Noninfectious pulmonary complications of infection with the human immunodeficiency virus. Am Rev Respir Dis 1989;140:1763.

MISCELLANEOUS INFILTRATIVE LUNG DISEASES

PULMONARY ANGIITIS & GRANULOMATOSIS

Wegener's granulomatosis is an idiopathic disease manifested by a combination of glomerulonephritis, necrotizing granulomatous vasculitis of the upper and lower respiratory tracts, and varying degrees of small vessel vasculitis. Complaints of chronic sinusitis are a common presentation; pulmonary symptoms occur less often. Arthralgias, fever, skin rash, and weight loss are frequent symptoms. Multiple nodular infiltrates, often with cavitation, are present on chest radiography. Tracheal stenosis and endobronchial disease are sometimes seen. Laboratory tests reveal no diagnostic abnormalities. Diagnosis depends on histologic identification of the characteristic necrotizing granulomatous vasculitis in biopsies of lung or sinus tissue; lung biopsy is more specific but is associated with greater morbidity.

Lymphomatoid granulomatosis is a systemic disease manifested by granulomatous angiitis and a polymorphic cellular infiltrate consisting of atypical lymphocytoid and plasmacytoid cells. Any organs may be involved, but lung, brain, and skin are the most frequently affected. In contrast to Wegener's granulomatosis, the upper airway and kidneys are rarely involved clinically, though histologic evidence of cellular infiltration of the kidneys is frequently seen. The glomeruli are spared. Radiographic manifestations may include multiple nodular infiltrates or diffuse reticular infiltrates. The diagnosis is suggested by the characteristic pattern of organ system involvement and is confirmed by histologic findings. Lymphomatoid granulomatosis has a poor prognosis, since it evolves into malignant lymphoma in nearly half of patients.

Allergic angiitis and granulomatosis (Churg-Strauss syndrome) is an idiopathic multisystem vasculitis of small and medium-sized arteries that occurs in patients with asthma. Histologic features include fibrinoid necrotizing epithelioid and eosinophilic granulomas. The skin and lungs are most often involved, but other organs, including the heart, gastrointestinal tract, liver, and peripheral nerves, may also be affected. Marked peripheral eosinophilia is the rule. Abnormalities on chest radiographs range from transient infiltrates to multiple nodules. This illness may be part of a spectrum that includes polyarteritis nodosa.

Treatment of these disorders consists of combination therapy with corticosteroids and cyclophosphamide. Oral prednisone (1 mg/kg/d initially, tapering slowly to alternate-day therapy over 3–6 months) is the corticosteroid of choice; in Wegener's granulomatosis, some clinicians may omit the use of steroids. For fulminant vasculitis, therapy may be initiated with intravenous methylprednisolone for several days. Cyclophosphamide (2 mg/kg/d initially, with dosage adjustments to avoid neutropenia) is given daily by mouth for at least 1 year after complete remission is obtained. Five-year survival rates in patients with these vasculitis syndromes have been improved to about 90% by the combination therapy.

Complete remissions can be achieved in over 90% of patients with Wegener's granulomatosis. The addition of daily trimethoprim-sulfamethoxazole to standard therapy is a promising new approach to treatment.

Cordier JF, et al: Pulmonary Wegener's granulomatosis: A clinical and imaging study of 77 cases. Chest 1990;97:906.

Leavitt RY, Fauci AS: Pulmonary vasculitis. Am Rev Respir Dis 1986;134:149.

ALVEOLAR HEMORRHAGE SYNDROMES

Diffuse alveolar hemorrhage may occur in a variety of immune and nonimmune disorders. Causes of **immune alveolar hemorrhage** have recently been classified as anti-basement membrane antibody disease (Goodpasture's syndrome), vasculitis and collagen vascular disease (systemic lupus erythematosus and others), idiopathic rapidly progressive glomerulonephritis, chemical or drug-related (penicillamine, trimellitic anhydride), and idiopathic (Leatherman, 1987). Hemoptysis, alveolar infiltrates on chest x-ray, anemia, dyspnea, and occasionally fever are characteristic. **Nonimmune disorders** causing diffuse hemorrhage include coagulopathy, mitral stenosis, and necrotizing pulmonary infection. Bronchoalveolar lavage is helpful to determine whether diffuse alveolar hemorrhage has an immune or an infectious basis.

Goodpasture's syndrome is idiopathic recurrent alveolar hemorrhage and rapidly progressive glomerulonephritis. The disease is mediated by anti-glomerular basement membrane antibodies detected as a linear fluorescent pattern on immunofluorescence studies of the lung and kidneys. Goodpasture's syndrome occurs mainly in men who are in their 30s and 40s. Hemoptysis is the usual presenting symptom, but pulmonary hemorrhage may be occult. Dyspnea, cough, hypoxemia, and diffuse bilateral alveolar infiltrates are typical features. Iron deficiency anemia and microscopic hematuria are usually present. The diagnosis is based on characteristic linear IgG deposits in glomeruli by immunofluorescence and on the presence of anti-glomerular basement membrane antibody in serum. The physician should attempt to distinguish Goodpasture's syndrome from other pulmonary-renal syndromes, which include systemic lupus erythematosus, idiopathic rapidly progressive glomerulonephritis, Wegener's granulomatosis, systemic necrotizing vasculitis, and drug-induced disease (penicillamine, trimellitic anhydride). Combinations of immunosuppressive drugs (methylprednisolone with cyclophosphamide) and plasmapheresis have yielded excellent results in recent years. The response to treatment is highly variable. Long-term remissions are occasionally observed.

Idiopathic pulmonary hemosiderosis is a disease of children or young adults characterized by recurrent pulmonary hemorrhage; in contrast to Goodpasture's syndrome, renal involvement and anti-glomerular basement membrane antibodies are absent. Treatment of acute episodes of hemorrhage with corticosteroids may be useful. Recurrent episodes of pulmonary hemorrhage may result in interstitial fibrosis.

Leatherman JW: Immune alveolar hemorrhage. Chest 1987;91:891.

PULMONARY ALVEOLAR PROTEINOSIS

Pulmonary alveolar proteinosis is a disease in which a phospholipid material similar to surfactant accumulates within alveolar spaces. The condition may be primary (idiopathic) or secondary (occurring in immune deficiency; following lung infections, including tuberculosis and viral infections). Progressive dyspnea is the usual presenting symptom, and chest x-ray shows bilateral alveolar infiltrates suggestive of pulmonary edema. The diagnosis is based on demonstration of characteristic intra-alveolar phospholipid on open lung biopsy. Analysis of bronchoalveolar lavage fluid holds promise as a less invasive diagnostic method.

The course of the disease varies; some patients experience spontaneous remission, whereas in others, progressive respiratory insufficiency develops. Pulmonary infection with *Nocardia* or fungi may occur. Therapy for alveolar proteinosis consists of periodic whole lung lavage, which is effective in reducing external dyspnea.

EOSINOPHILIC PNEUMONIA

The term "eosinophilic pneumonia" denotes a syndrome characterized by peripheral lung infiltrates shown to be eosinophilic by bronchoalveolar lavage or lung biopsy. Blood eosinophilia is present in most cases. Symptoms may be mild and transient and can include fever, cough, and wheezing (Lodffler's syndrome); or severe and progressive (chronic eosinophilic pneumonia). Fever, weight loss, and dyspnea may occur in chronic eosinophilic pneumonia. A severe acute form of eosinophilic pneumonia has recently been described, characterized by fever, respiratory failure, a high percentage of eosinophils in bronchoalveolar lavage fluid, rapid response to treatment with erythromycin and corticosteroids, and lack of recurrence.

Eosinophilic pneumonia may be associated with exposure to various drugs or infestation with roundworm parasites such as filariae, *Ascaris* (Lodffler's syndrome), or *Strongyloides*. No precipitating cause may be apparent in as many as one-third of cases. If an extrinsic cause is identified, therapy consists of removal of the offending drug or treatment of the underlying parasitic infestation. Corticosteroid treatment should be instituted if no treatable extrinsic cause is discovered. The response to corticosteroids is usually dramatic. Recurrences are common.

Allen JN et al: Acute eosinophilic pneumonia as a reversible cause of noninfectious respiratory failure. N Engl J Med 1989;321:569. (Two of 4 patients required mechanical ventilation. A hypersensitivity basis is proposed.)

AMYLOIDOSIS

Amyloid may accumulate in the lungs of patients with primary amyloidosis. Tracheobronchial, parenchymal nodular, and diffuse interstitial patterns of pulmonary involvement are seen. The tracheobronchial form may present with airflow obstruction mimicking asthma or with focal obstruction leading to atelectasis. The nodular form is usually asymptomatic. The diffuse interstitial form usually presents with dyspnea. The diagnosis requires the demonstration of amyloid deposits in tissue. Treatment is unsatisfactory; the prognosis of the diffuse interstitial form is poor.

Cordier JF, Loire R, Brune J: Amyloidosis of the lower respiratory tract: Clinical and pathologic features in a series of 21 patients. Chest 1986;90:827.

DISORDERS OF THE PULMONARY CIRCULATION

PULMONARY THROMBOEMBOLISM

Essentials of Diagnosis
- Predisposition to venous thrombosis, usually of the lower extremities.
- Abrupt onset of dyspnea, chest pain, apprehension, hemoptysis, or syncope.
- Acute respiratory alkalosis and hypoxemia in most patients.
- Characteristic defects on ventilation-perfusion lung scan.
- Diagnostic findings on pulmonary angiogram.

General Considerations
Pulmonary emboli arise from thrombi in the venous circulation or right side of the heart (thromboembolism), from tumors that have invaded the venous circulation (tumor emboli), or from other sources (amniotic fluid, air, fat, bone marrow, and foreign intravenous material).

Pulmonary thromboembolism is associated with as many as 200,000 deaths per year; about 10% of victims die within the first hour. Fewer than 10% of patients who die of pulmonary embolism have received treatment for the condition, a fact underscoring the difficulty encountered in diagnosis.

More than 90% of pulmonary emboli originate as clots in the deep veins of the lower extremities. Most deep venous thrombi originate in the calves, and some 80% of these spontaneously resolve without embolizing. The remainder may propagate into the iliofemoral veins. Fracture of the propagating thrombus in these proximal veins allows a clot to migrate into the inferior vena cava and ultimately to the lungs. One-third to one-half of patients with deep venous thrombosis of the iliofemoral system have clinically significant pulmonary embolism.

Physiologic risk factors for venous thrombosis include venous stasis, venous endothelial injury, and hypercoagulability (eg, oral contraceptives, cancer, protein C or S deficiency, and antithrombin III deficiency). Clinical risk factors include prolonged bed rest or inactivity, surgery, childbirth, advanced age, stroke, myocardial infarction, congestive heart failure, obesity, and fractures of the hip or femur. Occasionally, in situ thrombosis in the pulmonary arteries occurs without embolization; predisposing factors include sickle cell anemia, chest trauma, and certain congenital cardiac anomalies.

Discharge of thrombus into the pulmonary artery has both hemodynamic and pulmonary consequences. The hemodynamic consequences of pulmonary thromboembolism are related to mechanical obstruction of the pulmonary vascular bed and obscure neurohumoral reflexes causing vasoconstriction. Both factors result in increased pulmonary vascular resistance and, in severe cases, pulmonary hypertension and right ventricular failure. The pulmonary consequences of thromboembolism result from reflex bronchoconstriction in the embolized lung zone, wasted ventilation (increased physiologic dead space), and loss of alveolar surfactant. Frank pulmonary infarction is uncommon.

Clinical Findings

A. Symptoms and Signs: The clinical findings in pulmonary thromboembolism depend on the size of the embolus and the patient's preexisting cardiopulmonary status. In pulmonary embolism that is less than massive, clot obstructs less than two-thirds of the pulmonary arterial tree. In *massive* pulmonary embolism, acute right ventricular failure and systemic hypotension result. Recognizing pulmonary thromboembolism is more difficult in patients with underlying cardiopulmonary disease, and the cardiovascular effects of pulmonary emboli are usually more profound in these patients.

Symptoms of pulmonary thromboembolism include chest pain, which is often pleuritic, dyspnea, apprehension, cough, hemoptysis, and diaphoresis. In massive embolization, pulmonary embolism occasionally presents as syncope.

The signs of pulmonary thromboembolism include tachycardia, tachypnea, crackles, and accentuation of the pulmonic component of the second heart sound. Low-grade fever occurs in about 40% of cases. Thrombophlebitis, diaphoresis, and right-sided cardiac gallop each are noted in about a third of cases. The clinician should be alert to other conditions that mimic thrombophlebitis of the calf, including cellulitis, muscle strain or rupture, lymphangitis, and rupture of a Baker's cyst. Cyanosis, wheezing, and cardiac arrhythmias are noted in fewer than one-fourth of cases. Shock is unusual. Signs and symptoms do not generally differ between massive and less severe thromboembolism. Pulmonary embolism may mimic pneumonia, myocardial infarction, pneumothorax, and even rib fractures.

B. Laboratory Findings: The results of routine laboratory tests are not helpful in diagnosing pulmonary thromboembolism. Arterial blood gas measurements usually reveal acute respiratory alkalosis due to hyperventilation. About 90% of patients with proved pulmonary embolism have an arterial Po_2 under 80 mm Hg. Electrocardiographic findings are likewise not diagnostic. Nearly all patients with pulmonary thromboembolism have an abnormal ECG; tachycardia and nonspecific ST–T wave changes are the most common abnormalities. A pattern of acute right heart strain (S_1Q_3, S_{1-3}, T wave inversion in leads V_{1-3}) is more characteristic but uncommon. Pulmonary function tests are not specific.

C. Imaging and Special Examinations:

1. Chest radiography–The chest radiograph is usually abnormal in patients with pulmonary embolism, but the abnormalities are often related to chronic pulmonary or cardiac disease. No pathognomonic findings are present. Elevation of a hemidiaphragm and pulmonary infiltration are the most common abnormalities. Platelike atelectasis, oligemia in the embolized lung zone (Westermark sign), and prominence of the pulmonary artery are sometimes seen. A small unilateral pleural effusion is occasionally present. A homogeneous, wedge-shaped density based in the pleura and pointing toward the hilum (Hampton's hump) is highly suggestive of pulmonary infarction but is uncommon.

2. Lung scanning–Most if not all patients with suspected pulmonary embolism should undergo a perfusion scan. Though perfusion lung scans may be abnormal in other diseases, including COPD, asthma, pneumonia, and heart failure, their results may be used to direct subsequent pulmonary arteriography and reduce the load of contrast media in these patients. A ventilation scan may be performed prior to the perfusion scan if concurrent disease of the airways or lung parenchyma is present. It is important to recognize that a "low-probability" ventilation/perfusion scan does *not* rule out pulmonary thromboembolism. However, a high probability (85–90%) of pulmonary embolism exists when there is a lobar perfusion defect with ventilation mismatch.

The following are additional important considerations in the interpretation of lung scans looking for pulmonary emboli.

(1) A normal perfusion scan rules out clinically important pulmonary embolism, and no further diagnostic studies are necessary.

(2) A *single* segmental or subsegmental defect on the perfusion scan is unlikely to represent pulmonary embolism.

(3) *Multiple* segmental or larger perfusion defects are more likely to represent pulmonary emboli.

(4) Mismatched ventilation-perfusion defects (hypoperfusion with normal ventilation) involving segments or larger amounts of lung are likely to represent pulmonary embolism; this is least likely to be the case in subsegmental defects, more likely in segmental defects, and most likely in lobar defects.

(5) Perfusion defects in locations matching abnormalities on chest x-ray do not reliably predict either the presence or the absence of pulmonary embolism. If the infiltrate on chest x-ray is substantially larger than the perfusion defect, however, the likelihood of pulmonary embolism is low. If the defect on chest x-ray is substantially smaller than the perfusion defect, however, the likelihood of pulmonary embolism is high.

(6) Perfusion defects persist 7–14 days after pulmonary embolism, so a follow-up perfusion-ventilation scan is sometimes helpful in diagnosis. Resolution

of a perfusion defect in less than 5 days suggests an alternative diagnosis.

Intravenous digital subtraction angiography has been shown to compare favorably with ventilation-perfusion lung scanning in patients with suspected pulmonary embolism.

3. Venous thrombosis studies–Because the history and physical examination are neither sensitive nor specific in detecting thrombi in the deep veins of the lower extremities, specific tests such as contrast venography, impedance plethysmography, and duplex ultrasonography are necessary (see Chapter 9). None of these tests is ideal, and there is no consensus about which should be used. However, documentation of deep venous thrombosis in a patient with suspected pulmonary thromboembolism may preclude the need for pulmonary angiography.

Because of its high sensitivity and specificity, contrast venography remains the "gold standard" in testing for venous thrombosis. However, about 30% of patients with angiographically proved pulmonary embolism have negative contrast venograms. An intraluminal filling defect is pathognomonic of venous thrombosis. Disadvantages of contrast venography include discomfort, difficulty in interpretation expense, difficult technical requirements, and complications such as phlebitis in 3–4% of patients. It is less accurate below the knee. Impedance plethysmography has both a sensitivity and a specificity of about 95% in the detection of thrombi in the popliteal, femoral, and iliac veins. Serial impedance plethysmography is a safe, effective, noninvasive, and inexpensive approach to detection of proximal thrombi in outpatients with suspected acute deep venous thrombosis. Duplex ultrasonography is an alternative approach with similar sensitivity and specificity. Impedance plethysmography and duplex ultrasonography may not detect proximal vein thrombi if obstruction is not complete, and neither method is sensitive in detection of thrombi in calf veins. However, either study may be used to follow the patient for propagation of a calf vein thrombus into the popliteal vein. [125]I fibrinogen leg scanning is very sensitive in detecting fresh thrombi in calf, popliteal, and lower thigh veins. It is not sensitive to thrombi above the mid thigh and requires 24 hours for interpretation. For these reasons it has become less popular than the 2 major noninvasive studies, impedance plethysmography and duplex ultrasonography. Bilateral radionuclide venography has a sensitivity similar to that of contrast venography but lacks its specificity. This procedure may be combined with perfusion lung scanning and does not cause phlebitis.

If the physician suspects deep venous thrombosis, intravenous heparin should be started and a noninvasive study ordered. Impedance plethysmography and duplex ultrasonography are currently the noninvasive methods of choice. If either is positive, continued treatment is advised. If the noninvasive study is negative, it should be repeated serially until a positive result is obtained; if the results are repeatedly negative, therapy may be terminated. Contrast venography is advised if the noninvasive study yields equivocal results.

The sensitivity and specificity of various studies for the detection of deep venous thrombosis depend upon the expertise of the team performing the studies. Thus, practitioners should be aware of which studies are most likely to be accurate in the setting of their own practice.

4. Pulmonary angiography–Pulmonary angiography—which can detect emboli as small as 3 mm in diameter—remains the definitive test for diagnosis of pulmonary embolism because of its high sensitivity and specificity. Emboli smaller than 3 mm in diameter are unlikely to be of clinical significance. The finding of an intraluminal defect or an arterial cutoff on the pulmonary angiogram is diagnostic. Oligemia and asymmetry of blood flow are suggestive but not specific. After 5 days, negative results on angiography do not rule out the possibility that an embolism has occurred.

Pulmonary angiography is expensive and invasive, occasionally difficult to interpret, and may be associated with complications; in experienced hands, however, the procedure is associated with a morbidity and mortality rate of less than 1%. The procedure is advised when the diagnosis of pulmonary embolism must be established with certainty, as in situations where anticoagulation is considered especially risky. Ventilation-perfusion lung scans of "intermediate" probability for pulmonary thromboembolism are frequently encountered. Moreover, lung scans of suboptimal quality because of patient performance and technical limitations are commonplace. In these situations, pulmonary angiography is often valuable. Pulmonary angiography is required if any type of surgical procedure for prevention of recurrent thromboemboli is planned, eg, interruption of the inferior vena cava. It is indicated in patients with suspected embolism whenever the diagnosis remains in doubt after preliminary studies (clinical evaluation, lung scans, tests for deep venous thrombosis) have been performed. Allergy to the contrast medium is an absolute contraindication to pulmonary angiography. Relative contraindications include severe pulmonary hypertension, ventricular arrhythmias, left bundle branch block, and renal failure.

As in the use of radiocontrast materials for any purpose, precautions must be taken to prevent radiocontrast-induced acute renal failure.

Prevention

Prevention of deep venous thrombosis and pulmonary thromboembolism may be accomplished by using physical measures, low-dose heparin, and antiplatelet drugs in patients at risk.

Postoperative intermittent external pneumatic compression of the legs is recommended for patients undergoing neurosurgery, urologic surgery, or major knee surgery. Early ambulation after surgery, elevation of the legs for immobilized patients, and active and passive leg exercises are reasonable approaches to preventing deep venous thrombosis.

Low-dose heparin is of proved benefit in reducing the risk of deep vein thrombosis and fatal pulmonary embolism in general surgery patients; in patients undergoing surgery of the thorax, abdomen, or extremities; in patients who have suffered myocardial infarction, respiratory failure, and acute spinal cord injury; and in patients with stroke. If low-dose heparin is indicated, 5000 units subcutaneously is given every 8–12 hours, beginning 2 hours before surgery or upon admission to the hospital and continuing until the risk for deep vein thrombosis has lessened. Continuous monitoring of clotting studies is not necessary, though the partial thromboplastin time should be checked occasionally, since some patients show increased sensitivity to heparin. Low-dose heparin is not effective in preventing pulmonary embolism in patients with major long bone fractures or those undergoing hip surgery or above-the-knee amputation. Intravenous dextran, adjusted-dose heparin, and moderate-dose warfarin are effective approaches to prophylaxis against postoperative venous thrombosis in these high-risk patients. The *adjusted-dose* heparin regimen is to administer just enough heparin subcutaneously every 8 hours to maintain the activated partial thromboplastin time, measured 6 hours after injection, at 31.5–36 seconds. The *moderate-dose* warfarin protocol raises the prothrombin time to an international normalized ratio (INR) of 2.0–3.0 (1.3–1.5 times control, using rabbit brain thromboplastin). Antiplatelet drugs such as aspirin are not recommended for the prevention (or treatment) of venous thrombosis or pulmonary thromboembolism.

The reader is referred to a recent summary of recommendations for prevention and treatment of venous thromboembolic disease (Dalen and Hirsh, 1989).

Treatment

A. Anticoagulation: Anticoagulation for established pulmonary embolism is preventive rather than definitive therapy. For acute pulmonary thromboembolism or proximal (thigh) deep venous thrombosis, heparin is the anticoagulant of choice. Distal (calf) deep venous thrombosis does not require systemic anticoagulation *if* coexisting proximal deep venous thrombosis has been excluded by noninvasive studies or contrast venography. In the absence of such evidence, anticoagulation for 3 months is advised for isolated calf vein thrombosis. Heparin inhibits thrombin and other clotting factors by potentiating antithrombin III; it does not dissolve established thrombi but does prevent their distal propagation. Heparin reduces the rate of recurrence of pulmonary embolism; it may reduce the incidence of death due to recurrence.

Heparin is given intravenously by continuous infu-

sion. Intermittent subcutaneous heparin is clearly less effective in patients with acute proximal deep vein thrombosis. After a loading dose of 5000–10,000 units by bolus intravenous injection, the drug is given at a rate of 1000–1500 units/h. The activated partial thromboplastin time is determined 4–6 hours after therapy has been started and is maintained at 1.5–2 times the pretreatment control value until it has stabilized; the requirements for heparin are greater early in the clinical course. The platelet count is monitored every 2–3 days, because heparin may induce thrombocytopenia.

Oral anticoagulant therapy with warfarin may be started concurrently with heparin. A recent study suggests that institution of warfarin on the first day of anticoagulation with heparin is as effective as the old practice of instituting it several days later. Earlier hospital discharge and cost savings under diagnosis-related group financing should occur from this change in practice. Heparin is usually continued for at least 5 days in order to allow time for warfarin to exert its full anticoagulant effects. Warfarin alters the synthesis of vitamin K-dependent procoagulants (factors II, VII, IX, and X) and proteins C and S and requires 6–7 days to achieve full effectiveness. Begin treatment with 10 mg of warfarin daily (usually for 3–5 days) until the prothrombin time is 1.3–1.5 times control (using North American thromboplastin), which corresponds to an international normalized ratio (INR) of 2.0–3.0. Maintenance therapy with warfarin may require 2–15 mg daily, the required dose varying widely among patients. If warfarin is contraindicated or inconvenient, subcutaneous heparin may be substituted for warfarin, the dose being adjusted to maintain an activated partial thromboplastin time of 11/2 times the control value at the mid-dosing interval. Warfarin is contraindicated in pregnancy.

The duration of warfarin therapy after thromboembolic disease has been diagnosed depends on the individual patient's clinical situation, and insufficient data have accrued to define the optimal duration of therapy for each circumstance. If risk factors such as oral contraceptive use or immobility following a bone fracture have been eliminated, warfarin therapy for 1–3 months is reasonable. A minimum of 3 months of therapy is advised if risk factors cannot be quickly eliminated, as in patients with congestive heart failure, prolonged immobility, or venous stasis. If the patient has continuing, unresolvable risk factors, such as cancer, antithrombin III deficiency, or protein C deficiency, or a second pulmonary embolism after discontinuance of warfarin, permanent anticoagulant therapy is recommended.

The major risk of anticoagulant therapy is bleeding. Major hemorrhage occurs in about 5% of patients receiving intravenous heparin, and the death rate is 0.6%. The risk of hemorrhage is increased in women over 60 years of age and in patients taking aspirin. The rate of major hemorrhage is similar for warfarin

(2–10%), but serious hemorrhage is unusual in patients with adequately controlled prothrombin times (1.3–1.5 × control value, or INR 2.0–3.0). Longer prothrombin times invite more bleeding complications without enhancing efficacy. Subcutaneous heparin, administered in adjusted doses, may be as effective as warfarin in long-term treatment of deep venous thrombosis and is less likely to cause bleeding.

B. Thrombolytic Therapy: Lysis of pulmonary thromboemboli in situ represents the only available definitive medical treatment and is achieved by use of streptokinase and urokinase, which enhance endogenous fibrinolysis by activating plasmin. Plasmin directly lyses thrombi both in the pulmonary artery and in the venous circulation and also has a secondary anticoagulant effect. Thrombolytic therapy, when compared to heparin alone, accelerates the resolution of pulmonary emboli, reduces pulmonary artery and right heart pressures, and improves right and left ventricular function in patients with established pulmonary embolism. Thrombolytic therapy may also protect the pulmonary microcirculation and preserves the anatomy and function of the valves in deep veins of the lower extremities. It has not been shown to affect the mortality rate from pulmonary thromboembolism, however.

The use of thrombolytic therapy in clinical practice is controversial. Most physicians reserve its use for patients with acute massive pulmonary embolism confirmed by pulmonary angiography and for selected patients with established deep venous thrombosis. Suitable candidates for thrombolytic therapy include patients with hemodynamic compromise due to pulmonary embolism, those with underlying severe cardiopulmonary disease, and those who fail to show hemodynamic improvement after heparin therapy.

Care and expertise in monitoring therapy, managing bleeding, and controlling subsequent anticoagulation are essential. The duration of symptoms prior to starting thrombolytic therapy should be less than 7 days. Puncture of noncompressible arteries or veins, or intramuscular injections are not permitted during thrombolytic therapy. Anticoagulants and antiplatelet drugs should not be given concurrently. Absolute contraindications to thrombolytic therapy include active internal bleeding and recent (within 2 months) cerebrovascular accident. Other major contraindications include severe hypertension, recent trauma, gastrointestinal bleeding, and major surgical or obstetric procedures. Hemorrhage is the major complication of thrombolytic therapy and can usually be avoided by strict adherence to treatment guidelines.

Urokinase or streptokinase is given as a continuous intravenous infusion by an infusion pump. Streptokinase is usually preferred because it is less expensive, but development of antibodies may prevent future use of the drug. Streptokinase, 250,000 units intrave-

nously over 30 minutes as a loading dose, is followed by a maintenance dose of 100,000 units/h for 24–72 hours. The effectiveness of therapy is monitored by measuring the thrombin time 4 hours after initiation of therapy to ensure the presence of a fibrinolytic state. Too high a dose may produce a paradoxic normalization of the thrombin time, so that use of this test must be correlated with clinical assessment of bleeding. Some authorities suggest that monitoring the bleeding time during thrombolytic therapy gauges the risk of hemorrhagic complications. Administration of intravenous heparin is resumed upon completion of thrombolytic therapy.

Preliminary studies suggest that **tissue plasminogen activator,** a product of recombinant DNA technology that is useful as a thrombolytic agent in the early treatment of patients with acute myocardial infarction (see Chapter 8), is effective in the treatment of patients with documented pulmonary thromboembolism and those with deep venous thrombosis. Hemorrhagic complications and expense have tempered enthusiasm for the use of this drug. Recommendations for its use must await the conclusion of large clinical trials.

C. Additional Measures: Surgical interruption of the inferior vena cava is indicated when recurrent pulmonary embolism would be life-threatening in a patient with major contraindications to anticoagulation or failure or complications of anticoagulant or thrombolytic therapy. Life-threatening paradoxic thromboembolism or septic thromboembolism may also justify surgical interruption, which may be achieved by ligation, plication, clipping, and insertion of intraluminal filters in the inferior vena cava just below the renal veins. Percutaneous transjugular placement of a filter has become the preferred mode of inferior vena cava interruption when the patient is at continued risk for recurrent pulmonary thromboembolism from pelvic or lower extremity thrombi. The risks of recurrent pulmonary thromboembolism and inferior vena cava occlusion after filter placement are low (2–3%).

Surgical removal of acute pulmonary embolism (pulmonary embolectomy) is now rarely performed. The mortality rate of this procedure approaches 50%.

Prognosis

Pulmonary embolism may cause sudden death, though the prognosis for survivors is generally favorable. The prognosis depends on the underlying disease and on proper diagnosis and treatment. The mortality rate in patients with undiagnosed pulmonary thromboembolism is about 30%, compared to 10% when appropriate therapy for definitively diagnosed pulmonary embolism is initiated—though these figures do not reflect controlled studies. Perfusion defects resolve in most survivors. Pulmonary hypertension may be a complication of chronic recurrent pulmonary thromboembolism.

Dalen JE, Hirsh J (editors): American College of Chest Physicians: Second ACCP Conference on Antithrombotic Therapy. Chest 1989;95(Suppl):S1. [Entire issue.]

Goldhaber SZ (editor): Thrombolysis in cardiopulmonary disease. Chest 1990;97(Suppl):115 S. [Entire issue.]

Hull RD, et al: Clinical validity of a normal perfusion lung scan in patients with suspected pulmonary embolism. Chest 1990;97:23.

Moser KM: Venous thromboembolism. Am Rev Respir Dis 1990;141:235.

PULMONARY HYPERTENSION

Essentials of Diagnosis

- Dyspnea, fatigue, chest pain, and occasionally syncope on exertion.
- Narrow splitting of second heart sound with loud pulmonic component; findings of right ventricular hypertrophy and cardiac failure in advanced disease.
- Hypoxemia: wasted ventilation on pulmonary function tests in most cases.
- Electrocardiographic evidence of right ventricular strain or hypertrophy and right atrial enlargement.
- Enlarged central pulmonary arteries on chest x-ray.

General Considerations

The pulmonary circulation is unique because of its high blood flow, low pressure (normally 25/8 mm Hg, mean 12), and low resistance (normally 200–250 dynes/sec/cm^{-5}). It can accommodate large increases in blood flow during exercise with only modest increases in pressure because of its ability to recruit and distend blood vessels. The normal pulmonary circulation is also largely passive, since its pressures are determined mainly by the function of the right and left ventricles. Contraction of smooth muscle in the walls of pulmonary arteriolar resistance vessels becomes an important factor in numerous pathologic states.

Pulmonary hypertension is present when pulmonary artery pressure rises to a high level inappropriate for a given level of cardiac output. **Primary (idiopathic) pulmonary hypertension** (see Chapter 8) is a rare disorder of the pulmonary circulation occurring mostly in young and middle-aged women; it is characterized by progressive dyspnea, a rapid downhill course, and invariably fatal outcome. This condition is also called plexogenic pulmonary arteriopathy, in reference to the characteristic histopathologic plexiform lesion found in muscular pulmonary arteries. Secondary pulmonary hypertension is more common.

Selected mechanisms responsible for pulmonary hypertension and examples of corresponding clinical conditions are set forth in Table 7–16. Pulmonary hypertension is usually caused by reduction of the cross-sectional area of the pulmonary vasculature at the arterial, capillary, or venous level. Hypoxia of

Table 7–16. Mechanisms of pulmonary hypertension and examples of corresponding clinical conditions.

Reduction in cross-sectional area of pulmonary arterial bed
Vasoconstriction
  Hypoxia of any cause
  Acidosis
Loss of vessels
  Lung resection
  Emphysema
  Vasculitis
  Pulmonary fibrosis
  Connective tissue disease
Obstruction of vessels
  Pulmonary embolism (thromboemboli, tumor emboli, foreign body emboli, etc)
  In situ thrombosis
  Schistosomiasis
Narrowing of vessels
  Secondary structural changes due to pulmonary hypertension
Increased pulmonary venous pressure
Constrictive pericarditis
Left ventricular failure or reduced compliance
Mitral stenosis
Left atrial myxoma
Pulmonary veno-occlusive disease
Mediastinal diseases compressing pulmonary veins
Increased pulmonary blood flow
Congenital left-to-right intracardiac shunts
Increased blood viscosity
Polycythemia
Miscellaneous
Pulmonary hypertension occurring in association with hepatic cirrhosis and portal hypertension

any cause is the most important and potent stimulus of pulmonary arterial vasoconstriction. The mechanisms by which hypoxia causes pulmonary hypertension are poorly understood. Factors operating at the alveolar level and direct stimulation of arteriolar smooth muscle have been implicated. Hypoxia is partially or fully responsible for the pulmonary hypertension observed in chronic bronchitis, infiltrative lung disease due to various causes, kyphoscoliosis, obesity-hypoventilation syndrome, chronic mountain sickness, obstructive sleep apnea, and neuromuscular disease. Acidosis is also a potent stimulus of pulmonary hypertension and exerts a synergistic vasoconstrictive effect with hypoxia.

Extensive obliteration and obstruction of the pulmonary arterial tree may cause pulmonary hypertension. Once present, pulmonary hypertension is self-perpetuating. It introduces secondary structural abnormalities in pulmonary vessels, including smooth muscle hypertrophy and intimal proliferation, and these may eventually stimulate atheromatous changes and in situ thrombosis, leading to further narrowing of the arterial bed.

Increased pulmonary venous pressure, when sustained, may cause "postcapillary" pulmonary hypertension; left ventricular failure is the most common cause.

Pulmonary veno-occlusive disease is a rare cause of postcapillary pulmonary hypertension occurring in children and young adults. The cause is unknown. The disease is characterized by progressive fibrotic occlusion of pulmonary veins and venules. Nodular areas of pulmonary congestion, edema, hemorrhage, and hemosiderosis are found. Chest radiography reveals prominent, symmetric interstitial markings, Kerley B lines, pulmonary artery dilatation, and normally sized left atrium and left ventricle. Premortem diagnosis is often difficult but is occasionally established by open lung biopsy. There is no effective therapy, and most patients die within 2 years as a result of progressive pulmonary hypertension.

Pulmonary hypertension is readily recognized when an obvious cause, such as severe COPD, is present. In adults, pulmonary hypertension in the absence of COPD is often caused by chronic pulmonary thromboembolism, interstitial fibrosis, sleep apnea, or obesity-hypoventilation syndrome. Other disorders listed in Table 7–16 should be excluded before the diagnosis of primary pulmonary hypertension is entertained.

Clinical Findings

A. Symptoms and Signs: Secondary pulmonary hypertension is difficult to recognize clinically in the early stages, when symptoms and signs are primarily those of the underlying disease. Pulmonary hypertension may cause or contribute to dyspnea, which is present initially on exertion and later at rest. Dull, retrosternal chest pain resembling angina pectoris may be present. Fatigue and syncope on exertion also occur.

The signs of pulmonary hypertension include narrow splitting of the second heart sound, accentuation of the pulmonic component of the second heart sound, and a systolic ejection click. In advanced cases, tricuspid and pulmonic valve insufficiency and signs of right ventricular failure and cor pulmonale are found.

B. Laboratory Findings: Polycythemia is found in many cases of pulmonary hypertension that are associated with chronic hypoxemia. Electrocardiographic changes are those of right axis deviation, right ventricular hypertrophy, right ventricular strain, or right atrial enlargement.

C. Imaging and Special Examinations: Radiographic findings depend on the cause of pulmonary hypertension. In chronic disease, dilatation of the right and left main and lobar pulmonary arteries and enlargement of the pulmonary outflow tract are seen; in advanced disease, right ventricular and right atrial enlargement are seen. Peripheral "pruning" of large pulmonary arteries is characteristic of pulmonary hypertension in severe emphysema.

Echocardiography is helpful in evaluating patients thought to have mitral stenosis, left atrial myxoma, and pulmonary valvular disease. Echocardiography may also reveal right ventricular enlargement and paradoxic motion of the interventricular septum.

Doppler ultrasonography is a reliable noninvasive means of estimating systolic pulmonary artery pressure. However, other precise hemodynamic measurements can only be obtained with right heart catheterization, which is often helpful when postcapillary pulmonary hypertension, intracardiac shunting, or thromboembolic disease is considered as part of the differential diagnosis.

Routine pulmonary function tests reveal no findings diagnostic of pulmonary hypertension. Diminution of the pulmonary capillary bed may cause reduction in the single breath diffusing capacity.

Depending upon the suspected cause of pulmonary hypertension, ventilation-perfusion lung scanning, pulmonary angiography, and open lung biopsy are occasionally helpful. Ventilation-perfusion lung scanning is very helpful in identifying patients with pulmonary hypertension caused by recurrent pulmonary thromboemboli. Transbronchial biopsy carries an increased risk of bleeding.

Treatment

Treatment of primary pulmonary hypertension is discussed in Chapter 8. Treatment of secondary pulmonary hypertension consists mainly of treating the underlying disorder, such as COPD, sleep apnea, obesity-hypoventilation syndrome, and mitral stenosis. Early recognition of pulmonary hypertension is crucial to interrupt the self-perpetuating cycle responsible for the rapid progression of this disorder. By the time most patients present with signs and symptoms of pulmonary hypertension, however, the condition is far advanced. If hypoxemia or acidosis is detected, corrective measures should be started immediately. Supplemental oxygen administered for at least 15 hours per day has been demonstrated to be of benefit in patients with hypoxemic COPD.

Other disorders responsible for pulmonary hypertension should be treated appropriately. Patients with documented recurrent pulmonary thromboembolism should receive permanent anticoagulation therapy; some clinicians employ this therapy in pulmonary hypertension of unknown cause, since multiple, very small pulmonary emboli may produce this picture and be difficult to recognize clinically. Postcapillary pulmonary hypertension usually responds to treatment of the underlying cardiac disease.

Vasodilator therapy using various pharmacologic agents (eg, calcium antagonists, hydralazine, isoproterenol, diazoxide, nitroglycerin) has been tried in primary pulmonary hypertension and a few patients with secondary pulmonary hypertension with inconsistent results. Short-term benefits have been demonstrated with some of these agents, but improved outcome has not been documented. Complications of pulmonary vasodilator therapy have occurred, including systemic hypotension, hypoxemia, and even death. Routine clinical use of these agents is not currently recommended. Continuous long-term infusion of prostacyclin (PGI_2), a potent pulmonary vasodilator, shows some promise in preliminary studies of patients with primary pulmonary hypertension, but recommendations for its use must await the completion of large clinical trials.

It is important to distinguish primary pulmonary hypertension with pulmonary vasoconstriction, a potentially reversible condition, from fixed obstruction of the pulmonary vascular bed. Patients most likely to benefit from long-term pulmonary vasodilator therapy are those who respond favorably to a vasodilator challenge at right heart catheterization. Recent data suggest that the acute hemodynamic response to intravenous prostacyclin (PGI_2) in primary pulmonary hypertension may predict the long-term hemodynamic response to long-acting oral pulmonary vasodilators, but the clinical benefit of such testing has not been established. It is clear that long-term vasodilator therapy should be employed only if hemodynamic benefit is documented.

Patients with marked polycythemia (hematocrit > 60%) should undergo repeated phlebotomy in an attempt to reduce blood viscosity. Cor pulmonale complicating pulmonary hypertension is treated by managing the underlying pulmonary disease and by using diuretics, salt restriction, and, in appropriate patients, supplemental oxygen. The use of digitalis in cor pulmonale remains controversial. Pulmonary thromboendarterectomy may benefit selected patients with pulmonary hypertension secondary to chronic thrombotic obstructions of major pulmonary arteries.

Combined heart-lung transplantation (see Chapter 8) has been performed on patients with end-stage primary pulmonary hypertension as well as those with Eisenmenger's complex. The operative mortality rate is about 25%, and bronchiolitis obliterans is common in those who survive the operation.

Prognosis
The prognosis in secondary pulmonary hypertension depends on the course of the underlying disease. Patients with pulmonary hypertension due to fixed obliteration of the pulmonary vascular bed generally respond poorly to therapy; development of cor pulmonale in these cases implies a poor prognosis. The prognosis is favorable when pulmonary hypertension is detected early and the conditions leading to it are readily reversed.

Reeves JT, Groves BM, Turkevich D: The case for treatment of selected patients with primary pulmonary hypertension. Am Rev Respir Dis 1986;134:342.

Rich S, Levitsky S, Brundage BH: Pulmonary hypertension from chronic pulmonary thromboembolism. Ann Intern Med 1988;108:425. (Value of perfusion lung scanning and warfarin therapy; thromboendarterectomy in selected patients.)

Rubin LJ: Approach to the diagnosis and treatment of pulmonary hypertension. Chest 1989;96:659.

Rubin LJ et al: Treatment of primary pulmonary hyperten-

sion with continuous intravenous prostacyclin (epoprostenol): Results of a randomized trial. Ann Intern Med 1990;112:485.

Voelkel NF (editor): Pulmonary circulation and pulmonary hypertension. Chest 1988;93(Suppl):79S. [Entire issue.]

DISORDERS DUE TO CHEMICAL & PHYSICAL AGENTS

INHALATION OF AIR POLLUTANTS & TOXIC SUBSTANCES

The respiratory tract is exposed to numerous potentially harmful substances in the environment, including air pollutants and toxic gases and fumes. Whereas air pollutants are ubiquitous, particularly in urban areas, toxic gases and fumes are usually encountered in the workplace or as the result of an environmental accident. Respiratory tract defense mechanisms protect the lung from noxious substances, but when these defenses are breached, serious respiratory tract injury may result.

Clinical Findings
Exposure to low levels of air pollutants is usually inconsequential; exposure to higher levels produces symptoms of upper and lower respiratory tract irritation, particularly in patients with asthma and COPD. Exposure to the toxic substances listed in Table 7–17 results in profound illness characterized by upper respiratory complaints (sneezing, irritation of the eyes and nose, stridor) and features of tracheobronchitis (cough, wheezing, dyspnea). Systemic symptoms such as nausea and vomiting, headache, and fever are common; in severe disease, pulmonary edema may develop. Chest radiographs may be normal; however, bilateral diffuse infiltrates progressing to consolidation, atelectasis, and pulmonary edema can occur.

Treatment
Healthy persons exposed to the usual ambient levels of air pollutants need not observe special precautions. Patients with severe COPD or asthma should be advised to stay indoors and not engage in strenuous activity when high concentrations of air pollutants are present. If exposure to toxic chemicals is documented or suspected, patients should be observed carefully for as long as 24 hours after exposure. Respiratory distress may be absent initially, only to appear after a 12- to 24-hour delay.

If admitted to the hospital, the patient should be followed closely with oximetry after initial arterial blood gas measurements. Hypoxemia may occur before clinical and radiographic evidence of pulmonary

Table 7–17. Major air pollutants and toxic gases and fumes, their sources, and adverse effects.

Noxious Agent	Sources	Adverse Effects
Air pollutants		
Oxides of nitrogen	Automobile exhaust; gas stoves and heaters, wood-burning stoves, kerosene space heaters.	Respiratory tract irritation, bronchial hyperreactivity, impaired lung defenses, bronchiolitis fibrosa obliterans.
Hydrocarbons	Automobile exhaust, cigarette smoke.	Lung cancer.
Ozone	Automobile exhaust, high-altitude aircraft cabins.	Cough, substernal discomfort, bronchoconstriction, decreased exercise performance, respiratory tract irritation.
Sulfur dioxide	Power plants, smelters, oil refineries, kerosene space heaters.	Exacerbation of asthma and COPD, respiratory tract irritation. Hospitalization may be necessary, and death may occur in severe exposure.
Toxic gases and fumes		
Carbon monoxide	Cigarette smoke, incomplete combustion of organic fuels.	Headache, nausea and vomiting, dyspnea, dizziness, ataxia, convulsions, coma, death.
Sulfur dioxide	Leakage from storage tanks.	Airway irritation, exacerbation of COPD and asthma.
Ozone	Arc welding.	Cough, chest pain, eye and nose irritation.
Oxides of nitrogen (NO_2, N_2O_4)	Silage; arc welding, chemical industry.	Silo-filler's disease, pulmonary edema, hypotension, bronchiolitis fibrosa obliterans.
Cyanide	Production of synthetic rubber; extraction of gold and silver; electroplating.	Severe, rapidly progressive systemic toxicity with coma, convulsions, death within 4 hours.
Phosgene	Plastics and chemical industry.	Pulmonary edema after asymptomatic period.
Ammonia	Leakage from storage containers and railroad cars.	Severe inflammation of respiratory tract, laryngeal edema.
Cadmium	Welding, smelting of ores.	Pulmonary edema, tracheobronchitis, metal fume fever.
Chlorine	Spillage from storage containers; chemical and plastics industry.	Bronchitis, pulmonary edema.

edema develops and should be managed appropriately with supplemental oxygen. Because laryngeal edema and severe, exudative tracheobronchitis are common following inhalation of toxic substances, maintaining the patency of the airway is of paramount importance. Respiratory therapy may be required to clear the airway of tenacious secretions and sloughed fragments of mucosa. Acute respiratory failure is common and should be managed appropriately. Intubated patients require frequent suctioning to remove airway secretions. Intravenous fluids and vasopressor agents are necessary in some patients, but excessive amounts of fluids should be avoided because of the tendency to worsen pulmonary edema. Antibiotics are administered only if lower respiratory tract infection develops; bronchodilators are administered if bronchospasm is apparent. The use of corticosteroids in the management of acute lung injury due to inhalation of toxic substances is controversial; most authorities feel they are contraindicated in burn patients with smoke inhalation because of the risk of secondary infection.

Prognosis

The prognosis following acute lung injury from inhalation of toxic substances depends on the severity of exposure and the nature of the toxic substance.

Death may occur as a result of acute respiratory failure. Survivors have an excellent prognosis, with full recovery of lung function expected in most cases. Bronchiolitis obliterans may occur 1–6 weeks after apparent recovery from inhalation of nitrogen dioxide and should be managed with oral corticosteroids.

Samet JM, Marbury MC, Spengler JD: Health effects and sources of indoor air pollution. (2 parts.) Am Rev Respir Dis 1987;136:1486 and 137:221.

Schwartz DA, Smith DD, Lakshminarayan S: The pulmonary sequelae associated with accidental inhalation of chlorine gas. Chest 1990;97:820.

Wald PH, Balmes JR: Respiratory effects of short-term, high-intensity toxic inhalations: Smoke, gases, and fumes. J Intensive Care Med 1987;2:260.

SMOKE INHALATION

The inhalation of products of combustion may cause serious respiratory complications. As many as one-third of patients admitted to burn treatment units have pulmonary injury from smoke inhalation. Morbidity and deaths due to smoke inhalation exceed those attributed to the burns themselves. The death rate of patients with both severe body burns and smoke inhalation exceeds 50%. All patients with suspected smoke inhalation should be admitted to the hospital for observation and treatment.

It is important to look for and recognize 3 consequences of smoke inhalation: impaired tissue oxygenation, thermal upper airway injury, and chemical injury to the lung. Impaired tissue oxygenation results from inhalation of carbon monoxide or cyanide and is an immediate threat to life. The management of patients with carbon monoxide poisoning and cyanide poisoning is discussed in Chapter 33. The clinician must recognize that patients with carbon monoxide poisoning display a normal partial pressure of oxygen in arterial blood (Pa_{O_2}) but have a low *measured* oxyhemoglobin saturation (Sa_{O_2}). Immediate treatment with 100% oxygen is essential and should be continued until the measured carboxyhemoglobin level falls to less than 10% and concomitant metabolic acidosis has resolved.

Thermal injury to the mucosal surfaces of the upper airway occurs from inhalation of hot gases. Complications become evident by 18–24 hours. These include impaired ability to clear oral secretions and airway obstruction, producing inspiratory stridor. Respiratory failure with hypercapnia and hypoxemia occurs in severe cases. Early management (see also Chapter 32) includes the use of a high-humidity face mask with supplemental oxygen, gentle suctioning to evacuate oral secretions, elevation of the head 30 degrees to promote clearing of secretions, and topical epinephrine to reduce edema of the oropharyngeal mucous membrane. Helium-oxygen gas mixtures may reduce labored breathing. Close monitoring with arterial blood gases and later with oximetry is important. Examination of the upper airway with a fiberoptic laryngoscope or bronchoscope is superior to routine physical examination. Endotracheal intubation is often necessary to establish airway patency and is likely to be necessary in patients with deep facial burns, oropharyngeal or laryngeal edema, or respiratory failure. Tracheostomy should be avoided if possible because of an increased risk of pneumonia and death from sepsis.

Chemical injury to the lung results from inhalation of toxic gases and products of combustion, including aldehydes and organic acids. The site of lung injury depends upon the solubility of the gases inhaled, the duration of exposure, and the size of inhaled particles that transport noxious gases to distal lung units. Bronchorrhea and bronchospasm are seen early after exposure along with dyspnea, tachypnea, and tachycardia. Labored breathing and cyanosis may follow. Physical examination at this stage reveals diffuse wheezing and rhonchi. Bronchiolar edema and high-permeability pulmonary edema (ARDS) may develop within 1–2 days after exposure. Sloughing of the bronchiolar

mucosa may occur within 2–3 days, leading to airway obstruction, atelectasis and worsening hypoxemia. Bacterial colonization and pneumonia are common by 5–7 days after the exposure.

Treatment of the pulmonary component of smoke inhalation consists of supplemental oxygen, bronchodilators, suctioning of mucosal debris and mucopurulent secretions via an indwelling endotracheal tube, chest physical therapy to aid clearance of secretions, and adequate humidification of inspired gases. Positive end-expiratory pressure (PEEP) has been advocated to treat bronchiolar edema. Judicious fluid management and close monitoring for secondary bacterial infection with daily sputum Gram stains round out the management protocol.

The routine use of corticosteroids for chemical lung injury from smoke inhalation has been shown to be ineffective and may even be harmful. Routine or prophylactic use of antibiotics is not recommended.

Those patients who survive should be watched for the development of late bronchiolitis obliterans.

Haponik EF, Summer WR: Respiratory complications in burned patients: Pathogenesis and spectrum of inhalation injury. J Crit Care 1987;2:49. (Mechanisms and complications.)

Haponik EF et al: Smoke inhalation. Am Rev Respir Dis 1988;138:1060. (Pathogenesis and management.)

PULMONARY ASPIRATION SYNDROMES

Aspiration of foreign material into the tracheobronchial tree results from various disorders that impair normal deglutition, especially disturbances of consciousness and esophageal dysfunction.

Aspiration of Inert Material

Aspiration of inert material may cause asphyxia if the amount aspirated is massive and if cough is impaired, in which case immediate tracheobronchial suctioning is necessary. Most patients suffer no serious sequelae from aspiration of inert material.

Aspiration of Toxic Material

Aspiration of toxic material into the lung usually results in clinically evident pneumonia. **Hydrocarbon pneumonitis** is caused by ingestion of petroleum distillates, eg, gasoline, kerosene, furniture polish, and other household petroleum products. Lung injury results mainly from vomiting and secondary aspiration. Therapy is supportive. The lung should be protected from repeated aspiration with a cuffed endotracheal tube if necessary. **Lipid pneumonia** is a chronic syndrome related to the repeated aspiration of oily materials, eg, mineral oil, cod liver oil, and oily nose drops; it often occurs in elderly patients with impaired swallowing. Patchy infiltrates in dependent lung zones and lipid-laden macrophages in expectorated sputum are characteristic findings.

"Café Coronary"

Acute obstruction of the upper airway by food usually occurs in intoxicated individuals. Other predisposing factors include difficulty in swallowing, old age, poor dentition, dental problems that impair chewing, and use of sedative drugs. The Heimlich procedure may be lifesaving.

Retention of an Aspirated Foreign Body

Retention of an aspirated foreign body in the tracheobronchial tree may produce various acute and chronic conditions, including recurrent pneumonia, bronchiectasis, lung abscess, atelectasis, and postobstructive hyperinflation. Children are at greater risk than adults for foreign body aspiration. Occasionally, a misdiagnosis of asthma, COPD, or lung cancer is made in adult patients who have aspirated a foreign body. The plain chest x-ray usually suggests the site of the foreign body. In some cases, an expiratory film, demonstrating regional hyperinflation due to a check-valve effect, is helpful. Bronchoscopy is usually necessary to establish the diagnosis and attempt removal of the foreign body.

Chronic Aspiration of Gastric Contents

Chronic aspiration of gastric contents may result from primary disorders of the esophagus, eg, achalasia, esophageal stricture, scleroderma, esophageal carcinoma, esophagitis, and gastroesophageal reflux. In the last condition, relaxation of the tone of the lower esophageal sphincter allows reflux of gastric contents into the esophagus and predisposes to chronic pulmonary aspiration, especially at night. Cigarette smoking, consumption of alcohol, and use of theophylline are known to relax the lower esophageal sphincter. Pulmonary disorders linked to gastroesophageal reflux and chronic aspiration include bronchial asthma, idiopathic pulmonary fibrosis, bronchiectasis, and, in young children, apnea. Even in the absence of aspiration, acid in the esophagus may trigger bronchospasm through reflex mechanisms.

The diagnosis of chronic aspiration is difficult. Barium swallow is usually necessary to rule out esophageal disease. Management consists of elevation of the head of the bed, cessation of smoking, weight reduction, and antacids or H_2 receptor antagonists (eg, cimetidine, 300–400 mg) at night. Metoclopramide (10–20 mg at bedtime) or bethanechol (10–25 mg at bedtime) is helpful in some patients with gastroesophageal reflux, as they elevate pressure in the lower esophageal sphincter.

Acute Aspiration of Gastric Contents (Mendelson's Syndrome)

Acute aspiration of gastric contents is often catastrophic. The pulmonary response depends on the characteristics and amount of the gastric contents aspirated. The more acidic the material, the greater the degree of chemical pneumonitis. Aspiration of pure gastric acid (pH < 2.5) causes extensive desquamation of the bronchial epithelium, bronchiolitis, hemorrhage, and pulmonary edema. Acute gastric aspiration is one of the commonest causes of adult respiratory distress syndrome. The clinical picture is one of abrupt onset of respiratory distress, with cough, wheezing, fever, and tachypnea. Crackles are audible at the bases of the lungs. Hypoxemia may be noted immediately after aspiration occurs. Radiographic abnormalities, consisting of patchy alveolar infiltrates in dependent lung zones, appear within a few hours. If particulate food matter has been aspirated along with gastric acid, radiographic features of bronchial obstruction may be observed. Even without superinfection, fever and leukocytosis occur.

Treatment of acute aspiration of gastric contents consists of supplemental oxygen, measures to maintain the airway, and the usual measures for treatment of acute respiratory failure. There is no evidence to support the routine use of corticosteroids or prophylactic antibiotics after gastric aspiration has occurred. Secondary pulmonary infection, which occurs in about one-fourth of patients, typically appears 2–3 days after aspiration. Management of this complication depends upon the observed flora of the tracheobronchial tree (Table 7–11). Hypotension secondary to alveolocapillary membrane injury and intravascular volume depletion is common and is managed with the judicious administration of intravenous fluids.

Allen CJ, Newhouse MT: Gastroesophageal reflux and chronic respiratory disease. Am Rev Respir Dis 1984; 129:645. (Techniques of detection of reflux.)

Ducolone A et al: Gastroesophageal reflux in patients with asthma and chronic bronchitis. Am Rev Respir Dis 1987;135:327. (Most patients have reflux.)

Hoyt J: Aspiration pneumonitis: Patient risk factors, prevention, and management. J Intensive Care Med 1990; 5(Suppl):S2.

Limper AH, Prakash UBS: Tracheobronchial foreign bodies in adults. Ann Intern Med 1990;112:604.

Weissberg D, Schwartz I: Foreign bodies in the tracheobronchial tree. Chest 1987;91:730.

OCCUPATIONAL PULMONARY DISEASES

Many acute and chronic pulmonary diseases are directly related to inhalation of noxious substances encountered in the workplace; those disorders that are due to chemical agents may be classified as follows: (1) pneumoconioses, (2) hypersensitivity pneumonitis, (3) obstructive airway disorders, (4) toxic lung injury, (5) lung cancer, (6) pleural diseases, and (7) miscellaneous disorders.

Pneumoconioses

Pneumoconioses are chronic fibrotic lung diseases caused by the inhalation of coal dust and various inert, inorganic, or silicate dusts (Table 7–18). Pneumoconioses due to inhalation of inert dusts are usually asymptomatic disorders with diffuse nodular infiltrates on chest x-ray. Clinically important pneumoconioses include coal workers' pneumoconiosis, silicosis, and asbestosis. Treatment for each is supportive.

A. Coal Worker's Pneumoconiosis: In coal worker's pneumoconiosis, ingestion of inhaled coal dust by alveolar macrophages leads to the formation of coal macules, usually 2–5 mm in diameter, which appear on chest x-ray as small opacities throughout the lungs but are especially prominent in the upper lung. Simple coal worker's pneumoconiosis is usually asymptomatic; pulmonary function abnormalities are unimpressive. Cigarette smoking does not increase the prevalence of coal worker's pneumoconiosis but may have an additive detrimental effect on ventilatory function. In complicated coal worker's pneumoconiosis ("progressive massive fibrosis"), conglomeration and contraction in the upper lung zones occur, with radiographic and clinical features resembling complicated silicosis. **Caplan's syndrome** is a rare condition characterized by the presence of necrobiotic rheumatoid nodules (1–5 cm in diameter) in the periphery of the lung in coal workers with rheumatoid arthritis.

B. Silicosis: In silicosis, extensive or prolonged inhalation of free silica (silicon dioxide) particles in the respirable range (0.3–5 μm) causes the formation of small rounded opacities (silicotic nodules) throughout the lung. Calcification of the periphery of hilar lymph nodes ("eggshell" calcification) is an unusual finding that strongly suggests silicosis. Simple silicosis is usually asymptomatic and has no effect on routine pulmonary function tests; in complicated silicosis, large conglomerate densities appear in the upper lung and are accompanied by dyspnea and obstructive and restrictive pulmonary dysfunction. The incidence of tuberculosis is increased in patients with chronic silicosis. All patients with silicosis should have a tuberculin skin test. Chemoprophylaxis with isoniazid is recommended for silicotic patients who are tuberculin-reactive.

C. Asbestosis: Asbestosis, a nodular interstitial fibrosis occurring in asbestos workers and miners, is characterized by dyspnea, inspiratory crackles, and in some cases, clubbing and cyanosis. The radiographic features include interstitial fibrosis, thickened pleura, and calcified plaques (pleural) on the diaphragms or lateral chest wall. The lower lungs are more often involved than the upper. High-resolution CT scanning is emerging as the best imaging method in asbestosis because of its ability to detect parenchymal fibrosis and define the presence of coexisting pleural plaques. Cigarette smoking in asbestos workers increases the prevalence of radiographic pleural and parenchymal changes. It may also interfere with the clearance of short asbestos fibers from the lung. Pulmonary function studies show restrictive dysfunction and reduced diffusing capacity.

Hypersensitivity Pneumonitis

The term "hypersensitivity pneumonitis" (or "extrinsic allergic alveolitis") denotes nonatopic, nonasthmatic, allergic pulmonary disease. Hypersensitivity pneumonitis is manifested mainly as occupational disease (Table 7–19), in which exposure to inhaled organic agents leads to acute and eventually chronic pulmonary disease. Antibodies directed against the inhaled agent can be identified in serum. Acute illness is characterized by sudden onset of malaise, chills, fever, cough, dyspnea, and nausea 4–8 hours after exposure to the offending agent. This may occur after the patient has left work or even at night and thus may mimic paroxysmal nocturnal dyspnea. Bibasilar crackles, tachypnea, tachycardia, and

Table 7–18. Selected pneumoconioses.

Disease	Agent	Occupational Source
Metal dusts		
Siderosis	Metallic iron or iron oxide	Mining, welding, foundry work.
Stannosis	Tin, tin oxide	Mining, tinwork, smelting.
Baritosis	Barium salts	Glass and insecticide manufacturing.
Coal dust		
Coal worker's pneumoconiosis	Coal dust	Coal mining.
Inorganic dusts		
Silicosis	Free silica (silicon dioxide)	Rock mining, quarrying, stone cutting, tunneling, sandblasting, pottery, diatomaceous earth.
Silicate dusts		
Asbestosis	Asbestos	Mining, insulation, construction, shipbuilding.
Talcosis	Magnesium silicate	Mining, milling, rubber industry.
Kaolin pneumoconiosis	Sand, mica, aluminum silicate	Mining of china clay; pottery and cement work.
Shaver's disease	Aluminum powder	Manufacture of corundum.

Table 7-19. Selected causes of hypersensitivity pneumonitis.

Disease	Antigen	Source
Farmer's lung	*Micropolyspora faeni, Thermoactinomyces vulgaris.*	Moldy hay.
"Humidifier lung"	Thermophilic actinomycetes.	Contaminated humidifiers, heating systems, or air conditioners.
Bird-fancier's lung ("pigeon-breeder's disease")	Avian proteins.	Bird serum and excreta.
Bagassosis	*Thermoactinomyces sacchari* and *T vulgaris.*	Moldy sugarcane fiber (bagasse).
Sequoiosis	*Graphium, Aureobasidium,* and other fungi.	Moldy redwood sawdust.
Maple bark stripper's disease	*Cryptostroma (Coniosporium) corticale.*	Rotting maple tree logs or bark.
Mushroom picker's disease	Same as farmer's lung.	Moldy compost.
Suberosis	*Penicillium frequentans.*	Moldy cork dust.
Detergent worker's lung	*Bacillus subtilis* enzyme.	Enzyme additives.

(occasionally) cyanosis are noted. Small nodular densities sparing the apexes and bases of the lungs are noted on chest x-ray. Pulmonary function studies reveal *restrictive* dysfunction and reduced diffusing capacity. Laboratory studies reveal an increase in the white blood cell count with a shift to the left, hypoxemia, and the presence of precipitating antibodies to the offending agent in serum. Hypersensitivity pneumonitis antibody panels against common fungal antigens (cost approximately $50.00) are available.

A subacute hypersensitivity pneumonitis syndrome has been described that is characterized by the insidious onset of chronic cough and slowly progressive dyspnea, anorexia, and weight loss. Chronic respiratory insufficiency and the appearance of pulmonary fibrosis on radiographs may or may not occur after repeated exposure to the offending agent. Acute hypersensitivity pneumonitis is characterized by interstitial infiltrates of lymphocytes and plasma cells, with noncaseating granulomas in the interstitium and air spaces. Diffuse fibrosis is the hallmark of the subacute and chronic phases.

Treatment of hypersensitivity pneumonitis consists of identification of the offending agent, avoidance of further exposure, and, in severe acute or protracted cases, oral corticosteroids (prednisone, 0.5 mg/kg daily as a single morning dose, tapered to nil over

4–6 weeks). Change in occupation is advisable in some cases.

Obstructive Airway Disorders

Occupational pulmonary diseases manifested as obstructive airway disorders include occupational asthma, industrial bronchitis, and byssinosis.

A. Occupational Asthma: It has been estimated that from 2% to 5% of all cases of asthma are related to occupation. Offending agents include grain dust, tobacco, pollens, enzymes, gum arabic, synthetic dyes, isocyanates (particularly toluene diisocyanate), wood dust, rosin (soldering flux), inorganic chemicals (salts of nickel, platinum, and chromium), trimellitic anhydride, phthallic anhydride, formaldehyde, and various pharmaceutical agents, including penicillin, cimetidine, and sulfonamides. Diagnosis of occupational asthma depends on a high index of suspicion, an appropriate history, spirometric studies before and after exposure to the offending substance, and peak flow rate measurements in the workplace. Bronchial provocation testing (a pulmonary function laboratory test demonstrating bronchial hyperreactivity to pharmacologic or antigenic agents) is helpful in some cases. Treatment consists of avoidance of further exposure to the offending agent and bronchodilators Table 7–8), but symptoms may persist for years after workplace exposure has been terminated.

B. Industrial Bronchitis: Industrial bronchitis is chronic bronchitis found in coal miners and others exposed to cotton, flax, or hemp dust. Chronic disability does not often occur from industrial bronchitis.

C. Byssinosis: Byssinosis is an asthmalike disorder in textile workers caused by inhalation of cotton dust. The pathogenesis is obscure. Chest tightness, cough, and dyspnea are characteristically worse on Mondays or the first day back at work, with symptoms subsiding later in the week. Repeated exposure leads to chronic bronchitis.

Toxic Lung Injury

Toxic lung injury from inhalation of irritant gases is discussed in the section on smoke inhalation. **Silo-filler's disease** is acute toxic noncardiogenic pulmonary edema caused by inhalation of nitrogen dioxide encountered in recently filled silos. Bronchiolitis obliterans is a common late complication, which perhaps can be prevented by early treatment of the acute reaction with corticosteroids. Extensive exposure to silage gas may cause sudden death.

Lung Cancer

Many industrial pulmonary carcinogens have been identified, including asbestos, radon gas, arsenic, iron, chromium, nickel, coal tar fumes, petroleum oil mists, isopropyl oil, mustard gas, and printing ink. Cigarette smoking acts as a cocarcinogen with asbestos and radon gas to cause bronchogenic carcinoma. Asbestos alone causes malignant mesothelioma. Almost all histologic types of lung cancer have been associated with these carcinogens. Chloromethylmethyl ether specifically causes small-cell carcinoma of the lung.

Pleural Diseases

Occupational diseases of the pleura may result from exposure to asbestos (see above) or talc. Inhalation of talc causes pleural plaques that are similar to those caused by asbestos. Benign asbestos pleural effusion occurs in some asbestos workers and may cause chronic blunting of the costophrenic angle on chest x-ray.

Other Occupational Pulmonary Diseases

Occupational agents are also responsible for other pulmonary disorders. These include **berylliosis,** an acute or chronic pulmonary disorder related to exposure to beryllium, which is absorbed through the lungs or skin and widely disseminated throughout the body. Acute berylliosis is a toxic, ulcerative tracheobronchitis and chemical pneumonitis following intense and severe exposure to beryllium. Chronic berylliosis, a systemic disease closely resembling sarcoidosis, is more common. Chronic pulmonary beryllium disease is thought to be an alveolitis mediated by the proliferation of beryllium-specific helper-inducer T cells in the lung. Exposure to beryllium now occurs in machining and handling of beryllium products and alloys. Beryllium miners are not at risk for berylliosis. Beryllium is no longer used in fluorescent lamp production, which was a source of exposure before 1950.

Chan-Yeung M, Lam S: Occupational asthma. Am Rev Respir Dis 1986;133:686.

Cullen MR, Cherniack MG, Rosenstock L: Occupational medicine. (Two parts.) N Engl J Med 1990;322:594, 675.

Kriebel D et al: The pulmonary toxicity of beryllium. Am Rev Respir Dis 1988;137:464. (A state-of-the-art review of berylliosis.)

Mossman BT, Gee JBL: Asbestos-related diseases. N Engl J Med 1989;320:1721.

Saltini C et al: Maintenance of alveolitis in patients with chronic beryllium disease by beryllium-specific helper T cells. N Engl J Med 1989;320:1103.

DRUG-INDUCED LUNG DISEASE

Typical patterns of pulmonary response to various drugs implicated in drug-induced respiratory disease are summarized in Table 7–20. Pulmonary injury due to drugs occurs as a result of allergic reactions, idiosyncratic reactions, overdose, or undesirable side effects. In most patients, the mechanism of pulmonary injury is unknown.

Precise diagnosis of drug-induced pulmonary dis-

Table 7–20. Pulmonary manifestations of selected drug toxicities.

Asthma	**Pulmonary edema**
Propranolol and other beta	Noncardiogenic[1]
blockers	Aspirin
Aspirin	Chlordiazepoxide
Nonsteroidal anti-inflam-	Cocaine
matory drugs	Ethchlorvynol
Histamine	Cardiogenic
Methacholine	Propranolol
Acetylcysteine	**Pleural effusion**
Any nebulized medication	Bromocriptine
Cough	Nitrofurantoin
Captopril	Any drug inducing sys-
Enalapril	temic lupus erythemato-
Inhaled beclomethasone	sus
Inhaled cromolyn	Methysergide
Pulmonary infiltration	Chemotherapeutic agents
Without eosinophilia	**Mediastinal widening**
Amitriptyline	Phenytoin
Azathioprine	Corticosteroids
Amiodarone	Methotrexate
With eosinophilia	**Respiratory failure**
Sulfonamides	Neuromuscular blockade
L-Tryptophan	Aminoglycosides
Nitrofurantoin	Succinylcholine
Penicillin	Gallamine
Methotrexate	Dimethyltubocurarine
Drug-induced systemic	(metocurine)
lupus erythematosus	Central nervous system
Hydralazine	depression
Procainamide	Sedatives
Isoniazid	Hypnotics
Chlorpromazine	Narcotics
Phenytoin	Alcohol
Interstitial fibrosis	Tricyclic antidepressants
Nitrofurantoin	Oxygen
Bleomycin	
Busulfan	
Cyclophosphamide	
Methysergide	

[1] Heroin overdose also causes noncardiogenic pulmonary edema.

ease is often difficult, because results of routine laboratory studies are not helpful and radiographic findings are not specific. A high index of suspicion and a thorough medical history of drug usage are critical to establishing the diagnosis of drug-induced lung disease. The clinical response to cessation of the suspected offending agent is also helpful. Acute episodes of drug-induced pulmonary disease usually disappear 24–48 hours after the drug has been discontinued, but chronic syndromes may take longer to resolve. Challenge tests to confirm the diagnosis are risky and rarely performed.

Treatment of drug-induced lung disease consists of discontinuing the offending agent immediately and managing the pulmonary symptoms appropriately.

Cooper JAD Jr, White DA, Matthay RA: Drug-induced pulmonary disease. (2 parts.) Am Rev Respir Dis 1986;133:321, 488.

RADIATION LUNG INJURY

The lung is a radiosensitive organ that can be affected by external beam radiation therapy. The pulmonary response is determined by the volume of lung radiated, the dose and rate of therapy, and potentiating factors, eg, concurrent chemotherapy, previous radiation therapy in the same area, and simultaneous withdrawal of corticosteroid therapy. Symptomatic radiation lung injury occurs in about 10% of patients treated with megavoltage therapy for carcinoma of the breast, 5–15% of patients treated for carcinoma of the lung, and 5–35% of patients treated for lymphoma. Two phases of the pulmonary response to radiation are apparent: an acute phase (radiation pneumonitis) and a chronic phase (radiation fibrosis).

Radiation Pneumonitis

Radiation pneumonitis usually occurs 2–3 months (range 1–6 months) after completion of radiotherapy and is characterized by insidious onset of dyspnea, intractable dry cough, chest fullness or pain, weakness, and fever. Physical findings are usually absent, but inspiratory crackles may be heard in the involved area. In severe disease, respiratory distress and cyanosis occur that are characteristic of adult respiratory distress syndrome (ARDS). An increased white blood cell count and elevated sedimentation rate are common. Pulmonary function studies reveal reduced lung volumes, reduced lung compliance, hypoxemia, reduced diffusing capacity, and reduced maximum voluntary ventilation. Chest x-ray, which correlates poorly with the presence of symptoms, usually demonstrates an alveolar or nodular infiltrate with a ground-glass opacification limited to the irradiated area. Air bronchograms are often observed. The sharp borders of the infiltrate help distinguish radiation pneumonitis from other conditions, eg, infectious pneumonia, lymphangitic spread of carcinoma, and recurrent tumor. Treatment consists of aspirin, cough suppressants, and bed rest. Acute respiratory failure, if present, is treated appropriately. Although there is no proof that corticosteroids are effective in radiation pneumonitis, prednisone (1 mg/kg/d orally) is usually given immediately and tapered slowly over several weeks. Radiation pneumonitis usually resolves in 2–3 weeks. Death from ARDS is unusual.

Pulmonary Radiation Fibrosis

Pulmonary radiation fibrosis occurs in nearly all patients who receive a full course of radiation therapy for cancer of the lung and breast. Patients who experience radiation pneumonitis develop pulmonary fibrosis after an intervening period (6–12 months) of well-being. Most patients are asymptomatic, though slowly progressive dyspnea occurs in some. Radiation fibrosis may occur with or without antecedent radiation pneumonitis. Cor pulmonale and chronic respiratory

failure are rare. Radiographic findings include obliteration of normal lung markings, dense interstitial and pleural fibrosis, reduced lung volumes, tenting of the diaphragm, and sharp delineation of the irradiated area. No specific therapy is necessary, and corticosteroids have no value.

Other Complications of Radiation Therapy

Other complications of radiation therapy directed to the thorax include pericardial effusion, constrictive pericarditis, tracheoesophageal fistula, esophageal candidiasis, radiation dermatitis, and rib fractures. Small pleural effusions, radiation pneumonitis outside the irradiated area, spontaneous pneumothorax, and complete obstruction of central airways are unusual occurrences.

DISORDERS OF VENTILATION

The principal influences on ventilatory control are arterial PCO_2, pH, and PO_2. These variables are monitored by **peripheral and central chemoreceptors.** Under normal conditions, the ventilatory control system maintains arterial pH and PCO_2 within narrow limits; arterial PO_2 is more loosely controlled.

PRIMARY ALVEOLAR HYPOVENTILATION

Primary alveolar hypoventilation ("Ondine's curse") is an uncommon syndrome of unknown cause characterized by inadequate alveolar ventilation despite normal neurologic function and normal airways, lungs, chest, wall, and ventilatory muscles. Hypoventilation is even more marked during sleep. Individuals with this disorder are usually nonobese males in their third or fourth decades who present with lethargy, headache, and somnolence. Dyspnea is absent. Physical examination may reveal cyanosis and evidence of pulmonary hypertension and cor pulmonale. Hypoxemia and hypercapnia are present and improve with voluntary hyperventilation. Erythrocytosis is common. Results of pulmonary function tests are normal, but responses to induced hypercapnia and hypoxemia are reduced or absent. Central sleep apnea (see below) may occur and lead to severe nocturnal hypoxemia. Treatment with ventilatory stimulants such as medroxyprogesterone acetate, theophylline, acetazolamide, or methylphenidate may be of benefit. Augmentation of ventilation by mechanical methods (phrenic nerve stimulation, rocking bed, mechanical ventilators) has been helpful to some patients. Adequate oxygenation should be maintained with supplemental oxygen, but nocturnal oxygen therapy should be prescribed only if diagnostic nocturnal polysomnography has demonstrated its efficacy. Some patients show longer apneic intervals and increased CO_2 retention during sleep when given supplemental oxygen. Primary alveolar hypoventilation resembles—but should be distinguished from—**central alveolar hypoventilation,** in which impaired ventilatory drive with chronic respiratory acidemia and hypoxemia follows an insult to the brain stem (eg, bulbar poliomyelitis).

OBESITY-HYPOVENTILATION SYNDROME (Pickwickian Syndrome)

A few obese individuals demonstrate waking hypoventilation, which is distinguished from primary alveolar hypoventilation by the presence of extreme obesity. Symptoms, physical findings, and laboratory data are otherwise similar in the 2 syndromes. Hypercapnia, hypoxemia, and elevated hematocrit are characteristic features. Having the patient voluntarily hyperventilate for about 1 minute normalizes the P_{CO_2} and the P_{O_2}, in contrast to lung diseases causing chronic respiratory failure such as COPD. In obesity-hypoventilation syndrome, hypoventilation appears to result from a synergistic combination of blunted ventilatory drives and the mechanical load imposed upon the ventilatory apparatus by obesity. Most patients with obesity-hypoventilation syndrome also suffer from obstructive sleep apnea (see below). Therapy of obesity-hypoventilation syndrome consists mainly of weight loss, which improves hypercapnia and hypoxemia as well as the ventilatory responses to hypoxia and hypercapnia; and medroxyprogesterone acetate, 10–20 mg every 8 hours orally. Marked improvement in hypoxemia, hypercapnia, erythrocytosis, and cor pulmonale may result. The obesity-hypoventilation syndrome should not be confused with **narcolepsy,** a disorder of excessive daytime sleepiness and irresistible sleep attacks (see Chapter 19).

SLEEP-RELATED BREATHING DISORDERS

Abnormal ventilation during sleep is manifested by apnea (breath cessation for at least 10 seconds) or hypopnea (decrement in airflow with drop in oxyhemoglobin saturation of at least 4%). Episodes of apnea are **central** if ventilatory effort is absent for the duration of the apneic episode, **obstructive** if ventilatory effort persists throughout the apneic episode but no airflow occurs because of transient obstruction of the upper airway, and **mixed** if absent ventilatory effort precedes upper airway obstruction during the apneic episode. Pure central sleep apnea is uncommon; it may occur in normals, in patients with primary alveolar hypoventilation, or in patients with lesions of the brain stem. Cheyne-Stokes respiration, an accentuated form of periodic breathing with apnea, is indistinguishable from central sleep apnea. Obstructive and mixed sleep apneas are more common and may be associated with life-threatening cardiac arrhythmias, severe hypoxemia during sleep, and nocturnal consequences of daytime hypoxemia, including congestive heart failure, pulmonary hypertension, cor pulmonale, and secondary erythrocytosis.

Definitive diagnostic evaluation may include otolaryngologic examination and polysomnography, the monitoring of multiple physiologic factors during sleep. Electroencephalography, electro-oculography, electromyography, electrocardiography, oximetry, and measurement of respiratory effort and airflow are performed in a complete evaluation, but screening may be performed using oximetry and electrocardiography only. Indications for polysomnography include a history of nocturnal breath cessation, restless sleep, and loud snoring from a bed partner, daytime hypersomnolence, unexplained erythrocytosis, pulmonary hypertension, or cor pulmonale, and nocturnal cardiac arrhythmias (particularly bradycardia) noted on Holter monitoring.

Obstructive Sleep Apnea

Upper airway obstruction during sleep occurs when loss of normal pharyngeal muscle tone allows the pharynx to collapse passively during inspiration. Patients with anatomically narrowed upper airways (eg, micrognathia, macroglossia, obesity, tonsillar hypertrophy) are predisposed to the development of obstructive sleep apnea. Alcohol or sedatives before sleeping may precipitate or worsen the condition. Before making the diagnosis of obstructive sleep apnea, a drug history should be obtained and a seizure disorder, narcolepsy, or psychiatric depression excluded.

Most patients with obstructive or mixed sleep apnea are obese middle-aged men. Systemic hypertension is common. Patients complain of excessive daytime somnolence, morning sluggishness and headaches, daytime fatigue, cognitive impairment, recent weight gain, and impotence. Bed partners usually report loud cyclical snoring, breath cessation, restlessness, and often thrashing movements of the extremities during sleep. Personality changes, poor judgment, work-related problems, and intellectual deterioration may also be observed. Physical examination may be normal or may reveal systemic and pulmonary hypertension with cor pulmonale. The oronasopharynx is sometimes found to be narrowed by facial deformities, macroglossia, septal deviation, tumors, enlarged adenoids, or excessive pharyngeal soft tissue. Erythrocytosis is common. A hemoglobin level, blood glucose concentration, and thyroid function tests should be obtained. Observation of the sleeping patient reveals loud snoring interrupted by episodes of increasingly vigorous ventilatory effort that fail to produce airflow. A loud snort accompanies the first breath following an apneic episode. Polysomnography reveals apneic episodes associated with continued ventilatory effort of increasing vigor lasting as long as 1–2 minutes. Oxygen saturation falls, often to very low levels. Bradyarrhythmias such as sinus bradycardia, sinus arrest, or atrioventricular block may occur. Tachyarrhythmias, including paroxysmal supraventricular tachycardia, atrial fibrillation, and ventricular tachycardia, are common once airflow is reestablished.

Weight loss and strict avoidance of alcohol and hypnotic medications are the first steps in management and may be curative, but few patients can lose weight successfully. Nasal continuous positive airway pressure (nasal CPAP) is very helpful in such circumstances. Polysomnography is necessary to determine what level of CPAP (usually 5 or 10 cm H_2O) is necessary to abolish obstructive apneas. Patients must use the nasal CPAP system nightly. Unfortunately, only about 75% of patients continue to use nasal CPAP after 1 year. Pharmacologic therapy for obstructive sleep apnea is disappointing. Protriptyline (10–20 mg orally at bedtime) is helpful in a small number of patients. Supplemental oxygen may lessen the severity of nocturnal desaturation but may also lengthen apneas. Polysomnography is necessary to assess the effects of oxygen therapy; it should not be routinely prescribed. Mechanical devices inserted into the mouth at bedtime to hold the jaw forward and prevent pharyngeal occlusion appear promising in preliminary studies.

Uvulopalatopharyngoplasty, a procedure consisting of resection of pharyngeal soft tissue and amputation of approximately 15 mm of the free edge of the soft palate and uvula, may be helpful in selected patients with retropalatal airway occlusion during sleep. Identifying patients who will benefit is difficult. Only about half of these operations are successful. **Nasal septoplasty** is performed if gross anatomic nasal septal deformity is present. **Tracheostomy** relieves upper airway obstruction and its physiologic consequences and represents the definitive treatment for obstructive sleep apnea. However, it has adverse effects on speech and the sense of smell. Furthermore, the long-term care of the tracheostomy tube, especially in obese patients, can be difficult. These and other surgical approaches are reserved for patients with life-threatening arrhythmias or severe disability who have failed to respond to conservative therapy. In severe cases, it is prudent to combine tracheostomy with uvulopalatopharyngoplasty and attempt decannulation at a later time. This avoids the risk of acute airway obstruction due to postoperative edema.

American Thoracic Society: Indications and standards for cardiopulmonary sleep studies. Am Rev Respir Dis 1989;139:559.

Kales A, Vela-Bueno A, Kales JD: Sleep disorders: Sleep apnea and narcolepsy. Ann Intern Med 1987;106:434.
Katsantonis GP et al: Management of obstructive sleep apnea: Comparison of various treatment modalities. Laryngoscope 1988;98:304.
Weil JV et al: Respiratory disorders of sleep: Pathophysiology, clinical implications, and therapeutic approaches. Am Rev Respir Dis 1987;136:755.

HYPERVENTILATION SYNDROME

Hyperventilation is an increase in alveolar ventilation that is excessive for metabolic requirements (amount of CO_2 production). It may be caused by a variety of organic disorders. Functional hyperventilation may be acute or chronic. Acute hyperventilation presents with hyperpnea, paresthesias, carpopedal spasm, tetany, and anxiety. Chronic hyperventilation may present with various nonspecific symptoms, including fatigue, dyspnea, anxiety, palpitations, and dizziness. The diagnosis of chronic hyperventilation syndrome is established if symptoms are reproduced during voluntary hyperventilation. Once organic causes of hyperventilation have been excluded, treatment of acute hyperventilation consists of rebreathing expired gas from a paper bag held over the face in order to decrease respiratory alkalemia and its associated symptoms.

ACUTE RESPIRATORY FAILURE

Respiratory failure is defined as respiratory dysfunction resulting in abnormalities of oxygenation or CO_2 elimination severe enough to impair or threaten the function of vital organs. Arterial blood gas criteria

Acronyms in This Section	
A/C	Assist/control
AMV	Assisted mechanical ventilation
ARDS	Adult respiratory distress syndrome
CMV	Continuous mechanical ventilation
COPD	Chronic obstructive pulmonary disease
CPAP	Continuous positive airway pressure
DLV	Differential lung ventilation
EMMV	Extended mandatory minute ventilation
HFV	High-frequency ventilation
IMV	Intermittent mandatory ventilation
IRV	Inverse ratio ventilation
PEEP	Positive end expiratory pressure
PSV	Pressure support ventilation
SIMV	Synchronized intermittent mandatory ventilation

Table 7–21. Selected causes of acute respiratory failure in adults.

Airway disorders
  Asthma
  Chronic bronchitis or emphysema in acute
    exacerbation
Parenchymal lung disorders
  Adult respiratory distress syndrome
  Congestive heart failure
  Pneumonia
  Hypersensitivity pneumonitis
Pulmonary vascular disorders
  Pulmonary thromboembolism
Chest wall and pleural disorders
  Flail chest
  Pneumothorax
Neuromuscular disorders
  Narcotic or sedative-hypnotic overdose
  Guillain-Barré syndrome
  Botulism
  Spinal cord injury
  Myasthenia gravis
  Poliomyelitis

---

for respiratory failure are not absolute but may be arbitrarily established as a P_{O_2} under 60 mm Hg and a P_{CO_2} over 50 mm Hg. Acute respiratory failure may occur in both pulmonary and nonpulmonary disorders (Table 7–21). Respiratory failure may be considered a failure of oxygenation, failure of ventilation, or both. Appropriate treatment is guided by assessment of the relative contributions of each of these components to the overall clinical picture.

Clinical Findings

Symptoms and signs of acute respiratory failure are those of the underlying disease combined with those of hypoxemia and hypercapnia. The chief symptom of hypoxemia is dyspnea, though profound hypoxemia may exist in the absence of complaints. Signs of hypoxemia include cyanosis, restlessness, confusion, anxiety, delirium, tachypnea, tachycardia, hypertension, cardiac arrhythmias, and tremor. Dyspnea and headache are the cardinal symptoms of hypercapnia. Signs of hypercapnia include peripheral and conjunctival hyperemia, hypertension, tachycardia, tachypnea, impaired consciousness, papilledema, and asterixis. The symptoms and signs of acute respiratory failure are both insensitive and nonspecific; therefore, the physician must maintain a high index of suspicion and request an arterial blood gas analysis if respiratory failure is suspected.

Treatment

Treatment of the patient with acute respiratory failure consists of (1) specific therapy directed toward the underlying disease; (2) respiratory supportive care directed toward the maintenance of adequate gas exchange; and (3) general supportive care. Only the last 2 aspects are discussed below.

A. Respiratory Support: Respiratory support has both nonventilatory and ventilatory aspects.

1. Nonventilatory aspects–_The main therapeutic goal in acute hypoxemic respiratory failure is to ensure adequate oxygenation of vital organs._ Inspired oxygen concentration should be the lowest value that results in an oxygen saturation of $\geq$ 90% (P_{aO_2} about 60 mm Hg). Higher arterial oxygen tensions are of no benefit and may cause hypoventilation in patients with chronic hypercapnia; however, _oxygen therapy should not be withheld for fear of causing progressive respiratory acidemia._ Hypoxemia in patients with obstructive airway disease is usually easily corrected by administering low-flow oxygen by nasal cannula (1–3 L/min) or Venturi mask (24–28%). Higher concentrations of oxygen are necessary to correct hypoxemia in patients with adult respiratory distress syndrome (ARDS), pneumonia, and other parenchymal lung diseases and may be administered without fear of causing hypoventilation in these disorders.

2. Ventilatory aspects–Ventilatory support consists of maintaining patency of the airway and ensuring adequate alveolar ventilation. Tracheal intubation and mechanical ventilation are often required.

a. Tracheal intubation–Indications for tracheal intubation are (1) hypoxemia which is not quickly reversed by supplemental oxygen, (2) upper airway obstruction, (3) impaired airway protection, (4) poor handling of secretions, and (5) need for positive pressure mechanical ventilation. The trachea may be intubated by means of the oral or the nasal route. In general, orotracheal intubation is preferred in urgent or emergency situations because it is easier, faster, and less traumatic. Nasotracheal tubes are more comfortable and may be preferable if prolonged intubation is anticipated. The largest tube that can be easily passed through the glottis should be used. Successful intubation may be enhanced by preoxygenation and preventilation with a bag and mask before intubation and use of adequate topical anesthesia. The position of the tip of the endotracheal tube at the level of the aortic arch should be verified by chest x-ray immediately following intubation, and auscultation should be performed to verify that both lungs are being inflated. Only tracheal tubes with "floppy" (high-volume, low-pressure) air-filled or foam cuffs should be used.

b. Mechanical ventilation–Indications for mechanical ventilation include (1) apnea, (2) acute hypercapnia that is not quickly reversed by appropriate specific therapy, and (3) progressive patient fatigue despite appropriate conservative treatment. In general, positive-pressure, volume-cycled ventilators should be used to provide mechanical ventilatory support. Critical ventilator settings include mode of ventilation, tidal volume, frequency, inspiratory flow rate, sensitivity, and inspired oxygen concentration. Although all ventilator settings must be modified to fit the clinical situation, general guidelines for initial

Table 7–22. Typical initial ventilator settings in acute respiratory failure.

Mode of ventilation	Assist/control
Tidal volume	10–15 mL/kg ideal weight
Frequency	12–14/min
Inspiratory flow rate	50 L/min
Sensitivity	−3 cm water
Inspired O_2 concentration	100%

ventilator settings are for adult patients listed in Table 7–22. Patients with hyperinflation caused by airflow obstruction should be ventilated at the lower end of the indicated range for tidal volume, whereas patients with disease characterized by alveolar filling and collapse should be ventilated toward the higher end of this range. After about 20 minutes of mechanical ventilation, arterial blood gas analysis should be performed to guide subsequent ventilator settings. The inspired oxygen concentration should be quickly reduced to the lowest value compatible with an acceptable arterial oxygen tension or saturation. Arterial pH reflects the appropriateness of minute ventilation. Ventilation should be directed toward a pH within the normal range rather than toward normal arterial P_{CO_2}. Changes in minute ventilation are accomplished mainly by manipulating ventilatory frequency rather than tidal volume.

Several modes of ventilation are available. Assisted mechanical ventilation (AMV), or assist/control (A/C), is a ventilatory mode in which the ventilatory frequency set on the ventilator serves as a backup rate, but the patient may trigger the ventilator to deliver additional positive-pressure breaths. Continuous mechanical ventilation (CMV) provides ventilation at a specified rate for patients who are apneic. Intermittent mandatory ventilation (IMV) is a ventilatory technique in which the rate set on the ventilator serves as a backup rate, but the patient is able to augment the minute ventilation by taking spontaneous breaths through a one-way valve from a reservoir. Ventilator breaths are customarily delivered between spontaneous breaths (synchronized IMV, or SIMV). Intermittent mandatory ventilation may be of value for patients whose breathing cannot be synchronized with the ventilator; for tachypneic or agitated patients who develop respiratory alkalemia on assist/control ventilation; and for patients in whom strictly positive-pressure ventilation results in a reduction of cardiac output and in whom the occasional negative-pressure breaths of intermittent mandatory ventilation produce an improvement in cardiac output. New modes of mechanical ventilation include pressure support ventilation (PSV), high-frequency ventilation (HFV), inverse ratio ventilation (IRV), differential lung ventilation (DLV), and extended mandatory minute ventilation

(EMMV). All require the use of new, expensive, microprocessor-based mechanical ventilators.

Positive end-expiratory pressure (PEEP) is useful in improving oxygenation in patients with diffuse parenchymal lung disease such as ARDS. It should be used cautiously, especially in patients with localized parenchymal disease, hyperinflation, or very high airway pressure requirements during mechanical ventilation.

c. Weaning from mechanical ventilation– Predictors of successful termination of mechanical ventilation include clinical stability or improvement and the patient's ability to meet certain "weaning criteria" that test the reserve of the ventilatory system (Table 7–23). Judgment about overall respiratory status is always more important than numerical criteria. Improvement in function of the central nervous system (level of alertness, mental status) and other organ systems usually portends weaning success.

Patients capable of adequate spontaneous ventilation can be identified through the use of the "T-piece trial," in which the patient first undergoes thorough suctioning and then breathes humidified and oxygen-enriched gas spontaneously through the tracheal tube while in the sitting position. After 30 minutes, arterial blood gas measurements are obtained. If ventilation and oxygenation are adequate, the trial is prolonged and a second analysis is performed. If oxygenation and ventilation remain adequate, mechanical ventilation may be discontinued. If the patient has no other indications for intubation, the tracheal tube may be removed. Microatelectasis leading to hypoxemia without hypercapnia may occur when mechanical ventilation using large tidal volumes is replaced by spontaneous breathing. Continuous positive airway pressure (CPAP) applied through the tracheal tube during spontaneous ventilation may prevent this.

Rapid shallow breathing is an early predictor of weaning failure and results in impaired gas exchange. Those patients who fail one or more T-piece trials

Table 7–23. Predictors of successful termination of mechanical ventilation.

Forced vital capacity	≥ 10 mL/kg
Tidal volume	≥ 5 mL/kg
Spontaneous resting minute ventilation	≤ 10 L
Maximum voluntary ventilation	≥ Twice spontaneous resting minute ventilation
Peak inspiratory pressure	More negative than −20 cm water
"T"-piece trial	No evidence of rapid, shallow breathing; adequate ventilation and oxygenation

may require a more prolonged weaning process. Repeated episodes of spontaneous T-piece breathing of increasing duration are instituted and continued until the patient can maintain spontaneous ventilation. An alternative method is to ventilate the patient using SIMV and gradually reduce the frequency of mechanical breaths. Although convenient, IMV weaning may actually slow the weaning process and increase the patient's work of breathing against the demand valve of the ventilator. Weaning with PSV, which reduces the patient's work of breathing, is an alternative approach to weaning. Repeated failure to wean from mechanical ventilatory support is usually caused by failure of the respiratory muscles (the ventilatory "pump") to meet ventilatory requirements. Malnutrition, metabolic imbalance, inadequate systemic oxygen transport, cardiac failure, and inadequate ventilatory drive are other causes of weaning failure. Some patients also display psychologic dependence on ventilator support.

Potential complications of mechanical ventilation are numerous. Migration of the tip of the endotracheal tube into the right main bronchus can cause atelectasis of the left lung and overdistention of the right lung. **Barotrauma,** manifested by subcutaneous emphysema, pneumomediastinum, subpleural air cysts, pneumothorax, or systemic gas embolism, may occur in patients whose lungs are overdistended by excessive tidal volumes, especially those with hyperinflation caused by airflow obstruction or PEEP. Subtle parenchymal lung injury due to overdistention of alveoli is another potential hazard. In order to minimize the risk of barotrauma, alveolar inflation pressures and minute ventilation must be kept as low as possible consistent with adequate gas exchange. Acute respiratory alkalosis caused by overventilation is common. Hypotension induced by elevated intrathoracic pressure that results in decreased return of systemic venous blood to the heart may occur in patients treated with PEEP, those with severe airflow obstruction (an "auto-PEEP" effect), and those with intravascular volume depletion.

Negative pressure ventilation with chest cuirass and similar devices and continuous positive-pressure ventilation via tracheostomy tubes are acceptable approaches to treatment of chronic ventilatory failure when repeated attempts at weaning have failed. Mechanical problems are enormous. Nocturnal positive-pressure ventilation via nasal mask is a new experimental approach to management of patients with nocturnal hypoventilation from neuromuscular disease.

B. General Supportive Care: Patients with acute respiratory failure are seriously ill, and careful attention must be paid to general supportive measures. Maintenance of adequate nutrition is vital; parenteral nutrition should be used only when conventional feeding methods are not possible. Overfeeding, especially with carbohydrate, should be avoided, because it increases CO_2 production and may potentially worsen

or induce hypercapnia in patients with limited ventilatory reserve; however, failure to provide adequate nutrition is more common. Hypokalemia and hypophosphatemia may worsen hypoventilation due to muscle weakness. The hematocrit should be determined regularly and transfusions given if necessary. Sedative-hypnotics and narcotic analgesics are avoided if possible. If sedation is necessary, short-acting drugs such as triazolam, lorazepam, or oxazepam are preferred. Psychologic and emotional support, skin care to avoid decubitus ulcers, and meticulous avoidance of nosocomial infection and complications of tracheal tubes are vital aspects of comprehensive care for patients with acute respiratory failure.

Attention must also be paid to preventing complications associated with serious illness. Stress gastritis and ulcers may be avoided by administering sucralfate, antacids, or histamine H_2 receptor antagonists. The risk of deep venous thrombosis and pulmonary embolism may be reduced by subcutaneous administration of heparin (5000 units every 12 hours).

Course & Prognosis

The course and prognosis of acute respiratory failure vary and depend on the underlying disease. The prognosis of acute respiratory failure caused by uncomplicated sedative or narcotic drug overdose is excellent. Acute respiratory failure in patients with COPD who do not require intubation and mechanical ventilation has a good immediate prognosis. On the other hand, ARDS associated with sepsis has an extremely poor prognosis, with mortality rates of about 90%.

Plummer AL, O'Donohue WJ Jr, Petty TL: Consensus conference on problems in home mechanical ventilation. Am Rev Respir Dis 1989;140:555.

Sporn PH, Morganroth ML: Discontinuation of mechanical ventilation. Clin Chest Med 1988;9:113.

Slutsky AS: Nonconventional methods of ventilation. Am Rev Respir Dis 1988;138:175. (Review of low-frequency and high-frequency mechanical ventilation.)

Tobin MJ: Respiratory monitoring in the intensive care unit. Am Rev Respir Dis 1988;138:1625.

Weinberger SE, Schwartzstein RM, Weiss JW: Hypercapnia. N Engl J Med 1989;321:1223.

ADULT RESPIRATORY DISTRESS SYNDROME (ARDS)

Essentials of Diagnosis

- History of systemic or pulmonary insult.
- Respiratory distress.
- Diffuse pulmonary infiltrates.

- Severe hypoxemia refractory to treatment with supplemental oxygen.
- Normal pulmonary capillary wedge pressure.

General Considerations

Adult respiratory distress syndrome denotes acute respiratory failure following a systemic or pulmonary insult; it is characterized by respiratory distress, diffuse infiltrates, hypoxemia, noncompliant lungs, and normal pulmonary capillary wedge pressure. ARDS may follow a wide variety of catastrophic clinical events (Table 7–24). Common risk factors for ARDS include sepsis, aspiration of gastric contents, shock, trauma, severe pneumonia, and multiple blood transfusions. About one-third of ARDS patients initially have sepsis syndrome. Pro-inflammatory cytokines (tumor necrosis factor, interleukin-1) released from stimulated lymphocytes and macrophages appear to be pivotal in lung injury. Although the mechanism of lung injury varies with the cause, damage to capillary endothelial cells and alveolar epithelial cells (type I pneumocytes) is common to ARDS regardless of cause. Damage to these cells causes increased vascular permeability and inactivation of surfactant; both of these lead to interstitial and alveolar pulmonary edema and alveolar collapse.

Clinical Findings

ARDS is marked by the rapid onset of profound dyspnea that usually occurs 12–48 hours after the initiating event. Labored breathing, tachypnea, intercostal retractions, and crackles are noted on physical examination. Chest radiograph shows diffuse or patchy bilateral infiltrates that are initially interstitial

Table 7–24. Selected disorders associated with ARDS.

Systemic Insults	Pulmonary Insults
Trauma	Embolism of thrombus, fat, or
Sepsis	amniotic fluid
Pancreatitis	Miliary tuberculosis
Shock	Aspiration of gastric contents
Multiple transfusions	Diffuse pneumonia
Disseminated intravascular	Viral
coagulation	*Mycoplasma*
Burns	Legionnaire's
Drugs	(*Legionella*
Narcotics	*pneumophila*)
Aspirin	*Pneumocystis*
Chlordiazepoxide	Near-drowning
Phenylbutazone	Toxic gas inhalation
Colchicine	Nitrogen dioxide
Ethchlorvynol	Chlorine
Hydrochlorothiazide	Sulfur dioxide
Paraldehyde	Ammonia
Lidocaine	Smoke inhalation
Thrombotic thrombocytopenic	Oxygen toxicity
purpura	Lung contusions
Cardiopulmonary bypass	Radiation
Venous air embolism	High altitude
Head injury	Hanging
Paraquat	Reexpansion

but rapidly become alveolar; these characteristically spare the costophrenic angles. Air bronchograms occur in about 80% of cases. Upper lung zone venous engorgement (flow inversion) is distinctly uncommon. Heart size is normal, and pleural effusions are small or nonexistent. Marked hypoxemia occurs that is refractory to treatment with supplemental oxygen, indicating shunting. Most patients with ARDS demonstrate evidence of failure of other organ systems, particularly the kidneys, liver, gut, central nervous system, and cardiovascular system.

Differential Diagnosis

Since ARDS is a physiologic and radiographic syndrome rather than a specific disease, the concept of differential diagnosis does not strictly apply. Normal-permeability ("cardiogenic") pulmonary edema must be ruled out, however, because specific therapy is available for that disorder. Measurement of pulmonary capillary wedge pressure by means of a flow-directed pulmonary artery catheter may be required, though routine use of the Swan-Ganz catheter in ARDS is discouraged.

Prevention

No measures that effectively prevent ARDS have been identified; specifically, prophylactic use of PEEP in patients at risk for ARDS has not been shown to be effective. Intravenous methylprednisolone does not prevent ARDS when given early to patients with sepsis syndrome or septic shock.

Treatment

Treatment of ARDS must include identification and specific treatment of the underlying condition (eg, sepsis). Aggressive supportive care must then be provided to compensate for the severe dysfunction of the respiratory system associated with ARDS. Supportive therapy almost always includes tracheal intubation and mechanical ventilation. The use of positive end expiratory pressure (PEEP) usually improves oxygenation in patients with ARDS but does not affect the natural history of this condition. PEEP should be used to minimize pulmonary oxygen toxicity if the F_{IO_2} required to produce an acceptable level of oxygenation exceeds 0.6. The lowest level of PEEP that produces adequate oxygenation combined with an acceptable F_{IO_2} should be used. High levels of PEEP may improve arterial P_{O_2} but may depress cardiac output and reduce oxygen delivery. Cardiac output must be monitored with a thermodilution pulmonary artery catheter whenever there is concern about adequacy of systemic oxygen transport (a product of cardiac output and arterial oxygen content) or the fluid balance of the patient. Cardiac output that falls when PEEP is used may be improved by reducing the level of PEEP or by administering inotropic drugs (eg, dopamine); administering fluids to increase intravascular volume should be done only with great caution, because doing so may worsen alveolar edema.

Elevated pulmonary capillary pressure worsens pulmonary edema in the presence of increased capillary permeability; therefore, the goal of fluid management is to maintain pulmonary capillary wedge pressure at the lowest possible level compatible with adequate cardiac output. Crystalloid solutions should be used when intravascular volume expansion is necessary. Diuretics should be used to reduce intravascular volume if pulmonary capillary wedge pressure is elevated. Packed red blood cell transfusions (see Chapter 10) are given to keep the hematocrit above 25%, a practice that maintains a reasonable arterial oxygen content.

Oxygenation in patients with ARDS may sometimes be improved by turning them from the supine to the prone position.

Extracorporeal membrane oxygenation, PEEP, corticosteroids, and prostaglandin E_1 have been shown not to improve survival. Corticosteroid therapy may benefit patients with ARDS due to radiation pneumonitis and possibly fat embolism syndrome. However, in patients with sepsis syndrome and ARDS, intravenous methylprednisolone has been shown to impede reversal of ARDS and increase its mortality rate.

Broad-spectrum antimicrobial treatment should be started promptly when infection is known or suspected.

New treatment approaches *under investigation* include surfactant supplementation, ibuprofen, monoclonal antibodies against endotoxins, pentoxifylline, and extracorporeal CO_2 removal.

Course & Prognosis

The mortality rate associated with ARDS exceeds 50%. If ARDS is accompanied by sepsis, the mortality rate may reach 90%. The major cause of death in ARDS is nonpulmonary multiple organ system failure, often with sepsis. Median survival is about 2 weeks. Most survivors are asymptomatic within a few months, though abnormalities of oxygenation, diffusing capacity, and lung mechanics may persist in some.

Bernard GR et al: High-dose corticosteroids in patients with the adult respiratory distress syndrome. N Engl J Med 1987;317:1565. (No benefit from intravenous methylprednisolone in ARDS due to sepsis, aspiration, or mixed causes.)
Murray JF et al: An expanded definition of the adult respiratory distress syndrome. Am Rev Respir Dis 1988;138:720.

PLEURAL DISEASES

PLEURITIS

Pain due to acute pleural inflammation is caused by irritation of the parietal pleura. Such pain is localized, sharp, and fleeting and is made worse by cough, sneezing, deep breathing, or movement. When the central portion of the diaphragmatic parietal pleura is irritated, pain may be referred to the shoulder. There are numerous causes of pleuritis. The setting in which pleuritic pain develops helps to narrow the differential diagnosis; eg, in young, otherwise healthy individuals, pleuritis is usually caused by viral respiratory infections or pneumonia. The presence of pleural effusion, pleural thickening, or air in the pleural space requires further diagnostic and therapeutic measures. It should also be recalled that simple rib fracture may cause severe pleurisy.

Treatment of pleuritis consists of treating the underlying disease. Simple analgesics and anti-inflammatory drugs (eg, indomethacin, 25 mg orally 2 or 3 times daily) are often helpful for pain relief. Codeine (30–60 mg orally every 8 hours) may be used to control cough associated with pleuritic chest pain if retention of airway secretions is not a likely complication. Intercostal nerve blocks are sometimes helpful.

PLEURAL EFFUSION

Essentials of Diagnosis

- Asymptomatic in many cases; pleuritic chest pain if pleuritis is present; dyspnea if effusion is large.
- Decreased tactile fremitus; dullness to percussion; distant breath sounds; egophony if effusion is large.
- Radiographic evidence of pleural effusion.
- Diagnostic findings on thoracentesis.

General Considerations

Pleural fluid is formed in the normal individual mostly on the parietal pleural surface at the rate of about 0.1 mL/kg/h. Absorption of this fluid on the visceral pleural surface is thought to occur, keeping the pleural space nearly dry. However, the parietal pleura may also contribute to absorption. Up to 25 mL of pleural fluid is normally present in the pleural space, an amount not detectable on conventional chest radiographs. Movement of fluid into and out of the pleural space is dependent mostly on hydrostatic and osmotic forces in parietal and visceral pleural capillaries. **Pleural effusion** is an abnormal accumulation of fluid in the pleural space. The 5 major types of pleural effusion are transudates, exudates, empyema, hemorrhagic pleural effusion or hemothorax, and chylous or chyliform effusion.

Pleural effusions are classified as **transudates** or **exudates** to help in differential diagnosis. An exudate is a pleural fluid having *one or more* of the following features:

(1) Pleural fluid protein to serum protein ratio greater than 0.5.

(2) Pleural fluid LDH to serum LDH ratio greater than 0.6.

(3) Pleural fluid LDH greater than two-thirds the upper limit of normal serum LDH.

Transudates have none of these features.

Causes of transudates and exudates are listed in Table 7–25. Congestive heart failure accounts for most transudates and is the most common cause of pleural effusion. Bacterial pneumonia and cancer are the commonest causes of exudative effusion. Mechanisms (and examples) leading to formation of transudates include increase in hydrostatic pressure (congestive heart failure), decreased oncotic pressure (hypoalbuminemia), and greater negative intrapleural pressure (acute atelectasis). Exudates form as a result of disease of the pleura itself in association with increased capillary permeability (pneumonia) or reduced lymphatic drainage (carcinoma obstructing lymphatic drainage).

The gross appearance of pleural fluid helps to identify the other major types of pleural effusion. **Empyema** is an exudative pleural effusion caused by direct infection of the pleural space, causing the pleural fluid to appear purulent or turbid. **Hemothorax** is the presence of gross blood in the pleural space, usually a result of chest trauma. **Hemorrhagic pleural effusion** is a mixture of blood and pleural fluid. About 10,000 red blood cells per microliter are necessary to create blood-tinged pleural fluid;

Table 7–25. Causes of pleural fluid transudates and exudates.

Transudates	Exudates
Congestive heart failure	Parapneumonic effusion
Cirrhosis with ascites	Cancer
Nephrotic syndrome	Pulmonary embolism
Peritoneal dialysis	Empyema
Myxedema	Tuberculosis
Acute atelectasis	Connective tissue disease
Constrictive pericarditis	Viral infection
Superior vena cava obstruction	Fungal infection
Pulmonary embolism	Rickettsial infection
	Parasitic infection
	Asbestos pleural effusion
	Meigs' syndrome
	Pancreatic disease
	Uremia
	Chronic atelectasis
	Trapped lung
	Chylothorax
	Sarcoidosis
	Drug reaction
	Postmyocardial infarction syndrome

100,000 red blood cells per microliter make pleural fluid appear grossly bloody. If the hematocrit of pleural fluid is more than 50% of the hematocrit of peripheral blood, hemothorax is present. In the absence of trauma, grossly bloody pleural fluid suggests cancer or, less commonly, pulmonary embolism.

Pleural fluid that is milky in appearance should be centrifuged. Clearing of the milky appearance from the supernatant suggests empyema, whereas persistent cloudy or turbid supernatant signifies **chylous** or **chyliform pleural effusion.** Chylous pleural effusion occurs acutely in chylothorax as a result of disruption of the thoracic duct. Chyliform pleural effusion occurs in pseudochylothorax as a result of accumulation of cholesterol complexes in a chronically thickened pleural space, a phenomenon sometimes seen in cases of trapped lung (entrapment of lung by a fibrous "peel" on the visceral pleura), tuberculous pleuritis (especially with previous therapeutic pneumothorax), or rheumatoid pleural effusion. Chylous pleural effusion may be distinguished from chyliform pleural effusion on the basis of lipid analysis of the fluid. A chylous pleural effusion has chylomicrons and a high triglyceride level, usually above 100 mg/dL.

Clinical Findings

A. Symptoms and Signs: Small pleural effusions are usually asymptomatic, whereas large pleural effusions may cause dyspnea, particularly in the presence of underlying cardiopulmonary disease. Pleuritic chest pain and dry cough may occur; any pleural fluid found in association with pleuritic chest pain is invariably an exudate. Physical findings are absent if less than 200–300 mL of pleural fluid is present. Findings consistent with the presence of a larger pleural effusion include decrease in tactile fremitus, dullness to percussion, and diminution of breath sounds over the effusion. In large effusions that compress the lung, accentuation of breath sounds and egophony may be noted just above the effusion. A pleural friction rub indicates pleuritis. A massive pleural effusion with high intrapleural pressure may cause contralateral shift of the trachea and bulging of the intercostal spaces.

B. Laboratory Findings: Diagnostic thoracentesis should be performed whenever a pleural effusion is detected and no cause for the effusion is clinically apparent. More than 1 cm of free pleural fluid should be evident on a lateral decubitus x-ray before diagnostic thoracentesis is attempted. Not all pleural effusions require diagnostic thoracentesis.

Transudates lack the distinguishing protein and LDH findings described above and are usually identified on the basis of other characteristics (white blood cell count $< 1000/\mu L$, predominance of mononuclear cells in the differential, glucose level in pleural fluid equal to that of serum, and normal pH). Laboratory findings in exudative pleural effusions are more variable and are summarized in Table 7–26. If an exudate

Table 7–26. Characteristics of important exudative pleural effusions.

Etiology or Type of Effusion	Gross Appearance	White Blood Cell Count (cells/μL)	Differential[1]	Red Blood Cell Count (cells/μL)	Glucose	Comments
Malignant effusion	Turbid to bloody; occasionally serous.	1000– <100,000	M	100 to several hundred thousand.	Equal to serum levels; <60 mg/dL in 15% of cases.	Eosinophilia uncommon; positive results on cytologic examination.
Uncomplicated para- pneumonic effusion	Clear to turbid.	5000–25,000	P	<5000	Equal to serum levels.	Tube thoracostomy unnecessary.
Empyema	Turbid to purulent.	25,000–100,000	P	<5000	Less than serum levels; of- ten very low.	Drainage necessary; putrid odor suggests anaerobic infection.
Tuberculosis	Serous to serosanguineous.	5000–10,000	M	<10,000	Equal to serum levels; occasionally <60 mg/dL.	Protein may exceed 5 g/dL; eosinophils (>10%) or mesothelial cells (>5%) make diagnosis un- likely.
Rheumatoid effusion	Turbid; greenish-yellow.	1000–20,000	M or P	<1000	<40 mg/dL.	Secondary empyema common; high LDH, low complement, high rheumatoid factor, high cholesterol levels or cholesterol crystals are characteristic.
Pulmonary infarction	Serous to grossly bloody.	1000–50,000	M or P	100 to >100,000	Equal to serum levels.	Variable findings; no pathognomonic features.
Esophageal rupture	Turbid to purulent; red- brown.	<5000– >50,000	P	. . .	Usually low.	High amylase level (salivary origin); pneumothorax in 25% of cases; effusion usually on left side; pH <6.0 strongly suggests diagnosis.
Pancreatitis	Turbid to serosanguineous.	1000–50,000	P	1000–10,000	Equal to serum levels.	Usually left-sided; high amylase level.

[1] M = mononuclear cell predominance; P = polymorphonuclear leukocyte predominance.

is suspected, thoracentesis should be performed. One should have a low threshold for performing pleural biopsy at this time. This procedure is particularly useful in the diagnosis of tuberculosis and cancer. The presence of malignant cells or positive results on smear or culture are pathognomonic findings in pleural fluid; determination of other causes depends on a constellation of findings on gross examination and laboratory studies or on biopsy results. Routine laboratory tests of pleural fluid should include total and differential white blood cell count, protein, glucose, and LDH. Additional tests may be ordered as required after thoracentesis. Pleural fluid pH is helpful in narrowing the differential diagnosis of exudative effusions. A pH less than 7.30 indicates cancer, complicated parapneumonic effusion, lupus or rheumatoid effusion, tuberculosis, or esophageal rupture. A high percentage of lymphocytes in pleural fluid suggests tuberculosis or cancer. Low levels of glucose in pleural fluid point toward cancer, empyema, tuberculosis, esophageal rupture, or connective tissue disease (rheumatoid pleuritis or systemic lupus erythematosus). Elevated levels of amylase in pleural fluid suggest one of 4 diagnoses: pancreatitis, pancreatic pseudocyst, cancer, or esophageal rupture.

C. Imaging: About 250 mL of pleural fluid must be present before effusion can be detected on conventional erect posteroanterior chest x-ray. Lateral decubitus views can detect much smaller amounts of free (nonloculated) pleural fluid. Free pleural fluid collects in the subpulmonic area. Larger amounts of fluid spill over into the costophrenic sulcus to form a meniscus. Thickening of major and minor fissures is common. Atypical collections of pleural fluid are frequently seen. Lateral displacement of the apex of the diaphragm and abrupt obliteration of lung markings at the level of the diaphragm are features of subpulmonic effusion. Round or oval collections of fluid in fissures resemble tumors ("pseudotumors"). Ultrasound is useful to locate loculated or small effusions. Massive pleural effusion (opacification of an entire hemithorax) is usually caused by cancer but has been observed in tuberculosis and other diseases. CT scanning is sensitive in the detection of small amounts of free or loculated pleural fluid, but this imaging method is costly.

Treatment

Treatment addresses the disease causing the pleural effusion as well as the effusion itself. Because a specific diagnosis can be established in most cases of pleural effusion, a diagnosis of "idiopathic" effusion may delay or even prevent successful therapy.

A. Transudative Pleural Effusion: Transudative pleural effusions generally respond to treatment of the underlying condition; therapeutic thoracentesis is indicated only if massive effusion causes dyspnea. Pleurodesis and tube thoracostomy are rarely if ever indicated. When bilateral pleural effusions are de-

tected in a patient with congestive heart failure, neither diagnostic nor therapeutic thoracentesis is routinely indicated. Such effusions are likely to be transudates and will resolve with treatment of the underlying cardiac disease.

B. Malignant or Paramalignant Pleural Effusion: Pleural effusion in a patient with known cancer may be either malignant or paramalignant. In patients with **malignant pleural effusion,** the pleural surface is directly invaded by malignant cells (pleural fluid cytology or pleural tissue biopsy reveals evidence of malignancy). In such cases the tumor causing the effusion is unresectable, and treatment with chemotherapy or radiotherapy is directed at the underlying cancer. In patients with **paramalignant pleural effusion,** the pleural space is not directly invaded by tumor, and repeated thoracentesis and needle biopsy of the pleura give negative results. In this situation, the underlying tumor may or may not be resectable. Chemical **pleurodesis** (obliteration of the pleural space by producing fibrous adhesion between the visceral and the parietal pleura) is advised for selected patients with symptomatic malignant pleural effusion who fail to respond to chemotherapy or mediastinal radiation or who are not candidates for these forms of therapy. Intrapleural tetracycline is now the method of choice for chemical pleurodesis. An intercostal tube is inserted in a low interspace and placed on suction or water-seal drainage until as much fluid as possible has been removed, and 20 mg/kg of tetracycline dissolved in 50 mL of saline is then injected into the pleural cavity through the tube, which is clamped for 6 hours. The patient's position is changed frequently to distribute the tetracycline within the pleural space. The tube is unclamped and continued on water-seal drainage until drainage has decreased to less than 60 mL in 24 hours. This will usually occur within 5–6 days. Transient reaction to the tetracycline such as pleural pain or low-grade fever is treated symptomatically. Intrapleural instillation of 20 mL of 1% lidocaine may prevent pleural pain. Repeated therapeutic thoracentesis and surgical pleurectomy are alternative approaches for certain patients with rapidly recurring malignant pleural effusion.

C. Parapneumonic Pleural Effusion: Pleural effusion in the setting of pneumonia ("parapneumonic effusion") usually responds to systemic antibiotic therapy. Management steps include sputum Gram stain and culture, blood cultures, diagnostic thoracentesis, antibiotic therapy, and a decision regarding closed chest drainage (tube thoracostomy). *Effective therapy requires early intervention* to avoid progression of the effusion from the exudative to subsequent (fibrinopurulent and organized) stages. Loculation of pleural fluid collections is likely once organization has occurred. Laboratory findings—especially the pH, glucose concentration, and the white cell count of pleural fluid—are important in guiding additional therapy. In "uncomplicated" parapneumonic effusion, no pleural infection is present, and the pleural fluid glucose and pH are normal. Such effusion is likely to resolve spontaneously, and chest tube drainage is not required. In "complicated" parapneumonic effusion, pleural fluid is either frank empyema or has the potential to organize into a fibrous "peel." A low pH (< 7.2), low glucose (< 50 mg/dL), and high LDH (> 1000 IU/L)—but not pleural fluid white blood cell count or protein concentration—help to separate complicated from uncomplicated parapneumonic effusions.

Tube thoracostomy is required for parapneumonic effusion if any of the following are present: (1) the fluid resembles frank pus, (2) an organism is evident on Gram stain, (3) glucose < 40 mg/dL, or (4) pH < 7.0. If the pleural fluid pH is between 7.0 and 7.2 or the LDH is > 1000 IU/L, the physician should strongly consider chest tube placement or should monitor the effusion carefully with serial thoracenteses. A thick pleural "peel" developing after treatment of complicated parapneumonic effusion may resolve slowly over several months. Surgical decortication should be reserved for selected patients with established fibrothorax.

D. Hemothorax: Hemothorax is generally managed by the immediate insertion of one or more large chest tubes in order to control bleeding by causing apposition of pleural surfaces; chest tubes help the physician determine the amount of bleeding and decrease the risk of complications such as empyema and eventual fibrothorax. As much blood as possible should be drained before the chest tube is removed. Thoracotomy is occasionally required to control bleeding, remove large volumes of blood clots, and treat coexisting complications of trauma such as bronchopleural fistula. A very small hemothorax that is stable or improving on chest x-ray can be managed without tube drainage.

E. Other Types of Pleural Effusion: Management of patients with exudative pleural effusion due to other causes consists mainly of treating the underlying disease. Pleural fluid acidosis outside the setting of pneumonia is not an automatic indication for chest tube drainage. Patients with rheumatoid pleural effusions should be watched closely for the development of secondary empyema.

Prognosis

The prognosis of patients with pleural effusion depends on the prognosis of the underlying disease. The prognosis of patients with documented malignant pleural effusion is poor, particularly if pleural fluid pH or glucose levels are low.

American College of Physicians: Diagnostic thoracentesis and pleural biopsy in pleural effusions. Ann Intern Med 1985;103:799.

Gravelyn TR et al: Tetracycline pleurodesis for malignant pleural effusions: A 10-year retrospective study. Cancer 1987;59:1973.

Jacobs RF et al: Parapneumonic effusions and empyema. Am Rev Respir Dis 1987;136:1030.

Leslie WK, Kinasewitz GT: Clinical characteristics of the patient with nonspecific pleuritis. Chest 1988;94:603. (Conservative management in the absence of clinical features of cancer or tuberculosis.)

Sahn SA: The pleura. Am Rev Respir Dis 1988;138:184. (Review of pleural disease and effusions.)

SPONTANEOUS PNEUMOTHORAX

Essentials of Diagnosis

- Acute onset of ipsilateral chest pain and dyspnea, often of several days' duration.
- Minimal physical findings in mild cases; unilateral chest expansion, decreased tactile fremitus, hyperresonance, diminished breath sounds, mediastinal shift, cyanosis in tension pneumothorax.
- Presence of pleural air on chest x-ray.

General Considerations

Pneumothorax, or accumulation of air in the pleural space, is classified as spontaneous (primary or secondary) or traumatic. Primary pneumothorax occurs in the absence of an underlying cause, whereas secondary pneumothorax is a complication of preexisting pulmonary disease. Traumatic pneumothorax results from penetrating or nonpenetrating trauma and is often iatrogenic.

Secondary pneumothorax occurs as a complication of COPD, asthma, cystic fibrosis, tuberculosis, and a wide variety of infiltrative lung diseases, including *P carinii* pneumonia. Pneumothorax in association with menstruation (catamenial pneumothorax) is another well-established form of secondary pneumothorax. Because of underlying disease, secondary pneumothorax is usually a more serious condition than primary spontaneous pneumothorax.

The incidence of primary pneumothorax is about 9 per 100,000 per year; the disease affects mainly tall, thin men between the ages of 20 and 40 years. Primary pneumothorax is thought to occur from rupture of subpleural apical blebs in response to high negative intrapleural pressures. Familial factors and cigarette smoking may also be important.

Clinical Findings

A. Symptoms and Signs: Chest pain on the affected side and dyspnea occur in nearly all patients. Symptoms usually begin during rest or sleep. Many patients wait for several days before seeking medical attention. Alternatively, this may be present with life-threatening respiratory failure if underlying COPD or asthma is present; this is true irrespective of the size of the pneumothorax.

If pneumothorax is small, physical findings, other than mild tachycardia, are unimpressive. If pneumothorax is large, diminished breath sounds, decreased tactile fremitus, and hyperresonance are noted. Tension pneumothorax should be suspected in the presence of severe tachycardia, hypotension, and mediastinal or tracheal shift.

B. Laboratory Findings: Arterial blood gas analysis reveals hypoxemia in most patients but is often unnecessary. Left-sided primary pneumothorax may produce QRS axis and precordial T wave changes on the ECG.

C. Imaging: Demonstration of a visceral pleural line is diagnostic and is best revealed on an expiratory film. A few patients have secondary pleural effusion that demonstrates a characteristic air-fluid level on chest radiography. In tension pneumothorax, the pressure of air in the pleural space exceeds ambient pressure throughout the respiratory cycle. A check-valve mechanism allows air to enter the pleural space on inspiration and prevents egress of air on expiration. In supine patients, pneumothorax on a conventional chest x-ray may appear as an abnormally radiolucent costophrenic sulcus (the "deep sulcus" sign). In patients with tension pneumothorax, chest x-rays show a large amount of air in the affected hemithorax and contralateral shift of mediastinal structures. Tension pneumothorax usually occurs in the setting of penetrating trauma, lung infection, cardiopulmonary resuscitation, or positive-pressure mechanical ventilation.

Differential Diagnosis

If the patient is a young, tall, thin, cigarette-smoking man, the diagnosis of primary spontaneous pneumothorax is usually obvious and can be confirmed by chest x-ray. In secondary pneumothorax, it is sometimes difficult to distinguish loculated pneumothorax from an emphysematous bleb. Occasionally, pneumothorax may mimic myocardial infarction, pulmonary embolization, or pneumonia.

Complications

Tension pneumothorax may result in acute respiratory failure. Cardiopulmonary arrest and death are extremely rare. Pneumomediastinum may occur as a complication of spontaneous pneumothorax. If this is detected, rupture of the esophagus or a bronchus should be considered.

Treatment

Treatment depends upon the severity of pneumothorax. A patient with a small pneumothorax that has been observed to be stable in size for several days to a week can be followed closely with serial chest x-rays without hospitalization. The patient with a new small ($< 15\%$) pneumothorax should be hospitalized and placed at bed rest, treated symptomatically for cough and chest pain, and followed with serial chest x-rays every 12–24 hours. Observation in the hospital for 2 days is adequate in most cases. Many small pneumothoraces resolve spontaneously as air is absorbed from the pleural space; however, pneumothorax may unpredictably progress to tension pneumotho-

rax. In this situation, or in patients who are severely symptomatic or who have a larger pneumothorax ($> 15\%$), chest tube placement (tube thoracostomy) is performed. The chest tube is placed under water-seal drainage, and suction is applied until the lung expands. Intravenous catheters and emergency pneumothorax treatment tubes should not be used in the hospital setting because of a high rate of technical failures. Air leaks persisting after 3 days are unusual. Tube thoracostomy alone does not cause enough pleural scarification to prevent recurrence of spontaneous pneumothorax. Pulmonary edema on the affected side may follow abrupt evacuation of pneumothorax. If tension pneumothorax is suspected, a large-bore needle should be inserted immediately in the affected side; tube thoracostomy may be performed thereafter.

Chemical pleurodesis with instillation of tetracycline into the pleural space by chest tube has been recommended by some authorities for management of a first episode of spontaneous pneumothorax, but this procedure causes considerable pain.

All patients should be advised to discontinue smoking and warned that the risk of recurrence is 50%. Exposure to high altitudes, flying in unpressurized aircraft, and scuba diving should be avoided. If spontaneous pneumothorax recurs, the second episode should be managed in a manner similar to that of the first episode. Some experts advocate thoracotomy for any recurrence.

Indications for open thoracotomy include recurrences of spontaneous pneumothorax (the minimum number of episodes being controversial), any occurrence of bilateral pneumothorax, and failure of tube thoracostomy for the first episode (failure of lung to reexpand or persistent air leak). Open thoracotomy permits oversewing of the ruptured blebs responsible for the pneumothorax and greatly reduces the risk of recurrence. Pleural symphysis may be obtained by scarification from abrasion of the pleural surface. Pleurectomy is of no particular value.

Prognosis

About half of patients with spontaneous pneumothorax experience recurrence of the disorder after either observation or tube thoracostomy for the first episode. Recurrence after open thoracotomy is rare. Following successful therapy, there are no long-term complications.

Baumann MH, Sahn SA: Medical management and therapy of bronchopleural fistulas in the mechanically ventilated patients. Chest 1990;97:721.

Miller KS, Sahn SA: Chest tubes: Indications, technique, management, and complications. Chest 1987;91:258.

O'Rourke JP, Yee ES: Civilian spontaneous pneumothorax: Treatment options and long-term results. Chest 1989; 96:1302.

REFERENCES

Chang HK, Paiva M (editors): *Respiratory Physiology: Lung Biology in Health and Disease,* Vol 40. Marcel Dekker, 1989.

Crystal RG, West JB (editors): *The Lung: Scientific Foundations.* Raven Press, 1990.

Phelan PD, Landau LI, Olinsky A: *Respiratory Illness in Children,* 3rd ed. Blackwell, 1989.

Sexton DL (editor): *Nursing Care of the Respiratory Patient.* Appleton & Lange, 1989.

West JB: *Pulmonary Pathophysiology: The Essentials,* 3rd ed. Williams & Wilkins, 1987.

Baum GL, Wolinsky E (editors): *Textbook of Pulmonary Diseases,* 4th ed. Little, Brown, 1989.

Bone RC, George RB, Hudson LD (editors): *Acute Respiratory Failure.* Churchill Livingstone, 1987.

Burton GG, Hodgkin JE (editors): *Respiratory Care: A Guide to Clinical Practice,* 2nd ed. Lippincott, 1984.

Cherniak RM (editor): *Current Therapy in Respiratory Disease-3.* BC Decker, 1988.

Clausen JL (editor): *Pulmonary Function Testing Guidelines and Controversies: Equipment, Methods, and Normal Values.* Grune & Stratton, 1984.

Comroe J: *Physiology of Respiration,* 2nd ed. Year Book, 1974.

du Bois RM, Clarke SW (editors): *Fiberoptic Bronchoscopy in Diagnosis and Management.* Grune & Stratton, 1987.

Enright PL, Hyatt RE: *Office Spirometry: A Practical Guide to the Selection and Use of Spirometers.* Lea & Febiger, 1987.

Fairbanks DNF et al: *Snoring and Obstructive Sleep Apnea.* Raven Press, 1987.

Felson B: *Chest Roentgenology.* Saunders, 1973.

Fishman AP (editor): *Pulmonary Diseases and Disorders,* 2nd ed. McGraw-Hill, 1988.

Fishman AP (editor): *Handbook of Physiology, Section 3: The Respiratory System.* American Physiological Society and Williams & Wilkins, 1985.

Fraser RG et al: *Diagnosis of Diseases of the Chest,* 3rd ed. Saunders, 1988.

Kryger MH, Roth T, Dement WC: *Principles and Practice of Sleep Medicine.* Saunders, 1989.

Hodgkin JE, Petty TL (editors): *Chronic Obstructive Pulmonary Disease: Current Concepts.* Saunders, 1987.

Light RW: *Pleural Diseases.* Lea & Febiger, 1983.

Luce JM, Tyler ML, Pierson DJ: *Intensive Respiratory Care.* Saunders, 1984.

Morgan WKC, Seaton A (editors): *Occupational Lung Diseases,* 2nd ed. Saunders, 1984.

Mountain CF, Carr CT (editors): *Lung Cancer: Current Status and Prospects for the Future.* University of Texas Press, 1987.

Murray JF: *The Normal Lung,* 2nd ed. Saunders, 1986.

Murray JF, Nadel JA: *Textbook of Respiratory Medicine,* Saunders, 1988.

Netter FH: *The Ciba Collection of Medical Illustrations: Volume 7, Respiratory System.* Ciba, 1979.

Oho K, Amemiya R: *Practical Fiberoptic Bronchoscopy.* Igaku-Shoin, 1980.

Rippe JM et al (editors): *Intensive Care Medicine,* 2nd ed. Little, Brown, 1989.

Schwarz MI, King TE Jr (editors): *Interstitial Lung Disease.* BC Decker, 1988.

Shoemaker WC, et al: *The Society of Critical Care Medicine: Textbook of Critical Care,* 2nd ed. Saunders, 1988.

Spencer H: *Pathology of the Lung,* 4th ed. Pergamon, 1985.

Thurlbeck WM (editor): *Pathology of the Lung.* Thieme Medical Publishers, 1988.

West JB: *Respiratory Physiology: The Essentials,* 3rd ed. Williams & Wilkins, 1985.

Wilson AF (editor): *Pulmonary Function Testing Indications and Interpretations.* Grune & Stratton, 1985.

Zagelbaum GL, Welch MA Jr, Doyle PR: *Basic Arterial Blood Gas Interpretation.* Little, Brown, 1988.

8

Heart & Great Vessels

Barry M. Massie, MD, & Maurice Sokolow, MD

Evaluation of cardiovascular disease requires (1) identification of the physiologic abnormality, (2) delineation of the underlying structural abnormality and its cause, and (3) determination of the need for treatment and the type of treatment.

COMMON SYMPTOMS

The most common symptoms of heart disease are dyspnea, chest pain, palpitations, presyncope or syncope, and fatigue. None are specific, and interpretation depends on the entire clinical picture and, in many cases, diagnostic testing. These are discussed in greater detail under the diseases themselves.

Dyspnea

Dyspnea due to heart disease is precipitated by exertion and results from elevated left atrial and pulmonary venous pressures or hypoxia. The former are most commonly caused by left ventricular systolic dysfunction, left ventricular diastolic dysfunction (due to hypertrophy, fibrosis, or pericardial disease), or valvular obstruction. The acute onset or worsening of left atrial hypertension may result in **pulmonary edema.** Hypoxia may be due to pulmonary edema or intracardiac shunting. Dyspnea should be quantified by the amount of activity that precipitates it. Dyspnea is also a common symptom of pulmonary disease, and the etiologic distinction may be very difficult. Shortness of breath is also found in deconditioned or obese individuals, anxiety states, and many illnesses.

Orthopnea is dyspnea that occurs in recumbency and results from an increase in central blood volume. Orthopnea may also result from pulmonary disease. **Paroxysmal nocturnal dyspnea** is relieved by sitting up or standing; this symptom is more specific for cardiac disease.

Chest Pain

Chest pain is a common symptom that can occur as a result of pulmonary or musculoskeletal disease, esophageal or other gastrointestinal disorders, cervicothoracic nerve root irritation, or anxiety states, as well as many cardiovascular diseases. The commonest cause of cardiac chest pain is myocardial ischemia. This is usually described as dull, aching, or as a sensation of "pressure," "tightness," "squeezing," or "gas," rather than as sharp or spasmodic; and it is often perceived as an uncomfortable sensation rather than "pain." **Ischemic pain** usually subsides within 30 minutes but may last longer. Protracted episodes often represent **myocardial infarction.** The pain is commonly accompanied by a sense of anxiety or uneasiness. The location is usually retrosternal or left precordial. Though the pain may radiate to or be localized in the throat, lower jaw, shoulders, inner arms, upper abdomen, or back, it nearly always also involves the sternal region. Ischemic pain is often precipitated by exertion, cold temperature, meals, stress, or combinations of these factors and is usually relieved by rest. It is not related to position or respiration and is usually not elicited by chest palpation.

Hypertrophy of either ventricle and aortic valvular disease may also give rise to ischemic pain or pain with less typical features. Myocarditis and mitral valve prolapse are associated with chest pain of a more atypical nature. Pericarditis may produce pain that changes with position or respiration. Aortic dissection produces an instantaneous tearing pain of great intensity that often radiates to the back.

Palpitations, Dizziness, Syncope

Awareness of the heartbeat may be a normal phenomenon or may reflect increased cardiac or stroke output in patients with many noncardiac conditions (eg, exercise, thyrotoxicosis, anemia, anxiety). It may also be due to cardiac abnormalities that increase stroke volume (regurgitant valvular disease, bradycardia) or may be a manifestation of cardiac arrhythmias. Ventricular premature beats may be sensed as extra or "missed" beats. Supraventricular or ventricular tachycardia may be felt as rapid, regular or irregular palpitations or fluttering; many patients are asymptomatic, however.

If the abnormal rhythm is associated with a sufficient decline in arterial pressure or cardiac output, it may—especially in the upright position—impair cerebral blood flow, causing dizziness, blurring of vision, loss of consciousness (syncope), or other symptoms.

Cardiogenic syncope most commonly results from loss of sinus node impulse formation, atrioventricular conduction block, or ventricular tachycardia or fibrillation. It is associated with few prodromal symptoms and may thus be an occasion for injuries. The absence of premonitory symptoms helps distinguish cardiogenic syncope from vasovagal faint, postural hypotension, or seizure. Although recovery is often immediate, some patients may exhibit seizurelike movements. Aortic valve disease and hypertrophic obstructive cardiomyopathy may also cause syncope, which is usually exertional or postexertional.

Edema

Subcutaneous fluid collections appear first in the lower extremities in ambulatory patients or in the sacral region of bedridden individuals. In heart disease, edema results from elevated right atrial pressures. Right heart failure most commonly results from left heart failure, although the right-sided signs may predominate. Other cardiogenic causes of edema include pericardial disease, right-sided valve lesions, and cor pulmonale. Edema may also be due to peripheral venous insufficiency, venous obstruction, nephrotic syndrome, cirrhosis, or premenstrual fluid retention, or it may be idiopathic. Advanced right heart failure can produce ascites, always in conjunction with edema.

FUNCTIONAL CLASSIFICATION OF HEART DISEASE

As a means of quantifying the limitation on activity of cardiac patients imposed by their symptoms, the classification system of the New York Heart Association is commonly employed. In following individual patients, it is important to document specific activities that produce symptoms.

Class I: No limitation of physical activity. Ordinary physical activity does not cause undue fatigue, dyspnea, or anginal pain.

Class II: Slight limitation of physical activity. Ordinary physical activity results in symptoms.

Class III: Marked limitation of physical activity. Comfortable at rest, but less than ordinary activity causes symptoms.

Class IV: Unable to engage in any physical activity without discomfort. Symptoms may be present even at rest.

SIGNS OF HEART DISEASE

Although the cardiovascular examination centers on the heart, peripheral signs are often invaluable.

Cyanosis, Pallor

Cyanosis may be central, due to arterial desaturation, or peripheral, reflecting impaired tissue delivery of adequately saturated blood in low-output states, polycythemia, or peripheral vasoconstriction. Central cyanosis may be caused by pulmonary disease, left heart failure, or right-to-left shunting; the latter will not be improved by increasing the inspired oxygen concentration. **Pallor** usually indicates anemia but may be a sign of low cardiac output.

Peripheral Pulses & Venous Pulsations

Diminished peripheral pulses most commonly result from arteriosclerotic peripheral vascular disease and may be accompanied by localized bruits. Asymmetry of pulses should also arouse suspicion of coarctation of the aorta or aortic dissection; previous cardiac catheterization may also be responsible. Exaggerated pulses may indicate aortic regurgitation, coarctation, patent ductus arteriosus, or other conditions that increase stroke volume. The carotid pulse is a valuable aid to assessment of left ventricular ejection. It has a delayed upstroke in aortic stenosis and a bisferiens quality (2 palpable peaks) in mixed aortic valvular disease or hypertrophic obstructive cardiomyopathy. **Pulsus paradoxus** (a decrease in systolic blood pressure during inspiration greater than the normal 10 mm Hg) is a valuable sign of pericardial tamponade, though it also occurs in asthma and chronic obstructive pulmonary disease.

Jugular venous pulsations provide insight into right atrial pressure. They indicate (1) elevated central venous pressure if they are more than 3 vertical centimeters above the angle of Louis, (2) increased central blood volume if they rise more than 1 cm with sustained upper abdominal pressure (**hepatojugular reflux**), (3) tricuspid obstruction or pulmonary hypertension if the *a* wave is exaggerated, and (4) tricuspid regurgitation if large *cv* waves are seen. The latter may be associated with hepatic pulsations. Atrioventricular dissociation due to conduction block or ventricular arrhythmia can be recognized by intermittent cannon *a* waves.

Pulmonary Examination

Crackles heard at the lung bases are a sign of congestive heart failure but may be caused by similarly localized pulmonary disease. Wheezing and rhonchi suggest obstructive pulmonary disease but may occur in left heart failure. Pleural effusions with bibasilar percussion dullness and reduced breath sounds are common in congestive heart failure.

Precordial Pulsations

A parasternal lift usually indicates right ventricular hypertrophy, pulmonary hypertension (systolic pressure > 50 mm Hg), or left atrial enlargement; pulmonary artery pulsations may also be visible. The left ventricular apical impulse, if sustained and enlarged, suggests myocardial hypertrophy or dysfunction. If forceful but not sustained, the apical impulse may indicate volume overload or high-output states. Additional precordial pulsations may reflect regional abnormalities of left ventricular contraction.

Heart Sounds & Murmurs

Auscultation is diagnostic of—or helpful in diagnosis of—many heart diseases, including cardiac failure. Specific findings are discussed under diagnostic headings.

The first heart sound (S_1) may be diminished with severe left ventricular dysfunction or accentuated in mitral stenosis or short PR intervals. S_2 is usually split, with the 2 components (aortic preceding pulmonary) being separated more during inspiration; splitting is fixed in atrial septal defect, wide with right bundle branch block, and absent or reversed **(paradoxic splitting)** with aortic stenosis, left ventricular failure, or left bundle branch block. With normal splitting, an accentuated P_2 is an important sign of pulmonary hypertension. Third and fourth heart sounds (ventricular and atrial gallops, respectively) indicate ventricular volume overload or impaired compliance and may be heard over either ventricle. An apical S_3 is a normal finding in younger individuals and in pregnancy. Additional auscultatory findings include sharp, high-pitched sounds classified as "clicks." These may be early systolic and represent ejection sounds (as with a bicuspid aortic valve or pulmonary stenosis) or may occur in mid or late systole, indicating myxomatous changes in the mitral valve.

While many murmurs indicate valvular disease, a soft, short systolic murmur, usually localized along the left sternal border or toward the apex, may be innocent, reflecting pulmonary flow. Systolic murmurs are pansystolic (holosystolic) when they merge with the first sound and persist through all of systole or "ejection" murmurs when they begin after the first sound and end before the second sound, with a peak in early or mid systole. The former represent mitral regurgitation if maximal at the apex or in the axilla and tricuspid regurgitation or ventricular septal defect if best heard at the sternal border. Association of murmurs with palpable vibrations ("thrills") is always clinically significant, as are diastolic murmurs.

Lembo NJ et al: Bedside diagnosis of systolic murmurs. N Engl J Med 1988;318:1572.

DIAGNOSTIC TESTING

The chest radiograph will provide information about heart size, the pulmonary circulation (with characteristic signs suggesting both pulmonary artery or pulmonary venous hypertension), primary pulmonary disease, and aortic abnormalities. The echocardiogram has replaced the radiograph in Western countries in the assessment of individual chamber size and valvular disease. The electrocardiogram (ECG) indicates cardiac rhythm, reveals conduction abnormalities, and provides evidence of ventricular hypertrophy, myocardial infarction, or ischemia. Nonspecific ST segment and T wave changes may reflect these processes but are also noted with electrolyte imbalance, drug effects, and many other conditions.

SPECIAL DIAGNOSTIC PROCEDURES

Echocardiography

M-mode echocardiography yields quantitative measurements of left ventricular size, function, and thickness and qualitative information about aortic and mitral stenosis. It may be diagnostic of hypertrophic cardiomyopathy, pericardial effusion, mitral valve prolapse, valvular vegetations, and cardiac tumors. **Two-dimensional echocardiograms** visualize more of the heart. Left ventricular segmental wall motion can be assessed, and the size of both atria and the right ventricle can be determined. **Doppler ultrasound** now permits the quantitative estimation of transvalvular gradients and pulmonary artery pressure and qualitative evaluation of valvular regurgitation and intraventricular shunts. **Color Doppler** visually demonstrates patterns and directionality of flow; it has been particularly useful in evaluating congenital heart disease. **Transesophageal echocardiography** is used in an increasing number of centers to improve the quality of echocardiograms, to derive information about posterior structures and prosthetic valves, and to monitor patients during surgery.

Belkin RN, Kisslo J: Clinical applications of echocardiography in myocardial and valvular heart disease. Prog Cardiovasc Dis 1986;29:81.

Feigenbaum H: *Echocardiography*, 4th ed. Lea & Febiger, 1986.

Ritter SB: Application of Doppler color-flow mapping in the assessment and evaluation of congenital heart disease. Echocardiography 1987;4:543.

Sahn DJ, Valdes-Cruz LM: New advances in two-dimensional Doppler echocardiography. Prog Cardiovasc Dis 1986;28:367.

Seward JB et al: Transesophageal echocardiography: Technique, anatomic correlations, implementation, and clinical applications. Mayo Clin Proc 1988;63:649. (State-of-the-art review of this new procedure.)

Exercise Electrocardiography

The resting ECG is often insensitive to ischemia, but horizontal or downsloping exercise-induced ST segment depression, particularly when it exceeds 0.1 mV, is strongly suggestive. Exercise-induced chest pain and hypotension also suggest coronary disease. Exercise testing has a sensitivity of 60—80% and a specificity of 80—90%, and these figures increase with thallium scintigraphy. This procedure helps to diagnose or exclude disease, to estimate its severity, and to provide guidelines for activity in patients with known ischemic heart disease.

Detrano R, Froelicher VF: Exercise testing: Uses and limitations considering recent studies. Prog Cardiovasc Dis 1988;31:173.

Detrano R et al: The diagnostic accuracy of the exercise electrocardiogram: A meta-analysis of 22 years of research. Prog Cardiovasc Dis 1989;32:173.

Goldschlager N, Sox HC Jr: The diagnostic and prognostic value of the treadmill exercise test in the evaluation of chest pain, in patients with recent myocardial infarction, and in asymptomatic individuals. Am Heart J 1988; 116:523. (Editorialized review.)

Sox HC et al: The role of exercise testing in screening for coronary artery disease. Ann Intern Med 1989; 110:456. (Not currently indicated.)

Ambulatory Electrocardiographic Monitoring

Ambulatory electrocardiographic (Holter) monitoring is most useful for determining the need for therapy in patients with symptoms consistent with arrhythmia. Since these symptoms are often nonspecific, their temporal association with a conduction or rhythm disturbance provides a definitive indication for treatment. Documentation of asymptomatic "premonitory" abnormalities such as second-degree atrioventricular block, transient sinus node arrest, or nonsustained ventricular tachycardia may by association suggest the basis for previous symptomatic episodes. Ambulatory monitoring may assess the benefit of treatment, but its use in the evaluation of asymptomatic individuals should be limited. There is growing interest in the use of this technique for diagnosing asymptomatic ischemic episodes, but the interpretation of these episodes in patients without known coronary disease is uncertain.

Kennedy HL, Wiens RD: Ambulatory (Holter) electrocardiography and myocardial ischemia. Am Heart J 1989: 117:164. (Monitoring of ischemia, a newer application of ambulatory ECG monitoring.)

Knoebel SB et al: Guidelines for ambulatory electrocardiography: A report of the American College of Cardiology–American Heart Association joint task force on assessment of diagnostic and therapeutic cardiovascular procedures. Circulation 1989;79:206. (Position paper on role of ambulatory monitoring.)

Radionuclide Techniques

Several nuclear medicine studies are useful in the assessment of heart disease.

Thallium-201 scintigraphy demonstrates relative myocardial perfusion. It is most commonly employed in conjunction with exercise testing to detect ischemia, which appears as a perfusion defect. After 3–24 hours, the defect will fill in or "redistribute" with reversible ischemia but will remain fixed in regions of infarction. Thallium scintigraphy following dipyridamole-induced vasodilatation provides similar information in patients unable to exercise. The sensitivity and specificity of exercise thallium scintigraphy are in the 80–90% range, which is somewhat superior to the exercise ECG, but its expense should limit its use to situations in which ordinary exercise testing needs corroboration or is not accurate (eg, bundle branch block, digitalis

effect, baseline repolarization changes). Newer technetium-based perfusion markers should be available soon and should improve the quality of myocardial images.

Radionuclide angiography provides accurate measurements of left and, in some laboratories, right ventricular ejection fractions. Segmental wall motion may be examined, and semiquantitative estimates of valvular regurgitation are possible. Radionuclide angiography may be performed during exercise, so that changes in global or segmental left ventricular function can be employed to diagnose ischemia or impaired functional reserve. Thallium scintigraphy is a more accurate test for evaluating ischemic heart disease. Radionuclide angiography can also be used to quantify the pulmonary-to-systemic flow ratio in left-to-right shunts. Ratios above 1.3–1.5 can be accurately detected.

Technetium-99m pyrophosphate scintigraphy produces radiotracer uptake in areas of recent infarction. Its usefulness is limited by an 18- to 24-hour lag time after acute infarction before the test becomes positive and a limited sensitivity for small, especially nontransmural infarctions. This technique is most useful when the ECG and cardiac enzymes are nondiagnostic, such as after cardiac surgery or when chest pain has occurred more than 48 hours prior to assessment.

Rozanski A, Berman DS: The efficacy of cardiovascular nuclear medicine exercise studies. Semin Nucl Med 1987;17:104.

Newer Imaging Modalities

Many new imaging techniques have been developed, but their application in cardiovascular disease remains to be determined. **Computed tomography (CT scan)** can image the heart and, with contrast medium, the vascular system, but the relatively slow speed of most instruments limits its utility. The main application of CT is the evaluation of pericardial disease and aortic dissection. **Ultrafast** or **cine CT** involves a specially designed instrument with high temporal resolution. Its availability is limited, but early reports indicate that it will provide accurate assessment of cardiac size and function and bypass graft patency, as well as useful data on myocardial perfusion.

Magnetic resonance imaging (MRI) is an evolving modality that provides high-resolution images of the heart and vascular bed without radiation exposure or use of contrast media. It provides excellent anatomic definition, permitting assessment of pericardial disease, neoplastic disease of the heart, myocardial thickness, chamber size, and many congenital heart defects. Rapid acquisition sequences can produce excellent cine-mode images demonstrating left ventricular function and wall motion.

Positron emission tomography (PET) can provide

both qualitative and quantitative information concerning myocardial metabolism and blood flow, but its availability is limited, and a nearby cyclotron is required for many applications. Recent data indicate that PET can accurately distinguish between myocardium which is transiently dysfunctional ("stunned") due to ischemia and infarcted myocardium—a distinction that is important in considering revascularization.

Council on Scientific Affairs, AMA: Magnetic resonance imaging of the cardiovascular system: Present state of the art and future potential. JAMA 1988;259:253.

Ehman RL, Julgrud PR: Magnetic resonance imaging of the heart: Current status. Mayo Clin Proc 1989;64:1134. (Reviews all applications.)

Lipton MJ et al: Clinical applications of dynamic computed tomography. Prog Cardiovasc Dis 1986;28:349.

Schelbert HR, Buxton D: Insights into coronary artery disease gained from metabolic imaging. Circulation 1988;78:496. (Potential role of positron emission tomography.)

Cardiac Catheterization

Right heart catheterization is convenient to perform and allows measurement of right atrial, right ventricular, pulmonary artery and pulmonary capillary wedge pressures (the latter an indicator of left atrial pressure), oxygen saturation, and cardiac output. These data may diagnose intracardiac shunts, physiologically significant pericardial disease, and right-sided valve lesions and can distinguish between cardiac and pulmonary disease. Balloon flotation catheters permit hemodynamic measurements and continuous monitoring at the bedside. These data can be critical in the evaluation of shock, heart failure, myocardial infarction, respiratory failure, postoperative state, and many other situations. Complications include bleeding, pneumothorax, sepsis, arrhythmias, and pulmonary emboli.

Left heart catheterization permits quantitative assessment of mitral and aortic stenosis. With contrast angiography, valvular regurgitation and global and regional left ventricular function can be examined. Its main application is to produce selective coronary arteriograms.

Grossman W (editor): *Cardiac Catheterization and Angiography,* 3rd ed. Lea & Febiger, 1986.

Matthay MA, Chatterjee K: Bedside catheterization of the pulmonary artery: Risks compared with benefits. Ann Intern Med 1988;109:826. (A sobering perspective on the role of hemodynamic monitoring.)

McGrath RB: Invasive bedside hemodynamic monitoring. Prog Cardiovasc Dis 1986;29:129.

Pepine CJ: *Diagnostic and Therapeutic Catheterization.* Williams & Wilkins, 1989. (Current monograph with good coverage of interventional procedures.)

Electrophysiologic Testing

Intracardiac electrocardiographic recording and stimulation studies have revolutionized the diagnosis and treatment of severe arrhythmias. Electrophysiologic testing is important for evaluating unexplained syncope. The location and severity of atrioventricular conduction disturbances and sinus node dysfunction can be assessed in symptomatic patients in whom diagnostic information cannot be obtained by ambulatory monitoring. The mechanism and optimal therapy of complex supraventricular arrhythmias—particularly those associated with accessory conduction pathways—can be elucidated and the approach to ventricular arrhythmias similarly refined.

ACC/AHA Task Force Report: Guidelines for clinical intracardiac electrophysiologic studies. J Am Coll Cardiol 1989;14:1827.

Zipes DP, Rahimtoola SH (editors): State of the art consensus conference on electrophysiologic testing in the diagnosis and treatment of patients with cardiac arrhythmias. Circulation 1987;75(Suppl 3). (Entire issue.) (Consensus on methodology of, indications for, and significance of electrophysiologic testing.)

CONGENITAL HEART DISEASES

Congenital lesions account for only about 2% of heart disease in adults. Only the most common acyanotic lesions are discussed here. The reader is referred to the following references for full discussions:

Beekman RH, Rocchini AP: Transcatheter treatment of congenital heart disease. Prog Cardiovasc Dis 1989;32:1. (Discusses valve stenosis, coarctation, ASD, and VSD.)

Cheitlin MD: Congenital heart disease in the adult. Mod Concepts Cardiovasc Dis 1986;55:20.

Perloff JK: *The Clinical Recognition of Congenital Heart Disease,* 3rd ed. Saunders, 1987.

Roberts WC (editor): *Adult Congenital Heart Disease.* Davis, 1986.

PULMONARY STENOSIS

Essentials of Diagnosis

- No symptoms in patients with mild or moderately severe lesions.
- Severe cases may present with right-sided heart failure and cause sudden death.
- High-pitched systolic ejection murmur maximal in the second left interspace. S_2 delayed and soft or absent. Ejection click often present. Increased right ventricular impulse.
- Right ventricular hypertrophy on ECG; pulmonary artery dilatation on x-ray. Echo-Doppler diagnostic.

General Considerations

Stenosis of the pulmonary valve or infundibulum

increases the resistance to outflow, raises the right ventricular pressure, and limits pulmonary blood flow. In the absence of associated shunts, arterial saturation is normal, but severe stenosis causes peripheral cyanosis by reducing cardiac output. Clubbing and polycythemia do not develop unless a patent foramen ovale or atrial septal defect is present, permitting right-to-left shunting.

Clinical Findings

A. Symptoms and Signs: Mild cases (right ventricular-pulmonary artery gradient < 59 mm Hg) are asymptomatic. Moderate to severe stenosis (gradients > 80 mm Hg) may cause dyspnea on exertion, syncope, chest pain, and eventually right ventricular failure.

There is a palpable parasternal lift. A loud, harsh systolic murmur and a prominent thrill are present in the left second and third interspaces parasternally; the murmur is in the third and fourth interspaces in infundibular stenosis. The second sound is obscured by the murmur in severe cases; the pulmonary component is diminished, delayed, or absent. Both components are audible in mild cases. A right-sided S_4 and a prominent a wave in the venous pulse are present in severe cases.

B. ECG and Chest X-Ray: Right axis deviation or right ventricular hypertrophy is noted; peaked P waves provide evidence of right atrial overload. Heart size may be normal on radiographs, or there may be a prominent right ventricle and atrium or gross cardiac enlargement, depending upon the severity. There is often poststenotic dilatation of the pulmonary artery. Pulmonary vascularity is normal or diminished.

C. Diagnostic Studies: Echocardiography usually demonstrates the anatomic abnormality and assesses right ventricular size and function. Doppler ultrasound can measure the gradient accurately, which is usually confirmed by cardiac catheterization.

Prognosis & Treatment

Patients with mild stenosis may have a normal life expectancy. Severe stenosis is associated with sudden death and can cause heart failure in the 20s and 30s. Moderate stenosis may be asymptomatic in childhood and adolescence, but symptoms increase as patients grow older.

Symptomatic patients or those with evidence of right ventricular hypertrophy and resting gradients over 75–80 mm Hg require correction in most cases. Percutaneous balloon valvuloplasty has proved successful and is often the treatment of choice. Surgery can be performed with an operative mortality rate of 2–4% and an excellent long-term result in most cases.

Cooke JP, Seward JB, Holmes DR Jr: Transluminal balloon valvotomy for pulmonic stenosis in an adult. Mayo Clin Proc 1987;62:306. (Positive results with new procedure.)
Kopecky SL et al: Long-term outcome of patients undergoing surgical repair of isolated pulmonary valve stenosis. Follow-up at 20–30 years. Circulation 1988;78:1150. (Good results.)

COARCTATION OF THE AORTA

Essentials of Diagnosis

- Infants may have severe heart failure; children and adults are usually asymptomatic, presenting with hypertension.
- Absent or weak femoral pulses.
- Systolic pressure higher in upper extremities than in lower extremities; diastolic pressures are similar.
- Harsh systolic murmur heard in the back.
- ECG shows left ventricular hypertrophy; x-ray shows rib notching. Echo-Doppler is diagnostic.

General Considerations

Coarctation of the aorta consists of localized narrowing of the aortic arch just distal to the origin of the left subclavian artery. A bicuspid aortic valve is present in 25% of cases. Blood pressure is elevated in the aorta and its branches proximal to the coarctation and decreased distally. Collateral circulation develops through the intercostal arteries and branches of the subclavian arteries.

Clinical Findings

A. Symptoms and Signs: If cardiac failure does not occur in infancy, there are usually no symptoms until the hypertension produces left ventricular failure or cerebral hemorrhage; the latter may also occur from associated cerebral aneurysms. Strong arterial pulsations are seen in the neck and suprasternal notch. Hypertension is present in the arms, but the pressure is normal or low in the legs. This difference is exaggerated by exercise. Femoral pulsations are weak and are delayed in comparison with the brachial pulse. Patients with large collaterals may have relatively small gradients but still have severe coarctation. Late systolic ejection murmurs at the base are often heard better posteriorly, especially over the spinous processes. There may be an associated aortic insufficiency murmur due to a bicuspid aortic valve.

B. ECG and Chest X-Ray: The ECG usually shows left ventricular hypertrophy. Radiography shows scalloping of the ribs due to enlarged collateral intercostal arteries, dilatation of the left subclavian artery and poststenotic aortic dilatation, and left ventricular enlargement.

C. Diagnostic Studies: Measurement of the gradient across the lesion by catheterization and aortography remain the primary methods of diagnosis. Doppler ultrasound can also estimate the severity of obstruction.

Prognosis & Treatment

Cardiac failure is common in infancy and in older untreated patients; it is uncommon in late childhood and young adulthood. Most untreated patients with the adult form of coarctation die before age 40 from the complications of hypertension, rupture of the aorta, infective endarteritis, or cerebral hemorrhage (congenital aneurysms). Aortic dissection also occurs with increased frequency in coarctation.

Resection of the coarcted site has a surgical mortality rate near 1–4%. The risks of the disease are such, however, that all coarctations in patients up to age 20 years should be resected. In patients under 40 years of age, surgery is advisable if the patient has refractory hypertension or significant left ventricular hypertrophy. The surgical mortality rate rises considerably in patients over age 50 and is of doubtful value. Balloon angioplasty of the stenosis has been accomplished successfully and may become the procedure of choice, but aortic tears have been described. About one-fourth of corrected patients continue to be hypertensive years after surgery and they have all the complications associated with hypertension.

ATRIAL SEPTAL DEFECT

Essentials of Diagnosis

- Usually asymptomatic until middle age.
- Right ventricular lift; S$_2$ widely split and fixed.
- Grade I–III/VI systolic ejection murmur at pulmonic area.
- ECG shows right ventricular conduction delay; x-ray shows dilated pulmonary arteries and increased vascularity. Echo-Doppler usually diagnostic.

General Considerations

The most common form of atrial septal defect (80% of cases) is persistence of the ostium secundum in the mid septum; less commonly, the ostium primum (which is low in the septum) persists, in which case mitral or tricuspid abnormalities may also be present. A third form is the sinus venosus defect of the upper part of the septum. This is often associated with partial anomalous drainage of the pulmonary veins into the superior vena cava. In all cases, normally oxygenated blood from the left atrium passes into the right atrium, increasing right ventricular output and pulmonary blood flow.

Clinical Findings

A. Symptoms and Signs: Most patients with small or moderate defects are asymptomatic. With large shunts, exertional dyspnea or cardiac failure may develop, most commonly in the fourth decade or later. Prominent right ventricular and pulmonary artery pulsations are readily visible and palpable. A moderately loud systolic ejection murmur can be heard in the second and third interspaces parasternally as a result of increased pulmonary artery flow. S$_2$ is widely split and does not vary with breathing.

B. ECG and Chest X-Ray: Right axis deviation or right ventricular hypertrophy may be present in ostium secundum defects. Incomplete or complete right bundle branch block is present in nearly all cases of atrial septal defect, and superior axis deviation is noted in ostium primum defect. With sinus venosus defects, the P axis is leftward of +15 degrees. The chest radiograph shows large pulmonary arteries (with vigorous pulsations fluoroscopically), increased pulmonary vascularity, an enlarged right atrium and ventricle, and a small aortic knob.

C. Diagnostic Studies: Echocardiography can demonstrate right ventricular volume overload with a large right ventricle and atrium, and sometimes the defect itself. Echocardiography with contrast and Doppler flow studies can demonstrate shunting and increased pulmonary flow. Radionuclide flow studies quantify left-to-right shunting, and MRI can also elucidate the anatomy. Cardiac catheterization remains the definitive diagnostic procedure, since it can demonstrate an oxygen saturation "step-up," quantify the shunt, and measure pulmonary vascular resistance. Right and left ventricular contrast angiography may demonstrate associated valvular abnormalities or anomalous pulmonary venous drainage.

Prognosis & Treatment

Patients with small shunts may live a normal life span. Large shunts cause disability by age 40. Raised pulmonary vascular resistance secondary to pulmonary hypertension rarely occurs in childhood or young adult life in secundum defects but is more common in primum defects; after age 40, pulmonary hypertension, cardiac arrhythmias, and heart failure may occur in secundum defects. Infective endocarditis does not occur with increased frequency.

Small atrial septal defects do not require surgery. The risks are now sufficiently low so that patients with pulmonary to systemic flow ratios between 1.5 and 2.0 may be operated on if the total clinical picture warrants. Ratios exceeding 2.0 are an indication for surgical closure of the defect.

Surgery should be withheld from patients with pulmonary hypertension with reversed (right-to-left) shunt because of the risk of acute right heart failure. Relocation of pulmonary veins is required in patients with partial anomalous venous drainage. In ostium primum defects, in addition to closure of the defect, suture of the valve clefts—especially those of the mitral valve—is advisable if mitral regurgitation of any significant degree is present. The surgical mortality rate is low (< 1%) in patients under age 45, those who are not in cardiac failure, and those who have systolic pulmonary artery pressures less than 60 mm Hg. It increases to 5–10% in patients over age 40, with cardiac failure, or with systolic pulmonary artery pressures greater than 60 mm Hg.

Feldman T, Borow KM: Atrial septal defects in adults: Diagnosis and management. Cardiovasc Med (March) 1986;11:19.

PATENT DUCTUS ARTERIOSUS

Essentials of Diagnosis

- Adults with small or moderately large patent ductus are usually asymptomatic at least until middle age.
- Widened pulse pressure; loud S_2.
- Continuous murmur over pulmonary area; thrill common.
- Echo-Doppler is helpful, but the lesion is best visualized by aortography.

General Considerations

The embryonic ductus arteriosus fails to close normally and persists as a shunt connecting the left pulmonary artery and aorta, usually near the origin of the left subclavian artery. Prior to birth, the ductus is kept patent by the effect of circulating prostaglandins; in early infancy, a patent ductus can often be closed by administration of intravenous indomethacin. Blood flows continuously from the aorta through the ductus into the pulmonary artery in both systole and diastole; the defect is a form of arteriovenous fistula, increasing the work of the left ventricle. If it remains open, obliterative changes in the pulmonary arterioles can cause pulmonary hypertension. Then the shunt is bidirectional or right-to-left (Eisenmenger's syndrome). This complication does not correlate with shunt size.

Clinical Findings

A. Symptoms and Signs: There are no symptoms unless left ventricular failure or pulmonary hypertension develops. The heart is of normal size or slightly enlarged, with a hyperdynamic apical impulse. The pulse pressure is wide, and diastolic pressure is low. A continuous rough "machinery" murmur, accentuated in late systole at the time of S_2, is heard best in the left first and second interspaces at the left sternal border. Thrills are common.

B. ECG and Chest X-Ray: A normal tracing or left ventricular hypertrophy is found, depending upon the magnitude of shunting. On chest radiographs, the heart is normal in size and contour, or there may be left ventricular and left atrial enlargement. The pulmonary artery, aorta, and left atrium are prominent.

C. Diagnostic Studies: Echocardiography quantifies left ventricular and atrial size. The magnitude of the shunt can also be determined by radionuclide flow studies. Cardiac catheterization establishes the presence and severity of a left-to-right shunt and whether pulmonary hypertension is present; angiography can define its anatomy.

Prognosis & Treatment

Large shunts cause a high mortality rate from cardiac failure early in life. Smaller shunts are compatible with long survival, congestive heart failure being the most common complication. Infective endocarditis or endarteritis may also occur, and antibiotic prophylaxis is required. A small percentage of patients develop pulmonary hypertension and reversal of shunt (right-to-left shunting), such that the lower legs, especially the toes, appear cyanotic and clubbed in contrast to normally pink fingers. At this stage, the patient is inoperable.

Surgical correction is recommended for children or adults with symptoms or large shunts. Asymptomatic adults with no left ventricular hypertrophy and small left-to-right shunts are at low risk of developing pulmonary hypertension or congestive heart failure. The indications for ligation or division of a patent ductus arteriosus in the presence of pulmonary hypertension are controversial. Opinion favors ligation whenever the pulmonary vascular resistance is low and the flow through the ductus is from left to right.

VENTRICULAR SEPTAL DEFECT

Essentials of Diagnosis

- Adults asymptomatic if defect is small to moderate.
- Grade II–VI/VI pansystolic murmur maximal at the left sternal border; associated thrill common.
- ECG may show left or right ventricular hypertrophy if shunt is reversed; x-ray shows increased pulmonary vascularity. Echo-Doppler is diagnostic.

General Considerations

In this lesion, a persistent opening in the upper interventricular septum resulting from failure of fusion with the aortic septum permits blood to pass from the high-pressure left ventricle into the low-pressure right ventricle. The subsequent natural history and pathophysiology depend on the size of the defect and the magnitude of left-to-right shunting. Large defects are associated with early left ventricular failure. Chronic but more moderate left-to-right shunts may lead to pulmonary vascular disease and right-sided failure. Many ventricular defects close spontaneously in early childhood.

Clinical Findings

A. Symptoms and Signs: The clinical features are dependent upon the size of the defect and the presence or absence of a raised pulmonary vascular resistance. Large shunts are associated with loud, harsh holosystolic murmurs in the left third and fourth interspaces along the sternum and, in some cases, middiastolic flow murmurs and an S_3 at the apex. Smaller shunts may produce only an early systolic murmur or a diamond-shaped murmur. A systolic thrill is common. Clinical evidence of pulmonary hypertension is often more informative than the murmur itself. High defects may be associated with aortic regurgitation owing to prolapse of a valve leaflet.

B. ECG and Chest X-Ray: The ECG may be normal or may show right, left, or biventricular hypertrophy, depending on the size of the defect and the pulmonary vascular resistance. With large shunts, the right or left ventricle (or both), the left atrium, and the pulmonary arteries are enlarged, and pulmonary vascularity is increased on chest radiographs. If pulmonary vascular disease evolves, an enlarged pulmonary artery with diminished distal vascularity is seen.

C. Diagnostic Studies: Echocardiography can demonstrate chamber size and may demonstrate the defect. Doppler ultrasound can qualitatively assess the magnitude of shunting and the pulmonary artery pressure. Magnetic resonance imaging can often visualize the defect, while radionuclide flow studies quantify pulmonary-to-systemic flow ratios. Cardiac catheterization permits definitive diagnosis in all but the most trivial defects; it is the only technique that can measure pulmonary vascular resistance.

Prognosis & Treatment

Patients with the typical murmur as the only abnormality have a normal life expectancy except for the threat of infective endocarditis. The latter is more typical of smaller shunts. Antibiotic prophylaxis is mandatory. With large shunts, congestive heart failure may develop early in life, and survival beyond age 40 is unusual. Shunt reversal occurs in an estimated 25%, producing Eisenmenger's syndrome.

Small shunts (pulmonary-to-systemic flow ratio > 1.5) in asymptomatic patients do not require surgery. Defects causing large shunts should be repaired to prevent irreversible pulmonary vascular disease or late heart failure. When severe pulmonary hypertension is present (systolic pulmonary arterial pressures > 85 mm Hg) and the left-to-right shunt is small, the surgical mortality risk is at least 50%. If the shunt is reversed, surgery is contraindicated. If surgery is required because of unrelenting cardiac failure in infancy due to a large left-to-right shunt, early closure of the defect is now the preferred procedure. The surgical mortality rate is 2–3% for primary repair. Some defects (perhaps as many as 30%) close spontaneously. Therefore, surgery should be deferred until late childhood unless the disability is severe or unless pulmonary hypertension is observed to develop or progress.

ACUTE RHEUMATIC FEVER & RHEUMATIC HEART DISEASE

Essentials of Diagnosis

- Uncommon in USA except in immigrants.
- Peak incidence ages 5–15 years.
- Diagnosis based on Jones criteria (see text) and confirmation of streptococcal infection.
- May involve mitral and other valves acutely, rarely leading to heart failure.

General Considerations

Rheumatic fever is a systemic immune process which is a sequela to hemolytic streptococcal infection. It may be self-limited or may lead to slowly progressive valvular deformity. It had become uncommon in the USA, except in recent immigrants. However, there have been recent reports of new outbreaks in several regions of the USA. The peak incidence is between ages 5 and 15; rheumatic fever is rare before age 4 and after age 40. The characteristic lesion is a perivascular granulomatous reaction with vasculitis. The mitral valve is attacked in 75–80% of cases, the aortic valve in 30%, and the tricuspid and pulmonary valves in under 5%.

Clinical Findings

The presence of 2 major criteria—or one major and one minor criterion—establishes the diagnosis.

A. Major Criteria:

1. Carditis–Carditis is most likely to be evident in children and adolescents. Any of the following signs establishes the presence of carditis. (1) Pericarditis, which is uncommon in adults and diagnosed by detection of a friction rub or evidence of effusion by echocardiogram. (2) Cardiomegaly, detected by physical signs, radiography, or echocardiography. (3) Congestive failure, right–or left-sided—the former perhaps more prominent in children, with painful liver engorgement due to tricuspid regurgitation. (4) Mitral or aortic regurgitation murmurs, indicative of dilatation of a valve ring with or without associated valvulitis. The Carey-Coombs short middiastolic mitral murmur may be present.

In the absence of any of the above definitive signs, the diagnosis of carditis depends upon the following less specific abnormalities. (1) Electrocardiographic changes: The most significant abnormality is PR prolongation greater than 0.04 s above the patient's normal. Changing contour of P waves or inversion of T waves is less useful. (2) Changing quality of heart sounds. (3) Sinus tachycardia persisting during sleep and markedly increased by slight activity. (4) Arrhythmias, shifting pacemaker, ectopic beats.

2. Erythema marginatum and subcutaneous nodules–The former begin as rapidly enlarging macules that assume the shape of rings or crescents with clear centers. They may be raised, confluent, and either transient or persistent.

Subcutaneous nodules are uncommon except in children. They are small (≤ 2 cm in diameter), firm, and nontender and are attached to fascia or tendon sheaths over bony prominences. They persist for days or weeks, are recurrent, and are indistinguishable from rheumatoid nodules.

3. Sydenham's chorea–Sydenham's chorea—involuntary choreoathetoid movements primarily of the face, tongue, and upper extremities—may be the sole manifestation; half of cases have other overt signs of rheumatic fever. Girls are more frequently affected, and occurrence in adults is rare. This is the least common (3% of cases) but most diagnostic of the manifestations of rheumatic fever.

4. Arthritis–This is a migratory polyarthritis that involves the large joints sequentially. In adults, only a single joint may be affected. The arthritis lasts 1–5 weeks and subsides without residual deformity. Prompt response of arthritis to therapeutic doses of salicylates is characteristic.

B. Minor Criteria: These include fever, polyarthralgias, reversible prolongation of the PR interval, rapid erythrocyte sedimentation rate, evidence of an antecedent β-hemolytic streptococcal infection, or a history of rheumatic fever.

C. Laboratory Findings: There is nonspecific evidence of inflammatory disease, as shown by a rapid sedimentation rate. High or increasing titers of antistreptococcal antibodies, especially antistreptolysin O (ASO), are used to confirm recent infection; 10% of cases lack this serologic evidence.

Differential Diagnosis

Rheumatic fever may be confused with the following: rheumatoid arthritis, osteomyelitis, endocarditis, chronic meningococcemia, systemic lupus erythematosus, Lyme disease, sickle cell anemia, "surgical abdomen," and many other diseases.

Complications

Congestive heart failure occurs in severe cases. In the longer term, the development of rheumatic heart disease is the major problem. Other complications include arrhythmias, pericarditis with effusion, and rheumatic pneumonitis.

Primary Prevention

Rheumatic fever can usually be prevented by early and complete treatment of streptococcal infections. Oral penicillin V (250 mg 3 times daily for 10 days) or benzathine penicillin (600,000 units intramuscularly for patients weighing less than 60 lb; 1.2 million units intramuscularly for those weighing more than 60 lb) should be given. Oral erythromycin (40 mg/kg up to a maximum of 1 g in 2–4 doses) can be substituted in penicillin-allergic patients.

Treatment

A. Medical Measures:

1. Salicylates–The salicylates markedly reduce fever and relieve joint pain and swelling. They have no effect on the natural course of the disease. Adults may require aspirin, 0.6–0.9 g every 4 hours; children are treated with lower doses. Toxicity includes tinnitus, vomiting, and gastrointestinal bleeding.

2. Penicillin–Penicillin (benzathine penicillin, 1.2 million units intramuscularly daily for 10 days, or procaine penicillin, 600,000 units intramuscularly daily for 10 days) is employed to eradicate streptococcal infection if present. Erythromycin (dosage as above) may be substituted.

3. Corticosteroids–There is no proof that cardiac damage is prevented or minimized by corticosteroids. A short course of corticosteroids (prednisone, 40–60 mg orally daily, with tapering over 2 weeks) usually causes rapid improvement and is indicated when response to salicylates has been inadequate.

B. General Measures: Bed rest should be enforced until: return of temperature to normal without medications; normal sedimentation rate; normal resting pulse rate (< 100/min in adults); and return of ECG to baseline.

Prevention of Recurrent Rheumatic Fever

The goals of prevention are to avoid β-hemolytic streptococcal infections or to treat them promptly. Recurrences of rheumatic fever are most common in patients who have had carditis during their initial episode and in children, 20% of whom will have a second episode within 5 years. Recurrences are uncommon after 5 years and infrequent in patients over 25 years of age. Prophylaxis is usually discontinued after these times except in groups with a high risk of streptococcal infection—parents of young children, nurses, military recruits, etc.

A. Penicillin: The preferred method of prophylaxis is with benzathine penicillin G, 1.2 million units intramuscularly every 4 weeks. Oral penicillin (200,000–250,000 units twice daily) is less reliable.

B. Sulfonamides or Erythromycin: If the patient is allergic to penicillin, sulfadiazine (or sulfisoxazole), 1 g daily throughout the year, may be substituted, as may erythromycin, 250 mg orally twice daily.

Prognosis

Initial episodes of rheumatic fever last months in children and weeks in adults. The immediate mortality rate is 1–2%. Persistent rheumatic carditis with cardiomegaly, heart failure, and pericarditis imply a poor prognosis; 30% of children thus affected die within 10 years after the initial attack. Eighty percent of affected children attain adult life, and half of these have little if any limitation of activity. After 10 years, two-thirds of surviving patients will have detectable valvular disease. In adults, residual heart damage occurs in less than 20%, with mitral insufficiency the commonest; aortic insufficiency is more common than in children. In underdeveloped countries, acute rheumatic fever appears earlier in life, and the evolution to chronic valvular disease is accelerated.

Dajani AS et al: Prevention of rheumatic fever. Circulation 1988;78:1082. (American Heart Association consensus statement on who needs prophylaxis and what to give.)

Gotsman MS: Rheumatic fever in the 80's. (2 parts.) Cardiovasc Rev Rep 1985;6:861, 935.

Jones criteria (revised) for guidance in the diagnosis of rheumatic fever. Circulation 1984;69:A204. (American Heart Association consensus statement.)

Veasy LG et al: Resurgence of acute rheumatic fever in the intermountain area of the United States. N Engl J Med 1987;316:421. (Reminder that acute rheumatic fever still occurs.)

RHEUMATIC HEART DISEASE

Chronic rheumatic heart disease results from single or repeated attacks of rheumatic fever that produce rigidity and deformity of valve cusps, fusion of the commissures, or shortening and fusion of the chordae tendineae. Stenosis or insufficiency results, and the two often coexist. The mitral valve alone is affected in 50–60% of cases; combined lesions of the aortic and mitral valves occur in 20%; pure aortic lesions are seen in only 10%. Tricuspid involvement occurs only in association with mitral or aortic disease in about 10% of cases. The pulmonary valve is rarely affected. A history of rheumatic fever is obtainable in only 60% of patients with rheumatic heart disease.

The first clue to organic valvular disease is a murmur. Physical examination permits accurate diagnosis of most valve lesions. Echocardiography will reveal valve cusp thickening with decreased opening in stenosis, estimate the magnitude of regurgitation, and demonstrate the earliest stages of specific chamber enlargement.

Recurrences of acute rheumatic fever can be prevented (see above). The patient should also receive prophylactic antibiotics preceding dental extraction, urologic and surgical procedures, etc, to prevent endocarditis. With mitral valve disease, it is important to identify the onset of atrial fibrillation in order to institute anticoagulation. The important findings in each of the major valve lesions are summarized in Table 8–1. The hemodynamic changes, symptoms, associated findings, and course are discussed below.

VALVULAR HEART DISEASE

While most cases of valvular disease were at one time due to rheumatic heart disease (still true in underdeveloped countries), other causes are now more common. The typical findings of each lesion are described in Fig 8–1 and Table 8–1.

MITRAL STENOSIS

Essentials of Diagnosis
- Dyspnea, orthopnea, and paroxysmal nocturnal dyspnea.
- Symptoms often precipitated by onset of atrial fibrillation or pregnancy.
- Prominent mitral first sound, opening snap (usually), and apical crescendo diastolic rumble.
- ECG shows left atrial abnormality and, commonly, atrial fibrillation. Echo-Doppler confirms diagnosis and quantitates severity.

General Considerations
Nearly all patients with mitral stenosis have underlying rheumatic heart disease, though a history of rheumatic fever is often absent.

Clinical Findings
A. Symptoms and Signs: A characteristic finding of mitral stenosis is a localized middiastolic murmur low in pitch whose duration varies with the severity of the stenosis and the heart rate (Table 8–1). Because it is thickened, the valve opens in early diastole with an opening snap. The sound is sharp, is widely distributed over the chest, and occurs early after A_2 in severe and later in milder varieties of mitral stenosis. In severe mitral stenosis with low flow across the mitral valve, the murmur may be soft and difficult to find, but the opening snap can usually be heard. If the patient has both mitral stenosis and mitral insufficiency, the dominant features may be the systolic murmur of mitral regurgitation with or without a short diastolic murmur and a delayed opening snap.

When the valve has narrowed to less than 1.5 cm^2 (normal, 4–6 cm^2), the left atrial pressure must rise to maintain normal flow across the valve and a normal cardiac output. This results in a pressure difference between the left atrium and left ventricle during diastole. The pressure gradient and the length of the diastolic murmur reflect the severity of mitral stenosis; they persist throughout the diastole when the lesion is severe or when the ventricular rate is rapid.

In mild cases, left atrial pressure and cardiac output may be essentially normal and the patient asymptomatic, but in moderate stenosis (valve area < 1.5

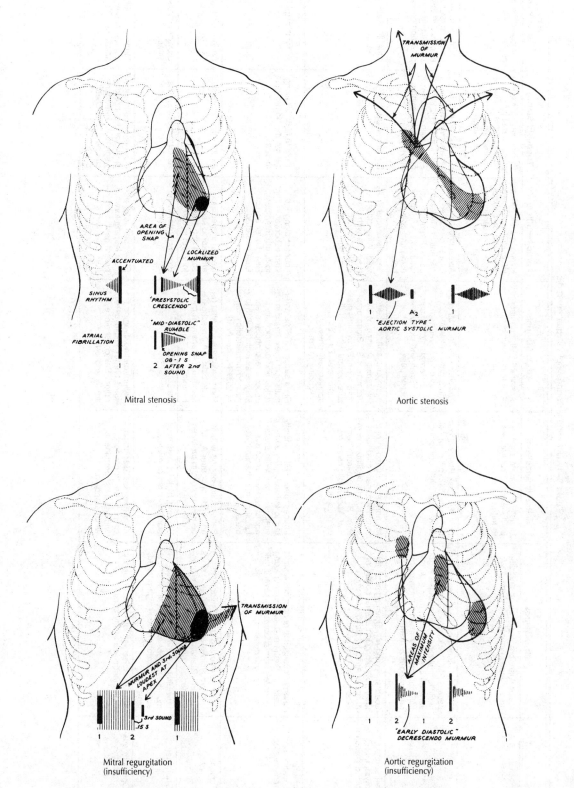

Figure 8–1. Murmurs and cardiac enlargement in common valve lesions.

Table 8-1. Differential diagnosis of valvular heart disease.

	Mitral Stenosis	Mitral Insufficiency	Aortic Stenosis	Aortic Insufficiency	Tricuspid Stenosis	Tricuspid Insufficiency
Inspection	Malar flush, precordial bulge and diffuse pulsation in young patients.	Usually prominent and hyperdynamic apical impulse to left of MCL.	Sustained PMI, prominent atrial filling wave.	Hyperdynamic PMI to left of MCL and down. Visible carotid pulsations. Capillary pulsations.	Giant a wave in jugular pulse with sinus rhythm. Often olive-colored skin (mixed jaundice and local cyanosis).	Large v wave in jugular pulse.
Palpation	"Tapping" sensation over area of expected PMI. Middiastolic and/or presystolic thrill at apex. Small pulse. Right ventricular pulsation left third to fifth ICS parasternally when pulmonary hypertension is present.	Forceful, brisk PMI; systolic thrill over PMI. Pulse normal, small, or slightly collapsing.	Powerful, heaving PMI to left and slightly below MCL. Systolic thrill over aortic area, sternal notch, or carotids. Small and slowly rising carotid pulse.	Apical impulse forceful and displaced significantly to left and down. Prominent carotid pulses. Rapidly rising and collapsing pulses.	Middiastolic thrill between lower left sternal border and PMI. Presystolic pulsation of liver (sinus rhythm only).	Right ventricular pulsation. Occasionally systolic thrill at lower left sternal edge. Systolic pulsation of liver.
Heart sounds, rhythm, and blood pressure	Loud snapping M_1. Opening snap following A_2 along left sternal border or at apex. Atrial fibrillation common. Blood pressure normal.	M_1 normal or buried in murmur. Prominent third heart sound. Atrial fibrillation common. Blood pressure normal. Midsystolic clicks may be present.	A_2 normal, soft, or absent. Paradoxic splitting of S_2. Prominent S_4. Blood pressure normal or systolic pressure normal with high diastolic level. Ejection click occasionally present just preceding murmur.	Sounds normal or A_2 loud. Wide pulse pressure with diastolic pressure < 60 mm Hg.	M_1 often loud.	Atrial fibrillation usually present.
Murmurs: Location and transmission	Sharply localized at or near apex, short diastolic (Graham Steell) murmur along lower left sternal border in severe pulmonary hypertension.	Loudest over PMI; transmitted to left axilla, left infrascapular area. With posterior papillary muscle dysfunction, may transmit to base.	Right second ICS parasternally or at apex; heard in carotids and occasionally in upper interscapular area. May be associated with low-pitched middiastolic murmur at apex (Austin Flint).	Loudest along left sternal border in third to fourth interspace. Heard over aortic area and apex.	Third to fifth ICS along left sternal border out to apex.	As for tricuspid stenosis.
Timing	Onset at opening snap ("middiastolic") with presystolic accentuation if in sinus rhythm. Graham Steell begins with P_2 (immediate diastolic).	Pansystolic: begins with M_1 and ends at or after A_2. May be late systolic in prolapse.	Midsystolic: begins after M_1, ends before A_2, reaches maximum intensity in mid systole.	Begins immediately after aortic second sound and ends before first sound.	As for mitral stenosis.	As for mitral insufficiency.
Character	Low-pitched, rumbling; presystolic murmur merges with loud M_1 in a "crescendo." Graham Steell high-pitched, blowing.	Blowing, high-pitched; occasionally harsh or musical.	Harsh, rough.	Blowing, often faint.	As for mitral stenosis.	Blowing, coarse, or musical.
Optimum auscultatory conditions	After exercise, left lateral recumbency. Bell chest piece lightly applied.	After exercise; diaphragm chest piece. In prolapse, findings most prominent while standing.	Patient resting, leaning forward, breath held in full expiration. Bell chest piece lightly applied.	Slow heart rate; patient leaning forward, breath held in expiration. Diaphragm chest piece.	Murmur usually louder during and at peak of inspiration. Patient recumbent. Bell chest piece.	Murmur usually becomes louder during inspiration.

X-ray	Straight left heart border. Large left atrium sharply indenting esophagus. Elevation of left bronchus. Large right ventricle and pulmonary artery if pulmonary hypertension present. Calcification occasionally seen in mitral valve.	Enlarged left ventricle and left atrium.	Concentric left ventricular hypertrophy. Prominent ascending aorta, small knob. Calcified valve common.	Moderate to severe left ventricular enlargement. Prominent aortic knob.	Enlarged right atrium only.	Enlarged right atrium and ventricle.
ECG	Broad P waves in standard leads; broad negative phase of diphasic P in V_1. If pulmonary hypertension is present, tall peaked P waves, right axis deviation, or right ventricular hypertrophy appears.	Left axis deviation or frank left ventricular hypertrophy. P waves broad, tall, or notched in standard leads; broad negative phase of diphasic P in V_1.	Left ventricular hypertrophy.	Left ventricular hypertrophy.	Tall, peaked P waves. Normal axis.	Right axis usual.
Echocardiography M mode	Thickened, immobile mitral valve with anterior and posterior leaflets moving together. Slow early diastolic filling slope, left atrial enlargement, normal to small left ventricle.	Thickened mitral valve in rheumatic disease; mitral valve prolapse; flail leaflet or vegetations may be seen. Enlarged left ventricle with above—normal, normal, or decreased function.	Dense persistent echoes from the aortic valve with poor leaflet excursion, left ventricular hypertrophy with preserved contractile function.	Diastolic vibrations of the anterior leaflet of the mitral valve and septum, early closure of the mitral valve when severe, dilated left ventricle with normal or decreased contractility.	Tricuspid valve thickening, decreased early diastolic filling slope of the tricuspid valve. Mitral valve also usually abnormal.	Enlarged right ventricle, prolapsing valve, mitral valve often abnormal.
Two-dimensional	Maximum diastolic orifice size reduced, subvalvular apparatus foreshortened, variable thickening of other valves.	Same as M-mode but more reliable.	Above plus poststenotic dilatation of the aorta, restricted opening of the aortic leaflets, bicuspid aortic valve in about 30%.	Above plus may show vegetations in endocarditis, bicuspid valve, root dilatation.	Above plus enlargement of the right atrium.	Same as above.
Doppler	Prolonged pressure half-time across mitral valve; indirect evidence of pulmonary hypertension.	Regurgitant flow mapped into left atrium; indirect evidence of pulmonary hypertension.	Increased transvalvular flow velocity, yielding calculated gradient.	Demonstrates regurgitation and qualitatively estimates severity.	Prolonged pressure half-time across tricuspid valve.	Regurgitant flow mapped into right atrium and venae cavae; right ventricular systolic pressure estimated.

A_2 = Aortic second sound
ICS = Intercostal space
M_1 = Mitral first sound

MCL = Midclavicular line
P_2 = Pulmonary second sound
PMI = Point of maximal impulse

cm^2)—especially with tachycardia, which shortens diastole and increases mitral flow rate—dyspnea and fatigue appear as the left atrial pressure rises. With severe stenosis, the left atrial pressure is high enough to produce pulmonary venous congestion at rest and reduce cardiac output, with resulting dyspnea, fatigue, and right heart failure. Recumbency at night further increases the pulmonary blood volume, causing orthopnea, paroxysmal nocturnal dyspnea, or actual transudation of fluid into the alveoli, leading to acute pulmonary edema. Severe pulmonary congestion may also be initiated by any acute respiratory infection, excessive salt and fluid intake, endocarditis, or recurrence of rheumatic carditis. As a result of long-standing pulmonary venous hypertension, anastomoses develop between the pulmonary and bronchial veins in the form of bronchial submucosal varices. These often rupture, producing mild or severe hemoptysis.

Fifty to 80% of patients develop paroxysmal or chronic atrial fibrillation that, until the ventricular rate is controlled, may precipitate dyspnea or pulmonary edema. Twenty to 30% of these patients will have major emboli in the cerebral, visceral, or peripheral arteries.

In a few patients, the pulmonary arterioles become narrowed; this greatly increases the pulmonary artery pressure and accelerates the development of right ventricular hypertrophy and failure. These patients have relatively little dyspnea but experience fatigue on exertion.

B. Diagnostic Studies: Echocardiography is the most valuable technique for assessing mitral stenosis. The valve is thickened, opens poorly, and closes slowly. The anterior and posterior leaflets are fixed and move together, rather than in opposite directions. Left atrial size can be determined by echocardiography: increased size denotes an increased likelihood of atrial fibrillation or systemic emboli. The mitral valve area can be measured, and the gradient and pulmonary artery pressure can be estimated by Doppler techniques. Echocardiography also detects atrial myxoma, which sometimes presents clinically in a fashion resembling mitral stenosis.

Because echocardiography provides most of the needed information, cardiac catheterization is employed primarily to detect associated valve, coronary, or myocardial disease—usually preoperatively.

Treatment & Prognosis

Mitral stenosis may be present for a lifetime with few or no symptoms, or it may become severe in a few years. In most cases, there is a long asymptomatic phase, followed by subtle limitation of activity. The onset of atrial fibrillation often precipitates more severe symptoms, although with return to sinus rhythm (using digoxin and, often, class I antiarrhythmic agents) or ventricular rate control, the patient may improve. Conversion to and subsequent maintenance of sinus rhythm is most commonly successful when

the duration of atrial fibrillation is brief ($<$ 6–12 months) and the left atrium is not severely dilated (diameter $<$ 4.5 cm). Once atrial fibrillation occurs, the patient should receive anticoagulation therapy. Systemic embolization in the presence of only mild to moderate disease is not an indication for surgery but should be treated with anticoagulants.

Indications for relieving the stenosis include the following: (1) uncontrollable pulmonary edema; (2) limiting dyspnea and intermittent pulmonary edema; (3) evidence of pulmonary hypertension with right ventricular hypertrophy or hemoptysis; (4) limitation of activity despite ventricular rate control and medical therapy; and (5) recurrent systemic emboli despite anticoagulation with moderate or severe stenosis.

Open mitral commissurotomy may be effective in patients without substantial mitral regurgitation. Replacement of the valve is indicated when combined stenosis and insufficiency are present or when the mitral valve is so distorted and calcified that a satisfactory valvulotomy is not possible. Operative mortality rates are low: 1–5% in most institutions. Balloon valvuloplasty is becoming increasingly popular. Initial success rates are high, especially if valve calcification is not excessive. The rate of restenosis is not yet known but appears to be lower than that with aortic stenosis. In most centers, surgery remains the procedure of choice except in patients with contraindications.

Problems associated with prosthetic valves are thrombosis (especially at the mitral position), paravalvular leak, endocarditis, and degenerative changes in tissue valves. Anticoagulant therapy is mandatory with mechanical prostheses and is usually employed for at least the initial 3 months with bioprostheses, especially if the patient has significant left atrial enlargement and remains in atrial fibrillation.

Keren G et al: Atrial fibrillation and atrial enlargement in patients with mitral stenosis. Am Heart J 1987;114:1146. (Current discussion of age-old problem.)

Palacios I et al: Percutaneous balloon valvotomy for patients with severe mitral stenosis. Circulation 1987:75:778.

Rahimtoola SH: Catheter balloon valvuloplasty of aortic and mitral stenosis in adults. Circulation 1987;75:895.

MITRAL REGURGITATION
(Mitral Insufficiency)

Essentials of Diagnosis

- Variable causes determine clinical presentation.
- May be asymptomatic for many years (or for life) or may cause left-sided heart failure.
- Pansystolic murmur at the apex, radiating into the axilla; associated with S_3.
- ECG shows left atrial abnormality and left ventricular hypertrophy; x-ray shows left atrial and ventricular enlargement. Echo-Doppler confirms diagnosis and estimates severity.

General Considerations

Mitral regurgitation may result from many processes. Rheumatic disease is associated with a thickened valve with reduced mobility and often a mixed picture of stenosis and regurgitation. Rheumatic disease has been replaced as the commonest cause of mitral regurgitation in most developed countries by other processes, which include myxomatous degeneration (eg, **mitral valve prolapse** with or without connective tissue diseases such as Marfan's syndrome), infective endocarditis, and subvalvular dysfunction (due to papillary muscle dysfunction or ruptured chordae tendineae). Cardiac tumors, chiefly left atrial myxoma, are a rare cause of mitral regurgitation.

Clinical Findings

A. Symptoms and Signs: During left ventricular systole, the mitral leaflets do not close normally, and blood is ejected into the left atrium as well as through the aortic valve. The net effect is an increased volume load on the left ventricle, and the presentation depends on the rapidity with which the lesion develops. In acute regurgitation, left atrial pressure rises abruptly, leading to pulmonary edema if severe. When it is chronic, the left atrium enlarges progressively, but the pressure in pulmonary veins and capillaries rises only transiently during exertion. Exertional dyspnea and fatigue progress gradually over many years.

Mitral regurgitation, like mitral stenosis, predisposes to atrial fibrillation; but this arrhythmia is less likely to provoke acute pulmonary congestion, and fewer than 5% of patients have peripheral arterial emboli. Mitral regurgitation more often predisposes to infective endocarditis.

Clinically, mitral regurgitation is characterized by a pansystolic murmur maximal at the apex, radiating to the axilla and occasionally to the base; a hyperdynamic left ventricular impulse and a brisk carotid upstroke; and a prominent third heart sound. Left atrial enlargement is usually considerable in chronic mitral regurgitation; the degree of left ventricular enlargement usually reflects the severity of regurgitation. Calcification of the mitral valve is less common than in pure mitral stenosis. The same is true of enlargement of the main pulmonary artery on radiographs. Hemodynamically, left ventricular volume overload may ultimately lead to left ventricular failure and reduced cardiac output, but for many years the left ventricular end-diastolic pressure and the cardiac output may be normal at rest, even with considerable increase in left ventricular volume.

Nonrheumatic mitral regurgitation may develop abruptly, such as with papillary muscle dysfunction following myocardial infarction, valve perforation in infective endocarditis, or ruptured chordae tendineae in mitral valve prolapse. In acute mitral insufficiency, patients are in sinus rhythm rather than atrial fibrillation, have little or no enlargement of the left atrium, no calcification of the mitral valve, no associated mitral stenosis, and in many cases little left ventricular dilatation.

Myxomatous mitral valve ("floppy" or "billowing" mitral valve, or mitral valve prolapse) is usually asymptomatic but may be associated with nonspecific chest pain, dyspnea, fatigue, or palpitations. Most patients are female, many are thin, and some have minor chest wall deformities. There are characteristic midsystolic clicks, which may be multiple, often but not always followed by a late systolic murmur. These findings are accentuated in the standing position. The diagnosis is primarily clinical but can be confirmed echocardiographically. Its significance is in dispute because of the frequency (up to 10%) with which it is diagnosed in healthy young men and women, but in occasional patients this lesion is not benign. Patients who have only a midsystolic click usually have no sequelae, but patients with a late or pansystolic murmur may develop significant mitral insufficiency, often due to rupture of chordae tendineae. The need for valve replacement is commonest in men and increases with aging, so that approximately 2% of patients with clinically significant regurgitation over age 60 will require surgery. Infective endocarditis may occur, chiefly in patients with murmurs; such patients should have antibiotic prophylaxis prior to dental work and surgical procedures. Sudden death is rare and is probably related to ventricular tachycardias; β-adrenergic blocking agents are often effective for supraventricular arrhythmias. If symptomatic ventricular tachycardia or fibrillation is present, antiarrhythmic therapy and, in many cases, electrophysiologic studies are indicated. An association between mitral prolapse and embolic cerebrovascular events has also been reported.

Papillary muscle dysfunction or infarction following acute myocardial infarction is less common. When mitral regurgitation is due to papillary dysfunction, it may subside as the infarction heals or left ventricular dilatation diminishes. If severe regurgitation persists, these patients have a poor prognosis with or without surgery and a natural history that reflects their underlying heart disease.

B. Diagnostic Studies: Echocardiography is useful in demonstrating the underlying pathologic process (rheumatic, prolapse, flail leaflet) but provides only estimates of its severity, even by Doppler techniques. The accompanying information concerning left ventricular size and function, left atrial size, pulmonary artery pressure, and right ventricular function can be invaluable in planning treatment as well as in recognizing associated lesions. Nuclear medicine techniques permit measurement of left ventricular function and estimation of the severity of regurgitation.

Cardiac catheterization provides the best assessment of regurgitation and, additionally, of left ventricular function and pulmonary artery pressure. Coronary arteriography is often indicated to determine the cause of the lesion and for preoperative evaluation.

Treatment & Prognosis

Acute mitral regurgitation due to endocarditis, myocardial infarction, and ruptured chordae tendineae often requires emergency surgery. Some patients can be stabilized with vasodilators or intra-aortic balloon counterpulsation, which reduces the amount of regurgitant flow by lowering systemic vascular resistance. Patients with chronic lesions may remain asymptomatic for many years. Operation is necessary when activity becomes limited or if left ventricular function deteriorates progressively. When left ventricular function is poor (ejection fraction < 40%), due either to chronic volume overload or to another process, the surgical risk is high and the subsequent outcome poor. There has been growing success with valve repair in nonrheumatic lesions, which avoids the complications of prosthetic valves described earlier. In addition, left ventricular function appears to be better preserved when the subvalvular structures can be maintained intact by valve repair.

Ansari A: Syndrome of mitral valve prolapse: Current perspectives. Prog Cardiovasc Dis 1989;32:31.

Hochreiter C et al: Mitral regurgitation: Relationship of noninvasive descriptors of right and left ventricular performance to clinical and hemodynamic findings and to prognosis in medically and surgically treated patients. Circulation 1986;73:900. (Left ventricular size and function are main determinants.)

Kirklin JW: Mitral valve repair for mitral incompetence. Med Concepts Cardiovasc Dis 1987;56:7. (Important alternative to valve replacement.)

MacMahon SW, Devereux RB, Schron E (guest editors): Proceedings of a National Heart, Lung, and Blood Institute symposium: Clinical and epidemiological issues in mitral valve prolapse. Am Heart J 1987;113:1265. (Consensus conference on prognosis and management of this problem. Covers all of the important management issues.)

Wilcken DE, Hickey AJ: Lifetime risk for patients with mitral valve prolapse of developing severe valve regurgitation requiring surgery. Circulation 1988;78:10.

AORTIC STENOSIS

Essentials of Diagnosis

- Usually asymptomatic until middle or old age.
- Delayed and diminished carotid pulses.
- Soft, absent, or paradoxically split S_2.
- Harsh systolic murmur and thrill along left sternal border, often radiating to the neck; may be louder at apex in older patients.
- ECG usually shows left ventricular hypertrophy; calcified valve on x-ray or fluoroscopy. Echo-Doppler is diagnostic in most cases.

General Considerations

Aortic valvular stenosis may follow rheumatic fever but is more commonly caused by progressive valvular calcification superimposed upon a congenitally bicuspid valve, or in the elderly, a previously normal valve. Aortic stenosis has become the commonest surgical valvular lesion in developed countries. Over 80% of patients are men. Valvular stenosis must be distinguished from supravalvular obstruction and from outflow obstruction of the left ventricular infundibulum.

Clinical Findings

A. Symptoms and Signs: Slightly narrowed, thickened, or roughened valves (aortic sclerosis) or aortic dilatation may produce the typical murmur and thrill without causing significant hemodynamic effects. In mild or moderate cases, the characteristic signs are a systolic ejection murmur at the aortic area transmitted to the neck and apex; in severe cases, a palpable left ventricular heave or thrill, a weak to absent aortic second sound, or reversed splitting of the second sound are present (see Table 8–1). When the valve area is less than 0.8–1 cm^2 (normal, 3–4 cm^2), ventricular systole becomes prolonged and the typical carotid pulse pattern of delayed upstroke and low amplitude is present. Left ventricular hypertrophy increases progressively, with resulting elevations in diastolic pressure. Cardiac output is maintained until the stenosis is severe (with a valve area < 0.8 cm^2). Patients may present with left ventricular failure, angina pectoris, or syncope.

Symptoms of failure may be sudden in onset or may progress gradually. Angina pectoris frequently occurs in aortic stenosis. One-half of patients with calcific aortic stenosis and angina have significant associated coronary artery disease, whereas coronary disease is noted at only half this rate in the absence of angina. Syncope is typically exertional and may be due to arrhythmias (usually ventricular tachycardia but sometimes sinus bradycardia), hypotension, or decreased cerebral perfusion resulting from increased blood flow to exercising muscle without compensatory increase in cardiac output. Sudden death may occur even in previously asymptomatic individuals.

B. Diagnostic Studies: The clinical assessment of aortic stenosis may be difficult, especially in older patients. The ECG reveals left ventricular hypertrophy or suggestive repolarization changes in most patients but may be normal in up to 10%. The chest radiograph may show a normal or enlarged cardiac silhouette, calcification of the aortic valve, and dilatation and calcification of the ascending aorta. Echocardiography can visualize the aortic valve gradient with considerable accuracy and can reliably exclude or diagnose severe stenosis. In patients with moderate obstruction, especially with low cardiac output or concomitant regurgitation, these evaluations may be inaccurate.

Cardiac catherization is the definitive diagnostic procedure. The valve gradient is measured and the valve area calculated; a valve area below 0.8 cm^2 indicates severe stenosis. Aortic regurgitation can be quantified by aortic root angiography. Coronary arteriography should be performed in most older patients with aortic stenosis, especially if angina is present.

Prognosis & Treatment

Following the onset of heart failure, angina, or syncope, the prognosis without surgery is poor (50% 3-year mortality rate). Medical treatment may stabilize patients in heart failure, but surgery is indicated for all symptomatic patients, including those with left ventricular dysfunction, which often improves postoperatively. Even asymptomatic patients are at risk for sudden death, although this is uncommon; valve replacement should be considered in them only when the gradient is severe (> 60 mm Hg) or left ventricular hypertrophy is advanced.

The surgical mortality rate for valve replacement is 2–5%, but it rises to 10% above the age of 70. Severe coronary lesions are usually bypassed at the same time. Anticoagulation is required for mechanical prostheses but is not essential with bioprostheses. The latter undergo degenerative changes and often require reoperation in 5–10 years. Many patients continue to exhibit conduction system disease or ventricular arrhythmias postoperatively.

The stenosis can be relieved in the majority of subjects, but the mortality rate of the procedure approaches that of surgery and restenosis occurs in up to 50% of cases within the first 6–12 months. This approach should be considered an alternative limited to individuals who are poor candidates for surgery or as an intermediate procedure to stabilize high-risk patients prior to surgery.

Brady ST et al: Percutaneous aortic balloon valvuloplasty in octogenarians: Morbidity and mortality. Ann Intern Med 1989;110:761. (Palliative at best.)

Craver JM et al: Predictors of mortality, complications, and length of stay in aortic valve replacement for aortic stenosis. Circulation 1988;78(Suppl 1):85. (Results in over 1000 patients.)

Lombard JT, Selzer A: Valvular aortic stenosis: A clinical and hemodynamic profile of patients. Ann Intern Med 1987;106:292. (Review of changing presentations.)

Pellikka PA et al: Natural history of adults with asymptomatic hemodynamically significant aortic stenosis. J Am Coll Cardiol 1990;15:1012. (While many become symptomatic, sudden death is rare.)

Richards KL et al: Calculation of aortic valve area by Doppler echocardiography: A direct application of the continuity equation. Circulation 1986;73:964. (Methods and results.)

Safian RD et al: Balloon aortic valvuloplasty in 170 consecutive patients. N Engl J Med 1988;319:125. (Large experience, sobering results. See editorial on p 169.)

AORTIC REGURGITATION
(Aortic Insufficiency)

Essentials of Diagnosis

- Usually asymptomatic until middle age; presents with left-sided failure or chest pain.
- Wide pulse pressure with associated peripheral signs.
- Hyperactive, enlarged left ventricle.
- Diastolic murmur along left sternal border.
- ECG shows left ventricular hypertrophy; x-ray shows left ventricular dilatation. Echo-Doppler confirms diagnosis and estimates severity.

General Considerations

Rheumatic aortic regurgitation has become less common than in the preantibiotic era, but nonrheumatic causes are frequent and are the major cause of isolated aortic regurgitation. These include congenitally bicuspid valves, infective endocarditis, and hypertension. Some patients have aortic regurgitation secondary to aortitis or aortic root disease, such as cystic medial necrosis (especially Marfan's syndrome), aortic dissection, ankylosing spondylitis, Reiter's syndrome, and syphilis.

Clinical Findings

A. Symptoms and Signs: The clinical presentation is determined by the rapidity with which regurgitation develops. In chronic regurgitation, the only sign for many years may be a soft aortic diastolic murmur. As the valve deformity increases, larger amounts regurgitate, diastolic blood pressure falls, and the left ventricle progressively enlarges. Most patients remain asymptomatic even at this point, and an often prolonged plateau phase, characterized by stable left ventricular dilatation, occurs. Left ventricular failure is a late event and may be sudden in onset. Exertional dyspnea and fatigue are the most frequent symptoms, but paroxysmal nocturnal dyspnea and pulmonary edema may also occur. Angina pectoris or atypical chest pain may be present. Associated coronary artery disease and syncope are less common than in aortic stenosis.

Hemodynamically, because of compensatory left ventricular dilatation, patients eject a large stroke volume which is adequate to maintain forward cardiac output until late in the course of the disease. Left ventricular diastolic pressure remains normal also but may abruptly rise when heart failure occurs. Abnormal left ventricular systolic function, as manifested by reduced ejection fraction and increasing end-systolic left ventricular volume, is a late sign.

The major physical findings relate to the wide arterial pulse pressure. The pulse has a rapid rise and fall (Corrigan's pulse), with an elevated systolic and low diastolic pressure, owing to the large stroke volume and rapid diastolic runoff back into the left ventricle, respectively. The large stroke volume is also responsible for characteristic findings such as Quincke's pulses (subungual capillary pulsations) and Duroziez's sign (diastolic murmur over a partially compressed peripheral artery, commonly the femoral). The apical impulse is prominent, laterally displaced, and usually hyperdynamic and may be sustained. The murmur itself may be quite soft and localized; it is high-pitched and decrescendo. A mid or late diastolic low-pitched mitral murmur (Austin Flint murmur) may be heard in advanced aortic insufficiency, owing to obstruction of mitral flow produced by partial closure of the mitral valve by the regurgitant jet.

When aortic insufficiency develops acutely (as in aortic dissection or infective endocarditis), left ventricular failure, manifested primarily as pulmonary edema, may develop rapidly, and surgery is urgently required. Patients with acute aortic insufficiency do not have the dilated left ventricle of chronic aortic insufficiency. In the same way, the diastolic murmur is shorter and may be minimal in intensity, making clinical diagnosis difficult.

B. Diagnostic Studies: The ECG usually shows moderate to severe left ventricular hypertrophy. Radiographs show cardiomegaly with left ventricular prominence.

Echocardiography can demonstrate diastolic fluttering of the anterior mitral leaflet or septum produced by the regurgitant jet. Serial assessments of left ventricular size and function are critical in determining the timing for valve replacement. Doppler techniques can qualitatively estimate the severity of regurgitation. Scintigraphic studies can quantify left ventricular function and functional reserve during exercise—a useful predictor of prognosis.

Cardiac catheterization can help quantify severity and is used to evaluate the coronary anatomy preoperatively.

Treatment & Prognosis

Aortic regurgitation that appears or worsens during or after an episode of infective endocarditis or aortic dissection may lead to acute severe left ventricular failure or subacute progression over weeks or months. The former usually presents as pulmonary edema; surgical replacement of the valve is indicated even during active infection. These patients may be transiently improved or stabilized by vasodilators.

Chronic regurgitation has a long natural history, but the prognosis without surgery becomes poor when significant symptoms occur. Vasodilators, such as hydralazine and angiotensin-converting enzyme inhibitors, can reduce the severity of regurgitation, and prophylactic treatment may postpone or avoid surgery in asymptomatic patients with severe regurgitation and dilated left ventricles. In symptomatic patients, medical therapy with diuretics, vasodilators, and digoxin can stabilize or improve symptoms but should usually be employed only as a preliminary to surgical

correction. Surgery is also indicated for those with few or no symptoms who present with significant left ventricular dysfunction (ejection fraction < 45–50%) or who exhibit progressive deterioration of left ventricular function, irrespective of symptoms.

The operative mortality rate is usually in the 3-5% range. Aortic regurgitation due to aortic root disease requires repair or replacement of the root, a more difficult operation. Following surgery, left ventricular size usually decreases and left ventricular function improves, except where dysfunction has been present chronically.

Greenberg B et al: Long-term vasodilator therapy of chronic aortic insufficiency: A randomized double-blinded, placebo-controlled clinical trial. Circulation 1988;78:92. (Large trial indicating value of prophylactic therapy.)

Nishimura RA et al: Chronic aortic regurgitation: Indications for operation, 1988. Mayo Clin Proc 1988;63:270.

Roman MJ et al: Aortic root dilatation as a cause of isolated, severe aortic regurgitation: Prevalence, clinical and echocardiographic patterns, and relation to left ventricular hypertrophy and function. Ann Intern Med 1987;106:800.

Siemienczuk D et al: Chronic aortic insufficiency: Factors associated with progression to aortic valve replacement. Ann Intern Med 1989;110:587. (Left ventricular size and function determine outcome.)

TRICUSPID STENOSIS

Tricuspid stenosis is usually rheumatic in origin. It should be suspected when "right heart failure" appears in the course of mitral valve disease, marked by hepatomegaly, ascites, and dependent edema. The typical diastolic rumble along the lower left sternal border mimics mitral stenosis. In sinus rhythm, a presystolic liver pulsation may be found.

Hemodynamically, a diastolic pressure gradient of 5–15 mm Hg is found across the tricuspid valve in conjunction with raised pressure in the right atrium and jugular veins, with prominent a waves and a slow y descent because of slow right ventricular filling.

Echocardiography usually demonstrates the lesion, and Doppler flow studies can measure the gradient; accompanying valve lesions can also be detected. Right heart catheterization is diagnostic.

Acquired tricuspid stenosis may be amenable to valvotomy under direct vision, but it usually requires a prosthetic valve replacement. There may be a role for balloon valvuloplasty.

TRICUSPID REGURGITATION

Tricuspid regurgitation may occur in a variety of situations other than disease of the tricuspid valve itself. The most common is right ventricular overload resulting from left ventricular failure due to any cause. Tricuspid insufficiency occurs in association with right ventricular and inferior myocardial infarction. Tricuspid valve endocarditis and resulting regurgitation are common in intravenous drug abusers. Other causes include the carcinoid syndrome, lupus erythematosus, and myxomatous degeneration of the valve. The symptoms and signs are identical to those resulting from right ventricular failure due to any cause. In the presence of mitral valve disease, the tricuspid valvular lesion can be suspected on the basis of early onset of right heart failure and a harsh systolic murmur along the lower left sternal border which is separate from the mitral murmur and which often increases in intensity during and just after inspiration.

Hemodynamically, tricuspid insufficiency is characterized by a prominent regurgitant systolic (v) wave in the right atrium and jugular venous pulse, with a rapid y descent and a small or absent x descent. The regurgitant wave, like the systolic murmur, is increased with inspiration, and its size depends upon the size of the right atrium. In tricuspid regurgitation, especially with right ventricular failure, an inspiratory S_3 may be present.

Replacement of the tricuspid valve is infrequently done now. Tricuspid insufficiency secondary to severe mitral valve disease or other left-sided lesions may regress when the underlying disease is corrected. When surgery is required, valve repair or valvuloplasty of the tricuspid ring is often preferable to valve replacement.

General References
on Valvular Heart Disease

Christakis GT et al: Predictors of operative survival after valve replacement. Circulation 1988;78(Suppl 1):25. (Results in 2500 patients operated on in the 1980s. Covers all valve lesions.)

Hammermeister KE et al: Comparison of outcome after valve replacement with a bioprosthesis versus a mechanical prosthesis. Initial 5 year results of a randomized trial. J Am Coll Cardiol 1987;10:719. (Similar survival rate early, but more complications with mechanical valves.)

Lee RT et al: Assessment of valvular heart disease with Doppler echocardiography. JAMA 1989;262:2131. (Clinically relevant review.)

Nishimura RA et al: Percutaneous balloon valvuloplasty. Mayo Clin Proc 1990;65:198. (Covers all lesions.)

Peller OG et al: Role of Doppler and imaging echocardiography in selection of patients for cardiac valvular surgery. Am Heart J 1987;114:1445. (Review of major diagnostic procedure.)

Rahimtoola SH: Perspective on valvular heart disease: An update. J Am Coll Cardiol 1989;14:1. (Excellent clinical review.)

INFECTIVE ENDOCARDITIS

Essentials of Diagnosis

- Preexisting organic heart lesion (not necessary in intraveous drug users).
- Persistent fever, nonspecific systemic symptoms.
- New or changing heart murmur.
- Evidence of systemic emboli.
- Leukocytosis, elevated erythrocyte sedimentation rate, positive blood culture.

General Considerations

Endocarditis has traditionally been classified as acute or subacute based upon the pathogenic organism and the clinical presentation, but this distinction has become less clear and the less specific term "infective endocarditis" is now more commonly used. Important factors that determine the clinical presentation are (1) the nature of the infecting organism; (2) whether the infection is superimposed upon preexisting abnormal cardiac structures; and (3) the source of infection, since endocarditis in intravenous drug abusers and infections acquired during open heart surgery have special features.

More virulent organisms—*Staphylococcus aureus* in particular—tend to produce a more rapidly progressive and destructive infection. Patients are more likely to present with acute febrile illnesses, early embolization, and acute valvular regurgitation and myocardial abscess formation. Still, these organisms can produce a more gradual illness, and more indolent organisms can occasionally cause the acute presentation. *Streptococcus viridans*, enterococci, and a variety of other gram-positive and gram-negative bacilli, yeasts, and fungi tend to cause a more subacute picture. Streptococcal infection tends to be more chronic, though the average incubation period is 1–2 weeks. Systemic and peripheral manifestations may predominate, but acute deterioration due to valve perforations or large emboli may supervene at any time.

Most patients who develop infective endocarditis have underlying cardiac disease, although this is frequently not the case with intravenous drug abusers and hospital-acquired infections. Abnormal valves or endocardial changes due to jet flow effects in congenital lesions (most commonly ventricular septal defect, tetralogy of Fallot, coarctation of the aorta, or patent ductus arteriosus) provide a nidus for infection during bacteremic episodes. Predisposing valvular abnormalities include rheumatic involvement of any valve, bicuspid aortic valves, calcific aortic valves, hypertrophic subaortic stenosis, and mitral valve prolapse. Because of its high prevalence, the latter condition is the most controversial. Most experts use antibiotic prophylaxis only in patients with a mitral insufficiency murmur. Although in the past rheumatic disease was the commonest predisposing condition, this is no longer the case in developed countries. Many patients with endocarditis do not have preexisting cardiac disease. This is especially true in drug abusers but may be the case in any patient.

The initiating event in infective endocarditis is intravascular contamination by pathogenic organisms. Contamination may occur directly or may result from transient or persistent bacteremia. Transient bacteremia is common during dental, upper respiratory, urologic, and lower gastrointestinal diagnostic and surgical procedures. It is less common during upper gastrointestinal and gynecologic procedures, though a high incidence has been reported during suction abortion. Intravenous drug abuse is a major cause of endocarditis and is the commonest source of right-sided (especially tricuspid) lesions. Although staphylococcal infections are most frequent, these patients may be infected by unusual organisms such as gram-negative bacilli, yeasts, and fungi, and multiple pathogens are not infrequently involved. Intravenous drug abusers with fever of obscure origin should be investigated by blood culture and treated for presumptive endocarditis. Hospital-acquired endocarditis may be related to infected intravascular or urinary catheters. Endocarditis may complicate prosthetic valve replacement—either early, as a result of surgical contamination, or late, as a result of bacteremia from other sources. Although the spectrum of pathogens has been associated with infections in the first 2 months after surgery, late prosthetic valve endocarditis is most commonly caused by *S viridans,* with *Staphylococcus epidermidis* also increased in frequency.

Clinical Findings

A. Symptoms and Signs: Most patients present with a febrile illness that has lasted several days to 2 weeks. Nonspecific symptoms are common. Cough, dyspnea, arthralgias or arthritis, diarrhea, and abdominal or flank pain may occur as a result of embolization or immunologically mediated phenomena. The initial symptoms or signs of endocarditis may be caused by arterial emboli or cardiac damage, described below under complications.

Most patients have readily documented fever, though fever may be absent in older individuals. Ninety percent have heart murmurs, but murmurs may be absent in patients with right-sided infections. A changing murmur is common only in acute endocarditis. The characteristic peripheral lesions—petechiae (on the palate or conjunctiva or beneath the fingernails); subungual ("splinter") hemorrhages; Osler nodes (painful, violaceous raised lesions of the fingers, toes, or feet); Janeway lesions (painless erythematous lesions of the palms or soles); and Roth spots (exudative lesions in the retina)—occur in a substantial minority of patients. Pallor and splenomegaly are other helpful signs.

In acute endocarditis, leukocytosis is common; in subacute cases, anemia and a normal white count are the rule. Hematuria and proteinuria as well as renal dysfunction may result from emboli or immunologically mediated glomerulonephritis.

B. Diagnostic Studies: Blood cultures are the definitive diagnostic procedure and are essential to guide antibiotic therapy. At least 6 cultures should be run to increase the probability of establishing the diagnosis. The optimal time to obtain cultures is just before a temperature rise. Cultures should be obtained in duplicate to permit recognition of contaminants, and blood should be cultured anaerobically and aerobically. Special procedures and media may be required to detect unusual organisms, such as *Coxiella, Chlamydia,* and certain fungi. Extended growth periods are required for *Brucella* and *Aspergillus,* among other organisms.

Positive cultures are usually readily obtainable in acute endocarditis and infections caused by gram-positive cocci, but cultures may fail to grow organisms in certain gram-negative or anaerobic bacterial infections and in fungal infections. Prior antibiotic therapy may temporarily sterilize the blood for up to a week. If initial cultures are negative and antibiotics have been given, cultures should be obtained every 24–48 hours for 7–10 days in suspected cases. Negative blood cultures have been reported in up to 30% of proved infective endocarditis cases, but with adequate numbers of cultures and optimal techniques, this number should be below 10%.

The chest x-ray may show evidence for the underlying cardiac abnormality and, in right-sided lesions, scattered lung infiltrates and multiple abscesses. The ECG is nondiagnostic. Changing conduction abnormalities suggest myocardial abscess formation.

The echocardiogram is useful in demonstrating underlying valvular lesions and in quantifying their severity (see sections on congenital and valvular disease). The echocardiogram is less accurate in diagnosing endocarditis. Characteristic vegetations are strongly suggestive of the diagnosis, but they are present only in a minority of cases.

Complications

The clinical course of infective endocarditis is determined by the degree of damage to the heart, by the site of infection (right- versus left-sided, aortic versus mitral valve), by whether embolization from the site of infection occurs, and by immunologically mediated processes. Destruction of infected heart valves is especially common and precipitous with *S aureus* and often enterococci but can occur with any organism. The resulting regurgitation can be mild or severe and can progress even after bacteriologic cure. The infection can also extend into the myocardium, resulting in abscesses leading to conduction disturbances, and can also involve the wall of the aorta, creating sinus of Valsalva aneurysms. Rarely, a picture resembling acute myocarditis dominates.

Peripheral embolization can occur with any organism. The most catastrophic are cerebral and myocardial embolizations, with resulting infarctions. The spleen and kidneys are also common sites. Peripheral emboli may initiate metastatic infections or may become established in vessel walls, leading to mycotic aneurysms. Right-sided endocarditis, which usually involves the tricuspid valve, often leads to septic pulmonary emboli, causing infarction and lung abscesses.

Prevention

Some cases of endocarditis arise after dental procedures or surgery of the upper respiratory, genitourinary, or intestinal tracts. Patients with predisposing congenital or valvular anomalies (see list under Pathophysiology) who are to have any of these procedures should be prepared according to the guidelines of the American Heart Association (Circulation 1984;70:1123A), though failures sometimes occur.

A. For Dental and Upper Respiratory Tract Procedures:

1. Oral–Penicillin V, 2 g 1 hour before the procedure and 1 g 6 hours later. In patients with penicillin allergy, give erythromycin, 1 g 1 hour before the procedure and 0.5 g 6 hours later.

2. Parenteral–Ampicillin, 1 g, or penicillin G, 2 million units, intramuscularly or intravenously, plus gentamicin, 1.5 mg/kg intramuscularly or intravenously, each given 1 hour before the procedure and again 8 hours later. In patients with penicillin allergy, give vancomycin, 1 g intravenously as a 1-hour infusion beginning 1 hour before the procedure, and repeat once 8 hours later.

B. For Gastrointestinal or Genitourinary Tract Procedures:

1. Parenteral–Ampicillin, 2 g intravenously or intramuscularly, plus gentamicin, 1.5 mg/kg intravenously or intramuscularly, each given 1 hour before the procedure and once 8 hours later. In patients with penicillin allergy, give vancomycin alone or with gentamicin as above.

2. Oral–Oral prophylaxis (amoxicillin, 3 g 1 hour before the procedure and 1.5 g 6 hours later) is probably less desirable than parenteral prophylaxis.

C. Alternative Regimens: Many alternative regimens have been proposed. For none of them is there absolute proof of efficacy. Any form of antimicrobial prophylaxis may favor the selection of resistant organisms in the normal flora, which may lead to more resistant infections.

Treatment

Antimicrobial treatment of endocarditis is outlined in Chapter 26.

While most cases can be successfully treated medically, operative management is sometimes required. Valvular regurgitation resulting in acute heart failure that does not resolve promptly after institution of medical therapy is an indication for valve replacement even if active infection is present, especially if the aortic valve is involved. Infections that do not respond to appropriate antimicrobial therapy after 7–10 days are more likely to be eradicated if the valve is replaced. Surgery is nearly always required for fungal endocarditis and is more often necessary with gram-negative bacilli. Surgery is also indicated when the infection involves the sinus of Valsalva or produces septal abscesses. Recurrent infection with the same organism often indicates that surgery is necessary, especially with infected prosthetic valves. Continuing embolization presents a difficult problem when the infection is otherwise responding but may be an indication for surgery when large vegetations are detected by echocardiography. Embolization after bacteriologic cure, however, does not necessarily imply recurrence of endocarditis. Some authors suggest that anticoagulation may be helpful to prevent emboli, but there is no good evidence to support this procedure, which increases the risk of catastrophic intracerebral hemorrhage.

Bisno AL et al: Antimicrobial treatment of infective endocarditis due to viridans streptococci, enterococci, and staphylococci. JAMA 1989;261:1471.

Brandenburg RO et al: Infective endocarditis: a 25-year overview of diagnosis and therapy. J Am Coll Cardiol 1983;1:280.

Kaye D: Prophylaxis for infective endocarditis: An update. Ann Intern Med 1986;104:419.

MacMahon SW et al: Risk of infective endocarditis in mitral valve prolapse with and without precordial systolic murmurs. Am J Cardiol 1987;59:105.

Marantz PR et al: Inability to predict diagnosis in febrile intravenous drug abusers. Ann Intern Med 1987;106:823. (Endocarditis unless proved otherwise.)

McKinsey DS, Ratts TE, Bisno AL: Underlying cardiac lesions in adults with infective endocarditis: The changing spectrum. Am J Med 1987;82:681. (More normal valves, fewer rheumatic valves.)

Reys TF: Infective endocarditis: A continuing challenge. Update on the causes, presentation, treatment and prophylaxis. J Crit Ill 1987;2:18.

Robbins MJ et al: Right-sided valvular endocarditis: Etiology, diagnosis, and an approach to therapy. Am Heart J 1986;111:128.

Terpenning MS, Buggy BP, Kauffman CA: Infective endocarditis: Clinical features in young and elderly patients. Am J Med 1987;83:626.

SYSTEMIC HYPERTENSION

Hypertension is an important preventable cause of cardiovascular disease; untreated, it increases the incidence of cardiac failure, coronary heart disease with angina pectoris and myocardial infarction, hemorrhagic and thrombotic stroke, and renal failure. Only about half of the hypertensive population are aware they have the condition, and only half of those who are aware of it have their pressure normalized by treatment.

Because cardiovascular morbidity and mortality rates increase as both systolic and diastolic blood pressures rise, defining a normal range for blood pressure is necessarily a somewhat arbitrary exercise. The American Joint National Committee on Detection, Evaluation, and Treatment of High Blood Pressure considers patients with diastolic blood pressures above 90 mm Hg to be hypertensive, though it does not recommend treatment for all such persons. Individuals with diastolic pressures between 85 and 89 mm Hg are classified as "high normal," indicating their added risk. Patients with systolic pressures above 160 mm Hg but normal diastolic pressures are said to have isolated systolic hypertension. Systolic pressures between 140 and 159 mm Hg in the presence of normal diastolic pressures are considered borderline, but as a rule of thumb patients under age 60 with systolic pressures above 100 mm Hg plus their age and "high normal diastolic pressure" can be considered hypertensive.

The World Health Organization has adopted more conservative criteria, classifying patients with pressures over 160/95 mm Hg as hypertensive and those with pressures between 140/90 and 160/95 mm Hg as borderline.

Because blood pressure readings in many individuals are highly variable, the diagnosis of hypertension should be made only after 3 readings on different occasions are elevated. Transient elevation of blood pressure caused by excitement or apprehension does not constitute hypertensive disease but may indicate a propensity toward its evolution.

Continued hypertension does not necessarily indicate the need for pharmacologic treatment. Nonpharmacologic approaches and individualized assessment of the benefit-to-risk ratio of drug therapy should precede pharmacologic management in patients with mild hypertension (diastolic pressure < 105 mm Hg).

Etiology & Classification

A. Primary (Essential) Hypertension: In about 95% of cases, no cause can be established. The condition occurs in 10–15% of white adults and 20–30% of black adults in the USA. The onset of essential hypertension is usually between ages 25 and 55. Hypertension is uncommon before age 20. In young people it is commonly caused by renal insufficiency, renal artery stenosis, or coarctation of the aorta.

Elevations in pressure are transient early in the course of the disease but eventually become permanent. Even in established cases, the blood pressure fluctuates widely in response to emotional stress and physical activity. Blood pressures taken by the patient at home or during daily activities using a portable apparatus are lower than those recorded in the office, clinic, or hospital and may be more reliable in estimating prognosis.

The pathogenesis of essential hypertension is multifactorial. Genetic factors play an important role. Children with one—and even more so with two—hypertensive parents tend to have higher blood pressures. Abnormal cation exchange in red blood cells has been suggested to be a potential marker of a genetic defect.

Environmental factors also appear to play an important role. Increased salt intake has long been incriminated as a pathogenic factor in essential hypertension. Increased salt intake alone is probably not sufficient to elevate blood pressure to abnormal levels; a combination of too much salt plus a genetic predisposition is required. Cl^- may be as important as Na^+ in the pathogenesis of hypertension. Other factors that may be involved in the pathogenesis of essential hypertension are the following:

1. Sympathetic nervous system hyperactivity–Sympathetic nervous system hyperactivity is most apparent in younger hypertensives, who may exhibit tachycardia and an elevated cardiac output. However, this is usually transient, and correlations between plasma catecholamines and blood pressure have generally been poor. Sympathetic activation may also play a role in "labile" hypertension, characterized by marked blood pressure fluctuations under differing, or even similar, circumstances.

2. Renin-angiotensin system–Renin, a proteolytic enzyme, is secreted by the juxtaglomerular cells surrounding afferent arterioles in response to a number of stimuli, including reduced renal perfusion pressure, diminished intravascular volume, circulating catecholamines, increased sympathetic nervous system activity, increased arteriolar stretch, and hypokalemia. Renin acts on angiotensinogen or renin substrate to cleave off the 10-amino-acid peptide angiotensin I. This peptide is then acted upon by angiotensin-converting enzyme to create the 8-amino-acid peptide angiotensin II, a potent vasoconstrictor and a major stimulant of aldosterone release from the adrenal glands. Despite the important role of this system in the regulation of blood pressure, it probably does not play a primary role in the pathogenesis of essential hypertension in most individuals. Black hypertensives and older patients tend to have lower plasma renin activity. Patients with low plasma renin activity may have higher intravascular volumes. Plasma renin activity levels can be best classified in relation to dietary sodium intake or urinary sodium excretion. Approximately 10% of essential hypertension patients have relatively high levels, 60% have essentially normal levels, and 30% have relatively low levels. Although such measurements have contributed to our understanding of the pathophysiology of hypertension, there is little clinical utility to measuring plasma renin activity.

3. Defect in natriuresis–Normal individuals increase their renal sodium excretion in response to elevations in arterial pressure and to a sodium or volume load. Hypertensive patients, particularly when their blood pressure is normal, exhibit a diminished ability to excrete a sodium load. This defect may result in increased plasma volume and hypertension. However, during chronic hypertension, a sodium load is usually handled normally.

4. Intracellular sodium and calcium–There is growing evidence that intracellular Na^+ is elevated in blood cells and other tissues in essential hypertension. This may result from abnormalities in Na^+-K^+ exchange and other Na^+ transport mechanisms. Circulating ''digitalislike'' substances may be responsible. An increase in intracellular Na^+ may lead to increased intracellular Ca^{2+} plus concentrations as a result of facilitated exchange. This could explain the increase in vascular smooth muscle tone that is characteristic of established hypertension.

5. Exacerbating conditions–A number of conditions exacerbate or precipitate hypertension in predisposed individuals. The best-documented of these is **obesity,** which is associated with an increase in intravascular volume and an appropriately high output. Weight reduction in the obese lowers blood pressure slightly. Excessive use of **alcohol** also raises blood pressure by increasing plasma catecholamines. Hypertension can be difficult to control in people with high alcohol intake. **Cigarette smoking** acutely raises blood pressure, again by increasing plasma norepinephrine, but the long-term effect of smoking in essential hypertension is less clear. The relationship of **exercise** to hypertension is also uncertain, although exercise training can lower blood pressure modestly. **Polycythemia** increases the viscosity, whether it be primary or due to diminished plasma volume. This may raise blood pressure.

B. Secondary Hypertension: With complete evaluation, approximately 5% of patients with hypertension can be found to have specific causes. These are labeled secondary hypertension.

1. Estrogen use–The most common definable cause is the chronic use of oral contraceptive pills. A small increase in blood pressure occurs in most women taking oral contraceptives, but considerable rises may occur. This is caused by volume expansion due to increased activity of the renin-angiotensin-aldosterone system. The primary abnormality is an increase in the hepatic synthesis of renin substrate. Approximately 5% of women taking oral contraceptives chronically will exhibit a rise in blood pressure above 140/90 mm Hg; this represents twice the expected prevalence. Contraceptive-related hypertension is more common in women over 35 years of age and in the obese. It is less common in those taking low-dose estrogen tablets. In most cases, hypertension is reversible by discontinuing the contraceptive, but it may take several weeks. There is no evidence that hypertension is related to postmenopausal estrogen use.

2. Renal disease–Virtually any disease of the renal parenchyma can produce secondary hypertension. The mechanism of renal hypertension is multifaceted, but most instances are related to increased intravascular volume or increased activity of the renin-angiotensin-aldosterone system. Hypertension exaggerates progression of renal insufficiency, so its early recognition and vigorous treatment is important. Hypertension may be reversed if plasma volume is controlled by drugs or dialysis or after bilateral nephrectomy (rarely necessary) and is often improved by renal transplantation. However, posttransplantation hypertension is also a problem; this is now recognized to be in part precipitated by immunosuppressive therapy with cyclosporine.

3. Renal vascular hypertension–Renal artery stenosis is a common cause of secondary hypertension and is present in 1–2% of hypertensive patients. The cause in younger individuals is most commonly fibromuscular hyperplasia. This accounts for approximately 30% of renal vascular disease, though it is more common in women under 50. The remainder of renal vascular disease is due to atherosclerotic stenoses of the proximal renal arteries. The mechanism of renal vascular hypertension is excessive renin release due to reduction in renal blood flow and perfusion pressure. Renal vascular hypertension may occur when a single branch of the renal artery is obstructed, but in as many as 25% of patients both arteries are obstructed.

Renal vascular hypertension may present in the same manner as essential hypertension but should be suspected in the following circumstances: (1) if the onset is below age 20 or after age 50, (2) if there are epigastric or renal artery bruits, (3) if there is atherosclerosis elsewhere, or (4) if there is abrupt deterioration in renal function after administration of angiotensin-converting enzyme inhibitors. Renal angiograms may be indicated if anatomic stenosis is strongly suggested by the history and signs and if the hypertensive disease is difficult to control medically.

There is no ideal ''screening'' test for renal vascular hypertension. All tests are sufficiently nonspecific so that in populations with a low incidence of the disease, false-positive results will exceed true-positives. In addition, none of these tests have more than 80% sensitivity. Additional diagnostic testing is appropriate only in the high-risk populations described in the previous paragraph. If the suspicion of renal vascular hypertension is sufficiently high, renal arteriography, the definitive diagnostic test, is the best approach. Where this procedure is not readily available, an intravenous urogram is an alternative but less satisfactory diagnostic procedure. Radioisotope renography, particularly following a test dose of captopril, has shown decreased renal blood flow and smaller kidney size on the side of the lesion. Measurement of plasma renin activity in the renal veins has been used to identify and lateralize physiologically significant renal artery stenosis, but there are both false-positive and false-negative results; therefore, these studies are now performed infrequently.

The treatment of patients with recognized renal vascular hypertension is controversial. Young individuals and good-risk patients of any age who have not responded to medical therapy should have the lesion corrected. Although the surgical results from renal artery reconstruction are generally good, percutaneous transluminal angioplasty is now the preferred approach for fibromuscular hyperplasia and for discrete stenotic arteriosclerotic lesions that do not involve the renal artery ostium. Older individuals, particularly if they have bilateral disease or other risk factors, may be managed medically if renal function does not deteriorate. The use of converting enzyme inhibitors has improved the success rate of medical therapy, but these have been associated with marked hypotension and deterioration of renal function in individuals with bilateral renal artery stenosis.

4. Primary hyperaldosteronism–Most patients with adrenal hypertension have excess aldosterone secretion as the underlying pathophysiologic process. They make up less than 0.5% of all cases of hypertension. The usual lesion is an adrenal adenoma, although a minority of patients have bilateral adrenal hyperplasia. The diagnosis should be suspected when patients present with hypokalemia prior to diuretic therapy and when this is associated with excessive urinary potassium excretion and suppressed levels of plasma renin activity. Aldosterone concentrations in urine and blood are elevated. The lesion can be demonstrated by CT scanning as well as by MRI and abdominal ultrasound. Even less commonly, patients with **Cushing's syndrome** (glucocorticoid excess) may manifest hypertension as a first sign (see Chapter 20).

5. Pheochromocytoma–Pheochromocytoma is an often sought but uncommonly found cause of hypertension. Blood pressure elevations result from excessive catecholamine secretion by the adrenal medulla or from extra-adrenal chromaffin tissue. The lesion is usually an adrenal tumor, which is bilateral in 10% of cases. Approximately 10% are malignant. The clinical presentation characteristically includes fluctuating blood pressure associated with headache, palpitations, pallor, sweating, orthostatic hypotension, and hyperglycemia. Severe hypertensive episodes may accompany anesthesia induction, surgery, ingestion of phenothiazines or tricyclic antidepressants, or beta-blocker therapy (which leaves alpha-adrenergic stimulation unopposed). However, many patients exhibit sustained rather than episodic hypertension, often associated with one or more of these features. Screening for pheochromocytoma is by measurement of metabolites of norepinephrine such as urinary metanephrine excretion, although urinary vanillylmandelic acid (VMA) assays are still performed. Plasma catecholamine levels provide valuable confirmatory information, especially during hypertensive episodes, but they may be elevated in some individuals without pheochromocytoma and are not continuously elevated in all patients with that disorder. Nonspecifically elevated plasma norepinephrine levels are usually suppressed after an oral dose of clonidine. The tumors can usually be demonstrated by CT scanning or by uptake of adrenal specific radionuclides such as metaiodobenzylguanidine (MIBG). Surgical excision is usually successful in nonmalignant cases. Secondary renal disease is more common in blacks than whites.

6. Coarctation of the aorta–This uncommon cause of hypertension has been discussed previously.

7. Hypertension associated with pregnancy–Hypertension occurring de novo or worsening during pregnancy is one of the commonest causes of maternal and fetal morbidity and mortality (see Chapter 13).

8. Other causes of secondary hypertension–Hypertension has also been associated with hyperparathyroidism, hypercalcemia due to any cause, acromegaly, hyperthyroidism, hypothyroidism, and a variety of neurologic disorders causing increased intracranial pressure.

Complications of Untreated Hypertension

Complications of hypertension are related either to sustained elevations of blood pressure, with consequent changes in the vasculature and heart, or to atherosclerosis that accompanies and is accelerated by long-standing hypertension. The excess morbidity and mortality related to hypertension are progressive over the whole range of systolic and diastolic blood pressures. However, end-organ damage varies markedly between individuals with similar levels of office hypertension. Ambulatory pressures are more closely related to end-organ damage. In general, blacks of both sexes and white males have a higher incidence of complications from hypertension. Specific complications include the following:

A. Hypertensive Cardiovascular Disease: Left ventricular hypertrophy is found in 10–30% of chronic hypertensives, depending on the level of blood pressure, the duration of hypertension, the technique of diagnosis (echocardiography is more sensitive than electrocardiography), and additional factors that remain poorly understood. Once established, left ventricular hypertrophy is an indication of increased risk for morbidity and mortality; for any level of blood pressure, its presence is associated with a several-fold increase in risk. In the past, hypertension was the major cause of congestive heart failure, but this complication is rare in patients receiving adequate treatment and is decreasing in prevalence. Hypertension remains an important exacerbating factor in patients with congestive heart failure due to other causes.

B. Hypertensive Cerebrovascular Disease: Hypertension is the major predisposing cause of stroke, especially intracerebral hemorrhage but also cerebral infarction. Cerebrovascular complications are more closely correlated with the systolic than the diastolic blood pressure. The incidence of these complications is markedly reduced by antihypertensive therapy.

C. Hypertensive Renal Disease: Chronic hypertension leads to nephrosclerosis, a common cause of renal insufficiency. Hypertensive renal damage is limited or prevented by successful therapy.

D. Aortic Dissection: Hypertension is a major cause and exacerbating factor in many patients with dissection of the aorta. The diagnosis and treatment of aortic dissection are discussed in Chapter 9.

E. Atherosclerotic Complications: The linkage between hypertension and atherosclerotic cardiovascular disease is much less close than that with the previously discussed complications. This reflects the multifactorial origin of atherosclerosis. Effective antihypertensive therapy is thus less successful in preventing coronary heart disease. Furthermore, because the duration of antihypertensive therapeutic trials has been relatively short, it is likely that most coronary events occurred in patients with preexisting coronary artery disease. Most patients with hypertension in the USA die of complications of atherosclerosis.

F. Malignant and Accelerated Hypertension: Any form of sustained hypertension, primary or secondary, may abruptly become accelerated, with resulting encephalopathy, nephropathy, retinopathy, heart failure, or myocardial ischemia. These complications are discussed below in the section on Hypertensive Urgencies and Emergencies.

Clinical Findings

The clinical and laboratory findings are mainly referable to involvement of the "target organs": heart, brain, kidneys, eyes, and peripheral arteries.

A. Symptoms: Mild to moderate essential hypertension is usually associated with normal health and well-being for many years. Vague symptoms often appear after patients learn they have "high blood pressure." Suboccipital pulsating headaches, characteristically occurring early in the morning and subsiding during the day, are common, but any type of headache may occur. Accelerated hypertension may be associated with somnolence, headache, confusion,

visual disturbances, and nausea and vomiting (hypertensive encephalopathy).

Patients with pheochromocytomas that secrete predominantly norepinephrine usually have sustained hypertension but may have intermittent hypertension. Attacks (lasting minutes to hours) of anxiety, palpitation, profuse perspiration, pallor, tremor, and nausea and vomiting occur; blood pressure is markedly elevated, and angina or acute pulmonary edema may occur. In primary aldosteronism, patients may have recurrent episodes of generalized muscular weakness or paralysis as well as paresthesias, polyuria, and nocturia due to associated hypokalemia; malignant hypertension, however, is rare.

Chronic hypertension often leads to left ventricular hypertrophy, which may be associated with diastolic or, in late stages, systolic dysfunction. Exertional and paroxysmal nocturnal dyspnea may result. Severe left ventricular hypertrophy predisposes to myocardial ischemia (especially when concomitant coronary artery disease is present), ventricular arrhythmias, and sudden death.

Renal involvement may not produce symptoms, but hematuria is frequent in the malignant phase.

Cerebral involvement causes (1) stroke due to thrombosis or (2) small or large hemorrhage from microaneurysms of small penetrating intracranial arteries. Hypertensive encephalopathy is probably caused by acute capillary congestion and exudation with cerebral edema. The findings are usually reversible if adequate treatment is given promptly. Although there is no strict correlation of diastolic blood pressure with hypertensive encephalopathy, it usually exceeds 130 mm Hg.

B. Signs: Physical findings depend upon the cause of hypertension, its duration and severity, and the degree of effect on target organs.

1. Blood pressure–A diagnosis of hypertension is not warranted in patients under age 50 unless the blood pressure exceeds 140/90 mm Hg on at least 3 separate occasions after the patient has rested 10 or more minutes in familiar, quiet, warm surroundings. On the initial observation, pressure should be examined in both arms and, if lower extremity pulses are diminished, in the legs to exclude coarctation of the aorta. Supine and standing measurements should be made to detect postural changes. Elderly patients may have falsely elevated readings by sphygmomanometry because of noncompressible vessels. This may be suspected in the presence of Osler's sign—a palpable brachial or radial artery when the cuff is inflated above systolic pressure.

2. Retinas–The Keith-Wagener (KW) classification of retinal changes in hypertension, in spite of deficiencies, has prognostic significance (see Table 5–2).

3. Heart and arteries–A loud aortic second sound and an early systolic ejection click may occur. Left ventricular enlargement with a left ventricular heave indicates well-established disease. A presystolic (S_4) gallop is due to increased compliance of the left ventricle; it is quite common.

4. Pulses–Direct bilateral comparison should be made of both carotid, radial, femoral, popliteal, and pedal pulses; and the presence or absence of bruits over major vessels, including the abdominal aorta and iliacs, should be determined.

C. Laboratory Findings: Most laboratory examinations are normal in uncomplicated essential hypertension. Testing is recommended to detect secondary hypertension and important associated conditions. Thus, standard testing should include measurements of hemoglobin (to detect anemia or polycythemia), complete urinalysis (to detect hematuria, proteinuria, and casts, which may signify primary renal disease or nephrosclerosis), renal function testing (for the same reasons), measurement of serum K^+ (to detect hyperaldosteronism), measurement of fasting blood sugar (to detect diabetes and as evidence for pheochromocytoma), and measurement of plasma lipids (as an indicator of atherosclerosis risk).

D. ECG and Chest X-Ray: Electrocardiographic criteria are highly specific but not very sensitive for left ventricular hypertrophy. The "strain" pattern of ST–T wave changes is a sign of more advanced disease and associated with a poor prognosis. In aldosteronism and Cushing's disease, the QT interval is prolonged and the ST segment may be depressed (hypokalemia). The chest x-ray often does not yield additional information in the uncomplicated hypertensive patient but may show aortic dilatation or calcification. It may demonstrate left ventricular enlargement or congestive heart failure. Rib notching and a small aortic knob suggest coarctation of the aorta.

E. Diagnostic Studies: Only if the clinical presentation or routine tests suggest secondary or complicated hypertension are additional diagnostic studies indicated. These may include blood and urinary tests for endocrine causes of hypertension, intravenous urograms, or renal ultrasound to diagnose primary renal disease (polycystic kidneys, obstructive uropathy) or renovascular abnormalities, and isotope renograms for the latter diagnosis. Further evaluation may include abdominal imaging studies (CT scan, or MRI) or renal arteriography.

Though not mandatory in uncomplicated essential hypertension, echocardiography can assess cardiac function and the severity of left ventricular hypertrophy. This information can be helpful in assessing cardiovascular symptoms and choosing therapy.

F. Summary: Since most hypertension is "primary," an extensive diagnostic evaluation is not indicated before starting therapy. Most clinicians obtain only a blood count, renal function test, electrolyte panel and urinalysis, and ECG after establishing the diagnosis. If conventional therapy is unsuccessful or if symptoms suggest a secondary cause, further studies are indicated.

Who Should Be Treated?

Recommendations concerning which patients should be treated remain controversial. Factors that unfavorably influence the prognosis in chronic arterial hypertension and so determine the threshold for drug therapy include the following: (1) the level of diastolic and systolic blood pressure, (2) a family history of hypertension-related complications, (3) male gender, (4) early age at onset, (5) black race, (6) retinal abnormalities, (7) cardiac abnormalities (eg, electrocardiographic changes, cardiomegaly, angina), (8) renal dysfunction, and (9) stroke.

Appropriate drug treatment of severe (diastolic pressure > 115 mm Hg) and moderate (> 105 mm Hg) asymptomatic chronic hypertension results in significantly lower morbidity and mortality rates from cardiovascular disease (heart failure, hemorrhagic stroke, renal failure) than occur in untreated control patients. In patients with diastolic pressure under 100–105 mm Hg, the data are less clear, largely because the above complications are less frequent, but most authorities feel they are reduced by treatment of patients with diastolic pressures over 95 mm Hg. The conclusion that treatment of hypertension decreases the incidence of clinical coronary disease has been suggested but not established. Current insurance data have shown that even slight increases in blood pressure reduce longevity, especially by causing premature atherosclerosis, but the reversibility of this risk in borderline and mild hypertension is established only with respect to strokes.

Most recommendations are based upon the diastolic blood pressure, although the systolic pressure is at least as good an indicator of risk. Virtually all patients should have 3 or more blood pressure measurements on different occasions prior to a final decision on therapy, since many patients will exhibit lower pressures. There is agreement that individuals with diastolic blood pressures greater than 100 mm Hg warrant treatment. At present, most authorities recommend treatment for patients who consistently exhibit diastolic pressures above 95 mm Hg despite nonpharmacologic measures. In these—and in individuals with blood pressures between 90 and 95 mm Hg—the presence of the additional risk factors noted above lowers the threshold for instituting therapy. White women tend to develop fewer complications, and a therapeutic threshold of 100 mm Hg may be appropriate in otherwise low-risk members of this group.

Nonpharmacologic Therapy

Because of growing appreciation of the adverse effects of antihypertensive drugs, more serious attempts at nonpharmacologic therapy of mild hypertension are being made. Approaches of proved but modest value include weight reduction, reduced alcohol consumption, and in some patients reduced salt intake. Exercise conditioning programs also appear to be somewhat effective. Calcium and potassium supplements have been advocated, but their ability to lower blood pressure is limited and probably not applicable to most patients.

Antihypertensive Drug Therapy

An ideal antihypertensive drug would be effective as a single agent or in combination with other agents in all classes of patients; would lower blood pressure by a physiologic mechanism; would reduce morbidity and mortality rates; would have no long-term toxicity or unpleasant side effects that affect life-styles; could be taken once a day; would not require multiple-dose titration steps; and would be of moderate cost. No such agent currently exists, but the growing number of available drugs has allowed the physician to tailor treatment to the needs of individual patients. These agents are listed in Table 8–2.

A. The Stepped Care Approach: Over the past 2 decades, the "stepped care" approach to treatment of hypertension has been advocated. Patients were initially started on a diuretic agent, or beta-blocker, and other drugs were added later if required. This approach has been highly effective, with approximately 80% of compliant patients exhibiting adequate blood pressure control. It has also been relatively inexpensive and straightforward.

However, a number of considerations have led experts to question this as a universal treatment plan. These include recognition of the frequency of adverse effects with diuretics and beta-blockers, concern over the long-term implications of the metabolic changes (especially unfavorable changes in plasma lipids) induced by these agents, realization that patients not controlled by one agent may be controlled by another without moving directly to combined therapy, and the more recent availability of other effective and well-tolerated agents with different mechanisms of action.

B. Potential Initial Medications: These considerations have led to the new Joint National Committee recommendation that 4 major classes of agents are effective and suitable for initial antihypertensive therapy: diuretics, beta-blockers, angiotensin-converting enzyme (ACE) inhibitors, and calcium channel blockers. These drugs produce comparable lowering of blood pressure in large populations but not in all demographic subgroups. Selection is based upon individual factors, which include age, race, life-style, accompanying illnesses, cost, and the experience of the physician. In addition, the alpha-adrenergic blockers and central sympatholytic agents are sometimes employed as single therapy.

C. Current Antihypertensive Agents: (See Table 8–2 for dosages.)

1. Diuretics–The diuretics remain the most widely used hypertensive medications. They are effective in patients with all levels of blood pressure and in all demographic groups. Relative to the beta-blockers and the ACE inhibitors, they are more potent in

blacks, older individuals, the obese, and other subgroups with increased plasma volume or low plasma renin activity. Overall, the diuretics administered alone, control blood pressure in 50–60% of patients and can be used effectively with all other agents.

Diuretics lower blood pressure initially by decreasing plasma volume (by suppressing tubular reabsorption of sodium, thus increasing the excretion of sodium and water) and cardiac output, but during chronic therapy their major hemodynamic effect is reduction of peripheral vascular resistance by an as yet unknown mechanism. It is now generally appreciated that most of the antihypertensive effect of these agents is achieved at lower dosages than used previously but that their biochemical effects are dose-related. The thiazide diuretics are the most widely used. The loop diuretics (such as furosemide) may lead to electrolyte and volume depletion more readily than the thiazides and have short durations of action; therefore, they are not ordinarily used in hypertension except in the presence of renal dysfunction (serum creatinine above 2.5 mg/dL).

Combinations of thiazide diuretics and potassium-sparing agents (spironolactone, triamterene, amiloride) are often employed, but these medications are considerably more expensive, have additional side effects, impose a risk of hyperkalemia if potassium supplements are given, are often unnecessary in patients receiving low diuretic dosages, and are dangerous in the presence of oliguria. Their use should be restricted to individuals demonstrating hypokalemia (serum $K^+ < 3.5$ mmol/L or a reduction greater than 0.6 mmol/L from baseline) and to patients at special risk from hypokalemia (those taking digitalis or having arrhythmias).

The adverse effects of diuretics relate chiefly to the metabolic changes listed in Table 8–2. Impotence, skin rashes, and photosensitivity are also relatively frequent. Hypokalemia may lead to decreased renal blood flow with a potential rise in serum creatinine, especially in older patients. Hypokalemia can be minimized by employing very low doses (hydrochlorothiazide, 12.5–25 mg daily), eating a high-potassium diet, and limiting salt intake. Diuretics also increase serum uric acid and may precipitate acute gout. Increases in blood glucose, triglycerides, and low-density lipoprotein cholesterol also are common and may be deleterious in the long term. These changes may be blunted by time and by a shift to a low-cholesterol, low-saturated fat diet, but their long-term consequences are unknown. Some experts feel that these lipid changes may limit the beneficial effect of blood pressure reduction on the progression of atherosclerosis.

2. Beta-adrenergic blocking agents–(Table 8–3.) These drugs are effective in hypertension because they decrease the heart rate and cardiac output. Even after continued use of beta-blockers for a number of years, cardiac output remains decreased and sys-

Table 8–2. Antihypertensive medications.

Class (Drug)	Initial Dosage	Usual Range	Common Adverse Effects	Comments
Diuretics			$\downarrow$ K$^+$, $\downarrow$ Mg^{2+}, $\uparrow$ glucose, $\uparrow$ Ca^{2+}, $\uparrow$ LDL cholesterol, $\uparrow$ uric acid Rash, impotence, metabolic changes	Concern over long-term consequences of metabolic changes; K$^+$ replacement often necessary
Hydrochlorothiazide	12.5–25 mg daily	12.5–100 mg daily		
Other thiazides	Various	Various		
Chlorthalidone	12.5–25 mg	12.5–50 mg daily		
Metolazone	2.5 mg daily	2.5–5 mg daily		
Indapamide	2.5 mg	2.5–5 mg daily		
Combination agents			Same as diuretics plus gastrointestinal disturbances	Hydrochlorothiazide 25 mg and triamterene 50 mg
Dyazide	1–2 capsules daily	1–4 capsules in 1 or 2 doses		
Maxzide	½ tablet daily	½–2 tablets daily		Hydrochlorothiazide 50 mg and triamterene 75 mg (half-dose pills available
Moduretic	½ tablet daily	½–2 tablets daily		Hydrochlorothiazide 50 mg and amiloride 5 mg
Beta-blockers			Bradycardia, fatigue, bronchospasm, sleep disturbances, cold extremities, impotence, $\uparrow$ triglycerides, $\downarrow$ HDL cholesterol	See Table 8–3.
Acebutolol	400 mg daily	400–1200 mg in 1 or 2 doses		
Atenolol	25 mg daily	25–200 mg daily		
Metoprolol	50 mg once daily	50–200 mg in 1 or 2 doses		
Nadolol	20 mg daily	20–160 mg daily		
Pindolol	5 mg twice daily	5–20 mg twice daily		
Propranolol	20 mg twice daily	20–160 mg twice daily		
Timolol	5 mg twice daily	5–20 mg twice daily		
Labetalol	100 mg twice daily	100–600 mg twice daily		Combined beta- and alpha-blocker
ACE inhibitors			Skin rash, taste disturbances, cough, angioneurotic edema, hypotension, renal insufficiency	
Captopril	12.5–25 mg twice daily	50–300 mg in 2 or 3 doses		
Enalapril	5 mg daily	5–40 mg in 1 or 2 doses		
Lisinopril	10 mg daily	10–40 mg daily		
Calcium blockers				
Verapamil SR	240 mg daily	240–480 mg in 1 or 2 doses	Constipation, headache, edema, bradycardia	Slow-release form
Diltiazem SR	120 mg twice daily	180–360 mg in 2 doses	Headache, bradycardia, edema	Slow-release form
Nifedipine GITS	30 mg daily	30–90 mg daily	Headache, palpitations, edema	Better tolerated than capsules
Nicardipine	20 mg 3 times daily	20–40 mg 3 times daily	Same as nifedipine	
Nitrendipine	5 mg twice daily	5–20 mg twice daily	Same as nifedipine	Approval pending
Central sympatholytics			Sedation, dry mouth, sexual dysfunction	Rebound hypertension
Clonidine	0.1 mg twice daily	0.1–0.3 twice daily		
Guanabenz	4 mg twice daily	4–16 mg twice daily	Same as clonidine	
Guanfacin	1 mg daily	1–3 mg daily	Same as clonidine	
Methyldopa	250 mg twice daily	250 mg–1 g twice daily	Sedation, dry mouth, sexual dysfunction, hemolytic anemia, hepatitis	
Peripheral sympatholytics			First dose syncope, palpitations, headaches	Tachyphylaxis may occur
Prazosin	1 mg twice daily	1–10 mg twice daily		
Terazosin	1 mg daily	1–20 mg in 1 or 2 doses		
Guanethidine	10 mg daily	10–100 mg daily	Orthostatic hypotension, diarrhea, sexual dysfunction	
Guanadrel	5 mg twice daily	5–20 mg twice daily	Same as guanethedine	
Reserpine	0.1 mg daily	0.1–0.25 mg daily	Depression, peptic disease	
Arteriolar dilators			Gastrointestinal intolerance, headache, tachycardia, positive ANA and SLE	
Hydralazine	25 mg twice daily	25–200 mg twice daily		
Minoxidil	5 mg daily	5–20 mg twice daily	Headache, fluid retention, hirsutism	

Table 8–3. Pharmacologic properties of beta-blockers.

	Cardio-selec-tivity	Intrinsic Sympatho-mimetic Activity	Lipid Solubility	Dosing
Propranolol	0	0	++	BID[1]
Metoprolol	+	0	++	OD or BID
Nadolol	0	0	0	OD
Atenolol	+	0	0	OD
Timolol	0	0	+	BID
Pindolol	0	++	+	BID
Acebutolol	+	+	+	OD or BID
Penbutolol	0	+	0	OD
Carteolol	0	+	0	OD
Labetalol[2]	0	0	++	BID

0 = absent; + = moderate; ++ = marked
OD = once daily; BID = twice daily.
[1] Propranolol is available also in a sustained-release formulation for administration once a day.
[2] Labetalol has additional alpha-adrenergic blocking properties.

temic vascular resistance increased with most agents. The beta-blockers also decrease renin release, and they are in general more efficacious in populations likely to have elevated plasma renin activity, such as younger white patients. They neutralize the reflex tachycardia caused by vasodilators such as hydralazine and prazosin in the treatment of hypertension. The beta-blockers are especially useful in patients with associated conditions that benefit from this mode of therapy. These include patients with angina pectoris, patients with previous myocardial infarction, and individuals with migraine headaches and somatic manifestations of anxiety.

Although all beta-blockers appear to be approximately equivalent in antihypertensive potency, they differ in a number of pharmacologic properties (these differences are summarized in Table 8–3). They differ with respect to whether their effect is relatively specific to the cardiac β_1 receptors (cardioselectivity) or whether they also block the β_2 receptors in the bronchi and vasculature; at higher dosages, however, all agents are nonselective. The beta-blockers also differ in their pharmacokinetics, lipid solubility— which determines whether they enter the brain and cause cerebral symptoms—and mechanisms of elimination. The effect on the pulse rate varies; pindolol or acebutolol, with intrinsic sympathetic activity, may be preferable in patients who develop more pronounced bradycardia (< 45/min) when given other beta-blockers. Labetalol is a combined alpha- and beta-blocker and, unlike most beta-blockers, decreases peripheral resistance more than the other agents.

The side effects of all beta-blockers include development of bronchial asthma in predisposed patients; bradycardia; atrioventricular conduction defects; left ventricular failure, because of the negative inotropic action of the sympatholytic action of the drugs; nasal congestion; Raynaud's phenomenon, especially in women; and central nervous system symptoms with nightmares, excitement, and confusion. Fatigue, lethargy, and impotence may occur. All beta-blockers tend to increase plasma triglycerides. The nonselective and, to a lesser extent, the cardioselective beta-blockers tend to depress the protective HDL fraction of plasma cholesterol. This is not seen in agents with intrinsic sympathomimetic activity, and as with diuretics, the changes are blunted with time and dietary changes. Some experts believe that these lipid changes may have an adverse effect on coronary artery disease.

These agents are contraindicated in patients with congestive heart failure, symptomatic bronchospasm, and peripheral vascular disease. Beta-blockers are relatively contraindicated in insulin-dependent diabetes, since they inhibit gluconeogenesis and may prolong hypoglycemic episodes.

3. Angiotensin-converting enzyme (ACE) inhibitors–These drugs are being increasingly used in mild to moderate hypertension, often as the initial medication. Their primary mode of action is inhibition of the renin-angiotensin-aldosterone system, but they also inhibit bradykinin degradation, stimulate vasodilating prostaglandin synthesis, and, sometimes, reduce sympathetic nervous system activity. These latter actions may explain why they exhibit some effect even in patients with low plasma renin activity. The ACE inhibitors appear to be most effective in younger individuals, whites, and those with increased plasma renin activity. They are relatively less effective in blacks and in the elderly. While as single therapy they achieve adequate antihypertensive control in only about 40–50% of patients, the combination of an ACE inhibitor and a diuretic or calcium channel blocker is potent.

The major advantage of the ACE inhibitors is their relative freedom from troublesome side effects. Severe hypotension can occur in patients with bilateral renal artery stenosis; acute renal failure may ensue. A chronic dry cough due to bronchial or laryngeal irritation is seen in approximately 5–10% of patients and may require stopping the drug. Skin rashes and taste alterations are seen more often with captopril than with the non-sulfhydryl-containing agents (enalapril and lisinopril) but often disappear with continued therapy. Angioneurotic edema is an uncommon but potentially dangerous side effect of all agents of this class. Proteinuria and neutropenia are very uncommon at the lower dosages now employed except in individuals with preexisting renal insufficiency or autoimmune disease. ACE inhibitors do not produce impotence or fatigue and therefore, unlike many other medications, do not impair quality of life.

4. Calcium channel blockers–All the agents of this class reduce blood pressure, and a number of new agents are becoming available specifically for this indication. They do so by peripheral vasodilation, which is associated with less reflex tachycardia, increase in myocardial contractility, or fluid retention than other vasodilators. These agents are effective as single-drug therapy in 50–60% of patients and appear to be beneficial in all demographic groups and all grades of hypertension. As a result, they may be preferable to beta-blockers and ACE inhibitors in blacks and older subjects. Calcium channel blockers and diuretics are less additive when given together than when either is combined with beta-blockers or ACE inhibitors. However, verapamil and diltiazem should be combined cautiously with beta-blockers because of their potential for depressing atrioventricular conduction and sinus node automaticity.

The most common side effects of calcium channel blockers are headache, peripheral edema, bradycardia, and constipation (especially with verapamil in the elderly). The dihydropyridine agents, such as nifedipine, nicardipine, and nitrendipine, are more likely to produce symptoms of vasodilation, such as headache, flushing, and palpitations. All calcium channel blockers have negative inotropic effects and may cause heart failure in patients with cardiac dysfunction. Most of these agents are now available in preparations that can be administered once or twice daily.

5. Drugs with central sympatholytic action–Methyldopa, clonidine, guanabenz, and guanfacine lower blood pressure by stimulating alpha-adrenergic receptors in the central nervous system, thus reducing efferent peripheral sympathetic outflow. These agents may be effective as single therapy in some patients, but they are often associated with fluid retention and subsequent "pseudotolerance." They are thus most useful in combination with diuretics or ACE inhibitors. In addition, these agents produce frequent side effects, including sedation, fatigue, dry mouth, postural hypotension, and impotence. An important concern is rebound hypertension following abrupt withdrawal. Methyldopa also causes hepatitis and hemolytic anemia and should be avoided except in individuals who have already tolerated chronic therapy.

6. Alpha-receptor antagonists–Prazosin and terazosin block postsynaptic alpha receptors, relax smooth muscle, and reduce blood pressure by lowering peripheral vascular resistance. These agents are effective as single-drug therapy in some individuals, but tachyphylaxis may appear during long-term therapy, and side effects are relatively common. The major side effects are marked hypotension and syncope after the first dose, which, therefore, should be small and be given at bedtime. Palpitations, headache, and nervousness may continue to occur after dosing. Unlike the beta-blockers and diuretics, the alpha-blockers have no adverse effect on serum lipid levels—in fact, they increase high-density lipoprotein cholesterol while reducing total cholesterol. Whether this is beneficial in the long term has not been established. These drugs are most useful in combination with diuretics or in multidrug combinations in refractory patients.

7. Arteriolar dilators–Hydralazine and minoxidil relax vascular smooth muscle and produce peripheral vasodilation. When given alone, they stimulate reflex tachycardia, increase myocardial contractility, and cause headache, palpitations, and fluid retention. They are usually given in combination with diuretics and beta-blockers in resistant patients. Hydralazine produces frequent gastrointestinal disturbances and may induce a lupuslike syndrome. Minoxidil causes hirsutism and marked fluid retention; this agent is reserved for the most refractory of patients.

8. Peripheral sympathetic inhibitors–These agents are now used infrequently. Reserpine remains an effective antihypertensive agent and a cost-effective one. Its reputation for inducing mental depression and its other side effects—sedation, nasal stuffiness, sleep disturbances, and peptic ulcers—have made it unpopular, though these problems are uncommon at low dosages. Guanethidine and guanadrel inhibit catecholamine release from peripheral neurons but frequently cause orthostatic hypotension (especially in the morning or after exercise), diarrhea, and fluid retention. These agents are used chiefly in refractory hypertension.

9. Combination therapy–Most patients with hypertension can be controlled with one agent or with 2-drug combinations such as (1) a diuretic plus a beta-blocker, (2) a diuretic plus an ACE inhibitor, (3) a diuretic plus a calcium channel blocker, or (4) a calcium channel blocker plus an ACE inhibitor. A minority may require triple-drug therapy. Patients who are compliant with their medications and who do not respond to these combinations should usually be evaluated for secondary hypertension before proceeding to more complex regimens.

Particularly useful multidrug regimens are (1) a

diuretic plus a beta-blocker plus a vasodilator or a calcium channel blocker; (2) a diuretic plus an ACE inhibitor plus either a calcium channel blocker or a sympatholytic (or both); and (3) a calcium channel blocker plus an ACE inhibitor plus either a sympatholytic or a beta-blocker (or both).

Goal of Treatment

The goal of treatment should be to reduce blood pressure to normal levels (ie, less than 140/90 mm Hg) with minimal side effects. Since there may be additional benefits from further lowering of blood pressure, most authorities also seek to achieve a minimum of 10 mm Hg reduction in diastolic pressure in patients with mild hypertension (90–99 mm Hg). In older patients with predominantly systolic hypertension, a systolic pressure of 150–160 mm Hg is a satisfactory end point. However, a significant decrease in hypertension-related morbidity from blood pressure reduction is possible even if these therapeutic goals are not achieved. Thus, a compromise between goal blood pressure and an adequately tolerated therapeutic regimen may be necessary in some individuals.

Prognosis

Although many patients with slight elevation of blood pressure live a normal life span, most patients with untreated moderate or severe hypertension die of complications within 20 years. Before effective antihypertensive drugs were available, 70% of patients died of heart failure or coronary artery disease, 15% of cerebral hemorrhage, and 10% of uremia.

Hypertensive Urgencies & Emergencies

Hypertensive emergencies have become less frequent in recent years but still require prompt recognition and aggressive but careful management. A spectrum of acute presentations exists, and the appropriate therapeutic approach varies.

Hypertensive urgencies are situations in which blood pressure must be reduced within a few hours. Examples are asymptomatic severe hypertension (systolic pressure > 240 mm Hg, diastolic pressure > 130 mm Hg) and symptomatic moderately severe hypertension (systolic pressure > 200 mg Hg, diastolic pressure > 120 mm Hg, or even lower levels) associated with headache, heart failure, or angina or occurring in the perioperative period. Parenteral therapy is rarely required, and partial reduction of blood pressure with relief of symptoms is the goal.

Hypertensive emergencies require substantial reduction of blood pressure within 1 hour to avoid serious morbidity or death. Although blood pressure is usually strikingly elevated (diastolic pressure > 130 mm Hg), the correlation between pressure and end-organ damage is often poor. It is the latter that determines the seriousness of the emergency and the approach to treatment. Emergencies include hypertensive encephalopathy (which presents with headache, irritability, confusion, and altered mental status due to cerebrovascular spasm), hypertensive nephropathy (which presents with hematuria, proteinuria, and progressive renal dysfunction due to arteriolar necrosis and intimal hyperplasia of the interlobular arteries), intracranial hemorrhage, dissecting aneurysm, preeclampsia-eclampsia, pulmonary edema, unstable angina, or myocardial infarction.

Malignant hypertension is a specific emergent syndrome characterized by encephalopathy or nephropathy with accompanying papilledema. Progressive renal failure usually ensues without therapy.

Parenteral therapy is indicated in most hypertensive emergencies, especially if encephalopathy is present. The initial goal of treatment should be rapid reduction of systolic and diastolic pressure by at least 20–40 mm Hg and 10–20 mm Hg, respectively, to levels below 180–200/110–120 mm Hg. A subsequent more gradual reduction to near-normal levels is appropriate.

A. Parenteral Agents: Several agents are available for management of acute hypertensive problems (Table 8–4). Sodium nitroprusside is the agent of choice for the most serious emergencies because of its rapid and easily controllable action, but continuous monitoring is essential when this agent is used. In the presence of myocardial ischemia, intravenous nitroglycerin or an intravenous beta-blocker, such as labetalol or esmolol, is preferable.

1. Nitroprusside sodium–0.5–10 μg/kg/min is given by controlled intravenous infusion gradually titrated to the desired effect. It lowers the blood pressure within seconds by direct arteriolar and venous dilatation. Monitoring with an intra-arterial line is essential to avoid hypotension. Nitroprusside—in combination with a beta-blocker—is especially useful in patients with aortic dissection.

2. Nitroglycerin, intravenous–This agent is a less potent antihypertensive than nitroprusside and should be reserved for patients with accompanying acute ischemic syndromes.

3. Trimethaphan–The ganglionic blocking agent trimethaphan (1–5 mg/min intravenously) is titrated with the patient sitting; its activity depends upon this. The patient can be placed supine if the hypotensive effect is excessive. The effect occurs within a few minutes and persists for the duration of the infusion.

4. Diazoxide–Diazoxide, 75–300 mg intravenously in a single dose or in multiple smaller doses, acts promptly as a vasodilator without decreasing renal blood flow. It has been used often in preeclampsia-eclampsia. Side effects include hypotension, which may be severe; this necessitates starting with a smaller dose in elderly patients or administering by slow infusion over 30 minutes, which is usually just as effective and better tolerated. Hyperglycemia and sodium and water retention may occur. The drug should be used

Table 8–4. Drugs for hypertensive crises.

Agent	Action	Dosage	Onset	Duration	Adverse Effects	Comments
Parenteral agents (intravenously unless noted)						
Nitroprusside	Vasodilator	0.5–10 µg/kg/min	Seconds	3–5 minutes	Gastrointestinal, central nervous system	Most effective treatment. Use with beta-blocker in aortic dissection.
Diazoxide	Vasodilator	15–30 mg/min to 300 mg	1–5 minutes	4–12 hours	Nausea, excessive hypotension, tachycardia, headache	Avoid in coronary artery disease and dissection. Use with beta-blocker and diuretic.
Trimethaphan	Ganglionic blocker	1–5 mg/min	1–3 minutes	10 minutes	Hypotension, ileus	Useful in aortic dissection.
Esmolol	Beta-blocker	Loading dose 500 µg/kg over 1 minute; maintenance 25–200 µg/kg/min	1–2 minutes	10–30 minutes	Bradycardia, nausea	Avoid in congestive heart failure, asthma.
Labetalol	Beta- and alpha-blocker	20 mg every 10 minutes to 300 mg	5 minutes	3–6 hours	Gastrointestinal, hypotension	Avoid in congestive heart failure, asthma. May be continued orally.
Hydralazine	Vasodilator	5–20 mg intravenously or intramuscularly	10–30 minutes	2–6 hours	Tachycardia, headache, gastrointestinal	Avoid in coronary artery disease, dissection.
Enalaprilat	ACE inhibitor	1.25 mg every 6 hours	15 minutes	6 hours or more	Excessive hypotension	Additive with diuretics; may be continued orally.
Furosemide	Diuretic	10–80 mg	15 minutes	4 hours	Hypokalemia	Adjunct to vasodilator.
Oral agents						
Nifedipine	Ca^{2+} channel blocker	10 mg initially; may be repeated after 30 minutes	15 minutes	2–6 hours	Excessive hypotension, tachycardia, headache	Response variable. May precipitate angina
Clonidine	Central sympatholytic	0.2 mg initially; 0.1 mg every hour to 0.8 mg	30–60 minutes	6–8 hours	Sedation	Rebound may occur.
Captopril	ACE inhibitor	6.25–25 mg	15–30 minutes	4–6 hours	Excessive hypotension	

only for short periods and is best combined with a powerful diuretic such as furosemide.

5. Esmolol–This rapidly acting beta-blocker is approved by the FDA only for treatment of supraventricular tachycardia, but it is useful in acutely lowering blood pressure, especially when combined with a vasodilator such as nitroprusside, nitroglycerin, or hydralazine. Esmolol is especially useful during myocardial ischemia or dissecting aneurysm. A loading dose of 500 mg/kg is given over 1 minute and may be repeated after 5 minutes. The maintenance infusion rate ranges from 25 to 200 mg/kg/min.

6. Labetalol–This combined beta–and alpha-adrenergic blocking agent is the only other beta-blocker that can lower blood pressure rapidly enough for emergency treatment. The usual intravenous dose is 20 mg over 5–10 minutes, followed by additional 20-mg increments every 10–20 minutes to a maximum of 300 mg.

7. Hydralazine–Hydralazine can be given in-

travenously or intramuscularly in 10-mg increments, but its effect is less predictable than that of other drugs in this group. It produces reflex tachycardia and should not be given without beta-blockers in patients with possible coronary disease or aortic dissection. Hydralazine is valuable in children and pregnant women.

8. Enalaprilat–This is the active form of the oral ACE inhibitor enalapril. The most widely studied dosage is 1.25 mg intravenously every 6 hours. The onset of action is usually within 15 minutes, but the peak effect may be delayed for up to 6 hours. Therefore, enalaprilat is useful primarily as an adjunctive agent.

9. Diuretics–Intravenous loop diuretics can be very helpful when the patient has signs of heart failure or fluid retention. Low dosages should be used initially (furosemide, 20 mg; or bumetanide, 0.5 mg). They facilitate the response to vasodilators, which often stimulate fluid retention.

B. Oral Agents: Patients with less severe acute hypertensive syndromes can often be treated with oral therapy. They should be closely monitored until a therapeutic end point is achieved.

1. Clonidine–Clonidine, 0.2 mg orally initially, followed by 0.1 mg every hour to a total of 0.8 mg, will usually lower blood pressure over a period of several hours. Sedation is frequent, and rebound hypertension may occur if the drug is stopped.

2. Nifedipine–Nifedipine, 5–10 mg orally or sublingually, will reduce blood pressure within 5–20 minutes in most patients. An additional 10-mg dose may be needed. Excessive hypotensive responses may occur, and reflex tachycardia may induce angina.

3. Captopril–Captopril, 12.5–25 mg orally, will also lower blood pressure in 15–30 minutes. The response is variable and may be excessive.

C. Subsequent Therapy: When the blood pressure has been brought under control, combinations of oral antihypertensive agents can be added as parenteral drugs are tapered off over a period of 2–3 days. Most subsequent regimens should include a diuretic.

Hypertension in the Presence of Renal Failure

In the presence of renal failure, hypertension is highly dependent on blood volume. If the blood pressure is not reduced by vigorous use of antihypertensive drugs—including furosemide, beta-blocking drugs, minoxidil, or diazoxide—dialysis should be employed; in most instances, the blood pressure will be reduced as the patient achieves a dry weight state. The presence of renal failure is an adverse prognostic sign, but vigorous therapy often can prolong life.

General

Applegate WB: Hypertension in elderly patients. Ann Intern Med 1989;110:901.

Frohlich ED et al: Recommendations for human blood pressure determinations by sphygmomanometers. Hypertension 1988;11:209A. (Pitfalls and guidelines.)

Gifford RW et al: Office evaluation of hypertension. Circulation 1989;79:721. (How to approach the initial evaluation.)

Kaplan NM: *Clinical Hypertension*, 4th ed. Williams & Wilkins, 1986. (Concise, clinically oriented.)

Pickering TG et al: How common is white coat hypertension? JAMA 1988; 259:225. (Discusses frequency and implications of "office hypertension.")

The 1988 report of the Joint National Committee on detection, evaluation, and treatment of high blood pressure. Arch Intern Med 1988;148:1023. (Comprehensive consensus statement covering definitions and guidelines for work-up and treatment of hypertension.)

Zachariah PK et al: Clinical use of home and ambulatory blood pressure monitoring. Mayo Clin Proc 1989; 64:1436. (How and when.)

Secondary Causes

Hollenberg NK: The treatment of renovascular hypertension: Surgery, angioplasty, and medical therapy with converting-enzyme inhibitors. Am J Kidney Dis 1987;10(Suppl 1):52. (Review of current approaches, including angioplasty.)

Sheps SG et al: Recent developments in the diagnosis and treatment of pheochromocytomas. Mayo Clin Proc 1990;65:88.

Working Group on Renovascular Hypertension: Detection, evaluation and treatment of renovascular hypertension. Arch Intern Med 1987;147:820. (Consensus guidelines.)

Young WF et al: Primary aldosteronism: Diagnosis and treatment. Mayo Clin Proc 1990;65:960.

Complications of Untreated Hypertension

Levy D et al: Echocardiographically detected left ventricular hypertrophy: Prevalence and risk factors. The Framingham Heart Study. Ann Intern Med 1988; 108:7. (LVH is a poor prognostic indicator.)

Massie BM et al: Hypertensive heart disease: The critical role of left ventricular hypertrophy. J Cardiovasc Pharmacol 1989;13(Suppl 1):S18. (Speculative review.)

O'Kelly BF et al: Coronary morbidity and mortality, pre-existing silent coronary artery disease and mild hypertension. Ann Intern Med 1989;110:1017. (Therapy should focus on reducing coronary complications.)

Perloff D, Sokolow M, Cowan R: The prognostic value of ambulatory blood pressures. JAMA 1983;249:2792. (First study demonstrating that ambulatory pressure is a better predictor of outcome.)

Rutan GH et al: Mortality associated with diastolic hypertension and isolated systolic hypertension among men screened for the Multiple Risk Factor Intervention Trial. Circulation 1988;77:504. (Important prognostic data.)

Phillips SJ: Pathogenesis, diagnosis, and treatment of hypertension-associated stroke. Am J Hypertens 1989;2:493.

Samuelsson O et al: Cardiovascular morbidity in relation to change in blood pressure and serum cholesterol levels in treated hypertension: Results from the primary prevention trial in Goteborg, Sweden. JAMA 1987;258:1768. (To decrease morbidity rate, must lower both.)

White WB et al: Average daily blood pressure, not office blood pressure, determines cardiac function in patients with hypertension. JAMA 1989;261:873. (Title indicates conclusion of this important study.)

Who Should Be Treated?

Littenberg B et al: Screening for hypertension. Ann Intern Med 1990;112:192. (Valuable and cost-effective.)

MacMahon SW et al: The effects of drug treatment for hypertension on morbidity and mortality from cardiovascular disease: A review of randomized controlled trials. Prog Cardiovasc Dis 1986;29(Suppl 1):99. (Comprehensive review.)

Sambhi MP et al: University of California, Davis, Conference: Mild hypertension. Am J Med 1988;85:675. (Excellent discussion of whom to treat and how to treat by 5 experts.)

1986 Guidelines for the treatment of mild hypertension: Memorandum from the WHO/ISH. Hypertension 1988;8:957. (Conservative guidelines.)

Nonpharmacologic Therapy

Australian Dietary Salt Study: Fall in blood pressure

with modest reduction in dietary salt intake in mild hypertension. Lancet 1989;1:399. (Feasible and effective.)

Nonpharmacologic approaches to the control of high blood pressure. Hypertension 1986;8:444. (Consensus statement by Joint National Committee.)

Antihypertensive Drug Therapy

Massie B et al: Diltiazem and propranolol in mild to moderate essential hypertension as monotherapy or with hydrochlorothiazide. Ann Intern Med 1987; 107:150. (Large study illustrates the equivalent efficacy of these 2 classes of drugs.)

Massie BM: Demographic considerations in the selection of antihypertensive therapy. Am J Cardiol 1987; 60: 121I. (Review of role of age, race and gender in choice of medication.)

Wikstrand J et al: Primary prevention with metoprolol in patients with hypertension: Mortality results from MAPHY Study. JAMA 1988;259:1976. (Controversial study suggesting that beta-blockers reduce cardiovascular complications more than diuretics.)

Williams GH: Converting-enzyme inhibitors in the treatment of hypertension. N Engl J Med 1988;319:1517.

Hypertensive Urgencies & Emergencies

Ferguson RK, Vlasses PH: Hypertensive emergencies and urgencies. JAMA 1986;255:1607.

Houston MC: Pathophysiology, clinical aspects, and treatment of hypertensive crises. Prog Cardiovasc Dis 1989;32:99.

CORONARY HEART DISEASE
(Arteriosclerotic Coronary Artery Disease; Ischemic Heart Disease)

Coronary atherosclerotic heart disease is the commonest cause of cardiovascular disability and death in the USA. Men are more often affected than women by an overall ratio of 4:1, but before age 40 the ratio is 8:1, and beyond age 70 it is 1:1. In men, the peak incidence of clinical manifestations is at age 50–60; in women, at age 60–70. Altered lipid metabolism or excessive intake of cholesterol and saturated fats, together with changes in the vascular endothelium and smooth muscle proliferation, lead to localized subintimal accumulations of fatty and fibrous tissue that progressively obstruct the coronary arteries and their main branches. Elevated total serum cholesterol and low-density lipoproteins are involved in the development of atherosclerosis and are markers of high risk. High-density lipoproteins play an equally important protective role. The total cholesterol to HDL cholesterol ratio is a useful predictor of coronary risk.

While atherosclerosis is a chronic process occurring over decades, plaque ulceration, intimal hemorrhage and dissection, and vascular thrombosis accelerate the process and are responsible for most acute ischemic syndromes, such as infarction and unstable angina.

Additional risk factors for the development of ischemic heart disease include age, male gender, genetic predisposition, arterial hypertension, cigarette smoking, and diabetes mellitus. Other factors of less certain importance include obesity, physical inactivity, and personality type.

Prevention
of Ischemic Heart Disease

Patients with clinical manifestations of coronary disease before age 50 tend to have predisposing risk factors, but this is often not the case in older individuals. It is not clear to what extent treating risk factors will prevent further progression of disease once it has started, but favorable trends are becoming clear. Discontinuance of smoking reduces cardiovascular morbidity. The treatment of hyperlipidemia has decreased the incidence of coronary events and has caused regression of atherosclerosis in peripheral arteries. Recent data suggest a beneficial effect even in individuals with only moderately elevated plasma lipids (cholesterol above 240 mg/dL), but an improvement in mortality rates remains to be demonstrated.

A recent study has indicated that prophylactic aspirin (325 mg every other day) in males over the age of 50 reduces the incidence of myocardial infarction. Whether this approach should be employed in the general population or only in those at higher risk is unclear, and the optimal dosage is not known. A prudent approach would be to administer 325 mg daily to men with at least one risk factor if no contraindication is present. The value of other platelet-inhibiting agents or dietary supplements, such as fish oil or omega-3 fats, is unknown.

Control of blood pressure has had less established impact on coronary morbidity but remains an important goal. The role of exercise remains controversial. The decrease in number of coronary deaths over the last 2 decades may be due to a decrease in the prevalence of risk factors but probably reflects also the role of coronary care units, better treatment of angina, arrhythmias, and heart failure, and improved survival after coronary revascularization in some patient subsets.

AHA Conference Report on Cholesterol: Circulation 1989;80:715. (Six workshop summaries on pathogenesis of atherosclerosis, dietary and drug therapy, and atherosclerosis regression.)

Anderson KM, Castelli WP, Levy D: Cholesterol and mortality: 30 years follow-up from the Framingham Study. JAMA 1987;257:2156.

Blankenhorn DH et al: Beneficial effects of combined colestipol-niacin therapy on coronary atherosclerosis and coronary venous bypass grafts. JAMA 1987;257:3233. (First study showing atherosclerosis can be reversed.)

Cleeman JJ: Report of the National Cholesterol Education

Program Expert Panel on Detection, Evaluation, and Treatment of High Blood Cholesterol in Adults. Arch Intern Med 1988;148:36. (Detailed consensus report.)

Dietary guidelines for healthy American adults: A statement for physicians and health professionals by the Nutrition Committee, American Heart Association. Circulation 1988;77:721A. (Guidelines for healthy diet.)

Final report on the aspirin component of the ongoing Physician's Health Study. N Engl J Med 1989;321:129.

Garber AM: Screening asymptomatic adults for cardiac risk factors: The serum cholesterol level. Ann Intern Med 1989;110:622. (Whom to screen and how to do it.)

Hennekins CH et al: Aspirin and other platelet agents in the secondary and primary prevention of cardiovascular disease. Circulation 1989;80:749.

McIntosh HD: Risk factors for cardiovascular disease and death: A clinical perspective. J Am Coll Cardiol 1989;14:24.

Ross R: The pathogenesis of atherosclerosis: An update. N Engl J Med 1986;314:488.

Stein B et al: Antithrombotic therapy in cardiac disease: An emerging approach based on pathogenesis and risk. Circulation 1989;80:1501.

Steinberg D: Lipoproteins and the pathogenesis of atherosclerosis. Circulation 1987;76:508. (Excellent review of pathophysiology.)

Yusuf S, Wittes J, Friedman L: Overview of results of randomized clinical trials in heart disease. 2. Unstable angina, heart failure, primary prevention with aspirin, and risk factor modification. JAMA 1988;260:2259. (Reviews potential for prevention of coronary artery disease by antihypertensive and hyperlipidemia and antiplatelet agents.)

Pathophysiology of Ischemia

Advanced stages of atherosclerotic coronary artery disease—even complete occlusion—may remain clinically silent. There is only a modest correlation between the clinical symptoms and the extent of disease. At present, the only means of determining the location and extent of narrowing is coronary arteriography, although ischemia can be recognized by other less invasive studies. Functional myocardial ischemia may be documented even in asymptomatic individuals by electrocardiographic stress tests, by reversible thallium-201 perfusion defects, by reversible segmental wall motion abnormalities at echocardiography, or by ambulatory ECG monitoring. Some episodes of myocardial ischemia are painful, causing angina pectoris; others are completely silent. Many silent episodes are brought on by emotional and mental stress. In patients with diagnosed coronary disease, as evidenced by prior myocardial infarction or angina, silent ischemic episodes have the same prognostic import as painful ones. The prognosis for patients with only silent ischemia is not well established.

Cohn PF: Silent myocardial ischemia. Ann Intern Med 1988;109:312.

Epstein SE, Quyyumi AA, Bonow RO: Myocardial ischemia: Silent or symptomatic. N Engl J Med 1988; 318:1038. (Physiology and implications of ischemia.)

Kennedy HL, Wiens RD: Ambulatory (Holter) electrocardiography and myocardial ischemia. Am Heart J 1989; 117:164. (Comprehensive review.)

Muller JE et al: Circadian variation and triggers of onset of acute cardiovascular disease. Circulation 1989;79:733. (More common in early morning.)

Rocco MB et al: Prognostic importance of myocardial ischemia detected by ambulatory monitoring in patients with stable coronary artery disease. Circulation 1988;78:877. (Ambulatory ischemia, whether or not symptomatic, predicts outcome better than exercise testing.)

Rozanski A et al: Mental stress and the induction of silent myocardial ischemia in patients with coronary artery disease. N Engl J Med 1988;318:1005. (Stress can cause ischemia. See also next item: editorial on p 1058 of same issue.)

Selwyn AP, Ganz P: Myocardial ischemia in coronary disease. (Editorial.) N Engl J Med 1988;318:1058.

SUDDEN DEATH

Sudden death may be the first clinical manifestation of coronary disease in as many as one-fourth of patients but is more likely to occur in patients with prior infarction and moderate to severe left ventricular dysfunction. In addition, 20% of patients with acute myocardial infarction will die before reaching a hospital. Most of these deaths are caused by ventricular fibrillation. See p 288 for management of patients at risk for sudden death and the management of survivors.

Gomes JA et al: The role of silent ischemia, the arrhythmic substrate and the short-long sequence in the genesis of sudden cardiac death. J Am Coll Cardiol 1989;14:1618. (Ventricular fibrillation not usually associated with ischemia.)

Kannel WB, Cupples LA, D'Agostino RB: Sudden death risk in overt coronary heart disease: The Framingham Study. Am Heart J 1987;113:799. (Best longitudinal follow-up. Fifty percent of coronary deaths are sudden.)

ANGINA PECTORIS

Essentials of Diagnosis

- Precordial chest pain, usually precipitated by stress or exertion.
- Electrocardiographic evidence of ischemia during pain or on exercise testing.
- Angiographic demonstration of significant obstruction of major coronary vessels.

General Considerations

Angina pectoris is usually due to atherosclerotic heart disease. Less commonly, other causes of coronary artery obstruction such as congenital anomalies, spasm, arteritis, or dissection may cause ischemia or infarction. Angina may also occur in the absence of coronary artery obstruction as a result of severe myocardial hypertrophy, severe aortic stenosis or insufficiency, or in response to increased metabolic demands, as in hyperthyroidism, marked anemia, or paroxysmal tachycardias with rapid ventricular rates. The underlying mechanism is a discrepancy between the myocardial requirements for oxygen and the amount delivered through the coronary arteries resulting from either increased demand (as in exercise) or diminished coronary flow (increased vascular tone or platelet deposition) or both.

Clinical Findings

A. History: The diagnosis of angina pectoris depends principally upon the history, which should specifically include the following information.

1. Circumstances that precipitate and relieve angina–Angina occurs most commonly during activity and is relieved by resting. Exertion that involves straining the thoracic or upper extremity muscles (eg, lifting) or walking rapidly uphill precipitates attacks most consistently. Patients prefer to remain upright rather than lie down. The amount of activity required to produce angina may be relatively consistent under comparable physical and emotional circumstances but may vary from day to day. It is usually less after meals, during excitement, or on exposure to cold. The threshold for angina is often lower in the morning or after strong emotion; the latter can provoke attacks in the absence of exertion. In addition, discomfort may occur during sexual activity, at rest, or at night as a result of coronary spasm.

2. Characteristics of the discomfort–Patients often do not refer to angina as "pain" but as a sensation of tightness, squeezing, burning, pressing, choking, aching, bursting, "gas," indigestion, or an ill-characterized discomfort. It is often characterized by clenching a fist over the mid chest. The distress of angina is never sharply localized and is not spasmodic.

3. Location and radiation–The distribution of the distress may vary widely in different patients but is usually the same for each patient unless unstable angina or myocardial infarction supervenes. In 80–90% of cases, the discomfort is felt behind or slightly to the left of the mid sternum. When it begins farther to the left or, uncommonly, on the right, it characteristically moves centrally to include the sternum. Although angina may radiate to any dermatome from C8 to T4, it radiates most often to the left shoulder and upper arm, frequently moving down the inner volar aspect of the arm to the elbow, forearm, wrist, or fourth and fifth fingers. Radiation to the right shoulder and distally is less common, but the characteristics are the same. Occasionally, angina may be felt initially in the lower jaw, the back of the neck, the interscapular area, high in the left back, or in the volar aspect of the wrist. If the patient identifies the site of pain by pointing to the area of the apical impulse with one finger, angina is unlikely.

4. Duration of attacks–Angina is of short dura-

tion and subsides completely without residual discomfort. If the attack is precipitated by exertion and the patient promptly stops to rest, it usually lasts less than 3 minutes. Attacks following a heavy meal or brought on by anger often last 15–20 minutes. Attacks lasting more than 30 minutes are unusual and suggest the development of unstable angina, myocardial infarction, or an alternative diagnosis.

5. Effect of nitroglycerin–The diagnosis of angina pectoris is strongly supported if sublingual nitroglycerin invariably shortens an attack and if prophylactic nitrates permit greater exertion or prevent angina entirely.

6. Risk factors–The presence of risk factors described previously makes the diagnosis of angina more likely, but their absence does not exclude angina since most patients do not have a risk profile markedly different from that of the general population.

B. Signs: Examination during a spontaneous or induced attack frequently reveals a significant elevation in systolic and diastolic blood pressure, although hypotension may also occur; occasionally, a gallop rhythm and an apical systolic murmur are present during pain only. Supraventricular or ventricular arrhythmias may be present, either as the precipitating factor or as a result of ischemia.

It is important to detect signs of diseases that may contribute to or accompany atherosclerotic heart disease, eg, diabetes mellitus (retinopathy or neuropathy), xanthelasma, tendinous xanthomas, hypertension, thyrotoxicosis, myxedema, or peripheral vascular disease. Aortic stenosis or regurgitation, hypertrophic cardiomyopathy, and mitral valve prolapse should be sought, since they may produce angina or other forms of chest pain.

C. Laboratory Findings: It is important to evaluate risk factors associated with the development of atherosclerosis, particularly serum cholesterol. Contributing factors such as anemia, renal disease, thyrotoxicosis, or myxedema should be sought if suggested by the history and physical examination.

D. Electrocardiography: The resting ECG is normal in about a quarter of patients with angina. In the remainder, abnormalities include old myocardial infarction, nonspecific ST–T changes, atrioventricular or intraventricular conduction defects, and changes of left ventricular hypertrophy. During anginal episodes, the characteristic electrocardiographic change is horizontal or downsloping ST segment depression that reverses after the ischemia disappears. T wave flattening or inversion may also occur. Less frequently, ST segment elevation is observed; this finding suggests severe (transmural) ischemia and often occurs with coronary spasm.

E. Exercise Electrocardiography: Exercise testing is the most useful readily available procedure to assess the patient with angina. Ischemia that is not present at rest is detected by precipitation of typical chest pain or ST segment depression (or, rarely, elevation). Exercise testing is often combined with scintigraphic studies (see below), but in patients without baseline ST segment abnormalities or in whom anatomic localization is not necessary, the exercise ECG should be the initial procedure because of considerations of cost and convenience.

Exercise testing can be done on a motorized treadmill or with a bicycle ergometer. A variety of exercise protocols are utilized, the most common being the Bruce protocol, which increases the treadmill speed and elevation every 3 minutes until limited by symptoms. At lease 2 electrocardiographic leads should be monitored continuously.

1. Precautions and risks–The usually quoted risk of exercise testing is one infarction or death per 1000 tests, but individuals with unstable angina or pain at rest or minimal activity are at higher risk and should not be tested. Many of the traditional exclusions, such as recent myocardial infarction or congestive heart failure, are no longer employed *if the patient is stable and ambulatory,* but aortic stenosis remains a contraindication. A physician should monitor the test, and full resuscitation equipment should be available. While most tests are carried to a symptom-limited end point (except submaximal testing early postinfarction), the test should be terminated when hypotension, significant ventricular or supraventricular arrhythmias, more than mild to moderate angina, or more than 3- to 4-mm ST segment depression occurs.

2. Indications–Exercise testing is employed (1) to confirm the diagnosis of angina; (2) to determine the severity of limitation of activity due to angina; (3) to assess prognosis in patients with known coronary disease, including those recovering from myocardial infarction, by detecting groups at high or low risk; (4) to evaluate responses to therapy; and (5) less successfully, to screen asymptomatic populations for silent coronary disease. The latter application is controversial. Because false-positive tests often exceed true positives, leading to much patient anxiety and self-imposed or mandated disability, exercise testing of asymptomatic individuals should be done only for those at high risk (usually a strong family history of premature coronary disease or hyperlipidemia), those whose occupations place them or others at special risk (eg, airline pilots), and older individuals commencing strenuous activity.

3. Interpretation–The usual electrocardiographic criterion for a positive test is 1 mm (0.1 mV) horizontal or downsloping ST segment depression (beyond baseline) measured 80 ms after the J point. By this criterion, 60–80% of patients with anatomically significant coronary disease will have a positive test, but 10–20% of those without significant disease will also be positive. False-positives are uncommon when a 2-mm depression is present. Additional information is inferred from the time of onset and duration of the electrocardiographic changes, their magnitude and configuration, blood pressure and heart rate changes, the duration of exercise, and the presence of associated symptoms. In general, patients exhibiting more severe ST segment depression (> 2 mm) at low workloads (< 6 min on the Bruce protocol) or heart rates (< 85% of age-predicted maximum)—especially when the duration of exercise and rise in blood pressure are limited or when hypotension occurs during the test—have more severe disease and a poorer prognosis. Depending on symptom status, age, and other factors, such patients should be referred for coronary arteriography and possible revascularization. On the other hand, less impressive positive tests in asymptomatic patients are often ''false-positives.'' Therefore, exercise testing results that do not conform to the clinical picture should be confirmed by scintigraphic study (see below).

F. Scintigraphic Assessment of Ischemia: Two nuclear medicine studies provide additional information about the presence, location, and extent of coronary disease.

1. Thallium-201 scintigraphy–This test provides images in which radionuclide uptake is proportionate to blood flow at the time of injection. Areas of diminished uptake reflect relative hypoperfusion (compared to other myocardial regions). If the radiotracer is injected during exercise or dipyridamole (Persantine)-induced coronary vasodilation, thallium-201 defects indicate a zone of ischemia or hypoperfusion. Over time, as relative blood flow equalizes, these defects tend to ''fill in'' if the abnormality is transient, indicating reversible ischemia. Defects observed when the radiotracer is injected at rest or still present 3–4 hours after an injection during exercise of dipyridamole vasodilatation usually indicate myocardial infarction (old or recent) but may be present with severe ischemia. Occasionally, other conditions, including infiltrative diseases (sarcoidosis, amyloidosis), left bundle branch block, and dilated cardiomyopathy, may produce resting or persistent perfusion defects.

In experienced laboratories, thallium-201 scintigraphy is positive in 75–90% of patients with anatomically significant coronary disease and in only about 10% of those without it. False-positive tests in women may be due to attenuation through breast tissue.

Thallium-201 scintigraphy is indicated (1) when the resting ECG makes an exercise ECG difficult to interpret (LBBB, baseline ST-T changes, low voltage, etc); (2) for confirmation of the results of the exercise ECG when they are contrary to the clinical impression (eg, a positive test in an asymptomatic patient); (3) to localize the region of ischemia; (4) to distinguish ischemic from infarcted myocardium; (5) to assess the completeness of vascularization following bypass surgery or coronary angioplasty; or (6) as a prognostic indicator in patients with known coronary disease.

2. Radionuclide angiography–This procedure

images the left ventricle and measures its ejection fraction and wall motion. In coronary disease, resting abnormalities usually represent infarction, and those that occur with exercise usually indicate stress-induced ischemia. Normal subjects usually exhibit an increase in ejection fraction with exercise or no change; patients with coronary disease may exhibit a decrease. Exercise radionuclide angiography has approximately the same sensitivity as thallium-201 scintigraphy, but it is less specific in older individuals and those with other forms of heart disease. The indications are similar to those for thallium-201 scintigraphy.

G. Echocardiography: Echocardiography can image the left ventricle and reveal segmental wall motion abnormalities, which may indicate ischemia or prior infarction. It is a convenient technique for assessing left ventricular function, which is an important indicator of prognosis and determinant of therapy. An increasing number of laboratories are performing echocardiograms during supine exercise or immediately following upright exercise; exercise-induced segmental wall motion abnormalities are used as an additional indicator of ischemia. This technique requires considerable expertise, however.

H. Coronary Angiography: Selective coronary arteriography is the definitive diagnostic procedure for coronary artery disease. It can be performed with low mortality (about 0.2%) and morbidity (1–7%), but the cost is high, and with currently available noninvasive techniques it is rarely indicated solely for diagnosis.

Coronary arteriography should be performed in the following groups:

(1) Patients being considered for coronary artery revascularization because of limiting stable angina who have failed to improve on an adequate medical regimen.

(2) Patients in whom coronary revascularization is being considered because the clinical presentation (unstable angina, postinfarction angina, etc) or noninvasive testing suggests high-risk disease (see Indications for Revascularization).

(3) Patients with aortic valve disease who also have angina pectoris, in order to determine whether the angina is due to accompanying coronary disease. Coronary angiography is also performed in asymptomatic older patients undergoing valve surgery so that concomitant bypass may be done if the anatomy is propitious.

(4) Patients who have had coronary revascularization with subsequent recurrence of symptoms, to determine whether bypass grafts or native vessels are occluded.

(5) Patients with cardiac failure in whom a surgically correctable lesion, such as left ventricular aneurysm, mitral insufficiency, or reversible ischemic dysfunction, is suspected.

(6) Patients surviving sudden death or with symptomatic or life-threatening arrhythmias in whom coronary artery disease may be a correctable cause.

(7) Patients with chest pain of uncertain cause or cardiomyopathy of unknown cause.

Coronary arteriography visualizes the location and severity of stenoses. Narrowing greater than 50% of the luminal diameter is considered clinically significant, although most lesions producing ischemia are associated with narrowing in excess of 70%. This information has important prognostic value, since mortality rates are progressively higher in patients with one-, 2-, and 3-vessel disease and those with left main coronary artery obstruction (ranging from 1% per year to 25% per year). Among stable patients, 20%, 30%, and 50% have one-, 2-, and 3-vessel involvement, respectively, while left main disease is present in 10%. In those with strongly positive exercise ECGs or scintigraphic studies, 3-vessel or left main disease may be present in 75–95% depending upon the criteria employed. Coronary arteriography also shows whether the obstructions are amenable to bypass surgery or percutaneous transluminal coronary angioplasty (PTCA).

I. Left Ventricular Angiography: Left ventricular angiography is usually performed at the same time as coronary arteriography. Global and regional left ventricular function are visualized, as well as mitral regurgitation if present. Left ventricular function is the major determinant of prognosis in stable coronary disease and of the risk of bypass surgery.

Armstrong WF: Echocardiography in coronary artery disease. Prog Cardiovasc Dis 1988;30:267.

Beller GA, Gibson RS: Sensitivity, specificity, and prognostic significance of noninvasive testing for occult or known coronary disease. Prog Cardiovasc Dis 1987; 29:241.

Califf RM et al: Importance of clinical measures of ischemia in the prognosis of patients with documented coronary artery disease. J Am Coll Cardiol 1988;11:20.

Cheitlin MD: Finding the high-risk patient with coronary artery disease. JAMA 1988;259:2271.

Eagle KA et al: Dipyridamole-thallium scanning in patients undergoing vascular surgery: Optimizing preoperative evaluation of cardiac risk. JAMA 1987;257:2585. (High-risk patients are detected.)

Lam JY et al: Safety and diagnostic accuracy of dipyridamole-thallium imaging in the elderly. J Am Coll Cardiol 1988;11:585. (Role of an increasingly used test.)

Ross J Jr, Fisch C: Guidelines for coronary angiography. J Am Coll Cardiol 1987;10:935. (Consensus report covering indications and procedures.)

Shub C: Stable angina pectoris: 1. Clinical patterns. 2. Cardiac evaluation and diagnostic testing. Mayo Clin Proc 1990;65:233, 243.

Silverman KJ, Grossman W: Angina pectoris: Natural history and strategies for evaluation and management. N Engl J Med 1984;310:1712.

Weiner DA et al: The role of exercise testing in identifying patients with improved survival after coronary artery bypass surgery. J Am Coll Cardiol 1986;8:741. (Revascularization better in patients with very positive tests.)

Coronary Vasospasm

Although most symptoms of myocardial ischemia result from fixed stenosis of the coronary arteries or thrombosis or hemorrhage at the site of lesions, some ischemic events may be precipitated by coronary vasoconstriction.

Spasm of the large coronary arteries with resulting decreased coronary blood flow may occur spontaneously or may be induced by mechanical irritation from a coronary catheter, by exposure to cold, or by ergot derivative drugs. Spasm may occur both in normal and in stenosed coronary arteries and may be silent or result in angina pectoris. Even myocardial infarction may occur as a result of spasm in the absence of visible obstructive coronary heart disease, although most instances of coronary spasm occur in the presence of coronary stenosis.

Cocaine-induced myocardial infarction is a growing problem. While coronary artery vasoconstriction plays a role in many patients, coronary thrombosis and increased myocardial energy requirements may also be important factors.

Prinzmetal's (variant) angina is a clinical syndrome in which chest pain occurs without the usual precipitating factors and is associated with ST segment elevation rather than depression. It often affects women under 50 years of age. It characteristically occurs in the early morning, awakening patients from sleep, tends to involve the right coronary artery, and is apt to be associated with arrhythmias or conduction defects. There may be no fixed stenoses.

Patients with this pattern of pain or any chest pain syndrome associated with ST segment elevation should usually undergo coronary arteriography to determine whether fixed stenotic lesions are present. If they are, aggressive medical therapy or revascularization is indicated, since this may represent an unstable phase of the disease. If significant lesions are not seen and spasm is suspected, ergonovine may be administered intravenously to precipitate vasospasm. This must be done cautiously and with nitroglycerin prepared for intracoronary administration, since irreversible spasm may lead to infarction. Episodes respond well to nitrates or calcium channel blockers, and both drugs are effective prophylactically. Beta-blockers have exacerbated coronary vasospasm, but they may have a role in management of patients in whom spasm is associated with fixed stenoses.

Frishman WH et al: Cocaine induced coronary artery disease: Recognition and treatment. Med Clin North Am 1989;73:475.

Lange RA et al: Cocaine-induced coronary-artery vasoconstriction. N Engl J Med 1989;321:1557.

Maseri A: Role of coronary artery spasm in symptomatic and silent myocardial ischemia. J Am Coll Cardiol 1987;9:249.

Walling A et al: Long-term prognosis of patients with variant angina. Circulation 1987;76:990.

Differential Diagnosis

With an appropriate history, the diagnosis of angina pectoris is more than 90% certain. When atypical features are present—such as prolonged duration (hours or days); or darting, knifelike pains at the apex or over the precordium—ischemia is less likely.

"Anterior chest wall syndrome" is characterized by sharply localized tenderness of intercostal muscles. Sprain or inflammation of the chondrocostal junctions, which may be warm, swollen, and red, may result in diffuse chest pain that is also reproduced by local pressure (Tietze's syndrome). Intercostal neuritis (herpes zoster, diabetes mellitus, etc) also mimics angina.

Cervical or thoracic spine disease involving the dorsal roots produces sudden sharp, severe chest pain suggesting angina in location and "radiation" but related to specific movements of the neck or spine, recumbency, and straining or lifting. Pain due to cervical or thoracic disk disease involves the outer or dorsal aspect of the arm and the thumb and index fingers rather than the ring and little fingers.

Peptic ulcer, chronic cholecystitis, esophageal spasm, and functional gastrointestinal disease may produce pain suggestive of angina pectoris. Reflux esophagitis is characterized by lower chest and upper abdominal pain after heavy meals, occurring in recumbency or upon bending over. The pain is relieved by antacids or H_2 receptor antagonists. The picture may be especially confusing because ischemic pain may also be associated with upper gastrointestinal symptoms, and esophageal motility disorders may be improved by nitrates and calcium channel blockers. Detailed assessment of esophageal motility may be necessary.

Degenerative and inflammatory lesions of the left shoulder, cervical rib, and the scalenus anticus syndrome differ from angina in that the pain is precipitated by movement of the arm and shoulder; paresthesias are present in the left arm, and postural exercises and pillow support to the shoulders in bed give relief.

Spontaneous pneumothorax may cause chest pain as well as dyspnea and may create confusion with angina as well as myocardial infarction. The same is true of pneumonia and pulmonary embolization. Dissection of the thoracic aorta can cause severe "tearing" chest pain that is commonly felt in the back; it is sudden in onset, reaches maximum intensity immediately, and may be associated with changes in pulses. Other cardiac disorders such as mitral valve prolapse, hypertrophic cardiomyopathy, myocarditis, pericarditis, aortic valve disease, or right ventricular hypertrophy may cause atypical chest pain or even myocardial ischemia. Noninvasive testing and, in many cases, cardiac catheterization may be required to establish the diagnosis.

Magarian GJ, Hickam DH: Noncardiac causes of angina-like chest pain. Prog Cardiovasc Dis 1986;29:65.

Treatment

A. Treatment of Acute Attack: Sublingual nitroglycerin is the drug of choice; it acts in about 1–2 minutes. Nitrates decrease arteriolar and venous tone, reduce preload and afterload, and lower the oxygen demand of the heart. Nitrates may also improve myocardial blood flow by dilating collateral channels and, in the presence of increased vasomotor tone, coronary stenoses. As soon as the attack begins, one fresh tablet is placed under the tongue. This may be repeated at 3- to 5-minute intervals. The dosage (0.3, 0.4, or 0.6 mg) and the number of tablets to be used before seeking further medical attention must be individualized. Nitroglycerin should also be used prophylactically before activities likely to precipitate angina. Pain not responding to 3–4 tablets or lasting more than 20 minutes may represent evolving infarction, and the patient should be instructed to seek medical attention.

B. Prevention of Further Attacks:

1. Aggravating factors–Angina may be aggravated by hypertension, left ventricular failure, arrhythmia (usually tachycardias), strenuous activity, cold temperatures, and emotional states. These factors should be identified and treated or avoided where possible.

2. Nitroglycerin–Nitroglycerin, 0.3–0.6 mg sublingually, should be taken just before activity which is likely to precipitate angina. Sublingual isosorbide dinitrate (2.5–10 mg) is only slightly longer-acting than sublingual nitroglycerin.

3. Long-acting nitrates–A number of longer-acting nitrate preparations are available. These include isosorbide dinitrate (Isordil, Sorbitrate), 10–40 mg orally 4 times daily; oral sustained-release nitroglycerin preparations, 6.25–12.5 mg 2–4 times daily; nitroglycerin ointment, 6.25–25 mg applied 2–4 times daily; and transdermal nitroglycerin patches that deliver nitroglycerin at a predetermined rate (usually 5–20 mg/24 h). Continuous nitrate blood levels are associated with tolerance, so it is best to design a regimen with daily nitrate-free intervals, depending upon the patient's pattern of pain.

Nitrate therapy is often limited by headache; if the dosage is too large and the patient remains erect, hypotension occurs.

4. Beta-blockers–The beta-blockers prevent angina by reducing myocardial oxygen requirements during exertion and stress. This is accomplished by reducing the heart rate, cardiac muscle contractility, and, to a lesser extent, blood pressure. All available beta-blockers appear to be effective for angina, but those with intrinsic sympathomimetic activity are less preferable because they may exacerbate angina in some individuals and have not been effective in secondary prevention trials. The pharmacology of the beta-blockers is discussed under Hypertension (Table 8–3).

Because beta-blockers improve survival after myocardial infarction, they are a reasonable initial choice for chronic antianginal therapy. The side effects of the beta-blockers have been discussed, but most importantly, they should be avoided in patients with bronchospasm and heart failure.

5. Calcium entry-blocking agents–(Table 8–5.) Verapamil, diltiazem, nifedipine, and nicardipine are chemically and pharmacologically heterogeneous agents that prevent angina by reducing myocardial oxygen requirements and by inducing coronary artery vasodilatation. Myocardial oxygen demand is lessened by reducing blood pressure, left ventricular wall stress, and, in the case of verapamil and diltiazem, resting or exercise heart rate. Though these agents are all potent coronary vasodilators, it is unclear whether they improve myocardial blood flow in most patients with stable exertional angina. In those with coronary vasospasm, the calcium entry blockers may be the agent of choice.

The currently available calcium channel blockers all have negative inotropic, chronotropic, and dromotropic properties in vitro, but the reflex sympathetic response may obscure these effects in vivo (except in the presence of beta blockade or severely depressed left ventricular function). Several additional calcium channel blockers of the dihydropyridine class, of which nifedipine is the prototype, are now available or will be in the near future. These include nicardipine, isradipine, nisoldipine, and felodipine. All are potent

Table 8–5. Oral calcium entry-blocking drugs.

Agent	Inhibition of Atrioventricular Conduction	Coronary Vasodilatation	Negative Inotropic Action	Hypotension, Edema	Dosage Initial (Range)
Verapamil	+++	++	+++	++	80 mg 3 times daily (240–480 mg daily)[1]
Diltiazem	+ to ++	++	+	+	60 mg 3 times daily (180–480 mg daily)[1]
Nifedipine	0 to +	+++	+	+++	10 mg 3 times daily (30–120 mg daily)[1]
Nicardipine	0 to +	+++	+ or ++	+++	20 mg 3 times daily (60–120 mg daily)

[1] Available also in sustained-release preparation.

peripheral and coronary vasodilators, but the absence of a negative inotropic effect has not been demonstrated. Each of the calcium channel blockers must be titrated upward at intervals of at least several days, since the range of dosages employed is wide.

6. Combination therapy–Patients remaining symptomatic when given one class of preventive agent should be treated with combinations. A beta-blocker and a long-acting nitrate or a beta-blocker and a calcium channel blocker (other than verapamil, where the risk of atrioventricular block or heart failure is higher) are the most appropriate combinations. A few patients will have a further response to a regimen including all 3 agents.

7. Platelet-inhibiting agents–Coronary thrombosis is responsible for most episodes of myocardial infarction and many unstable ischemic syndromes. Several studies have demonstrated the benefit of antiplatelet drugs following unstable angina and infarction, and a recent trial has demonstrated a reduction in myocardial infarctions in previously healthy men over 40. Therefore, unless contraindicated, small doses of aspirin (80 mg daily or 325 mg daily or every other day) should be prescribed for patients with angina.

8. Revascularization–The indications for coronary artery revascularization and the choice of procedure are discussed below.

Prognosis

The prognosis of angina pectoris has improved with advances in the understanding of its pathophysiology and in pharmacologic therapy. Mortality rates range from 1% to 25% per year depending on the number of vessels diseased, the severity of obstruction, the status of left ventricular function, and the presence of complex arrhythmias. In patients with stable symptoms and normal ejection fractions ($>55\%$, depending on the laboratory), the mortality rate is less than 4% per year. However, the outlook in individual patients is unpredictable, and nearly half of the deaths are sudden. Therefore, risk stratification is often attempted. Patients with accelerating symptoms have a poorer outlook. Among stable patients, those whose exercise tolerance is severely limited by ischemia (less than 6 minutes on the Bruce treadmill protocol) and those with extensive ischemia by exercise electrocardiography or scintigraphy have more severe anatomic disease and a poorer prognosis.

Abrams J: A reappraisal of nitrate therapy. JAMA 1988; 259:396.

Chan P et al: The role of nitrates, beta blockers, and calcium antagonists in stable angina pectoris. Am Heart J 1988; 116:838.

Fuster V et al: Platelet-inhibitor drugs' role in coronary artery disease. Prog Cardiovasc Dis 1987;29:325.

Packer M: Combined beta-adrenergic and calcium entry blockade in angina pectoris. N Engl J Med 1989;320:709. (Two drugs not always better than one.)

Parker JO: Nitrate therapy in stable angina pectoris. N Engl J Med 1987;316:1635. (Review with discussion of nitrate tolerance.)

Shub C: Stable angina pectoris: 3. Medical treatment. Mayo Clin Proc 1990;65:256.

REVASCULARIZATION PROCEDURES FOR PATIENTS WITH ANGINA PECTORIS

Indications

The indications for coronary artery revascularization in patients with stable angina pectoris are often debated. There is general agreement that otherwise healthy patients in the following groups should undergo revascularization. (1) Patients with unacceptable symptoms despite maximally tolerated medical therapy. (2) Patients with left main coronary artery stenosis greater than 50% with or without symptoms. (3) Patients with 3-vessel disease with moderate left ventricular dysfunction (ejection fraction 30–50%). (4) Patients with unstable angina who after symptom control by medical therapy continue to exhibit ischemia on exercise testing or monitoring. (5) Post-myocardial infarction patients with continuing angina or ischemia on noninvasive testing, particularly if they have received thrombolytic treatment (see sections on Unstable Angina and Myocardial Infarction).

In addition, many cardiologists feel that patients with less severe symptoms should be revascularized if they have anatomically critical lesions ($>90\%$ proximal stenoses, especially of the left anterior descending artery) or physiologic evidence of significant ischemia (early positive exercise tests, large exercise-induced thallium scintigraphic defects, or frequent episodes of ischemia on ambulatory monitoring). This trend toward aggressive intervention has accelerated as a result of the growing availability of coronary angioplasty. While such patients are at increased risk, it has not been proved that the prognosis is better after coronary revascularization by either surgery or angioplasty.

Type of Procedure

A. Coronary Artery Bypass Grafting (CABG): CABG can be accomplished with a very low mortality rate (1–3%) in otherwise healthy patients with preserved cardiac function. However, the mortality rate of this procedure has increased to 4–8% or higher in recent years because the surgical population includes a greater proportion of high-risk and older patients. Increasingly, younger individuals with focal lesions of one or several vessels are undergoing coronary angioplasty as the initial revascularization procedure.

Grafts employing one or both internal mammary

arteries (usually to the left anterior descending artery or its branches) provide the best long-term results in terms of patency and flow. Segments of the saphenous vein (or, less optimally, other veins) interposed between the aorta and the coronary arteries distal to the obstructions are also utilized. One to 5 distal anastomoses are commonly performed. After successful surgery, symptoms generally abate. The need for antianginal medications diminishes, and left ventricular function may improve.

The operative mortality rate is increased in patients with poor left ventricular function or those requiring other procedures (valve replacement or ventricular aneurysmectomy). Patients over 70 years of age, patients undergoing repeat procedures, or those with severe noncardiac disease also have higher operative mortality and morbidity rates, and full recovery is slow. Thus, CABG should be reserved for more severely symptomatic patients in this group. Early (1–6 months) graft patency rates average 85–90% (higher for internal mammary grafts), and subsequent graft closure rates are about 4% annually. Early graft failure is common in vessels with poor distal flow, while late closure is more frequent in patients who continue smoking and those with untreated hyperlipidemia. Antiplatelet therapy with aspirin alone or combined with dipyridamole improves graft patency rates. Long-term dipyridamole therapy is expensive, inconvenient, and of uncertain value. Repeat CABG or angioplasty (see below) is often necessitated by progressive native vessel disease and graft occlusions. Reoperation is technically demanding and less often fully successful than the initial operation.

B. Percutaneous Transluminal Coronary Angioplasty (PTCA): Coronary artery stenoses can be effectively dilated by inflation of a balloon under high pressure. This procedure is performed in the cardiac catheterization laboratory under local anesthesia either at the same time as diagnostic coronary arteriography or at a later time. The mechanism of dilation is rupture of the atheromatous plaque, with subsequent resorption of intraluminal debris.

This procedure was at one time reserved for proximal single-vessel disease, but now it is widely employed in multivessel disease with multiple lesions, though only rarely in left main disease. PTCA is also effective in CABG stenoses. Optimal lesions for PTCA are relatively proximal, noneccentric, free of plaque dissection, and removed from the origin of large branches. In the USA, the number of PTCA procedures now exceeds that of CABG operations. With improved catheter systems, experienced operators are able to manipulate the balloon catheter across approximately 90% of approachable lesions and successfully dilate 90% of those. The major early complication is intimal dissection with vessel occlusion. This can sometimes be treated by repeat PTCA, but urgent CABG is required in 3–5% of cases, and mor-

bidity and mortality rates are high. Therefore, these procedures must be done in a laboratory where surgery is available on short notice.

The major limitation with PTCA has been restenosis, which occurs in the first 6 months in 20–30% of vessels dilated. The mechanism of restenosis is unclear, and it can often be treated successfully by repeat PTCA.

C. Investigational Revascularization Procedures: There is considerable interest in the use of laser energy to "vaporize" atherosclerotic plaques and catheter devices to remove atheromatous material. These approaches are technically feasible and have been employed in peripheral arteries and investigationally in coronary arteries. Current data do not indicate a significant improvement in either initial success or restenosis rates with these experimental techniques, but the technologies are evolving.

Results

The mortality rates of PTCA and CABG are comparable in stable angina. Recovery after PTCA is obviously faster, but the early success rate of CABG is probably higher. The increasing popularity of PTCA primarily reflects its lower cost, shorter hospitalization, the perception that CABG is best done only once and can be reserved for later, and the preference of patients for less invasive treatment.

ACC/AHA Task Force Report: Guidelines for percutaneous transluminal coronary angiography. J Am Coll Cardiol 1988;12:529.

Bourassa MG et al: Long-term fate of bypass grafts. Circulation 1985;72(Suppl):V71. (Largest experience with serial angiography.)

Bourassa MG et al: Report of the Joint ISFC/WHO Task Force on coronary angioplasty. Circulation 1988;78:780. (Consensus statement on indications and results.)

Califf RM et al: The evolution of medical and surgical therapy for coronary artery disease: A 15-year perspective. JAMA 1989;261:2077. (Large series suggesting that survival with surgery may be better in most patient groups.)

Elayda MA et al: Coronary revascularization in the elderly patient. J Am Coll Cardiol 1984;3:1398. (Surgery more problematic over age 70.)

Forrester JS: Laser angioplasty: Now and in the future. Circulation 1988;78:777. (Editorial perspective.)

Foster ED: Reoperation for coronary artery disease. Circulation 1985;72(Suppl):V59. (Good discussion of difficult problem.)

Frye RL et al: Randomized trials in coronary artery bypass surgery. Prog Cardiovasc Dis 1987;30:1.

Henderson WG et al: Antiplatelet or anticoagulant therapy after coronary artery bypass surgery. Ann Intern Med 1989;111:743. (Aspirin increases graft patency.)

Holmes DR Jr et al: The effect of medical and surgical treatment on subsequent sudden cardiac death in patients with coronary artery disease: A report from the Coronary Artery Surgery Study. Circulation 1986;73:1254. (Major results of a key study.)

Holmes DR, Vliestra RE: Balloon angioplasty in acute and

chronic coronary artery disease. JAMA 1989;261:2109. (Concise review.)

Loop FD et al: Influence of the internal-mammary-artery graft on 10 year survival and other cardiac events. N Engl J Med 1986;314:1. (Results of large series indicate superiority of this procedure.)

Popma JJ, Dehmer GJ: Care of the patient after coronary angioplasty. Ann Intern Med 1989;110:547. (Management of acute complications and restenosis.)

Ryan TS: Guidelines for percutaneous transluminal coronary angioplasty. Circulation 1988;78:486. (Position paper reviewing indications, techniques, and results.)

Varnauskas E et al: Twelve-year follow-up of survival in the randomized European Coronary Surgery Study. N Engl J Med 1988;319:332. (Initial advantage of CABG disappears with time.)

See also Cheitlin and Weiner references on p 468.

UNSTABLE ANGINA

Most clinicians use the term "unstable angina" to denote an accelerating or "crescendo" pattern of pain in cases where previously stable angina occurs with less exertion or at rest, lasts longer, and is less responsive to medication. Coronary angioscopy has shown that a high proportion of patients with this pattern of symptoms have "complex" coronary stenosis characterized by plaque ulceration, hemorrhage, or thrombosis. This inherently unstable situation may progress to complete occlusion and infarction or may heal, with reendothelialization and a return to a stable though possibly more severe pattern of ischemia.

Diagnosis

Most patients with unstable angina will exhibit electrocardiographic changes during pain—commonly ST segment depression or T wave flattening or inversion but sometimes, and more ominously, ST segment elevation. They may exhibit signs of left ventricular dysfunction during pain and for a time thereafter.

Treatment

A. General Measures: Treatment of unstable angina should be multifaceted and vigorous. Patients should be hospitalized, maintained at bed rest or at very limited activity, monitored, and given supplemental oxygen. Sedation with a benzodiazepine agent is usually indicated. The systolic blood pressure is usually maintained at 100–120 mm Hg, except in previously severe hypertensives. Patients with heart rates above 70–80/min should be given beta-blockers unless heart failure or other medical contraindications are present.

B. Nitroglycerin: The nitrates are first-line therapy for unstable angina. Nonparenteral therapy with sublingual or oral agents or nitroglycerin ointment is usually sufficient. If pain persists despite the addition of other agents, intravenous nitroglycerin should be started. The usual initial dosage is 10 mg/min. The dosage should be titrated to 1–2 μg/kg/min over 30–60 minutes and further increased as tolerated if pain recurs. Dosages up to 10 μg/kg/min or higher may be used. Tolerance to continuous nitrate infusion is common. Careful—usually continuous—blood pressure monitoring is required when intravenous nitroglycerin is used.

C. Calcium Entry Blockers: Since alterations in coronary vasomotor tone more frequently play a role in unstable ischemic syndromes, these agents are commonly employed. In the presence of nitrates and without accompanying beta-blockers, diltiazem or verapamil is preferred, since nifedipine is more likely to cause reflex tachycardia or hypotension. The initial dosage should be low, but upward titration should proceed rapidly. (See Table 8–5.)

D. Beta-Blockers: These agents are effective in unstable angina, particularly when tachycardia is present or precipitated by other medications. The goal of acute treatment is to reduce the heart rate below 60–70/min. Again, the dosage can be titrated upward at intervals of several hours with careful monitoring.

E. Anticoagulation, Antiplatelet, and Thrombolytic Therapy: As noted above, intravascular thrombosis plays a prominent role in the pathophysiology of unstable angina and its progression to myocardial infarction. Therefore, most authorities recommend low-dose aspirin (325 mg daily) and commence intravenous heparin if ischemia persists. Several studies have demonstrated beneficial results with thrombolytic therapy, but the timing of and need for this approach remain to be determined.

F. Intra-aortic Balloon Counterpulsation (IABC): If pain persists with accompanying electrocardiographic changes despite the above measures, IABC should be considered both to reduce myocardial energy requirements (systolic unloading) and to improve diastolic blood flow. While this approach is often effective, other experts will proceed directly to coronary arteriography and revascularization. Intra-aortic balloon counterpulsation is best applied only if CABG or PTCA is planned. Aortic insufficiency is a contraindication, and IABC must be used cautiously in patients with peripheral vascular disease.

Prognosis & Indications for Revascularization

Patients who do not become ischemia-free on medical therapy should have early coronary arteriography and revascularization. Over 90% of patients can be rendered pain-free with these measures. Controlled trials have not shown any advantage in increased survival or lower infarction rates with CABG compared to medical therapy, although many patients treated medically will need surgery later for recurrent symptoms. However, these studies are from the early era of surgery and precede the availability of PTCA; furthermore, more sophisticated medical regimens are now available. Depending on the stringency of the definition of unstable angina, 10–30% of patients will have an early infarction, and the 1-year mortality rate is 10–20%. Recent data from ambulatory monitoring indicate that many patients without pain continue to have "silent" episodes of ST segment depression or, less commonly, elevation. These individuals have a poorer prognosis.

Because the outlook is poor following relief of unstable angina, most cardiologists recommend either (1) coronary arteriography before discharge or when the patient is stabilized or (2) early exercise testing to identify high-risk subsets for further invasive evaluation. The artery responsible for the ischemia can usually be determined from electrocardiographic or scintigraphic changes during pain, and the lesion is often amenable to PTCA. If revascularization is not performed, long-term management is the same as that outlined for stable angina pectoris.

Ambrose JA, Hjemdahl-Monsen CE: Arteriographic anatomy and mechanisms of myocardial ischemia in unstable angina. J Am Coll Cardiol 1987;9:1397. (Tight stenoses, complex lesions.)

De Feyter P et al: Coronary angioplasty for unstable angina: Immediate and late results in 200 consecutive patients with identification of risk factors for unfavorable early and late outcome. J Am Coll Cardiol 1988;12:324. (Favorable results in 200 patients.)

Fuster V, Chesebro JH: Mechanisms of unstable angina. (Editorial.) N Engl J Med 1986;315:1023.

Gotoh K et al: The role of intracoronary thrombus in unstable angina: Angiographic assessment and thrombolytic therapy during ongoing anginal attacks. Circulation 1988; 77:526. (Rationale and results of thrombolytic therapy.)

Gottlieb SO et al: Silent ischemia predicts infarction and death during 2-year follow-up of unstable angina. J Am Coll Cardiol 1987;10:756.

Luchi RJ, Scott SM, Deupree RH: Comparison of medical and surgical treatment for unstable angina pectoris: Results of a Veterans Administration cooperative study. N Engl J Med 1987;316:977. (No advantage to acute CABG, but many patients will need revascularization later.)

Munger T, Jae KO: Unstable angina. Mayo Clin Proc 1990;65:384. (Comprehensive review.)

Sherman CT et al: Coronary angioscopy in patients with unstable angina pectoris. N Engl J Med 1986;315:913. (Reveals frequent thrombus or plaque changes.)

Theroux P et al: Aspirin, heparin, or both to treat acute unstable angina. N Engl J Med 1988;319:1105. (Excellent study showing benefit of heparin with or without aspirin.)

ACUTE MYOCARDIAL INFARCTION

Essentials of Diagnosis

- Sudden but not instantaneous development of prolonged (> 30 minutes) anterior chest discomfort (sometimes felt as "gas") that may produce arrhythmias, hypotension, shock, or cardiac failure.
- Rarely painless, masquerading as acute congestive heart failure, syncope, cerebral vascular accident, or "unexplained" shock.
- Electrocardiography: ST segment elevation or depression, evolving Q waves, symmetric inversion of T waves.
- Elevation of cardiac enzymes (CK-MB, LDH fraction 1).
- Appearance of segmental wall motion abnormality.

General Considerations

Myocardial infarction results from prolonged myocardial ischemia, precipitated in most cases by an occlusive coronary thrombus at the site of a preexisting (though often not severe) atherosclerotic stenosis. More rarely, infarction may result from prolonged vasospasm, inadequate myocardial blood flow (eg, hypotension), or excessive metabolic demand. These processes also occur most commonly in patients with atherosclerotic disease. Very rarely, myocardial infarction may be caused by embolic occlusion, vasculitis, aortic root or coronary artery dissection, or aortitis. Cocaine is an increasingly common cause of infarction.

The location and extent of infarction depend upon the anatomic distribution of the occluded vessel, the presence of additional stenotic lesions, and the adequacy of collateral circulation. Thrombosis in the anterior descending branch of the left coronary artery results in infarction of the anterior left ventricle and interventricular septum. Occlusion of the left circumflex artery produces anterolateral or posterolateral infarction. Right coronary thrombosis leads to infarction of the posteroinferior portion of the left ventricle and may involve the right ventricular myocardium and interventricular septum. The arteries supplying the atrioventricular node and the sinus node more commonly arise from the right coronary; thus, atrioventricular block at the nodal level and sinus node dysfunction occur more frequently during inferior infarctions. However, because there are great individual variations in coronary anatomy and because associated lesions and collaterals may confuse the picture, prediction of coronary anatomy from the infarct location may be inaccurate.

Infarctions are often classified as transmural, if the classic electrocardiographic evolution of ST segment elevation to Q waves is observed; or nontransmural or subendocardial, if pain, enzyme elevations, and ST–T wave changes occur in the absence of new Q waves. However, on pathologic examination, most infarctions involve the subendocardium predominantly, and some transmural extension is common even in the absence of Q waves. Thus, the better classification is Q wave versus non-Q wave infarction. The latter may result from spontaneous lysis of the thrombus and often signifies the presence of additional jeopardized myocardium; it is associated with a higher incidence of reinfarction and recurrent ischemia.

The size and anatomic location of the infarction determines the acute clinical picture, the early complications, and the long-term prognosis. The hemodynamic findings are related directly to the extent of necrosis (together with the amount of damage from previous infarctions). In small infarctions, cardiac function is normal, whereas with more extensive damage, early heart failure and hypotension (cardiogenic shock) may appear. Additional myocardium beyond that initially infarcted is often threatened, being maintained by collateral circulation or by blood flow through a partially recanalized vessel. Thus, preventing extension of the infarct is one of the major goals of early management. The complications of acute infarction are discussed below.

Clinical Findings

A. Symptoms:

1. Premonitory pain—One-third of patients give a history of alteration in the pattern of angina, recent onset of typical or atypical angina, or unusual "indigestion" felt in the chest.

2. Pain of infarction—Most infarctions occur at rest unlike anginal episodes, and more commonly in the early morning. The pain is similar to angina in location and radiation but is more severe, and it builds up rapidly or in waves to maximum intensity over a few minutes or longer. Nitroglycerin has little effect; even narcotics may not relieve the pain. Patients may break out in a cold sweat, feel weak and apprehensive, and move about, seeking a position of comfort. They prefer not to lie quietly. Light-headedness, syncope, dyspnea, orthopnea, cough, wheezing, nausea and vomiting, or abdominal bloating may be present singly or in any combination.

3. Painless infarction—In a minority of cases, pain is absent or minor and is overshadowed by the immediate complications. As many as 25% of infarctions are detected on routine ECG without there having been any recallable acute episode.

4. Sudden death and early arrhythmias—Approximately 20% of patients with acute infarction will die before reaching the hospital; these deaths are usually in the first hour and are chiefly due to ventricular fibrillation.

B. Signs:

1. General—Patients usually appear anxious and are often sweating profusely. The heart rate may range from marked bradycardia (most commonly in inferior infarction) to tachycardia resulting from increased sympathetic nervous system activity, low cardiac output, or arrhythmia. The blood pressure may be high, especially in former hypertensives, or low in patients with shock. Respiratory distress usually indicates heart failure. Fever, usually low-grade, may appear after 12 hours and persist for several days.

2. Chest—Clear lung fields are a good prognostic sign, but basilar rales are common and do not necessarily indicate heart failure. More extensive rales or diffuse wheezing may indicate pulmonary edema.

3. Heart—The cardiac examination may be unim-

pressive or very abnormal. An abnormally located ventricular impulse often represents the dyskinetic infarcted region. Soft heart sounds may indicate left ventricular dysfunction. Atrial gallops (S_4) are the rule, whereas ventricular gallops (S_3) are less common and indicate significant left ventricular dysfunction. Mitral regurgitation murmurs are not uncommon and usually indicate papillary muscle dysfunction or, rarely, rupture. Pericardial friction rubs are uncommon in the first 24 hours but may appear later.

4. Extremities—Edema is usually not present. Cyanosis and cold temperature indicate low output. The peripheral pulses should be noted, since later shock or emboli may alter the examination.

C. Laboratory Findings: Leukocytosis of 10,000–20,000/μL often develops on the second day and disappears within a week. The most valuable diagnostic test is serial measurement of cardiac enzymes, of which creatine kinase (CK or CPK) rises the earliest and is the most specific for infarction. The MB isoenzyme is very specific for the heart. The peak CK value correlates with the size of the infarction. Serum lactic acid dehydrogenase may remain elevated for 5–7 days, and fraction l is relatively specific for myocardial damage. Serial determinations may be helpful in equivocal instances.

D. Electrocardiography: Most patients with acute infarction have ECG changes, and a normal tracing is rare. The extent of the electrocardiographic abnormalities provides only a crude estimate of the magnitude of infarction. The classic evolution of changes is from peaked ("hyperacute") T waves, to ST segment elevation, to Q wave development, to T wave inversion. This may occur over a few hours to several days. The evolution of new Q waves (> 30 ms in duration and 25% of the R wave amplitude) is diagnostic, but Q waves do not occur in 30–50% of acute infarctions (subendocardial or non-Q wave infarctions). If these patients have an appropriate clinical presentation, characteristic cardiac enzymes, and ST segment changes (usually depression) or T wave inversion lasting at least 48 hours, they are classified as having non-Q wave infarctions.

E. Chest X-Ray: The chest x-ray may demonstrate signs of congestive heart failure, but these changes often lag behind the clinical findings. Signs of aortic dissection should be sought as a possible alternative diagnosis.

F. Echocardiography: Echocardiography provides convenient bedside assessment of left ventricular global and regional function. This can help with the diagnosis and management of infarction; echocardiography has been used successfully to make judgments about admission and management of patients with suspected infarction, since normal wall motion makes an infarction unlikely. Doppler echocardiography is probably the most convenient procedure for diagnosing postinfarction mitral regurgitation or ventricular septal defect.

G. Scintigraphic Studies: Technetium-99m pyrophosphate scintigraphy can be used to diagnose acute myocardial infarction. When injected at least 18 hours postinfarction, the radiotracer complexes with calcium in necrotic myocardium to provide a "hot spot" image of the infarction. This test is insensitive to small infarctions, and false-positive studies occur, so its use is limited to patients in whom the diagnosis by electrocardiography and enzymes is not possible—principally those who present several days after the event or have intraoperative infarctions.

Thallium-201 scintigraphy will demonstrate "cold spots" in regions of diminished perfusion, which usually represent infarction when the radio-tracer is administered at rest, but abnormalities do not distinguish recent from old damage.

Radionuclide angiography demonstrates akinesis or dyskinesis in areas of infarction and also measures ejection fraction, which can be valuable. Right ventricular dysfunction may indicate infarction of this chamber.

H. Hemodynamic Measurements: These can be invaluable in managing the complicated patient. Their use is described below and in Table 8–7.

Cheitlin MD, McAllister HA, de Castro CM: Myocardial infarction without atherosclerosis. JAMA 1975;231:951. (Best review and pathologic discussion.)

DeWood MA et al: Coronary arteriographic findings soon after non-Q-wave myocardial infarction. N Engl J Med 1986;315:417. (Infarct-related vessel more often patent with non-Q wave myocardial infarction.)

Forrester JS et al: A perspective of coronary disease seen through the arteries of living man. Circulation 1987;75:505. (Acute thrombus is present in myocardial infarction.)

Pasternack PF, Calvin SB, Baumann FG: Cocaine-induced angina pectoris and acute myocardial infarction in patients younger than 40 years. Am J Cardiol 1985;55:847.

Treatment

A. Thrombolytic Therapy: Thrombolytic therapy reduces the mortality rate and limits infarct size in many patients when started within 3–6 hours after the onset of infarction. A recent large trial (ISIS-2) has suggested that it may have a lesser effect in some patients (probably those with extensive collateral circulation) for up to 24 hours, but this is controversial. The benefit is greatest in patients with potentially large infarcts, ie, those with anterior or multifocal electrocardiographic changes, but also occurs with inferior infarctions, who have a relatively good prognosis in any case. Patients with non-Q wave infarctions generally have incomplete or partially recanalized occlusions and have not benefited from thrombolysis. Serious bleeding complications occur in 0.5–5% of patients. Contraindications include known bleeding diatheses, a history of any cerebrovascular disease, uncontrolled hypertension ($> 190/$ 110 mm Hg), pregnancy, and recent trauma or surgery of the head or spine. Relative contraindications include recent major thoracoabdominal surgery or biopsies, gastrointestinal or genitourinary bleeding, diabetic retinopathy, current oral anticoagulant therapy, prolonged cardiopulmonary resuscitation, and noncompressible puncture sites. Older patients have a higher complication rate.

Therefore, the current recommendation is to administer thrombolytic therapy to patients under 70 years of age with ST elevation or Q waves who present within 6 hours after onset of pain unless otherwise contraindicated. Adjunctive aspirin causes a significant further reduction in mortality rate and should therefore be administered acutely. Therapy can be initiated in the emergency room or ambulance if personnel are appropriately trained and equipped.

Because of the shorter delays and fewer complications, the intravenous route is preferable to intracoronary. Prior to initiating thrombolytic therapy, 2 large-bore peripheral intravenous lines should be established and not removed until 6 hours after the thrombolytic agent is discontinued. Arterial punctures and other invasive procedures should be avoided if possible. Samples should be drawn for baseline coagulation tests (prothrombin time, partial thromboplastin time, and fibrinogen levels), blood typing, and other blood tests. Automated blood pressure monitoring (preferably noninvasive) should be instituted.

Four thrombolytic agents are now available and are described in Table 8–6. All are associated with higher reperfusion rates when administered within 3 hours after onset of infarction. **Tissue plasminogen activator (tPA)** is a naturally occurring thrombolytic factor that is theoretically the most thrombus-specific, but bleeding complications have not been less frequent with tPA, even though fibrinogen levels are better maintained, and hemorrhagic strokes may be more frequent. Incomplete data suggest that tPA produces higher reperfusion rates, especially if given more than 3 hours after the onset of pain. Reocclusion rates are higher with tPA because of its shorter half-life. Since tPA is significantly more expensive than alternative agents and has not been demonstrated to reduce mortality more strikingly or to preserve left ventricular function better than other agents, it should be reserved for patients in whom streptokinase is relatively contraindicated (by previous exposure, hypotension, or potential need for early surgery).

Streptokinase is much more likely to produce allergic reactions, including fever, chills, rashes, and anaphylaxis. Patients should be pretreated with steroids (hydrocortisone, 100 mg intravenously) and antihistamines (diphenhydramine, 25–50 mg intravenously), and this agent should be avoided if the patient has received it previously. Streptokinase also has a tendency to produce severe hypotension and therefore must be administered slowly. Hypotension should be treated by slowing or interrupting the infusion,

Table 8–6. Thrombolytic therapy for acute myocardial infarction.

	Streptokinase	Urokinase	tPA	Anistreplase (APSAC)
Source	Group C *Streptococcus*	Human urine or fetal culture	Recombinant DNA	Group C *Streptococcus*
$T_{1/2}$	10–12 minutes	11–16 minutes	5 minutes	90 minutes
Usual dose	1.5 million units	2 million units	100 mg	30 units
Administration	750,000 units over 20 minutes followed by 750,000 units over 40 minutes	Infuse over 1 hour	60 mg over first hour followed by 10 mg/h for 4 hours	Infuse over 2–5 minutes
Anticoagulation after infusion	Heparin, 1000 units/h adjusted to keep PTT 1.5 times control; aspirin, 325 mg daily.	Same as streptokinase	Heparin, 5000 units as bolus, followed by same procedure as streptokinase.	Same as streptokinase
Clot selectivity	Low	Moderate	High	Moderate to high
Fibrinogenolysis	+++	++	+	++
Bleeding	+	+	+[1]	+
Hypotension	+++	+	+	++
Allergic reactions	++	0	0	++
Reperfusion (%)[2]	55–60%	60%	70%	60%
Reocclusion (%)	5–10%	?	10–15%	?
Approximate cost	$200	$1300	$2400	$1700

tPA = tissue plasminogen activator.
[1] tPA may cause a higher incidence of cerebral hemorrhage than other agents.
[2] Estimated reperfusion rates when administered in first 3 hours. After 3 hours, tPA reperfusion rate is higher than that of streptokinase.

placing the patient in the Trendelenburg position, and administering fluids.

Urokinase has not been specifically approved for acute myocardial infarction, but small studies have demonstrated that it induces coronary thrombolysis.

Recently, anisoylated plasminogen streptokinase activator complex (**anistreplase; APSAC**) has received regulatory approval in the USA. This conjugate of streptokinase is inactive until the anisoyl group is hydrolyzed, which occurs gradually after injection (half-time, 90 minutes). The drug is concentrated at the site of the thrombus and is activated locally. Thus, it can be injected as a bolus but will provide continuing thrombolytic activity. A recent multicenter trial with APSAC demonstrated a 48% reduction in the acute mortality rate. A trial comparing it with tPA and streptokinase is ongoing.

After completion of the thrombolytic infusion, aspirin should be continued. Anticoagulation with heparin is advocated by most authorities, but its risk/benefit ratio has been questioned. Prophylactic treatment with antacids and an H_2 blocker is indicated.

Reperfusion rates of 40–80% can be expected, determined primarily by the interval between onset of the infarction and treatment. Reperfusion is recognized clinically by the abrupt cessation of pain, ventricular arrhythmias (most characteristically accelerated idioventricular rhythm), rapid evolution of the ECG to Q waves, and an early peak of CK (by 12 hours); however, all of these signs may be mislead-

ing. Even with anticoagulation, 10–20% of reperfused vessels will reocclude during hospitalization. This is usually recognized by the recurrence of pain and ST segment elevation and is treated by readministration of a thrombolytic agent or immediate angiography and PTCA.

The optimal management of myocardial infarction after thrombolysis is controversial and is under intense investigation. Patients with recurrent ischemic pain prior to discharge should undergo catheterization and, if indicated, revascularization. Some authorities recommend angiography for all potential candidates for revascularization and PTCA where anatomically feasible, while others reserve intervention for those with ischemia during predischarge exercise testing. Several recent trials in postthrombolytic patients (most particularly TIMI 2) have failed to show an advantage in mortality rate or left ventricular function with early PTCA compared with elective PTCA.

B. Acute PTCA: A number of centers are now performing immediate coronary arteriography in patients presenting within 3 hours after infarction. Either with or without the aid of thrombolytic agents, the occlusion can often be opened and the residual stenosis, if significant, dilated. However, several studies suggest that this approach offers no advantage over acute thrombolytic therapy followed by elective catheterization and PTCA 5–10 days later in selected patients. Patients with acute pump failure may be an exception.

C. General Measures: CCU monitoring should be instituted as soon as possible. Uncomplicated patients can be transferred to less intensively monitored settings after 24–48 hours. Activity should initially be limited to bed rest, with the availability of a nearby toilet or commode in more stable patients. Progressive ambulation should be started after 48–72 hours if tolerated. Low-flow oxygen therapy (2–4 L/min) is usually given. A liquid diet is recommended during the initial 24 hours.

D. Analgesia: An initial attempt should be made to relieve pain with sublingual nitroglycerin. However, if no response occurs after 2 or 3 tablets, intravenous opiates provide the most rapid and effective analgesia. Morphine sulfate, 4–8 mg, or meperidine, 50–75 mg, should be given. Subsequent small doses can be given every 15 minutes until pain abates.

E. Antiarrhythmic Prophylaxis: The incidence of ventricular fibrillation in hospitalized patients is approximately 5%, with 80% of episodes occurring in the first 12–24 hours. Prophylactic lidocaine infusions (1–2 mg/min) prevent most episodes; however, the value of routine lidocaine infusions in a monitored setting has been questioned, since the overall mortality rate is not reduced and asystole may be more frequent.

F. Beta-Adrenergic Blocking Agents: Several studies have shown modestly improved short-term survival when intravenous beta-blockers are given immediately after acute myocardial infarction. These agents reduce the duration of ischemic pain and the incidence of ventricular fibrillation. A favorable effect appears to persist even after thrombolytic therapy. However, the survival benefit is small, so beta-blockers should not be given to patients with relative contraindications. Long-term beta-blocker therapy is discussed below.

G. Anticoagulation: With the exception of patients undergoing thrombolysis and subsequent heparin therapy, the use of full anticoagulation remains controversial. Patients who will be at bed rest or on limited activity status for some time should be given 5000 units of heparin subcutaneously every 8–12 hours unless contraindicated. Aspirin, 325 mg daily, should be given unless contraindicated.

AIMS Trial Study Group: Long-term effects of intravenous anistreplase in acute myocardial infarction. Lancet 1990;335:427. (Markedly improved early and late survival.)

Gorlin R: Balancing the benefits, risks and unknowns of thrombolytic therapy in acute myocardial infarction. J Am Coll Cardiol 1988;11:1349. (Balanced view.)

ISIS-2 Collaborative Group: Randomised trial of intravenous streptokinase, oral aspirin, both, or neither among 17,187 cases of suspected acute myocardial infarction. Lancet 1988;2:349. (Strikingly positive trial for both agents.)

MacMahon S et al: Effects of prophylactic lidocaine in suspected acute myocardial infarction: An overview of results from the randomized, controlled trials. JAMA 1988;260:1910. (No apparent benefit overall.)

Marder VJ, Sherry S: Thrombolytic therapy: Current status. (2 parts.) N Engl J Med 1988;318:1512, 1585.

O'Neill W, Topol EJ, Pitt B: Reperfusion therapy of acute myocardial infarction. Prog Cardiovasc Dis 1988; 30:235.

Sleight P: Use of beta adrenoceptor blockade during and after acute myocardial infarction. Annu Rev Med 1986;37:415.

TIMI Study Group: Comparison of invasive and conservative strategies after treatment with intravenous tissue plasminogen activator in acute myocardial infarction: Results of the thrombolysis in myocardial infarction. N Engl J Med 1989;320:618. (Definitive trial demonstrating that PTCA can be reserved for those with predischarge evidence of ischemia.)

Topol EJ: Coronary angioplasty for acute myocardial infarction. Ann Intern Med 1988;109:970. (Acute angioplasty usually not warranted.)

White HD et al: Effect of intravenous streptokinase as compared with that of tPA on left ventricular function after first myocardial infarction. N Engl J Med 1989;320:817. (No difference in outcome.)

Complications

Most patients have one or more complications of myocardial infarction, although the response to treatment is usually prompt.

A. Infarct Extension and Postinfarction Ischemia: Recurrent infarction in the region of infarction (infarct extension) in the first 10–14 days occurs in approximately 10% of patients. It may be associated with prolonged or intermittent episodes of chest pain. In many cases, the process is relatively silent, being detected on routine ECG, by laboratory testing, or by onset or worsening of heart failure. Infarct extension is at least twice as common in non-Q wave infarcts and is more likely to occur after successful thrombolytic therapy owing to residual jeopardized myocardium. Diltiazem has been shown to reduce the rate of extension following non-Q wave infarction.

Approximately 30% of patients will have anginal episodes postinfarction. These are more common in patients with angina prior to infarction and in non-Q wave infarction. Postinfarction angina is associated with increased short- and long-term mortality rates. The underlying mechanism is usually inadequate blood flow through a recanalized vessel or reocclusion. Vigorous medical therapy should be instituted, including nitrates, calcium channel blockers, and beta-blockers, as well as aspirin and heparin. Thrombolytic therapy may also be helpful. Most patients with postinfarction angina—and all who are refractory to medical therapy—should undergo early catheterization and revascularization by PTCA or CABG.

B. Arrhythmias: Abnormalities of rhythm and conduction are common.

1. Sinus bradycardia—This is most common in inferior infarctions or may be precipitated by medications. Observation or withdrawal of the offending agent is usually sufficient. If accompanied by signs of low cardiac output, atropine, 0.5–1 mg intravenously, is usually effective. Temporary pacing is rarely required.

2. Supraventricular tachyarrhythmias–Sinus tachycardia is common and may reflect either increased adrenergic stimulation or hemodynamic compromise due to hypovolemia or pump failure. If the latter, beta blockade is contraindicated. Supraventricular premature beats are common and may be premonitory for atrial fibrillation. Electrolyte abnormalities and hypoxia should be corrected and causative agents (especially aminophylline) stopped. Atrial fibrillation should be rapidly controlled or converted to sinus rhythm. Intravenous verapamil (given cautiously in 2- to 5-mg increments up to 20 mg) or the short-acting beta-blocker esmolol (500 μg/kg, followed by 50–200 μg/kg/min) are the agents of choice if cardiac function is adequate. Digoxin (0.5 mg initial dosage; 0.25 mg every 90–120 minutes up to 1–1.25 mg) is preferable if heart failure is present with atrial fibrillation, but it takes longer. Cardioversion may be necessary if atrial fibrillation is complicated by hypotension, heart failure, or ischemia, but the arrhythmia often recurs. A class Ia agent such as procainamide or quinidine may be required in addition to verapamil, a beta-blocker, or digoxin to maintain sinus rhythm.

3. Ventricular arrhythmias–Ventricular arrhythmias are most common in the first few hours after infarction. Ventricular premature beats (VPBs) may be premonitory for ventricular tachycardia or fibrillation. Prophylactic lidocaine should be started (1 mg/kg bolus followed by an infusion of 2 mg/min) if more than 6 VPB/min, early (R on T wave) VPB, or couplets are observed. Additional boluses of 0.5 mg/kg followed by an increased infusion rate (up to 4 mg/min) may be necessary, but toxicity (tremor, anxiety, confusion, seizures) is common, especially in older patients and those with hypotension, heart failure, or liver disease. The infusion rate should be reduced after 3–4 hours, since blood levels tend to rise, but generally, once initiated, lidocaine should be continued for at least 24 hours.

Ventricular tachycardia should be treated with a 1 mg/kg bolus of lidocaine if the patient is stable or by electrical cardioversion (100–200 J) if not. If the arrhythmia cannot be suppressed with lidocaine, procainamide should be initiated (100-mg boluses over 1–2 minutes every 5 minutes to a cumulative dose of 750–1000 mg, followed by an infusion of 20–80 μg/kg/min). Hypotension may occur acutely, and depression of myocardial function or conduction may complicate maintenance therapy. Refractory ventricular arrhythmias may rarely respond to beta blockade (esmolol [500 μg/kg intravenously, followed by 50–200 μg/kg/min] is recommended because of its rapid onset and short duration of action), phenytoin (loading dose: boluses of 100 mg over 5 minutes every 5–10

minutes to a total of 1000 mg; maintenance 300–500 mg/d in divided doses), or bretylium tosylate (5 mg/kg intravenously over 3–5 minutes, repeated after 20 minutes if necessary, followed by an infusion of 1–2 mg/min). Ventricular fibrillation is treated electrically (300–400 J). Unresponsive ventricular fibrillation should be treated by bretylium and repeat cardioversion while CPR is administered. Accelerated idioventricular rhythm is a regular, wide complex rhythm at a rate of 70–100/min. It often follows reperfusion after thrombolytic therapy. The need for treating it in the absence of other ventricular arrhythmias is controversial.

4. Conduction disturbances–All degrees of atrioventricular block may occur in the course of acute myocardial infarction. Block at the level of the atrioventricular node is more common than infranodal block and occurs in approximately 20% of inferior myocardial infarctions. First-degree block is the most usual and requires no treatment. Second-degree block is usually of the Mobitz type I form (Wenckebach), is often transient but may be intermittent, and requires treatment only if associated with a heart rate slow enough to cause symptoms. Complete atrioventricular block occurs in up to 5% of acute inferior infarctions, usually is preceded by second-degree block, and usually resolves spontaneously, though it may persist for hours to several weeks. The escape rhythm originates in the distal atrioventricular node or atrioventricular junction and hence has a narrow QRS complex and is reliable, albeit often slow (30–50 beats/min). Treatment is often necessary because of resulting hypotension and low cardiac output. Intravenous atropine (1 mg) usually restores atrioventricular conduction temporarily, but if the escape complex is wide or if repeated atropine treatments are needed, temporary ventricular pacing is indicated. The prognosis for these patients is only slightly worse than that of patients who do not develop atrioventricular block.

In anterior infarctions, the site of block is distal, below the atrioventricular node, and usually a result of extensive damage of the His-Purkinje system and bundle branches. New first-degree block (prolongation of the PR interval) is unusual in anterior infarction; Mobitz type II atrioventricular block or complete heart block may be preceded by intraventricular conduction defects or may occur abruptly. The escape rhythm, if present at all, is an unreliable wide-complex idioventricular rhythm. Urgent ventricular pacing is mandatory, but even with successful pacing, mortality rates following the onset of complete heart block approach 80% because of the associated extensive myocardial change. New conduction abnormalities such as right or left bundle branch block or posterior or anterior fascicular blocks may presage progression, often sudden, to second–or third-degree atrioventricular block. Prophylactic temporary ventricular pacing is recommended for new-onset alternating bilateral bundle branch block, bifascicular block, or bundle branch block with worsening first-degree atrioventricular block. Patients with anterior infarction who progress to second–or third-degree block even transiently should be considered for insertion of a prophylactic permanent ventricular pacemaker before discharge.

C. Myocardial Dysfunction: The severity of cardiac dysfunction is proportionate to the extent of myocardial necrosis but is exacerbated by preexisting dysfunction and ongoing ischemia. Patients who have no signs of heart failure, normal blood pressure, and normal urine output have a good prognosis. Patients with hypotension or evidence of more than mild heart failure should have bedside right heart catheterization and continuous measurements of arterial pressure. These measurements permit the accurate assessment of cardiac function, facilitate the correct choice of therapy, and provide important prognostic information. Table 8–7 categorizes patients based upon these hemodynamic findings.

1. Left ventricular failure—Basilar rales are common in acute myocardial infarction, but dyspnea, more diffuse rales, and arterial hypoxemia usually indicate left ventricular failure. Since both the physical examination and chest x-ray correlate poorly with hemodynamic measurements and since the central venous pressure does not correlate with the pulmonary capillary wedge pressure (PCWP), right heart catheterization may be essential in monitoring therapy. General measures include supplemental oxygen to increase arterial saturation to above 95% and elevation of the trunk. Diuretics are usually the initial therapy unless right ventricular infarction is present. Intravenous furosemide (10–40 mg) or bumetanide (0.5–1 mg) is preferred because of the reliably rapid onset and short duration of action of these drugs. Higher dosages can be given if an inadequate response occurs. Morphine sulfate (4 mg intravenously followed by increments of 2 mg) is valuable in acute pulmonary edema.

Diuretics are usually effective; however, since most patients with acute infarction are not volume overloaded, the hemodynamic response may be limited and may be associated with hypotension. Vasodilators will reduce PCWP and improve cardiac output by a combination of venodilation (increasing venous capacitance) and arteriolar dilation (reducing afterload and left ventricular wall stress). In mild heart failure, sublingual isosorbide dinitrate (2.5–10 mg every 2 hours) or topical nitroglycerin ointment (6.25–25 mg every 4 hours) may be adequate to lower PCWP. In more severe failure, especially if cardiac output is reduced, sodium nitroprusside is the preferred agent. It should be initiated only with hemodynamic monitoring; the initial dosage should be low (0.25 μg/kg/min) to avoid excessive hypotension, but the dosage can be increased by increments of 0.5 μg/kg/min every 5–10 minutes up to 5–10 μg/kg/min until the desired hemodynamic response (PCWP lesser 18 mm Hg, CI > 2.5) is obtained. Excessive hypotension (mean blood pressure lesser 65–75 mm Hg) or tachycardia (> 10/min increase) should be avoided. Combi-

Table 8–7. Hemodynamic subsets in acute myocardial infarction.

Category	CI or SWI	PCWP	Treatment	Comment
Normal	> 2.2, > 30	< 15	None	Mortality rate < 5%.
Hyperdynamic	> 3.0, > 40	< 15	Beta-blockers	Characterized by tachycardia; mortality rate < 5%.
Hypovolemic	< 2.5, < 30	< 10	Volume expansion	Hypotension, tachycardia, but preserved left ventricular function by echocardiography; mortality rate 4–8%.
Left ventricular failure	< 2.2, < 30	> 15	Diuretics	Mild dyspnea, rales, normal blood pressure; mortality rate 10–20%.
Severe failure	< 2.0, < 20	> 20	Diuretics, vasodilators	Pulmonary edema, mild hypotension; inotropic agents, IABC may be required; mortality rate 20–40%.
Shock	< 1.8, < 20	> 18	Inotropic agents, IABC	IABC early unless rapid reversal; mortality rate > 60%.

CI = cardiac index (L/min/m²); SWI = stroke work index (g-m/m², calculated as [mean arterial pressure—PCWP] × stroke volume index × 0.0136); PCWP = pulmonary capillary wedge pressure (in mm Hg; pulmonary artery diastolic pressure may be used instead); IABC = intra-aortic balloon counterpulsation.

nation of nitroprusside with inotropic agents may be necessary to preserve blood pressure or maximize benefit.

Intravenous nitroglycerin (starting at 10 mg/min and titrating up to 10 µg/kg/min) is usually less effective but may lower PCWP with less hypotension. Oral or nonparenteral vasodilator therapy with nitrates or angiotensin-converting enzyme inhibitors is often necessary after the initial 24–48 hours (see below).

Inotropic agents should be avoided if possible, because they often increase heart rate and myocardial oxygen requirements. Dobutamine has the best hemodynamic profile, increasing cardiac output and modestly lowering PCWP, usually without excessive tachycardia, hypotension, or arrhythmias. The initial dosage is 2.5 µg/kg/min, and it may be increased by similar increments up to 15–20 µg/kg/min at intervals of 5–10 minutes. Dopamine is more useful in the presence of hypotension (see below), since it produces peripheral vasoconstriction, but it has a less beneficial effect on PCWP. Amrinone is a positive inotrope and vasodilator that produces hemodynamic effects similar to those of dobutamine but with a greater decrease in PCWP. However, its longer duration of action makes it less useful in unstable situations. Milrinone is a more potent and newer congener of amrinone with fewer side effects, but it remains investigational and its safety during long-term therapy has been questioned. Digoxin has not been helpful in acute infarction except to control the ventricular response in atrial fibrillation, but it may be beneficial if chronic heart failure persists.

2. Hypotension and shock–Patients with hypotension (systolic blood pressure < 100 mm Hg, individualized depending on prior blood pressure) and signs of diminished perfusion (low urine output, confusion, cold extremities) should be hemodynamically monitored. Up to 20% will have findings indicative of intravascular hypovolemia (due to diaphoresis, vomiting, decreased venous tone, medications—such as diuretics, nitrates, morphine, beta-blockers, calcium channel blockers, and thrombolytic agents—and lack of oral intake). These should be treated with successive boluses of 100 mL of normal saline until PCWP reaches 15–18 mm Hg to determine whether cardiac output and blood pressure respond. Right ventricular infarction, characterized by a normal PCWP but elevated right atrial pressure, can produce hypotension. This is discussed below.

Most hypotensive patients will have moderate to severe left ventricular dysfunction; pathologic studies indicate that more than 20% of the left ventricle is infarcted (> 40% in cardiogenic shock). If hypotension is only modest (systolic pressure > 90 mm Hg) and the PCWP is elevated, diuretics and an initial trial of nitroprusside (see above for dosing) are indicated. If the blood pressure falls, inotropic support will need to be added or substituted. Such patients may also be treated with intra-aortic balloon counter-

pulsation. This device unloads the left ventricle during systole and increases diastolic coronary artery filling pressure. It often facilitates the use of vasodilators in patients who previously did not tolerate them.

Dopamine is the most appropriate pressor for cardiogenic hypotension. It should be initiated at a rate of 2 µg/kg/min and increased at 5-minute intervals to the appropriate hemodynamic end point. At low dosages (< 5 µg/kg/min), it improves renal blood flow; at intermediate dosages (2.5–10 µg/kg/min), it stimulates myocardial contractility; at higher dosages (> 8 µg/kg/min), it is a potent α_1-adrenergic agonist. In general, blood pressure and cardiac index rise, but PCWP does not fall. Dopamine may be combined with nitroprusside or dobutamine (see above for dosing), or the latter may be used in its place if hypotension is not severe. Amrinone has hemodynamic effects similar to those of dobutamine, but its longer duration of action precludes rapid dosage adjustment. Norepinephrine is the usual pressor of last resort, since isoproterenol and epinephrine produce less vasoconstriction, do not increase coronary perfusion pressure (aortic diastolic pressure), and tend to worsen the balance between myocardial oxygen delivery and utilization.

Patients with cardiogenic shock have a poor prognosis. If they do not respond rapidly, the previously described measure—intra-aortic balloon counterpulsation—should be instituted. Operation to repair mechanical defects (see below), revascularize ischemic myocardium, and resect aneurysms should be considered. Cardiac transplantation is indicated in appropriate individuals.

D. Right Ventricular Infarction: Right ventricular infarction is present in one-third of patients with inferior wall infarction but is clinically significant in less than 50% of these. It presents as hypotension with relatively preserved left ventricular function and should be considered whenever patients with inferior infarction exhibit signs of low cardiac output and raised venous pressure. Hypotension is often exacerbated by medications that decrease intravascular volume or produce venodilation, such as diuretics, nitrates, and narcotics. Right atrial pressure and jugular venous pulsations are high, while PCWP is normal or low and the lungs are clear. The diagnosis is suggested by right precordial ST segment elevation and confirmed by echocardiography or hemodynamic measurements. When hypotension is present, hemodynamic measurements are necessary to monitor therapy. Treatment consists of fluid loading to improve left ventricular filling; inotropic agents may also be useful.

E. Mechanical Defects: Partial or complete rupture of a papillary muscle or of the interventricular septum occurs in less than 1% of acute myocardial infarctions and carries a poor prognosis. These complications occur in both anterior and inferior infarctions, usually 3–7 days after the acute event. They are detected by the appearance of a new systolic murmur and clinical deterioration, often with pulmonary edema. The 2 lesions are distinguished by the location of the murmur (apical versus parasternal) and by Doppler echocardiography. Hemodynamic monitoring is essential for appropriate management and demonstrates an increase in oxygen saturation between the right atrium and pulmonary artery in ventricular septal defect and, often, a large v wave with mitral regurgitation. Treatment by nitroprusside and, preferably, intra-aortic balloon counterpulsation reduces the regurgitation or shunt, but surgical correction is mandatory. There is controversy over whether this should be done acutely or after a period of stabilization; the better surgical results with the latter approach primarily reflect preoperative mortality in the highest-risk patients.

F. Myocardial Rupture: Complete rupture of the left ventricular free wall occurs in less than 1% of patients and usually results in immediate death. It occurs 2–7 days postinfarction, usually involves the anterior wall, and is more frequent in older women. Incomplete or gradual rupture may be sealed off by the pericardium, creating a **pseudoaneurysm.** It may be recognized by echocardiography, radionuclide angiography, or left ventricular angiography, often as an incidental finding. It demonstrates a narrow-neck connection to the left ventricle. Early surgical repair is indicated, since delayed rupture is common.

G. Left Ventricular Aneurysm: Ten to 20% of patients surviving an acute infarction develop a left ventricular aneurysm, a sharply delineated area of scar that bulges paradoxically during systole. This usually follows anterior Q wave infarctions. Aneurysms are recognized by persistent ST segment elevation (beyond 4–8 weeks), and a wide neck from the left ventricle can be demonstrated by echocardiography, scintigraphy, or contrast angiography. They rarely rupture but may be associated with arterial emboli, ventricular arrhythmias, and congestive heart failure. Surgical resection may be performed for these indications if other measures fail. The best results are obtained when the residual myocardium contracts well and when significant coronary lesions supplying adjacent regions are bypassed.

H. Pericarditis: The pericardium is involved in approximately 50% of infarctions, but pericarditis is often not clinically significant. Twenty percent of patients with Q wave infarctions will have an audible friction rub if examined repetitively. Pericardial pain occurs in approximately the same proportion after 2–7 days and is recognized by its variation with respiration and position (improved by sitting). Often, no treatment is required, but aspirin (650 mg every 4–6 hours) or indomethacin (25 mg 3–4 times daily) will usually relieve the pain. Anticoagulation should be avoided, since hemorrhagic pericarditis may result. From 1 to 12 weeks after infarction, Dressler's

syndrome (post-myocardial infarction syndrome) occurs in less than 5% of patients. This is an autoimmune phenomenon and presents as pericarditis with associated fever, leukocytosis, and, occasionally, pericardial or pleural effusion. It may recur over months. Treatment is the same as for other forms of pericarditis. A short course of corticosteroids may help if nonsteroidal agents do not relieve symptoms.

I. Mural Thrombus: Mural thrombi are common in large anterior infarctions but not in infarctions at other locations. Arterial emboli occur in approximately 5% of patients with known infarction, usually within 6 weeks. Anticoagulation with heparin followed by short-term (3-month) warfarin therapy prevents most emboli and should be considered in all patients with large anterior infarctions. Mural thrombi can be detected by echocardiography or MRI but with only moderate reliability, so these procedures should not be relied upon for determining the need for anticoagulation.

Barbour DJ, Roberts WC: Rupture of a left ventricular papillary muscle during acute myocardial infarction: Analysis of 22 necropsy patients. J Am Coll Cardiol 1986;8:558.

Bosch X et al: Early postinfarction ischemia: Clinical, angiographic, and prognostic significance. Circulation 1987; 75:988. (High incidence of events.)

Feigl D, Ashkenazy J, Kishon Y: Early and late atrioventricular block in acute inferior myocardial infarction. J Am Coll Cardiol 1984;4:35.

Forman MB et al: Determinants of left ventricular aneurysm formation after anterior myocardial infarction: A clinical and angiographic study. J Am Coll Cardiol 1986;8:1256. (Who develops an aneurysm.)

Goldberger M, Tabak SW, Shah PK: Clinical experience with intra-aortic balloon counterpulsation in 112 consecutive patients. Am Heart J 1986;111:497.

Hands ME et al: The in-hospital development of cardiogenic shock after myocardial infarction: Incidence, predictors of occurrence, outcome and prognostic factors. J Am Coll Cardiol 1989;14:40.

Isner JM: Right ventricular myocardial infarction. JAMA 1988;259:712.

Josephson ME: Treatment of ventricular arrhythmias after myocardial infarction. Circulation 1986;74:653.

Left ventricular thrombosis and stroke following myocardial infarction. (Editorial.) Lancet 1990;335:759.

Lo YS, Lesch M, Kaplan K: Postinfarction angina. Prog Cardiovasc Dis 1987;30:111.

Nishimura RA et al: Early repair of mechanical complications after acute myocardial infarction. JAMA 1986; 256:47.

Pohjola-Sintonen S et al: Ventricular septal and free wall rupture complicating acute myocardial infarction. Am Heart J 1989;117:809.

Scheinman MM, Gonzalez RP: Fascicular block and acute myocardial infarction. JAMA 1980;244:2646. (Still current management guidelines.)

Schreiber TL, Miller DH, Zola B: Management of myocardial infarction shock; Current status. Am Heart J 1989; 117:435.

Stratton JR, Resnick AD: Increased embolic risk in patients

with left ventricular thrombi. Circulation 1987;75:1004. (Emboli may occur quite late.)

Tofler GH et al: Pericarditis in acute myocardial infarction: Characterization and clinical significance. Am Heart J 1989;117:86.

Volpi A et al: In-hospital prognosis of patients with acute myocardial infarction complicated by primary ventricular fibrillation. N Engl J Med 1987;317:257. (Prognosis still relates to infarct size.)

Weisman HF, Healy B: Myocardial infarct expansion, infarct extension, and reinfarction: Pathophysiologic concepts. Prog Cardiovasc Dis 1987;30:73.

Postinfarction Prognosis

Twenty percent of patients with acute myocardial infarction die before they reach the hospital. Mortality rates in hospitalized patients range from 5% to 15% and are determined chiefly by the size of the infarction. Patients developing heart failure or hypotension have high early mortality rates. Several classification criteria have been developed to estimate early prognosis for survival. The most accurate is hemodynamic subsetting (Table 8–7). The prognosis after discharge is determined by 3 major factors: the degree of left ventricular dysfunction, the extent of residual ischemic myocardium, and the presence of ventricular arrhythmias. The mortality rate in the first year after discharge is approximately 6–8%, with over half of deaths occurring in the first 3 months, chiefly in patients with postinfarction heart failure. Subsequently, the mortality rate averages 4% per year.

A. Risk Stratification: A number of findings indicate increased risk after infarction. These include: (1) postinfarction angina; (2) non-Q wave infarction; (3) heart failure; (4) left ventricular ejection fraction less than 40%; (5) exercise-induced ischemia, diagnosed by electrocardiography or scintigraphy; and (6) ventricular ectopy (> 10 VPBs/h).

Patients with postinfarction angina should undergo coronary arteriography. Authorities differ about which tests should be performed routinely in other patients. Significant left ventricular dysfunction is most likely with anterior infarction or multiple infarctions. In these, noninvasive assessment of left ventricular function by echocardiography or scintigraphy will help assess prognosis and facilitate medical management. Submaximal exercise testing before discharge or a maximal test after 3–6 weeks helps patients and physicians plan the return to normal activity. Scintigraphy in conjunction with exercise testing adds additional sensitivity for ischemia and provides localizing information. Both exercise thallium scintigraphy and radionuclide angiography are used. Predischarge dipyridamole thallium scintigraphy is useful, since maximal exercise is not advisable; this approach is being used increasingly following thrombolytic therapy to determine which patients should undergo coronary arteriography and revascularization.

Ambulatory electrocardiographic monitoring for arrhythmias is of less clear value; though it has some prognostic value beyond measurements of left ventricular function, no benefit from antiarrhythmic therapy for asymptomatic patients has been demonstrated. Ischemia detected during ambulatory monitoring is an indicator of poor prognosis, but it is unclear how much additional information is obtained in patients who undergo exercise testing or scintigraphic studies.

A conservative approach to postinfarction evaluation would include measurement of left ventricular function in patients with signs of heart failure or large infarctions and a test for ischemia in patients without recurrent chest pain. The latter should occur before discharge if the patient has undergone thrombolytic therapy but may be delayed in most other patients.

B. Prophylactic Therapy: Many drugs have been studied, and some have been shown to be beneficial in preventing death or reinfarction. However, their usefulness in the era of thrombolysis and revascularization is unclear. Beta-blockers improve survival rates, primarily by reducing the incidence of sudden death in high-risk subsets of patients. Beta-blockers should be given to such individuals, except those with overt heart failure, but are of limited value in uncomplicated patients with small infarctions and normal exercise tests. No advantage of one preparation over another has been demonstrated except that those with intrinsic sympathomimetic activity have not proved beneficial in postinfarction patients. Calcium channel blockers have not been shown to improve prognosis overall, but both diltiazem and verapamil appear to reduce mortality rates in patients with preserved left ventricular function. Diltiazem prevents reinfarction after non-Q wave infarction. Antiplatelet agents are beneficial; low-dose aspirin (325 mg daily) is recommended. Anticoagulants have not been shown to improve prognosis, though they do reduce peripheral emboli in the early postdischarge phase (see above). Rigorous treatment of risk factors is recommended. Antiarrhythmic therapy other than with beta-blockers has not been shown to be effective except in patients with symptomatic arrhythmias and, in fact, class Ic agents increase the mortality rate in postinfarction patients. Cardiac rehabilitation programs and exercise training can be of considerable psychologic benefit, but it is not known whether they alter prognosis.

C. Revascularization: Because of the increasing use of thrombolytic therapy and accumulating experience with PTCA, the indications for revascularization are rapidly evolving. Postinfarction patients who appear likely to benefit from early revascularization if the anatomy is appropriate are (1) those who have undergone thrombolytic therapy and have residual symptoms or laboratory evidence of ischemia; (2) patients with left ventricular dysfunction and evidence of ischemia; (3) patients with non-Q wave infarction and evidence of more than mild ischemia; and (4) patients with markedly positive exercise tests and multivessel disease. The value of revascularization in the following groups is less clear: (1) patients treated with thrombolytic agents, with little evidence of reperfusion or residual ischemia; (2) patients with left ventricular dysfunction but no detectable ischemia; and (3) patients with preserved left ventricular function who have mild ischemia and are not symptom-limited. Patients who survive infarctions without complications, have preserved left ventricular function (ejection fraction > 50%), and have no exercise-induced ischemia have an excellent prognosis and do not require invasive evaluation.

American College of Physicians Position Paper: Evaluation of patients after recent acute myocardial infarction. Ann Intern Med 1989;110:485. (Concise guidelines.)

Debusk RF: Specialized testing after recent acute myocardial infarction. Ann Intern Med 1989;110:470. (Emphasis on identifying low- and high-risk groups.)

Gibson RS et al: Prognostic significance and beneficial effect of diltiazem on the incidence of early recurrent ischemia after non-Q-wave myocardial infarction: Results from the Multicenter Diltiazem Reinfarction Study. Am J Cardiol 1987;60:203. (Diltiazem reduces reinfarction rate.)

Gottlieb SO et al: Silent ischemia on Holter monitoring predicts mortality in high-risk postinfarction patients. JAMA 1988;259:1030. (Especially in patients who are not exercised.)

Greenland P, Chu JS: Efficacy of cardiac rehabilitation services: With emphasis on patients after myocardial infarction. Ann Intern Med 1988;109:650. (Comprehensive review with accompanying position paper.)

Josephson ME: Treatment of ventricular arrhythmias after myocardial infarction. Circulation 1986;74:653.

Kostis JB et al: Prognostic significance of ventricular ectopic activity in survivors of acute myocardial infarction. J Am Coll Cardiol 1987;10:231. (Ectopy is a marker of poor risk.)

Moss AJ, Benhorn J: Prognosis and management after a first myocardial infarction. N Engl J Med 1990;322:743.

Siegel D et al: Risk factor modification after myocardial infarction. Ann Intern Med 1988;109:213. (Often forgotten in the high-tech world.)

Topol EJ et al: A randomized controlled trial of hospital discharge 3 days after myocardial infarction in the era of reperfusion. N Engl J Med 1988;318:1083. (Safe in selected patients, but only 80 of 507 screened were randomized.)

Yusuf S, Wittes J, Friedman L: Overview of results of randomized clinical trials in heart disease: 1. Treatments following myocardial infarction. JAMA 1988;260:2088. (Includes thrombolysis, beta-blockers, nitrates, calcium channel blockers, antiarrhythmics, anticoagulants, and antiplatelet drugs.)

DISTURBANCES OF RATE & RHYTHM

Arrhythmias are harmful to the extent that they reduce cardiac output, lower blood pressure, and interfere with perfusion of the brain and myocardium, or tend to deteriorate into more serious arrhythmias with these consequences. Patients with otherwise normal hearts may tolerate rapid rates with few symptoms, but prolonged attacks may cause weakness, exertional dyspnea, and precordial aching. Whether slow heart rates produce symptoms at rest or on exertion depends upon the underlying state of the cardiac muscle and its ability to increase its stroke output. If the heart rate abruptly slows, as with the onset of complete heart block or transient standstill, syncope or convulsions may result.

Arrhythmias can usually be detected and diagnosed from the surface ECG and ambulatory electrocardiographic monitoring. In complex and life-threatening arrhythmias, invasive electrophysiologic studies aid in the diagnosis and evaluation of treatment.

Mechanisms of Arrhythmias

Electrophysiologic studies have greatly increased our understanding of the mechanisms underlying most arrhythmias. These include (1) disorders of impulse formation or automaticity, (2) abnormalities of impulse conduction, (3) reentry, and (4) triggered activity. Altered automaticity is the mechanism for sinus node arrest, many premature beats, and automatic rhythms as well as an initiating factor in reentry arrhythmias. Abnormalities of impulse conduction can occur at the sinus or atrioventricular node, in the intraventricular conduction system, and within the atria or ventricles. These are responsible for sinoatrial exit block, for atrioventricular block at the node or below, and for establishing reentry circuits.

Reentry is the underlying mechanism for many arrhythmias, including premature beats, most paroxysmal supraventricular tachycardias, and atrial flutter. For reentry to occur, there must be an area of unidirectional block with an appropriate delay to allow repeat depolarization at the site of origin. Reentry is confirmed if the arrhythmia can be terminated by interruption of the circuit by a spontaneous or induced premature beat. Triggered activity occurs when afterdepolarizations (abnormal electrical activity persisting after repolarization) reach the threshold level required to trigger a new depolarization. This may be the mechanism of ventricular tachycardia in the prolonged QT syndrome and in some cases of digitalis toxicity.

Mandel WJ: Cardiac Arrhythmias, 2nd ed. Lippincott, 1986.

Wit AL: Cellular electrophysiologic mechanisms of cardiac arrhythmia. Ann NY Acad Sci 1984;432:1.

Zipes DP: Cardiac electrophysiology: Promises and contributions. J Am Coll Cardiol 1989;13:1329. (Mechanisms, diagnosis, and treatment of arrhythmias.)

Electrophysiologic Testing

Electrophysiologic testing employing intracardiac electrocardiographic recordings and programmed atrial or ventricular (or both) stimulation has become increasingly important in the diagnosis and management of complex arrhythmias. The primary indications for electrophysiologic testing are (1) evaluation of recurrent syncope of possible cardiac origin, when the ambulatory ECG has not provided the diagnosis; (2) evaluation of the efficacy of pharmacotherapy in survivors of aborted sudden death or other patients with symptomatic or life-threatening ventricular tachycardia; (3) differentiation of supraventricular from ventricular arrhythmias; (4) evaluation of therapy in patients with accessory atrioventricular pathways; and (5) evaluation of patients for antitachycardia pacing devices and surgical or catheter ablation procedures.

Hamill SC et al: Clinical intracardiac electrophysiologic testing: Technique, diagnostic indications, and therapeutic uses. Mayo Clin Proc 1986;61:478.

Horowitz LN et al: Risks and complications of clinical cardiac electrophysiologic studies: A prospective analysis of 1000 consecutive patients. J Am Coll Cardiol 1987;9:1261. (Safe procedure in experienced laboratories.)

Wellens HJ, Brugada P, Stevenson WG: Programmed electrical stimulation: Its role in the management of ventricular arrhythmias in coronary heart disease. Prog Cardiovasc Dis 1986;29:165.

Zipes DP, Rahimtoola SH (editors): State-of-the-art consensus conference on electrophysiologic testing in the diagnosis and treatment of patients with cardiac arrhythmias. Circulation 1987;75(Suppl):III-1. (Entire issue.) (Guidelines and results.)

Antiarrhythmic Drugs
(Table 8–8)

Antiarrhythmic drugs have limited efficacy and produce frequent side effects. They are often divided into 4 classes based upon their electropharmacologic actions.

Class I agents block membrane sodium channels. Three subclasses are further defined by the effect of agents on the Purkinje fiber action potential. Class Ia drugs slow the rate of rise of the action potential (V_{max}) and prolong its duration, thus slowing conduction and increasing refractoriness. Class Ib agents do not affect but shorten action potential duration; they do not affect conduction or refractoriness. Class Ic agents prolong V_{max} and slow repolarization, thus slowing conduction and prolonging refractoriness, but more so than class Ia drugs.

Class II agents are the beta-blockers, which decrease automaticity, prolong atrioventricular conduction, and prolong refractoriness.

Class III agents block potassium channels and prolong repolarization, widening the QRS and prolonging the QT interval. They decrease automaticity and conduction and prolong refractoriness.

Class IV agents are the slow calcium channel blockers, which decrease automaticity and atrioventricular conduction.

Although the in vitro electrophysiologic effects of most of these agents have been defined, their use remains largely empirical. All can exacerbate arrhythmias (proarrhythmic effect), and most depress left ventricular function.

The risk of antiarrhythmic agents has recently been highlighted by the Coronary Arrhythmia Suppression Trial (CAST), in which 2 class Ic agents (flecainide and encainide) *increased* mortality rates in patients with asymptomatic ventricular ectopy after myocardial infarction. Therefore, class Ic agents should not be used except for life-threatening arrhythmias and refractory supraventricular tachyarrhythmias in patients with structurally normal hearts. The decision to treat asymptomatic ventricular ectopy with any antiarrhythmic agent should be carefully considered.

The use of antiarrhythmic agents is discussed below.

Belardinelli L, Lerman BB: Electrophysiologic basis for the use of adenosine in the diagnosis and treatment of cardiac arrhythmias. Br Heart J 1990;63:34.

CAST Investigators: Preliminary report: Effect of encainide and flecainide on mortality in a randomized trial of arrhythmia suppression after myocardial infarction. N Engl J Med 1989;321:406. (Increased mortality rate with therapy; related editorial on p 386.)

Funck-Brentano C et al: Propafenone. N Engl J Med 1990;322:518. (A new agent very popular abroad.)

Ruder M et al: Clinical experience with sotalal in patients with drug-refractory ventricular arrhythmias. J Am Coll Cardiol 1989;13:134.

Stanton MS et al: Arrhythmogenic effects of anti-arrhythmic drugs: A study of 506 patients treated for ventricular tachycardia or fibrillation. J Am Coll Cardiol 1989; 14:209.

Vaughn Williams EM: A classification of antiarrhythmic actions reassessed after a decade of new drugs. J Clin Pharmacol 1984;24:129. (Description and justification of standard classification system.)

Wellens HJJ, Brugado P: Treatment of cardiac arrhythmias: When, how, and where? J M Coll Cardiol 1989;14:14–17. (Important questions in the post-CAST era.)

SUPRAVENTRICULAR ARRHYTHMIAS

1. SINUS ARRHYTHMIA

Sinus arrhythmia is a cyclic increase in normal heart rate with inspiration and decrease with expiration. It results from reflex changes in vagal influence on the normal pacemaker and disappears with breath holding or increase of heart rate due to any cause. It has no clinical significance. It is common in both the young and the elderly.

2. SINUS BRADYCARDIA

Sinus bradycardia is a heart rate slower than 50/min due to increased vagal influence on the normal

Table 8–8. Antiarrhythmic drugs.

	Intravenous Dosage	Oral Dosage	Therapeutic Plasma Level	Route of Elimination	Mechanism	Indications	Side Effects
Quinidine	6–10 mg/kg (IM or IV) over 20 min (rarely used parenterally)	325–650 mg every 6–8 h	2–6 µg/mL	Hepatic	CLASS Ia: sodium channel blockers: Depress phase 0 depolarization; slow conduction; prolong repolarization.	APB, VPB, SVT, VT, prevent VF	GI, ↓ LVF, ↑ Dig
Procainamide	100 mg/1–3 min to 500–1000 mg; maintain at 2–6 mg/min	500–1500 mg every 3–6 h	4–10 µg/mL	Renal			Systemic lupus erythematosus, hypersensitivity; ↓ LVF
Disopyramide	—	100–200 mg every 6–8 h	2–6 µg/mL	Renal			Urinary retention, dry mouth, markedly ↓↓ LVF
Lidocaine	1–2 mg/kg at 50 mg/min; maintain at 1–4 mg/min	—	1–5 µg/mL	Hepatic	CLASS Ib: Shorten repolarization.	VPB, VT, prevent VF	CNS, GI
Tocainide	—	200–300 mg every 6–8 h	0.5–2 µg/mL	Hepatic			CNS, GI, leukopenia
Mexiletine	—	400–600 mg every 6–8 h	6–12 µg/mL	Hepatic			CNS, GI, leukopenia
Phenytoin	100 mg/5 min to 1000 mg; maintain at 100–500 mg/d	200–400 mg every 12–24 h	10–20 µg/mL	Hepatic			CNS, GI
Flecainide	—	50–200 mg twice daily	0.2–0.8 µg/mL	Hepatic	CLASS Ic: Depress phase 0 repolarization; slow conduction; prolong refractoriness; propafenone is a weak Ca^{2+} channel blocker.	Life-threatening ventricular, refractory SVT	CNS, GI, ↓↓ LVF, sudden death
Encainide	—	25–75 mg every 6–8 h	0.5–1 µg/mL	Hepatic			
Propafenone	—	150–300 mg every 8–12 h	—	Hepatic			
Esmolol	500 µg/kg over 1–2 min; maintain at 25–200 µg/kg/min	Other beta-blockers may be used.	—	Hepatic	CLASS II: Beta-blocker, slows AV conduction.	SVT; may prevent VF	↓ LVF, bronchospasm
Amiodarone	Same as oral	1200 mg/d for 7–14 days; maintain at 200–800 mg/d	1–5 µg/mL	Hepatic	CLASS III: Prolong action potential.	Refractory VT, SVT, prevent VT, VF	Pulmonary fibrosis, thyroid abnormalities, corneal and skin deposits, hepatitis, ↑ Dig
Sotalol	—	80–240 mg every 12 h	—	Renal		VT	↓ LVF; bradycardia, fatigue
Bretylium	5–10 mg/kg over 5–10 min; maintain at 0.5–2 mg/min	—	0.5–1.5 µg/mL	Renal		VF, VT	Hypotension, nausea
Verapamil	10–20 mg over 2–20 min; maintain at 5 µg/min	80–120 mg every 6–8 h	0.1–0.15 µg/mL	Hepatic	Class IV: Slow calcium channel blocker	SVT	↓ LVF, constipation, ↑ Dig

APB = atrial premature beats; CNS = central nervous system (dizziness, tremor); ↑ Dig = elevation of serum digoxin level; GI = gastrointestinal (nausea, vomiting, diarrhea); ↓ LVF = reduced left ventricular function; SVT = supraventricular tachycardia; VF = ventricular fibrillation; VPB = ventricular premature beats; VT = ventricular tachycardia.

pacemaker or organic disease of the sinus node. The rate usually increases during exercise or administration of atropine. Slight degrees have no significance, especially in youth or in athletes; it is of more concern if there is underlying heart disease. Elderly patients may develop weakness, confusion, or even syncope with slow heart rates due to degenerative disease of the sinus node. Atrial and ventricular ectopic rhythms are more apt to occur with slow ventricular rates. Rarely, pacing is required if symptoms correlate with the bradycardia.

Tresch DD, Fleg JL: Unexplained sinus bradycardia: Clinical significance and long-term prognosis in apparently healthy persons older than 40 years. Am J Cardiol 1986;58:1009. (Most do well.)

3. SINUS TACHYCARDIA

Sinus tachycardia is defined as a heart rate faster than 100 beats/min that is caused by rapid impulse formation from the normal pacemaker; it occurs with fever, exercise, emotion, anemia, heart failure, shock, thyrotoxicosis, or drug effect. The onset and termination are usually gradual, in contrast to paroxysmal supraventricular tachycardia due to reentry. The rate may reach 180/min in young persons but infrequently exceeds 160/min. The rhythm is basically regular, but serial 1-minute counts of the heart rate indicate that it varies 5 or more beats per minute with changes in position, with breath holding or sedation.

4. ATRIAL PREMATURE BEATS
   (Atrial Extrasystoles)

Atrial premature beats occur when an ectopic focus in the atria fires before the next sinus node impulse or a reentry circuit is established. The contour of the P wave usually differs from the patient's normal complex. Ventricular systole occurs prematurely, and the compensatory pause following this is only slightly longer than the normal interval between beats. Such premature beats occur frequently in normal hearts and are never a sufficient basis for a diagnosis of heart disease. Speeding of the heart rate by any means usually abolishes most premature beats. Early atrial premature beats may cause aberrant QRS complexes (wide and bizarre) or may be nonconducted to the ventricles because the latter are still refractory.

5. PAROXYSMAL SUPRAVENTRICULAR
   TACHYCARDIA
   (Atrial or Junctional Tachycardia)

This is the commonest paroxysmal tachycardia. It occurs more often in young patients with normal hearts. Attacks begin and end abruptly and may last several hours or longer. The heart rate may be 140–240/min (usually 160–220/min) and is perfectly regular (despite exercise or change in position). The P wave usually differs in contour from sinus beats. Patients may be asymptomatic except for awareness of rapid heart action, but some experience mild chest pain or shortness of breath, especially when episodes are prolonged, even in the absence of associated cardiac abnormalities. Paroxysmal supraventricular tachycardia may result from digitalis toxicity and then is commonly associated with atrioventricular block.

The most common mechanism for paroxysmal supraventricular tachycardia is reentry. In addition to the atrioventricular node, the reentry circuit may include the sinoatrial node, the atrium, or an accessory bypass tract (see below). Recent evidence indicates that about one-third of patients have aberrant pathways to the ventricles. A single fortuitously timed atrial or ventricular premature beat may set up the reentry circuit or may terminate it.

Treatment of the Acute Attack
In the absence of heart disease, serious effects are rare. Most attacks break spontaneously, and the physician should not use remedies that are more dangerous than the disease. Particular effort should be made to terminate the attack quickly if cardiac failure, syncope, or anginal pain develops or if there is underlying cardiac or (particularly) coronary disease. Because reentry is the most common mechanism for paroxysmal atrial tachycardia, effective therapy requires that conduction be interrupted at some point in the reentry circuit.

A. Mechanical Measures: A variety of methods have been used to interrupt attacks, and patients may learn to perform these themselves. These include Valsalva's maneuver, stretching the arms and body, lowering the head between the knees, coughing, and breath holding. These maneuvers, as is true also of carotid sinus pressure (see below), stimulate the vagus, delay atrioventricular conduction, and block the reentry mechanism, terminating the arrhythmias.

B. Vagal Stimulation With Carotid Sinus Pressure: *Caution: This procedure should not be performed if the patient has carotid bruits or a history of transient cerebral ischemic attacks.* With the patient relaxed in the semirecumbent position, firm but gentle pressure and massage are applied first over one carotid sinus for 10–20 seconds and then over the other. *Pressure should not be exerted on both carotid sinuses at the same time.* Continuous electrocardiographic or auscultatory monitoring of the heart rate is required so that carotid sinus pressure can be relieved as soon as the attack ceases or if excessive slowing occurs. Carotid sinus pressure will interrupt up to half the attacks, especially if the patient has been digitalized or sedated. Eyeball pressure has been recommended by some, but it should be avoided because of the danger of retinal detachment.

C. Drug Therapy: If mechanical measures fail, 2 rapidly acting intravenous agents will terminate more than 90% of episodes. Verapamil is given as a 2.5-mg bolus, followed by additional 2.5- to 5-mg doses every 1–3 minutes up to a total of 20 mg if blood pressure and rhythm are stable. If the rhythm recurs, further doses can be given. Oral verapamil, 80–120 mg every 4–6 hours, can be used as well in stable patients who are tolerating the rhythm without difficulty. A newer agent, intravenous adenosine, is equally effective and has a briefer duration of action. Adenosine has a less profound effect on myocardial contractility and blood pressure, so it is preferred in patients with poor left ventricular function or hypotension. A 6-mg bolus is administered. If no response is observed after 1–2 minutes, a second and third 12-mg bolus should be given. Since the half-life of adenosine is less than 10 seconds, the drug must be given rapidly (in 1–2 seconds from a proximal intravenous port). Adenosine is very well tolerated, but nearly 20% of patients will experience transient flushing, and some patients experience severe chest discomfort.

Esmolol, a short-acting beta-blocker, is also highly effective; the initial dose is 500 μg/kg intravenously over 1 minute followed by an infusion of 50–200 μg/min. Parasympathetic stimulating drugs such as edrophonium (Tensilon), 5–10 mg intravenously, which delay atrioventricular conduction, may break the reentry mechanism. Because it frequently causes nausea and vomiting, it should be used only if the previously discussed agents fail. Metaraminol or phenylephrine, alpha-adrenergic stimulants that activate the baroreceptors by raising the blood pressure and causing vagal stimulation, can break attacks but should be used cautiously because they may provoke excessive hypertension. Digoxin is effective, but it often requires several hours to safely administer an adequate dose. An initial dose of 0.5–0.75 mg intravenously, followed by 0.25 or 0.125 increments every 2–4 hours up to a total of 1–1.25 mg, is used. Outpatients who are tolerating the rhythm can be treated with oral digitalis. Intravenous procainamide may terminate supraventricular tachycardia; however, since it facilitates atrioventricular conduction and an initial increase in rate may occur, it is usually not given until after digoxin, verapamil, or a beta-blocker has been administered. In patients with Wolff-Parkinson-White syndrome, in which an accessory pathway is involved, these agents may be contraindicated (see below).

D. Cardioversion: If the clinical situation is severe enough to warrant immediate termination and adenosine and verapamil are contraindicated or ineffective, synchronized electrical cardioversion (beginning at 50–100 J) is almost universally successful. If digitalis toxicity is present or strongly suspected, as in the case of paroxysmal tachycardia with block, electrical cardioversion should be avoided.

Prevention of Attacks

A. Drugs: Digoxin orally is the usual drug of first choice because of its convenience and efficacy. Verapamil, alone or in combination with digitalis, is a second choice, though oral therapy is not as effective as intravenous therapy. (*Note:* Verapamil increases digoxin serum levels.) Beta-blockers are also effective. Patients who do not respond to these agents should be treated with a class Ia agent such as quinidine, perhaps in combination with digoxin or another agent that inhibits atrioventricular conduction. In patients taking quinidine, digoxin levels also increase by about 30%.

Procainamide and disopyramide are also effective. The newer class Ic agents, flecainide, encainide, and propafenone, are especially successful in patients with bypass tracts. Amiodarone is highly effective, but because of its toxicity it should be employed only in refractory and symptomatic patients.

B. His Bundle Ablation: In patients with repeated or near-incessant symptomatic attacks that are difficult to control despite aggressive therapy guided by electrophysiologic studies, interruption of the His bundle or accessory pathways has been accomplished by delivering electrical or radiofrequency energy via a properly positioned intracardiac catheter or by surgical section. A ventricular pacemaker is necessary, because complete atrioventricular block is often produced.

C. Antitachycardia Pacemakers: Specially programmed permanent pacemakers have been employed to sense the appearance of supraventricular tachycardia and pace to interrupt the reentry circuit and stop the arrhythmia. This approach requires the involvement of highly specialized electrophysiologists.

Garratt C et al: Comparison of adenosine and verapamil for termination of paroxysmal junctional tachycardia. Am J Cardiol 1989;64:1310. (Adenosine more effective.)

Keefe DL, Miura D, Somberg JC: Supraventricular tachyarrhythmias: Their evaluation and therapy. Am Heart J 1986;111:1150.

Langberg JJ et al: Catheter ablation of the atrioventricular junction with radiofrequency energy. Circulation 1989; 80:1527. (Promising approach to blocking atrioventricular conduction.)

Manolis AS, Estes NA: Supraventricular tachycardia: Mechanisms and therapy. Arch Intern Med 1987;147:1706.

6. ATRIAL FIBRILLATION

Atrial fibrillation is the commonest chronic arrhythmia. It occurs in rheumatic heart disease, dilated cardiomyopathy, atrial septal defect, hypertension, mitral valve prolapse, and hypertrophic cardiomyopathy. Atrial fibrillation may be the initial presenting sign in thyrotoxicosis, which should always be excluded. Atrial fibrillation often appears paroxysmally before becoming the established rhythm. Pericarditis, chest trauma or surgery, or excessive alcohol intake may cause attacks in patients with normal hearts.

Atrial fibrillation is the only common arrhythmia in which the ventricular rate is rapid and the rhythm very irregular. The atrial rate is 400–600/min, but most impulses are blocked at the atrioventricular node. The ventricular response is completely irregular, ranging from 80 to 180/min in the untreated state. Because of the varying stroke volumes resulting from varying periods of diastolic filling, not all ventricular beats produce a palpable peripheral pulse. The difference between the apical rate and the pulse rate is the "pulse deficit"; this deficit is greater when the ventricular rate is high.

The major morbidity from atrial fibrillation (other than precipitation of cardiac failure or ischemia) is arterial emboli from the poorly contracting and often enlarged left atrium. Because atrial fibrillation is associated with a significantly increased risk of stroke and other embolic complications, conversion to normal sinus rhythm is preferred. If conversion is not possible, anticoagulation should be initiated in patients with atrial fibrillation and mitral valve disease. Recent studies have indicated that atrial fibrillation of other causes, including "lone" atrial fibrillation (in which no cardiac pathology can be identified), is also associated with a higher risk of arterial emboli. Anticoagulation with warfarin reduces thromboembolic complications in patients less than 75 years of age. In a large ongoing trial, aspirin (325 mg daily) also appears to be beneficial.

Acute Ventricular Rate Control

The initial goal of therapy is to control the ventricular response. This should be accomplished rapidly if the patient manifests ischemia, hypotension, or heart failure but can be accomplished more gradually and on an outpatient basis in those who are tolerating the rhythm. Intravenous verapamil is the agent of choice and will control the ventricular response in 90% of patients. It selectively increases atrioventricular block and slows the ventricular rate. The short-acting beta-blocker esmolol is an alternative approach. Digoxin remains highly effective, albeit control takes longer to accomplish. For outpatients, digoxin is the usual drug of choice. An initial oral dose of 0.5 mg can be followed by 2 or 3 additional 0.25-mg doses every 6 hours. None of these agents should be given to patients with Wolff-Parkinson-White syndrome conducting antegrade through the accessory pathway (wide ventricular complexes), since conduction may accelerate (see below).

Cardioversion

Immediate cardioversion is required for patients with hypotension, heart failure, or angina. Other pa-

tients should be controlled medically; however, even when the ventricular rate is controlled medically, a decision must be made about whether to attempt conversion to sinus rhythm. In general, if atrial fibrillation is of recent onset (< 6 months), conversion is recommended. In patients with mitral valve disease or with a dilated left atrium, the risk of embolization is high, so most authorities initiate anticoagulation with warfarin for 2–4 weeks prior to electrical cardioversion. Conversion can be accomplished medically on an outpatient basis with quinidine (or other class Ia or Ic agent). Quinidine can be started at a dosage of 200 mg every 6 hours and increased to 300 mg and 400 mg in 2-day intervals. Since quinidine increases digoxin levels, these should be checked beforehand. Electrical conversion can be also performed on an ambulatory basis. Quinidine, 300 mg every 6 hours, is often given for 24 hours before the procedure to prevent recurrence. In some patients, conversion will occur. If it does not, synchronized DC shock should be employed, with the initial dosage being 100 J, though more current may be needed. Although digoxin alone often maintains sinus rhythm, the addition of a class Ia may be required. Amiodarone is perhaps the most effective agent, but its use is limited by its toxicity.

Treatment of Chronic Atrial Fibrillation

Digoxin is the preferred drug for chronic ventricular rate control in the absence of preexcitation. Higher than normal dosages and serum levels are often required to maintain the resulting ventricular response in the 60- to 80/min range and to prevent excessive rise with modest exertion. Often a second agent, such as verapamil or a beta-blocker, facilitates ventricular rate control, especially with activity.

Kopecky SL et al: The natural history of lone atrial fibrillation: A population-based study over three decades. N Engl J Med 1987;317:669. (Relatively benign prognosis.)

Mancini JGB, Goldberger AL: Cardioversion of atrial fibrillation: Consideration of embolization, anticoagulation, prophylactic pacemaker, and long-term success. Am Heart J 1982;104:617.

Petersen P et al: Placebo-controlled, randomized trial of warfarin and aspirin for prevention of thromboembolic complications in chronic atrial fibrillation. Lancet 1989;1:175. (Best study so far showing fewer events on warfarin.)

Stroke Prevention in Atrial Fibrillation Study Group Investigators: Preliminary report of the Stroke Prevention in Atrial Fibrillation Study. N Engl J Med 1990;322:863. (Ongoing study in which aspirin and warfarin were superior to placebo in nonrheumatic atrial fibrillation.)

Wolf PA, Abbott RD, Kamel WB: Atrial fibrillation: A major contributor to stroke in the elderly. The Framingham Study. Arch Intern Med 1987;147:1561.

7. ATRIAL FLUTTER

Atrial flutter is less common than fibrillation and usually occurs in patients with COPD, rheumatic or coronary heart disease, congestive heart failure, or atrial septal defect. Ectopic impulse formation occurs at atrial rates of 250–350/min, with transmission of every second, third, or fourth impulse through the atrioventricular node to the ventricles. When the ventricular rate is 75 (4:1 block), standing or exercise may cause sudden doubling of the rate to 150 (2:1 block). Because the risk of embolization is lower with atrial flutter than fibrillation, anticoagulation should be reserved for patients with mitral valve disease.

Atrial flutter is often not responsive to pharmacologic therapy. Unlike paroxysmal supraventricular tachycardia, atrial flutter does not respond to adenosine, but verapamil may transiently slow the ventricular rate by increasing atrioventricular block, and a combination of digoxin and quinidine may cause the rhythm to revert to sinus rhythm. In contrast, the rhythm is exquisitely sensitive to electrical cardioversion, which can often be accomplished with less than 50 J and is therefore the treatment of choice for acute episodes. Class Ia or Ic agents should be avoided unless an agent that delays atrioventricular conduction (eg, digoxin, verapamil, or a beta-blocker) has been administered, because they can lead to increased atrioventricular conduction. The same approaches discussed under atrial fibrillation are used to prevent further episodes.

Benditt DG et al: Atrial flutter, atrial fibrillation, and other primary atrial tachycardias. Med Clin North Am 1984; 68:895.

8. MULTIFOCAL (CHAOTIC) ATRIAL TACHYCARDIA

This is a rhythm characterized by varying P-wave morphology and markedly irregular PP intervals. The rate is usually between 100 and 140/min, and atrioventricular block is unusual. Most patients have severe associated illnesses, especially COPD. Treatment of the underlying condition is the most effective approach; verapamil is also of value.

Scher DL, Arsura EL: Multifocal atrial tachycardia: Mechanisms, clinical correlates, and treatment. Am Heart J 1989;118:574.

9. ATRIOVENTRICULAR JUNCTIONAL RHYTHM

The atrial-nodal junction or the nodal-His bundle junctions may assume pacemaker activity for the heart, usually at a rate of 40–60/min. This may occur in patients with myocarditis, coronary artery disease, and digitalis toxicity as well as in individuals with normal hearts. The rate responds normally to exercise, and the diagnosis is often an incidental finding on electrocardiographic monitoring, but it can be suspected if the jugular venous pulse shows cannon waves. Junctional rhythm is often an escape rhythm because of depressed sinus node function with sinoatrial block or delayed conduction in the atrioventricular node. **Nonparoxysmal junctional tachycardia** results from increased automaticity of the junctional tissues in digitalis toxicity or ischemia and is associated with a narrow QRS complex and a rate usually less than 120–130/min. It is usually considered benign when it occurs in acute myocardial infarction, but the ischemia that induces it may also induce ventricular tachycardia and ventricular fibrillation.

10. DIFFERENTIATION OF ABERRANTLY CONDUCTED SUPRAVENTRICULAR BEATS FROM VENTRICULAR BEATS

This distinction can be very difficult in patients with a wide QRS complex; it is important because of the differing prognostic and therapeutic implications of each type. Findings favoring a ventricular origin include (1) a QRS duration exceeding 0.14 s; (2) left axis deviation; (3) atrioventricular dissociation; (4) capture or fusion beats (infrequent); (5) monophasic (R) or biphasic (qR, QR, or RS) complexes in V_1; and (6) a qR or QS complex in V_6. Supraventricular origin is favored by (1) a triphasic QRS complex, especially if there was initial negativity in leads I and V_6; (2) ventricular rates exceeding 170/min; (3) QRS duration longer than 0.12 s but not longer than 0.14 s; and (4) the presence of preexcitation syndrome.

The relationship of the P waves to the tachycardia complex is helpful. A 1:1 relationship usually means a supraventricular origin, except in the case of ventricular tachycardia with retrograde P waves. If the P waves are not clearly seen, Lewis leads—in which the right arm electrode is placed in the V_1 position 2 interspaces higher than usual and the left arm electrode is placed in the usual V_1 position—may be employed. This accentuates the size of the P waves. Esophageal leads, in which the electrode is placed directly posterior to the left atrium, achieve the same effect even more clearly. Right atrial electrograms may also help to clarify the diagnosis by accentuating the P waves.

Akhtar M et al: Wide QRS complex tachycardia: Reappraisal of a common clinical problem. Ann Intern Med 1988;109:905. (Most wide-complex arrhythmias are ventricular tachycardia.)

11. SUPRAVENTRICULAR TACHYCARDIAS DUE TO ACCESSORY ATRIOVENTRICULAR PATHWAYS (Preexcitation Syndromes)

Pathophysiology & Clinical Findings

Accessory pathways between the atria and the ventricle which avoid the conduction delay of the atrioventricular node predispose to reentry tachycardias, such as paroxysmal supraventricular tachycardia and atrial flutter, and to atrial fibrillation. These may be wholly or partly within the node (Mahaim fibers), yielding a short PR interval and normal QRS morphology **(Lown-Ganong-Levine syndrome)**. More commonly, they make direct connections between the atria and ventricle through Kent Bundles **(Wolff-Parkinson-White syndrome)**. This produces a short PR interval but an early delta wave at the onset of the wide, slurred QRS complex owing to early ventricular depolarization of the region adjacent to the pathway. While the morphology and polarity of the delta wave can suggest the location of the bypass tract, mapping by intracardiac recordings is required for precise anatomic localization.

Accessory pathways occur in 0.1–0.3% of the population and facilitate reentry arrhythmias owing to the disparity in refractory periods of the atrioventricular node and accessory pathway. Whether the tachycardia is associated with a narrow or wide QRS complex is determined by whether antegrade conduction is through the node (narrow) or the bypass tract (wide). Many patients with Wolff-Parkinson-White syndrome never conduct antegrade through the bypass tract which is therefore "concealed." Although reentry supraventricular tachycardias involving the AV node are commonest, 20–30% of patients with tachyarrhythmias have atrial fibrillation or flutter. Many have no arrhythmia. A minority of patients conduct antegrade through the accessory pathway, but these individuals may develop very fast rates, especially during atrial fibrillation. Patients with RR intervals less than 220 ms are at highest risk. Digoxin and, to a lesser extent, verapamil and beta-blockers may decrease accessory pathway refractoriness and increase ventricular response and should be avoided in atrial fibrillation with accessory pathways.

Pharmacologic Therapy

Narrow complex reentry rhythms can be managed as discussed for paroxysmal supraventricular tachycardias other than atrial fibrillation or flutter. Adenosine has proved to be very effective; digoxin is best avoided in patients with known Wolff-Parkinson-White syndrome. The class Ia antiarrhythmics, as well as the newer class Ic and class III agents, will increase the refractoriness of the bypass tract and are the drugs of choice for wide-complex tachycardias. If hemodynamic compromise is present, cardioversion is warranted.

Long-term therapy often involves a combination of agents that increase refractoriness in the bypass tract (class Ia or Ic agents) and in the atrioventricular node (verapamil, digoxin, and beta-blockers), provided that atrial fibrillation or flutter with short RR cycle lengths is not present (see above). Amiodarone is effective in refractory cases. Patients who are difficult to manage should undergo electrophysiologic evaluation.

Electrophysiologic Evaluation & Specialized Treatment

Patients with preexcitation syndromes who have episodes of atrial fibrillation or flutter should be tested by induction of atrial fibrillation in the electrophysiologic laboratory, noting duration of the RR cycle; if it is less than 220 ms, a short refractory period is present, and these individuals are at highest risk for sudden death. Patients with frequent tachycardia, especially if refractory to therapy, and those who conduct antegrade through the accessory pathway should also be evaluated by electrophysiologic studies. These can determine the location of the accessory pathway, assess the risk of excessively rapid conduction, and facilitate appropriate drug selection. The accessory pathway can be localized and its refractory period determined. In difficult patients, if the bypass tract is accessible, either radiofrequency or electrical ablation or surgical interruption is the treatment of choice. Some patients can be managed with antitachycardia pacemakers that deliver properly timed impulses to interrupt the reentry cycle.

Arai A, Kron J: Current management of the Wolff-Parkinson-White syndrome. West J Med 1990;152:383.

Fischell TA et al: Long-term follow-up after surgical correction of Wolff-Parkinson-White syndrome. J Am Coll Cardiol 1987;9:283. (Excellent long-term results.)

Waspe LE et al: Susceptibility to atrial fibrillation and ventricular tachyarrhythmia in the Wolff-Parkinson-White syndrome: Role of the accessory pathway. Am Heart J 1986;112:1141. (Who is at risk for these complications.)

Wellens HJJ et al: The management of preexcitation syndromes. JAMA 1987;257:2325. (Diagnosis, localization of bypass tract, medical therapy, and surgery.)

VENTRICULAR ARRHYTHMIAS

1. VENTRICULAR PREMATURE BEATS (Ventricular Extrasystoles)

Ventricular premature beats are similar to atrial premature beats in mechanism and manifestations but are more common. They are characterized by wide QRS complexes that differ in morphology from the patient's normal beats. They are usually not preceded by a P wave, although retrograde ventriculoatrial conduction may occur. Unless the latter is present, there is a fully compensatory pause. Bigeminy and trigeminy are arrhythmias in which every second or third beat is premature. Exercise generally abolishes premature beats in normal hearts, and the rhythm becomes regular. The patient may or may not sense the irregular beat, usually as a skipped beat.

Premature beats have questionable significance in the absence of heart disease. Sudden death occurs more frequently (presumably as a result of ventricular fibrillation) when ventricular premature beats occur in the presence of organic heart disease but not in individuals with no known cardiac disease.

Ambulatory electrocardiographic monitoring or continuous electrocardiography during graded exercise reveals more frequent and complex ventricular premature beats than occur in a single routine ECG. Premature beats induced by a low level of exercise may have a worse prognosis than those which occur spontaneously. Devices that provide computer-assisted recording of the signal-averaged ECG have recently become available. Some investigators feel that patients with prolonged electrical depolarization (delayed after-depolarizations) are at higher risk for life-threatening arrhythmias, but this has not been confirmed adequately to guide therapy.

If no associated cardiac disease is present and if the ectopic beats are asymptomatic, no specific therapy is indicated. If they are frequent, electrolyte abnormalities and occult heart disease should be excluded. Treatment is probably indicated only for patients who are symptomatic. The value of ventricular premature beat suppression in asymptomatic patients is unknown even when they occur as couplets or brief runs. Recent data from the Coronary Arrhythmia Suppression Trial (CAST) suggest that at least in the setting of coronary artery disease and with class Ic agents, the risk-benefit ratio of such prophylactic therapy is unfavorable. If the underlying condition is mitral prolapse, hypertrophic cardiomyopathy, left ventricular hypertrophy, or coronary disease—or if the QT interval is prolonged—a trial of a beta-blocker may be worthwhile even though these agents are often unsuccessful. The class Ia and Ib agents (see Table 8–8) are all effective in reducing ventricular premature beats but often cause side effects and may exacerbate arrhythmias in 5–20% of patients. Class Ic agents, though highly effective, should not be used because of their potential for increased mortality rates. Amiodarone should not be given to patients unless more severe arrhythmias are present, because of its toxicity.

Kennedy HL et al: Long-term follow-up of asymptomatic healthy subjects with frequent and complex ventricular ectopy. N Engl J Med 1985;312:193. (Most do well.)

2. VENTRICULAR TACHYCARDIA

Ventricular tachycardia is defined as 3 or more consecutive ventricular premature beats. The usual rate is 160–240/min and is moderately regular but less so than atrial tachycardia. Carotid sinus pressure has no effect. The distinction from aberrant conduction of supraventricular tachycardia may be difficult and is discussed above. The usual mechanism is reentry, but abnormally triggered rhythms occur. Ventricular tachycardia is either nonsustained (lasting less than 30 seconds) or sustained. It may be asymptomatic or associated with syncope or milder symptoms of impaired cerebral perfusion.

Ventricular tachycardia is a frequent complication of acute myocardial infarction and dilated cardiomyopathy but may occur in hypertrophic cardiomyopathy, mitral valve prolapse, myocarditis, and in most other forms of myocardial disease. Torsade de pointes, a form of ventricular tachycardia in which QRS morphology varies, may occur spontaneously or after quinidine or any drug that prolongs the QT interval and has a particularly poor prognosis. In nonacute settings, most patients with ventricular tachycardia have known or easily detectable cardiac disease, and the finding of ventricular tachycardia is an unfavorable prognostic sign.

Treatment

A. Acute Ventricular Tachycardia: The treatment of acute ventricular tachycardia is determined by the degree of hemodynamic compromise and the duration of the arrhythmia. The management of ventricular tachycardia in acute infarction has been discussed. In other patients, if severe hypotension, heart failure, or angina is present, synchronized DC cardioversion with 100–400 J should be performed immediately. If the patient is tolerating the rhythm, lidocaine can be infused first and may terminate it. If the patient is stable and lidocaine is not effective, a trial of intravenous procainamide or bretylium may be successful; flecainide and encainide have also proved to be effective. Ventricular tachycardia can be terminated by ventricular overdrive pacing, and this approach is useful when the rhythm is recurrent.

Amiodarone takes time to achieve a therapeutic level, but intravenous or oral loading with 1000–2000 mg/d may deliver a therapeutic response in 24–72 hours or even earlier in refractory patients.

B. Chronic Recurrent Ventricular Tachycardia: The treatment of recurrent, nonsustained ventricular tachycardia (runs of 3 or more beats lasting less than 30 seconds) not associated with symptoms is controversial. In subjects without heart disease, this rhythm is not clearly associated with a poor prognosis, whereas in patients with organic heart disease, it is a marker for increased mortality rates from the underlying disease and, in some studies, from arrhythmias. Whether antiarrhythmic therapy is beneficial in these patients with **nonsustained ventricular tachycardia** is unclear, but it is usually recommended. Class Ia agents are usually employed, but class Ib and Ic drugs are alternatives (Table 8–8). Again, class Ic agents should be reserved for life-threatening arrhythmias. Beta-blockers are occasionally beneficial. The efficacy of treatment is assessed by ambulatory electrocardiographic monitoring. Some authorities recommend ventricular stimulation; if sustained tachycardia of similar morphology is induced, they undertake more aggressive management with the goal of complete suppression of the arrhythmia. Amiodarone should probably not be used for asymptomatic, nonsustained tachycardia unless sustained ventricular tachycardia is inducible and not suppressible with less toxic agents.

Patients with symptomatic or asymptomatic **sustained ventricular tachycardia** require effective suppressive therapy. To develop a therapeutic regimen, the rhythm either must be present spontaneously or be induced by programmed stimulation in the electrophysiology laboratory. Various antiarrhythmic drugs can then be given in sequence to determine which agents prevent ventricular tachycardia. Drugs that prevent the electrical induction of ventricular tachycardia in the laboratory or suppress its occurrence during monitoring are more likely to be effective in vivo for long-term therapy; long-term use of a particular drug may still be effective even if the arrhythmia is not fully prevented in the laboratory. This is the case especially with amiodarone, which has emerged as a very effective though toxic agent for this select group of patients. The potential of all antiarrhythmia drugs to exacerbate ventricular arrhythmias in some patients should be kept in mind in initiating and monitoring therapy.

Patients with sustained ventricular tachycardia who do not respond to or tolerate antiarrhythmic medications are candidates for an automatic implantable cardiac defibrillator (AICD), which can be programmed to sense tachycardias above a predetermined rate and deliver a shock after a predetermined latent period (sufficient to allow charging and for many patients to lose consciousness). Because of the risks and poor tolerability of antiarrhythmic therapy, many experts are using these devices earlier in patients with symptomatic ventricular tachycardia, but their high cost (over $20,000) and associated psychologic disability in many patients should be kept in mind. Another approach in specialized centers is to determine the site of origin of the ventricular tachycardia by mapping studies in the electrophysiology laboratory. In selected patients, this site can be surgically excised or isolated.

Gallagher JJ et al: Surgical treatment of arrhythmias. Am J Cardiol 1988;61:27A. (Deals with ventricular and supraventricular arrhythmias.)

Green HL: The efficacy of amiodarone in the treatment of ventricular tachycardia or ventricular fibrillation. Prog Cardiovasc Dis 1989;31:319.

Haines DE et al: Surgical ablation of ventricular tachycardia with sequential map-guided subendocardial resection: Electrophysiologic assessment and long-term follow-up. Circulation 1988;77:131.

Manolis AS et al: Automatic implanted cardioverter defibrillator. JAMA 1989;262:1362.

Manolis AS et al: Surgical therapy for drug-refractory ventricular tachycardia: Results with mapping-guided subendocardial resection. J Am Col Cardiol 1989;14:199. (Fully successful in 50–60% of cases.)

McGovern BA, Ruskin JN: Ventricular tachycardia: Initial assessment and approach to treatment. Mod Concepts Cardiovasc Dis 1987;56:13.

Mitchell LB et al: A randomized clinical trial of the noninvasive and invasive approaches to drug therapy of ventricular tachycardia. N Engl J Med 1987;317:1681. (Invasive approach better.)

Morady F et al: Catheter ablation of ventricular tachycardia with intracardiac shocks: Results in 33 patients. Circulation 1987;75:1037. (Still experimental but should get better.)

Scheinman M: Catheter and surgical treatment of cardiac arrhythmias. JAMA 1990;263:79. (Review dealing with ventricular and supraventricular arrhythmias.)

Vrobel JR et al: A general overview of amiodarone toxicity: Its prevention, detection, and management. Prog Cardiovasc Dis 1989;31:319.

3. VENTRICULAR FIBRILLATION

The management of ventricular fibrillation is discussed under complications of myocardial infarction and is similar in all clinical settings.

4. ACCELERATED IDIOVENTRICULAR RHYTHM

Accelerated idioventricular rhythm is a relatively regular wide complex rhythm with a rate of 60–120/min, usually with a gradual onset. Because the rate is often similar to the sinus rate, fusion beats and alternating rhythms are common. Two mechanisms have been invoked: (1) an escape rhythm due to suppression of higher pacemakers resulting from sinoatrial and atrioventricular block or from depressed sinus node function; and (2) slow ventricular tachycardia due to increased automaticity or, less frequently, reentry. It occurs commonly in acute infarction and following reperfusion after thrombolytic drugs. The incidence of associated ventricular fibrillation is much less than that of ventricular tachycardia with a rapid rate, and treatment is not indicated unless there is hemodynamic compromise or more serious arrhythmias. This rhythm also is common in digitalis toxicity.

Accelerated idioventricular rhythm must be distinguished from the idioventricular or junctional rhythm with rates less than 40–45/min that occurs in the presence of complete atrioventricular block. Atrioventricular dissociation—where ventricular rate exceeds sinus—but not atrioventricular block occurs in most cases of accelerated idioventricular rhythm.

5. LONG QT SYNDROME

Idiopathic long QT syndrome is an uncommon disease that was first described in deaf siblings. It is characterized by recurrent syncope, a long QT interval (usually 0.5–0.7 s), documented ventricular arrhythmias, and sudden death. The sympathetic nervous system (especially the left stellate ganglion) may be important in pathogenesis.

Beta-blockers are the most effective therapy for "congenital" long QT syndrome, though phenytoin and the class Ib agents have also been beneficial. Agents that prolong the QT (classes Ia, Ic, and III) are contraindicated. Refractory acute arrhythmic episodes may be treated by local anesthetic block of the left stellate ganglion, and recurrent episodes can be treated by resection of this ganglion as well as of the first 3–5 thoracic ganglia.

Acquired long QT. Acquired prolongation of the QT interval secondary to use of antiarrhythmic agents or antidepressant drugs, electrolyte abnormalities, myocardial ischemia, or significant bradycardia may result in ventricular tachycardia (torsade de pointes, ie, twisting about the baseline into varying QRS morphology). The role of a prolonged QT interval is difficult to evaluate because classes Ia, Ic, and III antiarrhythmic agents increase the QT interval and yet are effective in treating the ventricular tachyarrhythmias; it may be the reason that these drugs paradoxically cause ventricular tachycardia in some patients. Acquired QT interval prolongation requires further study, but prudence speaks against continuing therapy that prolongs the QT interval beyond 500 ms. The management of torsade de pointes differs from that of other forms of ventricular tachycardia. Class I, Ic, or III antiarrhythmics, which prolong the QT interval, should be avoided—or withdrawn immediately if being used. Intravenous beta-blockers may be effective, especially in the congenital form; intravenous magnesium has also worked. An effective approach is temporary ventricular or atrial pacing, which can both break and prevent the rhythm.

Jackman WM et al: The long QT syndromes: A critical review, new clinical observations, and a unifying hypothesis. Prog Cardiovasc Dis 1988;31:115.

Stratmann HG, Kennedy HL: Torsades de pointes associated with drugs and toxins: Recognition and management. Am Heart J 1987;113:1470.

CONDUCTION DISTURBANCES

Abnormalities of conduction can occur between the sinus node and atrium, within the atrioventricular node, and in the intraventricular conduction pathways.

SINOATRIAL EXIT BLOCK

Sinoatrial exit block produces a pause of duration equal to a multiple of the underlying PP interval. Often there is progressive shortening of the PP interval prior to the pause (sinoatrial Wenckebach). This disturbance may be due to excessive vagal tone, ischemia, fibrosis or calcification of the conduction fibers, or drug effect (especially digitalis, calcium channel blockers, antiarrhythmic agents, and sympatholytic medications). Sinoatrial exit block is usually asymptomatic, though prolonged pauses equivalent to sinus arrest rarely occur as part of the sick sinus syndrome and are treated as outlined below.

SICK SINUS SYNDROME

This imprecise diagnosis is applied to patients with sinus arrest, sinoatrial exit block, or persistent sinus bradycardia. These rhythms are often caused or exacerbated by drug therapy (digitalis, calcium channel blockers, beta-blockers, sympatholytic agents, antiarrhythmics), and agents that may be responsible should be withdrawn prior to making the diagnosis. Another presentation is of recurrent supraventricular tachycardias (paroxysmal reentry tachycardias, atrial flutter, and atrial fibrillation), associated with bradyarrhythmias ("tachy-brady syndrome"). The long pauses that often follow the termination of tachycardia cause the associated symptoms.

Pathologic causes of the syndrome include degenerative fibrotic lesions of the cardiac conduction system and other conditions in which sclerotic or granulomatous lesions may occur, including scleroderma, Chagas' disease, and various cardiomyopathies. Coronary disease is an uncommon cause.

Most patients with electrocardiographic evidence of sick sinus syndrome are asymptomatic, but rare individuals may experience syncope, dizziness, confusion, palpitations, heart failure, or angina. Because these symptoms are either nonspecific or have other causes, it is essential that they be demonstrated to coincide with arrhythmias. This may require prolonged ambulatory monitoring or the use of an event recorder. When the symptoms are associated with bradyarrhythmias, permanent pacing is indicated; since atrioventricular node disease is often also present, ventricular or dual chamber pacing is preferred unless electrophysiologic studies indicate normal atrioventricular conduction. Treatment of associated tachyarrhythmias is often difficult without first instituting pacing, since digoxin and other antiarrhythmic agents may exacerbate the bradycardia. Unfortunately, symptomatic relief following pacing has not been consistent, largely because of inadequate documentation of the etiologic role of bradyarrhythmias in producing the symptom. Furthermore, many of these patients may have associated ventricular arrhythmias that may require treatment; however, carefully selected patients may become asymptomatic with permanent pacing alone.

Crossen KJ, Cain ME: Assessment and management of sinus node dysfunction. Mod Concepts Cardiovasc Dis 1986;55:43.

Rosenqvist M et al: Clinical and electrophysiologic course of sinus node disease: Five-year follow-up study. Am Heart J 1985;109:513.

Tresch DD, Fleg JL: Unexplained sinus bradycardia: Clinical significance and long-term prognosis in apparently healthy persons older than 40 years. Am J Cardiol 1986;58:1009.

Atrioventricular Block

Atrioventricular block is categorized as first-degree (PR interval > 0.21 s with all atrial impulses conducted), second-degree (intermittent blocked beats), or third-degree (complete heart block, in which no supraventricular impulses are conducted to the ventricles).

Second-degree block is subclassified. In **Mobitz type I (Wenckebach)** atrioventricular block, the atrioventricular conduction time (PR interval) progressively lengthens, with the RR interval shortening, before the blocked beat; this phenomenon is almost always due to abnormal conduction within the atrioventricular node. **Mobitz type II** atrioventricular block is abrupt and is not preceded by a lengthening atrioventricular conduction time; it is usually due to block within the His bundle system. The classification as Mobitz type I or Mobitz type II is only partially reliable, because patients may appear to have both types on the surface ECG, and one cannot predict the site or origin of the 2:1 atrioventricular block from the ECG. The width of the QRS complexes assists in determining whether the block is nodal or infranodal. When they are narrow, the block is usually nodal; when they are wide, the block is usually infranodal. His bundle readings may be necessary for accurate localization. Management of atrioventricular block in acute myocardial infarction has already been discussed. This section deals with patients in the nonacute setting.

First-degree and **Mobitz type I block** may occur in normal individuals with heightened vagal tone. They may also occur as a drug effect (especially digitalis, calcium channel blockers, beta-blockers, or other sympatholytic agents), often superimposed on organic disease. These disturbances also occur transiently or chronically due to ischemia, infarction, inflammatory processes, fibrosis, calcification, or infiltration. The prognosis is usually good, since reliable alternative pacemakers arise from the atrioventricular junction below the level of block if higher degrees of block occur.

Mobitz type II block is almost always due to organic disease involving the infranodal conduction system. In the event of progression to complete heart block, alternative pacemakers are not reliable. Thus, prophylactic ventricular pacing is required.

Complete (third-degree) heart block is a more advanced form of block often due to a lesion distal to the His bundle and associated with bilateral bundle branch block. The QRS is wide and the ventricular rate is slower, usually less than 50/min. Transmission of atrial impulses through the atrioventricular node is completely blocked, and a ventricular pacemaker maintains a slow, regular ventricular rate, usually less than 45/min. Exercise does not increase the rate. The first heart sound varies in intensity; wide pulse pressure, a changing systolic blood pressure level, and cannon venous pulsations in the neck are also present. Patients may be asymptomatic or may complain of weakness or dyspnea if the rate is less than 35/min; symptoms may occur at higher rates if the left ventricle cannot increase its stroke output. During periods of transition from partial to complete heart block, some patients have ventricular asystole that lasts several seconds to minutes. Syncope occurs abruptly.

Patients with episodic or chronic infranodal complete heart block require permanent pacing, and temporary pacing is indicated if implantation is delayed.

Mymin D et al: The natural history of primary first-degree atrioventricular heart block. N Engl J Med 1986; 315:1183. (Relatively benign.)

Strasberg B et al: Natural history of chronic second-degree atrioventricular nodal block. Circulation 1981;63:1043. (Not so benign, depending on type and associated cardiac abnormalities.)

ATRIOVENTRICULAR DISSOCIATION

When a ventricular pacemaker is firing at a rate faster than or close to the sinus rate (accelerated idioventricular rhythm, ventricular premature beats, or ventricular tachycardia), atrial impulses arriving at the atrioventricular node when it is refractory may not be conducted. This phenomenon is atrioventricular dissociation but does not necessarily indicate atrioventricular block. No treatment is required aside from management of the causative arrhythmia.

INTRAVENTRICULAR CONDUCTION DEFECTS

Intraventricular conduction defects, including bundle branch block, are common in individuals with otherwise normal hearts and in many disease processes, including ischemic heart disease, inflammatory disease, infiltrative disease, cardiomyopathy, and postcardiotomy. Below the atrioventricular node and bundle of His, the conduction system trifurcates into a right bundle and anterior and posterior fascicles of the left bundle. Conduction block in each of these fascicles can be recognized on the surface ECG. Although such conduction abnormalities are often seen in normal hearts, they are more commonly due to organic heart disease—either an isolated process of fibrosis and calcification (Lev's or Lenegre's disease) or more generalized myocardial disease. Bifascicular block is present when 2 of these—right bundle, left anterior and posterior hemibundle—are involved. Trifascicular block is defined as right bundle branch block with alternating left hemiblock, alternating right and left bundle branch block, or bifascicular block with documented prolonged infranodal conduction (long HV interval).

The prognosis of intraventricular block is generally that of the underlying myocardial process. Even in bifascicular block, the incidence of occult complete heart block or progression to it is low, and pacing is not usually warranted. In patients with symptoms (eg, syncope) consistent with heart block and intraventricular block, pacing should be reserved for those with documented concomitant complete heart block on monitoring or those with a very prolonged HV interval (> 90 ms) with no other cause for symptoms. Even in the latter group, prophylactic pacing has not improved the prognosis significantly, probably because of the high incidence of ventricular arrhythmias in the same population.

Flowers NC: Left bundle branch block: A continuously evolving concept. J Am Coll Cardiol 1987;9:684. (Not benign but heart block uncommon.)

Kreger BE et al: Prevalence of intra-ventricular block in the general population: The Framingham Study. Am Heart J 1989;117:903. (Common in older patients.)

Scheinman MM et al: Electrophysiologic studies in patients with bundle branch block. PACE 1983;6:1157. (Follow-up study with suggested guidelines on when to measure HV and when to pace.)

PERMANENT PACING

The indications for permanent pacing have been discussed: symptomatic bradyarrhythmias, asymptomatic Mobitz II AV block, or complete heart block. The versatility of pacemaker generator units has increased markedly, and dual-chamber multiple programmable units are readily available. A newer development is rate-responsive pacing, in which the rate increases with activity, as sensed by increased motion or changes in body temperature. Conceptually, a pacemaker that senses and paces in both chambers is the most physiologic approach to pacing patients who remain in sinus rhythm. However, because of the substantially increased cost and complexity of dual-chamber pacing and the shorter projected battery life, their use should be limited to patients in whom atrial contraction produces a substantial increment in stroke volume and in those in whom sensing the atrial rate to provide rate-responsive ventricular pacing is useful. Dual-chamber pacing is most useful for individuals with left ventricular systolic or—perhaps more importantly—diastolic dysfunction and for physically active individuals. In patients with single-chamber pacemakers, the lack of an atrial kick may lead to the so-called pacemaker syndrome, in which the patient experiences signs of low cardiac output while upright. Patients with intermittent or potential bradyarrhythmias or conduction disturbances in whom pacing is primarily prophylactic should undergo ventricular pacing. Follow-up after pacemaker implantation, usually by telephonic monitoring, is essential. All pulse generators and lead systems have an early failure rate that is now below 5% as well as a finite life expectancy varying from 4 to 10 years.

Fearnot NE, Smith HJ, Geddes LA: A review of pacemakers that physiologically increase rate: The DDD and rate-responsive pacemakers. Prog Cardiovasc Dis 1986; 29:145. (High-tech pacing.)

Furman S, Hayes DL, Holmes DR Jr: A Practice of Cardiac Pacing, 2nd ed. Futura, 1989.

Luceri RM et al: The arrhythmias of dual-chamber cardiac pacemakers and their management. Ann Intern Med 1983;99:354. (New pacing modalities have their own problems.)

Parsonnet V, Bernstein A: Pacing in perspective: Concepts and controversies. Circulation 1986;73:1087.

EVALUATION OF SYNCOPE & SURVIVORS OF SUDDEN DEATH

SYNCOPE

Syncope—transient loss of consciousness due to inadequate cerebral blood flow—is a common clinical problem, especially in the elderly. More common still are episodes of dizziness, feeling "faint" (ie, a perception that loss of consciousness is imminent), seizures, and transient neurologic deficits associated with impaired consciousness. Thus, before a diagnosis of syncope can be established, epileptic seizures, transient ischemic attacks, and episodes of vertigo, hypoglycemia, and anxiety attacks (often accompanied by hyperventilation) must be excluded.

Syncope usually *does not have* the following features: premonitory aura, preceding autonomic signs and symptoms characteristic of hypoglycemia, vertigo, hyperventilation, gradual onset, convulsive movements and incontinence (though these may occur inconsistently), confusion postrecovery, and residual neurologic deficits.

Syncope is more likely to occur in patients with known heart disease, older men, and young women (who are prone to vasovagal episodes). Syncopal episodes are characteristically abrupt in onset (so much so that they frequently cause traumatic injuries), transient (lasting for seconds to a few minutes), and followed by prompt recovery of full consciousness.

Vasomotor syncope may be due to excessive vagal tone or impaired reflex control of the peripheral circulation. The most frequent type of vasodepressor syncope is vasovagal hypotension or the "common faint," which is often initiated by stressful, painful, or claustrophobic experience, especially in young women. Premonitory symptoms, such as nausea, diaphoresis, tachycardia, and loss of color, are usual. Episodes can be aborted by lying down or removing the inciting stimulus. Enhanced vagal tone with resulting hypotension is the cause of syncope in carotid sinus hypersensitivity and postmicturition syncope; vagal-induced sinus bradycardia, sinus arrest, and atrioventricular block are common accompaniments and may themselves be the cause of syncope. Carotid sinus massage under carefully monitored conditions may be diagnostic. Treatment consists largely of counseling patients to avoid predisposing situations. Permanent pacing may benefit patients with documented bradycardiac responses.

Orthostatic (postural) hypotension is another common cause of vasomotor syncope, especially in the elderly, in diabetics or other patients with autonomic neuropathy, in patients with blood loss or hypovolemia, and in patients taking vasodilators, diuretics, and adrenergic blocking drugs. In addition, a syndrome of chronic idiopathic orthostatic hypotension exists primarily in older men. In most of these conditions, the normal vasoconstrictive response to assuming upright posture, which compensates for the abrupt decrease in venous return, is impaired. A greater than normal decline (20 mm Hg) in blood pressure on arising from the supine to the standing position is observed, with or without tachycardia depending on the status of autonomic (baroreceptor) function. Studying patients with a tilt table can establish the diagnosis with more certainty. Autonomic function can be assessed by observing blood pressure and heart rate responses to Valsalva's maneuver.

Cardiogenic syncope can occur on a mechanical or arrhythmic basis. Mechanical problems that can cause syncope include aortic stenosis (where syncope may occur from autonomic reflex abnormalities or

ventricular tachycardia), pulmonary stenosis, hypertrophic obstructive cardiomyopathy, congenital lesions associated with pulmonary hypertension or right-to-left shunting, and left atrial myxoma obstructing the mitral valve. Episodes are commonly exertional or postexertional. More commonly, cardiac syncope is due to disorders of automaticity (sick sinus syndrome), conduction disorders (atrioventricular block), or tachyarrhythmias (especially ventricular tachycardia and supraventricular tachycardia with rapid ventricular rate).

The evaluation for syncope depends heavily on a careful history and physical examination (especially orthostatic blood pressure evaluation, examination of carotid and other arteries, cardiac examination, and, if appropriate, carotid sinus massage). The resting ECG may reveal arrhythmias, evidence of accessory pathways, prolonged QT interval, and other signs of heart disease (such as infarction or hypertrophy). If the history is consistent with syncope, ambulatory electrocardiographic monitoring is essential. This may need to be repeated several times. Event recorder and transtelephone electrocardiographic monitoring may be helpful in patients with intermittent presyncopal episodes. Electrophysiologic studies to assess sinus node function and atrioventricular conduction and to induce supraventricular or ventricular tachycardia are indicated in patients with recurrent episodes and nondiagnostic ambulatory ECGs. They reveal an arrhythmic cause in 20–50% of patients, depending on the study criteria, and are most often diagnostic when the patient has had multiple episodes and has identifiable cardiac abnormalities.

Day SC et al: Evaluation and outcome of emergency room patients with transient loss of consciousness. Am J Med 1982;73:15. (What to look for. Most do well.)
Kapoor WN et al: Prolonged electrocardiographic monitoring in patients with syncope: Importance of frequent or repetitive ventricular ectopy. Am J Med 1987;82:20.
Onrot J et al: Management of chronic orthostatic hypotension. Am J Med 1986;80:454.
Radack KL: Syncope: Cost-effective patient workup. Postgrad Med (July) 1986;80:169. (Practical approach.)
Strasberg B: Carotid sinus hypersensitivity and the carotid sinus syndrome. Prog Cardiovasc Dis 1989;31:379.
Strasberg B et al: The noninvasive evaluation of syncope of suspected cardiovascular origin. Am Heart J 1989;117:160.
Teichman SL et al: The value of electrophysiologic studies in syncope of undetermined origin: Report of 150 cases. Am Heart J 1985;100:469. (Results of a large series.)

SURVIVORS OF SUDDEN DEATH

Sudden cardiac death is defined as unexpected nontraumatic death in clinically well or stable patients who die within 1 hour after onset of symptoms. The causative rhythm in most cases is ventricular fibrillation, which is usually preceded by ventricular tachycardia; complete heart block and sinus node arrest may also cause sudden death. A disproportionate number of sudden deaths occur in the early morning hours. Over 75% of victims of sudden cardiac death have had severe coronary artery disease. Many have old infarctions. Sudden death may be the initial manifestation of coronary disease in up to 20% of patients and accounts for approximately 50% of deaths from coronary disease. When ventricular fibrillation occurs in the initial 24 hours after infarction, long-term management is no different from that of other patients with acute infarction. Other conditions that predispose to sudden death include severe left ventricular hypertrophy, hypertrophic cardiomyopathy, congestive cardiomyopathy, aortic stenosis, pulmonary stenosis, primary pulmonary hypertension, cyanotic congenital heart disease, mitral valve prolapse, hypoxia, electrolyte abnormalities, prolonged QT interval syndrome, and conduction system disease. Recent studies suggest that detection of late potentials (after the QRS complex) on a signal averaged surface ECG may identify a group of patients at risk of ventricular arrhythmias and sudden death.

Unless ventricular fibrillation occurred early postmyocardial infarction or an unusual correctable process was present (such as an electrolyte abnormality, drug toxicity, or aortic stenosis), these patients should undergo intensive investigation. Exercise testing or coronary arteriography should be performed to exclude coronary disease as the underlying cause. Conduction disturbances should be managed as described above. If serious prodromal ventricular arrhythmias such as sustained or nonsustained ventricular tachycardia or frequent ventricular premature beats are found by monitoring, their elimination by therapy may prevent further episodes—the evidence is conflicting. Most experts believe that ventricular stimulation studies are also indicated, especially if monitoring does not reveal significant arrhythmias. If inducibility cannot be prevented by the usual agents or if monitored arrhythmias are not obliterated, amiodarone may still be effective. Alternatively, either surgical or catheter ablation or implantation of an automatic implantable defibrillator may be attempted. Patients in whom ventricular tachycardia cannot be detected or induced are usually treated empirically with beta-blockers and antiarrhythmic therapy.

Patients who have recurrent sudden death, syncope due to ventricular arrhythmias, or documented sustained ventricular tachycardia despite these measures should be referred for ablation of foci or implantation of an automatic defibrillator.

DeLuna AB, Coumel P, Leclercq JF: Ambulatory sudden cardiac death: Mechanisms of production of fatal arrhythmia on the basis of data from 157 cases. Am Heart J 1989;117:151. (Most are due to ventricular fibrillation.)

Eldar M, Sauve MJ, Scheinman MM: Electrophysiologic testing and follow-up of patients with aborted sudden death. J Am Coll Cardiol 1987;10:291. (High incidence of ventricular arrhythmias.)

Epstein SE, Maron BJ: Sudden death and the competitive athlete: Perspectives on preparticipation screening studies. J Am Coll Cardiol 1986;7:220. (Review with focus on role of screening.)

Fogoros RN, Fiedler SB, Elson JJ: The automatic implantable cardioverter-defibrillator in drug-refractory tachyarrhythmias. Ann Intern Med 1987;107:635.

Hall PA et al: The signal averaged surface electrocardiogram and the identification of late potentials. Prog Cardiovasc Dis 1989;31:295. (Review of hot area of investigation.)

Kannel WB, Cupples LA, D'Agostino RB: Sudden death risk in overt coronary heart disease: The Framingham Study. Am Heart J 1987;113:799. (Provides demography of victims.)

Morady F et al: Role of myocardial ischemia during programmed stimulation in survivors of cardiac arrest with coronary artery disease. J Am Coll Cardiol 1987;9:1004.

Muller JE et al: Circadian variation in the frequency of sudden cardiac death. Circulation 1987;75:131. (Frequency highest from 7 to 11 AM.)

Saksena S, Camm AJ: Clinical investigation of implantable antitachycardia devices: Report of the policy conference of the North American Society of Pacing and Electrophysiology. J Am Coll Cardiol 1987;10:225. (Consensus statement.)

Wilber DJ et al: Out-of-hospital cardiac arrest: Use of electrophysiologic testing in the prediction of long-term outcome. N Engl J Med 1988;318:19. (Electrophysiologic studies valuable in determining prognosis.)

CARDIAC FAILURE

Essentials of Diagnosis

Left ventricular failure:

● Exertional dyspnea, cough, fatigue, orthopnea, paroxysmal nocturnal dyspnea, cardiac enlargement, rales, gallop rhythm, and pulmonary venous congestion.

Right ventricular failure:

● Elevated venous pressure, hepatomegaly, dependent edema.

Both:

● Combination of above.

General Considerations

Systolic function of the heart is governed by 4 major determinants: the contractile state of the myocardium, the preload of the ventricle (the end-diastolic volume and the resultant fiber length of the ventricles prior to onset of the contraction), the afterload applied to the ventricles (the impedance to left ventricular ejection), and the heart rate.

Cardiac function may be inadequate as a result of alterations in any of these determinants. In most instances, the primary derangement is depression of myocardial contractility caused either by loss of functional muscle (due to myocardial infarction, etc) or by processes diffusely affecting the myocardium. However, the heart may fail as a pump because preload is excessively elevated, such as in valvular regurgitation, or when afterload is excessive, such as in aortic stenosis or in severe hypertension. Pump function may also be inadequate when the heart rate is too slow or too rapid. While the normal heart can tolerate wide variations in preload, afterload, and heart rate, the diseased heart often has limited reserve for such alterations. Finally, cardiac pump function may be supranormal but nonetheless inadequate when metabolic demands or requirements for blood flow are excessive. This situation is termed high-output heart failure and, though uncommon, tends to be specifically treatable. Causes of high output include thyrotoxicosis, beriberi, severe anemia, arteriovenous shunting, and Paget's disease of bone.

Manifestations of cardiac failure can also occur as a result of isolated or predominant diastolic dysfunction of the heart. In these cases, filling of the left or right ventricle is impaired because the chamber is noncompliant ("stiff") due to excessive hypertrophy or changes in composition of the myocardium. Even though contractility may be preserved, diastolic pressures are elevated and cardiac output may be reduced.

Pathophysiology

When the heart fails, a number of adaptations occur both in the heart and systemically. If the stroke volume of either ventricle is reduced by depressed contractility or excessive afterload, end-diastolic volume and pressure in that chamber will rise. This increases end-diastolic myocardial fiber length, resulting in a greater systolic shortening (Starling's law of the heart). If the condition is chronic, ventricular dilatation will occur. While this may restore resting cardiac output, the resulting chronic elevation of diastolic pressures will be transmitted to the atria and to the pulmonary and systemic venous circulation. Ultimately, increased capillary pressure may lead to transudation of fluid with resulting pulmonary or systemic edema. Reduced cardiac output, particularly if associated with reduced arterial pressure or perfusion of the kidneys, will also activate several neural and humoral systems. Increased activity of the sympathetic nervous system will stimulate myocardial contractility, heart rate, and venous tone; the latter change results in a rise in the effective central blood volume, which serves to further elevate preload. Though these adaptations are designed to increase cardiac output, they may themselves be deleterious. Thus, tachycardia and increased contractility may precipitate ischemia in patients with underlying coronary artery disease, and the rise in preload may worsen pulmonary congestion. Sympathetic nervous system activation also increases peripheral vascular resistance; this adaptation is designed to maintain perfusion to vital organs, but when it is excessive it may itself reduce renal and other tissue blood flow. Peripheral vascular resistance is also a major determinant of left ventricular afterload, so that excessive sympathetic activity may further depress cardiac function.

One of the more important effects of lower cardiac output is reduction of renal blood flow and glomerular filtration rate, which leads to sodium and fluid retention. The renin-angiotensin-aldosterone system is also activated, leading to further increases in peripheral vascular resistance and left ventricular afterload as well as sodium and fluid retention. Heart failure is associated with increased circulating levels of arginine vasopressin, which also serves as a vasoconstrictor and inhibitor of water excretion. While release of atrial natriuretic peptide is increased in heart failure owing to the elevated atrial pressures, there is evidence of resistance to its natriuretic and vasodilating effects.

Hemodynamic Alterations

Myocardial failure is characterized by 2 hemodynamic derangements, and the clinical presentation is determined by their severity. Resting cardiac output or—in cases where compensatory mechanisms are relatively effective—the ability to increase cardiac output in response to increased demands imposed by exercise or even ordinary activity (cardiac reserve) is usually reduced. The second abnormality, elevation of ventricular diastolic pressures, is primarily a result of the compensatory processes.

Heart failure may be right-sided or left-sided. Patients with the picture of **left heart failure** have symptoms of low cardiac output and elevated pulmonary venous pressure; dyspnea is the predominant feature. Signs of fluid retention predominate in **right heart failure,** with the patient exhibiting edema, hepatic congestion, and, on occasion, ascites. Most patients exhibit signs of both right–and left-sided failure, and left ventricular dysfunction is the primary cause of right ventricular failure. Surprisingly, some individuals with severe left ventricular dysfunction will display few signs of left heart failure and appear to have isolated right heart failure. Indeed, they may be clinically indistinguishable from patients with cor pulmonale, who have right heart failure secondary to pulmonary disease.

Although this section concerns cardiac failure due to systolic left ventricular dysfunction, patients with diastolic dysfunction experience many of the same symptoms and may be difficult to distinguish clinically. Diastolic pressures are elevated even though diastolic volumes are normal or small. These pressures are transmitted to the pulmonary and systemic venous systems, resulting in dyspnea and edema. The commonest cause of diastolic cardiac dysfunction is left ventricular hypertrophy, but conditions such as hypertrophic or restrictive cardiomyopathy, diabetes, and pericardial disease can produce the same clinical picture. While diuretics are often useful in these patients, the other therapies discussed in this section (digitalis, vasodilators, inotropic agents) may be inappropriate.

Causes of Cardiac Failure

The syndrome of cardiac failure can be produced by many diseases. In developed countries, coronary artery disease with resulting myocardial infarction and loss of functioning myocardium (ischemic cardiomyopathy) is the commonest cause. A number of processes may present with dilated or congestive cardiomyopathy, which is characterized by left ventricular or biventricular dilatation and generalized systolic dysfunction. These are discussed elsewhere in this chapter, but the most common are alcoholic cardiomyopathy, viral myocarditis (including infections by HIV), and dilated cardiomyopathies with no obvious underlying cause (idiopathic cardiomyopathy). Rare causes of dilated cardiomyopathy include infiltrative diseases (hemochromatosis, sarcoidosis, amyloidosis, etc), other infectious agents, metabolic disorders, cardiotoxins, and drug toxicity.

Systemic hypertension remains an important cause of congestive heart failure and, even more commonly in the USA, an exacerbating factor in patients with cardiac dysfunction due to other causes. Patients with chronic volume overload of the left ventricle, such as mitral or aortic regurgitation, may develop progressive myocardial dysfunction and have a picture of cardiomyopathy even after the underlying condition is corrected. This form of congestive heart failure is preventable by early diagnosis and treatment of the valvular lesion.

Clinical Findings

A. Symptoms: The symptoms of cardiac failure have been discussed in part in earlier sections. The most common complaint is shortness of breath often chiefly exertional dyspnea at first and progressing to orthopnea, paroxysmal nocturnal dyspnea, and rest dyspnea. A more subtle and often overlooked symptom of heart failure is a chronic nonproductive cough, which is often worse in the recumbent position. Nocturia due to excretion of fluid retained during the day and increased renal perfusion in the recumbent position is a common nonspecific symptom of heart failure. Patients with heart failure also complain of fatigue and weakness, which result from reduced blood flow to skeletal muscle and the central nervous system. These symptoms may be exacerbated by electrolyte changes induced either by the heart failure or by diuretic treatment. Patients with right heart failure may experience right upper quadrant pain due to passive congestion of the liver, loss of appetite and nausea due to edema of the gut or impaired gastrointestinal perfusion, and peripheral edema.

Cardiac failure may present acutely in a previously asymptomatic patient. Causes include myocardial infarction, myocarditis, and acute valvular regurgitation

due to endocarditis or other conditions. These patients usually present with pulmonary edema. The management of acute heart failure has been discussed under myocardial infarction and centers around initial stabilization with diuretics and parenteral vasodilators or inotropic agents.

Patients may also present with acute exacerbations of chronic, stable heart failure. Exacerbations are usually caused by alterations in therapy (or patient noncompliance), excessive salt and fluid intake, arrhythmias, excessive activity, pulmonary emboli, intercurrent infection, or progression of the underlying disease.

B. Signs: Many patients with heart failure, including some with severe symptoms, appear comfortable at rest. Others will be dyspneic during conversation or minor activity, and those with long-standing severe heart failure may appear cachectic or cyanotic. The vital signs may be normal, but tachycardia, hypotension, and reduced pulse pressure may be present. Patients often show signs of increased sympathetic nervous system activity, including cold extremities and diaphoresis. Important peripheral signs of heart failure can be detected by examination of the neck, the lungs, the abdomen, and the extremities. Right atrial pressure may be estimated through the height of the pulsations in the jugular venous system. In addition to the height of the venous pressure, abnormal pulsations such as regurgitant v waves should be sought. Examination of the carotid pulse allows estimation of pulse pressure as well as detection of aortic stenosis. The thyroid examination is important, since occult hyperthyroidism and hypothyroidism are readily treatable causes of heart failure. In the lungs, crackles at the bases reflect transudation of fluid into the alveoli. Pleural effusions may cause bibasilar dullness to percussion. Expiratory wheezing and rhonchi may be signs of heart failure. Patients with severe right heart failure may have hepatic enlargement— tender or nontender—due to passive congestion. Systolic pulsations may be felt in tricuspid regurgitation. Sustained moderate pressure on the liver may increase jugular venous pressure (a positive hepatojugular reflux is an increase of > 1 cm). Ascites may also be present. Peripheral pitting edema is a common sign in patients with right heart failure and may extend into the thighs and abdominal wall.

The cardiac examination has been discussed. Cardinal signs in heart failure are a parasternal lift, indicating pulmonary hypertension; an enlarged and sustained left ventricular impulse, indicating left ventricular dilatation and hypertrophy; a diminished first heart sound, suggesting impaired contractility; and S_3 gallops originating in the left and sometimes the right ventricle. Murmurs should be sought to exclude primary valvular disease; secondary mitral regurgitation and tricuspid regurgitation murmurs are common in patients with dilated ventricles.

C. Laboratory Findings: A blood count may reveal anemia, a cause of high-output failure and an exacerbating factor in other forms of cardiac dysfunction, or polycythemia. Biochemical studies may show renal insufficiency as a possible compounding factor. Renal function tests also determine whether cardiac failure is associated with azotemia, with serum urea nitrogen elevated disproportionately to serum creatinine. Electrolytes may disclose heightened neuroendocrine activity with resultant hyponatremia. Particularly in older patients and those with atrial fibrillation or accompanying pericardial effusion, thyroid function should be assessed to detect occult thyrotoxicosis or myxedema. Rectal, gingival, or skin biopsies may be performed to exclude amyloidosis. The additional diagnostic assessment of patients with dilated cardiomyopathy may include iron studies to exclude hemochromatosis. Other studies, including myocardial biopsy, may be appropriate to exclude specific causes of dilated cardiomyopathy.

D. ECG and Chest X-Ray: Electrocardiography may indicate an underlying or secondary arrhythmia, myocardial infarction, or nonspecific changes that often include low voltage, intraventricular conduction defects, left ventricular hypertrophy, and nonspecific repolarization changes. Chest radiographs provide information about the size and shape of the cardiac silhouette. Cardiomegaly is an important finding. Evidence of pulmonary venous hypertension includes relative dilatation of the upper lobe veins, perivascular edema (haziness of vessel outlines), interstitial edema, and alveolar fluid. In acute heart failure, these findings correlate moderately well with pulmonary venous pressure, and when present in chronic failure they indicate elevated pressures. However, patients with chronic heart failure may show relatively normal pulmonary vasculature and have markedly elevated pressures. Pleural effusions are common and tend to be bilateral or right-sided.

E. Diagnostic Studies: Most patients with heart failure should undergo noninvasive cardiac testing because many of the symptoms are nonspecific and many studies have indicated that the clinical diagnosis of systolic myocardial dysfunction is often inaccurate. The primary confounding conditions are diastolic dysfunction of the heart with decreased relaxation and filling of the left ventricle (particularly in hypertension and in hypertrophic states) and pulmonary disease.

The most useful test is the echocardiogram. This will reveal the size and function of both ventricles and of the atria. It will also allow detection of pericardial effusion, valvular abnormalities, intracardiac shunts, and segmental wall motion abnormalities suggestive of old myocardial infarction as opposed to more generalized forms of dilated cardiomyopathy.

Radionuclide angiography measures left ventricular ejection fraction and permits analysis of regional wall motion. This test is especially useful when echocardiography is technically suboptimal, such as in patients with severe pulmonary disease.

F. Cardiac Catheterization: Cardiac catheterization is not necessary in most patients with heart failure. Clinical examination and noninvasive tests can determine left ventricular size and function well enough to confirm the diagnosis. Left heart catheterization is necessary when valvular disease must be excluded and when the presence and extent of coronary artery disease must be determined. The latter is particularly important when surgery to excise a left ventricular aneurysm is contemplated or when it is believed that left ventricular dysfunction may be partially reversible by revascularization. Right heart catheterization may be useful to select and monitor therapy in patients refractory to standard therapy.

Treatment

A. Correction of Reversible Causes: The major reversible causes have been discussed earlier and include thyrotoxicosis, myxedema, valvular lesions, intracardiac shunts, high-output states, arrhythmias, and alcohol–or drug-induced myocardial depression. Some metabolic and infiltrative cardiomyopathies may be partially reversible, or their progression may be slowed; these include hypercalcemia, hemochromatosis, sarcoidosis, and primary amyloidosis. Acute myocarditis may respond to immunosuppressive therapy and corticosteroids. Reversible causes of diastolic dysfunction include pericardial disease and left ventricular hypertrophy due to hypertension. Once it is established that there is no reversible component to the heart failure and that the underlying pathophysiologic process is impaired contractility of the left ventricle, the measures outlined below are appropriate.

B. Diet and Activity: Patients should routinely be under moderate sodium (1.5–2 g) restriction. More severe sodium restriction is usually difficult to achieve and unnecessary because of the availability of potent diuretic agents. Alterations in life-style reduce symptoms and the need for additional medications. In severe heart failure, restriction of activity, including bed rest if necessary, often facilitates temporary recompensation. With such limitations, these patients may exhibit profound diuresis even though fluid retention was previously refractory. There is no convincing evidence that prolonged bed rest alters the natural history of congestive heart failure.

C. Diuretic Therapy: Diuretics are the most effective means of providing symptomatic relief to patients with moderate to severe congestive heart failure. When fluid retention is mild, thiazide diuretics or a similar type of agent (hydrochlorothiazide, 25–100 mg; metolazone, 2.5–10 mg; chlorthalidone, 25–100 mg; etc) may be sufficient. These agents block sodium reabsorption in the cortical diluting segment at the terminal portion of the loop of Henle and in the proximal portion of the distal convoluted tubule. The result is natriuresis and kaliuresis. These agents also have weak carbonic anhydrase inhibitor activity, which results in proximal tubule inhibition of sodium reabsorption.

The thiazides are generally ineffective when the glomerular filtration rate falls below 30 mL/min, a not infrequent occurrence in patients with severe heart failure. Metolazone maintains its efficacy down to a glomerular filtration rate of approximately 10 mL/min. Adverse reactions to the thiazide diuretics include hypokalemia and intravascular volume depletion with resulting prerenal azotemia, skin rashes, neutropenia and thrombocytopenia, hyperglycemia, hyperuricemia, and hepatic dysfunction.

Patients with more severe heart failure should be treated with one of the "loop diuretics." These include furosemide (20–320 mg daily in single or divided doses), bumetanide (1–8 mg daily in single or divided doses), and ethacrynic acid (25–200 mg daily in single or divided doses). These agents have a rapid onset and short duration of action. In acute situations or when gastrointestinal absorption is in doubt, they should be given intravenously. The loop diuretics inhibit chloride reabsorption in the ascending limb of the loop of Henle, which results in natriuresis, kaliuresis, and metabolic alkalosis. They are active even in severe renal insufficiency, though very large doses (up to 500 mg of furosemide or equivalent) may be required. The major adverse reactions to loop diuretics relate to their potency; patients often develop excessive diuresis with resultant intravascular volume depletion, prerenal azotemia, and hypotension. Hypokalemia, particularly with accompanying digitalis therapy, is a major problem. Less common side effects include skin rashes, gastrointestinal distress, and ototoxicity (the latter more common with ethacrynic acid and possibly less common with bumetanide).

The potassium-sparing agents spironolactone, triamterene, and amiloride are often useful in combination with the loop diuretics and thiazides. Triamterene and amiloride act on the distal tubule to reduce potassium secretion. Their diuretic potency is only mild and not adequate for most patients with heart failure, but they may minimize the hypokalemia induced by more potent agents. Side effects include hyperkalemia, gastrointestinal symptoms, and renal dysfunction. Spironolactone is a specific inhibitor of aldosterone, which is often increased in congestive heart failure. Its onset of action is slower than the other potassium-sparing agents, and its side effects include gynecomastia. Combinations of potassium supplements or angiotensin converting enzyme inhibitors and potassium-sparing drugs can produce hyperkalemia.

Patients with refractory edema may respond to combinations of a loop diuretic and thiazidelike agents. Metolazone, because of its continued activity with renal insufficiency, is the most useful agent for such a combination. Extreme caution must be observed with this approach, since massive diuresis and electrolyte imbalances often occur; 2.5 mg of metolazone should be added to the previous dosage of loop diuretic. In many cases this is necessary only once or twice a week, but dosages up to 10 mg daily have been used in some patients.

D. Digitalis Glycosides: Although digitalis was once the mainstay of treatment in congestive heart failure, it is now used somewhat more judiciously. Nonetheless, the efficacy of digitalis has recently been reconfirmed in several large studies.

1. Mechanism of action–Digitalis has a number of effects on the heart. Its positive inotropic effect is accomplished by increasing intracellular calcium and enhancing actin-myosin cross-bridge formation. Digitalis binds to the sodium-potassium ATPase on the cell membrane and inhibits the sodium pump. The resulting increase in intracellular sodium facilitates sodium-calcium exchange, resulting in increasing intracellular calcium concentrations.

The digitalis glycosides have electrophysiologic effects that may be beneficial or deleterious in individual patients. These effects are primarily the result of enhancement of the cardiac effects of the parasympathetic nervous system. Its primary therapeutic effect is inhibition of atrioventricular conduction. This decreases the ventricular response to supraventricular arrhythmias, such as atrial fibrillation or flutter. In addition, digitalis decreases sinus node automaticity. The increase in intracellular calcium and sodium may enhance automaticity of latent pacemakers. This increased excitability of ventricular myocardium underlies many of the arrhythmias associated with digitalis toxicity. Digitalis effect and toxicity are increased by reduced intracellular potassium concentrations and increased extracellular calcium concentrations.

2. Pharmacokinetics–Digitalis glycosides are available in a variety of preparations, but of these only digoxin (intravenously and orally) and digitoxin (primarily orally) are usually employed. The intravenous route is preferable if a rapid effect is desired; this is necessary chiefly in the setting of rapid supraventricular arrhythmias when early control of the ventricular rate is desirable. Intravenous digoxin begins to have an effect after 15–30 minutes, and the peak effect is seen after 1½–3 hours. The usual initial dose is 0.5 mg given slowly over 10–20 minutes to avoid an immediate hypertensive response. Additional 0.25- mg or 0.125-mg doses may be administered after 3 hours. A total dosage of 1–1.25 mg is usually required to achieve full digitalis effect, but smaller dosages are sometimes adequate in older patients and in individuals with small lean body masses.

Therapeutic concentrations may also be achieved by the oral route. If a full effect is desired fairly rapidly, 1–1.25 mg are administered in divided dosages over the initial 24 hours. An additional 0.5 mg is added during the second 24 hours. In most instances, maximum effect is accomplished more gradually by administering 0.5 mg daily for 3 days, followed by the usual maintenance dosage. Digoxin is excreted principally by the kidneys and has a half-life ranging from 36 to 48 hours. The oral maintenance dose may range from 0.125 to 0.5 mg daily, depending on renal function, body size, age, thyroid function, and gastrointestinal absorption (ordinarily, approximately 60–70% of the oral dose is absorbed). Smaller doses are necessary in the presence of renal insufficiency. Unless the end point of therapy is control of the ventricular response in atrial fibrillation, it is worthwhile to measure serum digoxin levels after approximately 1 week of maintenance therapy; individual absorption rates and excretion rates may vary considerably. Digitoxin is less frequently used because of its long half-life (4–6 days), which will prolong the duration of toxicity if it occurs. Digitoxin is excreted by the liver, so blood levels may fluctuate less in patients with varying degrees of renal insufficiency.

A number of drugs have been found to affect digoxin pharmacology. Cholestyramine, some broad-spectrum oral antibiotics, antacids, and kaolin-pectin mixtures (eg, Kaopectate) may decrease absorption of digoxin. Quinidine, verapamil, amiodarone, and propafenone increase plasma levels of digoxin by reducing both the volume of distribution and the renal excretion of the agent. As noted previously, hypokalemia, hypercalcemia, and hypomagnesemia enhance the digitalis effect and potentiate its toxicity.

3. Digitalis toxicity–The therapeutic-to-toxic ratio of digitalis is quite narrow, and digitalis toxicity remains a potential problem. Its frequency has diminished as a result of improved understanding of its pharmacology, a trend toward employing lower dosages, and the availability of measurements of digoxin levels. Digoxin toxicity is uncommon with serum levels below 1.4 ng/mL and is present in approximately 50% of patients with levels above 3 ng/mL. Symptoms of digitalis toxicity include anorexia, nausea and vomiting, headache, visual symptoms (changes in color perception, halos, and scotomas), and disorientation. These symptoms may precede cardiotoxic effects.

Cardiac toxicity may take many forms, the most common being atrioventricular conduction disturbances, arrhythmias reflecting increased automaticity, and reentry arrhythmias. Arrhythmias due to digitalis toxicity include sinus node arrest, Mobitz type I second-degree atrioventricular block, ventricular premature beats or bigeminy, atrioventricular junctional tachycardia, paroxysmal supraventricular tachycardia with associated atrioventricular block, and ventricular tachycardia or fibrillation. When these arrhythmias are seen, digitalis toxicity should be suspected and the medication withheld. This, together with electrocardiographic monitoring, is adequate for many arrhythmias. Hypokalemia, if present, should be corrected, and any associated tachyarrhythmias may resolve after blood potassium levels increase to the high-normal range. Potassium administration may

exacerbate atrioventricular block, however. Ventricular tachycardia and very frequent ventricular premature beats should be treated with lidocaine or phenytoin. Class Ia and Ib agents are often less effective, and quinidine may exacerbate toxicity. Second-degree atrioventricular block usually does not require treatment, but complete heart block should be managed with atropine followed by temporary transvenous pacing. Electrical cardioversion for tachyarrhythmias should be avoided if possible, since digitalis toxicity may predispose to intractable ventricular fibrillation or cardiac standstill. If it cannot be avoided, patients should be pretreated with lidocaine (1 mg/kg) and low energy levels (10 J) should be employed initially.

Life-threatening episodes of digitalis toxicity or massive overdosages are characterized by severe hyperkalemia. They can be treated with digoxin-specific Fab antibody fragments. These are now commercially available and will rapidly reverse all manifestations of digitalis toxicity.

E. Vasodilators: Agents that dilate arteriolar smooth muscle and lower peripheral vascular resistance reduce left ventricular afterload. Medications that diminish venous tone and increase venous capacitance reduce the preload of both ventricles as their principal effect. Since, as noted earlier, most patients with moderate to severe heart failure have both elevated preload and reduced cardiac output, the maximum benefit of vasodilator therapy can be achieved by an agent or combination of agents with both actions. Many patients with heart failure have mitral or tricuspid regurgitation; agents that reduce resistance to left or right ventricular outflow tend to redirect regurgitant flow in a forward direction.

Several trials have indicated that vasodilator therapy with either the combination of hydralazine and nitrates or with angiotensin-converting enzyme inhibitors prolongs life in patients with moderate to severe heart failure. This evidence, plus many studies that show improvement in symptoms, has led to a wider use of these drugs.

The intravenous vasodilating drugs and their dosages have been discussed in the section on complications in acute myocardial infarction.

1. Nitrates–Sodium nitroprusside is a potent dilator of both the arteriolar resistance and venous capacitance vessels, and it consistently increases cardiac output and reduces ventricular filling pressures. It is only occasionally employed in the management of chronic heart failure, usually during episodes of acute decompensation. In such cases it may produce excessive hypotension, and it has been combined with dopamine or dobutamine to produce optimal hemodynamic improvement. Intravenous nitroglycerin is less useful in chronic heart failure, since it produces only a limited increase in cardiac output.

Long-term, nonparenteral vasodilator therapy has become a standard approach in patients with congestive heart failure. A number of medications with vasodilating activity have been studied in this setting. The longest experience has been with the various nitrate preparations. Isosorbide dinitrate, 20–80 mg orally every 6–8 hours, has proved effective in several small studies. Nitroglycerin ointment, 12.5–50 mg (1–4 in) every 6 hours, appears to be equally effective although somewhat inconvenient for long-term therapy. The optimal nitrate regimen probably consists of oral isosorbide dinitrate during the daytime and nitroglycerin applied overnight, since the latter has a longer duration of action. The nitrates are moderately effective in relieving shortness of breath, especially in patients with mild to moderate symptoms, but less successful—probably because they have little effect on cardiac output—in advanced heart failure. Nitrate therapy is generally well tolerated, but headaches and hypotension may limit the dose of all agents. The development of tolerance to chronic nitrate therapy is now generally acknowledged. This is minimized by intermittent therapy, especially if a daily 8- to 12-hour nitrate-free interval is employed, but probably develops to some extent in most patients receiving these agents. Transdermal nitroglycerin patches have no sustained effect in patients with heart failure and should not be employed for this indication.

2. Hydralazine—Oral hydralazine is a potent arteriolar dilator and markedly increases cardiac output in patients with congestive heart failure. However, as a single agent, it has not been shown to improve symptoms or exercise tolerance during chronic treatment. The combination of nitrates and oral hydralazine does appear to be effective, and this combination may improve survival in patients with mild to moderate symptoms.

Hydralazine therapy is frequently limited by side affects. Approximately 30% of patients are unable to tolerate the relatively high doses required to produce hemodynamic improvement in heart failure (200–400 mg daily in divided doses). The major side effect is gastrointestinal distress, but headaches, tachycardia, hypotension, and the drug-induced lupus syndrome are also relatively common.

3. Prazosin—Oral prazosin, a postsynaptic alpha-adrenergic blocking agent, was previously thought to be beneficial in patients with heart failure, but long-term benefits have not been demonstrated. The same can be said for the newer related agent terazosin.

4. Angiotensin-converting enzyme (ACE) inhibitors—The ACE inhibitors, of which 3 are now available in the USA (captopril, enalapril, and lisinopril), are the most effective vasodilators for congestive heart failure. These agents block the renin-angiotensin-aldosterone system, producing vasodilatation by blocking angiotensin II-induced vasoconstriction and decreasing sodium retention by reducing aldosterone secretion. They also inhibit the degradation of bradykinin, increase the production of vasodilating prostaglandins, and indirectly inhibit the adrenergic nervous system. Although the other vasodilators tend to stimulate the renin-angiotensin system and often lose part of their effect due to the resulting fluid retention, tolerance to the ACE inhibitors is uncommon.

Acute hemodynamic studies show that these agents reduce left ventricular filling pressure and right atrial pressure and moderately increase cardiac output. During long-term follow-up, these hemodynamic benefits are maintained or increased. ACE inhibitors lessen symptoms and increase exercise tolerance. They also correct the electrolyte abnormalities that characterize severe heart failure, such as hyponatremia and diuretic-induced hypokalemia, which may reduce the propensity to arrhythmias. Survival rates are improved by ACE inhibitor therapy in patients with severe heart failure and may be favorably altered in milder cases.

Because the ACE inhibitors may produce significant hypotension in some patients with congestive heart failure, particularly after the initial doses, they must be started with caution. Hypotension is most prominent in patients with hypovolemia, prerenal azotemia (especially if it is diuretic-induced), and hyponatremia (an indicator of activation of the renin-angiotensin system). Before therapy with the ACE inhibitors is started, other vasodilators should be discontinued and the dosages of diuretics should be reduced or the drugs withheld for 24 hours. Captopril is the preferred agent for beginning ACE inhibitor therapy because of its predictable onset and short duration of action (peak effect in 30–90 minutes). Treatment should be started with a low dose: either 12.5 mg or, in patients with hyponatremia or preexisting low blood pressure, 6.25 mg. The blood pressure should be monitored for the first 2 hours after dosing; if symptomatic or clinically significant hypotension does not occur, the patient may be sent home on a dosage of 12.5 mg 3 times daily. In patients with borderline blood pressure, renal function should be checked during the first week. The chronically effective dose of captopril appears to be 25 to 50 mg 3 times daily, although some patients will not tolerate this high a dose because of hypotension.

Enalapril and lisinopril are less convenient for initiating ACE inhibitor therapy in heart failure because their onset of action may be delayed beyond the time of convenient observation, and hypotension, if it occurs, may be prolonged. Because enalapril must be deesterified in the liver, which may be affected by passive congestion, its pharmacokinetics are less predictable in heart failure. However, maintenance therapy with enalapril or lisinopril in patients who do not develop hypotension has been very effective. The chronic dosage of enalapril ranges from 2.5 to 20 mg twice daily and that of lisinopril from 10 to 40 mg once daily.

The major limitation to ACE inhibitor therapy in heart failure is hypotension and renal insufficiency due to inadequate renal perfusion pressures. Other side effects such as skin rashes, taste alterations, cough, neutropenia, and proteinuria are less serious or very uncommon. The ACE inhibitors tend to increase serum potassium concentrations. Potassium-sparing agents should be withdrawn before ACE inhibitor therapy is started; and although potassium supplements may be required in individuals receiving diuretics and digitalis, their dosage should be decreased and subsequently adjusted as needed.

Vasodilator therapy was at one time reserved for patients not helped by digitalis and diuretics, but ACE inhibitors have been studied as adjuncts to diuretics and are at least as effective as digoxin. Many experts now consider them a second line of therapy after diuretics because of their potential to increase longevity. Studies are under way to determine whether vasodilator therapy, particularly with the ACE inhibitors, is indicated in patients with mild symptoms or those with asymptomatic left ventricular dysfunction.

F. Newer Positive Inotropic Agents: The digitalis derivatives are the only available oral inotropic agents at this time in the USA. However, a number of drugs that increase myocardial contractility in experimental preparations are under investigation. These include beta-adrenergic agonists, dopaminergic agents, and a group of nondigitalis, noncatecholamine agents that increase myocardial contractility by inhibiting myocardial phosphodiesterase. One of the latter class, amrinone, has been approved for intravenous use, but the value and safety of the newer positive inotropic agents for chronic treatment are in doubt.

G. Beta-Blocker Therapy: A number of investigators have suggested that beta-blockers in very low dosages may produce symptomatic improvement in patients with chronic congestive heart failure. This approach runs counter to the usual practice of avoiding beta-blockers in heart failure but has been justified by the potentially harmful effects of circulatory catecholamines and because it offers a means of reversing the "down-regulation" of myocardial beta receptors. Metoprolol has been the most studied, but agents with partial agonist effects may be equally or more effective. Obviously, this approach carries the risk of worsening heart failure; however, in patients with dilated cardiomyopathy of nonischemic origin with persistent tachycardia (> 100 beats/min), some data suggest a beneficial effect. These agents must be started at extremely low dosages (2.5 mg of metoprolol daily). The efficiency and safety of beta-blockers are now under investigation in multicenter trials.

H. Anticoagulation: Patients with severe left ventricular failure are prone to development of systemic arterial emboli, particularly when they are in atrial fibrillation. While these may be catastrophic, the routine use of anticoagulants is controversial, since these patients have short life expectancies and are taking multiple medications that may interfere with optimal regulation of anticoagulation. Most experts prescribe anticoagulants only to appropriate patients who have had embolic episodes and those with atrial fibrillation. Some also anticoagulate patients with dilated cardiomyopathy in normal sinus rhythm.

I. Antiarrhythmic Therapy: Patients with moderate to severe heart failure have a high incidence of both symptomatic and asymptomatic arrhythmias. Although fewer than 10% of patients have syncope or presyncope resulting from ventricular tachycardia, ambulatory monitoring reveals that up to 70% of patients have asymptomatic episodes of nonsustained ventricular tachycardia. These arrhythmias indicate a poor prognosis independent of the severity of left ventricular dysfunction, but many of the deaths are probably not arrhythmia-related, and there is no evidence that antiarrhythmic therapy improves prognosis in asymptomatic patients.

Patients with symptomatic ventricular arrhythmias should be treated vigorously as outlined elsewhere in this chapter. Whether patients with asymptomatic nonsustained ventricular tachycardia warrant therapy remains controversial, largely because such treatment is not without risk. Most effective antiarrhythmic agents may depress left ventricular function or may themselves worsen the arrhythmia. While most experts do not initiate treatment for frequent ventricular premature beats, they will attempt to suppress frequent episodes of nonsustained ventricular tachycardia. The first approach is usually with a class Ia agent (procainamide or quinidine; disopyramide should be avoided because of its negative inotropic effect). The class Ib agents (mexiletine, tocainide) have proved less effective; the class Ic drugs (encainide, flecainide, propafenone) may be effective but are more likely to depress left ventricular function and worsen the arrhythmia. Amiodarone is perhaps the most active agent, but because of its toxicity it should probably be reserved for symptomatic individuals.

Prognosis

Despite advances in treatment of patients with congestive heart failure, their prognosis remains poor, with annual mortality rates ranging from 10% in stable patients with mild symptoms to over 50% in patients with advanced, progressive symptoms. Poorer prognosis is associated with severe left ventricular dysfunction (ejection fractions < 20%), severe symptoms and limitation of exercise capacity (maximal oxygen consumption < 10 mL/kg/min), and secondary renal insufficiency, hyponatremia, and elevated plasma catecholamine levels. About 40–50% of patients with heart failure die suddenly, presumably due to ventricular arrhythmias. Nonsustained ventricular tachycardia is a poor prognostic sign, but its prevalence is so high that it cannot be used to predict which individuals are at risk of sudden death.

Bigger JT Jr: Why patients with congestive heart failure die: Arrhythmias and sudden cardiac death. Circulation

1987;75 (Suppl):IV28. (Electrophysiologically oriented review.)

Captopril-Digoxin Multicenter Research Group: Comparative effects of therapy with captopril and digoxin in patients with mild to moderate heart failure. JAMA 1988;259:539. (Improved symptoms, less deterioration than placebo, indicating diuretics alone are not optimal therapy.)

Cleland JG et al: Clinical, haemodynamic, and antiarrhythmic effects of long-term treatment with amiodarone of patients in heart failure. Br Heart J 1987;57:436. (Favorable trends with amiodarone.)

Cohn JN: Current therapy of the failing heart. Circulation 1988;78:1099. (General review with emphasis on vasodilators.)

Colucci WS, Wright RF, Braunwald E: New positive inotropic agents in the treatment of congestive heart failure: Mechanisms of action and recent clinical developments. (2 parts.) N Engl J Med 1986;314:290, 349.

Consensus Trial Study Group: Effects of enalapril on mortality in severe congestive heart failure: Results of the Cooperative North Scandinavian Enalapril Survival Study (CONSENSUS). N Engl J Med 1987;316:1429. (Improved survival with treatment.)

DiBianco R et al: A comparison of oral milrinone, digoxin, and their combination in the treatment of patients with chronic heart failure. N Engl J Med 1989;320:627. (Important study raising doubt about new inotropes but demonstrating digoxin efficacy.)

Geltman EM: Mild heart failure: Diagnosis and treatment. Am Heart J 1989;118:1278. (When and how to treat left ventricular dysfunction.)

Harizi RC, Bianco JA, Alpert JS: Diastolic function of the heart in clinical cardiology. Arch Intern Med 1988;148:99.

Kulick D et al: Resistance to isosorbide dinitrate in patients with severe chronic heart failure: Incidence and attempt at hemodynamic prediction. J Am Coll Cardiol 1988; 12:1023.

Kiyingi A et al: Metolazone in treatment of severe refractory congestive cardiac failure. Lancet 1990;335:29. (Extremely effective.)

Lant A: Diuretics: Clinical pharmacology and therapeutic use. (2 parts.) Drugs 1985;29:57, 620.

Little WC, Downes TR: Clinical evaluation of left ventricular diastolic performance. Prog Cardiovasc Dis 1990; 32:273. (How to determine when symptoms are due to diastolic dysfunction.)

Massie BM: Exercise tolerance in congestive heart failure: Role of cardiac function, peripheral blood flow and muscle metabolism and effect of treatment. Am J Med 1988;84 (Suppl 3A):75. (Pathophysiology of exercise limitation. Is it the heart or the periphery?)

Massie BM: New trends in the use of angiotensin converting enzyme inhibitors in chronic heart failure. Am J Med 1988;84(Suppl 4A):36.

Massie BM, Conway M: Survival of patients with congestive heart failure: Past, present, and future prospects. Circulation 1987;75(Suppl):IV-11.

Mulrow CD et al: Relative efficacy of vasodilator therapy in chronic congestive heart failure: Implications of randomized trials. JAMA 1988;259:3422.

Packer M: Neurohormonal interactions and adaptations in congestive heart failure. Circulation 1988;77:721.

Packer M: Therapeutic options in the management of chronic

heart failure: Is there a drug of first choice? Circulation 1989;79:198.

Parmley WW: Pathophysiology and current therapy of congestive heart failure. J Am Coll Cardiol 1989;13:771.

Pfeffer MA et al: Effect of captopril on progressive ventricular dilatation after anterior myocardial infarction. N Engl J Med 1988;319:80. (ACE inhibitor prevents ventricular enlargement. Would this approach be useful to delay progression of CHF?)

Smith TW: Digitalis: Mechanisms of action and clinical use. N Engl J Med 1988;318:358.

Stevenson LW, Perloff JK: The limited reliability of physical signs for estimating hemodynamics in chronic heart failure. JAMA 1989;261:884. (Left ventricular filling pressure cannot be estimated by examination.)

Wilson JR: Use of antiarrhythmic drugs in patients with heart failure: Clinical efficacy, hemodynamic results and relation to survival. Circulation 1987;75(Suppl):IV64. (Excellent review from a nonelectrophysiologic viewpoint.)

Woosley RL, Echt DS, Roden DM: Effects of congestive heart failure on the pharmacokinetics and pharmacodynamics of antiarrhythmic agents. Am J Cardiol 1986; 57:25B. (Problems can occur in using these agents.)

Cardiac Transplantation

Because of the poor prognosis in patients with advanced heart failure, cardiac transplantation is now performed in many centers throughout the world. Since the advent of cyclosporine immunosuppressive therapy and more careful screening of donor hearts, the survival of patients after cardiac transplantation has increased considerably. Many centers now have 1-year survival rates exceeding 80–90%, and 5-year survival rates are likely to exceed 70% in the future. Infections, hypertension and renal dysfunction caused by cyclosporine, rapidly progressive coronary atherosclerosis, and immunosuppressant-related cancers have been the major complications. Clearly, cardiac transplantation is effective in selected individuals, but the high cost and limited number of donor organs require careful patient selection. Patients who are candidates for transplantation should be assessed early in their course, since the incidence of sudden death is high once they exhibit advanced symptoms.

Copeland JG et al: Selection of patients for cardiac transplantation. Circulation 1987;75:2. (How to deal with this difficult problem.)

Schroeder JS, Hunt S: Cardiac transplantation: Update 1987. JAMA 1987;258:3142.

ACUTE PULMONARY EDEMA

Essentials of Diagnosis

- Acute onset or worsening of dyspnea at rest.
- Tachycardia, diaphoresis, cyanosis.
- Pulmonary rales, rhonchi; expiratory wheezing.
- X-ray shows interstitial and alveolar edema with or without cardiomegaly.
- Arterial hypoxemia.

General Considerations

The most common causes of cardiogenic pulmonary edema are acute myocardial infarction, acute volume overload of the left ventricle (valvular regurgitation or ventricular septal defect), and mitral stenosis.

Clinical Findings

Acute pulmonary edema presents with a characteristic clinical picture of severe dyspnea, the production of pink, frothy sputum, and diaphoresis and cyanosis. Examination of the lungs reveals rales in all lung fields or generalized wheezing and rhonchi. Pulmonary edema may appear suddenly in the setting of chronic heart failure or may be the first manifestation of cardiac disease, usually acute myocardial infarction, which may be painful or silent.

While most cases of pulmonary edema are due to left ventricular failure or mitral valve disease, a number of noncardiac conditions can also produce pulmonary edema. This occurs either because of imbalance in the Starling forces (such as can occur from a decrease in plasma proteins or an increase in pulmonary venous pressure) or a functional or anatomic abnormality of the alveolar-capillary membrane. Causes of noncardiogenic pulmonary edema include intravenous narcotics, increased intracerebral pressure, high altitude, sepsis, several medications, inhaled toxins, transfusion reactions, shock, and disseminated intravascular coagulation. These are usually distinguished from cardiogenic pulmonary edema by the clinical setting, the history, and the physical examination. Conversely, in most patients with cardiogenic pulmonary edema, an underlying cardiac abnormality can usually be detected clinically or by the ECG, chest x-ray, or echocardiogram.

The chest radiograph reveals signs of pulmonary vascular redistribution, blurriness of vascular outlines, increased interstitial markings, and, characteristically, the butterfly pattern of alveolar edema. The heart may be enlarged or normal in size depending on whether heart failure was previously present. An acute assessment of cardiac function by echocardiography or right heart catheterization is helpful in determining the cause. In cardiogenic pulmonary edema, the pulmonary capillary wedge pressure is universally elevated, usually over 25 mm Hg. Cardiac output may be normal or depressed. In noncardiogenic pulmonary edema, as in the acute respiratory distress syndrome, or severe pulmonary disease masquerading as pulmonary edema. the wedge pressure may be normal or even low.

Treatment

The patient should be placed in a sitting position with legs dangling over the side of the bed; this facilitates respiration and reduces venous return. Oxygen should be delivered by mask to obtain an arterial Po_2 greater than 60 mm Hg. If respiratory distress is severe, endotracheal intubation and mechanical ventilation may be necessary.

Morphine sulfate is highly effective in pulmonary edema. The initial dosage should be 4–8 mg intravenously (subcutaneous administration is effective in milder cases), and this may be repeated after 2–4 hours. Morphine increases venous capacitance, lowering left atrial pressure, and relieves anxiety, which can reduce the efficiency of ventilation. However, morphine may lead to CO_2 retention and reduce the ventilatory drive. Morphine should be avoided in patients with narcotic-induced pulmonary edema, who may improve with narcotic antagonists, and in those with neurogenic pulmonary edema.

Intravenous diuretic therapy (furosemide, 40 mg, or bumetanide, 1 mg—or higher doses if the patient has been receiving chronic diuretic therapy) is usually indicated even if the patient has not exhibited prior fluid retention. These agents produce immediate venodilation even prior to the onset of diuresis. Other approaches to therapy include further measures to reduce left ventricular preload. This may be accomplished by the administration of sublingual or intravenous nitrates and, in otherwise refractory cases, phlebotomy of approximately 500 mL of blood or plasmapheresis. Intravenous aminophylline may relieve the associated bronchospasm. The usual dose is 5 mg/kg intravenously over approximately 10 minutes, followed by a constant infusion of 0.1–0.6 mg/kg/h, with the appropriate rate being lower in older patients and those with severe heart failure. Aminophylline may exacerbate tachycardia or tachyarrhythmias, however. Particularly in patients with elevated arterial pressures, vasodilators such as intravenous nitroprusside may be worthwhile. In patients with low-output states, particularly when hypotension is present, positive inotropic agents are indicated. These approaches to treatment have been discussed previously.

Bernard GR, Brigham RL: Pulmonary edema: Pathophysiologic mechanisms and new approaches to therapy. Chest 1986;89:594. (Good review of pathophysiology and treatment.)

Braun S, Massie BM: Pulmonary edema. Page 398 in: *Current Therapy in Emergency Medicine*. Callaham ML (editor). BC Decker, 1987.

MYOCARDITIS & THE CARDIOMYOPATHIES

ACUTE MYOCARDITIS

Acute myocarditis is focal or diffuse inflammation of the myocardium. Most cases are infectious, caused by viral, bacterial, rickettsial, spirochetal, fungal, or parasitic agents; but toxins, drugs, and immunologic reaction can also cause myocarditis.

1. INFECTIOUS MYOCARDITIS

Essentials of Diagnosis

- Often follows respiratory infection.
- May present with chest pain (pleuritic or nonspecific), signs of heart failure, or arrhythmias.
- ECG may show sinus tachycardia, nonspecific repolarization changes, intraventricular conduction abnormalities.
- Echocardiogram documents cardiomegaly and contractile dysfunction.
- Myocardial biopsy may reveal a characteristic inflammatory pattern.

General Considerations

Viral myocarditis is the most common form and is usually caused by coxsackieviruses, but a host of other agents have also been responsible. Rickettsial myocarditis occurs with scrub typhus, Rocky Mountain spotted fever, and Q fever. Diphtheritic myocarditis is caused by the toxin and often is manifested by conduction abnormalities as well as heart failure.

A prevalent form of infectious myocarditis is that due to trypanosomiasis (Chagas' disease), an insect-borne protozoan infection caused by *Trypanosoma cruzi*. An acute inflammatory process may occur, but the major clinical manifestations appear after a latent period of more than a decade. At this stage, patients present with cardiomyopathy, congestive heart failure, conduction disturbances, and sudden death. Associated gastrointestinal involvement (megaesophagus and megacolon) is the rule. Toxoplasmosis causes myocarditis that is usually asymptomatic but can lead to heart failure. Among parasitic infections, trichinosis is the most common cause of cardiac involvement. The potential for the HIV virus to cause myocarditis is now well recognized, though the prevalence of this complication is not known, and it is an uncommon cause of morbidity and mortality in AIDS. In addition, other infectious myocarditides are more common in patients with AIDS.

Clinical Findings

A. Symptoms and Signs: Patients may present several days to a few weeks after the onset of acute febrile illness or a respiratory infection or with heart failure without antecedent symptoms. Pleural-pericardial chest pain is common. Nonspecific systemic symptoms are often present. Examination often reveals tachycardia, gallop rhythm, and other evidence of heart failure or conduction defect.

B. ECG and Chest X-Ray: Nonspecific ST–T changes and conduction disturbances are common. Ventricular ectopy may be the initial and only clinical finding. Chest x-ray is nonspecific.

C. Diagnostic Studies: Echocardiography provides the most convenient way of evaluating cardiac function and can exclude many other processes. Gallium-67 scintigraphy has been reported to yield cardiac uptake in acute or subacute myocarditis. Paired serum viral titers and serologic tests for other agents may indicate the cause.

D. Endomyocardial Biopsy: Pathologic examinations may reveal a round cell inflammatory reaction and patchy necrosis. This picture defines an "active" inflammatory stage and may persist for many months.

Treatment & Prognosis

Specific antimicrobial therapy is indicated if an infecting agent can be identified. Uncontrolled observations have suggested that immunosuppressive therapy with corticosteroids and other agents may improve the outcome when the process is acute (< 6 months) and the biopsy suggests acute inflammation. The value of routine myocardial biopsies in patients presenting with an acute myocarditic picture has not been established. However, empiric immunosuppressive therapy without histologic confirmation is probably unwarranted. Otherwise, treatment is directed toward the manifestations of heart failure and arrhythmias.

Many cases resolve spontaneously, but in others cardiac function deteriorates progressively and may evolve into dilated cardiomyopathy.

Acierro LJ: Cardiac complications in acquired immunodeficiency syndrome (AIDS): A review. J Am Coll Cardiol 1989;13:1144.

Acquatella H et al: Long-term control of Chagas disease in Venezuela: Effects on serologic findings, electrocardiographic abnormalities, and clinical outcome. Circulation 1987;76:556. (Current review of a common worldwide problem.)

Dec GW Jr et al: Active myocarditis in the spectrum of acute dilated cardiomyopathies: Clinical features, histologic correlates, and clinical outcome. N Engl J Med 1985;312:885. (Discusses the potential evolution from myocarditis to cardiomyopathy.)

Reyes MP, Lerner AM: Coxsackievirus myocarditis: With special reference to acute and chronic effects. Prog Cardiovasc Dis 1985;27:373.

2. DRUG-INDUCED & TOXIC MYOCARDITIS & MYOCARDIAL DYSFUNCTION

A variety of medications, illicit drugs, and toxic substances can produce acute inflammatory myocardial reactions or more chronic damage. The clinical presentation may vary widely, so this brief section will serve only to alert the physician to potential causative agents. Doxorubicin and other cytotoxic agents used for treatment of neoplasm, emetine (an antiparasitic agent for amebiasis), and catecholamines (especially with pheochromocytoma) can produce a pathologic picture of inflammation and necrosis together with clinical heart failure and arrhythmias;

toxicity of the first 2 is dose-related. The phenothiazines, lithium, chloroquine, disopyramide, antimony-containing compounds, and arsenicals can also cause electrocardiographic changes, arrhythmias, or heart failure. Hypersensitivity reactions to sulfonamides, penicillins, and aminosalicylic acid as well as other drugs can result in cardiac dysfunction. Radiation can cause an acute inflammatory reaction as well as a chronic fibrosis, usually in conjunction with pericarditis.

The incidence of cocaine cardiotoxicity has increased markedly. Cocaine can cause coronary artery spasm, myocardial infarction, arrhythmias, and myocarditis. Because many of these processes are believed to be mediated by cocaine's inhibitory effect on norepinephrine reuptake by sympathetic nerves, betablockers have been used therapeutically. In coronary spasm, calcium channel blockers are more appropriate.

Cregler LL, Mark H: Cardiovascular dangers of cocaine abuse. Am J Cardiol 1986;57:1185. (The spectrum of complications.)

Kantrowitz NE, Bristow MR: Cardiotoxicity of antitumor agents. Prog Cardiovasc Dis 1984;27:195. (A major limitation on treatment with some agents.)

THE CARDIOMYOPATHIES

The cardiomyopathies are a heterogeneous group of entities affecting the myocardium primarily and not associated with the major causes of cardiac disease, ie, ischemic heart disease, hypertension, valvular disease, or congenital defects. While some have specific causes, many cases are idiopathic. There is now general agreement on a classification of the cardiomyopathies into 3 categories based upon general features of their presentation and pathophysiology. Table 8–9 outlines this classification. Some patients have overlapping features, but this classification is of use in planning diagnostic evaluation and therapy.

Role of Myocardial Biopsy

The use of myocardial biopsy to make specific diagnoses in patients with cardiomyopathies is increasing. The indications for the procedure remain controversial, but it is essential for the early detection of transplant rejection. Biopsies have also been helpful in distinguishing restrictive cardiomyopathy from pericardial constriction, an often difficult problem. Occasionally, a specific diagnosis of amyloidosis, sarcoidosis, hemochromatosis, or an unusual infection can be made, but in most cases these conditions are suggested by other cardiac or systemic findings. Biopsies can reveal evidence of acute myocarditis and, if immunosuppressive therapy is contemplated, should be performed in appropriate patients.

Chow LC, Dittrich HC, Shabetai R: Endomyocardial biopsy in patients with unexplained congestive heart failure. Ann Intern Med 1988;109:535. (Low incidence of myocarditis and other diagnostic findings in a large series.)

Mason JW, O'Connell JB: Clinical merit of endomyocardial biopsy. Circulation 1989;79:971.

Table 8–9. Classification of the cardiomyopathies.

	Dilated	Hypertrophic	Restrictive
Frequent causes	Idiopathic, alcoholic, myocarditis, postpartum, doxorubicin, endocrinopathies, genetic diseases	Hereditary syndrome, possibly chronic hypertension	Amyloidosis, postradiation, post-open heart surgery, diabetes, endomyocardial fibrosis
Symptoms	Left or biventricular CHF	Dyspnea, chest pain, syncope	Dyspnea, fatigue, right-sided CHF
Physical examination	Cardiomegaly, S_3, elevated JVP, rales	Sustained PMI, S_4, variable systolic murmur, bisferiens carotid pulse	Elevated JVP, Kussmaul's sign
ECG	ST-T changes, conduction abnormalities, ventricular ectopy	LVH, exaggerated septal Q waves	ST-T changes, conduction abnormalities, low voltage
Chest x-ray	Enlarged heart, pulmonary congestion	Mild cardiomegaly	Mild to moderate cardiomegaly
Echocardiogram, nuclear studies	LV dilatation and dysfunction	LVH, asymmetric septal hypertrophy, small LV size, normal or supranormal function, systolic anterior mitral motion, diastolic dysfunction	Small or normal LV size, normal or mildly reduced LV function
Cardiac catheterization	LV dilatation and dysfunction, high diastolic pressures, low cardiac output	Small, hypercontractile LV, dynamic outflow gradient, diastolic dysfunction	High diastolic pressures, "square root" sign, normal or mildly reduced LV function

1. DILATED CARDIOMYOPATHY

Essentials of Diagnosis

- Symptoms and signs of heart failure.
- ECG may show low QRS voltage, nonspecific repolarization abnormalities, intraventricular conduction abnormalities.
- X-ray shows cardiomegaly.
- Echocardiogram usually indicated and confirms left ventricular dilatation, thinning, and dysfunction.

General Considerations

Dilated cardiomyopathies usually present with symptoms and signs of congestive heart failure (most commonly dyspnea). Left ventricular dilatation and systolic dysfunction are essential for diagnosis. Often no cause can be identified, but chronic alcohol abuse and myocarditis are probably frequent causes. Indeed, many believe that idiopathic dilated cardiomyopathy often represents the end stage of myocarditis. Histologically, the picture is one of extensive fibrosis.

Clinical Findings

A. Symptoms and Signs: In most patients, symptoms of heart failure develop gradually. They may be recognized because of asymptomatic cardiomegaly, electrocardiographic abnormalities, or ventricular ectopy. The initial presentation may be severe biventricular failure. The physical examination reveals cardiomegaly, S_3 gallop rhythm, and often a murmur of functional mitral regurgitation. Signs of left–and right-sided failure may be present on initial examination.

B. ECG and Chest X-Ray: The major findings are included in Table 8–9.

C. Diagnostic Studies: Laboratory tests should be performed to exclude treatable causes of cardiomyopathy. The role of myocardial biopsy has been discussed. An echocardiogram is indicated to exclude unsuspected valvular or other lesions and confirm the presence of dilated cardiomyopathy. Exercise thallium-201 scintigraphy may suggest the possibility of underlying coronary disease if a large reversible defect is found, but false-positives occur in cardiomyopathy. Cardiac catheterization is seldom of specific value unless myocardial ischemia or left ventricular aneurysm is suspected.

Treatment

Few cases of cardiomyopathy are amenable to specific therapy. Alcohol use should be discontinued. There is often marked recovery of cardiac function following a period of abstinence in alcoholic cardiomyopathy. Endocrine causes (thyroid dysfunction, acromegaly, pheochromocytoma) should be treated. Immunosuppressive therapy is not indicated in chronic dilated cardiomyopathy. The management of con-gestive heart failure is outlined in the section on heart failure.

Prognosis

The prognosis of dilated cardiomyopathy without clinical heart failure is variable, with some patients remaining stable, some deteriorating gradually, and others declining rapidly. Once heart failure is manifest, the natural history is similar to that of other causes of heart failure. Arterial and pulmonary emboli are more common in dilated cardiomyopathy than in ischemic cardiomyopathy; suitable candidates may benefit from chronic anticoagulation.

Abelmann WH, Lorell BH: The challenge of cardiomyopathy. J Am Coll Cardiol 1989;13:1219.

Johnson RA, Palacios I: Dilated cardiomyopathies of the adult. (2 parts.) N Engl J Med 1982;307:1051, 1119. (Still current review.)

Keren A et al: Mildly dilated congestive cardiomyopathy. Circulation 1985;72:302. (Outcome of patients diagnosed before onset of CHF.)

Regan TJ: Alcoholic cardiomyopathy. Prog Cardiovasc Dis 1984;27:141. (Pathophysiology and clinical course.)

Urbano-Marquez A et al: The effects of alcoholism on skeletal and cardiac muscle. N Engl J Med 1989;320:409. (Mechanism of alcohol toxicity.)

Wiener RS, Lockhart JT, Schwartz RG: Dilated cardiomyopathy and cocaine abuse: Report of two cases. Am J Med 1986;81:699. (Perhaps this occurs more frequently than is realized.)

Zarich SW, Nesto RW: Diabetic cardiomyopathy. Am Heart J 1989;118:1000.

2. HYPERTROPHIC CARDIOMYOPATHY

Essentials of Diagnosis

- May present with dyspnea, chest pain, syncope.
- Examination shows sustained apical impulse, S_4, systolic ejection murmur.
- ECG shows left ventricular hypertrophy.
- Echocardiogram shows hypertrophy, which may be asymmetric; usually shows normal or enhanced contractility and signs of dynamic obstruction.

General Considerations

In hypertrophic cardiomyopathy, there is inappropriate—ie, unrelated to any pressure or volume overload—myocardial hypertrophy that tends to impinge upon the left ventricular cavity. Characteristically, the interventricular septum is disproportionately involved (asymmetric septal hypertrophy), but in some cases the hypertrophy is localized to the apex. The left ventricular outflow tract is often narrowed during systole between the bulging septum and an anteriorly displaced anterior mitral valve leaflet, causing a dynamic obstruction (hence the name idiopathic hypertrophic subaortic stenosis; IHSS). The obstruction is worsened by factors that increase myocardial contractility (sympathetic stimulation, digoxin, postextrasystolic beat) or that decrease left ventricular filling (Valsalva's maneuver, peripheral vasodilators).

Hypertrophic cardiomyopathy is in some cases inherited as an autosomal dominant trait with variable penetrance. These patients usually present in early adulthood. Others are elderly, and many of those patients have a long history of hypertension. Some cases occur sporadically.

Except in late stages, hypertrophic cardiomyopathy is characterized by a small, hypercontractile left ventricle. Although dyspnea is a common symptom, it results primarily from markedly impaired diastolic compliance rather than systolic dysfunction or outflow obstruction.

Clinical Findings

A. Symptoms and Signs: The most frequent symptoms are dyspnea and chest pain. Syncope is also common and is typically postexertional, when diastolic filling diminishes while outflow obstruction remains increased. Arrhythmias are an important problem. Atrial fibrillation is a long-term consequence of chronically elevated left atrial pressures and is a poor prognostic sign. Ventricular arrhythmias are also common, and sudden death may occur, often in athletes after extraordinary exertion.

Features on physical examination are a bisferiens carotid pulse, triple apical impulse (due to the prominent atrial filling wave and early and late systolic impulses), and a loud S_4. In cases with outflow obstruction, a loud systolic murmur is present that increases with upright posture or Valsalva's maneuver and decreases with squatting.

B. ECG and Chest X-Ray: Left ventricular hypertrophy is nearly universal. Exaggerated septal Q waves inferolaterally may suggest myocardial infarction. The chest x-ray is often unimpressive.

C. Diagnostic Studies: The echocardiogram is diagnostic, revealing asymmetric left ventricular hypertrophy, systolic anterior motion of the mitral valve, early closing followed by reopening of the aortic valve, a small and hypercontractile left ventricle, and delayed relaxation and filling of the left ventricle during diastole. Doppler ultrasound reveals turbulent flow and a dynamic gradient across the aortic valve and, commonly, mitral regurgitation. Cardiac catheterization may confirm the gradient but adds little to echocardiographic studies.

Treatment

Beta-blockers should be the initial drug in symptomatic individuals, especially when dynamic outflow obstruction is noted on the echocardiogram. Dyspnea, angina, and arrhythmias respond in about 50% of patients. Calcium channel blockers, especially verapamil, have also been effective in symptomatic patients. Their effect may be due primarily to improved diastolic function, but their vasodilating actions may also increase outflow obstruction. Excision of part of the myocardial septum has been successful in patients with severe symptoms when performed by surgeons experienced with the procedure. Antiarrhythmic agents may be valuable because of the frequency of ventricular arrhythmias and their possible relation to sudden death.

Prognosis

The natural history of hypertrophic cardiomyopathy is highly variable. Some patients remain asymptomatic for many years or for life. Sudden death, especially during exercise, may be the initial event. Indeed, hypertrophic cardiomyopathy is the pathologic feature most frequently associated with sudden death in athletes. Other patients have a history of gradually progressive symptoms. A final stage may be a transition into dilated cardiomyopathy. Amiodarone, in particular, has been advocated in these patients.

Lewis JF, Maron BJ: Elderly patients with hypertrophic cardiomyopathy: A subset with distinctive left ventricular morphology and progressive clinical course late in life. J Am Coll Cardiol 1989;13:36.

Maron BJ et al: Hypertrophic cardiomyopathy: Interrelations of clinical manifestations, pathophysiology, and therapy, (2 parts.) N Engl J Med 1987;316:780, 844.

McIntosh CL, Maron BJ: Current operative treatment of obstructive hypertrophic cardiomyopathy. Circulation 1988;78:487. (Technique and results, which are excellent in selected patients.)

Wigle ED: Hypertrophic cardiomyopathy: A 1987 viewpoint. (Editorial.) Circulation 1987;75:311.

3. RESTRICTIVE CARDIOMYOPATHY

Restrictive cardiomyopathy is characterized by impaired diastolic filling with preserved contractile function. This condition is relatively uncommon, with the most frequent causes being amyloidosis, radiation, and myocardial fibrosis after open heart surgery. In Africa, endomyocardial fibrosis, a specific entity in which there is severe fibrosis of the endocardium, often with eosinophilia (Loffler's syndrome) is common. Other causes of a restrictive picture are infiltrative cardiomyopathies (eg, sarcoidosis, hemochromatosis) and connective tissue diseases (eg, scleroderma).

Amyloidosis can affect the heart in several ways. Although it is a frequent cause of restrictive cardiomyopathy, it more frequently produces dilated cardiomyopathy with congestive heart failure. Almost invariably, conduction disturbances are present. Rectal, abdominal fat, or gingival biopsies—as well as myocardial biopsy—can be diagnostic.

The primary diagnostic problem with restrictive cardiomyopathy is differentiation from constrictive pericarditis. The clinical picture often strongly suggests the diagnosis, but the status of left ventricular function (usually normal with pericarditis, slightly depressed with restrictive cardiomyopathy) can be helpful, as can be evidence of a thickened pericardium. Myocardial biopsies are usually negative with pericarditis but not in restrictive cardiomyopathy. In some cases, only surgical exploration can make the diagnosis.

Unfortunately, little useful therapy is available for either the causative conditions or the syndrome itself. Diuretics can help, but excessive diuresis can produce worsening symptoms.

Benotti JR, Grossman W: Restrictive cardiomyopathy. Annu Rev Med 1984;35:113. (Pathophysiology, etiology, and diagnosis.)

Sleisenger MH, Havlir D, Tierney LM Jr: Biochemical and clinical aspects of amyloidosis. West J Med 1987; 147:65.

DISEASES OF THE PERICARDIUM

ACUTE PERICARDITIS

The pericardium consists of 2 layers: the inner visceral layer, which is attached to the epicardium; and an outer parietal layer. The pericardium stabilizes the heart in anatomic position and reduces contact between the heart and surrounding structures. It is composed of fibrous tissue, and while it is loose enough to permit moderate changes in cardiac size, it cannot stretch rapidly enough to accommodate rapid dilatation of the heart or accumulation of fluid without increasing intrapericardial (and, therefore, intracardiac) pressure.

The pericardium is often involved by processes that affect the heart, but it may also be affected by diseases of adjacent tissues and may itself be a primary site of disease.

INFLAMMATORY PERICARDITIS

Acute inflammation of the pericardium may be infectious in origin or may be due to systemic diseases (autoimmune syndromes, uremia), neoplastic invasion, radiation effects, drug toxicity, leakage of blood into the pericardial space, or extension of inflammatory processes from the myocardium or lung. In many of these conditions, the pathologic process involves both the pericardium and the myocardium, and they often are associated with varying degrees of cardiac dysfunction.

The presentation and course of inflammatory pericarditis depend on its cause, but all syndromes are often (not always) associated with chest pain, which is usually pleuritic and postural (relieved by sitting).

The pain is substernal but may radiate to the neck, shoulders, back, or epigastrium. Dyspnea may also be present. A pericardial friction rub is characteristic, with or without evidence of fluid accumulation or constriction (see below). Fever and leukocytosis are often present. The ECG usually shows ST and T wave changes and may manifest a characteristic progression beginning with generalized ST elevation, followed by a return to baseline and then to T wave inversion. The chest x-ray may show cardiac enlargement if fluid has collected, as well as signs of related pulmonary disease. The echocardiogram may disclose pericardial effusions and indicate their hemodynamic significance, but it is often normal in inflammatory pericarditis.

Several of the specific pericarditis syndromes are discussed below.

Viral Pericarditis

Viral infections (especially infections with coxsackieviruses and echoviruses but also influenza, Epstein-Barr, varicella, hepatitis, mumps, and HIV viruses) are the commonest cause of acute pericarditis and probably are responsible for many cases classified as idiopathic. Males—usually under age 50—are most commonly affected. Pericardial involvement often follows upper respiratory infection. The diagnosis is usually clinical, but rising viral titers in paired sera may be obtained for confirmation. Cardiac enzymes may be slightly elevated, reflecting a myocarditic component. The differential diagnosis is primarily with myocardial infarction.

Treatment is generally symptomatic. Aspirin (650 mg every 3–4 hours) or other nonsteroidal agents (eg, indomethacin, 100–150 mg daily in divided doses) are usually effective. Corticosteroids may be beneficial in unresponsive cases. In general, symptoms subside in several days to weeks. The major early complication is tamponade, which occurs in fewer than 5% of patients. There may be recurrences in the first few weeks or months. Rare patients will continue to experience recurrences chronically, sometimes leading to constrictive pericarditis. Pericardial resection may be required.

Tuberculous Pericarditis

Tuberculous pericarditis has become rare in developed countries but remains common in other areas. It results from direct lymphatic or hematogenous spread; clinical pulmonary involvement may be absent or minor, although associated pleural effusions are common. The presentation tends to be subacute, but nonspecific symptoms (fever, night sweats, fatigue) may be present for days to months. Pericardial effusions are usually small or moderate but may be large. The diagnosis can be inferred if evidence of acid-fast bacilli are found elsewhere. The yield of organisms by pericardiocentesis is low; pericardial biopsy has a higher yield but may also be negative, and pericardiectomy may be required. Standard antituberculous drug therapy is usually successful, but constrictive pericarditis can occur.

Other Infectious Pericarditides

Bacterial pericarditis has become rare and usually results from direct extension from pulmonary infections. Signs and symptoms are similar to those of other types of inflammatory pericarditides, but patients appear toxic—often critically ill.

Uremic Pericarditis

This syndrome is a common complication of renal failure whose pathogenesis is uncertain; it occurs both with untreated uremia and in otherwise stable dialysis patients. The pericardium is characteristically "shaggy," and the effusion is hemorrhagic and exudative. Uremic pericarditis can present with or without symptoms; fever is absent. The pericarditis usually resolves with the institution of—or with more aggressive—dialysis. The role of anti-inflammatory agents is unclear, especially since most have antiplatelet activity. Tamponade is fairly common, and partial pericardiectomy (pericardial window) may be necessary.

Neoplastic Pericarditis

Spread of adjacent lung cancer as well as invasion by breast cancer, Hodgkin's disease, and lymphomas are the commonest neoplastic processes involving the pericardium and have become the most frequent cause of pericardial tamponade in many countries. Often the process is painless, and the presenting symptoms relate to hemodynamic compromise or the primary disease. The diagnosis can usually be made by cytologic examination of the effusion or by biopsy, but it may be difficult to establish clinically if the patient has received mediastinal radiation within the previous year. MRI and CT scan can visualize neighboring tumor when present. The prognosis with neoplastic effusion is dismal, with only a small minority surviving 1 year. If it is compromising the patient, the effusion is initially drained. Instillation of chemotherapeutic agents or tetracycline may also prevent recurrence. Pericardial windows are rarely effective, but partial pericardiectomy from a subxiphoid incision may be successful; patients may be too ill to tolerate this.

Postmyocardial Infarction or Cardiotomy Pericarditis (Dressler's Syndrome)

Pericarditis may occur 2–5 days after infarction due to an inflammatory reaction to myocardial necrosis. It usually presents as a recurrence of pain with pleural-pericardial features. A rub is often audible, and repolarization changes may be confused with ischemia. Large effusions are uncommon, and spontaneous resolution usually occurs in a few days. As-

pirin or nonsteroidal agents provide symptomatic relief.

Dressler's syndrome occurs weeks to several months after myocardial infarction or open heart surgery, may be recurrent, and probably represents an autoimmune syndrome. Patients present with typical pain, fever, malaise, and leukocytosis. The sedimentation rate is usually high. Large pericardial effusions and accompanying pleural effusions are frequent. Tamponade is rare with Dressler's syndrome after infarction but not when it occurs postoperatively. Nonsteroidal agents are given, but recurrences are common; corticosteroids are effective but may be difficult to withdraw without relapse.

Radiation Pericarditis

Radiation can initiate a fibrinous and fibrotic process in the pericardium, presenting as subacute pericarditis or constriction. The clinical onset is usually within the first year but may be delayed for many years. Radiation pericarditis usually follows treatments of more than 4000 cGy delivered to ports including more than 30% of the heart. Symptomatic therapy is the initial approach, but recurrent effusions and constriction often require surgery.

Other Causes of Pericarditis

These include connective tissue diseases, such as lupus erythematosus, rheumatoid arthritis, and drug-induced pericarditis (minoxidil, penicillins), and myxedema.

Ginzton LE, Laks MM: The differential diagnosis of acute pericarditis from the normal variant: New electrocardiographic criteria. Circulation 1982;65:1004.

Permanyer-Miralda G, Sagrista-Sauleda J, Soler-Soler J: Primary acute pericardial disease: A prospective series of 231 consecutive patients. Am J Cardiol 1985;56:623. (Large series showing diverse spectrum of disease.)

PERICARDIAL EFFUSION

Pericardial effusion can develop during any of the processes discussed in the preceding paragraphs. The speed of accumulation determines the physiologic importance of the effusion. Because the pericardium stretches, large effusions (> 1000 mL) that develop slowly may produce no hemodynamic effects. Smaller effusions that appear rapidly can cause tamponade. Tamponade is characterized by elevated intrapericardial pressure (> 15 mm Hg), which restricts venous return and ventricular filling. As a result, the stroke volume and pulse pressure fall, and the heart rate and venous pressure rise. Shock and death may result.

Clinical Findings

A. Symptoms and Signs: Pericardial effusions may be associated with pain if they occur as part of an acute inflammatory process or may be painless, as is often the case with neoplastic or uremic effusion. Dyspnea and cough are common, especially with tamponade. Other symptoms may result from the primary disease.

A pericardial friction rub may be present even with large effusions. In cardiac tamponade, tachycardia, tachypnea, a narrow pulse pressure, and a relatively preserved systolic pressure are characteristic. Pulsus paradoxus—a greater than 10 mm Hg decline in systolic pressure during inspiration due to further impairment of left ventricular filling—is the classic finding, but it may also occur with obstructive lung disease. Central venous pressure is elevated, and edema or ascites may be present; these signs favor a more chronic process.

B. Laboratory Findings: Laboratory tests tend to reflect the underlying processes.

C. Diagnostic Studies: Chest x-ray can suggest effusion by an enlarged cardiac silhouette with a "water-bottle" configuration. The ECG often reveals nonspecific T wave changes and low QRS voltage. Electrical alternans may be present. Echocardiography, however, is the primary method for demonstrating pericardial effusion. Tamponade presents a characteristic picture of inadequate ventricular filling (diastolic collapse of the right ventricle or right atrium). The echocardiogram readily discriminates pericardial effusion from congestive heart failure. Diagnostic pericardiocentesis or biopsy is often indicated for microbiologic and cytologic studies; a pericardial biopsy may be performed relatively simply through a small subxiphoid incision.

Treatment

Small effusions can be followed clinically and with the aid of echocardiograms. When tamponade is present, urgent pericardiocentesis is required. Removal of a small amount of fluid often produces immediate hemodynamic benefit, but complete drainage with a catheter is preferable. Continued drainage may be indicated.

Additional therapy is determined by the nature of the primary process. Recurrent effusion in neoplastic disease and uremia, in particular, may require partial pericardiectomy.

Kralstein J, Frishman W: Malignant pericardial diseases: Diagnosis and treatment. Am Heart J 1987;113:785.

Press OW, Livingston R: Management of malignant pericardial effusion and tamponade. JAMA 1987;257:1088.

Singh S et al: Usefulness of right ventricular diastolic collapse in diagnosing cardiac tamponade and comparison to pulsus paradoxus. Am J Cardiol 1986;57:652. (Evaluation of a commonly used sign of hemodynamic compromise.)

Spodick DH: The normal and diseased pericardium: Current concepts of pericardial physiology, diagnosis, and treatment. J Am Coll Cardiol 1983;1:240.

CHRONIC CONSTRICTIVE PERICARDITIS

Chronic inflammation can lead to a thickened, fibrotic, adherent pericardium that restricts diastolic filling and produces chronically elevated venous pressures. In the past, tuberculosis was the most common cause of constrictive pericarditis, but the process now more often occurs after radiation therapy, cardiac surgery, or viral pericarditis.

The principal symptoms are slowly progressive dyspnea, fatigue, and weakness. Chronic edema, hepatic congestion, and ascites are usually present. The examination reveals these signs and a characteristically elevated jugular venous pressure with a rapid y descent. Kussmaul's sign—an increase in jugular venous pressure during inspiration—occurs in constrictive pericarditis and restrictive cardiomyopathy. Pulsus paradoxus is unusual. Atrial fibrillation is common.

The chest x-ray may show normal heart size or cardiomegaly. Pericardial calcification is best seen on the lateral view and is common. Echocardiography can demonstrate a thick pericardium and small chambers. CT scans and MRI are helpful in revealing pericardial thickening and may be more sensitive than echocardiography.

The primary differential diagnoses are restrictive cardiomyopathy and tamponade. The former distinction can be difficult and is best made by evaluating left ventricular function (more consistently depressed in cardiomyopathy), measuring hemodynamics (which show more complete equalization of diastolic pressures in all 4 chambers in constrictive pericarditis), and demonstrating pericardial thickening and calcification.

Acute treatment consists of gentle diuresis. Surgical removal of the pericardium, which should be complete, is usually required in symptomatic patients but is associated with a relatively high mortality rate.

Cameron J et al: The etiologic spectrum of constrictive pericarditis. Am Heart J 1987;113:354.

Killian DM et al: Constrictive pericarditis after cardiac surgery. Am Heart J 1989;118:563. (Not a rare problem.)

Nishimura RA et al: Constrictive pericarditis: Assessment of current diagnostic procedures. Mayo Clin Proc 1985;60:397.

Seifert FC et al: Surgical treatment of constrictive pericarditis: Analysis of outcome and diagnostic error. Circulation 1986;72(Suppl II):264. (Problems, but success in appropriate patients.)

PULMONARY HYPERTENSION & HEART DISEASE

PRIMARY PULMONARY HYPERTENSION

Primary pulmonary hypertension is defined as pulmonary hypertension and elevated pulmonary vascular resistance in the absence of other disease of the lungs or heart. Pathologically, it is characterized by diffuse narrowing of the pulmonary arterioles. Circumstantial evidence suggests that unrecognized recurrent pulmonary emboli or in situ thrombosis may play a role in some cases. Primary pulmonary hypertension must be distinguished from chronic pulmonary heart disease (cor pulmonale), recurrent pulmonary emboli, mitral stenosis, congenital heart disease, and occult mitral stenosis. Exclusion of secondary causes by echocardiography and lung scanning—and, if necessary, pulmonary angiography—is essential.

The clinical picture is similar to that of pulmonary hypertension from other causes. Patients—characteristically young women—present with evidence of right heart failure that is usually progressive, leading to death in 2–8 years. Patients have manifestations of low cardiac output, with weakness and fatigue, as well as edema and ascites as right heart failure advances. Peripheral cyanosis is present, and syncope on effort may occur.

The chest x-ray shows enlarged main pulmonary arteries with reduced peripheral branches. The right ventricle is enlarged. The ECG shows right ventricular and atrial hypertrophy.

Some authorities advocate chronic oral anticoagulation. The efficacy of vasodilator drugs is controversial, in part because the responses are variable. The calcium channel blockers nifedipine and diltiazem appear to be the preferred agents. The best response may be in patients in the earlier stages of the disease, when a more reversible vasoconstrictive component is present. A recent trial with chronic home infusions of prostacyclin showed both hemodynamic and clinical benefit in patients with advanced disease.

The prognosis in primary pulmonary hypertension is poor. Although most patients have a downhill course within a few years, some patients survive for 5 to 6 years. Heart-lung transplantation is being employed more frequently now with encouraging successes, resulting primarily from the availability of cyclosporine to decrease rejection.

Burke CM et al: Twenty-eight cases of human heart-lung transplantation. Lancet 1986;1:517. (Primary pulmonary hypertension a major indication.)

Rich S: Primary pulmonary hypertension. Prog Cardiovasc Dis 1988;31:205. (Emphasis on treatment.)

Rubin LJ et al: Treatment of primary pulmonary hypertension with continuous intravenous prostacyclin (epoprostenol): Results of a randomized trial. Ann Intern Med 1990;112:485.

PULMONARY HEART DISEASE (Cor Pulmonale)

Essentials of Diagnosis

- Symptoms and signs of chronic bronchitis and pulmonary emphysema.
- Elevated jugular venous pressure, parasternal lift, edema, hepatomegaly, ascites.
- ECG shows tall, peaked P waves (P pulmonale), right axis deviation, and right ventricular hypertrophy.
- Chest x-ray: Enlarged right ventricle and pulmonary artery.
- Echocardiogram or radionuclide angiography excludes primary left ventricular dysfunction.

General Considerations

The term "cor pulmonale" denotes right ventricular hypertrophy and eventual failure resulting from pulmonary disease. Its clinical features depend upon both the primary disease and its effects on the heart.

Cor pulmonale is most commonly caused by chronic obstructive pulmonary disease. Rare causes include pneumoconiosis, pulmonary fibrosis, kyphoscoliosis, primary pulmonary hypertension, repeated episodes of subclinical or clinical pulmonary embolization, Pickwickian syndrome, schistosomiasis, and obliterative pulmonary capillary or lymphangitic infiltration from metastatic carcinoma. Hypoxia is the common denominator of these conditions which ultimately lead to cor pulmonale.

Clinical Findings

A. Symptoms and Signs: The predominant symptoms of compensated cor pulmonale are related to the pulmonary disorder and include chronic productive cough, exertional dyspnea, wheezing respirations, easy fatigability, and weakness. When the pulmonary disease causes right ventricular failure, these symptoms may be intensified. Dependent edema and right upper quadrant pain may also appear. The signs of cor pulmonale include cyanosis, clubbing, distended neck veins, right ventricular heave or gallop (or both), prominent lower sternal or epigastric pulsations, an enlarged and tender liver, and dependent edema.

B. Laboratory Findings: Polycythemia is often present in cor pulmonale secondary to COPD. The arterial oxygen saturation is below 85%; P_{CO_2} may or may not be elevated.

C. ECG and Chest X-Ray: The ECG may show right axis deviation and peaked P waves. Deep S waves are present in lead V_6. Right axis deviation and low voltage may be noted in patients with pulmonary emphysema. Frank right ventricular hypertrophy is uncommon except in "primary pulmonary hypertension." The ECG often mimics myocardial infarction; Q waves may be present in leads II, III, and aVF because of the vertically placed heart, but they are rarely deep or wide, as in inferior myocardial infarction. Supraventricular arrhythmias are frequent and nonspecific.

The chest radiograph discloses the presence or absence of parenchymal disease and a prominent or enlarged right ventricle and pulmonary artery.

D. Diagnostic Studies: Pulmonary function tests usually confirm the underlying lung disease. The echocardiogram should show normal left ventricular size and function but right ventricular dilatation. Perfusion lung scans are rarely of value, but, if negative, they exclude pulmonary emboli, an occasional cause of cor pulmonale. Pulmonary angiography is the most specific method of diagnosis for the pulmonary emboli, but it carries increased risk when performed in patients with pulmonary hypertension.

Differential Diagnosis

In its early stages, cor pulmonale can be diagnosed on the basis of radiologic, echocardiographic, or electrocardiographic evidence. Catheterization of the right heart will establish a definitive diagnosis but is usually performed to exclude left-sided heart failure, which may in some patients be an inapparent cause of right-sided failure. Differential diagnostic considerations relate chiefly to the specific pulmonary disease that has produced right ventricular failure (see above).

Treatment

The details of the treatment of chronic pulmonary disease (chronic respiratory failure) are discussed in Chapter 7. Otherwise, therapy is directed at the pulmonary process responsible for right heart failure. Oxygen, salt and fluid restriction, and diuretics are mainstays; digitalis has no place in right heart failure unless atrial fibrillation is present.

Prognosis

Compensated cor pulmonale has the same outlook as the underlying pulmonary disease. Once congestive signs appear, the average life expectancy is 2–5 years, but survival is significantly longer when uncomplicated emphysema is the cause.

NEOPLASTIC DISEASES OF THE HEART

Primary cardiac tumors are rare and constitute only a small fraction of all tumors that involve the heart or pericardium. Metastases from malignant tumors elsewhere are more frequent. Tumors involving the heart are bronchogenic carcinoma, carcinoma of the breast, malignant melanoma, the lymphomas, renal cell carcinoma, and, in patients with AIDS, Kaposi's sarcoma. These are often "silent" but may lead to pericardial tamponade, arrhythmias and conduction disturbances, heart failure, and peripheral emboli. The diagnosis is often made by echocardiography, but MRI and CT scanning are also helpful. The prognosis is dismal; effective treatment is not available.

The commonest primary tumors of the heart are atrial myxomas. These tend to occur in middle age, more often in women than in men. They usually originate in the intraventricular septum, with over 80% growing into the left atrium. Myxomas are benign tumors, but they can metastasize by embolization.

Patients with myxoma can present with a picture of a systemic illness, obstruction of blood flow through the heart, or signs of peripheral embolization. The characteristic picture includes fever, malaise, weight loss, leukocytosis, elevated sedimentation rate, and emboli (peripheral or pulmonary, depending on the location of the tumor). This picture is often confused with infective endocarditis, lymphoma, other cancers, or autoimmune diseases. In other cases, the tumor may grow to considerable size and produce symptoms by obstructing mitral flow. Episodic pulmonary edema (classically occurring when an upright posture is assumed) and signs of low output may result. Physical examination may reveal a diastolic sound related to motion of the tumor ("tumor plop") or a diastolic murmur similar to that of mitral stenosis. Right-sided myxomas may cause symptoms of right-sided failure. The diagnosis is established by echocardiography or by pathologic study of embolic material. MRI is also useful. Contrast angiography is usually not necessary. Surgical excision is usually curative.

Other primary cardiac tumors include rhabdomyomas, fibrous histiocytomas, hemangiomas, and a variety of unusual sarcomas. The diagnosis may be supported by an abnormal cardiac contour on x-ray. Echocardiography is usually helpful but may miss tumors infiltrating the ventricular wall. It is likely that MRI will be useful as well.

Fyke FE III et al: Primary cardiac tumors: Experience with 30 consecutive patients since the introduction of two-dimensional echocardiography. J Am Coll Cardiol 1985;5:1465.

Kapoor AS (editor): Cancer and the Heart. Springer-Verlag, 1986.

THE CARDIAC PATIENT & SURGERY

Patients with known or suspected cardiac disease undergoing general surgery present a common management problem. Anesthesia and surgery are often associated with marked fluctuations of heart rate and blood pressure, changes in intravascular volume, myocardial ischemia or depression, arrhythmias, decreased oxygenation, increased sympathetic nervous system activity, and alterations in medical regimens and pharmacokinetics. Even with careful monitoring and management, the perioperative period can be very stressful to cardiac patients.

The risk of surgery in patients with heart disease depends primarily on 3 factors: the type of operation, the nature of the heart disease, and the degree of preoperative stability. The type of anesthesia is less important, though halothane, enflurane, and barbiturates are more severe myocardial depressants, while narcotics have little depressive effect. Spinal and epidural anesthesia were previously thought to be preferable in patients with heart disease, but this has not proved to be the case.

The highest-risk procedures are surgery of the aorta and vascular procedures, in part because these patients often have associated severe coronary disease but also because marked blood pressure and volume changes are common. Major abdominal and thoracic surgery are also associated with substantial cardiovascular risk.

Numerous studies have evaluated the excess risk of surgery in patients with various cardiac diseases. Recent (within 3 months) myocardial infarction, unstable angina, congestive heart failure, significant aortic stenosis, uncontrolled hypertension ($> 180/110$ mm Hg), and complex ventricular arrhythmias all are associated with substantial increases in operative morbidity and mortality rates. Any degree of instability in these conditions magnifies the potential risk. Although less common, cyanotic congenital heart disease and severe primary or secondary pulmonary hypertension pose great risks during major surgery. In patients with any of these problems, the risk-to-benefit ratio of the planned surgery should be carefully examined. If the procedure is necessary but elective, consideration should be given to delaying it until full recovery postinfarction and correction or optimal stabilization of the other conditions are achieved. Hypertension should be at least moderately controlled. Patients with severe angina should have increased medical therapy or be considered for revascularization before noncardiac surgery. Symptomatic arrhythmias, nonsustained ventricular tachycardia, or high-grade atrioventricular block and cardiac failure should be treated optimally.

Clinical assessment is usually adequate to determine preoperative risk. In appropriate patients, noninvasive assessment of cardiac function can not only help estimate risk but also facilitate postoperative management. Possibly significant valve lesions can be evaluated by echocardiography and Doppler studies. The clinical severity of coronary disease is an important factor, especially in patients undergoing vascular procedures, and it can be evaluated by exercise stress test or thallium scintigraphy. In patients unable to exercise, dipyridamole-thallium scintigraphy can identify ischemia. Prophylactic coronary revascularization may be advised in patients slated for major vascular operations who have evidence of moderate or severe ischemia. Others advocate careful monitoring (including hemodynamics) and preventive antianginal therapy unless the patient is clinically unstable, in which case surgery should usually be deferred.

Once the decision to operate is made, careful management is essential. Most cardiac medications should be continued preoperatively and postoperatively. Monitoring is the best prophylactic measure; hemodynamic monitoring is critical for patients with heart failure, severe valve disease, or easily induced myocardial ischemia. Excessive hypertension, hypotension, and arrhythmias should be searched for and appropriately treated using rapidly acting agents. Transesophageal echocardiography provides another useful technique for continuous monitoring of cardiac function and detection of ischemic episodes. Ischemic events, whether symptomatic or silent, should be vigorously treated.

Detsky AS et al: Cardiac assessment for patients undergoing noncardiac surgery: A multifactorial clinical risk index. Arch Intern Med 1986;146:2131. (Includes discussion of all risk features.)

Deron SJ, Kotler MN: Noncardiac surgery in the cardiac patient. Am Heart J 1988;116:831.

Eagle KA et al: Combining clinical and thallium data optimizes preoperative assessment of cardiac risk before major vascular surgery. Ann Intern Med 1989;110:859.

Goldman L: Multifactional index of cardiac risk in noncardiac surgery: Ten year status report. J Cardiothorac Anesth 1987;1:237.

Massie BM: Cardiac disease and the surgical patient. In: *Current Surgical Diagnosis & Treatment*, 9th ed. Way LW (editor). Appleton & Lange, 1990.

Raby KE et al: Correlation between preoperative ischemia and major cardiac events after peripheral vascular surgery. N Engl J Med 1989;321:1296. (Ischemia on ambulatory ECG predicts events. Accompanying editorial [p 1330] discusses relative advantages of electrocardiography and scintigraphic techniques.)

THE CARDIAC PATIENT & PREGNANCY

The management of cardiac disease in pregnancy is discussed in detail in the references listed below. Only a few major points can be covered in this brief section.

CARDIOVASCULAR CHANGES DURING PREGNANCY

Normal physiologic changes during pregnancy can exacerbate symptoms of underlying cardiac disease even in previously asymptomatic individuals. Maternal blood volume rises progressively until the end of the sixth or seventh month. Stroke volume increases over the same time course as a result of the volume change and an increase in ejection fraction. The latter reflects predominantly a decline in peripheral resistance due to vasodilatation and the low-resistance shunting through the placenta. The heart rate tends to rise in the third trimester. Overall, cardiac output increases by 30–50%; systolic blood pressure tends to decline slightly or remain unchanged, but diastolic pressure falls significantly.

High cardiac output causes alterations in the cardiac examination. A third heart sound is prominent and normal, and a pulmonic flow murmur is common. Electrocardiographic changes include rate-related decreases in PR and QT intervals, a leftward axis shift, inferior Q waves due to the more horizontal position of the heart, and nonspecific ST–T wave changes.

MANAGEMENT OF PREEXISTING CONDITIONS

The physiologic changes imposed by pregnancy can cause cardiac decompensation in patients with any significant cardiac abnormality, but the most severe problems are encountered in patients with valvular stenosis (especially mitral and aortic stenosis), congenital or acquired abnormalities associated with pulmonary hypertension or right-to-left shunting, congestive heart failure due to any cause, coronary heart disease, and hypertension. Valvular insufficiency or left-to-right shunting often diminishes because of the fall in peripheral resistance and is better tolerated.

Mitral stenosis becomes more hemodynamically severe owing to the increase in diastolic flow and the rate-related shortening of diastole. Left atrial pressures rise, and dyspnea or pulmonary edema can occur in previously asymptomatic individuals. The onset of atrial fibrillation often leads to acute decompensation. Patients with moderate to severe stenosis should be discouraged from becoming pregnant or should have surgery before pregnancy. Patients who become symptomatic can undergo successful surgery, preferably in the third trimester. Balloon valvuloplasty is an attractive alternative, though radiation exposure to the fetus is unavoidable. Coarctation is usually well tolerated, but patients with symptoms should have corrective surgery before pregnancy. Patients with severe pulmonary hypertension and cyanotic congenital heart disease and those with severe aortic stenosis are at extremely high risk and should not become pregnant unless surgical correction is undertaken.

Asymptomatic arrhythmias should be closely observed unless underlying heart disease is present, in which case they should be treated with drugs. Paroxysmal supraventricular arrhythmias are quite common. Patients with Wolff-Parkinson-White syndrome often have more problems during pregnancy. Therapy is similar to that required for nonpregnant women.

Preexisting systemic hypertension is usually well tolerated and controllable, though the fetal morbidity rate is slightly increased. The incidence of preeclampsia and eclampsia (see Chapter 13) is increased.

Most experts discourage treatment with diuretics because hypovolemia may reduce uterine blood flow. Hydralazine and methyldopa have been well tolerated. Beta-blockers may retard fetal growth, but experience with them has been generally favorable. Little is known about the safety of most other antihypertensive agents.

CARDIOVASCULAR COMPLICATIONS OF PREGNANCY

Pregnancy-related hypertension (eclampsia and preeclampsia) is discussed in Chapter 13.

Cardiomyopathy of Pregnancy (Peripartum Cardiomyopathy)

In approximately one out of 4000–15,000 patients, dilated cardiomyopathy develops in the final month of pregnancy or within 6 months after delivery. The cause is unclear, but immune and viral causes have been postulated. The course of the disease is variable; many cases improve or resolve completely over several months, but others progress to refractory heart failure. Immunosuppressive therapy has been advocated, but few supportive data are available. Recently, beta-blockers have been administered judiciously to these patients, with at least anecdotal success. Recurrence in subsequent pregnancies has been reported.

Aortic Dissection

Pregnancy predisposes to aortic dissection, perhaps because of the accompanying connective tissue changes. Dissection usually occurs near term or shortly postpartum and is managed as it is in other patients; it may occur in the arteries in addition to the aorta, including the coronary arteries.

SPECIAL PROBLEMS

Prophylaxis for Infective Endocarditis

Although there is not universal agreement, many authorities recommend antibiotic prophylaxis during labor for patients at risk for endocarditis, especially if forceps or an episiotomy is employed. Ampicillin and gentamicin are the preferred regimen.

Management of Labor

While vaginal delivery is usually well tolerated, unstable patients (including patients with severe hypertension and worsening heart failure) should have cesarean section. An increased risk of aortic rupture has been noted during delivery in patients with coarctation of the aorta and severe aortic root dilatation with Marfan's syndrome, and vaginal delivery should be avoided in these conditions.

Cardiovascular Drugs During Pregnancy

Experience during pregnancy with many drugs is limited, and the effect on the fetus is often not well defined. Drugs with known potential for teratogenicity include phenytoin and warfarin (self-administered heparin should be substituted prior to conception if possible). Drugs that appear to be safe are hydralazine, methyldopa, digitalis, quinidine, procainamide, lidocaine, and short-term verapamil. Diuretics and beta-blockers are relatively safe but may have undesirable physiologic effects.

Ben-Ismail M et al: Cardiac valve prostheses, anticoagulation, and pregnancy. Br Heart J 1986;55:101. (How to manage difficult problem.)

Douglas PS: *Heart Disease in Women.* Davis, 1989. (Six chapters deal with problems related to pregnancy.)

Elkayam U, Gleicher N: *Cardiac Problems in Pregnancy: Diagnosis and Management of Maternal and Fetal Diseases,* 2nd ed. Alan R. Liss, 1989.

Julian DH, Szekely P: Peripartum cardiomyopathy. Prog Cardiovase Dis 1985;27:223.

Metcalfe J, McAnulty JH, Ueland K: *Burwell and Metcalfe's Heart Disease and Pregnancy: Physiology and Management,* 2nd ed. Little, Brown, 1986.

Midei MG et al: Peripartum myocarditis and cardiomyopathy. Circulation 1990;81:922. (Myocarditis may be the cause of peripartum myopathy, and immunosuppression may be effective.)

O'Connell JB et al: Peripartum cardiomyopathy: Clinical, hemodynamic, histologic and prognostic characteristics. J Am Coll Cardiol 1986;8:52.

Shapiro EP et al: Safety of labor and delivery in women with mitral valve prolapse. Am Heart J 1985;56:806. (One of the commonest questions.)

Sullivan JM, Ramanathan KB: Management of medical problems in pregnancy: Severe cardiac diseases. N Engl J Med 1985;313:304.

UCLA Conference: Pregnancy and congenital heart disease. Ann Intern Med 1990;112:445.

REFERENCES

Alpert JS, Rippe JM: *Manual of Cardiovascular Diagnosis and Therapy,* 3rd ed. Little, Brown, 1988. (Helpful but simple manual.)

Braunwald E (editor): *Heart Disease: A Textbook of Cardiovascular Medicine,* 3rd ed. Saunders, 1987. (Most chapters excellent. References up to 1987.)

Califf RM, Mark DB, Wagner GS: *Acute Coronary Care in the Thrombolytic Era.* Year Book, 1988. (Comprehensive and current.)

Constant J: *Bedside Cardiology,* 3rd ed. Little, Brown, 1986. (Very pragmatic monograph with emphasis on history and examination.)

Dalen JE, Alpert JE: *Valvular Heart Disease,* 2nd ed. Little, Brown, 1987. (Comprehensive multi-authored book.)

Eighteenth Bethesda Conference Report: Cardiovascular disease in the elderly. J Am Coll Cardiol 1987; 10(Suppl):A7. (Entire issue.) (Discusses special issues and manifestations of disease in elderly.)

Goldschlager N, Goldman MJ: *Principles of Clinical Electrocardiography,* 13th ed. Lange, 1989. (Excellent, comprehensive book.)

Hanson P: *Exercise and the Heart.* Cardiology Clinics (Vol 5, No 2). Saunders, 1987.

Hurst JW et al (editors): *The Heart,* 7th ed. McGraw-Hill, 1990. (Recently updated standard textbook.)

Maron BJ, Epstein SE, Mitchell JH (co-chairmen): 16th Bethesda Conference: Cardiovascular abnormalities in the athlete: Recommendations regarding eligibility for competition. J Am Coll Cardiol 1985;6:1189. (Consensus conference on managing heart disease in athletes and other active individuals.)

Marriot HJ: *Practical Electrocardiography,* 8th ed. Williams & Wilkins, 1988. (Excellent first book.)

Miller D et al: *Clinical Cardiac Imaging.* McGraw-Hill, 1988. (Current multi-authored book.)

Parmley WW, Chatterjee K (editors): *Cardiology.* 2 vols. Lippincott, 1987. (Many chapters excellent. Loose-leaf with regular updates and additions.)

Sokolow M, McIlroy MB, Cheitlin MD: *Clinical Cardiology,* 5th ed. Appleton & Lange, 1990. (More compact and practical book for the student, resident, and primary care physician.)

Standards and guidelines for cardiopulmonary resuscitation and emergency cardiac care. Circulation 1986;74(Suppl IV). (Entire supplement covering current guidelines and controversies.)

Blood Vessels & Lymphatics

Lawrence M. Tierney, Jr., MD, & John M. Erskine, MD

Atherosclerosis causes most degenerative arterial disease. Its incidence increases with age; although manifestations of the disease may appear in the fourth decade, people over 40 (particularly men) are most commonly affected. Risk factors include hypercholesterolemia, diabetes mellitus, smoking, and hypertension. Atherosclerosis tends to be a generalized disease, with some degree of involvement of all major arteries, but it produces its clinical manifestations by critical involvement of a limited number of arteries. Narrowing and occlusion of the artery are the most common manifestations of the disease, but weakening of the arterial wall from a loss of elastin and collagen, resulting in aneurysmal dilatation, also occurs, and both processes may be present in the same individual. Less common arterial diseases include vasculitis (of both large and small arteries), thromboangiitis obliterans (Buerger's disease), fibrodysplasia of visceral arteries, syphilitic aortitis, and radiation arteritis.

DISEASES OF THE AORTA

ANEURYSMS OF THE ABDOMINAL AORTA

Essentials of Diagnosis

- Most aneurysms are asymptomatic, detected at incidental physical examination or sonography.
- Back or abdominal pain often precedes rupture.
- Atherosclerotic occlusive disease not usually associated.

General Considerations

More than 90% of abdominal atherosclerotic aneurysms originate below the renal arteries, and many involve the bifurcation of the aorta. Aneurysms of the upper aorta are much less common. The infrarenal aorta is normally 2 cm in diameter; an aneurysm is considered present when the diameter exceeds 4 cm.

Clinical Findings

A. Symptoms and Signs:

1. Asymptomatic–A pulsating mid and upper abdominal mass may be discovered on a routine physical examination, most frequently in men over 50. Also, sonography done for other purposes often detects asymptomatic aneurysms. It is also the most cost-effective test for confirming a suspicion of aneurysm raised by physical examination.

2. Symptomatic–Pain is present in some form in one-fourth to one-third of cases and varies from mild to severe midabdominal or lower back discomfort. The pain may be constant or intermittent. Peripheral emboli may occur, even from small aneurysms, and symptomatic arterial insufficiency in the legs may result.

3. Rupture–Aortic aneurysm rupture results in death before hospitalization in 25–50% of patients, and others die before they reach the operating room. Those with bleeding confined to the retroperitoneal area may have severe pain in the abdomen, flank, or back and a pulsating abdominal mass without clinical evidence of rapid blood loss, and these are the patients that require emergency aneurysm resection, which has an operative mortality rate of 50% or more. Altogether, only 10–20% survive the acute rupture of an abdominal aortic aneurysm.

B. Laboratory Findings: Electrocardiography and renal function studies should be obtained to assess potential concomitant dysfunction in those systems.

C. Imaging: Abdominal ultrasonography is the diagnostic study of choice and is also valuable for following aneurysm size in patients not immediately treated surgically. Curvilinear calcifications outlining portions of the aneurysm wall may be visible on plain films of the aortic area in approximately three-fourths of those with an aneurysm, but this study is less sensitive than ultrasonography. Contrast-enhanced CT scanning may define the extent of the aneurysm, though some surgeons prefer preoperative aortography, MRI is probably as sensitive and specific as CT, but its use for this purpose is not widespread.

Treatment

Surgical excision and grafting is the treatment of choice for most aneurysms of the distal abdominal aorta. Aneurysms usually progressively enlarge and ultimately rupture if left untreated. The size of the aneurysm correlates best with the risk of rupture: In asymptomatic patients, surgery is advised when the aneurysm is 5 or 6 cm in diameter; in symptomatic patients, repair is indicated irrespective of size. Opinion differs about whether asymptomatic aneurysms in poor-risk patients should be removed or followed closely by means of ultrasound measurements to detect signs of expansion. Long-term beta-blockade appears to be associated with a decreased rate of growth of aneurysms that are being followed. Patients with significant symptomatic coronary or carotid disease may be more likely to suffer myocardial infarction or stroke during and following aneurysm resection; surgery or coronary angioplasty (or both) to lessen this risk prior to elective aneurysm repair is advocated by some. Other experienced vascular surgeons, however, believe the aneurysms should be treated first or there may be a higher rate of rupture in patients postoperative for major surgery such as coronary artery bypass grafting. Likewise, it is unclear whether prophylactic carotid artery surgery is even indicated. Finally, individuals over age 80 with good preoperative risk factors can undergo elective surgery with an acceptable mortality rate; those with significant associated disease generally should not undergo operation without compelling indications.

Complications

Irreversible renal injury can occur if hemodynamic instability is allowed to persist through surgery. Ischemia of the distal colon and of one or both legs occasionally occurs following this surgery; in most cases, it can be prevented by meticulous attention to detail before and during surgery. As noted above, these patients are susceptible to intra- and postoperative stroke and myocardial infarction.

Prognosis

The mortality rate following elective surgical resection is 3–8%, though in certain clinics it has recently approached 1%; clinicians must be aware of surgical success rates in their own institutions before making the often difficult decision to operate, especially in high-risk patients. Of those who survive surgery, approximately 60% are alive 5 years later, and in those who die, myocardial infarction is the leading cause of death. Among unoperated patients, less than 20% survive 5 years, and aneurysm rupture is the cause of 60% of the deaths. In general, a patient with an aortic aneurysm has a 3-fold greater chance of dying as a consequence of rupture of the aneurysm than of dying from surgical resection. If coronary or carotid artery surgery is done preoperatively, the added morbidity and mortality of these procedures must be considered in the overall approach to the patient.

Fortner G, Johansen K: Abdominal aortic aneurysm. Surg Clin North Am 1989;69:4.

ANEURYSMS OF THE THORACIC AORTA

Thoracic aortic aneurysms are most commonly due to atherosclerosis; syphilis is now a rare cause. Vasculitis and annuloaortic ectasia (with or without Marfan's syndrome) may also result in thoracic aneurysm. Traumatic aneurysms may occur just beyond the origin of the left subclavian artery when the wall of the aorta is incompletely torn as a result of a rapid deceleration accident. Less than 10% of aortic aneurysms are thoracic.

Clinical Findings

Manifestations depend largely on the size and position of the aneurysm and its rate of growth.

A. Symptoms and Signs: There may be no symptoms or signs if the aneurysm has been diagnosed by chest x-ray done for other reasons. Substernal, back, or neck pain may occur, as well as symptoms and signs due to pressure on (1) the trachea (dyspnea, stridor, a brassy cough), (2) the esophagus (dysphagia), (3) the left recurrent laryngeal nerve (hoarseness), or (4) the superior vena cava (edema in the neck and arms, distended neck veins). Aortic insufficiency may be present.

B. Imaging: In addition to chest x-rays, aortography may be necessary to substantiate the diagnosis and to delineate the precise location and extent of the aneurysm and its relation to the vessels arising from the arch. CT scan is of more use than ultrasound in scanning thoracic aneurysms and may be as sensitive and specific as aortography. Digital subtraction angiography or magnetic resonance imaging, if available, may be of value. The coronary vessels and the aortic valve should also be studied if the ascending aorta is involved.

Differential Diagnosis

It may be difficult to determine whether a mass in the mediastinum is an aneurysm, a neoplasm, or a cyst. The x-ray studies mentioned above will distinguish an aneurysm. Radioactive isotope studies (^{125}I) may be helpful in diagnosing a substernal goiter.

Treatment

Aneurysms of the thoracic aorta often progress, with increasing symptoms, and finally rupture. Resection of aneurysms is now considered the treatment of choice if a skilled surgical team is available and if the patient's general condition is such that the major surgical procedure usually required can be done with an acceptable risk. Small asymptomatic aneurysms, especially in poor-risk patients, are perhaps better treated only if progressive enlargement occurs. Control of hypertension may slow progression. The overall mortality rate of thoracic aneurysmectomy, however, is considerably higher than the 3–5% rate for abdominal aneurysms.

If the aortic valve is involved, an aortic valve replacement may be necessary, and reattachment of the coronary arteries or aortocoronary bypass grafts may also be indicated. Paraplegia due to anterior spinal artery compromise is a dreaded complication of excision and graft replacement of aneurysms involving the descending thoracic aorta (3% of cases).

Prognosis

Small aneurysms may change very little over a period of years, and death may result from causes other than rupture. If the aneurysm is large, symptomatic, and associated with hypertension or arteriosclerotic cardiovascular disease, the prognosis is poor. Saccular aneurysms, those distal to the left subclavian artery, and those limited to the ascending aorta can now be removed with an acceptable mortality rate. Resection of aneurysms of the transverse aortic arch involves major technical problems that can be dealt with only by skilled surgical teams using hypothermia to protect the nervous system.

Crawford ES et al: Thoracoabdominal aortic aneurysms: Preoperative and intraoperative factors determining immediate and long term results of operations in 605 patients. J Vasc Surg 1986;3:389.

PERIPHERAL ARTERY ANEURYSMS (Popliteal & Femoral)

Popliteal artery aneurysms rank third in frequency among aneurysmal lesions; most of the other peripheral aneurysms are femoral. Almost all are atherosclerotic and occur in men. They are often multiple and bilateral, and aneurysmal disease of the aortoiliac vessels is commonly associated with the more peripheral aneurysms, with elastin and collagen loss contributing to the arterial dilatation.

Popliteal Aneurysms

Almost half are asymptomatic when diagnosed, and they are generally discovered in the popliteal fossa as a pulsating mass 2 cm or more in diameter. When a popliteal aneurysm is diagnosed, abdominal aneurysm may be present and should be excluded by ultrasonography. Most aneurysms present with symptoms generally related to varying degrees of arterial insufficiency to the lower leg and foot, ie, intermittent claudication if insufficiency develops slowly, or severe ischemic manifestations with rest pain, pregangrene, or gangrene if sudden thrombosis of the aneurysm has developed or, less commonly, if distal embolization has occurred (see below). When complete thrombosis has occurred, a nonpulsatile popliteal mass is noted. The large aneurysms may be associated with a degree of venous obstructive manifestations or pain from pressure on the nerves; thrombophlebitis is infrequent, and rupture is rare.

Angiography is of value in defining the distal arterial tree and the collateral vessels. The actual size of the aneurysm is more clearly determined by ultrasound examination.

Popliteal aneurysms rank second to abdominal aortic aneurysms in the incidence of potentially serious complications. Even small aneurysms (2 cm in size) can become thrombosed or give rise to emboli, particularly if laminated clot exists within the lumen of the aneurysm. When thrombosis occurs, amputation may be required. Thus, surgery is advisable, and a reversed saphenous vein bypass graft with proximal and distal ligation of the aneurysm is generally employed. In large aneurysms with manifestations of vein or nerve compression, resection of the aneurysm with grafting of the arterial defect may be necessary.

Femoral Aneurysms

Femoral aneurysms, as manifested by a pulsatile mass in the femoral area on one or both sides, have the potential for the same complications as popliteal aneurysms, although rupture is a more frequent complication and limb-threatening episodes are less frequent in femoral aneurysms. Because the incidence of serious complications in the asymptomatic group seems to be considerably less than for popliteal aneurysms, there is more reason to follow rather than operate on smaller, asymptomatic femoral aneurysms and to deal first with aortoiliac and then popliteal aneurysms in preference to femoral aneurysms when aneurysmal disease exists in all of these areas.

Anton GE et al: Surgical management of popliteal aneurysms: Trends in presentation, treatment and results from 1952 to 1984, J Vasc Surg 1986;3:1986.
Melliere D et al: Should all spontaneous popliteal aneurysms be operated on? J Cardiovasc Surg 1986;27:273.

ACUTE AORTIC DISSECTION

Essentials of Diagnosis

- Sudden severe chest pain with radiation to the back, occasionally migrating to the abdomen and hips.
- Patient appears to be in shock, but blood pressure is normal or elevated.
- A history of hypertension is usually present. Aortic insufficiency may be present.

General Considerations

Extravasation of blood into and along the wall of the aorta may occur, resulting in aortic dissection. Dissection generally begins either in the proximal aorta just above the aortic valve or at a site just beyond the origin of the left subclavian artery. If the ascending aorta is involved, it is referred to as type A; all others are type B. The initial intimal tear probably results from the constant movement of the ascending and proximal descending aorta that occurs at these 2 points associated with the pulsatile blood flow from the heart. Dissection occurs on rare occasions in an aorta even without an intimal tear; these aortas invariably show histologic abnormalities of the media. Proximal dissections are more often in aortas involved with abnormalities of the smooth muscle, elastic tissue, or collagen; distal dissections occur in older patients with long-standing hypertension and is a relatively rare complication of long-standing hypertension. Pregnancy (types A and B), bicuspid aortic valves and coarctation (types A and B), and Marfan's syndrome (type A) are associated with dissection in younger individuals. Both hypertension and a forceful pulse are important in progression of dissection, which may extend from the ascending aorta distally to the abdominal aorta or beyond. Alternatively, dissection may remain limited to the ascending aorta and the aortic valve area, especially if hypertension is not present or is controlled early; furthermore, distal dissection may progress not only distally but also proximally. Death may occur after hours, days, or weeks and is usually due to rupture of the aorta into the pericardial sac (with cardiac tamponade), into the left pleural cavity, or into the retroperitoneal area. Dissection may rupture back into the true lumen of the aorta (recanalization) with blood flow through both the true and false lumens; long-term survival can thus occur.

Clinical Findings

A. Symptoms and Signs: Severe, persistent chest pain of sudden onset, nearly always anterior but often also posterior, which may later progress to the abdominal and hip areas, is characteristic. Radiation down the arms or into the neck may or may not occur. Usually there is only a mild decrease in the prerupture hypertensive level. Partial or complete occlusion of the arteries arising from the aortic arch or of the intercostal and lumbar arteries may lead to such central nervous system findings as syncope, hemiplegia, or paralysis of the lower extremities. Peripheral pulses and blood pressures may be diminished or unequal. Murmurs may appear over arteries along with signs of acute arterial insufficiency. An aortic diastolic murmur may develop as a result of dissection close to the aortic valve, resulting in secondary valvular insufficiency, heart failure, and cardiac tamponade.

B. Laboratory Findings: Electrocardiographic changes indicating left ventricular hypertrophy are often present; acute changes may not develop unless the dissection involves the coronary ostium. In that case, inferior wall abnormalities predominate, since dissection leads to compromise of the right rather than the left coronary artery. In some, the ECG may be perfectly normal.

C. Imaging: Chest radiographs often reveal an abnormal aortic contour or a wide superior mediasti-

num, with changes in the configuration and thickness of the aortic wall in successive films. There may be findings of pleural or pericardial effusion. CT scan with contrast enhancement and magnetic resonance imaging (MRI) are both sensitive studies but are too time-consuming if dissection is clinically likely. Such patients should have immediate angiography, because emergency surgery may be lifesaving in type A dissection and because most surgeons require angiographic confirmation preoperatively. MRI or CT scanning is best employed when dissection is considered possible but unlikely; a normal image by either technique is strong evidence against dissection.

Differential Diagnosis

Aortic dissection is most commonly confused with myocardial infarction (see Chapter 8) as well as other causes of chest pain, such as pulmonary embolization. However, it may simulate numerous neurologic lesions and even various abdominal conditions related to renal-visceral ischemia.

Treatment

A. Medical Measures: If hypertension is present, aggressive measures to lower the pressure should probably be initiated even before diagnostic studies have been completed. Treatment generally includes the simultaneous reduction of the systolic blood pressure to 100 mm Hg and reduction of the pulsatile aortic flow by means of the following:

(1) A rapid-acting antihypertensive agent as an intravenous infusion at a flow rate regulated by very frequent blood pressure determinations. Nitroprusside and trimethaphan are the most commonly used drugs and may be given as follows: (a) Nitroprusside (50 mg in 1000 mL of 5% dextrose in water) is started at a rate of 0.5 mL/min and the infusion rate increased by 0.5 mL every 5 minutes until adequate control of the pressure has been achieved. Thiocyanate levels should be obtained, and the infusion should be stopped if the drug level reaches 10 mg/dL; (b) Trimethaphan (1 or 2 mg/mL) may be infused with the patient in the semi-Fowler position.

(2) Intravenous propranolol, 0.15 mg/kg given over a 5-minute period and repeated as necessary to maintain the pulse rate at 60/min. The rapid-acting beta-blocker esmolol may be tried first in patients in whom adverse effects are considered more likely to occur. Intravenous reserpine may be used if beta-blockers are contraindicated.

Failure of this pharmacologic approach and the need for urgent surgery is suggested if chest pain is not relieved or if it reappears; if significant compromise or occlusion of a major branch of the aorta develops; or if progressive aortic enlargement, suggesting impending rupture, occurs.

B. Surgical Measures: The emphasis in treatment has shifted toward surgery, as a result of increased proficiency in handling these very difficult technical problems. If a skilled cardiovascular team is available, all acute dissections involving the ascending aorta (type A) should be treated promptly with surgery to relieve or to prevent aortic valve insufficiency and to prevent rupture. The ascending aorta and, if necessary, the aortic valve and arch may be replaced with reattachment of the coronaries and brachiocephalic vessels.

Surgical treatment is increasingly popular for dissections arising in the descending thoracic aorta (type B); it may be delayed until the hypertension and dissection have been stabilized by medical means. The origin of the dissection is then removed; the false lumen is closed; and a graft is inserted to deliver all blood flow through the normal lumen, thus relieving the occlusive pressure on the aortic branches.

Since patients with type B dissections tend to be poor surgical risks, permanent medical therapy may be offered. Regimens should include beta-blockers and antihypertensive drugs; vasodilators are contraindicated unless used with beta-blockers.

Prognosis

Without treatment, the mortality rate at 3 months is over 90%. Twenty percent are dead in 24 hours and 60% in 2 weeks. Survival without treatment, usually due to recanalization, does occasionally occur. Intensive pharmacologic methods to lower the pulse wave and blood pressure have led to healing of the dissected aorta in patients with acute dissection and will convert others to a subacute or chronic form, which may then be treated by surgery.

Cooke JP, Kazmier FJ, Orszulak TA: The penetrating aortic ulcer: Pathologic manifestations, diagnosis, and management. Mayo Clin Proc 1988;63:718.

Weingarten J, Tierney LM Jr: Aortic dissection. West J Med 1986;144:728.

ATHEROSCLEROTIC OCCLUSIVE DISEASE

Occlusive disease of the aorta and its branches is a common cause of disability. It is essential for the primary physician to emphasize its prevention, particularly in light of what is known about etiologic factors. Smoking must be interdicted in all individuals, and serum cholesterol should be determined in all adults under the care of physicians. Discontinuance of smoking and dietary or pharmacologic management when the serum cholesterol exceeds 200 mg/dL are prudent measures likely to reduce morbidity from atherosclerosis (see Chapters 1 and 21).

OCCLUSIVE DISEASE OF THE AORTA & ILIAC ARTERIES

Occlusive disease of the aorta and the iliac arteries begins most frequently just proximal to the bifurcation of the common iliac arteries and at or just distal to the bifurcation of the aorta. Atherosclerotic changes occur in the intima and media, often with associated perivascular inflammation and calcified plaques in the media. Progression involves the complete occlusion of one or both common iliac arteries and then the abdominal aorta up to the segment just below the renal vessels. Although atherosclerosis is a generalized disease, occlusion tends to be segmental in distribution, and when the involvement is in the aortoiliac vessels there may be minimal atherosclerosis in the more distal external iliac and femoral arteries. The best candidates for arterial reconstructive surgery procedures are those with localized occlusions at or just beyond the aortic bifurcation with relatively normal vessels proximally and distally. Conversely, patients with multisegmented arterial disease usually have more symptoms, are more difficult to treat, and are at greater risk of losing a limb.

Clinical Findings

Intermittent claudication is almost always present in the calf muscles and is usually present in the thighs and buttocks. It is most often bilateral and progressive. Some complain only of weakness in the legs when walking or a feeling of "tiredness" in the buttocks. Impotence is a common complaint in men. Rest pain is infrequent.

Femoral pulses are absent or very weak, and distal pulses are absent. A bruit may be heard over the aorta or over the iliac or femoral arteries. Atrophic changes of the skin, subcutaneous tissues, and muscles of the distal leg are usually minimal, as are dependent rubor and coolness of the skin, unless distal arterial disease is also present. Aortography including oblique views of the thigh and leg arteries demonstrates the level and extent of the occlusion and the condition of the vessels distal to the block. Doppler ultrasound offers noninvasive quantitation of blood pressure in pedal pulses.

Treatment

Surgical or angioplastic treatment is indicated if claudication interferes appreciably with the patient's essential activities or work. Discontinuation of smoking is essential; some surgeons insist on it as a prerequisite for operation.

Because many of these patients have coexisting ischemic heart disease, their medical management should be maximized preoperatively. The roles of exercise testing and coronary angiography have not been established. Some clinicians obtain these studies with an eye toward prophylactic bypass grafting or coronary angioplasty; this has not been conclusively shown to be of benefit in this situation if patients are minimally symptomatic.

A. Arterial Graft (Prosthesis): An arterial prosthesis bypassing the occluded segment is effective treatment for aortoiliac occlusive disease. In general, the bifurcation graft extends from the infrarenal abdominal aorta, usually by means of an end-to-end anastomosis, to the distal external iliac or common femoral arteries as end-to-side anastomoses. A patient may also be treated surgically with less risk but also less favorable results by means of a graft from the axillary artery to one or both femoral arteries or, in the case of iliac unilateral disease, from the femoral artery with normal blood flow to the contralateral femoral artery distal to the stenotic iliac vessel.

B. Thromboendarterectomy: This procedure, which avoids the use of a prosthesis, is generally used when the occlusion is limited to the common iliac arteries and when the external iliac and common femoral arteries are free of significant occlusive disease.

C. Endovascular Surgical Techniques: Occlusive lesions that were formerly dealt with entirely by methods as described in paragraphs A and B, above, are now being treated by percutaneous transluminal angioplasty with increasing frequency, and the stenotic areas of the aortic bifurcation and the iliac arteries may often be treated with greater safety and fewer complications using balloon angioplasty or atherectomy instruments to eliminate the stenotic area. (See below for further details.)

Prognosis

The operative mortality rate is 2–6%—a great deal less for the angioplastic procedure. The immediate and long-term benefits are often impressive. In patients with no distal occlusive disease, improvement is both subjective and objective, with relief of all or most of the claudication and, usually, return of all the pulses in the extremities. Late occlusions in this group of patients are infrequent, and if proper judgment is used in patient selection, results are comparable for angioplasty, endarterectomy, and arterial grafting techniques.

Szilagyi DE et al: A thirty year survey of the reconstructive surgical treatment of aortoiliac occlusive disease. J Vasc Surg 1986;3:421.

OCCLUSIVE DISEASE OF THE FEMORAL & POPLITEAL ARTERIES

In the region of the thigh and knee, the vessels most frequently blocked by occlusive disease are the superficial femoral artery and the popliteal artery. Atherosclerotic changes usually appear first at the most distal point of the superficial femoral artery, where it passes through the adductor magnus tendon into the popliteal space. In time, the whole superficial femoral artery may become occluded; the disease progresses into the popliteal artery less frequently. The common femoral and deep femoral arteries are usually patent and relatively free of disease, although the origin of the profunda femoris is sometimes narrowed. The distal popliteal and its 3 terminal branches may also be relatively free of occlusive disease.

Clinical Findings

A. Symptoms and Signs: Intermittent claudication is confined to the calf and foot. Atrophic changes in the lower leg and foot are distinct, with loss of hair, thinning of the skin and subcutaneous tissues, and diminution in the size of the muscles. Dependent rubor and blanching on elevation of the foot are usually present. When the leg is lowered after elevation, venous filling on the dorsal aspect of the foot may be slowed to 15–20 seconds or more. The foot is usually cool. The common femoral pulsations are usually of fair or good quality, although a bruit may be heard. No popliteal or pedal pulses can be felt. Pressure measurements in the distal leg, using ultrasound, will supply an objective functional assessment of the circulation and will aid in the decision to go on to x-ray studies and possibly surgery.

B. Imaging: A femoral arteriogram will show the location and extent of the block as well as the status of the distal vessels, and lateral or oblique views will reveal whether the origin of the profunda femoris is narrow. It is important to know the condition of the aortoiliac vessels also, since a relatively normal inflow as well as an adequate distal "run-off" is important in determining the likelihood of success of an arterial procedure. Added oblique and leg and foot views at aortography will supply important information.

Treatment

Walking is the most effective way to develop collateral circulation, and walking up to the point of claudication, followed by a 3-minute rest, should be done at least 8 times a day. Smoking must be discontinued.

Surgery is indicated (1) if intermittent claudication is progressive or incapacitating, interfering significantly with the patient's essential physical activities such as ability to work; or (2) if there is rest pain or pregangrenous or gangrenous lesions on the foot.

A. Arterial Graft: An autogenous vein graft using a reversed segment of the great saphenous vein can be placed, bypassing the occluded segment. The distal anastomosis is usually to the popliteal artery, below the site of major occlusive disease. Another approach is to destroy the valves in the in situ saphenous vein before making the bypass anastomosis. When the entire popliteal artery is occluded and gangrene or advanced ischemic changes are present in the foot, it is generally better to perform an amputation below the knee rather than an anastomosis to one of the leg arteries, though bypass anastomosis to a tibial or peroneal artery is being done by skilled vascular surgeons with increasing success. Synthetic arterial prostheses, with the possible exception of the PTFE (polytetrafluoroethylene) grafts, have not proved to be very successful in this area because of the relatively high incidence of early or late thrombosis.

B. Thromboendarterectomy: Thromboendarterectomy with removal of the central occluding core may be successful if the occluded and stenotic segment is very short.

When significant aortoiliac or common femoral occlusive disease exists as well as superficial femoral and popliteal occlusions, it is usually better to relieve the obstructions in the larger, proximal arteries and deliver more blood flow to the profunda femoris than to operate on the smaller distal vessels, where the chances of success are less. If the origin of the profunda femoris is narrowed, a limited procedure at that site—a profundoplasty—may be successful in improving blood flow to the leg and foot and may be used, especially in poor-risk patients with rest pain.

C. Endovascular Surgery: A dramatic change in methods of treating stenotic and occlusive lesions of the distal arterial tree has occurred in the last few years, so that an increasing number of patients are now being treated not by open surgical procedures but via a percutaneous transluminal approach. Endovascular surgical procedures call for the services of a skilled interventional radiologist, and a vascular surgeon must be available in case complications develop from the percutaneous procedure. A vascular laboratory should be available to aid in evaluation and follow-up of patients.

In such a setting, occlusive lesions may be treated using one or more approaches, which include (1) balloon angioplasty, using balloon-tipped catheters capable of forcefully dilating narrow or occluded areas of the aortoiliac, femoral-popliteal, and tibial peroneal vessels; (2) mechanical atherectomy devices to remove the occluding atheroma from the lumen of the artery; and (3) laser or thermal angioplasty equipment that can vaporize the occlusive material.

These techniques require arteriography. Anticoagulants, thrombolytics, antiplatelet drugs, and agents to counteract arterial spasm are frequently employed along with the procedure. By such means, very encouraging results are being obtained at reduced risk even in the small vessels distal to the popliteal artery, and there is no doubt that increasing numbers of patients will be selected for management by this technique as the results continue to improve. Recurrent stenosis can often be re-treated by these techniques, or bypass surgery may be elected.

The most favorable lesions include the single, short discrete stenosis in medium-sized arteries such as the iliac-femoral-popliteal vessels. Less favorable lesions include multiple stenosis in series, those longer than 5 cm, complete occlusions less than 5 cm long,

lesions in the smaller arteries, and stenotic arterial anastomoses or grafts, particularly if the patient has diabetes or is a smoker.

After any of these procedures, the patient is generally maintained on permanent antiplatelet medication.

Prognosis

Thrombosis of the "bypass" graft or of the endarterectomized vessel either in the immediate postoperative period or months or years later is relatively frequent in the superficial femoral-popliteal area. This is particularly true if iliac arterial stenosis exists or if one or more of the 3 terminal branches of the distal popliteal artery are badly diseased. It is also observed after endarterectomy, when a synthetic prosthesis is used, or after an angioplastic procedure. For this reason, operation is usually not recommended for mild or moderate claudication, and approximately 80% of these patients will have relatively stable symptoms and will go for years without much progression. Some may improve as collateral circulation develops. The chances of improvement after surgery are less in patients with ischemia or early gangrene, but surgery or angioplasty is often justified because some limbs can be saved from amputation. The 5-year overall patency rate for the saphenous vein bypass grafts is in the range of 60–80%, or less if the bypass is to a tibial artery. The 2-year patency rate after transluminal angioplasty is over 80% and thus compares favorably with the venous bypass results over that period, although the long-term results may not be as good. Only about 50% of these patients survive 5 years; most deaths are due to complications of atherosclerosis, especially myocardial infarction. After 5 years, the yearly mortality rate exceeds the rate of loss of patency of the graft.

Barry R et al: Prognostic indicators in femoropopliteal and distal bypass grafts. Surg Gynecol Obstet 1985;161:129.

Moore WS et al: Endovascular Surgery. Saunders, 1989. (State of the art in a rapidly developing field.)

OCCLUSIVE DISEASE OF THE ARTERIES IN THE LOWER LEG & FOOT

Occlusive processes in the lower leg and foot may involve, in order of incidence, the tibial and common peroneal arteries, the pedal vessels, and occasionally the small digital vessels. Symptoms depend upon the vessels that are narrowed or thrombosed, the suddenness and extent of the occlusion, and the status of the proximal and collateral vessels. The clinical picture may be a rather stable or a slowly progressive form of vascular insufficiency that over months or years may ultimately result in atrophy, ischemic pain, and, occasionally, gangrene.

Clinical Findings

Although all of the possible manifestations of vas-

INFECTIONS, ULCERS, & GANGRENE OF THE TOES OR FEET

Early Treatment of Acute Infections

The patient is placed at bed rest with the leg in a horizontal or slightly depressed position. An open or discharging lesion should be covered with a light gauze dressing, but tape should not be used on the skin. If advancing infection is present, an appropriate antibiotic should be started immediately. Dicloxacillin, a cephalosporin, and clindamycin are good choices.

Ulcerations covered with necrotic tissue can often be prepared for spontaneous healing or grafting with wet dressings of sterile saline changed 3-4 times a day. Petrolatum gauze and a bacitracin-neomycin ointment may also help soften crusted infected areas and aid drainage.

Early Management of Established Gangrene

In most instances an area of gangrene will progress to a point where the circulation provided by the inflammatory reaction is sufficient to prevent further necrosis. The process will at least temporarily demarcate at that level. This can be encouraged by measures similar to those outlined in the preceding section on the treatment of acute infection. If the skin is intact and the gangrene is dry and due only to arterial occlusion, antibiotics should be withheld. If infection is present or if the gangrene is moist, antibiotics should be used in an effort to limit the process and prevent septicemia.

If the gangrene involves only a segment of skin and the underlying superficial tissue, angioplasty or arterial grafting may be possible. If not, sympathectomy may be considered. The necrotic tissue can then be removed and the ulcer grafted or allowed to heal. If amputation is required, it can sometimes be carried out at a more distal level because of those procedures.

Amputations for Gangrene

(1) A toe that is gangrenous to its base can sometimes be amputated through the necrotic tissue and left open; this procedure may be employed to establish adequate drainage of purulent material when active infection is associated with the gangrene.

(2) When the distal part of the toe is gangrenous and there is sufficient circulation in the proximal toe, closed amputation can be carried out after the area has become well demarcated and inflammation has subsided.

(3) Transmetatarsal amputation can be considered if the gangrene involves one or more toes down to but not into the foot and if the circulation in the distal foot seems adequate to support healing.

(4) Below the knee is the amputation level of choice when gangrene or ischemia in the foot is so distributed that local amputation is not possible. The preservation of the knee and proximal part of the lower leg is most important in that a more useful prosthesis can be applied and the patient can walk. Even when the circulation below the knee is quite poor, successful healing of the stump is often achieved by the use of a meticulous and gentle technique and often a rigid cast to support a well-padded stump dressing. Amputation below the knee should be attempted if there is a chance of success. Amputation through the knee joint will sometimes succeed when a below-knee amputation would fail and provides a much more useful stump than the above-knee amputation.

(5) Amputation above the knee (through the distal thigh in the supracondylar area) is indicated in patients with very advanced peripheral vascular disease requiring amputation because of gangrene, particularly if the leg as well as the foot is extensively involved with infection. It is also employed if an attempted below-knee amputation has failed to heal. Even if the femoral artery is obliterated, there will be sufficient collateral circulation to allow healing provided gentle technique with good hemostasis is used. Few of these patients have the strength and coordination to walk with a prosthesis; most are limited to wheelchair and bed.

(6) Guillotine amputation: Infection with bacteremia or septicemia occasionally develops secondary to gangrene of the lower extremity. This usually requires emergency amputation. In such a situation, it is often wise to leave the stump open so that it can heal by second intention or be revised or reamputated when the infection has been controlled. The mortality rate of a major amputation in this group of poor-risk patients is approximately 10%.

cular disease in the lower leg and foot cannot be described here, there are certain significant clinical aspects that enter into the evaluation of these patients.

A. Symptoms and Signs: Intermittent claudication is the commonest presenting symptom. Aching fatigue during exertion usually appears first in the calf muscles; in more severe cases, a constant or cramping pain may be brought on by walking only a short distance. Less commonly, the feet are the site of most of the pain. The distance the patient can walk before onset of pain is indicative of the degree of circulatory inadequacy: 2 blocks (360–460 meters) or more is mild, one block is moderate, and one-half block or less is severe. Rest pain may occur at night and is a dull, persistent ache. As in the case of femoral and popliteal disease, rest pain implies severe involvement. A degree of relief can often be obtained by uncovering the foot and letting it hang over the side of the bed.

On examination, although the popliteal pulse may be present, both pedal pulses are usually absent. Exercise may make pedal pulses disappear in some patients. Dependent rubor is prominent. The skin is cool, atrophic, and hairless. Again, these findings may be indistinguishable from those of occlusive disease higher in the leg. The presence of a popliteal pulse points to more distal occlusion when these symptoms and signs are present.

B. Imaging: Films of the lower leg and foot may show calcification of the vessels. If there is a draining sinus or an ulcer close to a bone or joint, osteomyelitis may be apparent on the film. If fairly strong popliteal pulses can be felt, arteriography is of little value. Doppler ultrasonography provides an accurate blood pressure assessment in the pedal pulses.

Treatment

A. Medical Measures: Low-dose aspirin has theoretical value and is innocuous as an antiplatelet agent; it should be given to all patients with severe peripheral vascular disease. Pentoxifylline is a drug that affects vessel rheology and may allow more exercise before claudication develops but does not affect the natural history of the disease.

B. Circulatory Insufficiency in the Foot and Toes: Lumbar sympathectomy may be indicated when ischemic or pregangrenous changes are present in the distal foot or when small ulcers are present in a foot with diminished circulation. There is no change in the circulation to the muscles and thus no relief from claudication. Patients who cannot tolerate the surgical procedure may be considered for chemical sympathectomy with 6% phenol. Vasodilator drugs are of little or no value. The general care of the feet is most important (see Chapter 21.)

ARTERIAL DISEASE IN DIABETIC PATIENTS

Atherosclerosis develops more often and earlier in patients with diabetes mellitus, especially if the patient smokes. Either the large or small vessels may be involved, but occlusion of the smaller vessels is more frequent than in the nondiabetic, and diabetics thus more often have the form of the disease that may not be suitable for arterial surgery. Cigarette smoking is particularly harmful and must be strongly interdicted. Ulcers, when present, are more likely to be moist and infected; healing, if it occurs at all, may be very slow, and healed areas may break down easily.

Diabetic neuropathy with diminished or absent sensation of the toes or feet may occur, predisposing to injury or pressure ulcerations that may be neglected because of the absence of pain. These patients may not necessarily have diminished circulation to the feet.

Poor vision due to diabetic retinopathy makes the care of the feet more difficult and injury more likely. The best approach to diabetic lower limb loss is prevention, and the incidence can be reduced by up to 50% in communities with diabetic foot clinics. See Chapter 21 for instructions on care of the feet.

Samson RH et al: Combined segment arterial disease. Surgery 1985;97:385.

OCCLUSIVE CEREBROVASCULAR DISEASE

Although episodes of weakness or dizziness, blurred vision, or sudden complete hemiplegia may be due to a variety of causes, atherosclerotic occlusive or ulcerative disease accounts for many of these problems (see Chapter 18). Single or multiple segmental lesions are often located in the extracranial arteries and account for ischemic stroke syndromes in over half of cases. The extracranial areas most often involved are (1) the common carotid bifurcation, including the origins of the internal and external carotid arteries (approximately 90%); (2) the origin of the vertebral artery; and (3) the intrathoracic segments of the aortic arch branches.

Clinical Findings

A. Symptoms: Transient ischemic attacks (TIAs) may be the earliest manifestation of carotid arterial stenosis or ulceration. Episodes usually last for only a few minutes but may continue for up to 24 hours. Significant carotid artery stenosis with temporary diminished blood flow to the brain or ulcerations with microemboli from the ulcer to the brain or the ipsilateral retinal artery are responsible for many TIAs and may precede a complete stroke in half of these patients. The classic manifestations include contralateral weakness or sensory changes, speech alterations, and visual disturbance (usual temporary partial or complete loss of vision in the ipsilateral eye, known as amaurosis fugax). Vertebrobasilar TIAs are characterized by brain stem and cerebellar symptoms, including dysarthria, diplopia, vertigo, ataxia, and alternating hemiparesis or quadriparesis.

Dizziness and unsteadiness, particularly when associated with a quick change in position, are nonspecific and more often the result of postural hypotension than of vertebrobasilar problems. Atypical neurologic symptoms or personality changes are seldom symptoms of cerebral ischemia.

B. Signs: Bruits in the lower neck, diminished or absent pulsations in the neck or arms, and a blood pressure difference in the 2 arms of more than 10 mm Hg may be indications of occlusive disease in the brachiocephalic arteries. The most significant bruit is one that is sharply localized high in the lateral neck close to the angle of the jaw (overlying the common carotid bifurcation), but a major stenosis of 75% or more and thus sufficient to reduce the blood flow through the vessel is present in a minority of patients with these bruits. The murmur of aortic stenosis may be heard as a bruit over the subclavian and carotid arteries; when there is no such heart murmur, the bruit generally denotes disease in these arteries. Bruits are often present without symptoms, and the absence of a bruit does not exclude the possibility of carotid artery stenosis. Thus, bruits heard over the carotid arteries are neither sensitive nor specific enough to alter the diagnostic approach in this patient group. Microemboli can arise from ulcerations of arteries to the brain without stenosis or bruit, particularly if the ulcer is large. Only the common carotid and superficial temporal pulses can be felt with accuracy; the internal carotid pulses cannot usually be palpated.

Additional Studies

Diagnostic studies of the cerebral circulation are both noninvasive and invasive. Of the former, duplex ultrasonography, when available, is now the investigation of choice. In duplex ultrasound, 2 ultrasonic techniques are used in concert, and the clinician is provided with both physiologic and anatomic information; indeed, ulcerating plaques, hemorrhage into an atherosclerotic lesion, and other abnormalities may be observed in images comparable to those obtained by angiography. Results in combined studies show high specificity and sensitivity for this test—in excess of any other current noninvasive technique. In addition, the hemodynamic degree of stenosis may be accurately determined. At present, this is an expensive study because of the complexity of the instrumentation, but it can be expected to achieve increasing popularity. When duplex ultrasonography is unavailable, Doppler ultrasound provides an excellent alternative, though the information gleaned concerns mainly changes in blood flow caused by stenosis. Doppler ultrasound is not as sensitive as duplex ultrasonography; it has comparable specificity. When combined with the indirect information obtained by periorbital Doppler ultrasound—which detects collaterals in the periorbital circulation—its sensitivity may be increased. Doppler ultrasound does not identify anatomic abnormalities, however, as reliably as duplex ultrasound.

Arteriographic visualization of the cerebral vessels confirms the location and degree of stenoses and plaques, the presence of arterial occlusions, and the nature of collateral flow. Most often, both carotid and

vertebral-basilar systems are studied through a transfemoral percutaneous approach.

Treatment

A. Medical Measures: Acute strokes, most progressive or evolving strokes, and those with major neurologic deficits are treated by medical means as discussed in the section on cerebrovascular accidents in Chapter 18. Patients with transient ischemic attacks may be treated with antiplatelet drugs (aspirin, 100–325 mg/d, perhaps combined with dipyridamole, 50–75 mg/d) or with oral anticoagulants (see p 472), though there is now some evidence that the former are both safer and more effective than the latter, particularly in men.

B. Surgical Measures: Carotid endarterectomy, when expertly performed, may be offered for properly evaluated transient ischemic attacks. It is crucial that symptoms be specific for anterior circulation cerebral ischemia of recent origin and that the vascular surgeon be one who performs carotid endarterectomies regularly with a mortality-complication rate of less than 3%.

Recent studies indicate that the operative approach may now be more widely used than is warranted, considering the overall operative mortality and complication rates, and that it is often offered on marginal indications. It should be emphasized, therefore, that the best therapeutic approach to cerebral ischemia related to extracranial artery disease is still being formulated, and prospective double-blind studies now in progress in a number of centers may ultimately resolve these questions.

Considerable controversy exists as to whether surgery should be offered to patients with asymptomatic carotid bruits. Many surgeons believe that with increasing ability to evaluate stenosis noninvasively, it is possible to easily identify patients with high-grade stenosis who might theoretically be helped by prophylactic carotid endarterectomy. The best data available, however, indicate that with few exceptions, the risk of stroke in untreated patients with asymptomatic carotid bruits is less than the combined risk of carotid angiography and surgery if preventing stroke is the aim. About 2% of patients per year with such a bruit suffer a stroke; this approximates 3% if the stenosis exceeds 75%. Thus, the risk of causing stroke from angiography and surgery should be less than 3% if surgery is to be offered at all. The widespread variability in the skill of surgical teams has perhaps contributed to the nature of the controversy. It should also be noted that prophylactic carotid endarterectomy does not appear to alter the incidence of stroke complicating coronary artery bypass grafting. Stroke in this clinical setting may result from cardiac embolization and not from carotid disease.

Endarterectomy may be indicated as an emergency procedure in patients with very early and fluctuating neurologic deficits with significant carotid stenosis. It is not indicated in acute stroke or progressing stroke or when there is also severe intracranial disease.

Prognosis

The prognosis and results of therapy are related to the number of vessels involved, the degree of stenosis in each, and the collateral flow in the circle of Willis. Expertly performed surgery may have a mortality rate of 1–2% and with 1–4% permanent major or minor neurologic complications; there is wide institutional variation in these figures. Transient ischemic attacks known to be secondary to significant carotid artery stenosis or ulceration can often be eliminated by surgery, and although future strokes can occur in such patients, other arterial lesions, such as a contralateral carotid stenosis or intracranial arterial lesions, are often responsible. Concomitant coronary artery disease results in an overall mortality rate that is similar in operated and unoperated groups. In the best hands, the operative procedure in patients with transient ischemic attacks may reduce the chance of developing a permanent neurologic deficit within 5 years from 34–35% to 10%. The incidence of later stroke after uncomplicated endarterectomy is around 5–15%, and although restenosis may occur in the operated artery, it may not be clinically symptomatic. Significant carotid artery stenosis without symptoms entails no more than a 5–20% stroke risk over 3–5 years.

Feussner JR, Matchar DB: When and how to study the carotid arteries. Ann Intern Med 1988;109:805. (Superb overall review of the subject, recommending a conservative approach.)

Winslow CM et al: The appropriateness of carotid endarterectomy. N Engl J Med 1988;318:721. (A study indicating widespread overapplication of this operation and a high rate [10%] of major complications.)

VISCERAL ARTERY INSUFFICIENCY

Chronic intestinal ischemia generally results from atherosclerotic occlusive lesions at or close to the origins of the superior mesenteric, celiac, and inferior mesenteric arteries, leading to a significant reduction of blood flow to the intestines. Symptoms consist of epigastric or periumbilical postprandial pains that last for 1–3 hours. To avoid pain, the patient limits oral intake, and weight loss results; at this stage of the illness, pain may be absent. Diarrhea may be present. Such a history in a person over 45 years of age who appears chronically ill and who has peripheral arterial disease is probably an indication for arteriography if the patient is felt to be a candidate for surgery.

Acute intestinal ischemia results from (1) embolic occlusions of the visceral branches of the abdominal aorta, generally in patients with valvular heart disease or atrial fibrillation, or left ventricular mural thrombus; (2) thrombosis of one or more of the visceral vessels involved with arteriosclerotic occlusive changes, sometimes in patients with a history of abdominal angina as described in Chapter 11; or (3) nonocclusive mesenteric vascular insufficiency, generally in patients with congestive heart failure receiving digitalis therapy or in patients in shock. The acute onset of crampy or steady epigastric and periumbilical abdominal pain combined with minimal or no findings on abdominal examination and often a high leukocyte count should suggest one of these 3 events in the superior mesenteric system. Lactic acidosis, hypotension, and abdominal distention suggests bowel infarction rather than ischemia. Angiography of the superior mesenteric artery is essential for early diagnosis and should be performed promptly if surgery is contemplated. Mesenteric duplex scanning is a noninvasive technique for the anatomic and physiologic assessment of the visceral vessels and may be helpful in selecting patients for arteriography. If occlusion is present, antibiotics specific for intestinal flora should be instituted (eg, ampicillin and aminoglycoside plus clindamycin or metronidazole) and laparotomy should be performed to reestablish blood flow to the intestine if possible and remove necrotic bowel if at least some viable bowel exists.

Through early diagnosis and aggressive treatment, the very poor prognosis of the past should yield somewhat lower morbidity and mortality rates.

Ischemic colitis develops when the diminished circulation is most prominent in the distribution of the inferior mesenteric artery. Because of the nature of the collaterals, infarction is uncommon in this instance. However, the patient may have episodic bouts of crampy lower abdominal pain associated with mild diarrhea, often bloody. This picture may be indistinguishable from inflammatory bowel disease. Colonoscopy may reveal segmental inflammatory changes, most often in the rectosigmoid and the splenic flexure where the collateral circulation is most active. Because adequate collateral circulation usually develops, the prognosis is better than when the vascular insufficiency involves the superior mesenteric circulation, and maintenance of hydration may be all that is necessary (see also Chapter 11).

Jaxheimer EC et al: Chronic intestinal ischemia. Surg Clin North Am 1985;65:123.

Rapp JH et al: Durability of endarterectomy and antegrade grafts in the treatment of chronic visceral ischemia. J Vasc Surg 1986;3:799.

ACUTE ARTERIAL OCCLUSION

Essentials of Diagnosis

- Symptoms and signs depend on the artery occluded, the organ or region supplied by the artery, and the adequacy of the collateral circulation to the area primarily involved.

- Occlusion in an extremity usually results in pain, numbness, tingling, weakness, and coldness.
- There is pallor or mottling; motor, reflex, and sensory alteration; and collapsed superficial veins.
- Pulsations are absent in arteries distal to the occlusion. Occlusions in other areas result in such conditions as cerebrovascular accidents, intestinal ischemia and gangrene, and renal or splenic infarcts.

Differential Diagnosis

The primary differentiation is between arterial embolism and thrombosis. In an older individual with both arteriosclerotic vascular disease and cardiac disease, the differentiation may be very difficult, and in 10–20% a definite diagnosis either cannot be made or turns out to be incorrect. Arterial trauma may result in either occlusion or spasm.

1. ARTERIAL EMBOLISM

Arterial embolism is generally a complication of heart disease; a minority of those with embolism have rheumatic heart disease, but most have ischemic heart disease, with or without myocardial infarction. Atrial fibrillation is often present. Other forms of heart disease and miscellaneous causes account for the rest. In 10%, there is more than one embolism, and recurrent emboli after initial successful treatment may occur.

Emboli tend to lodge at the bifurcation of major arteries, with over half going to the aortic bifurcation or the vessels in the lower extremities; the carotid system is involved in 20%, and the upper extremity and the mesenteric arteries in the remainder. Emboli from arterial ulcerations are usually small, giving rise to transient symptoms in the toes or brain.

Clinical Findings

In an extremity, the initial symptoms are usually pain (sudden or gradual in onset), numbness, coldness, and tingling. Signs include absence of pulsations in the arteries distal to the block, coldness, pallor or mottling, hypesthesia or anesthesia, and weakness, muscle spasm, or paralysis. The superficial veins are collapsed. Later, blebs and skin necrosis may appear, and gangrene may occur.

Treatment

Immediate embolectomy is the treatment of choice in almost all early cases of emboli in extremities. It is best done within 4–6 hours after the embolic episode; it is occasionally successful after longer delays if the supplied tissue remains viable.

A. Emergency Preoperative Care:

1. Heparin–Heparin sodium, 5000 units intravenously, should be given as soon as the diagnosis is made or suspected in an effort to prevent distal thrombosis and continued until the time of surgery, maintaining the partial thromboplastin time (PTT) at twice

the normal level. It may also help relieve associated spasm.

2. Protect the part–The extremity is kept at or below the horizontal plane, and neither heat nor cold is applied. The limb must be protected from hard surfaces and overlying bedclothes.

3. Imaging–Arteriography is often of value either before or during surgery. There may be more than one embolus in an extremity. Echocardiography may confirm the source.

B. Surgical Measures: Local anesthesia is generally used if the occlusion is in an artery to an extremity. After the embolus is removed through the arteriotomy, the proximal and distal artery should be explored for additional emboli or secondary thrombi by means of a specially designed catheter with a small inflatable balloon at the tip (Fogarty catheter). An embolus at the aortic bifurcation or in the iliac artery can often be removed under local anesthesia through common femoral arteriotomies with the use of these same catheters. Laparotomy is necessary for emboli to the mesenteric circulation. Heparinization for a week or more postoperatively is indicated, and prolonged anticoagulation with warfarin is usually desirable after that to prevent recurrence.

Delayed embolectomy carried out more than 12 hours following the embolism or when there is ischemia or necrosis—as evidenced by mottled cyanosis, muscle rigidity, anesthesia, or markedly elevated serum CPK—involves a high risk of acute respiratory distress syndrome or acute renal failure. Anticoagulation rather than surgery or catheter embolectomy is the proper initial therapy under such circumstances, accepting urgent or elective amputation as the necessary lifesaving procedure in most instances.

Prognosis

Arterial embolism is a threat not only to the limb (5–25% amputation rate) but also to the life of the patient (25–30% hospital mortality rate, with the underlying heart disease responsible for over half of these deaths).

Emboli in the aortoiliac area are more dangerous than more peripheral emboli, and the mortality rate rises if there are multiple peripheral emboli or carotid or visceral emboli, approaching 100% if all 3 areas are involved. Emboli associated with hypertensive or arteriosclerotic heart disease have a poorer prognosis than those arising from rheumatic valvular disease.

In patients with atrial fibrillation, an attempt may be made to restore normal rhythm pharmacologically or by cardioversion after the patient has been anticoagulated; restoration of normal rhythm tends to be permanent only in patients with recent onset or transitory fibrillation. Long-term anticoagulant therapy diminishes the danger of further emboli and in the majority of patients is the only long-term prophylactic measure that can be instituted.

If no heart disease exists, arteriography may reveal

an arteriosclerotic ulcer or small aneurysm to be the origin of the embolus; depending upon location, these may be treated surgically. Three-fourths of the patients that do survive the embolic episode and the associated hospital stay may then have a good quality of life.

2. ACUTE ARTERIAL THROMBOSIS

Acute arterial thrombosis generally occurs in an artery in which the lumen has become narrow as a result of arteriosclerotic changes in the wall of the artery. Blood flowing through such a narrow, irregular, or ulcerated lumen may clot, leading to a sudden, complete occlusion of the narrow segment. The thrombosis may then propagate either up or down the artery to a point where the blood is flowing rapidly through a somewhat less diseased artery (usually to a significant arterial branch proximally or one or more functioning collateral vessels distally). Occasionally, the thrombosis is precipitated when the bloodstream dissects and displaces an arteriosclerotic plaque, blocking the lumen; trauma to the artery may precipitate a similar event. Inflammatory involvement of the arterial wall will also lead to acute thrombosis. Chronic mechanical irritation of the subclavian artery compressed by a cervical rib may also lead to a complete occlusion. Thrombosis in a diseased artery may be secondary to an episode of hypotension or cardiac failure. Polycythemia and dehydration also increase the chance of thrombosis, as do repeated arterial punctures.

Chronic, incomplete arterial obstruction usually results in the establishment of some collateral flow, and further flow will develop relatively rapidly through the collaterals once complete occlusion has developed. The extremity may be threatened for hours or days, however, while the additional collateral circulation develops around the block.

Clinical Findings

The local findings in the extremity are usually very similar to those described in the section on arterial embolism. The following differential points should be checked: (1) Are there manifestations of advanced occlusive arterial disease in other areas, especially the opposite extremity (bruit, absent pulses, secondary changes)? Is there a history of intermittent claudication? These clinical manifestations are suggestive but not diagnostic of thrombosis. (2) Is there a history or are there findings of rheumatic heart disease or of a recent episode of atrial fibrillation or myocardial infarction? If so, an embolism is more likely than a thrombosis. (3) Electrocardiography, echocardiography, and serum enzyme studies may give added information regarding the presence of a silent myocardial infarction and its likelihood as a source of an embolus. Ultimately, arteriography is necessary for accurate differential diagnosis and for planning therapy.

Treatment

Whereas emergency embolectomy is the usual approach in the case of an early occlusion from an embolus, a nonoperative approach is generally used in the case of thrombosis for 2 reasons: (1) The segment of thrombosed artery may be quite long, requiring rather extensive and difficult surgery (thromboendarterectomy or artery graft). The removal of a single embolus in a normal or nearly normal artery is, by comparison, relatively easy and quick. (2) The extremity is more likely to survive without development of gangrene because some collateral circulation has usually formed during the stenotic phase before acute thrombosis. With an embolism, this is not usually the case; the block is most often at a major arterial bifurcation, occluding both branches, and the associated arterial spasm is usually more acute. Treatment—particularly if tissue necrosis may be present—is as described for emergency preoperative care for arterial embolism. Thrombolytic therapy using streptokinase or the more expensive urokinase or tissue plasminogen activator (tPA) may be tried; if no tissue necrosis exists and in acute thrombosis, lysis may be achieved in 50–80% of cases, and direct arterial infusion has fewer bleeding complications than systemic therapy with these drugs. A complication and amputation rate of almost 20% and a mortality rate of 2% dictates caution in the use of this form of therapy. If successful thrombolysis occurs, rethrombosis may be prevented by angioplasty (see p 497). Otherwise, treatment is as outlined under emergency preoperative care for arterial embolism.

Prognosis

Limb survival usually occurs with acute thrombosis of the iliac or superficial femoral arteries; gangrene is more likely if the popliteal is suddenly occluded, especially if the period between occlusion and treatment is long or if there is considerable arterial spasm or proximal arterial occlusive disease. If the limb does survive the acute occlusion, significant functional recovery may occur gradually over a number of weeks. The later treatment and prognosis are outlined above in the section on occlusive disease of the iliac, femoral, and popliteal arteries.

THROMBOANGIITIS OBLITERANS (Buerger's Disease)

Essentials of Diagnosis

- Almost always in young men who smoke.
- Extremities involved with inflammatory occlusions of the more distal arteries, resulting in circulatory insufficiency of the toes or fingers.

● Thromboses of superficial veins may also occur.
● Course is intermittent and amputation may be necessary, especially if smoking is not stopped.

General Considerations

Buerger's disease is an episodic and segmental inflammatory and thrombotic process of the arteries and veins, principally in the limbs. The cause is not known. It is seen most commonly in men under 40 who smoke. The effects of the disease are almost solely due to occlusion of the arteries. The symptoms are primarily due to ischemia, complicated in the later stages by infection and tissue necrosis. The inflammatory process is intermittent, with quiescent periods lasting weeks, months, or years.

The arteries most commonly affected are the plantar and digital vessels in the foot and those in the lower leg. The arteries in the hands and wrists may also become involved. Different arterial segments may become occluded in successive episodes; a certain amount of recanalization occurs during quiescent periods. Superficial migratory thrombophlebitis is a common early indication of the disease.

Clinical Findings

The signs and symptoms are primarily those of arterial insufficiency, and the differentiation from arteriosclerotic peripheral vascular disease may be difficult; however, the following findings suggest Buerger's disease:

(1) The patient is a man under 40 who smokes.

(2) There is a history or finding of small, red, tender cords resulting from migratory superficial segmental thrombophlebitis, usually in the saphenous tributaries rather than the main vessel. A biopsy of such a vein often gives microscopic proof of Buerger's disease.

(3) Intermittent claudication is common and is frequently noted in the palm of the hand or arch of the foot. Rest pain is frequent and persistent. It tends to be more pronounced than in the patient with atherosclerosis. Numbness, diminished sensation, and pricking and burning pains may be present as a result of ischemic neuropathy.

(4) The digit or the entire distal portion of the foot may be pale and cold, or there may be rubor that may remain relatively unchanged by posture; the skin may not blanch on elevation, and on dependency the intensity of the rubor is often more pronounced than that seen in the atherosclerotic group. The distal vascular changes are often asymmetric, so that not all of the toes are affected to the same degree. Absence or impairment of pulsations in the dorsalis pedis, posterior tibial, ulnar, or radial artery is frequent.

(5) Trophic changes may be present, often with painful indolent ulcerations along the nail margins.

(6) There is usually evidence of disease in both legs and possibly also in the hands and lower arms.

There may be a history or findings of Raynaud's phenomenon in the finger or distal foot.

(7) The course is usually intermittent, with acute and often dramatic episodes followed by rather definite remissions. When the collateral vessels as well as the main channels have become occluded, an exacerbation is more likely to lead to gangrene and amputation. The course in the patient with atherosclerosis tends to be less dramatic and more persistent.

Differential Diagnosis

Differences between thromboangiitis obliterans and arteriosclerosis obliterans are discussed above.

Raynaud's disease causes symmetric bilateral color changes, primarily in young women. There is no impairment of arterial pulsations. Livedo reticularis and acrocyanosis are vasospastic diseases that do not affect peripheral pulsations; they do not show the early blanching of the digits seen in Raynaud's disease.

Treatment

The principles of therapy are the same as those outlined for atherosclerotic peripheral vascular disease, but the long-range outlook is better in patients with Buerger's disease, so that when possible the approach should be more conservative and tissue loss kept to a minimum.

A. General Measures: Smoking must be stopped; the physician must insist on it. The disease is almost sure to progress if this advice is not followed.

See the discussion of instructions in the care of the feet in Chapter 21.

B. Surgical Measures:

1. Sympathectomy–Sympathectomy may be useful in eliminating the vasospastic manifestations of the disease and aiding in the establishment of collateral circulation to the skin. It may also relieve the mild or moderate forms of rest pain. If amputation of a digit is necessary, sympathectomy may aid in healing of the surgical wound.

2. Amputation–The indications for amputation are similar in many respects to those outlined for the atherosclerotic group, although the approach should be more conservative from the point of view of preservation of tissue. Most patients with Buerger's disease who are managed carefully and who stop smoking do not require amputation of the fingers or toes. It is almost never necessary to amputate the entire hand, but amputation below the knee is occasionally necessary because of gangrene or severe pain in the foot.

Prognosis

Except in the case of the rapidly progressive form of the disease—and provided the patient stops smoking and takes good care of the feet—the prognosis for survival of the extremities is good.

IDIOPATHIC ARTERITIS OF TAKAYASU ("Pulseless Disease")

Pulseless disease, most frequent in young women, is an occlusive polyarteritis of unknown cause with a special predilection for the branches of the aortic arch. It occurs most commonly in Asians. Manifestations, depending upon the vessel or vessels involved, may include evidence of cerebrovascular insufficiency, with transient ischemic attacks and visual disturbances; and absent pulses in the arms, with a rich collateral flow in the shoulder, chest, and neck areas. The extent of the vascular involvement may be defined by angiography.

Pulseless disease must be differentiated from vascular lesions of the aortic arch due to atherosclerosis. Histologically, the arterial lesions are indistinguishable from those of giant cell arteritis. In the early stage of the disease, the progression of the vascular stenosis may be reversed by steroids; in the more advanced forms, bypass arterial grafts are necessary.

GIANT CELL ARTERITIS

This disorder is discussed in Chapter 15.

CHOLESTEROL ATHEROEMBOLIC DISEASE

In some patients with severe atherosclerosis involving the aorta and its branches, a distinct syndrome resulting from repeated microembolization has been observed. This syndrome occurs spontaneously following transfemoral aortographic procedures. Patients complain of pain in the abdomen and legs and of mottled lower extremities. Physical examination reveals cholesterol plaques in the optic fundi, livedo reticularis, and reduced arterial pulses (with or without bruits). Laboratory investigations disclose microhematuria, renal insufficiency, eosinophilia, and an accelerated sedimentation rate. Biopsies of the kidney and other tissues show cholesterol clefts in the small vessels.

Although no specific therapy exists, it is important to recognize this disease, since misdiagnosis of systemic vasculitis may result in inappropriate use of immunomodulating drugs.

VASOMOTOR DISORDERS

RAYNAUD'S DISEASE & RAYNAUD'S PHENOMENON

Essentials of Diagnosis

- Paroxysmal bilateral symmetric pallor and cyanosis followed by rubor of the skin of the digits.
- Precipitated by cold or emotional upset; relieved by warmth.
- Primarily a disorder of young women.

General Considerations

Raynaud's disease is the primary, or idiopathic, form of paroxysmal digital cyanosis. Raynaud's phenomenon, which is more common than Raynaud's disease, may be due to a number of regional or systemic disorders. In Raynaud's disease the digital arteries respond excessively to vasospastic stimuli. The cause is not known, but some abnormality of the sympathetic nervous system seems to be active in this entity.

Clinical Findings

Raynaud's disease and Raynaud's phenomenon are characterized by intermittent attacks of pallor or cyanosis—or pallor followed by cyanosis—in the fingers (and rarely the toes), precipitated by cold or occasionally by emotional upsets. In early attacks of Raynaud's phenomenon, only 1–2 fingertips may be affected; as it progresses, all the fingers down to the distal palm may be involved. The thumbs are rarely affected. During recovery there may be intense rubor, throbbing, paresthesia, and slight swelling. Attacks usually terminate spontaneously or upon returning to a warm room or putting the extremity in warm water. Between attacks there are no abnormal findings. Sensory changes that often accompany vasomotor manifestations include numbness, stiffness, diminished sensation, and aching pain. The condition may progress to atrophy of the terminal fat pads and the digital skin, and gangrenous ulcers may appear near the fingertips; they may heal during warm weather.

Raynaud's disease appears first between ages 15 and 45, almost always in women. It tends to be progressive, and, unlike Raynaud's phenomenon (which may be unilateral and may involve only 1–2 fingers), symmetric involvement of the fingers of both hands is the rule. Spasm becomes more frequent and prolonged.

Raynaud's disease may be diagnosed if the phenomenon persists for greater than 3 years without evidence of an associated disease (see below). There are no specific laboratory abnormalities; the diagnosis is a clinical one, though studies to exclude the conditions associated with Raynaud's disease are warranted.

Differential Diagnosis

Raynaud's disease must be differentiated from the numerous disorders that may be associated with Raynaud's phenomenon. The history and examination lead to the diagnosis of rheumatoid arthritis, systemic sclerosis, systemic lupus erythematosus, and mixed connective tissue disease, with which Raynaud's phenomenon is commonly associated. Raynaud's phenomenon is occasionally the first manifestation of these disorders.

The differentiation from thromboangiitis obliterans is usually not difficult, since thromboangiitis obliterans is generally a disease of men; peripheral pulses are often diminished or absent; and, when Raynaud's phenomenon occurs in association with thromboangiitis obliterans, it is usually in only one or 2 digits.

Raynaud's phenomenon may occur in patients with the thoracic outlet syndromes. In these disorders, involvement is generally unilateral, and symptoms referable to brachial plexus compression tend to dominate the clinical picture. Carpal tunnel syndrome should also be considered, and nerve conduction tests are appropriate in selected cases.

In acrocyanosis, cyanosis of the hands is permanent and diffuse. Frostbite may lead to chronic Raynaud's phenomenon. Ergot poisoning, particularly due to prolonged or excessive use of ergotamine, must also be considered.

Finally, Raynaud's phenomenon may be mimicked by cryoglobulinemia, in which serum proteins aggregate in the cooler distal circulation. Cryoglobulinemia may be idiopathic or associated with multiple myeloma and other hyperglobulinemic states.

Treatment

A. General Measures: The body should be kept warm, and the hands especially should be protected from exposure to cold; gloves should be worn when out in the cold. The hands should be protected from injury at all times; wounds heal slowly, and infections are consequently hard to control. Softening and lubricating lotion to control the fissured dry skin should be applied to the hands frequently. Smoking should be stopped.

B. Vasodilators: Vasodilators drugs are of limited value but may be of some benefit in those patients who are not adequately controlled by general measures and when there is peripheral vasoconstriction without significant organic vascular disease. With the relatively large doses used, side effects are troublesome. Shortening of temperature recovery time may occur with the use of reserpine, methyldopa, topical nitroglycerin (Transderm-Nitro 5) or a longer-acting oral nitrate, or phenoxybenzamine. Recently, nifedipine has been employed with good effect in the treatment of Raynaud's phenomenon and disease. It may be preferable to other medical measures.

C. Surgical Measures: Sympathectomy may be indicated when attacks have become frequent and severe, interfering with work and well-being—and particularly if trophic changes have developed and medical measures have failed. In the lower extremities, complete and permanent relief may result, whereas dorsal sympathectomies generally result in only temporary improvement in most patients treated with operation. Although vascular tone of the vessels in the hands usually ultimately reappears, the symptoms in the fingers that may thus recur in 1–5 years are usually milder and less frequent. Sympathectomies are of very limited value in far-advanced cases, particularly if significant digital artery obstructive disease with scleroderma is present.

Prognosis

Raynaud's disease is usually benign, causing mild discomfort on exposure to cold and progressing very slightly over the years. In a few cases rapid progression does occur, so that the slightest change in temperature may precipitate color changes. It is in this situation that sclerodactyly and small areas of gangrene may be noted, and such patients may become quite disabled by severe pain, limitation of motion, and secondary fixation of distal joints. The prognosis of Raynaud's phenomenon is that of the associated disease.

LIVEDO RETICULARIS

Livedo reticularis is an uncommon vasospastic disorder of unknown cause that results in constant mottled discoloration on large areas of the extremities, generally in a fishnet pattern with reticulated cyanotic areas surrounding a paler central core. It occurs primarily in young women. It may be associated with an occult malignant neoplasm, polyarteritis nodosa, or atherosclerotic microemboli to the skin.

Livedo reticularis is most apparent on the thighs and forearms and occasionally on the lower abdomen and is most pronounced in cold weather. The color may change to a reddish hue in warm weather but does not entirely disappear. A few patients complain of paresthesias, coldness, or numbness in the involved areas. Recurrent ulcers in the lower extremities may occur in severe cases.

Bluish mottling of the extremities is diagnostic. The peripheral pulses are normal. The extremity may be cold, with increased perspiration.

Treatment consists of protection from exposure to cold; use of vasodilators is seldom indicated. In most instances, livedo reticularis is entirely benign. The rare patient who develops ulcerations or gangrene should be studied for underlying systemic disease.

ACROCYANOSIS

Acrocyanosis is an uncommon symmetric condition that involves the skin of the hands and feet and, to a lesser degree, the forearms and legs. It is associated with arteriolar vasoconstriction combined with dilatation of the subpapillary venous plexus of the skin, through which deoxygenated blood slowly circulates. It is worse in cold weather but does not completely disappear during the warm season. It occurs in either sex, is most common in the teens and 20s, and usually improves with advancing age or during pregnancy. It is characterized by coldness, sweating, slight edema, and cyanotic discoloration of the involved areas. Pain, trophic lesions, and disability do not occur, and the peripheral pulses are present. The individual may thus be reassured and encouraged to dress warmly in cold weather.

ERYTHROMELALGIA

Erythromelalgia is a paroxysmal bilateral vasodilative disorder of unknown cause. Idiopathic (primary) erythromelalgia occurs in otherwise healthy persons, rarely in children, and affects men and women equally. A secondary type is occasionally seen in patients with polycythemia vera, hypertension, gout, and organic neurologic diseases.

The chief symptom is bilateral burning distress that lasts minutes to hours, involving circumscribed areas on the soles or palms first and, as the disease progresses, the entire extremity. The attack occurs in response to stimuli producing vasodilatation (eg, exercise, warm environment), especially at night when the extremities are warmed under bedclothes. Reddening or cyanosis as well as heat may be noted. Relief may be obtained by cooling the affected part and by elevation.

No findings are generally present between attacks. With onset of an attack, heat and redness are noted in association with the typical pain. Skin temperature and arterial pulsations are increased, and the involved areas may sweat profusely.

In primary erythromelalgia, aspirin may give excellent relief. The patient should avoid warm environments. In severe cases, if medical measures fail, section or crushing of peripheral nerves may be necessary to relieve pain.

Primary idiopathic erythromelalgia is uniformly benign.

POSTTRAUMATIC SYMPATHETIC DYSTROPHY (Causalgia)

Essentials of Diagnosis

- Burning or aching pain following trauma to an extremity of a severity greater than that expected from the initiating injury.
- Manifestations of vasomotor instability are generally present and include temperature, color, and texture alterations of the skin of the involved extremity.

General Considerations

Pain—usually burning or aching—in an injured extremity is the single most common finding, and the disparity between the severity of the inciting injury and the degree of pain experienced is the most charac-

teristic feature. Crushing injuries with lacerations and soft tissue destruction are the most common causes, but closed fractures, simple lacerations, burns (especially electric), and elective operative procedures are also responsible for this syndrome. It is rare in children. The manifestations of pain and the associated objective changes may be relatively mild or quite severe, and the initial manifestations often change if the condition proceeds to a chronic stage.

Clinical Findings

In the early stages, the pain, tenderness, and hyperesthesia may be strictly localized to the injured area, and the extremity may be warm, dry, swollen, and red or slightly cyanotic. The involved extremity is held in a splinted position by the muscles, and the nails may become ridged and the hair long. In advanced stages, the pain is more diffuse and worse at night; the extremity becomes cool and clammy and intolerant of temperature changes (particularly cold); and the skin becomes glossy and atrophic. The joints become stiff, generally in a position that makes the extremity useless. The bones become osteoporotic. The dominant concern of the patient may be to avoid the slightest stimuli to the extremity and especially to the trigger points that may develop.

Prevention

During operations on an extremity, peripheral nerves should be handled only when absolutely necessary and then with utmost gentleness. Splinting of an injured extremity for an adequate period during the early, painful phase of recovery, together with adequate analgesics, may help prevent this condition.

Treatment & Prognosis

A. Conservative Measures: It is most important that the condition be recognized and treated in the early stages, when the manifestations are most easily reversed and major secondary changes have not yet developed. In mild, early cases with minimal skin and joint changes, physical therapy involving active and passive exercises combined with diazepam, 2 mg twice daily, may relieve symptoms. Protecting the extremity from irritating stimuli is important, and the use of nonaddicting analgesics may be necessary.

B. Surgical Measures: If the condition fails to respond to conservative treatment or if there are more severe or advanced objective findings, sympathetic blocks (stellate ganglion or lumbar) may be helpful. Intensive physical therapy may be used during the pain-free periods following effective blocks. Patients who achieve significant temporary relief of symptoms after sympathetic blocks but fail to obtain permanent relief by the blocks may be cured by sympathectomy. In the advanced forms—particularly in association with major local changes and emotional reactions—the prognosis for a useful life is poor. The newer neurosurgical approaches using implantable electronic biostimulator devices to block pain impulses in the cervical spinal cord have met with some success.

Garrett WV et al: Posttraumatic pain syndromes: Causalgia and mimocausalgia. In: *Vascular Surgery: Principles and Practice.* Wilson SE, Williams RA (editors). McGraw-Hill, 1987.

VENOUS DISEASES

VARICOSE VEINS

Essentials of Diagnosis
- Dilated, tortuous superficial veins in the lower extremities.
- May be asymptomatic or may be associated with fatigue, aching discomfort, or pain.
- Edema, pigmentation, and ulceration of the skin of the distal leg may develop.
- Increased frequency after pregnancy.

General Considerations
Varicose veins develop predominantly in the lower extremities. They consist of abnormally dilated, elongated, and tortuous alterations in the saphenous veins and their tributaries. These vessels lie immediately beneath the skin and superficial to the deep fascia; they therefore do not have as adequate support as the veins deep in the leg, which are surrounded by muscles. An inherited defect seems to play a major role in the development of varicosities in many instances, but it is not known whether the basic valvular incompetence that exists is secondary to defective valves in the saphenofemoral veins or to a fundamental weakness of the walls of the vein, resulting in dilatation of the vessel. Periods of high venous pressure related to prolonged standing or heavy lifting are contributing factors, and the highest incidence is in women who have been pregnant. Fifteen percent of adults develop varicosities.

Secondary varicosities can develop as a result of obstructive changes and valve damage in the deep venous system following thrombophlebitis, or occasionally as a result of proximal venous occlusion due to neoplasm. Congenital or acquired arteriovenous fistulas are also associated with varicosities.

The long saphenous vein and its tributaries are most commonly involved, but the short saphenous vein may also be affected. There may be one or many incompetent perforating veins in the thigh and lower leg, so that blood can reflux into the varicosities not only from above, by way of the saphenofemoral junction, but also from the deep system of veins through the incompetent perforators in the mid thigh or lower leg. Largely because of these valvular defects in the most proximal valve of the long saphenous vein or in the distal communicating veins, venous pressure in the superficial veins does not fall appreciably on walking; over the years, the veins progressively enlarge, and the surrounding tissue and skin develop secondary changes such as fibrosis, chronic edema, and skin pigmentation and atrophy.

Clinical Findings
A. Symptoms: The severity of the symptoms caused by varicose veins is not necessarily correlated with the number and size of the varicosities; extensive varicose veins may produce no subjective symptoms, whereas minimal varicosities may produce many symptoms, especially in women. Dull, aching heaviness or a feeling of fatigue brought on by periods of standing is the most common complaint. Cramps may occur, often at night, and elevation of the legs typically relieves symptoms. One must be careful to distinguish between the symptoms of arteriosclerotic peripheral vascular disease, such as intermittent claudication and coldness of the feet, and symptoms of venous disease, since occlusive arterial disease usually contraindicates the operative treatment of varicosities distal to the knee. Itching from an associated eczematoid dermatitis may occur above the ankle.

B. Signs: Dilated, tortuous, elongated veins beneath the skin in the thigh and leg are generally readily visible in the standing individual, although in very obese patients palpation may be necessary to detect their presence and location. Secondary tissue changes may be absent even in extensive varicosities; but if the varicosities are of long duration, brownish pigmentation and thinning of the skin above the ankle are often present. Swelling may occur, but signs of severe chronic venous stasis such as extensive swelling, fibrosis, pigmentation, and ulceration of the distal lower leg usually denote the postphlebitic state. Doppler ultrasonography or the duplex scanner is useful diagnostically in detecting the precise location of incompetent valves, allowing reflux of blood from the femoral, popliteal, or more peripheral deep veins into the superficial veins; such knowledge allows more precise corrective surgery with better results.

Differential Diagnosis
Primary varicose veins should be differentiated from those secondary to (1) chronic venous insufficiency of the deep system of veins (the postphlebitic syndrome); (2) retroperitoneal vein obstruction from extrinsic pressure or fibrosis; (3) arteriovenous fistula (congenital or acquired)—a bruit is present and a thrill is often palpable; and (4) congenital venous malformation. Pain or discomfort secondary to arthritis, radiculopathy, or arterial insufficiency should be distinguished from symptoms associated with coexistent varicose veins.

Complications

If thin, atrophic, pigmented skin has developed at or above the ankle, secondary ulcerations may occur—often as a result of little or no trauma. An ulcer will occasionally extend into the varix, and the resulting fistula will be associated with profuse hemorrhage unless the leg is elevated and local pressure is applied to the bleeding point.

Chronic stasis dermatitis with fungal and bacterial infection may be a problem.

Thrombophlebitis may develop in the varicosities, particularly in postoperative patients, pregnant or postpartum women, or those taking oral contraceptives. Local trauma or prolonged periods of sitting may also lead to superficial venous thrombosis. Extension of the thrombosis into the deep venous system by way of the perforating veins or through the saphenofemoral junction may occur, resulting in deep thrombophlebitis and the risk of pulmonary embolism.

Treatment

A. Nonsurgical Measures: The use of elastic stockings (medium or heavy weight) to give external support to the veins of the proximal foot and leg up to but not including the knee is the best nonoperative approach to the management of varicose veins. These may be useful in early varicosities as well, in preventing progression of disease. When elastic stockings are worn during the hours that involve much standing and when this is combined with the habit of elevation of the legs when possible, reasonably good control can be maintained and progression of the condition and the development of complications can often be avoided. This approach may be used in elderly patients, in those who refuse or wish to defer surgery, sometimes in women with mild or moderate varicosities who plan to have more children, and in those with mild asymptomatic varicosities.

B. Surgical Measures: The surgical treatment of varicose veins consists of interruption or removal of the varicosities and the incompetent perforating veins. Accurate delineation and division of the latter are required to prevent formation of recurrent varicosities in previously uninvolved veins. Venous segments that are not demonstrated to be incompetent and varicosed should not be ligated or removed; they may be needed as artery grafts later in the patient's life.

Varicose ulcers that are small generally heal with local care, frequent periods of elevation of the extremity, and compression bandages or some form of compression boot dressing for the ambulatory patient. It is best to defer a stripping procedure until healing has been achieved and stasis dermatitis has been controlled. Some ulcers require skin grafting.

C. Compression Sclerotherapy: Sclerotherapy to obliterate and produce permanent fibrosis of the involved veins is generally reserved for the treatment of residual small varicosities following definitive varicose vein surgery. The injection of the sclerosing solution into the varicosed vein is followed by a period of compression of the segment, resulting in obliteration of the vein. Complications such as phlebitis, tissue necrosis, or infection may occur, and vary in incidence with the skill of the operator.

Prognosis

Patients should be informed that even extensive and carefully performed surgery may not prevent the development of additional varicosities and that further (though usually more limited) surgery or scleropathy may become necessary. Good results with relief of symptoms are usually obtained in most patients. If extensive varicosities reappear after surgery, the completeness of the high ligation should be questioned, and reexploration of the saphenofemoral area may be necessary. Even after adequate treatment, secondary tissue changes may not regress.

THROMBOPHLEBITIS

Thrombophlebitis is partial or complete occlusion of a vein by a thrombus with secondary inflammatory reaction in the wall of the vein. Trauma to the endothelium of the vein wall resulting in exposure of subendothelial tissues to platelets in the venous blood may initiate thrombosis, especially if a degree of venous stasis also exists. Platelet aggregates form on the vein wall followed by the deposition of fibrin, leukocytes, and finally erythrocytes; a thrombus results that can then propagate along the veins as a free-floating clot. Within 7–10 days, this thrombus becomes adherent to the vein wall, and secondary inflammatory changes develop, although a free-floating tail may persist. The thrombus is ultimately invaded by fibroblasts, resulting in scarring of the vein wall and destruction of the valves. Central recanalization may occur later, with restoration of flow through the vein; however, because the valves do not recover function, directional flow is not reestablished, leading in turn to secondary functional and anatomic problems.

1. THROMBOPHLEBITIS OF THE DEEP VEINS

Essentials of Diagnosis

- Pain in the calf or thigh, occasionally associated with swelling; alternatively, there may be no symptoms.
- History of congestive heart failure, recent surgery, neoplasia, oral contraceptive use, or varicose veins; prolonged inactivity also predisposes.
- Physical signs unreliable.
- Ultrasound and plethysmography are abnormal; venography is diagnostic.

General Considerations

The deep veins of the lower extremities and pelvis are most frequently involved. The process begins approximately 80% of the time in the deep veins of the calf, although it can arise in the femoral or iliac veins. When the process begins in the calf, propagation into the popliteal and femoral veins takes place in approximately 10% of these cases. About 3% of patients undergoing major general surgical procedures will develop clinical manifestations of thrombophlebitis, which may develop up to 2 weeks postoperatively; many others with the process will have no detectable findings. Certain operations, such as total hip replacement, are associated with appreciably higher incidences of thromboembolic complications. Illnesses that involve periods of bed rest, such as cardiac failure or stroke, are associated with a high incidence of thrombophlebitis. Use of oral contraceptive drugs, especially by women over 30 and by those who smoke, may be associated with hypercoagulability, resulting in thrombophlebitis in some women. These drugs should not be prescribed for women with a history of phlebitis. Hypercoagulability is also observed in cancer, particularly adenocarcinoma.

Clinical Findings

Approximately half of patients with thrombophlebitis have no symptoms or signs in the extremity in the early stages. The patient may suffer a pulmonary embolism, presumably from the leg veins, without symptoms or demonstrable abnormalities in the extremities.

A. Symptoms: The patient may complain of a dull ache, a tight feeling, or frank pain in the calf or, in more extensive cases, the whole leg, especially when walking.

B. Signs: Typical findings, though variable and unreliable and in about half of cases absent, are as follows: slight swelling in the involved calf, distention of the superficial venous collaterals; and slight fever and tachycardia. Any of these signs may occur without deep vein thrombosis. When the femoral and iliac veins are also involved, there may be tenderness over these veins, and the swelling in the extremity may be marked. The skin may be cyanotic if venous obstruction is severe, or pale and cool if a reflex arterial spasm is superimposed.

C. Diagnostic Techniques: Because of the difficulty in making a precise diagnosis by history and examination and because of the morbidity associated with treatment, diagnostic studies are essential.

1. Ascending contrast venography, the most accurate method of diagnosis, will define the location, extent, and degree of attachment of the thrombosis (thrombi in the profunda femoris and internal iliac veins will not be demonstrated). Because of the time, expense, and discomfort involved, this test is not used as a screening study and is unsuitable for repeated monitoring. It is particularly useful when the clinical picture strongly suggests calf vein thromboses but noninvasive tests are equivocal. It may on occasion produce or exacerbate a thrombotic process, but this occurs in less than 5% of patients.

2. The Doppler ultrasound blood flow detector allows the major veins in an extremity to be examined for thrombosis. This test is of value as a rapid screening procedure for the detection of thrombosis in large veins in high-risk patients, and it may be particularly helpful in detecting an extension of small thrombi in the calf veins into the popliteal and femoral veins. This test is inexpensive but operator-dependent; it relies on sonic differences in flow rates that occur with inspiration in normal veins. Incompetent venous valves in the legs may also be inferred from this investigation. Impedance plethysmography may similarly be used to detect the alteration of venous flow by obstruction of thrombi. High-resolution real time B-mode ultrasonography for detection of thrombosis may be used rather than phlebography to confirm positive or equivocal findings of plethysmography. These examinations may miss small thrombi in the calf veins when collateral channels are present. Because the accuracy of these methods in detecting main channel deep venous obstruction approaches 85–95%, the decision to start anticoagulation therapy can be based in most cases on one or more of these tests.

3. Radionuclide venography may be performed at the time of lung scanning. The isotope may be injected into a foot vein and immediate views obtained as the radionuclide moves up the circulation. In venous thrombosis, isotope accumulates at the clot and is not cleared. This test may also detect intra-abdominal venous thrombi—an advantage over Doppler ultrasound and plethysmography.

Differential Diagnosis

Calf muscle strain or contusion may be difficult to differentiate from thrombophlebitis; phlebography may be required to determine the correct diagnosis.

Cellulitis may be confused with thrombophlebitis; with infection, there is usually an associated wound, and inflammation of the skin is more marked.

Obstruction of the lymphatics or the iliac vein in the retroperitoneal area from tumor or irradiation may lead to unilateral swelling, but it is usually more chronic and painless. An acute arterial occlusion is more painful, the distal pulses are absent, there is usually no swelling, and the superficial veins in the foot fill slowly when emptied.

Bilateral leg edema is more likely to be due to heart or kidney disease.

Occasionally, a ruptured Baker cyst may produce unilateral pain and swelling in the calf. A history of arthritis in the knee of the same leg is a clue to diagnosis, and the patient may report disappearance of the popliteal cyst at the time symptoms develop.

Complications

A. Pulmonary Thromboembolism: See p 346.

B. Chronic Venous Insufficiency: Chronic venous insufficiency with or without secondary varicosities is a late complication of deep thrombophlebitis. (See Chronic Venous Insufficiency.)

Prevention

Prophylactic measures may diminish the incidence of venous thrombosis in hospitalized patients.

A. Nonpharmacologic Means: Venous stasis may be avoided by the following measures-

1. Elevation of the foot of the bed 15–20 degrees will encourage venous flow from the legs, particularly if the head of the bed is kept low or horizontal. Slight flexion of the knees is desirable. This position is also maintained on the operating table and in the recovery room. Sitting in a chair in the early postoperative period should be avoided.

2. Leg exercises, carried out by the surgical team immediately following major surgery and during the early postoperative period and practiced by the patient when in bed, are important. Intermittent pneumatic compression of the legs may be used prophylactically and may be the preventive measure of choice in patients in whom all anticoagulants are contraindicated, such as in patients undergoing neurosurgery.

3. Elastic antiphlebitic stockings may be employed, particularly in patients with varicose veins or a history of phlebitis who will require bed rest for a number of days. Walking for brief but regular periods postoperatively and during long airplane and automobile trips should be encouraged.

B. Anticoagulation: Anticoagulants may be used in patients considered at high risk for venous thrombosis.

1. Low-dose heparin, 5000 units every 12 hours subcutaneously 2 hours preoperatively and during the postoperative period of bed rest and limited ambulation, appears to be effective in reducing the incidence of thromboembolic complications in moderate-risk patients, although its effectiveness in major pelvic and hip procedures has been disappointing for these high-risk patients. Adjusted-dose heparin to a PTT in the upper half of the normal range—or warfarin to a PT 1.3–1.5 times control—is recommended.

2. Aspirin, 150 mg daily, may have a prophylactic value when used both pre- and postoperatively.

Treatment

A. Local Measures: As for prophylaxis, the legs should be elevated 15–20 degrees, the trunk should be kept horizontal, and the head and shoulders may be supported with pillows. The legs should be slightly flexed at the knees. Bed rest should be maintained until local tenderness and swelling have disappeared, by which time the thrombus has generally become adherent to the vein wall; a week may be adequate for calf thrombosis and 10–14 days for thigh or pelvic thrombosis. Walking but not standing or sitting is then permitted; the time out of bed and walking is increased each day.

B. Medical Measures (Anticoagulants): Therapy with anticoagulants is considered to be the preferred treatment in most cases of deep thrombophlebitis with or without pulmonary embolism. There is evidence that the incidence of fatal pulmonary embolism secondary to venous thrombosis is reduced by adequate anticoagulant therapy, and the incidence of death from additional emboli following an initial embolism is reduced. Progressive thrombosis with its associated morbidity is also reduced considerably, and the chronic secondary changes in the involved leg are probably also less severe. Heparin acts rapidly and must be considered the anticoagulant of choice for short-term therapy; hospitalization is generally necessary. After the initial phase of therapy with heparin, and if a prolonged period of anticoagulation is advisable, an oral drug can be used.

Treatment with heparin does not affect thrombi that have already developed but stops propagation and allows fibrinolysis to occur. The duration of therapy is purely an empirical decision—most clinicians administer heparin for 7–10 days and oral anticoagulants for at least 12 weeks, but data to support these regimens are sparse. Permanent anticoagulation may be considered if the stimulus to thrombosis is chronic—eg, congestive heart failure, postphlebitic syndrome—or if previous episodes have occurred. As experience with thrombolysis develops (see below), it may replace heparin as the treatment of first choice.

1. Heparin—Before starting heparin therapy, baseline coagulation studies should be obtained that should include a prothrombin time, a partial thromboplastin time, a bleeding time, a blood urea nitrogen measurement, and a platelet count. The therapeutic range of the commonly used partial thromboplastin time (PTT) is considered to be 1 1/2–2 times the baseline pretreatment value. Because the test can be done easily, any necessary adjustment in the heparin dose can be made immediately. Serious bleeding complications, such as bleeding into the brain or retroperitoneum, are more likely to occur in patients with other serious concomitant illnesses; in patients over age 60 (especially women); in patients with hypertension, uremia, hemostatic defects, or duodenal ulcer; or in patients who have had recent trauma or surgery.

The dose of heparin required to maintain the PTT at a therapeutic level may vary considerably with individuals or even in the same patient at different times during the course of treatment. The required dose is typically highest within the first days of therapy. Platelet counts should be performed every 2–3 days, and if thrombocytopenia develops, heparin should be discontinued. A hematocrit and a test on urine and stool for occult blood every 2–3 days may help detect bleeding. Aspirin and similar anti-inflammatory drugs and intramuscular medication should be avoided during heparin therapy.

Continuous intravenous infusion of heparin by means of a reliable infusion pump is favored over intermittent intravenous or subcutaneous therapy. Before starting the constant infusion, an initial loading dose of heparin should be given intravenously as a bolus (100 units/kg is often used). The constant infusion may then be started so that the average-sized adult receives 1000 units of heparin per hour (250–500 mL of 5% dextrose solution containing 100 units/mL is a convenient concentration), and the hourly dose is subsequently adjusted depending on laboratory determinations performed every 2–3 hours on blood drawn from the arm not being infused. A heparin algorithm combined with an easily interpreted flow-chart giving specific instructions with respect to the volume per hour required to deliver the desired dose of heparin is a great help to personnel who administer this potentially dangerous drug. After a stable infusion rate has been achieved, as determined by at least 2 successive PTTs in the therapeutic range, subsequent laboratory control may be repeated every 8–12 hours or possibly less often if a stable state develops. The therapeutic dose of heparin usually becomes less within 2–4 days. If longer-term anticoagulation is being contemplated, warfarin in doses of 10 mg daily may be given during the last 4 days of heparin use.

Rare patients may develop paradoxic hypercoagulability when treated with heparin.

2. Oral anticoagulants–The shift to the prothrombin depressant drugs usually occurs after the symptoms and signs of thrombosis have largely or completely subsided and after the patient becomes ambulatory. Prothrombin depressant drugs include coumarin and indandione derivatives; of these, warfarin sodium (Coumadin) is most commonly used now. The dose during the first 48 hours of therapy is usually 10–15 mg/d. The usual maintenance dose is 2.5–7.5 mg daily and must be determined for each individual patient. The approximate duration of effect of the drug is 2–3 days. A pretreatment prothrombin time should be determined, and if it is prolonged as compared with the control value, less drug should be used. Smaller doses should be used in the elderly, in patients with kidney or liver disease, and in those with congestive heart failure or chronic illness. These drugs are contraindicated during pregnancy. Interaction with many other drugs does occur, and the anticoagulant effect may be either potentiated or reduced; this possibility must be considered if the individual is already receiving other drugs at the time the anticoagulant is started. Attention to the maintenance dose is also required when a new drug which enhances or inhibits the anticoagulant effect is added or one which was in use is withdrawn. Many of the drugs that increase and decrease the sensitivity to coumarins are listed in Table 9–1.

A good therapeutic effect can usually be achieved

Table 9–1. Some drugs affecting prothrombin time (Quick one-stage test) of patients receiving anticoagulant therapy with coumarin or phenindione derivatives.

Prothrombin Time Increased By	Prothrombin Time Decreased By
Acetaminophen	Aminoglutethimide
Allopurinol	Antihistamines
p-Aminosalicyclic acid	Azathioprine
Amiodarone	Barbiturates
Androgens	Carbamazepine
Antibiotics (tetracyclines,	Contraceptives, oral
some cephalosporins [es-	Cyclophosphamide
pecially cefamandole, cefa-	Digitalis (in cardiac failure)
perazone, moxalactam],	Diuretics
erythromycin, chloram-	Ethchlorvynol
phenicol, metronidazole,	Glutethimide
sulfonamides)	Griseofulvin
Chloral hydrate	Mercaptopurine
Cholestyramine	Phenytoin
Cimetidine	Rifampin
Clofibrate	Vitamin K (in polyvitamin prep-
Disulfiram	arations and some diets)
Glucagon	Xanthines (eg, caffeine)
Heparin (Quick test increased;	
no effect on prothrombin-	
proconvertin [P and P] test)	
Hydroxyzine	
Indomethacin	
Mefenamic acid	
Methimazole	
Metronidazole	
Nalidixic acid	
Naproxen	
Oxyphenbutazone	
Phenylbutazone	
Phenyramidol	
Phenytoin	
Propylthiouracil	
Quinidine	
Quinine	
Salicylates (>3 to 5 g/d)	
Sulfinpyrazone	
Thyroid hormones	
Tricyclic antidepressants	

in 3–5 days and exists when the prothrombin time is around 1.3–1.5 times the control value. Further prolongation of the prothrombin time may result in bleeding complications (ie, hematuria, ecchymosis, epistaxis, gastrointestinal bleeding); even within the therapeutic range, complications are less common when prothrombin time is near 11/2 times control, without loss of benefit in most circumstances. At the beginning of treatment, daily prothrombin times should be determined and the subsequent dose withheld until the report is received. In well-stabilized patients, weekly to monthly determination may be adequate.

3. Treatment of bleeding and overdosage– Any new development that occurs in a patient receiving anticoagulant therapy should be considered to be a complication of the anticoagulant until proved otherwise. Bleeding complications will occur in at least 3% and death will result in 0.3% of patients receiving oral anticoagulants; the incidence of complications is higher with heparin. Complications appear most frequently after the first 3 days of heparin; they are infrequent when heparin is being given while diagnostic studies are in progress to determine whether thrombophlebitis or pulmonary embolization is present. The vitamin K analogue phytonadione (Mephyton (oral) or AquaMephyton (intravenous)) will counteract the effect of prothrombin depressant drugs, and if transfusion is necessary, fresh frozen plasma should be used. When the vitamin K analogues are given subcutaneously, their duration of action may be very long. Thus, if reanticoagulation is contemplated, intravenous phytonadione in low dosage (1 mg) should be used. When gastrointestinal or urologic bleeding occurs in a patient receiving anticoagulant therapy, investigation for a responsible anatomic lesion is mandated.

4. Thrombolytic therapy–The ideal treatment for thrombophlebitis involving the iliac, femoral, or popliteal veins or for a major pulmonary embolism would involve removal of the thrombus and restoration of blood flow through vessels that have been cleaned of the thrombus with little or no damage to their walls or valves. Heparin will not remove a thrombus and only serves to halt an ongoing thrombotic process. Streptokinase and urokinase are potent thrombolytic agents and may clear the vessels of fresh clots and restore them to normal function. As experience with these drugs increases, it appears that their safety approaches that of heparin. Since streptokinase is much less expensive than urokinase, it is preferable; however, since it is antigenic, subsequent use may not be possible. Also potentially valuable but expensive is tissue plasminogen activating factor. Treatment of deep venous thrombophlebitis with thrombolytic agents preserves valvular function in a fashion superior to heparin, and it may be less likely that patients so treated will develop postphlebitic syndrome. Complete resolution of the thrombosis occurs in about half of patients treated in the early stages, and protection against pulmonary embolism is not achieved. The presence of cerebral vascular disease is a contraindication to this therapy. After the initial treatment, anticoagulation is maintained with warfarin (see above). A loading dose of 250,000 units of streptokinase is administered over a 30-minute period, and 100,000 units per hour is given for 72 hours. The thrombin time (TT) is monitored for efficacy and kept a 2–5 times control. After discontinuance—and until TT is less than twice normal—heparin is begun until therapeutic levels of concomitantly given warfarin are achieved as outlined.

C. Surgical Measures: Inferior vena cava interruption may be necessary in cases where anticoagulants are contraindicated, such as where there is danger of intracranial hemorrhage from recent head trauma or surgery or from uncontrolled hypertension or in early postoperative period following major surgery.

Interruption may also be necessary if emboli occur in the face of anticoagulant therapy or if septic phlebitis is present. The preferred means of preventing pulmonary embolism in patients requiring mechanical control is the Greenfield vena cava filter. This device in inserted into the inferior vena cava through the right internal jugular vein under local anesthesia, and its placement involves fluorescent guidance. Percutaneous transfemoral placement is now also being used. Freedom from further emboli and patency of the mechanical filter is in the 95% range, and the mortality rate is much lower than when inferior vena caval ligation or plication is utilized.

Prognosis

With adequate treatment the patient usually returns to normal health and activity within 3–6 weeks. The prognosis in most cases is good once the period of danger of pulmonary embolism has passed. Occasionally, recurrent episodes of phlebitis will occur in spite of good local and anticoagulant management. Such cases may even have recurrent pulmonary emboli as well. Chronic venous insufficiency may result, with its associated complications; this is less likely when thrombolytics are used to treat acute phlebitis.

Hyers JM, Hull RD, Weg JG: Antithrombotic therapy for venous thromboembolic disease. Chest 1989;95(Suppl): 37S. (Consensus conference of experts in the field.)

2. THROMBOPHLEBITIS OF THE SUPERFICIAL VEINS

Essentials of Diagnosis

- Induration, redness, and tenderness along a superficial vein.
- Often a history of recent intravenous line or trauma. No significant swelling of the extremity.

General Considerations

Superficial thrombophlebitis may occur spontaneously, as in pregnant or postpartum women or in individuals with varicose veins or thromboangiitis obliterans; or it may be associated with trauma, as in the case of a blow to the leg or following intravenous therapy with irritating solutions. It may also be a manifestation of abdominal cancer such as carcinoma of the pancreas and may be the earliest sign. The long saphenous vein is most often involved. Superficial thrombophlebitis may be associated with occult deep vein thrombosis in about 20% of cases. Pulmonary emboli are rare.

Short-term plastic venous catheterization of superficial arm veins is now in routine use. The catheter should be observed daily for signs of local inflammation. It should be removed if a local reaction develops in the veins. Serious thrombotic or septic complications can occur if this policy is not followed. The steel intravenous needle with the anchoring flange (butterfly needle) is less likely to be associated with phlebitis and infection than the plastic catheter, but this may be due to its remaining in place for shorter periods.

Clinical Findings

The patient usually experiences a dull pain in the region of the involved vein. Local findings consist of induration, redness, and tenderness along the course of a vein. The process may be localized, or it may involve most of the long saphenous vein and its tributaries. The inflammatory reaction generally subsides in 1–2 weeks; a firm cord may remain for a much longer period. Edema of the extremity and deep calf tenderness are absent unless deep thrombophlebitis has also developed. Chills and high fever suggest septic phlebitis.

Differential Diagnosis

The linear rather than circular nature of the lesion and the distribution along the course of a superficial vein serve to differentiate superficial phlebitis from cellulitis, erythema nodosum, erythema induratum, panniculitis, and fibrositis. Lymphangitis and deep thrombophlebitis must also be considered.

Treatment

If the process is well localized and not near the saphenofemoral junction, local heat and bed rest with the leg elevated are usually effective in limiting the thrombosis. Nonsteroidal anti-inflammatory drugs relieve symptoms.

If the process is very extensive or is progressing upward toward the saphenofemoral junction, or if it is in the proximity of the saphenofemoral junction initially, ligation and division of the saphenous vein at the saphenofemoral junction are indicated. The inflammatory process usually regresses following this procedure, though removal of the involved segment of vein (stripping) may result in a more rapid recovery.

Anticoagulation therapy is usually not indicated unless the disease is rapidly progressing. It is indicated if there is extension into the deep system.

Septic thrombophlebitis requires excision of the involved vein up to its junction with an uninvolved vein in order to control bacteremia.

Prognosis

The course is generally benign and brief, and the prognosis depends on the underlying pathologic process. Phlebitis of a saphenous vein occasionally extends to the deep veins, in which case pulmonary embolism may occur.

CHRONIC VENOUS INSUFFICIENCY

Essentials of Diagnosis

- History of phlebitis or leg injury.
- Ankle edema is the earliest sign.
- Stasis pigmentation, dermatitis, subcutaneous induration, and often varicosities occur later.
- Ulceration at or above the ankle is common (stasis ulcer).

General Considerations

Chronic venous insufficiency generally results from changes secondary to deep thrombophlebitis, although a definite history of phlebitis is not obtainable in about 25% of these patients. There is often a history of leg trauma. It can also occur in association with varicose veins and as a result of neoplastic obstruction of the pelvic veins or congenital or acquired arteriovenous fistula.

When insufficiency is secondary to deep thrombophlebitis (the postphlebitic syndrome), the valves in the deep venous channels of the lower leg have been damaged or destroyed by the thrombotic process. The recanalized, nonelastic deep veins are functionally inadequate because of the damaged valves in the deep and perforating veins. The antegrade venous flow ensured by the valves and the calf muscle pump is lost, resulting in bidirectional flow and abnormally high ambulatory venous pressures in the calf veins in particular. The high ambulatory venous pressure transmitted through the communicating veins to the subcutaneous veins and tissues of the calf and ankle areas results in a series of deleterious secondary changes, including edema, fibrosis of subcutaneous tissue and skin, pigmentation of skin, and, later, dermatitis, cellulitis, and ulceration. Dilatation of the superficial veins may occur, leading to varicosities. Whereas primary varicose veins with no abnormality of the deep venous system may be associated with some similar changes, the edema is more pronounced in the postphlebitic extremities, and the secondary changes are more extensive and encircling.

Clinical Findings

Chronic venous insufficiency is characterized first by progressive edema of the leg (particularly the lower leg) and later also by secondary changes in the skin and subcutaneous tissues. The usual symptoms are itching, a dull discomfort made worse by periods of standing, and pain if an ulceration is present. The skin is usually thin, shiny, atrophic, and cyanotic; and a brownish pigmentation often develops. Eczema may be present, with superficial weeping dermatitis. The subcutaneous tissues become thick and fibrous. Recurrent ulcerations may occur, usually just above the ankle, on the medial or anterior aspect of the leg; healing results in a thin scar on a fibrotic base that often breaks down with minor trauma. Varicosities frequently appear that are associated with incompetent perforating veins.

Differential Diagnosis

Congestive heart failure and chronic renal disease

may result in bilateral edema of the lower extremities, but generally there are other clinical or laboratory findings of heart or kidney disease.

Lymphedema is associated with a brawny thickening in the subcutaneous tissue that does not respond readily to elevation; varicosities are absent, and there is often a history of recurrent cellulitis.

Primary varicose veins may be difficult to differentiate from the secondary varicosities that often develop in this condition, as discussed above. It may be impossible to exclude superimposed acute phlebitis from chronic venous insufficiency without diagnostic tests.

Other conditions associated with chronic ulcers of the leg include autoimmune diseases (eg, Felty's syndrome), arterial insufficiency (often very painful), sickle cell anemia, erythema induratum (bilateral and usually on the posterior aspect of the lower part of the leg), and fungal infections (cultures specific; no chronic swelling or varicosities).

Prevention

Irreversible tissue changes and associated complications in the lower legs can be minimized through early and energetic treatment of acute thrombophlebitis with anticoagulants that may minimize the occlusive and valve damage, particularly in the calf, and specific measures to avoid chronic edema in subsequent years, as described in A, below. Thrombolytic therapies of acute phlebitis may be of greater value than other anticoagulants in prevention.

Treatment

A. General Measures: Bed rest, with the legs elevated to diminish chronic edema, is fundamental in the treatment of the acute complications of chronic venous insufficiency. Measures to control the tendency toward edema include (1) intermittent elevation of the legs during the day and elevation of the legs at night (kept above the level of the heart with pillows under the mattress); (2) avoidance of long periods of sitting or standing; and (3) the use of well-fitting, heavy-duty elastic supports worn from the mid foot to just below the knee during the day and evening if there is any tendency for swelling to develop.

B. Stasis Dermatitis: Eczematous eruption may be acute or chronic; treatment varies accordingly.

1. Acute weeping dermatitis–

a. Wet compresses for 1 hour 4 times daily of solutions containing boric acid, buffered aluminum acetate (Burow's solution), or isotonic saline.

b. Compresses are followed with a local corticosteroid such as 0.5% hydrocortisone cream in a water-soluble base. (Neomycin and nystatin may be incorporated into this cream.)

c. Systemic antibiotics are indicated only if active infection is present.

2. Subsiding or chronic dermatitis–

a. Continue hydrocortisone cream for 1–2 weeks or until no further improvement is noted. Cor-

dran tape, a plastic tape impregnated with flurandrenolide, is a convenient way to apply both medication and dressing.

b. Zinc oxide ointment with ichthammol (Ichthyol), 3%, 1–2 times a day, cleaned off as desired with mineral oil.

c. Broad-spectrum antifungal such as clotrimazole cream (1%) or miconazole cream (2%) may be used.

3. Energetic treatment of chronic edema, as outlined in sections A and C, with almost complete bed rest is important during the acute phase of stasis dermatitis.

C. Ulceration: Ulcerations are preferably treated with compresses of isotonic saline solution, which aid the healing of the ulcer or may help prepare the base for a skin graft. A lesion can often be treated on an ambulatory basis by means of a semirigid boot applied to the leg after much of the swelling has been reduced by a period of elevation. The pumping action of the calf muscles on the blood flow out of the lower extremity is enhanced by a circumferential nonelastic bandage on the ankle and lower leg. The boot must be changed every 1–2 weeks, depending to some extent on the amount of drainage from the ulcer. The ulcer, tendons, and bony prominences must be adequately padded. Special ointments on the ulcer are not necessary. The semirigid boot may be made with Unna's paste (Gelocast, Medicopaste) or Gauztex bandage (impregnated with a nonallergenic self-adhering compound). After the ulcer has healed, heavy below-the-knee elastic stockings are used in an effort to prevent recurrent edema and ulceration. Occasionally, the ulcer is so large and chronic that total excision of the ulcer, with skin graft of the defect, is the best approach. This is often combined with ligation of all incompetent perforating veins.

D. Secondary Varicosities: Varicosities secondary to damage to the deep system of veins may in turn contribute to undesirable changes in the tissues of the lower leg. Varicosities should occasionally be removed and the incompetent veins connecting the superficial and deep system ligated, but the tendency toward edema will persist, because the chronic high venous pressure is usually not effectively lowered during walking by the procedure, and thus the measures outlined above (¶A) will be required for life. Varicosities can often be treated along with edema by elastic stockings and other nonoperative measures, and only about 15–20% require surgery. If the obstructive element in the deep system appears to be severe, B-mode ultrasonography, bidirectional Doppler velocity studies, or phlebography may be of value in mapping out the areas of venous obstruction or incompetence in the deep system as well as the number and location of the damaged perforating veins. A decision about whether to treat with surgery may be influenced by such a study; if the varicosities furnish the chief route of venous return, they should not be removed. Venous valvular reconstructive surgery is now in an investigative stage.

Prognosis

Individuals with chronic venous insufficiency often have recurrent problems, particularly if measures to counteract persistent venous hypertension, edema, and secondary tissue changes are not conscientiously adhered to throughout life. Additional episodes of acute thrombophlebitis may occur, and in reliable patients permanent anticoagulation is a reasonable therapeutic objective.

SUPERIOR VENA CAVAL OBSTRUCTION

Partial or complete obstruction of the thin-walled superior vena cava is a relatively rare condition that is usually secondary to the neoplastic or inflammatory process in the superior mediastinum. The most frequent causes are (1) neoplasms, such as lymphomas, primary malignant mediastinal tumors, or carcinoma of the lung with direct extension (over 80%); (2) chronic fibrotic mediastinitis, either of unknown origin or secondary to tuberculosis, histoplasmosis, or pyogenic infections; (3) thrombophlebitis, often by extension of the process from the axillary or subclavian vein into the innominate vein and vena cava and often associated with catheterization of these veins for central venous pressure measurements or for hyperalimentation; (4) aneurysm of the aortic arch; and (5) constrictive pericarditis.

Clinical Findings

A. Symptoms and Signs: The onset of symptoms is acute or subacute. Symptoms include swelling of the neck and face, headache, dizziness, visual disturbances, stupor, and syncope. There is progressive obstruction of the venous drainage of the head, neck, and upper extremities. The cutaneous veins of the upper chest and lower neck become dilated, and flushing of the face and neck develops. Brawny edema of the face, neck, and arms occurs later, and cyanosis of these areas then appears. Cerebral and laryngeal edema ultimately results in impaired function of the brain as well as respiratory insufficiency. Bending over or lying down accentuates the symptoms; sitting quietly is generally preferred. The manifestations are more severe if the obstruction develops rapidly and if the azygos junction or the vena cava between that vein and the heart is obstructed.

B. Laboratory Findings: The venous pressure is elevated (often > 20 cm of water) in the arm and is normal in the leg.

C. Imaging: Chest radiographs and a CT scan will define the location and often the nature of the obstructive process, and phlebography will map out the extent and degree of the venous obstruction and the collateral circulation. Brachial venography or radionuclide scanning following intravenous injection of technetium Tc 99m pertechnetate demonstrates a block to the flow of contrast material into the right heart and enlarged collateral veins. These techniques also allow estimation of blood flow around the occlusion as well as serial evaluation of the response to therapy.

Treatment

Though empiric therapy for neoplasm is occasionally warranted, the clinician should be aware of benign causes, especially histoplasmosis.

Emergency treatment for neoplasm consists of (1) intravenous administration of cyclophosphamide (1 g/m^2) through a central venous catheter or a lower extremity vein (to initiate tumor shrinkage); (2) intravenous diuretics; and (3) mediastinal irradiation, starting within 24 hours, with a treatment plan designed to give a high daily dose but a short total course of therapy to rapidly shrink the local tumor even further. Intensive combined therapy will palliate the process in up to 90% of patients. In patients with a subacute presentation, radiation therapy alone usually suffices.

Surgical procedures to bypass the obstruction are complicated by bleeding relating to high venous pressure. In cases secondary to mediastinal fibrosis or pericardial constriction, excision of the fibrous tissue around the great vessels may reestablish flow.

Prognosis

The prognosis depends upon the nature and degree of obstruction and its speed of onset. Slowly developing forms secondary to fibrosis may be tolerated for years. A high degree of obstruction of rapid onset secondary to cancer is often fatal in a few days or weeks, but treatment of the tumor with radiation and chemotherapeutic drugs may result in significant palliation for considerable periods of time.

Sculier JP, Feld R: Superior vena cava obstruction syndrome: Recommendations for management. Cancer Treat Rev 1985;12:209.

DISEASES OF THE LYMPHATIC CHANNELS

LYMPHANGITIS & LYMPHADENITIS

Essentials of Diagnosis

- Red streak from wound or area of cellulitis toward regional lymph nodes, which are usually enlarged and tender.
- Chills, fever, and malaise may be present.

General Considerations

Lymphangitis and lymphadenitis are common manifestations of a bacterial infection that is usually caused by hemolytic streptococci and usually arises from an area of cellulitis, generally at the site of an infected wound. The wound may be very small or superficial, or an established abscess may be present, feeding bacteria into the lymphatics. The involvement of the lymphatics is often manifested by a red streak in the skin extending in the direction of the regional lymph nodes, which are, in turn, generally tender and enlarged. Systemic manifestations include fever, chills, and malaise. The infection may progress rapidly, often in a matter of hours, and may lead to septicemia and even death.

Clinical Findings

A. Symptoms and Signs: Throbbing pain is usually present in the area of cellulitis at the site of bacterial invasion. Malaise, anorexia, sweating, chills, and fever of 37.8–40 °C (100–104 °F) develop rapidly. The red streak, when present, may be definite or may be very faint and easily missed, especially in dark-skinned patients. It is not usually tender or indurated, as is the area of cellulitis. The involved regional lymph nodes may be significantly enlarged and are usually quite tender. The pulse is often rapid.

B. Laboratory Findings: Leukocytosis with a leftward shift is usually present. Later, a blood culture may be positive. Culture and sensitivity studies on the wound exudate or pus may be helpful in treatment of the more severe or refractory infections.

Differential Diagnosis

Lymphangitis may be confused with superficial thrombophlebitis, but the erythematous reaction associated with thrombosis overlies the induration of the inflammatory reaction in and around the thrombosed vein. Venous thrombosis is not associated with lymphadenitis, and a wound of entrance with the secondary cellulitis is generally absent. Superficial thrombophlebitis frequently arises as a result of intravenous therapy, particularly when the needle or catheter is left in place for more than 2 days; if bacteria have also been introduced, suppurative thrombophlebitis may develop.

Cat-scratch fever should be considered when lymphadenitis is present in which the nodes, though often very large, are relatively nontender. Exposure to cats is common, but the scratch may be forgotten by the patient.

It is extremely important to differentiate cellulitis from soft tissue infections that require early and aggressive incision and often resection of necrotic infected tissue, eg, acute streptococcal hemolytic gangrene, necrotizing fasciitis, gram-negative anaerobic cutaneous gangrene, and progressive bacterial synergistic gangrene. These are deeper infections that are more anatomically extensive; patients appear more seriously ill.

Treatment

A. General Measures: Prompt treatment should include heat (hot, moist compresses or heating pad), elevation when feasible, and immobilization of the infected area. Analgesics may be prescribed for pain.

B. Specific Measures: Antibiotic therapy should always be instituted when local infection becomes invasive, as manifested by cellulitis and lymphangitis. A culture of any purulent discharge available should be obtained (often there is nothing to culture), and antibiotic therapy should be started in full doses at once. The initial drug may have to be replaced by a second antibiotic if a clinical response is not apparent in 36–48 hours or if the culture and sensitivity studies indicate that it is not effective. Because the causative organism is so frequently the streptococcus, penicillin is usually the drug of choice. If the patient is allergic to penicillin, erythromycin may be substituted. (See Chapter 31.)

C. Wound Care: Drainage of pus from an infected wound should be carried out, generally after the above measures have been instituted and only when it is clear that there is an abscess associated with the site of initial infection. An area of cellulitis should not be incised, because the infection may be spread by attempted drainage when pus is not present.

Prognosis

With proper therapy and particularly with the use of an antibiotic effective against the invading bacteria, control of the infection can usually be achieved in a few days. Delayed or inadequate therapy can still lead to overwhelming infection with septicemia.

LYMPHEDEMA

Essentials of Diagnosis

- Painless edema of one or both lower extremities, primarily in young women.
- Initially, pitting edema, which becomes brawny and often nonpitting with time.
- Ulceration, varicosities, and stasis pigmentation do not occur. There may be episodes of lymphangitis and cellulitis.

General Considerations

The underlying mechanism in lymphedema is impairment of the flow of lymph from an extremity. When due to congenital developmental abnormalities consisting of hypo- or hyperplastic involvement of the proximal or distal lymphatics, it is referred to as the primary form. The obstruction may be in the pelvic or lumbar lymph channels and nodes when the disease is extensive and progressive. The secondary form results when an inflammatory or mechanical obstruction of the lymphatics occurs from trauma, regional lymph node resection or irradiation, or extensive involvement of regional nodes by malignant disease or filariasis. Secondary dilatation of the lymphatics that occurs in both forms leads to incompetence of the valve system, disrupting the orderly flow along the lymph vessels, and results in progressive stasis of a protein-rich fluid, with secondary fibrosis. Episodes of acute and chronic inflammation may be superimposed, with further stasis and fibrosis. Hypertrophy of the limb results, with markedly thickened and fibrotic skin and subcutaneous tissue and diminution in the fatty tissue.

Lymphangiography and radioactive isotope studies are often useful in defining the specific lymphatic defect.

Treatment

The treatment of lymphedema is often not very satisfactory. The majority of patients can be treated conservatively with some of the following measures: (1) The flow of lymph out of the extremity, with a consequent decrease in the degree of stasis, can be aided through intermittent elevation of the extremity, especially during the sleeping hours (foot of bed elevated 15–20 degrees, achieved by placing pillows beneath the mattress); the constant use of elastic bandages or carefully fitted heavy-duty elastic stockings; and massage toward the trunk—either by hand or by means of pneumatic pressure devices designed to milk edema out of an extremity. (The Wright linear pump delivers sequential pressure cycles that effectively milk fluid out of the foot and leg and then out of the thigh.) (2) Secondary cellulitis in the extremity should be avoided by means of good hygiene and treatment of any trichophytosis of the toes. Once an infection starts, it should be treated by adequate periods of rest, elevation, and antibiotics. Infection can be a serious and recurring problem and is often difficult to control. Intermittent prophylactic antibiotics may occasionally be necessary. (3) Intermittent courses of diuretic therapy, especially in those with premenstrual or seasonal exacerbations. (4) In carefully selected cases, there are operative procedures that may give satisfactory functional results. Lymphaticovenous anastomosis using microsurgery has yielded some satisfactory cosmetic and functional results, particularly if lymph channels can be localized by lymphoscintigraphy and several lymphovenous anastomoses are made. This technique may replace the more deforming procedures and those aimed at introducing lymphatic bridges or lymphatic venous connections. Amputation is used as a last resort in very severe forms or when lymphangiosarcoma develops in the extremity.

Gloviczi P et al: Microsurgical lymphovenous anastomosis for treatment of lymphoedemas: A critical review. J Vasc Surg 1988;7:647.

Savage RC: The surgical management of lymphedema. Surg Gynecol Obstet 1985;160:283.

HYPOTENSION & SHOCK

Essentials of Diagnosis

- Low systemic blood pressure and tachycardia.
- Peripheral hypoperfusion and, in most, vasoconstriction.
- Altered mental status.
- Oliguria or anuria.
- Metabolic acidosis in many.

General Considerations

Shock occurs when the circulation of arterial blood is inadequate to meet tissue metabolic needs. Treatment must be directed both at the manifestations of shock and at its cause.

Classification

See Table 9–2.

A. Hypovolemic Shock: Decreased intravascular volume resulting from loss of blood, plasma, or fluids and electrolytes may be obvious (eg, external hemorrhage) or subtle (eg, sequestration in a "third space," as in pancreatitis). Compensatory vasoconstriction temporarily reduces the size of the vascular bed and may temporarily maintain the blood pressure, but if fluid is not replaced, hypotension occurs, peripheral resistance increases, capillary and venous beds collapse, and the tissues become progressively more hypoxic. Even a moderate sudden loss of circulating fluids can result in severe damage to vital centers.

B. Cardiogenic Shock: (See Chapter 8.) Inadequate cardiac function may result from disorders of the heart muscle, valves, or the electrical pacing system. Shock associated with myocardial infarction or other serious cardiac disease still carries a very high mortality rate (75–80%).

C. Obstructive Shock: (See Chapter 8.) Obstruction of the systemic or pulmonary circulation, the aortic and mitral valves, or venous inflow, as in pericardial disease, may reduce cardiac output sufficiently to cause shock. Cardiac tamponade, tension pneumothorax, and massive pulmonary embolism are medical emergencies requiring prompt diagnosis and treatment. Tamponade calls for immediate echocardiography and pericardiocentesis. The prognosis for patients with massive pulmonary embolism is guarded despite therapy with anticoagulants or thrombolytics; surgical embolectomy adds little. A less common cause of obstructive shock is myxoma with pulmonary hypertension.

D. Distributive Shock: Reduction in systemic vascular resistance from such diverse causes as sepsis,

Table 9–2. Classification of shock.[1]

Hypovolemic shock
  Loss of blood (hemorrhagic shock):
    External hemorrhage:
      Trauma
      Gastrointestinal tract bleeding
    Internal hemorrhage:
      Hematoma
  Loss of plasma:
    Burns
  Loss of fluid and electrolytes:
    External:
      Vomiting
      Diarrhea
      Excessive sweating
      Hyperosmolar states (diabetic ketoacidosis)
    Internal ("third-spacing"):
      Pancreatitis
      Ascites
      Bowel obstruction
Cardiogenic shock
  Dysrhythmia
    Tachyarrhythmia (nearly always ventricular tachycardia)
    Bradyarrhythmia
  "Pump failure" (secondary to myocardial infarction or other cardiomyopathy)
  Acute valvular dysfunction (especially regurgitant lesions)
  Rupture of ventricular septum or free ventricular wall
Obstructive shock
  Pericardial disease (tamponade, constriction)
  Disease of pulmonary vasculature (massive pulmonary emboli, tension pneumothorax, pulmonary hypertension)
  Cardiac tumor (atrial myxoma)
  Obstructive valvular disease (aortic or mitral stenosis)
Distributive shock
  Septic shock
  Anaphylactic shock
  Neurogenic shock
  Vasodilator drugs
  Acute adrenal insufficiency

[1] Adapted from Trunkey DD, Salber PR, Mills J: Shock. In: *Current Emergency Diagnosis & Treatment,* 3rd ed. Ho MT, Saunders CE (editors). Appleton & Lange, 1989.

anaphylaxis, or acute adrenal insufficiency may result in inadequate cardiac output despite normal circulatory volume.

1. Septic shock–(See Chapter 23.) Most commonly, vascular shock is due to gram-negative bacteremia (so-called septic shock). In overwhelming infection, there is an initial short period of vasoconstriction followed by vasodilatation, with venous pooling of blood in the microcirculation. The mortality rate is high (40–80%). Responsible organisms are most commonly gram-negative rods (*Escherichia coli, Klebsiella, Proteus,* and *Pseudomonas*) as well as gram-positive cocci *(Staphylococcus, Streptococcus)* and gram-negative anaerobes (eg, *Bacteroides*). Septic shock occurs more often in the very young and the very old; in diabetes, hematologic cancers, and diseases of the genitourinary, hepatobiliary, and intestinal tracts; and in association with immunosuppressive therapy. Immediate precipitating factors may be urinary, biliary, or gynecologic manipulations.

Septic shock is suspected when a febrile patient has chills associated with hypotension. Early, the skin may be warm and the pulse full ("warm shock"). Hyperventilation results in respiratory alkalosis. The sensorium and urinary output are often initially normal, with classic signs of shock becoming manifest later. The symptoms and signs of the inciting infection are not invariably present.

2. Neurogenic shock–Neurogenic or psychogenic factors, eg, spinal cord injury, pain, trauma, fright, gastric dilatation, or vasodilator drugs, may also cause distributive shock due to reflex vagal stimulation with decreased cardiac output, hypotension, and decreased cerebral blood flow.

Diagnosis of Shock & Impending Shock

Shock may be impending if the following signs are present.

A. Hypotension: Hypotension in adults is traditionally defined as a systolic blood pressure of 90 mm Hg or less. However, some normal adults may have levels that low without ill effects, and some hypertensive persons develop shock with what would ordinarily be considered normal blood pressures.

B. Orthostatic Changes in Vital Signs: Patients who are not clearly hypotensive when tested in the supine position should have blood pressures measured and pulses counted while sitting up with the legs dangling. If no change occurs when this is done, repeat the measurements with the patient standing. Three to 5 minutes between measurements are allowed to permit the pulse and blood pressure to stabilize. A drop in systolic pressure of 10–20 mm Hg or more associated with an increase in pulse rate of more than 15 beats/min suggests depleted intravascular volume. Some normovolemic patients with peripheral neuropathies or those taking certain medications (eg, some antihypertensive drugs) may demonstrate an orthostatic fall in blood pressure, but without associated increase in pulse rate.

C. Peripheral Hypoperfusion: Patients in shock often have cool or mottled extremities and weak or absent peripheral pulses.

D. Altered Mental Status: Patients may demonstrate normal mental status or may be restless, agitated, confused, lethargic, or comatose as a result of inadequate perfusion of the brain.

Treatment

Treatment depends upon prompt assessment of the cause, type, severity, and duration of shock as well as an accurate appraisal of underlying conditions that may influence the onset or maintenance of shock.

A. Position: The patient is placed in the Trendelenburg or supine position with legs elevated to maximize cerebral blood flow.

B. Oxygenation: Shock—especially septic shock—may result in hypoxia caused by pulmonary ventilation-perfusion mismatch or, in severe cases, by adult respiratory distress syndrome. Pathophysiology and treatment are discussed on pp 382 and 383.

C. Analgesics: Severe pain is treated promptly with analgesic drugs. Morphine sulfate, 8–15 mg subcutaneously, is appropriate for severe pain; since subcutaneous absorption is poor in patients in shock, 4-8 mg slowly intravenously may be used as an alternative. Morphine should not be given to unconscious patients, to those who have head injuries, to those with severe hypotension or unstable blood pressure, or to those with respiratory depression.

D. Laboratory Studies: A complete blood count is obtained immediately, and a blood specimen is sent for typing and cross-matching. Arterial blood gases (or finger oximeter oxygen saturation) and electrolytes are obtained routinely.

E. Urine Flow: Both oliguric and nonoliguric renal failure may occur in shock. In the patient without preexisting renal disease, urine output is a reliable indication of organ perfusion. An indwelling catheter to monitor urine flow (which should be kept above 0.5 mL/kg/h) may be indicated. Urine flow of less than 25 mL/h indicates inadequate renal perfusion, which, if not corrected, can result in renal tubular necrosis.

F. Monitor Cardiac Rhythm: Periodic electrocardiography or continuous automated monitoring will permit early detection and prompt treatment of myocardial ischemia from hypoperfusion, and arrhythmias from similar causes or from electrolyte and acid-base disturbances.

G. Central Venous Pressure (CVP) or Pulmonary Capillary Wedge Pressure (PCWP): Monitoring of central venous pressure or pulmonary capillary wedge pressure is helpful in treating shock. Central venous pressure determination is relatively simple but is not as reliable as the pulmonary capillary wedge pressure (PCWP) measured by the Swan-Ganz catheter technique, which provides a better index of left ventricular function. Determination of PCWP is indicated in patients in whom there is uncertainty about the role of cardiac function in the genesis of shock or in myocardial infarction with shock. It is also useful in guiding volume resuscitation in shock patients with a history of heart disease or in such patients in whom pulmonary disease has produced high central venous pressure.

In central venous pressure determination, a catheter is inserted percutaneously (or by cutdown) through a major vein. Normal values range from 5 to 8 cm of water. A low central venous pressure suggests the need for fluid replacement. A high central venous pressure (above 15 cm of water) suggests volume expansion exceeding the upper limit of normal but also cardiac tamponade or bronchospasm. The PCWP catheter is inserted in a similar fashion, with localization of its tip determined by monitoring the morphology of the pressure tracing as it is advanced. A PCWP over 14 mm Hg may serve as a warning of impending pulmonary edema. Catheter insertion requires a skilled and experienced physician and is expensive; the catheter itself costs about $175.00. Surveillance for the catheter-induced complications of hemorrhage, sepsis, pneumothorax, arrhythmias, and pulmonary infarction is an important part of intensive care.

H. Volume Replacement: Initial or emergency needs may be determined by the history, general appearance, vital signs, and hematocrit. There is no simple technique by which to accurately judge the fluid requirements. An estimate of total fluid losses is an essential first step. Response to therapy—particularly the effect of carefully administered, gradually increasing amounts of intravenous fluids on the central venous pressure or PCWP—is a valuable index.

Selection of the proper fluid for restoration and maintenance of hemodynamic stability is often difficult and controversial. It will depend upon the type of fluid that has been lost (whole blood, plasma, water, electrolytes), associated medical problems, availability of the various replacement solutions, clinical and laboratory monitoring facilities, and, in some circumstances, expense. The most effective replacement fluid in case of hemorrhage is packed red cells with saline, but other available fluids should be given immediately pending return of laboratory studies.

Rapid volume replacement in blood loss will often prevent shock. If central venous pressure or PCWP is low and the hematocrit greater than 35%—and if there is no clinical evidence to suggest occult blood loss—blood volume should be supported with crystalloid solutions or colloids.

1. Crystalloid solutions–Crystalloid fluids include sodium chloride (physiologic saline, 0.9%) or lactated Ringer's injection. Five hundred to 2000 mL of the selected solution is given rapidly intravenously—ideally under central venous pressure or pulmonary capillary wedge pressure monitoring. The crystalloids are readily available for emergencies and mass casualties. They may obviate the need for blood or colloids. They are often effective, at least temporarily, when given in adequate doses.

2. Colloids–Colloids are high-molecular-weight substances that do not diffuse readily across normal capillary membranes. Colloidal solutions increase the plasma oncotic pressure and thus in theory can draw fluid from the interstitial space into the intravascular space to cause additional fluid volume expansion. Capillary membranes in the lungs are often damaged in the patient in shock, so that larger molecules may leak from the intravascular space into the interstitium and have an adverse effect on pulmonary function (adult respiratory distress syndrome).

a. Blood–Packed or frozen red cells are preferred to whole blood, since remaining blood products may be used for other purposes. The amount of blood given depends on the clinical course, the hematocrit, and hemodynamic findings.

Screening of blood donors for hepatitis B infection and for AIDS virus antibodies has reduced the frequency of those infections following transfusion. The risk of AIDS infection from transfused blood is now estimated at approximately 1:40,000 in industrialized countries that screen appropriately. The risk for contracting hepatitis B is somewhat greater. Non-A, non-B hepatitis remains the commonest infectious complication of transfusion, with an incidence of 2–5%.

b. Plasma fractions–Group-specific frozen plasma is a satisfactory colloidal volume expander and occasionally can correct specific coagulation defects. Because of its expense, risk (same as blood transfusion), and relative ineffectiveness, however, its use should be limited. Unit-bagged plasma is preferable to pooled plasma. Albumin 5% in saline, albumin 25% in concentrate, or plasma protein fraction (containing 80–85% albumin) may be rapidly set up for emergencies, and blood typing is not required. These substances have been heat-treated to minimize the risk of infectious hepatitis.

c. Dextrans–Dextrans are high-molecular-weight polysaccharide colloids that are fairly effective plasma expanders. Because they can impair blood coagulation and interfere with blood typing and because they may cause anaphylactoid reactions, dextrans are used very infrequently now.

I. Vasoactive Drugs: Some adrenergic drugs can be useful in the adjunctive therapy of shock. *The adrenergic drugs should not be considered a primary form of therapy in shock.* Simple blood pressure elevation produced by the vasopressor drugs has little beneficial effect on the underlying disturbance, and in many instances the effect may be detrimental. Pressors are given only when hypotension persists after volume deficits are corrected and obstructive causes excluded or remedied.

1. Dopamine hydrochloride has an advantage over other adrenergic drugs because it has a beneficial effect on renal blood flow (at low dose) and because it increases cardiac output and blood pressure. Dopamine hydrochloride, 200 mg in 500 mL of sodium chloride injection USP (400 μg/mL), is given initially at a rate of 1–2 μg/kg/min. This dosage stimulates both the dopaminergic receptors, which increase the renal blood flow and urinary output, and the β-adrenergic cardiac receptors, which increase the cardiac output. If shock persists, gradually increasing doses of dopamine may be required. If dopamine alone fails to maintain adequate perfusion pressure, it may sometimes be necessary to use it in combination with another appropriate adrenergic drug.

Adverse reactions include ventricular arrhythmias, anginal pain, nausea and vomiting, headache, hypotension, azotemia, and rare cases of peripheral gangrene. Special care should be exercised when dopamine is used in the treatment of shock following myocardial infarction, because the drug's inotropic effect may increase myocardial oxygen demand. Do-

pamine should not be used in patients with pheochromocytoma or uncorrected tachyarrhythmias or in those who are receiving monoamine oxidase inhibitors.

2. Dobutamine, a synthetic catecholamine similar to dopamine but with greater inotropic effect, may be useful when filling pressures are high because of fluid overload or heart failure. Though dopamine at higher doses is a vasoconstrictor, dobutamine has no net effect on peripheral vascular resistance.

J. Corticosteroids: Corticosteroids are lifesaving in the treatment of shock associated with acute adrenal insufficiency (see Chapter 20). In other types of shock, however, corticosteroids are of no benefit.

K. Diuretics: Diuretics are not employed until volume deficits are corrected or obstructive causes remedied. The cautious early administration of mannitol as a 10–25% solution in 500–1000 mL of normal saline or Ringer's injection has been recommended in selected patients in whom oliguria is present despite volume replacement. Furosemide, 20 mg intravenously, is often given concomitantly. Prior to administration of diuretics, it may be helpful to determine the urinary sodium; values greater than 30 meq/L suggest acute tubular necrosis and the possible advantage of diuretic therapy in converting oliguric to nonoliguric expression of the disorder. There is no evidence that diuretics reduce the overall incidence of renal failure, though some believe they may convert oliguric renal insufficiency to a nonoliguric type.

L. Heparin: See Disseminated Intravascular Coagulation, p 714.

M. Fluid and Electrolyte Balance: Abnormalities of fluid, electrolyte, and acid-base balance are addressed. There is growing evidence that vigorous treatment with sodium bicarbonate should not be used as standard therapy. Its use should be reserved for cases of acidosis that fail to respond to adequate fluid resuscitation.

N. Treatment of Cardiac Disorders: Digitalis glycosides are indicated only for those patients with preexisting or presenting evidence of cardiac failure or digitalis-responsive arrhythmias. Atropine may be of value in treating selected bradycardias. The use of vasopressor drugs in myocardial infarction is reserved for patients with hypotension and elevated left ventricular filling pressure. Continuous cardiac monitoring is required. The hemodynamic effectiveness of vasodilator drugs in reducing preload and outflow resistance in patients with left ventricular failure has been established, but the mortality rate of cardiogenic shock is unchanged.

Further discussion of cardiogenic shock is found in Chapter 8.

Bone RC et al: A controlled clinical trial of high-dose methylprednisolone in the treatment of severe sepsis and septic shock. N Engl J Med 1987;317:653. (Most recent of several current studies concluding that steroids are of no benefit in the treatment of septic shock.)

Ognibene FD et al: Depressed left ventricular performance: Response to volume infusion in patients with sepsis and septic shock. Chest 1988;93:903. (Left ventricular stroke work index response to volume infusion was significantly less in 14 patients with septic shock when compared to 14 other critically ill patients without sepsis, suggesting altered ventricular performance in septic shock.)

Robin ED: The cult of the Swan-Ganz catheter: Overuse and abuse of pulmonary flow catheters. Ann Intern Med 1985;103:445.

Schreiber JL et al: Management of myocardial infarction shock: Current status. Am Heart J 1989;117:435.

REFERENCES

Bergan JJ, Yao JS (editors): *1986 Year Book of Vascular Surgery*. Year Book, 1986.

Kempczinski RF (editor): *The Ischemic Leg*. Year Book, 1985.

Moore WS (editor): *Vascular Surgery: A Comprehensive Review*, 2nd ed. Grune & Stratton, 1986.

Wilson SE, Williams RA (editors): *Vascular Surgery: Principles and Practice*. McGraw-Hill, 1987.

10

Blood

Charles A. Linker, MD

ANEMIAS

General Approach to Anemias

Anemia is a common problem in clinical medicine. Anemias should be characterized initially as to type and evaluated subsequently to determine the underlying cause. Anemia is said to be present in adults if the hematocrit is less than 41% in males or 37% in females. In taking the history, one should consider the possibility of congenital anemia based on the patient's personal and family history. One should consider whether the patient has been anemic in the past or has received treatment for anemia. The dietary history may help explain iron deficiency or folic acid deficiency. The possibility of prior or ongoing bleeding should always be considered. Physical examination should include careful attention to signs of primary hematologic diseases (lymphadenopathy, hepatosplenomegaly, or bone tenderness). Mucosal changes such as a smooth tongue raise the possibility of megaloblastic anemia.

Initial laboratory evaluation consists of obtaining a complete blood count, including measurement of red cell indices—chiefly the mean corpuscular volume (MCV). The reticulocyte count on the peripheral blood smear is an index of red blood cell production. Further laboratory tests may be ordered depending on the diagnostic possibilities in individual cases.

Anemias are classified according to their pathophysiologic basis, ie, whether related to diminished production or accelerated loss of red blood cells (Table 10–1); or according to cell size (Table 10–2). The diagnostic possibilities in microcytic anemia are iron deficiency, thalassemia, and anemia of chronic disease. A severely microcytic anemia (MCV < 70 fL) is always due either to iron deficiency or to thalassemia. Macrocytic anemia may be due to megaloblastic (folate or vitamin B_{12} deficiency) or nonmegaloblastic causes. A severely macrocytic anemia (MCV > 125 fL) is almost always due to megaloblastic causes, rare exceptions are the myelodysplastic syndromes, either before or after chemotherapy.

IRON DEFICIENCY ANEMIA

Essentials of Diagnosis

- Both pathognomonic: absent bone marrow iron stores or serum ferritin < 12 pg/L.

Table 10–1. Classification of anemias by pathophysiology.

Decreased production
  Hemoglobin synthesis: Iron deficiency, thalassemia, anemia of chronic disease
  DNA synthesis: Megaloblastic anemia
  Stem cell: Aplastic anemia, myeloproliferative leukemia
  Bone marrow infiltration: Carcinoma, lymphoma
  Pure red cell aplasia
Increased destruction
  Blood loss
  Hemolysis (intrinsic)
    Membrane: Hereditary spherocytosis, elliptocytosis
    Hemoglobin: Sickle cell, unstable hemoglobin
    Glycolysis: Pyruvate kinase, etc
    Oxidation: G6PD deficiency
  Hemolysis (extrinsic)
    Immune: Warm antibody, cold antibody
    Microangiopathic: Thrombotic thrombocytopenic purpura, hemolytic-uremic syndrome, valve
    Infection: Clostridial
    Hypersplenism

Table 10–2. Classification of anemias by MCV.

  Microcytic
    Iron deficiency
    Thalassemia
    Anemia of chronic disease
  Macrocytic
    Megaloblastic
      Vitamin B_{12} deficiency
      Folate deficiency
    Nonmegaloblastic
      Myelodysplasia, chemotherapy
      Liver disease
      Increased reticulocytosis
      Myxedema
  Normocytic
    Many causes

- Microcytic anemia (all cases).
- Response to iron therapy.

General Considerations

Iron deficiency is the most common cause of anemia worldwide. The anemia is usually mild, but it may become moderate or even severe. It is important to make the diagnosis so that the underlying cause (usually gastrointestinal blood loss) can be identified and treated (Table 10–3).

Iron is necessary for the formation of heme and other enzymes. Total body iron stores range between 2 and 4 g: approximately 50 mg/kg in men and 35 mg/kg in women. The vast majority (70–95%) of total body iron is present in hemoglobin in circulating red blood cells. One milliliter of packed red blood cells (not whole blood) contains approximately 1 mg of iron. In men, red blood cell volume is approximately 30 mL/kg. A 70-kg man will therefore have approximately 2100 mL of packed red blood cells and consequently 2100 mg of iron in his circulating blood. In women, the red cell volume is about 27 mL/kg; a 50-kg woman will thus have 1350 mg of iron circulating in her red blood cells. Only 200–400 mg of iron is present in myoglobin and nonheme enzymes. The amount of iron present in plasma is negligible. Aside from circulating red blood cells, the major location of iron in the body is the storage pool. Iron is deposited either as ferritin or as hemosiderin and is located largely in macrophages. Iron stores are normally 0.5–2 g, larger in men than in women. However, the range for storage iron is wide; approximately 25% of women in the USA have no storage iron.

The average American diet contains 10–15 mg of iron per day. About 10% of this amount is absorbed, which means that the net daily intake is 1–2 mg. Absorption occurs in the stomach, duodenum, and upper jejunum. Dietary iron present as heme is efficiently absorbed (10–20%) but nonheme iron less so (1–5%), largely because of interference by phosphates, tannins, and other food constituents. Small amounts of iron—approximately 1 mg/d—are normally lost though exfoliation of skin and mucosal cells. There is no mechanism for increasing normal body iron losses.

Menstrual blood loss in women plays a major role in iron metabolism. The average monthly menstrual blood loss is approximately 50 mL, or about 0.7 mg/d. However, menstrual blood loss may be 5 times the average. In order to maintain adequate iron stores, women with heavy menstrual losses must absorb 3–4 mg of iron from the diet each day. This strains the upper limit of what may reasonably be absorbed, and women with menorrhagia of this degree will almost always become iron-deficient.

In general, iron metabolism is balanced between absorption of 1 mg/d and loss of 1 mg/d. Pregnancy may also upset the iron balance, since requirements

Table 10–3. Causes of iron deficiency.

Deficient diet
Decreased absorption
Increased requirements
  Pregnancy
  Lactation
Blood loss
  Gastrointestinal
  Menstrual
  Blood donation
Hemoglobinuria
Iron sequestration
  Pulmonary hemosiderosis

increase to 2–5 mg of iron per day during pregnancy and lactation. Normal dietary iron cannot supply these requirements, and medicinal iron is needed during pregnancy.

It is possible to become iron-deficient because of dietary deficiency, though this is uncommon in adults. Decreased iron absorption can cause iron deficiency and is usually due to gastric surgery. Repeated pregnancy (especially with breast feeding) is a common cause of iron deficiency if increased requirements are not met with supplemental medicinal iron.

By far the most important cause of iron deficiency anemia is blood loss, especially gastrointestinal blood loss. Chronic aspirin use may cause chronic iron loss even without a documented structural lesion. It cannot be overemphasized that iron deficiency should prompt a search for a potential source of gastrointestinal bleeding unless another cause is identified. Other sources of blood loss include menorrhagia or other uterine bleeding and repeated blood donation.

Chronic hemoglobinuria may lead to iron deficiency, since more than 1 mg/d or iron can be lost by this route. The most common cause is traumatic hemolysis due to an abnormally functioning cardiac valve. Other causes of intravascular hemolysis (eg. paroxysmal nocturnal hemoglobinuria) should also be considered if hemoglobinuria is documented.

Rare causes of iron deficiency include sequestration of iron in pulmonary macrophages in the syndrome of idiopathic pulmonary hemosiderosis.

Clinical Findings

A. Symptoms and Signs: As a rule, the only symptoms of iron deficiency anemia are those of the anemia itself (easy fatigability, tachycardia, palpitations and tachypnea on exertion). Severe iron deficiency (uncommon in the USA) causes progressive skin and mucosal changes. These include a smooth tongue, brittle nails, and cheilosis. Advanced iron deficiency may cause dysphagia because of the formation of esophageal webs (Plummer-Vinson syndrome). Many iron-deficient patients develop pica, an unusual craving for specific foods (ice cubes, etc).

B. Laboratory Findings: Laboratory data are important in diagnosis and often reflect the severity of the anemia.

Iron deficiency develops slowly and in stages. The first stage is depletion of iron stores. At this point, there is anemia and no changes in red blood cell size. Iron stores in the marrow will become depleted and eventually disappear. The serum ferritin will become abnormally low. Ferritin values less than 30 µg/L usually indicate absent iron stores. The serum total iron-binding capacity (TIBC) will gradually rise.

After iron stores have been depleted, red blood cell formation will continue with deficient supplies of iron. Serum iron values will begin to fall to less than 30 µg/dL, and transferrin saturation will fall to less than 15%.

Eventually, anemia will develop. In the mildest state of anemia, the MCV remains normal. With progressive development of anemia, MCV will fall and the blood smear will show hypochromic microcytic cells. With further progression, anisocytosis (variations in red blood cell size) followed by poikilocytosis (variation in shape of red cells) will develop. Severe iron deficiency will produce a bizarre peripheral blood smear, with severely hypochromic cells, target cells, hypochromic pencil-shaped cells, and occasionally small numbers of nucleated red blood cells. The platelet count is usually normal in mild iron deficiency anemia but is typically elevated in more severe cases.

Differential Diagnosis

Other causes of microcytic anemia that need to be excluded include anemia of chronic disease, thalassemia, and (less commonly) sideroblastic anemia. Anemia of chronic disease is characterized by normal or increased iron stores in the bone marrow and a normal ferritin level. The TIBC is either normal or low. Thalassemia characteristically produces a greater degree of microcytosis (lower MCV) for any given level of anemia than does iron deficiency. Red blood cell morphology on the peripheral smear becomes abnormal earlier in the evolution of anemia, and iron parameters should be normal.

Treatment

To make the diagnosis of iron deficiency anemia, one can either demonstrate an iron-deficient state or evaluate the response to a therapeutic trial of iron replacement.

Since the anemia itself is rarely life-threatening, the most important part of treatment is identification of the cause—especially a source of occult blood loss. Iron deficiency cannot be overcome by increasing dietary iron; medicinal iron is always required.

A. Oral Iron: There is no better treatment than ferrous sulfate, 325 mg 3 times daily, which provides 180 mg of iron daily of which 10–20 mg is usually absorbed (though absorption may exceed this amount in cases of severe deficiency). Although ferrous sulfate is optimally taken 3 times a day on empty stomach, compliance is often improved by introducing the medicine more slowly in a gradually escalating dose. Patients who cannot tolerate iron on an empty stomach should take it with food. An appropriate response is a return of the hematocrit level halfway toward normal within 3 weeks. It is advisable to see the patient after 3 weeks both to monitor the hematologic response and to answer questions about the medication that may improve compliance. In general, hematologic values return to normal after 2 months of treatment. Iron therapy should continue for 3–6 months after restoration of normal hematologic values in order to replenish iron stores. Failure of response to iron therapy is usually due to noncompliance, although occasional patients may absorb iron poorly. Other reasons for failure to respond include incorrect diagnosis (anemia of chronic disease, thalassemia) and ongoing gastrointestinal blood loss that exceeds the rate of new erythropoiesis.

B. Parenteral Iron: The indications are intolerance to oral iron, refractoriness to oral iron (poor absorption), gastrointestinal disease precluding the use of oral iron, continued blood loss, and replacement of depleted iron stores when oral iron fails. Because of the possibility of severe and even fatal hypersensitivity reactions, parenteral iron therapy should be used only in cases of clinically significant documented iron deficiency after every reasonable attempt has been made to use oral therapy.

The dose may be calculated by estimating the decrease in volume of red blood cell mass and then supplying 1 mg of iron for each milliliter of volume of red blood cells below normal. One should then add approximately 1 g for storage iron. The entire dose may be given as an intravenous infusion over 4–6 hours. A test dose of a dilute solution is given first, and the patient should be observed closely during the entire infusion in a setting in which anaphylaxis can be treated.

Cook JD: Clinical evaluation of iron deficiency. Semin Hematol 1982;19:6.

Finch CA, Huebers H: Perspectives in iron metabolism. N Engl J Med 1982;306:1520.

ANEMIA OF CHRONIC DISEASE

Many chronic systemic diseases are associated with mild or moderate anemia. Common causes include chronic infection or inflammation, cancer, and liver disease. The anemia of chronic renal failure is somewhat different in pathophysiology and is usually more severe.

Red blood cell survival is modestly reduced, and the bone marrow fails to compensate adequately by increasing red blood cell production. Failure to increase red cell production is largely due to sequestration of iron within the reticuloendothelial system.

Decrease in erythropoietin is rarely an important cause of underproduction of red cells except in renal failure, when decreased erythropoietin is the rule.

Clinical Findings

A. Symptoms and Signs: The clinical features are those of the anemia, which is usually modest. The diagnosis should be suspected in cases of modest anemia in patients with known chronic diseases; it is confirmed by the findings of low serum iron, low TIBC, and normal or increased serum ferritin (or normal or increased bone marrow iron stores). In cases of significant anemia, coexistent iron deficiency or folic acid deficiency should be suspected. Decreased dietary intake of folate or iron is common in these ill patients, and many will also have ongoing gastrointestinal blood losses. Patients undergoing hemodialysis regularly lose both iron and folate during dialysis.

B. Laboratory Findings: The hematocrit rarely falls below 25% (except in renal failure). The MCV is usually normal but may be slightly reduced, though rarely to less than 70 fL. Red blood cell morphology is nondiagnostic, and the reticulocyte count is neither strikingly reduced nor increased. Characteristically, both the serum iron values and the TIBC are reduced. Serum iron values may be unmeasurable, and transferrin saturation may be extremely low. A mistaken diagnosis of iron deficiency anemia may be made if overemphasis is placed on the reduced serum iron and reduced transferrin saturation. A low serum iron and percentage saturation are diagnostic of iron deficiency only when the TIBC is also increased. In contrast to iron deficiency, serum ferritin values should be normal or increased. A serum ferritin value of less than 25 μg/L should suggest coexistent iron deficiency. A Prussian blue stain of the bone marrow should show normal or increased amounts of iron in macrophages.

Treatment

In most cases no treatment is necessary. In some, however—especially with severe renal insufficiency—red blood cell transfusions are required for symptomatic anemia. Purified recombinant erythropoietin has recently been shown to be safe and effective for treatment of the anemia of renal failure and other secondary anemias such as anemia related to cancer or inflammatory disorders (eg, rheumatoid arthritis). Erythropoietin is now commercially available as epoetin alfa (Epogen); however, it must be injected subcutaneously 3 or more times weekly and is very expensive. This agent should be used to alleviate anemia only when the patient is transfusion-dependent or when the quality of life is clearly improved by the hematologic response.

Eschbach JW et al: Correction of the anemia of end-stage renal disease with recombinant human erythropoietin: Results of a combined phase I and II clinical trial. N Engl J Med 1987;316:73.

Eschbach JW et al: Treatment of the anemia of progressive renal failure with recombinant human erythropoietin. N Engl J Med 1989;321:158.

Lee GR: The anemia of chronic disease. Semin Hematol 1983;20:61.

THE THALASSEMIAS

Essentials of Diagnosis

- Microcytosis out of proportion to the degree of anemia.
- Positive family history or lifelong personal history of microcytic anemia.
- Abnormal red blood cell morphology with microcytes, acanthocytes, and target cells.
- In beta thalassemia, elevated levels of hemoglobin A_2 or F.

General Considerations

The thalassemias are hereditary disorders characterized by reduction in the synthesis of globin chains (alpha or beta). Reduced globin chain synthesis causes reduced hemoglobin synthesis and eventually produces a hypochromic microcytic anemia because of defective hemoglobinization of red blood cells. Thalassemias can be considered among the hypoproliferative anemias, the hemolytic anemias, and the anemias related to abnormal hemoglobin, since all of these factors may play a role.

Normal adult hemoglobin is primarily hemoglobin A, which represents approximately 98% of circulating hemoglobin. Hemoglobin A is formed from a tetramer—2 alpha chains and 2 beta chains—and can be designated $\alpha_2\beta_2$. Two copies of the α-globin gene are located on chromosome 16, and there is no substitute for α-globin in the formation of hemoglobin. The β-globin gene resides on chromosome 11 adjacent to genes encoding the beta-like globin chains, delta and gamma. The tetramer of $\alpha_2\delta_2$ forms a hemoglobin A_2, which normally comprises 1–2% of adult hemoglobin. The tetramer a 2 g 2 forms hemoglobin F, which is the major hemoglobin of fetal life but which comprises less than 1% of normal adult hemoglobin.

Alpha thalassemia is due primarily to gene deletion directly causing reduced α-globin chain synthesis (Table 10–4). Since all adult hemoglobins are alpha-containing, alpha thalassemia produces no change in the percentage distribution of hemoglobins A, A_2, and F. In severe forms of alpha thalassemia, excess beta chains may form a β_4 tetramer called hemoglobin H. Hemoglobin H has high oxygen affinity and delivers oxygen to tissues poorly. It is also unstable and subject to oxidative denaturation under conditions of infection or exposure to oxidative drugs (sulfonamides, etc).

Beta thalassemias are usually caused by point muta-

Table 10–4. Alpha thalassemia syndromes.

Alpha Globin Genes	Syndrome	Hematocrit	MCV
4	Normal	Normal	
3	Silent carrier	Normal	
2	Thalassemia minor	32–40%	60–75 fL
1	Hemoglobin H disease	22–32%	60–70 fL
0	Hydrops fetalis		

tions rather than large deletions (Table 10–5). These mutations result in premature chain termination or in problems with transcription of RNA and ultimately result in reduced or absent β-globin chain synthesis. The molecular defects leading to beta thalassemia are numerous and heterogeneous. Defects that result in absent globin chain expression are termed β^0, whereas defects causing reduced synthesis are termed β^+. The reduced β-globin chain synthesis in beta thalassemia results in a relative increase in the percentages of hemoglobins A_2 and F compared to hemoglobin A, as the beta-like globins (gamma and delta) substitute for the missing beta chains. In the presence of reduced beta chains, the excess alpha chains are unstable and precipitate, leading to damage to red blood cell membranes. This damage causes marked intramedullary hemolysis (destruction of developing erythroid cells within the bone marrow) as well as hemolysis in the peripheral blood. The bone marrow becomes markedly hyperplastic under the drive of severe anemia and the ineffective erythropoiesis that results from destruction of the developing erythroid cells. This marked expansion of the erythroid element in the bone marrow causes severe bony deformities, osteopenia, and pathologic fractures.

Clinical Findings

A. Symptoms and Signs: The alpha thalassemia syndromes are seen primarily in persons from southeast Asia and China, and, less commonly, in blacks. Normally, adults have 4 copies of the α-globin chain. When 3 α-globin genes are present, the patient is hematologically normal and is called a silent carrier. When 2 α-globin genes are present, the patient is said to have alpha thalassemia trait, one form of thalassemia minor. These patients are clinically nor-

mal and have normal life expectancy and performance status. They have a very mild microcytic anemia with no harmful consequences. When only one α-globin chain is present, the patient has hemoglobin H disease. This is a chronic hemolytic anemia of variable severity (thalassemia minor or intermedia). Physical examination will reveal pallor and splenomegaly. Although affected individuals do not usually require transfusions, they may need transfusions during periods of hemolytic exacerbation caused by infection or other stresses. When all 4 α-globin genes are deleted, the affected fetus is stillborn as a result of hydrops fetalis.

Beta thalassemia affects persons of Mediterranean origin (Italian, Greek) and to a lesser extent Chinese, other Asians, and blacks. Patients homozygous for beta thalassemia have the syndrome of thalassemia major, formerly called Cooley's anemia. Affected children are normal at birth but during the first year of life develop severe anemia requiring transfusion. Signs of thalassemia typically develop after 6 months of age, because this is the time when hemoglobin synthesis switches from hemoglobin F to hemoglobin A. Numerous clinical problems ensue, including growth failure, bony deformities (abnormal facial structure, pathologic fractures), hepatosplenomegaly, and jaundice. The clinical course has been modified significantly by transfusion therapy. Children with severe thalassemia may grow normally until puberty, when they experience hypogonadism, growth failure, and clinical consequences of iron overload from years of transfusion. The transfusional iron overload (hemosiderosis) results in cardiomyopathy, progressive hepatomegaly, and numerous endocrine dysfunctions. Death from cardiac failure usually occurs between ages 20 and 30.

Patients homozygous for a milder form of beta thalassemia (allowing a higher rate of globin gene synthesis) may have the syndrome of thalassemia intermedia. These patients have chronic hemolytic anemia but usually do not require transfusions except under periods of stress. These patients develop iron overload because of increased gut absorption of iron and periodic transfusion. They survive into adult life but with hepatosplenomegaly and bony deformities.

Patients heterozygous for beta thalassemia have thalassemia minor. These patients have a mild microcytic anemia that is not clinically significant.

Prenatal diagnosis is available for couples at risk

Table 10–5. Beta thalassemia syndromes.

	Beta Globin Genes	Hgb A	Hgb A_2	Hgb F
Normal	Homozygous β	97–99%	1–3%	<1%
Thalassemia major	Homozygous β^0	0	4–10%	90–96%
	Homozygous β^+		4–10%	
Thalassemia intermedia	Homozygous β^+ (mild)	0–30%	0–10%	6–100%
Thalassemia minor	Heterozygous β^0	80–95%	4–8%	1–5%
	Heterozygous β^+	80–95%	4–8%	1–5%

of producing a child with one of the severe thalassemia syndromes. Asian couples whose parents on both sides have alpha thalassemia trait are at risk of producing an infant with hydrops fetalis. Mediterranean people (and, less commonly, Chinese or blacks) with 2 parents heterozygous for beta thalassemia are at risk of producing a child with Cooley's anemia. Genetic counseling should be offered, and the opportunity for prenatal diagnosis should be discussed.

B. Laboratory Findings:

1. Alpha thalassemia trait–Patients with 2 α-globin genes have mild anemia, with hematocrits between 28% and 40%. The MCV is strikingly low (60–75 fL) despite the modest degree of anemia, and the red blood count is usually normal. The peripheral blood smear shows mild abnormalities, including microcytes, hypochromia, occasional target cells, and acanthocytes (cells with irregularly spaced bulbous projections). The reticulocyte count and iron parameters are normal. Hemoglobin electrophoresis will show no increase in the percentage of hemoglobins A_2 or F and no hemoglobin H. Alpha thalassemia trait is usually diagnosed by exclusion in a patient with modest anemia, significant microcytosis, and no elevation of hemoglobins A_2 or F. Definitive diagnosis depends upon hemoglobin gene mapping demonstrating a reduced number of α-globin genes, but this procedure is not commonly available and should not be necessary for clinical diagnosis.

2. Hemoglobin H disease–These patients have a variably severe hemolytic anemia, with hematocrits between 22% and 32%. The MCV is strikingly low (69–70 fL). The peripheral blood smear is markedly abnormal, with hypochromia, microcytosis, target cells, and poikilocytosis. The reticulocyte count is elevated. Hemoglobin electrophoresis will show the presence of a fast migrating hemoglobin (hemoglobin H), which comprises 10–40% of the hemoglobin. A peripheral blood smear can be stained with supravital dyes to demonstrate the presence of hemoglobin H.

3. Beta thalassemia minor–Like patients with alpha thalassemia trait, these patients have a modest anemia with hematocrit between 28% and 40%. The MCV ranges from 55 to 75 fL, and the red blood cell count is usually normal. The peripheral blood smear is mildly abnormal, with hypochromia, microcytosis, and target cells. In contrast to alpha thalassemia, basophilic stippling may be present. The reticulocyte count may be normal or slightly elevated. Hemoglobin electrophoresis (using quantitative techniques) may show an elevation of hemoglobin A_2 to 4–8% and occasional elevations of hemoglobin F to 1–5%.

4. Beta thalassemia major–Beta thalassemia major produces a severe life-threatening anemia, and without transfusion the hematocrit may fall to less than 10%. The peripheral blood smear is bizarre, showing severe poikilocytosis, hypochromia, microcytosis, target cells, basophilic stippling, and nucleated red blood cells. Little or no hemoglobin A is present. Variable amounts of hemoglobin A_2 are seen, and the major hemoglobin present is hemoglobin F.

Differential Diagnosis

Mild forms of thalassemia must be differentiated from iron deficiency. Compared to iron deficiency anemia, patients with thalassemia have a lower MCV, a more normal red blood count, and a more abnormal peripheral blood smear at modest levels of anemia. Iron parameters are normal. The diagnosis of beta thalassemia can be shown by demonstrating increased levels of hemoglobin A_2 (or, less commonly, hemoglobin F), while the diagnosis of alpha thalassemia is made by exclusion. Severe forms of thalassemia may be confused with other hemoglobinopathies. The diagnosis will be made by hemoglobin electrophoresis.

Treatment

Patients with mild thalassemia (alpha thalassemia trait or beta thalassemia minor) are clinically normal and require no treatment. Most importantly, patients with microcytosis should be identified so that they will not be subjected to repeated evaluations for iron deficiency and inappropriately given supplemental iron. Patients with hemoglobin H disease should take folate supplementation and avoid medicinal iron and oxidative drugs such as sulfonamide drugs. They may occasionally need transfusion during pregnancy or under periods of stress. Patients with severe thalassemia should be maintained on a regular transfusion schedule and should receive folate supplementation. Splenectomy is occasionally performed when hypersplenism causes a marked increase in the transfusion requirement. Deferoxamine is routinely given as an iron-chelating agent to avoid or postpone hemosiderosis. Oral iron chelators are now undergoing testing in an investigational setting and may have a major impact.

Recently, allogeneic bone marrow transplantation has been investigated as treatment for beta thalassemia major. Young children who have not yet experienced iron overload and chronic organ toxicity do fairly well, and approximately 70% appear to do well. The role of transplantation is currently the subject of debate.

Kazazian HH, Boehm CD: Molecular basis and prenatal diagnosis of β-thalassemia. Blood 1988;72:1107.

Nienhuis AW, Anagnou NP, Ley TJ: Advances in thalassemia research. Blood 1984;63:738.

Steinberg MH, Embury SH: α-Thalassemia in blacks: Genetic and clinical aspects and interactions with the sickle hemoglobin gene. Blood 1986;68:985.

SIDEROBLASTIC ANEMIA

The sideroblastic anemias are a heterogeneous group of disorders in which hemoglobin synthesis is reduced because of failure to incorporate heme into protoporphyrin to form hemoglobin. Iron accumulates, particularly in the mitochondria. A Prussian blue stain of the bone marrow will reveal ringed sideroblasts, cells with iron deposits (in the mitochondrium) encircling the red cell nucleus. Rare cases are congenital, but the disorder is usually acquired. Sometimes it represents a stage in evolution of a generalized bone marrow disorder that may ultimately terminate in acute leukemia. Other important causes include chronic alcoholism, drug toxicity (antituberculous agents, chloramphenicol), and lead poisoning.

Patients have no specific clinical features other than those related to anemia. The anemia is usually moderate, with hematocrits of 20–30%, but transfusions may occasionally be required. Although the MCV is usually normal or slightly increased, it may occasionally be low, leading to confusion with iron deficiency. The peripheral blood smear characteristically shows a dimorphic population of red blood cells, one normal and one hypochromic. It is the presence of hypochromic cells on peripheral smear combined with a low MCV that may raise the consideration of iron deficiency. In cases of lead poisoning, coarse basophilic stippling of the red cells is seen.

The diagnosis is made by examination of the bone marrow. Characteristically, there is marked erythroid hyperplasia, a sign of ineffective erythropoiesis (expansion of the erythroid compartment of the bone marrow that does not result in the production of reticulocytes in the peripheral blood). The iron stain of the bone marrow shows a generalized increase in iron stores and the presence of ring sideroblasts. Other characteristic laboratory features include a high serum iron and a high transferrin saturation. In the presence of lead poisoning, serum lead levels will be elevated.

When lead toxicity is causative, it may be treated with chelation therapy. Occasional patients will respond to pharmacologic doses of folate or pyridoxine, but most patients do not respond to therapy. Occasionally, the anemia is so severe that support with red cell transfusion is required. These patients appear not to respond to erythropoietin therapy.

Cazzola M et al: Natural history of idiopathic refractory sideroblastic anemia. Blood 1988;71:305.

VITAMIN B$_{12}$ DEFICIENCY

Essentials of Diagnosis
- Macrocytic anemia.
- Macro-ovalocytes and hypersegmented neutrophils on peripheral blood smear.
- Serum vitamin B$_{12}$ level less than 100 pg/mL.

General Considerations

Vitamin B$_{12}$ belongs to the family of cobalamins and serves as a cofactor for 2 important reactions in humans. As methylcobalamin, it serves as a cofactor for methionine synthetase in the conversion of homocysteine to methionine. As adenosylcobalamin, it serves as a cofactor for the conversion of methylmalonyl-CoA to succinyl-CoA. All vitamin B$_{12}$ comes from the diet, and vitamin B$_{12}$ is present in all foods of animal origin. We absorb approximately 5 μg/d of vitamin B$_{12}$ from the diet.

After being ingested, vitamin B$_{12}$ becomes bound to intrinsic factor, a protein secreted by gastric parietal cells. Other cobalamin-binding proteins (called R factors) compete with intrinsic factor for vitamin B$_{12}$. Vitamin B$_{12}$ bound to R factors cannot be absorbed. The vitamin B$_{12}$-intrinsic factor complex travels through the intestine and is absorbed in the terminal ileum by cells with specific receptors for the complex. It is then transported through plasma and stored in the liver. Three plasma transport proteins have been identified. Transcobalamins I and III (differing only in carbohydrate structure) are secreted by white blood cells. Although approximately 90% of plasma vitamin B$_{12}$ circulates bound to these proteins, only transcobalamin II is capable of transporting vitamin B$_{12}$ into cells. The liver contains 2000–5000 μg of stored vitamin B$_{12}$. Since daily losses are 3–5 μg/d, the body usually has sufficient stores of vitamin B$_{12}$ so that vitamin B$_{12}$ deficiency develops more than 3 years after vitamin B$_{12}$ absorption ceases.

Since vitamin B$_{12}$ is present in all foods of animal origin, dietary vitamin B$_{12}$ deficiency is extremely rare and seen only in vegans—strict vegetarians who avoid all dairy products as well as meat and fish (Table 10–6). Abdominal surgery may lead to vitamin B$_{12}$ deficiency in several ways. Gastrectomy will eliminate that site of intrinsic factor production; blind loop syndrome will cause competition for vitamin B$_{12}$ by bacterial overgrowth in the lumen of the intestine; and surgical resection of the ileum will eliminate the site of vitamin B$_{12}$ absorption. Rare causes of vitamin B$_{12}$ deficiency include Scandinavian fish tapeworm (*Diphyllobothrium latum*) disease (rarely seen in the United States) and severe Crohn's disease caus-

Table 10–6. Causes of vitamin B$_{12}$ deficiency.

Dietary deficiency (rare)
Decreased production of intrinsic factor
Pernicious anemia
Gastrectomy
Competition for vitamin B$_{12}$ in gut
Blind loop syndrome
Fish tapeworm (rare)
Decreased ileal absorption of vitamin B$_{12}$
Surgical resections
Crohn's disease
Transcobalamin II deficiency (rare)

ing sufficient destruction of the ileum to retard vitamin B_{12} absorption.

By far the most common cause of vitamin B_{12} deficiency is that associated with **pernicious anemia.** This is a hereditary autoimmune disorder historically seen chiefly in patients of Scandinavian or northern European ancestry but now seen with increased frequency in young black and Hispanic women. Although the disease is hereditary, it is rarely manifested before age 35. Pernicious anemia produces a number of clinical findings in addition to vitamin B_{12} deficiency. Atrophic gastritis is invariably present and results in histamine-fast achlorhydria. These patients may also have a number of other autoimmune diseases, including IgA deficiency, rheumatoid arthritis, Graves' disease, and polyglandular endocrine insufficiency. Over time, the atrophic gastritis is associated with an increased risk of gastric carcinoma.

Clinical Findings

A. Symptoms and Signs: The hallmark of vitamin B_{12} deficiency is megaloblastic anemia. The anemia may be severe, with hematocrits as low as 10–15%. The megaloblastic state also produces changes in mucosal cells, leading to glossitis, as well as other vague gastrointestinal disturbances such as anorexia and diarrhea. Vitamin B_{12} deficiency also leads to a complex neurologic syndrome. Peripheral nerves are usually affected first, and patients complain initially of paresthesias. The posterior columns next become impaired, and patients complain of difficulty with balance. In more advanced cases, cerebral function may be altered as well, though on occasion dementia may precede hematologic changes.

On examination, patients are usually pale and may be mildly icteric. Neurologic examination will reveal decreased vibration and position sense.

B. Laboratory Findings: The megaloblastic state produces an anemia of variable severity that on occasion may be very severe. The MCV is usually strikingly elevated, between 110 and 140 fL. However, it is possible to have vitamin B_{12} deficiency with a normal MCV. Occasionally, the normal MCV may be explained by coexistent thalassemia or iron deficiency, but in other cases the reason for the normal MCV is obscure. Patients with neurologic signs or symptoms that suggest possible vitamin B_{12} deficiency should be thoroughly evaluated for the possibility of that deficiency despite a normal MCV and the absence of anemia. The peripheral blood smear is usually strikingly abnormal, with anisocytosis and poikilocytosis. A characteristic finding is the macroovalocyte, but numerous other abnormal shapes are usually seen. Because of the strikingly abnormal red blood cell morphology, it is often mistakenly assumed that the anemia is hemolytic. The neutrophils are hypersegmented. Typical features include a mean lobe count greater than 4 or the finding of nonlobed neutrophils. The reticulocyte count is reduced. Because vita-

min B_{12} deficiency affects all hematopoietic cell lines, in severe cases the white blood cell count and platelet count are reduced, and pancytopenia is present.

Bone marrow morphology is characteristically abnormal. Marked erythroid hyperplasia is present as a response to defective red blood cell production (ineffective erythropoiesis). Characteristic megaloblastic changes in the erythroid series include abnormally large cell size and asynchronous maturation of the nucleus and cytoplasm—ie, cytoplasmic maturation continues while impaired DNA synthesis causes retarded nuclear development. In the myeloid series, giant metamyelocytes are characteristically seen.

Other laboratory abnormalities include markedly elevated LDH and a modest increase in indirect bilirubin. These 2 findings are a reflection of intramedullary destruction of developing erythroid cells (ineffective erythropoiesis).

The diagnosis of vitamin B_{12} deficiency is made by finding an abnormally low vitamin B_{12} serum level. Whereas the normal vitamin B_{12} level is 150–350 pg/mL, most patients with overt vitamin B_{12} deficiency will have serum levels less than 100 pg/mL. The Schilling test is used to document the decreased absorption of oral vitamin B_{12} characteristic of pernicious anemia. Initially, a large intramuscular dose of vitamin B_{12} is given to saturate plasma transport proteins. Radiolabeled vitamin B_{12} is given orally, and a 24-hour urine collection is performed to determine how much vitamin B_{12} is absorbed and subsequently excreted. Normally, more than 7% of an administered dose is present in the urine; most patients with impaired absorption will have less than 3% of the dose present in the urine. The second stage of the Schilling test is to administer radiolabeled vitamin B_{12} together with intrinsic factor. If pernicious anemia (a lack of intrinsic factor) is the case of vitamin B_{12} deficiency, the combined use of vitamin B_{12} and intrinsic factor should correct the abnormally low absorption. However, the full-blown megaloblastic state causes abnormalities in intestinal epithelium that may lead to generalized malabsorption. In these cases, the second stage of the Schilling test will remain abnormal until the intestinal mucosal defect is first corrected by vitamin B_{12} replacement (in approximately 2 months).

Differential Diagnosis

Vitamin B_{12} deficiency should be differentiated from folic acid deficiency, the other common cause of megaloblastic anemia. The differentiation is based on a low serum vitamin B_{12} level and a normal serum folate level. Differentiation of vitamin B_{12} deficiency from myelodysplasia (the other common cause of macrocytic anemia with abnormal morphology) is based on the characteristic morphology and the low vitamin B_{12} level.

It should be emphasized that any neurologic signs or symptoms suggestive of vitamin B_{12} deficiency should be evaluated for that disorder even in the absence of anemia or macrocytosis.

Treatment

Patients with pernicious anemia cannot absorb oral vitamin B_{12} and require parenteral therapy. Intramuscular injections of 200 μg are adequate for each dose. Replacement is usually given daily for the first week, weekly for the first month, and then monthly for life. It should be stressed that pernicious anemia is a lifelong disorder and that if patients discontinue their monthly therapy, the vitamin deficiency will recur.

Patients respond to therapy with an immediate improvement in their sense of well-being. Hypokalemia may complicate the first several days of therapy, particularly if the anemia is severe. A brisk reticulocytosis occurs in 5–7 days, and the hematologic picture normalizes in 2 months. Central nervous system symptoms and signs are reversible if they are of relatively short duration (less than 6 months), but they may be permanent if treatment is not initiated promptly.

Carmel R, Johnson CS: Racial patterns in pernicious anemia: Early age at onset and increased frequency of intrinsic-factor antibody in black women. N Engl J Med 1978; 298:647.

Green R et al: Masking of macrocytosis by alpha-thalassemia in blacks with pernicious anemia. N Engl J Med 1982;307:1322.

Kapadia CP, Donaldson RM Jr: Disorders of cobalamin (vitamin B_{12}) absorption and transport. Annu Rev Med 1985;36:93.

FOLIC ACID DEFICIENCY

Essentials of Diagnosis

- Macrocytic anemia.
- Macro-ovalocytes and hypersegmented neutrophils on peripheral blood smear.
- Normal serum vitamin B_{12} levels.
- Reduced folate levels in red blood cells or serum.

General Considerations

Folic acid is the term commonly used for pteroylmonoglutamic acid. In its reduced form of tetrahydrofolate, it serves as an important mediator of many reactions involving one-carbon transfers. Important reactions include the conversion of homocysteine to methionine and of deoxyuridylate to thymidylate, an important step in DNA synthesis.

Folic acid is present in most fruits and vegetables (especially citrus fruits and green leafy vegetables) and daily requirements of 50–100 μg/d are usually met in the diet. Total body stores of folate are approximately 5000 μg, enough to supply requirements for 2–3 months.

By far the most common cause of folate deficiency

Table 10–7. Causes of folate deficiency.

Dietary deficiency
Decreased absorption
Tropical sprue
Drugs: Phenytoin, sulfasalazine
Increased requirement
Chronic hemolytic anemia
Pregnancy
Exfoliative skin disease
Loss: Dialysis
Inhibition of reduction to active form
Methotrexate

is inadequate dietary intake (Table 10–7). Alcoholics, anorectic cancer patients, elderly persons who do not buy fresh fruits and vegetables, and persons who overcook their food are candidates for folate deficiency. Reduced folate absorption is rarely seen except in the case of tropical sprue. However, drugs such as phenytoin or sulfasalazine may interfere with folate absorption. Folic acid requirements are increased in pregnancy, chronic hemolytic anemia, and exfoliative skin disease, and in these cases the increased requirements (5–10 times normal) may not be met by a normal diet. Patients with increased folate requirements should receive oral medicinal supplementation with 1 mg/d of folic acid.

Clinical Findings

A. Symptoms and Signs: The clinical features are similar to those of vitamin B_{12} deficiency, with megaloblastic anemia and megaloblastic changes in mucosa. However, there are none of the neurologic abnormalities associated with vitamin B_{12} deficiency.

B. Laboratory Findings: The megaloblastic anemia is identical to that resulting from vitamin B_{12} deficiency (see above). However, the serum vitamin B_{12} level is normal. In contrast, the serum folic acid level is low, usually less than 3 ng/mL (normal: > 6 ng/mL). However, serum folate levels are often misleading, since one meal containing folate will cause a transient correction of the low serum level. For these reasons, the red blood cell folate level, which reflects folic acid intake over the previous months, is often more reliable and should replace serum folate as the appropriate test. A red blood cell folate level of less than 150 ng/mL is diagnostic of folate deficiency.

Differential Diagnosis

The megaloblastic anemia of folate deficiency should be differentiated from vitamin B_{12} deficiency by the finding of a normal vitamin B_{12} level and a reduced serum folate or red blood cell folate level. Alcoholics, who often have folate deficiency, may also have anemia of liver disease. This latter macrocytic anemia does not cause megaloblastic morphologic changes but rather produces target cells in the peripheral blood. Patients with HIV-related illnesses being treated with zidovudine frequently develop macrocytosis but do not manifest typical megaloblastic morphology.

Treatment

Folic acid deficiency is treated with folic acid, 1 mg/d orally. The response is similar to that seen in the treatment of vitamin B_{12} deficiency, with rapid improvement and a sense of well-being, reticulocytosis in 5–7 days, and total correction of hematologic abnormalities within 2 months. Large doses of folic acid may produce hematologic responses in cases of vitamin B_{12} deficiency but will allow neurologic damage to progress. This error must be avoided.

Lindenbaum J: Status of laboratory testing in the diagnosis of megaloblastic anemia. Blood 1983;61:624.
Lindenbaum J et al: Neuropsychiatric disorders caused by cobalamin deficiency in the absence of anemia or macrocytosis. N Engl J Med 1988;318:1720.
Talley NJ: Risk for colorectal adenocarcinoma in pernicious anemia: A population-based cohort study. Ann Intern Med 1989;111:738.

PURE RED CELL APLASIA

Adult acquired pure red cell aplasia is extremely rare. It appears to be an autoimmune disease in which an IgG antibody specifically attacks erythroid precursors. A congenital form (Diamond-Blackfan syndrome) has been identified. In adults, the disease is usually idiopathic. However, cases have been seen in association with systemic lupus erythematosus, chronic lymphocytic leukemia, lymphomas, or thymoma. Some drugs (phenytoin, chloramphenicol) may cause red cell aplasia. Transient episodes of red cell aplasia are probably common in response to viral infections, especially parvovirus infections. However, these acute episodes will go unrecognized unless the patient has a chronic hemolytic disorder, in which case the hematocrit may fall precipitously.

Clinically, the only signs are those of anemia, unless the patient has an associated autoimmune or lymphoproliferative disorder. The anemia is often severe and is normochromic. Reticulocytes are very low or absent. Red blood cell morphology is normal, and the myeloid and platelet lines are unaffected. The bone marrow is normocellular. All elements present are normal, but erythroid precursors are markedly reduced or absent.

Occasionally, other signs of autoimmune disorder such as hypogammaglobulinemia or a positive antinuclear antibody test are seen. In some cases, the chest radiograph will reveal a thymoma.

The disorder should be distinguished from aplastic anemia (in which the marrow was generally hypocellular and other cell lines are affected) and from myelodysplasia. This latter disorder is recognized by the presence of morphologic abnormalities that should not be present in pure red cell aplasia.

If the thymoma is present, it should be resected, and in some cases the anemia will remit. In other cases, suppression of the autoimmune phenomenon with prednisone, cyclophosphamide, and plasmapheresis should be considered. High-dose intravenous gamma globulin has produced excellent responses in a small number of cases. The duration of response remains to be determined, and more experience is needed before this treatment can be generally recommended. Antithymocyte globulin, useful in aplastic anemia, has also been reported to be of value.

Clark DA, Dessypris EN, Krantz SB: Studies on pure red cell aplasia. 11. Results of immunosuppressive treatment of 37 patients. Blood 1984;63:277.
McGuire WA et al: Treatment of antibody-mediated pure red cell aplasia with high-dose intravenous gammaglobulin. N Engl J Med 1987;317:1004.

HEMOLYTIC ANEMIAS

The hemolytic anemias are a group of disorders in which red blood cell survival is reduced, either episodically or continuously. The bone marrow has the ability to increase erythroid production up to 8-fold in response to reduced red cell survival, so anemia will be present only when the ability of the bone marrow to compensate is outstripped. This will occur when red cell survival is extremely short or when the ability of the bone marrow to compensate is impaired for some second reason.

Hemolysis is an uncommon cause of anemia. In assessing whether hemolytic anemia is present, one must determine whether the rate of fall of the hematocrit is faster than can be accounted for by lack of production alone. Since red blood cell survival is normally 120 days, in the absence of red cell production the hematocrit will fall at the rate of approximately 1/100 of the hematocrit per day, which translates to a decrease in the hematocrit reading of approximately 3% per week. For example, a fall of hematocrit from 45% to 36% over 3 weeks' time need not indicate hemolysis, since this rate of fall would result simply from cessation of red blood cell production. If the hematocrit is falling at a faster rate than that due to decreased production, blood loss or hemolysis is the cause. Consequently, hemolysis can be defined as a hematocrit falling at a rate faster than can be accounted for by lack of production alone in the absence of bleeding.

Reticulocytosis is an important clue to the presence of hemolysis, since in most hemolytic disorders the bone marrow will respond with increased red blood cell production. However, hemolysis can be present without reticulocytosis when a second disorder (infection, folate deficiency) is superimposed on hemolysis; in these circumstances, the hematocrit will fall rapidly. However, reticulocytosis also occurs during recovery from hypoproliferative anemia or bleeding. Hemolysis is correctly diagnosed (when bleeding is excluded) when the hematocrit is either falling or stable despite reticulocytosis.

Hemolytic disorders are generally classified according to whether the defect is intrinsic to the red cell or due to some external factor (Table 10–8). Intrinsic defects have been described in all components of the red blood cell, including the membrane, glycolytic and other enzymes, and hemoglobin. Most of these disorders are hereditary. The vast majority of hemolytic anemias due to external factors are the immune hemolytic anemias.

Certain laboratory features are common to all the hemolytic anemias. Haptoglobin, a normal plasma protein that binds and clears hemoglobin released into plasma, may be depressed in hemolytic disorders. However, haptoglobin levels are influenced by many factors and, by themselves, are not a reliable indicator of hemolysis. When intravascular hemolysis occurs, transient hemoglobinemia occurs. Hemoglobin is filtered through the glomerulus and usually reabsorbed by tubular cells. Hemoglobinuria will be present only when the capacity for reabsorption of hemoglobin by these cells is exceeded. In the absence of hemoglobinuria, evidence for prior intravascular hemolysis is the presence of hemosiderin in shed renal tubular cells (positive urine hemosiderin). With severe intravascular hemolysis, hemoglobinemia and methemalbuminemia may be present. Hemolysis increases the indirect bilirubin, and the total bilirubin may rise to as high as 4 mg/dL. Bilirubin levels higher than this indicate some degree of hepatic dysfunction. Serum LDH levels are strikingly elevated in cases of microangiopathic hemolysis (thrombotic thrombocytopenic purpura, hemolytic-uremic syndrome) and may be elevated in other hemolytic anemias. Iron levels are usually not affected by hemolysis, since the iron from

sequestered red cells is recycled through the reticuloendothelial system. Only causes of intravascular hemolysis will lead to iron deficiency due to hemoglobinemia.

HEREDITARY SPHEROCYTOSIS

Essentials of Diagnosis

- Spherocytes and increased reticulocytes on peripheral blood smear.
- Negative Coombs test.
- Positive family history.

General Considerations

Hereditary spherocytosis is a disorder of the red blood cell membrane, leading to chronic hemolytic anemia. Normally, the red blood cell is a biconcave disk with a diameter of 7–8 μm. The red blood cells must be both strong and deformable—strong to withstand the stress of circulating for 120 days and deformable so as to pass through capillaries 3 mm in diameter and splenic fenestrations in the cords of the red pulp of approximately 2 μm. The red blood cell skeleton, made up primarily of the proteins spectrin and actin, gives the red cells these characteristics of strength and deformability.

The membrane defect in hereditary spherocytosis has not been defined but is most likely an abnormality in spectrin. The result is a decrease in surface-to-volume ratio that results in a spherical shape of the cell. These spherical cells are less deformable and unable to pass through 2-μm fenestrations in the splenic red pulp. Hemolysis takes place because of trapping of red blood cells within the spleen.

Family members should be screened to detect those with spherocytosis (see laboratory findings).

Clinical Findings

A. Symptoms and Signs: Hereditary spherocytosis is an autosomal dominant disease of variable severity. It is often diagnosed during childhood, but milder cases may be discovered incidentally late in adult life. Anemia may or may not be present, since the bone marrow may be able to compensate for shortened red cell survival. Severe anemia (aplastic crisis) may occur when bone marrow compensation is impaired by infection or folate deficiency. Chronic hemolysis may cause jaundice and pigment gallstones, leading to attacks of cholecystitis. Examination may reveal icterus and a palpable spleen.

B. Laboratory Findings: The anemia is of variable severity, and the hematocrit may be normal. Reticulocytosis is always present. The peripheral blood smear shows the presence of spherocytes, small cells that have lost their central pallor. Spherocytes usually make up only a small percentage of red blood cells on the peripheral smear. Hereditary spherocytosis is one of the few disorders associated with increased

Table 10–8. Classification of hemolytic anemias.

Intrinsic
 Membrane defects: Hereditary spherocytosis, hereditary elliptocytosis, paroxysmal nocturnal hemoglobinuria
 Glycolytic defects: Pyruvate kinase deficiency, severe hypophosphatemia
 Oxidation vulnerability: G6PD deficiency, methemoglobinemia
 Hemoglobinopathies: Sickle syndromes, unstable hemoglobins, methemoglobinemia
Extrinsic
 Immune: Autoimmune, lymphoproliferative disease, drug toxicity
 Microangiopathic: Thrombotic thrombocytopenic purpura, hemolytic-uremic syndrome, disseminated intravascular coagulation, valve hemolysis, metastatic adenocarcinoma, vasculitis
 Infection: *Plasmodium, Clostridium, Borrelia*
 Hypersplenism
 Burns

MCHC, often greater than 36 g/dL. As with other hemolytic disorders, there may be an increase in indirect bilirubin. The Coombs test is negative.

The presence of spherocytes may be confirmed by the osmotic fragility test. Spherocytes are red cells that have lost some membrane surface and are abnormally vulnerable to swelling induced by hypotonic media. Increased osmotic fragility merely reflects the presence of spherocytes and does not distinguish hereditary spherocytosis from other spherocytic hemolytic disorders such as autoimmune hemolytic anemia.

Treatment

These patients should receive uninterrupted supplementation with folic acid, 1 mg/d. The treatment of choice is splenectomy, which will not correct the membrane defect or correct the spherocytosis but will eliminate the site of hemolysis. In very mild cases discovered late in adult life, splenectomy may not be necessary.

Friedman EW: Hereditary spherocytosis in the elderly. Am J Med 1988;84:513.
Palek J, Lux SE: Red cell membrane skeletal defects in hereditary and acquired hemolytic anemias. Semin Hematol 1983;20:189.

HEREDITARY ELLIPTOCYTOSIS

Hereditary elliptocytosis is a congenital disorder of the red blood cell membrane and probably is due to abnormalities in spectrin tetramer formation. The disorder is autosomal dominant and of variable severity. In the most common form of hereditary elliptocytosis, the mild hemolytic disorder is well compensated, and there is little or no anemia. However, more severe varieties do produce anemia, splenomegaly, and pigment gallstones.

In the common mild variety, the hallmark of the disorder is the elliptical shape of the majority of red blood cells on peripheral blood smear. Reticulocytosis may be present. In the rare severe varieties of the disorder (hereditary pyropoikilocytosis), the peripheral blood smear is extremely bizarre; and in addition to elliptocytes, microspherocytes and a variety of unusually shaped red cells are present.

No treatment is usually indicated. Severe variants are treated with splenectomy and folate supplementation.

PAROXYSMAL NOCTURNAL HEMOGLOBINURIA

Paroxysmal nocturnal hemoglobinuria is an acquired clonal stem cell disorder that results in abnormal sensitivity of the red blood cell membrane to lysis by complement. The exact nature of the defect is unknown but involves both increased binding of C3b and increased vulnerability to lysis by complement. Paroxysmal nocturnal hemoglobinuria is a very rare disorder and should be suspected in confusing cases of hemolytic anemia.

The best screening test for paroxysmal nocturnal hemoglobinuria is the sucrose hemolysis test. The diagnosis can be confirmed by Ham's (acidified serum) test.

Clinical Findings

A. Symptoms and Signs: The anemia is of variable severity and may be severe. Classically, patients report episodic hemoglobinuria resulting in reddish brown urine. Hemoglobinuria may be present in the first morning urine, since the mild respiratory acidosis of sleep leads to enhanced complement activity. In addition to anemia, these patients may be affected by thrombosis, especially mesenteric and hepatic vein thromboses. The reason for thrombus formation is unclear but may be related to platelet activation by complement. As this is a stem cell disorder, paroxysmal nocturnal hemoglobinuria may progress either to aplastic anemia or to acute myeloid leukemia.

B. Laboratory Findings: Anemia is of variable severity, and reticulocytosis may or may not be present. Abnormalities on the blood smear are nondiagnostic and may include macro-ovalocytes. As with other hemolytic disorders, haptoglobin may be decreased or absent. Since the episodic hemolysis in paroxysmal nocturnal hemoglobinuria is intravascular, the finding of urine hemosiderin is a useful test. Serum LDH is characteristically elevated. Iron deficiency is commonly present and is related to chronic iron loss from hemoglobinuria, since hemolysis is primarily intravascular.

The white blood cell count and platelet count may be decreased. A decreased leukocyte alkaline phosphatase—evidence for qualitative abnormality in the myeloid series—is good evidence for paroxysmal nocturnal hemoglobinuria. Bone marrow morphology is variable and may show either hypoplasia or erythroid hyperplasia.

Treatment

Iron replacement is often indicated for treatment of iron deficiency. This may improve the anemia but may also cause a transient increase in hemolysis. For unclear reasons, prednisone is effective in decreasing hemolysis, and some patients can be managed effectively with alternate-day steroids. In severe cases, bone marrow transplantation has been used to correct the disorder.

Nicholson-Weller A et al: Deficiency of the complement regulatory protein, "DK accelerating factor," on membranes of granulocytes, monocytes and platelets in paroxysmal nocturnal hemoglobinuria. N Engl J Med 1985; 312:1091.

PYRUVATE KINASE DEFICIENCY

The red blood cell obtains 90% of its energy from anaerobic glycolysis. Defects in glycolytic enzymes produce a chronic hemolytic anemia because of depletion of ATP. Severe hypophosphatemia may result in hemolysis for the same reason.

Pyruvate kinase deficiency is a very rare autosomal recessive disorder that causes chronic hemolytic anemia, usually with onset in childhood. In addition to the anemia, splenomegaly and pigment gallstones may be present. The red blood cell smear is normal, and the diagnosis is made by specific enzyme assays available only in specialized laboratories. Splenectomy is the treatment of choice.

Valentine WN, Tanaka KR, Paglia DE: Hemolytic anemias and erythrocyte enzymopathies. Ann Intern Med 1985; 103:245.

GLUCOSE-6-PHOSPHATE DEHYDROGENASE DEFICIENCY

Essentials of Diagnosis
- X-linked recessive disorder seen commonly in American black men.
- Episodic hemolysis in response to oxidant drugs or infection.
- Minimally abnormal peripheral blood smear.
- Reduced levels of G6PD between hemolytic episodes.

General Considerations
Glucose-6-phosphate dehydrogenase (G6PD) deficiency is a hereditary enzyme defect that causes episodic hemolytic anemia because of decreased ability of red blood cells to deal with oxidative stresses. The hexose monophosphate shunt is not an important source of energy generation in red cells but is important in generating reduced glutathione, which protects hemoglobin from oxidative denaturation. The first step in this pathway is the generation of NADPH by the action of G6PD on glucose 6-phosphate. NADPH serves as a cofactor for glutathione reductase in generating reduced glutathione, which detoxifies hydrogen peroxide. In the absence of reduced glutathione, hemoglobin may become oxidized. Oxidized hemoglobin denatures and forms precipitants called Heinz bodies. These Heinz bodies cause membrane damage, which leads to removal of these cells by the spleen.

Numerous types of G6PD enzymes have been described. The normal type found in Caucasians is designated G6PD-B. Most American blacks have G6PD-A, which is normal in function. Ten to 15% of American blacks have the variant G6PD designated A⁻, in which there is only 15% of normal enzyme activity, and enzyme activity declines rapidly as the red blood cell ages past 40 days. It is the fact that enzyme activity declines with red blood cell age that explains many of the clinical findings in this disorder. Many other G6PD variants have been described, including some Mediterranean variants with extremely low enzyme activity.

Clinical Findings
G6PD deficiency is an X-linked recessive disorder affecting 10–15% of American black males. Female carriers are rarely affected—only when an unusually high percentage of cells producing the normal enzyme are inactivated.

A. Symptoms and Signs: Patients are usually healthy, without chronic hemolytic anemia or splenomegaly. Hemolysis occurs as a result of oxidative stress on the red blood cells, generated either by infection or exposure to certain drugs. Common drugs initiating hemolysis include primaquine, quinidine, quinine, sulfonamides, and nitrofurantoin. When hemolysis occurs, the patient may become jaundiced and have dark urine. Even with continuous use of the offending drug, the hemolytic episode is usually self-limited because older red blood cells (with low enzyme activity) are removed and replaced with a population of young red blood cells with adequate functional levels of G6PD.

Severe G6PD deficiency (as in Mediterranean variants) may produce a chronic hemolytic anemia, and hemolytic crises may be severe or even fatal.

B. Laboratory Findings: Between hemolytic episodes, the blood is normal. During episodes of hemolysis, there is reticulocytosis and increased serum indirect bilirubin. The red blood cell smear is not diagnostic but may reveal a small number of "bite" cells—cells that appear to have had a bite taken out of their periphery. This in fact indicates pitting of hemoglobin aggregates by the spleen. Heinz bodies may be demonstrated by staining a peripheral blood smear with crystal violet. (They are not visible on the usual Wright-stained blood smear.) Specific enzyme assays for G6PD may reveal a low level. Results for G6PD assays may be misleading if they are performed during a hemolytic episode when the enzyme-deficient cohort of cells has been removed and replaced with a young cohort with nearly normal enzyme activity. In these cases, the enzyme assays should be repeated after hemolysis has resolved. In severe cases of G6PD deficiency, enzyme levels are always low.

Treatment
No treatment is necessary except to avoid known oxidant drugs.

Luzzatto L: Inherited hemolytic states: Glucose-6-phosphate dehydrogenase deficiency. Clin Haematol 1975;4:83.
Valentine WM, Tanaka KR, Paglia DE: Hemolytic anemias and erythrocyte enzymopathies. Ann Intern Med 1985; 103:245.

SICKLE CELL ANEMIA & RELATED SYNDROMES

Essentials of Diagnosis

- Irreversibly sickled cells on peripheral blood smear.
- Positive family history and lifelong history of hemolytic anemia.
- Recurrent painful episodes.
- Hemoglobin S is the major hemoglobin seen on electrophoresis.

General Considerations

Sickle cell anemia is an autosomal dominant disorder in which an abnormal hemoglobin (hemoglobinopathy) leads to chronic hemolytic anemia with a variety of severe clinical consequences. The disorder is a classic example of disease caused by a point mutation in DNA. A single DNA base change leads to an amino acid substitution of valine for glutamine in the sixth position on the β-globin chain. The abnormal beta chain is designated β^s and the tetramer of $\alpha_2\beta^s_2$ is designated hemoglobin S.

When in the deoxy form, hemoglobin S forms polymers that damage the red blood cell membrane. Both polymer formation and early membrane damage are reversible. However, red blood cells that have undergone repeated sickling are damaged beyond repair and become irreversibly sickled cells.

The rate of sickling is influenced by a number of factors, most importantly by the concentration of hemoglobin S in the individual red blood cell. Red cell dehydration makes the cell quite vulnerable to sickling. Sickling is also strongly influenced by the presence of other hemoglobins within the cell. Hemoglobin F cannot participate in polymer formation, and its presence markedly retards sickling. Other factors that increase sickling are those which lead to formation of deoxyhemoglobin S, eg, acidosis and hypoxemia, either systemic or locally in tissues.

Prenatal diagnosis is now available for couples at risk of producing a child with sickle cell anemia. DNA from fetal cells can be directly examined, and the presence of the sickle cell mutation can be accurately and definitively diagnosed. Genetic counseling should be made available to such couples.

Clinical Findings

A. Symptoms and Signs: The hemoglobin S gene is carried in 8% of American blacks, and one birth out of 400 in American blacks will produce a child with sickle cell anemia. The disorder has its onset during the first year of life, when hemoglobin F levels fall as a signal (of unknown nature) is sent to the bone marrow to switch from γ-globin to β-globin production.

Chronic hemolytic anemia produces jaundice, pigment gallstones, splenomegaly, and poorly healing ulcers over the lower tibia. The chronic anemia may become life-threatening when severe anemia is produced by hemolytic or aplastic crises. Aplastic crises occur when the ability of the bone marrow to compensate is reduced by viral or other infection or by folate deficiency. Hemolytic crises may be related to splenic sequestration of sickled cells (primarily in childhood, before the spleen has been infarcted) or with coexistent disorders such as G6PD deficiency.

Acute painful episodes due to acute vaso-occlusion may occur spontaneously or be provoked by infection, dehydration, or hypoxia. Clusters of sickled red cells occlude the microvasculature of the organs involved. These episodes last hours to days and produce acute pain and low-grade fever. Common sites of acute painful episodes include the bones (especially the back and long bones) and the chest. Acute vaso-occlusion may also cause strokes and priapism. Vaso-occlusive episodes are not associated with increased hemolysis.

Repeated episodes of vascular occlusion cause chronic organ damage affecting a large number of organs, especially the heart and liver. Ischemic necrosis of bone occurs, rendering the bone susceptible to osteomyelitis due to staphylococci or (less commonly) salmonellae. In adult life, the spleen is infarcted. Infarction of the papillae of the renal medulla causes renal tubular defects and gross hematuria. Retinopathy is often present and may lead to blindness.

These patients are prone to delayed puberty and may rarely have an increased incidence of infection. Infections are related to hyposplenism as well as to defects in the alternative pathway of complement.

On examination, patients are often chronically ill and jaundiced. There is hepatomegaly, but the spleen is not palpable in adult life. The heart is enlarged, with a hyperdynamic precordium and systolic murmurs. Nonhealing ulcers of the lower leg and retinopathy may be present.

Sickle cell anemia becomes a chronic multisystem disease, with death from organ failure commonly occurring between ages 20 and 40.

B. Laboratory Findings: Chronic hemolytic anemia is present. The hematocrit is usually 20–30%. The peripheral blood smear is characteristically abnormal, with irreversibly sickled cells comprising 5–50% of red cells. Other findings include reticulocytosis (10–25%), nucleated red blood cells, and hallmarks of hyposplenism such as Howell-Jolly bodies and target cells. The white blood cell count is characteristically elevated to 12,000–15,000/μL, and thrombocytosis may occur. Indirect bilirubin levels are high and haptoglobin is absent.

The presence of hemoglobin S can be demonstrated by a screening test. The sodium metabisulfite test has now largely been replaced by a solubility test in high-ionic-strength media. Normal hemoglobin will produce a clear solution, whereas hemoglobin S will produce a turbid solution. The diagnosis of sickle cell anemia may be confirmed by hemoglobin electro-

Table 10–9. Hemoglobin distribution in sickle cell syndromes.

Genotype	Diagnosis	Hgb A	Hgb S$_3$	Hgb A$_2$	Hgb F
AA	Normal	97–99%	0	1–2%	< 1%
AS	Sickle trait	60%	40%	1–2%	< 1%
SS	Sickle cell anemia	0	85–98%	1–3%	5–15%
SB^0 thal	Sickle B thalassemia	0	70–80%	3–5%	10–20%
SB$^+$ thal	Sickle B thalassemia	10–20%	60–75%	3–5%	10–20%
AS, α thalassemia	Sickle trait	70–75%	25–30%	1–2%	< 1%

phoresis (Table 10–9). Hemoglobin S has an abnormal migration pattern on electrophoresis and will usually comprise 85–98% of hemoglobin. In homozygous S disease, no hemoglobin A will be present. Hemoglobin F levels are variably increased, and high hemoglobin F levels are associated with a more benign clinical course.

Treatment

No specific treatment is available for the primary disease. However, both longevity and quality of life may be improved by comprehensive medical management by a concerned physician. Patients are maintained chronically on folic acid supplementation and should not routinely be given transfusions. Transfusions are indicated for aplastic or hemolytic crises and during the third trimester of pregnancy.

When acute painful episodes occur, precipitating factors should be identified and infections treated if present. The patient should be kept well hydrated, and oxygen should be given if the patient is hypoxic. Otherwise, treatment is supportive (hydration and analgesics).

Acute vaso-occlusive crises can be treated with exchange transfusion, in which the patient's blood containing a sickled hemoglobin is removed and replaced with normal blood. However, this should not be performed as a routine procedure, because of risks of transfusion including iron overload and stimulation of alloantibody production. Exchange transfusions are indicated for the treatment of intractable crises, priapism, and stroke and as a preventive measure for patients undergoing general anesthesia.

Cytotoxic agents such as hydroxyurea have recently been shown to increase hemoglobin F levels (by stimulating erythropoiesis in more primitive erythroid precursors). Clinical trials are being conducted to evaluate whether this will ameliorate clinical disease. Pending results of these studies, the use of hydroxyurea cannot be recommended.

Kark JA: Sickle cells trait as a risk factor for sudden death in physical training. N Engl J Med 1987;317:781.

Koshy M et al: Prophylactic red cell transfusions in pregnant patients with sickle cell disease: A randomized cooperative study. N Engl J Med 1988;319:1447.

Rodgers GP et al: Hematologic responses of patients with sickle cell disease to treatment with hydroxyurea. N Engl J Med 1990;322:1037.

Steinberg MH, Hebbel RP: Clinical diversity of sickle cell anemia: Genetic and cellular modulation of disease severity. Am J Hematol 1983;14:405.

SICKLE CELL TRAIT

Patients with the heterozygous genotype (AS) have sickle cell trait. These persons are clinically normal and have acute painful episodes only under extreme conditions such as vigorous exertion at high altitudes (or in unpressurized aircraft). The patients are hematologically normal, with no anemia and normal red blood cells on peripheral blood smear. They may, however, have a defect in renal tubular function, causing an inability to concentrate the urine. A screening test for sickle hemoglobin (sodium metabisulfite or solubility test) will be positive, and hemoglobin electrophoresis will reveal that approximately 40% of hemoglobin is hemoglobin S (Table 10–9).

No treatment is necessary. These patients should be considered normal in all respects.

SICKLE THALASSEMIA

Patients with homozygous sickle cell anemia and alpha thalassemia have a somewhat milder form of hemolysis because of a slower rate of sickling related to reduced hemoglobin concentration (MCHC) within the red blood cell.

Patients who are double heterozygotes for sickle cell anemia and beta thalassemia are clinically affected with sickle cell syndromes. Sickle β^0 thalassemia is clinically very similar to homozygous SS disease. Vaso-occlusive crises may be somewhat less severe, and the spleen is usually not infarcted. Hematologically, the MCV is usually low-in contrast to the normal MCV of sickle cell anemia—and the smear usually reveals fewer irreversibly sickled cells. Hemoglobin electrophoresis (Table 10–9) reveals no hemoglobin A but will show an increase in hemoglobin A$_2$ which is not present in sickle cell anemia.

Sickle β^+ thalassemia is a milder disorder than homozygous SS disease, with fewer crises. The spleen is usually palpable. The hemolytic anemia is less severe, and the hematocrit is usually 30–38%, with reticulocytes of 5–10%. Hemoglobin electrophoresis shows the presence of some hemoglobin A.

HEMOGLOBIN C DISORDERS

Hemoglobin C is formed by a single amino acid substitution at the same site of substitution as in sickled hemoglobin but with lysine instead of valine substituted for glutamine at the β_6 position. Hemoglobin C is nonsickling but may participate in polymer formation in association with hemoglobin S. Homozygous hemoglobin C disease produces a mild hemolytic anemia with splenomegaly, mild jaundice, and pigment gallstones. The peripheral blood smear shows numerous target cells as well as occasional cells with rectangular crystals of hemoglobin C. Persons heterozygous for hemoglobin C are clinically normal.

Patients with hemoglobin SC disease are double heterozygotes for beta S and beta C. These patients, like those with sickle β^+ thalassemia, have a milder hemolytic anemia and milder clinical course than those with homozygous SS disease. There are fewer vaso-occlusive events, and the spleen remains palpable in adult life. However, persons with hemoglobin SC disease have more retinopathy and more ischemic necrosis of bone than those with SS disease. The hematocrit is usually 30–38%, with 5–10% reticulocytes and few irreversibly sickled cells on the blood smear. Target cells are more numerous than in SS disease. Hemoglobin electrophoresis will show approximately 50% hemoglobin C, 50% hemoglobin S, and no increase in hemoglobin F levels.

UNSTABLE HEMOGLOBINS

Unstable hemoglobins are prone to oxidative denaturation even in the presence of a normal G6PD system. The disorder is autosomal dominant and of variable severity. Most patients have a mild chronic hemolytic anemia with splenomegaly, mild jaundice, and pigment gallstones. Less severely affected patients are not anemic except under conditions of oxidative stress.

The diagnosis is made by the finding of Heinz bodies and a normal G6PD level. Hemoglobin electrophoresis is usually normal, since these hemoglobins characteristically do not have a change in their migration pattern. These hemoglobins can be shown to precipitate in isopropanol. Usually no treatment is necessary. Patients with chronic hemolytic anemia should receive folate supplementation and avoid known oxidative drugs. In rare severe cases, splenectomy may be required.

AUTOIMMUNE HEMOLYTIC ANEMIA

Essentials of Diagnosis
- Acquired hemolytic anemia.
- Spherocytes and reticulocytosis on peripheral blood smear.
- Positive Coombs test.

General Considerations
Autoimmune hemolytic anemia is an acquired disorder in which an IgG autoantibody is formed that binds to the red blood cell membrane. The antibody is most commonly directed against a basic component of the Rh system and is present on virtually all human red blood cells. When IgG antibodies coat the red blood cell, the Fc portion of the antibody is recognized by macrophages (with Fc receptor) present in the spleen and other portions of the reticuloendothelial system. The interaction between splenic macrophage and the antibody-coated red blood cell results in removal of red blood cell membrane and the formation of a spherocyte because of the decrease in surface-to-volume ratio of the red blood cell. These spherocytic cells have decreased deformability and become trapped in the red pulp of the spleen because of their inability to squeeze through the 2-μm fenestrations. When large amounts of IgG are present on red blood cells, complement may be fixed. Direct lysis of cells is rare, but the presence of C3b on the surface of red blood cells allows Kupffer cells in the liver to participate in the hemolytic process because of the presence of C3b receptors on Kupffer cells.

Approximately half of all cases of autoimmune hemolytic anemia are idiopathic. The disorder may also be seen in association with systemic lupus erythematosus, chronic lymphocytic leukemia, or diffuse lymphomas. It must be distinguished from drug-induced hemolytic anemia. Methyldopa commonly stimulates the production of an autoantibody with the same specificity as that in idiopathic autoimmune hemolytic anemia. Other drugs (penicillin, quinidine) become associated with the red blood cell membrane, and the antibody is directed against the membrane-drug complex.

The Coombs antiglobulin test forms the basis for diagnosis of these immune hemolytic disorders. The Coombs reagent is a rabbit IgM antibody raised against human IgG or human complement. The direct Coombs test is performed by mixing the patient's red blood cells with the Coombs reagent and looking for agglutination. Agglutination (a positive test) indicates the presence of antibody on the red blood cell surface. The indirect Coombs test is performed by mixing the patient's serum with a panel of type O red blood cells. After incubation of the test serum and panel red blood cells, the Coombs reagent is added. Agglutination in this system indicates the presence of free antibody in the patient's serum. Because the traditional Coombs test relies on visible agglutination as an end point, the test is not very sensitive and will not detect immune hemolytic anemias, in which only a small amount of IgG is present on red blood cells. More sensitive tests (micro-Coombs) are now available.

Clinical Findings

A. Symptoms and Signs: Autoimmune hemolytic anemia typically produces an anemia of rapid onset that may be life-threatening in severity. Patients complain of fatigue and may present with angina or congestive heart failure. On examination, jaundice and splenomegaly are usually present. If the patient has an underlying disorder such as systemic lupus erythematosus or chronic lymphocytic leukemia, features of these diseases may be present.

B. Laboratory Findings: The anemia is of variable severity but may be severe, with hematocrit of less than 10%. Reticulocytosis is usually present, and spherocytes are seen on the peripheral blood smear. In cases of severe hemolysis, the stressed bone marrow may also release nucleated red blood cells. As with other hemolytic disorders, indirect bilirubin is increased. Approximately 10% of patients with autoimmune hemolytic anemia have coincident immune thrombocytopenia (Evans's syndrome).

The direct Coombs test is positive for IgG and possibly for complement as well. The indirect Coombs test may or may not be positive. A positive indirect Coombs test indicates the presence of a large amount of autoantibody that has saturated binding sites in the red blood cell and consequently appears in the serum. A patient with acquired spherocytic hemolytic anemia that may be of the autoimmune variety who has a negative Coombs test should be tested with a micro-Coombs test (which is necessary to make the diagnosis in approximately 10% of cases). Because the patient's serum usually contains the autoantibody, it may be difficult to obtain a compatible cross-match with donor's cells. Suitable donors may be selected by special laboratory methods.

Treatment

Initial treatment is with prednisone, 1–2 mg/kg/d in divided doses. If anemia is life-threatening, transfusions should be given cautiously. Most transfused blood will survive no more poorly than the patient's own red blood cells. However, because of difficulty in performing the cross-match, it is possible that incompatible blood will be given, and patients must be monitored carefully during transfusion. Decisions regarding transfusions should be made in consultation with a hematologist (or blood bank physician). If prednisone is ineffective or if the disease recurs on tapering the dose of prednisone to an acceptable chronic dose, splenectomy should be performed. Patients with autoimmune hemolytic anemia refractory to prednisone and splenectomy may be treated with a variety of immunosuppressive agents. Large doses

of intravenous IgG (400 mg/kg) may be temporarily effective in halting hemolysis.

The long-term prognosis for patients with this disorder is good. Splenectomy is often successful in controlling or at least ameliorating the disorder.

Ahn YS et al: Danazol therapy for autoimmune hemolytic anemia. Ann Intern Med 1985;102:298.
Frank MM et al: pathophysiology of immune hemolytic anemia. Ann Intern Med 1977;87:210.
Petz LD, Garratty G: Churchill Livingstone, 1980.
Sokol RJ, Hewitt S, Stamps BK: Autoimmune haemolysis: An 18-year study of 865 cases referred to a regional transfusion centre. Br Med J 1981;282:2023.

COLD AGGLUTININ DISEASE

Essentials of Diagnosis

- Increased reticulocytes and spherocytes on peripheral blood smear.
- Coombs test positive only for complement.
- Positive cold agglutinin test.

General Considerations

Cold agglutinin disease is an acquired hemolytic anemia due to an IgM autoantibody usually directed against the I antigen on red blood cells. These IgM autoantibodies characteristically will not react with cells at 37 °C but only at lower temperatures. Since the blood temperature (even in the most peripheral parts of the body) rarely goes lower than 20 °C, only antibodies active at higher temperatures than this will produce clinical effects. In the cooler parts of the body (fingers, nose, ears), agglutination of red blood cells by the IgM antibodies will transiently occur. Hemolysis results indirectly from attachment of IgM, which in the cooler parts of the circulation binds and fixes complement. When the red blood cell returns to a warmer temperature, the IgM antibody dissociates, leaving complement on the cell. Lysis of cells rarely occurs. Rather, C3b present on the red cells is recognized by Kupffer cells (which have receptors for C3b), and red blood cell sequestration ensues.

Most cases of chronic cold agglutinin disease are idiopathic. Others occur in association with Waldenstrodm's macroglobulinemia, an indolent lymphoproliferative disease in which a monoclonal IgM paraprotein is produced. Acute postinfectious cold agglutinin disease occurs following mycoplasmal pneumonia or infectious mononucleosis (with antibody directed against antigen i rather than I).

Clinical Findings

A. Symptoms and Signs: In chronic cold agglutinin disease, symptoms related to red blood cell agglutination occur on exposure to cold, and patients may complain of mottled or numb fingers or toes. Hemolytic anemia is rarely severe, but episodic hemoglobinuria may occur on exposure to cold. The hemolytic anemia in acute postinfectious syndromes is rarely severe.

B. Laboratory Findings: Mild anemia is present with reticulocytosis and spherocytes. The direct Coombs test will be positive for complement only. Occasionally, a micro-Coombs test is necessary to reveal bound complement (low-titer cold agglutinin disease).

Treatment

Treatment is largely symptomatic, based on avoiding exposure to cold. Patients with severe involvement may be treated with alkylating agents such as chlorambucil. Splenectomy is ineffective, since hemolysis takes place in the liver. Prednisone is ineffective in reducing Kupffer cell function.

Schreiber AD, Herskovitz BS, Goldwein M: Low-titer cold-hemagglutinin disease: Mechanism of hemolysis and response to corticosteroids. N Engl J Med 1977;296:1490.
Silberstein LE: Cold hemagglutinin disease associated with IgG coloreactive antibody. Ann Intern Med 1987;106: 238.

MICROANGIOPATHIC HEMOLYTIC ANEMIAS

The microangiopathic hemolytic anemias are a group of disorders in which red blood cell fragmentation takes place. The anemia is intravascular, producing hemoglobinemia, hemoglobinuria, and, in severe cases, methemalbuminemia. The hallmark of the disorder is the finding of fragmented red blood cells (schistocytes, helmet cells) on the peripheral blood smear.

These fragmentation syndromes can be caused by a variety of disorders (Table 10–8). Thrombotic thrombocytopenic purpura is the most important of these and is discussed below. Clinical features of the fragmentation syndromes are variable and depend on the underlying disorder. Coagulopathy and thrombocytopenia are variably present.

Chronic microangiopathic hemolytic anemia (such as is present with a malfunctioning cardiac valve prosthesis) may cause iron deficiency anemia because of continuous low-grade hemoglobinuria. This can be diagnosed by measuring 24-hour excretion of iron in the urine.

HEMOLYSIS RELATED TO INFECTION

Clostridial infections may cause severe intravascular hemolysis, presumably because of the action of a clostridial toxin on the red blood cell membrane. Malaria may cause intravascular hemolysis because of parasitism of red blood cells; falciparum malaria causes the severest form (blackwater fever).

Other infections associated with hemolysis are bartonellosis and babesiosis.

APLASTIC ANEMIA

Essentials of Diagnosis
- Pancytopenia.
- No abnormal cells seen.
- Hypocellular bone marrow.

General Considerations

All hematopoietic cells are derived from a pluripotent stem cell that gives rise to precursors of erythroid, myeloid, and platelet forms. Injury to or suppression of this hematopoietic stem cell will result in pancytopenia—reduction in all 3 hematopoietic cell lines (red blood cells, neutrophils, and platelets). Aplastic anemia is a condition of bone marrow failure that arises from injury to or abnormal expression of the stem cell. The bone marrow becomes hypoplastic, and pancytopenia develops.

There are a number of causes of aplastic anemia (Table 10–10). Direct stem cell injury may be caused by radiation, chemotherapy, toxins, or pharmacologic agents. Systemic lupus erythematosus may rarely cause suppression of the hematopoietic stem cell by an IgG autoantibody directed against the stem cell. However, the most common pathogenesis of aplastic anemia appears to be autoimmune suppression of hematopoiesis by a T cell-mediated cellular mechanism.

Clinical Findings

A. Symptoms and Signs: Patients come to medical attention because of the consequences of bone marrow failure. Anemia leads to symptoms of weakness and fatigue; neutropenia causes vulnerability to bacterial infections; and thrombocytopenia results in mucosal and skin bleeding. Physical examination may reveal signs of pallor, purpura, and petechiae. Other abnormalities such as hepatosplenomegaly, lymphadenopathy, or bone tenderness should *not* be present, and their presence should lead one to question the diagnosis of aplastic anemia.

B. Laboratory Findings: The hallmark of aplas-

Table 10–10. Causes of aplastic anemia.

Congenital (rare)
"Idiopathic" (probably autoimmune)
Systemic lupus erythematosus
Chemotherapy, radiotherapy
Toxins: Benzene, toluene, insecticides
Drugs: Chloramphenicol, phenylbutazone, gold salts, sulfonamides, phenytoin, carbamazepine, quinacrine, tolbutamide
Posthepatitis
Pregnancy
Paroxysmal nocturnal hemoglobinuria

tic anemia is pancytopenia. However, early in the evolution of aplastic anemia, only one or 2 cell lines may be reduced.

Anemia may be severe and is always associated with decreased reticulocytes. Red blood cell morphology is remarkable. The MCV is usually normal but occasionally may be increased. Neutrophils and platelets are reduced in number, and no immature or abnormal forms are seen. The bone marrow aspirate and the bone marrow biopsy appear hypocellular, with only scant amounts of normal hematopoietic progenitors. No abnormal cells are seen.

Differential Diagnosis

The diagnosis of aplastic anemia is made in cases of pancytopenia with a hypocellular marrow biopsy containing no abnormal cells. Aplastic anemia must be differentiated from other causes of pancytopenia (Table 10–11). Myelodysplastic disorders or acute leukemia may occasionally be confused with aplastic anemia. These are differentiated by the presence of morphologic abnormalities or increased blasts. Hairy cell leukemia has been misdiagnosed as aplastic anemia and should be recognized by a high incidence of splenomegaly and by the presence of abnormal lymphoid cells on the bone marrow biopsy. Pancytopenia in the presence of a normal bone marrow is usually due to systemic lupus erythematosus, disseminated infection, or hypersplenism. Isolated thrombocytopenia may occur early as aplastic anemia develops and be confused with immune thrombocytopenia.

Treatment

Mild cases of aplastic anemia may be treated with supportive care. Red blood cell transfusions and platelet transfusions are given as necessary, and antibiotics are used to treat infections.

Severe aplastic anemia is defined by the presence of neutrophils less than 500/μL, platelets less than 20,000/μL, reticulocytes less than 1%, and bone marrow cellularity less than 20%. When this constellation (or 3 of the 4) of features is present, the median survival is approximately 3 months, and only 20% of patients will survive 1 year. Severe aplastic anemia

Table 10–11. Causes of pancytopenia.

Bone marrow disorders
  Aplastic anemia
  Myelodysplasia
  Acute leukemia
  Myelofibrosis
  Infiltrative disease: Lymphoma, myeloma, carcinoma, hairy
    cell leukemia
  Megaloblastic anemia
Nonmarrow disorders
  Hypersplenism
  Systemic lupus erythematosus
  Infection: Tuberculosis, AIDS, leishmaniasis, brucellosis

is a life-threatening condition that requires urgent treatment. The treatment of choice for adults under age 20 who have HLA-matched siblings is allogeneic bone marrow transplantation. The best results occur in younger patients who have not been previously transfused. Prior transfusion increases the risk of graft rejection, apparently because of poor sensitization to antigens present on hematopoietic progenitors. Young patients may tolerate severe anemia and thrombocytopenia and should not be transfused unless there is imminent bleeding or cardiorespiratory distress. These patients and their siblings should be HLA-typed promptly and referred for further evaluation by a hematologist.

For adults over age 30 or those without HLA-matched siblings, the treatment of choice for severe aplastic anemia is antithymocyte globulin (ATG). ATG is a horse serum containing polyclonal antibodies against human T cells. The success of this form of treatment has helped confirm the notion that most cases of aplastic anemia are immunologically mediated rather than caused by irreversible stem cell injury. ATG is given in the hospital over 5–8 days in conjunction with transfusion and antibiotic support. Responses usually occur in 4–12 weeks. Responses to ATG are usually only partial, but the blood counts rise high enough to give patients a safe and transfusion-free life.

Androgens have been widely used in the past, with a low response rate. However, a few patients can be maintained successfully with this form of treatment. One regimen is oxymethalone, 2–3 mg/kg orally daily. In the rare syndrome of systemic lupus erythematosus causing humorally mediated aplastic anemia, the combination of plasmapheresis and high-dose prednisone may be successful.

Course & Prognosis

Patients with severe aplastic anemia have a rapidly fatal illness if left untreated. Allogeneic bone marrow transplantation is highly successful in young adults with HLA-matched siblings. For this group of patients, the durable complete response rate is 80%. For older adults or those who have previously been exposed to blood products, long-term survival rates are between 40% and 70%. ATG treatment leads to partial response in approximately 60% of adults, and the long-term prognosis of responders appears to be very good.

Camitta BM, Storb R, Thomas ED: Aplastic anemia: Pathogenesis, diagnosis, treatment, and prognosis. (2 parts.) N Engl J Med 1982;306:645, 712.

Champlin RE et al: Graft failure following bone marrow transplantation for severe aplastic anemia: Risk factors and treatment results. Blood 1989;73:606.

McGlave PB: Therapy of severe aplastic anemia in young adults and children with allogeneic bone marrow transplantation. Blood 1987;70:1325.

Storb R et al: Marrow transplantation with or without donor

buffy coat cells for 65 transfused aplastic patients. Blood 1982;59:236.

Vadhan-Raj S et al: Stimulation of myelopoiesis in patients with aplastic anemia by recombinant human granulocyte-macrophage colony stimulating factor. N Engl J Med 1988;319:1628.

Young N et al: A multicenter trial of anti-thymocyte globulin in aplastic anemia and related diseases. Blood 1988; 72:1861.

NEUTROPENIA

Neutropenia exists when the neutrophil count falls below 1500/μL. However, blacks and other specific population groups may normally have neutrophil counts as low as 1200/μL. The neutropenic patient is increasingly vulnerable to infection by gram-positive and gram-negative bacteria and by the fungi *Candida* and *Aspergillus*. The risk of infection is related to the severity of neutropenia. Patients with "chronic benign neutropenia" are free of infection for years despite very low neutrophil levels.

A variety of bone marrow disorders and nonmarrow conditions may cause neutropenia (Table 10–12). All the causes of aplastic anemia (Table 10–10) and pancytopenia (Table 10–11) may cause neutropenia as part of their overall picture. Isolated neutropenia is often due to an idiosyncratic reaction to a drug, and agranulocytosis (complete absence of neutrophils in the peripheral blood) is almost always due to a drug reaction or to exposure to a variety of chemicals (eg, pesticides). In these cases, examination of the bone marrow shows virtual absence of myeloid precursors, with other cell lines undisturbed. Pure white cell aplasia is a rare condition in which an autoantibody is formed against myeloid progenitors. Neutropenia in the presence of a normal bone marrow may be due to immunologic peripheral destruction, sepsis, or hypersplenism.

Table 10–12. Causes of neutropenia.

Bone marrow disorders
Aplastic anemia
Pure white cell aplasia
Congenital (rare)
Cyclic neutropenia
Drugs: Sulfonamides, chlorpromazine, procainamide, penicillin, cephalosporins, cimetidine, methimazole, phenytoin, chlorpropamide
Benign chronic
Peripheral disorders
Hypersplenism
Sepsis
Immune
Felty's syndrome

Clinical Findings

Neutropenia results in stomatitis and in infections. Infections are usually due to gram-positive or gram-negative aerobic bacteria or to fungi such as *Candida* or *Aspergillus*. The most common infections are septicemia, cellulitis, and pneumonia. It should be emphasized that in the presence of severe neutropenia the usual signs of inflammatory response to infection may be absent. Infection (especially septicemia) in the presence of severe neutropenia is a medical emergency, and death may occur within hours without appropriate antibiotic therapy.

Felty's syndrome is a combination of neutropenia with seropositive rheumatoid arthritis. The bone marrow is usually normal, and the neutropenia appears to be related to antineutrophil antibodies causing peripheral destruction of these cells. The disorder is clinically manifested as repeated infections and nonhealing ulcers on the lower legs. For unclear reasons, the severity of clinical problems does not correlate well with the degree of neutropenia.

Treatment

Infections in a neutropenic patient should be treated on an emergent basis. Many combinations of broad-spectrum antibiotics can be used, but particular attention should be paid to enteric gram-negative bacteria. Combined treatment with aminoglycosides and a semisynthetic penicillin is commonly used. Offending drugs should be immediately discontinued, but third-generation cephalosporins such as ceftazidime are effective as single-agent therapy and obviate the need for an aminoglycoside.

When Felty's syndrome leads to repeated bacterial infections, splenectomy is the treatment of choice. Splenectomy usually leads to healing of leg ulcers and to reduction in the rate of infection whether or not the neutrophil count rises.

The prognosis of patients with neutropenia depends on the underlying cause. Most patients with drug-induced agranulocytosis can be supported with broad-spectrum antibiotics and will recover completely.

Blumfelder TM, Logue GL, Shimm DS: Felty's syndrome: Effects of splenectomy upon granulocyte count and granulocyte-associated IgG. Ann Intern Med 1981;94:623.

Dale DC et al: Chronic neutropenia. Medicine 1979;58:128.

LEUKEMIAS & OTHER MYELOPROLIFERATIVE DISORDERS

Myeloproliferative disorders are due to acquired clonal abnormalities of the hematopoietic stem. Since the stem cell gives rise to myeloid, erythroid, and

Table 10–13. Classification of myeloproliferative disorders.

Myeloproliferative syndromes
Polycythemia vera
Myelofibrosis
Essential thrombocytosis
Chronic myeloid leukemia
Myelodysplastic syndromes
Acute myeloid leukemia

Table 10–15. Causes of polycythemia.

Spurious polycythemia
Secondary polycythemia
Hypoxia: Cardiac disease, pulmonary disease, high altitude
Carboxyhemoglobin: Smoking
Renal lesions
Erythropoietin-secreting tumors (rare)
Abnormal hemoglobins (rare)
Polycythemia vera

platelet cells, one sees qualitative and quantitative changes in all these cell lines. In some disorders (chronic myeloid leukemia), specific characteristic chromosomal changes are seen. In others, although the disorder is presumed to be related to a defect in DNA, no characteristic cytogenetic abnormalities are seen.

Classically, the myeloproliferative disorders produce characteristic syndromes with well-defined clinical and laboratory features (Tables 10–13 and 10–14). However, these disorders are grouped together because the disease may evolve from one form into another and because hybrid disorders are commonly seen. All of the myeloproliferative disorders may progress to acute myeloid leukemia.

POLYCYTHEMIA VERA

Essentials of Diagnosis

- Increased red blood cell mass.
- Splenomegaly.
- Normal arterial oxygen saturation.
- Usually elevated white blood count and platelet count.

General Considerations

Polycythemia vera is an acquired myeloproliferative disorder that causes overproduction of all 3 hematopoietic cell lines, most prominently the red blood cells. The hematocrit is elevated (at sea level) when values exceed 54% in males or 51% in females (Table 10–15).

When the hematocrit is elevated, the red blood cell mass should be measured to determine whether true polycythemia or relative polycythemia exists. Normal values for red blood cell mass are 26–34 mL/kg in men and 21–29 mL/kg in women. Relative (''spurious'') polycythemia characteristically presents in middle-aged men who are overweight and hypertensive; the hematocrit is almost always less than 60%.

If the red blood cell mass is increased, one must determine whether the increase is primary or secondary. Primary polycythemia (polycythemia vera) is a bone marrow disorder characterized by autonomous overproduction of erythroid cells. Erythroid production is independent of erythropoietin, and the serum erythropoietin level is low. In vitro, erythroid progenitor cells grow without added erythropoietin, a finding not seen in normal individuals.

Polycythemia vera is a relatively common disorder. Sixty percent of patients are male, and the median age at presentation is 60. Polycythemia vera rarely occurs in adults under age 40.

Clinical Findings

A. Symptoms and Signs: Most patients present with symptoms related to expanded blood volume and increased blood viscosity. Common complaints include headache, dizziness, tinnitus, blurred vision, and fatigue. Generalized pruritus, especially that occurring following a warm shower or bath, may be a striking symptom and is related to histamine release from the increased number of basophils present. Patients may also initially complain of epistaxis. This is probably related to engorgement of mucosal blood vessels in combination with abnormal hemostasis due to qualitative abnormalities in platelet function.

Physical examination reveals plethora and engorged

Table 10–14. Laboratory features of myeloproliferative disorders.

	White Count	Hematocrit	Platelet Count	Red Cell Morphology
Chronic myeloid leukemia	↑ ↑	Normal	Normal or ↑	Normal
Myelofibrosis	Normal or ↓ or ↑	Normal or ↓	↓ or normal or ↑	Abnormal
Polycythemia vera	Normal or ↑	↑	Normal or ↑	Normal
Essential thrombocytosis	Normal or ↑	Normal	↑ ↑	Normal

retinal veins. The spleen is palpably enlarged in 75% of cases, but splenomegaly is nearly always present when imaged. Less commonly, the liver is mildly enlarged.

Thrombosis is the most common complication of polycythemia vera and the major cause of morbidity and death in this disorder. Thrombosis appears to be related to increased blood viscosity and abnormal platelet function. Uncontrolled polycythemia leads to a very high incidence of thrombotic complications of surgery, and elective surgery should be deferred until the condition has been treated. Paradoxically, in addition to thrombosis, increased bleeding also occurs. There is a high incidence of peptic ulcer disease as well as gastrointestinal bleeding. Overproduction of uric acid may lead to gout.

B. Laboratory Findings: The hallmark of polycythemia vera is a hematocrit above normal, at times greater than 60%. Red blood cell morphology is normal. The white blood count is characteristically elevated to 10,000–20,000/μL and the platelet count is variably elevated, sometimes with counts exceeding 1,000,000/μL. Platelet morphology is usually normal, but large hypogranular forms may be seen. White blood cells are usually normal, but basophilia is frequently present. By definition, the red blood cell mass is elevated.

The bone marrow is hypercellular, with panhyperplasia of all hematopoietic elements. A characteristic finding is increased numbers of megakaryocytes. Iron stores are usually absent from the bone marrow, having been transferred to the increased circulating red blood cell mass. Iron deficiency may result from chronic gastrointestinal blood loss. Bleeding may lower the hematocrit to the normal range (or lower), creating diagnostic confusion.

Vitamin B_{12} levels are strikingly elevated because of increased levels of transcobalamin III (secreted by white blood cells). The leukocyte alkaline phosphatase is characteristically elevated as a marker of qualitative abnormalities in the myeloid line. Uric acid levels may be increased. There is no characteristic chromosomal abnormality in this disorder.

Although red blood cell morphology is usually normal at presentation, microcytosis, hypochromia, and poikilocytosis may result from iron deficiency following treatment by phlebotomy (see below). Progressive hypersplenism may also lead to elliptocytosis.

Differential Diagnosis

Spurious polycythemia, in which an elevated hematocrit is due to contracted plasma volume rather than increased red cell mass, may be related to diuretic use or may occur without obvious cause.

A secondary cause of polycythemia should be suspected if splenomegaly is absent and the high hematocrit is not accompanied by increases in other cell lines. Arterial oxygen saturation should be measured to determine if hypoxia is the cause. A smoking history should be taken and carboxyhemoglobin levels measured when indicated. An intravenous urogram or renal sonogram may be indicated to evaluate the kidneys for abnormalities. A positive family history should lead to investigation for congenital high-affinity hemoglobin.

Polycythemia vera should be differentiated from other myeloproliferative disorders (Table 10–14). Marked elevation of the white blood count above 30,000/μL) should lead to consideration of chronic myeloid leukemia. This disorder is confirmed by the finding of a low leukocyte alkaline phosphatase and by the presence of the Philadelphia chromosome. Abnormal red blood cell morphology and nucleated red blood cells in the peripheral blood should lead to the consideration of myelofibrosis. This condition is diagnosed by bone marrow biopsy showing fibrosis of the marrow. Essential thrombocytosis is diagnosed when the platelet count is strikingly elevated and the red blood cell count is normal.

Treatment

The treatment of choice is phlebotomy. One unit of blood (approximately 500 mL) is removed weekly until the hematocrit is less than 45%; the hematocrit is maintained at less than 45% by repeated phlebotomy as necessary. Because repeated phlebotomy produces iron deficiency, the requirement for phlebotomy should gradually decrease. It is important to avoid medicinal iron supplementation, as this can thwart the goals of a phlebotomy program. It is not necessary to manipulate the diet to decrease iron intake. Patients will usually feel much better as soon as the hematocrit is lowered. Maintaining the hematocrit at normal levels has been shown to decrease the incidence of thrombotic complications.

Occasionally, myelosuppressive therapy is indicated. Indications include a high phlebotomy requirement, marked thrombocytosis, and intractable pruritus. Alkylating agents and radiophosphorus (^{32}P) have been shown to increase the risk of conversion of this disease to acute leukemia. Hydroxyurea is now being widely used when myelosuppressive therapy is indicated because of the presumption that antimetabolites will not be leukemogenic. Busulfan may also be used.

The role of antiplatelet agents such as aspirin in preventing thrombotic complications is controversial. High doses of aspirin (325 mg 3 times daily) plus dipyridamole (25 mg 3 times daily) cause a marked increase in gastrointestinal bleeding and should not be given routinely. However, antiplatelet treatment may be warranted in selected patients who have recurrent thromboses despite control of their plate counts with myelosuppressive therapy. One aspirin tablet daily (325 mg) may be effective therapy.

Allopurinol may be indicated for hyperuricemia. Antihistamine therapy with diphenhydramine and cimetidine may be helpful for control of pruritus.

Prognosis

Polycythemia is an indolent disease with median survival of 10–15 years. The major cause of morbidity and mortality is arterial thrombosis. Over time, polycythemia vera may convert to myelofibrosis or to chronic myeloid leukemia. In approximately 10% of cases, the disorder progresses to acute myeloid leukemia, which is usually refractory to therapy.

Berk PD et al: Therapeutic recommendations in polycythemia vera based on Polycythemia Vera Study Group protocols. Semin Hematol 1986;23:132.

MYELOFIBROSIS

Essentials of Diagnosis

- Teardrop poikilocytosis on peripheral smear.
- Leukoerythroblastic blood picture; giant abnormal platelets.
- Hypercellular bone marrow with reticulin or collagen fibrosis.

General Considerations

Myelofibrosis (myelofibrosis with myeloid metaplasia, agnogenic myeloid metaplasia) is a myeloproliferative disorder characterized by fibrosis of the bone marrow, splenomegaly, and a leukoerythroblastic peripheral blood picture with teardrop poikilocytosis. It is widely believed that fibrosis occurs in response to increased secretion of platelet-derived growth factor (PDGF). In response to bone marrow fibrosis, extramedullary hematopoiesis (hematopoietic cell development outside the bone marrow) takes place in the liver, spleen, and lymph nodes. In these sites, mesenchymal cells responsible for fetal hematopoiesis can be reactivated.

Clinical Findings

A. Symptoms and Signs: Myelofibrosis develops in adults over age 50 and is usually insidious in onset. Patients most commonly present with fatigue related to their anemia or abdominal fullness related to splenomegaly. Uncommon presentations include bleeding and bone pain. On examination, splenomegaly is almost invariably present and is sometimes massive. The liver is enlarged in more than half of cases.

Later in the course of the disease, progressive bone marrow failure takes place as the marrow becomes progressively more fibrotic. Anemia becomes severe, and red cell transfusion becomes necessary. Progressive thrombocytopenia leads to bleeding. The spleen continues to enlarge, which leads to early satiety. Painful episodes of splenic infarction may occur. Late in the course of the disease, the patient becomes cachectic and may experience severe bone pain, especially in the lower legs. Hematopoiesis in the liver

leads to portal hypertension with ascites, esophageal varices, and eventually liver failure.

B. Laboratory Findings: Patients are almost invariably anemic at presentation. The white blood count is variable—either low, normal, or elevated—and may be increased to $50,000/\mu L$. The platelet count is variable. The peripheral blood smear is characteristic, consisting of significant poikilocytosis with numerous teardrop forms. Immature myeloid and erythroid forms are present (leukoerythroblastic blood picture). Nucleated red blood cells are present and the myeloid series is less strikingly shifted, with immature forms including a small percentage of promyelocytes or myeloblasts. Platelet morphology may be bizarre, and giant degranulated platelet forms (megakaryocyte fragments) may be seen. The triad of teardrop poikilocytosis, leukoerythroblastic blood, and giant abnormal platelets is almost diagnostic of myelofibrosis.

The bone marrow is usually inaspirable (dry tap). Early in the course of the disease, the bone marrow is hypercellular, with a marked increase in megakaryocytes. Fibrosis at this stage is detected only by a silver stain demonstrating increased reticulin fibers. Later in the course of the disease, bone marrow biopsy reveals that fibrosis becomes more severe, with eventual replacement of hematopoietic precursors by collagen fibrosis. There is no characteristic chromosomal abnormality.

Differential Diagnosis

A leukoerythroblastic blood picture may be seen in response to severe infection or inflammation. However, teardrop poikilocytosis and giant abnormal platelet forms will not be present. Bone marrow fibrosis may be seen in metastatic carcinoma, Hodgkin's disease, and hairy cell leukemia. These disorders are diagnosed by characteristic tissue morphology.

Myelofibrosis is distinguished from other myeloproliferative disorders by the characteristic constellation of findings (Table 10–14). Chronic myeloid leukemia is diagnosed when there is marked elevation of the white blood count, a low leukocyte alkaline phosphatase, normal red blood cell morphology, and the presence of the Philadelphia chromosome. Polycythemia vera is characterized by an elevated hematocrit, and patients with essential thrombocytosis should have normal red blood cell morphology. Ultimately, the diagnosis is made by examination of the bone marrow biopsy.

Treatment

There is no specific treatment for this disorder. Anemic patients are supported with red blood cells in transfusion. Androgens such as oxymetholone or testosterone may help reduce the transfusion requirement but are poorly tolerated by women. Recombinant erythropoietin (epoetin alfa; Epogen) has been reported to be of value in a small number of cases.

Splenectomy is not routinely performed but is indicated for splenic enlargement that causes recurrent painful episodes, severe thrombocytopenia, or an unacceptably high red blood cell transfusion requirement.

Course & Prognosis

It is often hard to date the onset of myelofibrosis, but the median survival from time of diagnosis is approximately 5 years. End-stage myelofibrosis is a wasting illness characterized by generalized debility, liver failure, and bleeding from thrombocytopenia. Some cases may terminate in acute myeloid leukemia.

Demory JL: Cytogenetic studies and their prognostic significance in agnogenic myeloid metaplasia: A report on 47 cases. Blood 1988;72:855.

Varki A et al: The syndrome of idiopathic myelofibrosis: A clinicopathologic review with emphasis on the prognostic variables predicting survival. Medicine 1983; 62:353.

CHRONIC MYELOID LEUKEMIA

Essentials of Diagnosis

- Markedly elevated white blood count.
- Markedly left-shifted myeloid series with a low percentage of promyelocytes and blasts.
- Presence of Philadelphia chromosome.

General Considerations

Chronic myeloid leukemia is a myeloproliferative disorder characterized by overproduction of myeloid cells. These myeloid cells retain the capacity for differentiation, and normal bone marrow function is retained during the early phases. The disease usually remains stable for years and then transforms to a more overtly malignant disease.

Chronic myeloid leukemia is associated with a characteristic chromosomal abnormality, the Philadelphia chromosome, and was the first disease associated with a specific karyotypic abnormality. The Philadelphia chromosome is now recognized to be a reciprocal translocation between the long arms of chromosomes 9 and 22. A large portion of 22q is translocated to 9q, and a smaller piece of 9q is moved to 22q. This translocation is thought to be pathogenically significant, based on recent evidence that oncogene activation occurs. The portion of 9q that is translocated contains *abl,* a proto-oncogene that is the cellular homolog of the Ableson murine leukemia virus. The *abl* gene is received at a specific site on 22q, the break point cluster (bcr). The fusion gene *abl*-bcr produces a novel protein that differs from the normal transcript of the *abl* gene in that it possesses tyrosine kinase activity (a characteristic activity of transforming genes).

Usually at the time of diagnosis, the Philadelphia

chromosome-positive clone dominates and may be the only one detected. However, a normal clone is present and may express itself either in vivo, after certain forms of therapy, or in vitro, in long-term bone marrow cultures. Approximately 5% of cases of chronic myeloid leukemia are Philadelphia chromosome-negative. In some cases, although the characteristic karyotype is not seen at the light microscopic level, gene mapping demonstrates translocation of *abl* to 22q. In other cases of Philadelphia-negative chronic myeloid leukemia, the disease is atypical and is better described as chronic myelomonocytic leukemia. Philadelphia chromosome-negative disease has a poor prognosis.

Early chronic myeloid leukemia ("chronic phase") does not behave like a malignant disease. Normal bone marrow function is retained, white blood cells differentiate, and, despite some qualitative abnormalities (low leukocyte alkaline phosphatase), the neutrophils combat infection normally. However, chronic myeloid leukemia is inherently unstable, and the disease progresses to accelerated phase and finally after several years, to blast crisis. This progression of the disease is often associated with added chromosomal defects superimposed on the Philadelphia chromosome. Blast crisis chronic myeloid leukemia is an overtly malignant process that becomes indistinguishable from acute leukemia.

Clinical Findings

A. Symptoms and Signs: Chronic myeloid leukemia is a disorder of middle age (median age at presentation is 42 years). Patients usually present with fatigue, night sweats, and low-grade fever related to the hypermetabolic state caused by overproduction of white blood cells. At other times, the patient complains of abdominal fullness related to splenomegaly, or an elevated white blood count is discovered incidentally. Rarely, the patient will present with a clinical syndrome related to leukostasis with blurred vision, respiratory distress, or priapism. The white blood count in these cases is usually greater than 500,000/μL.

On examination, the spleen is enlarged (often markedly so), and sternal tenderness may be present as a sign of marrow overexpansion.

Acceleration of the disease is often associated with fever in the absence of infection, bone pain, and splenomegaly. In blast crisis, patients may experience bleeding and infection related to bone marrow failure.

B. Laboratory Findings: The hallmark of chronic myeloid leukemia is an elevated white blood count; the median white blood count at diagnosis is 150,000/μL. The peripheral blood is characteristic. The myeloid series is left-shifted, with mature forms dominating and with cells usually present in proportion to their degree of maturation. Blasts are usually less than 5%. Basophilia of granulocytes may be present. The peripheral blood smear gives the impression that the bone marrow has spilled over into the blood. At presentation, the patient is usually not anemic. Red blood cell morphology is normal, and nucleated red blood cells are rarely seen. The platelet count may be normal or elevated (sometimes to strikingly high levels). Platelet morphology is usually normal, but abnormally large forms may be seen.

The bone marrow is hypercellular, with markedly left-shifted myelopoiesis. Myeloblasts comprise less than 5% of marrow cells.

The leukocyte alkaline phosphatase score is invariably low and is a sign of qualitative abnormalities in neutrophils. The vitamin B_{12} level is usually markedly elevated because of increased secretion of transcobalamin III. Uric acid levels may be high.

The Philadelphia chromosome is almost invariably present and may be detected in the peripheral blood or bone marrow.

With progression to the accelerated and blast phases, progressive anemia and thrombocytopenia occur, and the percentage of blasts in the blood and bone marrow increases. Blast phase chronic myeloid leukemia is diagnosed when blasts comprise more than 30% of bone marrow cells.

Differential Diagnosis

Early chronic myeloid leukemia must be differentiated from the reactive leukocytosis associated with infection, inflammation, or cancer. In these reactive disorders, the white blood count is usually less than 50,000/μL, splenomegaly is absent, the leukocyte alkaline phosphatase is normal or increased, and the Philadelphia chromosome is not present. If one is in doubt whether leukocytosis is due to chronic myeloid leukemia or a reactive condition, the patient should be observed, since there is no advantage to early therapy for asymptomatic patients.

Chronic myeloid leukemia must be distinguished from other myeloproliferative disease (Table 10–14). The hematocrit should not be elevated, the red blood cell morphology should be normal, and nucleated red blood cells should be rare or absent. Definitive diagnosis is made by finding the Philadelphia chromosome.

Treatment

Treatment is usually not an emergent necessity even with white blood counts over 200,000/μL, since the majority of circulating cells are mature myeloid cells that are smaller and more deformable than primitive leukemic blasts. In the rare instances in which extreme hyperleukocytosis (priapism, respiratory distress, visual blurring, altered mental status), leukapheresis should be performed on an emergency basis in conjunction with myelosuppressive therapy.

The usual treatment is palliative and improves the patient's sense of well-being without altering the natural history of the disease. Myelosuppressive therapy consists of giving either busulfan or hydroxyurea in combination with allopurinol. When busulfan is used, the usual dose is 4–8 mg daily for 4–8 weeks. One aims to lower the white count to 10,000–20,000/μL. Busulfan has a notoriously prolonged duration of action, and it is important not to lower the white blood count too much because this will expose the patient to an unnecessary risk of infection. Because of these problems, hydroxyurea is more commonly used. The initial dose is usually 2–4 g/d orally, and the maintenance dose varies between 0.5 and 2 g/d as necessary to maintain the white blood count at 10,000–20,000/μL. Hydroxyurea must be given without interruption, since the white blood count will rise within days after discontinuing this medication. The response to hydroxyurea is usually gratifying. The white blood count decreases, the spleen decreases in size, and the patient becomes asymptomatic. Most patients in the chronic phase of chronic myeloid leukemia will have no symptoms either from the disease or their chemotherapy.

Recombinant alpha interferon has been used in the treatment of the chronic phase with good results. Sixty percent of patients have a good hematologic response. With prolonged treatment (12–18 months), a proportion of those responders lose the Philadelphia chromosome. Clinical trials are under way to evaluate whether this treatment will alter the natural history of the disease.

Although the response to myelosuppressive therapy of the chronic phase is gratifying, the treatment is only palliative, and the disease is invariably fatal. Curative therapy is available with high-dose chemotherapy in association with allogeneic bone marrow transplantation. This treatment is available for adults under age 50 who have HLA-matched siblings. Approximately 50% of adults have long-term disease-free survival following bone marrow transplantation and appear to be cured of their disease, with the better results in younger patients. All young patients should be given the opportunity for allogeneic bone marrow transplantation in the chronic phase if they have suitable bone marrow donors. For young patients without sibling donors, HLA-matched unrelated donors may be located through computer-based registries of volunteer bone marrow donors. This type of therapy is currently being evaluated.

Blast crisis of chronic myeloid leukemia is a notoriously difficult form of acute leukemia to treat. Lymphoid blast crisis (present in one-third of cases) should be identified because chemotherapy for this disorder is less toxic and more effective. Therapy with daunorubicin, vincristine, and prednisone (used in treatment of acute lymphoblastic leukemia) will lead to remission—usually short-lived—in 70% of these cases.

Course & Prognosis

Median survival is 3–4 years. Once the disease has progressed to the accelerated or blast phase, survival is measured in months. Approximately 60%

of young adults who have successful allogeneic bone marrow transplantation appear to be cured.

Champlin R et al: Chronic leukemias: Oncogenes, chromosomes and advances in therapy. Ann Intern Med 1986; 104:671.

Champlin RE, Golde DW: Chronic myelogenous leukemia: Recent advances. Blood 1985;65:1039.

Goldman JM et al: Bone marrow transplantation for chronic myelogenous leukemia in chronic phase. Ann Intern Med 1988;108:806.

Sokal JE et al: Prognostic discrimination in "good risk" chronic granulocytic leukemia. Blood 1984;63:789.

Talpaz M et al: Hematologic remission and cytogenetic improvement induced by recombinant human interferon-alpha in chronic myelogenous leukemia. N Engl J Med 1986;314:1065.

Thomas ED, Clift RA: Indications for marrow transplantation in chronic myelogenous leukemia. Blood 1989; 73:861.

Thomas ED et al: Marrow transplantation for the treatment of chronic myelogenous leukemia. Ann Intern Med 1986;104:155.

MYELODYSPLASTIC SYNDROMES

Essentials of Diagnosis

- Cytopenias with a hypercellular bone marrow.
- Morphologic abnormalities in 2 or more hematopoietic cell lines.

General Considerations

The myelodysplastic syndromes are a group of acquired clonal disorders of the hematopoietic stem cell. They are characterized by the constellation of cytopenias, a hypercellular marrow, and a number of morphologic abnormalities. The disorders are usually idiopathic but may be seen after cytotoxic chemotherapy—especially procarbazine for Hodgkin's disease and melphalan for multiple myeloma or ovarian carcinoma.

Despite the presence of adequate numbers of hematopoietic progenitor cells, "ineffective hematopoiesis" occurs, resulting in various cytopenias. Ultimately, the disorder may evolve into frank acute myeloid leukemia, and the term "preleukemia" has been used to describe these disorders. Although no specific chromosomal abnormality is seen in myelodysplasia, there are frequently abnormalities involving the long arm of chromosome 5, which contains a number of genes encoding both growth factors and receptors involved in myelopoiesis.

Clinical Findings

A. Symptoms and Signs: Elderly patients are usually affected except in cases of postchemotherapy myelodysplasia. Patients usually present with fatigue, infection, or bleeding related to bone marrow failure. The course may be indolent, and the disease may present as a wasting illness with fever, weight loss, and general debility. On examination, splenomegaly may be present in combination with pallor, bleeding, and various signs of infection.

B. Laboratory Findings: Anemia may be severe and may require transfusion support. The MCV is normal or increased, and macro-ovalocytes may be seen on the peripheral blood smear. The reticulocyte count is usually reduced. The white blood cell count is usually normal or reduced, and neutropenia is common. The neutrophils may exhibit morphologic abnormalities, including deficient numbers of granules or a bilobed nucleus (Pelger-Huet). The myeloid series may be left-shifted, and small numbers of promyelocytes or blasts may be seen. The platelet count is normal or reduced, and hypogranular platelets may be present.

The bone marrow is characteristically hypercellular. Erythroid hyperplasia is common, and signs of abnormal erythropoiesis include megaloblastic features, nuclear budding, or multinucleated erythroid precursors. The Prussian blue stain may demonstrate ringed sideroblasts. The myeloid series is often left-shifted, with variable increases in blasts. Deficient or abnormal granules may be seen. A characteristic abnormality is the presence of dwarf megakaryoctyes with a unilobed nucleus.

Differential Diagnosis

As the number of blasts increase in the bone marrow, myelodysplasia is arbitrarily separated from acute myeloid leukemia by the presence of less than 30% blasts.

Treatment

Patients affected primarily by anemia are best supported with red blood cell transfusions. Patients with severe neutropenia or thrombocytopenia or those with marked constitutional symptoms may be treated with low-dose chemotherapy, although results of such treatment are poor.

Young patients (under age 50) with matched sibling donors can be successfully treated with ablative chemotherapy and allogeneic bone marrow transplantation. Cure rates are approximately 50%.

Course & Prognosis

Myelodysplasia is an ultimately fatal disease. Patients most commonly succumb to infections or bleeding. The risk of transformation to acute myeloid leukemia depends on the percentage of blasts in the bone marrow. Patients with more than 5% blasts in the bone marrow will almost invariably develop leukemia if they do not die of their cytopenias first. Allogeneic bone marrow transplantation is the only definitive therapy.

Appelbaum FR et al: Treatment of preleukemic syndromes with marrow transplantation. Blood 1987;69:92.

Bennett JM et al: Proposals for the classification of the myelodysplastic syndromes. Br J Haematol 1982;51:189.

Feneaux P et al: Prognostic factors in adult chronic myelomonocytic leukemia: An analysis of 107 cases. J Clin Oncol 1988;6:1417.

Thompson JA et al: Subcutaneous granulocyte macrophage colony-stimulating factor in patients with myelodysplastic syndrome: Toxicity, pharmacokinetics and hematologic effects. J Clin Oncol 1989;7:629.

ACUTE LEUKEMIA

Essentials of Diagnosis

- Cytopenias or pancytopenia.
- Bone marrow failure causing infection, bleeding, or fatigue.
- More than 30% blasts in the bone marrow.

General Considerations

Acute leukemia is a malignancy of the hematopoietic progenitor cell. The malignant cell loses its ability to mature and differentiate. These cells proliferate in an uncontrolled fashion and ultimately replace normal bone marrow elements. Most cases arise with no clear cause. However, radiation and some toxins (benzene) are clearly leukemogenic. In addition, a number of chemotherapeutic agents (especially procarbazine, melphalan, and other alkylating agents) may cause leukemia. The leukemias seen after toxin or chemotherapy exposure often develop from a myelodysplastic prodrome and are associated with abnormalities in chromosomes 5 and 7. Although a number of other cytogenetic abnormalities are seen in certain types of acute leukemia, their exact role in pathogenesis remains unclear.

Most of the clinical findings in acute leukemia are due to bone marrow failure, which results from replacement of normal bone marrow elements by the malignant cell. Less common manifestations include direct organ infiltration (skin, gastrointestinal tract, meninges).

Acute leukemia is one of the outstanding examples of a once invariably fatal disease that is now treatable and potentially curable with combination chemotherapy.

Acute lymphoblastic leukemia (ALL) comprises 80% of the acute leukemias of childhood. The peak incidence is between 3 and 7 years of age. However, ALL is also seen in adults and comprises approximately 20% of adult acute leukemias. Acute myeloid leukemia (AML; acute nonlymphocytic leukemia [ANLL]) is chiefly an adult disease with a median age at presentation of 50 years and an increasing incidence with advanced age. However, it is also seen in young adults and children.

Clinical Findings

A. Symptoms and Signs: Most patients with acute leukemia present with an acute illness and have been ill only for days or weeks. The most common presenting complaints are those due to bone marrow failure: fatigue, bleeding, and infection. Bleeding (usually due to thrombocytopenia) is usually in the skin and mucosal surfaces, manifested as gingival bleeding, epistaxis, or menorrhagia. Less commonly, widespread severe bleeding is seen in patients with disseminated intravascular coagulation (seen in acute promyelocytic leukemia and monocytic leukemia). Infection is due to neutropenia, with the risk of infection becoming high as the neutrophil count falls below 500/μL. Patients with neutrophil counts less than 100/μL almost invariably become infected within several days. The most common pathogens are gram-negative bacteria (E coli, Klebsiella, Pseudomonas) or fungi (Candida, Aspergillus). Common presentations include cellulitis, pneumonia, and perirectal infections. Septicemia in severely neutropenic patients is a medical emergency and can cause death within a few hours if treatment with appropriate antibiotics is delayed.

Patients may also seek medical attention because of gum hypertrophy and bone and joint pain. The most dramatic presentation is hyperleukocytosis, in which a markedly elevated circulating blast count (usually > 200,000/μL) leads to impaired circulation, presenting as headache, confusion, and dyspnea. Leukostasis is a medical emergency, and patients require emergent leukapheresis and chemotherapy.

On examination, patients are usually pale and have purpura, petechiae, and various signs of infection. Stomatitis and gum hypertrophy may be seen in patients with monocytic leukemia. There is variable enlargement of the liver, spleen, and lymph nodes. Bone tenderness, particularly in the sternum and tibia, may be present.

B. Laboratory Findings: The hallmark of acute leukemia is the combination of pancytopenia with circulating blasts. However, blasts may be absent from the peripheral smear in as many as 10% of cases ("aleukemic leukemia").

The bone marrow is usually hypercellular and dominated by blasts. More than 30% blasts are required to make a diagnosis of acute leukemia.

A number of other laboratory abnormalities may be present. Hyperuricemia and hypokalemia may be seen. If disseminated intravascular coagulation is present, the fibrinogen level will be reduced, the prothrombin time prolonged, and fibrin degradation products present. Patients with acute lymphoblastic leukemia (especially T cell) may have a mediastinal mass visible on chest radiograph. Patients with meningeal leukemia will have blasts present in the spinal fluid. This is seen in approximately 5% of cases at diagnosis and is more common in monocytic types of acute myeloid leukemia.

The diagnosis of acute leukemia is made by finding more than 30% blasts in the bone marrow. Acute leukemia should then be classified as either acute lymphoblastic or acute myeloid leukemia, also called acute nonlymphocytic leukemia. Patients with acute myeloid leukemia may have granules visible in the blast cells. The Auer rod, an eosinophilic needlelike inclusion in the cytoplasm, is pathognomonic of acute myeloid leukemia. To confirm the myeloid nature of the cells, histochemical stains demonstrating myeloid enzymes such as peroxidase or chloroacetate esterase may be useful. Monocytic lineage can be demonstrated by the finding of butyrate esterase. Acute lymphoblastic leukemia should be considered when there is no morphologic or histochemical evidence of myeloid or monocytic lineage. The diagnosis is confirmed by demonstrating surface markers characteristic of primitive lymphoid cells. Terminal deoxynucleotidal transferase (TdT) is present in 95% of cases of acute lymphoblastic leukemia. A variety of monoclonal antibodies have been used to define other phenotypes of acute lymphoblastic leukemia. Primitive B lymphocyte antigens include CALLA, B1, and BA1. T cell acute lymphoblastic leukemia is diagnosed by the finding of rosette formation with sheep erythrocytes or identification of cell markers by monoclonal antibodies such as Leu-1 or Leu-9.

Acute myeloid leukemia is usually so categorized on the basis of morphology and histochemistry as follows: Acute myeloblastic leukemia (M1), acute myeloblastic leukemia with differentiation (M2), acute promyelocytic leukemia (M3), acute myelomonocytic leukemia (M4), acute monoblastic leukemia (M5), and erythroleukemia (M6).

Acute lymphoblastic leukemia is most usefully classified by immunologic phenotype as follows: common, early B lineage, and T cell.

Differential Diagnosis

Acute myeloid leukemia must be distinguished from other myeloproliferative disorders, chronic myeloid leukemia, and myelodysplastic syndromes. The diagnosis is made by finding more than 30% blasts in the bone marrow. It is important to distinguish acute leukemia from a left-shifted bone marrow that is recovering from a previous toxic insult. If the question is in doubt, a bone marrow study should be repeated in several days to see if maturation has taken place. Acute lymphoblastic leukemia must be distinguished from other lymphoproliferative disease such as chronic lymphocytic leukemia, lymphomas, and hairy cell leukemia. It may also be confused with the atypical lymphocytosis of mononucleosis. An experienced observer can distinguish these entities based on morphology.

Treatment

Acute leukemia may present as a medical emergency. Sepsis in a neutropenic patient must be treated immediately with broad-spectrum antibiotics. Leukostasis must be treated immediately with leukapheresis and chemotherapy. Disseminated intravascular coagulation must be treated with replacement of platelets, coagulation factors, and fibrinogen in combination with heparin (discussed below).

Most young patients with acute leukemia are treated with the objective of effecting a cure. The first step in treatment is to obtain complete remission, defined as normal peripheral blood with resolution of cytopenias, normal bone marrow with no excess in blasts, and normal clinical status. However, complete remission is not synonymous with cure, and leukemia will invariably recur if no further treatment is given.

Acute myeloid leukemia is treated initially with intensive combination chemotherapy, including daunorubicin and cytarabine. Effective treatment produces aplasia of the bone marrow, which takes 2–3 weeks to recover. During this period, intensive supportive care, including transfusion and antibiotic therapy, is required. Once complete remission has been achieved, several different types of postremission therapy are potentially curative. Options include repeated intensive chemotherapy, high-dose chemoradiotherapy with allogeneic bone marrow transplantation, and high-dose chemotherapy with autologous bone marrow transplantation.

Acute lymphoblastic leukemia is treated initially with combination chemotherapy, including daunorubicin, vincristine, prednisone, and sometimes asparaginase. Remission induction therapy for acute lymphoblastic leukemia is less myelosuppressive than treatment for acute myeloid leukemia and does not necessarily produce marrow aplasia. After achieving complete remission, patients receive central nervous system prophylaxis with cranial irradiation and intrathecal methotrexate so that meningeal sequestration of leukemic cells does not develop. As with acute myeloid leukemia, patients may be treated with either chemotherapy or high-dose chemotherapy plus bone marrow transplantation.

Prognosis

Approximately 70–80% of adults with acute myeloid leukemia under age 50 achieve complete remission. Chemotherapy leads to long-term disease-free survival in 20–30% of cases. Allogeneic bone marrow transplantation (for younger adults with HLA-matched siblings) is curative in approximately 50% of cases. The role of autologous bone marrow transplantation remains to be defined, but preliminary results suggest that this may be the treatment of choice. Older adults with acute myeloid leukemia achieve complete remission approximately 50% of the time. A selected older patient may be treated with intensive chemotherapy with curative intent.

Eighty percent of adults with acute lymphoblastic leukemia achieve complete remission. Subsequent postremission chemotherapy is curative in 30–50% of adults. Acute lymphoblastic leukemia in children is much more responsive to therapy, with 95% achieving complete remission and 50–60% of these being cured with postremission treatment that is far less toxic than that necessary for adults.

Applebaum FR et al: Chemotherapy versus marrow transplantation for adults with acute nonlymphocytic leukemia: A five-year follow-up. Blood 1988;72:179.

Champlin R, Gale RP: Acute myelogenous leukemia: Recent advances in therapy. Blood 1987;69:1551.

Hoelzer D et al: Prognostic factors in a multicenter study for treatment of acute lymphoblastic leukemia in adults. Blood 1988;71:123.

Jacobs AD, Gale RP: Recent advances in the biology and treatment of acute lymphoblastic leukemia in adults. N Engl J Med 1984;311:1219.

Linker CA et al: Improved results of treatment of adult acute lymphoblastic leukemia. Blood 1987;69:1242.

CHRONIC LYMPHOCYTIC LEUKEMIA

Essentials of Diagnosis

- Lymphocytosis > 15,000/μL.
- "Mature" appearance of lymphocytes.

General Considerations

Chronic lymphocytic leukemia is a clonal malignancy of B lymphocytes (rarely T lymphocytes). The disease is usually indolent, with slowly progressive accumulation of long-lived small lymphocytes. These cells are immunoincompetent and respond poorly to antigenic stimulation.

Chronic lymphocytic leukemia is manifested clinically by immunosuppression, bone marrow failure, and organ infiltration with lymphocytes. Immunosuppression, bone marrow failure, and infiltration of organs account for most clinical manifestation. Immunodeficiency is also related to inadequate antibody production by the abnormal B cells. With advanced disease, chronic lymphocytic leukemia may cause damage by direct tissue infiltration.

Clinical Findings

A. Symptoms and Signs: Chronic lymphocytic leukemia is a disease of the elderly, with 90% of cases occurring after age 50 and a median age at presentation of 65. Many patients will be incidentally discovered to have lymphocytosis. Others present with fatigue or lymphadenopathy. On examination, 80% of patients will have lymphadenopathy and half will have enlargement of the liver or spleen.

A prognostically useful staging system has been developed as follows: stage 0, lymphocytosis only; stage I, lymphocytosis plus lymphadenopathy; stage II, organomegaly; stage III, anemia; stage IV, thrombocytopenia. Chronic lymphocytic leukemia usually pursues an indolent course but occasionally will present as a rapidly progressive disease. These patients usually have larger, less mature-appearing lymphocytes and are said to have "prolymphocytic" leukemia. In 5–

10% of cases, chronic lymphocytic leukemia may be complicated by autoimmune hemolytic anemia or autoimmune thrombocytopenia. In approximately 5% of cases, while the systemic disease remains stable, an isolated lymph node will be transformed into an aggressive large cell lymphoma (Richter's syndrome).

B. Laboratory Findings: The hallmark of chronic lymphocytic leukemia is isolated lymphocytosis. The white blood count is usually greater than 20,000/μL and may be markedly elevated. Usually 75–98% of the circulating cells are lymphocytes. Lymphocytes appear small and "mature," with condensed nuclear chromatin, and are morphologically indistinguishable from normal small lymphocytes. The hematocrit and platelet count are usually normal at presentation. The bone marrow is variably infiltrated with small lymphocytes. The malignant cells weakly express surface immunoglobulin, and the monoclonal nature of the cells can be demonstrated by the finding of a single light chain type on the surface.

Hypogammaglobulinemia is present in half of cases and becomes more common with advanced disease. In some instances, a small amount of IgM paraprotein is present in the serum. Pathologic changes in lymph nodes are the same as in diffuse small cell lymphocytic lymphoma.

Differential Diagnosis

A few syndromes can be confused with chronic lymphocytic leukemia. Viral infections producing lymphocytosis should be obvious from the presence of fever and other clinical findings. Other lymphoproliferative diseases such as Waldenstrodm's macroglobulinemia, hairy cell leukemia, or lymphoma in the leukemic phase are distinguished on the basis of the morphology of circulating lymphocytes and bone marrow.

Treatment

Most cases of early indolent chronic lymphocytic leukemia require no specific therapy. Indications for treatment include progressive fatigue, troublesome lymphadenopathy, or the development of anemia or thrombocytopenia. Initial therapy includes chlorambucil and prednisone. A common regimen is chlorambucil, 0.6–1 mg/kg, in combination with 4 days of prednisone every 3 weeks. Complications such as autoimmune hemolytic anemia or immune thrombocytopenia may be treated with high-dose prednisone but often require splenectomy for control. Fludarabine is a promising new experimental agent which is useful in treating disease refractory to other agents.

Prognosis

Median survival is approximately 6 years, and 25% of patients live more than 10 years. Patients with stage 0 or I disease have a median survival of 10 years. It is important to reassure these patients that despite the frightening diagnosis of "leukemia" they can live a normal life for many years. Patients with stage III or IV disease have a median survival of less than 2 years. Chronic lymphocytic leukemia is managed in palliative fashion. Patients with advanced disease benefit only briefly from intensive therapy.

French Cooperative Group on Chronic Lymphocytic Leukemia: Effects of chlorambucil and therapeutic decision in initial forms of chronic lymphocytic leukemia (stage A): Results of a randomized clinical trial on 612 patients. Blood 1990;75:1414.

Gale RP, Foon KA: Chronic lymphocytic leukemia: Recent advances in biology and treatment. Ann Intern Med 1985;103:101.

Keating MJ: Fludarabine: A new agent with major activity against chronic lymphocytic leukemia. Blood 1989; 74:19.

Lee JS et al: Prognosis of chronic lymphocytic leukemia: A multivariate regression analysis of 325 untreated patients. Blood 1987;69:929.

HAIRY CELL LEUKEMIA

Essentials of Diagnosis
- Pancytopenia.
- Splenomegaly, often massive.
- Hairy cells present on blood smear and bone marrow biopsy.

General Considerations
Hairy cell leukemia, an uncommon form of leukemia, is an indolent cancer of B lymphocytes.

Clinical Findings
A. Symptoms and Signs: The disease characteristically presents in middle-aged men. The median age at presentation is 55 years, and there is a striking 5:1 male predominance. Most patients present with gradual onset of fatigue, but others complain of symptoms related to markedly enlarged spleen and still others come to attention because of infection.

On physical examination, splenomegaly is almost invariably present and may be massive. The liver is enlarged in half of cases, but lymphadenopathy is uncommon.

B. Laboratory Findings: The hallmark of hairy cell leukemia is pancytopenia. Anemia is nearly universal, and 75% of patients have thrombocytopenia and neutropenia as well. The "hairy cells" are usually present in small numbers on the peripheral blood smear and have a characteristic appearance with numerous cytoplasmic projections. Less commonly, a "leukemic form" of the disorder exists in which large numbers of hairy cells dominate the peripheral blood smear. The bone marrow is usually inaspirable (dry tap), and the diagnosis is made by characteristic morphology on bone marrow biopsy. The hairy cells have a characteristic histochemical staining pattern, with tartrate-resistant acid phosphatase (TRAP). Patho-

logic examination of the spleen shows marked infiltration of the red pulp with hairy cells. This is in marked contrast to the usual predilection of lymphomas to involve the white pulp of the spleen.

Hairy cell leukemia is usually an indolent disorder whose course is dominated by pancytopenia and recurrent infections, including mycobacterial infections.

Differential Diagnosis
Hairy cell leukemia should be distinguished from other lymphoproliferative diseases such as chronic lymphocytic leukemia, Waldenström's macroglobulinemia, and non-Hodgkin's lymphomas.

Treatment
Many patients with indolent disease require no specific therapy. In the past, the treatment of choice has been splenectomy, indicated for severe cytopenias or recurrent infections. More recently, interferon has produced responses in a high proportion of patients and has led to disappearance of the disease for some time. Two experimental drugs, deoxycoformycin and 2-chlorodeoxyadenosine, appear very promising. Both appear to produce complete remissions which last for several years. Their ultimate role in treatment remains to be defined.

Course & Prognosis
The development of new effective therapies (interferon and deoxycoformycin) appears to have changed the prognosis of this disease. Formerly, median survival was 6 years, and only one-third of patients survived longer than 10 years. Although longer follow-up will be required, it now appears that most patients with hairy cell leukemia will live longer than 10 years. With current trends in treatment, the prognosis appears open-ended at this time.

Golomb HM et al: Report of a multi-institutional study of 193 patients with hairy cell leukemia treated with interferon-alpha 2B. Semin Oncol 1988;15:7.

Kraut EH et al: Pentostatin in the treatment of advance hair cell leukemia. J Clin Oncol 1989;7:168. Piro LD et al: Lasting remissions in hair cell leukemia induced by a single infusion of 2-chlorodeoxyadenosine. N Engl J Med 1990;322:1117.

Ratain MJ et al: Prognostic variables in hair cell leukemia after splenectomy as initial therapy. Cancer 1988;62:2420

LYMPHOMAS

NON-HODGKIN'S LYMPHOMAS

Essentials of Diagnosis
- Pathologic diagnosis of lymphoma is by biopsy of lymph nodes or other tissues.

General Considerations

The non-Hodgkin's lymphomas are a heterogeneous group of cancers of lymphocytes. The disorders are variable in clinical presentation and course, varying from indolent disease to rapidly progressive devastating illnesses.

Results of studies using techniques of molecular biology have provided clues to the pathogenesis of these disorders. The best-studied example is Burkitt's lymphoma, in which a characteristic cytogenetic abnormality of translocation between the long arms of chromosomes 8 and 14 has been identified. The proto-oncogene c-*myc* is translocated from its normal position on chromosome 8 to the heavy chain locus on chromosome 14. Cells committed to B cell differentiation are likely to have enhanced expression of this heavy chain locus, and it is likely that overexpression of c-*myc* (in its new anomalous position) is related to malignant transformation. In the follicular lymphomas, translocations of a possible oncogene *bcl*-2 from the chromosome to the heavy chain locus on chromosome 14 may play a similar role.

Classification of the lymphomas is a controversial area still undergoing evolution. Recently, the National Cancer Institute has sponsored a "working formulation" that characterizes these lymphomas according to their biologic behavior, whether indolent or aggressive (Table 10–16).

Clinical Findings

A. Symptoms and Signs: Patients with indolent lymphomas usually present with painless lymphadenopathy, which may be isolated or widespread. Involved lymph nodes may be present in the retroperitoneum, mesentery, and pelvis. However, the indolent lymphomas are often disseminated at the time of diagnosis, and bone marrow involvement is frequent.

Patients with high-grade lymphomas may present

Table 10–16. Classification of lymphomas; "working formulation."

Low-grade
  Small lymphocytic
  Small lymphocytic, plasmacytoid
  Follicular, small cleaved cell
  Follicular mixed cell
Intermediate-grade
  Follicular large cell
  Diffuse small cleaved cell
  Diffuse mixed cell
  Diffuse large cell
High-grade
  Immunoblastic
  Small noncleaved (Burkitt's)
  Small noncleaved (non-Burkitt's)
  Lymphoblastic
  True histiocytic
Other
  Cutaneous T cell (mycosis fungoides)
  Adult T cell leukemia/lymphoma
  T γ lymphocytosis

with adenopathy or with constitutional symptoms such as fever, drenching night sweats, or weight loss. On examination, lymphadenopathy may be isolated, or extranodal sites of disease (skin, gastrointestinal tract) may be found. Patients with Burkitt's lymphoma frequently present with abdominal pain or abdominal fullness because of the predilection of the disease for the abdomen.

Patients should be evaluated to determine the site and extent of disease. Physical examination should be supplemented by chest x-ray and CT scan of the abdomen and pelvis. The bone marrow should be biopsied, and—in selected cases such as high-risk morphology—a lumbar puncture should be performed.

B. Laboratory Findings: The peripheral blood is usually normal, but a number of lymphomas may present in a "leukemic" phase. In these situations, the distinction between leukemia and lymphoma is arbitrary, as the malignant cell has the same characteristics. Examples of the diseases that may present as lymphoma or leukemia are small cell lymphoma versus chronic lymphocytic leukemia, small cell plasmacytic lymphoma versus Waldenstrodm's macroglobulinemia, follicular small cleaved cell lymphoma versus lymphosarcoma cell leukemia, cutaneous T cell lymphoma versus Sézary syndrome, lymphoblastic lymphoma versus T cell acute lymphoblastic leukemia, and Burkitt's lymphoma versus B cell acute lymphoblastic leukemia.

Bone marrow involvement is usually manifested as paratrabecular lymphoid aggregates. In some high-grade lymphomas, the meninges may be involved and the spinal fluid may contain malignant cells. The chest radiograph may show a mediastinal mass in lymphoblastic lymphoma.

The serum LDH level is useful in evaluating the extent of disease and the aggressiveness of tumor behavior.

The diagnosis of lymphoma is made by tissue biopsy. Needle aspiration may yield suspicious results, but usually a lymph node biopsy (or biopsy of involved extranodal tissue) is required.

Treatment

Once a pathologic diagnosis is established, the patient should be evaluated ("staged") to determine the extent of disease. The primary purpose of staging is to determine whether regional therapy such as surgery or radiation therapy is appropriate or whether the disease must be approached in a systemic fashion with chemotherapy.

The indolent lymphomas are usually not curable and are approached with palliative therapy. If patients are asymptomatic, no initial treatment may be necessary. However, in 1–3 years, the disease will usually progress and require treatment. Treatment decisions are individualized depending on the patient's age and performance status and the extent of disease. Initial therapy is based on the alkylating agents. Appropriate regimens include chlorambucil, 0.6–1 mg/kg every 3 weeks, or combination therapy with cyclophosphamide, vincristine, and prednisone (CVP). Patients with more aggressive or resistant disease may require more intensive therapy. Those with apparently localized disease may be treated initially with local radiation.

Patients with high-grade lymphomas should be treated with curative intent. Local irradiation is occasionally used (supplemented by brief intensive chemotherapy) but the mainstay of therapy is aggressive combination chemotherapy. The traditional treatment regimen has been cyclophosphamide, Adriamycin (doxorubicin), Oncovin (vincristine), and prednisone (CHOP). More recent regimens appear to generate superior results, and clinical trials to confirm this impression are under way.

Patients who relapse following initial response have been successfully treated with intensive chemotherapy and autologous bone marrow transplantation.

Prognosis

The median survival of patients with indolent lymphomas is 6–8 years. These diseases ultimately become refractory to chemotherapy. This often occurs at the time of histologic progression of the disease to a more aggressive form of lymphoma. The prognosis of patients with high-grade lymphomas depends on their response to chemotherapy. Depending on the initial pathologic subtype and initial bulk of disease, these patients are variably curable.

With appropriate therapy, approximately 50% of patients with disseminated large-cell lymphomas may be cured. Results are better in those who are young, are in good clinical, condition, and have less advanced stages of disease. Salvage therapy with autologous bone marrow transplantation may be effective in 50% of cases if the disease is still responsive to chemotherapy and the patient comes to transplant in good condition and with minimal tumor bulk.

Armitage JO, Cheson BD: Interpretation of clinical trials in diffuse large cell lymphoma. J Clin Oncol 1988; 6:1335.

Cheson BD et al: Low-grade, non-Hodgkin's lymphomas revisited. Cancer Treat Rep 1986;70:1051.

Freedman AS et al: Autologous bone marrow transplantation in B-cell non-Hodgkin's lymphoma: Very low treatment-related mortality in 100 patients in sensitive relapse. J Clin Oncol 1990;8:784.

Klimo P, Connors JM: MACOP-B chemotherapy for the treatment of diffuse large cell lymphomas. Ann Intern Med 1985;102:596.

Petersen FB et al: Autologous bone marrow transplantation for malignant lymphoma: A report of 101 cases from Seattle. J Clin Oncol 1990;8:638.

Velasquez WS et al: Risk classification as the basis for clinical staging of diffuse large cell lymphoma derived from 10-year survival data. Blood 1989;74:551.

HODGKIN'S DISEASE

Essentials of Diagnosis
- Painless lymphadenopathy.
- Constitutional symptoms may be present.
- Pathologic diagnosis by lymph node biopsy.

General Considerations

Hodgkin's disease is a group of cancers characterized by Reed-Sternberg cells in an appropriate reactive cellular background. The nature of the malignant cell is a subject of controversy, but recent evidence suggests that it is of macrophage origin.

Clinical Findings

There is a bimodal age distribution, with one peak in the 20s and a second peak over age 50. Most patients present because of a painless mass, commonly in the neck. Others may seek medical attention because of constitutional symptoms such as fever, weight loss, or drenching night sweats, or because of generalized pruritus. An unusual symptom of Hodgkin's disease is pain in an involved lymph node following alcohol ingestion.

An important clinical feature of Hodgkin's disease is its tendency to arise within lymph node areas and to spread in an orderly fashion to contiguous areas of lymph nodes. Only late in the course of the disease will vascular invasion lead to widespread hematogenous dissemination.

The diagnosis is made by examination of lymph node tissue by an experienced hematopathologist. Hodgkin's disease is divided into several subtypes: lymphocyte predominance, nodular sclerosis, mixed cellularity, and lymphocyte depletion. Hodgkin's disease should be distinguished pathologically from other malignant lymphomas. It may also occasionally be confused with reactive lymph nodes seen in infectious mononucleosis, cat-scratch disease, or drug reactions (phenytoin).

Patients should initially undergo a "staging" evaluation to determine the extent of disease. The purpose of this evaluation is to determine whether localized treatment (radiotherapy) is indicated or if systemic chemotherapy must be given. The staging nomenclature is as follows: stage I, one lymph node region involved; stage II, involvement of 2 lymph node areas on one side of the diaphragm; stage III, lymph node region involved on both sides of the diaphragm; Stage IV, disseminated disease with bone marrow or liver involvement. In addition, patients are designated stage A if they lack constitutional symptoms and stage B if significant weight loss, fever, or night sweats are present.

Treatment

Patients with localized disease (stages IA, IIA) are treated with radiation therapy. Patients with disseminated disease (IIIB, IV) are treated with aggressive combination chemotherapy. The treatment of choice appears to be Adriamycin (doxorubicin), bleomycin, vincristine, dacarbazine (ABVD) or ABVD alternating with mechlorethamine, Oncovin (vincristine), procarbazine, and prednisone (MOPP). The optimal management of patients with stages IIB or IIIA is controversial, but current evidence suggests an advantage to combination chemotherapy.

Prognosis

Hodgkin's disease is no longer invariably fatal, and patients with both localized and disseminated disease should be treated with curative intent. The prognosis of patients with stage IA or IIA disease treated by radiotherapy is excellent, with 10-year survival rates in excess of 80%. Patients with disseminated disease (IIIB, IV) have 5-year survival rates of 20–50%. The poorer results are seen in patients who are elderly, those who have bulky disease, and those with lymphocyte depletion or mixed cellularity on histologic examination. The prognosis of patients with stage IIB or stage IIIA disease is intermediate, with 5-year survival rates between 30% and 60%.

Bonadonna G, Valagussa P, Santoro A: Alternating non-cross-resistant combination chemotherapy or MOPP in stage IV Hodgkin's disease: A report of 8-year results. Ann Intern Med 1986;104:739.

Carde P et al: Clinical stages I and II Hodgkin's disease: A specifically tailored therapy according to prognostic factors. J Clin Oncol 1988;6:239.

MULTIPLE MYELOMA

Essentials of Diagnosis

- Monoclonal paraprotein by serum or urine protein electrophoresis or immunoelectrophoresis.
- Bone pain and destruction.
- Replacement of bone marrow by malignant plasma cells.

General Considerations

Multiple myeloma is a malignancy of plasma cells characterized by replacement of the bone marrow, bone destruction, and paraprotein formation. Myeloma is a complex disease that causes clinical signs and symptoms through a variety of mechanisms.

Replacement of the bone marrow (and perhaps humoral suppression of myelopoiesis) leads initially to anemia and later to general bone marrow failure. Bone destruction causes bone pain, osteoporosis, lytic lesions, and pathologic fractures. Hypercalcemia is common and appears to be mediated by osteoclast activating factor (OAF) or similar lymphokines. The malignant plasma cells can form tumors (plasmacytomas) that have a predilection for causing spinal cord compression.

The paraproteins secreted by the malignant plasma cells may cause problems in their own right. Very high paraprotein levels (either IgG or IgA) may cause the hyperviscosity syndrome. The light chain component of the immunoglobulin may cause renal failure (often aggravated by hypercalcemia). Paraproteins may become catabolized into amyloid, worsening renal failure and causing a vast array of systemic symptoms.

Myeloma patients are prone to recurrent infections for a number of reasons, including neutropenia and the immunosuppressive effects of chemotherapy. Additionally, there is a failure of antibody production in response to antigen challenge, and myeloma patients are especially prone to infections with encapsulated organisms such as *Streptococcus pneumoniae* and *Haemophilus influenzae*.

Clinical Findings

A. Symptoms and Signs: Myeloma is a disease of older adults (median age at presentation, 60 years). The classic picture of myeloma is anemia, back pain, and an elevated sedimentation rate in an older man, and the most common presenting complaints are those related to anemia, bone pain, and infection. Bone pain is most common in the back or ribs or may present as a pathologic fracture, especially of the femoral neck. Patients may also come to medical attention because of renal failure; spinal cord compression, or the hyperviscosity syndrome (mucosal bleeding, vertigo, nausea, visual disturbances, alterations in mental status). Occasionally, patients are diagnosed as having myeloma because of initial laboratory findings of hypercalcemia, proteinuria, elevated sedimentation rate, or abnormalities on serum protein electrophoresis.

Examination may reveal pallor, bone tenderness, and soft tissue masses. Patients may have neurologic signs related to neuropathy or spinal cord compression. Patients with amyloidosis may have an enlarged tongue, neuropathy, or congestive heart failure.

B. Laboratory Findings: Anemia is nearly universal. Red blood cell morphology is normal, but rouleau formation is common and may be marked. The neutrophil and platelet counts are usually normal at presentation. Only rarely will plasma cells be visible on peripheral smear (plasma cell leukemia).

The hallmark of myeloma is the finding of a paraprotein on serum protein electrophoresis (SPEP). The majority of patients will have a monoclonal spike visible in the beta or gamma globulin region. Immunoelectrophoresis (IEP) will reveal this to be a monoclonal protein. Approximately 20% of patients will have no demonstrable paraprotein in the serum. SPEP or IEP of the urine will reveal either complete immunoglobulin or light chains. Overall, approximately 60% of myeloma patients will have an IgG paraprotein, 25% an IgA, and 15% light chains only.

The bone marrow will be infiltrated by variable

numbers of plasma cells ranging from 5% to 100%. Occasionally, the plasma cells may be morphologically indistinguishable from normal cells but more commonly will appear abnormal. Bone radiographs are important in establishing the diagnosis of myeloma. Lytic lesions are most commonly seen in the axial skeleton: skull, spine, proximal long bones, and ribs. At other times, only generalized osteoporosis is seen. The radionuclide bone scan is not useful in detecting bone lesions in myeloma, as there is usually no osteoblastic component.

Other laboratory features include hypercalcemia, renal failure, and an elevated erythrocyte sedimentation rate. Some patients have proximal renal tubular acidosis, with phosphaturia, glucosuria, and uricosuria. The urinalysis may reveal proteinuria, but the dipstick test (which detects primarily albumin) is unreliable for light chains. Often there is a narrow anion gap when the paraprotein is cationic. On occasion, the abnormal protein is cryoprecipitatable, resulting in positive studies for cryoglobulins.

Differential Diagnosis

When a patient is discovered to have a monoclonal paraprotein, the distinction between myeloma and benign monoclonal gammopathy must be made. Benign monoclonal gammopathy can be considered an adenoma of plasma cells and is present in 1% of all adults and 3% of adults over age 70. Thus, if one considers all patients with paraproteins, benign monoclonal gammopathy is far more common than myeloma. Most commonly, patients with benign monoclonal gammopathy will have a monoclonal IgG spike less than 2.5 g/dL, and the height of the spike remains stable. In approximately 25% of cases, benign monoclonal gammopathy progresses to overt malignant disease, but this may take years or even decades.

Myeloma is distinguished from benign monoclonal gammopathy by findings of replacement of the bone marrow, bone destruction, and progression over time. Although the height of the paraprotein spike should not be used by itself to distinguish benign from malignant disease, in practice all patients with IgG spikes greater than 3.5 g/dL prove to have myeloma. An IgA spike of greater than 2 g/dL is almost always due to myeloma. If there is doubt about whether paraproteinemia is benign or malignant, the patient should be observed without therapy, since there is no advantage to early treatment of asymptomatic multiple myeloma.

Myeloma should be distinguished from polyclonal hypergammaglobulinemia seen in reactive conditions. The distinction is made by finding the polyclonal as opposed to the monoclonal spike. Myeloma may also need to be distinguished from other malignant lymphoproliferative diseases such as Waldenström's macroglobulinemia, lymphomas, and primary amyloidosis.

Treatment

The goal of treatment of myeloma is palliation. Patients with minimal disease or in whom the diagnosis of malignancy is in doubt should be observed without treatment. Most commonly, patients require treatment at diagnosis because of bone pain or other symptoms related to the disease. In the past, standard therapy has been melphalan plus prednisone; more recently, combination chemotherapy with alkylating agents has been used. The optimal chemotherapy regimen has not been determined. The height of the paraprotein spike on SPEP is a useful marker for monitoring response to therapy. Patients who fail to respond to standard therapy may be effectively salvaged with low-dose continuous infusion therapy, the VAD (vincristine, Adriamycin (doxorubicin), dexamethasone) regimen.

A number of other ancillary measures are important in the treatment of myeloma. Localized radiotherapy may be useful for palliation of bone pain or for eradicating tumor at the site of pathologic fracture. Hypercalcemia should be treated aggressively and prolonged immobilization and dehydration avoided. Recently, allogeneic bone marrow transplantation has been tried for the few young patients with multiple myeloma. Initial results appear promising, but this is currently experimental treatment.

Prognosis

The median survival of patients with myelomas is 3 years. The prognosis is markedly affected by a number of prognostic features, with shorter survivals in those with high paraprotein spikes, renal failure, hypercalcemia, or extensive bony disease. Patients are said to have a "low tumor burden" if the IgG spike is less than 5 g/dL and there is no more than one lytic bone lesion and no evidence of severe anemia, hypercalcemia, or renal failure. These patients have a median survival of 5–6 years. Conversely, patients with a "high tumor burden" have an IgG spike greater than 7 g/dL, hematocrit less than 25%, calcium greater than 12 mg/dL, or more than 3 lytic bone lesions. Median survival for this group is approximately 1 year.

Barlogie B et al: Plasma cell myeloma: New biological insights and advances in therapy. Blood 1989;73:865.

Cavo M et al: Prognostic variables and clinical staging in multiple myeloma. Blood 1989;74:1774.

Fermand J et al: Treatment of aggressive multiple myeloma by high-dose chemotherapy and total body irradiation followed by blood stem cell autologous graft. Blood 1988;73:20

WALDENSTRÖM'S MACROGLOBULINEMIA

Essentials of Diagnosis

- Monoclonal IgM paraprotein.

- Infiltration of bone marrow by plasmacytic lymphocyte.
- Absence of lytic bone disease.

General Considerations

Waldenström's macroglobulinemia is a malignant disease of B cells that appear to be a hybrid of lymphocytes and plasma cells. These cells characteristically secrete an IgM paraprotein, and many clinical manifestations of the disease are related to this macroglobulin.

Clinical Findings

A. Symptoms and Signs: This disease characteristically presents insidiously in patients in their 60s or 70s. Patients usually present with fatigue related to anemia. Hyperviscosity of serum may be manifested in a number of ways. Mucosal and gastrointestinal bleeding is related to engorged blood vessels and platelet dysfunction. Other complaints include nausea, vertigo, and visual disturbances. Alterations in consciousness vary from mild lethargy to stupor and coma. The IgM paraprotein may also cause symptoms of cold agglutinin disease or peripheral neuropathy.

On examination, there may be hepatosplenomegaly or lymphadenopathy. The retinal veins are characteristically engorged. Purpura may be present. There should be no bone tenderness.

B. Laboratory Findings: Anemia is nearly universal, and rouleau formation is common. The anemia is related in part to expansion of the plasma volume by 50–100% due to the presence of the paraprotein. Other blood counts are usually normal. The abnormal plasmacytic lymphocyte usually appears in small numbers on the peripheral blood smear. The bone marrow is characteristically infiltrated by the plasmacytic lymphocytes.

The hallmark of macroglobulinemia is the presence of a monoclonal IgM spike seen on serum protein electrophoresis (SPEP) in the beta or gamma globulin region. The serum viscosity is usually increased above the normal of 1.4–1.8 times that of water. Symptoms of hyperviscosity usually develop when the serum viscosity is over 4 times that of water, and marked symptoms usually arise when the viscosity is over 6 times that of water. Because paraproteins vary in their physicochemical properties, there is no strict correlation between the concentration of paraprotein and serum viscosity. However, after a certain threshold, viscosity rises exponentially with small increments in paraprotein amounts.

The IgM paraprotein may cause a positive Coombs test or have cold agglutinin or cryoglobulin properties. If one suspects macroglobulinemia but the SPEP shows only hypogammaglobulinemia, one should repeat the test while taking special measures to maintain the blood at 37 °C, since the paraprotein may precipitate out at room temperature.

Bone radiographs should be normal, and there should be no evidence of renal failure.

Differential Diagnosis

Waldenström's macroglobulinemia is differentiated from benign monoclonal gammopathy by the finding of bone marrow infiltration. It is differentiated from chronic lymphocytic leukemia and multiple myeloma by bone marrow morphology and the finding of thecharacteristic IgM spike.

Treatment

Patients who present with marked hyperviscosity syndrome (stupor or coma) should be treated on an emergency basis with plasmapheresis. Pheresis will usually rapidly reduce the paraprotein level below the threshold required to produce symptoms. On a chronic basis, some patients can be managed with periodic plasmapheresis alone. Others are treated with intermittent chemotherapy with chlorambucil or cyclophosphamide.

Prognosis

Waldenström's macroglobulinemia is an indolent disease with a median survival rate of 3–5 years. However, patients may survive 10 years or longer.

Dellagi K et al: Waldenström's macroglobulinemia and peripheral neuropathy: A clinical and immunologic study of 25 patients. Blood 1983;62:280.
Kantarjian HM et al: Fludarabine therapy in macroglobulinemic lymphoma. Blood 1990;75:1928.

DISORDERS OF HEMOSTASIS

Disorders of hemostasis may be due to defects in either platelet number or function or to problems in formation of a fibrin clot (coagulation). Bleeding due to platelet disorders is typically mucosal or skin bleeding. Common problems include epistaxis, gum bleeding, menorrhagia, gastrointestinal bleeding, purpura, and petechiae. Petechiae are seen almost exclusively in conditions of thrombocytopenia and not platelet dysfunction. Bleeding due to coagulopathy may occur as deep muscle hematomas as well as skin bleeding. Spontaneous hemarthroses are seen only in severe hemophilia.

IDIOPATHIC (AUTOIMMUNE) THROMBOCYTOPENIC PURPURA

Essentials of Diagnosis

- Isolated thrombocytopenia.
- Other hematopoietic cell lines normal.

- No systemic illness.
- Spleen not palpable.
- Normal bone marrow with normal or increased megakaryocytes.

General Considerations

Idiopathic thrombocytopenic purpura is an autoimmune disorder in which an IgG autoantibody is formed that binds to platelets. It is not clear which antigen on the platelet surface is involved. Although the antiplatelet antibody may bind complement, platelets are not destroyed by direct lysis. Rather, destruction takes place in the spleen, where splenic macrophages with Fc receptors bind to antibody-coated platelets. Since the pathogenesis of this disorder is now well understood, the term idiopathic is no longer appropriate, but the term idiopathic thrombocytopenic purpura is deeply entrenched in the literature (ITP).

The spleen plays a major role in the pathogenesis of idiopathic thrombocytopenic purpura. The spleen is the major site both of antibody production and platelet sequestration. This explains the high degree of effectiveness of splenectomy in treating this disorder.

Clinical Findings

A. Symptoms and Signs: Idiopathic thrombocytopenic purpura occurs commonly in childhood, frequently precipitated by viral infection and usually self-limited. In contrast, the adult form is usually a chronic disease and only infrequently follows a viral infection. It is a disease of young persons, with peak incidence between ages 20 and 50, and there is a 2:1 female predominance.

Patients are systemically well and not febrile. The presenting complaint is mucosal or skin bleeding. Common types of bleeding are epistaxis, oral bleeding, menorrhagia, purpura, and petechiae.

On examination, the patient appears well, and there are no abnormal findings other than those related to bleeding. An enlarged spleen should lead one to doubt the diagnosis. Common signs of bleeding are purpura, petechiae, and hemorrhagic bullae in the mouth.

B. Laboratory Findings: The hallmark of the disease is thrombocytopenia, which may be severe. This is one of the few disorders that will produce a platelet count less than 10,000/μL. The other blood counts are usually normal except for mild anemia, which can be explained by bleeding. Peripheral blood cell morphology is normal except that platelets are slightly enlarged (megathrombocytes). These larger platelets are young platelets produced in response to enhanced platelet destruction. Approximately 10% of patients will have coexistent autoimmune hemolytic anemia, and in these cases one will see anemia, reticulocytosis, and spherocytes on peripheral smear. Red blood cell fragmentation should not be seen.

The bone marrow will appear normal, with a normal or increased number of megakaryocytes. Coagulation studies will be entirely normal. Tests now available to quantitate platelet-associated IgG may help in the diagnosis. At present, although these tests are highly sensitive (95%), they are very nonspecific, and 50% of all patients with thrombocytopenia from any cause may have increased levels of IgG on the platelet.

Differential Diagnosis

Thrombocytopenia may be produced either by abnormal bone marrow function or by peripheral destruction (Table 10–17). Although most bone marrow disorders produce abnormalities in addition to isolated thrombocytopenia, diagnoses such as myelodysplasia can only be excluded by examining the bone marrow. Most causes of thrombocytopenia resulting from peripheral destruction can be ruled out by initial evaluation. Disorders such as disseminated intravascular coagulation, thrombotic thrombocytopenic purpura, hemolytic-uremic syndrome, hypersplenism, and sepsis are easily excluded by the absence of systemic illness. Thus, patients with isolated thrombocytopenia with no other abnormal findings almost certainly have immune thrombocytopenia. Patients should be questioned regarding drug use, especially sulfonamides, quinidine, quinine, thiazides, cimetidine, gold, and heparin. Heparin is now the most common cause of drug-induced thrombocytopenia in hospitalized patients. Systemic lupus erythematosus and chronic lymphocytic leukemia are common causes of secondary idiopathic thrombocytopenic purpura.

Treatment

Few adults with idiopathic thrombocytopenic purpura will have spontaneous remissions, and most will require treatment. Initial treatment is with prednisone, 1–2 mg/kg/d. Prednisone works primarily by decreasing the affinity of splenic macrophages for antibody-coated platelets. High-dose prednisone therapy also reduces the binding of antibody to the platelet surface,

Table 10–17. Causes of thrombocytopenia.

Bone marrow disorders
Aplastic anemia
Hematologic malignancies
Myelodysplasia
Megaloblastic anemia
Chronic alcoholism
Nonmarrow disorders
Immune disorders
Idiopathic thrombocytopenic purpura
Drug-induced
Secondary
Posttransfusion purpura
Hypersplenism
Disseminated intravascular coagulation
Thrombotic thrombocytopenic purpura
Hemolytic-uremic syndrome
Sepsis
Hemangiomas
Viral infection, AIDS

and long-term therapy may decrease antibody production. Bleeding will often diminish within 1 day after beginning prednisone—even before the platelet count begins to rise. This effect has been attributed to "enhanced vascular stability" produced by prednisone. The platelet count will usually begin to rise within a week, and responses are almost always seen within 3 weeks. About 80% of patients will respond to prednisone therapy, and the platelet count will usually return to normal. High-dose prednisone therapy should be continued until the platelet count is normal, and the dose should then be gradually tapered. In most patients, thrombocytopenia will recur if prednisone is completely withdrawn, and one aims to find a low prednisone dose that will maintain an adequate platelet count. It is not necessary for the platelet count to be entirely normal; the risk of bleeding is small with platelet counts above 50,000/μL.

Splenectomy is the most definitive treatment for idiopathic thrombocytopenic purpura, and most adult patients will ultimately undergo splenectomy. High-dose prednisone therapy should not be prolonged unduly in an attempt to avoid surgery. Splenectomy is indicated if patients do not respond to prednisone initially or require unacceptably high doses to maintain an adequate platelet count. Other patients may be intolerant of prednisone or may simply prefer the surgical alternative. Splenectomy can be performed safely even with platelet counts less than 10,000/μL. Approximately 80% of patients benefit from splenectomy with either complete or partial remission.

High-dose intravenous immunoglobulin, 400 mg/kg/d for 3–5 days, is highly effective in rapidly raising the platelet count. The response rate is approximately 90%, and the platelet count rises within 1–5 days. However, this treatment is very expensive (approximately $5000), and the beneficial effect lasts only 1–2 weeks. Immunoglobulin treatment should be reserved for emergency situations such as preparing a severely thrombocytopenic patient for surgery.

For patients who fail to respond to prednisone and splenectomy, danazol, 600 mg/d, has been used, with responses obtained in about half of cases. Immunosuppressive agents employed in refractory cases include vincristine, vinblastine infusions, azathioprine, and cyclophosphamide. In using any of these more toxic treatments, one must carefully balance the risks against the anticipated benefits.

Platelet transfusions are rarely used in the treatment of idiopathic thrombocytopenic purpura, since exogenous platelets will survive no better than the patient's own platelets and in many cases will survive less than a few hours. Platelet transfusion should be reserved for cases of life-threatening bleeding in which enhanced hemostasis for even an hour may be of benefit.

Prognosis

The prognosis for remission is good. In most cases, the disease is initially controlled with prednisone, and splenectomy offers definitive therapy for most patients. The major concern during the initial phases is cerebral hemorrhage, which becomes a risk when the platelet count is less than 5000/μL. These patients usually exhibit warning signs of mucosal bleeding. However, at these very low platelet counts, fatal bleeding is rare. Chronic disease that has failed to respond to prednisone and splenectomy has a waxing and waning course over years and usually requires continued management. However, bleeding is rarely life-threatening.

Ahn YS et al: Long-term danazol therapy in autoimmune thrombocytopenia: Unmaintained remission and age-dependent response in women. Ann Intern Med 1989; 111:723.

Berchtold P, McMillan R: Therapy of chronic idiopathic thrombocytopenic purpura in adults. Blood 1989;74: 2309.

Bussel JB et al: Maintenance treatment of adults with chronic refractory immune thrombocytopenic purpura using repeated intravenous infusions of gammaglobulin. Blood 1988;72:121.

THROMBOTIC THROMBOCYTOPENIC PURPURA

Essentials of Diagnosis

- Microangiopathic hemolytic anemia and thrombocytopenia.
- Neurologic abnormalities.
- Fever in the absence of infection.
- Normal coagulation tests.

General Considerations

Thrombotic thrombocytopenic purpura is an uncommon syndrome characterized by the triad of microangiopathic hemolytic anemia, thrombocytopenia, and neurologic abnormalities, as well as fever and renal abnormalities. The cause is unknown. A platelet-agglutinating factor has recently been identified in the plasma of these patients. Its role in pathogenesis remains controversial.

Thrombotic thrombocytopenic purpura is seen primarily in young adults between ages 20 and 50, and there is a slight female predominance. The syndrome is occasionally precipitated by estrogen use or pregnancy and has recently been seen as a late complication of AIDS.

Clinical Findings

A. Symptoms and Signs: Patients come to medical attention because of anemia, bleeding, or neurologic abnormalities. The neurologic signs and symptoms are unusual in that they may wax and wane over minutes. Neurologic symptoms include headache, confusion, aphasia, and alterations in consciousness from lethargy to coma. With more advanced disease, one may see hemiparesis and seizures.

On examination, the patient appears acutely ill and is usually febrile. One may detect pallor, purpura, petechiae, and signs of neurologic dysfunction. Patients may have abdominal pain and tenderness due to pancreatitis.

B. Laboratory Findings: Anemia is universal and may be extremely severe. There is usually marked reticulocytosis and occasional circulating nucleated red blood cells. The hallmark of thrombotic thrombocytopenic purpura is a microangiopathic blood picture with fragmented red blood cells (schistocytes, helmet cells, triangle forms) on the smear. One cannot make the diagnosis without significant red blood cell fragmentation. Thrombocytopenia is invariably present and may be severe. White blood cells may show increased band neutrophils.

Hemolysis may be manifested by increasing indirect bilirubin, absent haptoglobin, and occasionally hemoglobinemia and hemoglobinuria. In severe cases, methemalbuminemia may impart a brown color to the plasma. The LDH is usually markedly elevated in proportion to the severity of hemolysis. The Coombs test should be negative.

Coagulation tests (prothrombin time, partial thromboplastin time, fibrinogen) are normal. Elevated fibrin degradation products may be seen, as in other acutely ill patients. Renal insufficiency may be present, and the urinalysis may be abnormal.

Pathologically, one may see the characteristic hyaline thrombus in capillaries and small arteries.

Differential Diagnosis

The normal values of coagulation tests differentiate thrombotic thrombocytopenic purpura from disseminated intravascular coagulation (DIC). Other conditions causing microangiopathic hemolysis (Table 10–18) should be excluded. Evans's syndrome is characterized by the combination of autoimmune thrombocytopenia and autoimmune hemolytic anemia, but the peripheral smear will show spherocytes and not red blood cell fragments. Skin or muscle biopsy is usually not necessary for diagnosis but may be helpful when vasculitis is a consideration.

Treatment

Thrombotic thrombocytopenic purpura should be treated on an emergency basis with large-volume plas-

Table 10–18. Causes of microangiopathic hemolytic anemia.

Thrombotic thrombocytopenic purpura
Hemolytic-uremic syndrome
Disseminated intravascular coagulation
Prosthetic valve hemolysis
Metastatic adenocarcinoma
Malignant hypertension
Vasculitis

mapheresis. Sixty to 80 mL/kg of plasma should be removed and replaced with fresh-frozen plasma. Treatment should be continued daily until the patient is in complete remission. Prednisone and antiplatelet agents (aspirin and dipyridamole) have been used in addition to plasmapheresis, but their role is unclear.

Patients who do not respond to plasmapheresis or who have rapid recurrences require splenectomy. The combination of splenectomy, steroids, and dextran has been used with success.

Prognosis

With the advent of plasmapheresis, the formerly dismal prognosis of thrombotic thrombocytopenic purpura has been dramatically changed. Eighty to 90% of patients now recover completely. Most complete responses are durable, but in 10–20% of cases, the disease will be chronic and relapsing.

Lichtin AE et al: Efficacy of intense plasmapheresis in thrombotic thrombocytopenic purpura. Arch Intern Med 1987;147:2122.

Liu ET, Linker CA, Shuman MA: Management of treatment failures in thrombotic thrombocytopenic purpura. Am J Hematol 1986;23:347.

Shepard KV, Bukowski RM: The treatment of thrombotic thrombocytopenic purpura with exchange transfusions, plasma infusions and plasma exchange. Semin Hematol 1987;24:178.

HEMOLYTIC-UREMIC SYNDROME

Essentials of Diagnosis

- Microangiopathic hemolytic anemia, thrombocytopenia, and renal failure.
- Normal coagulation test.
- Absence of neurologic abnormalities.

General Considerations

Hemolytic-uremic syndrome is an uncommon disorder consisting of microangiopathic hemolytic anemia, thrombocytopenia, and renal failure due to microangiopathy (with decreased glomerular filtration, proteinuria, and hematuria). The cause is unclear. The disease is similar to thrombotic thrombocytopenic purpura except that different vascular beds are involved. The pathogenesis of the 2 disorders is probably similar, and a platelet-agglutinating factor found in plasma may be involved. In children, hemolytic-uremic syndrome frequently occurs after a diarrheal illness secondary to infections with *Shigella, Salmonella, E coli* strain 0157:H7, or viral agents. The mortality rate of this form is low (< 5%). In adults, this syndrome is frequently precipitated by estrogen use or pregnancy (especially postpartum) or occurs as a complication of malignant hypertension or renal transplantation. A familial (hereditary) type has been identified in which members of a family have recurrent episodes over several years.

Clinical Findings

A. Symptoms and Signs: Patients present with anemia, bleeding, or renal failure. The renal failure may or may not be oliguric. In contrast to thrombotic thrombocytopenic purpura, there are no neurologic manifestations other than those due to the uremic state.

B. Laboratory Findings: As in thrombotic thrombocytopenic purpura, there is microangiopathic hemolytic anemia and thrombocytopenia, but the thrombocytopenia is often less severe. The peripheral blood smear should show striking red blood cell fragmentation, and the diagnosis of hemolytic-uremic syndrome is untenable without this finding. The LDH is usually strikingly elevated in proportion to the severity of hemolysis, and the Coombs test is negative. Coagulation tests are normal with the exception of elevated fibrin degradation products.

Renal insufficiency is invariably present, and anuric renal failure requiring dialysis may be seen. Kidney biopsy will show endothelial hyaline thrombi in the afferent arterioles and glomeruli. Ischemic necrosis in the renal cortex may occur with obstruction from intravascular coagulation.

Differential Diagnosis

Disseminated intravascular coagulation is excluded by normal coagulation results. Other causes of microangiopathic hemolytic anemia (Table 10–18) should be considered. Occasionally, vasculitis or acute glomerulonephritis is considered, and in these cases renal biopsy may be necessary to establish the diagnosis if the platelet count will allow it.

Hemolytic-uremic syndrome is arbitrarily distinguished from thrombotic thrombocytopenic purpura by the presence of renal failure and the lack of neurologic findings.

Treatment

In children, hemolytic-uremic syndrome is almost always self-limited and requires only conservative management of acute renal failure. In adults, however, without treatment, there is a high rate of permanent renal insufficiency and death. Persistent thrombocytopenia and microangiopathic hemolytic anemia and worsening renal failure with hypertension are indications for more aggressive treatment. The treatment of choice (as in thrombotic thrombocytopenic purpura) is large-volume plasmapheresis with fresh-frozen replacement (exchange of up to 80 mL/kg), repeated daily until remission or until lack of success is clearly evident. Heparin, antiplatelet agents (dipyridamole, aspirin), and corticosteroids (prednisone) have all been employed with some success.

Prognosis

The prognosis of hemolytic-uremic syndrome in adults remains unclear. Without effective therapy, up to 40% of patients have died, and 80% have had chronic renal insufficiency. Early institution of aggressive therapy with plasmapheresis promises to be beneficial.

Hakim RM: Successful management of thrombocytopenia, microangiopathic anemia and acute renal failure by plasmapheresis. Am J Kidney Dis 1985;5:170.
Kaplan BS, Proesman W: The hemolytic uremic syndrome of childhood and its variants. Semin Hematol 1987;24:148.
Siegler RL: Management of hemolytic uremic syndrome. J Pediatr 1988;112:1014.

CONGENITAL QUALITATIVE PLATELET DISORDERS

Bleeding disorders characterized by prolonged bleeding times despite a normal platelet count are called qualitative platelet disorders. Patients have a positive family history or lifelong personal history of the defect. The disorders may be classified as (1) acquired and congenital disorders intrinsic to the platelet and (2) von Willebrand's disease (see next section), a disorder of a plasma protein necessary for platelet adhesion (Table 10–19). When an intrinsic qualitative platelet disorder is suspected, platelet aggregation studies should be evaluated to make a specific diagnosis.

Glanzmann's Thrombasthenia

This is a rare autosomal recessive intrinsic platelet disorder causing bleeding. Platelets are unable to aggregate because of lack of receptors (containing glycoproteins IIb and IIa) for fibrinogen, which forms the bridges between platelets during aggregation. Clinically, it is manifested chiefly as mucosal bleeding (epistaxis, gingival bleeding, menorrhagia) and postoperative bleeding. The bleeding defect is of variable severity but may be severe.

Platelet numbers and morphology are normal, but the bleeding time is markedly prolonged. Platelets fail to aggregate in response to typical agonists (ADP, collagen, thrombin) but aggregate normally in response to ristocetin, which causes platelet clumping by a separate mechanism.

Patients are treated with platelet transfusions when necessary. Platelet transfusion therapy is limited by the tendency of these patients to develop multiple alloantibodies.

Bernard-Soulier Syndrome

This is a rare autosomal recessive intrinsic platelet disorder causing bleeding. Platelets cannot adhere to subendothelium because they lack receptors (composed of glycoprotein Ib) for von Willebrand factor, which mediates platelet adhesion. This is often a severe bleeding disorder with mucosal and postoperative bleeding.

Thrombocytopenia may be present, and platelets on smear are abnormally large. The bleeding time is markedly prolonged. Platelet aggregation is normal in response to standard agonists (collagen, ADP, thrombin), but platelets fail to aggregate in response to ristocetin. Measurements of von Willebrand factor in the plasma are normal. Patients are treated with platelet transfusion when necessary.

Storage Pool Disease

This is a group of mild bleeding disorders characterized by defective secretion of platelet granule contents (especially ADP) that stimulate platelet aggregation. Most patients are mildly affected and have increased bruising and postoperative bleeding.

Platelets are normal in number and morphology, but the bleeding time is slightly prolonged. In some cases, the baseline bleeding time is normal, but it becomes markedly prolonged after aspirin. There are variable abnormalities in platelet aggregation studies.

Most patients do not require treatment but should avoid aspirin. Platelet transfusions transiently correct the bleeding tendency. Some patients respond to infusions of cryoprecipitate, and some respond transiently to desmopressin acetate (DDAVP), 0.3 μg/kg.

George JN, Nurden AT, Phillips DR: Molecular defects in interactions of platelets with the vessel wall. N Engl J Med 1984;311:1084.

Ruggieri ZM, Zimmerman TS: von Willebrand factor and von Willebrand disease. Blood 1987;70:895.

VON WILLEBRAND'S DISEASE

Essentials of Diagnosis

- Family history with autosomal dominant pattern of inheritance.
- Prolonged bleeding time, either at baseline or after challenge with aspirin.
- Reduced levels of factor VIII antigen or ristocetin cofactor.
- May have reduced levels of factor VIII coagulant activity.

General Considerations

Von Willebrand's disease is the most common congenital disorder of hemostasis. It is transmitted in an autosomal dominant pattern. It is a group of disorders characterized by deficient or defective von Willebrand factor (vWF), a protein that mediates platelet adhesion. Adhesion is a process separate from platelet aggregation. Platelets adhere to the subendothelium via vWF, which is bound to a specific receptor composed of glycoprotein Ib (and missing in Bernard-Soulier syndrome). Platelets aggregate via fibrinogen, which binds to a different receptor composed of glycoproteins IIb and IIIa (deficient in Glanzmann's throm-

basthenia). The platelet aggregation system is entirely normal in von Willebrand's disease.

Von Willebrand factor is synthesized in megakaryocytes and endothelial cells and circulates in plasma as multimers of varying size. Only the large multimeric forms are functional in mediating platelet adhesion. Von Willebrand factor has a separate function of binding the factor VIII coagulant protein and protecting it from degradation. The factor VIII coagulant protein (factor VIII:C), a protein encoded by a gene on the × chromosome, is the protein deficient in classic hemophilia. Any of the multimeric forms of vWF can bind and protect factor VIII:C. Von Willebrand's disease, which is primarily a disorder of platelet function, may secondarily cause a coagulation disturbance because of deficient levels of factor VIII:C. However, this coagulopathy is rarely severe.

There are several subtypes of von Willebrand's disease. The most common type (type I, 80% of all cases) is caused by a quantitative decrease in vWF. Type IIa is caused by a qualitative abnormality in protein that prevents multimer formation. Only small multimers are present, and both intermediate and large forms that mediate platelet adhesion are missing. Type IIb von Willebrand's disease is caused by a qualitative abnormality in the protein that causes rapid clearance of the large multimeric forms. Type III von Willebrand's disease is a rare autosomal recessive disorder in which vWF is nearly absent. Pseudo-von Willebrand disease is a rare disorder in which an abnormal platelet membrane has excessive avidity for the large multimeric forms of vWF, causing their clearance from plasma.

Clinical Findings

A. Symptoms and Signs: Von Willebrand's disease is a common disorder affecting both men and women. Most cases are mild. Most bleeding is mucosal (epistaxis, gingival bleeding, menorrhagia), but gastrointestinal bleeding may occur. In most cases, incisional bleeding occurs after surgery or dental extractions. Von Willebrand's disease is rarely as severe as hemophilia, and spontaneous hemarthroses do not occur.

The bleeding tendency is exacerbated by aspirin. Characteristically, bleeding decreases during pregnancy or estrogen use.

B. Laboratory Findings: Platelet number and morphology are normal, and the bleeding time is usually (not always) prolonged. The bleeding time should be ascertained whenever this diagnosis is considered and correlates most closely with the clinical bleeding tendency. When the bleeding time is normal, it is prolonged markedly by aspirin. Normal persons will prolong their bleeding time to a minor extent with aspirin but rarely out of the normal range. In the most common form of von Willebrand's disease (type I), vWF levels in plasma are reduced. This may be measured by factor VIII antigen, which mea-

Table 10–19. Qualitative platelet disorders.

Congenital
  Glanzmann's thrombasthenia
  Bernard-Soulier syndrome
  Storage pool disease
Acquired
  Myeloproliferative disorders
  Uremia
  Drugs: Aspirin, anti-inflammatory agents
  Autoantibody
  Paraproteins
  Acquired storage pool
  Fibrin degradation products
Von Willebrand's disease

---

sures the immunologic presence of vWF, or by ristocetin cofactor activity, which measures functional properties of vWF in mediating platelet adhesion.

When factor VIII antigen is reduced, one may also see a decrease in factor VIII coagulant (factor VIII:C) levels. When factor VIII:C levels are less than 25%, the partial thromboplastin time (PTT) will be prolonged. Platelet aggregation studies with standard agonists (ADP, collagen, thrombin) are normal, but platelet aggregation in response to ristocetin is usually subnormal.

In difficult cases, it may be helpful to assay directly the multimeric composition of vWF.

Table 10–20. Causes of prolonged partial thromboplastin time.

Congenital factor deficiencies
  Contact factors
  Factor XII
  Factor XI
  Factor IX
  Factor VIII
    Hemophilia
    Von Willebrand's disease
Anticoagulants
  Anti-VIII
  Lupus
  Heparin

Differential Diagnosis

When patients present with a prolonged bleeding time, one must distinguish von Willebrand's disease from other qualitative platelet disorders (Table 10–19). Acquired qualitative platelet disorders can usually be diagnosed by recent onset of the bleeding tendency and other characteristic clinical features. Congenital intrinsic platelet disorders may present with a positive family history and lifelong history of bleeding episodes. Von Willebrand's disease is diagnosed by the finding of abnormal measurements of vWF and by normal results of platelet aggregation.

When patients present with a prolonged PTT, measurements of factor VIII:C will distinguish von Willebrand's disease from all disorders except hemophilia (Table 10–20). Hemophilia is diagnosed when factor VIII:C is reduced but all measurements of vWF (factor VIII antigen, ristocetin cofactor activity) are normal.

Patients with a suspicious bleeding history but with normal bleeding time and PTT pose a diagnostic problem. On occasion, the postaspirin bleeding time can be used to unmask a bleeding disorder. At other times, one must perform further plasma assays of vWF to make the diagnosis. Von Willebrand's disease waxes and wanes in severity and may be difficult to diagnose, especially in a woman taking estrogens (which raise vWF levels).

It is often useful to distinguish between subtypes of von Willebrand's disease (Table 10–21), because only type I usually responds to desmopressin (DDAVP) and because type IIb may be aggravated by its use.

Treatment

The bleeding disorder is characteristically mild, and no treatment is routinely given other than avoidance of aspirin. However, patients often need to be prepared for surgical or dental procedures. The bleeding time is probably the best indicator of the likelihood of bleeding, and prophylactic therapy may be reasonably withheld if the procedure is minor and the bleeding time is normal.

Standard therapy for von Willebrand's disease is

Table 10–21. Types of Von Willebrand's disease.

	Bleeding Time	Factor VIII Antigen	Ristocetin Cofactor Activity	Factor VIII Coagulant Activity	Multimer
Type I	↑ or N	↓ or N	↓ or N	↓ or N	N
Type IIa	↑	↓ or N	0	↓ or N	Abn
Type IIb	↑	↓ or N	↓ or N	↓ or N	Abn
Type III	↑	0	0	0	—
Pseudo-vW disease	↑	↓ or N	↓ or N	↓ or N	Abn
Hemophilia A	N	N	N	↓	N

N = normal; Abn = abnormal.

transfusion of plasma cryoprecipitate. It should be noted that factor VIII concentrates (using the treatment of hemophilia A) cannot be used, as they do not contain functional vWF. Each unit of cryoprecipitate will raise vWF levels approximately 3%, and thus 10–15 units of cryoprecipitate are commonly used to raise vWF levels by 30–50%. Factor VIII antigen levels decline, with a half-life of 12–18 hours, but the duration of corrected bleeding time is usually shorter than this. In some instances the prolonged bleeding time may be completely corrected. Factor VIII coagulant levels may remain elevated for 24–48 hours following cryoprecipitate infusion (unlike the 12–hour half-life of factor VIII:C in classic hemophilia), but these levels are not useful in determining therapy. When replacement therapy is indicated, cryoprecipitate should be given every 12 hours—or more frequently if the bleeding tendency is severe. Only the bleeding time correlates with bleeding risk, but it is impractical to perform this test frequently.

Desmopressin acetate (DDAVP), Stimate) is a useful treatment for mild type I von Willebrand's disease. The dose is 0.3 μg/kg, after which vWF levels usually rise 2- to 3-fold in 30–90 minutes. Desmopressin acetate appears to cause release of stored vWF from endothelial cells. The treatment can be given only every 24 hours as stores of vWF become depleted. The drug is not effective in type IIa von Willebrand's disease, in which no endothelial stores are present, and may be harmful in type IIb or may lead to thrombocytopenia and increased bleeding.

The antifibrinolytic agents aminocaproic acid (EACA; Amicar) and tranexamic acid (Cyklokapron) is useful as adjunctive therapy during dental procedures. After either cryoprecipitate or desmopressin acetate, the patient is given 4 g orally every 4 hours for several days to reduce the likelihood of bleeding.

Prognosis

The prognosis is excellent. In most cases, the bleeding disorder is mild, and in the more serious cases replacement therapy is effective.

De la Fuente B et al: Response of patients with mild and moderate hemophilia A and von Willebrand's disease to treatment with desmopressin. Ann Intern Med 1985;103:6.

ACQUIRED QUALITATIVE PLATELET DISORDERS

A number of acquired disorders lead to abnormal platelet function (Table 10–19).

Uremia

Uremia causes abnormal platelet function by unknown mechanisms. The severity of the bleeding tendency is roughly proportionate to the degree of renal insufficiency. Bleeding is most commonly mucosal and gastrointestinal and may occasionally be severe. Dialysis is effective in reducing the bleeding tendency but may not completely eliminate it. Patients appear to respond to transfusion with cryoprecipitate, 10 units every 12 hours. Desmopressin acetate, 0.3 μg/kg every 24 hours, appears to be just as effective as cryoprecipitate.

Myeloproliferative Disorders

All the myeloproliferative disorders can produce abnormalities in platelet function. A number of biochemical abnormalities are present in these platelets, but the cause of the bleeding tendency is unclear. The severity of the bleeding tendency correlates roughly with the height of the platelet count. Bleeding decreases when the platelet count is controlled with myelosuppressive therapy. In cases of life-threatening bleeding with high platelet counts, plateletpheresis may be necessary to control bleeding. Platelet transfusion will also be helpful temporarily.

Other Disorders

Aspirin causes a mild bleeding tendency by irreversibly acetylating cyclooxygenase, an enzyme that participates in platelet aggregation. The effect lasts for the life of the platelet and may be manifest for 7–10 days, although the major effect lasts only 3–5 days. The effect is not dose-dependent, and 65 mg of aspirin is sufficient.

Aspirin by itself does not cause significant bleeding, but it may unmask bleeding disorders such as mild von Willebrand's disease or mild thrombocytopenia. Certain antibiotics (ticarcillin, some cephalosporins) cause a mild bleeding tendency, presumably by coating the surface of platelets. Nonsteroidal anti-inflammatory drugs cause a transient aspirin-like effect.

Patients with autoantibodies against platelets may have prolonged bleeding times even in the absence of thrombocytopenia. Platelet-associated IgG levels should be high, and the bleeding tendency responds quickly to modest doses of prednisone such as 20 mg/d. Acquired storage pool disease refers to the circulation of "exhausted platelets" that have been stimulated to release their granule contents and hence are no longer functional. Such granule release occurs in response to cardiopulmonary bypass and severe vasculitis.

Janson PA et al: Treatment of the bleeding tendency in uremia with cryoprecipitate. N Engl J Med 1980; 303:1318.

Livio M et al: Conjugated estrogens for the management of bleeding associated with renal failure. N Engl J Med 1986;315:731.

Mannucci PM: Desmopressin: A nontransfusional form of treatment for congenital and acquired bleeding disorders. Blood 1988;72:1449.

Weiss HJ et al: Acquired storage pool deficiency with increased platelet-associated IgG: Report of 5 Cases. Am J Med 1980;69:711.

HEMOPHILIA A

Essentials of Diagnosis

- X-linked recessive pattern of inheritance with only males affected.
- Low factor VIII coagulant activity.
- Normal factor VIII antigen.
- Spontaneous hemarthroses.

General Considerations

Hemophilia A (classic hemophilia, factor VIII deficiency hemophilia) is a hereditary disorder in which bleeding is due to deficiency of the coagulation factor VIII (VIII:C). In most cases, the factor VIII coagulant protein is quantitatively reduced, but in a small number of cases the coagulant protein is present by immunoassay but defective.

Hemophilia is a classic example of an X-linked recessive disease, and as a rule only males are affected. In rare instances, female carriers are clinically affected if their normal X chromosomes are disproportionately inactivated. Females may also become affected if they are the offspring of a hemophiliac father and carrier mother.

Hemophilia is classified as severe if factor VIII:C levels are less than 1%, moderate if levels are 1–5%, and mild if levels are greater than 5%. Families tend to breed true in the severity of hemophilia produced.

Clinical Findings

A. Symptoms and Signs: Hemophilia A is the most common severe bleeding disorder and after von Willebrand's disease is the most common congenital bleeding disorder overall. Approximately one in 10,000 males is affected. The bleeding tendency is related to factor VIII:C levels. Bleeding may occur anywhere. The most common sites of bleeding are into joints (knees, ankles, elbows), into muscles, and from the gastrointestinal tract. Spontaneous hemarthroses are so characteristic of severe hemophilia that they are almost diagnostic of the disorder. Patients with mild hemophilia bleed only in response to major trauma or surgery. Patients with moderately severe hemophilia bleed in response to mild trauma or surgery, and those with severe hemophilia bleed spontaneously.

Unfortunately, many hemophiliacs are now seropositive for HIV infection transmitted via factor VIII concentrate, and many have already developed AIDS. HIV-associated immune thrombocytopenia may aggravate the bleeding tendency.

B. Laboratory Findings: The partial thromboplastin time (PTT) is prolonged, and other measures of coagulation, including prothrombin time, bleeding time, and fibrinogen level, are normal. Levels of factor VIII:C are reduced, but measurements of von Willebrand factor are normal (Table 10–21).

If one mixes plasma from a hemophiliac patient with normal plasma, the PTT will become normal. Failure of the PTT to normalize in such a mixing test is diagnostic of the presence of a factor VIII inhibitor.

A low platelet count should raise a suspicion of HIV-associated immune thrombocytopenia.

Differential Diagnosis

The finding of a reduced factor VIII:C level will distinguish this disorder from other causes of prolonged PTT (Table 10–20). Clinically, factor VIII hemophilia is indistinguishable from factor IX hemophilia, and only specific factor assays can distinguish these disorders. In cases of mild hemophilia, the disorder needs to be distinguished from von Willebrand's disease by VIII:A assay, which shows normal levels of factor VIII antigen in the latter.

An important issue for the families of hemophiliac patients is identifying which females are carriers. Female carriers can usually be identified by the presence of low or normal levels of factor VIII:C with normal levels of factor VIII antigen.

Treatment

Patients with hemophilia should try to live as nearly normal lives as possible. Activities associated with a risk of trauma should be avoided, however, and aspirin should never be used.

Standard treatment is based on infusion of factor VIII concentrates, now heat-treated to reduce the likelihood of transmission of AIDS. The level of factor VIII one aims to achieve in plasma depends on the severity of the bleeding problem. In response to minor bleeding, it may be necessary only to raise factor VIII:C levels to 25% with one infusion. For moderate bleeding (such as deep muscle hematomas), it is adequate to raise the level initially to 50% and maintain the level at greater than 25% with repeated infusion for 2–3 days. When major surgery is to be performed, one raises the factor VIII:C level to 100% and then maintains the factor level at greater than 50% continuously for 10–14 days. Head injuries (with or without neurologic signs) should be emergently treated as though major bleeding were present.

The dose of factor VIII concentrate is calculated on the basis that one unit of factor VIII is the amount present in 1 mL of plasma. Plasma volume is 40 mL/kg, and the volume of distribution of factor VIII:C is 1.5 times the plasma volume. Thus, to raise the level 100%, the dose should be 40 × 1.5 + 60 units/kg, or approximately 4000 units. To raise the levels to 25% would require 1000 units. The half-life of factor VIII:C is approximately 12 hours. Thus, during major surgery, to achieve an initial level of 100% and maintain it continuously at greater than 50%, a dose of 60 units/kg (approximately 4000 units) initially followed by 30 units/kg (approximately 2000 units) every 12 hours should be adequate. During surgery, one should initially verify that these doses give the anticipated levels. If factor VIII levels fail to rise as expected, one should suspect an inhibitor. Patients with inhibitors require specialized therapy under direction of an experienced hematologist.

Mild hemophilia may be treated with cryoprecipitate in place of factor VIII concentrates. One unit of cryoprecipitate contains about 100 units of factor VIII:C. For mild hemophiliacs, desmopressin acetate, 0.3 µg/kg every 24 hours, may be useful in preparing for minor surgical procedures. Desmopressin acetate causes release of factor VIII:C and will raise the factor VIII:C levels 2- to 3-fold for several hours. In the management of persistent bleeding following use of either desmopressin acetate or factor VIII concentrate, patients may be treated with aminocaproic acid (EACA; Amicar), 4 g orally every 4 hours for several days.

The ongoing care of patient with hemophilia should be coordinated with an orthopedic surgeon who can help manage the chronic joint deformities of these patients.

Prognosis

The prognosis of patients with hemophilia has been transformed by the availability of factor VIII replacement. The major limiting factors are disability from recurrent joint bleeding and viral infections (hepatitis B, AIDS) from recurrent transfusion. Approximately 15% of patients develop inhibitors to factor VIII, and these patents may die of bleeding because they cannot be adequately supported with factor VIII.

Brettler DB, Levine PH: Factor concentrates for treatment of hemophilia: Which one to choose? Blood 1989; 73:2067.

Kasper CK, Dietrich SL: Comprehensive management of haemophilia. Clin Haematol 1985;14:489.

Kasper CK et al: Hematologic management of hemophilia A for surgery. JAMA 1985;253:1279.

Kitchens CS: Surgery in hemophilia and related disorders: A prospective study of 100 consecutive procedures. Medicine 1986;65:34.

White GC, Shoemaker CB: Factor VIII gene and hemophilia A. Blood 1989;73:1.

HEMOPHILIA B

Essentials of Diagnosis

- X-linked recessive inheritance, with only males affected.
- Low levels of factor IX coagulant activity.
- Spontaneous hemarthroses.

General Considerations

Hemophilia B (Christmas disease, factor IX hemophilia) is a hereditary bleeding disorder due to deficiency of coagulation factor IX. Most commonly, factor IX is quantitatively reduced, but in one-third of cases an abnormally functioning molecule is immu-

nologically present. Factor IX deficiency is one-seventh as common as factor VIII deficiency hemophilia but is otherwise clinically and genetically identical.

The PTT is prolonged, and factor IX levels are reduced when measured by specific factor assays. Other laboratory features are the same as for factor VIII hemophilia.

Treatment

Factor IX hemophilia is managed with factor IX concentrates. Factor VIII concentrates are ineffectual in this type of hemophilia; therefore it is imperative to distinguish between the two. The same dosing considerations apply as in factor VIII hemophilia, with the exception that the volume of distribution of factor IX is twice the plasma volume, so that 80 units/kg are necessary to achieve a 100% level. In addition, the half-life of factor IX is 18 hours. Thus, to maintain a patient through major surgery, the dosage should be 80 units/kg (approximately 6000 units) initially followed by 40 units/kg (3000 units) every 18 hours. Factor levels should be measured to ensure that expected levels are achieved and that an inhibitor is not present.

Unlike factor VIII concentrates, factor IX concentrates contain a number of other proteins, including activated coagulating factors that appear to contribute to a risk of thrombosis with recurrent usage of factor IX concentrates. Because of the risk of thrombosis, more care is needed in deciding to use these concentrates. Desmopressin acetate is not useful in this disorder.

Prognosis

The prognosis for these patients is the same as for those with factor VIII hemophilia.

OTHER CONGENITAL COAGULATION DISORDERS

Factor XI Deficiency

This disorder is seen primarily among Ashkenazi Jews and is autosomal recessive. The PTT may be markedly prolonged, and specific assays of factor XI will show reduced levels. This is usually a mild bleeding disorder manifested primarily by postoperative bleeding. Factor replacement is given with fresh-frozen plasma when necessary.

Afibrinogenemia

In this rare disorder, fibrinogen is absent and both prothrombin time and partial thromboplastin time are markedly prolonged. These patients may have a severe bleeding disorder similar to hemophilia. Fibrinogen is replaced with cryoprecipitate.

Other Coagulation Disorders

Bleeding disorders due to isolated deficiency of

factors II, V, X, or VII are extremely rare. Deficiencies of factor XII and the contact pathway factors cause a markedly prolonged PTT but are not associated with any increased bleeding.

Factor XIII deficiency results in delayed bleeding after trauma or surgery. All coagulation tests are normal. The disorder is diagnosed by showing instability of the fibrin clot in 8-molar urea. Factor XIII is replaced with cryoprecipitate or plasma.

COAGULOPATHY OF LIVER DISEASE

Essentials of Diagnosis
- Prothrombin time more prolonged than PTT.
- No response to Vitamin K.

General Considerations
The liver is the site of synthesis of all the coagulation factors except factor VIII. As hepatic insufficiency develops, the vitamin K-dependent factors (factors II, VII, IX, X) and factor V are the first to be affected. Because of its rapid turnover (half-life 6 hours), factor VII levels are the first to decline. Conversely, fibrinogen levels are remarkably well conserved, and decreased fibrinogen synthesis does not occur unless liver disease is very severe.

Liver disease has a number of other effects on the hemostatic system. Increased fibrinolysis occurs because the liver synthesizes α_2 antiplasmin (the main inhibitor of fibrinolysis), which is responsible for the clearance of plasminogen activator. Biliary tract disease may lead to malabsorption of vitamin K, and congestive splenomegaly may produce mild thrombocytopenia. A variety of chronic liver diseases cause abnormal posttranslation modification of fibrinogen with resultant dysfibrinogenemia.

Clinical Findings
A. Symptoms and Signs: The coagulopathy of liver disease may lead to bleeding at any site. Excessive fibrinolysis may lead to oozing at venipuncture sites.

B. Laboratory Findings: Hepatic coagulopathy produces a more marked abnormality in the prothrombin time (PT) than in the partial thromboplastin time (PTT). Early in the course of liver disease, only the PT will become affected. Fibrinogen levels should be normal, and the thrombin time should be normal unless dysfibrinogenemia is present. The platelet count should be normal unless production is suppressed by acute alcohol ingestion or unless hypersplenism is present. The peripheral blood smear may show target cells.

Differential Diagnosis
Hepatic coagulopathy can be distinguished from vitamin K deficiency only by demonstrating the failure of vitamin K to correct the abnormal values. Liver

Table 10–22. Causes of isolated prolonged prothrombin time.

Liver disease
Vitamin K deficiency
Warfarin therapy
Factor VII deficiency

Table 10–23. Causes of prolonged prothrombin time and partial thromboplastin time.

Liver disease
Vitamin K deficiency
Disseminated intravascular coagulation
Heparin
Warfarin
Isolated factor deficiencies (rare): II, V, X, I

disease is distinguished from disseminated intravascular coagulation by the normal fibrinogen level and lack of thrombocytopenia. End-stage liver disease almost invariably leads to some element of disseminated intravascular coagulation, and the disorders overlap (Tables 10–22 and 10–23).

Treatment
Long-term treatment of hepatic coagulopathy with factor replacement is usually ineffective. Fresh-frozen plasma is the treatment of choice, and volume overload will limit one's ability to maintain hemostatic factor levels. For example, to maintain factor levels greater than 25%, one must initially raise the level to 50% with 50% of the plasma volume (20 mL/kg) and then replace 10 mL/kg every 6 hours to maintain adequate factor VII levels. In average-sized persons, this will require transfusion of 1400 mL of plasma initially followed by 700 mL every 6 hours. Factor IX concentrates are contraindicated in liver disease because of their tendency to cause disseminated intravascular coagulation. If thrombocytopenia is present, platelet transfusion may be of some help, but platelet recovery is usually disappointing because of hypersplenism.

Prognosis
The prognosis is that of the underlying liver disease.

VITAMIN K DEFICIENCY

Essentials of Diagnosis
- Prothrombin time more prolonged than PTT.
- Rapid correction with vitamin K replacement.
- Underlying dietary deficiency or antibiotic use.

General Considerations
Vitamin K plays a role in coagulation by acting as a cofactor for the posttranslational g-carboxylation of zymogens II, VII, IX, and X. The modified zymogens (with γ-carboxyglutamic acid residues) are able

INTRINSIC SYSTEM

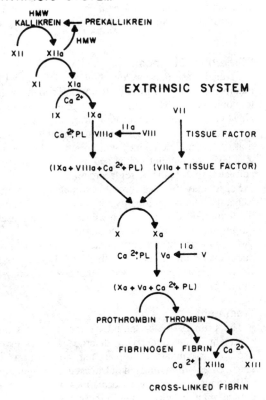

Figure 10–1. Cascade mechanism of blood coagulation. PL, phospholipid; Ca^{2+}, calcium ion; HMW, high-molecular-weight kininogen. (Adapted from Davie and Ratnoff. Reproduced, with permission, from Baugh RF, Hougie C: The chemistry of blood coagulation. Clin Haematol 1979;8:3.)

to bind to platelets in a calcium-dependent reaction and consequently better participate in the complex reactions that activate factors×and II (Fig 10–1). Without γ-carboxylation, these reactions on the platelet surface occur slowly and hemostasis is impaired.

Vitamin K is supplied in the diet primarily in leafy vegetables and endogenously from synthesis from intestinal bacteria. Factors that contribute to vitamin K deficiency include poor diet, malabsorption, and broad-spectrum antibiotics suppressing colonic flora. A characteristic setting for vitamin K deficiency is a postoperative patient who is not eating and who is receiving antibiotics. Body stores of vitamin K are small, and deficiency may develop in as little as 1 week.

Clinical Findings

A. Symptoms and Signs: There are no specific clinical features, and bleeding may occur at any site.

B. Laboratory Findings: The prothrombin time

is prolonged to a greater extent than the PTT, and with mild vitamin K deficiency only the PT is defective (Tables 10–22 and 10–23). Fibrinogen level, thrombin time, and platelet count are not affected.

Differential Diagnosis

Vitamin K deficiency can be distinguished from hepatic coagulopathy only by assessing the response to vitamin K therapy. Surreptitious warfarin use will produce laboratory features indistinguishable from those of vitamin K deficiency.

Vitamin K deficiency is distinguished from disseminated intravascular coagulation by the normal platelet count and normal fibrinogen level in the former.

Treatment

Vitamin K deficiency responds rapidly to subcutaneous vitamin K, and a single dose of 15 mg will completely correct laboratory abnormalities in 12–24 hours.

Prognosis

The prognosis is excellent, as vitamin K deficiency can be completely corrected with replacement.

Furie B, Furie BC: Molecular basis of vitamin K-dependent gamma carboxylation. Blood 1990;75:1753.

DISSEMINATED INTRAVASCULAR COAGULATION (DIC)

Essentials of Diagnosis

- Hypofibrinogenemia, thrombocytopenia, fibrin degradation products, and prolonged prothrombin time.
- Underlying serious illness.
- Microangiopathic hemolytic anemia may be present.
- Fibrin monomer may be present.

General Considerations

Coagulation is usually confined to a localized area by the combination of blood flow and circulating inhibitors of coagulation, especially antithrombin III. If the stimulus to coagulation is too great, these control mechanisms can be overwhelmed, leading to the syndrome of disseminated intravascular coagulation. In pathophysiologic terms, disseminated intravascular coagulation can be thought of as the consequence of the presence of circulating thrombin (normally confined to a localized area). The effects of thrombin are to cleave fibrinogen to fibrin monomer, stimulate platelet aggregation, activate factors V and VIII, and release plasminogen activator, which generates plasmin. Plasmin in turn cleaves fibrin, generating fibrin degradation products, and further inactivates factors V and VIII. Thus, the excess thrombin activity produces hypofibrinogenemia, thrombocytopenia, depletion of coagulation factors, and fibrinolysis.

Disseminated intravascular coagulation can be caused by a number of serious illnesses, including sepsis (especially with gram-negative bacteria but possible with any widespread bacterial or fungal infection), severe tissue injury (especially burns and head injury), obstetric complications (amniotic fluid embolus, septic abortion, retained dead fetus), cancer (acute promyelocytic leukemia, mucinous adenocarcinomas), and major hemolytic transfusion reactions.

Clinical Findings

A. Symptoms and Signs: Disseminated intravascular coagulation leads to both bleeding and thrombosis. Bleeding is far more common than thrombosis, but the latter may dominate if coagulation is activated to a far greater extent than fibrinolysis. Bleeding may occur at any site, but spontaneous bleeding and oozing at venipuncture sites or wounds are important clues to the diagnosis. Thrombosis is most commonly manifested by digital ischemia and gangrene, but catastrophic events such as renal-cortical necrosis and hemorrhagic adrenal infarction may occur. Disseminated intravascular coagulation may also secondarily produce microangiopathic hemolytic anemia.

Subacute disseminated intravascular coagulation is seen primarily in cancer patients and is manifested primarily as recurrent superficial and deep venous thromboses (Trousseau's syndrome).

B. Laboratory Findings: Disseminated intravascular coagulation produces a complex coagulopathy with the characteristic constellation of hyperfibrinogenemia, elevated fibrin degradation products, thrombocytopenia, and a prolonged prothrombin time. Hyperfibrinogenemia is the most important diagnostic laboratory feature, because few disorders (congenital hypofibrinogenemia, severe liver disease) will lower the fibrinogen level. In some cases of disseminated intravascular coagulation, when the patient's baseline fibrinogen level is markedly elevated, the initial fibrinogen level may be normal. However, since the half-life of fibrinogen is approximately 4 days, a noticeably falling fibrinogen level will confirm the diagnosis of disseminated intravascular coagulation.

Other laboratory abnormalities are variably present. The partial thromboplastin time may or may not be prolonged. Fibrin monomer is present in approximately one-third of cases. Although not very sensitive, its presence is highly specific for disseminated intravascular coagulation. In approximately one-fourth of cases, a microangiopathic hemolytic anemia is present, and fragmented red blood cells are seen on the peripheral smear. Antithrombin III levels may be markedly depleted. When fibrinolysis is activated, levels of plasminogen and a 2-antiplasmin may be low.

Subacute disseminated intravascular coagulation produces a very different laboratory picture. Thrombocytopenia and elevated fibrin degradation products are usually the only abnormalities. Fibrinogen levels are normal, and the PTT may be either normal or short.

Differential Diagnosis

Liver disease may prolong both the PT and PTT, but fibrinogen levels are usually normal, and the platelet count is usually normal or only slightly reduced. However, severe liver disease may be difficult to distinguish from disseminated intravascular coagulation. Vitamin K deficiency will not affect the fibrinogen level or platelet count and will be completely corrected by vitamin K replacement.

Sepsis may produce thrombocytopenia and digital ischemia, and coagulopathy may be present because of vitamin K deficiency. However, in these cases, the fibrinogen level should be normal.

Thrombotic thrombocytopenic purpura may produce fever and microangiopathic hemolytic anemia. However, fibrinogen levels and other coagulation tests should be normal.

Treatment

The primary focus should be the diagnosis and treatment of the underlying disorder that has given rise to disseminated intravascular coagulation. In many cases, disseminated intravascular coagulation will produce laboratory abnormalities with only mild clinical manifestations, and in these cases no specific therapy is required.

When the underlying cause of disseminated intravascular coagulation is rapidly reversible (such as in obstetric cases), replacement therapy alone may be indicated. The role of heparin in the treatment of disseminated intravascular coagulation is controversial. In some cases, when any increase in bleeding is unacceptable (neurosurgical procedures), heparin therapy is contraindicated. However, when disseminated intravascular coagulation is producing serious clinical consequences and the underlying cause is not rapidly reversible, heparin therapy may be necessary to control the syndrome. Such therapy is routinely used in the treatment of acute promyelocytic leukemia. In cases where disseminated intravascular coagulation causes thrombosis, heparin therapy is mandatory.

In replacement therapy, platelet transfusion should be used to maintain a platelet count greater than $50,000/\mu L$. Fibrinogen is replaced with cryoprecipitate, and one should aim for a level of 150 mg/dL. One unit of cryoprecipitate usually raises the fibrinogen level by 6–8 mg/dL, so that 15 units of cryoprecipitate will raise the level from 50 to 150 mg/dL. Coagulation factor deficiency may require replacement with fresh-frozen plasma.

Heparin therapy must be used in combination with replacement therapy, since administering heparin on its own will lead to an unacceptable increase in bleeding. Heparin therapy usually requires a dose of 500–750 units per hour. Heparin cannot be effective if antithrombin III levels are markedly depleted. Antithrombin III levels should be measured, and fresh-frozen plasma should be used to raise levels to greater than 50%. In using heparin, it is not necessary to prolong the PTT. Successful therapy is indicated by a rising fibrinogen level. Fibrin degradation products will decline over 1–2 days. Improvement in the platelet count may lag as much as 1 week behind control of the coagulopathy.

In some cases, when disseminated intravascular coagulation is complicated by excessive fibrinolysis, even the combination of heparin and replacement therapy may not be adequate to control bleeding. In these cases, aminocaproic acid, 1 g intravenously per hour, or tranexamic acid, 10 mg/kg intravenously every 8 hours, should be added to decrease the rate of fibrinolysis, raise the fibrinogen level, and control bleeding. *Caution:* It must be emphasized that aminocaproic acid can *never* be used without heparin in disseminated intravascular coagulation, since fatal thrombosis may occur.

Prognosis

The prognosis is that of the underlying disease. Severe disseminated intravascular coagulation can be lethal.

Feinstein DI: Diagnosis and management of disseminated intravascular coagulation: The role of heparin therapy. Blood 1982;60:284.

LUPUS ANTICOAGULANT

The lupus anticoagulant is an IgM or IgG immunoglobulin that produces a prolonged PTT by binding to the phospholipid used in the in vitro PTT assay. As such, it is a laboratory artifact and does not cause a clinical bleeding disorder. The "lupus anticoagulant" is seen in 5–10% of patients with systemic lupus erythematosus. More commonly, it is seen without an underlying disorder or in patients taking phenothiazines.

There is no bleeding defect unless a second disorder such as thrombocytopenia, hypoprothrombinemia, or a prolonged bleeding time is present. Paradoxically, the lupus anticoagulant has been associated with an increased risk of thrombosis and of recurrent spontaneous abortions.

The PTT is prolonged and fails to correct when the patient's plasma is mixed in a 1:1 dilution with normal plasma. The PT is either normal or slightly prolonged. The fibrinogen level and thrombin time are normal. The Russell viper venom (RVV) time is a more sensitive assay and is specifically designed to demonstrate the presence of a lupus anticoagulant.

An antiphospholipid, the lupus anticoagulant, will cause a false-positive VDRL test for syphilis.

Lupus anticoagulant should be suspected in cases of a markedly prolonged PTT without clinical bleeding (other causes are factor XII or contact factor deficiency). The plasma mixing test will demonstrate the presence of an inhibitor by the failure of normal plasma to correct the PTT. When acquired factor VIII inhibitors are being considered, a factor VIII:C level may be measured; this will be normal in patients with lupus anticoagulant.

No specific treatment is necessary. Prednisone will usually rapidly eliminate the lupus anticoagulant, and it has been suggested that prednisone therapy reduces spontaneous abortions in this syndrome. It is not clear whether prednisone has any effect on the thrombotic tendency associated with lupus anticoagulant. Patients with thromboses should be treated with anticoagulation in standard doses. Because of the artificially prolonged PTT, heparin therapy is difficult to monitor properly. The dose of warfarin administered may also be inadequate if the baseline PT is prolonged.

Asherson RA et al: The "primary" anti-phospholipid syndrome: Major clinical and serologic features. Medicine 1989;68:366.
Branch DW et al: Obstetric complications associated with the lupus anticoagulant. N Engl J Med 1985;313:1322.
Mueh JR, Herbst KD, Rapaport SI: Thrombosis in patients with the lupus anticoagulant. Ann Intern Med 1980; 92:156.

ACQUIRED FACTOR VIII ANTIBODIES

Antibodies to factor VIII may develop either postpartum or with no underlying illness. Factor VIII antibodies also develop in 15% of patients with factor VIII hemophilia who have received infusions of plasma concentrates.

Acquired factor VIII antibodies usually produce a severe bleeding disorder. The PTT is prolonged, and the fibrinogen level, prothrombin time, and platelet count are not affected. A plasma mixing test will usually reveal the presence of an inhibitor by the failure of normal plasma to correct the prolonged PTT. However, the mixing test may require incubation for 2–4 hours to reveal the inhibitor. Factor VIII coagulant levels are low.

Factor VIII antibodies should be suspected in any acquired severe bleeding disorder associated with a prolonged PTT. Factor VIII antibodies are distinguished from lupus anticoagulants both by the presence of clinical bleeding and more importantly by the reduced factor VIII:C level. The diagnosis is confirmed by mixing tests and in vivo by the failure of factor VIII concentrates to raise the factor VIII:C levels by the expected amount.

The treatment of choice is cyclophosphamide, usually combined with prednisone. In the interim, aggressive factor VIII replacement may be necessary. Plasmapheresis to reduce inhibitor levels may be useful. Treatment of factor VIII antibodies is complex and should be done in consultation with a hematologist.

The prognosis of these patients is variable, and many die of overwhelming bleeding.

Lian EC et al: Combination immunosuppressive therapy after factor VIII infusion for factor VIII inhibitor. Ann Intern Med 1989;110:774.

HYPERCOAGULABLE STATES

In many cases, thrombosis is related to local factors causing stasis of blood flow or damage to a blood vessel. Common examples are deep venous thrombosis in the legs following prolonged sitting in one position and thrombosis in the femoral and iliac veins following hip surgery. However, in other cases a systemic disorder causes a general increase in the risk of thrombosis (Table 10–24).

Cancer is associated with an increased risk of both venous and arterial thrombosis. In some cases, low-grade disseminated intravascular coagulation appears to be responsible. In unusual cases, a unique cancer procoagulant stimulates the clotting system. Myeloproliferative disorders such as polycythemia vera, essential thrombocytosis, and paroxysmal nocturnal hemoglobinuria are associated with a high incidence of thrombosis, caused by qualitative platelet abnormalities. For the indolent diseases polycythemia vera and essential thrombocytosis, thrombosis is the major cause of morbidity and deaths. Venous thrombosis may occur in unusual locations such as the mesenteric, hepatic, or splenic venous beds. Arterial thrombosis occurs as well and may be manifested as large vessel occlusion (stroke, myocardial infarction) or as microvascular events with painful burning in the hands and feet.

Table 10–24. Causes of hypercoagulability.

Acquired
Cancer
Inflammatory disorders: Ulcerative colitis
Myeloproliferative disorders
Postoperative
Estrogens, pregnancy
Lupus anticoagulant
Heparin-induced thrombocytopenia
Congenital
Antithrombin III deficiency
Protein C deficiency
Protein S deficiency
Dysfibrinogenemia
Abnormal plasminogen

Heparin is an uncommon but important cause of hypercoagulability. Heparin has been associated with thrombocytopenia in about 10% of treatment courses. Often the thrombocytopenia is modest and resolves spontaneously. However, in some cases severe thrombocytopenia occurs. It is most often in this setting that arterial thrombosis occurs as a complication. The arteries involved are often large ones, such as the iliac artery or even the aorta. It is imperative that heparin be discontinued in this setting, since continuing the drug almost always leads to a fatal outcome.

A number of congenital biochemical defects have also been associated with hypercoagulability (Table 10–24). A family history is usually present. The thromboses are almost always venous and may occur in the large veins of the abdomen. Thromboses often occur during early adulthood rather than in childhood and are often precipitated by factors such as trauma or pregnancy. Antithrombin III deficiency is by far the most common of these disorders. The diagnosis is made by demonstrating reduced levels of the factors in plasma. Dysfibrinogenemia is diagnosed by a prolonged reptilase time.

The syndrome of warfarin-induced skin necrosis may occur in patients with undiagnosed protein C deficiency. Protein C is vitamin K-dependent and has a shorter half-life than the coagulation proteins. Warfarin, by creating a vitamin K-dependent state, will transiently deplete protein C before it leads to anticoagulation. During the period of hypercoagulability due to unopposed protein C depletion, thrombosis of skin vessels may lead to infarction and necrosis. The syndrome can be prevented by the use of heparin for 5–7 days until warfarin induces anticoagulation.

Treatment

If a patient is recognized to be at increased risk of thrombosis, effective prophylactic therapy is usually available. Preoperatively, minidose heparin (5000 units every 8–12 hours) may be useful in reducing the risk of thrombosis in the perioperative period. The hypercoagulable state associated with cancer may benefit from treatment with heparin, 10,000 units subcutaneously every 12 hours. Warfarin is usually ineffective in preventing thrombosis in this situation, most likely because low-grade disseminated intravascular coagulation is the cause. In patients with myeloproliferative disease who have had symptoms of thrombosis, antiplatelet therapy may be helpful. However, such therapy should not be used indiscriminately, because these patients are also at increased risk of bleeding. For patients with erythromelalgia (painful redness and burning of the hands), aspirin, 325 mg daily, is almost always effective.

For patients with congenital biochemical defects such as deficiency of antithrombin III or the vitamin K-dependent proteins C and S, warfarin is effective and should probably be given for life. Family members should be screened for the presence of the defect so that their increased risk of thrombosis can be noted and acted upon.

Menache D et al: Evaluation of safety, recovery, half-life and clinical efficacy of antithrombin III (human) in patients with hereditary anti-thrombin III deficiency. Blood 1990;75:33.

Schafer AI: The hypercoagulable states. Ann Intern Med 1985;102:814.

BLOOD TRANSFUSIONS

RED BLOOD CELL TRANSFUSIONS

Red blood cell transfusions are given to raise the hematocrit levels in patients with anemia or to replace losses after acute bleeding episodes. Because of the inherent risks, blood transfusions should never be given to correct anemia when simpler measures such as administration of iron, folate, or vitamin B_{12} can be used instead. Several types of components containing red blood cells are available.

(1) Fresh whole blood: The major advantage of this component is the simultaneous presence of red blood cells, plasma, and fresh platelets. Fresh whole blood is never absolutely necessary, since all the above components are available separately. The major indications for use of whole blood are cardiac surgery or massive hemorrhage when more than 10 units of blood are required in a 24-hour period.

(2) Packed red blood cells: Packed red cells are the component most commonly used to raise the hematocrit. Each unit has a volume of about 300 mL, of which approximately 200 mL consists of red blood cells. One unit of packed red cells will usually raise the hematocrit by approximately 4%. The expected rise in hematocrit can be calculated using an estimated red blood cell volume of 200 mL/unit and a total blood volume of about 70 mL/kg. For example, a 70-kg man will have a total blood volume of 4900 mL, and each unit of packed red blood cells will raise the hematocrit by $200 \div 4900$ equals 4%.

(3) Leukopoor blood: Patients with severe leukoagglutinin reactions to packed red blood cells may require depletion of white blood cells and platelets from transfused units. White blood cells can be removed either by centrifugation or by washing. Preparation of leukopoor blood causes additional expense and leads to some loss of red cells.

(4) Frozen blood: Red blood cells can be frozen and stored for up to 3 years, but the technique is cumbersome and expensive, and frozen blood should be used sparingly. The major application is for the purpose of maintaining a supply of rare blood types.

Patients with very rare blood types may donate units for autologous transfusion should the need arise. Frozen red cells are also occasionally needed for patients with severe leukoagglutinin reactions or anaphylactic reactions to plasma proteins, since frozen blood has essentially all white blood cells and plasma components removed.

(5) Autologous packed red blood cells: Patients scheduled for elective surgery may donate blood for autologous transfusion. These units may be stored for up to 35 days.

Compatibility Testing

Before transfusion, the recipient's and the donor's blood are cross-matched to avoid hemolytic transfusion reactions. Although many antigen systems are present on red blood cells, only the ABO and Rh systems are specifically tested prior to all transfusions. The A and B antigens are the most important, because everyone who lacks one or both red cell antigens has isoantibodies against the missing antigen or antigens in his or her plasma. These antibodies activate complement and can cause rapid intravascular lysis of the incompatible red cells. In emergencies, type O blood can be given to any recipient, but only packed cells should be given to avoid transfusion of donor plasma containing anti-A or anti-B antibodies.

The other important antigen routinely tested for is the D antigen of the Rh system. Approximately 15% of the population lack this antigen. In patients lacking the antigen, anti-D antibodies are not naturally present, but the antigen is highly immunogenic. A recipient whose red cells lack D and who receives D-positive blood may develop anti-D antibodies that can cause severe lysis of subsequent transfusions of D-positive red cells.

Blood typing includes assay of recipient serum for unusual antibodies by mixing the serum with panels of red cells representing commonly occurring weak antigens. The screening is particularly important if the recipient has had previous transfusions.

Hemolytic Transfusion Reactions

Major hemolytic transfusion reactions are the most dread complication of transfusion and can be fatal. The most severe reactions are those involving mismatches in the ABO system. Most of these cases are due to clerical errors and mislabeled specimens. Hemolysis is rapid and intravascular, releasing free hemoglobin into the plasma. The severity of these reactions depends on the dose of red blood cells given. The most severe reactions are those seen in surgical patients under anesthesia. They will be unable to give early warning signs of myalgias and chills.

Hemolytic transfusion reactions caused by minor antigen systems are typically less severe. The hemolysis usually takes place at a slower rate and is extravascular. Sometimes these transfusion reactions may be delayed for 5–10 days after transfusion. In such cases, the recipient has received blood containing an immunogenic action, and in the time since transfusion, a new alloantibody has been formed. The most common antigens involved in such reactions are Duffy, Kidd, Kell, and C and E loci of the Rh system.

A. Signs and Symptoms: Major hemolytic transfusion reactions cause fever and chills and severe backache and headache. In severe cases, there may be apprehension, dyspnea, hypotension, and vascular collapse. Such symptoms will usually lead to recognition of a transfusion reaction. *The transfusion must be stopped immediately!* In severe cases, disseminated intravascular coagulation or acute renal failure from tubular necrosis can occur, or both may occur.

Patients under general anesthesia will not give such signs, and the first indication may be oliguria and generalized bleeding.

B. Laboratory Findings and Management:
1. Identification of the recipient and of the blood should be checked. The donor transfusion bag with its pilot tube must be returned to the blood bank, and a fresh sample of the recipient's blood must accompany the donor bag for retyping of donor and recipient blood samples and for repeat of the crossmatch.

2. The hematocrit will fail to rise by the expected amount. Coagulation studies will reveal evidence of renal failure and disseminated intravascular coagulation in severe cases. Hemoglobinuria will turn the plasma pink and eventually result in hemoglobinuria. In cases of delayed hemolytic reactions, the hematocrit will fall and the indirect bilirubin will rise. In these cases, the new offending alloantibody is easily detected in the patient's serum.

C. Treatment: If a hemolytic transfusion reaction is suspected, the transfusion should be stopped at once. A sample of anticoagulated blood from the recipient should be centrifuged to detect free hemoglobin in the plasma. If hemoglobinemia is present, the patient should be vigorously hydrated to prevent acute tubular necrosis. There is some evidence that forced diuresis with mannitol may help prevent renal damage.

Leukoagglutinin Reactions

Most transfusion reactions are not hemolytic but represent reactions to antigens present on white blood cells or platelets in patients who have been sensitized to the antigens through previous transfusions or pregnancy. Most commonly, patients will develop fever and chills within 12 hours after transfusion. In severe cases, cough and dyspnea may occur and the chest x-ray may show transient pulmonary infiltrates. Because no hemolysis is involved, the hematocrit rises by the expected amount despite the reaction.

Leukoagglutinin reactions may respond to acetaminophen and diphenhydramine. In severe cases, steroids may be of help. Patients with severe leukoag-glutinin reactions may require transfusion of leukopoor red blood cells in the future.

Anaphylactic Reactions

Rarely, patients will develop hives or bronchospasm during a transfusion. These reactions are almost always due to plasma proteins rather than white blood cells. Patients who are IgA-deficient may develop these reactions because of antibodies to IgA. Patients with such reactions may require transfusion of washed or even frozen red blood cells to avoid future severe reactions.

Contaminated Blood

Rarely, blood is contaminated with gram-negative bacteria. Transfusion can lead to septicemia and shock from endotoxin. If this is suspected, the offending unit should be cultured and the patient treated with antibiotics as indicated.

Diseases Transmitted Through Transfusion

Despite the use of only volunteer blood donors and the routine screening of blood, transfusion-associated hepatitis remains a problem. All blood products (red blood cells, platelets, plasma, cryoprecipitate) can transmit viral diseases. All blood is routinely screened for hepatitis B surface antigen. In addition, blood banks routinely test for antibodies to HIV and to hepatitis core antigen. Because of specific screening, hepatitis B accounts for less than 10% of cases of transfusion-associated hepatitis. The most common form is non-A, non-B hepatitis. Overt hepatitis occurs at a rate of approximately 1% for each unit of blood transfused, and subclinical hepatitis probably occurs 10 times as often. Methods of detecting non-A, non-B hepatitis have been developed and will probably be in clinical use within the year. This should markedly reduce the problem of transfusion-associated hepatitis. Because of more rigorous screening of blood associated with the recent recognition of the possibility of transfusion-associated AIDS, the risk of hepatitis may decrease in the future. It is currently estimated that with proper screening the risk of transmitting AIDS is less than 1:100,000 for each unit of blood transfused.

Platelet Transfusion

Platelet transfusions are indicated in cases of thrombocytopenia due to decreased platelet production. They are not useful in immune thrombocytopenia, since transfused platelets will last no longer than the patient's endogenous platelets. The risk of spontaneous bleeding rises when the platelet count falls to less than 20,000/μL, and the risk of life-threatening bleeding increases when the platelet count is less than 10,000/μL. Because of this, prophylactic platelet transfusions are often given at these very low levels. Platelet transfusions are also given prior to invasive procedures or surgery, and the goal should be to raise the platelet count to over 50,000/μL.

Platelets are most commonly derived from donated blood units. One unit of platelets (derived from 1 unit of blood) usually contains $5–7 \times 10^{10}$ platelets suspended in 35 mL of plasma. Ideally, 1 platelet unit will raise the recipient's platelet count by 10,000/μL, and transfused platelets will last for 2 or 3 days. However, responses are often suboptimal, with poor platelet increments and short survival times. This may be due to sepsis, splenomegaly, or alloimmunization. Most alloantibodies causing platelet destruction are directed at HLA antigens. Patients requiring long periods of platelet transfusion support should be monitored to document adequate responses to transfusions so that the most appropriate product can be used. Patients may benefit from HLA-matched platelets derived from either volunteer donors or family members, with platelets obtained by plateletpheresis. Recently, techniques of cross-matching platelets have been developed and appear to identify suitable platelet donors (nonreactive with the patient's serum) without the need for HLA typing. Such single-donor platelets usually contain the equivalent of 6 units of random platelets, or $30–50 \times 10^{10}$ platelets suspended in 200 mL of plasma. Ideally, these platelet concentrates will raise the recipient's platelet count by 60,000/μL. Preliminary reports suggest that leukocyte-depleted platelets may be less immunogenic and that their use may delay the onset of alloimmunization.

Granulocyte Transfusions

Granulocytes for transfusion may be procured by leukapheresis. Approximately $1–3 \times 10^{10}$ times granulocytes can be collected from the donor. However, this number of granulocytes represents less than 10% of normal daily granulocyte production, and granulocytes survive only for hours. There is usually no detectable increase in the number of recipient granulocytes after such transfusions. Hazards of granulocyte transfusions include transmission of CMV infection and severe leukoagglutinin reactions. Because of these considerations, prophylactic granulocyte transfusions are not used in severely neutropenic patients.

Granulocyte transfusions are seldom indicated. However, they may be beneficial in patients with profound neutropenia ($<100/μL$) who have gram-negative sepsis or progressive soft tissue infection despite optimal antibiotic therapy. In these cases, it is clear that progressive infection is due to failure of host defenses. In such situations, daily granulocyte transfusions should be given and continued until the neutrophil count rises to above 500/μL. Such granulocytes must be derived from ABO-matched donors. Although HLA matching is not necessary, it is preferred, since patients with alloantibodies to donor white blood cells will have severe reactions and no benefit.

The donor cells usually contain some immunocompetent lymphocytes capable of producing graft-versus-host disease in HLA-incompatible hosts whose immunocompetence may be impaired. Irradiation of the units of cells with 1500 cGy will destroy the lymphocytes without harm to the granulocytes or platelets.

TRANSFUSION OF PLASMA COMPONENTS

Fresh-frozen plasma is available in units of approximately 200 mL. Fresh plasma contains normal levels of all coagulation factors (about 1 unit/mL). Fresh frozen plasma is used to correct coagulation factors deficiency and to treat thrombotic thrombocytopenic purpura.

Cryoprecipitate is made from fresh plasma. One unit has a volume of approximately 20 mL and contains approximately 250 mg of fibrinogen and between 80 and 100 units of factor VIII and von Willebrand factor. Cryoprecipitate is used to treat factor VIII deficiency and von Willebrand's disease and to supplement fibrinogen in cases of congenital deficiency of fibrinogen or disseminated intravascular coagulation. One unit of cryoprecipitate will raise the fibrinogen level by about 8 mg/dL.

Mollison PL: *Blood Transfusions in Clinical Medicine.* Blackwell, 1988.

REFERENCES

Jandl JH (editor): *Blood: Textbook of Hematology.* Little, Brown, 1987.

Williams WJ et al (editors): *Hematology,* 4th ed. McGraw-Hill, 1990.

11   Alimentary Tract & Liver

C. Michael Knauer, MD, & Sol Silverman, Jr., DDS

NAUSEA & VOMITING

These intensely disagreeable symptoms may occur singly or concurrently and may be due to a wide variety of factors (see below). The pathophysiology of vomiting is not completely understood. Vomiting appears to involve 2 functionally distinct medullary centers: the vomiting center, which initiates and controls the act of emesis; and the chemoreceptor trigger zone, which is activated by many drugs and endogenous and exogenous toxins. The vomiting center may receive stimuli from the alimentary tract and other organs, from the cerebral cortex, from the vestibular apparatus, and from the chemoreceptor trigger zone. Two or more stimuli may coexist.

An oversimplified classification of causes of vomiting is as follows:

(1) Alimentary disorders: Irritation, inflammation, motility disorder, or mechanical disturbance at any level of the gastrointestinal tract.

(2) Hepatobiliary and pancreatic disorders.

(3) Acute systemic infection.

(4) Central nervous system disorders: Increased intracranial pressure, stroke, migraine, infection, toxins, radiation sickness.

(5) Labyrinthine disorders: Motion sickness, infection, Meniere's syndrome.

(6) Endocrine disorders: Diabetic acidosis, adrenocortical crisis, pregnancy, starvation, lactic acidosis.

(7) Genitourinary disorders: Uremia, infection, obstruction.

(8) Cardiovascular disorders: Acute myocardial infarction, congestive heart failure.

(9) Drugs: Morphine, meperidine, codeine, excess alcohol, anesthetics, anticancer drugs, many others.

(10) Psychologic disorders: Reaction to pain, fear, or displeasure, chronic anxiety reaction, anorexia nervosa, bulimia, psychosis.

Complications of vomiting include fluid and electrolyte disturbances, pulmonary aspiration of vomitus, gastroesophageal mucosal tear (Mallory-Weiss syndrome), malnutrition, and postemetic rupture of the esophagus (Boerhaave's syndrome).

Treatment

Simple acute vomiting such as occurs following dietary or alcoholic indiscretion or during morning sickness of early pregnancy may require little or no treatment. Avoiding known aggravating factors and taking simple corrective dietary measures usually suffice.

Severe or prolonged nausea and vomiting usually require careful medical management in the hospital. The following general measures may be used as adjuncts to specific medical or surgical treatment:

A. Fluids and Nutrition: Hypokalemia and metabolic alkalosis are common in patients with severe vomiting. Withhold food temporarily and give intravenously 5% dextrose in saline with appropriate KCl supplementation to maintain euvolemia. If vomiting continues, employ a nasogastric tube to intermittent suction for gastric decompression. When oral feedings are resumed, begin with dry foods in small quantities, eg, salted crackers, graham crackers. With "morning sickness," these foods may best be taken before arising. Later, change to frequent small feedings of simple palatable foods. Hot beverages (tea and clear broths) and cold beverages (iced tea and carbonated liquids, especially ginger ale) are tolerated quite early. Avoid lukewarm beverages.

B. Medical Measures: *Note:* Unless nausea and vomiting of pregnancy are severe or progressive, avoid using medication for this purpose. The possible teratogenic effects of many classes of drugs are now being investigated.

Antiemetic drugs are usually better for preventing vomiting, but they may be employed selectively if the cause of vomiting cannot be treated effectively. The drugs should be used cautiously to avoid masking the development of serious illness and should be avoided in pregnancy. The choice of drug treatment depends on the reasons for the vomiting, the needs of the patient, and the known pharmacology of the available drugs:

(1) Sedatives, alone or with anticholinergics, may be helpful in patients with psychogenic vomiting.

(2) Antihistamines, eg, dimenhydrinate, 50 mg orally or intramuscularly every 4 hours or 100 mg by suppository twice daily, may be useful for patients with vestibular disorders (eg, Meniere's syndrome, motion sickness).

(3) Phenothiazines, eg, prochlorperazine, 5–10 mg orally or intramuscularly 3 times daily or 25 mg by suppository twice daily, may be preferred for vomiting caused by drugs, radiation sickness, or surgery.

(4) Metoclopramide, 10 mg orally or intravenously,

is particularly helpful for the nausea and vomiting of diabetic gastroparesis and for the prevention of the nausea and vomiting of cancer chemotherapy.

(5) Tetrahydrocannabinol (from marihuana) may be helpful in the treatment of refractory vomiting induced by cancer chemotherapy.

C. Psychotherapy: Attempt to determine the possible psychic basis of prolonged nausea and vomiting, but avoid aggressive psychotherapy during the acute phase of the illness. Hospitalization and restricted visiting may be necessary.

Hanson JS et al: The diagnosis and management of nausea and vomiting: A review. Am J Gastroenterol 1985; 80:210.

Malagelada J-R, Camilleri M: Unexplained vomiting: A diagnostic challenge. Ann Intern Med 1984;101:211.

HICCUP
(Singultus)

Hiccup, although usually transient and benign, may be caused by or associated with a wide range of disorders. Of importance are disease processes just above and below the diaphragm, such as (1) inflammation (pneumonia, esophagitis, subphrenic abscess, pancreatitis); (2) gastric distention; (3) neoplasms; (4) myocardial infarction or pericardial disease; (5) metabolic derangements (azotemia); (6) central nervous system disorders (infection, tumors); and (7) idiopathic disorders. Correction of potentially remediable causes will be most effective in the management of hiccup. Occasionally, hiccup is unilateral; this may have implications for therapy in refractory cases.

Treatment

Countless measures have been suggested for interrupting the rhythmic reflex that produces hiccup. At times, however, none of these may be successful, and the symptom may be so prolonged and severe as to jeopardize the patient's life.

A. Simple Home Remedies: These measures probably act by diverting the patient's attention; they consist of distracting conversation, fright, painful or unpleasant stimuli, or of having the patient perform such apparently purposeless procedures as breath holding, sipping ice water, or inhaling strong fumes. Swallowing a teaspoon of dry cane sugar may be effective.

B. Medical Measures:

1. Sedation–Any of the common sedative drugs may be effective, eg, diazepam, 5 mg orally.

2. Stimulation of nasopharynx–A soft catheter introduced nasally to stimulate the nasopharynx and pharynx is often successful.

3. Local anesthetics–Viscous 2% lidocaine, 15 mL orally, may be of some use. General anesthesia may be tried in intractable cases.

4. CO$_2$ inhalations–Have the patient rebreathe into a paper bag for 3–5 minutes, or give 10–15% CO$_2$ mixture by face mask for 3–5 minutes.

5. Tranquilizers–Phenothiazine drugs have been used successfully for prolonged hiccup, eg, chlorpromazine, 25 mg.

6. Antacids.

C. Surgical Measures: Various phrenic nerve operations, including bilateral phrenicotomy, may be indicated in extreme cases that fail to respond to all other measures and are considered to be a threat to life.

CONSTIPATION

The frequency of defecation and the consistency and volume of stools vary so greatly from individual to individual that it is often difficult to determine what is "normal." Familial, social, and dietary customs may help determine individual differences in bowel habits. Normal bowel movements may range in frequency from 3 to 12 stools per week, and the weights may range from 35 to 200 g of stool per day. The complaint of constipation often reflects the attitude of the patient with respect to the expected pattern of bowel movements. The patient should be considered to be constipated only if defecation is unexplainably delayed for days or if the stools are unusually hard, dry, and difficult to express. Constipation may result from repeatedly ignoring the urge to defecate because of unwillingness to interrupt social, recreational, or occupational activities.

Because there are many specific organic causes of constipation (see below), it is essential to explore such possibilities in patients with unexplained constipation. Be especially suspicious of organic causes when there have been sudden and unaccountable changes in bowel habits, or blood in the stools.

Causes of Constipation

(1) Dietary factors: Highly refined and low-fiber foods, inadequate fluids.

(2) Physical inactivity: Inadequate exercise, prolonged bed rest.

(3) Pregnancy.

(4) Advanced age (often multifactorial).

(5) Drugs: Analgesics (codeine, oxycodone (Percodan)), anesthetics, antacids (aluminum and calcium salts), anticholinergics, anticonvulsants, antidepressants (tricyclics, monoamine oxidase inhibitors), antihypertensives (ganglionic blocking agents), antiparkinsonism drugs, antipsychotic drugs (phenothiazines), β-adrenergic blocking agents, bismuth salts, calcium channel blockers, diuretics, iron salts, laxatives and cathartics (chronic use), metallic intoxications (arsenic, lead, mercury), muscle relaxants, opiates.

(6) Metabolic abnormalities: Hypokalemia, hyperglycemia, uremia, porphyria, amyloidosis.

(7) Endocrine abnormalities: Hypothyroidism, hypercalcemia, panhypopituitarism, pheochromocytoma, glucagonoma.

(8) Lower bowel abnormality: (a) Colon: prediverticular disease, diverticulosis, diverticulitis of sigmoid colon, neoplasm, extrinsic obstruction, inflammatory disease, especially with stricture and motility disorders. (b) Rectum: Disturbances in the defecatory mechanism, rectal intussusception, aganglionosis, pelvic floor spasm, neoplasm, inflammation. (c) Anus: Stricture, fissure, neoplasm.

(9) Neurogenic abnormalities: Innervation disorders of the bowel wall (aganglionosis, autonomic neuropathy), spinal cord disorders (trauma, multiple sclerosis, tabes dorsalis), disorders of the splanchnic nerves (tumors, trauma), cerebral disorders (strokes, parkinsonism, neoplasm).

(10) Psychogenic disorders.

(11) Enemas (chronic use).

Diagnosis

The history is all-important in the evaluation of this problem. If the cause is not obvious (no tumors, no stricture, etc) and the patient does not respond to simple measures (see below), further workup may be indicated to determine whether the problem is decreased motility or "outlet obstruction."

A. Motility Disorders: Assess transit through the colon with radiopaque markers.

B. Obstruction: Barium enema to assess for possible distal aganglionic segment, rectal biopsy to assess the presence of ganglion cells, defecography to assess for rectal intussusception (usual mechanism for solitary rectal ulcer and pelvic floor relaxation), anorectal manometry.

C. Metabolic Disorders: Hypothyroidism and hypercalciuria should be considered.

Treatment

The patient should be told that a daily bowel movement is not essential to health or well-being and that many symptoms (eg, lack of "pep") attributed to constipation have no such relationship.

A. Reestablishment of Regular Evacuation: Cathartics and enemas should not be used for simple constipation, since they interfere with the normal bowel reflexes. If it seems inadvisable to withdraw such measures suddenly from a patient who has employed them for a long time, the milder laxatives and enemas (see below) can be used temporarily. Bulking agents (eg, psyllium seed, methylcellulose) can be used indefinitely. Cathartic and enema "addicts" often defy all medical measures, and treatment is especially difficult when there is a serious underlying psychiatric disturbance.

B. Diet: The diet may be modified to satisfy the following requirements:

1. Adequate volume—Often "constipation" is merely due to inadequate food intake.

2. Adequate bulk or residue—Food with high fiber content such as bran and raw fruits and vegetables may be helpful.

3. Vegetable irritants—Unless there is a specific contraindication (eg, intolerance), stewed or raw fruits (particularly prunes and figs) or vegetables may be of value, especially in the "atonic" type of constipation.

4. Adequate fluids—The patient should be encouraged to drink adequate quantities of fluids to permit passage of intestinal contents. Six to 8 glasses of fluid per day, in addition to the fluid content of foods, are ordinarily sufficient. A glass of hot water taken one-half hour before breakfast seems to exert a mild laxative effect.

C. Laxatives: Laxatives may be classified as (1) stimulants (irritants), (2) bulk-forming agents, (3) osmotic laxatives, (4) wetting agents, and (5) lubricants. They are intended for temporary use on a selective basis by patients with simple constipation. Laxatives should *never* be given to patients with undiagnosed abdominal pain or when there is a possibility of intestinal obstruction or fecal impaction. Prolonged use of laxatives is seldom justified unless definitive therapy for specific disease is not possible. Chronic laxative use interferes with normal bowel motility and reflexes, thereby setting up a pattern for persistent constipation. Habitual use may also result in damage to the myenteric plexus of the colon and rectum. Melanosis coli may occur with certain laxatives but is probably not functionally important. There are no advantages—and there may be serious disadvantages—to mixing various laxatives.

1. Stimulant (irritant) laxatives—

a. Docusate sodium (eg, Colace, Doxinate), 50–350 mg/d. This agent interferes with sodium resorption in the colon, leading to increased water content in stool. Docusate sodium is also an "irritant" that produces mucosal changes in the small bowel, but the effect of this action on stool character or frequency is unclear.

b. Cascara sagrada aromatic fluid extract, a mild agent; 4–8 mL acts within 6–12 hours.

c. Bisacodyl (Dulcolax, etc), a mild to moderate laxative that stimulates sensory nerve endings of the colon to produce parasympathetic reflexes; 10–15 mg acts within 6 hours. Efficacious in suppository form as well; particularly useful in patients with spinal cord injury.

d. Phenolphthalein, a potent over-the-counter laxative; 30–240 mg acts within 4–6 hours.

e. Glycerin suppository, an agent for lubricating hard fecal material and stimulating the rectocolic reflex; 3 g acts within 30 minutes.

2. Bulk-forming agents—

a. Psyllium hydrophilic mucilloid (Hydrocil, Konsyl, Metamucil), more than 14 g (1–2 rounded teaspoonfuls) 2–3 times daily after meals in a full glass of water, is probably one of the least harmful mild laxatives when administered with an adequate or high fluid intake. It is particularly useful in elderly patients and in those with irritable colon syndrome.

b. Unprocessed bran, one-fourth cup daily with cereal or in unsweetened applesauce.

3. Osmotic laxatives–

a. Milk of magnesia (magnesium hydroxide), 15–30 mL at bedtime, is a common mild-to-moderate generically available laxative. It should not be used by patients with impaired renal function, in whom hypermagnesemia may develop.

b. Citrate of magnesia, 120–240 mL. Avoid use for patients with renal impairment (see above).

c. Sodium phosphate, 4-8 g in hot water before breakfast.

d. Lactulose syrup, 15–60 mL daily (relatively inexpensive).

4. Wetting agents–Docusate sodium is a detergent; see ¶ 1(a) above.

5. Lubricants–Liquid petrolatum (mineral oil), 15–30 mL per rectum, may help soften stool. Administration orally should be avoided because of risk of aspiration with resulting lipid pneumonia, and because petrolatum may interfere with intestinal absorption of fat-soluble vitamins.

D. Enemas: Because they interfere with restoration of a normal bowel reflex, enemas should ordinarily be used only as a temporary expedient in chronic constipation or fecal impaction. Infrequently, it may be necessary to administer enemas for prolonged periods.

1. Saline enema (nonirritating)–Warm physiologic saline solution, 500–2000 mL.

2. Warm tap water (irritating)–500–1000 mL.

3. Soapsuds (SS) enema (irritating)–75 mL of soap solution per liter of water.

4. Oil retention enema–180 mL of mineral oil or vegetable oil instilled in the rectum in the evening, retained overnight, and evacuated the next morning.

E. Surgery: For the rare patient in whom all medical and dietary measures fail and in whom constipation continues to severely affect enjoyment of life, left or subtotal colectomy may prove beneficial.

Metcalf AM et al: Simplified assessment of segmental colonic transit. Gastroenterology 1987;92:40.
Pemberton J: Chronic constipation: Matching type to treatment. Contemp Intern Med (September) 1989, p 64. (Pathophysiology and management.)
Wald A, Hinds JP, Caruna BJ: Psychological and physiological characteristics of patients with severe idiopathic constipation. Gastroenterology 1989;97:932. (Management needs to be individualized.)

FECAL IMPACTION

Hardened or puttylike stools in the rectum or colon may interfere with the normal passage of feces; if the impaction is not removed manually, by enemas, or by surgery, it can cause partial or complete intestinal obstruction. The impaction may be due to organic causes (painful anorectal disease, tumor, or neurogenic disease of the colon) or to functional causes (bulk laxatives, antacids, residual barium from x-ray study, low-residue diet, starvation, drug-induced colonic stasis, or prolonged bed rest and debility). The patient may give a history of obstipation, but more frequently there is a history of watery diarrhea. There may be blood or mucus in the stool. Physical examination may reveal a distended abdomen, palpable "tumors" in the abdomen, and a firm stool in the rectum. The impaction may be broken up digitally or dislodged with a sigmoidoscope. Cleansing enemas (preferably in the knee-chest position) or, in the case of impaction higher in the colon, colonic irrigations may be of value. Daily oil retention enemas followed by digital fragmentation of the impaction and saline enemas may be necessary.

Wald A: Colorectal function and constipation in the elderly. Pract Gastroenterol 1989;13:36.

GASTROINTESTINAL GAS
(Flatulence)

The amount of gastrointestinal gas varies considerably from individual to individual. Subjective estimates by patients may be at considerable variance from observed findings, which indicate the average to be 17 passages of flatus per 24 hours. Five gases—nitrogen and oxygen from swallowed air, and carbon dioxide, hydrogen, and methane produced in the gut—constitue more than 99% of gastrointestinal gas. Excessive belching or eructation is usually due to air swallowed during eating or drinking, or it may be due to a nervous habit of sucking in air; the latter may be severe.

Excessive passage of flatus per rectum is due largely to gases formed by bacterial fermentation of maldigested carbohydrates and cellulose in the intestine. Rectal gas consists predominantly of H_2, CO_2, and CH_4—all odorless; there is little objective information on the malodorous gases. Many problems of abdominal bloating or distention with pain appear to be caused by disordered bowel motility rather than by excessive gas. Since excessive gastrointestinal gas may be due to both functional and organic disease, complaints of unusual belching, bloating, and flatulence may require search for specific causes.

Treatment

A. Correction of Aerophagia: Anxiety states are often associated with deep breathing and sighing and consequent swallowing of considerable quantities of air. Chewing gum contributes to swallowing of air.

B. Correction of Physical Defects: These sometimes interfere with normal swallowing or breathing: (1) Structural deformities of the nose and nasopharynx, eg, nasal obstruction and adenoids. (2) Spatial defects of the teeth or ill-fitting dentures.

C. Diet: The diet should be nutritious as tolerated and enjoyed by the patient, but eliminate foods that may lead to excessive flatulence in susceptible individuals. An initial trial of a lactose-free diet is often rewarding.

D. Medications: Drugs (including charcoal, simethicone, and antiflatulence tablets) are generally unsatisfactory and may be only of placebo value. Anticholinergic-sedative drugs serve to diminish the flow of saliva (which is often excessive in some patients), thereby reducing the aerophagia that accompanies swallowing; bowel motility is reduced.

Altman DF: Downwind update: A discourse on matters gaseous. (Medical Staff Conference.) West J Med 1986;145:502.

DIARRHEA

Diarrhea is defined as an increase in the frequency, fluidity, and volume (> 200 g/d) of bowel movements. Normal bowel function varies from individual to individual, and the definition of diarrhea must take this variation into account. Factors influencing stool consistency are poorly understood; water content is not the sole determinant. Thus, the definition of diarrhea in a clinical sense is an increase in frequency or increased fluidity of bowel movements in a given individual. In pathophysiologic terms, diarrhea results from the passage of stools containing excess water, ie, from malabsorption or secretion of water. Although daily stool weight or water is probably the best single index to diarrhea, "small-volume diarrhea" with frequent evacuations of blood, mucus, or exudate is a syndrome often signifying disease of the distal colon.

Pathophysiology
A. Types of Diarrhea:
1. With excess fecal water–
a. Osmotic diarrhea–Excess water-soluble molecules in the bowel lumen cause osmotic retention of intraluminal water. *Examples:* Magnesium hydroxide, undigested disaccharides, surreptitious use of laxatives.
b. Secretory diarrhea–Excessive active ion secretion by the mucosal cells of the intestine. *Examples:* Cholera, toxigenic *Escherichia coli*, Zollinger-Ellison syndrome, carcinoid syndrome, vipoma.
c. Exudative disease–Abnormal mucosal permeability, with intestinal loss of serum proteins, blood, mucus, or pus.
d. Impaired contact between intestinal chyme and absorbing surface–Rapid transit, short bowel syndromes.

2. Without excess fecal water–Frequent small, painful evacuations are usually a result of disease of the left colon or rectum.

B. Causes of Diarrhea: Most diarrheal states are self-limited and pose no special diagnostic problem. The following list of the causes of diarrhea is indicative of the extensive diagnostic evaluation that may be required in patients with unexplained, profound, or chronic diarrhea.
1. Psychogenic disorders–"Nervous" diarrhea.
2. Drugs–Magnesium-containing antacids, antibiotics, laxatives, sorbitol (excess diet drinks, sugarless gum, etc), metoclopramide.
3. Intestinal infections–
a. Viral infections–Enterovirus, Norwalk virus.
b. Bacterial infections–6Most common are *Campylobacter jejuni, Shigella, Salmonella,* and *Yersinia enterocolitica.*
c. Bacterial toxins–*Clostridium difficile,* enterotoxigenic *Escherichia coli, Staphylococcus, V parahaemolyticus,* and *V cholerae.*
4. Parasitic infections–*Giardia lamblia, Entamoeba histolytica, Cryptosporidium,* and *Isospora* are the most common.
5. Other intestinal factors–Fecal impaction, lactase deficiency (milk intolerance), antibiotic therapy, inflammatory bowel disease, catharsis habituation, vagotomy, carcinoma, heavy metal poisoning, gastrocolic fistula, and amyloidosis.
6. Cholestatic syndromes–Hepatitis and bile duct obstruction may result in steatorrhea and mild diarrhea.
7. Malabsorption states–Primary small bowel mucosal diseases (eg, celiac sprue), short small bowel states, and intestinal blind loop syndrome (eg, diverticula, afferent loop).
8. Pancreatic disease–Pancreatic insufficiency, diabetes mellitus, pancreatic endocrine tumors.
9. Reflex from other viscera–Pelvic disease (extrinsic to gastrointestinal tract).
10. Neurologic disease–Tabes dorsalis, diabetic neuropathy.
11. Metabolic disease–Hyperthyroidism.
12. Immunodeficiency disease–IgA deficiency, AIDS.
13. Malnutrition–Marasmus, kwashiorkor.
14. Food allergy.
15. Dietary factors–Excessive fresh fruit intake, caffeine-containing foods.
16. Factitious–Surreptitious laxative ingestion.
17. Unknown.

Diagnosis
A specific diagnosis can often be made on the basis of the history and physical examination alone. Otherwise, it is based on examination of diarrheal material for polymorphonuclear cells, parasites, and culture for bacterial pathogens. This is best accom-

plished at sigmoidoscopy prior to preparation with a cleansing enema. Cotton swabs should not be used in making slides, since both polymorphonuclear cells and parasites cling to cotton. The presence of polymorphonuclear cells indicates an inflammatory process. Rectal biopsy may prove helpful, particularly when *Entamoeba histolytica* is being considered and there is colitis. These studies should be performed prior to barium studies and before starting treatment. Assay for *Clostridium difficile* is highly accurate with current techniques.

Treatment

A. Correct Physiologic Changes Induced by Diarrhea:

1. Acid-base disturbance, fluid loss.

2. Electrolyte depletion (hyponatremia, hypokalemia, hypocalcemia, hypomagnesemia).

3. Malnutrition, vitamin deficiencies.

4. Psychogenic disturbances (eg, fixation on gastrointestinal tract or anxiety regarding incontinence in cases of long-standing diarrhea).

B. Diet:

1. Acute severe—Food should be withheld for the first 24 hours or restricted to lukewarm clear liquids—a physiologic glucose and salt solution, sipped slowly as needed to replace large fluid and electrolyte losses, may be especially useful in patients with severe watery diarrhea. Frequent small soft feedings are added as tolerated. Milk and milk products are the last foods to be added, since temporary lactase deficiency frequently is present after an ''insult'' to the small intestine.

2. Convalescent—Food should be incorporated into the diets of patients convalescing from acute diarrhea as tolerated. Nutritious food, preferably all cooked, in small frequent meals, is usually well tolerated. *Avoid* raw vegetables and fruits, fried foods, bran, whole grain cereals, preserves, syrups, candies, pickles, relishes, spices, coffee, and alcoholic beverages.

3. Chronic diarrhea—Chronic diarrhea is due to many causes. Nutritional disturbances range from none to marked depletion of electrolytes, water, protein, fat, and vitamins. Treat specific disease when known (eg, gluten-free diet in celiac sprue and enzyme replacement in pancreatic insufficiency). Give fat-soluble vitamins (vitamins A, D, E, K) when steatorrhea is present. Some patients are so ill that they require parenteral alimentation, sometimes at home.

C. Antidiarrheal Agents:

Antidiarrheal drugs must be used with great caution in inflammatory bowel disease and amebiasis because of the risk of ''toxic'' dilatation of the colon. They should usually be avoided in bacillary dysentery, since they may prolong or worsen the course of the acute illness.

1. Pepto-Bismol—Give 30 mL 3–6 times per day for symptomatic treatment of diarrhea. Remind the patient that this agent causes black stools.

2. Narcotic analogues—Avoid with possible acute infectious diarrhea, as they may worsen and prolong the course.

a. Diphenoxylate with atropine (Lomotil), 2.5 mg 3–4 times daily as needed. It must be used cautiously in patients with advanced liver disease and in those who are addiction-prone or who are taking sedatives.

b. Loperamide (Imodium), 2 mg 2–4 times daily, is effective in acute and chronic diarrhea.

3. Narcotics—Narcotics must be avoided in chronic diarrheas unless there is intractable diarrhea, vomiting, and colic. Always exclude the possibility of acute surgical abdominal disease before administering opiates, especially incomplete obstruction and diverticulitis. Give any of the following:

a. Paregoric, 4–8 mL after liquid movements as needed or with bismuth.

b. Codeine phosphate, 15–60 mg subcutaneously, if the patient is vomiting, after liquid bowel movements as needed.

c. Strong opiates— Morphine should be reserved for selected patients with severe acute diarrhea who fail to respond to more conservative measures.

4. Anticholinergic drugs, particularly when used in combination with sedatives, exert a mild antiperistaltic action in acute and chronic diarrheas associated with anxiety tension states. It may be necessary to administer the various drugs to a point near toxicity in order to achieve the desired effect.

D. Special Situations:

1. Clonidine, 1-mg patch, for managing diarrhea associated with diabetes, cryptosporidia, etc.

2. Somatostatin or analogues (Octreotide), 75 µg intravenously 2–4 times daily, for patients with diarrhea due to carcinoid tumor, vipoma, and perhaps diabetes.

E. Psychotherapy:

Source cases of chronic diarrhea are of psychogenic origin. A survey of anxiety-producing mechanisms should be made in all patients with this complaint. Antidepressant drug therapy may be useful, particularly since many of these agents have an anticholinergic effect.

F. Prophylaxis:

Traveler's diarrhea, most commonly due to enterotoxigenic *E coli* or *Shigella*, can frequently be prevented with the prophylactic use of doxycycline or trimethoprim-sulfamethoxazole. However, the low incidence and moderate morbidity among travelers to developing countries probably do not warrant the risks of prophylactic treatment of all travelers.

Black RE: Epidemiology of traveler's diarrhea and relative importance of various pathogens. Rev Infect Dis 1990;12(Suppl 1):73.

Cohen MB, Giannella RA: Bacterial diarrheal disease: Host and bacterial factors involved in intestinal infection. View Dig Dis (Sept) 1987;19:4.

Field M, Rao MR, Chang EB: Intestinal electrolyte transport

and diarrheal disease. (Two parts.) N Engl J Med 1989;321:800, 879. (Rational approach to management.)

Ogbounaya KI: Diabetic diarrhea: Pathophysiology, diagnosis, and management. Arch Intern Med 1990;150:262. (Clonidine and somatostatin analogues in treatment.)

Smith PD et al: Intestinal infections in patients with the acquired immunodeficiency syndrome (AIDS): Etiology and response to therapy. Ann Intern Med 1988;108:328.

Steffen R: Worldwide efficacy of bismuth subsalicylate in the treatment of traveler's diarrhea. Rev Infect Dis 1990;12(Suppl 1):80.

MASSIVE UPPER GASTROINTESTINAL HEMORRHAGE

Massive upper gastrointestinal hemorrhage is a common emergency. It may be defined as rapid loss of sufficient blood to cause hypovolemic shock. The actual volume of blood loss required to produce shock varies with the size, age, and general condition of the patient and with the rapidity of bleeding. Sudden loss of 20% or more of blood volume (blood volume is approximately 75 mL/kg of body weight) produces hypotension, tachycardia, and other signs of shock. For example, a previously well 70-kg man who develops shock as a result of gastrointestinal hemorrhage will have lost at least 1000–1500 mL of blood. The immediate objectives of management are (1) to restore an effective blood volume and (2) to establish a diagnosis on which definitive treatment can be based.

The major causes of upper gastrointestinal bleeding are peptic ulceration of the duodenum, stomach, or esophagus, esophageal varices, and gastritis. In addition, bleeding may be due to Mallory-Weiss syndrome and hemorrhagic gastritis due to ulcerogenic drugs such as aspirin, nonsteroidal anti-inflammatory drugs, or alcohol. Vascular lesions are a rare cause of massive upper gastrointestinal hemorrhage.

Clinical Findings

A. Symptoms and Signs: There is usually a history of sudden weakness or fainting associated with or followed by tarry stools or vomiting of blood. Melena occurs in most patients and hematemesis in over half. Hematemesis is especially common in esophageal varices (90%), gastritis, and gastric ulcer. The patient may or may not be in shock when first seen but will at least be pale and weak if major blood loss has occurred. If the patient is not vomiting, a nasogastric tube will often help determine if the bleeding is in the upper gastrointestinal tract. There may be a history of peptic ulcer, chronic liver disease, other predisposing disease, alcoholic excess, or severe vomiting.

There is usually no pain, and the pain of peptic ulcer disease often stops with the onset of bleeding. Abdominal findings are not remarkable except when hepatomegaly, splenomegaly, or a mass (neoplasm) is present. Bowel sounds may be increased due to blood in the gut.

The cause of bleeding should be established as promptly as possible, since management will in part be dependent on the findings. This is particularly true if emergency surgery is anticipated, so that surgical approach and type of procedure can be determined.

A history of peptic ulcer or of antacid ingestion suggests duodenal ulcer. Ingestion of aspirin or other nonsteroidal anti-inflammatory agents on a regular or intermittent basis suggests gastric ulcer or hemorrhagic erosive gastritis. A history of alcoholism or evidence of chronic liver disease, such as jaundice, hepatosplenomegaly, spider angioma, palmar erythema, ascites, or encephalopathy, indicates probable portal hypertension and possible variceal bleeding. Aspiration of gastric contents by nasogastric tube is diagnostically useful and permits estimation of the continued rate of bleeding.

The principal diagnostic procedures that should be carried out after necessary emergency treatment has been given are outlined below.

B. Laboratory Findings: In addition to the baseline studies of a complete blood count, urinalysis, and serum electrolyte and creatinine measurements, the following may prove helpful in selected patients.

1. Liver function studies–Serum bilirubin, aminotransferases, albumin:globulin ratio, alkaline phosphatase, and prothrombin time may help support a diagnosis of chronic liver disease with associated portal hypertension.

2. Coagulation studies–In addition to the prothrombin time, a platelet count and partial thromboplastin time are useful, especially when there is a history of excessive dental, gynecologic, or other bleeding. Bleeding times in azotemic patients and those with recent NSAID or aspirin use will indicate the status of platelet competency.

C. Endoscopy: Upper panendoscopy should be the first definitive examination performed if an experienced endoscopist is available. This procedure will allow identification of the bleeding site in 80–95% of patients with upper gastrointestinal bleeding. Furthermore, if bleeding is active, treatment through the endoscope is possible, including sclerotherapy for bleeding esophageal varices and thermal treatment (heater probe, multipolar electrocoagulation) of bleeding gastric and duodenal ulcers. When it is not certain that bleeding is from the upper gastrointestinal tract, sigmoidoscopy should be the first diagnostic procedure.

D. Imaging: If upper gastrointestinal endoscopy does not reveal the bleeding site, selective angiography should be considered if the bleeding persists. Arteriography may not be successful if the bleeding is less than 1 mL/min. Radionuclide scanning with technetium Tc 99m red cell labeling also has advocates. Upper gastrointestinal series may be useful when bleeding abates.

Treatment

A. General Measures: The patient should be under the observation of the primary care physician, a gastroenterologist, and a surgeon from the outset. Bed rest and charting of fluid intake, urine output, and temperature are ordered. Insert a large-bore nasogastric tube to verify the source of hemorrhage and to remove gastric contents (see below). If bleeding continues or if tachycardia or hypotension is present, monitor and treat the patient for shock (see Chapter 1). Insert a Foley catheter and 2 large-bore intravenous lines (18-gauge minimum). Blood is obtained immediately for complete blood count, hematocrit, and crossmatching of at least 4 units of packed red blood cells. In interpreting the hematocrit, it should be kept in mind that after acute blood loss, a period of 24–36 hours may be required for reequilibration of body fluids. In the interim, the hematocrit may not reflect the extent of blood loss. Frequent determination of vital signs, especially those associated with postural changes, is helpful in estimating acute blood loss. Replacement therapy is started immediately with normal saline. If shock is severe or if the patient has portal hypertension, fresh-frozen plasma is given while a blood transfusion is being prepared.

Aqueous vasopressin (Pitressin) by intravenous drip in 5% glucose in water at the rate of 0.2–0.4 units/min may cause temporary arteriolar vasoconstriction and lowering of the portal venous pressure for variceal bleeding. Its efficacy is unproved.

Water-soluble vitamin K (menadiol sodium diphosphate [Synkayvite]), 5–10 mg intramuscularly, is given empirically if hepatobiliary disease is suspected. Restlessness may be due to continued hemorrhage, shock, or hypoxia.

B. Blood Replacement: Treatment of shock by transfusion with blood cells or fresh-frozen plasma (or both) is begun without delay. Hematocrit determinations are done every few hours until they are stabilized. The objective of blood replacement is to relieve shock and restore blood volume. The amount of blood required is estimated on the basis of vital signs, measured loss, central venous pressure, and renal perfusion as measured by urine output. While a patient is actively bleeding, at least 6 units of packed red blood cells should be available for emergency transfusion; rapid administration will control shock. When blood pressure and pulse have been restored to relatively normal levels and clinical signs of hypovolemia are no longer present, the rate of transfusion can be slowed. The total volume of blood given is determined by the course of the disease. A poor response usually means continued bleeding (see below) or inadequate replacement. Venous pressure or pulmonary artery wedge pressure is useful in selected patients in gauging adequacy of blood replacement and detecting over-

transfusion and congestive heart failure. Rarely is it necessary to transfuse to a hematocrit of greater than 25–26%.

C. Medical Measures: Acid peptic digestion is a causative or aggravating factor in many cases of massive upper gastrointestinal hemorrhage, perhaps including varices. Feedings and oral medications for ulcer are begun as soon as shock and nausea have subsided. Continued slight bleeding is not a contraindication for the following regimen:

1. Diet–Liquid diet for the first 24 hours, followed by a soft or regular diet, depending on the clinical situation.

2. Acid reduction–While a nasogastric tube is still in place, antacids such as aluminum hydroxide-magnesium hydroxide mixtures can be administered hourly by mouth in a dose of 30 mL to protect the distal esophagus from reflux and to help neutralize gastric contents not suctioned by the tube. In the fasting patient, an H_2 antagonist by constant infusion (cimetidine, 37.5 mg/h; ranitidine, 8.3 mg/h; or famotidine, 1 mg/h) following an intravenous bolus (cimetidine, 300 mg; ranitidine, 50 mg; or famotidine, 20 mg) reduces acid output, although it does not appear to affect the incidence of acute rebleeding. Furthermore, higher doses per hour may need to be given to achieve the target of a constant intragastric pH of greater than 4.0. For the nonfasting patient with ulcer disease, the H_2 receptor antagonists (cimetidine, ranitidine, famotidine), antacids, and sucralfate are equally efficacious in inducing healing. Therapeutic doses of antacids, 1 and 3 hours after meals and at bedtime, may cause diarrhea. There is little evidence that antacid therapy of any type is useful in acute upper gastrointestinal bleeding.

3. A nasogastric tube may be useful to permit continued decompression of the stomach and evacuation of blood by lavage with saline. The tube is also useful to monitor the rate of continued bleeding. Whenever the tube is placed, the patient should be in a moderate reversed Trendelenburg position, if possible, to minimize reflux around the tube. See above concerning antacid use.

D. Management of Bleeding Esophageal Varices: When varices are the cause of bleeding, special measures are indicated (see p 467).

E. Indications for Emergency Operation: Emergency surgery to stop active bleeding should be considered under any of the following circumstances: (1) When the patient has received 6 units of packed cells or more of blood but shock is not controlled or recurs promptly. (2) When acceptable blood pressure and hematocrit cannot be maintained with a maximum of 2 units of packed red blood cells every 8 hours. (3) When bleeding is slow but persists more than 2–3 days. (4) When bleeding stops initially but recurs while the patient is receiving adequate medical treatment. (5) When the patient is over age 60. The death rate from exsanguination in spite of conservative measures is greater in those over age 60 and in those who have shock or recurrent hemorrhage.

Some patients will have a pigmented protuberance—often called a "visible vessel"—present in an ulcer base on endoscopy. About half of these patients will have uncontrolled or recurrent bleeding during their hospital stay and will require endoscopic hemostatic therapy (heater probe, multipolar electrocoagulation) or surgery.

Prognosis

The overall mortality rate of about 14% indicates the seriousness of massive upper gastrointestinal hemorrhage. Fatality rates vary greatly, depending upon the cause of bleeding and the presence of other serious systemic disease. The overall operative mortality rate for emergency surgery to stop bleeding is high, and best results are obtained when bleeding can be controlled medically and surgery deferred until the patient has recovered from the effects of bleeding. Hemorrhage from duodenal ulcer causes death in about 3% of treated cases, whereas in bleeding varices the mortality rate may be as high as 50%.

Changchien CS et al: Different implications of stigmata of recent hemorrhage in gastric and duodenal ulcers. Dig Dis Sci 1988;33:400. (Clinical refinements on basis of endoscopic criteria.)

Laine L: Multipolar electrocoagulation in the treatment of active upper gastrointestinal tract hemorrhage: A prospective controlled trial. N Engl J Med 1987;316:1613. (Decreases transfusion requirement, length of hospital stay, and need for surgery.)

Levy M et al: Major upper gastrointestinal tract bleeding: Relation to the use of aspirin and other nonnarcotic analgesics. Arch Intern Med 1988;148:281. (Increased risk.)

McClave SA et al: Dieulafoy's cirsoid aneurysm of the duodenum. Dig Dis Sci 1988;33:801. (A cause of upper gastrointestinal bleeding, particularly in the stomach.)

Wilcox CM, Truss CD: Gastrointestinal bleeding in patients receiving long-term anticoagulant therapy. Am J Med 1988;84:683. (Role of prothrombin time in diagnosis.)

MASSIVE LOWER GASTROINTESTINAL HEMORRHAGE

Massive lower gastrointestinal bleeding occurs most frequently in older, poor-risk patients and is always a *medical emergency*. Colonic diverticulosis and angiodysplasia (acquired arteriovenous malformation) are the most common causes of hemodynamically significant lower gastrointestinal bleeding, but other possibilities—including massive upper gastrointestinal hemorrhage—must be considered (see above).

Causes of Massive
Lower Abdominal Hemorrhage
A. Colonic Disorders:
1. Inflammatory–Ulcerative colitis, regional en-

teritis, infectious diarrhea (eg, shigellosis), radiation colitis.

2. Diverticular–Diverticulosis.

3. Vascular–Hemorrhoids, angiodysplasia (vascular ectasia), bowel ischemia, colonic varices, aortic aneurysm with enteric fistula.

4. Neoplastic–Benign and malignant disorders.

5. Hereditary–Telangiectasias, arteriovenous malformations.

6. Coagulopathies–Anticoagulant drugs, blood dyscrasias.

B. Upper Gastrointestinal Disorders:
1. Vascular–Esophageal varices, telangiectasias, aortoduodenal fistula.

2. Ulcerative–Peptic ulceration.

3. Neoplastic–Benign and malignant disorders.

Management of Hemorrhage

The patient usually has a sudden onset of weakness and fainting, combined with or followed by passage of grossly bloody stools (which may be either bright red or dark red according to the time elapsed since the beginning of the hemorrhage). There may be a history and physical findings of one or more of the disorders listed above; shock may be present.

If rectal bleeding is copious or if there is evidence of shock, the patient should be resuscitated with intravenous fluids and blood products before and during the diagnostic evaluation. Colonic bleeding stops spontaneously in about 75% of patients treated with bed rest and simple resuscitative measures.

A nasogastric tube should be inserted to rule out upper gastrointestinal bleeding (see above). However, unless bile is aspirated via this tube, one cannot be certain that bleeding is not duodenal in origin. Rectal examination and proctosigmoidoscopy may identify bleeding lesions of the anorectal region as well as of the sigmoid mucosa. Lesions may require biopsy so that appropriate therapy can be instituted.

If several blood transfusions are necessary, further definitive diagnostic study is warranted. Radionuclide localization of shed technetium Tc 99m-labeled red cells is proving to be helpful in localizing lower gastrointestinal bleeding. Pertechnetate Tc 99m scintigraphy can be used to localize ectopic gastric mucosa, such as in Meckel's diverticulum, with an accuracy of about 90%. Meckel's diverticulum is an occasional cause of lower gastrointestinal bleeding in young patients. Colonoscopy may sometimes be useful for identifying and fulgurating bleeding sites. Selective mesenteric angiography can sometimes demonstrate and localize the site of hemorrhage in patients who are actively bleeding. Once the bleeding site is identified, selective intra-arterial infusion of vasopressin into the affected portion may control the bleeding, at least temporarily, in 75–80% of cases. If no bleeding site can be determined, laparotomy and appropriate surgical treatment may be required.

Cello JP et al: Diagnosis and management of lower gastrointestinal tract hemorrhage: Medical Staff Conference UCSF. West J Med 1985;143:80.

Koval G et al: Aggressive angiographic diagnosis in acute lower gastrointestinal hemorrhage. Dig Dis Sci 1987; 32:248.

Richter JM et al: Angiodysplasia: Natural history and efficacy of therapeutic interventions. Dig Dis Sci 1989; 34:1542. (Rebleeding common, especially in the elderly.)

ACUTE PERITONITIS

Essentials of Diagnosis

- Abdominal pain, vomiting, fever, and prostration.
- Abdominal rigidity and diffuse or local tenderness (often rebound).
- Later, abdominal distention and paralytic ileus.
- Leukocytosis.

General Considerations

Localized or generalized peritonitis is the most important complication of a wide variety of acute abdominal disorders. Peritonitis may be caused by infection or chemical irritation. Perforation or necrosis of the gastrointestinal tract is the usual source of infection. Chemical peritonitis occurs in acute pancreatitis and in the early stages of gastroduodenal perforation. Spontaneous bacterial peritonitis may occur in decompensated cirrhotic patients with ascites. Sclerosing peritonitis may be associated with neoplastic disease and certain drugs (eg, beta-blockers, methysergide).

Clinical Findings

A. Systemic Reaction: Malaise, prostration, nausea, vomiting, septic fever, leukocytosis, and electrolyte imbalance are usually seen in proportion to the severity of the process. If infection is not controlled, toxemia is progressive, and septic shock may develop.

B. Abdominal Signs:

1. Pain and tenderness–Depending upon the extent of involvement, pain and tenderness may be localized or generalized. Abdominal pain on coughing, rebound tenderness referred to the area of peritonitis, and tenderness to light percussion over the inflamed peritoneum are characteristic. Pelvic peritonitis is associated with rectal and vaginal tenderness.

2. Muscle rigidity–The muscles overlying the area of inflammation usually become spastic. When peritonitis is generalized (eg, after perforation of a peptic ulcer), marked rigidity of the entire abdominal wall may develop immediately. Rigidity is frequently diminished or absent in the late stages of peritonitis,

in severe toxemia, and when the abdominal wall is weak.

3. Paralytic ileus–Intestinal motility is markedly inhibited by peritoneal inflammation. Diminished to absent peristalsis and progressive abdominal distention are the cardinal signs. Vomiting occurs as a result of pooling of gastrointestinal secretions and gas, most of which is swallowed air.

C. Imaging: Abdominal films show gas and fluid collections in both large and small bowel, usually with generalized rather than localized dilatation. The bowel walls, when shown in relief by the gas patterns, may appear to be thickened, indicating the presence of edema or peritoneal fluid. A gentle barium enema will determine whether large bowel obstruction is present or not.

D. Diagnostic Abdominal Tap: Recovery of ascitic fluid for amylase and protein measurements, culture, and cytologic examination—to include absolute number of polymorphonuclear neutrophils—is useful.

Differential Diagnosis

Peritonitis, which may present a highly variable clinical picture, must be differentiated from acute intestinal obstruction, acute cholecystitis with or without choledocholithiasis, pancreatitis, renal colic, gastrointestinal hemorrhage, lower lobe pneumonias, porphyria, periodic fever, hysteria, black widow spider bite, and central nervous system disorders (eg, tabes dorsalis).

Complications

The most frequent sequela of peritonitis is abscess formation in the pelvis, in the subphrenic space, between the leaves of the mesentery, or elsewhere in the abdomen. Antibiotic therapy may mask or delay the appearance of localizing signs of abscess. When fever, leukocytosis, toxemia, or ileus fails to respond to the general measures outlined for the management of peritonitis, a collection of pus should be suspected. This will usually require percutaneous ultrasound-guided or surgical drainage. Liver abscess and pylephlebitis are rare complications. Adhesions may cause early or, more frequently, late intestinal obstruction.

Treatment

The measures employed in peritonitis as outlined below are generally applicable as supportive therapy in most acute abdominal disorders. The objectives are (1) to control infection, (2) to minimize the effects of paralytic ileus, and (3) to correct fluid, electrolyte, and nutritional disorders.

A. Specific Measures: Operative procedures to close perforations, to remove sources of infection such as gangrenous bowel or an inflamed appendix, or to drain abscesses are frequently required.

B. General Measures: No matter what specific operative procedures are employed, their ultimate success will often depend upon the care with which the following general measures are performed:

1. Bed rest in the medium Fowler (semisitting) position is preferred.

2. Nasogastric suction is started as soon as peritonitis is suspected, to prevent gastrointestinal distention. Suction is continued until peristaltic activity returns and the patient begins passing flatus. A self-tending sump tube should be used, but it must be checked frequently for patency. In persistent paralytic ileus, the intestinal tract may be more adequately decompressed by means of a long intestinal tube (eg, Miller-Abbott), although passage of such a tube into the small bowel is frequently difficult because of poor intestinal motility. In rare cases, combined gastric and long intestinal tube suction may be necessary to relieve or prevent distention.

3. Give nothing by mouth. Oral intake can be resumed slowly after nasogastric suction is discontinued.

4. Fluid and electrolyte therapy and parenteral feeding are required.

5. Narcotics and sedatives should be used liberally to ensure comfort and rest.

6. Antibiotic therapy– Initial antibiotic therapy should be broad-spectrum, aimed at covering aerobic and anaerobic enteric flora. When cultures are available, antibiotics are chosen according to sensitivity studies.

7. Blood transfusions are used as needed to control anemia.

8. Septic shock, if it develops, requires intensive treatment.

Prognosis

If the cause of peritonitis can be corrected, the infection, accompanying ileus, and metabolic derangement can usually be managed successfully.

PERIODIC DISEASE
(Benign Paroxysmal Peritonitis, Familial Mediterranean Fever, Periodic Fever, Recurrent Polyserositis)

Periodic disease is a heredofamilial disorder of unknown pathogenesis, probably metabolic, characterized by recurrent episodes of abdominal or chest pain, fever, and leukocytosis. It is usually restricted to people of Mediterranean ancestry, primarily Armenians, Sephardic Jews, and Arabs and to some extent people of Egypto-Arabic origin living in Turkey, Greece, and Italy. The disease suggests surgical peritonitis, but the acute attacks are recurrent, self-limited, and not fatal. Secondary amyloidosis (serum amyloid protein A-derived) may occur, and death may result from renal or cardiac failure. Acute episodes may be precipitated by emotional upsets, alco-

hol, or dietary indiscretion. Treatment is symptomatic and supportive. A low-fat diet may reduce the number and severity of attacks. Daily administration of colchicine, 0.6–1.8 mg, strikingly reduces the number of attacks.

Zemer D et al: Colchicine in the prevention and treatment of the amyloidosis of familial Mediterranean fever. N Engl J Med 1986;314:1001.

DISEASES OF THE MOUTH

DISCOLORED TEETH

The most common causes of discolored teeth are food stains, bacteria, tobacco use, and drugs. These can be managed by altering habits and by practicing dental prophylaxis. There may be pulpal hemorrhage induced by trauma, resulting in a deposition of hemosiderin on the internal crown surface. This causes a darkening of the tooth, which usually remains sterile and asymptomatic but nonvital. These teeth can be effectively bleached for aesthetic reasons. Occasionally, however, discoloration is due to changes in tooth structure caused by tetracyclines, congenital defects of enamel or dentin, fluorosis, and erythroblastosis fetalis.

Tetracycline discoloration occurs in some patients when these antibiotics are given during the period of tooth development, particularly in the fetus and during the first 8 years of life. Since an entire layer of dentin may be calcified in a few days, a small dosage over a short period may be incorporated into and appear to involve an entire tooth. The discoloration is gray-brown or yellow-brown and is permanent. A typical yellow fluorescence is seen under ultraviolet light.

Dental fluorosis occurs most frequently when the fluoride in the water supply exceeds 2 ppm (1 ppm is the recommended concentration). Fluorosis can also be caused when the daily ingestion of fluoride-vitamin combinations exceeds the recommended levels (maximum of 1 mg of fluoride). The frequency and intensity of the discoloration are proportionate to the concentration in the water and the amount consumed during tooth development. The discoloration can vary from chalky-white to yellow-brown stains, often irregular in appearance. These teeth can be effectively bleached as required with 30% hydrogen peroxide.

Rare hereditary congenital defects may cause brownish discoloration of the teeth. Treatment is primarily for aesthetic reasons.

ABSCESSES OF THE TEETH
(Periapical Abscess)

Dental decay is not self-limiting; unless it is removed, it will lead to infection of the pulp and subsequent periapical abscess. Pulp infection may also result from physical and chemical trauma. The only treatment is root canal therapy (cleansing and filling of the canal) or extraction.

In the early stage of pulp infection, the symptoms may not be localized to the infected tooth. Intermittent throbbing pain is usually present and is intensified by local temperature change. In the later putrescent stage, the pain is extreme and continuous and may be accentuated by heat but is often relieved by cold. After the infection reaches the bone, the typical syndrome is localization, pain upon pressure, and looseness of the tooth. Symptoms may then disappear completely, and, if drainage occurs, a parulis (gumboil) may be the only finding. When drainage is inadequate, swelling, pain, lymphadenopathy, and fever are often present. At this stage, antibiotics are advisable before local therapy is undertaken. Diagnosis depends upon symptoms, pulp testing (hot, cold, electricity), percussion, x-rays (may not show the diagnostic periapical radiolucency), looseness, deep decay or fillings, parulis, and swelling. Rule out sinusitis, neuralgia, and diseases affecting the cervical lymph nodes.

Incision and drainage are indicated whenever possible. Antibiotics and analgesics may be given as necessary. Unless contraindicated from a history of hypersensitivity, penicillin is the antibiotic of choice. Do not use antibiotic troches.

If not eventually treated by root canal therapy or extraction, the abscess may develop into a more extensive osteomyelitis or cellulitis (or both) or may eventually become cystic, expand, and slowly destroy bone without causing pain.

PERIODONTAL DISEASE

Periodontal disease is related to accumulations of microorganisms and substrate (plaque) on tooth surfaces. These may calcify and be recognized as calculus. Food, bacteria, and calculi that are present between the gums and teeth in areas called "dental pockets" may cause an inflammatory process and the formation of pus (pyorrhea) with or without discomfort or other symptoms. If this continues unchecked, the involved teeth will become loose and eventually will be lost as a result of resorption of supporting alveolar bone. If there is no drainage, accumulation of pus will lead to acute swelling and pain (lateral abscess).

The diagnosis depends upon a combination of findings, including localized pain, loose teeth, dental pockets, erythema, and swelling or suppuration. Radiography may reveal destruction of alveolar bone.

As in periapical abscess, the severity of signs and symptoms will determine the advisability of antibiotics. Local drainage and oxygenating mouth rinses (3% hydrogen peroxide in an equal volume of warm water) will usually reverse the acute symptoms and allow for routine follow-up procedures. Curettage or gingivectomy (or both) to reduce excess gum tissue helps prevent formation of the "dental pockets" that predispose to acute periodontal infections. In some cases, because of the advanced nature of the lesion (bone loss) or the position of the tooth (third molars in particular), extraction is indicated.

In some cases, periodontal disease occurs even in the presence of good hygiene and without obvious cause. Chronic progressive periodontal disease is a common finding in AIDS and is often an early sign or symptom of HIV infection. Programs of regular dental care (periodic curettage and gingival or bone procedures) and home care (brushing, flossing, and rinsing) to remove dental plaque will at least slow alveolar bone destruction. Chlorhexidine (Peridex) is a useful antiseptic mouth rinse.

Ciancio SG et al: Nonsurgical antibacterial approaches to periodontal treatment. J Am Dent Assoc 1988;116:22.
Williams RC: Periodontal disease. N Engl J Med 1990; 322:373.
Winkler JR, Murray PA: AIDS update: Periodontal disease. J Calif Dent Assoc 1987;15:20.

VINCENT'S INFECTION
(Necrotizing Ulcerating Gingivitis, Trench Mouth)

Vincent's infection is an acute inflammatory disease of the gums that may be accompanied by pain, bleeding, fever, and lymphadenopathy. It often is found to be caused by a synergistic infection with fusiform bacilli and spirochetes. It is common in young adults and may occur as a response to many factors such as poor mouth hygiene, inadequate diet and sleep, alcoholism, immunosuppression, and found associated with various other diseases such as infectious mononucleosis, thrush, blood dyscrasias, and diabetes mellitus. There is superficial gingival necrosis, resulting in pain and halitosis.

Management depends upon ruling out underlying systemic factors and treating the signs and symptoms as indicated with penicillin, oxygenating mouth rinses (3% hydrogen peroxide in an equal volume of warm water), analgesics, rest, and appropriate dietary measures. Refer the patient to a dentist for further treatment (eg, curettage).

Melnick SL et al: Epidemiology of acute necrotizing ulcerative gingivitis. Epidemiol Rev 1988;10:191.

APHTHOUS ULCER
(Canker Sore, Ulcerative Stomatitis)

Aphthous ulcers (canker sores) are the most common form of ulcerative stomatitis. Lesions are usually 1–2 mm in diameter but may be up to 10 times larger. They occur on unkeratinized mucosa, commonly buccal and labial, and are not found on gingiva, palate, and the dorsal tongue, which are keratinized epithelia. Lesions typically present as flat, round ulcerations, with yellow fibrinoid centers and a red halo. The painful stage can last up to a week. One or more ulcers may be present, and they tend to be recurrent. It has never been adequately demonstrated that this lesion is due to a virus or any other specific chemical, physical, or microbial agent. Aphthous ulcers probably represent an autoimmune reaction. Nuts, chocolates, and irritants such as citrus fruits often cause flare-ups of aphthous ulceration, but abstinence will not prevent recurrence. Aphthous ulcers may be associated with other conditions such as inflammatory bowel disease, Behcset's syndrome, infectious mononucleosis, and prolonged fever. The diagnosis depends mainly upon ruling out similar but more readily identifiable disease, a history of recurrence, and inspection of the ulcer.

Bland mouth rinses and hydrocortisone-antibiotic ointments reduce pain and encourage healing. Fluocinonide ointment (Lidex 0.05%) mixed in equal parts in an adhesive base (Orabase) has been particularly useful. Sedatives and analgesics may be of help. Vaccines and gamma globulins have not proved significantly beneficial. Although caustics relieve pain by cauterizing the fine nerve endings, they also cause necrosis and scar tissue. Systemic antibiotics are contraindicated. Systemic prednisone (20–60 mg/d) for a short period of time will accelerate healing and diminish pain.

Healing of mild aphthous attacks usually occurs in 1–3 weeks. Occasionally, aphthous ulcers take a more severe form, in which they are larger, persist sometimes for months, and may leave a scar. This form can be confused with carcinoma.

Ulcerative stomatitis is a general term for multiple ulcerations on an inflamed oral mucosa. It may be secondary to blood dyscrasias, erythema multiforme (allergies), bullous lichen planus, acute herpes simplex infection, pemphigoid, pemphigus, and drug reactions. If the lesions cannot be classified clinically or by laboratory tests, biopsy may be required.

Olson JA, Greenspan JS, Silverman S Jr: Recurrent aphthous ulcerations. J Calif Dent Assoc 1982;10:53.

Silverman S Jr, Lozada-Nur F, Migliorati C: Clinical efficacy of prednisone in the treatment of patients with oral inflammatory ulcerative diseases: A study of fifty-five patients. Oral Surg 1985;59:360.

HERPETIC STOMATITIS

Herpetic infections of the mouth can be primary (one episode) or secondary (recurrent attacks).

Primary gingivostomatitis due to herpesvirus hominis type 1 occurs in about 90% of the population before age 10. The disease has diverse manifestations, ranging from mild, almost unrecognizable signs and symptoms to multiple yellow-gray intraoral and lip ulcerations, erythema, edema, fever, cervical lymphadenopathy, and malaise. The course of the illness usually entails an increase in signs and symptoms for 1 week and then 1 week of progressive improvement as antibodies are produced (serum antibody titers will increase at least 4-fold). Because of severe pain, young children may not eat and may require intravenous hydration for the 4– and 10-day self-limited course. Adults who have never been infected or who have not developed adequate immunity may develop similar disease. Increasing susceptibility is seen in patients on immunosuppressive drugs. Infection with herpesvirus confers permanent immunity.

Herpetic gingivostomatitis must be differentiated from aphthous stomatitis, which is not due to a virus. The lesions of herpetic stomatitis can occur on any mucosal surface and almost always include the gingiva and often the lips The diagnosis is established by the history (no prior attack and short duration), characteristic signs and symptoms, and a confirmatory cytologic smear (pathognomonic pseudogiant cells). Direct cultures for herpes simplex virus are positive but impractical. Monoclonal antibody techniques for identifying the herpes simplex virus are accurate and quick.

There is no evidence that the disease is contagious; however, this might be explained by existing immunologic resistance among the contacts.

Treatment is palliative (analgesics, bland mouth rinses, fluids, soft diet, and rest). In the differential diagnosis, erythema multiforme, infectious mononucleosis, and pemphigus must be considered.

Recurrent intraoral herpetic infections are extremely rare and only occur on the mucosa covering bone (gingiva and palate). The ulcers are small, shallow, and irregular in size and shape. They can be mistaken for traumatic abrasions. There is no effective therapy; the infection is self-limiting within 2 weeks.

Herpes labialis (cold sore) is due to recurrent herpesvirus infections. These lesions usually have a burning premonitory stage and are first manifested by small vesicles that soon rupture and scab. Factors that trigger herpesvirus migration by nerve pathways to the lip range from unidentifiable stimuli to temperature changes, chemical and physical irritants, or "stress."

The diagnosis is based on the history and appearance of the lesions. The differential diagnosis includes carcinoma, syphilitic chancre, and erythema multiforme. No method of treatment has been uniformly successful. Improvement has been claimed with the use of idoxuridine and acyclovir ointments, chloroform, ether applications, lysine, and vitamin C.

When any of the above herpetic infections are severe, acyclovir (200 mg orally 5–6 times daily) may be helpful in shortening the clinical course, decreasing postherpetic pain, and preventing recurrences. In immunocompromised patients (those with HIV infection or those receiving immunosuppressive drugs), herpesvirus reactivation can be frequent, severe, and progressive and may present as atypical stomatitis. For these individuals, acyclovir (1–2 g daily) is indicated.

There is no firm evidence that type 1 herpesvirus is associated with oral carcinoma.

Corey L, Spear PG: Infections with herpes simplex viruses. (2 parts.) N Engl J Med 1986;314:686, 749.
Molinari JA, Merchant VA: Herpesviruses: Manifestations and transmission. J Calif Dent Assoc 1989;17:24.

OTHER VIRAL CAUSES OF STOMATITIS

In children, **herpes zoster** (varicella) oral mucosal vesicles and ulcers are occasionally seen in association with chickenpox on the face and trunk. Varicella is more common in the winter months and in children under 10 years of age.

Herpangina is caused by coxsackieviruses types A and B. It affects children under 6 years old, usually in summer. Abrupt onset of fever and dysphagia is accompanied by white-gray vesicular and ulcerative lesions 1–2 mm in diameter with surrounding bright red halos limited to the tonsillar fossae and soft palate.

Hand-foot-and-mouth disease, also caused by one or more coxsackieviruses and also occurring in young children usually in summer, is characterized by vesicular-ulcerative lesions on the lips and buccal mucosa. It is distinguished from herpangina by the presence of lesions on the soles and palms, accompanied by a transient erythematous rash.

Guy JT: Oral manifestations of systemic disease. Page 1231 in: *Otolaryngology: Head and Neck Surgery.* Cummings CW, Frederickson J (editors). Mosby, 1986.
Scully C: Infectious diseases in oral medicine: Review of the literature. Pages 135–190 in: *Perspectives on 1988 World Workshop on Oral Medicine.* Millard HD, Mason DK (editors). Year Book, 1988.

CANDIDIASIS
(Moniliasis, Thrush)

Thrush is due to overgrowth of *Candida* species (*C albicans* in more than 90% of cases). It is characterized by creamy-white curdlike patches anywhere in the mouth. The adjacent mucosa is usually erythematous. The white membrane is easily scraped off with a tongue depressor—unlike lichen planus or leukopla-

kia—and doing so often uncovers a raw, bleeding surface. Quite commonly, a candidal lesion may appear as a slightly granular or irregularly eroded erythematous patch. Pain is commonly present, as is halitosis and dysgeusia; fever and lymphadenopathy are uncommon. This fungus appears in about half of normal-appearing mouths, but overgrowth does not occur unless the "balance" of the oral microbial flora is disturbed.

Candidiasis is most commonly seen in denture wearers, with the appliances serving as a nutrient reservoir to foster fungal growth. It is also frequently seen in patients with debilitating or acute illness or in those being treated with broad-spectrum antibiotics, chemotherapy, and corticosteroids. Candidal growth also is favored by xerostomia (eg, after head and neck irradiation or the use of saliva-altering drugs), diabetes mellitus, anemia, and immunosuppressed status. Unexplained thrush in a high-risk group for AIDS is a portent of HIV infection (see Chapter 24). Concomitant candidiasis of the gastrointestinal tract (including the pharynx and the esophagus) may occur.

The diagnosis is based upon the varied clinical picture of surface white patches or erythematous changes and may be confirmed by culture. A wet preparation using potassium hydroxide frequently will reveal characteristic spores and sometimes the more suggestive mycelia. Biopsy from active lesions will often reveal pseudomycelia of *Candida* invading surface epithelium.

Treatment

Treatment is usually successful; however, the infection will often return in spite of treatment as long as causative factors are present. Local treatment often should be prolonged well beyond the period of signs or symptoms. Mouth rinses made up of equal parts of hydrogen peroxide and saline solution, 0.12% chlorhexidine (Peridex), or Listerine may provide local relief and promote healing. Specific antifungal therapy consists of any of the following: nystatin mouth rinses, 500,000 units 3 times daily (100,000 units/mL in a flavored vehicle), held in the mouth and then swallowed; nystatin vaginal troches (100,000 units) to be dissolved orally 5 times daily; clotrimazole troches (Mycelex) (10 mg) to be dissolved orally 5 times a day; ketoconazole tablets (Nizoral), 200–400 mg with breakfast for 7–14 days; and fluconazole tablets (Diflucan), 100 mg daily for 1–2 weeks. In denture wearers, nystatin powder (100,000 units/g) applied to the dentures 3–4 times daily for several weeks, can be helpful in reversing signs and symptoms.

Chronic angular cheilitis is often a manifestation of candidiasis, but it is also frequent in nutritional deficiency. It is best treated with nystatin powder or Mycolog (nystatin-triamcinolone acetonide) cream or 2% ketoconazole cream. Mucocutaneous candidiasis is rare and frequently does not respond well to any form of treatment, including immunostimulation.

Klein RS et al: Oral candidiasis in high-risk patients as the initial manifestation of the acquired immunodeficiency syndrome. N Engl J Med 1984;311:354.

Samaranayke LP: Oral candidosis: Predisposing factors and pathogenesis. Pages 219–235 in: *The 1989 Dental Annual*. Derrick DD (editor). Wright, 1989.

Silverman S: Fungal infections: Candidiasis. Pages 16–32 in: *Silverman's Color Atlas of Oral Manifestations of AIDS*. BC Decker, 1989.

LEUKOPLAKIA

Leukoplakia (a white patch) of the oral mucous membranes is occasionally a sign of carcinoma; it is important to rule out cancer. The most common cause of leukoplakia is epithelial hyperplasia and hyperkeratosis, usually in response to an irritant. In many cases the etiology cannot be determined.

Leukoplakia is usually asymptomatic. It is often discovered upon routine examination or by patients feeling roughness in their mouths. Because there is no reliable correlation between clinical features and microscopic findings, a definitive diagnosis may be established only by histopathologic examination. However, because of the extensiveness of some intraoral leukoplakias, cytologic smears and application of vital staining techniques (1% aqueous toluidine blue) are helpful in supplementing both clinical and biopsy information.

Remove all irritants (eg, tobacco, ill-fitting dentures). If the leukoplakia is not reversible, perform excision when feasible. Since some leukoplakias occur so diffusely that complete excision is impractical, careful examination and follow-up are essential. The diagnosis must be reaffirmed periodically, since a leukoplakia may unpredictably be transformed into a malignant tumor. Electrodesiccation, cryosurgery, vitamin A, and proteolytic enzymes have not been predictably effective. Removal utilizing the CO_2 laser has been effective.

When erythema or ulceration is associated with leukoplakia, the risk for dysplasia and carcinoma increases. Additionally, the diagnosis becomes more difficult since vesiculoerosive inflammatory diseases must be considered in the differential diagnosis.

Chu FW, Silverman S Jr, Dedo HH: CO_2 laser treatment of oral leukoplakia. Laryngoscope 1988;98:125.

Silverman S Jr et al: Oral leukoplakia and malignant transformation: A follow-up study of 257 patients. Cancer 1984;53:563.

SIALADENITIS

Acute inflammation of a parotid or submandibular salivary gland is usually due to viral or bacterial infection or, less commonly, blockage of the duct. The gland is swollen and tender. Observation of Wharton's and Stensen's ducts may show absent or scanty secretion, with fluctuation of swelling, especially during meals, which indicates blockage; or a turbid secretion, which suggests infection. Clinical examination and x-ray may disclose ductal or glandular calcific deposits. Sialograms are of help in differentiating normal and diseased glands. Probing the ducts may reveal an inorganic plug or organic stenosis.

Dryness of the mouth (xerostomia) may be due to inflammation of the salivary glands as well as mouth breathing, dehydration, anticholinergic and psychotropic drugs, Sjodgren's syndrome, and radiation injury (see Glossodynia, Glossopyrosis, below).

Tumors may be confused with nonneoplastic inflammation. In these situations, biopsy (usually excisional) should be performed, but only after other diagnostic and therapeutic procedures have failed to yield a diagnosis. Fine-needle aspiration biopsies have been reliable and do not interfere with subsequent treatment. Neoplasms are usually not associated with an acute onset and, at least in the early phases, are not painful. The lymph nodes are intimately associated with the salivary glands, and consideration must be given to diseases in which lymphadenopathy is a prominent finding, eg, lymphomas and metastatic cancer. Salivary gland enlargement may also be due to autoimmune inflammation and hyperplasia, such as is Sjodgren's syndrome, diabetes, and HIV infection.

In the acute stage, antibiotics, heat, and analgesics are indicated. Ductal stones that are too large for removal by massage and manipulation must be removed surgically (when the acute phase has subsided). If calcification or infection of the gland recurs often, extirpation of the gland must be considered. Radiation therapy may be effective in curing acute or recurrent sialadenitis that does not respond to other types of therapy.

Blitzer A: Inflammatory and obstructive disorders of salivary glands. J Dent Res 1987;66:675.

Sreebny LM, Valdini A, Yu A: Xerostomia: Relationship to non-oral symptoms, drugs, and diseases. Oral Surg Oral Med Oral Pathol 1989;68:419.

GLOSSITIS

Inflammation of the tongue (usually associated with partial or complete loss of the filiform papillae, which creates a red, smooth appearance) may be secondary to anemia, nutritional deficiency, drug reactions, infections, dehydration, and physical or chemical irritations. Treatment is based on identifying and correcting the primary cause if possible and palliating the tongue symptoms as required. Many obscure cases are due to such conditions as geographic tongue and autoimmune reactions.

The diagnosis is usually based on the history and laboratory studies, including cultures as indicated.

Empiric therapy may be of diagnostic value in obscure cases.

When the cause cannot be determined and there are no symptoms, therapy is not indicated.

Dreizen S: The telltale tongue. Postgrad Med (March) 1984;75:150.

GLOSSODYNIA, GLOSSOPYROSIS
(Chronic Lingual Papillitis)

Burning and pain, which may involve the entire tongue or isolated areas and may occur with or without glossitis, may be associated findings in hypochromic or pernicious anemia, nutritional disturbances, or diabetes mellitus and may be the presenting symptoms. Xerostomia, drugs (frequently diuretics), and candidiasis may be responsible. Smoking can be a causative irritant. Allergens (eg, in dentifrices) are rare causes of tongue pain. Certain foods may cause flare-ups but are not the primary causes. Dental prostheses, caries, and periodontal disease are usually of not causative significance.

Although most cases occur in postmenopausal women, these disorders are neither restricted to this group nor indicative of hypoestrogenemia.

In most cases a primary cause cannot be identified. Cultures are of no value, since the offending organisms are usually present also in normal mouths. Many clinicians believe that these symptoms occur on a primarily functional basis.

Treatment is mainly empiric, since causative factors usually are not identified. Important approaches include ruling out systemic conditions sometimes associated with these symptoms, changing the drugs being given for other disorders, and reassuring patients that there is no evidence of infection or neoplasia. Ointments and mouth rinses are of no value.

Partial xerostomia may be remedied by sucking on nonmedicated sugarless troches or by the administration of pilocarpine, 10–20 mg daily in divided doses, or bethanechol, 100–200 mg daily in divided doses. Saliva substitutes have been of little value.

Gorsky M, Silverman S Jr, Chinn H: Burning mouth syndrome: A review of 98 cases. J Oral Med 1987;42:7.
Powell FC: Glossodynia and other disorders of the tongue. Dermatol Clin 1987;5:687.

PIGMENTATION OF GINGIVAE

Abnormal pigmentation of the gingiva is most commonly a racially controlled melanin deposition in the epithelial cytoplasm. It is most prevalent in nonwhite peoples. The color varies from brown to black, and the involvement may be in isolated patches or a diffuse speckling. Nongenetic causes include epithelial or dermal nevi (rare), drugs (eg, bismuth, arsenic, mercury, or lead), and amalgam fragments that become embedded in the gums during dental work. (Mercury from this source has not been determined to be a health hazard.) Similar lesions may also appear during the menopause or in Addison's disease, intestinal polyposis, neurofibromatosis, and several other disorders associated with generalized pigmentations.

The most important consideration is to rule out malignant melanoma (extremely rare in the mouth), which is suggested by rapid growth, slight elevation, and marked discoloration.

Buchner A, Hansen LS: Pigmented nevi of the oral mucosa: A clinicopathologic study of 32 new cases and review of 75 cases from the literature. Oral Surg 1980;49:55.

ORAL CANCER

Cancers of the lips, tongue, floor of the mouth, buccal mucosa, palate, gingivae, and oropharynx account for about 4% of all cancers. Carcinoma of the tongue is the most frequent site. Estimates from various surveys indicate that the average 5-year survival rate for all patients with oral cancer is less than 50%. However, with early detection, the 5-year survival rates and morbidity rates are markedly improved. (By definition, detection is "early" when lesions are less than 3 cm in size, without evidence of metastases.) Therefore, early diagnosis followed by adequate treatment appears to be the most effective means of controlling oral cancer.

Squamous cell carcinoma is the most common type, accounting for over 90% of all oral cancers. Oral cancer is a disease of older people; over 90% of all cases occur after age 45, and the average age is about 60. The male/female ratio is about 2:1.

The cause of oral cancer is not known. A genetic factor is not apparent. There is a definite increased risk with the use of tobacco and alcohol. Oral leukoplakia is an important precancerous lesion.

Red to purple mucosal lesions on the gingiva, palate, and tongue in patients with high-risk factors (homosexuals, bisexuals, intravenous drug abusers) may be due to Kaposi's sarcoma associated with AIDS. The oral cavity is a frequent site of Kaposi's sarcoma and may represent the only affected tissue. The lesions may be flat or nodular, the latter usually being symptomatic.

Clinical Findings
There are no reliable signs or symptoms in early oral carcinoma, although pain is the most frequent first complaint. An early cancer may appear as a small white patch (leukoplakia), an aphthouslike or traumatic ulcer, an erythematous plaque, or a small swelling. Biopsy is the only method of definitely diagnosing a carcinoma. However, immediate biopsy

of every ill-defined or innocuous-appearing lesion is impractical and not indicated. Exfoliative cytology is a simple, reliable, and acceptable means of differentiating benign and early malignant neoplasms. In the case of small lesions whose gross appearance would be altered by biopsy, the clinician who will give the treatment should see the lesion before the biopsy is taken in order to determine the extent of resection or radiation required. Staining with 1% toluidine blue, with subsequent binding to dysplastic and malignant epithelium, has been very helpful in early detection and selection of biopsy sites. Lymph nodes should not be incised for biopsy for fear of causing dissemination of tumor cells. Fine-needle aspiration biopsy is expedient and accurate.

Treatment

Curative treatment consists of surgery and radiation, alone or in combination. An attempt should be made to save the teeth necessary to support prostheses. The periodontium is maintained in optimal condition by periodic routine dental procedures. When areas that have been directly in the beam of irradiation are treated, extreme care is exercised and antibiotics may be selectively administered. Frequent fluoride applications appear to aid in minimizing tooth decalcification and caries. Alterations of taste and saliva may be permanent. Pilocarpine solution, 5 mg 2–4 times daily, or bethanechol, 25 mg tablets, 100–200 mg daily in divided doses, will often selectively increase salivation. Salivary substitutes may be of limited help in some patients.

Decker J, Goldstein JC: Current concepts in otolaryngology: Risk factors in head and neck cancer. N Engl Med 1982;306:1151.

Silverman S: HIV-associated malignancies. Pages 65-80 in: *Silverman's Color Atlas of Oral Manifestations of AIDS*. BC Decker, 1989.

Silverman S Jr: Early diagnosis of oral cancer. Cancer 1988;62:1796.

DISEASES OF THE ESOPHAGUS

REFLUX ESOPHAGITIS
(Peptic Esophagitis)

Essentials of Diagnosis

- Substernal burning, cramping, severe pain, or pressure (any or all).
- Symptoms aggravated by recumbency or increase of abdominal pressure; relieved by upright position.
- Nocturnal regurgitation, cough, dyspnea, aspiration may be present.

General Considerations

Reflux esophagitis results from regurgitation of gastric contents into the esophagus. Acid, pepsins, or bile reflux is essential in pathogenesis. Hyperemia or exudates with erosions are seen at endoscopy in 70% of those with biopsy-proved esophagitis. The pathophysiology includes a permanently or intermittently incompetent lower esophageal sphincter, frequency and duration of reflux, and the inability of the esophagus to generate secondary peristaltic waves that normally prevent prolonged contact of the mucosa with acid and pepsin. A hiatal hernia may or may not be present. The presence of a concentric or sliding hiatal hernia is of no consequence unless it is associated with reflux.

Clinical Findings

A. Symptoms and Signs: Pyrosis ("heartburn") is the most common symptom and is inconstantly indicative of the degree of esophagitis that is secondary to reflux. It is frequently severe, occurring 30–60 minutes after eating, and is initiated or accentuated by recumbency and relieved by sitting upright. Pain at the lower sternal level or xiphoid frequently radiates into the interscapular area, neck, jaw, or down the arms and may be indistinguishable from angina pectoris.

The symptoms are the result of reflux of acid or alkaline gastric contents into the esophagus because of an incompetent lower esophageal sphincter or some degree of gastric outlet obstruction. The conditions associated with an incompetent esophageal sphincter are hiatal hernia, pregnancy, obesity, recurring or persistent vomiting, nasogastric tubes, and Raynaud's phenomenon. Other symptoms include water brash (combination of regurgitation and increased salivation), hoarseness, globus, dysphagia, and odynophagia due to diffuse spasm, stricture, or ulceration; hematemesis; and melena. Iron deficiency anemia may occur with chronic occult bleeding. Aspiration may cause cough, dyspnea, and perhaps asthma or pneumonitis.

B. Imaging: Esophageal reflux may be seen at fluoroscopy at the time of barium study. Unless stricture, ulcer, or motor abnormalities are present, esophagitis usually cannot be diagnosed by x-ray. In some patients, reflux may be impossible to document by radiographic techniques.

C. Special Examinations: Most patients with reflux can be managed effectively with the usual measures set forth below. Patients who do not respond fully or have atypical or complicated presentations should be investigated further.

1. Acid perfusion test (Bernstein)–During perfusion of the distal esophagus with 0.1-N HCl, the patient's symptoms will be reproduced if due to esophagitis. Control perfusion with 0.9% saline solution should be performed first. This is best done in conjunction with esophageal manometry (see below).

2. Peroral endoscopy–Thirty percent of patients with symptoms of esophagitis will have normal-appearing mucosa upon endoscopic inspection of the esophagus. Biopsy of the mucosa (at least 3 cm proximal to the esophagogastric junction) will establish the diagnosis of esophagitis in most of these patients. Biopsy can identify those with Barrett's esophagus (see below). All patients with complaints of dysphagia should undergo esophagoscopy.

3. Esophageal manometry–This test is useful for assessing lower esophageal sphincter function, the ability of the esophagus to clear refluxed acid, and the presence of esophageal dysmotility. Symptomatic patients with no functioning lower esophageal sphincter are usually surgical candidates.

4. Esophageal pH monitoring–This is the most objective means of demonstrating esophageal reflux and the clearing time of refluxed acid—a determinant of esophagitis. pH is best monitored on a 24–hour basis with a portable "Holter-like" monitor. It is currently considered the "gold standard" for determining the frequency and duration of reflux and its relevance to the patient's symptoms.

Differential Diagnosis

The differentiation of the retrosternal chest pain of esophagitis from that of angina pectoris or myocardial infarction may require sequential ECGs, enzyme determinations, and close clinical observation. Gastroduodenal ulcer disease, presenting with similar symptoms, can usually be distinguished by radiographic or endoscopic study. Less common—but an important differential—- is the acute pain of localized esophagitis or an esophageal ulcer due to dry swallowing of medications: tetracyclines, quinidine, and aspirin, among others.

Complications

Esophagitis, stricture, and esophageal ulcer are the most common complications. Hoarseness, bronchospasm, and chronic pulmonary disease are being increasingly recognized as sequelae of esophageal reflux. Gastritis in the herniated portion of the stomach is sometimes a cause of occult bleeding and anemia.

Treatment

A. General Measures: Since obesity is often an associated or precipitating factor in esophagitis, weight reduction is essential. Other conditions that predispose to increased intra-abdominal pressure, eg, tight belts or corsets, should be avoided. The patient should also be advised to avoid lying down immediately after meals and to sleep with the head of the bed elevated 20–25 cm with wooden blocks. Medication should be taken with an ample amount of water, preferably when the patient is upright. Foods that decrease lower esophageal sphincter pressure should be avoided as much as possible, eg, dietary fat, chocolate, peppermint, and possibly caffeine. Tobacco and alcohol also decrease lower esophageal sphincter pressure and are best avoided. Many patients become symptomatic when they ingest citrus or tomato products or chocolate and should avoid these foods.

B. Medical Measures:

1. Antacids–One ounce taken 1 and 3 hours after meals and at bedtime is effective in neutralizing residual acidic peptic gastric contents. Combination antacids containing aluminum hydroxide, magnesium salts (hydroxide, carbonate, or trisilicate), or alginic acid, 1 or 2 tablets chewed thoroughly after meals and at bedtime, may be effective in relieving the effects of reflux.

2. Histamine H_2 receptor blockers–Ranitidine (Zantac) is the only H_2 receptor blocker approved for peptic esophagitis. The dose is 300 mg at dinnertime or twice daily.

3. Proton pump inhibitor (gastric)–Omeprazole, 20 mg/d, is a potent inhibitor of basal and stimulated gastric secretion and is the most effective drug to date for inducing healing of peptic esophagitis— 81% at 4 weeks versus 6% for placebo. Relapse rate after discontinuation of the medicine is high. The drug has FDA approval for only short-term (8-week) use.

4. Cholinergic agents–Bethanechol chloride, 10–20 mg at mealtime, may increase esophageal and gastric motility and speed gastric emptying, thereby decreasing reflux.

5. Gastrointestinal stimulants–Metoclopramide (Reglan), 10–20 mg/d, will increase the rate of gastric and esophageal emptying by stimulating the smooth muscle of the intestine. Metoclopramide may produce agitation in some patients.

C. Surgical Measures: Antireflux operations may be indicated in a small number of patients who have persistent or recurrent symptoms despite adequate medical therapy. The most commonly performed antireflux procedure is Nissen fundoplication, which produces good results though with some recurrences reported after 5 years. Placement of an Angelchik ring around the distal esophagus in the infradiaphragmatic region is still occasionally done. The long-term results of this procedure are unknown.

Prognosis

Most patients (85–90%) with esophagitis respond to management of weight reduction, antacids, elevation of the head of the bed, and other nonsurgical measures. Even those with strictures (see below) can usually be managed successfully with these measures plus bougienage. For those who cannot be managed medically, fundoplication produces good results in most instances.

Harvey RF et al: Effects of sleeping with the bed-head raised and of ranitidine in patients with severe peptic oesophagitis. Lancet 1987;2:1200.
Hetzel DJ et al: Healing and relapse of severe peptic

esophagitis after treatment with omeprazole. Gastroenterology 1988;95:903. (Very effective, but relapse occurs rapidly after treatment is discontinued.)

Irwin RS et al: Chronic cough as the sole presenting manifestation of gastroesophageal reflux. Am Rev Respir Dis 1989;140: 1294. (Increases the range of clinical concerns for patients with reflux.)

Smith JL et al: Sensitivity of the esophageal mucosa to pH in gastroesophageal reflux disease. Gastroenterology 1989;96:683.

Ward PH et al: Complications of gastroesophageal reflux. West J Med 1988;149:58.

BARRETT'S ESOPHAGUS

Barrett's esophagus is a disorder in which the esophagus is lined with columnar epithelium for varying lengths. It probably represents a response of the esophagus to reflux injury. The symptoms are pyrosis or dysphagia. The incidence of this condition is 3 times greater in males than in females. The entity should be thought of when there is radiographic evidence of a high, benign esophageal stricture or discrete "peptic ulcer." Esophagoscopy and biopsy are required to establish the histologic characteristics.

Treatment is the same as for esophagitis. These patients have about a 10% lifetime risk of developing adenocarcinoma in this abnormal epithelium. Criteria for follow-up are unclear, but upper endoscopy with biopsies—looking for neoplasm or dysplasia—at 1- to 2-year intervals appears reasonable at this time. The columnar epithelium may regress after successful antireflux surgery, possibly decreasing the chance of malignant degeneration.

Ovasak J, Miettinen M, Kivilaakso E: Adenocarcinoma arising in Barrett's esophagus. Dig Dis Sci 1989;34:1336.

Reid BJ et al: Endoscopic biopsy can detect high-grade dysplasia or early adenocarcinoma in Barrett's esophagus without grossly recognizable neoplastic lesions. Gastroenterology 1988;94:81.

Winters C Jr et al: Barrett's esophagus: A prevalent, occult complication of gastroesophageal reflux disease. Gastroenterology 1987;92:118.

INFECTIOUS ESOPHAGITIS

Infectious esophagitis usually occurs in immunosuppressed or immunodeficient patients and is manifested by odynophagia, which may be so severe that saliva cannot be swallowed. Self-limited herpes esophagitis has been reported in otherwise normal patients. Patients with candidal esophagitis usually have oral thrush; those with herpes or cytomegalovirus infection may have oral lesions.

The presence of oral thrush in the characteristic clinical setting requires no further diagnostic efforts unless concomitant cytomegalovirus, herpes, or cryptosporidial infection is considered a possibility, eg,

when therapy for candidiasis has been unsuccessful. Endoscopy with biopsy and brushings for culture is then indicated. In the absence of oral thrush, the diagnosis is best made by endoscopy with biopsy.

Treatment

A. For *Candida* Infection: Give ketoconazole, 400–600 mg orally daily for 6 weeks, followed by 200 mg orally daily for life (in immunocompromised patients). In many immunocompromised patients, ketoconazole absorption is poor secondary to low gastric acid output and can be enhanced by the co-administration of 100 mL of 0.1-N HCl. In treatment failures, low-dose amphotericin B, 10–15 mg intravenously over a 2-week period, may be effective.

B. For Herpes Simplex Infection: Give acyclovir, 350 mg intravenously every 8 hours for 7 days.

C. For Cytomegalovirus Infection: Give ganciclovir (DHPG), 5 mg/kg intravenously every 8 hours for 20 days, or longer if necessary.

D. For *Cryptosporidium* Infection: No effective treatment is available.

Course & Prognosis

The esophagitis can usually be controlled. The prognosis is that of the underlying disease.

Byard RW, Champion MC, Orizaga M: Variability in the clinical presentation and endoscopic findings of herpetic esophagitis. Endoscopy 1987;19:153.

Lake-Bakaar G et al: Gastropathy and ketoconazole malabsorption in the acquired immunodeficiency syndrome (AIDS). Ann Intern Med 1988;109:471. (0.1 N HCl with ketoconazole restored ketoconazole absorption to normal.)

CORROSIVE ESOPHAGITIS

Essentials of Diagnosis

- History of ingestion of corrosive substance.
- Oral, pharyngeal, or substernal pain.
- Odynophagia.
- Evidence of mucosal injury.

General Considerations

This disorder results from inadvertent or deliberate (suicidal) ingestion of a liquid or crystalline alkali (Plumber's Helper, Drano, etc) or acid (toilet bowl cleaners, hydrochloric acid, etc) substance.

Clinical Findings

There is usually an almost immediate sensation of severe burning pain of the oropharynx. Gagging secondary to spasm of the cricopharyngeus is common, and some of the material may be regurgitated. Much of the ingested material will traverse the esophagus, causing burning substernal pain that may last for days. The stomach is often affected as well.

Physical findings may include obvious mucosal

burns of the lips, mouth, or hypopharynx as well as acute distress due to the pain. Drooling is common. In severe cases, marked hypotension and a shocklike state may be present. With ammonia or formaldehyde ingestion, the odor will be apparent.

Treatment

Treatment is supportive, with fluids plus narcotics for pain relief. Avoid maneuvers that may induce vomiting, so that there will be no secondary mucosal exposure to the noxious material. Administration of water by mouth may help dilute the corrosive substance. No antidotes are available, and nasogastric tubes are to be avoided because of the risks of inducing retching and perforation.

Indications for peroral endoscopy are controversial. Perhaps endoscopy is most helpful in patients with a history of ingestion and a normal-appearing oropharynx, in whom endoscopy can help determine the extent of injury, if any. In patients with obvious oropharyngeal burns and substernal chest pain, little appears to be gained by endoscopy.

Although corticosteroids and antibiotics have been used in cases of acute corrosive esophagitis, there is no clear justification for these agents in the published reports. Severe injuries may require esophagogastrectomy with colon interposition.

Course & Prognosis

Mild to moderate burns of the esophagus usually heal without sequelae. Patients with more severe injuries have a small risk of perforation in the short term and a greater risk of stricture formation in the long term. If the stricture is localized, it can often be managed with bougienage. If it is long and tight, surgical replacement of the esophagus with colon interposition may be necessary.

Yakshe PN, Benjamin SB: An overview of caustic ingestion. Contemp Gastroenterol 1989;2:50.

BENIGN STRICTURE OF THE ESOPHAGUS

Healing of any inflammatory lesion of the esophagus may result in stricture formation. Common causes are peptic esophagitis secondary to gastroesophageal reflux, indwelling nasogastric tube, Barrett's epithelium and ulcer formation, ingestion of corrosive substances, acute viral or bacterial infectious diseases, sclerotherapy of varices, and, rarely, injuries caused by endoscopes.

The principal symptom is dysphagia, which may not appear for years after the initial result. Ability to swallow liquids is maintained the longest.

Odynophagia (painful swallowing) occurs not infrequently in association with dysphagia (difficult swallowing). The patient's description of the point at which the "hang-up" of food is perceived conforms with amazing accuracy to the level of the obstruction.

Radiographic demonstration of smooth narrowing with no evidence of mucosal irregularity is usually diagnostic. However, esophagoscopy, biopsy, and cytologic examination are mandatory in all cases to rule out the possibility of cancer.

Dilatation is the definitive form of treatment, using Puestow dilators, mercury-filled (Maloney or Savary) bougies, or balloon dilatation to attain a lumen size of 44–60F. However, both patient and physician must be prepared for continuing bougienage, since recurrence of stenosis may occur if dilatation is terminated once swallowing again becomes normal. Monthly passage of the largest bougie the patient can tolerate usually prevents regression. If dilatation is unsuccessful, surgical replacement of the esophagus with a segment of stomach, jejunum, or colon will be indicated.

Bonavina L et al: Drug-induced esophageal strictures. Ann Surg 1987;206:173. (Quinidine and tetracycline commonly implicated.)
Patterson DJ et al: Natural history of benign esophageal stricture treated by dilatation. Gastroenterology 1983; 85:346.

LOWER ESOPHAGEAL RING (Schatzki's Ring)

The finding of a static but distensible lower esophageal ring signifies the presence of a sliding hiatal hernia that may or may not be symptomatic. Most rings histologically represent the esophagogastric junction. Manometric studies have also confirmed that the lower esophageal ring physiologically represents the point at which the esophagus and stomach meet. Some rings can be purely esophageal in origin.

The classic ring is 4 mm or less in thickness, is composed of a connective tissue core with muscularis mucosae, and is covered on the upper side by squamous epithelium and on the lower side by columnar epithelium. Submucosal fibrosis is present, but esophagitis is usually absent. Significant gastroesophageal reflux is not present.

Not all lower esophageal rings are mucosal in nature. Some are due to muscular contractions of the esophagus. Distention of the lower esophagus with barium does not obliterate a mucosal ring but accentuates it. Dysphagia is usually present when the ring reduces the internal esophageal lumen to a diameter of 13 mm of less and is often present with a diameter of 18 mm or less.

Most rings can be seen at endoscopy with fiberoptic instruments and can frequently be successfully treated simply by passing an esophagoscope through the ring, thereby dilating it. With a tight ring, one or 2 biopsies can be taken around its circumference, followed either by endoscopic bougienage or bougienage with mer-cury-filled dilators.

Ott DJ et al: Review: Esophagogastric region and its rings. AJR 1984;142:281.

MOTILITY DISORDERS OF THE ESOPHAGUS

Motility disorders of the esophagus range from absent peristalsis (aperistalsis) to hyperperistalsis and spasm. Combinations of all of these with abnormal lower or upper esophageal sphincter function complete the clinical picture. The abnormalities as determined by radiography or esophageal manometry may be either symptomatic or asymptomatic.

Aperistalsis of the Esophagus

This is absence of motor activity of the esophagus as determined fluoroscopically and, more precisely, by esophageal motility/manometry studies. The clinical corollary may be a sensation of esophageal fullness, dysphagia, or symptoms of reflux with heartburn. Aperistalsis is commonly associated with Raynaud's phenomenon (80%) and thus is common in patients with scleroderma (about 80%), systemic lupus erythematosus (20–25%), and polymyositis (10–15%). Aperistalsis may also occur in the elderly.

The clinical consequences of aperistalsis are failure to clear refluxed gastric contents, leading to esophagitis, decreased lower esophageal sphincter function, and, in some cases, esophageal ulceration and stricture. The scleroderma patient, in addition to having aperistalsis, usually has dysfunction of the lower esophageal sphincter secondary to muscle displacement by the fibrosing process, leading to an incompetent sphincter and increased reflux.

Management is basically that of reflux esophagitis and should be anticipatory, ie, before symptoms appear, in patients likely to have aperistalsis and an incompetent lower esophageal sphincter (eg, patients with Raynaud's phenomenon or scleroderma).

Presbyesophagus

This refers to the radiographic demonstration of esophageal dysmotility as characterized by nonpropulsive contractions (tertiary contractions), usually as an incidental finding during an upper gastrointestinal study. Presbyesophagus is usually asymptomatic and requires no therapy.

Diffuse Esophageal Spasm

Symptomatic diffuse esophageal spasm is characterized by substernal pain or dysphagia or both. The pain may be indistinguishable from angina and may include radiation of pain into the neck, jaws, right arm, left arm, or to the back. There may be hypersalivation and reflux of recently swallowed food. A spe-cific cause is seldom found, but there may be associated reflux esophagitis. Very cold or very hot foods may trigger an episode. Diffuse esophageal spasm may be part of the spectrum of achalasia (see below).

Radiographically and endoscopically, vigorous nonpropulsive esophageal contractions are noted. Manometrically, they may be high-pressure sustained, nonpropulsive contractions. Diagnosis is essentially based on the clinical picture, since all of the objective findings can be seen in asymptomatic patients. A high resting lower esophageal sphincter pressure is common, but, as is not the case in achalasia, the sphincter will relax normally.

Sublingual nitroglycerin is usually effective for the acute episode, and long-acting nitroglycerin (isosorbide)—or both—are often effective. In severely symptomatic patients unresponsive to medical management, a long esophageal myotomy may prove helpful.

Nutcracker Esophagus

This condition presents similarly to diffuse esophageal spasm but manometrically is characterized by high-pressure (> 175 mm Hg) propulsive contractions that are often of prolonged duration. Medical management is as for symptomatic diffuse esophageal spasm.

Achalasia of the Esophagus

Achalasia is a motor disorder of the esophagus characterized by loss of primary peristalsis, presence of a hypertonic lower esophageal sphincter that does not relax in response to a swallow, and evidence of denervation of the esophagus as shown by an exaggerated esophageal response to cholinergic agents (Cannon's law of denervation). It is, in part, the result of impaired integration of parasympathetic stimulation. There is difficulty in swallowing both liquids and solids, at first of variable frequency and degree but later usually persistent and severe and characterized by dysphagia, occasional odynophagia, frequent regurgitation of food, and dilatation of the esophagus, as shown by radiography. Although achalasia may appear in infancy or old age, it most commonly afflicts patients in the third to fifth decades. It may predispose to esophageal carcinoma.

Two types of achalasia of the esophagus can be defined by differences in pathologic anatomy, symptoms, and radiographic findings. The first type (about 75% of cases) is characterized by a beaklike narrowing of the distal 2–4 cm of the esophagus. The more proximal portion is markedly dilated and tortuous, with the ultimate appearance of an elongated sigmoid configuration. Stasis of intraluminal contents is responsible for varying degrees of esophagitis. Patients with this form of achalasia characteristically experience dysphagia without chest pain. However, regurgitation may cause aspiration, with resultant pneumonitis, bronchiectasis, lung abscess, or pulmonary fibrosis.

The second form of achalasia, vigorous achalasia,

is characterized by recurring esophageal spasm, which may result in retrosternal and subxiphoid pain with frequent associated dysphagia or hypersalivation. The circular muscle of the esophagus appears hypertrophied, and the dilatation proximal to the lower esophageal sphincter is not as marked as with the first type of achalasia.

Dysphagia may initially be intermittent, with food apparently sticking at the level of the xiphoid cartilage, and is associated with variable discomfort in the retrosternal or subxiphoid areas. Precipitation or accentuation of difficult swallowing may inconstantly follow the ingestion of solids or cold beverages and may be related to emotionally stressful situations. Continued esophageal dilatation with retention of food and liquids results in a sensation of fullness behind the sternum. Pain (when present) may also radiate to the back, neck, and arms and may occur independently of swallowing. Increased hydrostatic pressure within the esophagus will overcome the high resting pressure of the lower esophageal sphincter, and patients should therefore drink extra water and perform the Valsalva maneuver so that the esophageal contents will more readily enter the stomach. However, prolonged impairment of alimentation may cause varying degrees of malnutrition.

Radiographic diagnosis is based on the characteristic tapering of the distal esophagus in a conical fashion to a markedly narrowed distal segment, 1–3 cm long, which usually lies above the diaphragm. Fluoroscopy, cinefluorography, and films of the proximal esophagus reveal purposeless and ineffectual contractions as well as varying degrees of dilatation. Esophageal fluid levels may be evident on routine chest x-ray. Recent studies indicate that as many as 50% of these patients have additional pharyngeal and upper esophageal sphincter abnormalities on videofluoroscopy. Esophageal motility and manometric studies provide characteristic findings and are usually required to establish a diagnosis of achalasia, particularly in the radiologically less well defined case.

After the patient has consumed a clear liquid diet for 24–36 hours and undergone preendoscopic aspiration and lavage, esophagoscopy needs to be performed at least once in every case of achalasia to ascertain the severity of esophagitis and to eliminate the possibility of occult carcinoma.

Passage of a pneumatic dilator under fluoroscopic guidance—designed to split muscle fibers of the lower esophageal sphincter—has been recommended as appropriate nonsurgical treatment. Passage of mercury-filled bougies is only a short-term palliative measure at best. Treatment of achalasia with long-acting nitrates (eg, isosorbide dinitrate) or calcium channel blockers (eg, nifedipine), which lower the resting pressure of the lower esophageal sphincter, has met with modest success. Esophagocardiomyotomy is ultimately required in approximately 20–25% of patients.

Upper Esophageal Sphincter Dysfunction

A hypotensive upper esophageal sphincter has on occasion been associated with the "lump in the throat" sensation as well as reflux of stomach contents into the mouth. Esophageal reflux is being increasingly associated with the globus sensation (lump in throat) as well as with hoarseness. In the elderly patient with cervical dysphagia, the upper esophageal sphincter usually functions normally, but there is ineffective swallowing, most likely due to a lacunar or larger cerebrovascular accident. The gag reflux in this latter setting is often decreased or absent.

The hypertensive upper esophageal sphincter, often with poor relaxation on deglutition, is associated with dysphagia and may well be the underlying abnormality that gives rise to Zenker's diverticulum—a posterior out-pouching of the cervical esophagus just cephalad to the upper esophageal sphincter. These diverticula may harbor inspissated food, giving rise to halitosis, regurgitation of food eaten 1 or 2 days before, and increasing dysphagia secondary to pressure on the esophagus. What appears to be a hypertensive upper esophageal sphincter may actually be related to poor pharyngeal contraction.

Management of these disorders is difficult. For the hypotensive upper esophageal sphincter, little but antireflux measures can be offered. For the stroke patient with dysphagia, a feeding tube (nasogastric or gastric) can be offered to provide nutrition until there is return of function. For the hypertensive upper esophageal sphincter that is symptomatic or with an associated Zenker's diverticulum, surgical myotomy is the treatment of choice. Lower esophageal sphincter dysfunction should be excluded first.

Chuong JJH et al: Achalasia as a risk factor for esophageal carcinoma: A reappraisal. Dig Dis Sci 1985;29:1105.

Csendes A et al: Late subjective and objective evaluation of the results of esophagomyotomy in 100 patients with achalasia of the esophagus. Surgery 1988;104:469. (Twenty percent had postoperative reflux.)

DiPalma JA, Meyer GW: A rational clinical approach to esophageal motor disorders. Dysphagia 1987;2:97.

Jones B et al: Pharyngeal findings in 21 patients with achalasia of the esophagus. Dysphagia 1987;2:87.

Kahrilas PJ et al: Upper esophageal sphincter functions during deglutition. Gastroenterology 1988;95:52. (Current understanding of physiology.)

Richter JE, Barish CF, Castell DO: Abnormal sensory perception in patients with esophageal chest pain. Gastroenterology 1986;91:845.

ESOPHAGEAL DIVERTICULA

Essentials of Diagnosis

- Dysphagia progressing as more is eaten; bad breath, foul taste in mouth.

- Regurgitation of undigested or partially digested food representing first portion of a meal.
- Radiography (barium) confirms diagnosis.

General Considerations

The clinical picture and pathologic effects of an esophageal diverticulum are to a large extent dictated by the location of the lesion. It is therefore convenient to distinguish pharyngoesophageal (pulsion or Zenker's), midesophageal (traction), and epiphrenic (traction-pulsion) diverticula by their locations. The first (pharyngoesophageal) develops through the space at the junction of the hypopharynx and esophagus just proximal to the cricopharyngeal sphincter, occurs chiefly in middle-aged men, and may attain large size. The second (midesophageal) type rarely is larger than 2 cm, may be multiple, frequently arises opposite the pulmonary hilar region, occurs with equal frequency in men and women, and usually causes no symptoms. The third and least common (epiphrenic) type occurs primarily in men in the esophageal segment immediately proximal to the hiatus, may be congenital in origin, and progressively enlarges, so that symptoms develop in middle age. Pharyngoesophageal and epiphrenic diverticula frequently produce nocturnal regurgitation and aspiration, with resultant bronchitis, bronchiectasis, and lung abscess.

Clinical Findings

A. Symptoms and Signs: The main symptoms of pharyngoesophageal (Zenker's) diverticula are dysphagia, regurgitation, gurgling sounds in the neck, nocturnal coughing, halitosis, and weight loss. Enlargement of the pouch results in its downward dissection between the postesophageal septum of the deep cervical fascia and the prevertebral fascia. When filled with food, the pouch may appear as a swelling at the side of the neck and internally may cause compression and obstruction of the proximal esophagus. There is occasionally so much compression of the esophagus that its entrance becomes slitlike, making it difficult to find endoscopically, and this readily explains the difficulty in swallowing and impaired nutrition.

Epiphrenic diverticula, which are occasionally associated with peptic strictures, usually cause no symptoms at first but ultimately may produce dysphagia, pain, and pulmonary complications.

Although midesophageal diverticula may rarely be responsible for mediastinal abscess or esophagobronchial fistulas and inconstantly may cause dysphagia, these lesions generally produce no symptoms.

B. Imaging: Barium swallow will usually demonstrate the 3 types of diverticula.

Differential Diagnosis

Regurgitation and difficult swallowing associated with diverticula must be distinguished from that caused by neoplasm, vascular anomalies, strictures, or motility dysfunction of the esophagus. Epiphrenic diverticula must also be differentiated from esophageal ulcer. Physical examination, radiography, and endoscopy will clarify the diagnosis.

Treatment & Prognosis

Large and symptom-producing pharyngoesophageal and epiphrenic diverticula should be treated surgically by amputation. Although recurrence or postoperative dysphagia is occasionally seen following operation for the former, long-term results are usually excellent. Cricopharyngeal sphincter myotomy has been advocated for pharyngoesophageal diverticula secondary to an abnormal sphincter. Since midesophageal pouches rarely produce complications or significant symptoms, therapy is usually not required.

Maran AG, Wilson JA, Al Muhanna AH: Pharyngeal diverticula. Clin Otolaryngol 1986;11:219.

CARCINOMA OF THE ESOPHAGUS

In the USA, carcinoma of the esophagus is predominantly a disease of men in the fifth to eighth decades. It usually arises from squamous epithelium. There is increased incidence of squamous cell carcinoma of the esophagus among smokers and in association with other otolaryngologic neoplasms. Stasis-induced inflammation such as is seen in achalasia or esophageal stricture and chronic irritation induced by excessive use of alcohol seemingly are etiologically important in the development of this neoplasm. Malignant tumors of the distal esophagus are frequently adenocarcinomas that originate in the stomach and spread cephalad. Conversely, squamous cell carcinoma of the esophagus rarely invades the stomach. Primary adenocarcinoma of the esophagus is much less common and probably arises in Barrett's epithelium. Regardless of cell type, the prognosis for cancer of the esophagus is usually poor.

Clinical Findings

A. Symptoms and Signs: Dysphagia, which is progressive and ultimately prevents swallowing of even liquids, is the principal symptom. Anterior or posterior chest pain that is unrelated to eating implies local extension of the tumor, whereas significant weight loss over a short period is an ominous sign.

B. Imaging: Barium swallow is positive for an irregular, frequently annular space-occupying lesion. CT scan of the esophagus can delineate extraesophageal involvement (eg, mediastinum, lymph nodes).

C. Special Examinations: Esophagoscopy, biopsy, and cytologic examination are confirmatory.

Differential Diagnosis

Achalasia can be differentiated by endoscopy, esophageal manometry, and cinefluorography. Since there is a significant association of stricture with malignant neoplasms, any narrowing of the lumen should be evaluated by esophagoscopy and biopsy.

Treatment & Prognosis

Although it was once considered a hopeless disease, improvements during the last 2 decades in anesthesia, surgical techniques, radiation therapy, and adjuvant chemotherapy have improved survival rates of patients with esophageal carcinoma. Adjuvant chemotherapy using cisplatin, vindesine, and bleomycin with radiation or surgery appears to improve the course and length of survival in this disease. After dilatation of tumor-bearing portions of the esophagus, effective palliation can often be accomplished by the use of prosthetic tubes that are inserted through the mouth to facilitate swallowing. Cure rates are still dismal, however, and do not exceed 5–10%.

Gastrostomy may improve nutrition but does not prolong survival, and the inability of completely obstructed patients to swallow even saliva makes the operation of questionable value for palliation. Anticancer drugs have not proved to be of value.

DeMeester TR, Barlow AP: Surgery and current management for cancer of the esophagus and cardia. Curr Probl Surg 1988;25:541.

Roth JA et al: Randomized clinical trial of preoperative and postoperative adjuvant chemotherapy with cisplatin, vindesine, and bleomycin for carcinoma of the esophagus. J Thorac Cardiovasc Surg 1988;96:242.

BENIGN NEOPLASMS OF THE ESOPHAGUS

Benign tumors of the esophagus are quite rare and are generally found accidentally by either the radiologist or endoscopist or the prosector in the lower half of the esophagus. The most common of the benign neoplasms is the leiomyoma, which arises from one of the smooth muscle coats of the esophagus. This lesion may be circumferential or multiple, gradually increases in size (up to 2–2.5 cm), and may ultimately compromise the esophageal lumen or normal peristalsis, producing dysphagia. Other uncommon benign tumors are fibromas, lipomas, myoblastomas, lymphangiomas, hemangiomas, and schwannomas. The diagnosis is made by barium swallow and esophagoscopy. Cytologic examination is not helpful, and biopsy may be inadequate because these lesions are submucosal. Surgical removal is curative.

ESOPHAGEAL WEBS

Esophageal webs are thin membranous structures that include in their substance only mucosal and submucosal coats. They are occasionally congenital but more commonly appear to be the sequelae of ulceration, local infection, hemorrhage, or mechanical

trauma. Cervical vertebral exostoses are sometimes mentioned as a common cause. Most webs are found in the proximal portion of the esophagus and produce significant dysphagia with occasional laryngospasm secondary to aspiration. Difficult swallowing secondary to a web—when combined with iron deficiency anemia, splenomegaly, glossitis, and spooning of the nails and occurring almost invariably in premenopausal women—is called Plummer-Vinson syndrome. In this condition, a diaphanous web is usually located immediately below the cricopharyngeus and is associated with an atrophic pharyngoesophagitis. Esophagoscopy (essential to rule out carcinoma) ameliorates dysphagia by disrupting the web. Bougienage with Maloney or Hurst dilators may occasionally be necessary.

MALLORY-WEISS SYNDROME (Mucosal Lacerations of the Esophagus or Cardioesophageal Junction)

Forceful or prolonged vomiting, retching, coughing, or other forceful Valsalva-like maneuver followed by the vomiting of bright red blood suggests Mallory-Weiss syndrome. The bleeding is due to a vertical tear involving the mucosa of the cardioesophageal junction or, more commonly, the most proximal portion of the stomach. A hiatal hernia is frequently present. The diagnosis is based on the history of vomiting followed by hematemesis and confirmed by endoscopic demonstration of the mucosal tear. Usually no active intervention is required, as most lesions stop bleeding spontaneously. If concomitant esophagitis or esophageal varices are present, the bleeding may be more prominent. In a third of cases, the classic history of bleeding after vomiting is not present. Endoscopic hemostatic techniques occasionally (heater probe, injection with 1:10,000 epinephrine) or surgery rarely may be required to control bleeding.

Sugawa C et al: Mallory-Weiss syndrome: A study of 224 patients. Am J Surg 1983;145:30.

DISEASES OF THE STOMACH

GASTRITIS

Gastritis is a descriptive term often used by clinicians for vague, self-limited illnesses characterized by nausea, anorexia, epigastric distress with or without vomiting, and some systemic symptoms. For the gastroenterologist, gastritis is an endoscopic finding of varying specificity seen both with and without associated clinical symptoms. For the pathologist, gastritis means the presence of inflammatory cells, acute or chronic (or both)—as well as the organism *Helicobacter pylori*—in the gastric mucosa with or without additional mucosal abnormalities.

There are many causes of gastritis.

Clinical Findings

A. Symptoms and Signs: The manifestations of gastritis are variable depending on the cause, but persistent anorexia is often a major feature. Epigastric fullness or easy satiety as well as nausea and vomiting may be present. Upper gastrointestinal bleeding, occasionally major, may occur, particularly with drug-, stress-, or corrosive-induced erosive hemorrhagic gastritis. In patients with gastritis secondary to acute infections or bacterial toxins (staphylococcal toxin), malaise, diarrhea, colic, fever, chills, and headache may be associated, with resultant dehydration. Examination may show epigastric tenderness.

B. Laboratory Findings: The laboratory findings may be normal or may reflect the underlying process—infectious, hemorrhagic, etc.

C. Special Examinations: For those who present with acute upper gastrointestinal hemorrhage, early endoscopy (within 24 hours) permits accurate identification of the source: hemorrhagic erosive gastritis, drug-induced ulcerations, etc. The clinical preendoscopic diagnosis of the source of bleeding is correct no more than half the time. In patients with corrosive gastritis, endoscopy permits determination of the extent of injury. In the dyspeptic patient with normal radiographic studies who is unresponsive to the usual treatment, peroral endoscopy may demonstrate the presence or absence of motility disorders or mucosal abnormalities.

Differential Diagnosis

Conditions such as peptic ulcer, neoplasms, cholecystitis, esophageal spasm, angina pectoris, abdominal angina, pancreatic disease, and psychologic gastrointestinal disorders must be considered.

Treatment & Prognosis

A. Drug-Induced Gastritis: Remove the offending agent. If bleeding is a major part of the clinical picture—ie, requiring transfusion—serious consideration must be given to administration of platelets, since the endogenous platelets are ineffective for up to 5 days after stopping aspirin. Sucralfate, 1 g 30–60 minutes before meals 3 times a day and at bedtime, or a liquid antacid, 30 mL, 60 minutes after a meal, is often effective. In the absence of ulcer disease, a week's course should be sufficient.

B. Gastric Ulcer-Associated Gastritis: Gastritis is almost always present in patients with peptic gastric ulcer. The treatment is that of the ulcer.

C. Stress Gastritis: This is best managed by prevention. In the stressed noneating patient (burn center, intensive care unit), gastric ulcer should be prevented by hourly titrations of the intragastric pH to at least 4.0–5.0. This is achieved by instillation of antacids or by continuous intravenous infusion of an H_2 antagonist (the usual bolus dose given by infusion) after an initial bolus dose or, in the enterally fed patient, by continuous nasogastric infusion of the liquid diet (Ensure, Osmolyte, etc). There is evidence that in the nonfed patient, sucralfate, 1 g every 4–6 hours, is equally effective, with a lower incidence of aspiration pneumonia, when compared to the gastric acid-suppressed patient.

Once the patient has developed erosive bleeding gastritis, support with transfusions and intragastric neutralization with antacids or H_2 antagonists seem reasonable. Sucralfate may be of benefit as well.

D. Gastritis Associated With Aging: Endoscopically, many individuals past age 65 have what is termed "chronic gastritis" or "atrophic gastritis," often verified by biopsy as a thinning of the mucosa and decrease in the glandular elements. These conditions are rarely symptomatic and require no treatment unless there is associated malabsorption of vitamin B_{12}.

E. Idiopathic Gastritis: Endoscopic evaluation of epigastric distress commonly discloses varying degrees of erythema and mucosal irregularities without erosions or bleeding. Biopsies often will show an increase in chronic inflammatory cells, occasionally polymorphonuclears, and the organism *Helicobacter pylori*. The role of *H pylori*, a gram-negative rod, is still unsettled, but increasing evidence suggests that it may be etiologic in antral gastritis and may play a role in peptic ulcer disease.

Rare causes of gastritis include sarcoidosis, tuberculosis, syphilis, eosinophilia, Crohn's disease, and Meaneatrier's disease.

F. Postgastrectomy Gastritis: Symptomatic postgastrectomy gastritis is uncommon, though acute gastritis (redness) is frequently seen by endoscopy at the anastomosis. When more extensive gastritis is seen, it is often associated with bile reflux (see below) or uncommonly with a bezoar. Owing to poor gastric motility there is a tendency after resection for vegetable bezoars to form, and this not only helps produce a mechanically induced gastritis but causes sensations of fullness, obstruction, and easy satiety. The bezoar can usually be broken with the endoscope. Kanulase tablets, which contain the enzyme cellulase (9 mg per tablet), are often helpful in breaking down the cellulose of a vegetable/fruit bezoar. Two tablets every 2–3 hours during the day for a week may be necessary. Avoidance of large quantities of cellulose-containing foods is important.

G. Bile Reflux: This is an occasional cause of severe gastritis after pyloroplasty or gastric resection, particularly following Billroth II anastomosis. It is characterized by almost constant epigastric pain, and endoscopy shows a fiery red mucosa. Although bile sequestrants have been tried, they have been at best only marginally successful. If symptoms persist, operation is necessary and consists of implanting the afferent loop 25–40 cm below the gastrojejunostomy so that bile does not bathe the gastric pouch. The success rate with this procedure is high but less than 100%.

H. Acute Corrosive Esophagitis and Gastritis: Ingestion of corrosive substances is most common in children but may occur in cases of attempted suicide. The substances most commonly swallowed are strong acids (sulfuric, nitric), alkalies (lye, potash), oxalic acid, iodine, bichloride of mercury, arsenic, silver nitrate, and carbolic acid. The esophagus is most severely injured. Gastric changes vary from superficial edema and hyperemia to deep necrosis and sloughing or even perforation.

Corrosion of the lips, tongue, mouth, and pharynx, along with pain and dysphagia due to esophageal lesions, is usually present. Nitric acid causes brown discoloration; oxalic acid causes white discoloration of mucous membranes. There is severe epigastric burning and cramping pain, nausea and vomiting, and diarrhea. The vomitus is often blood-tinged. Severe prostration with a shocklike picture and thirst may occur. Palpation of the abdomen may show epigastric tenderness or extreme rigidity. Leukocytosis and mild proteinuria are present.

Immediate treatment is supportive, including analgesics, intravenous fluids and electrolytes, sedatives, and antacids. Although the specific antidote (see Chapter 33) should be administered immediately, supportive measures must not be neglected. The benefit to be expected from the antidote appears minuscule if a large amount of corrosive has been ingested, and the benefit is doubtful considering that tissue damage occurs almost immediately. Avoid emetics and lavage if corrosion is severe, because of the danger of perforation.

The outcome depends upon the extent of tissue damage. Fiberoptic endoscopy may serve to determine the extent of injury. Emergency laparotomy may be indicated to resect the area of gangrene and potential perforation. If alkali has been ingested, prednisone, 20 mg every 8 hours started immediately, may prevent esophageal stricture. This dose should be tapered slowly over several weeks.

After the acute phase has passed, place the patient on a peptic ulcer regimen. If perforation has not occurred, recovery is the rule. However, pyloric stenosis may occur early or late, requiring gastric aspiration, parenteral fluid therapy, and surgical intervention.

The amount of the corrosive substance, its local and general effects, and the speed with which it is removed or neutralized determine the outcome. If the patient survives the acute phase, gastric effects are usually overshadowed by esophageal strictures, although chronic gastritis or stricture formation at the pylorus may follow.

Dilawari JB et al: Corrosive acid ingestion in man: Clinical and endoscopic study. Gut 1984;25:183.

Dooley CP et al: Prevalence of *Helicobacter pylori* infection and histologic gastritis in asymptomatic persons. N Engl J Med 1989;321:1526. (Clinical pertinence still unclear.)

Driks MR et al: Nosocomial pneumonia in intubated patients given sucralfate as compared with antacids or histamine type 2 blockers: The role of gastric colonization. N Engl J Med 1987;317:1376.

Katzka DA, Sunshine AG, Cohen S: The effect of nonsteroidal anti-inflammatory drugs on upper gastrointestinal tract symptoms and mucosal integrity. J Clin Gastroenterol 1987;9:142.

Niemelad S et al: Characteristics of reflux gastritis. Scand J Gastroenterol 1987;22:349.

PEPTIC ULCER

A peptic ulcer is an acute or chronic benign ulceration occurring in a portion of the digestive tract that is accessible to gastric secretions. An active peptic ulcer does not occur in the absence of acid-peptic gastric secretions. Other than the requirement for acid and pepsin, the cause of peptic ulcer at any level of the gut remains obscure.

Other factors in peptic ulceration (besides the presence of gastric acid) include hypersecretion of hydrochloric acid (in only one-third of duodenal ulcer patients) and decreased tissue resistance.

Peptic ulcer may occur during the course of drug therapy (salicylates and other nonsteroidal anti-inflammatory drugs, reserpine). It may occur as a result of critical illness or severe tissue injury such as extensive burns or intracranial surgery (stress ulcer), and may be associated with endocrine tumors producing gastrin, which stimulates hypersecretion of hydrochloric acid and results in a very refractory peptic ulcer diathesis (Zollinger-Ellison syndrome, gastrinoma).

Graham DY: Campylobacter pylori and peptic ulcer disease. Gastroenterology 1989;96:615. (A possible cause.)

Griffin MR, Ray WA, Schaffner W: Nonsteroidal anti-inflammatory drug use and death from peptic ulcer in elderly persons. Ann Intern Med 1988;109:359. (Increased risk in the elderly.)

1. DUODENAL ULCER

Essentials of Diagnosis

- Epigastric distress 45–60 minutes after meals, or nocturnal pain, both relieved by food, antacids, or vomiting. Epigastric tenderness and guarding.
- Chronic and periodic symptoms.
- Gastric analysis shows acid in all cases and hypersecretion in some.
- Ulcer crater or deformity of duodenal bulb on x-ray or with oral endoscopy.

General Considerations

The incidence of duodenal ulcer has been declining at a rate of about 8% per year for the past decade. It still remains a major health problem. Although the average age at onset is 33 years, duodenal ulcer may occur at any time from infancy to the later years. It is now almost equally common in males and females. Occurrence during pregnancy is unusual.

Duodenal ulcer is 2–3 times as common as benign gastric ulcer.

About 95% of duodenal ulcers occur in the duodenal bulb or cap. The remainder are between this area and the ampulla. Ulcers below the ampulla are rare. The ulceration varies from a few mm to 1–2 cm in diameter and extends at least through the muscularis mucosae, often through to the serosa and into the pancreas. The margins are sharp, but the surrounding mucosa is often inflamed and edematous. The base consists of granulation tissue and fibrous tissue, representing healing and continuing digestion.

Clinical Findings

A. Symptoms and Signs: Symptoms may be absent, or vague and atypical. In the typical case, pain is described as gnawing, burning, cramplike, or aching, or as "heartburn"; it is usually mild to moderate, located over a small area near the midline in the epigastrium near the xiphoid. The pain may radiate below the costal margins, into the back, or, rarely, to the right shoulder. Nausea may be present, and vomiting of small quantities of highly acid gastric juice with little or no retained food may occur. The distress usually occurs 45–60 minutes after a meal; is usually absent before breakfast; worsens as the day progresses; and may be most severe between 12 midnight and 2:00 AM It is relieved by food, milk, alkalies, and vomiting, generally within 5–30 minutes.

Spontaneous remissions and exacerbations are common. Precipitating factors are often unknown but may include trauma, infections, or physical or emotional distress.

Signs include superficial and deep epigastric tenderness, voluntary muscle guarding, and unilateral (rectus) spasm over the duodenal bulb.

B. Laboratory Findings: Bleeding, hypochromic anemia, and occult blood in the stools may occur in chronic ulcers; amylase may be elevated if there is posterior penetration. Gastric analysis shows acid in all cases and a basal and maximal gastric hypersecretion of hydrochloric acid in some.

C. Imaging: An ulcer crater is demonstrable by radiography in 50–70% of cases but may be obscured by deformity of the duodenal bulb. When no ulcer is demonstrated, the following are suggestive of ulceration: (1) irritability of the bulb, with difficulty in retaining barium there, (2) point tenderness over the bulb, (3) pylorospasm, (4) gastric hyperperistalsis, and (5) hypersecretion or retained secretions.

D. Special Examinations: Peroral endoscopy has proved a valuable adjunct in the diagnosis of duodenal ulcer not demonstrated radiographically. It may also reveal duodenitis, a disorder that may have a pathogenetic mechanism in common with duodenal ulcer.

Differential Diagnosis

When symptoms are typical, the diagnosis of peptic ulceration can be made with assurance; when symptoms are atypical, duodenal ulcer may be confused clinically with functional gastrointestinal disease, gastritis, gastric carcinoma, and irritable colon syndrome. The final diagnosis often depends upon x-ray or endoscopic observation.

Complications

A. Intractability to Treatment: Most cases of apparently intractable ulcer are probably due to an inadequate medical regimen or failure of cooperation on the part of the patient. The designation "intractable" should be reserved for patients who have received an adequate supervised trial of therapy. The possibility of gastrinoma as well as complications of the ulcer must always be considered.

B. Hemorrhage Due to Peptic Ulcer: Hemorrhage is caused either by erosion of an ulcer into an artery or vein or, more commonly, by bleeding from granulation tissue. Most bleeding ulcers are on the posterior wall. The sudden onset of weakness, faintness, dizziness, chills, thirst, cold moist skin, desire to defecate; and the passage of loose, tarry, or even red stools with or without coffee-ground vomitus are characteristic of acute duodenal ulcer hemorrhage.

The blood findings (hemoglobin, red cell count, and hematocrit) lag behind the blood loss by several hours and may give a false impression of the quantity of blood lost. Postural hypotension and tachycardiac and central venous pressure are more reliable indicators or hypovolemia than the hematocrit.

C. Perforation: Perforation occurs almost exclusively in men 25–40 years of age. The symptoms and signs are those of peritoneal irritation and peritonitis; ulcers that perforate into the lesser peritoneal cavity cause less dramatic symptoms and signs. A typical description of perforated peptic ulcer is an acute onset of epigastric pain, often radiating to the shoulder or right lower quadrant and sometimes associated with nausea and vomiting, followed by a lessening of pain for a few hours and then by boardlike rigidity of the abdomen, fever, rebound tenderness, absent bowel sounds, leukocytosis, tachycardia, and even signs of marked prostration. Radiographic demonstration of free air in the peritoneal cavity confirms the diagnosis.

D. Penetration: Extension of the crater beyond the duodenal wall into contiguous structures but not into the free peritoneal space occurs fairly frequently with duodenal ulcer and is one of the important causes of failure of medical treatment. Penetration usually occurs in ulcers on the posterior wall, and extension is usually into the pancreas; but the liver, biliary tract, or gastrohepatic omentum may be involved.

Radiation of pain into the back, night distress, inadequate or no relief from eating food or taking alkalies, and, in occasional cases, relief upon spinal flexion and aggravation upon hyperextension—any or all of these findings in a patient with a long history of duodenal ulcer usually signify penetration.

E. Obstruction: Minor degrees of pyloric obstruction are present in about 20–25% of patients with duodenal ulcer, but clinically significant obstruction is much less common. The obstruction is generally caused by edema and spasm associated with an active ulcer, but it may occur as a result of scar tissue contraction even in the presence of a healed ulcer.

The occurrence of epigastric fullness or heaviness and, finally, copious vomiting after meals—with the vomitus containing undigested food from a previous meal—suggests obstruction. The diagnosis is confirmed by the presence of an overnight gastric residual exceeding 50 mL containing undigested food, and x-ray evidence of obstruction, gastric dilatation, and hyperperistalsis. A succussion splash on pressure in the left upper quadrant may be present, and gastric peristalsis may be visible.

Treatment

Currently, antacids, histamine H_2 receptor antagonists, and sucralfate have all been shown to be equally effective in the treatment of duodenal ulcers when compared with placebos. These regimens provide symptomatic relief in the vast majority of patients. Less clear has been the therapeutic efficacy of various dietary measures. The limiting factor with existing therapies is that although the ulcers heal, the ulcer diathesis remains and recurrence rates are high.

A. Acute Phase:

1. General measures–The patient should be educated concerning the disease and encouraged to have adequate rest and sleep, and it may sometimes be necessary to recommend 2 or 3 weeks' rest from work if that can be managed. In some instances, if the home situation is unsuitable or if the patient is unable to cooperate, hospitalization is recommended.

Alcohol, a gastric secretagogue and irritant, should be strictly forbidden. The patient should also quit smoking, since smoking has been shown to markedly decrease the healing rate of duodenal ulcer even when optimal treatment is being given.

Reserpine, salicylates, and all other nonsteroidal anti-inflammatory analgesics may aggravate peptic ulcer or may even cause perforation and hemorrhage.

2. Diet–All controlled clinical studies have documented that neither the type nor the consistency of diet will affect the healing of ulcers. The important principles of dietary management of peptic ulcer are as follows: (1) nutritious diet; (2) regular meals; and

(3) restriction of coffee, tea, cola beverages, decaffeinated coffee, and alcohol.

In the acute phase, when there is partial gastric outlet obstruction, it is often useful to begin with a full liquid diet, provided that 1-hour postprandial gastric residuals are less than 100 mL.

It is doubtful that dietary measures other than elimination of known aggravating factors play a significant role in preventing ulcer recurrence.

3. Antacids–Antacids usually relieve ulcer pain promptly. Antacid dosage should be selected on the basis of neutralizing capacity. The response to antacids varies widely according to the preparation, the dosage, and the individual patient. Tablet preparations must be thoroughly chewed and dissolved to have effectiveness.

In order to be effective, antacids must be taken frequently. During the acute phase, a full dose 1 and 3 hours after meals and at bedtime should be sufficient. If pain relief is not achieved on this regimen, the stomach is emptying too rapidly or the patient is secreting more acid that the antacid can neutralize. (Suspect Zollinger-Ellison syndrome.)

Magnesium hydroxide-aluminum hydroxide mixtures (many preparations available) are effective and widely used antacids. The usual dose is 30 mL. When full therapeutic doses are given, the magnesium in the mixtures may produce diarrhea; it may be necessary to alternate with a straight aluminum hydroxide gel preparation (eg, Alternagel), which tends to be constipating. Prolonged ingestion of aluminum hydroxide gel may lead to phosphate depletion and osteoporosis. Magnesium salts should be used cautiously in patients with renal insufficiency.

Calcium carbonate has an excellent neutralizing action and may be used at times when the magnesium-aluminum gel antacids are inadequate. Antacid mixtures containing aluminum hydroxide, calcium carbonate, and magnesium hydroxide are available (Camalox), and the usual dose is 15–30 mL. A paradoxic calcium-induced gastric hypersecretion has been reported but probably has no clinical significance with this combination agent. However, when calcium carbonate (Tums) alone is used, there may be hypercalcemia and its attendant complications.

4. Sucralfate (Carafate)–This nonabsorbable aluminum salt of sucrose octasulfate is a mucosal protective agent that has antipepsin activity and tends to adhere to areas of gastric and duodenal mucosal injuries, eg, ulcers. It is as effective with duodenal ulcer as antacids or H_2 receptor blockers and has the advantage of being nonsystemic. The only side effect reported to date is mild constipation in about 5% of patients. Dosage is 1 g 30–60 minutes before meals and at bedtime or 2 g 30–60 minutes before breakfast and dinner. Antacids may be used when necessary but not within 1 hours of sucralfate.

5. Histamine H_2 receptor antagonists–

a. Cimetidine (Tagamet)–This drug markedly

inhibits gastric secretion stimulated by food, gastrin, histamine, and caffeine. Cimetidine is approved in the USA for short-term treatment of duodenal ulcer and gastric ulcer, for use in preventing recurrence of duodenal ulcer (up to 1 year), for management of Zollinger-Ellison syndrome, and for treatment of other hypersecretory states such as systemic mastocytosis. The dosage is 300 mg 4 times daily before meals and at bedtime or 800 mg after dinner. An alternative dosage is 400 mg twice daily. The dose must be reduced by half in patients with renal insufficiency. An intravenous form is available. The dosage, depending on the indication, is 50 mg/h after an initial 300-mg bolus dose.

Rare side effects have included gynecomastia, galactorrhea, impotence, skin rashes, leukopenia, agranulocytosis, hepatitis, elevated serum creatinine, decreased IgA and IgM, and confusion in the elderly. Of more concern are interactions between cimetidine and warfarin, theophylline, lidocaine, phenytoin, and other drugs, which occur via the P-450 cytochrome system of the liver.

b. Ranitidine (Zantac)–This H_2 receptor antagonist is more potent than cimetidine and interferes less than cimetidine with the metabolism of drugs that use the P-450 cytochrome system of the liver. Ranitidine is of value in treatment of duodenal ulcer, benign gastric ulcer, gastric reflux disease, and Zollinger-Ellison syndrome. The dosage is 150 mg every 12 hours or 300 mg at dinnertime. An intravenous form of ranitidine is available; the dosage is 8.3 mg/h by continuous infusion after an initial bolus dose of 50 mg. The dose must be reduced by half in patients with renal insufficiency.

Rare side effects have included mild serum transaminase elevation (more common with intravenous administration), decreases in white blood cell and platelet counts, false-positive tests for proteinuria with Multistix, and some increase in headaches. Gynecomastia and impotence secondary to cimetidine have reversed when ranitidine is substituted. There have been no reports of galactorrhea.

c. Famotidine (Pepcid)–This H_2 receptor antagonist is more potent than either ranitidine or cimetidine. The full therapeutic dose is 40 mg at dinnertime. Because of this agent's longer half-life, the intravenous dose of 20 mg every 12 hours is claimed to be equivalent to the same dose by constant infusion; however, in our experience, the drug is best given by constant infusion, ie, a 20-mg bolus followed by 2 mg/h.

d. Nizatidine (Axid)–Similar to the other H_2 antagonists. The dose for active disease is 300 mg after dinner.

6. Parasympatholytic (anticholinergic) drugs–Although the parasympatholytic drugs have been widely used over a long period of time for treatment of peptic ulcer, their effectiveness is questionable. The dosage necessary to produce significant gastric antisecretory effect may cause blurring of vision, constipation, urinary retention, and tachycardia. Anticholinergic drugs should be avoided in patients with glaucoma, esophageal reflux, gastric ulcer, pyloric obstruction, cardiospasm, gastrointestinal hemorrhage, bladder neck obstruction, or serious myocardial disease.

7. Proton pump inhibitor (gastric)–Omeprazole, 20 mg/d, induces achlorhydria or near achlorhydria in most ulcer patients and has been reported to hasten duodenal ulcer healing. Relapse rates are no different from those reported with other agents. The drug is not yet approved by the FDA for use in patients with peptic ulcer.

B. Convalescent Phase: Once the diagnosis is established, it is unnecessary to repeat the gastrointestinal series unless complications develop. The patient should be informed about the chronic and recurrent nature of the illness and warned about the consequences of inadequate treatment. Although the cause of ulcer recurrence is not known, it may be associated with use of alcohol, tobacco, emotional stress, and infections, particularly of the upper respiratory tract. The patient should be instructed to return to the ulcer regimen if symptoms recur or if conditions known to aggravate the ulcer cannot be avoided. Antacids or other medications should be readily available.

C. Treatment of Complications:

1. Hemorrhage–Institute immediate emergency measures for treatment of hemorrhage and shock (see p 403).

2. Perforation–Acute perforation constitutes a surgical emergency. Immediate surgical repair, preferably by simple surgical closure, is indicated. More extensive operations may be unwise at the time of the acute episode because of the increased operative hazard due to the patient's poor physical condition. If the patient has had no previous therapy or if previous therapy has been inadequate, conservative medical treatment should be instituted after the surgery.

The morbidity and mortality rates depend upon the amount of spillage and especially the time lapse between perforation and surgery. Surgical closure of the perforation is indicated as soon as possible. If surgery is delayed beyond 24 hours, gastric suction, antibiotics, and intravenous fluids are the treatment of choice.

3. Obstruction–Obstruction due to spasm and edema can usually be treated adequately by gastric decompression and ulcer therapy; obstruction due to scar formation requires surgery. It must be remembered that the obstruction may not represent a complication of an ulcer but may be due to a primary neoplastic disease, especially in those patients with no history or only a short history of peptic ulcer.

a. Medical measures (for obstruction due to spasm or edema) consist of bed rest, preferably in a hospital; continuous gastric suction for 72 hours; and parenteral administration of electrolytes and fluids.

After 72 hours, test the degree of residual obstruction with the saline load test. Instill 700 mL of normal saline into the stomach with the patient at least sitting, and aspirate the contents after 30 minutes. If less than 200 mL is recovered, begin liquid feeding. If the residual volume is greater than 200 mL, obstruction is still present and the patient is usually a surgical candidate. Do not use anticholinergic drugs, since they delay gastric emptying. Give sedative-tranquilizer drugs and a progressive diet as tolerated. Use antacids as with uncomplicated ulcer.

b. Surgical measures (for obstruction due to scarring) are indicated only after a thorough trial of conservative measures.

Prognosis

Duodenal ulcer tends to have a chronic course with remissions and exacerbations. Many patients can be adequately controlled by medical management. About 25% develop complications, and 5–10% ultimately require surgery for obstruction, uncontrollable pain, or recurrent bleeding. The recurrence rate is substantially reduced if the patient stops smoking and is given an H_2 receptor blocking agent at dinnertime or sucralfate twice a day for at least 1 year.

Collier DSJ, Pain JA: Non-steroidal anti-inflammatory drugs and peptic ulcer perforation. Gut 1985;26:359.

Gustavsson S et al: Trends in peptic ulcer surgery: A population-based study in Rochester, Minnesota, 1956–1985. Gastroenterology 1988;94:688.

Lam SK et al: Sucralfate overcomes adverse effect of cigarette smoking on duodenal ulcer healing and prolongs subsequent remission. Gastroenterology 1987;92:1193.

McQuaid KR, Isenberg JI: Duodenal ulcers: New views on pathophysiology and treatment. Contemp Intern Med (October) 1989, p 42.

Mulholland MW, Debas HT: Recent advances in the treatment of duodenal ulcer disease: A surgical perspective. West J Med 1987;147:301.

Sonnenberg A: Changes in physician visits for gastric and duodenal ulcer in the United States during 1958–1984 as shown by National Disease and Therapeutic Index (NDTI). Dig Dis Sci 1987;32:1. (Changes in incidence of these entities.)

2. ZOLLINGER-ELLISON SYNDROME (Gastrinoma)

Essentials of Diagnosis

- Severe peptic ulcer disease.
- Gastric hypersecretion.
- Elevated serum gastrin.
- Gastrinoma of pancreas, duodenum, or other ectopic site.

General Considerations

Zollinger-Ellison peptic ulceration syndrome, although uncommon, is not rare. Sixty percent of patients are males. Onset may be at any age from early childhood on but is most common in persons 20–50 years old. Most patients have the gastrin-secreting tumor in the pancreas; a few have tumors in the submucosa of the duodenum and stomach, the hilum of the spleen, and the regional lymph nodes. They may be either single or multiple. Approximately two-thirds of Zollinger-Ellison tumors are malignant with respect either to their biologic behavior or to their histologic appearance.

Clinical Findings

A. Symptoms and Signs: Pain is of the typical peptic ulcer variety but is more difficult to control by medical means. Diarrhea may occur secondary to the hypersecretion or as a result of inactivation of lipase when the intraluminal pH of the small bowel falls below 6.5, thus interfering with fat digestion. Hemorrhage, perforation, and obstruction occur commonly.

B. Laboratory Findings: The most reliable means of establishing the diagnosis of Zollinger-Ellison syndrome is measurement of serum gastrin by radioimmunoassay. Patients with Zollinger-Ellison syndrome usually have serum gastrin levels higher than 300 pg/mL—often considerably higher. Elevated gastrin levels are also observed in patients rendered achlorhydric by H_2 blockers. Serum calcium levels are useful in revealing hypercalcemia to evaluate the possibility of hyperparathyroidism and multiple endocrine adenomatosis. Gastric analysis reveals basal gastric hypersecretion (> 15 meq/h). Maximal acid output following stimulation with pentagastrin does not show the increased rate of gastric acid secretion as much as in normal people or in patients with peptic ulcer disease not of the Zollinger-Ellison type. In the Zollinger-Ellison patient, the basal acid output is greater than 60% of the maximal output, while in ordinary peptic ulcer disease the basal output is usually substantially less than 60% of the maximal. Intravenous secretin causes a marked elevation of serum gastrin in patients with gastrinomas and is essential in diagnosis.

C. Imaging: Gastrointestinal series reveal that 75% of the ulcers are in the first part of the duodenum and that the ulcers are usually not multiple. Ulcers occurring in the second, third, or fourth portion of the duodenum or in the jejunum are strongly suggestive of Zollinger-Ellison syndrome. Coarseness of the proximal jejunal folds and radiographic evidence of gastric hypersecretion also suggest Zollinger-Ellison syndrome.

Treatment

H_2 receptor blockers have been shown to markedly inhibit gastric acid secretion in patients with gastrinoma and have brought about healing of ulcers, but doses 4–10 times higher than conventional ones may be required. Omeprazole, a proton pump inhibitor, is also effective. In patients poorly controlled with

H_2 receptor blockers alone, vagotomy and pyloroplasty may also be necessary.

Wolfe MM, Jensen RT: Zollinger-Ellison syndrome: Current concepts in diagnosis and management. N Engl J Med 1987;317:1200. (Medical progress article.)

3. GASTRIC ULCER

Essentials of Diagnosis

- Epigastric distress on an empty stomach, relieved by food, antacids, or vomiting but with early recurrence after eating; weight loss common.
- Epigastric tenderness and voluntary muscle guarding.
- Anemia, occult blood in stool, gastric acid.
- Ulcer demonstrated by x-ray or gastroscopy.
- Acid present on gastric analysis.

General Considerations

Benign gastric ulcer is in many respects similar to duodenal ulcer. Acid gastric juice is necessary for its production, but decreased tissue resistance appears to play a more important role than hypersecretion. Most patients have a history of aspirin or other nonsteroidal anti-inflammatory drug use.

About 60% of benign gastric ulcers are found within 6 cm of the pylorus. The ulcers are generally located at or near the lesser curvature and most frequently on the posterior wall. Another 25% of the ulcers are located higher on the lesser curvature.

If the radiographic appearance of the ulcer is benign, the occurrence of carcinoma is about 3.3%. If it is indeterminate (features of both benignancy and malignancy), it is approximately 9.5%. With evidence of associated duodenal ulcer, it is about 1%.

Clinical Findings

A. Symptoms and Signs: There may be no symptoms, or only vague and atypical symptoms. The epigastric distress is typically described as gnawing, burning, aching, or "hunger pangs," referred at times to the left subcostal area. Episodes occur usually 45–60 minutes after a meal and are relieved by food, alkalies, or vomiting. Nausea and vomiting are frequent complaints. There may be a history of remissions and exacerbations, especially if patients are taking aspirin or other nonsteroidal analgesics. Weight loss and fatigue are common.

Epigastric tenderness or voluntary muscle guarding is usually the only finding.

B. Laboratory Findings: If bleeding has occurred, there may be hypochromic anemia or occult blood in the stool. The gastric analysis always shows an acid pH after pentagastrin and usually the presence of low normal to normal secretion.

C. Other Examinations: An upper gastrointestinal series is the usual initial diagnostic procedure for the non-actively bleeding patient suspected of having a gastric ulcer. When the radiographic appearance of the ulcer is not clearly benign or when an ulcer is not 75% healed by 8 weeks or completely healed by 12 weeks, peroral endoscopy with multiple biopsies (6–10) of the ulcer margin and base is indicated to rule out cancer.

Differential Diagnosis

The symptoms of gastric ulcer, especially if atypical, must be differentiated from those of gastritis and functional gastrointestinal distress.

Most important is the differentiation of benign from malignant gastric ulcer. A favorable response to adequate medical management is presumptive evidence that the lesion is not malignant. Malignant ulcers may respond initially, but residual changes at the site usually demonstrate the nature of the process.

Complications

Hemorrhage, perforation, and obstruction may occur.

Treatment

Ulcer treatment (as for duodenal ulcer) should be intensive. Aspirin and other nonsteroidal anti-inflammatory agents must be avoided. Repeat x-rays should be obtained to document healing at 8 weeks. Failure to respond in 12 weeks with complete healing may be an indication for surgical resection in the patient who has no contraindication to surgery. Gastroscopy and biopsy should be repeated. Histamine H_2 receptor antagonists and sucralfate are as effective as antacids in healing gastric ulcer. However, even a carcinoma may show improvement on an ulcer regimen, and clinical relief does not necessarily mean that the ulcer is benign. Follow-up at 3 and 6 months after apparently complete healing is therefore indicated. In the event of recurrence under intensive medical management, perforation, obstruction, or massive uncontrollable hemorrhage, surgery is mandatory.

Prognosis

Gastric ulcers tend to be recurrent. There is no evidence that malignant degeneration of gastric peptic ulceration ever occurs. Recurrent uncomplicated ulcer is not a serious event, and, in fact, it may heal more readily than the previous ulcer.

Adkins RB et al: The management of gastric ulcers: A current review. Ann Surg 1985;201:741.

Duggan JM et al: Peptic ulcer and nonsteroidal anti-inflammatory agents. Gut 1986;27:929. (Strong association with gastric ulcer; unclear as to duodenal ulcer.)

Lanza FL et al: Double-blind, placebo-controlled endoscopic comparison of the mucosal protective effects of misoprostol versus cimetidine on tolmetin-induced mucosal injury to the stomach and duodenum. Gastroenterology 1988;95:289. (Misoprostol highly protective, especially for gastric mucosa.)

Perrault J, Fleming CR, Dozois RR: Surreptitious use of salicylates: A cause of chronic recurrent gastroduodenal ulcers. Mayo Clin Proc 1988;63:337. (Consider determining salicylate level in these patients.)

Walan A et al: Effect of omeprazole and ranitidine on ulcer healing and relapse rates in patients with benign gastric ulcer. N Engl J Med 1989;320:69. (Omeprazole is superior and may soon be available for this indication.)

4. STOMAL (MARGINAL) ULCER
(Jejunal Ulcer)

Marginal ulcer should be suspected when there is a history of operation for an ulcer followed by recurrence of abdominal symptoms after a symptom-free interval of months to years. The marginal ulcer incidence after simple gastroenterostomy is 15–20%; after subtotal gastrectomy or vagotomy and antrectomy, about 2%. Nearly all of the ulcers are jejunal, and the others are located on the gastric side of the anastomosis.

Clinical Findings

The abdominal pain is burning or gnawing, often more severe than the preoperative ulcer pain, and is located lower in the epigastrium, even below the umbilicus and often to the left. The pain often covers a wider area and may radiate to the back.

The "food-pain rhythm" of peptic ulcer distress frequently occurs earlier (within an hour) in marginal ulcer as a result of more rapid emptying time; and relief with antacids, food, and milk may be incomplete and of short duration. Nausea, vomiting, and weight loss are common. Hematemesis occurs frequently. Low epigastric tenderness with voluntary muscle guarding is usually present. An inflammatory mass may be palpated. Anemia and occult blood in the stool are common. On radiography, the ulcer niche at the stoma is often difficult to demonstrate or differentiate from postsurgical defects, despite use of compression films. Peroral endoscopy is the most effective means of diagnosing stomal ulcer.

Differential Diagnosis

Stomal ulcer must be differentiated from functional gastrointestinal distress, especially in a patient concerned about the possibility of recurrence of an ulcer after surgery. Atypical symptoms must be differentiated from "bile" gastritis and from biliary tract or pancreatic disease. Consider the possibility of Zollinger-Ellison syndrome as well as the use of aspirin or other NSAIDs.

Complications

Complications include gross hemorrhage, perforation, stenosis of the stoma, and gastrojejunocolic fistula.

Treatment

Histamine H_2 receptor antagonists as used in treatment of duodenal and gastric ulcer often lead to healing. Occasionally, further surgical intervention is necessary, ie, repeat vagotomy, revision of the gastrojejunostomy, or further gastric resection.

Mosimann F, Donovan IA, Alexander-Williams J: Pitfalls in the diagnosis of recurrent ulceration after surgery for peptic ulcer disease. J Clin Gastroenterol 1985;7:133. (Endoscopy best for diagnosis; difficulties in differentiating etiologic roles of excess acid, bile reflux, or underlying mechanics.)

POSTGASTRECTOMY SYNDROMES

Dumping Syndrome

Postgastrectomy dumping syndrome probably occurs in about 10% of patients after partial gastrectomy. The pathogenesis is complex and incompletely understood. The disorder is provoked mainly by soluble hypertonic carbohydrates, which, when present in the small intestine, have an osmotic effect resulting in rapid flow of fluid into the small intestine; increase in free plasma kinins; increase in peripheral blood flow; and a modest drop in plasma volume with a corresponding increase in hematocrit and a mild decrease in serum potassium. Whether sympathetic vasomotor responses contribute to the syndrome is uncertain.

One or more of the following symptoms occur within 20 minutes after meals: sweating, tachycardia, pallor, epigastric fullness and grumbling, warmth, nausea, abdominal cramps, weakness, and, in severe cases, syncope, vomiting, or diarrhea. Nonspecific electrocardiographic changes may be noted. Plasma glucose is not low during an attack.

It is important to distinguish this syndrome from the reactive hypoglycemia that occurs in some postgastrectomy patients. This latter syndrome occurs much later after the meal (1–3 hours) and is relieved by the ingestion of food.

Changing the diet to frequent (6) small, equal feedings high in protein, moderately high in fat, and low in simple carbohydrates usually lessens the severity of symptoms. Fluids should not be taken with meals. Sedative and anticholinergic drugs may be of value.

Afferent (Blind) Loop Syndrome

The afferent loop syndrome occurs after a subtotal gastrectomy with Billroth II anastomosis or gastrojejunostomy. The syndrome may occur acutely early in the postoperative period or months to years following operation. An acute abdominal catastrophe (rare) may require emergency operation to release the obstruction and follow-up measures to prevent recurrence. More commonly, afferent loop syndrome is caused by chronic or recurring partial obstruction, although the exact etiologic mechanisms are not clear. The symptoms are caused by distention of and stasis within the afferent loop of the gastrojejunostomy. Typically, abdominal pain occurs 15–30 minutes after eating and is relieved by vomiting of bile fluid that does not contain food. Hyperamylasemia may be associated.

Poor emptying of the afferent loop may result in stasis of contents, leading to bacterial overgrowth. This in turn may lead to deficiency of vitamin B_{12} because of bacterial uptake of vitamin B_{12}. Deconjugation of bile salts may also occur, with subsequent impairment of micelle formation, leading to steatorrhea and its attendant complications. This complication is not usually associated with obstructive symptoms.

Avoidance of the Billroth II procedure will prevent the afferent loop from occurring. Surgical reconstruction of the afferent loop to produce better emptying is the treatment of choice. Bacterial overgrowth can be temporarily controlled with repeated 7- to 10-day courses of a broad-spectrum antibiotic, such as tetracycline, 250 mg 4 times daily. With vitamin B_{12} deficiency, vitamin B_{12} should be administered.

Bile Reflux

Bile reflux is one of the most debilitating complications following gastric surgery. Bile reflux may occur after cholecystectomy and occasionally with no prior surgery. Typically, the patient experiences nausea, substernal distress, and anorexia. Vomiting or reflux of clear bile-stained fluid may occur.

Medical management is unsatisfactory. The surgical approach is a diversion of bile from the stomach. The Roux-en-Y gastrojejunostomy procedure serves this end.

Other Postgastrectomy Syndromes

Other complications that may follow gastric surgery include reflux esophagitis, gastric retention, postvagotomy diarrhea, and the development of carcinoma in the gastric stump many years after surgery. Iron deficiency anemia occurs in 50% of patients 5 years or longer after a Billroth II gastrectomy, because of the bypassing of the duodenum, the major locus for iron absorption. The incidence of pulmonary tuberculosis is thought to be increased after gastrectomy.

Horowitz M, Collins PJ, Shearman DJC: Disorders of gastric emptying in humans and the use of radionuclide techniques. Arch Intern Med 1985;145:1467.
Meyer JH: Chronic morbidity after ulcer surgery. Chap 53, p 962, in: *Gastrointestinal Disease: Pathophysiology, Diagnosis, Management,* 4th ed. Sleisenger MH, Fordtran JS (editors). Saunders, 1989.

CARCINOMA OF THE STOMACH

Essentials of Diagnosis

- Upper gastrointestinal symptoms with weight loss in patients over age 40.
- Palpable abdominal mass (very late).
- Anemia, occult blood in stools, positive cytologic examination.
- Gastroscopic and x-ray abnormality.

General Considerations

Carcinoma of the stomach is a common cancer of the digestive tract. It occurs predominantly in males over 40 years of age. Delay of diagnosis is caused by absence of definite early symptoms and by the fact that patients treat themselves instead of seeking early medical advice. Further delays are due to the equivocal nature of early findings and to temporary improvement with symptomatic therapy.

A history of the following possibly precancerous conditions should alert the physician to the danger of stomach cancer:

(1) Atrophic gastritis of pernicious anemia: The incidence of adenomas and carcinomas is *significantly increased.*

(2) Chronic gastritis, particularly atrophic gastritis: There is a wide variation in the reported incidence of gastritis with cancer, and a definite relationship has not been proved.

(3) Gastric ulcer: The major problem is in the differentiation between benign and malignant ulcer.

(4) Achlorhydria: The incidence of lowered secretory potential in early life is higher in those patients who later develop carcinoma.

(5) Patients who have had a partial gastrectomy for peptic ulcer 10–15 years previously may have an increased risk of gastric cancer.

Carcinoma may originate anywhere in the stomach. Grossly, lesions tend to be of 4 types (Borrman):

Type I: Polypoid, intraluminal mass.

Type II: Noninfiltrating ulcer.

Type III: Infiltrating ulcer.

Type IV: Diffuse infiltrating process (to linitis plastica).

Gross typing generally correlates better with prognosis than the histologic grading of malignancy, ie, type I has a better prognosis than type II, etc.

Clinical Findings

A. Symptoms and Signs: Early gastric carcinoma, such as is detected in the mass surveys in Japan, causes no symptoms. The appearance of symptoms implies relatively advanced disease. The patient may complain of vague fullness, nausea, a sensation of pressure, belching, and heartburn after meals, with or without anorexia (especially for meat). These symptoms in association with weight loss and a decline in general health and strength in a man over age 40 years should suggest the possibility of stomach cancer. Diarrhea, hematemesis, and melena may be present.

Specific symptoms may be determined in part by the location of the tumor. A peptic ulcer-like syndrome generally occurs with ulcerated lesions (types

II and III) and in the presence of acid secretion but may occur with complete achlorhydria. Unfortunately, symptomatic relief from antacids tends to delay diagnosis. Symptoms of pyloric obstruction are progressive postprandial fullness to vomiting of almost all ingested foods. Lower esophageal obstruction causes progressive dysphagia and regurgitation. Early satiety usually occurs with linitis plastica but may be seen with other cancers.

Physical findings are usually limited to weight loss and, if anemia is present, pallor. In about 20% of cases, a palpable abdominal mass is present; this does not necessarily mean that the lesion is inoperable. Liver or peripheral metastases may also be present.

B. Laboratory Findings: Achlorhydria (gastric pH > 6.0) after stimulation with pentagastrin, 6 mg/kg intramuscularly or subcutaneously, in the presence of a gastric ulcer is virtually pathognomonic of cancer; but this finding is present in only about 20% of patients with gastric cancer. If bleeding occurs, there will be occult blood in the stool and mild to severe anemia. The anemia may be normochromic and normocytic even without bleeding.

C. Other Examinations: Endoscopic biopsy and directed cytology will provide the correct diagnosis in almost every case. These methods will also establish the important differential diagnosis between adenocarcinoma and the malignant lymphomas.

Differential Diagnosis

The symptoms of carcinoma of the stomach are often mistaken for those of benign gastric ulcer, chronic gastritis, irritable colon syndrome, or functional gastrointestinal disturbance; x-ray and gastroscopic findings must be differentiated from those of benign gastric ulcer or tumor. Nonhealing ulcers or ulcers that are enlarging with a strict ulcer regimen require surgery. Most of these will still be benign.

The clinical history of gastric leiomyosarcoma may be indistinguishable from that of carcinoma. Bleeding, particularly massive, is more common. These tumors account for approximately 1.5% of gastric cancers. A palpable mass is more frequent than in gastric carcinoma, and the x-ray picture is characteristically that of a well-circumscribed intramural mass with, frequently, a central crater.

With the decreasing incidence of carcinoma of the stomach in the USA, gastric lymphoma now accounts for about 10% of gastric malignant disease. It is an important consideration in patients presenting with enlarged gastric folds, masses, or ulcerations. Biopsy and cytologic examination are essential in establishing the diagnosis. The prognosis is much more favorable than in patients with carcinoma; cure may be anticipated in over half of patients if the tumor is confined to the stomach.

Treatment

Surgical resection is the only curative treatment.

Signs of metastatic disease include a hard, nodular liver, enlarged left supraclavicular (Virchow's) nodes, skin nodules, ascites, rectal shelf, and x-ray evidence of osseous or pulmonary metastasis. If none of these are present and there is no other contraindication to operation, exploration is indicated. The presence of an abdominal mass is not a contraindication to laparotomy, since bulky lesions can often be totally excised. Palliative resection or gastroenterostomy is occasionally helpful. Radiation may be of some value. Multiple-drug regimens are under study. Mitomycin C, 5-fluorouracil, doxorubicin, and cytarabine (cytosine arabinoside) in various combinations have been reported to be beneficial.

For gastric lymphoma, the treatment is surgical excision, radiation, or a combination of the two.

Prognosis

There is wide variation in the biologic malignancy of gastric carcinomas. In many, the disease is widespread before symptoms are apparent; in a fortunate few, slow growth may progress over years and be resectable even at a late date. Approximately 10% of all patients with gastric carcinoma will be cured by surgical resection.

Green PH et al: Increasing incidence and excellent survival of patients with early gastric cancer: Experience in a United States medical center. Am J Med 1988;85:658. (Survival rate similar to that of individuals of same age without gastric cancer and.)

Hockey MS et al: Primary gastric lymphoma. Br J Surg 1987;74:483.

Lundegardh G et al: Stomach cancer after partial gastrectomy for benign ulcer disease. N Engl J Med 1988; 319:195. (Risk greater for those operated on for gastric than for duodenal ulcer.)

Schein PS: Chemotherapy of gastric carcinoma. Eur J Surg Oncol 1987;13:3.

Yan C, Brooks JR: Surgical management of gastric adenocarcinoma. Am J Surg 1985;149:771.

BENIGN TUMORS OF THE STOMACH

Most benign tumors do not cause symptoms and often are so small that they are overlooked on x-ray examination. Their importance lies in the problem of differentiation from malignant lesions, their precancerous possibilities, and the fact that they occasionally cause symptoms.

These tumors may be of epithelial origin (eg, adenomas, papillomas) or mesenchymal origin (eg, leiomyomas, fibromas, hemofibromas, lipomas, hemangiomas). The mesenchymal tumors, which are intramural, rarely undergo malignant change. Most polyps of the stomach are hyperplastic ones with no malignant potential. Adenomas have a small but unknown potential for malignant change.

Clinical Findings

A. Symptoms and Signs: Large tumors may cause a vague feeling of epigastric fullness or heaviness; tumors located near the cardia or pylorus may produce symptoms of obstruction. If bleeding occurs, it will cause symptoms and signs of acute gastrointestinal hemorrhage (eg, tarry stools, syncope, sweating, vomiting of blood). Chronic blood loss will cause symptoms of anemia (fatigue, dyspnea). If the tumor is large, a movable epigastric mass may be palpable.

B. Laboratory Findings: The usual laboratory findings may be present.

C. Imaging: The radiograph is characterized by a smooth filling defect, clearly circumscribed, which does not interfere with normal pliability of peristalsis. Larger tumors may show a small central crater, especially leiomyomas.

Treatment & Prognosis

If symptoms occur (particularly hemorrhage), surgical resection is necessary. If there are no symptoms, the patient does not require surgery. These tumors may even regress spontaneously. Polyps may be excised by endoscopic electroresection.

Feczko PJ et al: Gastric polyps: Radiological evaluation and clinical significance. Radiology 1985;155:581.

Graham SM, Ballantyne GH, Modlin IM: Gastric epithelioid leiomyomatous tumors. Surg Gynecol Obstet 1987; 164:391.

DISEASES OF THE INTESTINES

REGIONAL ENTERITIS
(Regional Ileitis, Granulomatous Ileocolitis, Crohn's Disease)
(See also Granulomatous Colitis, Below.)

Essentials of Diagnosis

- Insidious onset.
- Intermittent bouts of diarrhea, low-grade fever, and right lower quadrant pain.
- Fistula formation or right lower quadrant mass and tenderness (late finding).
- Radiographic evidence of abnormality of the terminal ileum.

General Considerations

Regional enteritis is a chronic inflammatory disease that may involve the alimentary tract anywhere from the mouth to the anus. The ileum is the principal site of the disease, either alone or in conjunction with the colon and jejunum. It generally occurs in young adults and runs an intermittent clinical course with mild to severe disability and frequent complications.

There is marked thickening of the submucosa with lymphedema, lymphoid hyperplasia, nonspecific granulomas, and often ulceration of the overlying mucosa. A marked lymphadenitis occurs in the mesenteric nodes. The inflammatory involvement tends to be transmural.

The cause is unknown. Genetic factors appear to play a role. There is a higher than normal incidence in monozygotic twins and a greater than random familial incidence. The most common familial pattern involves 2 or more affected siblings. Regional enteritis and chronic ulcerative colitis occur in the same families. The possibility of an infectious origin for regional enteritis has been raised by studies demonstrating transmission of an agent from tissues with regional enteritis into immunologically deficient mice and rabbits, but no agent to date has been substantiated.

Clinical Findings

A. Symptoms and Signs: The disease is characterized by exacerbations and remissions. Colicky or steady abdominal pain is present in the right lower quadrant or periumbilical area at some time during the course of the disease and varies from mild to severe. Diarrhea may occur, usually with intervening periods of normal bowel function or constipation. Patients with these symptoms are often diagnosed as having irritable or functional bowel disease. Fever may be low-grade or, rarely, spiking with chills. Anorexia, flatulence, malaise, and weight loss are present. Milk products and chemically or mechanically irritating foods may aggravate symptoms.

Abdominal tenderness is usually present, especially in the right lower quadrant, with signs of peritoneal irritation and an abdominal or pelvic mass in the same area. The mass is tender and varies from a sausagelike thickened intestine to matted loops of intestine.

Regional enteritis may pursue various clinical patterns. In certain instances, the course is indolent and the symptomatology mild. In other instances, the course is toxic, with fever, toxic erythema, arthralgia, anemia, etc. Still other patients pursue courses complicated by stricture or perforations of the bowel and suppurative complications of intra-abdominal perforation.

B. Laboratory Findings: There is usually a hypochromic (occasionally macrocytic due to vitamin B_{12} malabsorption) anemia and occult blood in the stool. The small bowel x-ray may show mucosal irregularity, ulceration, stiffening of the bowel wall, and luminal narrowing. Barium enema may show fissures or deep ulcers. Eccentric involvement, skipped areas of involvement, and strictures suggest Crohn's disease of the colon. Sigmoidoscopic examination may show an edematous hyperemic mucosa or a discrete ulcer when the colon is involved.

Differential Diagnosis

Acute regional enteritis may simulate acute appendicitis. Location in the terminal ileum requires differentiation from intestinal tuberculosis, *Yersinia enterocolitica* infection, lymphomas, and, in the immunodeficient patient, *Mycobacterium avium-intracellulare*. Regional enteritis involving the colon must be distinguished from idiopathic ulcerative colitis, amebic colitis, ischemic colitis, and infectious disease of the colon. The sigmoidoscopic and x-ray criteria distinguishing these various entities may not be absolute, and definitive diagnosis may require cultures, examinations of the stool for parasites, and biopsy in selected instances.

Complications

Ischiorectal and perianal fistulas occur frequently. Fistulas may occur to the bladder or vagina and even to the skin in the area of a previous scar. Mechanical intestinal obstruction may occur. Nutritional deficiency caused by malabsorption and maldigestion (the latter caused by a decreased bile salt pool) may produce a spruelike syndrome. Generalized peritonitis is rare because perforation occurs slowly, is locally contained, or results in internal fistulization. The incidence of colorectal or small bowel cancer in regional enteritis patients is greater than in a control population, but less than for ulcerative colitis. Migratory peripheral synovitis and axial arthropathy indistinguishable from sporadic ankylosing spondylitis may occur.

Treatment & Prognosis

A. General Measures: The diet should be high in calories and vitamins and adequate in protein. Raw fruits and vegetables should be avoided in patients who have obstructive symptoms. These patients may benefit from a nonresidue, well-balanced diet to maintain nutrition until obstructive symptoms subside. Anemia, dehydration, diarrhea, and avitaminosis should be treated as indicated.

B. Antimicrobial Agents: In our present state of knowledge about this disease, antimicrobials are indicated only for specific infectious problems, ie, abscess, fistulas.

1. Sulfasalazine–Sulfasalazine (Azulfidine), 2–8 g/d orally, has been shown to be effective, especially for disease involving the colon. The salicylate moiety of sulfasalazine, 5-aminosalicylic acid, appears to be of equal efficacy without the side effects attributable to the sulfapyridine portion of sulfasalazine. 5-Aminosalicylic acid will soon be available for use.

2. Antibiotics–In cases of acute suppuration (manifested by tender mass, fever, leukocytosis) ampicillin, 2-4 g/d intravenously or orally, may be useful. Clindamycin or metronidazole (for anaerobes)

and aminoglycosides are also effective. In cases where internal fistulization has led to a defunctionalized loop with bacterial overgrowth or where stricture formation has led to small bowel stasis with malabsorption, tetracycline, 1–2 g/d orally, may be valuable in combating bacterial overgrowth in the bowel and correcting absorptive malfunction.

3. Metronidazole–Metronidazole, 15 mg/kg/d, is effective in colonic disease and for enterocutaneous fistulas.

C. Adrenocortical Hormones: These agents are often of use in the diffuse form of the disease and are particularly helpful in the toxic forms (arthritis, anemia, toxic erythemas). The complications of long-term therapy can be minimized by administering the drug on an alternate-day schedule (eg, prednisone, 15–40 mg every other day) once the patient's clinical symptoms have been brought under control. Sulfasalazine and prednisone are effective in the acute phase of the disease but do not exert a prophylactic effect. In a national cooperative study, azathioprine proved to be of no value, though perhaps the observation period may have been too short. Mercaptopurine, the active metabolite of azathioprine, has a beneficial effect on the fistulas of Crohn's disease as well as on other features of the disease.

D. Other Medical Measures: When terminal ileal disease is present, vitamin B_{12} supplementation is often necessary. Calcium supplementation in the form of calcium gluconate or Os-Cal will alleviate the frequent calcium deficiency seen in these patients and is also helpful in decreasing excessive oxalate absorption, resulting in lowered incidence of oxalate urinary tract stones.

E. Surgical Measures: Surgical treatment of this disease is best limited to the management of its complications. Resection of the small bowel, particularly the extensive resection often necessary in regional enteritis, leads to a "short bowel" syndrome (diminished absorptive surface), ie, malabsorption of vitamin B_{12} to varying degrees (loss of terminal ileum), hyperoxaluria, steatorrhea, osteomalacia, and macrocytic anemia (due to folic acid and vitamin B_{12} deficiency). Stricturoplasty may be helpful and preserve bowel. Short-circuiting operations may lead to blind loops (intestinal defunctionalization with bacterial overgrowth) with similar difficulties in absorption. When surgery is necessary in this disease, study of postsurgical bowel function is indicated to detect the possibility of impaired function.

Danzi JT: Extraintestinal manifestations of idiopathic inflammatory bowel disease. Arch Intern Med 1988; 148:297.

Dirks E et al: Clinical relapse of Crohn's disease under standardized conservative treatment and after excisional surgery. Dig Dis Sci 1989;34:1832. (Guidance for operation and benefits for selected patients.)

Farmer RG, Whelan G, Fazio VW: Long-term follow-up of patient with Crohn's disease: Relationship between the clinical pattern and prognosis. Gastroenterology 1985;88:1818.

Petras RE, Mir-Madjlessi SH, Farmer RG: Crohn's disease and intestinal carcinoma: A report of 11 cases with emphasis on associated epithelial dysplasia. Gastroenterology 1987;93:1307.

Prantera C et al: Prediction of surgery for obstruction in Crohn's ileitis: A study of 64 patients. Dig Dis Sci 1987;32:1363.

Schneebaum CW et al: Terminal ileitis associated with Mycobacterium avium-intracellulare infection in a homosexual man with acquired immune deficiency syndrome. Gastroenterology 1987;92:1127.

Søorensen VZ, Olsen BG, Binder V: Life prospects and quality of life in patients with Crohn's disease. Gut 1987;28:382.

TUMORS OF THE SMALL INTESTINE

Benign and malignant tumors of the small intestine are rare. There may be no symptoms or signs, but bleeding or obstruction (or both) may occur. The obstruction consists of either an intussusception with the tumor in the lead or a partial or complete occlusion in the lumen by growth of the tumor. Bleeding may cause weakness, fatigability, light-headedness, syncope, pallor, sweating, tachycardia, and tarry stools. Obstruction causes nausea, vomiting, and abdominal pains. The abdomen is tender and distended, and bowel sounds are high-pitched and active. Malignant lesions produce weight loss and extraintestinal manifestations (eg, pain due to stretching of the liver capsule, flushing due to carcinoid). In the case of a duodenal carcinoma, a peptic ulcer syndrome may be present. A palpable mass is rarely found.

If there is bleeding, melena and hypochromic anemia occur. X-ray (small bowel series, preferably by enteroclysis) may show the tumor mass or dilatation of the small bowel if obstruction is present; in the absence of obstruction, it is extremely difficult to demonstrate the mass.

Benign Tumors

Benign tumors may be symptomatic or may be incidental findings at operation or autopsy. Treatment consists of surgical removal.

Benign **adenomas** constitute 25% of all benign bowel tumors. **Lipomas** occur most frequently in the ileum; the presenting symptom is usually obstruction due to intussusception. **Leiomyomas** are usually associated with bleeding and may also cause intussusception. **Angiomas** behave like other small bowel tumors but have a greater tendency to bleed.

Multiple intestinal polyposis of the gastrointestinal tract (any level) associated with mucocutaneous pigmentation (Peutz-Jeghers syndrome) is a benign condition. Malignant change has been reported but is rare, and the entity becomes a problem only with complications such as obstruction or bleeding. The polyps are hamartomas, and the pigment is melanin. The pigment is most prominent over the lips and buccal mucosa.

Malignant Tumors

The treatment of malignant tumors and their complications is usually surgical.

Adenocarcinoma is the most common cancer of the small bowel, occurring most frequently in the duodenum and jejunum. Symptoms are due to obstructions or hemorrhage. The prognosis is very poor. **Lymphomas** are also first manifested by obstruction of bleeding. Perforation or malabsorption may also occur. Postoperative radiation therapy may occasionally be of value. **Sarcomas** occur most commonly in the mid small bowel and may first be manifested by mass, obstruction, or bleeding. The prognosis is guarded.

Carcinoid tumors arise from the argentaffin cells of the gastrointestinal tract. Ninety percent of these tumors occur in the appendix, and 75% of the remainder occur in the small intestine (usually the distal ileum). Carcinoids may arise in other sites, including the stomach, colon, bronchus, pancreas, and ovary. Most small bowel carcinoids do not produce carcinoid syndrome. The main problem is metastases. In general, carcinoid syndrome occurs only with malignant tumors that have metastasized. The tumor may secrete serotonin and bradykinin. The systemic manifestations may consist of (1) paroxysmal flushing and other vasomotor symptoms, (2) dyspnea and wheezing, (3) recurrent episodes of abdominal pain and diarrhea, and (4) symptoms and signs of right-sided valvular disease of the heart. The diagnosis is confirmed by finding elevated levels of 5-hydroxyindoleacetic acid in the urine. The primary tumor is usually small, and obstruction is unusual. The metastases are usually voluminous and surprisingly benign. Treatment is symptomatic and supportive; surgical excision may be indicated if the condition is recognized before widespread metastases have occurred. Response to treatment with serotonin antagonists has been irregular. Repeated administration of corticotropin or the corticosteroids may occasionally be of value. The prognosis for cure is poor, but long-term survival is not unusual.

Auger MJ, Allan NC: Primary ileocecal lymphoma. Cancer 1990;65:358.

Sachs JR, Bralow SP: Primary malignancies of the small bowel. Intern Med 1989;10:120.

MECKEL'S DIVERTICULITIS

Meckel's diverticulum, a remnant of the omphalomesenteric duct, is found in about 2% of persons, more frequently in males. It arises from the ileum 60–90 cm from the ileocecal valve and may or may not have an umbilical attachment. Most are silent, but various abdominal symptoms may occur. The blind pouch may be involved by an inflammatory process similar to appendicitis; its congenital bands or inflammatory adhesions may cause acute intestinal obstruction; it may induce intussusception; or, in the 16% that contain heterotopic islands of gastric mucosa, it may form a peptic ulcer.

The symptoms and signs of the acute appendicitis-like disease and the acute intestinal obstruction caused by Meckel's diverticulitis cannot be differentiated from other primary processes except by exploration. Ulcer type distress, if present, is localized near the umbilicus or lower and, more importantly, is not relieved by alkalies or food. If ulceration has occurred, blood will be present in the stool. Massive gastrointestinal bleeding and perforation may occur. The presence of Meckel's diverticulum can frequently be determined in patients with gastric mucosa by a technetium radioisotope scan.

Meckel's diverticulitis should be resected, either for relief or for differentiation from acute appendicitis. Surgery is curative.

Farr CM et al: Bleeding Meckel's diverticulum in an adult. J Clin Gastroenterol 1989;11:208. (Interesting case and brief review of the literature.)

MESENTERIC VASCULAR INSUFFICIENCY

1. CHRONIC MESENTERIC VASCULAR INSUFFICIENCY (Abdominal Angina)

Intestinal angina may be secondary to atherosclerosis and may precede vascular occlusion (see below). In some instances it may be caused by compression of the vessels either by the crura of the diaphragm or by anomalous bands.

Localized or generalized postprandial pain is the classic picture, often lasting 2–3 hours. The intensity of pain may be related to the size of the meal; the relationship to eating leads to a diminution in food intake and, eventually, weight loss. In some cases, the pain becomes less prominent as the patient diminishes caloric intake. An epigastric bruit may be heard. Laboratory evidence of mild malabsorption may be present. The small bowel series may reveal a motility disorder. Visceral angiograms are necessary to confirm narrowing of the celiac and mesenteric arteries. It is generally believed that 2 of the 3 main vessels must be involved in order for symptoms to occur. Patients almost invariably have clinical evidence of severe peripheral vascular disease.

Surgical revascularization of the bowel is the treatment of choice if the patient's condition permits. Small, frequent feedings may prove helpful.

Hunter GC, Guernsey JM: Mesenteric ischemia. Med Clin North Am 1988;72:1091.

2. ACUTE MESENTERIC VASCULAR INSUFFICIENCY

Essentials of Diagnosis
- Severe abdominal pain with unimpressive physical examination early.
- Often a history of vascular disease.
- Abdominal distention, tenderness, rigidity are late findings.
- Leukocytosis, hemoconcentration.

General Considerations
Mesenteric arterial or venous occlusion is a catastrophic abdominal disorder. Arterial occlusion is occasionally embolic but is more frequently thrombotic. Both occur more frequently in men and in the older age groups. Acute mesenteric vascular occlusion may also be a small vessel phenomenon, particularly in patients with vasculitis in association with a variety of collagen diseases. In patients with sudden onset of pain in the setting of recent myocardial infarction or in the presence of an arrhythmia, serious consideration must be given to the possibility of an embolic event.

Involvement of the superior mesenteric artery or its branches is common. The affected bowel becomes congested, hemorrhagic, and edematous, and may cease to function, producing intestinal obstruction. True ischemic necrosis then develops.

Intestinal infarction may occur in the absence of mesenteric vascular thrombosis; nonocclusive disease may in fact be a more common cause of infarction than is occlusion. Most patients have been in severe congestive heart failure or shock or in a state of hypoxia. Although many patients with this syndrome have been receiving digitalis glycosides, the relationship of this agent to the bowel problem is unclear. Occlusive vascular disease may also play a role in reducing perfusion of the bowel in these patients.

Clinical Findings
A. Symptoms and Signs: Generalized abdominal pain often comes on abruptly and is usually steady and severe, but it may begin gradually and may be intermittent, with colicky exacerbations. Nausea and vomiting occur; the vomitus is rarely bloody. Bloody diarrhea and marked prostration, sweating, and anxiety may occur. For a period following the occlusion, symptoms are severe but the physical findings meager.

Shock may be evident. Abdominal distention occurs well after pain begins, and audible peristalsis (evident early) may later disappear. As peritoneal irritation develops, diffuse tenderness, rigidity, and rebound tenderness appear; this is a late finding.

B. Laboratory Findings: Hemoconcentration,

leukocytosis ($> 15,000/\mu L$ with a shift to the left), and blood in the stool may be present; lactic acidosis may be a prominent feature.

C. Imaging: A plain film of the abdomen shows the nonspecific findings of moderate gaseous distention of the small and large intestines and evidence of peritoneal fluid. CT scan may be helpful in revealing atherosclerotic compromise of the celiac axis and superior mesenteric artery.

Differential Diagnosis

Acute pancreatitis or a perforated viscus may resemble bowel infarction. Free peritoneal air in perforation may help to differentiate this condition; however, serum amylase may be elevated in intestinal infarction.

Treatment & Prognosis

The treatment of acute mesenteric arterial thrombosis consists of the measures necessary to (1) restore fluid, colloid, and electrolyte balance; (2) decompress the bowel; and (3) prevent sepsis by administration of antimicrobial drugs. Angiography is performed if embolus is suspected. Unless there are absolute contraindications to surgery, laparotomy should be done as soon as possible and gangrenous bowel resected. If the infarction is due to an isolated thrombus or embolus or the superior mesenteric artery, embolectomy or thrombectomy may be possible. Anticoagulants are not indicated. The mortality rate is extremely high in the acute disease. The treatment of nonthrombotic intestinal infarction poses a therapeutic dilemma. Basically, the principles are the same, ie, maintenance of fluid, electrolyte, and colloid balance. Surgical resection of gangrenous bowel in a patient with congestive failure is a formidable undertaking but should be tried if at all possible. The prognosis in either event is grave; survival is unusual.

Hunter GC, Guernsey JM: Mesenteric ischemia. Med Clin North Am 1988;72:1091.

Odurny A, Sniderman KW, Colapinto RF: Intestinal angina: Percutaneous transluminal angioplasty of the celiac and superior mesenteric arteries. Radiology 1988; 167:59.

ACUTE ORGANIC SMALL INTESTINAL OBSTRUCTION

Essentials of Diagnosis

- Colicky abdominal pain, vomiting, constipation, borborygmus.
- Tender distended abdomen without peritoneal irritation.
- Audible high-pitched tinkling peristalsis or peristaltic rushes.
- Radiographic evidence of dilated loops of small intestine with or without fluid levels. Little or no leukocytosis.

General Considerations

Acute organic intestinal obstruction usually involves the small intestine, particularly the ileum. Major inciting causes are external hernia and postoperative adhesions. Less common causes are gallstones, neoplasms, granulomatous processes, intussusception, volvulus, internal hernia, and foreign bodies.

Clinical Findings

A. Symptoms and Signs: Colicky abdominal pain in the periumbilical area becomes more constant and diffuse as distention develops. Vomiting, at first of a reflex nature associated with the waves of pain, later becomes fecal in obstruction of the distal bowel. Borborygmus and consciousness of intestinal movement, obstipation, weakness, perspiration, and anxiety are often present. The patient is restless, changing position frequently with pain, and has sweating, tachycardia, and dehydration. Abdominal distention may be localized, with an isolated loop, but usually is generalized. The higher the obstruction, the less the distention; the longer the time of obstruction, the greater the distention. Audible peristalsis, peristaltic rushes with pain paroxysms, high-pitched tinkles, and visible peristalsis may be present. Moderate generalized abdominal tenderness may be present, and there are no signs of peritoneal irritation. Fever is absent or low-grade. A tender hernia may be present.

B. Laboratory Findings: Hemoconcentration may occur with true dehydration or may reflect sequestration of fluid in the obstructed loop or third space. Leukocytosis is absent or mild. Vomiting may cause electrolyte disturbances.

C. Imaging: Abdominal radiography reveals gas- and fluid-filled loops of bowel, and the gas does not progress downward on serial radiographs. Fluid levels may be visible.

Differential Diagnosis

The differential diagnosis includes other acute abdominal conditions such as inflammation and perforation of a viscus or renal or gallbladder colic. The absence of peritoneal signs, ie, rigidity and rebound tenderness, should aid in differentiating small bowel obstruction from ileus secondary to peritonitis, but the differential would then also include pseudo-obstruction. The absence of leukocytosis and the presence of high-pitched bowel sounds or intestinal rushes are also helpful. Similar also is mesenteric vascular disease and torsion of an organ (eg, ovarian cyst). In the late stages of obstruction it may be impossible to distinguish acute organic intestinal obstruction from the late stage of peritonitis with ileus.

Complications

Strangulation (necrosis of the bowel wall) occurs with impairment of the blood supply to the gut. Strangulation is difficult to determine clinically, but fever, marked leukocytosis, and signs of peritoneal irritation should alert the clinician to this possibility. Strangulation may lead to perforation, peritonitis, and sepsis. Strangulation increases the mortality rate of intestinal obstruction to about 25%.

Treatment

A. Supportive Measures:

1. Decompression of the intestinal tract by nasogastric suction should relieve vomiting, reduce intestinal distention, and prevent aspiration.

2. Correct fluid, electrolyte, and colloid deficits.

3. Give broad-spectrum antibiotics (gentamicin and ampicillin or clindamycin) if strangulation is suspected.

B. Surgical Measures:
Complete obstruction of the intestine is treated surgically after appropriate supportive therapy. Strangulation is always a danger as long as obstruction persists, and fever, leukocytosis, peritoneal signs, or blood in the feces means that strangulation may have occurred and that immediate surgery is required.

If the bowel is successfully decompressed during the preoperative preparation period, with cessation of pain and passage of flatus and feces, surgery may be delayed. Otherwise, surgical relief of the obstruction is indicated. Surgery consists of relieving the obstruction and removing gangrenous bowel with reanastomosis.

Prognosis

Prognosis varies with the causative factor and the presence of strangulation.

Mucha P Jr: Small intestine obstruction. Surg Clin North Am 1987;67:597.

FUNCTIONAL OBSTRUCTION
(Adynamic Ileus, Paralytic Ileus)

Essentials of Diagnosis

- Continuous abdominal pain, distention, vomiting, and obstipation.
- History of a precipitating factor (surgery, peritonitis, pain, anticholinergic drugs, pneumonia, inferior myocardial infarction).
- Minimal abdominal tenderness; decreased to absent bowel sounds.
- X-ray evidence of gas and fluid in bowel.

General Considerations

Adynamic ileus is a neurogenic or muscular impairment of peristalsis that may lead to intestinal obstruction. It is a common disorder that may be due to a variety of intra-abdominal causes, eg, gastrointestinal surgery, peritoneal irritation (hemorrhage, ruptured viscus, pancreatitis, peritonitis), or anoxic organic obstruction. Drugs with anticholinergic properties, renal colic, vertebral fractures, spinal cord injuries, severe infections, uremia, diabetic coma, and electrolyte abnormalities (especially hypokalemia) also may cause adynamic ileus.

Clinical Findings

A. Symptoms and Signs: There is mild to moderate abdominal pain, continuous rather than colicky, associated with vomiting (which may later become fecal) and obstipation. Borborygmus is absent. Symptoms of the initiating condition may also be present (eg, fever; prostration due to ruptured viscus).

Abdominal distention is generalized and may be massive, with nonlocalized minimal abdominal tenderness and no signs of peritoneal irritation unless due to the primary disease. Bowel sounds are decreased to absent. Dehydration may occur after prolonged vomiting or from sequestration of fluid in bowel loops. Other signs of the initiating disorder may be present.

B. Laboratory Findings: With prolonged vomiting, hemoconcentration and electrolyte imbalance may occur. Leukocytosis, anemia, and elevated serum amylase may be present, depending upon the initiating condition.

C. Imaging: Radiography of the abdomen shows distended gas-filled loops of bowel in the small and large intestines and even in the rectum. There may be evidence of air-fluid levels in the distended bowel. When the underlying clinical problem is unclear, a barium enema and subsequent small bowel x-ray will rule out organic obstruction.

Differential Diagnosis

The symptoms and signs of obstruction with absent bowel sounds and a history of a precipitating condition leave little doubt about the diagnosis. It is important to make certain that the adynamic ileus is not secondary to an organic obstruction, especially anoxic, where conservative management is harmful and immediate surgery may be lifesaving.

Treatment

Most cases of adynamic ileus are postoperative and respond to restriction of oral intake with gradual liberalization of the diet as the bowel function returns. Severe and prolonged ileus may require gastrointestinal suction and complete restriction of oral intake. Parenteral restoration of fluids and electrolytes is essential in such instances. A rectal tube or even a colonoscope may be helpful to decompress a dilated colon. When conservative therapy fails, it may be necessary to operate for the purpose of decompressing the bowel by enterostomy or cecostomy and to rule out mechanical obstruction.

Those cases of adynamic ileus secondary to other disorders (eg, electrolyte imbalance, severe infection, intra-abdominal or back injury, pneumonitis) are managed as above plus treatment of the primary disease.

Prognosis

The prognosis varies with that of the initiating disorder. Adynamic ileus may resolve without specific therapy when the cause is removed. Intubation with decompression is usually successful in causing return of function.

IDIOPATHIC INTESTINAL PSEUDO-OBSTRUCTION

This idiopathic disorder, usually seen in teenagers or young adults, is characterized by recurring symptoms of small bowel obstruction but no evidence of organic obstruction on x-ray or with surgical exploration. Ogilvie's syndrome, a similar problem, consists of primarily cecal dilatation in older patients who are bedfast and often have chronic obstructive pulmonary disease. In both, all previously mentioned causes of functional obstruction are absent. The patient is treated with nasogastric suction, intravenous fluids, and parenteral nutrition as required; colonoscopic decompression or cecostomy may be necessary in Ogilvie's syndrome.

Esquivel CO et al: Postoperative small bowel intussusception. West J Med 1985;143:108.
Fausel CS, Goff JS: Nonoperative management of acute idiopathic colonic pseudo-obstruction (Ogilvie's syndrome). West J Med 1985;143:50.
Krishnamurthy S, Schuffler MD: Pathology of neuromuscular disorders of the small intestine and colon. Gastroenterology 1987;93:610.

MALABSORPTION SYNDROMES (Primary Mucosal Disease)

Malabsorption syndromes may be associated with a wide variety of small intestine mucosal disease processes that have in common the malabsorption of nutrients by the gastrointestinal tract. These syndromes should be contrasted to states of maldigestion where intraluminal abnormalities result in failure to absorb nutrients, such as pancreatic insufficiency, bile salt deficiency, and a variety of postsurgical abnormalities. The clinical and laboratory manifestations are summarized in Table 11–1.

Targan SR et al: Immunologic mechanisms in intestinal diseases. Ann Intern Med 1987;106:853.

1. CELIAC SPRUE & TROPICAL SPRUE

Essentials of Diagnosis

- Bulky, pale, frothy, foul-smelling, greasy stools with increased fecal fat on chemical analysis of the stool.
- Weight loss and signs of multiple vitamin deficiencies. Impaired intestinal absorption of vitamins D, E, A, and K, as well as fat.

Table 11–1. Clinical and laboratory manifestations of malabsorption.[1]

Manifestation	Laboratory Findings	Malabsorbed Nutrient
Steatorrhea (bulky, light-colored)	Increased fecal fat; decreased serum cholesterol	Fat
Diarrhea (increased fecal water)	Increased fecal fat or positive bile salt breath test	Fatty acids or bile salts
Weight loss; malnutrition (muscle wasting); weakness, fatigue	Increased fecal fat and nitrogen; decreased glucose and xylose absorption	Calories (fat, protein, carbohydrates)
Abdominal distention		
Iron deficiency anemia	Hypochromic anemia; low serum iron	Iron
Megaloblastic anemia	Macrocytosis; decreased vitamin B_{12} absorption (^{67}Co-labeled B_{12}); decreased serum vitamin B_{12} and folic acid activity (microbiologic assay)	Vitamin B_{12} or folic acid
Paresthesia; tetany; positive Trousseau and Chvostek signs	Decreased serum calcium, magnesium, and potassium	Calcium, vitamin D, magnesium, potassium
Bone pain; pathologic fractures; skeletal deformities	Osteoporosis; osteomalacia on x-ray	Calcium, protein
Bleeding tendency (ecchymoses, melena, hematuria)	Prolonged prothrombin time	Vitamin K
Edema	Decreased serum albumin; increased fecal loss of α_1-antitrypsin	Protein (or protein-losing enteropathy)
Nocturia; abdominal distention	Increased small bowel fluid on x-ray	Water
Milk intolerance (cramps, bloating, diarrhea)	Flat lactose tolerance test; decreased mucosal lactase levels	Lactose

[1] Modified from Bayless TM: Malabsorption in the elderly. *Hosp Pract* (Aug) 1979;**14**:57.

● Hypochromic or megaloblastic anemia; small bowel x-ray pattern that of small bowel dilatation and dilution of barium.

General Considerations

Sprue syndromes are diseases of disturbed small intestine function characterized by impaired absorption, particularly of fats, and motor abnormalities. Celiac sprue responds to a gluten-free diet, whereas tropical sprue does not. The polypeptide gliadin is the offending substance in gluten. Although an infectious cause has not been conclusively demonstrated, tropical sprue behaves clinically like an infectious disease. It responds to folic acid and broad-spectrum antibiotics.

The clinical severity of sprue syndrome varies depending upon the extent of the lesion in the small intestine and the duration of the disease. Severe wasting, gastrointestinal protein loss, multiple vitamin deficiencies, and adrenal and pituitary deficiency may be associated with the severe forms of the disease. A flat intestinal mucosa without villi in the small intestine is noted, and some observers have described degenerative changes in the myenteric nerve plexuses. With the loss of villi, the microvilli are also lost, leading to disaccharidase deficiency, particularly lactase deficiency.

Rare secondary varieties of sprue syndrome in which the cause of the small intestine dysfunction is known include gastrocolic fistulas, obstruction of intestinal lacteals by lymphoma, Whipple's disease, extensive regional enteritis, and parasitic infections such as giardiasis, cryptosporidiasis, strongyloidiasis, and coccidiosis.

Clinical Findings

A. Tropical Sprue: Patients with tropical sprue are either residents of, or have had prolonged visits in, tropical regions. The main symptom is diarrhea; at first it is explosive and watery; later, stools are fewer and more solid and characteristically pale, frothy, foul-smelling, and greasy, with exacerbations on high-fat diet. Indigestion, flatulence, abdominal cramps, weight loss (often marked), pallor, asthenia, irritability, paresthesias, and muscle cramps may occur. Quiescent periods with or without mild symptoms may occur especially on leaving the tropics. Symptoms may appear years after the patient has left endemic areas.

Vitamin deficiencies cause glossitis, cheilosis, angular stomatitis, cutaneous hyperpigmentation, and dry, rough skin. Abdominal distention and mild tenderness are present. Edema occurs late.

Anemia is usually macrocytic, and, with blood loss or malabsorption of iron, may be hypochromic, microcytic, or mixed. The fecal fat is increased. Serum proteins, calcium, phosphorus, cholesterol, and prothrombin are low. Gastric hypochlorhydria is frequent. The pancreatic enzymes are normal.

Radiographs using nonflocculating barium show dilatation of the intestine and occasionally excess fluid and gas.

B. Celiac Sprue: This disorder is characterized by defective absorption of fat, protein, carbohydrates, iron, and water. Absorption of fat-soluble vitamins A, D, and K is impaired. Osteomalacia may ensue. Protein loss from the intestine may occur. Elimination of gluten from the diet causes dramatic improvement. Gluten is found in wheat, barley, oats, and rye and is used as a filler in many prepared foods and medications. Diligent elimination of this substance from the diet is important in achieving remission.

In one-third of patients with celiac sprue, symptoms begin in early childhood. Symptoms may persist into adult life, but there is usually a latent phase of apparent good health. The anemia is usually hypochromic and microcytic. The complications of impaired absorption are more severe: infantilism, dwarfism, tetany, vitamin deficiency signs, and even rickets may be seen. The definitive diagnosis of steatorrhea requires quantitative measurement of fecal fat, preferably on a known fat intake, and a characteristic small bowel biopsy.

Patients presenting with dermatitis herpetiformis frequently have associated celiac sprue, usually symptomatic. Both the sprue and the dermatitis herpetiformis are responsive to a gluten-free diet—the latter only after many months, and rechallenge with gluten results in recurrence of the rash within weeks.

A small group of patients with apparent celiac sprue are nonresponsive to a gluten-free diet. On closer inspection of the small bowel mucosal biopsy, a collagenous layer is found between the surface absorptive cells and the lamina propria. No consistently helpful medical therapy has yet been found. Other causes of nonresponsiveness may include the development of lymphoma, ulcerative jejunoileitis, or perhaps a steroid-responsive lesion.

Differential Diagnosis

It is necessary to differentiate between the various causes of malabsorption to permit selection of specific therapy, if any. Anatomic abnormalities such as fistulas, blind loops, and jejunal diverticulosis may be found on radiography. Regional enteritis usually has a characteristic radiographic appearance but must be distinguished from intestinal tuberculosis and lymphoma. The small bowel x-ray appearance in Whipple's disease, nodular lymphoid hyperplasia, intestinal lymphoma, and amyloidosis is abnormal but not specific or diagnostic. In primary diseases of the small intestine, mucosal suction biopsy is the most effective way of making the diagnosis. The pathologic response in some diseases is patchy, and multiple specimens may be required. Pancreatic insufficiency due to obstruction may be diagnosed by low-volume output by the pancreas in response to intravenous administration of secretin.

Treatment

A. Tropical Sprue: Folic acid, 10 -20 mg daily orally or intramuscularly for a few weeks, corrects diarrhea, anorexia, weight loss, glossitis, and anemia. Tetracycline, 250 mg orally 4 times daily, is given at the outset of treatment. When complete remission occurs, the patient may be maintained on 5 mg of folic acid daily. If the patient has achlorhydria, giving vitamin B_{12} intramuscularly should also be considered. Hypochromic anemia can be treated with oral iron. A high-calorie, high-protein, low-fat diet can be given.

B. Celiac Sprue: Strict elimination of gluten from the diet will lead to clinical recovery. If there is no response, inquire about other medications (many use gluten as a filler) and look for collagenous sprue. The diet must be gluten-free. In addition, the diet should be high in calories and protein and low in fat. Initially, the diet should also be lactose-free because of the loss of lactase-containing microvilli; once remission is induced, lactose-containing foods may be added. Prothrombin deficiency is treated by means of water-soluble vitamin K orally or, if urgent, parenterally. Treat hypocalcemia or tetany with calcium phosphate or gluconate, 2 g orally or intravenously 3 times daily, and vitamin D, 5–20 thousand units. Multiple vitamin supplements may also be advisable. Macrocytic anemia usually responds to vitamin B_{12}, 100 mg intramuscularly every month until the disease is in clinical remission.

The corticosteroids may be advantageous in certain patients with sprue, particularly the severely ill, since they increase the absorption of nitrogen, fats, and other nutrients from the gastrointestinal tract. They have a nonspecific effect in increasing appetite and inducing mild euphoria. Cortisol is best given in dosages of 100–300 mg/24 h intravenously and tapered off according to the patient's response.

Prognosis

With proper treatment, the response is good. Patients with celiac sprue have a late increased incidence of abdominal lymphoma and carcinomas. Patients who develop gastrointestinal symptoms while in remission on a gluten-free diet should be carefully evaluated for cancer.

Cooper BT, Read AE: Coeliac disease and lymphoma. Q J Med 1987;63:269.

Gawkrodger DJ et al: Dermatitis herpetiformis: Diagnosis, diet and dermography. Gut 1984;25:151.

Patel DG, Krogh CM, Thompson WG: Gluten in pills: A hazard for patients with celiac disease. Can Med Assoc J 1985;133:114. (Many common prescription and OTC drugs have gluten as a filler.)

Trier JS: Celiac sprue. Pages 1134–1157 in: *Gastrointestinal Disease: Pathophysiology, Diagnosis, Management,* 4th ed. Sleisenger MH, Fordtran JS (editors). Saunders, 1989.

2. DISACCHARIDASE DEFICIENCY

Lactase deficiency may occur in a congenital or adult-onset form. With the congenital form, the absence of lactase leads to acidic diarrhea (fecal pH 4.5–6.0). There are large amounts of lactic acid in the stool secondary to bacterial breakdown of lactose. The infant fails to thrive until lactose-containing foods are eliminated from the diet.

Lactase deficiency in the adult is common worldwide. It has been estimated from many studies that the incidence of lactase deficiency is 70–90% in Orientals, blacks, Native Americans, and Mediterranean populations. The incidence of lactase deficiency in northern and western Europeans is 10–15%. Symptoms may vary from minor abdominal bloating, distention, flatulence, and discomfort to markedly severe diarrhea in response to even small amounts of lactose. The diagnosis, although often established clinically, is confirmed by a lactose tolerance test; marked diarrhea usually occurs with this test. Onset in the adult may follow gastroduodenal surgery and may be associated with regional enteritis. The primary mucosal diseases of the small intestine usually have associated lactase deficiency.

Intercurrent acute illnesses, such as viral and bacterial enteritis, particularly in children, will frequently injure the microvilli of the mucosal cells of the small intestine, resulting in temporary lactase deficiency.

Other congenital defects described thus far are sucrose-isomaltose and glucose-galactose intolerance. Secondary disaccharidase deficiencies have been described in patients with giardiasis, celiac disease, ulcerative colitis, short bowel syndrome, and cystic fibrosis and postgastrectomy. Removal of the offending sugar from the patient's diet will often result in remission.

Dipalma J, Narvaez RM: Prediction of lactose malabsorption in referral patients. Dig Dis Sci 1988;33:303.

3. WHIPPLE'S DISEASE

Whipple's disease is an uncommon malabsorption disorder due to an infection of the gut with widespread systemic manifestations. Histologic examination of a small bowel mucosal biopsy specimen reveals characteristic large, foamy mononuclear cells filled with cytoplasmic material that gives a positive periodic acid-Schiff staining reaction. Electron microscopy reveals Whipple's bacilli in the intestines and in the eyes, heart, lungs, synovia, kidneys, and central nervous system. The disease occurs primarily in middle-aged men and is of insidious onset; without treatment, it is usually fatal. The manifestations include abdominal pain, diarrhea, steatorrhea, gastrointestinal bleeding, fever, lymphadenopathy, polyarthritis, edema, gray to brown skin pigmentation, and severe central nervous system manifestations. Anemia and hypoproteinemia are common.

Treatment programs are somewhat controversial but should be continued for at least 1 year and should include administration of agents that cross the blood-brain barrier. Current options are trimethoprim-sulfamethoxazole (TMP-SMZ) alone or parenteral penicillin and streptomycin followed by TMP-SMZ. Reappearance of symptoms after or during therapy suggests emergence of resistant organisms, and the antibiotic should be changed.

Keinath RD et al: Antibiotic treatment and relapse in Whipple's disease: Long-term follow-up of 88 patients. Gastroenterology 1985;88:1867.

PROTEIN-LOSING ENTEROPATHY

Leakage of plasma proteins into the intestinal lumen is an integral phase of the metabolism of plasma proteins. In certain intestinal disease states, excessive protein loss into the intestinal lumen may be responsible for the hypoproteinemia that occurs. Excessive loss of plasma protein may be due to increased mucosal permeability to protein, inflammatory exudation, excessive cell desquamation, or direct leakage of lymph from obstructed lacteals. Gastrointestinal diseases associated with protein-losing enteropathy include all of the primary mucosal diseases of the small bowel, as well as gastric carcinoma, lymphoma, gastric rugal hypertrophy, parasitic infections, and others.

Treatment consists of management of the primary disorder.

APPENDICITIS

Essentials of Diagnosis

- Early periumbilical discomfort, followed by right lower quadrant abdominal pain and tenderness with signs of peritoneal irritation.
- Anorexia, nausea and vomiting, and constipation.
- Low-grade fever and mild polymorphonuclear leukocytosis.

General Considerations

Appendicitis is initiated by obstruction of the appendiceal lumen by a fecalith, inflammation, foreign body, or neoplasm. Obstruction is followed by infection, edema, and, frequently, infarction of the appendiceal wall. Intraluminal tension develops rapidly and tends to cause early mural necrosis and perforation. All ages and both sexes are affected, but appendicitis is more common in males between 10 and 30 years of age.

Appendicitis is one of the most frequent causes of acute surgical abdomen. The symptoms and signs usually follow a fairly stereotyped pattern, but appendicitis is capable of such protean manifestations that it should be considered in the differential diagnosis of every obscure case of intra-abdominal sepsis and pain.

Clinical Findings

A. Symptoms and Signs: An attack of appendicitis usually begins with epigastric or periumbilical pain associated with 1–2 episodes of vomiting. Within 2–12 hours, the pain shifts to the right lower quadrant, where it persists as a steady soreness that is aggravated by walking or coughing. There is anorexia, moderate malaise, and slight fever. Constipation is usual, but diarrhea occurs occasionally, as does nausea and vomiting.

At onset there are no localized abdominal findings. Within a few hours, however, progressive right lower quadrant tenderness can be demonstrated; careful examination will usually identify a single point of maximal tenderness. The patient can often place a finger precisely on this area, especially if asked to accentuate the soreness by coughing. Light percussion over the right lower quadrant is helpful in localizing tenderness. Rebound tenderness and spasm of the overlying abdominal muscles are usually present. Psoas and obturator signs, when positive, are strongly suggestive of appendicitis. Rectal tenderness is common and, in pelvic appendicitis, may be more definite than abdominal tenderness. Peristalsis is diminished or absent. Slight to moderate fever is present.

B. Laboratory Findings: Moderate leukocytosis $(10,000–20,000/\mu L)$ with an increase in neutrophils is usually present. It is not uncommon to find microscopic hematuria and pyuria.

C. Imaging: There are no characteristic changes on plain films of the abdomen. However, visualization in the right lower quadrant of a radiopaque shadow consistent with fecalith in the appendix may heighten the suspicion of appendicitis. In uncertain cases, barium enemas are being used, as visualization of the entire appendix rules out acute appendicitis.

Factors That Cause Variations From the "Classic" Clinical Picture

A. Anatomic Location of Appendix: Abdominal findings are most definite when the appendix is in the iliac fossa or superficially located. When the appendix extends over the pelvic brim, abdominal signs may be minimal, greatest tenderness being elicited on rectal examination. Right lower quadrant tenderness may be poorly localized and slow to develop in retrocecal or retroileal appendicitis. Inflammation of a high-lying lateral appendix may produce maximal tenderness in the flank, and in the left lower quadrant in situs inversus. Bizarre locations of the appendix may rarely occur in association with a mobile or undescended cecum; in such cases, symptoms and signs may localize in the right upper or left lower quadrant.

B. Age:

1. Infancy and childhood–In infancy, appendicitis is relatively rare. When it does occur, history and physical findings are difficult to interpret. The disease tends to progress rapidly, and rupture results in generalized peritonitis.

2. Old age–Elderly patients frequently have few or no prodromal symptoms. Abdominal findings may be unimpressive, with slight tenderness and negligible muscle guarding, until perforation occurs. Fever and leukocytosis may also be minimal or absent. When the white count is not elevated, a shift to the left is significant evidence of inflammation.

C. Obesity: Obesity frequently increases the difficulty of evaluation by delaying the appearance of abdominal signs and by preventing sharp localization.

D. Pregnancy: See discussion in Chapter 13.

Differential Diagnosis

Acute gastroenteritis is the disorder most commonly confused with appendicitis. In rare cases it either precedes or is coincident with appendicitis. Vomiting and diarrhea are more common. Fever and the white blood count may rise sharply and may be out of proportion to abdominal findings. Localization of pain and tenderness is usually indefinite and shifting. Hyperactive peristalsis is characteristic. Gastroenteritis frequently runs an acute course. A period of observation usually serves to clarify the diagnosis.

Mesenteric adenitis may cause signs and symptoms identical with appendicitis. Usually, however, there are some clues to the true diagnosis. Mesenteric adenitis is more likely to occur in children or adolescents; respiratory infection is a common antecedent; localization of right lower quadrant tenderness is less precise and constant; and true muscle guarding is infrequent. In spite of a strong suspicion of mesenteric adenitis, it is often safer to advise appendectomy than to risk a complication of appendicitis by delay.

Meckel's diverticulitis may mimic appendicitis. The localization of tenderness may be more medial, but this is not a reliable diagnostic criterion. Because operation is required in both diseases, the differentiation is not critical. When a preoperative diagnosis of appendicitis proves on exploration to be erroneous, it is essential to examine the terminal 150 cm of ileum for Meckel's diverticulitis and mesenteric adenitis.

Regional enteritis, amebiasis, acute ileitis due to *Yersinia pseudotuberculosis,* perforated duodenal ulcer, ureteral colic, acute salpingitis, mittelschmerz, ruptured ectopic pregnancy, and twisted ovarian cyst may also be confused with appendicitis. Right lower lobe pneumonia sometimes is associated with prominent right lower quadrant pain.

Complications

A. Perforation: Appendicitis may rarely subside spontaneously, but it is an unpredictable disease with a marked tendency (about 95%) to progression and perforation. Because perforation rarely occurs within the first 8 hours, diagnostic observation during this period is relatively safe. Signs of perforation include increasing severity of pain, tenderness, and spasm in the right lower quadrant followed by evidence of generalized peritonitis or of a localized abscess. Ileus, fever, malaise, and leukocytosis become more marked. If perforation with abscess formation or generalized peritonitis has already occurred when the patient is first seen, the diagnosis may be quite obscure.

The treatment of perforated appendicitis is appendectomy unless a well-localized right lower quadrant or pelvic abscess has already walled off the appendix. Supportive measures are as for acute peritonitis.

1. Generalized peritonitis–Clinical findings and treatment are discussed elsewhere in this chapter.

2. Appendiceal abscess–Malaise, toxicity, fever, and leukocytosis vary from minimal to marked. Examination discloses a tender mass in the right lower quadrant or pelvis. Pelvic abscesses tend to bulge into the rectum or vagina.

Abscesses usually become noticeable 2–6 days after onset, but antibiotic therapy may delay their appearance. Appendiceal abscess is occasionally the first and only sign of appendicitis and may be confused with neoplasm of the cecum, particularly in older persons, who may have little or no systemic reaction to the infection.

Treatment of early abscess is by intensive combined antibiotic therapy (eg, ampicillin, gentamicin, and metronidazole or clindamycin). On this regimen, the abscess will frequently resolve. Appendectomy should be performed 6–12 weeks later. A well-established progressive abscess in the right lower quadrant should be drained without delay. Pelvic abscess requires drainage when it bulges into the rectum or vagina and has become fluctuant.

B. Pylephlebitis: Suppurative thrombophlebitis of the portal system with liver abscess is a rare but highly lethal complication. It should be suspected when septic fever, chills, hepatomegaly, and jaundice develop after appendiceal perforation. Intensive combined antibiotic therapy with surgical drainage of the abscesses is indicated.

C. Other Complications: These include subphrenic abscess and other foci of intra-abdominal sepsis. Intestinal obstruction may be caused by adhesions.

Treatment

A. Preoperative Care:

1. Observation for diagnosis–Within the first 8–12 hours after onset, the symptoms and signs of appendicitis are frequently indefinite. Under these circumstances a period of close observation is essential. The patient is placed at bed rest and given nothing by mouth. *Note:* Laxatives should not be prescribed when appendicitis or any form of peritonitis is suspected. Narcotic medications are avoided if possible, but sedation with tranquilizing agents is not contraindicated. Abdominal and rectal examinations, white blood count, and differential count are repeated periodically. Abdominal films and an upright chest film must be obtained as part of the investigation of all difficult diagnostic problems. In most cases of appendicitis, the diagnosis is clarified by localization of signs to the right lower quadrant within 12 hours after onset of symptoms.

2. Intubation–Preoperatively, a nasogastric tube is inserted if there is sufficient peritonitis or toxicity to indicate that postoperative ileus may be troublesome. In such patients the stomach is aspirated and lavaged if necessary, and the patient is sent to the operating room with the tube in place.

3. Antibiotics–In the presence of a marked systemic reaction with severe toxicity and high fever, preoperative administration of antibiotics (eg, the above-noted regimen, though many alternatives exist) is advisable.

B. Surgical Treatment: In uncomplicated appendicitis, appendectomy is performed as soon as fluid imbalance and other significant systemic disturbances are controlled. Little preparation is usually required. Early surgery has a mortality rate of a fraction of 1%. The morbidity and mortality rates associated with this disease reflect the occurrence of gangrene and perforation that occur when operation is delayed.

C. Postoperative Care: In uncomplicated appendicitis, postoperative gastric suction is usually not necessary. Ambulation is begun on the first postoperative day. The diet is advanced from clear liquids to soft solids during the second to fifth postoperative days depending upon the rapidity with which peristalsis and gastrointestinal function return. Parenteral fluid supplements are administered as required. Enemas are contraindicated. Milk of magnesia or a similar mild laxative may be given orally at bedtime daily from about the third day onward if necessary. Antibiotic therapy is advisable for 5–7 days, or longer if abdominal fluid at operation was purulent or malodorous, if culture was positive, or if the appendix was gangrenous. Primary wound healing is the rule, and the period of hospitalization is usually 1 week or less. Normal activity can usually be resumed in 2–3 weeks after surgery in uncomplicated cases.

D. Emergency Nonsurgical Treatment: When surgical facilities are not available, treat as for acute peritonitis. One such a regimen, acute appendicitis may subside, and complications will be minimized.

Prognosis

With accurate diagnosis and early surgical removal, mortality and morbidity rates are minimal. Delay of diagnosis produces significant mortality and morbidity rates if complications occur.

Recurrent acute attacks may occur if the appendix

is not removed. "Chronic appendicitis" does not exist.

Bongard F, Landers DV, Lewis F: Differential diagnosis of appendicitis and pelvic inflammatory disease: A prospective analysis. Am J Surg 1985;150:90.

Hoffman J, Rasmussen O: Aids in the diagnosis of acute appendicitis. Br J Surg 1989;76:774. (Most helpful are clinical observations, ultrasound, and barium enema.)

Puylaert JB et al: A prospective study of ultrasonography in the diagnosis of appendicitis. N Engl J Med 1987;317:666. (Led to correct diagnosis—nonappendiceal—in several patients in this series.)

INTESTINAL TUBERCULOSIS (Tuberculous Enterocolitis)

Gastrointestinal tuberculosis may occur anywhere along the gastrointestinal tract. Involvement of the intestine frequently complicates pulmonary tuberculosis but goes clinically unrecognized. Ingestion of milk containing tubercle bacilli is another means of infection. Many cases have neither association.

The mode of infection is by ingestion of tubercle bacilli, with the formation of ulcerating lesions in the intestine, particularly the ileocecal region, and involvement of the mesenteric lymph nodes; alternatively, reactivation of a primary intestinal focus may result in active intestinal tuberculosis.

Clinical Findings

Symptoms may be absent or minimal even with extensive disease. When present, they usually consist of fever, anorexia, nausea, flatulence, distention after eating, and food intolerance. There may be abdominal pain and mild to severe cramps, usually in the right lower quadrant and often after meals. Constipation may be present, but mild to severe diarrhea is more characteristic. Tuberculosis may involve the peritoneum. The disease of course is chronic and may be difficult to distinguish from inflammatory bowel disease, ameboma, or intestinal lymphoma or carcinoma.

Findings on abdominal examination are not characteristic, although there may be mild right lower quadrant tenderness. Fistula in ano may be evident. Weight loss occurs.

There are no characteristic laboratory findings. The presence of tubercle bacilli in the feces does not correlate with intestinal involvement.

Radiographic examination of the involved bowel reveals irritability and spasm, particularly in the cecal region; irregular hypermotility of the intestinal tract; ulcerated lesions and irregular filling defects, particularly in the right colon and ileocecal region; and usually pulmonary tuberculosis. Colonoscopy with biopsy may prove helpful in establishing the diagnosis.

Treatment & Prognosis

The prognosis varies with that of the pulmonary disease. The intestinal lesions usually respond to the same regimen as for pulmonary tuberculosis, ie, 4 drugs for 6–9 months. Operation may be required for intestinal obstruction or for diagnosis, though colonic lesions are readily accessible for endoscopic biopsy.

DISEASES OF THE COLON & RECTUM

IRRITABLE BOWEL SYNDROME

Irritable bowel syndrome is a term denoting a clinical entity characterized by some combination of (1) abdominal pain; (2) altered bowel function, constipation, or diarrhea; (3) hypersecretion of colonic mucus; (4) dyspeptic symptoms (flatulence, nausea, anorexia); and (5) varying degrees of anxiety or depression. This common group of disorders has many names, eg, nervous indigestion, functional dyspepsia, pylorospasm, irritable colon, spastic "colitis," functional "colitis," mucous "colitis," intestinal neurosis, and laxative or cathartic "colitis."

Pathogenesis

Three main factors appear significant in the pathogenesis of irritable bowel syndrome.

(1) Colonic motor activity: There is no abnormality of either motility or electrical activity of the colon specific to the irritable bowel syndrome. However, prediverticular disease can be frequently demonstrated and is characterized by increased width of the sigmoid circular muscles, increased segmentation, and increased nonpropulsive intraluminal pressures. Colonic motor activity is abnormally increased in patients with colonic pain, eg, after meals, after administration of cholecystokinin or cholinergic drugs, or after emotional stress. Altered small bowel motility may also occur and appears to be correlated with symptoms.

(2) Psychologic stress: Many patients with irritable bowel syndrome exhibit colonic symptoms at times of stress. The changes in colonic function are common manifestations of emotional tension. The reaction, however, may be more severe in patients with irritable bowel.

(3) Diet: A low-residue diet in some patients may be a prominent predisposing factor. Intolerance of lactose and other sugars may account for the irritable bowel syndrome in certain patients.

It is essential to eliminate the possibility of organic gastrointestinal disease. A history of "nervousness" and emotional disturbances can usually be obtained. Bowel consciousness and cathartic and enema habits are prominent features. There is a highly variable complex of gastrointestinal symptoms: nausea and vomiting, anorexia, foul breath, sour stomach, flatulence, cramps, and constipation or diarrhea; hysteria and depression are the most prevalent psychologic problems.

Nocturnal diarrhea, awakening the patient from a sound sleep, is frequently a result of organic disease of the bowel and is less prominent in irritable bowel syndrome.

Clinical Findings

Examination discloses variable abdominal tenderness, particularly along the course of the colon. Sigmoidoscopy often reveals marked spasm and mucus in the colonic lumen and will frequently provoke the patient's spontaneously occurring symptoms. Laboratory studies should include a complete blood count and stool examination to rule out the presence of occult blood, ova, parasites, and pathogenic bacteria. Gastrointestinal x-rays may show altered gastrointestinal motility without other evidence of abnormalities.

Treatment

A. Diet: No single diet is applicable to all patients with irritable bowel syndrome. Some patients may respond to an increase in dietary fiber. Exclusion of milk and milk products may prove helpful. Irrational fear of foods must be dispelled.

B. Psychotherapy: Reassurance is important. Once the diagnosis has been established, the patient should be reassured that the symptoms are not due to an organic disease. Anxiety or depression should be treated appropriately. Antidepressants may be helpful, in part because of their anticholinergic effect.

C. Vegetable Mucilages: Psyllium hydrophilic mucilloid (Metamucil) may be useful.

Kellow JE, Phillips SF: Altered small bowel motility in irritable bowel syndrome is correlated with symptoms. Gastroenterology 1987;92:1885.

Schuster MM: Irritable bowel syndrome. Pages 1402–1408 in: *Gastrointestinal Disease: Pathophysiology, Diagnosis, Management,* 4th ed. Sleisenger MH, Fordtran JS (editors). Saunders, 1989.

INFECTIOUS COLITIS

Bacterial infections are common causes of acute colitis and are usually associated with fever, cramps, and diarrhea with tenesmus and often with blood in the stool. The most common causes are *Campylobacter jejuni, Shigella, Salmonella,* and *Yersinia enterocolitica.* (See Chapter 26.) Diarrhea due to the toxins of *E coli* (a common cause of "turista") should be considered, but this is a secretory diarrhea without evidence of colitis. Anal intercourse may be responsible for additional infectious diseases of the rectum, including gonorrhea, syphilis, lymphogranuloma vene-reum, condyloma latum, herpes simplex, and AIDS.

AIDS (see Chapter 24) is a multisystem disorder, and the impaired immune function of the intestinal tract makes it particularly vulnerable to damage because of the large number of potential pathogens usually found in the intestinal lumen. Diarrhea and weight loss may precede the other manifestations of AIDS. Rectal and jejunal biopsies may show histologic abnormalities in AIDS patients with diarrhea.

Sigmoidoscopy will usually reveal acute colitis with small ulcerations; a mucus smear will reveal a preponderance of polymorphonuclear neutrophils; and cultures may reveal the organism. Tuberculosis is an uncommon cause.

Acute and chronic colitis caused by parasites such as the protozoan *Entamoeba histolytica* is common worldwide and not uncommon in the USA. It may be clinically indistinguishable from other types of acute and chronic colitis; differentiation can often be made by smears of aspirates at sigmoidoscopy, multiple stool examinations, and, in patients with sigmoidoscopic abnormalities, mucosal biopsy. In chronic forms, the areas of involvement are most commonly the cecum, sigmoid colon, or rectum. The chronic form may mimic granulomatous colitis or neoplasm. Complications include local abscess, liver abscess, and fistula formation. For treatment, see Chapter 28.

Cohen MB, Giannella RA: Bacterial diarrheal disease: Host and bacterial factors involved in intestinal infection. Viewpoints on Dig Dis 1987;19:(4):1.

Goodman LJ et al: Empiric antimicrobial therapy of domestically acquired acute diarrhea in urban adults. Arch Intern Med 1990;150:541.

Nostrant TT, Kumar NB, Appelman HD: Histopathology differentiates acute self-limited colitis from ulcerative colitis. Gastroenterology 1987;92:318.

Sachs MK, Dickinson GM: The infectious enteritides. Pract Gastroenterol 1989;13:47.

ANTIBIOTIC-ASSOCIATED COLITIS

Antibiotic-associated colitis may occur during antibiotic usage or up to 2 weeks subsequent to usage. The disease usually subsides when the offending antibiotic is withdrawn, but it is potentially lethal and diagnosis should be pursued.

Pseudomembranous colitis is characterized by profuse watery diarrhea with cramps, tenesmus, low-grade fever, and, rarely, blood per rectum. Current or recent antibiotic therapy is a usual part of the history. Almost all antibiotics have been implicated; clindamycin, ampicillin, and the cephalosporins are most common. Metronidazole is effective in treatment of pseudomembranous enterocolitis, but it has also been reported to be a cause of this disease. Uncommonly, the disease occurs without antibiotic usage.

There is evidence for person-to-person spread.

Diarrhea occurs secondary to selective overgrowth of the bacterium *Clostridium difficile*, which produces a toxin that causes the lesion of pseudomembranous colitis. Laboratory assays for detecting this toxin in stool are now available and are important in establishing the diagnosis.

Physical findings may be minimal but can include a distended, tender abdomen with a dilated bowel. Sigmoidoscopy may reveal a pseudomembrane characterized by adherent plaques (mushroom caps) of exudate with intervening normal mucosa. Occasionally the exudate is confluent. When the pseudomembrane is stripped away, capillary type bleeding will occur from the denuded mucosa. In a few patients, routine sigmoidoscopy is normal but colonoscopy shows involvement of the sigmoid colon or more proximal areas, sometimes only the right colon is involved.

Metronidazole, 0.5 g orally 3 times a day for 7–10 days, is the drug of choice and is curative in about 90% of cases. For those infections not cleared by metronidazole, the much more expensive vancomycin at a dosage of 500–1000 mg/d orally for 10 days is usually effective.

Complications of the untreated illness include dehydration with electrolyte imbalance, perforation, toxic megacolon, and death.

A similar colitis without pseudomembrane is clinically indistinguishable from pseudomembranous colitis and may be more common. It is usually (not always) *C difficile* toxin-related. Sigmoidoscopy and occasionally colonoscopy will show evidence of acute colitis, often right-sided. Ampicillin is often associated. All antibiotics should be withdrawn, and treatment should proceed as with pseudomembranous colitis if the toxin is demonstrated. Otherwise, treat expectantly.

Fekety R et al: Treatment of antibiotic-associated *Clostridium difficile* colitis with oral vancomycin: Comparison of two dose regimens. Am J Med 1989;86:15. (Efficacy of 125 mg/d is equal to that 500 mg/d.)

McFarland LV et al: Nosocomial acquisition of *Clostridium difficile* infection. N Engl J Med 1989;320:204.

Silva J: Update on pseudomembranous colitis. (Medical Staff Conference.) West J Med 1989;151:644.

NONSPECIFIC ULCERATIVE COLITIS

Essentials of Diagnosis

- Bloody diarrhea with lower abdominal cramps.
- Mild abdominal tenderness, weight loss, fever.
- Anemia; no stool pathogens.
- Specific x-ray and sigmoidoscopic abnormalities.

General Considerations

Ulcerative colitis is a chronic inflammatory disease

of the colon of unknown cause characterized by bloody diarrhea, a tendency to remissions and exacerbations, and involvement mainly of the left colon. It is primarily a disease of adolescents and young adults but may have its onset in any age group.

The pathologic process is that of acute nonspecific inflammation of the colonic mucosa, particularly the rectosigmoid area, with multiple irregular superficial ulcerations. Repeated episodes lead to thickening of the wall with scar tissue, and the proliferative changes in the epithelium may lead to polypoid structures. Pseudopolyps are usually indicative of severe ulceration. The cause is not known; it may be multiple.

Clinical Findings

A. Symptoms and Signs: This disease may vary from mild cases with relatively minimal symptoms to acute and fulminating, with severe diarrhea and prostration. Diarrhea is characteristic; there may be up to 10–25 discharges daily, with blood and mucus in the stools, or blood and mucus may occur without feces. Blood in the stool is the cardinal manifestation of ulcerative colitis. Constipation may occur instead of diarrhea. The small intestine is never involved.

Nocturnal diarrhea is usually present when daytime diarrhea is prominent. Rectal tenesmus may be severe, and anal incontinence may be present. Cramping lower abdominal pain often occurs but is generally mild. Anorexia, malaise, weakness, and fatigability may also be present. A history of intolerance to dairy products can sometimes be obtained, and there is a tendency toward remissions and exacerbations.

Fever, weight loss, and evidence of toxemia vary with the severity of the disease. Abdominal tenderness is generally mild and occurs without signs of peritoneal irritation. Abdominal distention may be present in the fulminating form and is a poor prognostic sign. Rectal examination may show perianal irritation, fissure, hemorrhoids, and, uncommonly, fistulas and abscesses.

B. Laboratory Findings: Hypochromic microcytic anemia due to blood loss is usually present. In acute disease, a polymorphonuclear leukocytosis may also be present. The sedimentation rate is usually elevated. Stools contain blood, pus, and mucus but no pathogenic organisms. Hypoproteinemia may occur. In the fulminating disease, electrolyte disturbances may be evident.

C. Imaging: As shown by air contrast barium enema, the involvement may be regional to generalized and may vary from irritability and fuzzy margins to pseudopolyps, decreased size of colon, shortening and narrowing of the lumen, and loss of haustral markings. When the disease is limited to the rectosigmoid area, the barium enema may even be normal. This study should be avoided when patients are actively symptomatic.

D. Special Examinations: Sigmoidoscopy discloses rectal involvement in over 95% of cases, with mucosal hyperemia, petechiae, and minimal granularity in mild cases and ulceration and polypoid changes in severe cases. The mucosa, even when it appears grossly normal, is friable when wiped with a cotton sponge. Colonoscopic examination may prove useful in defining the extent of ulcerative colitis but should be avoided when patients are actively symptomatic. It is recommended that colonoscopy with multiple biopsies looking for dysplasia and cancer be performed annually after the tenth year of disease.

Differential Diagnosis

Bacillary dysentery is excluded on the basis of culture for specific stool pathogens. Amebiasis is excluded by stool examination, the indirect hemagglutination test, and biopsy. When rectal strictures have developed, lymphogranuloma venereum is ruled out by history and complement fixation test. Other entities that must be distinguished are functional diarrhea, granulomatous colitis, intestinal neoplasm, and diverticulitis. It is imperative that any cultures and parasitology specimens be obtained before barium examinations are performed or before therapy is begun. Rectal abscesses and fistulas are considerably less frequent than in granulomatous colitis.

Complications

A. Colonic Complications: Complications include colonic perforation, toxic dilatation of the colon, carcinoma, and massive colonic hemorrhage.

The incidence of carcinoma is significantly greater in patients with ulcerative colitis. It appears to be related to 2 factors. The first is the extent of involvement. Involvement of the entire colon carries a greater risk than minimal disease; disease confined to the rectum, in fact, is unassociated with increased risk of cancer. The second factor is duration of the disease. The risk rises from approximately 0.2% at 19 years to 2.8% at 15 years, 4.5% at 20 years, and 13.5% at 30 years.

B. Systemic Complications: Systemic complications include pyoderma gangrenosum, erythema nodosum, polyarthritis, ankylosing spondylitis, ocular lesions (episcleritis, iritis, uveitis), oral ulcers, liver disease (pericholangitis, sclerosing cholangitis), anemia, pleuropericarditis, thrombophlebitis, and impaired growth and sexual development in children.

Treatment

Ulcerative colitis is characterized by recurrent exacerbations, varying degrees of damage to the colonic mucosa, and complications both intestinal and extraintestinal. The treatment programs should attempt to (1) terminate the acute attack, (2) prevent recurrent attacks, and (3) promote healing of the damaged mucosa. Long-term therapy may be modified by considerations relating to complications, eg, carcinoma and ocular disease. Symptomatic remission should not be the only index of therapeutic response.

The choice and intensity of therapy should be determined by the clinical severity of the disease.

A. Severe (Fulminant) Disease:

1. Hospitalization–Hospitalization is indicated. Patients with severe disease may deteriorate rapidly, with hemorrhage, perforation, toxic megacolon, and sepsis developing over a short period of time.

2. General measures–

a. Restore circulating blood volume with fluids, plasma, and blood as indicated.

b. Discontinue opiates and anticholinergics.

c. Correct electrolyte abnormalities. d. Discontinue all oral intake. Institute nasogastric suction if the colon has become dilated.

3. Antimicrobial therapy–The clinical course of fulminant ulcerative colitis is associated with extensive necrosis of colonic mucosa, and perforation with sepsis is not uncommon in this form of the disease. Intravenous antibiotics are given these patients for presumed or potential sepsis. Ampicillin, a cephalosporin, clindamycin, metronidazole, and gentamicin have been used singly, but more often in appropriate combinations.

4. Adrenocorticosteroids–Give intravenous hydrocortisone, 300 mg daily, or methylprednisolone, 48 mg daily, in divided doses at 6– to 8-hour intervals.

5. Surgery–If the patient with toxic colonic dilatation does not improve within 24 hours, colonic resection is usually indicated. In those patients who have fulminant disease but are not toxic, intravenous therapy is continued for 5–7 days. If the patient fails to respond or deteriorates, colectomy should be considered. Malnourished patients may be benefited by total parenteral nutrition during this phase.

B. Moderate Disease: This group of patients has substantial evidence of activity, ie, diarrhea, abdominal cramping, weight loss, and anemia, and hospitalization should be advised. However, they are not in a toxic condition, ie, they do not have severe hypoproteinemia, fever, or leukocytosis.

1. Diet–Food served should be appealing and contain adequate protein; foods known to exacerbate the individual patient's problems are avoided. Some patients appear to be lactase-deficient and should avoid milk and milk products.

2. Adrenocorticosteroids–Give prednisone, 20–60 mg orally daily, and reduce by 5 mg per day per week when there is clinical and sigmoidoscopic evidence of improvement. Hydrocortisone enemas, 100 mg each night, may provide additional benefit.

3. Sulfasalazine–Sulfasalazine, 4–8 g daily in divided doses, has been shown to be beneficial in reducing inflammation and in decreasing the frequency of recurrent attacks in this form of the disease. It has been suggested that mesalamine (5-aminosalicylic acid; Rowasa) is the active moiety of sulfasalazine and that it does not have the side effects attributed to the sulfonamide moiety; it is available as rectal suspension, and had equal efficacy when compared

to hydrocortisone enemas. An oral preparation is anticipated. Sulfasalazine has been shown to produce oligospermia and infertility in men during the treatment period.

C. Mild Disease: These patients have minimal evidence of inflammatory bowel disease, ie, asymptomatic rectal bleeding, minimal involvement by sigmoidoscopic examination, and no systemic signs.

1. Diet–See ¶ 1 above.

2. Sulfasalazine–Sulfasalazine, 2–4 g daily in divided doses, as prolonged maintenance therapy. Mesalamine (Rowasa; 5-aminosalicylic acid) is available as rectal suspension for administration by enema and avoids steroid side effects but costs considerably more than hydrocortisone enemas.

3. Adrenocorticosteroids–Hydrocortisone enemas or suppositories, 100 mg each night until lesion heals or treatment proves ineffective.

D. Surgical Measures: Surgical excision of the colon is required for patients with refractory disease, severe extracolonic complications (growth suppression), prolonged widespread colon disease, massive hemorrhage, or extensive perirectal disease. The usual procedure is total colectomy with a permanent ileostomy. With increasing frequency the rectum is preserved (stripped of its mucosa) and an ileoanal anastomosis performed with ileal mucosa replacing the stripped rectal mucosa. This allows intestinal continuity and avoids an ileostomy, but most of these patients will have 4–7 semiliquid stools per day.

Prognosis

The course may be characterized by remissions and exacerbations over a period of many years, or it may be fulminant. Permanent and complete cure on medical therapy is unusual, and life expectancy is shortened. The incidence of bowel cancer in patients with active disease rises with each decade after the diagnosis. Medical measures control the majority of cases but colectomy is often necessary for fulminant, refractory disease and for complications. Because of potential complications with chronic ulcerative colitis, close follow-up is indicated, particularly after the disease has been present for 8–10 years. It is recommended that after 10 years of disease, colonoscopy be performed annually, and that on these occasions multiple biopsies should be examined for dysplasia. Dysplasia is considered a precancerous lesion and if severe is thought to be an indication for colectomy.

Cangemi JR et al: Effect of proctocolectomy for chronic ulcerative colitis on the natural history of primary sclerosing cholangitis. Gastroenterology 1989;96:790.

Danish 5-ASA Group: Topical 5-aminosalicylic acid versus prednisolone in ulcerative proctosigmoiditis: A randomized, double-blind multicenter trial. Dig Dis Sci 1987; 32:598.

Danzi JT: Extraintestinal manifestations of idiopathic inflammatory bowel disease. Arch Inter Med 1988; 148: 297.

Gilat T et al: Colorectal cancer in patients with ulcerative colitis: A population study in central Israel. Gastroenterology 1988;94:870. (Incidence at 10, 20, and 30 years.)

Ginsberg AL et al: Treatment of left-sided ulcerative colitis with 4-aminosalicylic acid enemas: A double-blind, placebo-controlled trial. Ann Inter Med 1988;108:195.

Hendriksen C, Kreiner S, Binder V: Long-term prognosis in ulcerative colitis: Based on results from a regional patient group from the County of Copenhagen.

Gut 1985;26:158. Mulder CJ et al: Double-blind comparison of slow-release 5-aminosalicylate and sulfasalazine in remission maintenance in ulcerative colitis. Gastroenterology 1988;95:1449. (5-Aminosalicylate is better tolerated and just as effective.)

Malatjalian DA: Pathology of inflammatory bowel disease in colorectal biopsies. Dig Dis Sci 1987;32(December Suppl):55. Pemberton JH et al: Ileal pouch-anal anastomosis for chronic ulcerative colitis: Long-term results. Ann Surg 1987;206:504.

TOXIC DILATATION OF THE COLON
(Toxic Megacolon)

Toxic megacolon is a life-threatening complication of idiopathic ulcerative colitis or Crohn's disease of the colon. The disease has also been observed in amebiasis, pseudomembranous colitis, typhoid fever, and bacillary dysentery. It results from extensive damage to the mucosa, with areas of mucosal denudation and inflammation of the submucosal layers. Contributing factors include cathartics, opiates, anticholinergics, and hypokalemia. It is manifested clinically by evidence of systemic toxicity, fever, leukocytosis, tachycardia, and abdominal distention. Radiographically, the colon is dilated. Colonic dilatation per se without signs of systemic toxicity may be the result of potassium deficiency or anticholinergic or opiate therapy. The mortality rate of this fulminant complication is high, and treatment, both medical and surgical, should be instituted as soon as possible.

Treatment consists of the following urgent measures: (1) Decompress the bowel and pass an intestinal tube to prevent swallowed air from further distending the colon. (2) Replace lost fluids and electrolytes and restore colloid and blood volume. Remember that diarrhea and adrenal steroid therapy significantly reduce total body potassium and that this has an adverse effect on colonic function. (3) Suppress the inflammatory reaction with hydrocortisone, 100 mg intravenously every 8 hours. (4) Prevent sepsis with broad-spectrum antibiotics (eg, ampicillin, metronidazole, and gentamicin or other combinations).

Careful observation with frequent abdominal films during the period of 8–12 hours while the above therapy is being given determines whether or not the patient will require surgical treatment. If the colon decompresses, medical therapy is continued; if not, colectomy should be considered. These patients are desperately ill, and if surgery is necessary the procedure of choice is subtotal colectomy. This reduces operating time and the extent of operative trauma. Most of the patients who develop toxic dilatation of the colon but do not require emergency colectomy will require colectomy at a later time because of continuing disease.

Greenstein AJ et al: Outcome of toxic dilatation in ulcerative and Crohn's colitis. J Clin Gastroenterol 1985;7:137.

GRANULOMATOUS COLITIS
(Crohn's Disease of the Colon)

Granulomatous colitis (transmural colitis; Crohn's disease of the colon) may be difficult or impossible to distinguish from the mucosal form of colitis (idiopathic ulcerative colitis) by clinical criteria alone. The most distinguishing feature is transmural involvement in Crohn's colitis. Table 11–2 briefly summarizes the features of these 2 entities. However, the differential diagnostic criteria, when tested against the pathologic findings following colectomy, show a substantial overlap in clinical, radiographic, and histologic criteria.

The most common clinical manifestations are abdominal cramping, diarrhea, and weight loss. Extracolonic manifestations such as erythema nodosum, spondylitis, polyarthritis, and perirectal disease may antedate the colonic manifestations of the disease.

The treatment of granulomatous colitis is essentially the same as for idiopathic ulcerative colitis.

Hamilton SR: Colorectal carcinoma in patients with Crohn's disease. Gastroenterology 1985;89:398. (Increased incidence and younger patients.)

Table 11–2. Differential features of ulcerative colitis and granulomatous colitis.[1]

	Ulcerative Colitis	Granulomatous Colitis
Clinical		
Systemic toxicity	Occasional	Rare
Bleeding	Common	Rare
Perianal disease	Rare	Common
Fistula	Rare	Common
Perforation	Rare	Common
Sigmoidoscopy	Diffuse, friable superficial ulceration	Discrete, occasionally diffuse
X-ray		
Distribution	Continuous	Segmental
Mucosa	Serrated	Fissures to deep ulcers
Stricture	Rare	Common
Pathology	Mucosal microabscesses	Transmural involvement, granulomas

[1] Reference: Margulis AR et al: The overlapping spectrum of ulcerative and granulomatous colitis: A roentgenographic-pathologic study. *Am J Roentgenol* 1971;**113**:325.

Longo WE, Ballantyne GH, Cahow CE: Treatment of Crohn's colitis: Segmental or total colectomy? Arch Surg 1988;123:588. (In those with disease limited to the colon, proctocolectomy appears to have a strikingly lower recurrence rate.)

Heer M et al: Acute ischaemic colitis in a female long distance runner. Gut 1987;28:896.

Hunter GC, Guernsey JM: Mesenteric ischemia. Med Clin North Am 1988;72:1091.

ISCHEMIC COLITIS

Interference with blood flow to the colon causes ischemic colitis. The rectum is usually spared because of its dual blood supply from the inferior mesenteric artery and, via the rectal (hemorrhoidal) vessels, from the internal iliac artery. Most patients are over 50 years old and have a history of peripheral vascular disease. Previous aortic surgery, with inadvertent sacrifice of the inferior mesenteric artery, is a predisposing factor. Younger women taking oral contraceptives are also at risk. Other associations include long-distance running.

Presenting symptoms are lower abdominal pain of sudden onset, fever, vomiting, and the passage of bright red blood and clots per rectum. A neutrophil leukocytosis is usual. The sigmoidoscopic examination is often normal, since involvement is usually of the more proximal portions of the colon, particularly the cecum, splenic flexure, and sigmoid colon. When the sigmoid colon is involved, a demarcation in mucosal color can often be seen at the rectosigmoid junction. Involvement of the sigmoid colon or the rectum (rare) may have the appearance on sigmoidoscopy of nonspecific proctocolitis or multiple ulcers, polypoid or nodular lesions, or, in some instances, hemorrhagic or necrotic membrane formation.

Plain films of the abdomen may show generalized dilatation of the colon. Barium enema normally shows a segmental area of involvement occurring, in descending order of frequency, in the splenic flexure, sigmoid colon, and ascending colon. The involved area is characterized by a variable combination of thumbprinting (edematous mucosal folds), sawtoothed mucosal irregularity, tubular narrowing, and sacculation. Angiograms may be helpful in diagnosis, but most ischemic disease is nonocclusive. Inflammatory bowel involvement by Crohn's disease, idiopathic ulcerative colitis, and infection and stricture due to carcinoma must be ruled out.

Severe ischemia leading to gangrene is treated by replacement of blood volume, antibiotics (eg, ampicillin, clindamycin or metronidazole, and gentamicin), and excision of necrotic bowel. Less severe ischemia leading to stricture formation is treated by resection of the stricture. Transient ischemia requires no specific treatment.

The prognosis is good in transient proctocolitis. The mortality rate is high when gangrene occurs.

Brandt LJ et al: Simulations of colonic carcinoma by ischemia. Gastroenterology 1985;88:1137.

DIVERTICULAR DISEASE OF THE COLON

Essentials of Diagnosis

- Intermittent, cramping left lower abdominal pain.
- Constipation or alternating constipation and diarrhea.
- Tenderness in the left lower quadrant.
- X-ray evidence of diverticula, thickened interhaustral folds, narrowed lumen.

General Considerations

Diverticula of the colon occur with increasing frequency after age 40—5% in the fifth decade and 50% in the ninth decade. Although diverticula may occur throughout the gut, excluding the rectum, they are most common in the high-pressure areas of the colon (eg, sigmoid). They tend to dissect along the course of the nutrient vessels, and they consist of a mucosal layer and the serosa. The inflammatory complication, diverticulitis, probably affects 10–20% of patients at some time.

Inflammatory changes in diverticulitis vary from mild polymorphonuclear infiltration in the wall of the sac to extensive inflammatory change in the surrounding area (peridiverticulitis), with perforation or abscess formation. The changes are comparable to those that occur in appendicitis.

Clinical Findings

A. Symptoms and Signs: Left lower quadrant pain may be steady and severe and last for days or may be cramping and intermittent and relieved by a bowel movement. Constipation is usual, but diarrhea may occur. Occult blood is found in the stool in about 20% of cases. Diverticulosis coli (without inflammation) is the most common cause of colonic hemorrhage; lower gastrointestinal hemorrhage is uncommon in diverticulitis.

B. Laboratory Findings: Noncontributory in uncomplicated diverticular disease.

C. Imaging: Radiographic examination reveals diverticula and in some cases spasm, interhaustral thickening, or narrowing of the colonic lumen.

Complications

Diverticulitis is a complication of diverticular disease in which gross or microscopic perforation of the diverticulum has occurred. The clinical manifestations vary with the extent of the inflammatory process and may include pain, signs of peritoneal irritation, chills, fever, sepsis, ileus, and partial or complete colonic obstruction. Peritonitis and abscess formation may also occur. Urinary frequency and dysuria are associated with bladder involvement in the inflammatory process. Fistula formation usually involves the bladder (usually vesicosigmoid, with pneumaturia a characteristic symptom) but may also be to the skin, perianal area, or small bowel. The white blood count shows polymorphonuclear leukocytosis. Red and white blood cells may be seen in the urine and, with fistula, numerous bacteria. Blood and urine cultures may be positive.

Differential Diagnosis

The constrictive lesion of the colon seen on x-ray or at sigmoidoscopy must be differentiated from carcinoma of the colon. The appearance of a short lesion with abrupt transition to normal bowel suggests carcinoma. Colonoscopy with biopsy can be very useful in these instances.

Treatment

The treatment of uncomplicated diverticular disease consists primarily of increasing bulk in the diet by means of the following: (1) high-residue diet; (2) unprocessed bran, ¼ cup daily in fruit juice or muffins; or (3) bulk additives such as psyllium hydrophilic mucilloid (Hydrocil, Konsyl, Metamucil, and others). Other measures that may be helpful are (1) stool softeners such as docusate sodium (Colace and others), 240 mg/d; and (2) anticholinergic drugs to decrease "spasm" in the sigmoid colon.

The treatment of acute diverticulitis requires antibiotic therapy. Agents should be selected with the intention of eradicating aerobic and anaerobic intestinal flora, eg, combinations of broad-spectrum penicillins, cephalosporins, aminoglycosides, and clindamycin or metronidazole.

Recurrent attacks of diverticulitis or the presence of perforation, fistula formation, or abscess formation requires surgical resection of the involved portion of the colon.

Massive diverticular hemorrhage usually stops spontaneously. Adequate blood replacement and careful endoscopic and barium studies are indicated to rule out other causes of bleeding. In certain instances, selective arteriography may localize the site of the bleeding and make it possible to control the bleeding with vasopressin. Operation may be required for uncontrolled bleeding.

Diverticulitis most typically occurs in the left colon; hemorrhage is most often noted to originate from right-sided diverticula.

Prognosis

The usual case is mild and responds well to dietary measures and antibiotics.

Hackford AW, Veidenheimer MC: Diverticular disease of the colon: Current concepts and management. Surg Clin North Am 1985;65:347.

ANGIODYSPLASIA OF THE COLON

Angiodysplasia is a disorder characterized by abnormal clusters of arterioles and dilated vascular spaces and veins in the submucosa and mucosa. Angiodysplasia of the colon as a cause of acute and chronic lower gastrointestinal bleeding is being increasingly recognized. It is seen chiefly in patients over age 50 (most of them over 70) with a prevalence of approximately 2% and is characterized by painless, usually self-limited intermittent rectal bleeding. The bleeding is usually of dark red blood but may be occult. There may be tarry stools. Up to 30% of patients have a history of surgery for gastrointestinal bleeding—eg, vagotomy and pyloroplasty, gastrectomy. Most lesions of angiodysplasia are in the cecum and right colon.

Treatment

A. Medical Treatment: The patient must be stabilized with fluids and packed red cells as clinically dictated and then evaluated for bleeding diatheses. To rule out an upper gastrointestinal site, upper endoscopy should be seriously considered even when the gastric aspirate is negative for blood and positive for bile. The sequence of additional evaluation is controversial, partly depending upon the resources available, but would include the following:

1. Technetium-labeled red cell scan to attempt to localize the site of bleeding. This is more sensitive than angiography; it has been shown to identify bleeding at a rate of 0.05 mL/min in experimental settings and at a rate of 0.5 mL/min clinically.

2. Colonoscopy after appropriate cleansing of the colon. In some studies, over 80% of patients with angiographically proved angiodysplasia are identified in this way.

3. Angiography provides definitive diagnosis at centers where experts with the procedure are available.

B. Surgical Treatment: The major options are cautery or sclerosis of the vascular lesion via colonoscopy, or surgical resection.

Imperiale TF, Ransohoff DF: Aortic stenosis, idiopathic gastrointestinal bleeding, and angiodysplasia: Is there an association? Gastroenterology 1988;95:1670. (Probably not.)

Richter JM et al: Angiodysplasia: Clinical presentation and colonoscopic diagnosis. Dig Dis Sci 1984;29:481.

POLYPS OF THE COLON & RECTUM (Intestinal Polyps)

Adenomatous polyps of the colon and rectum are common benign neoplasms that are usually asymptomatic but may cause painless rectal bleeding. They may be single or multiple, occur most frequently in the sigmoid and rectum, and are found incidentally in about 9% of autopsies. The incidence of polyps increases with age. The diagnosis is established by sigmoidoscopy, double contrast barium enema, and colonoscopy. When a polyp is found in the rectum, the colon should be studied by x-ray or colonoscopy.

Whether polyps are precancerous is an important question. Pedunculated adenomatous polyps less than 1 cm in diameter have very slight malignant potential and can usually be managed by simple polypectomy through the colonoscope. Larger adenomatous polyps impose a greater cancer risk and must be removed. Villous adenomas are usually sessile and become malignant in 10% of cases if they are 2 cm in diameter or less and in up to 50% of cases if they are larger. These too require removal, which can often be accomplished with the colonoscope; if not, surgical resection is required. Because colonic polyps tend to recur and because of their malignant potential, colonoscopic surveillance should be scheduled at 1 year postpolypectomy. If no polyps are found at that time, a repeat examination is indicated 2 years later unless clinically indicated sooner. For polyps removed by colonoscopic polypectomy that are determined to be malignant, the sufficiency of polypectomy as the sole treatment is determined by the histologic characteristics of the cancer and the extent of invasion of the stalk and the mucosa.

There are several familial polyp syndromes, some of which have a strong predilection for carcinoma. These need to be identified and treated and genetic counseling provided. For polyps with high malignant potential, colectomy with ileostomy or ileoproctostomy—after stripping of the rectal mucosa—is indicated.

Achkar E, Carey W: Small polyps found during fiberoptic sigmoidoscopy in asymptomatic patients. Ann Intern Med 1988;109:880. (Suggests that even hyperplastic polyps are markers for potentially more serious lesions elsewhere in the colon. Controversial.)

Bulow S: Colorectal polyposis syndromes. Scand J Gastroenterol 1984;19:289.

Cranley JP et al: When is endoscopic polypectomy adequate therapy for colonic polyps containing invasive carcinoma? Gastroenterology 1986;91:419.

Stryker SJ et al: Natural history of untreated colonic polyps. Gastroenterology 1987;93:1009.

CANCER OF THE COLON & RECTUM

Essentials of Diagnosis

- Altered bowel function (constipation) and bright red rectal bleeding in distal lesions.
- Blood in the feces, unexplained anemia, weight loss in right-sided carcinomas.
- Palpable mass involving colon or rectum valuable when present.
- Endoscopic or radiographic evidence of neoplasm.

General Considerations

Carcinoma is the only common cancer of the colon and rectum. Lymphoma, carcinoid, melanoma, fibrosarcoma, and other types of sarcoma occur rarely. The treatment of all is essentially the same.

Carcinoma of the colon and rectum accounts for about 15% of cancer deaths, second only to cancer of the lung. Predisposing causes are listed in Table 11–3. Males are affected slightly more commonly than females. The highest incidence is in patients about 50 years of age, but occasional cases have been reported in younger persons and even in children. Previously reported distribution of cancer of the large bowel was approximately 16% in the cecum and ascending colon, 5% in the transverse colon, 9% in the descending colon, 20% in the sigmoid, and 50% in the rectum; many observers believe the incidence of more proximal lesions is increasing.

Many lesions of the rectum and colon lie within reach of the examining finger or sigmoidoscope and therefore can be biopsied on the first visit.

Clinical Findings

Symptoms vary depending upon whether the lesion is in the right or the left side of the colon. In either case, a persistent change in the customary bowel habits should invariably alert the physician to investigate the colon. Bleeding is a cardinal diagnostic point. An acute abdominal emergency may be precipitated by perforation or colonic obstruction (due to circumferential narrowing, not intussusception). The diagnosis of colonic and rectal cancer is established by sigmoidoscopy and colonoscopy with biopsy and barium enema. Polyps and carcinoma not detected by barium enema may be detected by colonoscopy.

A. Carcinoma of the Right Colon: Because the fecal stream is fluid and the bowel lumen large in the right half of the colon, symptoms of obstruction occur less frequently than in left-sided tumors. Vague abdominal discomfort is often the only initial complaint. This may progress to cramplike pain, occasionally simulating cholecystitis or appendicitis. Second-

Table 11–3. Factors associated with increased risk of colonic cancer.

Standard Risk	High Risk[1]
After age 40 (both men and women)	Rectocolonic polyps (familial polyposis, villous polyps, adenomatous polyps, history of juvenile polyps) Cancer elsewhere in the body Familial history of colon cancer Ulcerative colitis Granulomatous colitis Immunodeficiency disease

[1] Listed in approximate decreasing frequency or importance.

ary anemia with associated weakness and weight loss is found in half of patients with right colon lesions. The stools are usually positive for occult blood but rarely show gross blood. The patient is likely to have diarrhea. The first indication of cancer may be the discovery of a palpable mass in the right lower quadrant.

B. Carcinoma of the Left Colon: Obstructive symptoms predominate, particularly increasing constipation. There may be short bouts of diarrhea. Occasionally the first sign is acute colonic obstruction. A small amount of bright red blood with bowel movements is common, and anemia is found in about 20% of cases. At times a mass is palpable. About half of patients give a history of weight loss.

Differential Diagnosis

Diverticulitis is usually associated with fever and has a different x-ray appearance. Functional bowel distress may also simulate cancer of the colon symptomatically, as may hemorrhoids. Other causes of iron deficiency anemia also merit consideration.

Treatment

Treatment is primarily surgical and determined by the Dukes stage of the carcinoma: Dukes A (mucosal involvement only) and Dukes B disease (local invasion but without penetration of the serosa) have high cure rates following surgical resection. For patients with Dukes C disease (involvement of regional lymph nodes), surgical en bloc resection plus adjuvant chemotherapy with fluorouracil and levamisole provides a 60% 4-year survival rate. Patients with Dukes D disease (distant metastases), resection of the primary lesion is usually indicated for palliation. Occasionally, surgical pursuit of single metastases to the liver is warranted.

Radiation therapy appears useful for rectal carcinomas.

Prognosis

Over 90% of patients with carcinoma of the colon and rectum are suitable for either curative or palliative resection, with an operative mortality rate of 3–6%. The overall 5-year survival rate after resection is about 50%. If the lesion is confined to the bowel and there is no evidence of lymphatic or blood vessel invasion, the 5-year survival rate is 60–70%. Local recurrence of carcinoma in the anastomotic suture line or wound area occurs in 10–15% of cases. The incidence of local recurrence can be decreased if special precautions are taken at operation to avoid implantation of malignant cells. About 5% of patients develop multiple primary colon cancers. Early identification of resectable local recurrence of a new neoplasm depends upon careful follow-up with sigmoidoscopy and barium enema every 6 months for 2 years and yearly thereafter. Carcinoembryonic antigen (CEA) is also a marker for detection of recurrent tumor (levels in-

crease) in patients with falls to normal levels after resection and may prove useful if monitored at 6-month intervals.

Barry MJ, Mulley AG, Richter JM: Effect of workup strategy on the cost-effectiveness of fecal occult blood screening for colorectal cancer. Gastroenterology 1987;93:301.

Heule BV et al: Presentation of malignant lymphoma in the rectum. Cancer 1982;49:2602.

Minsky BD et al: Resectable adenocarcinoma of the rectosigmoid and rectum: 1. Patterns of failure and survival. 2. The influence of blood vessel invasion. Cancer 1988;61:1408, 1417.

Moertel CG et al: Levamisole and fluorouracil B for adjuvant therapy of resected colon carcinoma. N Engl J Med 1990;322:352.

Steinberg SM et al: Prognostic indicators of colon tumors. Cancer 1986;57:1866.

ANORECTAL DISEASES

HEMORRHOIDS

Essentials of Diagnosis

- Rectal bleeding, protrusion, and vague discomfort.
- Mucoid discharge from rectum.
- Characteristic findings on external anal inspection or anoscopic examination.

General Considerations

Internal hemorrhoids are varices of the portion of the venous hemorrhoidal plexus that lies submucosally just proximal to the dentate margin. External hemorrhoids arise from the same plexus but are located subcutaneously immediately distal to the dentate margin. There are 3 primary internal hemorrhoidal masses; right anterior, right posterior, and left lateral. Three to 5 secondary hemorrhoids may be present between the 3 primaries. Straining at stool, constipation, prolonged sitting, and anal infection are contributing factors and may precipitate complications such as thrombosis. The diagnosis is suspected on the history of protrusion, anal pain, or bleeding and is confirmed by proctologic examination.

Carcinoma of the colon or rectum not infrequently aggravates hemorrhoids or produces similar complaints. Polyps may be present as a cause of bleeding that is wrongly attributed to hemorrhoids. For these reasons, the treatment of hemorrhoids is always preceded by sigmoidoscopy and barium enema. When portal hypertension is suspected as a causative factor, investigations for liver disease should be carried out. Hemorrhoids that develop during pregnancy or parturition tend to subside thereafter and should be treated conservatively unless persistent.

Clinical Findings

The symptoms of hemorrhoids are usually mild and remittent, but a number of disturbing complications may develop and call for active medical or surgical treatment. These complications include pruritus; incontinence; recurrent protrusion requiring manual replacement by the patient; fissure, infection, or ulceration; prolapse and strangulation; and secondary anemia due to chronic blood loss. Carcinoma has been reported to develop very rarely in hemorrhoids.

Treatment

Conservative treatment suffices in most instances of mild hemorrhoids, which may improve spontaneously or in response to a high-roughage diet, psyllium seed preparation, or nonirritating laxatives to produce soft stools. Local pain and infection are managed with warm sitz baths and insertion of a soothing anal suppository 2 or 3 times daily. Benzocaine and similar types of anal ointments should be avoided so as not to sensitize the patient to these agents. Prolapsed or strangulated hemorrhoids may be treated conservatively by gentle reduction with a lubricated gloved finger; by rubber band ligation or cryosurgery, or both; or by surgical resection.

For severe symptoms or complications, complete internal and external hemorrhoidectomy is advisable and is a highly satisfactory procedure when properly done. Excision of a single external hemorrhoid, evacuation of a thrombosed pile, and the injection treatment of internal hemorrhoids fall within the scope of office practice. Injection therapy is effective, but there is a recurrence rate of more than 50%.

Evacuation of Thrombosed External Hemorrhoid

This condition is caused by the rupture of a vein at the anal margin, forming a clot in the subcutaneous tissue. The patient complains of a painful lump, and examination shows a tense, tender, bluish mass covered with skin. If the patient is seen after 24–48 hours when the pain is subsiding—or if symptoms are minimal—hot sitz baths are prescribed. If discomfort is marked, removal of the clot is indicated. With the patient in the lateral position, the area is prepared with antiseptic, and 1% lidocaine is injected intracutaneously around and over the lump. An ellipse of skin is then excised and the clot evacuated. A dry gauze dressing is held in place for 12–24 hours by taping the buttocks together, and daily sitz baths are then begun.

Guthrie JF: The current management of hemorrhoids. Pract Gastroenterol 1987;11:56.

CRYPTITIS & PAPILLITIS

Anal pain and burning of brief duration with defecation is suggestive of cryptitis and papillitis. Digital and anoscopic examination reveals hypertrophied papillae and indurated or inflamed crypts. Treatment consists of adding bulk agents, such as psyllium seed preparations, to the diet; sitz baths; and anal suppositories containing hydrocortisone after each bowel movement. Some recommend local application of 5% phenol in oil or carbolfuchsin compound to the crypts. If these measures fail, surgical excision of involved crypts and papillae should be considered.

Anorectal Infections

Anorectal infections are seen chiefly in homosexual men and can be divided into 2 clinical syndromes: proctitis and proctocolitis.

Proctitis is characterized by anorectal pain, mucopurulent or bloody discharge, tenesmus, constipation, and an inflamed, often mucopurulent rectal mucosa. The most common pathogens are *Neisseria gonorrhoeae*, chlamydiae, and herpesvirus. The diagnosis can be made on sigmoidoscopy, with specimens obtained for Gram's stain and culture as well as by biopsy. Syphilis may cause proctitis, with a chancre appearing 2–6 weeks after anal intercourse. Secondary syphilis may be characterized by condyloma latum, which must be differentiated from anal warts.

The differential diagnosis should include traumatic proctitis.

Treatment depends upon the cause.

Proctocolitis implies involvement beyond the rectum to include at least the sigmoid colon. The causes may include those of proctitis, but more commonly are due to *Shigella, Campylobacter,* or amebiasis. Symptoms usually include diarrhea, abdominal cramping, and fever—in addition to the symptoms of proctitis.

Ulcerative colitis and granulomatous colitis must be considered in the differential diagnosis.

Treatment depends upon the specific bacteriologic diagnosis.

Rectal Prolapse & Solitary Ulcer

Rectal prolapse is a not uncommon problem, particularly among the elderly, and is associated with a long history of constipation and straining. The support structures of the anorectal area have usually become weakened, leading to rectal intussusception with straining. An early manifestation may be solitary rectal ulcer—a painful condition with ulcerogenesis apparently secondary to the intussusception.

Management consists of surgical correction of the lax support system.

Metcalf AM, Loening-Baucke V: Anorectal functions and defecation dynamics in patients with rectal prolapse. Am J Surg 1988;155:206.

Womack NR et al: Pressure and prolapse: The cause of solitary rectal ulceration. Gut 1987;28:1228.

FISSURA IN ANO
(Anal Fissure)

Acute fissures represent linear disruption of the anal epithelium due to various causes. They usually clear if bowel movements are kept regular and soft (eg, with a bulk agent, bran, or psyllium seed preparation). The local application of a mild styptic such as 1–2% silver nitrate or 1% gentian violet solution may be of value.

Chronic fissure is characterized by (1) acute pain during and after defecation; (2) spotting of bright red blood at stool, with occasional more abundant bleeding; (3) tendency to constipation through fear of pain; and (4) the late occurrence of a sentinel pile, a hypertrophied papilla, and spasm of the anal canal (usually very painful on digital examination). Regulation of bowel habits with use of bran or psyllium seed preparation in the diet or use of stool softeners, sitz baths, or anal suppositories (eg, Anusol) twice daily should be tried. If these measures fail, the fissure, sentinel pile, or papilla and the adjacent crypt must be excised surgically. Postoperative care is along the lines of the preoperative treatment.

ANAL ABSCESS

Perianal abscess should be considered the acute stage of an anal fistula until proved otherwise. The abscess should be adequately drained as soon as localized. Hot sitz baths may hasten the process of localization. The patient should be warned that the fistula may persist after drainage of the abscess. It is painful and fruitless to search for the internal opening of a fistula in the presence of acute infection. The presence of an anal abscess should alert the clinician to the possibility of inflammatory bowel disease, especially Crohn's disease.

FISTULA IN ANO

About 95% of all anal fistulas arise in an anal crypt, and they are often preceded by an anal abscess. If an anal fistula enters the rectum above the pectinate line and there is no associated disease in the crypts, granulomatous colitis, regional ileitis, rectal tuberculosis, lymphogranuloma venereum, cancer, or foreign body should be considered in the differential diagnosis.

Acute fistula is associated with a purulent discharge from the fistulous opening. There is usually local itching, tenderness, or pain aggravated by bowel movements. Recurrent anal abscess may develop. The involved crypt can occasionally be located anoscopically with a crypt hook. Probing the fistula should be gentle because false passages can be made with ease, and in any case demonstration of the internal opening by probing is not essential to the diagnosis.

Treatment is by surgical incision or excision of the fistula under general anesthesia. If a fistula passes deep to the entire anorectal ring, so that all the muscles must be divided in order to extirpate the tract, a 2-stage operation must be done to prevent incontinence.

ANAL CONDYLOMAS
(Genital Warts)

These wartlike papillomas of the perianal skin and anal canal flourish on moist, macerated surfaces, particularly in the presence of purulent discharge. They are not true tumors but are infectious and autoinoculable, probably owing to a sexually transmitted papovavirus. They must be distinguished from condylomata lata caused by syphilis. The diagnosis of the latter rests on a positive serologic test for syphilis or discovery of *Treponema pallidum* on darkfield examination.

Treatment consists of cautious accurate application of liquid nitrogen or 25% podophyllum resin in tincture of benzoin to the lesion (with bare wooden or cotton-tipped applicator sticks to avoid contact with uninvolved skin). The compound should be washed off after 2–4 hours. Condylomas in the anal canal are treated through the anoscope and the painted site dusted with powder to localize the application and minimize discomfort. Electrofulguration under local anesthesia is useful if there are numerous lesions. Local cleanliness and the frequent use of a talc dusting powder are essential.

Condylomas tend to recur. The patient should be observed for several months and advised to report promptly if new lesions appear.

BENIGN ANORECTAL STRICTURES

Traumatic

Acquired stenosis is usually the result of surgery or trauma that denudes the epithelium of the anal canal. Hemorrhoid operations in which too much skin is removed or which are followed by infection are the commonest cause. Constipation, ribbon stools, and pain on defecation are the most frequent complaints. Stenosis predisposes to fissure, low-grade infection, and, occasionally, fistula.

Prevention of stenosis after radical anal surgery is best accomplished by local cleanliness, hot sitz baths, and gentle insertion of the well-lubricated finger twice weekly for 2–3 weeks beginning 2 weeks after surgery. When stenosis is chronic but mild, graduated anal dilators of increasing size may be inserted daily by the patient. For marked stenosis, a plastic operation on the anal canal is advisable.

Inflammatory

A. Lymphogranuloma Venereum: This disease is caused by certain immunotypes of Chlamydia and is the commonest cause of an infectious inflammatory stricture of the anorectal region. It is most common in women and in male homosexuals and occurs in about 3% of patients in sexually transmitted disease clinics. Acute proctitis due to lymphatic spread of the organism occurs early and may be followed by perirectal infections, sinuses, and formation of scar tissue (resulting in stricture). Swollen, often painful, purple discolored inguinal lymph nodes appear early in the course. Frei and complement fixation tests are positive but not highly sensitive.

The tetracycline drugs are curative in the initial phase of the disease. When extensive chronic secondary infection is present or when a stricture has formed, repeated biopsies are essential because epidermoid carcinoma develops in about 4% of strictures. Local operation on a stricture may be feasible, but a colostomy or an abdominoperineal resection is often required.

B. Granuloma Inguinale: This disease may cause anorectal fistulas, infections, and strictures. The Donovan body is best identified in tissue biopsy when there is rectal involvement. Epidermoid carcinoma develops in about 4% of cases with chronic anorectal granuloma.

The early lesions respond to tetracyclines. Destructive or constricting processes may require colostomy or resection.

Rompalo AM, Stamm WE: Anorectal and enteric infections in homosexual men. West J Med 1985;142:647.
Sohn N: The rectum in AIDS. Pract Gastroenterol 1988;12:50.

ANAL INCONTINENCE

Obstetric tears, anorectal operations (particularly fistulotomy), and neurologic disturbances are the most frequent causes of anal incontinence. Diarrhea due to any cause or fecal impaction may contribute to incontinence. When incontinence is due to surgery or trauma, surgical repair of the divided or torn sphincter is indicated. Repair of anterior childbirth lacerations should be delayed for 6 months or more. In those with manometrically demonstrated decreased anal sphincter tone, biofeedback therapy has been moderately successful in achieving continence.

Schoetz DJ Jr: Operative therapy for anal incontinence. Surg Clin North Am 1985;65:35.

SQUAMOUS CELL CARCINOMA OF THE ANUS

These tumors are relatively rare, comprising only 1–2% of all cancers of the anus and large intestine. Bleeding, pain, and local tumor are the commonest symptoms. The lesion is often confused with hemor-

rhoids or other common anal disorders. These tumors tend to become annular, invade the sphincter, and spread upward into the rectum; they are encountered regularly in AIDS patients.

Except for very small lesions (which can be adequately excised locally), treatment is by combined abdominoperineal resection. Radiation therapy is reserved for palliation and for patients who refuse or cannot withstand operation. Metastases to the inguinal nodes are treated by radical groin dissection when clinically evident. The 5-year survival rate after resection is about 50%.

DISEASES OF THE LIVER & BILIARY TRACT

JAUNDICE (Icterus)

Since antiquity, a yellowish appearance of the skin and scleras has been recognized as a manifestation of liver disease. Jaundice is evidence of accumulation of bilirubin—a red pigment product of heme metabolism—in the body tissues; it has extrahepatic as well as hepatic causes. Hyperbilirubinemia may be due to abnormalities in the formation, transport, metabolism, and excretion of bilirubin. Total serum bilirubin is normally 0.2–1.2 mg/dL, and jaundice may not be clinically recognizable until levels are about 3 mg/dL.

From an anatomic standpoint, elevation of serum bilirubin levels is prehepatic, hepatic, or posthepatic. Prehepatic jaundice is due to excess production of bilirubin (eg, hemolysis). In hepatic jaundice, elevated serum bilirubin may be caused by qualitative or quantitative dysfunction of liver cells (eg, faulty uptake, metabolism, or excretion of bilirubin). Posthepatic jaundice results from interference with the physiologic removal of bilirubin from the hepatobiliary system (eg, obstruction of the common bile duct).

Because of the great diversity of causes of jaundice, no classification is entirely satisfactory; one that includes anatomy, biochemistry, and etiology is presented in Table 11–4.

Gollan JL (editor): Pathobiology of bilirubin and jaundice. Semin Liver Dis 1988,8:105.

Manifestations of Diseases Associated With Jaundice
A. Prehepatic: Weakness or abdominal or back pain may occur with acute hemolytic crises. There is normal stool and urine color, mild jaundice, indirect

Table 11–4. Classification of jaundice.

Type of Hyperbilirubinemia	Location and Cause
Unconjugated hyperbilirubinemia (predominant indirect-acting bilirubin)	**PREHEPATIC**
	Increased bilirubin production (eg, hemolytic anemias, hemolytic reactions, hematoma, infarction).
	HEPATIC
	Impaired bilirubin uptake and storage (eg, posthepatitis hyperbilirubinemia, Gilbert's syndrome, drug reactions).
	Impaired glucuronyl transferase activity (eg, Crigler-Najjar syndrome, Gilbert's syndrome).
Conjugated hyperbilirubinemia (predominant direct-acting bilirubin)	Faulty excretion of bilirubin conjugates (eg, Dubin-Johnson syndrome, Rotor's syndrome).
	Biliary epithelial damage (eg, hepatitis, hepatic cirrhosis).
	Intrahepatic cholestasis (eg, viral hepatitis, alcoholic hepatitis, certain drugs, biliary cirrhosis).
	Hepatocellular damage or intrahepatic cholestasis resulting from miscellaneous causes (eg, viral hepatitis, spirochetal infections, infectious mononucleosis, cholangitis, sarcoidosis, lymphomas, industrial toxins).
	POSTHEPATIC
	Gallstones, biliary atresia, carcinoma of biliary duct, sclerosing cholangitis, choledochal cyst, external pressure on common duct, pancreatitis, pancreatic neoplasms.

(unconjugated) hyperbilirubinemia with no bilirubin in the urine, and splenomegaly, except in sickle cell anemia. Hepatomegaly is variable.

B. Hepatic:

1. Acquired–Malaise, anorexia, low-grade fever, and right upper quadrant discomfort are manifestations. Dark urine, jaundice, and amenorrhea occur. An enlarged, tender liver, vascular spiders; palmar erythema; ascites; gynecomastia; sparse body hair; fetor hepaticus; and asterixis may be present, depending on the cause and chronicity of the liver abnormality.

2. Congenital–This form may be asymptomatic; the intermittent cholestasis is often accompanied by pruritus, light-colored stools, and, occasionally, malaise.

C. Posthepatic: There is colicky right upper quadrant pain, weight loss (carcinoma), jaundice, dark urine, and light-colored stools. Fluctuating jaundice and intermittently colored stools indicate intermittent obstruction owing to stone or to carcinoma

of the ampulla or junction of the intrahepatic ducts. Blood in the stools suggests cancer. Hepatomegaly, visible and palpable gallbladder (Courvoisier's sign), ascites, rectal (Blumer's) shelf, and weight loss also suggest cancer. Chills and fever are more common in choledocholithiasis with cholangitis.

Diagnostic Methods
for Evaluation of Jaundice
(Table 11–5)

A. Laboratory Studies: AST (SGOT) is valuable in the assessment of liver disease. Diagnostic usefulness is enhanced when the test is combined with complementary studies such as alkaline phosphatase and serum bilirubin. ALT (SGPT) may be useful in differentiating alcoholic from viral hepatitis, because ALT levels are much lower than AST levels in alcoholic hepatitis. Serologic tests for viral hepatitis may be helpful when clinically indicated.

B. Liver Biopsy: Percutaneous liver biopsy is a safe and accurate way of diagnosing diffuse hepatic disease. It is of less value in differentiating intrahepatic from extrahepatic cholestasis and is moderately successful in defining liver metastases.

C. Imaging: When the cause of jaundice cannot be determined on the basis of the patient's history and clinical and laboratory findings, it may be possible to differentiate hepatocellular and obstructive jaundice in 80–90% of cases by ultrasonography, CT scan, or radionuclide imaging, all of which are noninvasive (but the latter 2 are expensive). Dilated bile ducts demonstrated by these techniques indicate biliary obstruction, which helps distinguish between obstructive and hepatocellular disease. Ultrasonography and CT scan can be used to demonstrate hepatomegaly, intrahepatic tumors, and dilated hepatic ducts. Ultrasonography can also identify gallbladders and detect even 2-mm gallstones and is more sensitive than CT for common duct disease.

If surgical (obstructive) jaundice is initially suspected, some clinicians proceed directly from clinical and laboratory findings to percutaneous transhepatic cholangiography; this fine-needle technique often pinpoints the cause, location, and extent of the biliary obstruction. Unusual complications may include fever, bacteremia, bile peritonitis, and intraperitoneal hemorrhage. More widely used is endoscopic retrograde cholangiopancreatography, which requires a skilled endoscopist; this technique is comparable in accuracy to percutaneous cholangiography. It may also be utilized to demonstrate pancreatic causes of jaundice or, if choledocholithiasis is present, to carry out papillotomy and stone extraction. Complications of the endoscopic procedure include pancreatitis and cholangitis, which occur in less than 3% of cases.

Gollan JL et al: Pathobiology of bilirubin and jaundice. Semin Liver Dis 1988;8:105.

Lieberman DA, Krishnamurthy GT: Intrahepatic versus ex-

Table 11–5. Liver function tests: Normal values and changes in 2 types of jaundice.

Tests	Normal Values	Hepatocellular Jaundice	Uncomplicated Obstructive Jaundice
Bilirubin Direct	0.1–0.3 mg/dL	Increased	Increased
Indirect	0.2–0.7 mg/dL	Increased	Increased
Urine bilirubin	None	Increased	Increased
Serum albumin/ total protein	Albumin, 3.5–5.5 Total protein, 6.5–8.4	Albumin decreased	Unchanged
Alkaline phosphatase	30–115 IU	Increased (++)	Increased (++++)
Cholesterol Total	100–250 mg/dL	Decreased if damage severe	Increased
Esters	60–70% of total	Decreased if damage severe	Normal
Prothrombin time	60–100%. After vitamin K, 15% increase in 24 hours.	Prolonged if damage severe and does not respond to parenteral vitamin K	Prolonged if obstruction marked but responds to parenteral vitamin K
ALT (SGPT) AST (SGOT)	ALT, 5–35 IU AST, 5–40 IU	Increased in hepatocellular damage, viral hepatitis	Minimally increased

trahepatic cholestasis: Discrimination with biliary scintigraphy combined with ultrasound. Gastroenterology 1986;90:734. (Discrimination was possible in 88% with combined studies.)

Muraca M, Fevery J, Blanckaert N: Relationships between serum bilirubins and production and conjugation of bilirubin: Studies in Gilbert's syndrome, Crigler-Najjar disease, hemolytic disorders, and rat models. Gastroenterology 1987;92:309.

Scharschmidt BF, Goldberg HI, Schmid R: Current concepts in diagnosis: Approach to the patient with cholestatic jaundice. N Engl J Med 1983;308:1515.

VIRAL HEPATITIS

Essentials of Diagnosis

- Anorexia, nausea, vomiting, malaise, symptoms of upper respiratory throat infection or "flu"-like syndrome, aversion to smoking.
- Fever; enlarged, tender liver, jaundice.
- Normal to low white cell count; abnormal liver tests, especially a markedly elevated transaminase early in the course.
- Liver biopsy shows characteristic hepatocellular necrosis and mononuclear infiltrate but is rarely indicated.

General Considerations

Hepatitis can be caused by many drugs and toxic agents as well as by numerous viruses, the clinical manifestations of which may be quite similar. The development of serologic tests has made possible the identification of a growing number of specific viruses causing viral hepatitis. The more common of these are (1) hepatitis A virus (HAV—causing "infectious" or short incubation period disease); (2) hepatitis B virus (HBV); (3) hepatitis C virus (mostly posttransfusion "NANB"); (4) hepatitis D virus (delta antigen); and (5) hepatitis E virus (an enterically transmitted hepatitis seen in epidemic form in Asia and North Africa).

A. Hepatitis A: (Fig 11–1.) Hepatitis A is a viral infection of the liver that may occur sporadically or in epidemics. The liver involvement is part of a generalized infection but dominates the clinical picture. Although transmission of the virus may occur by contaminated needles, it is usually by the fecal-oral route. The excretion of hepatitis A virus (HAV) as determined by immune electron microscopy of stool occurs up to 2 weeks prior to clinical illness. HAV is rarely demonstrated in feces after the first week

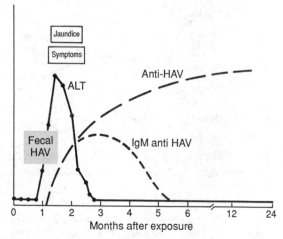

Figure 11–1. The typical course of acute type A hepatitis. HAV = hepatitis A antigen; anti-HAV = antibody to hepatitis A virus; ALT = alanine aminotransferase. (Reproduced, with permission, from Schafer DF, Hoofnagle JH: Viewpoints on Digestive Diseases 1982;14:5.)

of illness. There is no known carrier state with HAV. Blood and stools are infectious during the incubation period (2–6 weeks) and early illness until peak transaminase levels are achieved. Posttransfusion hepatitis due to HAV is rare. Although the mortality rate with hepatitis A is low, it may cause fulminant disease. Chronic hepatitis does not occur. The mortality rate (as with hepatitis B) appears to be age-related.

Antibodies to type A hepatitis appear early in the course of the illness and tend to persist in the serum. Both IgM and IgG antibodies are positive soon after the onset of the illness. Peak titers of IgG antibodies occur after 1 month of disease and may persist for years. Peak titers of IgM antibodies occur during the first week of clinical disease and usually disappear within an 8-week period; therefore, measurement of these antibodies is an excellent test for demonstrating acute hepatitis A infection. The presence of anti-HAV activity indicates (1) previous exposure to HAV, (2) noninfectivity, and (3) immunity to recurring HAV infection. It does not imply previous clinically apparent hepatitis, nor does it establish a relationship to ongoing liver disease unless seroconversion has been demonstrated.

B. Hepatitis B: (Fig 11–2.) Hepatitis B is a viral infection of the liver usually transmitted by inoculation of infected blood or blood products. However, the antigen has been found in most body secretions, and it is known that the disease can be spread by oral or sexual contact. Hepatitis B virus (HBV) is highly prevalent in homosexuals and intravenous drug abusers. Other groups at high risk include patients and staff at hemodialysis centers, physicians, dentists, nurses, and personnel working in clinical and pathology laboratories and blood banks. Approximately 5–10% of infected individuals become carriers, providing a substantial reservoir of infection. Forty to 70% of infants born to HBsAg-positive mothers will develop antigens to hepatitis B in the bloodstream. Fecal-oral transmission of virus B has also been documented. The incubation period of hepatitis B is 6 weeks to 6 months but may be prolonged by the administration of hyperimmune globulin. Clinical features of hepatitis A and B are similar; however, the onset in hepatitis B tends to be more insidious.

There are 3 distinct antigen-antibody systems that relate to HBV infection. In addition, DNA polymerase activity can be measured as a sensitive index of viral replication and infectivity.

1. HBsAg–The surface antigen (HBsAg) is the antigen routinely measured in blood. The presence of HBsAg is the first manifestation of HBV infection occurring before biochemical evidence of liver disease. HBsAg persists throughout the clinical illness. Persistence of HBsAg is usually associated with clinical and laboratory evidence of chronic hepatitis. The presence of HBsAg establishes infection with HBV and implies infectivity. Specific antibody to HBsAg (anti-HBs) occurs in most individuals after clearance of HBsAg. Anti-HBs is usually delayed after clearance of HBsAg. During this serologic gap, infectivity has been demonstrated. Development of anti-HBs signals recovery from HBV, noninfectivity, and protection from HBV infection.

2. HBcAg–Anti-HBc IgM appears shortly after HBsAg is detected. Its presence in the settings of acute clinical hepatitis is strongly supportive of hepatitis B virus as the etiologic agent, and it fills the serologic gap in patients who have cleared the HBsAg but do not yet have detectable amounts of anti-HBs. Anti-HBc IgM can be found alone or in any combination with HBsAg or Anti-HBs and persists for up to 1–2 years. Infectivity has been demonstrated in instances where donors are HBsAg-negative and positive for HBcAg IgM. Ultimately, Anti-HBc IgG becomes the marker for past infections, as does Anti-HBs also.

3. HBeAg–HBeAg is a soluble protein found only in HBsAg-positive sera. It appears during the incubation period shortly after the detection of HBsAg and only during HBsAg reactivity. HBe is detected as early as the fourth week of illness. The clinical usefulness of this antigen-antibody system lies in its predictive value of infectivity.

4. DNA polymerase–DNA polymerase activity is first detectable at the time of peak HBsAg titer, suggesting that this enzyme is a manifestation of viremia and viral replication. DNA polymerase activity is usually transient but may persist for years in chronic carriers and is an indication of continued infectivity.

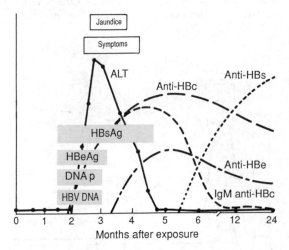

Figure 11–2. The typical course of acute type B hepatitis. HBsAg = hepatitis B surface antigen; anti-HBs = antibody to HBsAg; HBeAg = hepatitis Be antigen; anti-HBe = antibody to HBeAg; anti-HBc = antibody to hepatitis B core antigen; DNA p = DNA polymerase; ALT = alanine aminotransferase. (Reproduced, with permission, from Hoofnagle JH, Schafer DF: Semin Liv Dis 1986;6:1.)

C. Delta Agent: The delta agent is a defective viral agent RNA genome and has been identified only in association with hepatitis B infection and specifically only in the presence of HBsAg; it is cleared when the latter is cleared.

Clinically, the delta agent may increase the severity of an acute HBV infection, aggravate previously existing HBV liver disease, or cause new disease in asymptomatic HBsAg carriers. When the delta agent is coincident with an acute HBV infection, the infection appears to be more severe, and the delta agent has recently been found in up to 50% of fulminant HBV infections. In chronic active hepatitis B, presence of the delta agent appears to carry a more severe prognosis. Vertical transmission of this agent appears to be much less frequent than that of HBV.

At present, there are no unique preventive or therapeutic measures for delta agent infections.

D. Hepatitis C (HCV): Recently it has become possible to clone a portion of the non-A, non-B hepatitis agent responsible for the majority of cases of posttransfusion hepatitis. An assay has been developed to detect antibody against a major gene product of this agent, and this assay should soon be available. It appears to have high sensitivity and 100% specificity for HCV. HCV as now defined is responsible for approximately 80% of cases of posttransfusional hepatitis and some sporadic cases. The appearance of anti-HCV is delayed as much as 22 weeks after exposure (14–16 weeks after onset of hepatitis) and persists for at least 10 years. This new assay should significantly reduce the incidence of transfusions hepatitis, which currently is 4–7%.

E. Miscellaneous Causes: Other viral agents that cause hepatitis include Epstein-Barr virus and cytomegalovirus. About 15–20% of cases of transfusional hepatitis are not caused by HCV.

Clinical Findings

The clinical picture of viral hepatitis is extremely variable, ranging from asymptomatic infection without jaundice (common in non-A, non-B posttransfusion hepatitis) to a fulminating disease and death in a few days.

A. Symptoms:

1. Prodromal phase–The speed of onset varies from abrupt to insidious, with general malaise, myalgia, arthralgia and occasionally arthritis, easy fatigability, upper respiratory symptoms (nasal discharge, pharyngitis), and severe anorexia out of proportion to the degree of illness. Nausea and vomiting are frequent, and diarrhea or constipation may occur. Fever is generally present but is rarely over 39.5 °C (103.1 °F) save in occasional cases of hepatitis A. Defervescence often coincides with the onset of jaundice. Chills or chilliness may mark an acute onset.

Abdominal pain is usually mild and constant in the upper right quadrant or right epigastrium and is often aggravated by jarring or exertion. (On rare occa-

sions, upper abdominal pain may be severe enough to simulate cholecystitis or cholelithiasis.) A distaste for smoking, paralleling anorexia, may occur early.

2. Icteric phase–Clinical jaundice occurs after 5–10 days but may appear at the same time as the initial symptomatology. Some patients never develop clinical icterus. With the onset of jaundice, there is often an intensification of the prodromal symptoms, followed by progressive clinical improvement.

3. Convalescent phase–There is an increasing sense of well-being, return of appetite, and disappearance of jaundice, abdominal pain and tenderness, and fatigability.

4. Course and complications–The acute illness usually subsides rapidly over a 2– to 3-week period with complete clinical and laboratory recovery by 9 weeks in the case of hepatitis A and by 16 weeks for hepatitis B and hepatitis non-A, non-B. In 5–10% of cases, the course may be more protracted, and less than 1–3% will have an acute fulminant course.

B. Signs: Hepatomegaly—rarely marked—is present in over half of cases. Liver tenderness is usually present. Splenomegaly is reported in 15% of patients, and soft, enlarged lymph nodes—especially in the cervical or epitrochlear areas—may occur. Signs of general toxemia vary from minimal to severe.

C. Laboratory Findings: The white cell count is normal to low, especially in the preicteric phase. Large atypical lymphocytes, such as are found in infectious mononucleosis, may occasionally be seen. Mild proteinuria is common, and bilirubinuria often precedes the appearance of jaundice. Acholic stools are often present during the initial icteric phase. Blood and urine studies tend to reflect hepatocellular damage, with abnormal AST (SGOT) or ALT (SGPT) values. Bilirubin and alkaline phosphatase are elevated and, in a minority of patients, remain so after transaminase levels have normalized. HBsAg is usually positive in hepatitis B. The prothrombin time may be prolonged in severe hepatitis.

Differential Diagnosis

The differential diagnosis of viral hepatitis should include, in addition to infection with viruses A, B, C, and delta agent, other viral diseases such as infectious mononucleosis, cytomegalovirus infection, and herpes simplex virus infection; spirochetal diseases such as leptospirosis and secondary syphilis; brucellosis; rickettsial diseases such as Q fever; and drug-induced liver disease, particularly due to acetaminophen.

The prodromal phase of the nonicteric form of the disease must be distinguished from other infectious diseases such as influenza, upper respiratory infections, and the prodromal stages of the exanthematous diseases. In the obstructive phase of viral hepatitis, it is necessary to rule out choledocholithiasis, chlorpromazine toxicity, and carcinoma of the head of the pancreas. Prevention

Strict isolation of patients is not necessary, but hand washing after bowel movements is required. Thorough hand washing by medical attendants who come into contact with contaminated utensils, bedding, or clothing is essential. Disinfection of feces is not necessary when waterborne sewage disposal is available. Hepatitis B is for the most part transmitted by the parenteral route, but the possibility of fecal-oral infection as well as sexual transmission must be considered. Screening by means of HBsAg and AST (SGOT) determinations can remove potentially infectious individuals from blood donor lists. Unfortunately, there is increasing evidence that other viruses are responsible for similar clinical states. In blood donors, routine screening for HBsAg and elevated ALT has reduced the incidence of posttransfusion hepatitis. Testing for anti-HCV will soon be possible. In the USA, the avoidance of unnecessary transfusions and the exclusion of commercially obtained blood, along with clinical studies of the donor as well as the HBsAg and serum transaminase determinations, may be helpful in excluding potential sources of infectious blood. It may make possible the detection of one-third of infected donors. The use of disposable needles and syringes protects medical attendants as well as other patients.

A. Gamma Globulin: Gamma globulin should be routinely given to all *close* personal contacts of patients with hepatitis A. The recommended dose of 0.02 mL/kg body weight has been found to be protective for hepatitis A if administered during the incubation period. It is also desirable that individuals traveling to or residing in endemic regions receive gamma globulin within 2 weeks after arrival; if staying more than 2 months, the recommended dose is 5 mL for adults. In the event of prolonged residence, a second dose should be given after 5–6 months.

B. Hepatitis B Hyperimmune Globulin: Hepatitis B hyperimmune globulin may be protective if given in large doses within 7 days of exposure and again at 30 days (adult dose is 0.06 mL/kg body weight). At present, this preparation is recommended for individuals exposed to hepatitis B surface antigen-contaminated material via the mucous membranes or through breaks in the skin. Persons who have had sexual contact with patients with acute hepatitis B surface antigen-positive disease should also receive hepatitis B hyperimmune globulin. Hepatitis B hyperimmune globulin is also indicated for newborn infants of HBsAg-positive mothers; give 0.5 mL shortly after birth. In addition to the hyperimmune hepatitis B globulin in the above clinical situation, the vaccine series should be promptly initiated (see below). Hepatitis B hyperimmune globulin does not seem to be indicated in the prevention of transfusion-associated hepatitis.

C. Hepatitis B Vaccine: The currently used vaccine is recombinant-derived. Recipients must have a negative serologic test for HBsAg and HBcAb. Potential candidates are persons at high risk, including renal dialysis patients and attending personnel, patients requiring repeated transfusions, spouses of HBsAg-positive individuals, male homosexuals, and newborns of HBsAg-positive mothers. All entering medical and nursing students should be vaccinated, as well as all medical technologists. Better than 90% of recipients of the vaccine mount protective antibody to hepatitis B. The dose for adults is 1 mL initially and 1 mL again at 1 and 6 months; for greatest reliability of absorption, the deltoid muscle is the preferred site of injection. The newborn and pediatric dose is one-half the adult dose.

Treatment

A. General Measures: Bed rest should be at the patient's option during the acute initial phase of the disease, when symptoms are most severe. Bed rest beyond the most acute phase is not warranted. However, return to normal activity during the convalescent period should be gradual. If nausea and vomiting are significant problems, or if oral intake is substantially decreased, the intravenous administration of 10% glucose solution is indicated. If the patient shows signs of impending coma, protein should be temporarily interdicted and gradually reintroduced and increased as clinical improvement takes place. In general, dietary management consists of giving palatable meals as tolerated, without overfeeding. Patients with acute hepatitis should avoid strenuous physical exertion, alcohol, and hepatotoxic agents. While the administration of small doses of oxazepam is safe (not metabolized or excreted by the liver), it is recommended that morphine sulfate be avoided.

B. Corticotropin and Corticosteroids: In controlled studies, these agents have demonstrated no benefit in patients with viral hepatitis, including those with fulminant hepatitis.

Prognosis

The clinical course, morbidity, and mortality of viral hepatitis may vary considerably. In most cases of viral hepatitis, clinical recovery is complete in 3–16 weeks. Laboratory evidence of disturbed liver function may persist for a longer period, but most such patients go on to complete recovery. The overall mortality rate is less than 1%, but the rate is reportedly higher in older people (particularly postmenopausal women).

Hepatitis A does not progress to chronic liver disease, though persistent hepatitis A with anti-HAV IgM has been seen for up to 1 year. The mortality rate is less than 0.2%. About 10% of hepatitis B patients and perhaps an even higher percentage of hepatitis C patients develop chronic liver disease (see below). The mortality rates quoted for hepatitis B and hepatitis C infections (0.1–15%) are higher than for hepatitis A infections, but these figures may reflect other factors than virulence (eg, age, associated illness).

Chronic hepatitis, as characterized by transaminasemia for more than 6 months, occurs in 5–10% of patients. Some of this latter group develop chronic active hepatitis with or without cirrhosis. Liver biopsy is necessary to make this distinction.

Hepatitis tends to be more severe and potentially has a poorer prognosis in the elderly or in those with other complicating illnesses. Posttransfusion clinically apparent hepatitis occurs as a complication in 0.25–3% of blood transfusions and as high as 12% of those receiving pooled blood products. The asymptomatic carrier state and persistent viremia after acute disease make control of contamination in donor blood extremely difficult.

Alter HJ et al: Detection of antibody to hepatitis C virus in prospectively followed transfusion recipients with acute and chronic non-A, non-B hepatitis. N Engl J Med 1989;321:1495. (Evidence that hepatitis C is responsible for most cases of posttransfusion hepatitis.)

Bonino F, Smedile A: Delta agent (type D) hepatitis. Semin Liver Dis 1986;6:28.

Bradley DW, Maynard JE: Etiology and natural history of post-transfusions and enterically transmitted non-A, non-B hepatitis. Semin Liver Dis 1986;6:56.

Centers for Disease Control: Update on hepatitis B prevention: Recommendations of the Immunization Practices Advisory Committee. Ann Intern Med 1987;107:353.

Horowitz MM et al: Duration of immunity after hepatitis B vaccination: Efficacy of low-dose booster vaccine. Ann Intern Med 1988;108:185.

Lemon SM: Type A viral hepatitis: New developments in an old disease. N Engl J Med 1985;313:1059.

Rosina F, Saracco G, Rizzetto M: Risk of posttransfusion infection with the hepatitis delta virus: A multicenter study. N Engl J Med 1985;312:1488.

VARIANTS OF VIRAL HEPATITIS

Cholestatic Hepatitis

There is usually a cholestatic phase in the initial icteric phase of viral hepatitis, but in occasional cases, this is the dominant manifestation of the disease. The course tends to be more prolonged than that of ordinary hepatitis. The symptoms are often extremely mild, but jaundice is deeper, and pruritus is often present. Laboratory tests of liver function indicate cholestasis with hyperbilirubinemia, bilirubinuria, and elevated alkaline phosphatase and cholesterol.

Differentiation of this type of hepatitis from extrahepatic obstruction may be difficult. Percutaneous transhepatic cholangiography or endoscopic retrograde cholangiography may be necessary to make the distinction, though ultrasonography usually suffices.

Fulminant Hepatitis

Hepatitis may take a rapidly progressive course terminating in less than 10 days. Up to 75% of those due to viral hepatitis are due to hepatitis B (with about half of these associated with the delta antigen). Most of the remainder are due to hepatitis C, but hepatitis A can also—rarely—induce fulminant hepatitis. Extensive necrosis of large areas of the liver gives the typical pathologic picture of acute liver atrophy. Toxemia and gastrointestinal symptoms are more severe, and hemorrhagic phenomena are common. Neurologic symptoms of hepatic coma develop. Jaundice may be absent or minimal, but laboratory tests show extreme hepatocellular damage. A more insidious course of fulminant hepatitis is occasionally seen, characterized by progressive clinical deterioration over a 6- to 8-week period leading to encephalopathy and then usually death.

The treatment of fulminant hepatitis is directed toward those metabolic abnormalities associated with severe liver cell dysfunction. They include coagulation defects; disordered fluid, electrolyte, and acid-base balance; hypoglycemia; and nitrogenous intoxication. Monitoring of the patient, with vigorous correction of the deficits noted, provides the hope that some patients will survive who might otherwise succumb before liver regeneration can occur.

Adrenocorticosteroids, exchange transfusions, and perfusions through pig and baboon livers have not proved effective. Preliminary experiences with emergency liver transplantation have show promise.

Starzl TE, Demetris AJ, VanThiel D: Liver transplantation. (Two parts.) N Engl J Med 1989;321:1014, 1092.

CHRONIC HEPATITIS

Chronic hepatitis is defined as a chronic inflammatory reaction of the liver of more than 6 months' duration, as demonstrated by persistently abnormal liver tests. For proper treatment, it is crucial to determine whether the disease will resolve, remain static, or progress to cirrhosis. The causes of chronic hepatitis are only partially defined. It may be a sequela of infection resulting from hepatitis B virus, as well as a sequela of hepatitis C. Hepatitis A virus has not yet been shown to lead to chronic hepatitis. Additionally, identical clinical entities may be associated with drug reactions, including methyldopa and isoniazid. Wilson's disease and α_1-antitrypsin deficiency can also present as chronic liver disease, and α_1-antitrypsin deficiency is also associated with chronic liver disease.

1. CHRONIC PERSISTENT HEPATITIS

This form of chronic hepatitis represents an essentially benign condition with a good prognosis. The diagnosis is confirmed by liver biopsy. The biopsy may show portal tract infiltration with primarily mononuclear cells and occasional areas of focal inflammation in the parenchyma. The boundary between portal tracts and parenchyma remains sharp, and there is little or no "piecemeal necrosis" (a process in which the liver cells are gradually destroyed and replaced by fibrous tissue septa). In essence, the architecture of the hepatic lobule remains intact. The symptomatology varies from the asymptomatic state to various vague manifestations including fatigability, anorexia, malaise, and lassitude. Physical examination is usually normal. Laboratory findings are those of intermittent or persistent transaminasemia, usually in the range of 2–3 times normal.

Liver biopsy helps establish the diagnosis of persistent hepatitis. The treatment is reassurance of the patient. Corticosteroids and immunosuppressive drugs should not be given. Dietary restrictions, excessive vitamin supplementation, and prolonged bed rest are not necessary. The prognosis is excellent. Rarely does the disease progress to chronic active hepatitis.

2. CHRONIC ACTIVE HEPATITIS (Chronic Aggressive Hepatitis, Lupoid Hepatitis)

This form of chronic hepatitis is usually characterized by progression to cirrhosis, although milder cases may resolve spontaneously. Piecemeal necrosis refers to this inflammatory process at the interface of the portal area and the liver lobule. In severe cases, piecemeal necrosis may be associated with considerable hepatic fibrosis and ultimately with cirrhosis. In very mild cases, it may be difficult to distinguish this entity from chronic persistent hepatitis. Liver biopsies repeated at varying intervals may be necessary to make the distinction as well as to monitor therapy.

Clinical Findings
A. Symptoms and Signs
1. Chronic active hepatitis (lupoid type)–This is generally a disease of young people, particularly young women. However, the disease can occur at any age. The onset is usually insidious, but about 25% of cases present as an acute attack of hepatitis. Although the serum bilirubin is usually increased, 20% of these patients have anicteric disease. Examination often reveals a healthy-appearing young woman with multiple spider nevi, cutaneous striae, acne, and hirsutism. Amenorrhea may be a feature of this disease. Multisystem involvement, including kidneys, joints, lungs, and bowel, and Coombs-positive hemolytic anemia are associated with this clinical entity. Markers for hepatitis B are absent.

2. Chronic active hepatitis (HBsAg-positive type)–This type of hepatitis clinically resembles the lupoid type of disease. The histologic pictures of these 2 types of chronic active hepatitis are indistin-

guishable. The HBsAg form of chronic active hepatitis appears to affect males predominantly. It may be noted as a continuum of acute hepatitis or may be manifested only by biochemical abnormalities of liver function.

In the more active form, HBeAg or DNA polymerase (or both) may be present, indicative of active viral replications. HBc IgM is also present in about 70%. There are increased risks for the development of hepatoma in these patients.

3. Delta agent in hepatitis B–Acute delta infection superimposed on chronic HBV infection usually results in severe acute hepatitis; however, it may be subclinical and manifested only by a transient transaminase rise; in this setting, chronic delta infection ensues. Delta infection among HBsAg carriers is common and is associated with the presence of liver damage, characterized by chronic active hepatitis with or without cirrhosis.

4. Chronic active hepatitis (non-A, non-B type)–This type occurs in up to 5% of patients with posttransfusion hepatitis and in sporadic cases. It is clinically indistinguishable from chronic active hepatitis of other causes and may actually be the most common. The clinical setting, lack of hepatitis markers, absence of other potential causes (eg, drugs, Wilson's disease) and liver biopsy determine the category.

B. Laboratory Findings: The serum bilirubin is usually normal or only modestly increased (4.5–7 mg/dL); AST (SGOT), IgG, IgM, and gamma globulin levels are higher than normal. Late in the disease, serum albumin levels are usually decreased and prothrombin time may be significantly prolonged and will not respond to vitamin K therapy. Antinuclear and smooth muscle antibodies are positive 15–50% of the time but are nonspecific. Latex fixation tests for rheumatoid arthritis and anticytoplasmic and immunofluorescent antimitochondrial antibodies are positive in 25–50% of patients. Hepatitis B antigen is not found in the blood of patients with classic "lupoid" hepatitis.

The activity of chronic active hepatitis can be defined practically and accurately in terms of objective criteria. Thus, the magnitude of transaminase and gamma globulin elevations and the degree of hepatocellular necrosis are suitable means of defining quantitatively quite readily by establishing arbitrary biochemical standards. For example, either a 10-fold increase in serum transaminase level or a 5-fold elevation of AST with a 2-fold increase in gamma globulin concentration constitutes "high-grade" activity.

Differential Diagnosis
Chronic active hepatitis can be confused with 5 other chronic liver conditions: cholestatic viral hepatitis, chronic persistent hepatitis, subacute hepatic necrosis, postnecrotic cirrhosis, and Wilson's disease. Classically, Wilson's disease should be considered

in any patient under the age of 30 who has chronic active hepatitis; however, the initial diagnosis has been made as late as age 58. The differentiation is made on the basis of the clinical course, sequential laboratory testing, and liver biopsy.

Treatment

Prolonged or enforced bed rest has not been shown to be beneficial. Activity should be modified according to the patient's symptoms. The diet should be well balanced, without specific limitations other than sodium or protein restrictions as dictated by water retention or encephalopathy.

Prednisone has been shown to decrease the serum bilirubin, AST (SGOT), and gamma globulin levels and reduce the piecemeal necrosis in patients with non-B chronic active hepatitis. The mortality rate in those patients treated with corticosteroids is also significantly reduced. However, relapse after discontinuance of prednisone therapy occurs frequently. For patients with chronic active hepatitis due to HBV infection, the risks of increasing viral replication and infectiousness with the use of corticosteroids are considerable and are a relative contraindication to their use. Patients who are symptomatic owing to the chronic active hepatitis, are HbsAg-negative, and have severe histologic abnormalities are the most suitable candidates for corticosteroid therapy.

Prednisone or an equivalent drug is given initially in doses of 30 mg orally daily, with gradual reduction to the lowest maintenance level (usually 15–20 mg/d) that will control the symptomatology and reduce the abnormal liver function. If symptoms are not controlled, azathioprine or mercaptopurine, 50–150 mg/d orally, is added, with the primary benefit being that doses of corticosteroids can be much lower. Azathioprine at doses of more than 1.5 mg/kg body weight for a prolonged period imposes a significant hazard—occurring in 28% of patients—of bone marrow suppression with the initial finding of leukopenia. Doses in chronic active hepatitis are usually less, and the resulting side effects are much less serious; nevertheless, complete blood counts should be monitored weekly for the first 8 weeks of therapy and at less frequent intervals subsequently. A common regimen that gives therapeutic efficacy with few side effects is as follows: prednisone, 10–15 mg/d, and azathioprine (or mercaptopurine), 50 mg/d .

Prognosis

The course of chronic active hepatitis is variable and unpredictable. The sequelae of chronic active hepatitis secondary to hepatitis B include cirrhosis, liver cell failure, and hepatocellular carcinoma. It has been stated that 40–50% of patients with chronic active hepatitis die within 5 years of the onset of symptoms. Most patients die of hepatocellular failure and associated complications of portal hypertension.

Czaja AJ et al: Complete resolution of inflammatory activity following corticosteroid treatment of HBsAg-negative chronic active hepatitis. Hepatology 1984;4:622.

Dragosics B et al: Long-term follow-up study of asymptomatic HBsAg-positive voluntary blood donors in Austria: A clinical and histologic evaluation of 242 cases. Hepatology 1987;7:302.

Hay JE et al: The nature of unexplained chronic aminotransferase elevations of a mild to moderate degree in asymptomatic patients. Hepatology 1989;9:193. (Only histopathology will differentiate.)

Hoofnagle JH: Type D (delta) hepatitis. JAMA 1989; 261:1321.

Hoofnagle JH, Shafritz DA, Popper H: Chronic type B hepatitis and the "healthy" HBsAg carrier state. Hepatology 1987;7:758.

Weissberg JI et al: Survival in chronic hepatitis B: An analysis of 379 patients. Ann Intern Med 1984;101:613.

ALCOHOLIC HEPATITIS

Alcoholic hepatitis is an acute or chronic inflammation of the liver that occurs as a result of parenchymal necrosis induced by alcohol abuse. Although a variety of terms were used in the past to describe this type of hepatitis in chronic alcoholics, the term alcoholic hepatitis is now regarded as the most appropriate one to describe this injury, which is currently accepted as the precursor of alcoholic cirrhosis.

While alcoholic hepatitis is often a reversible disease, it is the most common cause of cirrhosis in the USA. This is especially significant, since cirrhosis ranks among the most common causes of death of adults in this country. Alcoholic hepatitis does not develop in all chronic heavy drinkers; the exact prevalence and incidence are not known but have been estimated to be about one-third. Women appear to be more susceptible than men.

Alcoholic hepatitis usually occurs after years of excessive drinking. Although it may not develop in many patients even after several decades of alcohol abuse, it appears in a few individuals within a year of excessive drinking. Over 80% of patients with alcoholic hepatitis were drinking 5 years or more before developing any symptoms that could be attributed to liver disease. In general, the longer the duration of drinking (10–15 or more years) and the larger the alcoholic consumption (usually more than 120 g of alcohol per day, which is equal to 8 oz of 100-proof whiskey, 30 oz of wine, or 100 oz of beer (eight 12-oz cans)), the greater the probability of developing alcoholic hepatitis and cirrhosis. It is also important to realize that while drinking large amounts of alcoholic beverages is essential for the development of alcoholic hepatitis, drunkenness is not. In drinking individuals, the rate of ethanol metabolism can be sufficiently high to permit the consumption of large quantities of spirits without raising the blood alcohol level over 80 mg/dL, the concentration at which the conventional breath analyzer begins to detect ethanol.

The roles of proteins, vitamins, and calories in the development of alcoholic hepatitis or in the progression of this lesion to cirrhosis are not understood.

Only liver biopsy can establish the diagnosis with certainty, since any of the manifestations of alcoholic hepatitis can be seen in other types of alcoholic liver disease such as fatty liver or cirrhosis, as well as liver disease due to other causes.

Clinical Findings

A. Symptoms and Signs: Alcoholic hepatitis is usually seen after a recent period of heavy drinking. That history in addition to complaints of anorexia and nausea and the objective demonstration of hepatomegaly and jaundice strongly suggest the diagnosis. Abdominal pain and tenderness, splenomegaly, ascites, fever, and encephalopathy support the diagnosis. The clinical presentation of alcoholic hepatitis can vary from an asymptomatic patient with an enlarged liver to a critically ill individual who dies quickly.

B. Laboratory Findings: Anemia is variable and usually macrocytic. Leukocytosis with shift to the left is common and is seen more frequently in patients with severe disease. Leukopenia is occasionally seen and disappears after cessation of drinking. About 10% of patients have thrombocytopenia that appears related to a direct toxic effect of alcohol on megakaryocyte production.

AST (SGOT) is normal in 15–25% of patients; when increased, it is usually under 300 units/mL. ALT (SGPT) is almost invariably less than the AST, often by a factor of 2–5 or more. Serum alkaline phosphatase is generally elevated, but rarely more than 3 times the normal value. Serum bilirubin is increased in 60–90% of patients, and when levels greater than 6 mg/dL are demonstrated it can be assumed that the process is severe. The serum albumin is depressed, and the gamma globulin is elevated in 50–75% of individuals with alcoholic hepatitis even in the absence of cirrhosis.

Liver biopsy is diagnostic and may reveal both cirrhosis and alcoholic hepatitis.

C. Special Procedures: Scintiphotographic evaluation (liver scanning) using ^{99m}Tc sulfur colloid will reveal patchy hepatic uptake of the isotope; marked bone marrow uptake, which is indicative of portal hypertension; and splenomegaly. Liver scanning is nonspecific and rarely indicated.

Differential Diagnosis

Alcoholic hepatitis may be closely mimicked by diseases of the hepatobiliary tree such as cholecystitis and cholelithiasis. A history of chronic insobriety and recent debauch is helpful but far from conclusive. Percutaneous liver biopsy, if there is no contraindication, is a reliable means of differentiation; alterna-

tively, various imaging procedures may indicate primary biliary tract disease.

Complications

Clinical deterioration and worsening abdominal pain and tenderness may result in the unfortunate decision to perform laparotomy. The postoperative mortality rate of acutely ill patients with alcoholic hepatitis is far greater than that of those who are operated on for intra– or extrahepatic cholestasis.

Treatment

A. General Measures: Discontinue all alcoholic beverages. During periods of anorexia, every effort should be made to provide sufficient amounts of carbohydrate and calories to reduce endogenous protein catabolism and gluconeogenesis and to prevent hypoglycemia. Although the clinical value of intravenous hyperalimentation has not been established, the judicious administration of parenteral fluids is most important. Caloric intake is gratifyingly improved by the use of palatable liquid formulas during the transition period between totally intravenous alimentation and normal feeding. The administration of vitamins, particularly folic acid, is an important part of treatment and is frequently associated with dramatic clinical improvement in patients with alcoholic liver disease.

B. Corticosteroids: The use of corticosteroids in this disorder has been evaluated over a period of more than 20 years, with conflicting reports of success. Recently, methylprednisolone was shown to be beneficial in patients with alcoholic hepatitis and either encephalopathy or very elevated bilirubin and prolonged prothrombin times. Anabolic steroids are not beneficial.

Prognosis

A. Short-Term: The severity of liver injury, which can be ascertained clinically, biochemically, and histologically, enables valid speculation about prognosis. The presence of asterixis seems to be associated with an increased likelihood of death. Biochemically, it has been shown that when the prothrombin time is short enough to permit performance of liver biopsy without risk, the 1-year mortality rate is 7.1%, rising to 18% if there is progressive prolongation of that parameter during hospitalization. Individuals in whom the prothrombin time is so prolonged that liver biopsy cannot be attempted have a 42% mortality rate at 1 year.

B. Long Term: In the USA, the mortality rate over a 3-year period of persons who recover from acute alcoholic hepatitis is 10 times greater than that of average individuals of comparable age. The histologically severe form of the disease is associated with continued excessive mortality rates after 3 years, whereas the death rate is not increased after the same period in those whose liver biopsies show only mild alcoholic hepatitis.

The most important prognostic consideration is the indisputable fact that continued excessive drinking is associated with reduction of life expectancy in these individuals. The prognosis is indeed poor if the patient is unable to abstain from drinking.

Carithers RL Jr et al: Methylprednisolone therapy in patients with severe alcoholic hepatitis: A randomized multicenter trial. Ann Intern Med 1989;110:685. (Striking decrease in short-term mortality rate.)
Maddrey WC: Alcoholic hepatitis: Clinicopathologic features and therapy. Semin Liver Dis 1988;8:91.

UNCOMMON HYPERBILIRUBINEMIA STATES

There are about a half-dozen hyperbilirubinemic states that must be distinguished from hemolytic disease, hepatitis, and surgical jaundice (Table 11–6). The disorders are benign, with the notable exception of the rate type I Crigler-Najjar syndrome, for which there is no known effective treatment. These hyperbilirubinemic states are very uncommon, with the exception of Gilbert's syndrome, which may occur in up to 5% of the population.

Gollan JL (editor): Pathobiology of bilirubin and jaundice. Semin Liver Dis 1988;8:105. (Entire issue.)

DRUG- & TOXIN-INDUCED LIVER DISEASE

The continuing synthesis, testing, and introduction of new drugs into clinical practice has resulted in an increase in toxic reactions of many types. Many widely used therapeutic agents may cause hepatic injury. The diagnosis of drug-induced liver injury is not always easy. Drug-induced liver disease can mimic viral hepatitis or biliary tract obstruction. The clinician must be aware of drug-induced liver disease and must question the patient carefully about the use of various drugs before dismissing this possibility.

Direct Hepatotoxic Group

The liver lesion caused by this group of drugs is characterized by (1) dose-related severity, (2) reproducibility in experimental animals, (3) a latent period following exposure, and (4) susceptibility in all individuals: acetaminophen, alcohol, carbon tetrachloride, chloroform, heavy metals, mercaptopurine, phosphorus, stilbamidine, tetracyclines, valproic acid, vitamin A.

Viral Hepatitis-Like Reactions

Reactions of this type are sporadic, suggesting host idiosyncrasy: amiodarone, aspirin, chloramphenicol, chlortetracycline, cinchophen, dantrolene, halothane, isoniazid, ketoconazole, methoxyflurane, methyl-

Table 11–6. Uncommon hyperbilirubinemic disorders.

	Nature of Defect	Type of Hyper-bilirubinemia	Clinical and Pathologic Characteristics
Constitutional hepatic dysfunction (Gilbert's syndrome)	Glucuronyl transferase deficiency	Unconjugated (indirect) bilirubin	Benign, asymptomatic hereditary jaundice. Hyperbilirubinemia increased by 24- to 36-hour fast. No treatment required. Prognosis excellent.
Crigler-Najjar syndrome			Severe, nonhemolytic hereditary jaundice of neonates. Type I cases sustain CNS damage (kernicterus). Milder cases (type II) may persist into adult life and may benefit from treatment with phenobarbital.
Familial chronic idiopathic jaundice (Dubin-Johnson syndrome)	Faulty excretory function of liver cells (hepatocytes)	Conjugated (direct) bilirubin	Benign, asymptomatic hereditary jaundice. BSP excretion impaired. Gallbladder does not visualize on oral cholecystography. Liver darkly pigmented on gross examination. Biopsy shows centrilobular brown pigment. Prognosis excellent.
Rotor's syndrome			Similar to Dubin-Johnson syndrome but liver is not pigmented and the gallbladder is visualized on oral cholecystography. Prognosis excellent.
Benign intermittent cholestasis	Cholestatic liver dysfunction	Unconjugated plus conjugated (total) bilirubin	Benign intermittent idiopathic jaundice, itching, and malaise. Onset in early life and may persist for lifetime. Alkaline phosphatase increased. Cholestasis found on liver biopsy. (Biopsy is normal during remission.) Prognosis excellent.
Recurrent jaundice of pregnancy			Benign cholestatic jaundice of unknown cause, usually occurring in the third trimester of pregnancy. Itching, gastrointestinal symptoms, and abnormal liver excretory function tests. Cholestasis noted on liver biopsy. Prognosis excellent, but recurrence with subsequent pregnancies or use of birth control pills is characteristic.

dopa, oxacillin, phenylbutazone, pyrazinamide, quinidine, streptomycin, sulfamethoxypyridazine, zoxazolamine.

Cholestatic Reactions

There are 2 general categories that differ in clinical presentation and histopathologic features. These reactions are dose-dependent, but marked differences in individual susceptibility exist:

A. Noninflammatory: Probable direct effect of agent on bile secretory mechanisms and on inflammatory reactions: azathioprine, mercaptopurine, mestranol, methyltestosterone, norethandrolone.

B. Inflammatory: Inflammation of portal areas, with allergic features, eg, eosinophilia: chlorothiazide, chlorpromazine, chlorpropamide, erythromycin, estolate, penicillamine, prochlorperazine, promazine, sulfadiazine, thiouracils.

Chronic Active Hepatitis

Clinically and histologically indistinguishable from postviral chronic active hepatitis: aspirin, chlorpromazine, dantrolene, halothane, isoniazid, methyldopa, nitrofurantoin, oxyphenisatin, sulfonamides.

Miscellaneous Reactions

A. Fatty Liver:

1. Large fatty inclusions–Alcohol, amiodarone, corticosteroids, methotrexate.

2. Small cytoplasmic droplets–Tetracyclines, valproic acid.

B. Granulomas: Allopurinol, quinidine, phenylbutazone, phenytoin.

C. Cirrhosis: Methotrexate.

D. Peliosis Hepatis: Anabolic steroids (Halotestin), azathioprine, oral contraceptive steroids.

E. Neoplasms: Oral contraceptive steroids.

FATTY LIVER

It was formerly believed that malnutrition rather than ethanol was responsible for steatosis (fatty metamorphosis) of the liver in the alcoholic. More recently, it has come to be agreed that the role of deficient nutrition in such individuals has been overemphasized. However, it cannot be ignored that inadequate diets—specifically, those deficient in choline, methionine, and dietary protein—can produce fatty liver (kwashiorkor) in children.

Other nonalcoholic causes of steatosis are obesity (the commonest cause), starvation, diabetes mellitus, corticosteroids, poisons (carbon tetrachloride and yellow phosphorus), endocrinopathies such as Cushing's syndrome, tetracycline toxicity, Reye's syndrome, TPN, and, rarely, pregnancy.

Regardless of the cause, there are apparently at least 5 factors, acting in varying combinations, that are responsible for the accumulation of fat in the liver: (1) increased mobilization of fatty acids from peripheral adipose depots; (2) decreased utilization or oxidation of fatty acids by the liver; (3) increased hepatic fatty acid synthesis; (4) increased esterification of fatty acids into triglycerides; and (5) decreased secretion or liberation of fat from the liver.

Liver function studies may show elevated transaminase and alkaline phosphatase levels. Percutaneous liver biopsy is diagnostic but seldom needed.

Treatment consists of removing or modifying the offending factor.

Prognosis depends on the underlying condition.

Heubi JE et al: Reye's syndrome: Current concepts. Hepatology 1987;7:155.

Powell EE et al: The natural history of nonalcoholic steatohepatitis: A follow-up study of forty-two patients. Hepatology 1990;11:74. (A probable cause of "cryptogenic cirrhosis.")

Riely CA et al: Acute fatty liver of pregnancy: A reassessment based on observations in 9 patients. Ann Intern Med 1987;106:703.

CIRRHOSIS

The current concept of cirrhosis includes only those cases in which hepatocellular injury leads to both fibrosis and nodular regeneration throughout the liver. These features delineate cirrhosis as a serious and irreversible disease—eighth leading cause of death in males, ninth in females in USA in 1981; rate of 12.3/100,000 per year; over 65% alcohol-related—that is characterized not only by variable degrees of hepatic cell dysfunction but also by portosystemic shunting and portal hypertension. Fibrosis alone, regardless of its severity, is excluded by the previous definition. Also excluded by definition are the early stages of chronic biliary obstruction, hemochromatosis, and primary biliary cirrhosis, none of which form regenerating nodules until late.

An important part of this concept is the realization that the histopathology of cirrhosis may change with the passage of time in any one patient. Terms such as "portal" and "postnecrotic" refer not so much to separate disease states with different causes as to different expressions of hepatic injury.

Attempts to classify cirrhosis on the basis of cause or pathogenesis are usually unsuccessful when applied to individual patients. Such persons often represent end-stage cirrhosis, enabling only speculation about the evolutionary process. The use of a purely anatomic and descriptive categorization facilitates easier and more practical classification. One such classification that is currently employed divides cirrhosis into micronodular, mixed, and macronodular forms. It is important, however, to remember that these are stages of development rather than separate diseases.

(1) Micronodular cirrhosis is the form in which the regenerating nodules are no larger than the original

lobules, ie, approximately 1 mm in diameter or less. It has been suggested that this feature results from the persistence of the offending agent (alcohol), a substance that prevents regenerative growth.

(2) Macronodular cirrhosis is characterized by larger nodules, which can measure several centimeters in diameter and often contain central veins. This form corresponds more or less to postnecrotic cirrhosis but does not necessarily follow episodes of massive necrosis and stromal collapse.

(3) Mixed macro- and micronodular cirrhosis points up the fact that the features of cirrhosis are highly variable and not always easy to classify. In any case, the configuration of the liver is determined by the mixture of liver cell death and regeneration as well as the deposition of fat, iron, and fibrosis.

Finally, it should be emphasized that there does exist a limited relationship between anatomic types and etiology as well as between anatomic types and prognosis. For example, alcoholics who continue to drink tend to have micronodular cirrhosis. The presence of fatty micronodular cirrhosis, although not an infallible criterion, is strongly suggestive of chronic alcoholism. On the other hand, there is a higher incidence of liver cell carcinoma in macronodular than in micronodular cirrhosis, although the latter is much more common in the USA because of the alcohol relationship. This propensity to malignancy is perhaps related either to the increased regeneration in macronodular cirrhosis or to the longer period required for the process to develop. Clinical Findings

A. Symptoms and Signs: Micronodular (Laennec's) cirrhosis may cause no symptoms for long periods, both at onset and later in the course (compensated phase). The onset of symptoms may be insidious or, less often, abrupt. Weakness, fatigability, and weight loss are common. In advanced cirrhosis, anorexia is usually present and may be extreme, with associated nausea and occasional vomiting. Abdominal pain may be present and is related either to hepatic enlargement and stretching of Glisson's capsule or to the presence of ascites. Menstrual abnormalities (usually amenorrhea), impotence, loss of libido, sterility, and painfully enlarged breasts in men (rare) may occur. Hematemesis is the presenting symptom in 15–25%. Oliguria is common.

In 70% of cases, the liver is enlarged, palpable, and firm if not hard and has a blunt or nodular edge; and the left lobe may predominate. Skin manifestations consist of spider nevi (usually only on the upper half of the body), palmar erythema (mottled redness of the thenar and hypothenar eminences), telangiectases of exposed areas, and evidence of vitamin deficiencies (glossitis and cheilosis). Weight loss, wasting, and the appearance of chronic illness are present. Jaundice—usually not an initial sign—is mild at first, increasing in severity during the later stages of the disease. Ascites, pleural effusion, peripheral edema, and purpuric lesions are late findings. Precoma (sleep

reversal, asterixis, tremor, dysarthrias, delirium, and drowsiness) and coma also occur very late except when precipitated by an acute hepatocellular insult or an episode of gastrointestinal bleeding. Fever may be present in 35% on presentation and usually reflects a complication such as alcoholic hepatitis. spontaneous bacterial peritonitis, cholangitis, or some other intercurrent event. Clinical splenomegaly is present in 35–50% of cases. The superficial veins of the abdomen and thorax are dilated and reflect the intrahepatic obstruction to portal blood flow.

B. Laboratory Findings: Laboratory abnormalities are either absent or minimal in latent or quiescent cirrhosis. Anemia, a frequent finding, is often macrocytic; causes include suppression of erythropoiesis by alcohol as well as folate deficiency, hemolysis, hypersplenism, and insidious or overt blood loss from the gastrointestinal tract. The white cell count may be low, elevated, or normal, reflecting hypersplenism or infection; thrombocytopenia may be secondary to alcoholic marrow suppression, sepsis, folate deficiency, or splenic sequestration. Coagulation abnormalities may also be a result of failure of synthesis of clotting constituents in the liver.

Blood chemical studies show primarily hepatocellular injury and dysfunction, reflected by elevations of AST (SGOT), alkaline phosphatase, and bilirubin. Serum albumin is low; gamma globulin is increased.

Liver biopsy shows cirrhosis.

C. Imaging: Plain films of the abdomen may reveal hepatic or splenic enlargement. Barium studies of the upper gastrointestinal tract may reveal the presence of esophageal or gastric varices. Ultrasound is helpful for determining the presence of occult ascites, liver size, presence of hepatic nodules, and, in very experienced hands, small hepatomas. Together with Doppler studies, ultrasound is increasingly used to evaluate patency of the splenic and portal veins, but splenoportography is still the "gold standard" in this regard. Hepatic scanning using ^{99m}Tc sulfur colloid may occasionally be helpful in documenting splenomegaly; however, this objective can be achieved at much less cost with a "flat plate" of the abdomen, and diffuse patchy uptake of the isotope in the liver makes the test useless in the evaluation of hepatoma.

D. Special Examinations: Esophagogastroscopy demonstrates or confirms the presence of varices and detects specific causes of bleeding in the esophagus, stomach, and proximal duodenum. Peritoneoscopy is helpful in judging the type of cirrhosis present though it is usually unnecessary for clinical purposes.

Differential Diagnosis

As previously noted, differentiation of one type of cirrhosis from another can be difficult, but determining the cause is important both for prognostic and, potentially, therapeutic reasons. Hemochromatosis may be associated with "bronzing" of the skin, arthritis, heart failure, and diabetes mellitus; special staining of liver biopsies will be positive for increased iron deposition in the hepatic parenchyma. Primary biliary cirrhosis tends to occur more frequently in women and is associated with marked pruritus, significant elevation of alkaline phosphatase, and positive antimitochondrial antibodies. Congestive heart failure and constrictive pericarditis may also be simulated by cirrhosis when ascites is prominent.

Complications

Upper gastrointestinal tract bleeding may occur from varices, hemorrhagic gastritis, or gastroduodenal ulcers. Hemorrhage may be massive, resulting in fatal exsanguination or portosystemic encephalopathy. Liver failure may also be precipitated by alcoholism, surgery, and infection. Carcinoma of the liver and portal vein thrombosis occur more frequently in patients with cirrhosis but are still uncommon. Lowered resistance often leads to serious infections, particularly of the lungs and peritoneum.

Treatment

A. General Measures: The principles of treatment include abstinence from alcohol and adequate rest, especially during the acute phase. The diet should be palatable, with adequate calories and protein (75–100 g/d) and, in the stage of fluid retention, sodium and fluid restriction. In the presence of hepatic precoma or coma, protein intake should be reduced or excluded. Vitamin supplementation is desirable.

B. Special Problems:

1. Ascites and edema due to sodium retention, hypoproteinemia, and portal hypertension– Paracentesis is usually indicated. Abdominal paracentesis is rarely associated with serious complications such as bleeding, infection, or bowel perforation.

In some patients, there is a rapid diminution of ascites on dietary sodium and fluid restriction alone. In individuals who pose more significant problems of fluid retention and who are considered to have "intractable" ascites, the urinary excretion of sodium is less than 10 meq/L. Mechanisms that have been postulated to explain sodium retention in cirrhosis include impaired liver inactivation of aldosterone and increased aldosterone secretion secondary to increased renin production, which is associated with decreased renal cortical blood flow of uncertain cause. If such persons are permitted unrestricted fluids, serum sodium progressively falls, representing impairment of free water excretion. With a 200-mg sodium diet and 500-mL allowance of oral fluids per day, ascites production ceases and the patient's abdominal discomfort abates; however, this regimen is unrealistic in most clinical situations.

a. Restoration of plasma proteins–This is dependent upon improving liver function and serves as a practical index of recovery. Therapeutic use of albumin intravenously is of little value.

b. Diuretics–Spironolactone should be used after documentation of secondary aldosteronism, as evidenced by markedly low urinary sodium. Starting with 50 mg twice daily and monitoring the aldosterone antagonist effect, reflected by the urinary sodium concentration, the dose is increased 100 mg every 3 days (up to a daily dosage of 1000 mg) until the urinary sodium excretion exceeds 60 meq/L. Monitoring for hyperkalemia is important. Diuresis commonly occurs at this point and may be augmented by the addition of a potent agent such as furosemide. This potent diuretic, however, will maintain its effect even with a falling glomerular filtration rate, with resultant prerenal azotemia. The dose of furosemide ranges from 40 to 120 mg/d, and the drug should be administered with careful monitoring of serum electrolytes, especially potassium.

The goal of weight loss in the nonedematous ascitic patient should be no more than 1–11/2 lb/d.

c. Large-volume paracentesis–Recently there has been increasing experience—still being debated—with large-volume paracentesis (4–6 L) in the management of symptomatic ascites; when this is done, it is safest to give intravenous albumin concomitantly at a dosage of 8–10 g/L of ascites fluid removed to protect the intravascular volume. This can be repeated daily until ascites is largely gone.

d. Peritoneovenous shunts–Peritoneovenous shunts have been advocated for use in patients with refractory ascites or hepatorenal syndrome. These shunts are frequently effective but carry a considerable complication rate: disseminated intravascular coagulation in 65% of patients (25% symptomatic; 5% severe), bacterial infections in 4–8%, congestive heart failure in 2–4%, and variceal bleeding from sudden expansion of intravascular volume.

2. Hepatic encephalopathy–Hepatic encephalopathy is the result of biochemical abnormalities associated with hepatocellular deficit or hepatic bypass of portal vein blood into the systemic circulation. Although disturbed ammonia metabolism is inherent in the clinical entity of hepatic encephalopathy, it is clear that ammonia per se is not solely responsible for the disturbed mental status. Hepatic encephalopathy may be aggravated by sepsis. Bleeding into the intestinal tract may significantly increase the amount of protein in the bowel and may precipitate rapid development of liver coma. Other factors that may precipitate hepatic encephalopathy include alkalosis, potassium deficiency induced by diuretics, narcotics, hypnotics, and sedatives; medications containing ammonium or amino compounds; paracentesis with attendant hypovolemia; and hepatic or systemic infection.

Dietary protein should be curtailed or completely withheld during acute episodes. Parenteral or enteral nutrition is usually indicated.

Gastrointestinal bleeding should be controlled if possible and blood purged from the gastrointestinal tract. This can be accomplished with 120 mL of magnesium citrate by mouth or nasogastric tube every 3–4 hours until the stool is free of gross blood.

Lactulose (Cephulac), a nonabsorbable synthetic disaccharide, is digested by bacteria in the colon to short-chain fatty acids, resulting in acidification of colon contents. This acidification favors the ammonium ion in the $NH_4^+ \rightarrow NH_3$ equation; NH_4^+ is not absorbable, and it is the NH_3 that is absorbable and thought to be neurotoxic. The acid pH induced by lactulose also inhibits the degradation of amino acids, protein, and blood. When given orally, the initial dose of lactulose for acute hepatic encephalopathy is 30 mL 3 or 4 times daily, or a dose that will produce no more than 2–3 soft stools per day. When rectal use is indicated because of the patient's inability to take medicines orally, the dose is 300 mL of lactulose in 700 mL of saline or sorbitol as a retention enema for 30–60 minutes; it may be repeated every 4–6 hours. One liter of nonfat milk may be used instead, because there is no lactase in the colon and the bacteria reduce the lactose to short-chain fatty acids. The end result is the same as what can be achieved with lactulose for a fraction of the cost.

The intestinal flora may also be controlled with neomycin sulfate, 0.5–1 g orally every 6 hours for 5–7 days. Side effects of neomycin include diarrhea, malabsorption, superinfection, ototoxicity, and nephrotoxicity, usually only after prolonged use.

If agitation is marked, give oxazepam, 10–30 mg orally or by nasogastric tube, cautiously as indicated. Avoid narcotics, tranquilizers, and sedatives metabolized or excreted by the liver.

3. Anemia–For iron deficiency anemia, give ferrous sulfate, 0.3 g enteric-coated tablets, one tablet 3 times daily after meals. Folic acid, 1 mg/d orally, is indicated in the treatment of macrocytic anemia associated with alcoholism.

4. Hemorrhagic tendency–A bleeding tendency due to hypoprothrombinemia may be treated with vitamin K preparations. This treatment is ineffective in the presence of severe hepatic disease when other coagulation factors are deficient. Transfusions with packed red blood cells may be necessary to replace blood loss. Correcting the prolonged prothrombin time in these situations requires large volumes of fresh-frozen plasma, and the effect is transient; for that reason, plasma infusions are not indicated. Menadione, 1–3 mg orally 3 times daily after meals, seldom helps but is often tried.

5. Hemorrhage from esophageal varices–When active variceal bleeding is evident, attempts should be made to sclerose the bleeding varices transendoscopically. If this procedure cannot be performed or is not successful, bleeding can often be controlled by use of the quadruple-lumen (Minnesota) tube. Unfortunately, there is a high incidence of recurrent variceal bleeding after balloon tamponade has been discontinued. Injection sclerotherapy has proved to be quite effective (80%) in stopping the acute episode of variceal bleeding. The advantages of this technique are simplicity and avoidance of a major surgical procedure in a poor-risk patient. Repeated injections may be necessary. If bleeding cannot be controlled by sclerotherapy, emergency surgical decompression of portal hypertension may be considered in selected patients. Morbidity and mortality rates are substantially lower when surgical shunting procedures are performed electively than when performed on an urgent basis. After the patient has been stabilized for 3–5 days, the beta-blocker propranolol can be given in an attempt to lower the portal pressure. The dosage is usually 20–80 mg twice daily, with the goal of reducing the pretreatment resting pulse by 25% but not below 60/min. The efficacy of beta-blockers is still controversial both for management of the patient with portal hypertension and varices after hemorrhage as well as prophylactically. Prophylactic sclerotherapy has been shown not to be beneficial.

6. Spontaneous bacterial peritonitis–This occurs in cirrhotic patients with ascites. Abdominal pain, increasing ascites, fever, and progressive encephalopathy suggest the possibility, although symptoms may be very mild. Paracentesis reveals an ascitic fluid with, most commonly, a total white cell count of more than 300 cells/mL with more than 250 PMNs/mL and a protein concentration of 1 g/dL or less. Cultures of ascites give the best results—80–90% positive—when aerobic and anaerobic blood culture bottles are inoculated at the bedside. Common organisms found are *E coli* and pneumococci. Pending culture results, if there are 250 or more PMNs/mL, intravenous antibiotic therapy should be initiated with antibiotics such as ampicillin or cefotetan. The mortality rate is high.

7. Hepatorenal syndrome–In patients with cirrhosis or severe alcoholic hepatitis, hepatorenal syndrome is often a preterminal event. Characterized by oliguria, hyponatremia, and low urinary sodium, it is diagnosed only when other causes of renal failure have been excluded. The cause is unknown; histologically, the kidneys are normal. Death is commonly due to complicating infection or hemorrhage.

Prognosis

The prognosis in advanced cirrhosis has shown little change over the years. A major factor for survival is the patient's ability to discontinue the use of alcohol. In established cases with severe hepatic dysfunction, only 50% survive 2 years and only about 35% survive 5 years. Hematemesis, jaundice, and ascites are unfavorable signs. In selected cases, liver transplantation is a consideration.

Bass NM: Preventing hemorrhage from esophageal varices. (Editorial.) N Engl J Med 1987;317:893.

Colombo M et al: b-Blockade prevents recurrent gastrointestinal bleeding in well-compensated patients with alcoholic cirrhosis: A multicenter randomized controlled trial. Hepatology 1989;9:433. (Propranolol is effective in those who survive 2 weeks after variceal bleeding and whose liver status is in the Child's A or B category.)

Gines P et al: Compensated cirrhosis: Natural history and prognostic factors. Hepatology 1987;7:122.

Henderson JM et al: Endoscopic variceal sclerosis compared with distal splenorenal shunt to prevent recurrent variceal bleeding in cirrhosis: A prospective randomized trial. Ann Intern Med 1990;112:262. (Most representative of current wisdom.)

LeVeen HH: The LeVeen shunt. Annu Rev Med 1985; 36:453.

Runyon BA: Spontaneous bacterial peritonitis: An explosion of information. Hepatology 1988;8:171.

Santangelo WC et al: Prophylactic sclerotherapy of large esophageal varices. N Engl J Med 1988;318:814.

Stassen WN, McCullough AS: Management of ascites. Semin Liver Dis 1985;5:291.

Westaby D et al: A controlled trial of oral propranolol compared with injection sclerotherapy for the long-term management of variceal bleeding. Hepatology 1990; 11:353. (Suggests equal efficacy.)

BILIARY CIRRHOSIS

1. PRIMARY BILIARY CIRRHOSIS

Primary biliary cirrhosis is a chronic disease of the liver manifested by cholestasis. It is insidious in onset, occurs usually in women aged 40–60, and is often detected by the chance finding of elevated alkaline phosphatase levels. The disease is progressive and complicated often by steatorrhea, xanthomatous neuropathy, osteomalacia, and portal hypertension.

Clinical Findings
A. Symptoms and Signs: The onset is insidious and is heralded by pruritus. Jaundice usually occurs within 2 years of onset of pruritus. Physical examination reveals hepatosplenomegaly. Xanthomatous lesions may occur in the skin and tendons and around the eyelids.

B. Laboratory Findings: Hemograms are normal early in the disease. Serologic tests reflect cholestasis with elevation of alkaline phosphatase, cholesterol, and bilirubin. Mitochondrial antibodies are present in an incidence reported to be 83–98% in different series.

Differential Diagnosis
The disease must be differentiated from chronic biliary tract obstruction (stone or stricture), carcinoma of the bile ducts, cholestatic liver disease associated with inflammatory bowel disease, and sarcoidosis.

Treatment
Treatment is symptomatic. Cholestyramine may be beneficial for the pruritus. Vitamins A, K, and D should be administered parenterally if steatorrhea is present. Calcium supplementation may be helpful for osteomalacia. Penicillamine, corticosteroids, and azathioprine have proved to be of no benefit. Colchicine, methotrexate, and ursodeoxycholic acid have had some reported benefit in early studies. Advanced primary biliary cirrhosis is a major indication for liver transplantation.

Berk PD (editor): Primary biliary cirrhosis. Semin Liver Dis 1989;9:103.

Bodenheimer H Jr, Schaffner F, Pezzullo J: Evaluation of colchicine therapy in primary biliary cirrhosis. Gastroenterology 1988;95:124. (Shows some promise.)

Esquivel CO et al: Transplantation for primary biliary cirrhosis. Gastroenterology 1988;94:1207. (The most rewarding group of patients for liver transplant.)

Maddrey WC, Van Thiel DH: Liver transplantation: An overview. Hepatology 1988;8:948.

Powell FC, Schroeter AL, Dickson ER: Primary biliary cirrhosis and the CREST syndrome: A report of 22 cases. Q J Med 1987;62:75.

2. SECONDARY BILIARY CIRRHOSIS

Secondary biliary cirrhosis follows chronic obstruction to bile flow. Superimposed infection may hasten the process. Bile flow is most commonly impaired in an extrahepatic site by calculus, neoplasm, stricture, or biliary atresia.

Clinical Findings
A. Symptoms and Signs: The clinical presentation is usually that of the underlying cause of the cholestasis (eg, carcinoma of the pancreas, choledocholithiasis, choledochal cysts).

B. Laboratory Findings: Hemograms are normal except insofar as they reflect the inciting lesion (eg, cholangitis associated with choledocholithiasis). Serologic tests reflect cholestasis with elevated alkaline phosphatase. The mitochondrial antibody is present in less than 1% of patients with secondary biliary cirrhosis.

C. Imaging: Ultrasound may reveal dilated ducts (especially intrahepatic), hilar or pancreatic masses, and occasionally common duct stones. CT scan is more accurate than ultrasound for lesions of the pancreas.

The more definitive procedures are the invasive ones: endoscopic retrograde cholangiography (ERCP) and percutaneous transhepatic cholangiography. Selection of one or the other is dictated by the expertise available and the anticipated problem: For choledocholithiasis, ERCP is clearly the procedure of choice, since papillotomy with stone extraction can usually be accomplished and is therapeutic. Either method allows placement of stents. For balloon dilation of ductal strictures, ERCP is preferable.

HEMOCHROMATOSIS

Hemochromatosis is a genetically transmitted disease characterized as autosomal recessive and HLA-related, with linkage to HLA-A3 and HLA-B14 or HLA-A3 and HLA-B7. This disorder of iron metabolism is characterized by increased accumulation of dietary iron, as hemosiderin in the liver, pancreas, heart, adrenals, testes, pituitary, and kidneys. Eventually the patient may develop hepatic, pancreatic, and cardiac insufficiency. The disease usually occurs in males and is rarely recognized before the fifth decade.

Clinical Findings

Clinical manifestations include arthropathy, hepatomegaly and evidence of hepatic insufficiency (late finding), occasional skin pigmentation (slate gray due to iron and brown due to melanin), cardiac enlargement with or without heart failure or conduction defects, diabetes mellitus with its complications, and impotence in the male. Bleeding from esophageal varices may occur, and in patients who develop cirrhosis, there is a 10% incidence of hepatic carcinoma. The disease should be considered in those with a family history and in patients with unexplained mild liver test abnormalities. The clinical disease appears in affected women 10–20 years postmenopause.

Laboratory findings include mildly abnormal liver tests, elevated plasma iron, increased percentage saturation of transferrin, elevated serum ferritin, and the characteristic liver biopsy that stains positive for iron.

Treatment

Early diagnosis and treatment in the precirrhotic phase of hemochromatosis is of great importance. Treatment consists initially of weekly phlebotomies of 500 mL of blood (about 250 mg of iron), perhaps continued for 2–3 years to achieve depletion of iron stores. This process is monitored by hematocrit and serum iron determinations. When iron store depletion is achieved, maintenance phlebotomies (every 2–4 months) are continued. The chelating agent, deferoxamine, administered intramuscularly to patients with hemochromatosis, has been shown to produce urinary excretion of up to 5–18 g of iron per year. This rate of urinary excretion compares favorably with the rate of 10–20 g of iron removed annually by weekly or biweekly phlebotomies. The treatment, however, is painful and not always practical. Active treatment of the complications of hemochromatosis—arthropathy, diabetes, heart and liver disease, and hypopituitarism—is important.

Although the long-term benefits of iron depletion therapy have not been completely established, available data indicate that the course of the disease may be favorably altered by chelation or bleeding. There appear to be fewer cardiac conduction defects and lower insulin requirements with these treatments.

Crosby WH: Hemochromatosis: Current concepts and management. Hosp Pract (Feb 15) 1987;22:173.

WILSON'S DISEASE

Wilson's disease (hepatolenticular degeneration) is a rare familial disorder that is inherited in an autosomally recessive manner and occurs in both males and females between the first and third decades. The condition is characterized by excessive deposition of copper in the liver and brain.

Awareness of the entity is important, since it may masquerade as chronic active hepatitis, psychiatric disorder, or neurologic disease. It is potentially reversible, and appropriate therapy will prevent neurologic and hepatic damage.

The major physiologic aberration in Wilson's disease is excessive absorption of copper from the small intestine and decreased excretion of copper by the liver, resulting in increased tissue deposition, especially in the liver, brain, cornea, and kidney. Ceruloplasmin, the plasma copper-carrying protein, is low. Urinary excretion of copper is high.

Clinical Findings

Wilson's disease can present primarily as a neurologic abnormality, with liver involvement appearing later; or the reverse may be true, with hepatic disease being the initial manifestation. It may first be clinically recognized when jaundice appears in the first few years of life. The diagnosis should always be considered in any child with manifestations of atypical hepatitis, splenomegaly with hypersplenism, hemolytic anemia, portal hypertension, and neurologic or psychiatric abnormalities. Wilson's disease should also be considered in young adults (under 40 years of age) with chronic active hepatitis as well as those with acute fulminant hepatitis.

The neurologic manifestations are related to basal ganglia dysfunction and are characterized by rigidity or parkinsonian tremor. Hepatic involvement is evidenced by signs of cirrhosis, portal hypertension, and biochemical confirmation of hepatocellular insufficiency. The pathognomonic sign of the condition is the Kayser-Fleischer ring, which represents fine pigmented granular deposits in Descemet's membrane in the cornea close to the endothelial surface. Scattering and reflection of light by these deposits give rise to the typically brownish or gray-green appearance of the ring. The ring itself is not always complete and is usually most marked at the superior and inferior poles of the cornea. It can frequently be seen with the naked eye and almost invariably by slit lamp examination.

The diagnosis is based on demonstration of increased urinary copper excretion ($> 100 \ \mu g/24 \ h$) or low serum ceruloplasmin levels ($< 20 \ \mu g/dL$), and elevated hepatic copper concentration (> 100

μg/g of dry liver). Early in the course of Wilson's disease, the serum alkaline phosphatase appears to be lower than for matched normals. Histologically, the disease may present as an acute viral hepatitis. In other patients, it may present clinically and histologically as chronic active hepatitis. Cirrhosis ultimately occurs.

Treatment

Early treatment is essential for removal of copper before it can produce neurologic or hepatic damage. Oral penicillamine (0.75–2 g/d in divided doses) is the drug of choice, making possible urinary excretion of chelated copper. Pyridoxine, 50 mg per week, is added, since penicillamine is an antimetabolite of this vitamin. If penicillamine treatment cannot be tolerated because of gastrointestinal, hypersensitivity, or autoimmune reactions, consider the use of trientine (Cuprid), 500 mg twice daily. Early in the treatment phase, restriction of dietary copper (shellfish, organ foods, legumes are rich in copper) may be of value.

Treatment should continue indefinitely. The prognosis is good in patients who are effectively treated before liver or brain damage has occurred.

Marsden CD: Wilson's disease. Q J Med 1987;65:959.

Rakela J et al: Fulminant Wilson's disease treated with postdilution hemofiltration and orthotopic liver transplantation. Gastroenterology 1986;90:2004. (Patient did well.)

Shaver WA, Bhatt H, Combes B: Low serum alkaline phosphatase activity in Wilson's disease. Hepatology 1986;6:859.

Walshe JM: Diagnosis and treatment of presymptomatic Wilson's disease. Lancet 1988;2:435. (Suggests autosomal recessive gene and benefits of early diagnosis.)

HEPATIC VEIN OBSTRUCTION (Budd-Chiari Syndrome)

This uncommon disorder is due to occlusion of the hepatic veins from a variety of causes. Hepatovenous obstructions may be associated with caval webs, right-sided heart failure or constrictive pericarditis, polycythemia, use of birth control pills, pyrrolizidine alkaloids ("bush teas"), neoplasms causing hepatic vein occlusions, paroxysmal nocturnal hemoglobinuria, and pregnancy. Approximately 30% are idiopathic.

Clinical manifestations may include tender, painful hepatic enlargement; jaundice; splenomegaly; and ascites. With advanced disease, bleeding varices and hepatic coma may be evident. Isotopic liver scan may show prominent caudate lobes, since its venous drainage may not come from the hepatic vein. Caval venogram can delineate caval webs and occluded hepatic veins. Percutaneous liver biopsy frequently shows a characteristic central lobular congestion.

Ascites should be treated with fluid and salt restriction and diuretics and efforts made to find treatable causes. Surgical decompression of the congested liver may be required. Liver transplantation is a consideration. Mean survival is about 12–18 months, with a range of a few weeks to more than 20 years.

Friedman AC et al: Magnetic resonance imaging diagnosis of Budd-Chiari syndrome. Gastroenterology 1986; 91: 1289.

NONCIRRHOTIC PORTAL HYPERTENSION

Noncirrhotic portal hypertension must be considered in the differential diagnosis of splenomegaly or upper gastrointestinal bleeding due to esophageal or gastric varices. This syndrome may be due to portal vein obstruction, splenic vein obstruction (gastric varices without esophageal varices), schistosomiasis, noncirrhotic intrahepatic portal sclerosis, or arterial-portal vein fistula. Consideration of the diagnosis is most important. Angiography of the portal system is confirmatory, as is needle biopsy of the liver, particularly for schistosomiasis and noncirrhotic intrahepatic portal sclerosis. Other than for splenomegaly, the physical findings are not remarkable, and the endoscopic findings are those of esophageal or gastric varices. The liver tests are usually normal, but there may be findings of hypersplenism.

If splenic vein thrombosis is the cause, splenectomy is curative. Surgical decompression of the portal hypertension may well be undertaken in those without splenic vein thrombosis.

Benhamon JP, Lebrel D: Noncirrhotic intrahepatic portal hypertension in adults. Clin Gastroenterol 1985;14:21.

Valla D et al: Etiology of portal vein thrombosis in adults: A prospective evaluation of primary myeloproliferative disorders. Gastroenterology 1988;94:1063. (Thirty-three patients with portal vein thrombosis, about half due to myeloproliferative disorders.)

HEPATIC ABSCESS

1. PYOGENIC ABSCESS

Single or multiple local collections of pus in the liver that are large enough to be seen with the naked eye are presently quite rare, principally because of the use of antibiotics and improved methods of diagnosis of appendicitis, which was formerly the most common precursor of liver abscess. Although the actual clinical incidence cannot be determined because the condition is aborted or modified by antimicrobial treatment, hepatic abscess is still reported in 0.5–1.5%

or autopsy specimens. It is equally distributed between men and women, usually in the sixth or seventh decade.

There are 5 ways in which the liver can be invaded by bacteria: (1) by way of the portal vein; (2) by way of ascending cholangitis in the common duct; (3) by way of the hepatic artery, secondary to bacteremia; (4) by direct extension from an infectious process; and (5) by traumatic implantation of bacteria through the abdominal wall.

Despite the use of antimicrobial drugs, 10% of cases of liver abscess are secondary to appendicitis. Another 10% have no demonstrable cause and are classified as idiopathic. At present, ascending cholangitis is the most common cause of hepatic abscess in the USA. Bacterial infection of the hepatobiliary tree is more likely to accompany obstruction by stone than obstruction by carcinoma of the head of the pancreas. The most frequently encountered organisms are *Escherichia coli, Proteus vulgaris, Enterobacter aerogenes,* and multiple anaerobic species.

Hepatic candidiasis is being reported with increasing frequency, particularly in immunocompromised patients.

Clinical Findings
Clinically, fever is almost always present and may antedate other symptoms or signs. Pain is prominent and is localized to the right hypochondrium or epigastric area. Jaundice, tenderness in the right upper abdomen, and either steady or swinging fever are the chief physical findings.

Laboratory examination reveals leukocytosis with a shift to the left. Chest roentgenograms will usually reveal elevation of the diaphragm if the abscess is on the right side. Left-sided abscess does not produce significant diaphragmatic elevation. Ultrasound or CT scan may reveal the presence of intrahepatic defects. Hepatic candidiasis is seen usually in the setting of systemic candidiasis, and on CT scan the characteristic appearance is that of multiple "bulls-eyes." Liver function studies are nonspecifically abnormal.

Treatment
Treatment should consist of antimicrobial agents that are effective against coliform organisms. If adequate response to therapy is not rapid, needle or surgical drainage should be undertaken. Failure to recognize and treat the condition is attended by mortality rates of about 60% in patients with multiple abscesses. Hepatic candidiasis often responds to intravenous amphotericin.

Gyorffy EJ et al: Pyogenic liver abscess: Diagnostic and therapeutic strategies. Ann Surg 1987;206:699. (Microabscesses may be treated medically; others used percutaneous or surgical drainage.)
Haron E et al: Hepatic candidiasis: An increasing problem in immunocompromised patients. Am J Med 1987;83:17.
Thaler M et al: Hepatic candidiasis in cancer patients: The evolving picture of the syndrome. Ann Intern Med 1988;108:88.
Webb TH et al: Liver abscess. Hosp Physician (April) 1989, p 46.

2. AMEBIC LIVER ABSCESS

Amebic abscess is more common as a primary presentation than is pyogenic abscess. Usual symptoms and signs, which may have been present for 1–30 days, are right upper quadrant pain, often with associated fever, and right pleuritic chest pain. Associated dysentery is uncommon, but 20% of patients will have had a significant recent diarrheal episode. Usually there is a history of travel to endemic areas.

Clinical Findings
Physical examination discloses fever in most cases, toxic appearance of varying degree, and a tender palpable liver with marked "punch" tenderness. Right lung base abnormalities and localized intercostal tenderness are common. Acute amebic appendicitis is not an uncommon precursor.

Laboratory findings usually consist of mild to moderate anemia, moderate leukocytosis with a shift to the left, and slightly abnormal liver tests. Serologic amebic gel diffusion tests or indirect hemagglutination tests for Entamoeba histolytica are positive in 95% of patients but may be nondiagnostic on presentation, with a marked rise in titer over the subsequent 3–4 weeks.

An elevated right hemidiaphragm is frequently seen on chest radiograph. Ultrasonography, liver scan with ^{99m}Tc sulfur colloid, or CT scan is helpful in delineating the location and number of abscesses. Most are in the right lobe.

Treatment
Metronidazole, 750 mg 3 times per day orally for 5–10 days, is the drug of choice. Occasionally, a second course is necessary. In the acutely toxic patient, percutaneous needle aspiration and decompression of the abscess bring about a greater feeling of well-being and also allow for demonstration of the ameba in over 50% of cases. Following completion of treatment for the abscess, the patient needs to take iodoquinol (Yodoxin), 650 mg 3 times a day for 20 days (for adults), to eradicate the intestinal cyst phase of amebiasis.

Fever usually subsides rapidly once treatment is initiated. The hepatic defect may persist for as long as 6 months.

Complications include rupture of the abscess transcutaneously, into the peritoneal cavity, pleural space, lungs, or pericardium, with a significant associated mortality rate if undiagnosed. Rarely, distal embolization has been reported.

Barnes PF et al: A comparison of amebic and pyogenic abscesses of the liver. Medicine 1987;66:472.

Kubitschek KR et al: Amebiasis presenting as pleuropulmonary disease. West J Med 1985;142:203.

NEOPLASMS OF THE LIVER

Neoplasms of the liver arise either in the hepatic parenchymal cells or biliary ductules. A tumor that arises from parenchymal cells is called a hepatocellular carcinoma; one that originates in the ductular cells is called a cholangiocarcinoma.

Hepatocellular carcinomas are associated with cirrhosis in general and hepatitis B in particular. The world over and especially in Africa and Asia, hepatitis B is of major etiologic significance. The association with *Clonorchis sinensis* may also be of importance in Asia. Other associations include hemochromatosis and alcoholic liver disease, the latter at a lower incidence but with a greater number of total cases.

Histologically, the tumor may be made up of cords or sheets of cells that roughly resemble the hepatic parenchyma or associated with a desmoplastic reaction. In the case of a cholangiocarcinoma, a fibrous stroma or tissue containing structures that simulate bile ducts will be seen. Blood vessels such as portal or hepatic veins are commonly involved by tumor.

The presence of a hepatocellular carcinoma may be unsuspected until there is deterioration in the condition of a cirrhotic patient who was formerly stable. Cachexia, weakness, and weight loss are associated symptoms. The sudden appearance of ascites, which may be bloody, suggests portal or hepatic vein thrombosis by tumor or bleeding from the necrotic tumor. In the chronic hepatitis B patient or chronic HBsAg carrier, surveillance for the development of hepatoma should be seriously considered.

Physical examination is positive for tender enlargement of the liver, with an occasionally palpable mass. Auscultation may reveal a bruit over the tumor, or a friction rub may be heard when the process has extended to the surface of the liver.

Laboratory tests may reveal leukocytosis, as opposed to the leukopenia that is frequently encountered in cirrhotic patients. A normal or elevated hematocrit may be found, owing to elaboration of erythropoietin by the tumor. Sudden and sustained elevation of the serum alkaline phosphatase in a patient who was formerly stable is a common finding. Hepatitis B surface antigen is present in more than 50% of cases. Alpha fetoprotein—not usually found in adults—is demonstrable in 30–50% of patients with hepatocellular carcinoma. Cytologic study of ascitic fluid may reveal malignant cells. For surveillance, careful ultrasound examination of the liver appears helpful. How often or after how many years of HBsAg positivity this should be done is unclear at this time.

Arteriography is frequently diagnostic, revealing a tumor "blush" that reflects the highly vascular nature of the tumor. Almost as helpful is the CT scan when done with and without intravenous contrast to characterize the location and vascularity of the tumor. Liver biopsy is diagnostic.

Attempts at surgical resection are fruitless if concomitant cirrhosis is present and if the tumor is multifocal. Surgical resection of solitary hepatocellular carcinomas may result in cure if the unaffected liver is normal. Chemotherapy has not been shown to prolong life.

1. LIVER NEOPLASMS IN WOMEN TAKING ORAL CONTRACEPTIVES

Benign and malignant neoplasms have been encountered in women taking oral contraceptives. Two distinct entities with characteristic clinical, radiologic, and histopathologic features have been described. Focal nodular hyperplasia occurs at all ages but is questionably related to oral contraceptives. It is usually asymptomatic and hypervascular on CT scan. Microscopically, focal nodular hyperplasia consists of hyperplastic units of hepatocytes with centrally placed proliferating bile ducts. Liver cell adenoma occurs most commonly in the third and fourth decades of life; the clinical presentation is one of acute abdominal disease due to necrosis of the tumor with hemorrhage. The tumor is hypovascular and reveals a cold defect on liver scan. Grossly, the cut surface appears structureless. As seen microscopically, the liver cell adenoma consists of sheets of hepatocytes without portal tracts or central veins. The only physical finding in focal nodular hyperplasia or liver cell adenoma is a palpable abdominal mass in some cases. Liver function is usually normal. Treatment of focal nodular hyperplasia is resection in the symptomatic patient. The prognosis is excellent. Liver cell adenoma often undergoes necrosis and rupture; resection is advised. Regression of benign hepatic tumors may follow cessation of oral contraceptives.

2. MISCELLANEOUS LIVER NEOPLASMS

The most common benign neoplasm of the liver is the cavernous hemangioma, often an incidental finding on CT scan. This lesion must be differentiated from other space-occupying intrahepatic lesions, usually by CT scan with contrast. MRI appears to be even more specific. Needle biopsy may be necessary to differentiate these lesions. They rarely require treatment.

Di Bisceglie AM et al: Hepatocellular carcinoma. Ann Intern Med 1988;108:390.

Dunk AA et al: Hepatocellular carcinoma and the hepatitis B virus: A study of British patients. Q J Med 1987; 62:109.

Ohnishi K et al: Prognosis of hepatocellular carcinoma smaller than 5 cm in relation to treatment: Study of 100 patients. Hepatology 1987;7:1285.

Regan LS: Screening for hepatocellular carcinoma in high-risk individuals: A clinical review. Arch Intern Med 1989;149:1741. (Emphasizes adjusting intensity of screening to the degree of risk of hepatocellular carcinoma.)

Welch TJ et al: Focal nodular hyperplasia and hepatic adenoma: Comparison of angiography, CT, US, and scintigraphy. Radiology 1985;156:593. (Scintigraphy separated these 2 groups most of the time.)

CHOLELITHIASIS
(Gallstones)

Gallstones are more common in women than in men and increase in incidence in both sexes and all races with aging. Data indicate that in the USA 10% of men and 20% of women between the ages of 55 and 65 have gallstones and that the total exceeds 15 million people. Although gallstones are less common in black people, cholelithiasis attributable to hemolysis has been encountered in over a third of individuals with sickle cell disease. Native Americans of both the Northern and Southern Hemispheres have a high rate of cholesterol cholelithiasis. As many as 75% of Pima women over the age of 25 years have cholelithiasis. A common threat among Native Americans is their high legume intake. The incidence of gallstones is also high in individuals with certain diseases such as regional enteritis. Approximately one-third of individuals with inflammatory involvement of the terminal ileum have cholesterol gallstones due to disruption of bile salt resorption that results in decreased solubility of the bile. The incidence of cholelithiasis is also increased in patients with diabetes mellitus. Pregnancy as a significant association with gallstones has been overemphasized.

Classification of Gallstones

The simplest classification of gallstones is according to chemical composition: stones containing predominantly cholesterol and stones containing predominantly calcium bilirubinate. The latter comprise less than 5% of the stones found in Europe or the USA but 30–40% of stones found in Japan.

Three compounds comprise 80–95% of the total solids dissolved in bile: conjugated bile salts, lecithin, and cholesterol. Cholesterol is a neutral sterol; lecithin is a phospholipid; and both are almost completely insoluble in water. However, bile salts are able to form multimolecular aggregates (micelles) that solubilize lecithin and cholesterol in an aqueous solution. Bile salts alone are relatively inefficient in solubilizing cholesterol (approximately 50 molecules of bile salt are necessary to solubilize 1 molecule of cholesterol), but the solubilization of lecithin in bile salt solutions results in a mixed micelle that is 7 times more efficient

in the solubilization of cholesterol. Precipitation of cholesterol microcrystals may come about through a simultaneous change in all 3 major components.

Treatment

Cholelithiasis is frequently asymptomatic and is discovered fortuitously in the course of routine radiographic study, operation, or autopsy.

There is disagreement about the desirability of cholecystectomy in patients with "silent" gallstones, including diabetics. Operation is usually indicated for symptomatic cholelithiasis. "Symptomatic" cholelithiasis may be quite diverse in its presentation but usually includes right upper quadrant discomfort and colicky pain. There must be careful consideration of other sources of the symptoms.

Cheno- and ursodeoxycholic acids are bile salts that on oral administration are able to cause dissolution of some cholesterol stones. Of these bile salts, chenodeoxycholic acid may induce diarrhea and mild liver test abnormalities, and ursodeoxycholic acid is quite expensive. They are probably effective only in patients with a functioning gallbladder, as determined by gallbladder visualization or oral cholecystography (represents not more than 15% of patients with gallstones). These agents may be most efficacious in terms of safety, cost, and rapidity of stone dissolution when used in combination, at a dose of 5 mg/kg body weight of each daily in 2 divided doses. Dissolution of gallstones may require 2 years or longer. In half of patients, gallstones recur within 5 years after treatment is stopped. Obesity may induce resistance to therapy. Intermittent therapy is ineffective.

Lithotripsy as a treatment modality for cholelithiasis has had some initial success in a limited number of patients. This procedure does require concomitant treatment with cheno– or ursodeoxycholic acid (or both).

Heiss FW et al: Common bile duct calculi. 1. Surgical therapy. 2. Nonsurgical therapy. Postgrad Med (Feb 15) 1984;75:88, 109. (Special issue.)

Podda M et al: Efficacy and safety of a combination of chenodeoxycholic acid and ursodeoxycholic acid for gallstone dissolution. Gastroenterology 1989;96:222. (Combinations appear better.)

Nervi F et al: Influence of legume intake on biliary lipids and cholesterol saturation in young Chilean men. Gastroenterology 1989;96:825. (Legume intake a risk factor.)

Sackmann M et al: Shock-wave lithotripsy of gallbladder stones: The first 175 patients. N Engl J Med 1988;318:393.

ACUTE CHOLECYSTITIS

Essentials of Diagnosis

- Steady, severe pain and tenderness in the right hypochondrium or epigastrium.
- Nausea and vomiting.

- Jaundice.
- Fever and leukocytosis.

General Considerations

Cholecystitis is associated with gallstones in over 90% of cases. It occurs when a calculus becomes impacted in the cystic duct and inflammation develops behind the obstruction. Vascular abnormalities of the bile duct or pancreatitis may rarely produce cholecystitis in the absence of gallstones. If the obstruction is not relieved, pressure builds up within the gallbladder as a result of continued secretion. Primarily as a result of ischemic changes secondary to distention, gangrene may develop, with resulting perforation. Although generalized peritonitis is possible, the leak usually remains localized and forms a chronic, well-circumscribed abscess cavity.

Clinical Findings

A. Symptoms and Signs: The acute attack is often precipitated by a large or fatty meal and is characterized by the relatively sudden appearance of severe, minimally fluctuating pain which is localized to the epigastrium or right hypochondrium and which in the uncomplicated case may gradually subside over a period of 12–18 hours. Vomiting occurs in about 75% of patients and in half of instances affords variable relief. Right upper quadrant abdominal tenderness is almost always present and is usually associated with muscle guarding and rebound pain. A palpable gallbladder is present in about 15% of cases. Jaundice is present in about 25% of cases and, when persistent or severe, suggests the possibility of choledocholithiasis. Fever is usually present.

B. Laboratory Findings: The white count is usually high (12,000–15,000/μL). Total serum bilirubin values of 1–4 mg/dL may be reported even in the absence of common duct obstruction. Serum transaminase and alkaline phosphatase are often elevated—the former as high as 300 mU/mL and even higher when associated with ascending cholangitis. Serum amylase may also be moderately elevated.

C. Imaging: Films of the abdomen may show gallstones in 15% of cases. ^{99m}Tc hepatobiliary imaging agents (iminodiacetic acid compounds), also known as HIDA scan, are useful in demonstrating an obstructed cystic duct, which is the cause of acute cholecystitis in most patients. This test is reliable if the bilirubin is under 5 mg/dL. Right upper quadrant abdominal ultrasound may show the presence of gallstones but is not specific for acute cholecystitis.

Differential Diagnosis

The disorders most likely to be confused with acute cholecystitis are perforated peptic ulcer, acute pancreatitis, appendicitis in a high-lying appendix, perforated carcinoma or diverticulum of the hepatic flexure, liver abscess, hepatitis and pneumonia with pleurisy on the right side. The definite localization of pain and tenderness in the right hypochondrium, with frequent radiation to the infrascapular area, strongly favors the diagnosis of acute cholecystitis. True cholecystitis without stones raises the question of polyarteritis nodosa (rarely), or acalculous cholecystitis. The latter is occasionally observed in acutely ill medical or surgical patients who have had no oral intake for prolonged periods.

Complications

A. Gangrene of the Gallbladder: Continuation or progression of right upper quadrant abdominal pain, tenderness, muscle guarding, fever, and leukocytosis after 24–48 hours suggests severe inflammation and possible gangrene of the gallbladder. Necrosis may occasionally develop without definite signs in either the obese or the elderly.

B. Cholangitis: Intermittently high fever and chills strongly suggest choledocholithiasis.

Treatment

Acute cholecystitis will usually subside on a conservative regimen (withholding of oral feedings, intravenous alimentation, analgesics and antibiotics if indicated). Cholecystectomy can be performed within 2–3 days after hospitalizing or can be scheduled for 6–8 weeks later, depending on the surgeon's preference and the clinical aspects of the individual case. If, as occasionally happens, recurrent acute symptoms develop during this waiting period, cholecystectomy is indicated without delay. If nonsurgical treatment has been elected, the patient (especially if diabetic or elderly) should be watched carefully for evidence of gangrene of the gallbladder or cholangitis.

Operation is mandatory if the patient is diabetic or when there is evidence of gangrene or perforation. Operation during the first 24 hours can be justified as a means of reducing overall morbidity in good-risk patients in whom the diagnosis is unequivocal. It is usually best to defer surgery, if possible, in the presence of acute pancreatitis, unless choledocholithiasis is suspected.

A. Medical Treatment: During the acute period, the patient should be observed frequently, with careful abdominal examination and sequential determination of the white cell count several times a day. Analgesics such as meperidine are preferred for pain control. Morphine derivatives in effective doses are known to produce spasm of the sphincter of Oddi and may cause spurious elevations of serum amylase. Meperidine may have the same effects but to a much lesser degree. Anticholinergic agents are rarely indicated for these patients, in part because they may mask the development of paralytic ileus or prolong its duration. Appropriate antimicrobial agents should be employed in all but the most mild and rapidly subsiding cases.

B. Surgical Treatment: When surgery is elected for acute cholecystitis, cholecystectomy is the procedure of choice. Cholangiography should be performed at the time of operation to ascertain the need for common duct exploration. In the poor-risk patient or when technical difficulties preclude cholecystectomy, cholecystostomy can be performed under local anesthesia.

Prognosis

Mild acute cholecystitis usually subsides, but recurrences are common. Symptomatic cholecystitis is a definite indication for surgery. Persistence of symptoms after removal of the gallbladder implies either mistaken diagnosis, functional bowel disorder, or technical error, since cholecystectomy is curative.

Addison NV, Finan PJ: Urgent and early cholecystectomy for acute gallbladder disease. Br J Surg 1988;75:141.

Dawson SL, Mueller PR: Nonoperative management of biliary obstruction. Annu Rev Med 1985;36:1.

Fink-Bennett D et al: The sensitivity of hepatobiliary imaging and realtime ultrasonography in the detection of acute cholecystitis. Arch Surg 1985;120:904.

Hickman MS, Schwesinger WH, Page CP: Acute cholecystitis in the diabetic: A case-control study of outcome. Arch Surg 1988;123:409.

Williamson RCN: Progress report: Acalculous disease of the gallbladder. Gut 1988;29:860.

CYSTIC DUCT SYNDROMES

Precholecystectomy

A small group of patients (mostly women) has been reported in whom right upper quadrant abdominal pain occurred frequently following meals. Conventional radiographic study of the upper gastrointestinal tract and gallbladder—including intravenous cholangiography—was unremarkable. Using cholecystokinin (CCK) as a gallbladder stimulant, contraction and evacuation of the viscus did not take place, as usually occurs in the 3- to 5-minute period after injection of the hormone. However, the gallbladder assumed a "golf ball" configuration, and biliary type pain was reproduced. At the time of cholecystectomy, the gallbladders were found to be enlarged and could not be emptied by manual compression. Anatomic and histologic examination of the operative specimens revealed obstruction of the cystic ducts either because of fibrotic stenosis at their proximal ends or because of adhesions and kinking. Additional diagnostic considerations are ampullary spasm and biliary dyskinesia. Biliary manometry (not generally available) during ERCP may prove helpful in making the diagnosis.

Postcholecystectomy

Following cholecystectomy, a variable group of patients complain of continuing symptoms, ie, right upper quadrant pain, flatulence, and fatty food intolerance. The persistence of symptoms in this group of patients suggests the possibility of an incorrect diagnosis prior to cholecystectomy, eg, esophagitis, pancreatitis, radiculitis, or functional bowel disease. It is important to rule out the possibility of choledocholithiasis or common duct stricture as a cause for persistent symptoms in the postoperative period.

Pain has been associated with dilatation of the cystic duct remnant, neuroma formation in the ductal wall, foreign body granuloma, or traction on the common duct by a long cystic duct. The clinical presentation of colicky pain, chills, fever, or jaundice should suggest biliary tract disease. Liver tests for cholestasis, abdominal ultrasonography, or retrograde cholangiography may be necessary to rule out biliary tract disease. Surgery, with common duct exploration for stones and removal of the cystic duct remnant, may be necessary.

Alberti-Flor JJ et al: Mirizzi syndrome. Am J Gastroenterol 1985;80:822.

Bode WE, Aust JB: Isolated cystic dilatations of the cystic duct. Am J Surg 1983;145:828.

Jennings SA et al: Management of retained cystic duct stone. Br J Surg 1982;69:91.

Steinberg WM: Sphincter of Oddi dysfunction: A clinical controversy. Gastroenterology 1988;95:1409.

CHRONIC CHOLECYSTITIS

The most common disability that results from cholelithiasis is chronic cholecystitis. It is characterized pathologically by varying degrees of chronic inflammation on gross inspection or microscopic examination of the gallbladder. In about 4–5% of cases, the villi of the gallbladder undergo polypoid enlargement due to deposition of cholesterol that may be visible to the naked eye ("strawberry gallbladder," cholesterolosis). In other instances, adenomatous hyperplasia of all or part of the gallbladder wall may be so marked as to give the appearance of a myoma (pseudotumor). Calculi are usually present. The diagnosis is often erroneously applied to collections of symptoms that are only vaguely or indirectly related to gallbladder dysfunction.

Clinical Findings

A. Symptoms and Signs:

1. Pain–Chronic cholecystitis is associated with discrete bouts of right hypochondriac and epigastric pain that is either steady or intermittent. Discomfort is usually persistent, but, if intermittent, the height of pain may be separated by 15- to 60-minute intervals.

The onset of pain is usually abrupt, with maximum intensity and plateau reached within 15 minutes to 1 hour. Attacks of biliary colic may persist for as long as several hours or be as brief as 15–20 minutes, the average duration being about 1 hour. Pain referral to the interscapular area is occasionally noted.

2. Chronic indigestion–Chronic indigestion is

considered by many to be commonly due to gallbladder disease. Fatty food intolerance, belching, flatulence, a sense of epigastric heaviness, upper abdominal pain of varying intensity, and pyrosis are some of the symptoms that have been erroneously considered to be suggestive of cholelithiasis and cholecystitis. Efforts have therefore been made to evaluate "dyspeptic" symptomatology in relationship to objective evidence of gallbladder disease. It can be assumed that the association of chronic indigestion and gallstones is fortuitous. If cholecystectomy is performed in patients with calculi who have complained of a constellation of "dyspeptic" symptoms, the results of operation may be unpredictable and unsatisfactory.

3. Physical examination–Physical examination is nonspecific, revealing abdominal tenderness which may be localized to the right hypochondrium and epigastric area but which may also be diffuse. Hydrops of the gallbladder results when subsidence of acute cholecystitis occurs but cystic duct obstruction persists, producing distention of the gallbladder with a clear mucoid fluid. The gallbladder in that circumstance is palpable in the right upper abdomen. The presence of jaundice obviously supports the diagnosis of cholecystitis with choledocholithiasis.

B. Laboratory Findings: Laboratory studies are usually not diagnostic.

C. Imaging: Films of the abdomen taken prior to oral cholecystography may reveal opacification of the gallbladder caused by high concentrations of calcium carbonate (limy bile) or radiopaque stones. Nonvisualization of the gallbladder implies cholecystitis (95% accuracy) provided there is radiologic evidence that the oral contrast material has been absorbed and excreted. It is important to remember the following technical reasons for nonvisualization: failure to ingest the dye, vomiting or diarrhea, gastric outlet obstruction or esophageal stricture, intestinal malabsorption, abnormal location of the gallbladder, liver disease (including preicteric hepatitis), Dubin-Johnson-Sprinz-Nelson syndrome, fat-free diet prior to cholecystography, and previous cholecystectomy.

Ultrasound examination of the gallbladder is a useful means of detecting stones. The accuracy of diagnosis of cholelithiasis (but not cholecystitis) in some centers is high (96%) and the incidence of false-positive results low (2%).

Differential Diagnosis

When nonspecific symptoms are present, it is necessary to consider the possibilities of gastroduodenal ulcer disease, chronic relapsing pancreatitis, irritable colon syndrome, and malignant neoplasms of the stomach, pancreas, hepatic flexure, or gallbladder. Barium enema and upper gastrointestinal series complement cholecystography. Microscopic examination of bile obtained by biliary drainage is occasionally helpful in demonstrating calculous disease of the gall-

bladder. (The test is valid only in the absence of hepatic disease.)

Complications

The presence of cholelithiasis with chronic cholecystitis can result in acute exacerbation of gallbladder inflammation, common duct stone, cholecystenteric fistulization, pancreatitis, and, rarely, carcinoma of the gallbladder. Calcified gallbladder has a high association with gallbladder carcinoma and is an indication for cholecystectomy.

Treatment

Although documented cholelithiasis and cholecystitis ideally should be managed surgically, significant metabolic and cardiovascular disease or other factors may preclude operation. Nonspecific "dyspeptic" symptoms (eg, heartburn, belching, abdominal pain, bloating, flatulence, constipation) frequently are ameliorated by careful use of low-fat diets and weight reduction. Anticholinergics and sedatives, along with antacids and hydrophilic agents, may prove helpful.

Surgical treatment is the same as for acute cholecystitis, with operative cholangiography employed if there is a possibility of choledocholithiasis.

Prognosis

The overall mortality rate of cholecystectomy is less than 1%, but hepatobiliary tract surgery is a more formidable procedure in the elderly and has a mortality rate of 5–10%. A technically successful surgical procedure in an appropriately selected patient is generally followed by complete cessation of symptoms.

Ramond MJ et al: Sensitivity and specificity of microscopic examination of gallbladder bile for gallstone recognition and identification. Gastroenterology 1988;95:1339. (Presence of crystals in gallbladder bile is highly predictive of gallstone disease.)

CHOLEDOCHOLITHIASIS

Essentials of Diagnosis

- Often a history of biliary colic or jaundice.
- Sudden onset of severe right upper quadrant or epigastric pain, which may radiate to the right scapula or shoulder.
- Occasional patients present with painless jaundice, however.
- Nausea and vomiting.
- Fever, often followed by hypothermia and gram-negative shock, jaundice, and leukocytosis.
- Abdominal films may reveal gallstones.

General Considerations

About 15% of patients with gallstones have choledocholithiasis. The percentage rises with age, and the incidence in elderly people may be as high as 50%. Common duct stones usually originate in the gallbladder but may also form spontaneously in the common duct postcholecystectomy. The stones are frequently "silent" as no symptoms result unless there is obstruction.

Clinical Findings

A. Symptoms and Signs: A history suggestive of biliary colic or prior jaundice can usually be obtained. The additional features that suggest the presence of a common duct stone are (1) frequently recurring attacks of right upper abdominal pain that is severe and persists for hours: (2) chills and fever associated with severe colic; and (3) a history of jaundice that was chronologically associated with abdominal pain. The combination of pain, fever (and chills), and jaundice represents Charcot's triad and denotes the classic picture of cholangitis. The presence of altered sensorium, lethargy, and septic shock connotes acute suppurative cholangitis accompanied by pus in the obstructed duct and represents a surgical emergency.

Biliary colic in choledocholithiasis is apparently caused by rapidly increasing biliary pressure that is secondary to sudden obstruction to the flow of bile. Radiation of pain into the interscapular area may be helpful in differentiating choledocholithiasis from cholecystolithiasis. Hepatomegaly may be present in calculous biliary obstruction, and tenderness is usually present in the right hypochondrium and epigastrium. Usually there are no specific physical findings.

B. Laboratory Findings: Bilirubinuria and elevation of serum bilirubin are present if the common duct is obstructed; levels commonly fluctuate. Serum alkaline phosphatase elevation is especially suggestive of obstructive jaundice. Not uncommonly, serum amylase elevations are present because of secondary pancreatitis. Because prolonged obstruction of the common duct results in hepatocellular dysfunction, AST (SGOT) will be abnormal, often strikingly. Prolongation of the prothrombin time occurs when there is disturbance of the normal enterohepatic circulation of bile, with its exclusion from the intestinal tract. When extrahepatic obstruction persists for more than a few weeks, differentiation of obstruction from primarily inflammatory disease becomes progressively more difficult.

C. Imaging: Although ultrasonography, CT scan, and radionuclide imaging may help to differentiate hepatocellular and obstructive jaundice, percutaneous transhepatic cholangiography or endoscopic retrograde cholangiography (ERCP) provides the most direct and accurate nonsurgical means of determining the cause, location, and extent of obstruction. If the obstruction is thought to be due to a stone, ERCP is the procedure of choice because of its therapeutic potential.

Differential Diagnosis

The most common cause of obstructive jaundice is common duct stone. Next in frequency is carcinoma of the pancreas, ampulla of Vater, or common duct. Metastatic carcinoma (usually from the gastrointestinal tract) and direct extension of gallbladder cancer are other important causes of obstructive jaundice. Hepatocellular jaundice can usually be differentiated by the history, clinical findings, and liver tests, but liver biopsy is necessary on occasion.

Complications

A. Biliary Cirrhosis: Common duct obstruction lasting longer than 30 days results in severe liver damage. Hepatic failure with portal hypertension occurs in untreated cases.

B. Hypoprothrombinemia: Patients with obstructive jaundice or liver disease may bleed excessively as a result of prolonged prothrombin times. When prothrombin response to parenteral versus oral administration of these agents is compared, the nature of the underlying lesion (hepatocellular versus obstructive) can be determined; obstructive jaundice will respond to parenteral vitamin K or water-soluble oral vitamin K.

Treatment

Common duct stone is usually treated by cholecystectomy and choledochostomy. In the postcholecystectomy patient with choledocholithiasis, endoscopic papillotomy with stone extraction is preferable to transabdominal surgery.

A. Preoperative Preparation: Emergency operation is rarely necessary unless severe ascending cholangitis is present. A few days devoted to careful evaluation and preparation will be well spent.

Liver function should be evaluated thoroughly. Prothrombin time should be restored to normal by parenteral administration of vitamin K preparations (see above). Nutrition should be restored by a high-carbohydrate, high-protein diet and vitamin supplementation. Cholangitis, if present, should be controlled with antimicrobials, but may necessitate more urgent surgical decompression.

B. Indications for Common Duct Exploration: At every operation for cholelithiasis, the advisability of exploring the common duct must be considered. Operative cholangiography via the cystic duct is a very useful procedure for demonstrating common duct stone.

1. Preoperative findings suggestive of choledocholithiasis include a history (or the presence) of obstructive jaundice; frequent attacks of biliary colic; cholangitis; a history of pancreatitis; and a percutaneous transhepatic cholangiogram showing stone, obstruction, or dilatation of the duct.

2. Operative findings of choledocholithiasis are palpable stones in the common duct; dilatation or thickening of the wall of the common duct; gallbladder stones small enough to pass through the cystic duct; and pancreatitis.

3. For the patient with a T tube and a common duct stone, manipulation with various special instruments via the T tube or T tube sinus tract is often successful in extracting the stone.

4. For the poor-risk patient, urgent endoscopic sphincterotomy has become the treatment of choice.

C. Postoperative Care:

1. Antibiotics–Postoperative antibiotics are not administered routinely after biliary tract surgery. Cultures of the bile are always taken at operation. If biliary tract infection was present preoperatively or is apparent at operation, ampicillin with gentamicin or a cephalosporin is administered postoperatively until the results of sensitivity tests on culture specimens are available.

2. Management of the T-tube–Following choledochostomy, a simple catheter or T tube is placed in the common duct for decompression. It must be attached securely to the skin or dressing because accidental removal of the tube may be disastrous. A properly placed tube should drain bile at the operating table and continuously thereafter; otherwise, it should be considered blocked or dislocated. The volume of bile drainage varies from 100 to 1000 mL daily (average, 200–400 mL). Above-average drainage may be due to obstruction at the ampulla (usually by edema), increased bile output, low resistance or siphonage effect in the drainage system, or a combination of these factors.

3. Cholangiography–A cholangiogram should be taken through the T tube on about the seventh or eighth postoperative day. Under fluoroscopic control, a radiopaque medium is aseptically and gently injected until the duct system is outlined and the medium begins to enter the duodenum. The injection of air bubbles must be avoided, since on x-ray they resemble stones in the duct system. Spot films are always taken. If the cholangiogram shows no stones in the common duct and the opaque medium flows freely into the duodenum, the tube is clamped overnight and removed by simple traction on the following day. A small amount of bile frequently leaks from the tube site for a few days. A rubber tissue drain is usually placed alongside the T tube at operation. This drain is partially withdrawn on the fifth day and shortened daily until it is removed completely on about the seventh day.

Gogel HK et al: Acute suppurative obstructive cholangitis due to stones: Treatment by urgent endoscopic sphincterotomy. Gastrointest Endosc 1987;33:210.

Greig JD, Krukowski ZH, Matheson NA: Surgical morbidity and mortality in 129 patients with obstructive jaundice. Br J Surg 1988;75:216.

Mitchell SE, Clark RA: A comparison of computed tomography and sonography in choledocholithiasis. AJR 1984; 142:729.

Siegman-Igra Y et al: Septicemia from biliary tract infection. Arch Surg 1988;123:366.

BILIARY STRICTURE

Benign biliary strictures are the result of surgical trauma in about 95% of cases. The remainder are caused by blunt external injury to the abdomen, pancreatitis, or erosion of the duct by a gallstone.

Signs of injury to the duct may or may not be recognized in the immediate postoperative period. If complete occlusion has occurred, jaundice will develop rapidly; but more often a tear has been accidentally made in the duct, and the earliest manifestation of injury may be excessive or prolonged loss of bile from the surgical drains. Bile leakage contributes to the production of localized infection, which in turn accentuates scar formation and the ultimate development of a fibrous stricture.

Cholangitis is the most common syndrome produced by stricture. Typically, the patient notices episodes of pain, fever, chills, and jaundice within a few weeks to months after cholecystectomy. With the exception of jaundice during an attack of cholangitis and right upper quadrant abdominal tenderness, physical findings are usually not significant.

Serum alkaline phosphatase is usually elevated. Hyperbilirubinemia is variable, fluctuating during exacerbations and usually remaining in the range of 5–10 mg/dL. Blood cultures may be positive during an episode of cholangitis. Percutaneous transhepatic cholangiography or endoscopic retrograde cholangiopancreatography can be valuable in demonstrating the stricture.

Differentiation from choledocholithiasis may require surgical exploration. Operative treatment of a stricture frequently necessitates performance of choledochojejunostomy or hepaticojejunostomy to reestablish bile flow into the intestine.

Biliary stricture is not a benign condition, since significant hepatocellular disease will inevitably occur if it is allowed to continue uncorrected. The death rate for untreated stricture ranges from 10 to 15%.

Braasch JW, Rossi RL: Reconstruction of the biliary tract. Surg Clin North Am 1985;65:273.

Shemesh E, Brook O, Bat L: Endoscopic Gruntzig balloon dilation of benign strictures in the biliary system. Isr J Med Sci 1985;21:889.

PRIMARY SCLEROSING CHOLANGITIS

Primary sclerosing cholangitis is a rare nonspecific inflammatory reaction of unknown cause involving both the intra- and extrahepatic biliary ducts. It is characterized by a diffuse inflammation of the biliary tract leading to fibrosis and strictures of the biliary system. The disease is closely associated with ulcerative colitis, which is present in approximately two-thirds of patients with primary sclerosing cholangitis; however, only 1% of patients with ulcerative colitis develop clinically significant sclerosing cholangitis. Primary sclerosing cholangitis appears to be often associated with increased HLA-B8 histocompatibility antigen. Primary sclerosing cholangitis may occur at any period of life and may initially simulate a slowly growing bile duct carcinoma. However, the chronicity of the process militates against neoplasm. The criteria for making the diagnosis of primary sclerosing cholangitis are as follows: (1) progressive obstructive jaundice; (2) absence of calculi in the gallbladder or biliary ducts; (3) absence of prior surgical injury to the biliary tract; (4) absence of diseases causing cholangitis; (5) absence of congenital biliary anomalies; (6) thickening and narrowing of the biliary ductal system, demonstrated by palpation at surgery, biopsy, or x-ray techniques; (7) absence of biliary cirrhosis; and (8) exclusion of cholangiocarcinoma by long-term follow-up and multiple liver biopsies. Endoscopic retrograde cholangiography is the best means of establishing the diagnosis of primary sclerosing cholangitis.

Clinically, the disease presents as progressively obstructive jaundice, frequently preceded by malaise, pruritus, anorexia, and indigestion. Treatment with corticosteroids and broad-spectrum antimicrobial agents has been employed with inconsistent and unpredictable results. Ursodeoxycholic acid and methotrexate are experimental therapies. Liver transplantation has been successful and should be considered. The prognosis is regarded as poor, with few individuals living more than a few years after the appearance of symptoms.

LaRusso NF, Wiesner RH, Ludwig J: Is primary sclerosing cholangitis a bad disease? (Editorial.) Gastroenterology 1987;92:2031.
Wiesner RH et al: Primary sclerosing cholangitis: Natural history, prognostic factors and survival analysis. Hepatology 1989;10:430.

CARCINOMA OF THE BILIARY TRACT

Carcinoma of the gallbladder occurs in approximately 2% of all people operated on for biliary tract disease. It is notoriously insidious, and the diagnosis is usually made unexpectedly at surgery. Spread of the cancer—by direct extension into the liver or to the peritoneal surface—may be the initial manifestation.

Carcinoma of the extrahepatic bile ducts accounts for 3% of all cancer deaths in the USA. It affects both sexes equally but is more prevalent in individuals age 50–70. There is a questionable increased incidence in patients with chronic nonspecific ulcerative colitis.

Clinical Findings

Progressive jaundice is the most common and is usually the first sign of obstruction of the extrahepatic biliary system. Pain is usually present in the right upper abdomen and radiates into the back. Anorexia and weight loss are common and are frequently associated with fever and chills. Rarely, hematemesis may be a confusing presentation that results from erosion of tumor into a blood vessel. Fistula formation between the biliary system and adjacent organs may also occur. The course is usually one of rapid deterioration, with death occurring within a few months.

Physical examination will reveal profound jaundice. A palpable gallbladder with obstructive jaundice usually signifies malignant disease (Courvoisier's law). This clinical generalization has been proved to be accurate only about 50% of the time. Hepatomegaly is usually present and is associated with liver tenderness. Ascites may occur with peritoneal implants. Pruritus and skin excoriations are common.

Laboratory examinations reveal hyperbilirubinemia, predominantly of the conjugated variety. Total serum bilirubin values range from 5 to 30 mg/dL. There is usually concomitant elevation of the alkaline phosphatase and serum cholesterol. AST (SGOT) is normal or minimally elevated.

The most helpful diagnostic studies before surgery are either percutaneous transhepatic or endoscopic retrograde cholangiography. One or both of these procedures may be required in order to define the pathologic anatomy of the ductal obstruction.

Treatment

Unless there are overwhelming contraindications, palliative surgery is indicated to decompress the hepatobiliary system and relieve jaundice. This can be accomplished by cholecystoduodenostomy or by T tube drainage of the common duct. The prognosis is poor, few patients surviving for more than 6 months after surgery.

Koga A et al: Diagnosis and operative indications for polypoid lesions of the gallbladder. Arch Surg 1988;123:26.
Nesbit GM et al: Cholangiocarcinoma: Diagnosis and evaluation of resectability by CT and sonography as procedures complementary to cholangiography. Am J Roentgenol 1988;151:933.

DISEASES OF THE PANCREAS

ACUTE PANCREATITIS

Essentials of Diagnosis

- Abrupt onset of dull epigastric pain, often with radiation to the back.

- Nausea, vomiting, sweating, weakness.
- Abdominal tenderness and distention, fever.
- Leukocytosis, elevated serum and urinary amylase, elevated serum lipase.
- History of previous episodes, often related to alcohol intake.

General Considerations

Acute pancreatitis is often a severe intra-abdominal disease due to acute inflammation of the pancreas and associated "escape" of pancreatic enzymes from acinar cells into surrounding tissues. Most cases are related to biliary tract disease or heavy alcohol intake. Among the more than 80 other causes or associations are hypercalcemia, hyperlipidemias (types I, IV, and V), abdominal trauma (including surgery), drugs (including sulfonamides and thiazides), vasculitis, and viral infections. The exact pathogenesis is not known but may include edema or obstruction of the ampulla of Vater with resultant reflux of bile into pancreatic ducts, stenosis of the accessory pancreatic duct (duct of Santorini), and direct injury to the acinar cells.

Pathologic changes vary from acute edema and cellular infiltration to necrosis of the acinar cells, hemorrhage from necrotic blood vessels, and intra– and extrapancreatic fat necrosis. All or part of the pancreas may be involved.

Clinical Findings

A. Symptoms and Signs: Epigastric abdominal pain, generally abrupt in onset, is steady and severe and is often made worse by walking and lying supine and better by sitting and leaning forward. The pain usually radiates into the back but may radiate to the right or left. Nausea and vomiting are usually present. Severe weakness, sweating, and anxiety are noted in severe attacks. There may be a history of alcohol intake or a heavy meal immediately preceding the attack, or a history of milder but otherwise similar episodes in the past, even suggestive of biliary colic.

The abdomen is tender mainly in the upper abdomen, most often without guarding, rigidity, or rebound. The abdomen may be distended, and bowel sounds may be absent in associated paralytic ileus. Fever of 38.4–39 °C (101.1–102.2 °F), tachycardia, hypotension (even true shock), pallor, and a cool clammy skin are often present. Mild jaundice is common. An upper abdominal mass may be present but is not characteristic. Acute renal failure may occur early in the course of acute pancreatitis, usually prerenal in character.

B. Assessment of Severity: Ranson's criteria are generally used in assessing the severity of acute alcoholic pancreatitis on presentation (pancreatitis due to other causes has similar criteria). When 3 or more of the following criteria are present on admission, a severe course can be accurately predicted:

1. Age over 55 years.
2. White blood cell count over 16,000/μL.

3. Blood glucose over 200 mg/dL.
4. Base deficit over 4 meq/L.
5. Serum LDH over 350 IU/L.
6. AST over 250 IU/L.

Development of the following in the first 48 hours indicates a worsening prognosis:

1. Hematocrit drop of more than 10 percentage points.
2. BUN rise greater than 5 mg/dL.
3. Arterial Po_2 of less than 60 mm Hg.
4. Serum calcium of less than 8 mg/dL.
5. Estimated fluid sequestration of more than 6 L.

When 5 or 6 of the 11 criteria are present, the mortality rate is about 40%—and higher if more criteria are present.

C. Laboratory Findings: Findings of leukocytosis (10,000–30,000/μL), proteinuria, casts (25% of cases), glycosuria (10–20% of cases), hyperglycemia, and elevated serum bilirubin may be present. Blood urea nitrogen and serum alkaline phosphatase may be elevated and coagulation tests abnormal. Decrease in serum calcium may reflect a decreased serum albumin (because fluids have collected in the third space) and correlates well with severity of disease. Levels lower than 7 mg/dL are associated with tetany and an unfavorable prognosis.

Serum amylase and lipase are elevated within 24 hours in 90% of cases, and return to normal is variable depending on the severity of disease. Urine amylase may be very high and may remain elevated longer than serum amylase. In those who develop ascites or left pleural effusions, amylase content is high and is indicative of the cause of these fluid collections.

D. Imaging: A 2-way view of the abdomen may show gallstones, a "sentinel loop" (a segment of air-filled small intestine most commonly in the left upper quadrant), the "colon cutoff sign" (a gas-filled segment of transverse colon abruptly ending at the area of pancreatic inflammation), or linear focal atelectasis of the left lower lobe of the lungs with or without pleural effusion. These findings suggest acute pancreatitis but are not diagnostic. CT scan is useful in demonstrating an enlarged pancreas, in detecting pseudocysts, and in determining the extent of phlegmons. Ultrasonography is less reliable, because the echoes are deflected by the gas-distended small intestine frequently associated with acute pancreatitis.

D. Electrocardiographic Findings: ST–T wave changes may occur, but they usually differ from those of myocardial infarction. Abnormal Q waves do not occur as a result of pancreatitis.

Differential Diagnosis

Acute pancreatitis may be difficult to differentiate from an acutely perforated duodenal ulcer. One must keep in mind that pancreatitis may be the presenting clinical picture of choledocholithiasis with or without cholangitis, as well as of a penetrating duodenal ulcer.

It may occur owing to infection by mumps virus, post-ERCP, or postoperatively owing to surgical manipulation in the area of the pancreas. Serum amylase may also be elevated in high intestinal obstruction, in mumps not involving the pancreas (salivary amylase), in ectopic pregnancy, after administration of narcotics, and after abdominal surgery. Other conditions to be differentiated are acute cholecystitis, acute intestinal obstruction, leaking aortic aneurysm, renal colic, and acute mesenteric vascular insufficiency or thrombosis.

Complications

Intravascular volume depletion secondary to leakage of fluids in the pancreatic bed and ileus with fluid-filled loops of bowel may result in prerenal azotemia and even acute tubular necrosis without overt shock. This usually occurs within 24 hours of the onset of acute pancreatitis and lasts 8–9 days. Some patients require peritoneal dialysis or hemodialysis.

One of the most serious complications of acute pancreatitis is adult respiratory distress syndrome (ARDS); cardiac dysfunction may be superimposed. It usually occurs 3–7 days after the onset of pancreatitis in patients who have required large volumes of fluid and colloid to maintain blood pressure and urine output. Most require assisted respiration with positive end-expiratory pressure.

Pancreatic abscess is a suppurative process in necrotic tissue, with rising fever, leukocytosis, and localized tenderness and epigastric mass. This may be associated with a left-sided pleural effusion or an enlarging spleen secondary to splenic vein thrombosis.

Pseudocysts, encapsulated fluid collections with high enzyme content, commonly appear in pancreatitis when CT scans are used to monitor the evolution of an acute attack. Although the natural history of pseudocysts is still not well delineated, it appears that those less than 6 cm in diameter are likely to resolve spontaneously. Pseudocysts most commonly are within or adjacent to the pancreas but can present most anywhere (eg, mediastinal, retrorectal), having extended along anatomic planes. Multiple pseudocysts occur in 14% of patients with pseudocysts. Pseudocysts may become secondarily infected, necessitating drainage as for an abscess. Erosion of the inflammatory process into a blood vessel can result in a major hemorrhage into the cyst.

Chronic pancreatitis develops in about 10% of cases.

Permanent diabetes mellitus and exocrine pancreatic insufficiency occur uncommonly after a single acute episode. Prevention

Potential causative factors should be removed or corrected, eg, biliary tract disease, alcohol intake, hyperlipidemia, hypercalcemia, duodenal ulcer, or certain offending drugs. The patient should be warned not to eat large meals or foods that are high in fat content and not to drink alcohol. The most common precipitating factor in acute pancreatitis is alcohol intake.

Treatment

A. Management of Acute Disease: The pancreatic rest program includes withholding food and liquids by mouth, bed rest, and in those with moderately severe pain or ileus, nasogastric suction. Pain is controlled with meperidine (Demerol), 100–150 mg intramuscularly every 3–4 hours as necessary. Other narcotics may be used if pain control is not achieved, but they may cause smooth muscle contractions (spasm of the ampulla of Vater).

In more severe pancreatitis, there may be considerable leakage of fluids, necessitating more than the normal amount of intravenous fluids to maintain intravascular volume. Saline is chiefly used, but fresh-frozen plasma or serum albumin may be necessary. With colloid solutions, there may be an increased risk of developing adult respiratory distress syndrome. If shock persists after adequate volume replacement (including packed red cells), pressors may be required. For the severe pancreatitis patient requiring a large volume of parenteral fluids, central venous pressure and blood gases should be monitored at regular intervals.

Calcium gluconate must be given intravenously if there is evidence of hypocalcemia with tetany. Antibiotics should be reserved for specific infections. For fever exceeding 39 °C (102.2 °F), institution of antibiotics has been recommended after cultures have been obtained of blood, urine, sputum, and pleural effusion (if present) and needle aspirations of the pancreatic phlegmon (with CT guidance).

The patient with severe pancreatitis requires attention in an intensive care unit. Close follow-up of blood count, hematocrit, serum electrolytes, and creatinine is required.

B. Follow-Up Care: Medical management is preferred; the patient is observed closely for evidence of continued inflammation of the pancreas or related structures. A surgeon should be consulted in all cases of suspected acute pancreatitis. If the diagnosis is in doubt and investigations indicate a strong possibility of a serious surgically correctable lesion (eg, perforated peptic ulcer, common duct stone), exploration is indicated.

Aggressive surgery and enteral or parenteral hyperalimentation may increase survival in patients with hemorrhagic or suppurative pancreatitis. Initially, enterostomy tubes and drainage are established. Subsequent surgery is performed to debride necrotic pancreas and surrounding tissue.

When acute pancreatitis is unexpectedly found on exploratory laparotomy, it is usually wise to close without intervention of any kind. If the pancreatitis appears mild and cholelithiasis is present, cholecystostomy or cholecystectomy may be justified. Patients with unsuspected pancreatitis who receive the least intra-abdominal manipulation have the lowest morbidity and mortality rates after laparotomy, except as noted above. Peritoneal lavage improves early survival in severe acute pancreatitis. Late septic complications are unaffected.

The development of a pancreatic abscess is an indication for prompt drainage, usually through the flank. In persistent pseudocyst, the role of surgery is unclear. Pseudocysts may require drainage, when infected or associated with persisting pain, pancreatitis, or common duct obstruction. Diagnosis of infection in a pseudocyst may be difficult; empirical broad-spectrum antibiotics are initiated, and the decision to explore surgically or drain percutaneously is mainly a clinical one.

No fluid or foods should be given orally until the patient is largely free of pain and has bowel sounds. Clear liquids are then given, and a gradual progression to a regular low-fat diet is pursued, guided by the patient's tolerance and by the absence of pain. Pancreatitis complicated by prolonged ileus (24 hours or more), abdominal distention, or vomiting requires nasogastric suction until they subside, along with parenteral nutrition. Intravenous fluids are given as needed to replace lost fluids, electrolytes, and blood.

Prognosis

Recurrences are common. The mortality rate for acute hemorrhagic pancreatitis is high, especially when hepatic, cardiovascular, or renal impairment is present. Surgery is indicated only when the diagnosis is in doubt, when the patient is desperately ill despite conservative therapy, or in the presence of an associated disorder such as stones in the biliary tract.

Gerzof SG et al: Early diagnosis of pancreatic infection by combined tomography-guided aspiration. Gastroenterology 1987;93:1315.

Grendell JH, Egan J: Acute pancreatitis. (Medical Staff Conference.) West J Med 1987;146:598.

Lee MJ et al: Endoscopic retrograde cholangiopancreatography after acute pancreatitis. Surg Gynecol Obstet 1986;163:354.

Moody FG: Pancreatitis. Gastroenterol Clin North Am 1988;17:433.

Reber HA: Surgical intervention in necrotizing pancreatitis. (Editorial.) Gastroenterology 1986;91:479.

Steinberg WM: Acute drug– and toxin-induced pancreatitis. Hosp Pract (May 15) 1985;20:95.

Wade JW: Twenty five year experience with pancreatic pseudocysts: Are we making progress? Am J Surg 1985;149:705.

Warshaw AL, Rutledge PL: Cystic tumors mistaken for pancreatic pseudocysts. Ann Surg 1987;205:393.

CHRONIC PANCREATITIS
(Chronic Relapsing Pancreatitis)

Chronic pancreatitis occurs most often in patients with alcoholism, hereditary pancreatitis, hypercalcemia, and hyperlipoproteinemias (types I, IV, and V). Progressive fibrosis and destruction of functioning glandular tissue occur as a result. Pancreaticolithiasis and obstruction of the duodenal end of the pancreatic duct are often present. Pancreatitis recurring after cholecystectomy for cholelithiasis should raise the suspicion of a retained or newly developed common duct stone.

Differentiation of chronic from recurrent pancreatitis is important in that recurrent pancreatitis is initiated by a specific event (eg, alcoholic binge, passage of a stone), whereas chronic pancreatitis is a self-perpetuating disease characterized by pain and pancreatic exocrine or endocrine insufficiency.

Clinical Findings

A. Symptoms and Signs: Persistent or recurrent episodes of epigastric and left upper quadrant pain with referral to the upper left lumbar region are typical. Anorexia, nausea, vomiting, constipation, flatulence, and weight loss are common. Abdominal signs during attacks consist chiefly of tenderness over the pancreas, mild muscle guarding, and paralytic ileus: Attacks may last only a few hours or as long as 2 weeks; pain may eventually be almost continuous. Steatorrhea (as indicated by bulky, foul, fatty stools) may occur.

B. Laboratory Findings: Serum amylase, lipase, and bilirubin may be elevated during acute attacks; normal amylase does not exclude the diagnosis, however. Glycosuria may be present. Excess fecal fat may be demonstrated on chemical analysis of the stool.

C. Imaging: Plain films often show pancreaticolithiasis and mild ileus. Right upper quadrant ultrasound may reveal cholelithiasis, and upper gastrointestinal series may demonstrate a widened duodenal loop. Endoscopic retrograde cholangiopancreatography is a technique that is widely used. It may show dilated ducts, intraductal stones, strictures, or tumor. Failure to cannulate the duct occurs in less than 20% of cases.

Complications

Narcotic addiction is common. Other frequent complications include diabetes mellitus, pancreatic pseudocyst or abscess, cholestatic liver disease with or without jaundice, steatorrhea, malnutrition, and peptic ulcer.

Treatment

Correctable coexistent biliary tract disease should be treated surgically.

A. Medical Measures: A low-fat diet should be

prescribed. Alcohol is forbidden because it frequently precipitates attacks. Mild sedatives or anticholinergics may be helpful. Narcotics should be avoided if possible. Steatorrhea is treated with pancreatic supplements that are selected on the basis of their lipase activity. Cotazym, Festal, Ilozyme, Ku-Zyme HP, Pancrease, and Viokase have high lipase activity. The usual dose is 2 capsules before, during, and after meals. Concurrent administration of H_2 receptor antagonists decreases the inactivation of lipase by acid and may thereby decrease steatorrhea further. Pain secondary to chronic pancreatitis may be benefited by the use of pancreatic enzymes. Treat associated diabetes as for any other insulinopenic patient. Every effort is made to manage the disease medically.

B. Surgical Treatment: The only indication for surgery in chronic pancreatitis, other than internal drainage of persistent pseudocysts or to treat other complications, is to attempt to relieve pain. The objectives of surgical intervention are to eradicate biliary tract disease, ensure a free flow of bile into the duodenum, and eliminate obstruction of the pancreatic duct. When obstruction of the duodenal end of the duct can be demonstrated by endoscopic retrograde cholangiopancreatography, dilatation of the duct or resection of the tail of the pancreas with implantation of the distal end of the duct by pancreaticojejunostomy may be successful. Anastomosis between the longitudinally split duct and a defunctionalized limb of jejunum without pancreatectomy may be in order. In advanced cases it may be necessary, as a last resort, to do subtotal or total pancreatectomy.

Prognosis

This is a serious disease and often leads to chronic invalidism. The prognosis is best when patients with acute pancreatitis are carefully investigated with their first attack and are found to have some remediable condition such as chronic cholecystitis and cholelithiasis, choledocholithiasis, stenosis of the sphincter of Oddi, or hyperparathyroidism. Medical management of the hyperlipidemias frequently associated with the condition may also prevent recurrent attacks. Surgical relief of these aggravating conditions may prevent recurrent pancreatic disease.

Bank S: Chronic pancreatitis: Clinical features and medical management. Am J Gastroenterol 1986;81:153.

Bradley EL Jr: Long-term results of pancreatojejunostomy in patients with chronic pancreatitis. Am J Surg 1987;153:207.

Lankisch PG et al: Pancreatic calcifications: No indicator of severe exocrine pancreatic insufficiency. Gastroenterology 1986;90:617.

Levy P et al: Mortality factors associated with chronic pancreatitis: Unidimensional and multidimensional analysis of a medical-surgical series of 240 patients. Gastroenterology 1989;96:1165. (Alcohol abstinence appears to have a favorable influence.)

Nealon WT et al: Operative drainage of the pancreatic duct delays functional impairment in patients with chronic pancreatitis: A prospective analysis. Ann Surg 1988;208:321. (A consideration.)

Rocca G et al: Increased incidence of cancer in chronic pancreatitis. J Clin Gastroenterol 1987;9:175.

CARCINOMA OF THE HEAD OF THE PANCREAS & THE PERIAMPULLARY AREA

Essentials of Diagnosis
- Obstructive jaundice (may be painless).
- Enlarged gallbladder may be painful.
- Upper abdominal pain with radiation to back, weight loss, and thrombophlebitis are usually late manifestations.

General Considerations
Carcinoma is the commonest neoplasm of the pancreas. About 75% are in the head and 25% in the body and tail of the organ. Carcinomas involving the head of the pancreas, the ampulla of Vater, the common bile duct, and the duodenum are considered together, because they are usually indistinguishable clinically; of these, carcinomas of the pancreatic head constitute over 90%. They comprise 3% of cancers and 5% of cancer deaths.

Clinical Findings
A. Symptoms and Signs: Pain is present in over 70% of cases and is often vague, diffuse, and located in the epigastrium. Radiation of pain into the back is common and sometimes predominates. Sitting up and leaning forward may afford some relief, and this usually indicates that the lesion has spread beyond the pancreas and is inoperable. The pain is rarely confused with biliary colic. Diarrhea, as a relatively early symptom, is seen occasionally. Migratory thrombophlebitis is a rare sign. Jaundice and weight loss are common but late findings. An uncommon occurrence but a useful clinical rule (Courvoisier's law) is that jaundice associated with a palpable gallbladder is indicative of obstruction by neoplasm. In addition, a hard, fixed, occasionally tender mass may be present.

B. Laboratory Findings: There may be mild anemia. Glycosuria, hyperglycemia, and impaired glucose tolerance or true diabetes mellitus are found in 10–20% of cases. The serum amylase or lipase level is occasionally elevated. Liver function tests are those of obstructive jaundice. Steatorrhea in the absence of jaundice is uncommon. The secretin test of exocrine secretion usually has a low volume with normal bicarbonate concentration. In about 60% of cases, duodenal cytologic studies have shown malignant cells. Occult blood in the stool is suggestive of carcinoma of the ampulla of Vater. The most helpful serologic marker to date for pancreatic carcinoma is

CA19–9, with a sensitivity of 70% and a specificity of 87%.

C. Imaging: Radiographic examination is usually noncontributory in involvement of the body and tail of the pancreas, except when the splenic vein is involved. With obstruction of the splenic vein, splenomegaly or gastric varices are present, the latter delineated by an upper gastrointestinal series, endoscopy, or angiography. With carcinoma of the head of the pancreas, the gastrointestinal series may show a widening of the duodenal loop, mucosal abnormalities in the duodenum ranging from edema to invasion or ulceration, or spasm or compression. Hypotonic duodenography and selective celiac and superior mesenteric arteriography may be most helpful by demonstrating either the encroachment of the duodenum or abnormal vessels in the region of the pancreas. Endoscopic retrograde cholangiopancreatography may delineate the pancreatic duct system and suggest carcinoma. Data are not available on how often this procedure leads to a therapeutic decision. CT scan is most helpful in delineating the extent of the pancreatic mass and allows for percutaneous aspiration of the mass for cytologic studies.

Treatment

Abdominal exploration is usually necessary when cytologic diagnosis cannot be made or if resection is to be attempted, which includes about 30% of patients. Radical pancreaticoduodenal resection is indicated for lesions strictly limited to the head of the pancreas, periampullary zone, and duodenum. When resection is not feasible, cholecystojejunostomy is performed to relieve the jaundice. A gastrojejunostomy is also done if duodenal obstruction is expected to develop later. High-voltage irradiation and combination drug chemotherapy should be considered, as should endoscopic stenting as well.

Prognosis

Carcinoma of the head of the pancreas has a very poor prognosis. Reported 5-year survival rates range from 2.3 to 5.2%. Lesions of the ampulla, common duct, and duodenum have a better prognosis, with reported 5-year survival rates of 20–40% after resection. The reported operative mortality rate of radical pancreaticoduodenectomy is 10–15%.

Freeny PC et al: Pancreatic ductal adenocarcinoma: Diagnosis and staging with dynamic CT. Radiology 1988; 166:125.

Kamisawa T et al: Carcinoma of the ampulla of Vater: Expression of cancer-associated antigens inversely correlated with prognosis. Am J Gastroenterol 1988; 83:1118. (Tissue CEA immunoreactivity may correlate with mean survival.)

Leese T et al: Tumours and pseudotumours of the region of the ampulla of Vater: An endoscopic, clinical and pathological study. Gut 1986;27:1186.

Pleskow DK et al: Evaluations of a serologic marker, CA19–9, in the diagnosis of pancreatic cancer. Ann Intern Med 1989;110:704.

CARCINOMA OF THE BODY & TAIL OF THE PANCREAS

About 25% of pancreatic cancers arise in the body or tail. Islet cell tumors arise in the pancreas, as do the non-B cell gastrin-secreting tumors associated with Zollinger-Ellison syndrome. There are no characteristic findings in the early stages. The initial symptoms are vague epigastric or left upper quadrant distress. Anorexia and weight loss usually occur. Later, pain becomes more severe and frequently radiates through to the left lumbar region. A mass in the mid or left epigastrium may be palpable. The spontaneous development of thrombophlebitis is suggestive. If suspected, the diagnosis can often be supported by CT scanning and confirmed by percutaneous aspiration of the mass for cytologic analysis. Sometimes, surgical exploration is necessary for diagnosis. Resection is rarely feasible, and cure is rarer still. The response to fluorouracil (5-FU) has been disappointing. Studies are under way to evaluate multiple-drug therapy. Serum determination of the monoclonal antigen CA19–9 raises a suspicion of the presence of pancreatic carcinoma in the setting of chronic pancreatitis.

Connolly MM et al: Survival in 1001 patients with carcinoma of the pancreas. Ann Surg 1987;206:366. Trede M: The surgical treatment of pancreatic carcinoma. Surgery 1985;97:28. Van Dyke JA, Stanley RJ, Berland LL: Pancreatic imaging. Ann Intern Med 1985;102:212.

REFERENCES

Berk JE et al (editors): *Bockus Gastroenterology*, 4th ed. 7 vols. Saunders, 1985.

DeDombal FT (editor): *Inflammatory Bowel Disease: Some International Data and Reflections*. Oxford Univ Press, 1986.

Dooley CP et al: Double-contrast barium meal and upper gastrointestinal endoscopy. Ann Intern Med 1984; 101:538.

Kirsner JB, Shorter RG: *Inflammatory Bowel Disease*, 3rd ed. Lea & Febiger, 1988.

Schiff L: *Diseases of the Liver*, 6th ed. Lippincott, 1987.

Sherlock S: *Diseases of the Liver and Biliary System*, 8th ed. Lippincott/Blackwell, 1989.

Silen W: *Cope's Early Diagnosis of the Acute Abdomen*, 17th ed. Oxford Univ Press, 1987.

Sleisenger MH, Fordtran JS (editors): *Gastrointestinal Dis-ease: Pathophysiology, Diagnosis, Management*, 4th ed. Saunders, 1989.

Toledo-Pereyra LH (editor): *The Pancreas: Principles of Medical and Surgical Practice*. Wiley, 1985.

Welch CE, Malt RA: Surgery of the stomach, duodenum, gallbladder, and bile ducts. N Engl J Med 1987;316:999.

Armando E. Giuliano, MD

CARCINOMA OF THE FEMALE BREAST

Essentials of Diagnosis

- Higher incidence in women who have delayed child bearing, those with a family history of breast cancer, and those with a personal history of breast cancer or some types of mammary dysplasia.
- Early findings: Single, nontender, firm to hard mass with ill-defined margins; mammographic abnormalities and no palpable mass.
- Later findings: Skin or nipple retraction; axillary lymphadenopathy; breast enlargement, redness, edema, pain, fixation of mass to skin or chest wall.
- Late findings: Ulceration; supraclavicular lymphadenopathy; edema of arm; bone, lung, liver, brain, or other distant metastases.

General Considerations

The breast is the most common site of cancer in women, and cancer of the breast has been the leading cause of death from cancer among women in the USA. However, in 1987, lung cancer accounted for more deaths in women than breast cancer. The probability of developing breast cancer increases throughout life. The mean and the median age of women with breast cancer is 60–61 years.

There will be about 142,000 new cases of breast cancer and about 43,000 deaths from this disease in women in the USA in 1989. At the present rate of incidence, one of every 11 American women will develop breast cancer during her lifetime. Women whose mothers or sisters had breast cancer are more likely to develop the disease than others. Risk is increased in patients whose mothers' or sisters' breast cancers occurred before menopause or was bilateral, or was present in 2 or more first-degree relatives. However, there is no history of breast cancer among female relatives in over 90% of patients with breast cancer. Nulliparous women and women whose first full-term pregnancy was after age 35 have a slightly higher incidence of breast cancer than multiparous women. Late menarche and artificial menopause are associated with a lower incidence of breast cancer, whereas early menarche (under age 12) and late natural menopause (after age 50) are associated with a slight increase in risk of developing breast cancer

as well. Mammary dysplasia (fibrocystic disease of the breast), when accompanied by proliferative changes, papillomatosis, or atypical epithelial hyperplasia, is associated with an increased incidence of cancer. A woman who has had cancer in one breast is at increased risk of developing cancer in the other breast. Women with cancer of the uterine corpus have a breast cancer risk significantly higher than that of the general population, and women with breast cancer have a comparably increased endometrial cancer risk. In the USA, breast cancer is more common in whites than in nonwhites. The incidence of the disease among nonwhites (mostly blacks), however, is increasing, especially in younger women. In general, rates reported from developing countries are low, whereas rates are high in developed countries, with the notable exception of Japan. Some of the variability may be due to underreporting in the developing countries, but a real difference probably exists. Dietary factors, particularly increased fat content, may account for some differences in incidence. There is some evidence that administration of estrogens to postmenopausal women may result in a slightly increased risk of breast cancer, but only with higher, long-term doses of estrogens. Alcohol consumption may increase the risk of breast cancer slightly.

Women who are at greater than normal risk of developing breast cancer (Table 12–1) should be identified by their physicians, taught the techniques of breast self-examination, and followed carefully. Screening programs involving periodic physical ex-

Table 12–1. Factors associated with increased risk of breast cancer.[1]

Race	White
Age	Older
Family history	Breast cancer in mother or sister (especially bilateral or premenopausal)
Previous medical history	Endometrial cancer Some forms of mammary dysplasia Cancer in other breast
Menstrual history	Early menarche (under age 12) Late menopause (after age 50)
Pregnancy	Late first pregnancy

[1] Normal lifetime risk in white women = 1 in 11.

amination and mammography of asymptomatic high-risk women increase the detection rate of breast cancer and may improve the survival rate. Unfortunately, most women who develop breast cancer do not have significant identifiable risk factors, and analysis of epidemiologic data has failed to identify women who are not at significant risk and would not benefit from screening. Therefore, virtually all women over about age 35 could possibly benefit from screening, although the cost-benefit ratio of screening programs to society as a whole is unclear. New, less expensive screening techniques, such as single-view mammography and the use of mobile vans, are being investigated in an attempt to reduce the cost of widespread screenings.

Growth potential of tumor and resistance of host vary over a wide range from patient to patient and may be altered during the course of the disease. The doubling time of breast cancer cells ranges from several weeks in a rapidly growing lesion to nearly a year in a slowly growing one. Assuming that the rate of doubling is constant and that the neoplasm originates in one cell, a carcinoma with a doubling time of 100 days may not reach clinically detectable size (1 cm) for about 8 years. On the other hand, rapidly growing cancers have a much shorter preclinical course and a greater tendency to metastasize to regional nodes or more distant sites by the time a breast mass is discovered.

The relatively long preclinical growth phase and the tendency of breast cancers to metastasize have led many clinicians to believe that breast cancer is a systemic disease at the time of diagnosis. Although it may be true that breast cancer cells are released from the tumor prior to diagnosis, variations in the host-tumor relationship may prohibit the growth of disseminated disease in many patients. For this reason, a pessimistic attitude concerning the management of localized breast cancer is not warranted, and many patients can be cured with proper treatment.

Staging

The extent of disease evident from physical findings and special preoperative studies is used to determine the clinical stage of the lesion. Histologic staging is performed after examination of the axillary specimen. The results of clinical staging are used in designing the treatment plan (Table 12–2). Both clinical and histologic staging are of prognostic significance.

Clinical Findings

The patient with breast cancer usually presents with a lump in the breast. Clinical evaluation should include assessment of the local lesion and a search for evidence of metastases in regional nodes or distant sites. After the diagnosis of breast cancer has been confirmed by biopsy, additional studies are often needed to complete the search for distant metastases or an occult primary in the other breast. Then, before any decision is made about treatment, all the available

Table 12–2. Clinical and histologic staging of breast carcinoma and relation to survival.

Clinical Staging (American Joint Committee)	5-Year Survival (%)
Stage I	85
Tumor <2 cm in diameter	
Nodes, if present, not felt to contain metastases	
Without distant metastases	
Stage II	66
Tumor <5 cm in diameter	
Nodes, if palpable, not fixed	
Without distant metastases	
Stage III	41
Tumor >5 cm or—	
Tumor any size with invasion of skin or attached to chest wall	
Nodes in supraclavicular area	
Without distant metastases	
Stage IV	10
With distant metastases	

	Survival (%)	
Histologic Staging	5 Years	10 Years
All patients	63	46
Negative axillary lymph nodes	78	65
Positive axillary lymph nodes	46	25
1–3 positive axillary lymph nodes	62	38
>4 positive axillary lymph nodes	32	13

clinical data are used to determine the extent or "stage" of the patient's disease.

A. Symptoms: When the history is taken, special note should be made of breast cancer risk factors, relation of mass to menstrual cycle, and previous breast problems. Back or other bone pain may be the result of osseous metastases. Systemic complaints or weight loss should raise the question of metastases, which may involve any organ but most frequently the bones, liver, and lungs. The more advanced the cancer in terms of size of primary, local invasion, and extent of regional node involvement, the higher the incidence of metastatic spread to distant sites.

The presenting complaint in about 70% of patients with breast cancer is a lump (usually painless) in the breast (Table 12–3). About 90% of breast masses are discovered by the patient herself. Less frequent symptoms are breast pain; nipple discharge; erosion, retraction, enlargement, or itching of the nipple; and redness, generalized hardness, enlargement, or shrinking of the breast. Rarely, an axillary mass, swelling of the arm, or bone pain (from metastases) may be the first symptom. Thirty-five to 50 percent of women with cancer involved in organized screening programs have cancers detected by mammography only and not physical examination.

B. Signs: The relative frequency of carcinoma in various anatomic sites in the breast is shown in Fig 12–1.

Inspection of the breast is the first step in physical examination and should be carried out with the patient

Table 12–3. Initial symptoms of mammary carcinoma.[1]

Symptom	Percentage of All Cases
Painless breast mass	66
Painful breast mass	11
Nipple discharge	9
Local edema	4
Nipple retraction	3
Nipple crusting	2
Miscellaneous symptoms	5

[1] Adapted from report of initial symptoms in 774 patients treated for breast cancer at Ellis Fischel State Cancer Hospital, Columbia, Missouri. Reproduced, with permission, from Spratt JS Jr, Donegan WL: *Cancer of the Breast.* Saunders, 1967.

sitting, arms at sides and then overhead. Abnormal variations in breast size and contour, minimal nipple retraction, and slight edema, redness, or retraction of the skin can be identified. Asymmetry of the breasts and retraction or dimpling of the skin can often be accentuated by having the patient raise her arms overhead or press her hands on her hips in order to contract the pectoralis muscles. Axillary and supraclavicular areas should be thoroughly palpated for enlarged nodes with the patient sitting (Fig 12–2). Palpation of the breast for masses or other changes should be performed with the patient both seated and supine with the arm abducted (Fig 12–3).

Breast cancer usually consists of a nontender, firm or hard lump with poorly delineated margins (caused by local infiltration). Slight skin or nipple retraction is an important sign. Minimal asymmetry of the breast

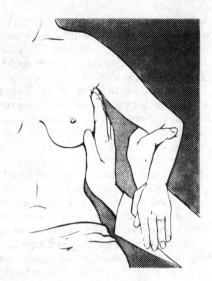

Figure 12–2. Palpation of axillary region for enlarged lymph nodes.

may be noted. Very small (1–2 mm) erosions of the nipple epithelium may be the only manifestation of Paget's carcinoma. Watery, serous, or bloody discharge from the nipple is an occasional early sign but is more often associated with benign disease.

A lesion smaller than 1 cm in diameter may be difficult or impossible for the examiner to feel and yet may be discovered by the patient. She should always be asked to demonstrate the location of the mass; if the physician fails to confirm the patient's suspicions, the examination should be repeated in 1 month, preferably 1–2 weeks after the onset of menses. During the premenstrual phase of the cycle, increased innocuous nodularity may suggest neoplasm or may obscure an underlying lesion. If there is any

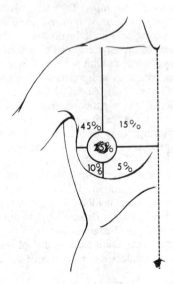

Figure 12–1. Frequency of breast carcinoma at various anatomic sites.

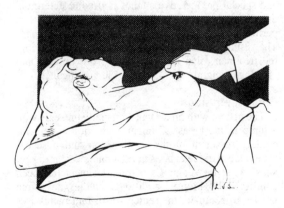

Figure 12–3. Palpation of breasts. Palpation is performed with the patient supine and arm abducted.

question regarding the nature of an abnormality under these circumstances, the patient should be asked to return after her period.

The following are characteristic of advanced carcinoma: edema, redness, nodularity, or ulceration of the skin; the presence of a large primary tumor; fixation to the chest wall; enlargement, shrinkage, or retraction of the breast; marked axillary lymphadenopathy; supraclavicular lymphadenopathy; edema of the ipsilateral arm; and distant metastases.

Metastases tend to involve regional lymph nodes, which may be clinically palpable. With regard to the axilla, one or 2 movable, nontender, not particularly firm lymph nodes 5 mm or less in diameter are frequently present and are generally of no significance. Firm or hard nodes larger than 5 mm in diameter usually contain metastases. Axillary nodes that are matted or fixed to skin or deep structures indicate advanced disease (at least stage III). Histologic studies show that microscopic metastases are present in about 30% of patients with clinically negative nodes. On the other hand, if the examiner thinks that the axillary nodes are involved, this will prove on histologic section to be correct in about 85% of cases. The incidence of positive axillary nodes increases with the size of the primary tumor and with the local invasiveness of the neoplasm.

Usually no nodes are palpable in the supraclavicular fossa. Firm or hard nodes of any size in this location or just beneath the clavicle (infraclavicular nodes) are suggestive of metastatic cancer and should be biopsied. Ipsilateral supraclavicular or infraclavicular nodes containing cancer indicate that the patient is in an advanced stage of the disease (stage IV). Edema of the ipsilateral arm, commonly caused by metastatic infiltration of regional lymphatics, is also a sign of advanced (stage IV) cancer.

C. Special Clinical Forms of Breast Carcinoma:

1. Paget's carcinoma–The basic lesion is usually an infiltrating ductal carcinoma, usually well differentiated. The nipple epithelium is infiltrated, but gross nipple changes are often minimal, and a tumor mass may not be palpable. The first symptom is often itching or burning of the nipple, with a superficial erosion or ulceration. The diagnosis is established by biopsy of the erosion.

Paget's carcinoma is not common (about 1% of all breast cancers), but it is important because it appears innocuous. It is frequently diagnosed and treated as dermatitis or bacterial infection, leading to unfortunate delay in detection. When the lesion consists of nipple changes only, the incidence of axillary metastases is about 5%, and the prognosis is excellent. When a breast tumor is also present, the incidence of axillary metastases rises, with an associated marked decrease in prospects for cure by surgical or other treatment.

2. Inflammatory carcinoma–This is the most malignant form of breast cancer and constitutes less than 3% of all cases. The clinical findings consist of a rapidly growing, sometimes painful mass that enlarges the breast. The overlying skin becomes erythematous, edematous, and warm. Often there is no distinct mass, since the tumor infiltrates the involved breast diffusely. The diagnosis should be made when the redness involves more than one-third of the skin over the breast and biopsy shows invasion of the subdermal lymphatics. The inflammatory changes, often mistaken for an infectious process, are caused by carcinomatous invasion of the dermal lymphatics, with resulting edema and hyperemia. If the physician suspects infection but the lesion does not respond rapidly (1–2 weeks) to antibiotics, a biopsy must be performed. Metastases tend to occur early and widely, and for this reason inflammatory carcinoma is rarely curable. Mastectomy is seldom, if ever, indicated. Radiation, hormone therapy, and anticancer chemotherapy are the measures most likely to be of value.

3. Occurrence during pregnancy or lactation–Only 1–2% of breast cancers occur during pregnancy or lactation. Breast cancer complicates approximately one in 3000 pregnancies. The diagnosis is frequently delayed, because physiologic changes in the breast may obscure the true nature of the lesion. This results in a tendency of both patients and physicians to misinterpret the findings and to procrastinate in deciding on biopsy. When the neoplasm is confined to the breast, the 5-year survival rate after mastectomy is about 70%. Axillary metastases are already present in 60–70% of patients, and for them the 5-year survival rate after mastectomy is only 30–40%. Pregnancy (or lactation) is not a contraindication to operation, and treatment should be based on the stage of the disease as in the nonpregnant (or nonlactating) woman. Overall survival rates have improved as cancers are now diagnosed in pregnant women earlier than in the past.

4. Bilateral breast cancer–Clinically evident simultaneous bilateral breast cancer occurs in less than 1% of cases, but there is a 5–8% incidence of later occurrence of cancer in the second breast. Bilaterality occurs more often in women under age 50 and is more frequent when the tumor in the primary breast is lobular. The incidence of second breast cancers increases directly with the length of time the patient is alive after her first cancer—about 0.5% per year.

In patients with breast cancer, mammography should be performed before primary treatment and at regular intervals thereafter, to search for occult cancer in the opposite breast. Routine biopsy of the opposite breast is usually not warranted.

D. Laboratory Findings:
A consistently elevated sedimentation rate may be the result of disseminated cancer. Liver or bone metastases may be associated with elevation of serum alkaline phosphatase. Hyper-

calcemia is an occasional important finding in advanced cancer of the breast. Carcinoembryonic antigen (CEA) may be used as a marker for recurrent breast cancer.

E. Imaging for Metastases: Chest radiographs may show pulmonary metastases. CT scan of liver and brain is of value only when metastases are suspected in these areas. Bone scans utilizing technetium Tc 99m-labeled phosphates or phosphonates are more sensitive than skeletal x-rays in detecting metastatic breast cancer. Bone scanning has not proved to be of clinical value as a routine preoperative test in the absence of symptoms, physical findings, or abnormal alkaline phosphatase levels. The frequency of abnormal findings on bone scan parallels the status of the axillary lymph nodes on pathologic examination.

F. Mammography: The 2 methods of mammography in common use are ordinary film radiography and xeroradiography. From the standpoint of diagnosing breast cancer, they give comparable results. It is now possible to perform a high-quality mammogram while delivering less than 1 rad to the mid breast.

Mammography is the only reliable means of detecting breast cancer before a mass can be palpated in the breast. Some breast cancers can be identified by mammography as long as 2 years before reaching a size detectable by palpation.

Although false-positive and false-negative results are occasionally obtained with mammography, the experienced radiologist can interpret mammograms correctly in about 90% of cases. Where mammography is employed proficiently, approximately 30–35% of lesions biopsied will be malignant.

Indications for mammography are as follows: (1) to evaluate each breast when a diagnosis of potentially curable breast cancer has been made, and at yearly intervals thereafter; (2) to evaluate a questionable or ill-defined breast mass or other suspicious change in the breast; (3) to search for an occult breast cancer in a woman with metastatic disease in axillary nodes or elsewhere from an unknown primary; (4) to screen women prior to cosmetic operations or prior to biopsy of a mass, to examine for an unsuspected cancer; (5) to screen at regular intervals a selected group of women who are at high risk for developing breast cancer (see below); and (6) for the purpose of following those who have been treated with breast-conserving surgery and radiation.

Patients with a dominant or suspicious mass must undergo biopsy despite mammographic findings. The mammogram should be obtained prior to biopsy so that other suspicious areas and can be noted and the contralateral breast can be checked. Mammography is never a substitute for biopsy, because it may not reveal clinical cancer in a very dense breast, as may be seen in young women with mammary dysplasia, and may not reveal medullary type cancer. Breast

ultrasonography can be used to differentiate a cystic from a solid mass.

G. Biopsy: The diagnosis of breast cancer depends ultimately upon examination of tissue removed by biopsy. Treatment should never be undertaken without an unequivocal histologic diagnosis of cancer. The safest course is biopsy examination of all suspicious masses found on physical examination and, in the absence of a mass, of suspicious lesions demonstrated by mammography. About 30% of lesions thought to be definitely cancer prove on biopsy to be benign, and about 15% of lesions believed to be benign are found to be malignant. These findings demonstrate the fallibility of clinical judgment and the necessity for biopsy.

The simplest method is needle biopsy, either by aspiration of tumor cells (fine-needle aspiration cytology) or by obtaining a small core of tissue with a Vim-Silverman or other special needle. A negative needle biopsy should be followed by open biopsy, because false-negative needle biopsies may occur in 15–20% of cancers.

The preferred method is open biopsy under local anesthesia as a separate procedure prior to deciding upon definitive treatment. The patient need not be admitted to the hospital. Decisions on additional workup for metastatic disease and on definitive therapy can be made and discussed with the patient after the histologic diagnosis of cancer has been established. This approach has the advantage of avoiding unnecessary hospitalization and diagnostic procedures in many patients, since cancer is found in the minority of patients who require biopsy for diagnosis of a breast lump. In addition, in situ cancers are not easily diagnosed cytologically.

As an alternative in patients in highly suspicious circumstances, the patient may be admitted directly to the hospital, where the diagnosis is made on frozen section of tissue obtained by open biopsy under general anesthesia. If the frozen section is positive, the surgeon could proceed immediately with operation. This one-step method should rarely be used today except perhaps when cytologic study has already suggested the presence of cancer.

In general, the 2-step approach—that is, outpatient biopsy followed by definitive operation at a later date—is preferred in the diagnosis and treatment of breast cancer, because patients can be given time to adjust to the diagnosis of cancer, can carefully consider alternative forms of therapy, and can seek a second opinion should they feel it important. Studies have shown no adverse effect from the short (1–2 weeks) delay of the 2-step procedure, and this is the current recommendation of the National Cancer Institute.

At the time of the initial biopsy of breast cancer, it is important for the physician to preserve a portion of the specimen for determination of estrogen and progesterone receptors.

H. Cytology: Cytologic examination of nipple discharge or cyst fluid may be helpful on rare occasions. As a rule, mammography (or ductography) and breast biopsy are required when nipple discharge or cyst fluid is bloody or cytologically questionable.

Early Detection

A. Screening Programs: A number of mass screening programs consisting of physical and mammographic examination of the breasts of asymptomatic women have been conducted. They are identifying more than 6 cancers per 1000 women. About 80% of these women have negative axillary lymph nodes at the time of surgery, whereas, by contrast, only 45% of patients found in the course of usual medical practice have uninvolved axillary nodes. Detecting breast cancer before it has spread to the axillary nodes greatly increases the chance of survival, and about 85% of such women will survive at least 5 years.

Both physical examination and mammography are necessary for maximum yield in screening programs, since about 40% of early breast cancers can be discovered only by mammography and another 40% can be detected only by palpation. Women 20–40 years of age should have a breast examination as part of routine medical care every 2–3 years. Women over age 40 should have yearly breast examinations.

The American College of Radiology and the American Cancer Society have published guidelines regarding use of mammography in asymptomatic women. A baseline mammogram should be performed on all women between ages 35 and 40 years. Women aged 40–49 years should have a mammogram every 1–2 years. Annual mammograms are indicated for women age 50 years or older. High-risk women—those whose mothers or sisters had bilateral or premenopausal breast cancer, those who have had cancer of one breast, and those with histologic abnormalities associated with subsequent cancer (eg, atypical epithelial hyperplasia, papillomatosis, lobular carcinoma in situ)—should have an annual mammogram and biannual examinations. The usefulness of screening mammography in young women without identifiable risk factors is not yet of proved value. However, in a recent large study of women under age 50, nearly half of all cancers were detected by mammography alone. Critics of screening question whether early detection actually improves survival sufficiently to justify its cost. Mammographic parenchymal patterns are not a reliable predictor of the risk of developing breast cancer.

Ductography is useful to evaluate the cause of nipple discharge. In this study, the radiologist injects contrast medium into the discharging duct and obtains a mammogram. The injected duct may contain a filling defect (most commonly an intraductal papilloma) or may have a dilated or cystic appearance.

Other modalities of breast imagery have been investigated. Automated breast ultrasonography is very useful in distinguishing cystic from solid lesions but should be used only as a supplement to physical examination and mammography in screening for breast cancer. Diaphanography (transillumination of the breasts) and thermography are of no proved screening value.

B. Self-Examination: All women over age 20 should be advised to examine their breasts monthly. Premenopausal women should perform the examination 7–8 days after the menstrual period. The breasts should be inspected initially while standing before a mirror with the hands at the sides, overhead, and pressed firmly on the hips to contract the pectoralis muscles. Masses, asymmetry of breasts, and slight dimpling of the skin may become apparent as a result of these maneuvers. Next, in a supine position, each breast should be carefully palpated with the fingers of the opposite hand. Physicians should instruct women in the technique of self-examination and advise them to report at once for medical evaluation if a mass or other abnormality is noted. Some women discover small breast lumps more readily when their skin is moist while bathing or showering. Most women do not practice self-examination, and its value is controversial. Clearly, however, it is not harmful and may be beneficial.

Differential Diagnosis

The lesions to be considered most often in the differential diagnosis of breast cancer are the following, in descending order of frequency: mammary dysplasia (cystic disease of the breast), fibroadenoma, intraductal papilloma, lipoma, and fat necrosis. The differential diagnosis of a breast lump should be established without delay by biopsy, by aspiration of a cyst, or by observing the patient until disappearance of the lump within a period of a few weeks.

Pathologic Types

Numerous pathologic subtypes of breast cancer can be identified histologically (Table 12–4). These pathologic types are distinguished by the histologic appearance and growth pattern of the tumor. In general, breast cancer arises either from the epithelial lining of the large or intermediate-sized ducts (ductal) or from the epithelium of the terminal ducts of the lobules (lobular). The cancer may be invasive or in situ. Most breast cancers arise from the intermediate ducts and are invasive (invasive ductal, infiltrating ductal), and most histologic types are merely subtypes of invasive ductal cancer with unusual growth patterns (colloid, medullary, scirrhous, etc). Ductal carcinoma that has not invaded the extraductal tissue is intraductal or in situ ductal. Lobular carcinoma may be either invasive or in situ.

Except for the in situ cancers, the histologic subtypes have only a slight bearing on prognosis when outcomes are compared after accurate staging. Vari-

Table 12–4. Histologic types of breast cancer.

	Percent Occurrence
Infiltrating ductal (not otherwise specified)	70–80
Medullary	5–8
Colloid (mucinous)	2–4
Tubular	1–2
Papillary	1–2
Invasive lobular	6–8
Noninvasive	4–6
Intraductal	2–3
Lobular in situ	2–3
Rare cancers	<1
Juvenile (secretory)	. . .
Adenoid cystic	. . .
Epidermoid	. . .
Sudoriferous	. . .

ous histologic parameters, such as invasion of blood vessels, tumor differentiation, invasion of breast lymphatics, and tumor necrosis have been examined, but they too seem to have little prognostic value.

The noninvasive cancers by definition lack the ability to spread. However, in patients whose biopsies show noninvasive intraductal cancer, associated invasive ductal cancers are present in about 1–3% of cases. Some clinicians consider lobular carcinoma in situ (LCIS) to be a premalignant lesion that is not a true cancer. It lacks the ability to spread but is associated with subsequent development of invasive cancer in at least 20% of cases. In LCIS, the subsequent cancer may occur in either breast regardless of the side of the original biopsy.

Hormone Receptor Sites

The presence or absence of estrogen and progesterone receptors in the cytoplasm of tumor cells is of paramount importance in managing patients with recurrent or metastatic disease. Up to 60% of patients with metastatic breast cancer will respond to hormonal manipulation if their tumors contain estrogen receptors. However, fewer than 5% of patients with metastatic, estrogen receptor-negative tumors can be successfully treated with hormonal manipulation.

Progesterone receptors may be an even more sensitive indicator than estrogen receptors of patients who may respond to hormonal manipulation. Up to 80% of patients with metastatic progesterone receptor-positive tumors seem to respond to hormonal manipulation. Receptors probably have no relationship to response to chemotherapy.

Some studies suggest that estrogen receptors are of prognostic significance. Patients whose primary

tumors are receptor-positive have a more favorable course than those whose tumors are receptor-negative.

Receptor status is not only valuable for the management of metastatic disease but may help in the selection of patients for adjuvant therapy. Some studies suggest that adjuvant hormonal therapy (tamoxifen) for patients with receptor-positive tumors and adjuvant chemotherapy for patients with receptor-negative tumors may improve survival rates even in the absence of lymph node metastases (see Adjuvant Therapy, p 494).

It is advisable to obtain an estrogen-receptor assay for every breast cancer at the time of initial diagnosis. Receptor status may change after hormonal therapy, radiotherapy, or chemotherapy. The specimen requires special handling, and the laboratory should be prepared to process the specimen correctly.

Curative Treatment

Treatment may be curative or palliative. Curative treatment is advised for clinical stage I and II disease (Table 12–2). Treatment can only be palliative for patients in stage IV and for previously treated patients who develop distant metastases or unresectable local recurrence.

A. Therapeutic Options: Radical mastectomy involves en bloc removal of the breast, pectoral muscles, and axillary nodes and was the standard curative procedure for breast cancer from the turn of the century until about 20 years ago. Radical mastectomy removes the primary lesion and the axillary nodes with a wide margin of surrounding tissue, including the pectoral muscles. **Extended radical mastectomy** involves, in addition to standard radical mastectomy, removal of the internal mammary nodes. It has been recommended by a few surgeons for medially or centrally placed breast lesions and for tumors associated with positive axillary nodes, because of the known frequency of internal mammary node metastases under these circumstances. **Modified radical mastectomy** (total mastectomy plus axillary dissection) consists of en bloc removal of the breast with the underlying pectoralis major fascia (but not the muscle) and axillary lymph nodes. Some surgeons remove the pectoralis minor muscle. Others retract or transect the muscle to facilitate removal of the axillary lymph nodes. Modified radical mastectomy gives superior cosmetic and functional results compared with standard radical mastectomy. **Simple mastectomy** (total mastectomy) consists of removing the entire breast, leaving the axillary nodes intact. Limited procedures such as **segmental mastectomy** (lumpectomy, quadrant excision, partial mastectomy) are becoming more popular as definitive treatment. The proved efficacy of **irradiation** in sterilizing the primary lesion and the axillary and internal mammary nodes has made radiation therapy with segmental mastectomy a reasonable option for primary treatment of most breast cancers.

B. Choice of Primary Therapy: The extent of

disease and its biologic aggressiveness are the principal determinants of the outcome of primary therapy. Clinical and pathologic staging help in assessing extent of disease (Table 12–2), but each is to some extent imprecise. Since about two-thirds of patients eventually manifest distant disease regardless of the form of primary therapy, there is a tendency to think of breast carcinoma as being systemic in most patients at the time they first present for treatment.

There is a great deal of controversy regarding the optimal method of primary therapy of stage I, II, and III breast carcinoma, and opinions on this subject have changed considerably in the past decade. Legislation initiated in California and Massachusetts and now adopted in numerous states requires physicians to inform patients of alternative treatment methods in the management of breast cancer.

Radical Mastectomy

For about three-quarters of a century, radical mastectomy was considered standard therapy for this disease. The procedure was designed to remove the primary lesion, the breast in which it arose, the underlying muscle, and, by dissection in continuity, the axillary lymph nodes that were thought to be the first site of spread beyond the breast. When radical mastectomy was introduced by Halsted, the average patient presented for treatment with advanced local disease (stage III), and a relatively extensive procedure was often necessary just to remove all gross cancer. This is no longer the case. Patients present now with much smaller, less locally advanced lesions. Most of the patients in Halsted's original series would now be considered incurable by surgery alone, since they had extensive involvement of the chest wall, skin, and supraclavicular regions.

Although radical mastectomy is extremely effective in controlling local disease, it has the disadvantage of being one of the most deforming of any of the available treatments for management of primary breast cancer. The surgeon and patient are both eager to find therapy that is less deforming but does not jeopardize the chance for cure. This operation as well as extended radical mastectomy is rarely performed now.

Less Radical Surgery & Radiation Therapy

A number of clinical trials have been performed during the past decade in which the magnitude of the surgical procedure has been varied, with and without the use of local and regional radiotherapy.

Radical mastectomy, modified radical mastectomy, and simple mastectomy have been compared in numerous clinical trials. It has not been demonstrated that more extensive surgery and more rigorous local control increase survival. Simple mastectomy has the highest regional recurrence rate, since the lymph nodes are not removed, and as many as 30% of patients

with clinically negative nodes will have metastatic breast cancer within the nodes. At least half of these patients subsequently develop regional recurrences. The addition of radiotherapy to mastectomy will also reduce the incidence of local recurrence, but radiotherapy does not improve overall survival rates. Even the removal of occult cancer in axillary lymph nodes is not reflected in improved overall survival rates, though regional failures will be much lower.

The most significant recent advance in the management of primary breast cancer has been the realization that less than total mastectomy combined with radiotherapy may be as effective as more radical operations alone for certain patients.

Radiation therapy alone (without surgery) in the treatment of primary breast cancer fails to achieve local control in about 50% of cases. However, the combination of limited surgery and radiation appears to be as effective as mastectomy in achieving local control without diminishing long-term survival.

The results of the Milan trial and a large randomized trial conducted by the National Surgical Adjuvant Breast Project (NSABP) in the USA showed that disease-free survival rates were similar for patients treated by partial mastectomy plus axillary dissection followed by radiation therapy and for those treated by modified radical mastectomy (total mastectomy plus axillary dissection). All patients whose axillary nodes contained tumor received adjuvant chemotherapy.

In the NSABP trial, patients were randomized to 3 treatment types: (1) "lumpectomy" (removal of the tumor with *confirmed* tumor-free margins) plus whole breast irradiation, (2) lumpectomy alone, and (3) total mastectomy. All patients underwent axillary lymph node dissection. Some patients in this study had tumors as large as 4 cm with (or without) palpable axillary lymph nodes. Few local treatment failures were observed in any group. The lowest local recurrence rate was among patients treated with lumpectomy and postoperative irradiation; the highest was among patients treated with lumpectomy alone. However, no statistically significant differences were observed in overall or disease-free survival among the 3 treatment groups. This study shows that lumpectomy and axillary dissection with postoperative radiation therapy is as effective as modified radical mastectomy for the management of patients with stage I and stage II breast cancer. A high local failure rate (nearly 40% at 8 years) was seen for lumpectomy without radiation therapy.

The results of these and other trials have demonstrated that much less aggressive surgical treatment of the primary lesion than has previously been thought necessary gives equivalent therapeutic results and may preserve an acceptable cosmetic appearance.

It is important to recognize that axillary dissection is valuable both in planning therapy and in staging of the cancer. Operation is extremely effective in preventing axillary recurrences. In addition, lymph nodes removed during the procedure can be pathologically assessed. This assessment is essential for the planning of adjuvant therapy, which is often recommended.

Current Recommendations

We believe that partial mastectomy (lumpectomy) plus axillary dissection and radiation therapy or total mastectomy plus axillary dissection (modified radical mastectomy) are the best initial treatments for most patients with potentially curable carcinoma of the breast. Radical mastectomy may rarely if ever be required. Similarly, extended radical mastectomy would rarely be appropriate. Treatment of the axillary nodes is not indicated for noninfiltrating cancers, because nodal metastases are rarely present.

Preoperatively, full discussion with the patient regarding the rationale for operation and alternative forms of treatment is essential. Women with small tumors (< 4 cm) with or without axillary lymph node involvement should have the option of treatment by partial mastectomy (lumpectomy) plus axillary dissection and radiotherapy. Breast reconstruction should be discussed with the patient. Time spent preoperatively in educating the patient and her family is time well spent.

Adjuvant Therapy

Chemotherapy or hormonal therapy is advocated for most patients with curable breast cancer. The objective of adjuvant therapy is to eliminate the occult metastases responsible for late recurrences while they are microscopic and theoretically most vulnerable to anticancer agents.

Numerous clinical trials with various adjuvant chemotherapeutic regimens have been completed. The most extensive clinical experience to date is with the CMF regimen (cyclophosphamide, methotrexate, and fluorouracil). The regimen should be continued for 6 months in patients with axillary metastases. Premenopausal women with positive axillary nodes definitely benefit from adjuvant chemotherapy. The recurrence rate in premenopausal patients who received no adjuvant chemotherapy was more than 11/2 times that of those who received therapy. No therapeutic effect with CMF has been shown in postmenopausal women with positive nodes, perhaps because therapy was modified so often in response to side effects that the total amount of drugs administered was less than planned. Other trials with different agents support the value of adjuvant chemotherapy; in some cases, postmenopausal women appear to benefit as well. Recently, a study from the same group (Milan) showed a beneficial effect for both premenopausal and postmenopausal women with negative nodes treated with CMF. Combinations of drugs are clearly superior to single drugs.

Adjuvant chemotherapy can be offered confidently to premenopausal women with metastases in axillary lymph nodes, but the use of adjuvant chemotherapy in postmenopausal women and patients with negative axillary lymph nodes is more controversial.

The addition of hormones may improve the results of adjuvant therapy. For example, tamoxifen has been shown to enhance the beneficial effects of melphalan and fluorouracil in postmenopausal women whose tumors are estrogen receptor-positive. Tamoxifen alone is the recommended treatment for postmenopausal women with estrogen receptor-positive tumors.

The length of time adjuvant therapy must be administered remains uncertain. Several studies suggest that shorter treatment periods may be as effective as longer ones. The Milan group has compared 6 versus 12 cycles of postoperative CMF and found 5-year disease-free survival rates to be comparable. One of the earliest adjuvant trials (Nissen-Meyer) used a 6-day perioperative regimen of intravenous cyclophosphamide alone; follow-up at 15 years shows a 15% improvement in disease-free survival rates for treated patients, suggesting that short-term therapy may be effective.

Patients with negative nodes have not been treated with adjuvant therapy until recently. The Milan group, however, has shown a significant beneficial effect using CMF as adjuvant therapy in women whose tumors are estrogen receptor-negative and whose lymph nodes show no metastases.

In May 1988, a *Clinical Alert* from the National Cancer Institute was mailed to practicing physicians advising them of the unpublished results of several studies of adjuvant therapy in node-negative women. These studies have now been published and show a beneficial effect of adjuvant chemotherapy or tamoxifen in delaying recurrence, but as of yet no effect has been seen on survival.

The recent recommendations for adjuvant chemotherapy can be summarized as follows (Table 12–5 and 12–6): (1) Premenopausal women with positive lymph nodes and either estrogen receptor-positive or estrogen receptor-negative tumors should be treated with adjuvant combination chemotherapy. (2) Premenopausal women with negative nodes whose tumors

Table 12–5. Adjuvant chemotherapy for premenopausal women. (Summary of NIH Consensus Conference and *Clinical Alert* [1988]).

Nodal Involvement	Estrogen Receptors	Adjuvant Systemic Therapy
Yes	Positive	Combination chemotherapy
Yes	Negative	Combination chemotherapy
No	Positive	Tamoxifen[1]
No	Negative	Combination chemotherapy[1]

[1] Effect on overall survival not yet clearly demonstrated.

Table 12–6. Adjuvant chemotherapy for postmenopausal women. (Summary of NIH Consensus Conference and *Clinical Alert* [1988]).

Nodal Involvement	Estrogen Receptors	Adjuvant Systemic Therapy
Yes	Positive	Tamoxifen
Yes	Negative	Combination chemotherapy[1]
No	Positive	Tamoxifen[1]
No	Negative	Combination chemotherapy[1]

[1] Effect on overall survival not yet clearly demonstrated.

are estrogen receptor-positive benefit from tamoxifen; premenopausal women with negative axillary nodes whose tumors are estrogen receptor-negative benefit from combination chemotherapy. (3) Postmenopausal patients with positive lymph nodes and positive hormone receptor tumors should receive tamoxifen. (4) Postmenopausal patients with positive lymph nodes whose tumors are estrogen receptor-negative benefit from adjuvant combination chemotherapy. (5) Postmenopausal women with negative axillary nodes whose tumors are estrogen receptor-positive may benefit from adjuvant tamoxifen; postmenopausal women with negative axillary lymph nodes whose tumors are estrogen receptor-negative may benefit from adjuvant chemotherapy.

The NIH concludes in the *Clinical Alert:* "Adjuvant hormonal or adjuvant cytotoxic chemotherapy can have a meaningful impact on the natural history of node-negative breast cancer patients." However, the short follow-up in the node-negative studies and the lack of a yet observed effect on survival has still not completely clarified the role of adjuvant therapy for these patients.

Important questions remaining to be answered are the timing and duration of adjuvant chemotherapy; which chemotherapeutic agents should be applied for which subgroups of patients; how best to coordinate adjuvant chemotherapy with postoperative radiation therapy; the use of hormonal therapy; and the use of combinations of hormonal therapy and chemotherapy. Adjuvant systemic therapy is not currently indicated in the favorable small, nonpalpable tumors that cannot be quantitatively tested for hormonal receptors.

Follow-Up Care

After primary therapy, patients with breast cancer should be followed for life for at least 2 reasons: to detect recurrences and to observe the opposite breast for a second primary carcinoma. Local and distant metastases occur most frequently within the first 3 years. During this period, the patient is examined every 3–4 months. Thereafter, examination is done every 6 months until 5 years postoperatively and then every 6–12 months. Special attention is given to the remaining breast, because of the increased risk of developing a second primary. The patient should examine her own breast monthly, and a mammogram should be obtained annually. In some cases, metastases are dormant for long periods and may appear up to 10–15 years or longer after removal of the primary tumor. Use of estrogen or progestational agents is probably inadvisable in patients free of disease after treatment of primary breast cancer, particularly those patients whose tumor was hormone receptor-positive. If topical estrogens are needed for senile vaginitis or urinary incontinence, periodic use of a topical testosterone preparation will usually suffice.

A. Local Recurrence: The incidence of local recurrence correlates with tumor size, the presence and number of involved axillary nodes, the histologic type of tumor, and the presence of skin edema or skin and fascia fixation with the primary. About 8% of patients develop local recurrence after total mastectomy and axillary dissection. When the axillary nodes are not involved, the local recurrence rate is 5%, but the rate is as high as 25% when they are involved. A similar difference in local recurrence rate was noted between small and large tumors. Factors that affect the rate of local recurrence in patients who had partial mastectomies are not yet determined. However, early studies show that such things as multifocal cancer, in situ tumors, positive resection margins, chemotherapy, and radiotherapy are important.

Chest wall recurrences usually appear within the first 2 years but may occur as late as 15 or more years after mastectomy. Suspect nodules should be biopsied. Local excision or localized radiotherapy may be feasible if an isolated nodule is present. If lesions are multiple or accompanied by evidence of regional involvement in the internal mammary or supraclavicular nodes, the disease is best managed by radiation treatment of the whole chest wall including the parasternal, supraclavicular, and axillary areas.

Local recurrence after mastectomy usually signals the presence of widespread disease and is an indication for bone and liver scans, posteroanterior and lateral chest x-rays, and other examinations as needed to search for evidence of metastases. Most patients with locally recurrent tumor will develop distant metastases within 2 years. After partial mastectomy, local recurrence does not have as serious a prognostic significance. Completion of the mastectomy should be done for local recurrence after partial mastectomy. When there is no evidence of metastases beyond the chest wall and regional nodes, irradiation for cure or complete local excision should be attempted. Patients with local recurrence may be cured with local resection or radiation. Systemic chemotherapy or hormonal treatment should be used for postmenopausal women who develop disseminated disease or those in whom local recurrence occurs following total mastectomy.

B. Edema of the Arm: Significant edema of the arm occurs in 10–30% of patients after radical mastectomy and in about 5% after modified radical mastectomy. Edema of the arm is less frequent after modified radical mastectomy than after radical mastectomy and occurs more commonly if radiotherapy has been given or if there was postoperative infection. Early trials suggest that partial mastectomy with radiation to the axillary lymph nodes is followed by chronic edema of the arm in 10–20% of patients. To avoid this complication, many authorities advocate axillary lymph node sampling rather than complete axillary dissection. Judicious use of radiotherapy, with treatment fields carefully planned to spare the axilla as much as possible, can greatly diminish the incidence of edema. Since axillary dissection is a more accurate staging operation than axillary sampling, we recommend axillary dissection, with removal of at least level I and II lymph nodes, in combination with partial mastectomy.

Late or secondary edema of the arm may develop years after treatment, as a result of axillary recurrence or of infection in the hand or arm, with obliteration of lymphatic channels. There is usually no obvious cause of late arm swelling.

C. Breast Reconstruction: Breast reconstruction, with the implantation of a prosthesis, is usually feasible after standard or modified radical mastectomy. Reconstruction should probably be discussed with patients prior to mastectomy, because it offers an important psychologic focal point for recovery. However, most patients who are initially interested in reconstruction decide later that they no longer wish to undergo the procedure. Reconstruction is not an obstacle to the diagnosis of recurrent cancer.

D. Risks of Pregnancy: Data are insufficient to definitely determine whether interruption of pregnancy improves the prognosis of patients who are discovered during pregnancy to have potentially curable breast cancer and who receive definitive treatment. Theoretically, the increasingly high levels of estrogen produced by the placenta as the pregnancy progresses could be detrimental to the patient with occult metastases of hormone-sensitive breast cancer. Moreover, occult metastases are present in most patients with positive axillary nodes, and treatment by adjuvant chemotherapy would be potentially harmful to the fetus. Under these circumstances, interruption of early pregnancy seems reasonable, with progressively less rationale for the procedure as term approaches. Obviously, the decision must be highly individualized and will be affected by many factors, including the patient's desire to have the baby and the generally poor prognosis when axillary nodes are involved.

Equally problematic and important is the advice regarding future pregnancy (or abortion in case of pregnancy) to be given to women of child-bearing age who have had a mastectomy or other definitive treatment for breast cancer. Under these circumstances, one must assume that pregnancy will be harmful if occult metastases are present, although this has not been shown. Patients whose tumors are ER-negative probably would not be affected by pregnancy. A number of studies have shown no adverse effect of pregnancy on survival of women who had breast cancer and subsequently become pregnant.

In patients with inoperable or metastatic cancer (stage IV disease), induced abortion is usually advisable, because of the possible adverse effects of hormonal treatment, radiotherapy, or chemotherapy upon the fetus.

Prognosis

The stage of breast cancer is the single most reliable indicator of prognosis. Patients with disease localized to the breast and no evidence of regional spread after microscopic examination of the lymph nodes have by far the most favorable prognosis. Estrogen and progesterone receptors appear to be an important prognostic variable, because patients with hormone receptor-negative tumors and no evidence of metastases to the axillary lymph nodes have a much higher recurrence rate than do patients with hormone receptor-positive tumors and no regional metastases. The histologic subtype of breast cancer (eg, medullary, lobular, comedo) seems to have little, if any, significance in prognosis once these tumors are truly invasive. Flow cytometry of cell suspensions from tumors to analyze DNA index and S-phase frequency aid in prognosis. Tumors with marked aneuploidy have a poor prognosis.

As mentioned above, several different treatment regimens achieve approximately the same results when given to the appropriate patient. Localized disease can be controlled with local therapy—either surgery alone or limited surgery in combination with radiation therapy.

Most patients who develop breast cancer will ultimately die of breast cancer. The mortality rate of breast cancer patients exceeds that of age-matched normal controls for nearly 20 years. Thereafter, the mortality rates are equal, although deaths that occur among breast cancer patients are often directly the result of tumor. Five-year statistics do not accurately reflect the final outcome of therapy.

When cancer is localized to the breast, with no evidence of regional spread after pathologic examination, the clinical cure rate with most accepted methods of therapy is 75–90%. Exceptions to this may be related to the hormonal receptor content of the tumor, tumor size, host resistance, or associated illness. Patients with small estrogen and progesterone receptor-positive tumors and no evidence of axillary spread probably have a 5-year survival rate of nearly 90%. When the axillary lymph nodes are involved with tumor, the survival rate drops to 40–50% at 5 years and probably less than 25% at 10 years. In general, breast cancer appears to be somewhat more malignant in younger than older women, and this may be related to the fact that fewer younger women have estrogen receptor-positive tumors.

General

Baines CJ: Breast self-examination. Cancer 1989; 64:2661. Bassett LW, Giuliano AE, Gold RH; Staging for breast carcinoma. Am J Surg 1989;157:250.

Bonadonna G: Conceptual and practical advances in the management of breast cancer. J Clin Oncol 1989; 7:1380.

Council on Scientific Affairs, AMA: Early detection of breast cancer. JAMA 1984;252:3008.

Fentiman IS, Rubens RD, Hayward JL: Control of pleural effusions in patients with breast cancers: A randomized trial. Cancer 1983;52:737.

Fisher B: The revolution in breast cancer surgery: Science or anecdotalism? World J Surg 1985;9:655.

Fisher B et al: Eight-year results of a randomized clinical trial comparing total mastectomy and lumpectomy with or without irradiation in the treatment of breast cancer. N Engl J Med 1989;320:822.

Fisher ER et al: Pathologic findings from the National Surgical Adjuvant Breast and Bowel Projects (NSABP): Prognostic discriminants for 8-year survival for node-negative invasive breast cancer patients. Cancer 1990;65:2121.

Hagelberg RS, Jolly PC, Anderson RP: Role of surgery in the treatment of inflammatory breast carcinoma. Am J Surg 1984;148:125.

Harris JR et al: Time course and prognosis of local recurrence following primary radiation therapy for early breast cancer. J Clin Oncol 1984;2:37.

Health and Public Policy Committee, American College of Physicians: The use of diagnostic tests for screening and evaluating breast lesions. Ann Intern Med 1985;103:143.

Hedley DW, Rugg CA, Gelber RD: Association of DNA with prognosis of nodes-positive early breast cancer. Cancer Res 1987;47:4729.

Henson DE, Ries LA: Progress in early breast cancer detection. Cancer 1990;65:2155.

Kurtz JM et al: Results of wide excision for mammary recurrence after breast-conserving therapy. Cancer 1988;61:1969.

Lagios MD et al: Paget's disease of the nipple: Alternative management in cases without or with minimal extent of underlying breast carcinoma. Cancer 1984;54:545.

Lipsztein R, Dalton JF, Bloomer WD: Sequelae of breast irradiation. JAMA 1985;253:3582.

Mansour EG et al: Tissue and plasma carcinoembryonic antigen in early breast cancer: A prognostic factor. Cancer 1983;51:1243.

Morrison AS: Review of evidence on the early detection and treatment of breast cancer. Cancer 1989;64:2651.

Mushlin AI: Diagnostic decision: Diagnostic tests in breast cancer: Clinical strategies based on diagnostic probabilities. Ann Intern Med 1985;103:79.

O'Malley MS, Fletcher SW: Screening for breast cancer with breast self-examination. JAMA 1987;257:2197.

Pigott J et al: Metastases to the upper levels of the axillary nodes in carcinoma of the breast and its implications for nodal sampling procedures. Surg Gynecol Obstet 1984;158:255.

Schnitt SJ et al: Ductal carcinoma in situ (intraductal carcinoma) of the breast. N Engl J Med 1988;318:898.

Seidman H, Stellman SD, Mushinski MH: A different perspective on breast cancer risk factors: Some implications of the nonattributable risks. CA 1982;32:301.

Skrabanek P: False premises and false promises of breast cancer screening. Lancet 1985;2:316.

Sunshine JA et al: Breast carcinoma in situ: A retrospective review of 112 cases with a minimum 10-year follow-up. Am J Surg 1985;150:44.

Veronesi U, Zucali R, Del Vecchio M: Conservative treatment of breast cancer with the QU.A.RT. technique. World J Surg 1985;9:676.

Veronesi U, Zucali R, Luini A: Local control and survival in early breast cancer: The Milan trial. Int J Radiat Oncol Biol Phys 1986;9:676.

Veronesi U, Zucali R, Luini A: Local control and survival in early breast cancer: The Milan trial. Int J Radiat Oncol Biol Phys 1985;12:717.

Willet WC: Moderate alcohol consumption and the risk of breast cancer. N Engl J Med 1987;316:1174.

Winchester DP et al: Surgical management of stages O, I, and IIA breast cancer. Cancer 1990;65: 2105.

Mammography

Boyd NF et al: Mammographic signs as risk factors for breast cancer. Br J Cancer 1982;45:185.

Carlile T et al: Breast cancer prediction and the Wolfe classification of mammograms. JAMA 1985;254: 1050.

Egan RL: Mammography: Current recommendations and their rationale. Consultant 1984;28:166.

Hall FM; Screening mammography: Potential problems on the horizon. N Engl J Med 1986;314:53.

Lamas AM, Horwitz RI, Peck D: Usefulness of mammography in the diagnosis and management of breast disease in postmenopausal women. JAMA 1984; 252:2999.

Mammography 1982: A statement of the American Cancer Society. CA 1982:32:226.

Mann BD et al: Delayed diagnosis of breast cancer as a result of negative mammogram. Arch Surg 1983; 118:23.

Sickles EA et al: Mammography after needle aspiration of palpable breast masses. Am J Surg 1983:145:395.

Hormone Receptors

Aamdal S et al: Estrogen receptors and long-term prognosis in breast cancer. Cancer 1984;53:2525.

Chevallier B et al: Prognostic value of estrogen and progesterone receptors in operable breast cancer: Results of a univariate and multivariate analysis. Cancer 1988;62:2517.

Manni A: Hormone receptors and breast cancer. N Engl J Med 1983;309:1383.

McCarty KS Jr et al: Relationship of age and menopausal status to estrogen receptor content in primary carcinoma of the breast. Ann Surg 1983;197:123.

Qazi R, Chuang JL, Drobyski W: Estrogen receptors and the patterns of relapse in breast cancer. Arch Intern Med 1984;144:2365.

Adjuvant Chemotherapy

Bonadonna G, Valagussa P: Adjuvant systemic therapy for resectable breast cancer. J Clin Oncol 1985;3:259.

Bonadonna G, Valagussa P: Review: Adjuvant systemic therapy for breast cancer. J Clin Oncol 1985;3:259.

Breast Cancer Trials Committee, Scottish Cancer Trials Office: Adjuvant tamoxifen in the management of operable breast cancer: The Scottish trial. Lancet 1987;2:171.

Cummings FJ et al: Adjuvant tamoxifen treatment of elderly women with stage II breast cancer: A double blind comparison with placebo. Ann Intern Med 1985;103:324.

DeVita VT Jr: Breast cancer therapy: Exercising all our options. (Editorial.) N Engl J Med 1989;320:527.

Early Breast Cancer Trialists' Collaborative Group: Effects of adjuvant tamoxifen and of cytotoxic therapy on mortality in early breast cancer: An overview of 61 randomized trials among 28,896 women. N Engl J Med 1988;319:1681.

Fisher B et al: A randomized clinical trial evaluating sequential methotrexate and fluorouracil in the treatment of patients with node-negative breast cancer who have estrogen receptor-negative tumors. N Engl J Med 1989;320:473.

Fisher B et al: A randomized clinical trial evaluating tamoxifen in the treatment of patients with node-negative breast cancer who have estrogen receptor-positive tumors. N Engl J Med 1989;320:479.

Henderson IC: Adjuvant chemotherapy of breast cancer: A promising experiment or standard practice. (Editorial.) J Clin Oncol 1985;3:140.

Henderson IC: Adjuvant systemic therapy for early breast cancer. Curr Probl Cancer 1987;11:127.

McGuire WL: Adjuvant therapy of node-negative breast cancer. (Editorial.) N Engl J Med 1989;320:525.

National Institutes of Health: Clinical Alert, May 18, 1988. National Institutes of Health Consensus Development Conference Statement: Adjuvant chemotherapy for breast cancer. Vol 5, No. 12, 1985.

Rose C et al: Anti-estrogen treatment of postmenopausal breast cancer patients with high risk of recurrence: 72 months of life table analysis and steroid hormone receptor status. World J Surg 1985;9:765.

Tancini G et al: Adjuvant CMF in breast cancer: Comparative 5-year results of 12 versus 6 cycles. J Clin Oncol 1983;1:2.

TREATMENT OF ADVANCED BREAST CANCER

This section covers palliative therapy of disseminated disease incurable by surgery (stage IV).

Radiotherapy

Palliative radiotherapy may be advised for locally advanced cancers with distant metastases in order to control ulceration, pain, and other manifestations in the breast and regional nodes. Irradiation of the breast and chest wall and the axillary, internal mammary, and supraclavicular nodes should be undertaken in an attempt to cure locally advanced and inoperable lesions when there is no evidence of distant metastases. A small number of patients in this group are cured in spite of extensive breast and regional node involvement. Adjuvant chemotherapy should be considered for such patients.

Palliative irradiation is also of value in the treatment of certain bone or soft tissue metastases to control pain or avoid fracture. Radiotherapy is especially useful in the treatment of isolated bony metastasis and chest wall recurrences.

Hormone Therapy

Disseminated disease may respond to prolonged endocrine therapy such as administration of hormones; ablation of the ovaries, adrenals, or pituitary; or administration of drugs that block hormone receptor sites (eg, antiestrogens) or drugs that block the synthesis of hormones (eg, aminoglutethimide). Hormonal manipulation is usually more successful in postmenopausal women. If treatment is based on the presence of estrogen receptor protein in the primary tumor or metastases, however, the rate of response is nearly equal in premenopausal and postmenopausal women. A favorable response to hormonal manipulation occurs in about one-third of patients with metastatic breast cancer. Of those whose tumors contain estrogen receptors, the response is about 60% and perhaps as high as 80% for patients whose tumors contain progesterone receptors as well. Because only 5–10% of women whose tumors do not contain estrogen receptors respond, they should not receive hormonal therapy except in unusual circumstances such as an elderly patient who could not tolerate chemotherapy.

Since the quality of life during a remission induced by endocrine manipulation is usually superior to a remission following cytotoxic chemotherapy, it is usually best to try endocrine manipulation first in cases where the estrogen receptor status of the tumor is unknown. However, if the estrogen receptor status is unknown but the disease is progressing rapidly or involves visceral organs, endocrine therapy is rarely successful, and introducing it may waste valuable time.

In general, only one type of systemic therapy should be given at a time, unless it is necessary to irradiate a destructive lesion of weight-bearing bone while the patient is on another regimen. The regimen should be changed only if the disease is clearly progressing but not if it appears to be stable. This is especially important for patients with destructive bone metastases, since minor changes in the status of these lesions are difficult to determine radiographically. A plan of therapy that would simultaneously minimize toxicity and maximize benefits is often best achieved by hormonal manipulation.

The choice of endocrine therapy depends on the menopausal status of the patient. Women within 1 year of their last menstrual period are considered to be premenopausal, while women whose menstruation ceased more than a year ago are postmenopausal. The initial choice of therapy is referred to as primary hormonal manipulation; subsequent endocrine treatment is called secondary or tertiary hormonal manipulation.

A. The Premenopausal Patient:

1. Primary hormonal therapy–Bilateral oophorectomy has been the first choice for primary hormonal manipulation in premenopausal women. It can be achieved rapidly and safely by surgery or, if the patient is a poor operative risk, by irradiation of the ovaries. Ovarian radiation therapy should be avoided in otherwise healthy patients, however, because of the high rate of complications and longer time necessary to achieve results. Oophorectomy presumably works by eliminating estrogens, progestins, and androgens, which stimulate growth of the tumor. The average remission is about 12 months.

The potent antiestrogen tamoxifen is an alternative to oophorectomy in the premenopausal patient. The response rate to tamoxifen is similar to that of oophorectomy, leading many authorities to recommend tamoxifen as the primary hormonal treatment of metastatic breast cancer in premenopausal women with estrogen receptor-positive tumors. However, tamoxifen appears to increase ovarian production of estrogen, which may oppose its antitumor effect.

Experience is presently insufficient to advocate tamoxifen in preference to oophorectomy. The operation is not associated with long-term endocrine dysfunction, as are adrenalectomy and hypophysectomy. Randomized trials are now being conducted, evaluating higher doses of tamoxifen in an attempt to replace oophorectomy. In general, there appears to be no advantage to combining tamoxifen with other hormones simultaneously.

2. Secondary or tertiary hormonal therapy– Although patients who do not respond to oophorectomy or tamoxifen should be treated with cytotoxic drugs, those who respond and then relapse may subsequently respond to another form of endocrine treatment. The initial choice for secondary endocrine manipulation has not been clearly defined. Adrenalectomy or hypophysectomy induces regression in approximately 30–50% of patients who have previously responded to oophorectomy. However, these procedures are rarely performed now.

Patients who respond initially to oophorectomy but subsequently relapse should receive tamoxifen. If this treatment fails, use of aminoglutethimide (Cytadren) or megestrol acetate (Megace) should be considered. Aminoglutethimide is an inhibitor of adrenal hormone synthesis and, when combined with a corticosteroid, provides a therapeutically effective "medical adrenalectomy." Megace is a progestational agent. Both drugs cause less morbidity and mortality than surgical adrenalectomy; can be discontinued once the patient improves; and are not associated with the many problems of postsurgical hypoadrenalism, so that patients who require chemotherapy are more easily managed.

B. The Postmenopausal Patient:
1. Primary hormonal therapy–Tamoxifen, 10 mg twice daily, is now the initial therapy of choice for postmenopausal women with metastatic breast cancer amenable to endocrine manipulation. It has fewer side effects than diethylstilbestrol, the former

therapy of choice, and is just as effective. The main side effects of tamoxifen are nausea, vomiting, and skin rash. Rarely, it may induce hypercalcemia.

2. Secondary or tertiary hormonal therapy– Postmenopausal patients who do not respond to primary endocrine manipulation should be given cytotoxic drugs. Postmenopausal women who respond initially to tamoxifen but later manifest progressive disease could be given diethylstilbestrol or megestrol acetate. Some authorities use aminoglutethimide. Megestrol has fewer side effects than either aminoglutethimide or diethylstilbestrol. Androgens have many side effects and should rarely be used. In general, hypophysectomy or adrenalectomy is rarely necessary.

Chemotherapy

Cytotoxic drugs should be considered for the treatment of metastatic breast cancer (1) if visceral metastases are present (especially brain or lymphangitic pulmonary); (2) if hormonal treatment is unsuccessful or the disease has progressed after an initial response to hormonal manipulation; or (3) if the tumor is estrogen receptor-negative. The most useful single chemotherapeutic agent to date is doxorubicin (Adriamycin), with a response rate of 40–50%. The remissions tend to be brief, and in general, experience with single-agent chemotherapy in patients with disseminated disease has not been encouraging.

Combination chemotherapy using multiple agents has proved to be more effective, with objectively observed favorable responses achieved in 60–80% of patients with stage IV disease. Various combinations of drugs have been used, and clinical trials are continuing in an effort to improve results and to reduce undesirable side effects. Doxorubicin and cyclophosphamide produced an objective response in 87% of 46 patients who had an adequate trial of therapy. Other chemotherapeutic regimens have consisted of various combinations of drugs, including cyclophosphamide, vincristine, methotrexate, and fluorouracil, with response rates ranging up to 60–70%. Prior adjuvant chemotherapy does not seem to alter response rates in patients who relapse. Few new drugs or combinations of drugs have been sufficiently effective in breast cancer to warrant wide acceptance.

Malignant Pleural Effusion

This condition develops at some time in almost half of patients with breast cancer (see Chapter 7).

Antman K, Gale P: Advanced breast cancer: High dose chemotherapy and bone marrow transplants. Ann Intern Med 1988;108:570.

Buzdar AU: Current status of endocrine treatment of carcinoma of the breast. Semin Surg Oncol 1990;6:77.

Henderson IC et al: New agents and new medical treatments for advanced breast cancer. Semin Oncol 1987;14:34.

Hortobagyi GN et al: Sequential cyclic combined hormonal

therapy for metastatic breast cancer. Cancer 1989; 64:1002.

Ingall JN: Principles of therapy in advanced breast cancer. Hematol Oncol Clin North Am 1989;3:743.

Ingle JN: Integration of hormonal agents and chemotherapy for the treatment of women with advanced breast cancer. Mayo Clin Proc 1985;59:232.

Manni A: Tamoxifen therapy of metastatic breast cancer. J Lab Clin Med 1987;109:290.

Nemoto T et al: Tamoxifen (Nolvadex) versus adrenalectomy in metastatic breast cancer. Cancer 1984;53: 1333.

Rose C, Mouridsen HT: Endocrine management of advanced breast cancer. Hormone Res 1989;1:189.

Swain SN et al: Fluorouracil and high dose leucovorin in previously treated patients with metastatic breast cancer. J Clin Oncol 1989;7:890.

CARCINOMA OF THE MALE BREAST

Essentials of Diagnosis

- A painless lump beneath the areola in a man usually over 50 years of age.
- Nipple discharge, retraction, or ulceration may occur.

General Considerations

Breast cancer in men is a rare disease; the incidence is only about 1% of that in women. The average age at occurrence is about 60—somewhat older than the commonest presenting age in women. The prognosis, even in stage I cases, is worse in men than in women. Blood-borne metastases are commonly present when the male patient appears for initial treatment. These metastases may be latent and may not become manifest for many years. As in women, hormonal influences are probably related to the development of male breast cancer. There is a high incidence of both breast cancer and gynecomastia in Bantu men, theoretically owing to failure of estrogen inactivation by a damaged liver associated with vitamin B deficiency.

Clinical Findings

A painless lump, occasionally associated with nipple discharge, retraction, erosion, or ulceration, is the chief complaint. Examination usually shows a hard, ill-defined, nontender mass beneath the nipple or areola. Gynecomastia not uncommonly precedes or accompanies breast cancer in men. Nipple discharge is an uncommon presentation for breast cancer in men, as it is in women. However, nipple discharge in a man is an ominous finding associated with carcinoma in nearly 75% of cases.

Breast cancer staging is the same in men as in women. Gynecomastia and metastatic cancer from another site (eg, prostate) must be considered in the differential diagnosis of a breast lesion in a man. Biopsy settles the issue.

Treatment

Treatment consists of modified radical mastectomy in operable patients, who should be chosen by the same criteria as women with the disease. Irradiation is the first step in treating localized metastases in the skin, lymph nodes, or skeleton that are causing symptoms.

Since breast cancer in men is frequently a disseminated disease, endocrine therapy is of considerable importance in its management. Castration in advanced breast cancer is the most successful palliative measure and more beneficial than the same procedure in women. Objective evidence of regression may be seen in 60–70% of men who are castrated—approximately twice the proportion in women. The average duration of tumor growth remission is about 30 months, and life is prolonged. Bone is the most frequent site of metastases from breast cancer in men (as in women), and castration relieves bone pain in most patients so treated. The longer the interval between mastectomy and recurrence, the longer the tumor growth remission following castration. As in women, there is no correlation between the histologic type of the tumor and the likelihood of remission following castration.

Bilateral adrenalectomy (or hypophysectomy) has been proposed as the procedure of choice when tumor has reactivated after castration. Aminoglutethimide therapy should replace adrenalectomy in men as it has in women. Corticosteroid therapy is considered by some to be efficacious but probably has no value when compared to major endocrine ablation.

Estrogen therapy—5 mg of diethylstilbestrol 3 times daily orally—may rarely be effective. Androgen therapy may exacerbate bone pain. Castration and corticosteroids are the main lines of therapy for advanced breast cancer in men at present. Tamoxifen is becoming increasingly popular and should replace castration as the initial therapy for metastatic disease. Chemotherapy should be administered for the same indications and using the same dose schedules as for women with metastatic disease.

Examination of the cancer for hormone receptor protein may prove to be of value in predicting response to endocrine ablation. Adjuvant chemotherapy for the same indications as in breast cancer in women may be useful, but experience with this form of treatment is lacking at present.

Prognosis

The prognosis of breast cancer is poorer in men than in women. The crude 5- and 10-year survival rates for clinical stage I breast cancer in men are about 58% and 38%, respectively. For clinical stage II disease, the 5- and 10-year survival rates are approximately 38% and 10%. The overall survival rates at 5 and 10 years are 36% and 17%.

Axelsson J, Andersson A: Cancer of the male breast. World J Surg 1983;7:281.

Kantarjian H et al: Hormonal therapy for metastatic male breast cancer. Arch Intern Med 1983;143:237.

Patel JK, Nemoto T, Dao TL: Metastatic breast cancer in males: Assessment of endocrine therapy. Cancer 1984; 53:1344.

Yap HY et al: Chemotherapy for advanced male breast cancer. JAMA 1980;243:1739.

MAMMARY DYSPLASIA
(Fibrocystic Disease)

Essentials of Diagnosis

- Painful, often multiple, usually bilateral masses in the breast.
- Rapid fluctuation in the size of the masses is common.
- Frequently, pain occurs or increases and size increases during premenstrual phase of cycle.
- Most common age is 30–50. Rare in postmenopausal women.

General Considerations

This disorder, also known as fibrocystic disease or chronic cystic mastitis, is the most frequent lesion of the breast. It is common in women 30–50 years of age but rare in postmenopausal women; this suggests that it is related to ovarian activity. Estrogen hormone is considered a causative factor. The term "mammary dysplasia," or "fibrocystic disease," is imprecise and encompasses a wide variety of pathologic entities. These lesions are always associated with benign changes in the breast epithelium, some of which are found so commonly in normal breasts that they are probably variants of normal breast histology but have unfortunately been termed a "disease."

The microscopic findings of fibrocystic disease include cysts (gross and microscopic), papillomatosis, adenosis, fibrosis, and ductal epithelial hyperplasia. Although mammary dysplasia has been considered to increase the risk of subsequent breast cancer, it is probable that only the variants in which proliferation of epithelial components is demonstrated represent true risk factors.

Clinical Findings

Mammary dysplasia may produce an asymptomatic lump in the breast that is discovered by accident, but pain or tenderness often calls attention to the mass. There may be discharge from the nipple. In many cases, discomfort occurs or is increased during the premenstrual phase of the cycle, at which time the cysts tend to enlarge. Fluctuation in size and rapid appearance or disappearance of a breast tumor are common in cystic disease. Multiple or bilateral masses are common, and many patients will give a history of transient lump in the breast or cyclic breast pain.

Differential Diagnosis

Pain, fluctuation in size, and multiplicity of lesions are the features most helpful in differentiation from carcinoma. However, if a dominant mass is present, the diagnosis of cancer should be assumed until disproved by biopsy. Final diagnosis often depends on biopsy. Mammography may be helpful, but the breast tissue in these young women is usually too radiodense to permit a worthwhile study. Sonography is useful in differentiating a cystic from a solid mass.

Treatment

Because mammary dysplasia is frequently indistinguishable from carcinoma on the basis of clinical findings, it is advisable to perform biopsy examination of suspicious lesions, which is usually done under local anesthesia. Surgery should be conservative, since the primary objective is to exclude cancer. Simple mastectomy or extensive removal of breast tissue is rarely, if ever, indicated for mammary dysplasia.

When the diagnosis of mammary dysplasia has been established by previous biopsy or is practically certain, because the history is classic, aspiration of a discrete mass suggestive of a cyst is indicated. The patient is reexamined at intervals thereafter. If no fluid is obtained or if fluid is bloody, if a mass persists after aspiration, or if at any time during follow-up a persistent lump is noted, biopsy should be performed.

Breast pain associated with generalized mammary dysplasia is best treated by avoiding trauma and by wearing (night and day) a brassiere that gives good support and protection. Hormone therapy is not advisable, because it does not cure the condition and has undesirable side effects. Recently, danazol, a synthetic androgen, has been used for patients with severe pain. This treatment suppresses pituitary gonadotropins and should be reserved for the unusual, severe case.

The role of caffeine consumption in the development and treatment of fibrocystic disease is controversial. Some studies suggest that eliminating caffeine from the diet is associated with improvement. Many patients are aware of these studies and report relief of symptoms after giving up coffee, tea, and chocolate. Similarly, many women find vitamin E helpful. However, these observations have been difficult to confirm.

Prognosis

Exacerbations of pain, tenderness, and cyst formation may occur at any time until the menopause, when symptoms usually subside, except in patients receiving estrogens. The patient should be advised to examine her own breasts each month just after menstruation and to inform her physician if a mass appears. The risk of breast cancer in women with mammary dysplasia showing proliferative or atypical changes in the epithelium is higher than that of women in general. Follow-up examinations at regular intervals should therefore be arranged.

Dupont WD, Page DL: Risk factor for breast cancer in women with proliferative breast disease. N Engl J Med 1985;312:146.

Humphrey LJ et al: Fibrocystic breast disease. Contemp Surg 1983;23:97.

Hutter RVP: Goodbye to "fibrocystic disease." (Editorial.) N Engl J Med 1985;312:179.

Leis HP Jr: Management of nipple discharge. World J Surg 1989;13:736.

Page DL: Cancer risk assessment in benign breast biopsies Hum Pathol 1986;17:871.

Wisbey JR et al: Natural history of breast pain. Lancet 1983;2:672.

FIBROADENOMA OF THE BREAST

This common benign neoplasm occurs most frequently in young women, usually within 20 years after puberty. It is somewhat more frequent and tends to occur at an earlier age in black than in white women. Multiple tumors in one or both breasts are found in 10–15% of patients.

The typical fibroadenoma is a round, firm, discrete, relatively movable, nontender mass 1–5 cm in diameter. The tumor is usually discovered accidentally. Clinical diagnosis in young patients is generally not difficult. In women over 30, cystic disease of the breast and carcinoma of the breast must be considered. Cysts can be identified by aspiration. Fibroadenoma does not normally occur after the menopause, but postmenopausal women may occasionally develop fibroadenoma after administration of estrogenic hormone.

Treatment is by excision under local anesthesia as an outpatient procedure, with pathologic examination of the specimen.

Cystosarcoma phyllodes is a type of fibroadenoma with cellular stroma that tends to grow rapidly. This tumor may reach a large size and if inadequately excised will recur locally. The lesion is rarely malignant. Treatment is by local excision of the mass with a margin of surrounding breast tissue. The treatment of malignant cystosarcoma phyllodes is more controversial. In general, complete removal of the tumor and a rim of normal tissue should avoid recurrence. Since these tumors may be large, simple mastectomy is sometimes necessary to achieve complete control.

Briggs RM, Walters M, Rosenthal D: Cystosarcoma phyllodes in adolescent female patients. Am J Surg 1983;146:712.

Hart J et al: Practical aspects in the diagnosis and management of cystosarcoma phyllodes. Arch Surg 1988;123:1079.

Wilkinson S, Forrest AP: Fibroadenoma of the breast. Br J Surg 1985;72:838.

DIFFERENTIAL DIAGNOSIS OF NIPPLE DISCHARGE

In order of increasing frequency, the following are the commonest causes of nipple discharge in the nonlactating breast: carcinoma, intraductal papilloma, mammary dysplasia with ectasia of the ducts. The important characteristics of the discharge and some other factors to be evaluated by history and physical examination are as follows:

(1) Nature of discharge (serous, bloody, or other).

(2) Association with a mass or not.

(3) Unilateral or bilateral.

(4) Single duct or multiple duct discharge.

(5) Discharge is spontaneous (persistent or intermittent) or must be expressed.

(6) Discharge produced by pressure at a single site or by general pressure on the breast.

(7) Relation to menses.

(8) Premenopausal or postmenopausal.

(9) Patient taking contraceptive pills, or estrogen for postmenopausal systems.

Unilateral, spontaneous serous or serosanguineous discharge from a single duct is usually caused by an intraductal papilloma or, rarely, by an intraductal cancer. In either case, a mass may not be present. The involved duct may be identified by pressure at different sites around the nipple at the margin of the areola. Bloody discharge is more suggestive of cancer but is usually caused by a benign papilloma in the duct. Cytologic examination may identify malignant cells, but negative findings do not rule out cancer, which is more likely in women over age 50. In any case, the involved duct, and a mass if present, should be excised. Ductography may identify a filling defect prior to excision of the duct system.

In premenopausal females, spontaneous multiple duct discharge, unilateral or bilateral, most marked just before menstruation, is often due to mammary dysplasia. Discharge may be green or brownish. Papillomatosis and ductal ectasia are usually seen on biopsy. If a mass is present, it should be removed.

Milky discharge from multiple ducts in the nonlactating breast may occur in certain syndromes (Chiari-Frommel syndrome, Argonz-Del Castillo (Forbes-Albright) syndrome), presumably as a result of increased secretion of pituitary prolactin. An endocrine workup may be indicated. Drugs of the chlorpromazine type and contraceptive pills may also cause milky discharge that ceases on discontinuance of the medication.

Oral contraceptive agents may cause clear, serous, or milky discharge from a single duct, but multiple duct discharge is more common. The discharge is more evident just before menstruation and disappears on stopping the medication. If it does not and is from a single duct, exploration should be considered.

Purulent discharge may originate in a subareolar abscess and require excision of the abscess and related lactiferous sinus.

When localization is not possible and no mass is palpable, the patient should be reexamined every week for 1 month. When unilateral discharge persists, even without definite localization or tumor, exploration must be considered. The alternative is careful follow-up at intervals of 1–3 months. Mammography should be done. Cytologic examination of nipple discharge for exfoliated cancer cells may be helpful in diagnosis.

Chronic unilateral nipple discharge, especially if bloody, is an indication for resection of the involved ducts.

Discharge from the nipple. (Editorial.) Lancet 1983;2: 1405.

FAT NECROSIS

Fat necrosis is a rare lesion of the breast but is of clinical importance, because it produces a mass, often accompanied by skin or nipple retraction, that is indistinguishable from carcinoma. Trauma is presumed to be the cause, although only about half of patients give a history of injury to the breast. Ecchymosis is occasionally seen near the tumor. Tenderness may or may not be present. If untreated, the mass associated with fat necrosis gradually disappears. As a rule, the safest course is to obtain a biopsy. The entire mass should be excised, primarily to rule out carcinoma. Fat necrosis is common after segmental resection and radiation therapy.

BREAST ABSCESS

During nursing, an area of redness, tenderness, and induration not infrequently develops in the breast. The organism most commonly found in these abscesses is *Staphylococcus aureus*. In the early stages, the infection can often be reversed while continuing nursing with that breast by administering an antibiotic (see Puerperal Mastitis, Chapter 13). If the lesion progresses to form a localized mass with local and systemic signs of infection, an abscess is present and should be drained, and nursing should be discontinued.

A subareolar abscess may develop (rarely) in young or middle-aged women who are not lactating. These infections tend to recur after incision and drainage unless the area is explored in a quiescent interval with excision of the involved lactiferous duct or ducts at the base of the nipple. Except for the subareolar type of abscess, infection in the breast is very rare unless the patient is lactating. In the nonlactating breast, inflammatory carcinoma must always be considered. Therefore, findings suggestive of abscess in the nonlactating breast require incision and biopsy of any indurated tissue.

REFERENCES

Bassett LW, Gold RH: Breast cancer detection: *Mammography and Other Methods in Breast Imaging*, 2nd ed. Grune & Stratton, 1987.
Haagensen CD: *Diseases of the Breast*, 3rd ed. Saunders, 1985.
Haagensen CD, Bodian C, Haagensen DE Jr: *Breast Carcinoma: Risk and Detection*. Saunders, 1981.

Harris JR et al: *Breast Diseases*. Lippincott, 1987.
McDivitt RW: *The Breast*. Williams & Wilkins, 1984.
Ragaz J, Ariel IM: *High Risk Breast Cancer*. Springer-Verlag, 1989.
Spratt JS, Donegan WL: *Cancer of the Breast*, 3rd ed. Saunders, 1988.

13   Gynecology & Obstetrics

Alan J. Margolis, MD, & Sadja Greenwood, MD, MPH

GYNECOLOGY

ABNORMAL PREMENOPAUSAL BLEEDING

Normal menstrual bleeding lasts an average of 4 days (range, 1–7 days), with a mean blood loss of 35 mL. Blood loss of over 80 mL per cycle is abnormal and frequently produces anemia. Excessive bleeding, often with the passage of clots, may occur at regular menstrual intervals (**menorrhagia**) or irregular intervals (**dysfunctional uterine bleeding**). When there are fewer than 21 days between the onset of bleeding episodes, the cycles are likely to be anovular. **Ovulation bleeding,** a single episode of spotting between regular menses, is quite common. Heavier or irregular intermenstrual bleeding warrants investigation.

Clinical Findings

A. Symptoms and Signs: The diagnosis of the disorders underlying the bleeding usually depends upon (1) a careful description of the duration and amount of flow, related pain, and relationship to the last menstrual period (LMP); (2) a history of pertinent illnesses; (3) a history of all medications the patient has taken in the past month, so that possible inhibition of ovulation or endometrial stimulation can be assessed; and (4) a careful pelvic examination to look for pregnancy, uterine myomas, adnexal masses, infection, or evidence of endometriosis.

B. Laboratory Studies: Cervical smears should be obtained as needed for cytologic and culture studies. Blood studies should include measurements of hemoglobin, hematocrit, white blood cell count and differential, sedimentation rate, and platelet count. Urinalysis and measurement of blood sugar levels should be performed to rule out diabetes. A test for pregnancy and studies of thyroid function and blood clotting should be considered in the clinical evaluation. Tests for ovulation in cyclic menorrhagia include basal body temperature records, serum progesterone measured 1 week before the expected onset of menses, and analysis of an endometrial biopsy specimen for secretory activity shortly before the onset of menstruation.

C. Imaging: Pelvic ultrasound may be useful to diagnose intrauterine or ectopic pregnancy, subserous or intrauterine myomas, endometriosis, or adnexal masses that may be related to abnormal bleeding. Hysterosalpingography can outline endometrial polyps, submucous myomas, or uterine synechias. MRI can definitively diagnose submucous myomas and adenomyosis.

D. Cervical Biopsy and Endometrial Curettage: Biopsy, curettage, or aspiration of the endometrium and curettage of the endocervix are often necessary to diagnose the cause of bleeding. These and other invasive gynecologic diagnostic procedures are described in Table 13–1, Polyps, tumors, and submucous myomas are commonly identified in this way. If cancer of the cervix is a possibility, multiple quadrant biopsies (colposcopically directed if possible) and endocervical curettage are indicated as first steps.

E. Hysteroscopy: Hysteroscopy can visualize endometrial polyps, submucous myomas, and exophytic endometrial cancers. It is useful immediately before D&C.

Treatment

A. Emergency Measures: For acute blood loss, employ the shock position and give sedation and intravenous fluids. Blood transfusions are rarely necessary. Hemostasis may require surgical D&C. Definitive treatment depends on the underlying cause.

B. Management of Dysfunctional Uterine Bleeding: Premenopausal patients with abnormal uterine bleeding include those with submucous myomas, infection, early abortion, or pelvic neoplasms. The history, physical examination, and laboratory findings should identify such patients, who require definitive therapy depending upon the cause of the bleeding. A large group of patients remains, most of whom have dysfunctional uterine bleeding on a hormonal basis.

Dysfunctional uterine bleeding is usually caused by overgrowth of endometrium due to estrogen stimulation without adequate progesterone to stabilize growth; this occurs in anovular cycles. Anovulation associated with high estrogen levels commonly occurs in teenagers, in women aged late 30s to late 40s, and in extremely obese women or those with polycys-

Table 13–1. Common gynecologic diagnostic procedures.

Colposcopy
Visualization of cervical, vaginal, or vulvar epithelium under 5–50× magnification to identify abnormal areas requiring biopsy. Used to identify genital warts on males as well as females. An office procedure.

D&C
Dilation of the cervix and curettage of the entire endometrial cavity, using a metal curet or suction cannula and often using forceps for the removal of endometrial polyps. Performed to diagnose endometrial disease and to stop heavy bleeding. Can usually be done in the office under local anesthesia.

Endometrial biopsy
Removal of one or more areas of the endometrium by means of a curet. Less accurate diagnostically than D&C. An office procedure performed under local anesthesia.

Endocervical curettage
Removal of endocervical epithelium with a small curet for diagnosis of cervical dysplasias and cancer. An office procedure performed under local anesthesia.

Hysteroscopy
Visual examination of the uterine cavity with a small fiberoptic endoscope passed through the cervix. Biopsies, excision of myomas, and other procedures can be performed. Can be done in the office under local anesthesia or in the operating room under general anesthesia.

Hysterosalpingography
Injection of radiopaque dye through the cervix to visualize the uterine cavity and oviducts. Mainly used in diagnosis of infertility.

Laparoscopy
Visualization of the abdominal and pelvic cavity through a small fiberoptic endoscope passed through a subumbilical incision. Permits diagnosis, tubal sterilization, and treatment of many conditions previously requiring laparotomy. General anesthesia is usually used.

---

tic ovaries. The use of synthetic estrogen without added progestin is another common cause. Prolonged low levels of unopposed estrogen can cause spotting; high levels can result in profuse or prolonged bleeding.

Such bleeding can usually be treated hormonally; progestins, which limit and stabilize endometrial growth, are generally effective. Office D&C is usually not necessary in women under age 40. Medroxyprogesterone acetate, 10 mg/d, or norethindrone acetate, 5 mg/d, should be given for 10–14 days starting on day 15 of the cycle, following which withdrawal bleeding (so-called medical curettage) will occur. The treatment is repeated for several cycles; it can be reinstituted if amenorrhea or dysfunctional bleeding recurs. In young women who are bleeding actively, oral contraceptives can be given 4 times daily for 5–7 days; after withdrawal bleeding occurs, pills are taken in the usual dosage for 3 cycles. In cases of intractable heavy bleeding, danazol in doses of 200 mg 4 times daily is sometimes used to create an atrophic endometrium. This drug generally stops bleeding and will allow the patient to build up her hemoglobin for a few months prior to definitive surgery.

If the abnormal bleeding is not controlled by hormonal treatment, a D&C is necessary to check for incomplete abortion, polyps, submucous myomas, or endometrial cancer. In women over age 40 with severe or persistent dysfunctional bleeding, a D&C or careful endometrial biopsy is generally indicated to rule out neoplasm before beginning hormonal therapy.

Endometrial ablation through the hysteroscope with laser or electrocautery photocoagulation is currently being used; this technique is designed to reduce or prevent any future menstrual flow.

Nonsteroidal anti-inflammatory drugs (ibuprofen, naproxen, mefenamic acid, etc) will often reduce blood loss in menorrhagia, even that associated with an IUD.

Prolonged use of a progestin, as in a minipill, in injectable contraceptives, or in the therapy of endometriosis, can also lead to intermittent bleeding, sometimes severe. In this instance, the endometrium is atrophic and fragile. If bleeding occurs, it should be treated with estrogen as follows: ethinyl estradiol, 20 μg, or conjugated estrogens, 1.25 mg/d for 7 days. In cases of heavy bleeding, intravenous conjugated estrogens, 25 mg every 4 hours for 3–4 doses, can be used, followed by oral estrogen for 1 week or a combination oral contraceptive. This will thicken the endometrium and control the bleeding.

It is useful for the patient and the physician to discuss stressful situations or life-styles that may contribute to anovulation and dysfunctional bleeding, such as prolonged emotional turmoil or excessive use of drugs or alcohol.

C. Use of Thyroid Hormone: Hypermenorrhea or menorrhagia is often noted in hypothyroidism. Oligomenorrhea or amenorrhea accompanies hyperthyroidism if the periods are altered. Thyroid hormone will improve menstrual function if a deficiency in thyroid hormone production is the only problem. It should not be used for all patients with abnormal menstrual periods.

Van Eijkeren MA et al: Menorrhagia: A review. Obstet Gynecol Surv 1989;44:421.

POSTMENOPAUSAL VAGINAL BLEEDING

Vaginal bleeding that occurs 6 months or more following cessation of menstrual function should be investigated. The most common causes are endometrial proliferation, hyperplasia, or cancer; cervical cancer; and administration of estrogens in a noncyclic manner or without added progestin. Other causes include atrophic vaginitis, trauma, endometrial polyps, trophic ulcers of the cervix associated with prolapse of the uterus, and blood dyscrasias. Uterine bleeding is usually painless, but pain will be present if the cervix is stenotic, if bleeding is severe and rapid, or if infection or torsion or extrusion of a tumor is present. The patient may report a single episode of spotting or profuse bleeding for days or months.

Diagnosis

The vulva and vagina should be carefully inspected for areas of bleeding, ulcers, or neoplasms. A cytologic smear of the cervix and vaginal pool should be taken; this may disclose exfoliated neoplastic cells. An unstained wet mount of vaginal fluid in saline and potassium hydroxide may reveal white blood cells, infective organisms, or free basal epithelial cells indicative of a low estrogen effect. Endocervical curettage and aspiration curettage of the endometrium should be performed next. These procedures often can be performed in the office with sedation and a paracervical block. A careful search for endometrial polyps should be made. The tissue obtained may reveal polyps, endometrial hyperplasia (with or without an atypical glandular pattern), or cancer.

Treatment

Aspiration curettage (with polypectomy if indicated) will frequently be curative. If simple endometrial hyperplasia is found, give cyclic progestin therapy (medroxyprogesterone acetate, 10 mg/d, or norethindrone acetate, 5 mg/d) for 21 days of each month for 3 months. A repeat D&C can then be performed, and if tissues are normal and estrogen replacement therapy is reinstituted, a progestin should be prescribed (as above) for the last 10–14 days of each estrogen cycle, followed by 5 days with no hormone therapy, so that the uterine lining will be shed. If endometrial hyperplasia with atypical cells or carcinoma of the endometrium is found, hysterectomy is necessary.

PREMENSTRUAL SYNDROME
(Premenstrual Tension)

The premenstrual syndrome is a recurrent, variable cluster of troublesome physical and emotional symptoms that develop during the 7–14 days before the onset of menses and subside when menstruation occurs. The syndrome intermittently affects about one-third of all premenopausal women, primarily those 25–40 years of age. In about 10% of affected women, the syndrome may be recurrent and severe. Although not every woman experiences all the symptoms or signs at one time, many describe bloating, breast pain, ankle swelling, a sense of increased weight, skin disorders, irritability, aggressiveness, depression, inability to concentrate, libido change, lethargy, and food cravings.

The pathogenesis of premenstrual syndrome is still uncertain. Suppression of ovarian function with GnRH has been shown to diminish all symptoms during therapy. Suppression of ovulation with the oral contraceptive is sometimes helpful, but the patient often complains that she still has premenstrual syndrome.

It is obvious that further investigation and well-controlled therapeutic studies of this heterogeneous syndrome will be necessary for rational treatment. Current treatment methods are mainly empiric. The physician should provide the best support possible for the patient's emotional and physical distress. This includes the following:

(1) Careful evaluation of the patient, with understanding, explanation, and reassurance, is of first importance.

(2) Advise the patient to keep a daily diary of all symptoms for 2–3 months, to help in evaluating the timing and characteristics of the syndrome. If her symptoms occur throughout the month rather than in the 2 weeks before menses, she may be depressed or may have other emotional problems in addition to premenstrual syndrome. Psychotherapy and self-help groups are helpful for many women or couples.

(3) A diet emphasizing complex carbohydrates (whole grains, vegetables, and fruits) can be recommended. Foods high in sugar content and alcohol should be avoided to minimize reactive hypoglycemia. Salt intake should be restricted to reduce fluid retention. Use of caffeine should be minimized whenever tension and irritability predominate.

(4) A variety of vitamins and minerals in relatively high doses have been suggested for this syndrome, but none have proved useful in double-blind studies, and some have undesirable side effects. If a supplement is desired, use a single daily dose of a multivitamin-multimineral containing the RDA for these substances.

(5) A program of regular conditioning exercise, such as jogging, has been found to decrease depression, anxiety, and fluid retention premenstrually in several studies.

(6) Natural progesterone taken daily or by vaginal suppositories in doses of 50–400 mg daily during the luteal phase is widely used for premenstrual syndrome. Double-blind studies have not confirmed its efficacy, nor has the safety of this treatment been evaluated.

(7) Danazol (100–200 mg daily during the luteal phase) has been reported to be helpful, as has mefenamic acid (250 mg 4 times daily in the luteal phase). Short-acting benzodiazepines have also been used, but the potential for addiction to these drugs makes their use problematic in this recurrent disorder.

Keye WR: *The Premenstrual Syndrome.* Saunders, 1988.

Rossignol AK et al: Tea and premenstrual syndrome in the People's Republic of China. Am J Public Health 1989;79:67. (Caffeine consumption in tea was strongly related to the prevalence of premenstrual syndrome; the effects were dose-dependent.)

Smith S, Schiff I: The premenstrual syndrome: Diagnosis and management. Fertil Steril 1989;52:527.

DYSMENORRHEA

1. PRIMARY DYSMENORRHEA

Primary dysmenorrhea is menstrual pain associated with ovular cycles in the absence of pathologic findings. The pain usually begins within 1–2 years after the menarche and may become more severe with time. The frequency of cases increases up to age 20 and then decreases with age and markedly with parity. Thirty to 50% of women are affected at some time, and 5–10% have severe pain.

Primary dysmenorrhea is low, midline, wavelike, cramping pelvic pain often radiating to the back or upper thighs. Cramps may last for 1 or more days and may be associated with nausea, syncope, diarrhea, headache, and flushing. The pain is produced by uterine vasoconstriction, anoxia, and sustained contractions mediated by prostaglandins.

Clinical Findings

The pelvic examination is normal between menses; examination during menses may produce more severe pain, but no pathologic findings are seen.

Treatment

Nonsteroidal anti-inflammatory drugs (ibuprofen, mefenamic acid, naproxen) are generally helpful. Ibuprofen is now available without a prescription. Drugs should be given at the onset of bleeding to avoid inadvertent drug use during early pregnancy. Ovulation can be suppressed and dysmenorrhea usually prevented by oral contraceptives. Women with less severe dysmenorrhea often get relief with aspirin or acetaminophen. A high fluid intake and avoidance of exposure to extreme cold can be helpful. Acupuncture has been reported to be helpful by some investigators.

2. SECONDARY DYSMENORRHEA

Secondary dysmenorrhea is menstrual pain for which an organic cause exists. It usually begins well after menarche, sometimes even as late as the third or fourth decade of life.

Clinical Findings

The history and physical examination commonly suggest endometriosis or pelvic inflammatory disease. Other causes may be submucous myoma, IUD use, cervical stenosis with obstruction, or blind uterine horn (rare).

Diagnosis

Laparoscopy is often needed to differentiate endometriosis from pelvic inflammatory disease. Submucous myomas can be detected most reliably by MRI but also by hysterogram, by hysteroscopy, or by passing a sound or curet over the uterine cavity during D&C. Cervical stenosis may result from induced abortion, creating crampy pain at the time of expected menses with no blood flow; this is easily cured by passing a sound into the uterine cavity after administering a paracervical block.

Treatment

A. Specific Measures: Periodic use of analgesics, including the nonsteroidal anti-inflammatory drugs given for primary dysmenorrhea, may be beneficial, and oral contraceptives may give relief, particularly in endometriosis and chronic salpingitis. Danazol is effective in the treatment of endometriosis.

B. Surgical Measures: If disability is marked or prolonged, laparoscopy or exploratory laparotomy is usually warranted. Definitive surgery depends upon the degree of disability and the findings at operation.

VAGINITIS

Inflammation and infection of the vagina are common gynecologic problems, resulting from a variety of pathogens, allergic reactions to vaginal contraceptives or other products, or the friction of coitus. The normal vaginal pH is 4.5 or less, and *Lactobacillus* is the predominant organism. At the time of the midcycle estrogen surge, clear, elastic, mucoid secretions from the cervical os are often profuse. In the luteal phase and during pregnancy, vaginal secretions are thicker, white, and sometimes adherent to the vaginal walls. These normal secretions can be confused with vaginitis.

Clinical Findings

When the patient complains of vaginal irritation, pain, or unusual discharge, a careful history should be taken, noting the onset of the menstrual period; recent sexual activity; use of contraceptives, tampons, or douches; and the presence of vaginal burning, pain, pruritus, or unusually profuse or malodorous discharge. The physical examination should include careful inspection of the vulva and speculum examination of the vagina and cervix. The cervix is cultured for gonococcus or *Chlamydia* if applicable. The vagina should be cultured for *S aureus* if toxic shock syndrome (see Chapter 26) is suspected or for *Candida* if yeast forms are not demonstrated by wet mount but are strongly suspected. A specimen of vaginal discharge is examined under the microscope in a drop of saline solution to look for trichomonads, bacteria, white blood cells, and clue cells (stippled or granulated epithelial cells whose cell borders are obscured by bacteria; see Bacterial Vaginosis, below). Discharge from the vaginal walls should be inspected in a drop of 10–20% potassium hydroxide to search for *Candida*. The vaginal pH can be tested; it is frequently greater than 4.5 in infections due to tricho-monads and anaerobic bacteria, including *Gardner-ella*. A bimanual examination to look for evidence of pelvic infection should follow.

A. *Candida albicans:* Pregnancy, diabetes, and use of broad-spectrum antibiotics or corticosteroids predispose to *Candida* infections. Heat, moisture, and occlusive clothing also contribute to the risk. Pruritus, vulvovaginal erythema, and a white curdlike discharge that is not malodorous are found. Micro-scopic examination with 10–20% potassium hydrox-ide reveals filaments and spores. Cultures with Nicker-son's medium may be used if *Candida* is suspected but not demonstrated.

B. *Trichomonas vaginalis:* This protozoan flag-ellate infects the vagina, Skene's ducts, and lower urinary tract in women and the lower genitourinary tract in men. It is transmitted through coitus. Pruritus and a malodorous discharge occur, along with diffuse vaginal redness and red macular lesions on the cervix in severe cases. Motile organisms with flagella are seen by microscopic examination of a wet mount with saline solution. The organism can sometimes be found in a first-morning specimen of urine from an infected male.

C. Bacterial Vaginosis: (Formerly *Gardnerella*, *Haemophilus*, or bacterial vaginitis.) An overgrowth of *Gardnerella* and other anaerobes is often associated with increased malodorous discharge without obvious vulvitis or vaginitis. The discharge is grayish and sometimes frothy, with a pH of 5.0–5.5. An aminelike (''fishy'') odor is present if a drop of discharge is alkalinized with 10–20% potassium hydroxide. On wet mount in saline, epithelial cells are covered with bacteria to such an extent that cell borders are obscured (clue cells). Vaginal cultures are generally not useful in diagnosis.

D. Atrophic Vaginitis: In the absence of estrogen stimulation, the vulvar and vaginal tissues shrink, the vaginal walls become thin and dry, and rugal folds disappear. Tenderness and pruritus, with result-ing dysuria and dyspareunia, may occur. Fissures and ulcerations of tissue with spotting or bleeding may result from coitus. The wet mount will reveal predominantly parabasal cells.

E. Condylomata Acuminata (Genital Warts): Warty growths on the vulva, perianal area, vaginal walls, or cervix are caused by various types of the human papillomavirus. They are sexually transmitted. Pregnancy and immunosuppression favor growth. Vulvar lesions may be obviously wartlike or may be diagnosed only after application of 4% acetic acid (vinegar) and colposcopy, when they appear whitish, with prominent papillae. Fissures may be present at the fourchette. Vaginal lesions may show diffuse hy-pertrophy or a cobblestone appearance. Cervical le-sions may be visible only by colposcopy after pretreat-ment with 4% acetic acid. These lesions are believed to be related to dysplasia and cervical cancer. Vulvar

cancer is also currently considered to be associated with the human papillomavirus.

Treatment

A. *Candida albicans:* Treatment with butacona-zole, clotrimazole, terconazole, or miconazole cream or suppositories nightly for 3–7 days is generally effective; nystatin suppositories, gentian violet solu-tion (1–2%), or boric acid capsules (600 mg twice daily) have also been successful. In recurrent cases, prophylaxis may be attempted with use of these fungi-cides twice weekly or with oral nystatin, 500,000–1,000,000 units 3 times daily for 3 weeks. The sexual partner may be treated with fungicidal creams.

B. *Trichomonas vaginalis:* Treatment of both partners simultaneously is necessary; metronidazole, 2 g as a single dose for 1 day or 250 mg 3 times daily for 7 days, is usually employed. In resistant cases, use 2 g of metronidazole taken as a single daily dose for 5 days, with a vaginal insert of a 500-mg oral tablet daily. If this is not effective in eradicating the organisms, laboratory sensitivity tests can be arranged with the Centers for Disease Control in Atlanta. Treatment of a confirmed resistant organ-ism is with metronidazole, 1 g 3 times daily for 14 days, with nightly vaginal suppository insertion of a 500-mg oral tablet. Metronidazole should be avoided in the first trimester of pregnancy.

Patients who refuse metronidazole may obtain relief with daily douches containing 4 tablespoons of vine-gar and 4 drops of detergent shampoo in 1 quart of water. The male partner should use a condom during sexual intercourse. Clotrimazole vaginal cream is also said to be useful.

C. Bacterial Vaginosis: In severe cases, treat with metronidazole, 500 mg twice daily for 7 days; or clindamycin, 300 mg twice daily for 7 days. In milder cases with minimal symptoms, patients can be reassured that the condition may disappear sponta-neously. They can douche with povidone-iodine solu-tion (1 tablespoon per quart of water), vinegar (3–4 tablespoons per quart of water), or a milky suspension of yogurt to restore *Lactobacillus* levels. The use of vaginal iodine solutions is not recommended in preg-nancy. Sexual partners should use condoms whenever bacterial vaginosis is treated.

D. Atrophic Vaginitis: Treatment consists of oral hormone replacement therapy or local applications of estrogen cream. Conjugated estrogen cream, one-eighth applicatorful (0.3 mg of conjugated estrogens), applied daily for 1 week and then every other day, will relieve most symptoms of dyspareunia with mini-mal systemic effects. Testosterone propionate cream 1% is helpful for individuals unable to use estrogen. For symptomatic relief, this treatment must be main-tained indefinitely.

E. Condylomata Acuminata: Both partners should be treated for warts anywhere on their bodies. Genital warts in the male may only be visible with magnification. Treatment for small vulvar warts is with podophyllum resin 25% in tincture of benzoin (do not use during pregnancy or on bleeding lesions) or 50–90% trichloroacetic acid, carefully applied to avoid the surrounding skin. The pain of trichloroacetic acid application can be lessened by a sodium bicarbonate paste applied immediately after treatment. Podophyllum resin must be washed off after 2–4 hours. Freezing with liquid nitrogen is also effective. Treatment of large warts (> 2 cm) and vaginal warts is with CO_2 laser or electrodesiccation and curettage of the base, following local or general anesthesia. Multiple vaginal warts may be treated with intravaginal applications of fluorouracil. Use one-half applicatorful of 5% fluorouracil cream nightly for 5 days. A tampon is inserted after cream insertion, and the introitus and vulva are further protected by application of zinc oxide ointment. In all cases, treat any other vaginal infections and sexually transmitted diseases.

Boden E et al: Clinical characteristics of papillomavirus-vulvovaginitis. Acta Obstet Gynecol Scand 1988;67:147.
Kaufman RH (editor): Vulvovaginal candidiasis: A symposium. J Reprod Med 1986;31(Suppl 7):639.
Eschenbach DA et al: Diagnosis and clinical manifestations of bacterial vaginosis. Am J Obstet Gynecol 1988; 158:819.

CERVICITIS

Infection of the cervix must be distinguished from physiologic ectopy of columnar epithelium, which is common in young women. True cervicitis is characterized by a red edematous cervix with purulent, often blood-streaked discharge and tenderness on cervical motion. The infection may follow tears during delivery or abortion or may result from a sexually transmitted pathogen such as *Neisseria gonorrhoeae*, *Chlamydia*, or herpesvirus (which presents with vesicles and ulcers on the cervix during a primary herpetic infection). Oral contraceptives, which induce hyperplasia of the endocervical epithelium, are associated with increased cervical infections with *Chlamydia*.

The symptoms of cervicitis include leukorrhea, low back pain, dyspareunia, dysmenorrhea, dysuria, urinary frequency and urgency, and spotting or bleeding. Yellow mucopurulent endocervical secretions and the presence of 10 or more polymorphonuclear leukocytes per oil immersion field are suggestive of chlamydial infection.

A culture for *N gonorrhoeae* should be taken from the endocervix as well as a test for *Chlamydia*. Appropriate antibiotics should be given to the patient and her partner. (See Chapter 26 for discussion.) Three months after treatment, approximately 20% of women will have persistent or recurrent mucopus in the cervix, not explained by relapse or reinfection. This may be related to cervical ectopy and an inflammatory

reaction caused by columnar cell contact with the vaginal environment.

Paavonen J et al: Randomized treatment of mucopurulent cervicitis with doxycycline or amoxicillin. Am J Obstet Gynecol 1989;161:128.

CYST & ABSCESS OF BARTHOLIN'S DUCT

Gonorrhea and other infections often involve Bartholin's duct, causing obstruction of the gland. Drainage of secretions is prevented, leading to pain, swelling, and abscess formation. The infections usually resolve and pain disappears, but stenosis of the duct outlet with distention often persists. Reinfection causes recurrent tenderness and further enlargement of the duct.

The principal symptoms are periodic painful swelling on either side of the introitus and dyspareunia. A fluctuant swelling 1–4 cm in diameter in the inferior portion of either labium minus is a sign of occlusion of Bartholin's duct. Tenderness is evidence of active infection.

Pus or secretions from the gland should be cultured for gonorrhea, *Chlamydia*, and other pathogens. Treat with appropriate antibiotics (see Chapter 26) and frequent warm soaks. If an abscess develops, aspiration or incision and drainage are the simplest forms of therapy, but the problem may recur. Marsupialization, incision and drainage with the insertion of an indwelling Word catheter, or laser treatment will establish a new duct opening. This can be done at the time of abscess formation or as an interval procedure.

Cheetham DR: Bartholin's cyst: Marsupialization or aspiration? Am J Obstet Gynecol 1985;152:569. (A simple technique of aspiration is described.)
Davis GD: Management of Bartholin duct cysts with the carbon dioxide laser. Obstet Gynecol 1985;65:279.

EFFECTS OF EXPOSURE TO DIETHYLSTILBESTROL IN UTERO

Between 1947 and 1971, diethylstilbestrol (DES) was widely used in the USA for diabetic women during pregnancy and to treat threatened abortion. It is estimated that 2–3 million fetuses were exposed. A relationship between fetal DES exposure and clear cell carcinoma of the vagina was later discovered, and a number of other related anomalies have since been noted. In one-third of all exposed women, there are changes in the vagina (adenosis, septa), cervix (deformities and hypoplasia of the vaginal portion of the cervix), or uterus (T-shaped cavity). In males exposed to DES in utero, testicular and epididymal abnormalities and an increase in oligospermia (although not carcinoma) have been reported.

At present, all exposed women are advised to have an initial colposcopic examination to outline vaginal and cervical areas of abnormal epithelium, followed by cytologic examination of the vagina (all 4 quadrants of the upper half of the vagina) and cervix at 6-month intervals. Lugol's iodine stain of the vagina and cervix will also outline areas of metaplastic squamous epithelium.

Many women are not aware of having been exposed to DES. Therefore, in the age groups at risk, examiners should pay attention to structural changes of the vagina and cervix that may signal the possibility of DES exposure and indicate the need for follow-up.

The incidence of clear cell carcinoma is approximately one in 1000 exposed women, and the incidence of cervical and vaginal intraepithelial neoplasia (dysplasia and carcinoma in situ) is twice as high as in unexposed women. DES daughters have more difficulty conceiving and have an increased incidence of early abortion, ectopic pregnancy, and premature births. In addition, mothers treated with DES in pregnancy appear to have a small increase in the incidence of breast cancer, beginning 20 years after exposure.

Bernstein J et al: Development of cervical and vaginal squamous cell neoplasia as a late consequence of in utero exposure to diethylstilbestrol. Obstet Gynecol Survey 1988;43:15.

Linn S et al: Adverse outcomes of pregnancy in women exposed to diethylstilbestrol in utero. J Reprod Med 1988;33:3.

CERVICAL INTRAEPITHELIAL NEOPLASIA (CIN; Dysplasia of the Cervix)

The squamocolumnar junction of the uterine cervix represents an area of active squamous cell proliferation. In childhood, this junction is located to a variable degree on the exposed vaginal portion of the cervix. At puberty, because of hormonal influence and possibly because of changes in the vaginal pH, the squamous margin begins to encroach on the single-layered, mucus-secreting epithelium, creating an area of metaplasia (transformation zone). Factors associated with coitus (see Prevention, below) may lead to cellular abnormalities, which over a period of time can result in the development of squamous cell dysplasia or cancer. There are varying degrees of dysplasia (Table 13–2), defined by the degree of cellular atypia; all types must be observed and treated if they persist or become more severe. At present, the malignant potential of a specific lesion cannot be predicted. Some lesions remain stable for long periods of time; some regress; and others advance.

Clinical Findings

There are no specific signs or symptoms of cervical intraepithelial neoplasia. The presumptive diagnosis

Table 13–2. Classification systems for Papanicolaou smears.

Classification	Dysplasia	Cervical Intraepithelial Neoplasia (CIN)
1	Benign	Benign
2	Benign with inflammation	Benign with inflammation
3	Mild dysplasia	CIN I
3	Moderate dysplasia	CIN II
3	Severe dysplasia	CIN III
4	Carcinoma in situ	CIN III
5	Invasive cancer	Invasive cancer

is made by cytologic screening of an asymptomatic population with no grossly visible cervical changes. All visibly abnormal cervical lesions should be biopsied.

Diagnosis

A. Cytologic Examination (Papanicolaou Smear): All specimens can be spread on one slide and fixed. For optimal screening, specimens should be taken from the vaginal pool, the squamocolumnar junction, and the endocervical canal using a plastic spatula or a special nylon brush.

Cytologic reports from the laboratory may describe findings in one of several ways (see Table 13–2). While use of class I–IV is decreasing, the CIN classification continues to be used along with a description of abnormal cells, including evidence of human papillomavirus (HPV). A new term, "squamous intraepithelial lesions (SIL)," low-grade or high-grade, will be used increasingly. Cytopathologists consider a Pap smear to be a medical consultation and will recommend further diagnostic procedures, treatment for infection, and comments on factors that prevent adequate evaluation.

B. Colposcopy: Viewing the cervix with 10–20 × magnification allows for assessment of the size and margins of an abnormal transformation zone and determination of extension into the endocervical canal. The application of 4% acetic acid (vinegar) dissolves mucus, and the acid's desiccating action sharpens the contrast between normal and actively proliferating thickened squamous epithelium. Abnormal changes include white patches and vascular atypia, which indicate areas of greatest cellular activity. Paint the cervix with Lugol's solution (strong iodine solution [Schiller's test]). Normal squamous epithelium will take the stain; nonstaining squamous epithelium should be biopsied. (The single-layered, mucus-secreting endocervical tissue will not stain either but can readily be distinguished by its darker pink, shinier appearance.)

C. Biopsy: Colposcopically directed punch biopsy and endocervical curettage are office procedures. If colposcopic examination is not performed, the normal-appearing cervix shedding atypical cells can be evaluated by endocervical curettage and multiple punch biopsies of nonstaining squamous epithelium or tissue from each quadrant of the cervix.

Microscopic examination of biopsy specimens will diagnose the degree of cellular atypia suggested by the cytologic examination. Endocervical curettage will confirm the presence of abnormalities in the endocervical canal. Data from both procedures are important in deciding on treatment.

Prevention

Current data suggest that cervical infection with the human papillomavirus (HPV) is associated with a high percentage of all cervical dysplasias and cancers. There are over 50 recognized HPV subtypes, of which types 6 and 11 tend to cause mild dysplasias, while types 15, 18, and 31 cause higher grade cellular changes. Herpes simplex virus may play a synergistic role but is not believed to be a major etiologic agent in human genital cancers.

Cervical cancer almost never occurs in virginal women; it is epidemiologically related to the number of sexual partners a woman has had and the number of other female partners a male partner has had. Use of the diaphragm or condom has been associated with a protective effect. Long-term oral contraceptive users develop more dysplasias and cancers of the cervix than users of other forms of birth control, and smokers are also more at risk. Preventive measures therefore include the following:

(1) Sexually active women should undergo regular cytologic screening to detect abnormalities.

(2) Women should limit the number of sexual partners.

(3) Use of a diaphragm by the woman or condom by the man will protect the cervix.

(4) Women should stop smoking.

(5) If a cytologic abnormality is found, the woman should stop using oral contraceptives or other contraceptive methods that leave the cervix exposed and should use a diaphragm or ask her male partner to use a condom.

(6) Prompt treatment of genital warts is advisable for men and women.

Treatment

Treatment varies depending on the degree and extent of cervical intraepithelial neoplasia. Biopsies should always precede treatment.

A. Cauterization or Cryosurgery: The use of either hot cauterization or freezing (cryosurgery) is effective for noninvasive small lesions visible on the cervix without endocervical extension.

B. CO₂ Laser: This well-controlled method minimizes tissue destruction. It is colposcopically directed and requires special training. It may be used with large visible lesions. In current practice it involves the vaporization of the transformation zone on the cervix and the distal 5–7 mm of endocervical canal.

C. Conization of the Cervix: Conization allows for complete histopathologic assessment and generally results in excision of the lesion. It should be reserved for cases of severe dysplasia or cancer in situ (CIN III), particularly those with endocervical extension. The procedure can be performed with the scalpel or CO_2 laser.

D. Examination of Male Partners: Male partners of women with cervical dysplasias or cancer should be examined; about 70% will have warts on the penile shaft or just within the urethra. Diagnosis is made by application of 4% acetic acid (vinegar) and examination under magnification, preferably with a colposcope. Treatment is with podophyllum resin, trichloroacetic acid, or liquid nitrogen.

E. Follow-Up: Because recurrence is possible—especially in the first 2 years after treatment—and because the false-negative rate of cervical cytologic tests is 20%, close follow-up is imperative. Vaginal cytologic examination should be repeated at 3-month intervals. After 2 years, yearly examinations suffice.

Krebs H-B: Management of human papillomavirus-associated genital lesions in men. Obstet Gynecol 1989;73:312.

National Cancer Institute Workshop: The 1988 Bethesda system for reporting cervical/vaginal cytological diagnoses. JAMA 1989;262:931.

CARCINOMA OF THE UTERINE CERVIX

Essentials of Diagnosis

- Abnormal uterine bleeding and vaginal discharge.
- Cervical lesion may be visible on inspection as a tumor or ulceration.
- Vaginal cytology usually positive; must be confirmed by biopsy.

General Considerations

Cancer appears first in the intraepithelial layers (the preinvasive stage, or carcinoma in situ). Preinvasive cancer (CIN III) is a common diagnosis in women 25–40 years of age and is etiologically related to infection with the human papillomavirus (subtypes 16, 18, and 31). Two to 10 years are required for carcinoma to penetrate the basement membrane and invade the tissues. After invasion, death usually occurs in 3–5 years in untreated or unresponsive patients.

Clinical Findings

A. Symptoms and Signs: The most common signs are metrorrhagia, postcoital spotting, and cervical ulceration. Bloody or purulent, odorous, nonpruritic discharge appears after invasion. Bladder and rectal dysfunction or fistulas and pain are late symptoms. Anemia, anorexia, and weight loss are signs of advanced disease.

B. Cervical Biopsy and Endocervical Curettage, or Conization: These procedures are necessary steps after a positive Papanicolaou smear to determine the extent and depth of invasion of the cancer. Even if the smear is positive, treatment is never justified until definitive diagnosis has been established through biopsy studies.

C. "Staging," or Estimate of Gross Spread of Cancer of the Cervix: The depth of penetration of the malignant cells beyond the basement membrane is a reliable clinical guide to the extent of primary cancer within the cervix and the likelihood of secondary to metastatic cancer. It is customary to stage cancers of the cervix under anesthesia as shown in Table 13–3. Further assessment may be carried out by abdominal and pelvic CT scanning or MRI.

Table 13–3. International classification of cancer of the cervix (1985).[1]

Preinvasive carcinoma	
Stage 0	Carcinoma in situ, intraepithelial carcinoma.
Invasive carcinoma	
Stage I	Carcinoma strictly confined to the cervix (extension to the corpus should be disregarded).
Ia	Preclinical carcinomas of the cervix, ie, those diagnosed only by microscopy.
Ia1	Minimal microscopically evident stromal invasion.
Ib2	Lesions detected microscopically that can be measured. The upper limits of the measurement should not show a depth of invasion of > 5 mm taken from the base of the epithelium, either surface or glandular, from which it originates; and a second dimension, the horizontal spread, must not exceed 7 mm. Larger lesions should be larger than 7 mm.
Stage II	Carcinoma extends beyond the cervix but has not extended onto the pelvic wall. The carcinoma involves the vagina, but not the lower third.
IIa	No obvious parametrial involvement. The vagina has been invaded, but not the lower third.
IIb	Obvious parametrial involvement.
Stage III	Carcinoma has extended onto the pelvic wall. On rectal examination, there is no cancer-free space between the tumor and the pelvic wall. The tumor involves the lower third of the vagina. All cases with hydronephrosis or nonfunctioning kidney.
IIIa	No extension onto the pelvic wall. Vaginal involvement, but not the lower third.
IIIb	Extension onto the pelvic wall and/or hydronephrosis or nonfunctioning kidney.
Stage IV	Carcinoma extended beyond the true pelvis or clinically involving the mucosa of the bladder or rectum. Do not allow a case of bullous edema as such to be allotted to stage IV.
IVa	Spread of growth to adjacent organs (that is, rectum or bladder with positive biopsy from these organs).
IVb	Spread of growth to distant organs.

[1] Approved by the International Federation of Gynecology and Obstetrics (FIGO). Adopted by American College of Obstetrics and Gynecology (1986).

Complications

Metastases to regional lymph nodes occur with increasing frequency from stage I to stage IV. Paracervical extension occurs in all directions from the cervix. The ureters are often obstructed lateral to the cervix, causing hydroureter and hydronephrosis and consequently impaired kidney function. Almost two-thirds of patients with carcinoma of the cervix die of uremia when ureteral obstruction is bilateral. Pain in the back and in the distribution of the lumbosacral plexus is often indicative of neurologic involvement. Gross edema of the legs may be indicative of vascular and lymphatic stasis due to tumor.

Pelvic infections may complicate cervical carcinoma. Vaginal fistulas to the rectum and urinary tract are severe late complications. Incontinence of urine and feces is a major late complication, particularly in debilitated individuals.

Hemorrhage is the cause of death in 10–20% of patients with extensive invasive carcinoma.

Treatment

A. Emergency Measures: Vaginal hemorrhage originates from gross ulceration and cavitation in stage II–IV cervical carcinoma. Ligation and suturing of the cervix are usually not feasible, but ligation of the uterine or hypogastric arteries may be lifesaving when other measures fail. Styptics such as negatol (Negatan), Monsel's solution, or acetone are effective, although delayed sloughing may result in further bleeding. Wet vaginal packing is helpful. Irradiation usually controls bleeding.

B. Specific Measures:

1. Noninvasive carcinoma (stage 0)–In a woman over 40 with in situ carcinoma of the cervix, total hysterectomy is the surgical treatment of choice; rarely, irradiation may be used alternatively in women who are poor operative risks. In a younger woman who wishes to retain her uterus, conization of the cervix may be acceptable. This is a calculated risk and imposes the absolute necessity of cytologic examinations every 6 months for an indefinite time.

2. Invasive carcinoma–Irradiation is generally the best treatment for invasive squamous cell carcinoma or adenocarcinoma of the cervix. The objectives of irradiation are (1) the destruction of primary and secondary carcinoma within the pelvis and (2) the preservation of tissues not invaded. Gamma emissions derived from x-rays, ^{60}Co, radium, the cyclotron, the linear accelerator, and comparable sources are employed. All stages of cancer may be treated by this method, and there are fewer medical contraindications to irradiation than to radical surgery. Selected stage I cases can be treated satisfactorily with radical surgical procedures by experienced pelvic surgeons.

Prognosis

The overall 5-year arrest rate for squamous cell carcinoma or adenocarcinoma originating in the cervix is about 45% in the major clinics. Percentage arrest rates are inversely proportionate to the stage of cancer: stage 0, 99%; stage I, 77%; stage II, 65%; stage III, 25%; stage IV, about 5%.

CARCINOMA OF THE ENDOMETRIUM (Corpus or Fundal Cancer)

Adenocarcinoma of the uterine corpus is the second most common cancer of the female genital tract. It occurs most often in women 50–70 years of age. Many patients with this problem will have taken unopposed estrogen in the past; their increased risk appears to persist for 10 or more years after stopping the drug. Obesity, nulliparity, diabetes, and polycystic ovaries with prolonged anovulation and the extended use of tamoxifen for the treatment of breast cancer are also risk factors.

Abnormal bleeding is the presenting sign in 80% of cases. Pyometra or hematometra may be due to carcinoma of the endometrium. Pain occurs late in the disease, with metastases or infection.

Papanicolaou smears of the cervix occasionally show atypical endometrial cells but are an inconsistent diagnostic tool. Endocervical curettage and endometrial curettage or aspiration are the only reliable means of diagnosis. Adequate specimens of each can usually be obtained during an office procedure performed following local anesthesia (paracervical block) and sedation. General anesthesia may sometimes be necessary for a satisfactory examination and safe diagnostic procedure. Simultaneous hysteroscopy can be a valuable addition in order to find localized growth or polyps within the uterine cavity.

Pathologic assessment is important in differentiating hyperplasias, which often can be treated with cyclic oral progestins.

Prevention

Periodic pelvic examinations and cervical smears and prompt D&C for patients who report abnormal menstrual bleeding or postmenopausal uterine bleeding will reveal many incipient as well as clinical cases of endometrial cancer. Postmenopausal women taking estrogens or younger women with prolonged anovulation can be given oral progestins for 10 days at the end of each estrogen cycle in order to promote periodic shedding of the uterine lining; this has been associated with a decreased incidence of uterine adenocarcinoma.

Staging

Examination under anesthesia, fractional D&C, chest x-ray, intravenous urography, cystoscopy, sigmoidoscopy, and MRI will help determine the extent of the disease and its appropriate treatment. The staging is based on the surgical and pathologic evaluation.

Treatment

Treatment consists of total hysterectomy and bilateral salpingo-oophorectomy. Peritoneal material for cytologic examination is routinely taken. Preliminary external irradiation or intracavitary radium therapy is indicated if the cancer is poorly differentiated or if the uterus is definitely enlarged in the absence of myomas. If invasion deep into the myometrium has occurred or if sampled preaortic lymph nodes are positive for tumor, postoperative irradiation is indicated.

Palliation of advanced or metastatic endometrial adenocarcinoma may be accomplished with large doses of progestins, eg, medroxyprogesterone, 400 mg intramuscularly weekly, or megestrol acetate, 80–160 mg daily orally.

Prognosis

With early diagnosis and treatment, the 5-year arrest rate is 80–85%.

Creasman WT: New gynecologic cancer staging. Obstet Gynecol 1990;75:287.

Rubin GL et al: Estrogen replacement therapy and the risk of endometrial cancer: Remaining controversies. Am J Obstet Gynecol 1990;162:148.

CERVICAL POLYPS

Cervical polyps commonly occur after the menarche and are occasionally noted in postmenopausal women. The cause is not known, but inflammation may play an etiologic role. The principal symptoms are discharge and abnormal vaginal bleeding. However, abnormal bleeding should not be ascribed to a cervical polyp without sampling the endocervix and endometrium. The polyps are visible in the cervical os on speculum examination.

Cervical polyps must be differentiated from polypoid neoplastic disease of the endometrium, small submucous pedunculated myomas, and endometrial polyps. Cervical polyps rarely contain malignant foci.

Treatment

Cervical polyps can generally be removed in the office by avulsion. If the cervix is soft, patulous, or definitely dilated and the polyp is large, surgical D&C is required (especially if the pedicle is not readily visible). Exploration of the cervical and uterine cavities with the polyp forceps and curet may reveal multiple polyps.

MYOMA OF THE UTERUS (Fibroid Tumor, Fibromyoma)

Essentials of Diagnosis

- Irregular enlargement of the uterus (may be asymptomatic).

- Heavy or irregular vaginal bleeding, dysmenorrhea.
- Acute and recurrent pelvic pain if the tumor becomes twisted on its pedicle or infarcted.
- Symptoms due to pressure on neighboring organs (large tumors).

General Considerations

Myoma is the most common benign neoplasm of the female genital tract. It is a discrete, round, firm, often multiple uterine tumor composed of smooth muscle and connective tissue. The most convenient classification is by anatomic location: (1) intramural, (2) submucous, (3) subserous, (4) intraligamentous, (5) parasitic (ie, deriving its blood supply from an organ to which it becomes attached), and (6) cervical. A submucous myoma may become pedunculated and descend through the cervix into the vagina.

Clinical Findings

A. Symptoms and Signs: In nonpregnant women, myomas are frequently asymptomatic. However, they can cause urinary frequency, dysmenorrhea, heavy bleeding (often with anemia), or other complications due to the presence of an abdominal mass. Occasionally, degeneration occurs, causing intense pain. Infertility may be due to a myoma that significantly distorts the uterine cavity.

In pregnant women, myomas occasionally cause additional hazards: abortion, malpresentation, failure of engagement, premature labor, localized pain (from red degeneration or torsion), dystocia, ineffectual labor, and postpartum hemorrhage.

B. Laboratory Findings: Hemoglobin levels may be decreased as a result of blood loss, but in rare cases polycythemia is present, presumably as a result of the production of erythropoietin by the myomas.

C. Imaging: Ultrasonography will confirm the presence of uterine myomas and can be used sequentially to monitor growth. When multiple subserous or pedunculated myomas are being followed, ultrasonography is important to exclude ovarian masses. MRI delineates intramural and submucous myomas accurately and can diagnosis adenomyosis. Hysterography or hysteroscopy can also confirm cervical or submucous myomas.

Differential Diagnosis

Irregular myomatous enlargement of the uterus must be differentiated from the similar but symmetric enlargement that may occur with uterine pregnancy or adenomyosis. Subserous myomas must be distinguished from ovarian tumors. Malignant leiomyosarcoma is a very rare tumor; the average age at onset is 55 years.

Treatment

A. Emergency Measures: Give blood transfusions if necessary. If the patient is markedly anemic as a result of long, heavy menstrual periods, preoperative treatment with depot medroxyprogesterone acetate or danazol will slow or stop bleeding, and medical treatment of anemia can be given prior to surgery. Emergency surgery is required for acute torsion of a pedunculated myoma. The only emergency indication for myomectomy during pregnancy is torsion; abortion is not an inevitable result.

B. Specific Measures:

1. Nonpregnant women–In women who are not pregnant, small asymptomatic myomas should be observed at 6-month intervals. Elective myomectomy can be done to preserve the uterus. Myomas do not urgently require surgery unless they cause significant pressure on the ureters, bladder, or bowel or severe bleeding leading to anemia or are undergoing rapid growth. Cervical myomas larger than 3–4 cm in diameter or pedunculated myomas that protrude through the cervix must be removed.

GnRH analogues are being used preoperatively for 2- to 3-month periods to induce reversible hypogonadism, which reduces the size of myomas, suppresses their further growth, and reduces surrounding vascularity. These effects are desirable before myomectomy or hysterectomy. Regrowth of myomas occurs within several months after termination of GnRH.

2. Pregnant patients–If the uterus is no larger than a 6-month pregnancy by the fourth month of gestation, an uncomplicated course may be anticipated. If the mass (especially a cervical tumor) is the size of a 5- or 6-month pregnancy by the second month, abortion will probably occur. If possible, defer myomectomy or hysterectomy until 6 months after delivery, at which time involution of the uterus and regression of the tumor will be complete.

C. Surgical Measures: Surgical measures available for the treatment of myoma are myomectomy and total or subtotal abdominal or vaginal hysterectomy. Myomectomy is the treatment of choice during the childbearing years. The ovaries should be preserved if possible in women under age 50.

Prognosis

Surgical therapy is curative. Future pregnancies are not endangered by myomectomy, although cesarean delivery may be necessary after wide dissection with entry into the uterine cavity.

Friedman AJ et al: A randomized, placebo-controlled, double blind study evaluating leuprolide acetate depot treatment before myomectomy. Fertil Steril 1989;52:728.
Katz VL et al: Complications of uterine leiomyomas in pregnancy. Obstet Gynecol 1989;73:593.

CARCINOMA OF THE VULVA

Essentials of Diagnosis

- History of genital warts.
- History of prolonged vulvar irritation, with pruri-

tus, local discomfort, or slight bloody discharge.
- Early lesions may suggest or include chronic vulvitis.
- Late lesions appear as a mass, an exophytic growth, or a firm, ulcerated area in the vulva.
- Biopsy is necessary to make the diagnosis.

General Considerations

The vast majority of cancers of the vulva are squamous lesions that classically have occurred in women over 50 years of age. Several subtypes (particularly 6, 16, and 18) of the human papillomavirus have been identified in vulvar cancer. As with squamous cell lesions of the cervix, dysplasias of varying severity are now recognized on the vulva. A grading system of vulvar intraepithelial neoplasia (VIN) from mild dysplasia to carcinoma in situ has been proposed.

Differential Diagnosis

Biopsy is essential for the diagnosis of vulvar cancer and should be performed with any localized atypical vulvar lesion, including white patches. Multiple skin-punch specimens can be taken in the office under local anesthesia, with care to include tissue from the edges of each lesion sampled.

Benign vulvar disorders that must be excluded in the diagnosis of carcinoma of the vulva include chronic granulomatous lesions (eg, lymphogranuloma venereum, syphilis), vulvar nodulations, condylomas, hidradenoma, or neurofibroma. Kraurosis, lichen sclerosis et atrophicus, or other associated leukoplakic changes in the skin should be biopsied but usually are not malignant.

Treatment

A. General Measures: Early diagnosis and treatment of irritative or other predisposing or contributing causes to carcinoma of the vulva should be pursued. Remove prominent or enlarging pigmented moles of the vulva before they become malignant.

B. Surgical Measures:

1. In situ squamous cell carcinoma of the vulva and small, invasive basal cell carcinoma of the vulva should be excised with a wide margin. If the squamous carcinoma in situ is extensive or multicentric, laser therapy or superficial surgical removal of vulvar skin may be required. In this way, the clitoris and uninvolved portions of the vulva may be spared. Skin grafting may be necessary, but mutilating vulvectomy is avoided.

2. Invasive carcinoma confined to the vulva without evidence of spread to adjacent organs or to the regional lymph nodes will necessitate radical vulvectomy and inguinal lymphadenectomy if the patient is able to withstand surgery. Debilitated patients may be candidates for palliative irradiation only.

Prognosis

Patients with vulvar carcinoma 3 cm in diameter or less without inguinal lymph node metastases who can sustain radical surgery have about a 90% chance of a 5-year arrest of the cancer. If the lesion is greater than 3 cm and has metastasized, the likelihood of 5-year survival is less than 25%.

ENDOMETRIOSIS

Aberrant growth of endometrium outside the uterus, particularly in the dependent parts of the pelvis and in the ovaries, is a common cause of abnormal bleeding and secondary dysmenorrhea. This condition is known as endometriosis. Depending on the location and extent of the endometrial implants, infertility, dyspareunia, or rectal pain with bleeding may result. Aching pain tends to be constant, beginning 2–7 days before the onset of menses to become increasingly severe until flow slackens. Pelvic examination may disclose tender indurated nodules in the cul-de-sac, especially if the examination is done at the onset of menstruation.

Endometriosis must be distinguished from pelvic inflammatory disease, ovarian neoplasms, and uterine myomas. In general, only in salpingitis and endometriosis are the symptoms aggravated by menstruation. Bowel invasion by endometrial tissue may produce clinical findings, including blood in the stool, that must be distinguished from bowel neoplasm. Differentiation in these instances depends upon proctosigmoidoscopy and biopsy.

Ultrasound examination will often reveal complex fluid-filled masses that cannot be distinguished from neoplasms. Barium enema may delineate colonic involvement of endometriosis. The clinical diagnosis of endometriosis is presumptive and must be confirmed by laparoscopy or laparotomy.

Treatment

A. Medical Treatment: The goal of medical treatment is to preserve the fertility of women wanting future pregnancies, ameliorate symptoms, and simplify future surgery or make it unnecessary. Medications are designed to inhibit ovulation over 4–9 months and lower hormone levels, thus preventing cyclic stimulation of endometriotic implants and decreasing their size.

1. The GnRH analogue nafarelin (Synarel) is used by nasal spray for 6 months to suppress ovulation. Side effects of hypoestrinism may occur, including hot flashes and vaginal dryness.

2. Danazol (Danocrine) is used for 6–9 months in the lowest dose necessary to suppress menstruation, usually 200–400 mg twice daily. Side effects are androgenic and include decreased breast size, acne, and hirsutism.

3. Combination estrogen-progestin oral contraceptives, one daily continuously for 6–9 months. Increase the dose only with the onset of breakthrough bleeding.

4. Medroxyprogesterone acetate (Depo-Provera), 100 mg intramuscularly every 2 weeks for 4 doses; then 100 mg every 4 weeks; add oral estrogen or estradiol valerate, 30 mg intramuscularly, for breakthrough bleeding. Use for 6–9 months.

5. Low-dose oral contraceptives can be given for 21 days out of each 28; prolonged suppression of ovulation will often inhibit further stimulation of residual endometriosis, especially if taken after one of the therapies mentioned above.

6. Analgesics, with or without codeine, may be needed during menses. Nonsteroidal anti-inflammatory drugs may be helpful.

B. Surgical Measures: The surgical treatment of moderately extensive endometriosis depends upon the patient's age and symptoms and her desire to preserve reproductive function. If the patient is under 35, resect the lesions, free adhesions, and suspend the uterus. At least 20% of patients so treated can become pregnant, although some must undergo surgery again if the disease progresses. If the patient is over 35 years old, is disabled by pain, and has involvement of both ovaries, bilateral salpingo-oophorectomy and hysterectomy will probably be necessary.

Foci of endometriosis can be treated at laparoscopy by bipolar coagulation or laser vaporization. Because pelvic endometriosis can take forms other than the classic powder burns and hemorrhagic cysts, a meticulous survey of the peritoneum is required.

Prognosis

The prognosis for reproductive function in early or moderately advanced endometriosis is good with conservative therapy. Bilateral ovariectomy is curative for patients with severe and extensive endometriosis with pain. Following hysterectomy and oophorectomy, estrogen replacement therapy is indicated.

Cramer DW et al: The relation of endometriosis to menstrual characteristics, smoking, and exercise. JAMA 1986; 255:1904.

Henzel MR et al: Administration of nasal nafarelin as compared with oral danazol for endometriosis. N Engl J Med 1988;318:485. (Nafarelin, A GnRH agonist, was as effective as danazol in treating endometriosis and enhancing posttreatment fertility. The 2 drugs had different side effects.)

Stripling MC et al: Subtle appearance of pelvic endometriosis. Fertil Steril 1988;49:427.

VAGINAL HERNIAS
(Cystocele, Rectocele, Enterocele)

Cystocele, rectocele, and enterocele are vaginal hernias commonly seen in multiparous women. Cystocele is a hernia of the bladder wall into the vagina,

causing a soft anterior fullness. Cystocele may be accompanied by urethrocele, which is not a hernia but a sagging of the urethra following its detachment from the symphysis during childbirth. Rectocele is a herniation of the terminal rectum into the posterior vagina, causing a collapsible pouchlike fullness. Enterocele is a vaginal vault hernia containing small intestine, usually in the posterior vagina and resulting from a deepening of the pouch of Douglas. Enterocele may also accompany uterine prolapse or follow hysterectomy, when weakened vault supports or a deep unobliterated cul-de-sac containing intestine protrudes into the vagina. One or more of the 3 types of hernias often occur in combination.

Supportive measures include a high-fiber diet for constipation and care to empty the bladder completely. Weight reduction in obese patients and limitation of straining and lifting are helpful. Pessaries may reduce cystocele, rectocele, or enterocele temporarily and are helpful in women who do not wish surgery or are chronically ill.

The only cure for symptomatic cystocele, rectocele, or enterocele is corrective surgery. The prognosis following an uncomplicated procedure is good. Hysterectomy without closure of a significant defect in the pelvic floor will be followed by enterocele.

UTERINE PROLAPSE

Uterine prolapse most commonly occurs as a delayed result of childbirth injury to the pelvic floor (particularly the transverse cervical and uterosacral ligaments). Unrepaired obstetric lacerations of the levator musculature and perineal body augment the weakness. Attenuation of the pelvic structures with aging and congenital weakness can accelerate the development of prolapse.

In slight prolapse, the uterus descends only part way down the vagina; in moderate prolapse, the corpus descends to the introitus and the cervix protrudes slightly beyond; and in marked prolapse (procidentia), the entire cervix and uterus protrude beyond the introitus and the vagina is inverted. Inability to walk comfortably because of protrusion or discomfort from the presence of a vaginal mass is an indication that surgical treatment should be considered.

Treatment

The type of surgery depends upon the extent of prolapse and the patient's age and her desire for menstruation, pregnancy, and coitus. The simplest, most effective procedure is vaginal hysterectomy with appropriate repair of the cystocele and rectocele. If the patient desires pregnancy, a partial resection of the cervix with plication of the cardinal ligaments can be attempted. For elderly women who do not desire coitus, partial obliteration of the vagina is surgically simple and effective. Abdominal uterine suspension or ventrofixation will fail in the treatment of prolapse.

A well-fitted vaginal pessary (eg, inflatable doughnut type, Gellhorn pessary) may give relief if surgery is refused or contraindicated.

PELVIC INFLAMMATORY DISEASE (PID; Salpingitis, Endoparametritis)

Essentials of Diagnosis

- Abdominal, cervical, and adnexal tenderness.
- One or more of the following:
  Temperature > 38 °C.
  White blood cell count > 10,000/μL.
  Purulent material on culdocentesis.
  Pelvic abscess or inflammatory mass on pelvic examination or ultrasound.
  Gonococci present in endocervix on culture or Gram stain.

General Considerations

Pelvic inflammatory disease has increased in incidence in recent years owing to the rise in sexually transmitted disease. It is most common in young, nulliparous, sexually active women with multiple partners. Use of an IUD is associated with a 2-fold increase in risk; condoms or diaphragms with a spermicide provide significant protection. Endoparametritis can result from induced abortion or any other instrumentation of the uterus.

Pelvic inflammatory disease is a polymicrobial infection caused by a variety of aerobic and anaerobic bacteria, including *N gonorrhoeae, Peptostreptococcus, Bacteroides,* and *Chlamydia.* Organisms present in the endocervix may not be the same ones present in the uterine tubes and peritoneal cavity.

Tuberculous salpingitis is rare in the USA but more common in developing countries; it is characterized by pain and irregular pelvic masses not responsive to antibiotic therapy. Spread of disease is not by sexual contact.

Clinical Findings

A. Symptoms and Signs: Patients with pelvic inflammatory disease often have lower abdominal pain, chills and fever, menstrual disturbances, purulent cervical discharge, and cervical and adnexal tenderness. Right upper quadrant pain may indicate perihepatitis (Fitz-Hugh and Curtis syndrome), which is localized peritonitis involving the anterior surface of the liver and the adjacent peritoneum of the anterior abdominal wall. However, since these findings are not always present and are not specific to pelvic inflammatory disease, the criteria for diagnosis remain as stated above. In chronic pelvic inflammatory disease, dysmenorrhea, dyspareunia, infertility, recurrent low-grade fever, and tender pelvic masses are common.

B. Laboratory Findings: The white blood cell count and sedimentation rate are not consistently elevated. Gram stains and cultures of endocervical material and fluid obtained from culdocentesis (if available) are valuable guides to therapy. Gram stains of urethral material and cultures from the sexual partner, if available, are also useful.

C. Ultrasonic Findings: Pelvic ultrasound may help to distinguish the masses of pelvic infection from those of endometriosis, uterine myomas, ovarian cysts or tumors, and ectopic pregnancy.

Differential Diagnosis

Appendicitis, ectopic pregnancy, septic abortion, hemorrhagic or ruptured ovarian cysts or tumors, twisted ovarian cyst, degeneration of a myoma, and acute enteritis must be considered. Pelvic inflammatory disease is more likely to occur when there is a history of pelvic inflammatory disease, recent sexual contact, recent onset of menses, or an IUD in place or if the partner has a sexually transmitted disease. Acute pelvic inflammatory disease is highly unlikely when recent intercourse has not taken place or an IUD is not being used. A sensitive serum pregnancy test should be obtained to rule out ectopic pregnancy. Culdocentesis will differentiate hemoperitoneum (ruptured ectopic pregnancy or hemorrhagic cyst) from pelvic sepsis (salpingitis, ruptured pelvic abscess, or ruptured appendix). Pelvic ultrasound is helpful in the differential diagnosis of ectopic pregnancy of over 6 weeks. Laparoscopy is often utilized to diagnose pelvic inflammatory disease, and it is imperative if the diagnosis is not certain or if the patient has not responded to antibiotic therapy after 48 hours. The appendix should be visualized at laparoscopy to rule out appendicitis. Cultures obtained at the time of laparoscopy are often specific and helpful.

Treatment

A. Hospitalization: Patients with acute pelvic inflammatory disease should be hospitalized if there is fever higher than 38 °C or a possible pelvic abscess, if they are pregnant, if diagnosis is uncertain, or if oral antibiotics are not tolerated.

B. Antibiotics: Early treatment with appropriate antibiotics effective against *N gonorrhoeae, Chlamydia,* and anaerobes is essential to preserve fertility. Treatment of the sexual partner with tetracycline, 500 mg 4 times daily for 7 days, to eradicate *N gonorrhoeae* and *Chlamydia* should be given if possible.

Various treatment regimes for acute pelvic inflammatory disease are effective. Hospitalized patients can be given one of the following regimens: (1) Cefoxitin, 2 g intravenously every 6 hours, or cefotetan, 2 g intravenously every 12 hours, plus doxycycline, 100 mg intravenously twice daily. Continue intravenous administration for at least 48 hours after fever has abated. Continue tetracycline, 500 mg 4 times daily, or doxycycline, 100 mg twice daily orally to complete 10–14 days of therapy (contraindicated in pregnancy). (2) Clindamycin, 600 mg intravenously every 6 hours, plus gentamicin or tobramycin, 2 mg/ kg intravenously followed by 1.5 mg/kg intravenously every 8 hours. Continue intravenous administration for at least 48 hours after temperature is normal. Continue clindamycin, 450 mg 4 times daily orally to complete 10–14 days of therapy. (3) Metronidazole, 1 g intravenously every 12 hours, plus doxycycline, 100 mg intravenously every 12 hours. Continue intravenous administration for at least 48 hours after fever has abated. Then continue both drugs orally at the same dosage to complete 10–14 days of therapy.

Outpatients with milder cases of pelvic inflammatory disease should receive one of the following regimens: (1) ceftriaxone, 250 mg intramuscularly, followed by doxycycline, 100 mg twice daily orally, or tetracycline, 500 mg 4 times daily orally, for 10–14 days; or (2) cefoxitin, 2 g intramuscularly, with probenecid, 1 g orally, followed by doxycycline or tetracycline as above; or (3) amoxicillin, 3 g orally, or aqueous procaine penicillin G, 4.8 units intramuscularly, either with probenecid, 1 g orally, followed by doxycycline or tetracycline as above. Amoxicillin may not be as effective in areas where there is a high incidence of β-lactamase-producing gonococci.

C. General Measures: Fluids, a nutritious diet, and bed rest are advisable. Pain is controlled with simple analgesics. Sexual intercourse should be delayed until recovery is complete, often 2–3 months. Subsequent use of condoms or a diaphragm with a spermicide will reduce the risk of reinfection. Women who have had pelvic inflammatory disease should ask new or promiscuous partners to use condoms with a spermicide and should avoid coitus during menses, when flare-ups are most common.

D. Surgical Measures: Tubo-ovarian abscesses may require surgical excision or transcutaneous or transvaginal aspiration. Unless rupture is suspected, institute high-dose antibiotic therapy in the hospital, and monitor therapy with ultrasound. In 70% of cases, antibiotics are effective; in 30%, there is inadequate response in 48–72 hours, and intervention is required. Unilateral adnexectomy in the presence of unilateral abscess is acceptable. Hysterectomy and bilateral salpingo-oophorectomy may be necessary for overwhelming infection or in cases of chronic disease with intractable pelvic pain.

Prognosis

One-fourth of women with acute disease develop long-term sequelae, including repeated episodes of infection, chronic pelvic pain, dyspareunia, ectopic pregnancy, or infertility. The risk of infertility increases with repeated episodes of salpingitis: it is estimated at 11% after the first episode, 23% after a second episode, and 54% after a third episode.

Wolner-Hanssen P et al: Decreased risk of symptomatic chlamydial pelvic inflammatory disease associated with oral contraceptive use. JAMA 1990;263:54.

OVARIAN TUMORS

Ovarian tumors are common forms of neoplastic disease in women. Most are benign, but some are malignant. The wide range of types and patterns of ovarian tumors is due to the complexity of ovarian embryology and differences in tissue of origin. Most systems of classification utilize largely the tumor histogenesis, but there may be advantages to employing other criteria such as clinical behavior—functional and nonfunctional, cystic or solid—and always macroscopic or microscopic appearance (Table 13–4).

The incidence of ovarian cancer is increased in women with breast cancer or a family history of ovarian cancer in a first-degree relative.

The history and physical examination may be supplemented by selected imaging studies to define the status of the pelvis by ultrasound and MRI: evaluate other sites by upper and lower intestinal studies and intravenous urography. Laparoscopy is often useful for preoperative evaluation. Routine pelvic ultrasound has not been found to be a satisfactory screening test for early ovarian cancer.

Treatment

The treatment of ovarian tumors must be individualized. Small unilocular tumors (as determined by ultrasound) in premenopausal women can be observed for a few months. A 2-month trial of suppression of ovulation with oral contraceptives usually causes functional cysts to disappear. If ultrasound suggests septation or solid components, a neoplasm is more likely, and surgical exploration should be prompt. If a plain film of the abdomen shows calcification, a benign teratoma is likely. Whenever possible in young women, ovarian cystectomy rather than total removal of the ovary is desirable. An enlarged ovary in a postmenopausal woman should be evaluated promptly. If ultrasound study shows enlargement to twice the size of the contralateral ovary, surgery is indicated.

The initial surgery is the optimum time for a complete evaluation of the extent of the tumor and for its definitive treatment. Operations for suspected ovarian cancer should be performed at hospitals with facilities for performing frozen section biopsy and by personnel familiar with extended surgery, including bowel and bladder procedures.

Treatment for ovarian cancer is surgery (excision or debulking of any visible neoplasia, hysterectomy and bilateral oophorectomy, appendectomy, omentectomy, selective lymphadenectomy) and chemotherapy.

Table 13–4. Ovarian functional and neoplastic tumors.

Tumor	Incidence	Size	Consistency	Menstrual Irregularities	Endocrine Effects	Potential For Malignancy	Special Remarks
Follicle cysts	Rare in childhood; frequent in menstrual years; never in postmenopausal years.	< 6 cm, often bilateral.	Moderate	Occasional	Occasional anovulation with persistently proliferative endometrium.	0	Often disappear after a 2-month regimen of oral contraceptives.
Corpus luteum cysts	Occasional, in menstrual years.	4–6 cm, unilateral.	Moderate	Occasional delayed period	Prolonged secretory phase.	0	Functional cysts. Intraperitoneal bleeding occasionally.
Theca lutein cysts	Occurs with hydatidiform mole, choriocarcinoma; also with gonadotropin or clomiphene therapy.	To 4–5 cm, multiple, bilateral. (Ovaries may be ≥ 20 cm in diameter.)	Tense	Amenorrhea	hCG elevated as a result of trophoblastic proliferation.	0	Functional cysts. Hematoperitoneum or torsion of ovary may occur. Surgery to be avoided.
Inflammatory (tubo-ovarian abscess)	Concomitant with acute salpingitis.	To 15–20 cm, often bilateral.	Variable, painful	Menometrorrhagia	Anovulation usual.	0	Unilateral removal indicated if possible.
Endometriotic cysts	Never in preadolescent or postmenopausal years. Most common in women age 20–40 years.	To 10–12 cm, occasionally bilateral.	Moderate to softened	Rare	0	Very rare	Associated pelvic endometriosis. Medical treatment or conservative surgery recommended.
Teratoid tumors: Benign teratomas (dermoid cysts)	Childhood to postmenopause.	< 15 cm; 15% are bilateral.	Moderate to softened	0	0	Rare	Torsion can occur. Partial oophorectomy recommended.
Malignant teratomas	< 1% of ovarian tumors. Usually in infants and young adults.	> 20 cm, unilateral.	Irregularly firm	0	0	All	Unresponsive to any therapy.
Cystadenoma, cystadenocarcinoma	Common in reproductive years.	Serous: < 25 cm, 33% bilateral. Mucinous; up to 1 meter, 10% bilateral.	Moderate to softened / Moderate to softened	0	0	> 50% for serous. About 5% for mucinous.	Peritoneal implants often occur with serous tumors, rarely occur with mucinous tumors. If mucinous tumor is ruptured, pseudomyxoma peritonei may occur.
Endometrioid carcinoma	15% of ovarian carcinomas.	Moderate, 13% bilateral.	Firm	0	0	All	Adenocarcinoma of endometrium coexists in 15–30% of cases.
Fibroma	< 5% of ovarian tumors.	Usually < 15 cm.	Very firm	0	0	Rare	Ascites in 20% (rarely, pleural fluid).
Arrhenoblastoma	Rare. Average age 30 years or more.	Often small (< 10 cm), unilateral.	Firm to softened	Amenorrhea	Androgens elevated.	< 20%	Recurrences are moderately sensitive to irradiation.
Theca cell tumor (thecoma)	Uncommon.	< 10 cm, unilateral.	Firm	Occasionally irregular periods	Estrogens or androgens elevated.	< 1%	. . .
Granulosa cell tumor	Uncommon. Usually in prepubertal girls or women older than 50 years.	May be very small.	Firm to softened	Menometrorrhagia	Estrogens elevated.	15–20%	Recurrences are moderately sensitive to irradiation.
Dysgerminoma	About 1–2% of ovarian tumors.	< 30 cm, bilateral in one-third of cases.	Moderate to softened	0	. . .	All	Very radiosensitive.
Brenner tumor	About 1% of ovarian tumors.	< 30 cm, unilateral.	Firm	0	. . .	Very rare	> 50% occur in postmenopausal years.
Secondary ovarian tumors	10% of fatal malignant disease in women.	Varies, often bilateral.	Firm to softened	Occasional	Very rare (thyroid, adrenocortical origin).	All	Bowel or breast metastases to ovary common.

Prognosis

The prognosis for benign ovarian tumors after surgical removal is excellent. The outlook for ovarian cancer, unless diagnosed in the earliest stages, is poor. There is no satisfactory screening test for ovarian cancer at present. The CA 125 blood test can be used to follow the possibility of recurrence after surgery or the response to chemotherapy.

Richardson GS et al: Common epithelial cancer of the ovary. N Engl J Med 1985;312:415.

PERSISTENT ANOVULATION (Polycystic Ovary Syndrome, Stein-Leventhal Syndrome)

Essentials of Diagnosis

- Chronic anovulation.
- Infertility.
- Elevated plasma LH values and a reversed FSH/ LH ratio.
- Hirsutism (in 70% of patients).

General Considerations

These patients have a relatively steady state of high estrogen, androgen, and LH levels, rather than the fluctuating condition seen in ovulating women. Increased levels of estrone come from obesity (conversion of ovarian and adrenal androgens to estrone in body fat) or from excessive levels of androgens seen in some women of normal weight. The high estrone levels are believed to cause a suppression of pituitary FSH and a relative increase in LH. Constant LH stimulation of the ovary results in anovulation, multiple cysts, and theca cell hyperplasia with excess androgen output. The polycystic ovary has a thickened, pearly white capsule.

Women with Cushing's syndrome, congenital adrenal hyperplasia, and androgen-secreting adrenal tumors also tend to have high circulating androgen levels and anovulation with polycystic ovaries.

Clinical Findings

Polycystic ovary syndrome is manifested by hirsutism (70% of cases), obesity (40%), and virilization (20%). Fifty percent of patients have amenorrhea, 30% have abnormal uterine bleeding, and 20% have normal menstruation. Additionally, they show insulin resistance and hyperinsulinemia when infused with glucose. The patients are generally infertile, although they may ovulate occasionally. They have an increased long-term risk of cancer of the breast and endome trium because of unopposed estrogen secretion.

Differential Diagnosis

Anovulation in the reproductive years may also be due to (1) premature menopause (high FSH and LH levels); (2) rapid weight loss or extreme physical exertion (normal FSH and LH levels for age); (3) discontinuation of oral contraceptives (anovulation for 6 months or more occasionally occurs); (4) pituitary adenoma with elevated prolactin (galactorrhea may or may not be present); (5) hyper- or hypothyroidism. Always check FSH, LH, prolactin, and TSH levels when amenorrhea has persisted for 6 months or more without a diagnosis. A 10-day course of progestin (eg, medroxyprogesterone acetate, 10 mg/ d) will cause withdrawal bleeding if estrogen levels are high. This will aid in the diagnosis and prevent endometrial hyperplasia. In long-term anovular patients over age 35, it is wise to search for an estrogen-stimulated cancer with mammography and endometrial aspiration.

Treatment

In obese patients with polycystic ovaries, weight reduction is often effective; a decrease in body fat will lower the conversion of androgens to estrone and thereby help to restore ovulation.

If the patient wishes to become pregnant, clomiphene or other drugs can be employed for ovulatory stimulation. Ovulation can also be restored in some patients with dexamethasone, 0.5 mg each night. Wedge resection of the ovary is often successful in restoring ovulation and fertility, although this procedure is used less commonly now that medical treatments are available.

If the patient does not desire pregnancy, give medroxyprogesterone acetate, 10 mg/d for the first 10 days of each month. This will ensure regular shedding of the endometrium so that hyperplasia will not occur. If contraception is desired, a low-dose combination oral contraceptive can be used; this is also useful in controlling hirsutism, for which treatment must be continued for 6–12 months before results are seen.

Hirsutism may be managed with epilation and electrolysis. Dexamethasone, 0.5 mg each night, is helpful in women with excess adrenal androgen secretion. If hirsutism is severe, some patients will elect to have a hysterectomy and bilateral oophorectomy followed by estrogen replacement therapy. Spironolactone, an aldosterone antagonist, is also useful for hirsutism in doses of 25 mg 3 or 4 times daily. The benefits of this drug in reducing hair growth must be weighed against its potential side effects of hyperkalemia, menstrual abnormalities, sedation, headache, ataxia, etc.

Nestler JE, Clore JN, Blackard WG: The central role of obesity (hyperinsulinemia) in the pathogenesis of the polycystic ovary syndrome. Am J Obstet Gynecol 1989;161:1095.

URINARY INCONTINENCE

Occasional loss of urine under a variety of circumstances occurs in 40% of women. Urinary frequency, nocturia, and urgency are sometimes associated with incontinence. A careful history of drinking and voiding habits, amount of leakage and timing of leakage, and evidence of urinary tract infection will help in diagnosis. The normal bladder holds up to 500 mL, and voiding generally occurs every 2–3 hours while awake.

Women with stress incontinence following childbirth have urethras displaced downward from the normal position above the urogenital diaphragm. Sudden increases in intra-abdominal pressure are transmitted to the otherwise normally functioning bladder but not to the prolapsed urethra, and so urine tends to leak at that moment. Estrogen-deprived postmenopausal women have similar urine loss due to decreased tone of the urethra and surrounding tissue.

Abnormal bladder muscle (detrusor) function can also cause incontinence. A hypotonic (neurogenic) bladder will have a large capacity and will empty spontaneously and incompletely by overflow. A hypertonic bladder with a small capacity and variable levels of high detrusor tone will also cause urine loss intermittently with or without increases in intra-abdominal pressure.

Symptoms, history, physical examination, and routine laboratory tests sometimes are insufficient for accurate diagnosis. When the cause of incontinence is unclear or when there are multiple symptoms, cystometric study of the bladder may be needed. Cystometry measures pressures within the bladder and along the urethra during bladder filling and with the patient in different positions and with different stress mechanisms such as coughing.

Treatment

Effective therapy for pure stress incontinence will increase the patient's ability to transmit intravesical pressure to the mid urethra but will not necessarily improve intraurethral pressure per se. A trial of medical treatment is always indicated before surgery is considered.

Medical disorders such as diabetes mellitus, extreme obesity, and chronic and recurrent urinary tract infections should be controlled if possible. Postmenopausal women should receive a trial of estrogen replacement (either cyclic oral medication or small doses of vaginal cream). Patients who do not have serious neurologic disorders and have not sustained severe physical injury can be taught to contract the pubococcygeus muscles repeatedly to help reestablish and increase control of the urogenital diaphragm and thus improve urinary function (Kegel isometric exercises). For maximum effect, sequences of exercises should be done 3–4 times a day for several months. Patients who fail to respond to exercises or medical treatment may be candidates for surgery, particularly when cystocele or prolapse of the bladder and uterus is present.

A study of bladder dynamics will identify abnormal detrusor activity as well as an unusually large or small bladder capacity. Measurement of closing pressures along the urethra will help in determining whether surgical procedures to lengthen and support the urethra will be successful. A voiding cystourethrogram will identify an excessively mobile prolapsing urethra. A useful surgical prognostic test is to elevate the anterior vaginal wall lateral to the urethra at the urethrovesical junction with a Smith-Hodge pessary. If loss of urine does not occur with cough, the surgical prognosis is good.

Medical therapy alone improves half of cases to some degree and should be tried before surgery in women with confirmed stress and urge incontinence. The overall cure rate in patients who require operation is about 85%. The most successful procedure is retropubic suspension of the paravaginal tissues (Burch procedure). Other types of urethral suspension (Pereyra operation) and vaginal urethral plication are occasional alternatives.

Patients with irritable bladders of decreased capacity who have annoying frequency and urge incontinence can be encouraged to retrain their bladders by scheduled voidings at increasing intervals. Initial improvement occurs within 2–4 weeks, and retraining should continue for 4–6 months. A variety of drugs with anticholinergic activity have also proved useful for frequency, nocturia, and urge incontinence. Among these are propantheline, 5 mg twice daily; dicyclomine, 10 mg daily or twice daily; oxybutynin, 5 mg twice daily; and flavoxate, 100 mg twice daily. Imipramine, 25 mg daily or twice daily, and amitriptyline, 25 mg daily or twice daily, can be used for their anticholinergic effects as well as their antidepressant activity. In older women, the risk of these drugs for precipitation of angle-closure glaucoma should be recognized. Indomethacin, 50 mg daily or twice daily, and nifedipine, 10 mg daily or twice daily, have also been tried.

PAINFUL INTERCOURSE (Dyspareunia)

Questions related to sexual functioning should be asked as part of the reproductive history. Two helpful questions are, "Are you sexually active?" and "Are you having any sexual difficulties at this time?" The physician should be able to provide sex counseling and should allow adequate time for a discussion of problems related to sexuality, personal relationships, contraception, and fears of pregnancy.

Painful intercourse may be caused by vulvovaginitis; vaginismus; an incompletely stretched hymen; insufficient lubrication of the vagina; vaginal atrophy; or tumors or other pathologic conditions. Careful history taking and a thorough pelvic examination are essential. During the pelvic examination, the patient should be placed in a half-sitting position and given a hand-held mirror and then asked to point out the site of pain and describe the type of pain.

Etiology

A. Vulvovaginitis: Vulvovaginitis is inflammation or infection of the vagina. Areas of marked tenderness in the vulvar vestibule without visible inflammation occasionally show lesions resembling small condylomas on colposcopy. For a detailed discussion of vaginitis, see that section of this chapter.

B. Vaginismus: Vaginismus is voluntary or involuntary contraction of muscles around the introitus. It results from fear, pain, sexual trauma, or having learned negative attitudes toward sex during childhood.

C. Remnants of the Hymen: The hymen is usually adequately stretched during initial intercourse, so that pain does not occur subsequently. In some women, the pain of initial intercourse may produce vaginismus. In others, a thin or thickened rim or partial rim of hymen remains after several episodes of intercourse, causing pain.

D. Insufficient Lubrication of the Vagina: Insufficient vaginal lubrication may be due to inadequate time for sexual arousal or to low estrogen effect during lactation or following menopause. When estrogen levels are normal (as evidenced by the occurrence of menstrual periods or the presence of moist, healthy-appearing vaginal mucosa with rugal folds), dyspareunia is probably due to inadequate sexual arousal prior to coitus. Low estrogen levels are evidenced by decreased introital diameter, dry vaginal mucosa, fewer rugal folds, and thinned, reddened epithelium.

E. Infection, Endometriosis, Tumors, or Other Pathologic Conditions: Pain occurring with deep thrusting during coitus is usually due to acute or chronic infection of the cervix, uterus, or adnexa; endometriosis; adnexal tumors; or adhesions resulting from prior pelvic disease or operation. Careful history taking and a pelvic examination will generally help in the differential diagnosis.

F. Dyspareunia Due to Unknown Cause: Occasionally, no organic cause of pain can be found. These patients may have psychosexual conflicts or a history of childhood sexual abuse.

Treatment

A. Vulvovaginitis: Infection or inflammation should be treated after careful diagnosis. Vestibular lesions resembling warts on colposcopy or biopsy should be treated in the appropriate way (see Vaginitis). The sexual partner should also be treated to prevent recurrence. Irritation from spermicides may be a factor. The couple may be helped by a discussion of noncoital techniques to achieve organism until the infection subsides.

B. Vaginismus: Sexual counseling and education on anatomy and sexual functioning may be appropriate. The patient can be instructed in self-dilation, using a lubricated finger or test tubes of graduated sizes. Before coitus (with adequate lubrication) is attempted, the patient—and then her partner—should be able to easily and painlessly introduce 2 fingers into the vagina. Penetration should never be forced, and the woman should always be the one to control the depth of insertion during dilation or intercourse.

C. Remnants of the Hymen: In rare situations, manual dilation of a remaining hymen under general anesthesia is necessary. Surgery should be avoided.

D. Insufficient Lubrication of the Vagina: If inadequate sexual arousal is the cause, sexual counseling for the woman—and her partner if possible—is helpful. Lubricants may be used during sexual foreplay. For women with low plasma estrogen levels, use of a lubricant during coitus is sometimes sufficient. If not, use conjugated estrogen cream, one-eighth applicatorful daily for 10 days and then every other day. Using the applicator or a finger, the patient can apply the cream directly to the most tender area, usually the hymenal ring. Testosterone cream 1–2% in a water-soluble base is also helpful.

E. Infection, Endometriosis, Tumors, or Other Pathologic Conditions: Medical treatment of acute cervicitis, endometritis, of salpingitis and temporary abstention from coitus usually relieve pain. Hormonal or surgical treatment of endometriosis may be helpful. Dyspareunia resulting from chronic pelvic inflammatory disease or any condition causing extensive adhesions or fixation of pelvic organs is difficult to treat without extirpative surgery. Couples can be advised to try coital positions that limit deep thrusting and to use manual and oral sexual techniques.

F. Dyspareunia Due to Unknown Cause: Colposcopy in discrete areas of pain without obvious lesions may be useful to rule out papilloma virus infections. Biopsies should be taken if there is an identifiable lesion. Supportive, understanding discussion may be helpful. Small amounts of topical remedies such as 1% testosterone cream, estrogen cream, or topical lidocaine gel may relieve pain. Resolution of psychosexual problems or problems relating to traumatic sexual experiences may be necessary.

Bachman GA, Leiblum SR, Grill J: Brief sexual inquiry in gynecologic practice. Obstet Gynecol 1989;73:425.

INFERTILITY

A couple is said to be infertile if pregnancy does not result after 1 year of normal sexual activity without contraceptives. About 14% of couples are infertile; the incidence of infertility increases with age. The male partner contributes to about 40% of cases of infertility. A combination of factors is common. Couples whose infertility is unexplained after evaluation have a 34% chance of conceiving within 6 months and a 76% chance by 2 years.

Diagnostic Survey

A basic infertility study can be performed, usually within a 3-month period, although timing can vary depending on convenience and the desires of the couple. Both partners are evaluated.

During the initial interview, the physician can present an overview of infertility and discuss a plan of study. Separate private consultations are then conducted, allowing appraisal of psychosexual adjustment without embarrassment or criticism. Pertinent details (eg, sexually transmitted disease or prior pregnancies) must be obtained. A complete medical, surgical, occupational, and obstetric history must be taken. The ill effects of excess caffeine, cigarettes, alcohol, and other recreational drugs on fertility in both men and women should be discussed. Prescription drugs that impair male potency should be noted. The gynecologic history should include queries regarding the menstrual pattern. The present history includes use and types of contraceptives, douches, libido, sex techniques, frequency and success of coitus, and correlation of intercourse with time of ovulation. Family history includes familial traits, illnesses, repeated abortions, maternal DES use, and abnormal children.

General physical and genital examinations are performed on both partners. Basic laboratory studies include complete blood count, urinalysis cervical culture for *Chlamydia,* serologic test for syphilis, rubella antibody determination, and thyroid function tests. Tay-Sachs screening should be offered if both parents are Jews and sickle cell screening if both parents are black. Screening mammography can also be offered to women over 35.

The woman is instructed to chart her basal body temperature orally daily on arising and to record on a graph episodes of coitus and days of menstruation. Self-performed urine tests for the midcycle LH surge can be used to enhance temperature observations relating to ovulation.

The man is instructed to bring a complete ejaculate for analysis. Sexual abstinence for at least 3 days before the semen is obtained is emphasized. A clean, dry, wide-mouthed bottle for collection is preferred. Condoms should not be employed, as the protective powder or lubricant may be spermicidal. Semen should be examined within 1–2 hours after collection. Semen is considered normal with the following minimum values; volume, 3 mL; concentration, 20 million sperm per milliliter; motility, 50% after 2 hours; and normal forms, 60%. If the sperm count is abnormal, further evaluation includes a search for exposure to environmental and workplace toxins, alcohol or drug abuse, and hypogonadism.

A. First Testing Cycle: A postcoital test (Sims-Huhner test) is scheduled for just before ovulation (eg, day 12 or 13 in an expected 28-day cycle). Preovulation timing can be enhanced by serial urinary LH tests or repeated measurement of ovarian follicle growth by ultrasound. The patient is examined within 6 hours after coitus. The cervical mucus should be clear, elastic, and copious owing to the influence of the preovular estrogen surge. (The mucus is scantier and more viscid before and after ovulation.) A good spinnbarkeit (stretching to a fine thread 4 cm or more in length) is desirable. A small drop of cervical mucus should be obtained from within the cervical os and examined under the microscope. The presence of 5 or more active sperm per high-power field constitutes a satisfactory postcoital test. If no spermatozoa are found, the test should be repeated (assuming that active spermatozoa were present in the semen analysis). Sperm agglutination and sperm immobilization tests should be considered if the sperm are immotile or show ineffective tail motility.

The presence of more than 3 white blood cells per high-power field in the postcoital test suggests cervicitis in the woman or prostatitis in the man. When estrogen levels are normal, the cervical mucus dried on the slide will form a fernlike pattern when viewed with a low-power microscope. This type of mucus is necessary for normal sperm transport.

The serum progesterone level should be measured at the midpoint of the secretory phase (21st day); a level of 10–20 ng/mL confirms adequate luteal function.

B. Second Testing Cycle: Hysterosalpingography using an oil dye is performed within 3 days following the menstrual period. This x-ray study will demonstrate uterine abnormalities (septa, polyps, submucous myomas) and tubal obstruction. A repeat x-ray film 24 hours later will confirm tubal patency if there is wide pelvic dispersion of the dye. This test has been associated with an increased pregnancy rate by some observers. If the woman has had prior pelvic inflammation, give tetracycline, 2 g/d, beginning immediately before and for 7 days after the x-ray study.

C. Further Testing:

1. Gross deficiencies of sperm (number, motility, or appearance) require repeat analysis. Zona-free hamster egg penetration tests are available to evaluate the ability of human sperm to fertilize an egg.

2. Obvious obstruction of the uterine tubes requires assessment for microsurgery or in vitro fertilization.

3. Absent or infrequent ovulation requires additional laboratory evaluation. Elevated FSH and LH levels indicate ovarian failure causing premature menopause (in women under age 30, karyotyping is indicated to rule out chromosomal abnormalities). Elevated LH levels in the presence of normal FSH levels confirm the presence of polycystic ovaries. Elevation of blood prolactin (PRL) levels suggests pituitary microadenoma.

4. Major histocompatibility antigen typing of both partners will confirm human leukocyte antigen-B locus homozygosity, which is found in greater than expected numbers among couples with unexplained infertility.

5. Ultrasound monitoring of folliculogenesis may reveal the occurrence of unruptured luteinized follicles. **6.** Endometrial biopsy in the luteal phase associated with simultaneous serum progesterone levels will rule out luteal phase deficiency.

D. Laparoscopy: Approximately 25% of women whose basic evaluation is normal will have findings on laparoscopy explaining their infertility (eg, peritubal adhesions, endometriotic implants).

Treatment

A. Medical Measures: Fertility may be restored by appropriate treatment in many patients with endocrine imbalance, particularly those with hypo- or hyperthyroidism. Antibiotic treatment of cervicitis is of value. After 6 months of condom protection during intercourse, an antigen-antibody reaction will usually resolve, and sperm agglutination or immobilization should cease to be a problem.

Women who engage in vigorous athletic training often have low sex hormone levels; fertility improves with reduced exercise and some weight gain.

B. Surgical Measures: Excision of ovarian tumors or ovarian foci of endometriosis can improve fertility. Microsurgical relief of tubal obstruction due to salpingitis or tubal ligation will reestablish fertility in a significant number of cases. In special instances of cornual or fimbrial block, the prognosis with newer surgical techniques has become much better. Peritubal adhesions or endometriotic implants often can be treated via laparoscopy or via laparotomy immediately following laparoscopic examination if prior consent has been obtained.

With varicocele in the male, sperm characteristics are often improved following surgical treatment.

C. Induction of Ovulation:

1. Clomiphene citrate (Clomid)–Clomiphene citrate stimulates gonadotropin release, especially LH. Consequently, plasma estrone (E_1) and estradiol (E_2) also rise, reflecting ovarian follicle maturation. If E_2 rises sufficiently, an LH surge occurs to trigger ovulation.

After a normal menstrual period or induction of withdrawal bleeding with progestin, give 50 mg of clomiphene orally daily for 5 days. If ovulation does not occur, increase the dose to 100 mg orally daily for 5 days. If ovulation still does not occur, repeat the course with 150 and then 200 mg daily for 5 days and add chorionic gonadotropin, 10,000 units intramuscularly, 7 days after clomiphene.

The rate of ovulation following this treatment is 90% in the absence of other infertility factors. The pregnancy rate is high. Twinning occurs in 5% of these patients, and 3 or more fetuses are found in rare instances (< 0.5% of cases). An increased incidence of congenital anomalies has not been reported. Painful ovarian cyst formation occurs in 8% of patients and may warrant discontinuation of therapy.

In the presence of increased androgen production (DHEA-S > 200 μg/dL), the addition of dexamethasone, 0.5 mg, or prednisone, 5 mg, at bedtime, improves the response to clomiphene. Dexamethasone should be discontinued after pregnancy is confirmed.

2. Bromocriptine (Parlodel)–Use only if PRL levels are elevated and there is no withdrawal bleeding following progesterone administration (otherwise use clomiphene). The usual dose is 2.5 mg twice daily. To minimize side effects (nausea, diarrhea, dizziness, headache, fatigue), bromocriptine should be taken with meals. Begin with 2.5 mg once daily and increase to 2–3 times daily in increments of 1.25 mg. The drug is discontinued once pregnancy has occurred.

3. Human menopausal gonadotropins (hMG) (Pergonal)–hMG is indicated in cases of hypogonadotropism and most other types of anovulation (exclusive of ovarian failure). Because of the complexities, laboratory tests, and expense associated with this treatment, patients who require hMG for the induction of ovulation should be referred to a specialist. Hypothalamic amenorrhea unresponsive to clomiphene will be reliably and successfully treated with subcutaneous pulsatile gonadotropin-releasing hormone (GnRH). Use of this substance will avoid the dangerous ovarian complications and the 25% incidence of multiple pregnancy associated with hMG.

4. Ovarian wedge resection–Wedge resection is indicated rarely and only when medical measures are not effective.

D. Treatment of Endometriosis: See p 515.

E. Treatment of Low Midluteal Progesterone Levels: Midluteal progesterone levels of less than 10 ng/mL can be treated with one of the following regimens:

1. Progesterone suppositories, 50 mg twice daily on days 17–31 of the ovarian cycle. If the woman becomes pregnant, continue for 8 weeks.

2. Clomiphene (see above) can also be used for luteal phase insufficiency.

F. Treatment of Inadequate Transport of Sperm:

1. Cervical mucus will provide better transport following administration of 0.3 mg of conjugated equine estrogens from days 5 to 15 of the ovarian cycle (ovulation may be delayed).

2. Intrauterine insemination of concentrated washed sperm has been used to bypass a poor cervical environment associated with scant or hostile cervical mucus. The sperm must be handled by sterile methods, washed in sterile saline or tissue culture solutions, and centrifuged. A small amount of fluid (0.5 mL) containing the sperm is then instilled into the uterus.

G. Artificial Insemination in Azoospermia: If azoospermia is present, artificial insemination by a donor usually results in pregnancy, assuming female function is normal. Both partners must consent to this method. The use of frozen sperm is currently preferable to fresh sperm because the frozen specimen can be held pending cultures and blood test results for sexually transmitted diseases, including AIDS.

H. New Reproductive Technologies—In Vitro Fertilization-Embryo Transfer: This technique is becoming a standard approach to fertility problems involving severe tubal disease, in couples with unexplained long-term infertility, and where the male is oligospermic. A highly organized team of specialists in reproductive function and sophisticated technology are required for successful results. Ultrasound-guided aspiration of oocytes has replaced laparoscopic retrieval in most cases. Two or 3 embryos are placed to maximize the chances of implantation. Cryopreservation of excess embryos has allowed repeated transfers if the initial attempt fails. Women with transmissible genetic diseases or those with premature ovarian failure are potential recipients of donated frozen embryos.

Data collected in 1987 showed that the in vitro fertilization pregnancy rate was 15% of completed transfer cycles, with 12% of these pregnancies resulting in living children with no excess of anomalies. Variations in the standard transcervical placement of embryos now include gamete or zygote intra-fallopian tube transfer (GIFT; ZIFT).

Prognosis

The prognosis for conception and normal pregnancy is good if minor (even multiple) disorders can be identified and treated; poor if the causes of infertility are severe, untreatable, or of prolonged duration (over 3 years).

It is important to remember that in the absence of severe causes of infertility (azoospermia, prolonged amenorrhea, or bilateral tubal obstruction), 30% of couples will achieve a pregnancy within 3 years. Most of these successes will be unrelated to therapy. Offering appropriately timed information about adoption is considered part of a complete infertility regimen.

Collins JA et al: Treatment-independent pregnancy among infertile couples. N Engl J Med 1983;309:1201.
Howe G et al: Effects of age, cigarette smoking, and other factors on fertility: Findings in a large prospective study. Br Med J 1985;290:1697.
Seibel MM: A new era in reproductive technology: In vitro fertilization, gamete intrafallopian transfer, and donated gametes and embryos. N Engl J Med 1988;318:828.

CONTRACEPTION

Voluntary control of childbearing benefits women, men, and the children born to them. Contraception should be available to all women and men of reproductive ages. Education about contraception and access to contraceptive pills or devices are especially important for sexually active teenagers and for women following childbirth or abortion.

Education about sexually transmitted disease, especially AIDS, should be given to all sexually active people, along with information that condoms with spermicide offer a high degree of protection (but not complete protection) to both sexes against sexually transmitted disease as well as pregnancy. The worldwide AIDS epidemic should cause a significant shift toward the use of condoms plus spermicide.

1. ORAL CONTRACEPTIVES

Combined Oral Contraceptives

A. Efficacy and Methods of Use: Oral contraceptives (birth control pills) have a theoretical failure rate of less than 0.5% if taken absolutely on schedule and a typical failure rate of 3%. Their primary mode of action is suppression of ovulation. The pills are initially started on the first or fifth day of the ovarian cycle and taken daily for 21 days, followed by 7 days of placebos or no medication, and this schedule is then continued for each cycle. The pills are often started on the first Sunday after the onset of menses, to help patients remember their starting day and to avoid menses on the weekend. If a pill is missed at any time, 2 pills should be taken the next day, and another method of contraception should be used for the rest of the cycle (eg, condoms or foam). A backup method should also be used during the first cycle if the pills are started later than the fifth day.

B. Benefits of Oral Contraceptives: Besides offering convenient, effective contraception, there are noncontraceptive advantages to oral contraceptives. Menstrual flow is lighter, resultant anemia is less common, and dysmenorrhea is relieved for most women. Functional ovarian cysts generally disappear with oral contraceptive use, and new cysts do not occur. Pain with ovulation and postovulatory aching are relieved. The risk of ovarian and endometrial cancer is decreased. The risks of salpingitis and ectopic pregnancy may be diminished. Acne is usually improved. The frequency of developing myomas is lower in long-term users (> 4 years).

C. Selection of an Oral Contraceptive: Most clinicians first prescribe 30–35 μg of estrogen combined with 1 mg or less of progestin. This low dose of estrogen provides highly effective contraception but is also associated with more spotting, breakthrough bleeding, and missed menstrual periods than higher doses, and the patient should be warned of these side effects. Patients taking pills containing more than 50 μg of estrogen should be switched to lower doses, since many adverse side effects of the pill are dose-related. The progestins vary in potency and androgenicity. When hirsutism or acne is a problem, it is best to use ethynodiol diacetate or norethindrone. When breakthrough bleeding or dysfunctional bleeding occurs, many clinicians use a compound with norgestrel. Low-dose oral contraceptives currently used in the USA are shown in Table 13–5.

D. Drug Interactions: Several drugs interact with

Table 13–5. Commonly used low-dose oral contraceptives.

Name	Type	Progestin	Estrogen (Ethinyl Estradiol)
Lo/Ovral	Combination	0.3 mg dl-norgestrel	30 μg
Nordette and Levlen	Combination	0.15 mg levonorgestrel	30 μg
Norinyl 1/35 and Or-tho-Novum 1/35	Combination	1 mg norethindrone	35 μg
Loestrin 1.5/30	Combination	1.5 mg norethindrone acetate	30 μg
Demulen 1/35	Combination	1 mg ethynodiol diacetate	35 μg
Brevicon and Modicon	Combination	0.5 mg norethindrone	35 μg
Ovcon 35	Combination	0.4 mg norethindrone	35 μg
Ortho-novum 10/11	Biphasic	0.5 mg norethindrone (days 1–10) 1 mg norethindrone (days 11–21)	35 μg
Ortho-novum 777	Triphasic	0.5 mg norethindrone (days 1–7) 0.75 mg norethindrone (days 8–14) 1 mg norethindrone (days 15–21)	35 μg
Tri-Norinyl	Triphasic	0.5 mg norethindrone (days 1–7) 1 mg norethindrone (days 8–16) 0.5 mg norethindrone (days 17–21)	35 μg
Triphasil and Tri-Levlen	Triphasic	0.05 mg levonorgestrel (days 1–6) 0.075 mg levonorgestrel (days 7–11) 0.125 mg levonorgestrel (days 12–21)	30 μg 40 μg 30 μg
Micronor and Nor-QD	Progestin-only minipill	0.35 mg norethindrone to be taken continuously	
Ovrette	Progestin-only minipill	0.075 mg dl-norgestrel to be taken continuously	

oral contraceptives to decrease their efficacy by caus-ing induction of microsomal enzymes in the liver, by increasing sex hormone-binding globulin, and by other mechanisms. Some commonly prescribed drugs in this category are the anticonvulsants phenytoin, phenobarbital (and other barbiturates), primidone, and carbamazepine and the antituberculous drug rifampin. Women taking these drugs should use another means of contraception for maximum safety.

E. Contraindications and Adverse Effects: Oral contraceptives have been associated with many adverse effects; they are contraindicated in some situa-tions and should be used with caution in others (Table 13–6).

1. Myocardial infarction–The risk of heart at-tack is higher with use of oral contraceptives, particu-larly with pills containing 50 mg of estrogen or more. Age over 44 years; cigarette smoking; obesity; or the presence of hypertension, diabetes, or hypercho-lesterolemia increases the risk. Young nonsmoking women have minimal increased risk. Smokers over age 30–35 and women with other cardiovascular risk factors should use other methods of birth control.

2. Thromboembolic disease–An increased rate of fatal and nonfatal venous thromboembolism is found in oral contraceptive users, especially if the dose of estrogen is 50 μg or more. Women who develop thrombophlebitis should stop using this method, as should those at risk of thrombophlebitis because of surgery, fracture, serious injury, or immo-bilization.

3. Cerebrovascular disease–An increased risk of thrombotic and hemorrhagic stroke and subarach-noid hemorrhage has been found; smoking is associ-ated with increased risk. Women who develop warn-ing symptoms such as severe headache, blurred or lost vision, or other transient neurologic disorders should stop using oral contraceptives. Women with hypertensive disease should not use the pill.

4. Carcinoma–A relationship between long-term (3–4 years) oral contraceptive use and occurrence of cervical dysplasia and cancer has been found in various studies. No confirmed relationship has been found between use of oral contraceptives and cancer of the breast. Birth control pills appear to protect against endometrial and ovarian cancer. Rarely, oral

Table 13–6. Contraindications to use of oral contraceptives.

Absolute contraindications
Pregnancy
Thrombophlebitis or thromboembolic disorders (past or present)
Stroke or coronary artery disease (past or present)
Cancer of the breast (known or suspected)
Undiagnosed abnormal vaginal bleeding
Estrogen-dependent cancer (known or suspected)
Benign or malignant tumor of the liver (past or present)
Relative contraindications
Age over 35 years and heavy cigarette smoking (> 15 cigarettes daily)
Cervical intraepithelial neoplasia
Migraine or recurrent persistent, severe headache
Hypertension
Cardiac or renal disease
Diabetes
Gallbladder disease
Cholestasis during pregnancy
Active hepatitis or infectious mononucleosis
Sickle cell disease (S/S or S/C type)
Surgery, fracture, or severe injury
Lactation
Significant psychologic depression

contraceptives have been associated with the development of benign or malignant hepatic tumors; this may lead to rupture of the liver, hemorrhage, and death. The risk increases with higher dosage, longer duration of use, and older age.

5. Gallbladder disease–There is an increased risk of gallbladder disease and subsequent cholecystectomy for cholesterol stones in pill users.

6. Metabolic disorders–A decrease in glucose tolerance and an increase in triglyceride levels is seen in pill takers, and women with diabetes should therefore rarely use this method.

7. Hypertension–Oral contraceptives may cause hypertension in some women; the risk is increased with longer duration of use and older age. Women who have or develop hypertension should use other contraceptive methods.

8. Headache–Migraine or other vascular headaches may occur or worsen with pill use. If severe or frequent, the pill should not be used.

9. Amenorrhea–Postpill amenorrhea lasting a year or longer occurs occasionally, sometimes with galactorrhea. PRL levels should be checked; if elevated, a pituitary prolactinoma may be present.

10. Disorders of lactation–Combined oral contraceptives can impair the quantity and quality of breast milk and should therefore not be given before the infant is weaned. Progestin-only minipills can be used during lactation.

11. Other disorders–Psychologic depression may occur or be worsened with oral contraceptive use. Fluid retention may occur. Asthma may be worsened. Patients who had cholestatic jaundice during pregnancy may develop jaundice while taking birth control pills. Contact lens use may become more difficult.

F. Minor Side Effects: Nausea and dizziness may occur in the first few months of pill use. A weight gain of 2–5 lb commonly occurs. Spotting or breakthrough bleeding between menstrual periods may occur, especially if a pill is skipped or taken late; this may be helped by switching to a pill of slightly greater potency (see ¶C, above). Missed menstrual periods may occur, especially with low-dose pills. A pregnancy test should be performed if pills have been skipped or if 2 or more menstrual periods are missed. Depression, fatigue, and decreased libido can occur. Chloasma may occur, as in pregnancy, and is increased by exposure to sunlight.

Progestin Minipill

A. Efficacy and Methods of Use: Formulations containing 0.35 mg of norethindrone or 0.075 mg of norgestrel are available in the USA. Their efficacy is slightly lower than that of combined oral contraceptives, with failure rates of 1–4% being reported. The minipill is believed to prevent conception by causing thickening of the cervical mucus to make it hostile to sperm, alteration of ovum transport (which may account for the higher rate of ectopic pregnancy with these pills), and inhibition of implantation. Ovulation is inhibited inconsistently with this method. The minipill is begun on the first day of a menstrual cycle and then taken continuously for as long as contraception is desired.

B. Advantages: The low dose and absence of estrogen make the minipill safe during lactation; it may increase the flow of milk. It is often tried by women who want minimal doses of hormones and by patients who are over age 35. The minipill can be used by women with uterine myomas or sickle cell disease (S/S or S/C). Like the combined pill, the minipill decreases the likelihood of pelvic inflammatory disease by its effect on cervical mucus.

C. Complications and Contraindications: Minipill users often have bleeding irregularities (eg, prolonged flow, spotting, or amenorrhea); such patients may need monthly pregnancy tests. Ectopic pregnancies are more frequent, and complaints of abdominal pain should be investigated with this in mind. The absolute contraindications and many of the relative contraindications listed in Table 13–6 apply to the minipill. Exceptions are mentioned in ¶B, above. Minor side effects of combination oral contraceptives such as weight gain and mild headache may also occur with the minipill.

Mishell DR: Contraception. N Engl J Med 1989;320:777.

2. CONTRACEPTIVE INJECTIONS & IMPLANTS (Long-Acting Progestins)

Injections of long-acting progestins such as medroxyprogesterone acetate or norethindrone enanthate are widely used in many countries. They are not approved for contraception in the USA because of FDA concerns about animal studies showing an increased incidence of associated breast and genital tract cancer. Injections are given at 3- to 6-month intervals. Pregnancy rates are as low as those of combined oral contraceptives taken conscientiously. Uterine bleeding may be irregular at first, and amenorrhea eventually occurs. Ovulation after the last injection may be delayed. Absolute and relative contraindications are similar to those of the minipill.

Norplant, a new contraceptive implant containing levonorgestrel, is available in over 40 countries worldwide. Thirty micrograms of levonorgestrel is released daily from 6 subcutaneously placed rods. The system is effective for 5 years. Contraceptive efficacy is very high, but 25% of patients request removal of the implants because of irregular bleeding.

3. INTRAUTERINE DEVICES (IUDs)

The only IUDs currently manufactured in the USA are the Progestasert (which secretes progesterone into the uterus) and the Copper T380A. Some all-plastic IUDs (Lippes Loop) are also still in use. Failure rates of most IUDs are 2–4%; the mechanism of action is thought to be prevention of implantation.

The all-plastic IUDs do not need to be replaced at a specific time, and some women use them for 10 years or more. The copper-bearing IUDs must be replaced every 4 years for maximum efficacy. The progesterone-secreting IUDs must be replaced yearly but have the advantage of causing decreased cramping and menstrual flow.

The IUD is often an excellent contraceptive method for parous women with one sexual partner. It is less desirable for young nulliparas because of the greater threat of pelvic inflammatory disease in young women and the possible impairment of future fertility.

Insertion

Insertion can be performed during or after the menses, at midcycle to prevent implantation, or later in the cycle if the patient has not become pregnant. Immediate postpartum insertion with IUDs designed to minimize expulsion has been successful in some studies; most clinicians wait until 8 weeks postpartum. When insertion is performed during lactation, there is greater risk of uterine perforation or embedding of the IUD. Insertion immediately following abortion is acceptable if there is no sepsis and if follow-up insertion a month later will not be possible; otherwise, it is wise to wait until 4 weeks postabortion.

Contraindications & Complications

Contraindications to use of IUDs are outlined in Table 13–7.

Table 13–7. Contraindications to IUD use.

Absolute contraindications
Pregnancy
Acute or subacute pelvic inflammatory disease or purulent cervicitis
Relative contraindications
Past history of pelvic inflammatory disease or ectopic pregnancy
Multiple sexual partners
Nulliparous woman concerned about future fertility
Lack of available follow-up care
Menorrhagia or severe dysmenorrhea
Cervical or uterine neoplasia
Abnormal size or shape of uterus, including myomas distorting cavity
Valvular heart disease
Diabetes

A. Pregnancy: An IUD can be inserted within 5 days following a single episode of unprotected midcycle coitus as a postcoital contraceptive. An IUD should not be inserted into a pregnant uterus. If pregnancy occurs as an IUD failure, there is a greater chance of spontaneous abortion if the IUD is left in situ (50%) than if it is removed (25%). Spontaneous abortion with an IUD in place is associated with a high risk of severe sepsis, and death can occur rapidly. Women using an IUD who become pregnant should have the IUD removed if the string is visible. It can be removed at the time of abortion if this is desired. If the string is not visible and the patient wants to continue the pregnancy, she should be informed of the serious risk of sepsis and, occasionally, death with such pregnancies. She should be informed that any flulike symptoms such as fever, myalgia, headache, or nausea warrant immediate medical attention for possible septic abortion.

Since the ratio of ectopic to intrauterine pregnancies is increased among IUD wearers, clinicians should search for adnexal masses in early pregnancy and should always check the products of conception for placental tissue following abortion.

B. Pelvic Inflammatory Disease: IUD use is associated with an increased risk of pelvic inflammatory disease, and therefore the IUD should rarely be used by teenagers, women desiring more children, women with multiple sexual partners, and women with a history of pelvic inflammatory disease or ectopic pregnancy. The IUD should never be inserted in the presence of cervicitis, endometritis, or salpingitis.

If pelvic infection develops, the signs and symptoms may be minimal at first. When infection is strongly suspected, the IUD should be removed and antibiotic treatment begun. With pelvic pain in IUD users, it is wise to consider ectopic pregnancy in the differential diagnosis.

C. Menorrhagia or Severe Dysmenorrhea: The IUD can cause heavier menstrual periods, bleeding between periods, and more cramping, so it is generally not suitable for women who already suffer from these problems. However, progesterone-secreting IUDs can be tried in these cases, as they often cause decreased bleeding and cramping with menses. Nonsteroidal anti-inflammatory drugs are also helpful in decreasing bleeding and pain in IUD users.

D. Complete or Partial Expulsion: Spontaneous expulsion of the IUD occurs in 10–20% of cases during the first year of use. Remove any IUD if the body of the device can be seen or felt in the cervical os.

E. Missing IUD Strings: If the transcervical tail cannot be seen, this may signify unnoticed expulsion, perforation of the uterus with abdominal migration of the IUD, or simply retraction of the string into the cervical canal or uterus owing to movement of the IUD or uterine growth with pregnancy. Once pregnancy is ruled out, one should probe for the IUD with a sterile sound or forceps designed for IUD removal, after administering a paracervical block. If the IUD cannot be detected, pelvic ultrasound will demonstrate the IUD if it is in the uterus. Alternatively, obtain anteroposterior and lateral x-rays of the pelvis with another IUD or a sound in the uterus as a marker, to confirm an extrauterine IUD. If the IUD is in the abdominal cavity, it should generally be removed by laparoscopy or laparotomy. Open-looped all-plastic IUDs such as the Lippes Loop can be left in the pelvis without danger, but ring-shaped IUDs may strangulate a loop of bowel and copper-bearing IUDs may cause tissue reaction and adhesions.

Perforations of the uterus are less likely if insertion is performed slowly, with meticulous care taken to follow directions applicable to each type of IUD.

Tatum HG, Connell EB: A decade of intrauterine contraception: 1976–1986. Fertil Steril 1986;46:173.

4. DIAPHRAGM & CERVICAL CAP

The diaphragm (with contraceptive jelly) is a safe and effective contraceptive method with features that make it acceptable to some women and not others. Failure rates range from 2 to 20%, depending on the motivation of the woman and the care with which the diaphragm is used. The advantages of this method are that it has no systemic side effects and gives significant protection against pelvic infection and cervical dysplasia as well as pregnancy. The disadvantages are that it must be inserted near the time of coitus and that pressure from the rim predisposes some women to cystitis after intercourse.

The cervical cap (with contraceptive jelly) is similar to the diaphragm but fits snugly over the cervix only (the diaphragm stretches from behind the cervix to behind the pubic symphysis). The cervical cap is more difficult to insert and remove than the dia-phragm. The main advantages are that it can be used by women who cannot be fitted for a diaphragm because of a relaxed anterior vaginal wall or by women who have discomfort or develop repeated bladder infections with the diaphragm.

Because of the small risk of toxic shock syndrome, a cervical cap or diaphragm should not be left in the vagina for over 12–18 hours, nor should these devices be used during the menstrual period (see above).

5. CONTRACEPTIVE SPONGE, FOAM, CREAM, JELLY, & SUPPOSITORY

These products are available without prescription, are easy to use, and are fairly effective, with reported failure rates of 2–29%. All contain the spermicides nonoxynol 9 or octoxynol 9, which also have some virucidal and bactericidal activity. The contraceptive sponge is inserted before intercourse and can be used for repeated acts of intercourse but should not be left in the vagina for longer than 12–18 hours, because of the risk of toxic shock syndrome (see Chapter 26). The sponge is more effective in nulliparous women than in parous women. Foams, creams, jellies, and suppositories also have the advantages of being simple to use and easily available. Their disadvantage is a slightly higher failure rate than with the diaphragm or condom.

6. CONDOM

The male sheath of latex or animal membrane affords good protection against pregnancy—equivalent to that of a diaphragm and spermicidal jelly; latex (but not animal membrane) condoms also offer protection against sexually transmitted disease and cervical dysplasia. Men and women seeking protection against AIDS transmission are advised to use a latex condom along with spermicide during vaginal or rectal intercourse. When a spermicide such as vaginal foam is used with the condom, the failure rate approaches that of oral contraceptives. Condoms coated with spermicide are now available in the USA. The disadvantages of condoms are dulling of sensation and spillage of semen due to tearing, slipping, or leakage with detumescence of the penis.

Rietmeijer CAM et al: Condoms as physical and chemical barriers against human immunodeficiency virus. JAMA 1988;259:1851.

7. CONTRACEPTION BASED ON AWARENESS OF FERTILE PERIODS

There is renewed interest in methods to identify times of ovulation and avoidance of unprotected intercourse at that time as a means of family planning. These methods are most effective when the couple restricts intercourse to the postovular phase of the cycle or uses a barrier method at other times. Women benefit from learning to identify their fertile periods. Well-instructed, motivated couples may achieve low pregnancy rates with fertility awareness, but in many field trials, the pregnancy rates were as high as 20%.

"Symptothermal" Natural Family Planning

The basis for this approach is patient-observed increase in clear elastic cervical mucus, brief abdominal midcycle discomfort ("mittelschmerz"), and a sustained rise of the basal body temperature about 2 weeks after onset of menstruation. Unprotected intercourse is avoided from shortly after the menstrual period, when fertile mucus is first identified, until 48 hours after ovulation, as identified by a sustained rise in temperature and the disappearance of clear elastic mucus.

Calendar Method

After the length of the menstrual cycle has been observed for at least 8 months, the following calculations are made: (1) The first fertile day is determined by subtracting 18 days from the shortest cycle; (2) the last fertile day is determined by subtracting 11 days from the longest cycle. For example, if the observed cycles run from 24 to 28 days, the fertile period would extend from the sixth day of the cycle (24 minus 18) through the 17th day (28 minus 11).

Basal Body Temperature Method

This method indicates the safe time after ovulation has passed. The temperature must be taken immediately upon awakening, before any activity. A slight drop in temperature often occurs 1–1½ days before ovulation, and a rise of about 0.4 °C (0.7 °F) occurs 1–2 days after ovulation. The elevated temperature continues throughout the remainder of the cycle. The second day after the rise marks the end of the fertile period.

8. POSTCOITAL CONTRACEPTION

If unprotected intercourse occurs in midcycle and the woman is certain she has not inadvertently become pregnant earlier in the cycle, the following regimens are effective in preventing implantation. The failure rate is less than 1.5%. These methods should be started within 72 hours after coitus. (1) Ethinyl estradiol, 2.5 mg twice daily for 5 days. (2) Ovral (50 μg of ethinyl estradiol with 0.5 mg of norgestrel, 2 tablets at once followed by 2 tablets 12 hours later. Antinausea medication may be necessary with these regimens. Bleeding should occur within 3–4 weeks. If pregnancy

occurs, abortion is advisable because of fetal exposure to possibly teratogenic doses of sex steroids.

IUD insertion within 5 days after one episode of unprotected midcycle coitus will also prevent pregnancy; copper-bearing IUDs have been tested for this purpose. The disadvantage of this method is possible infection, especially in rape cases; the advantage is ongoing contraceptive protection if this is desired in a patient for whom the IUD is a suitable choice.

9. ABORTION

Since the legalization of abortion in the USA in 1973, the related maternal mortality rate has fallen markedly, because illegal and self-induced abortions have been replaced by safer medical procedures. Abortions in the first trimester of pregnancy are performed by vacuum aspiration under local anesthesia. A similar technique, dilatation and evacuation, is often used in the second trimester, with general or local anesthesia. Techniques utilizing intra-amniotic instillation of hypertonic saline solution or prostaglandins are also occasionally used after 18 weeks from the LMP but are more difficult for the patient. Abortions are rarely performed after 20 weeks from the LMP. It is currently believed that fetal viability begins at about 24 weeks. Legal abortion has a mortality rate of 1:100,000. Rates of morbidity and mortality rise with length of gestation. Currently in the USA, 90% of abortions are performed before 12 weeks' gestation and only 3–4% after 17 weeks. Every effort should be made to continue the trend toward earlier abortion.

Complications resulting from abortion include retained products of conception (often associated with infection and heavy bleeding) and unrecognized ectopic pregnancy. Immediate analysis of the removed tissue for placenta can exclude or corroborate the diagnosis of ectopic pregnancy. Women presenting with fever, bleeding, or abdominal pain after abortion should be examined; use of broad-spectrum antibiotics and reaspiration of the uterus are frequently necessary. Hospitalization is advisable if acute salpingitis requires intravenous administration of antibiotics. Complications following illegal abortion often need emergency care for hemorrhage, septic shock, or uterine perforation.

Rh immune globulin should be given to all Rh-negative women following abortion. Contraception should be thoroughly discussed and contraceptive supplies or pills provided at the time of abortion. In women with a past history of pelvic inflammatory disease, prophylactic antibiotics are indicated: A one-dose regimen is doxycycline, 300 mg orally 1 hour before the procedure, or aqueous penicillin G, 1 million units intravenously 30 minutes before. In the second trimester, use cefazolin, 1 g intravenously 30 minutes before the procedure. Many clinics prescribe tetracycline, 500 mg 4 times daily for 5 days before the procedure for all patients.

Long-term sequelae of repeated induced abortions have been studied, but as yet there is no consensus on whether there are increased rates of fetal loss or premature labor. It is felt that such adverse sequelae can be minimized by performing early abortion with minimal cervical dilatation or by the use of *Laminaria* to induce gradual cervical dilatation.

10. STERILIZATION

In the USA, sterilization is the most popular method of birth control for couples who want no more children. Although sterilization is reversible in some instances, reversal surgery in both men and woman is costly, complicated, and not always successful. Therefore, patients should be counseled carefully before sterilization and should view the procedure as final.

Vasectomy is a safe, simple procedure in which the vas deferens is severed and sealed through a scrotal incision under local anesthesia. Long-term follow-up studies on vasectomized men show no excess risk of heart disease, cancer, or immune system problems.

Female sterilization is currently performed via laparoscopic bipolar electrocoagulation or plastic ring application of the uterine tubes or via minilaparotomy with Pomeroy tubal resection. The advantages of laparoscopy are minimal postoperative pain, small incisions, and rapid recovery. The advantages of minilaparotomy are that it can be performed with standard surgical instruments under local or general anesthesia. However, there is more postoperative pain and a longer recovery period. Failure rates after tubal sterilization are approximately 0.5%; this fact should be discussed with women preoperatively. There are recent reports that menstrual irregularities may increase after sterilization by unipolar tubal coagulation, but probably not after other techniques.

RAPE

Rape, or sexual assault, is legally defined in different ways in various jurisdictions. Physicians and emergency room personnel who deal with rape victims should be familiar with the laws pertaining to sexual assault in their own state. From a medical and psychologic viewpoint, it is essential that persons treating rape victims recognize the nonconsensual and violent nature of the crime. About 95% of reported rape victims are women. Penetration may be vaginal, anal, or oral and may be by the penis, hand, or a foreign object. The absence of genital injury does not imply consent by the victim. The assailant may be unknown to the victim or may be an acquaintance or even the spouse.

"Unlawful sexual intercourse," or statutory rape, is intercourse with a female before the age of majority even with her consent.

Rape represents an expression of anger, power, and sexuality on the part of the rapist. The rapist is usually a hostile man who uses sexual intercourse to terrorize and humiliate a woman. Women neither secretly want to be raped, nor do they expect, encourage, or enjoy rape.

Rape involves severe physical injury in 5–10% of cases and is always a terrifying experience in which most victims fear for their lives. Consequently, all victims suffer some psychologic aftermath. Moreover, some may acquire sexually transmissible disease or become pregnant.

Because rape is a personal crisis, each patient will react differently. The rape-trauma syndrome comprises 2 principal phases:

(1) Immediate or acute: Shaking, sobbing, and restless activity may last from a few days to a few weeks. The patient may experience anger, guilt, shame, and fear of revenge or may repress these emotions. Reactions vary depending on the victim's personality and the circumstances of the attack.

(2) Late or chronic: Problems related to the attack may develop weeks or months later. The life-style and work patterns of the individual may change. Sleep disorders or phobias often develop. Loss of self-esteem can rarely lead to suicide.

Physicians and emergency room personnel who deal with rape victims should work with community rape crisis centers whenever possible to provide ongoing supportive, skilled counseling.

General Office Procedures

The physician who first sees the alleged rape victim should be empathetic. Begin with a statement such as, "This is a terrible thing that has happened to you. I want to help."

(1) Secure written consent from the patient, guardian, or next of kin for gynecologic examination; for photographs if they are likely to be useful as evidence; and for notification of police. If police are to be notified, do so, and obtain advice on the transfer of evidence.

(2) Obtain and record the history in the patient's own words. The sequence of events, ie, the time, place, and circumstances, must be included. Note the date of the LMP, whether or not the woman is pregnant, and the time of the most recent coitus prior to the sexual assault. Note the details of the assault such as body cavities penetrated, use of foreign objects, and number of assailants.

Note whether the alleged victim is calm, agitated, or confused (drugs or alcohol may be involved). Record whether the patient came directly to the hospital or whether she bathed or changed her clothing. Record findings but do not issue even a tentative diagnosis lest it be erroneous or incomplete. Do not use the word "rape" in the recorded history.

(3) Have the patient disrobe while standing on a white sheet. Hair, dirt, and leaves; underclothing; and any torn or stained clothing should be kept as evidence. Scrape material from beneath fingernails and comb pubic hair for evidence. Place all evidence in separate clean paper bags or envelopes and label carefully.

(4) Examine the patient, noting any traumatized areas that should be photographed. Examine the body and genitals with a Wood light to identify semen, which fluoresces; positive areas should be swabbed with a premoistened swab and air-dried in order to identify acid phosphatase from prostatic secretions.

(5) Perform a pelvic examination, explaining all procedures and obtaining the patient's consent before proceeding gently with the examination. (In children, general anesthesia may be necessary during the pelvic examination or for repair of vaginal lacerations.) Use a narrow speculum lubricated with water only. Collect material with sterile cotton swabs from the vaginal walls and cervix and make 2 air-dried smears on clean glass slides. Swab the mouth (around molars and cheeks) and anus in the same way, if appropriate. Label all slides carefully. Collect secretions from the vagina, anus, or mouth with a premoistened cotton swab, place at once on a slide with a drop of saline, and cover with a coverslip. Look for motile or nonmotile sperm under high, dry magnification, and record the percentage of motile forms.

(6) Perform appropriate laboratory tests as follows. Culture the vagina, anus, or mouth (as appropriate) for *N gonorrhoeae* and *Chlamydia*. Perform a Papanicolaou smear of the cervix, a baseline pregnancy test, and VDRL test. A confidential test for HIV antibody can be obtained if desired by the patient and repeated in 2–4 months if initially negative. Repeat the pregnancy test if the next menses is missed, and repeat the VDRL test in 6 weeks. Obtain blood (10 mL without anticoagulant) and urine (100 mL) specimens if there is a history of forced ingestion or injection of drugs or alcohol.

(7) Transfer clearly labeled evidence, eg, laboratory specimens, directly to the clinical pathologist in charge or to the responsible laboratory technician, in the presence of witnesses (never via messenger), so that the rules of evidence will not be breached.

Treatment

(1) Give analgesics or tranquilizers if indicated.

(2) Administer tetanus toxoid if deep lacerations contain soil or dirt particles.

(3) Give ceftriaxone, 250 mg intramuscularly, to prevent gonorrhea. In addition, give tetracycline, 500 mg 4 times daily for 7 days, or doxycycline, 100 mg twice daily for 7 days, to increase the efficacy of treatment against penicillin-resistant gonococci and to treat chlamydial infection. Incubating syphilis will probably be prevented by these medications, but the VDRL test should be repeated 6 weeks after the assault.

(4) Prevent pregnancy by using one of the methods discussed under Postcoital Contraception, if necessary (see above).

(5) Make sure the patient and her family and friends have a source of ongoing psychologic support.

Green WM: *Rape: The Evidential Examination and Management of the Adult Female Victim.* Lexington Books, 1988.

MENOPAUSAL SYNDROME

Essentials of Diagnosis

- Cessation of menses due to aging or to bilateral oophorectomy.
- Elevation of FSH and LH levels.
- Hot flushes and night sweats (in 80% of women).
- Decreased vaginal lubrication; thinned vaginal mucosa with or without dyspareunia.

General Considerations

The term "menopause" refers to the final cessation of menstruation, either as a normal part of aging or as the result of surgical removal of both ovaries. In a broader sense, as the term is commonly used, it denotes a 1- to 3-year period during which a woman adjusts to a diminishing and then absent menstrual flow and the physiologic changes that may be associated—hot flushes, night sweats, and vaginal dryness or soreness with coitus.

The average age at menopause in Western societies today is 51 years. Premature menopause is defined as ovarian failure and menstrual cessation before age 40; this often has a genetic or autoimmune basis. Surgical menopause due to bilateral oophorectomy is common and can cause more severe symptoms owing to the sudden rapid drop in sex hormone levels.

There is no objective evidence that cessation of ovarian function is associated with increased emotional disturbance or personality changes. However, the time of menopause often coincides with other major life changes, such as departure of children from home, a midlife identity crisis, or divorce. These events, coupled with a sense of the loss of youth, may exacerbate the symptoms of menopause and cause psychologic distress.

Clinical Findings

A. Symptoms and Signs:

1. Cessation of menstruation–Menstrual cycles generally become irregular as menopause approaches. Anovular cycles occur more often, with irregular cycle length and occasional menorrhagia. Menstrual flow usually diminishes in amount owing to decreased estrogen secretion, resulting in less abundant endometrial growth. Finally, cycles become longer, with missed periods or episodes or spotting only. When no bleeding has occurred for one year, the menopausal transition can be said to have occurred. Any bleeding after this time warrants investigation by endometrial curettage or aspiration to rule out endometrial cancer.

2. Hot flushes–Hot flushes (feelings of intense heat over the trunk and face, with flushing of the skin and sweating) occur in 80% of women as a result of the decrease in ovarian hormones. Hot flushes can begin before the cessation of menses. An increase in pulsatile release of gonadotropin-releasing hormone from the hypothalamus is believed to trigger the hot flushes by affecting the adjacent temperature-regulating area of the brain. Hot flushes are more severe in women who undergo surgical menopause. Flushing is more pronounced late in the day, during hot weather, after ingestion of hot foods or drinks, or during periods of tension. Occurring at night, they often cause sweating and insomnia and result in fatigue on the following day.

3. Dyspareunia–With decreased estrogen secretion, thinning of the vaginal mucosa and decreased vaginal lubrication occur and may lead to dyspareunia. The introitus decreases in diameter. Pelvic examination reveals pale, smooth vaginal mucosa and a small cervix and uterus. The ovaries are not normally palpable after the menopause. Continued sexual activity will help prevent tissue shrinkage; use of lubricants, estrogen or testosterone cream, or oral estrogen therapy can prevent or relieve pain.

4. Osteoporosis–Osteoporosis may occur as a late sequela of menopause (see Chapter 20).

B. Laboratory Findings: Vaginal cytologic examination will show a low estrogen effect with predominantly parabasal cells. Serum FSH and LH levels are elevated.

Treatment

A. Natural Menopause: Education and support from health providers, midlife discussion groups, and reading material will help most women having difficulty adjusting to the menopause. Physiologic symptoms can be treated as follows:

1. Vasomotor symptoms–Give conjugated estrogens, 0.3 mg or 0.625 mg; (estradiol, 1 or 2 mg; or estrone sulfate, 0.625 mg) from day 1 to day 25 of each calendar month. Alternatively, estradiol can be given transdermally as skin patches that are changed twice weekly and secrete 0.05–0.1 mg of hormone daily (Estraderm). Use from day 1 to day 25 of the calendar month. When either form of estrogen is used, add a progestin (medroxyprogesterone acetate, 10 mg, or norethindrone acetate, 2.5–5 mg) on days 14–25, to prevent endometrial hyperplasia or cancer. Withhold hormones from day 26 until the end of the month, when the endometrium will be shed, producing a light, generally painless monthly period. If the patient has had a hysterectomy, a progestin need not be used. Explain to the patient that hot flushes will probably return if the hormone is discontinued. When women wish to stop hormone therapy, the dose should be tapered.

Clonidine, an α-adrenergic agonist, has been found to be effective in reducing hot flashes when given orally or transdermally in doses of 100–150 μg daily. Side effects include dry mouth, drowsiness, and blood pressure decrease, but the effects are usually mild at these low dosages.

2. Dyspareunia–This problem can be treated with hormone therapy as outlined above. Alternatively, topical use of hormone creams in small doses will often relieve pain with minimal systemic absorption. Use Premarin or Estrace vaginal cream, one-eighth applicatorful (0.3 mg of conjugated estrogen) nightly for 7–10 nights. Thereafter, use every other night or twice weekly. Testosterone propionate 1–2% in a vanishing cream base used in the same manner is also effective if estrogen is contraindicated. A bland lubricant such as unscented cold cream or water-soluble gel can be helpful at the time of coitus.

3. Osteoporosis–Women should ingest at least 800 mg of calcium daily throughout life. Nonfat or low-fat milk products, calcium-fortified orange juice, green leafy vegetables, corn tortillas, and canned sardines or salmon consumed with the bones are good dietary sources. In addition, 1 g of elemental calcium should be taken as a daily supplement at the time of the menopause and thereafter; calcium supplements should be taken with meals to increase their absorption. Vitamin D, 400 IU/d from food, sunlight, or supplements, is necessary to enhance calcium absorption. A daily program of energetic walking and exercise to strengthen the arms and upper body helps maintain bone mass.

Women most at risk for osteoporotic fractures should consider hormone replacement therapy. This includes Caucasian and Asian women, especially if they have a family history of osteoporosis; are thin, short, cigarette smokers, and physically inactive; or have had a low calcium intake in adult life. The dosage is usually the same as for treatment of vasomotor symptoms.

B. Surgical Menopause: The abrupt hormonal decrease resulting from oophorectomy generally results in severe vasomotor symptoms and rapid onset of dyspareunia and osteoporosis unless treated. Estrogen replacement is generally started immediately after surgery. Conjugated estrogen, 1.25 mg, estrone sulfate, 1.25 mg, or estradiol, 2 mg, is given for 25 days of each month. After age 45–50 years, this dose can be tapered to 0.3 mg or 0.635 mg of conjugated estrogen or equivalent.

C. Contraindications to Estrogen Therapy: Women with conditions listed in Table 13–8 should generally not use estrogen. Progestins can be substituted in some cases but are not advisable for patients with diabetes or circulatory disease. At present, certain studies suggest that long-term use of postmeno-

Table 13–8. Contraindications to estrogen therapy.

Cancer of the breast or uterus
Estrogen-dependent ovarian cancer
History of thromboembolic disease
Hepatic adenoma or other significant liver disease
Gallstones or gallbladder disease

pausal estrogens is associated with breast cancer development. Since epidemiologists are debating this question, women with strong risk factors for breast cancer should be so advised, and all women should be followed carefully with breast examination and mammography. Estrogens must be given with progestins as outlined above in women who have a uterus, to avoid endometrial cancer. Most authorities believe that estrogen in low doses will retard atherosclerosis by raising high-density lipoprotein levels, but progestins have the opposite effect. Since estrogen doubles the risk of gallbladder disease necessitating cholecystectomy, its use in women with gallstones or a history of cholecystitis is unwise. Estrogen may cause the growth of uterine myomas, which otherwise shrink after the menopause.

Ettinger B, Genant HK, Cann CE: Postmenopausal bone loss is prevented by treatment with low-dosage estrogen with calcium. Ann Intern Med 1987;106:40.

Holbrook TL, Barrett-Connor E, Wingard DL: Dietary calcium and risk of hip fracture: 14-year prospective population study. Lancet 1988;2:1046. (Supports the hypothesis that increased dietary calcium protects against hip fracture.

OBSTETRICS

DIAGNOSIS & DIFFERENTIAL DIAGNOSIS OF PREGNANCY

It is advantageous to diagnose pregnancy as promptly as possible when a sexually active woman misses a menstrual period or has symptoms suggestive or pregnancy. In the event of a wanted pregnancy, she can begin prenatal care early and discontinue use of recreational drugs (eg, alcohol, tobacco, marihuana) or potentially teratogenic medication in the critical weeks of embryogenesis in the first trimester. In the event of an unwanted pregnancy, she can consider termination of the pregnancy at an early stage.

Pregnancy Tests

Currently available tests (Table 13–9) permit very early diagnosis of pregnancy, sometimes even before the time of the missed menses. All urine or blood tests rely on the detection of hCG produced by the placenta. hCG levels increase shortly after implantation, double approximately every 48 hours, reach a peak at 50–75 days, and fall to lower levels in the second and third trimesters. The older slide tests for pregnancy, which are of lower sensitivity, become accurate 7–10 days after the missed period. Most laboratories (and newer home pregnancy tests) now use monoclonal antibodies specific for hCG; these tests are performed on urine or serum and are accurate at the time of the missed period or shortly after it, depending on their sensitivity.

Compared with intrauterine pregnancies, ectopic pregnancies may show lower levels of hCG, which level off or fall in serial determinations. Quantitative assays of hCG repeated at 48- to 72-hour intervals are used in the diagnosis of ectopic pregnancy, as well as in cases of molar pregnancy, threatened abortion, and missed abortion. Comparison of hCG levels between laboratories may be misleading in a given patient because different international standards produce results that vary by a factor of two.

Manifestations of Pregnancy

The following symptoms and signs are usually due to pregnancy, but none are diagnostic. A record or history of time and frequency of coitus may be of considerable value.

A. Symptoms: Amenorrhea, nausea and vomiting, breast tenderness and tingling, urinary frequency and urgency, "quickening" (may be noted at about the 18th week), weight gain.

Table 13–9. Selected diagnostic tests for pregnancy.

Test	Sensitivity (in mIU of hCG/mL)	Comments
Slide test with urine	500–2000	Latex inhibition tests to detect hCG. Convenient for office use. Accurate 4 weeks after conception. May cross-react with LH. Proteinuria, opiates, and psychotropic drugs may give false-positive results.
Monoclonal antibody test with urine	20–200	Colorimetric test. Designed for office and home use. Accurate 2–3 weeks after conception. Specific for hCG.
Radioimmunoassay (RIA)	5	Some tests accurate 1 week after conception. Specific for hCG. Also used for quantitative assays in abnormal pregnancies (molar, ectopic, threatened abortion).

B. Signs (in Weeks From LMP): Breast changes (enlargement, vascular engorgement, colostrum), abdominal enlargement, cyanosis of vagina and cervical portion (about the seventh week), softening of the cervix (seventh week), softening of the cervicouterine junction (eighth week), generalized enlargement and diffuse softening of the corpus (after eighth week).

By 14–15 weeks from the LMP, the uterine fundus is palpable above the pubic symphysis, and by 20–22 weeks, it has reached the umbilicus. By 28 weeks it is usually halfway between the umbilicus and the xiphoid process, and by 38 weeks it has reached the xiphoid process. The fetal heart can be heard at the end of the first trimester with an ultrasonic stethoscope and by 20 weeks with an ordinary fetoscope.

Differential Diagnosis

The nonpregnant uterus enlarged by myomas can be confused with the gravid uterus, but it is usually very firm and irregular. An ovarian tumor may be found midline, displacing the nonpregnant uterus to the side or posteriorly. Ultrasonography and a pregnancy test will help make an accurate diagnosis in these circumstances.

ESSENTIALS OF PRENATAL CARE

The first prenatal visit, occurring as early as possible after the diagnosis of pregnancy, should include the following:

History

Age, ethnic background, occupation. Onset of LMP and its normality, possible conception dates, bleeding after LMP, medical history, all prior pregnancies (duration, outcome, and complications), symptoms of present pregnancy. Use of drugs, alcohol, tobacco, caffeine, nutritional habits (Table 13–10). Family history of congenital anomalies and inheritable diseases.

Physical Examination

Height, weight, blood pressure, general physical examination. Abdominal and pelvic examination: (1) estimate uterine size or measure fundal height; (2) evaluate bony pelvis for symmetry and adequacy; (3) evaluate cervix for infection, effacement, dilatation; (4) detect fetal heart sounds with Doppler device (or ultrasound) after 10 weeks from LMP if fetal demise is suspected because of uterine bleeding or inadequate uterine growth.

Laboratory Tests

Urinalysis, complete blood count with red cell indices, serologic test for syphilis; rubella antibody titer, blood group, Rh type, atypical antibody screening, and HBsAg evaluation. If indicated clinically, cervical cultures for *Neisseria gonorrhoeae* and *Chlamydia;* Papanicolaou smear of the cervix, culture for

Table 13–10. Common drugs that are teratogenic or fetotoxic.[1]

Alcohol	Anticonvulsants
Amebicides	Aminoglutethimide, ethotoin, phenytoin, paramethadione, trimethadione, valproic acid
Carbarsone	
Analgesics and antipyretics	
Aspirin and other salicylates (in third trimester); narcotics (prolonged use)	Antidiabetics
	Oral hypoglycemics
	Antihypertensives
Antibiotics	Diazoxide, thiazide diuretics, reserpine
Aminoglycosides, chloramphenicol, tetracycline, trimethoprim, sulfonamides (in third trimester)	Antineoplastics
	All agents
	Antithyroid drugs
	Radioiodine, propylthiouracil, methimazole
Antifungal drugs	
Griseofulvin, ketoconazole	Disulfiram (Antabuse)
Antiparasitic drugs	Ergotamine
Lindane, mebendazole, Fansidar (sulfadoxine and pyrimethamine), and others	Hormones
	Estrogens, diethylstilbestrol, progestins, androgens
Antiviral drugs	Isotretinoin (Accutane)
Amantadine, ribavirin, and others	Nonsteroidal anti-inflammatory drugs in third trimester
Anticoagulants	Psychoactive drugs
Warfarin, dicumarol and other coumarin derivatives	Lithium, benzodiazepines, amitriptyline
	Tobacco smoking

[1] Additional drugs are also contraindicated during pregnancy. Evaluate any drug for its need and its potential adverse effects. Further information on any drug can be obtained by telephoning the drug manufacturer or by calling the Massachusetts Teratogen Information Service ([617] 787–4957).

herpes simplex if suspicious lesions are seen. Hemoglobin electrophoresis for anemic black (Hgb S, C, F) and Asian women (Hgb A_2). Women who may carry the AIDS virus should be offered confidential HIV antibody studies (intravenous drug users, prostitutes, partners of AIDS-ARC patients, women from Haiti or Africa, recipients of transfusions from 1978 to 1985). Tuberculosis skin tests when indicated. Chorionic villus sampling at 9–12 weeks or amniocentesis at 16 weeks from LMP if patient is over 35 or has had prior offspring with chromosomal abnormality; Tay-Sachs blood screening for Jewish women with Jewish partners; toxoplasmosis titers to determine susceptibility to the acute illness during pregnancy.

Prenatal HBsAg screening is recommended for women in the following high-risk groups if it is not done routinely:

Women of Asian, Pacific Island, or Alaskan Eskimo descent, whether immigrants or born in the USA

Women born in Haiti or sub-Saharan Africa

Women with histories of any of the following:
Acute or chronic liver disease

Work or treatment in hemodialysis unit

Work or residence in an institution for the mentally retarded

---

HIGH-RISK OBSTETRIC CATEGORIES
(After Wigglesworth)

History of Any of the Following:

Hereditary abnormality (osteogenesis imperfecta, Down's syndrome, etc)

Premature or small-for-dates neonate (most recent delivery)

Congenital anomaly, anemia, blood dyscrasia, preeclampsia-eclampsia, etc

Severe social problem (teen-age pregnancy, drug addiction, alcoholism, etc)

Long-delayed or absent prenatal care

Age less than 18 or over 35 years

Teratogenic viral illness or dangerous drug administration in the first trimester

A fifth or subsequent pregnancy, especially when the gravida is over 35 years of age

Prolonged infertility or essential drug or hormone treatment

Significant stressful or dangerous events in the present pregnancy (critical accident, excessive exposure to irradiation, etc)

Heavy cigarette smoking

Pregnancy within 2 months after a previous delivery

Diagnosis of Any of the Following:

Height under 60 inches or a prepregnant weight of 20% less than or over the standard for height and age

Minimal or no weight gain during the first half of pregnancy

Obstetric complications (preeclampsia-eclampsia, multiple pregnancy, hydramnios, etc)

Abnormal presentation (breech, presenting part unengaged at term, etc)

A fetus that fails to grow normally or is disparate in size from that expected

A fetus over 42 weeks of gestation.

Rejection as a blood donor

Blood transfusion on repeated occasions

Frequent occupational exposures to blood in medicodental settings

Household contact with a hepatitis B virus carrier or a patient undergoing hemodialysis

Multiple episodes of sexually transmitted disease

Intravenous drug abuse in patient or partners

Advice to Patients

(1) Take no medications unless prescribed by a doctor or a registered midwife.

(2) Avoid x-rays unless they are essential; inform the dentist or radiologist of pregnancy.

(3) Avoid all street drugs, alcohol, and tobacco.

(4) Decrease caffeine to 0–1 cup of coffee or tea daily.

(5) Avoid eating raw or rare meat. Wash hands after handling raw meat. Wash all fruits and vegetables before eating.

(6) Pay attention to good nutrition and take prenatal vitamins with iron and folate as directed. Do not diet to lose weight. Plan to gain about 11 kg during pregnancy.

(7) Get adequate daily rest; avoid exhausting work.

(8) Do not work where there are chemical or radiation hazards.

(9) Avoid excessive heat in saunas or hot tubs.

(10) Perform mild to moderate exercises daily; avoid exhausting or hazardous exercises or new athletic training programs. Keep heart rate below 150 beats/min during exercise, and conclude with a 5-minute slowdown. Swimming with moderate exertion provokes the least significant degree of uterine and fetal response.

(11) Wear gloves during gardening or while disposing of cat litter (if this risk cannot be avoided). Wash hands after performing these duties.

(12) Enroll with your partner in a class on preparation for childbirth optimally starting during the seventh month of pregnancy.

Schedule of Prenatal Visits for Normal Pregnancy

Up to 28 weeks: every 4 weeks.
Up to 36 weeks: every 2 weeks.
36 weeks to delivery: weekly.

Tests & Procedures in Second & Third Trimesters

A. Each Visit: Weight, blood pressure, fundal height, fetal heart rate, urine specimen for protein and sugar. Fetal position. Review of patient's concerns about pregnancy; health and nutritional advice.

B. 8–12 Weeks: Confirm uterine growth by pelvic examination. Fetal heart tones are generally audible with a Doppler stethoscope at 12 weeks of gestation. When indicated for genetic reasons, chorionic villous sampling is done between 9 and 12 weeks by transvaginal or transabdominal aspiration, depending on the location of the placenta.

C. 15–18 Weeks: Genetic amniocentesis for women over 35; or with family history of congenital anomalies; or with previous child with chromosomal abnormality, errors or metabolism, or neural tube defect; or with history of repeated spontaneous abortions. Questions relating to prenatal genetic counseling or ultrasound diagnosis may be referred to the Yale Prenatal Diagnostic Hotline: 1–800–627–5217.

D. 16–18 Weeks: Alpha-fetoprotein (AFP) determination on maternal blood in patients with history of fetuses with neural tube defects and in diabetics. In some states, this test has become mandatory for all women.

E. 14–26 Weeks: Ultrasound examination for determining pregnancy duration if LMP is unclear or uterine size is incompatible with dates.

F. 24–28 Weeks: Oral glucose tolerance test with

50 g glucose and 1-hour blood sugar (< 140 mg/dL is normal) to screen for gestational diabetes.

G. 28 Weeks: Rh immunoglobulin for unsensitized Rh-negative patients.

H. 28 Weeks On: Ultrasound examination for suspected intrauterine growth retardation (most accurate after 28 weeks); repeat every 3–4 weeks to assess changes. Ultrasound examination near term or postterm may be used for suspected macrosomia.

I. 28–32 Weeks: Repeat complete blood count. Baseline vaginal examination to detect cervical thinning and dilatation, suggesting premature onset of labor.

J. 36 Weeks to Delivery: Careful assessment of the presenting part to diagnose breech presentations so that external version with the aid of tocolytic drugs can be accomplished before labor. Daily regularly scheduled patient-monitored fetal kick counts to confirm fetal well-being (normal is 3 movements within 10 minutes of observation immediately following a snack or meal). Speculum examination to culture for genital herpes infection if active infection is suspected. At 38 weeks, culture the cervix for group B β-hemolytic streptococci; if positive, treat mother in labor.

K. Postterm to Beyond 41 Weeks: Review dates and milestones of pregnancy. Evaluate cervical status. Perform nonstress tests twice weekly and obtain ultrasound profile for fetal weight, breathing, and limb movements; fetal position and body tone; and amniotic fluid volume (biophysical profile). Perform ultrasound-directed amniocentesis for lung maturity tests and the presence of meconium. Consider induction of labor during confirmed 42nd week of gestation.

Nagey DA: The content of prenatal care. Obstet Gynecol 1989;74:516.

Prevention of perinatal transmission of Hepatitis B virus: prenatal screening of all pregnant women for Hepatitis B surface antigen. MMWR 1988;37 (Suppl):22.

Sokol RJ, Martier SS, Ager JW: the T-ACE questions: Practical prenatal detection of risk-drinking. Am J Obstet Gynecol 1989;160:863.

NUTRITION IN PREGNANCY

Nutrition in pregnancy significantly affects maternal health and infant size and well-being. Pregnant women should have nutrition counseling early in prenatal care and access to supplementary food programs if they lack funds for adequate nutrition. Counseling should stress abstention from alcohol, smoking, and drugs. Caffeine and artificial sweeteners should be used only in small amounts. ''Empty calories'' should be avoided, and the diet should contain the following foods: protein foods of animal and vegetable origin; milk and milk products; whole-grain cereals and breads; and fruits and vegetables, especially green leafy vegetables.

Weight gain in pregnancy should be at least 11 kg, which includes the added weight of the fetus, placenta, and amniotic fluid and of maternal reproductive tissues, fluid, blood, increased fat stores, and increased lean body mass. Maternal fat stores are a caloric reserve for pregnancy and lactation; weight restriction in pregnancy to avoid developing such fat stores may affect the development of other fetal and maternal tissues and is not advisable. Obese women can have adequate-sized infants with less weight gain but should be encouraged to eat high-quality foods. Normally, a pregnant woman gains 1–2 kg in the first trimester and slightly less than 0.5 kg/wk thereafter. She needs approximately an extra 200–300 kcal/d (depending on energy output) and 30 g/d of additional protein, for a total protein intake of about 75 g/d. Appropriate caloric intake in pregnancy helps prevent infants of low birth weight.

Rigid salt restriction is not necessary. While the consumption of highly salted snack foods and prepared foods is not desirable, 2–3 g/d of sodium is permissible. The increased calcium needs of pregnancy (1200 mg/d) can be met with milk, milk products, green vegetables, soybean products, corn tortillas, and calcium carbonate supplements.

The increased need for iron and folic acid should be met from foods as well as vitamin and mineral supplements. (See section on anemia in pregnancy.) Megavitamins should not be taken in pregnancy, as they may result in fetal malformation or disturbed metabolism. However, a balanced prenatal supplement containing 30–60 mg of elemental iron, 0.5–0.8 mg of folate, and the recommended daily allowances of various vitamins and minerals is widely used in the USA and is probably beneficial to many women with marginal diets. There is some evidence that periconceptional vitamin supplements decrease the risk of neural tube defects in the fetus. Lactovegetarians and ovolactovegetarians do well in pregnancy; vegetarian women who eat neither eggs nor milk products should have their diets assessed for adequate calories and protein and should take oral vitamin B 12 supplements during pregnancy and lactation.

Frentzen BH, Dimperio DL, Cruz AC: Maternal weight gain: Effect of infant birth weight among overweight and average-weight low-income women. Am J Obstet Gynecol 1988;159:1114.

TRAVEL DURING PREGNANCY

During an otherwise normal low-risk pregnancy, travel can be planned most safely between the 18th and 32nd weeks. Commercial flying in pressurized cabins does not pose a threat to the fetus. An aisle seat in the non-smoking section will allow frequent walks. Adequate fluids should be taken during the flight.

It is not advisable to travel to endemic areas of yellow fever in Africa or Latin America or to areas of Africa or Asia where there is chloroquine-resistant falciparum malaria, since severe complications of malaria are more common in pregnancy.

Ideally, all immunizations should precede pregnancy. Live virus products are contraindicated (measles, rubella, yellow fever). Inactivated poliovaccine (Salk) can be used instead of the oral vaccine. Vaccines against pneumococcal pneumonia and meningococcal meningitis can be used, but their safety during pregnancy has not been conclusively proved.

Pooled gamma globulin to prevent hepatitis A is safe and does not carry a risk of AIDS. Chloroquine can be used for malaria prophylaxis in pregnancy, and proguanil is also safe.

Water should be purified by boiling, since iodine purification may provide more iodine than is safe during pregnancy.

Do not use prophylactic antibiotics or bismuth subsalicylate during pregnancy to prevent diarrhea. Use oral rehydration fluids, and treat bacterial diarrhea with erythromycin or ampicillin if necessary.

Barry M, Bia F: Pregnancy and travel. JAMA 1989;261:728.

VOMITING OF PREGNANCY
(Morning Sickness)
& HYPEREMESIS GRAVIDARUM
(Pernicious Vomiting of Pregnancy)

Morning or evening nausea and vomiting usually begin soon after the first missed period and cease after the fourth to fifth months of gestation. At least half of women, most of them primiparas, complain of nausea and vomiting during early pregnancy. This problem exerts no adverse effects on the pregnancy and does not presage other complications, though it is common with multiple pregnancy and hydatidiform mole. Persistent severe vomiting during pregnancy— hyperemesis gravidarum—can be disabling and require hospitalization. Dehydration, acidosis, and nutritional deficiencies may develop with protracted vomiting.

The cause of vomiting during pregnancy is believed to be high estrogen levels.

Treatment
A. Mild Nausea and Vomiting Pregnancy: Reassurance and dietary advice are all that is required in most instances. Frequent small meals of nutritious, easily digested low-fat foods should be suggested. Begin prenatal vitamin and mineral supplements as soon as tolerated.

Because of possible teratogenicity, drugs used during the first half of pregnancy should be restricted

to those of major importance to life and health. Antiemetics, antihistamines, and antispasmodics are generally unnecessary to treat nausea of pregnancy. Vitamin B_6 (pyridoxine), 50–100 mg/d orally, is nontoxic and may be helpful in some patients.

B. Hyperemesis Gravidarum: Hospitalize the patient in a private room at bed rest. Give nothing by mouth for 48 hours, and maintain hydration and electrolyte balance by giving appropriate parenteral fluids and vitamin supplements as indicated. Rarely, total parenteral nutrition may become necessary. As soon as possible, place the patient on a dry diet consisting of 6 small feedings daily with clear liquids 1 hour after eating. Prochlorperazine rectal suppositories may be useful, and psychosocial consultation is advisable. After stabilization in the hospital, the patient can be maintained at home even if she requires intravenous fluids in addition to her oral intake.

Depue RH et al: Hyperemesis gravidarum in relation to estradiol levels, pregnancy outcome, and other maternal factors: A seroepidemiologic study. Am J Obstet Gynecol 1987;156:1137.

SPONTANEOUS ABORTION

Essentials of Diagnosis
- Vaginal bleeding in a pregnant woman before the 20th week of gestation.
- Uterine cramping.
- Disappearance of symptoms and signs of pregnancy.
- The products of conception may or may not be expelled.

General Considerations
Abortion is defined as termination of gestation before the 20th week of pregnancy. About three-fourths of spontaneous abortions occur before the 16th week of gestation; of these, three-fourths occur before the eighth week. Almost 20% of all clinically recognized pregnancies terminate in spontaneous abortion.

More than 60% of spontaneous abortions result from ovular defects due to maternal or paternal factors; about 15% are caused by maternal trauma, infections, dietary deficiencies, diabetes mellitus, hypothyroidism, or anatomic malformations. There is no reliable evidence that abortion may be induced by psychic stimuli such as severe fright, grief, anger, or anxiety. In about one-fourth of cases, the cause of abortion cannot be determined.

It is important to identify those cases of late abortion (after 16 weeks) that result from cervical incompetence, since this is treatable. Often these women will have a history of late abortions associated with spontaneous rupture of the membranes and minimal labor. Some will have a history of wide cervical dilatation during D&C. In the nonpregnant state, an incompetent cervix will easily admit a dilator 8 mm in diameter.

Clinical Findings

A. Symptoms and Signs:

1. Threatened abortion–Bleeding or cramping occurs, but the pregnancy continues.

2. Inevitable abortion–The passage of some or all of the products of conception is impending. Bleeding and cramping persist, and the cervix is effaced and dilated.

3. Complete abortion–The fetus and placenta are completely expelled. Pain ceases but spotting may persist.

4. Incomplete abortion–A significant portion of the pregnancy (usually a placental fragment) remains in the uterus. Only mild cramps are reported, but bleeding is persistent and often excessive.

5. Missed abortion–The pregnancy has ceased to develop for at least 1 month, but the conceptus has not been expelled. Symptoms of pregnancy disappear. There is a brownish vaginal discharge but no free bleeding. Pain does not develop. The cervix is semifirm and slightly patulous; the uterus becomes smaller and irregularly softened; the adnexa are normal.

B. Laboratory Findings: Pregnancy tests show low or falling levels of hCG. A complete blood count should be obtained if bleeding is heavy. Determine Rh type, and give Rh immune globulin if the type is Rh-negative. All tissue recovered should be assessed by a pathologist.

C. Ultrasonographic Findings: An expert ultrasonographer can identify a gestational sac at 6 weeks from the LMP and a fetal pole at 7 weeks. Serial observations are often required to evaluate changes in size of the embryo. A small, irregular sac without a fetal pole is diagnostic of an inevitable abortion.

Differential Diagnosis

The bleeding that occurs in abortion of a uterine pregnancy must be differentiated from the abnormal bleeding of an ectopic pregnancy and anovular bleeding in a nonpregnant woman. The passage of hydropic villi in the bloody discharge is diagnostic of the abortion of a hydatidiform mole.

Treatment

A. General Measures:

1. Threatened abortion requires 24–48 hours of bed rest followed by gradual resumption of usual activities, with abstinence from coitus and douching. Hormonal treatment is contraindicated. Antibiotics should be used only if there are signs of infection.

2. Missed or inevitable abortion requires counseling regarding the fate of the pregnancy and planning for its elective termination at a time chosen by the patient and physician. Insertion of *Laminaria* to dilate the cervix followed by aspiration is the method of choice. Prostaglandin vaginal suppositories are an effective alternative.

B. Surgical Measures:

1. Incomplete abortion requires prompt removal of any products of conception remaining within the uterus. Analgesia and a paracervical block are useful, followed by uterine exploration with ovum forceps or uterine aspiration.

2. Spontaneous abortion in the second trimester of pregnancy due to an incompetent cervix can sometimes be prevented by cerclage using a 5-mm woven Dacron strip (Shirodkar method) or circumsuture with braided silk (McDonald method).

Wilcox AJ et al: Incidence of early loss of pregnancy. N Engl J Med 1988;319:189.

RECURRENT (HABITUAL) ABORTION

Recurrent, or habitual, abortion has been defined for years as the loss of 3 or more previable (< 500 g) pregnancies in succession. Recurrent or chronic abortion occurs in about 0.4–0.8% of all pregnancies. Abnormalities related to repeated abortion can be identified in approximately half of the couples. If a woman has lost 3 previous pregnancies without identifiable cause, she still has a 70–80% chance of carrying a fetus to viability. If she has aborted 4 or 5 times, the likelihood of a successful pregnancy is 65–70%.

Recurrent abortion is a clinical rather than pathologic diagnosis. The clinical findings are similar to those observed in other types of abortion (see above).

Treatment

A. Preconception Therapy: Preconception therapy is aimed at detection of maternal or paternal defects that may contribute to abortion. A thorough general and gynecologic examination is essential. Cervical cultures for *Chlamydia*, herpesvirus, and cytomegalovirus and endometrial cultures for *Ureaplasma urealyticum* and *Toxoplasma gondii* should be taken. A random blood glucose test, thyroid function studies, lupus anticoagulant, and an antinuclear antibody test are indicated. Endometrial tissue should be examined in the postovulation stage of the cycle to determine the adequacy of the response of the endometrium to hormones. The competency of the cervix must be determined and hysteroscopy or hysterography used to exclude submucous myomas and congenital anomalies. Chromosomal (karyotype) analysis of both partners rules out balanced translocations (found in 5% of infertile couples). Every attempt should be made to restore and maintain good physical and emotional health.

Recent experiments have focused on the major histocompatibility complex (MHC) of chromosome 6, which carries HLA loci and other genes that may influence reproductive success. Many couples who experience habitual abortion share a significant number of HLA antigens, and some women demonstrate a lack of maternal antibody response to paternal lymphocytes, which is customarily found in normal women after successful childbearing. Centers where HLA typing can be performed will identify couples whose unusual gene sharing may play a role in habitual abortion. The immunologic approach of enhancing maternal antibody response to paternal lymphocytes is still experimental.

B. Postconception Therapy: Provide early prenatal care and schedule frequent office visits. Complete bed rest is justified only for bleeding or pain. Empiric steroid sex hormone therapy is contraindicated.

Prognosis

The prognosis is excellent if the cause of abortion can be corrected.

Sargent IL et al: Maternal immune response to the fetus in early pregnancy and recurrent miscarriage. Lancet 1988;2:1099.

ECTOPIC PREGNANCY

Essentials of Diagnosis

- Abnormal vaginal bleeding with symptoms suggestive of pregnancy.
- Cramping pains in the lower abdomen. A tender mass palpable outside the uterus.
- Pelvic ultrasound finding of empty uterus after seventh week from LMP.
- Failure to recover placental tissue at the time of induced abortion.

General Considerations

Any pregnancy arising from implantation of the ovum outside the cavity of the uterus is ectopic. Ectopic implantation occurs in about one out of 150 live births. About 98% of ectopic pregnancies are tubal. Other sites of ectopic implantations are the peritoneum or abdominal viscera, the ovary, and the cervix. Any condition that prevents or retards the migration of the fertilized ovum to the uterus can predispose to an ectopic pregnancy, including a history of infertility, pelvic inflammatory disease, ruptured appendix, and prior tubal surgery. Combined intra- and extrauterine pregnancy (heterotopic) may occur rarely. In the USA, undiagnosed or undetected ectopic pregnancy is currently the most common cause of maternal death in pregnancies with abortive outcomes.

Clinical Findings

A. Symptoms and Signs: The cardinal symptoms and signs of tubal pregnancy are (1) amenorrhea or irregular bleeding and spotting, followed by (2) pelvic pain, and (3) pelvic (adnexal) mass formation. They may be acute or chronic.

1. Acute (about 40% of tubal ectopic pregnancies)–Severe lower quadrant pain occurs in almost every case. It is sudden in onset, lancinating, intermittent, and does not radiate. Backache is present during attacks. Collapse and shock occur in about 10%, often after pelvic examination. At least two-thirds of patients give a history of abnormal menstruation; many have been infertile.

2. Chronic (about 60% of tubal ectopic pregnancies)–Blood leaks from the tubal ampulla over a period of days, and considerable blood may accumulate in the peritoneum. Slight but persistent vaginal spotting is reported, and a pelvic mass can be palpated. Abdominal distention and mild paralytic ileus are often present.

B. Laboratory Findings: Blood studies may show anemia and slight leukocytosis. Quantitative serum pregnancy tests will show levels generally lower than expected for normal pregnancies of the same duration. If pregnancy tests are followed over a few days, there may be a slow rise or a plateau rather than the doubling every 2 days associated with normal early intrauterine pregnancy or the falling levels that occur with spontaneous abortion.

C. Imaging: Ultrasonography can reliably demonstrate a gestational sac 6 weeks from the LMP and a fetal pole at 7 weeks if located in the uterus. An empty uterine cavity raises a strong suspicion of extrauterine pregnancy, which can occasionally be revealed by endovaginal ultrasound.

D. Special Examinations: Aspiration of the pouch of Douglas (culdocentesis) with an 18-gauge spinal needle will confirm hemoperitoneum. Laparoscopy to confirm an ectopic pregnancy is of great value prior to laparotomy.

Differential Diagnosis

Clinical and laboratory findings suggestive or diagnostic of pregnancy will distinguish ectopic pregnancy from many acute abdominal illnesses such as acute appendicitis, acute pelvic inflammatory disease, ruptured corpus luteum cyst or ovarian follicle, and urinary calculi. Uterine enlargement with clinical findings similar to those found in ectopic pregnancy is also characteristic of an aborting uterine pregnancy or hydatidiform mole. Doctors performing induced abortions must always suspect ectopic pregnancy when postabortal tissue examination fails to reveal placenta. They must take steps for immediate diagnosis, including prompt microscopic tissue examination, ultrasonography, and serial hCG titers every 48 hours. Patients must be warned of possible ectopic pregnancy problems and followed very closely.

Treatment

Hospitalize the patient if there is a reasonable likelihood of ectopic pregnancy. Type and cross-match blood. Ideally, diagnosis and operative treatment should precede frank rupture of the tube and intraabdominal hemorrhage.

Surgical treatment is definitive. Generally, salpingectomy will be required if the tube has ruptured. If the condition of the patient permits, assessment of the other tube is important at the time of laparotomy. Patency of the contralateral tube can be established by the injection of indigo carmine into the uterine cavity with appropriate compression of the lower uterine segment.

When the ectopic pregnancy is unruptured, it can often be removed via the laparoscope. Methotrexate—given systemically or by local injection into the ectopic pregnancy—is being used experimentally.

Iron therapy for anemia may be necessary during convalescence. Give Rh_o (D) immune globulin to Rh-negative patients.

Prognosis

Repeat tubal pregnancy occurs in about 12% of cases. This should not be regarded as a contraindication to future pregnancy, but the patient requires careful observation and early ultrasound confirmation of an intrauterine pregnancy.

Marchbanks PA et al: Risk factors for ectopic pregnancy. JAMA 1988;259:1823.

PREGNANCY-INDUCED HYPERTENSION (Preeclampsia-Eclampsia)

Essentials of Diagnosis

- Onset of symptoms in the third trimester of pregnancy.
- Blood pressure >140/90 mm Hg, or a rise of 30 mm Hg systolic or 15 mm Hg diastolic, noted on 2 occasions 6 hours apart, associated with the following:

    Significant proteinuria (500 mg/dL/24 h).

    Generalized edema, headache, visual disturbances, and epigastric pain.

    Increasing symptoms and signs preceding convulsions.

General Considerations

Preeclampsia-eclampsia usually occurs in the last trimester of pregnancy. It is often first observed during labor or in the first 24 hours after delivery. The term preeclampsia denotes the nonconvulsive form; with the development of convulsions and coma, the disorder is termed eclampsia. About 5% of pregnant women in the USA develop preeclampsia. Primiparas are most commonly affected. The incidence of preeclampsia is increased with multiple pregnancies, essential hypertension, diabetes mellitus, chronic renal disease, collagen disorders, and hydatidiform mole. Uncontrolled eclampsia is a significant cause of mater-

nal death. Five percent of cases of preeclampsia progress to eclampsia. Perinatal survival is very low when severe preeclampsia develops before the 28th week of pregnancy.

The basic cause is not known. Recent laboratory investigations suggest that it is an endothelial disorder resulting from poorly perfused placenta, which releases a factor—perhaps lipid peroxide—that injures the endothelium. Although changes are initiated in the first trimester, the problem is not seen clinically until the second half of pregnancy. Before the syndrome is clinically manifested, there is generalized vasospasm, causing increased total peripheral resistance and reduction of plasma volume and blood flow. The longer vasospasm continues, the greater the likelihood of associated pathologic changes in maternal organs, including the placenta; this indirectly affects the fetus.

None of the interventions recommended to reduce the incidence or severity of the process have proved to be of significant value when studied objectively, including diuretics, dietary restriction or enhancement, sodium restriction, and vitamin-mineral supplements. The only cure is termination of the pregnancy at a time as favorable as possible for fetal survival in the light of the medical condition of the mother.

A recent clinical investigation suggests that low-dose aspirin (100 mg daily starting in the third trimester) reduces the incidence of preeclampsia in women at high risk for developing the problem.

Clinical Findings

A. Preeclampsia:

1. Mild–Symptoms are absent. Diastolic blood pressure is elevated to 90–100 mm Hg. There is minimal proteinuria and no evidence of intrauterine growth retardation.

2. Severe–Headache, visual changes, and upper abdominal pain due to liver enlargement are present, as is oliguria. Intrauterine growth retardation is present. Blood pressure exceeds 160/110 mm Hg. Ophthalmoscopic examination reveals arteriolar spasm, occasional edema of the optic disks, and cotton-wool exudates. Laboratory findings include proteinuria (> 2000 mg/dL/24 h), evidence of azotemia (increased serum creatinine, uric acid, or urea nitrogen), disseminated intravascular coagulation (thrombocytopenia, decreased fibrinogen, and increased fibrin split products), and hepatocellular damage, including hyperbilirubinemia.

B. Eclampsia: The symptoms of eclampsia usually are engrafted on those of severe preeclampsia and include the following: (1) generalized tonic-clonic convulsions; (2) coma followed by amnesia and confusion; (3) 3–4+ proteinuria; (4) marked hypertension preceding a convulsion, and hypotension thereafter (during coma or vascular collapse); and (5) oliguria or anuria.

Differential Diagnosis

The combination of renal, neurologic, and hypertensive findings in a previously normal pregnant woman distinguishes a preeclampsia-eclampsia from primary hypertensive, renal, or neurologic disease.

Treatment

A. Preeclampsia: This condition should be recognized as early as possible by meticulous prenatal care. The objectives of treatment are (1) to prevent eclampsia, abruptio placentae, hepatic rupture, and ocular or vascular accidents; and (2) to deliver a normal baby that will survive. Place the patient at bed rest and give small doses of a benzodiazepine if necessary to make bed rest more acceptable. Delivery should be delayed, if possible, until the disease is under control and the fetus is mature ($\geq$ equal 34 weeks of gestation).

1. Home management–Most patients can be managed at home (at bed rest) under alert supervision, including frequent blood pressure readings performed by the patient or a relative, daily urine protein determinations, and careful recording of fluid intake and output. Mild sodium restriction ($<$ 3 g of salt per day) is advisable. If improvement does not occur in 48 hours, transfer the patient to a hospital.

2. Hospital care–Determine blood pressure, serum electrolytes, and urine protein at frequent intervals. Examine the ocular fundi every day, noting particularly arteriolar spasm, edema, hemorrhages, and exudates. The diet should be high in calcium, low in fat, high in complex carbohydrate, and moderate in protein content. Sedatives to promote quiet rest are indicated. Intravenous hydralazine is the antihypertensive of choice if diastolic blood pressure goes above 110 mm Hg. When labor ensues, parenteral magnesium sulfate is required to prevent seizures.

3. Observation of the fetus–With stabilization of preeclampsia, an optimal time for delivery minimizes perinatal illness and death. Deliver the fetus after 37 weeks by appropriate induction of labor, with cesarean section reserved for obstetric indications. Earlier in the third trimester, the status of the fetus can be followed with nonstress tests and oxytocin challenge tests done at 48-hour intervals. Regular maternal observations of fetal movements ("kick counts") are also useful. Estriol and human placental lactogen determinations are not necessary.

B. Eclampsia:

1. Emergency care–If the patient is convulsing, turn her on her side to prevent aspiration and to prevent the caval syndrome. Insert a padded tongue blade or plastic airway between the teeth. Aspirate fluid and food from the glottis or trachea. Give oxygen by nasal prongs. Give magnesium sulfate, 4 g (20 mL of a 20% solution) intravenously over a 4-minute period. At the same time, give 10 g of magnesium sulfate (20 mL of a 50% solution), one-half (10 mL) deep in each buttock (1 mL of 2% lidocaine may be added to each syringe to minimize pain). Thereafter, every 4 hours give 5 g of magnesium sulfate (10 mL of a 50% solution) in alternate buttocks as long as (1) knee jerk is present, (2) respirations are regular in rate (not $<$ 16/min), and (3) urine output was at least 100 mL in the previous 4 hours. In cases of overdosage, give calcium gluconate (or equivalent), 20 mL of a 10% aqueous solution intravenously slowly, and repeat every hour until urinary, respiratory, and neurologic depression have cleared.

2. General care–Hospitalize the patient in a darkened, quiet room at absolute bed rest, lying on her side, with side rails for protection during convulsions. Allow no visitors. Do not disturb the patient for unnecessary procedures (eg, baths, enemas), and leave the blood pressure cuff on her arm. Typed and crossmatched blood must be available for immediate use, because patients with eclampsia often develop premature separation of the placenta with hemorrhage and are susceptible to shock.

3. Laboratory evaluation–Insert a retention catheter for accurate measurement of the quantity of urine passed. Determine the protein content of each 24-hour specimen until the fourth or fifth postpartum day. Blood tests to evaluate clotting factors, liver function, and electrolytes should be obtained as often as the severity and progression of the disease indicate.

4. Physical examination–Check blood pressure frequently during the acute phase and every 2–4 hours thereafter. Monitor the fetal heart constantly, if possible. Perform ophthalmoscopic examination once a day. Examine the face, extremities, and especially the sacrum (which becomes dependent when the patient is in bed) for edema.

5. Diet and fluids–If the patient is convulsing, give nothing by mouth. Record fluid intake and output for each 24-hour period. If she can eat and drink, give a high-carbohydrate, moderate-protein, low-fat diet. If the urine output exceeds 700 mL/d, replace the output plus visible fluid loss with isotonic fluid. If the output is less than 700 mL/d, allow no more than 2000 mL of fluid per day (including parenteral fluid).

6. Diuretics–Because maternal hypovolemia is the rule in patients with preeclampsia-eclampsia, diuretics should be avoided. Hypertonic solutions are also unnecessary. Furosemide may be used in cases of pulmonary edema.

7. Sedatives–Use these agents sparingly if at all.

8. Antihypertensives–Hydralazine given in 5- to 10-mg increments intravenously every 20 minutes is used whenever the diastolic pressure is above 100 mm Hg. A satisfactory response is a decrease to 90–100 mm Hg. Further lowering may impair placental perfusion.

9. Delivery–Because severe hypertensive disease, renal disease, and preeclampsia-eclampsia are usually aggravated by continuing pregnancy, the best method of treatment of any of these disorders is termination of pregnancy, preferably after definite fetal viability. Control eclampsia before attempting induction of labor or delivery. Vaginal delivery is preferred. Induce labor, preferably by amniotomy alone, when the patient's condition permits. Use oxytocin to stimulate labor if necessary. Monitor the fetus carefully. Regional anesthesia is the technique of choice. Nitrous oxide (70%) and oxygen (30%) may be given with contractions, but 100% oxygen should be administered between contractions during the second stage.

Elective cesarean section may be considered if the patient is not at term or if labor is not inducible. Convulsions or coma must be absent for 12 or more hours before cesarean section is performed.

Prognosis

The maternal mortality rate in eclampsia is 10–15%. Most patients improve strikingly in 24–48 hours with appropriate therapy, but early termination of pregnancy is usually required.

Babies of mothers with preeclampsia-eclampsia are usually small for gestational age (probably because of placental malfunction). Their perinatal mortality rate is 4–5 times that of infants of nonpreeclamptic women.

Roberts JM et al: Preeclampsia: An endothelial cell disorder. Am J Obstet Gynecol 1989;161:1200.

Schiff E et al: The use of aspirin to prevent pregnancy-induced hypertension and lower the ratio of thromboxane A$_2$ to prostacyclin in relatively high risk pregnancies. N Engl J Med 1989;321:351.

GESTATIONAL TROPHOBLASTIC NEOPLASIA
(Hydatidiform Mole & Choriocarcinoma)

Essentials of Diagnosis

- Uterus sometimes larger than expected for duration of pregnancy.
- Excessively elevated levels of hCG.
- Vesicles passed from vagina.
- Ultrasound findings characteristic of mole.
- Uterine bleeding in pregnancy.

General Considerations

Gestational trophoblastic neoplasia is a spectrum of disease that includes hydatidiform mole, invasive mole, and choriocarcinoma. Cytogenetics has demonstrated that complete hydatidiform moles develop from androgenetic conceptions, which are almost always euploid (46 chromosomes). Partial moles are from conceptions in which sets of paternal chromosomes exceed maternal sets and thus are generally polyploid (23 × 3 or more chromosomes). Partial moles generally show evidence of an embryo or gestational sac, are slower growing and less symptomatic, and are often present clinically as a missed abortion.

Partial moles tend to follow a benign course, while complete moles have a greater tendency to become choriocarcinomas.

The highest rates of gestational trophoblastic neoplasia occur in some developing countries, with rates of 1:125 pregnancies in certain areas of the Orient. In the USA, the frequency is 1:1500 pregnancies. Risk factors include low socioeconomic status, a history of mole, and age below 18 or above 40. Approximately 10% of women require further treatment after evacuation of the mole; 5% develop choriocarcinoma.

Clinical Findings

A. Symptoms and Signs: Excessive nausea and vomiting occur in over one-third of patients with hydatidiform mole. Uterine bleeding, beginning at 6–8 weeks, is observed in virtually all instances and is indicative of threatened or incomplete abortion. In about one-fifth of cases, the uterus is larger than would be expected in a normal pregnancy of the same duration. Intact or collapsed vesicles may be passed through the vagina. These grapelike clusters or enlarged villi are diagnostic. Bilaterally enlarged cystic ovaries are sometimes palpable. They are the result of ovarian hyperstimulation due to excess of hCG.

Preeclampsia-eclampsia, frequently of the fulminating type, may develop during the second trimester of pregnancy, but this is unusual.

Choriocarcinoma may be manifested by continued or recurrent uterine bleeding after evacuation of a mole or following a delivery, abortion, or ectopic pregnancy. The presence of an ulcerative vaginal tumor, pelvic mass, or evidence of distant metastatic tumor may be the presenting observation. The diagnosis is established by pathologic examination of curettings or by biopsy.

B. Laboratory Findings: A serum hCG β-subunit value above 40,000 mIU/mL or a urinary hCG value in excess of 100,000 IU/24 h increases the likelihood of hydatidiform mole, although such values are occasionally seen with a normal pregnancy (eg, in multiple gestation).

C. Ultrasonography: Ultrasound has virtually replaced all other means of preoperative diagnosis of hydatidiform mole. The multiple echoes indicating edematous villi within the enlarged uterus and the absence of a fetus and placenta are pathognomonic.

D. Imaging: A preoperative chest film is indicated to rule out pulmonary metastases of trophoblast.

Treatment

A. Specific (Surgical) Measures: Empty the uterus as soon as the diagnosis of hydatidiform mole is established, preferably by suction. Do not resect ovarian cysts or remove the ovaries; spontaneous regression of theca lutein cysts will occur with elimination of the mole.

If malignant tissue is discovered at surgery or during

the follow-up examination, chemotherapy is indicated.

Thyrotoxicosis indistinguishable clinically from that of primary thyroid or pituitary origin may occur. Surgical removal of the mole promptly corrects the thyroid overactivity.

B. Follow-up Measures: Effective contraception (preferably birth control pills) should be prescribed. Weekly quantitative hCG level measurements are initially required. Moles show a progressive decline in hCG. After 2 negative weekly tests (< 5 mIU/mL), the interval may be increased to monthly for 6 months and then to every 2 months for a year. If levels plateau or begin to rise, the patient should be evaluated by repeat chest film and D&C before the initiation of chemotherapy.

C. Antitumor Chemotherapy: For low-risk patients with a good prognosis, give methotrexate, 0.4 mg/kg intramuscularly over a 5-day period, or dactinomycin, 10–12 μg/kg/d intravenously over a 5-day period (see Tables 3–2 and 3–3). Refer patients with a poor prognosis to a tumor center, where multiple-agent chemotherapy probably will be given. The side effects—anorexia, nausea and vomiting, stomatitis, rash, diarrhea, and bone marrow depression—usually are reversible in about 3 weeks. They can be ameliorated by the administration of folic acid. Death occurs occasionally from agranulocytosis or toxic hepatitis. Repeated courses of methotrexate 2 weeks apart generally are required to destroy the trophoblast and maintain a zero chorionic gonadotropin titer, as indicated by hCG β-subunit determination.

D. Supportive Measures: Replace blood, give iron, and encourage good nutrition. If infection is suspected, give broad-spectrum antibiotics for 24 hours before and 3–4 days after surgery. Prescribe oral contraceptives (if acceptable) or another reliable birth control method to avoid the hazard and confusion of elevated hCG from a new pregnancy. hCG levels should be negative for a year before pregnancy is again attempted. In the pregnancy following a mole, the hCG level should be checked 6 weeks postpartum.

Prognosis

A 5-year arrest after courses of chemotherapy, even when metastases have been demonstrated, can be expected in at least 85% of cases of choriocarcinoma.

THIRD-TRIMESTER BLEEDING

Five to 10% of women have vaginal bleeding in late pregnancy. Multiparas are more commonly affected. The clinician must distinguish between placental causes of obstetric bleeding (placenta previa, premature separation of the placenta) and nonplacental causes (systemic disease or disorders of the lower genital tract).

The approach to the problem of bleeding in late pregnancy should be conservative and expectant.

The patient should be hospitalized at once and placed at complete bed rest. Perform a gentle abdominal examination. Significant degrees of premature separation of the placenta (abruptio placentae) cause uterine tetany and tenderness, whereas placenta previa is associated with painless bleeding, abnormal fetal position (breech, transverse lie), and a high presenting part. Inspect the vagina and cervix with a speculum for cancer or infection. Avoid digital rectal or vaginal examination, which may result in excessive bleeding. Typed and cross-matched blood should be ready in case of need during the examination. Ultrasonography is accurate in detecting placental location. Over 90% of patients with third-trimester bleeding will stop bleeding in 24 hours with bed rest alone, although the bleeding may recur at a later time. If bleeding is profuse and persistent, and especially if there are persistent uterine contractions, vaginal examination is indicated after preparation for cesarean section and blood replacement.

If the patient is less than 36 weeks pregnant, it may be necessary to keep her in the hospital or at home at bed rest until the chances of delivering a viable infant improve and amniotic fluid tests confirm lung maturity.

When a diagnosis of placenta previa has been made and cesarean section is anticipated, the banking of autologous blood from the patient should be considered.

McVay PA et al: Safety and use of autologous blood donation during the third trimester of pregnancy. Am J Obstet Gynecol 1989;160:1479.

MEDICAL CONDITIONS COMPLICATING PREGNANCY

Anemia

Plasma volume increases approximately 50% during pregnancy, while red cell volume increases 25%, causing hemodilution with lowered hemoglobin and hematocrit values, which are maximally changed around the 24th week. True anemia in pregnancy is often defined as a hemoglobin measurement below 10 g/dL or hematocrit below 30%. Anemia is very common in pregnancy, causing fatigue, anorexia, dyspnea, and edema. Prevention through optimal nutrition and iron and folic acid supplementation is desirable. The basic laboratory examination is a complete blood count with red cell indices and a stool test for occult blood.

A. Iron Deficiency Anemia: Many women enter pregnancy with low iron stores resulting from heavy menstrual periods, previous pregnancies, or poor nutrition. It is difficult to meet the increased requirement for iron through diet, so that anemia often develops unless iron supplements are given. Red cells may not become hypochromic and microcytic until the hematocrit has fallen far below normal levels. The reticulocyte count is low. A serum iron level below 40 μg/dL and a transferrin saturation less than 16% suggest iron deficiency anemia. Treatment consists of a diet containing iron-rich foods and 60 mg of elemental iron (eg, 300 mg of ferrous sulfate) times a day with meals. Iron is best absorbed if taken with a source of vitamin C (raw fruits and vegetables, lightly cooked greens). For prevention of anemia, all pregnant women should take daily iron supplements containing 60 mg of elemental iron.

B. Folic Acid Deficiency Anemia: Folic acid deficiency anemia is the main cause of macrocytic anemia in pregnancy, since vitamin B 12 deficiency anemia is rare in the childbearing years. The daily folate requirement doubles from 400 μg to 800 μg in pregnancy. Twin pregnancies, acute infections, malabsorption syndromes, and use of anticonvulsant drugs such as phenytoin can precipitate folic acid deficiency. The anemia may first be seen in the puerperium owing to the increased need for folate during lactation.

The diagnosis is made by finding macrocytic red cells and hypersegmented neutrophils in a blood smear. However, blood smears in pregnancy may be difficult to interpret, since they frequently show iron deficiency changes as well. Because the deficiency is hard to diagnose and folate intake is inadequate in some socioeconomic groups, 0.8–1 mg of folic acid is routinely given as a supplement in pregnancy. Treat an established deficiency with 1–5 mg/d.

Good sources of folate in food are leafy green vegetables, orange juice, peanuts, and beans. Cooking and storage of food destroy folic acid. Strict vegetarians who eat no eggs or milk products should take vitamin B 12 supplements during pregnancy and lactation.

C. Sickle Cell Anemia: Women with sickle cell anemia are subject to serious complications in pregnancy. The anemia becomes more severe, and crises may occur more frequently. Complications include infections, bone pain, pulmonary infarction, congestive heart failure, and preeclampsia. There is an increased rate of spontaneous abortion and higher maternal and perinatal mortality rates. Newer methods of intensive medical treatment have improved the outcome for mother and fetus. Frequent transfusions of packed cells or leukocyte-poor washed red cells are used to lower the level of hemoglobin S and elevate the level of hemoglobin A; this minimizes the severity of anemia and the risk of sickle cell crises. Folic acid supplements should be given, and analgesics and adequate hydration are important.

Parent with sickle cell disease or sickle cell trait may wish to undergo first-trimester chorionic villus biopsy or second-trimester amniocentesis to determine whether sickle cell anemia has been passed on to the fetus. Genetic counseling should be available before pregnancy and postpartum for all patients with hemoglobinopathies and their partners. Elective sterilization and therapeutic abortion should be available if desired. IUDs and oral contraceptives are contraindicated for these patients, but progestin-only contraceptives may be used.

Women with sickle cell trait alone generally have an uncomplicated gestation. Sickle cell-hemoglobin C disease in pregnancy is similar to sickle cell anemia and is treated similarly.

Asthma

The effect of pregnancy on asthma is unpredictable. About 50% of patients have no change, 25% improve, and 25% get worse. For acute attacks of bronchospasm, subcutaneous epinephrine is the treatment of choice. For mild episodes, theophylline or ephedrine can be used; cromolyn for prevention is also considered safe. For severe cases, 5–7 days of prednisone (30–50 mg/d) can be helpful, with inhaled beclomethasone dipropionate being used to permit a gradual decrease in oral corticosteroids.

Greenberger PA, Patterson R: Current concepts: Management of asthma during pregnancy. N Engl J Med 1985;312:897.

AIDS During Pregnancy

In the USA at present, 78% of women with AIDS are intravenous drug users or partners of drug users. Prostitutes, women partners of hemophiliacs and recipients of HIV-contaminated blood transfusions (1978–1985) represent smaller groups of infected women. The prevalence of AIDS among heterosexual women without identified risks is estimated to be 0.02%. Asymptomatic HIV infection is not associated with a decreased pregnancy rate or increased risk of adverse pregnancy outcomes. There is no evidence that pregnancy causes AIDS progression.

The rates of transplacental transmission of AIDS have varied from 20% to 50%, apparently related to the stage of the mother's illness. HIV-infected women should be advised not to breast-feed their infants.

Prenatal HIV testing is voluntary in the USA and should be encouraged in the high-risk groups. Appropriate counseling of HIV antibody-positive pregnant women includes the option of pregnancy termination.

Obstetric caregivers should meticulously observe the established protocols for skin and eye protection against blood and internal secretions, particularly at the time of delivery.

Shapiro CN et al: Review of human immunodeficiency virus infection in women in the United States. Obstet Gynecol 1989;74:800.

Diabetes Mellitus

During pregnancy there is increased tissue resistance to insulin with resultant increased levels of blood insulin as well as glucose and triglycerides. These changes result from secretion of human placental lactogen and increasing levels of estrogen and progesterone. The prevention of common hazards of diabetes, such as hypoglycemia, ketosis, and diabetic coma, requires great effort and attention to detail on the part of both the physician and the patient. Although pregnancy does not appear to alter the ultimate severity of diabetes, retinopathy and nephropathy may appear or become worse during pregnancy. Over the years, the White classification of diabetes during pregnancy (Table 13–11) has allowed for uniform description and comparison of diabetic pregnant women.

Even in carefully managed diabetics, the incidence of obstetric complications such as hydramnios, preeclampsia-eclampsia, infections, and prematurity is increased. The infants are larger than those of nondiabetic women. There is an increase in the number of unexplained fetal deaths in the last few weeks of pregnancy as well as a high rate of neonatal deaths. There is general agreement that the outcome of diabetic pregnancies is best among women served at regional centers where teams of clinicians regularly manage significant numbers of patients.

Prepregnancy metabolic evaluation of diabetic women is crucial to ensure a problem-free pregnancy, decreased risk of spontaneous abortion, and a normal healthy newborn. Glycosylated hemoglobin (HbA_{1c}) levels will define the quality of glucose control in the preceding weeks and months. Fair to good control is generally associated with levels of HbA_{1c} less than 9.5%. Euglycemia should be established before conception and should be maintained during pregnancy with patient-performed blood glucose monitoring at home 4 times daily and frequent small meals (6 per day). Recent data confirm that perinatal problems for mother and newborn are decreased as fastidious diabetic control increases.

The maintenance of euglycemia is improved by patient-performed blood sugar monitoring at home 4 times daily with added postmeal observations once or twice a week. Attempts are under way to decrease the number of congenital anomalies associated with diabetic pregnancies. Prepregnancy evaluation and adjustment of insulin control based on glycosylated hemoglobin will maintain strict euglycemia in early pregnancy when organogenesis is occurring. The use of a continuous insulin pump is under study for its effect in lowering the frequency of anomalies. Time of delivery is dictated by deterioration of diabetic control, the onset of preeclampsia, decreased fetal reactivity as judged by nonstress or oxytocin challenge tests, or confirmation of lung maturity at or about 38 weeks of pregnancy. Cesarean sections are performed for obstetric indications.

Because 50% of gestational diabetics go on to develop overt diabetes mellitus and because the infants of gestational diabetics suffer risks similar to those borne by infants of diabetic mothers, screening of all pregnant women for glucose intolerance has been recommended between the 24th and 28th weeks of pregnancy (Table 13–12). Nutritional advice, blood glucose monitoring, and obstetric surveillance should be meticulous.

Gestational diabetes should be evaluated 6–8 weeks postpartum by a 2-hour oral glucose tolerance test (75 g glucose load).

Damm P, Mosted-Pedersen L: Significant decrease in congenital malformations in newborn infants of an unselected population of diabetic women. Am J Obstet Gynecol 1989;161:1163.

Table 13–11. Modified White classification of diabetes mellitus.[1]

Class A: Chemical diabetes diagnosed *before pregnancy;* managed by diet *alone;* any age of onset or duration.
Class B: Insulin treatment necessary *before* pregnancy; onset after age 20; duration of less than 10 years.
Class C: Onset at age 10–19; or duration of 10–19 years.
Class D: Onset before age 10; or duration of 20 or more years; or chronic hypertension; or background retinopathy.
Class F: Renal disease.
Class H: Coronary artery disease.
Class R: Proliferative retinopathy.
Class T: Renal transplant.

[1] Reproduced, with permission, from Pernoll ML, Benson RC (editors): *Current Obstetric & Gynecologic Diagnosis & Treatment,* 6th ed. Appleton & Lange, 1987.

Table 13–12. Screening and diagnostic criteria for gestational diabetes mellitus.

Screening for gestational diabetes
1. 2 hour postprandial glucose. . . . Glucose measurement in blood.
2. 50-g oral glucose load, administered between the 24th and 28th weeks, without regard to time of day or time of last meal, to all pregnant women who have not been identified as having glucose intolerance before the 24th week.
3. Venous plasma glucose measured 1 hour later.
4. Value of 140 mg/dL (7.8 mmol/L) or above in venous plasma indicates the need for a full diagnostic glucose tolerance test.

Diagnosis of gestational diabetes mellitus
1. 100-g oral glucose load, administered in the morning after overnight fast lasting at least 8 hours but not more than 14 hours, and following at least 3 days of unrestricted diet (> 150 g carbohydrate) and physical activity.
2. Venous plasma glucose is measured fasting and at 1, 2, and 3 hours. Subject should remain seated and not smoke throughout the test.
3. Two or more of the following venous plasma concentrations must be equaled or exceeded for positive diagnosis: fasting, 105 mg/dL (5.8 mmol/L); 1 hour, 190 mg/dL (10.6 mmol/L); 2 hours, 165 mg/dL (9.2 mmol/L); 3 hours, 145 mg/dL (8.1 mmol/L).

Heart Disease

Most cases of heart disease complicating pregnancy in the USA now are of congenital origin. About 5% of maternal deaths are due to heart disease. Pregnancy causes a significant increase in pulse rate, an increase of cardiac output of more than 30%, and a rise in plasma volume greater than red cell mass with relative hemodilution. Both vital capacity and oxygen consumption rise only slightly.

For practical purposes, the functional capacity of the heart is the best single measurement of cardiopulmonary status.

Class I: Ordinary physical activity causes no discomfort (perinatal mortality rate about 5%).

Class II: Ordinary activity causes discomfort and slight disability (perinatal mortality rate 10–15%).

Class III: Less than ordinary activity causes discomfort or disability; patient is barely compensated (perinatal mortality rate about 35%).

Class IV: Patient decompensated; any physical activity causes acute distress (perinatal mortality rate over 50%).

In general, patients with class I or class II functional disability (80% of pregnant women with heart disease) do well obstetrically. Over 80% of maternal deaths due to heart disease occur in women with class III or IV cardiac disability. Congestive failure is the usual cause of death. Three-fourths of these deaths occur in the early puerperium. Pregnancy is contraindicated in Eisenmenger's complex; in severe mitral stenosis if there is pulmonary hypertension; in Marfan's syndrome, in which the aorta is prone to rupture; and in primary pulmonary hypertension. In addition, pregnancy is poorly tolerated in patients with aortic stenosis (uncorrected), aortic coarctation, tetralogy of Fallot, active rheumatic carditis, and any other lesion with class III or class IV symptoms.

Therapeutic abortion and elective sterilization should be offered to patients with significant cardiac disease. Cesarean section should be performed only upon obstetric indications. Appropriate antibiotic prophylaxis against infective endocarditis is indicated after delivery or termination of pregnancy.

Sullivan JM, Ramanathan KB: Current concepts: Management of medical problems of pregnancy: Severe cardiac disease. N Engl J Med 1985;313:304.

Herpes Genitalis
(See also Chapter 4.)

Infection of the lower genital tract by herpes simplex virus type 2 (HSV-2) is a common sexually transmitted disease of potential seriousness to pregnant women and their newborn infants. Even though one series in the USA reports that 20% of women in an obstetric practice are positive for HSV-2 antibodies, a history of the infection is unreliable and the incidence of neonatal infection is extremely low (1:20,000–1:3000 live births). Most infected neonates are born to women with no history, signs, or symptoms of infection.

Cesarean section is indicated at the time of labor if there are definite prodromal symptoms, active genital lesions, or a positive cervical culture obtained within the preceding week. Abdominal delivery is protective to the baby even several hours after rupture of the membranes.

Women who have had primary herpes infection late in pregnancy are at high risk of shedding virus at delivery. They should be screened by means of weekly cultures during the last month of pregnancy, because the neonatal attack rate is 50%.

Woman with a history of recurrent genital herpes have a neonatal attack rate of 8% and should be followed by clinical observation and culture of any suspicious lesions. Since asymptomatic viral shedding is not predictable by antepartum cultures, current recommendations do not include routine cultures in individuals with a history of herpes but with no active disease. However, when labor begins, vulvar and cervical cultures should be taken. Prompt treatment of a potentially infected newborn after a positive maternal herpes culture should permit successful management of the baby.

For treatment, see Chapter 31. The safety of acyclovir in pregnancy has not been established.

Prober CG et al: Use of routine viral cultures at delivery to identify neonates exposed to herpes simplex virus. N Engl J Med 1988:318:887.

Hypertensive Disease

Hypertensive disease in women of childbearing age is usually essential hypertension. Other less common but important causes should be looked for: coarctation of the aorta, pheochromocytoma, aldosteronism, and renovascular and renal hypertension.

Preeclampsia is superimposed on 20% of pregnancies in women with hypertensive disease, and in such patients it appears earlier, is more severe, and is more often associated with intrauterine growth retardation. It may be difficult to determine whether or not hypertension in a pregnant woman precedes or derives from the pregnancy if she is not examined until after the 20th week and there is no reliable medical history. When in doubt, treat for preeclampsia. The hypertension of preeclampsia usually recedes 6 weeks after delivery. If it persists for 3 months postpartum, it is probably essential hypertension.

Pregnant women with probable hypertensive disease require antihypertensive drugs only if the diastolic pressure is sustained at or above 110 mm Hg. One should strive to keep the diastolic pressure between 90 and 100 mm Hg. However, if the pressure is over 110 mm Hg, do not attempt to lower it quickly by more than 25%.

If a hypertensive woman is being managed successfully by medical treatment when she registers for antenatal care, one may generally continue the antihypertensive medication. Diuretics can be continued in pregnancy; propranolol is best replaced by a more selective β-adrenergic antagonist that is less lipid-soluble (eg, metoprolol). For initiation of treatment, one may begin with hydralazine, 25 mg orally daily, and increase the dosage as indicated. If the response is unsatisfactory or if the patient is not near term, give methyldopa, 250 mg orally twice daily, again building in divided doses as needed to as much as 2 g daily.

The incidence or severity of preeclampsia and the increased perinatal mortality rate associated with hypertensive syndromes are reduced slightly by long-term drug therapy.

Therapeutic abortion may be indicated in cases of severe hypertension during pregnancy. If pregnancy is allowed to continue, the risk to the fetus must be assessed periodically in anticipation of early delivery. An early second-trimester ultrasound examination will confirm the duration of pregnancy, and follow-up examinations after 28 weeks will evaluate intrauterine growth retardation.

Maternal Hepatitis B Carrier State

There are an estimated 200 million chronic carriers of hepatitis B virus worldwide. Among these people there is an increased incidence of chronic active hepatitis, cirrhosis, and hepatocellular carcinoma. The frequency of the hepatitis B carrier state varies from 1% in the USA and Western Europe to 35% in parts of Africa and Asia. All pregnant women should be screened for hepatitis B surface antigen (HBsAg). The mother who will transmit the virus to her baby after delivery can be recognized by positive blood tests for hepatitis B surface antigen (HBsAg) and hepatitis B e antigen (HBeAg). Vertical transmission can be blocked by the immediate postdelivery administration to the newborn of 0.5 mL of hepatitis B immunoglobulin and 10 mg of hepatitis B vaccine intramuscularly. The vaccine dose is repeated at 1 and 6 months of age.

Prevention of perinatal transmission of hepatitis B virus: Prenatal screening of all pregnant women for hepatitis B surface antigen. MMWR 1988;37:341.

Seizure Disorders

Women contemplating pregnancy who have not had a seizure for 5 years should consider a prepregnancy trial of withdrawal from seizure medication. Those with recurrent epilepsy should use a single drug with blood level monitoring. Trimethadione and valproic acid are contraindicated during pregnancy;

phenytoin is also considered teratogenic and should not be used unless absolutely necessary. Phenobarbital is considered the drug of choice in pregnancy. Anticonvulsant serum levels should be measured at least monthly and dosage adjustments made to keep serum levels in the low normal therapeutic range. Pregnant women taking these drugs should receive vitamin supplements, including folic acid, throughout pregnancy and vitamin K, 20 mg/d, during the last month to help prevent coagulation problems in the newborn.

Newborns of mothers taking phenobarbital or phenytoin are at risk of bleeding tendencies due to decreased levels of vitamin K-dependent clotting factors. Such infants should receive an injection of vitamin K_1, 1 mg given subcutaneously immediately after delivery, and should have clotting studies 2–4 hours later. Breast-feeding is not contraindicated.

Yerby MS: Problems and management of the pregnant woman with epilepsy. Epilepsia 1987;28 (Suppl 3):529.

Syphilis, Gonorrhea, & *Chlamydia trachomatis* Infection (See also Chapters 26 and 27.)

These sexually transmitted diseases have significant consequences for mother and child. Untreated syphilis in pregnancy will cause late abortion or transplacental infection with congenital syphilis. Gonorrhea will produce large-joint arthritis by hematogenous spread as well as newborn eye damage. Maternal chlamydial infections are largely asymptomatic but are manifested in the newborn by inclusion conjunctivitis and, at age 2–4 months, by pneumonia. The diagnosis of each can be reliably made by appropriate laboratory tests, which should be included in all prenatal care. The sexual partners of women with sexually transmitted diseases should be identified and treated also if that can be done.

Thyrotoxicosis

Thyrotoxicosis during pregnancy may result in fetal anomalies, late abortion, or preterm labor and fetal hyperthyroidism with goiter. Thyroid storm in late pregnancy or labor is a life-threatening emergency.

Radioactive isotope therapy must never be given during pregnancy. The thyroid inhibitor of choice is propylthiouracil, which acts to prevent further thyroxine formation by blocking iodination of tyrosine. There is a 2- to 3-week delay before the pretreatment hormone level begins to fall. The initial dose of propylthiouracil is 100–150 mg 3 times a day; the dose is lowered as the euthyroid state is approached. It is desirable to keep thyroxine (T_4) in the high normal range during pregnancy. A maintenance dose of 100 mg/d minimizes the chance of fetal hypothyroidism and goiter. Elective thyroidectomy is recommended by some in preference to medical management during and even after pregnancy (see Chapter 20).

Recurrent postpartum thyroiditis is a newly recognized entity occurring 3–6 months after delivery. A hyperthyroid state of 1–3 months' duration is followed by hypothyroidism, sometimes misdiagnosed as depression. Microsomal thyroid antibodies and thyroglobulin antibodies are present. Recovery is spontaneous in over 90% of cases after 3–6 months.

Burrow GN: Current concepts: The management of thyrotoxicosis in pregnancy. N Engl J Med 1985;313:562.

Tuberculosis

The diagnosis of tuberculosis in pregnancy is made by history taking, physical examination, and skin testing, with special attention to women from ethnic groups with a high prevalence of the disease (such as women from southeast Asia). Chest films should not be obtained as a routine screening measure in pregnancy but should be used only patients with a skin test that has converted from negative to positive or with suggestive findings in the history and physical examination. Use abdominal shielding if a chest film is obtained.

If adequately treated, tuberculosis in pregnancy has an excellent prognosis. There is no increase in spontaneous abortion, fetal problems, or congenital anomalies in patients receiving antitubercular chemotherapy.

Treatment is with isoniazid and ethambutol or isoniazid and rifampin. Because isoniazid therapy may result in vitamin B_6 deficiency, a supplement of 50 mg/d of vitamin B_6 should be given simultaneously. Streptomycin, ethionamide, and most other antituberculous drugs should be avoided in pregnancy.

Urinary Tract Infection

The urinary tract is especially vulnerable to infections during pregnancy because the altered secretions of steroid sex hormones and the pressure exerted by the gravid uterus upon the ureters and bladder cause hypotonia and congestion and predispose to urinary stasis. Labor and delivery and urinary retention postpartum also may initiate or aggravate infection. *Escherichia coli* is the offending organism in over two-thirds of cases.

From 2% to 8% of pregnant women have asymptomatic bacteriuria, which some believe to be associated with increased risk of prematurity. It is estimated that 20–40% of these women will develop pyelonephritis during pregnancy.

A first-trimester urine culture is indicated in women with a history of recurrent or recent episodes of urinary tract infection. If the culture is positive, treatment should be initiated as a prophylactic measure. Sulfisoxazole, nitrofurantoin, penicillins, and cephalosporins are acceptable medications for 7–10 days. Sulfonamides should not be given in the third trimester. If bacteriuria returns, suppressive medication (one daily dose of an appropriate antibiotic) for the remainder of the pregnancy is indicated. Acute pyelonephritis requires hospitalization for intravenous administration of antibiotics until the patient is afebrile; this is followed by a full course of oral antibiotics.

SURGICAL COMPLICATIONS DURING PREGNANCY

Elective major surgery should be avoided during pregnancy. However, normal, uncomplicated pregnancy has no debilitating effect and does not alter operative risk except as it may interfere with the diagnosis of abdominal disorders and increase the technical problems of intra-abdominal surgery. Abortion is not a serious hazard after operation unless peritoneal sepsis or other significant complication occurs.

During the first trimester, congenital anomalies may be induced in the developing fetus by hypoxia. Avoid surgical intervention during this period; if surgery does become necessary, the greatest precautions must be taken to prevent hypotension and hypoxia.

The second trimester is usually the optimal time for elective operative procedures.

Appendicitis

Appendicitis occurs in about one of 5000 pregnancies. Diagnosis is more difficult when the disease occurs in pregnant persons, since the appendix is carried high and to the right, away from McBurney's point, as the uterus enlarges, and localization of pain and infection does not usually occur. Nausea, vomiting, fever, and leukocytosis occur regularly. Any right-sided pain associated with these symptoms should raise a suspicion of appendicitis. In at least 20% of obstetric patients, the diagnosis of appendicitis is not made until the appendix has ruptured and peritonitis has become established. Such a delay may lead to premature labor or abortion. With early diagnosis and appendectomy, the prognosis is good for mother and baby.

Carcinoma of the Breast

Cancer of the breast (see also Chapter 12) is diagnosed approximately once in 3500 pregnancies. Pregnancy may accelerate the growth of cancer of the breast; however, delay in diagnosis affects the outcome of treatment more significantly. Inflammatory carcinoma is an extremely virulent type of breast cancer that occurs most commonly during lactation. Prepregnancy mammography should be encouraged for women over age 35 who are anticipating a pregnancy.

Breast enlargement during pregnancy obscures parenchymal masses, and breast tissue hyperplasia decreases the accuracy of mammography. Any perceived discrete mass should be promptly evaluated by aspiration to verify cystic structure and then by fine-needle biopsy if it is solid. A definitive diagnosis may require excisional biopsy under local anesthesia. If breast biopsy confirms the diagnosis of cancer, surgery should be done regardless of the stage of the pregnancy. If spread to the regional glands has occurred, irradiation or chemotherapy should be considered. Under these circumstances, termination of an early pregnancy or delay of therapy for fetal maturation is indicated.

Choledocholithiasis, Cholecystitis, & Idiopathic Cholestasis of Pregnancy

Severe choledocholithiasis and cholecystitis are not common during pregnancy despite the fact that women tend to form gallstones. When they do occur, it is usually in late pregnancy or in the puerperium. About 90% of patients with cholecystitis have gallstones; 90% of stones will be visualized by ultrasonography.

Symptomatic relief may be all that is required.

Gallbladder surgery in pregnant women should be attempted only in extreme cases (eg, obstruction), because it increases the perinatal mortality rate to about 15%. Cholecystostomy and lithotomy may be all that is feasible during advanced pregnancy, cholecystectomy being deferred until after delivery. On the other hand, withholding surgery when it is definitely needed may result in necrosis and perforation of the gallbladder and peritonitis. Cholangitis due to impacted common duct stone requires surgical removal of gallstones and establishment of biliary drainage.

Idiopathic cholestasis of pregnancy is due to a hereditary metabolic (hepatic) deficiency aggravated by the high estrogen levels of pregnancy. It causes intrahepatic biliary obstruction of varying degrees. The rise in bile acids is sufficient in the third trimester to cause severe, intractable, generalized itching and sometimes clinical jaundice. There may be mild elevations in blood bilirubin and alkaline phosphatase levels. The fetus is generally unaffected, although an increased prematurity rate has been reported. Resins such as cholestyramine (4 g 3 times a day) absorb bile acids in the large bowel and relieve pruritus but are difficult to take and may cause constipation. Their use requires vitamin K supplementation. The disorder is relieved once the infant has been delivered, but it recurs in subsequent pregnancies and sometimes with the use of oral contraceptives.

Ovarian Tumors

The most common adnexal mass in early pregnancy is the corpus luteum, which may become cystic and enlarge to 6 cm in diameter. Any persistent mass over 5 cm should be evaluated by ultrasound examination; unilocular cysts are likely to be corpus luteum cysts, whereas septated or semisolid tumors are likely to be neoplasms. Ovarian tumors may undergo torsion and cause abdominal pain and nausea and vomiting and must be differentiated from appendicitis, other bowel disease, and ectopic pregnancy. Patients with suspected ovarian cancer should be referred to a gynecologic oncologist to determine whether the pregnancy can progress to fetal viability or whether treatment should be instituted without delay.

Mazze R, Kallen B: Reproductive outcome after anesthesia and operation during pregnancy: A registry study of 5405 cases. Am J Obstet Gynecol 1989;161:1178.

PREVENTION OF HEMOLYTIC DISEASE OF THE NEWBORN (Erythroblastosis Fetalis)

The antibody anti-Rh_o (D) is responsible for most severe instances of hemolytic disease of the newborn (erythroblastosis fetalis). About 15% of whites and much lower proportions of blacks and Asians are Rh_o (D)-negative. If an Rh_o (D)-negative woman carries an Rh_o (D)-positive fetus, she may develop antibodies against Rh_o (D) when fetal red cells enter her circulation at delivery (or during abortion, ectopic pregnancy, abruptio placentae, or other antepartum bleeding problems). This antibody, once produced, remains in the woman's circulation and poses a serious threat of hemolytic disease for subsequent Rh-positive fetuses.

Passive immunization against hemolytic disease of the newborn now is possible with Rh_o (D) immune globulin, a purified concentrate of antibodies against Rh_o (D) antigen. To be maximally effective, the Rh_o (D) immune globulin should be given within 72 hours after delivery (or spontaneous or induced abortion or ectopic pregnancy). The antibodies in the immune globulin destroy fetal Rh-positive cells so that the mother will not produce anti-Rh_o (D). During her next Rh-positive gestation, erythroblastosis will be prevented.

The usual dose of Rh_o (D) immune globulin for prevention of isoimmunization is 1 vial (300 mg) intramuscularly.

It has recently been demonstrated that a rare Rh-negative woman will become sensitized by small fetomaternal bleeding episodes in the early third trimester. An additional safety measure is the administration of the immune globulin at the 28th week of pregnancy. The antibody molecules are too large to pass through the placenta and affect an Rh-positive fetus. The maternal clearance of the globulin is slow enough that protection will continue for 12 weeks.

Mild to moderate degrees of hemolytic disease continue to occur in association with Rh subgroups (C, c, or E) or the Kell (k) factor. Therefore, atypical antibodies should be checked in the third trimester of all pregnancies.

PREVENTION OF PRETERM (PREMATURE) LABOR

Preterm (premature) labor is labor that begins before the 37th week of pregnancy; it is responsible for 85% of neonatal illnesses and deaths. The onset of labor is a result of a complex sequence of biologic events involving regulatory factors that are still poorly understood. It is theorized that the delicate balance of hormones and other agents which maintain pregnancy may be upset by maternal changes such as alteration in estrogen-progesterone-prostaglandin production or by fetal factors such as increases in fetal ACTH and cortisol. If these events occur too early, preterm labor may ensue. The most significant risk factors for the onset of preterm labor are a past history of preterm delivery, premature rupture of the membranes, urinary tract infection, or exposure to diethylstilbestrol. In the current pregnancy, multiple gestation and abdominal or cervical surgery are especially important. To estimate the clinical risk, see Table 13–13.

Low rates of preterm delivery are associated with success in educating patients to identify regular, frequent uterine contractions and in alerting medical and nursing staff to evaluate these patients early and initiate treatment if cervical changes can be identified. Cessation of work or physical activities that seem related to increased uterine activity is mandatory. Resting at home will often suffice to slow contractions. Portable light-weight monitors of uterine contractions are being evaluated for home use. If successful, they will permit a woman to record uterine activity at will or on a schedule and to transmit the data by telephone to a central terminal for analysis.

In more acute situations, sedation with opiates and hydration with oral or intravenous fluids, if given before uterine contractions have changed the cervix appreciably, will often avert the need for specific drug therapy. Intravenous magnesium sulfate in doses

Table 13–13. Risk of preterm delivery.[1]

Score[2]	Socioeconomic Status	Past History	Daily Habits	Current Pregnancy	
				Mother	Fetus
1	2 children at home. Low socioeconomic status.	One first trimester abortion. Less than 1 year since last birth.	Work outside home.	Unusual fatigue.	. . .
2	Under 20 years of age. Over 40 years of age. Single parent.	Two first trimester abortions.	More than 10 cigarettes per day.	Less than 12 lb weight gain by 32 weeks. Albuminuria. Hypertension. Bacteriuria.	. . .
3	Very low socioeconomic status. Malnourished. Shorter than 150 cm (5 ft). Weighs less than 45 cm (100 lb).	Three first trimester abortions.	Unusual anxiety. Heavy work. Long, tiring travel. Long commute distance.	Weight loss of 2 kg. Febrile illness. Leiomyomas.	Head engaged before 34 weeks.
4	Under 18 years of age.	Pyelonephritis.	. . .	Uterine bleeding after 12 weeks. Effacement or dilation of cervix before 36 weeks. Uterine irritability.	. . .
5	. . .	Uterine anomaly. Second trimester abortion. Cone biopsy.	. . .	Placenta previa. Hydramnios.	. . .
10	. . .	Premature delivery. DES exposure. Repeated second trimester abortion.	. . .	Abdominal surgery. Cervical surgery.	Twins. Small-for-dates fetus.

[1] Modified and reproduced, with permission, from Zuspan FK, Quilligan EJ (editors): *Practical Manual of Obstetric Care.* Mosby, 1982. (Modified from Creasy R: Personal communication.)
[2] Score is computed by addition of the number of points given any item in any column. 0–5 = minimal risk; 6–9 = moderate risk; 10 or more = high risk.

similar to those used for the treatment of preeclampsia is an effective tocolytic and can be used before intravenous beta-adrenergic drugs are initiated. Magnesium sulfate can be given initially as a 4-g bolus and followed by a continuous infusion of 2 g/h. The rate may be increased by 1 g/h every 30 minutes until contractions cease or a blood magnesium concentration of 6–8 mg/dL is reached. Samples of magnesium levels are drawn at 1, 6 and 12 hours and each time the infusion rate is increased. After contractions have ceased for 12 hours, ritodrine can be started.

Uterine smooth muscle is largely under sympathetic nervous system control, and stimulation of b 2 receptors relaxes the myometrium. Consequently, inhibition of uterine contractility often can be accomplished by the administration of β-adrenergic drugs such as ritodrine (Yutopar).

Ritodrine can be administered by intravenous infusion in lactated Ringer's injection, beginning at a rate of 50 μg/min and increasing by 50 μg/min every 20 minutes until contractions cease or become less frequent than every 10 minutes or until an infusion rate of 350 μg/min is reached. After 1 hour of satisfactory tocolysis, the infusion rate can be decreased by 50 μg/min every 30 minutes to a rate that continues inhibition. If labor recurs, the step-up and step-down regimen can be reinstituted. Oral therapy is started 30 minutes before stopping intravenous ritodrine and is continued in a dose of 10–20 mg every 4–6 hours. A dose-related elevation of heart rate of 20–40 beats/min may occur. An increase of systolic blood pressure up to 10 mm Hg is likely, and the diastolic pressure may fall 10–15 mm Hg during the infusion. Nonetheless, cardiac output increases considerably. Transient elevation of blood glucose, insulin, and fatty acids together with slight reduction of serum potassium have been reported. Fetal tachycardia may be slight or absent. No drug-caused perinatal deaths have been reported. Maternal side effects requiring dose limitation are tachycardia ($\geq$ 140 beats/min), palpitations, and nervousness. Fluids should be limited to 2500 mL/24 h. Serious side effects (pulmonary edema, chest pain with or without electrocardiographic changes) are often idiosyncratic, not dose-related, and warrant termination of therapy.

One must identify cases in which untimely delivery is the sole threat to the life or health of the infant. An effort should be made to eliminate (1) maternal conditions that compromise the intrauterine environment and make premature birth the lesser risk, eg, preeclampsia-eclampsia; (2) fetal conditions that either are helped by early delivery or render attempts to stop premature labor meaningless, eg, severe erythroblastosis fetalis; and (3) clinical situations in which it is likely that an attempt to stop labor will be futile, eg, ruptured membranes, cervix fully effaced and dilated more than 3 cm, strong labor in progress.

In pregnancies of less than 34 weeks' duration, betamethasone (12 mg intramuscularly repeated in 24 hours) is administered to hasten fetal lung maturation and permit delivery 48 hours after initial treatment when prolongation of pregnancy is contraindicated.

Caritis SN: A pharmacologic approach to the infusion of ritodrine. Am J Obstet Gynecol 1988;158:380.
Hollander DI, Nagey DA, Pupkin MJ: Magnesium sulfate and ritodrine hydrochloride: A randomized comparison. Am J Obstet Gynecol 1987;156:631.

LACTATION

Breast feeding should be encouraged by educative measures throughout pregnancy and the puerperium. Mothers should be told the benefits of breast feeding—it is emotionally satisfying, promotes mother-infant bonding, is economical, and gives significant immunity to the infant. Breast feeding also helps women lose some of the extra fat gained during pregnancy. If the mother must return to work, even a brief period of nursing is beneficial.

Transfer of immunoglobulins in colostrum and breast milk protects the infant against many systemic and enteric infections. Macrophages and lymphocytes transferred to the infant from breast milk play an immunoprotective role. The intestinal flora of breast-fed infants have fewer bacterial and viral infections, less severe diarrhea, fewer allergy problems, and less subsequent obesity than bottle-fed infants.

Frequent breast feeding on an infant demand schedule enhances milk flow and successful breast feeding. Mothers breast-feeding for the first time need help and encouragement from physicians, nurses, and other nursing mothers of lay groups such as the La Leche League. Milk supply can be increased by increased suckling and increased rest.

Nursing mothers should have a fluid intake of over 2 L/d. The United States RDA calls for 24 g of extra protein (over the 44 g/d baseline for an adult woman) and 550 extra kcal/d in the first 6 months of nursing. Calcium intake should be 1200–1500 mg/d. Continuation of a prenatal vitamin and mineral supplement is wise. Strict vegetarians who eschew both milk and eggs should always take vitamin B 12 supplements during pregnancy and lactation.

Effects of Drugs in a Nursing Mother

Drugs taken by a nursing mother may accumulate in milk and be transmitted to the infant. The amount of a drug entering the milk depends on the drug's lipid solubility, mechanism of transport, and degree of ionization (Table 13–14).

Suppression of Lactation

A. Mechanical Suppression: The simplest and safest method of suppressing lactation after it has started is to gradually transfer the baby to a bottle

Table 13–14. Common drugs or substances to be used cautiously or not at all by nursing mothers.[1] (Additional drugs are also contraindicated during pregnancy and lactation. Evaluate any drug for its need and its potential adverse effects.)

Drugs or Substances	Effect on Nursing Infant
Alcohol	No harmful effects unless taken in excess, when it can be associated with decreased linear growth and sedation.
Antibiotics Aminoglycosides	Not advised; will alter infant's bowel flora.
Nitrofurantoin	May cause hemolytic anemia in infant with glucose-6-phosphate dehydrogenase (G6PD) deficiency.
Tetracycline	Effects are dose-related; amount infant receives from milk is too small to cause discoloration of teeth. Safe.
Chloramphenicol[2]	Neonate may be unable to conjugate the drug; potential harm to bone marrow, leading to anemia, shock, and death.
Sulfonamides[2]	May cause jaundice in the neonatal period; may cause hemolytic anemia in infant with glucose-6-phosphate dehydrogenase (G6PD) deficiency.
Metronidazole	Nursing may be resumed 48 hours after last dose.
Anticoagulants Phenindione[2]	Can use heparin or warfarin instead.
Antihistamines	Contraindicated because of increased sensitivity of newborns and infants to antihistamines.
Antineoplastics[2]	Suspend nursing if these drugs are taken.
Antithyroids Thiouracil;[2] methimazole[2]	Contraindicated; may cause goiter or agranulocytosis.
Propylthiouracil	Considered safe.
Cardiac drugs Quinidine[2]	Contraindicated; may cause arrhythmia in infant.
Cimetidine[2] ranitidine	Concentrated in breast milk; may suppress gastric acidity and cause central nervous system stimulation.
Ergot alkaloids Ergotamine (in doses to treat migraine)[2]	Causes vomiting, diarrhea, convulsions. May suppress lactation.
Bromocriptine[2]	Suppresses lactation.
Gold salts[2]	Contraindicated.
Hormones Oral contraceptives	Contraindicated; may cause reduction of milk supply. Progestin-only minipill may be used.
Laxatives Cascara, senna	Can cause diarrhea in infant.
Lithium carbonate[2]	Contraindicated because of toxicity.
Nicotine	Increased respiratory disease in infants exposed to smoke.
Radioactive materials for testing[2] ^{67}Ga	Insignificant amount excreted in milk; no nursing for 2 weeks.
^{125}I	Discontinue nursing for 48 hours.
^{131}I	After a test dose, nursing may be resumed after 24–36 hours; after a treatment dose, nursing may be resumed after 2–3 weeks.
^{99m}Tc	Discontinue nursing for 72 hours (half-life, 6 hours)
Sedatives and tranquilizers	Can cause sedation in infant. Benzodiazepines should be avoided.
Other drugs Caffeine	Irritability, poor sleep pattern with large amounts.
Cannabis;[2] cocaine;[2] polyhalogenated biphenyls[2] (eg, PCBs, PBBs); D-lysergic acid[2] (LSD)	Contraindicated; may interfere with mother's caretaking abilities and nutrition.

[1] Modified and reproduced, with permission, from Sahu S: Drugs and the nursing mother. *Am Fam Physician* (Dec) 1981;24:137.
[2] Absolutely contraindicated.

or a cup over a 3-week period. Milk supply will decrease with decreased demand, and minimal discomfort ensures. If nursing must be stopped abruptly, the mother should avoid nipple stimulation, refrain from expressing milk, and use a snug brassiere. Ice packs and analgesics can be helpful. If suppression is desired before nursing has begun, use this same technique. Engorgement will gradually recede over a 2- to 3-day period.

B. Hormonal Suppression: Oral and long-acting injections of hormonal preparations are available to suppress lactation. They are all effective if begun at the time of delivery but have occasional side effects—increased thromboembolic episodes (estrogens), hair growth (androgens), changes in blood pressure, and temporary emotional changes (bromocriptine).

1. Suppression with estrogens–Ethinyl estradiol, 0.05 mg, is administered as follows:

a. Four tablets (0.2 mg) twice daily on first postpartum day.

b. Three tablets (0.15 mg) twice daily on second day.

c. Two tablets (0.1 mg) twice daily on third day.

d. One tablet (0.05 mg) twice daily on fourth to seventh days.

2. Suppression with estrogen and androgens–Testosterone enanthate, 180 mg/mL, and estradiol valerate, 8 mg/mL, 2 mL injected intramuscularly immediately after delivery, are very effective.

3. Suppression with bromocriptine–Bromocriptine (Parlodel), 2.5 mg orally twice daily with meals for 10–14 days, will suppress lactation in women who do not wish to nurse their infants or after stillbirth or abortion. Rebound lactation may occur when the drug is discontinued. The drug should not be started until 4 hours postpartum, when vital signs are stable. Postural hypotension, nausea, headache, dizziness, nasal congestion, and mild constipation have been noted as side effects. These symptoms can be allayed by reducing the dose of the drug temporarily. Hypertension, seizures, stroke, and myocardial infarctions have also been reported in a small number of women. Because of this possibility, the drug should not be used in patients with pregnancy-induced hypertension and should be discontinued if severe headache or visual disturbances occur. Blood pressure should be monitored carefully throughout the duration of bromocriptine use.

Watson DL et al: Bromocriptine mesylate for lactation suppression: A risk for postpartum hypertension? Obstet Gynecol 1989;74:573.

PUERPERAL MASTITIS
(See also Chapter 12.)

Postpartum mastitis occurs sporadically in nursing mothers shortly after they return home, or it may occur in epidemic form in the hospital. Hemolytic *Staphylococcus aureus* is usually the causative agent. Inflammation is generally unilateral, and women nursing for the first time are more often affected.

Mastitis frequently begins within 3 months after delivery and may start with a sore or fissured nipple. There is obvious cellulitis in an area of breast tissue, with redness, tenderness, local warmth, and fever. Treatment consists of antibiotics effective against penicillin-resistant organisms (dicloxacillin or a cephalosporin) and regular emptying of the breast by nursing followed by expression of any remaining milk by hand or with a mechanical suction device.

If the mother begins antibiotic therapy before suppuration begins, infection can usually be controlled in 24 hours. If delay is permitted, breast abscess can result. Incision and drainage are required for abscess formation. Despite puerperal mastitis, the baby usually thrives without prophylactic antimicrobial therapy.

REFERENCES

Briggs GG et al: *Drugs in Pregnancy and Lactation: A Reference Guide to Fetal and Neonatal Risk,* 2nd ed. Williams & Wilkins, 1986.

Callen P: *Ultrasonography in Obstetrics and Gynecology,* 2nd ed. Saunders, 1988.

Cunningham FG, Macdonald PC, Gant NF: *Williams Obstetrics,* 18th ed. Appleton & Lange, 1989.

Cutler WB, Garcia CR: *The Medical Management of Menopause and Premenopause.* Lippincott, 1984.

Gleicher N (editor): *Principles of Medical Therapy in Pregnancy.* Plenum, 1985.

Hatcher RA et al: *Contraceptive Technology, 1990–1992,* 15th rev ed. Irvington, 1990.

Kaplan HS et al: *The Evaluation of Sexual Disorders: Psychological and Medical Aspects.* Brunner-Mazel, 1983.

Pernoll M, Benson RC (editors): *Current Obstetric & Gynecologic Diagnosis & Treatment,* 6th ed. Appleton & Lange, 1987.

Ryan KJ, Berkowitz R, Barbieri RL: *Kistner's Gynecology: Principles and Practice,* 5th ed. Year Book, 1990.

Scott JR et al: *Danforth's Obstetrics and Gynecology,* 6th ed. Lippincott, 1990.

Speroff L, Glass R, Kase N: *Clinical Gynecologic Endocrinology and Infertility,* 4th ed. Williams & Wilkins, 1989.

Worthington-Roberts BS, Vermeersch J, Williams SL: *Nutrition in Pregnancy and Lactation,* 3rd ed. Mosby, 1984.

Allergic & Immunologic Disorders

14

Abba Terr, MD, & Daniel P. Sites, MD

A wide variety of diseases in humans are associated with disorders of the immune response. Knowledge of immunoglobulin structure and function and of the cellular basis of immunity has resulted in a better understanding of these disorders. Diseases of immunity are usually caused by pathologic imbalances resulting from either excesses or deficiencies of immunocompetent cells or their products that disrupt normal homeostasis. This chapter provides a brief overview of basic and clinical immunology as an approach to the patient with immunologic disease.

IMMUNOGLOBULINS & ANTIBODIES

IMMUNOGLOBULIN STRUCTURE & FUNCTION

Immunoglobulins, which represent about 25% of plasma proteins, are specialized molecules that possess antibody activity. The basic unit of all immunoglobulins consists of 4 polypeptide chains linked by disulfide bonds. There are 2 identical heavy chains (MW 55,000–70,000) and 2 identical light chains (MW about 23,000). Both heavy and light chains have a C-terminal constant (C) region and an N-terminal variable (V) region. A hypervariable portion of the V regions of heavy and light chains folded together in a 3-dimensional conformation form the combining site, which is responsible for the specific interaction with antigen.

Antibodies contain one of 5 classes of heavy chains (γ, α, μ, δ, and ϵ) and one of 2 types of light chains (and). Either type of light chain can be associated with each of the heavy chain classes. Approximately 60% of human immunoglobulins have light chains, and 40% have light chains. About 10 million different antibody specificities are thought to exist in a given individual.

Immunoglobulin Classes

A. Immunoglobulin M (IgM): IgM is made up of 5 identical basic immunoglobulin units. These units are connected to one another by disulfide bonds and a small polypeptide known as J chain. The molecular weight of IgM is about 900,000. The IgM molecule is found predominantly in the intravascular compartment and on the surface of B lymphocytes and does not normally cross the placenta. IgM antibody predominates early in immune responses; carbohydrate antigens such as blood group substances predominantly stimulate IgM.

B. Immunoglobulin A (IgA): IgA is present in the blood and relatively high concentration in saliva, colostrum, tears, and secretions of the bronchi and the gastrointestinal tract. Serum IgA is a single immunoglobulin unit, whereas secretory IgA is made up of 2 units connected to each other by a J chain. A 70,000-MW molecule called secretory component is attached to the Fc portions. It is necessary to transport IgA into the lumens of exocrine glands, and it confers resistance to enzymatic destruction. Secretory IgA plays an important role in host defense against viral and bacterial infections by blocking transport of microbes across mucosa.

C. Immunoglobulin G (IgG): IgG is a single immunoglobulin unit of MW 150,000 that comprises about 85% of total serum immunoglobulins. IgG is distributed in the extracellular fluid and is the only immunoglobulin that normally crosses the placenta. IgG binds complement via an Fc receptor present in the constant region of the heavy chain. IgG binds to the surface of cells and microbes, which allows them to be phagocytosed or killed by cytotoxic cells.

D. Immunoglobulin E (IgE): IgE is present in serum in very low concentrations as a single immunoglobulin unit with heavy chains. Approximately 50% of patients with allergic diseases have increased serum IgE levels. IgE is a skin-sensitizing or reaginic antibody by virtue of attachment to mast cells. The specific interaction between antigen and IgE bound to the surface of mast cells results in the release of inflammatory products such as histamine, leukotriene, and chemotactic factors. These mediators can result in bronchospasm, vasodilation, smooth muscle contraction, and chemoattraction of other inflammatory and immune cells.

E. Immunoglobulin D (IgD): IgD is present in the serum in very low concentrations as a single basic immunoglobulin unit with δ heavy chains. IgD is found on the surface of most B lymphocytes in association with IgM, where it probably serves as a receptor for antigen.

Goodman JW: Immunoglobulins: Structure and function. Chapter 9 in: *Basic & Clinical Immunology,* 7th ed. Stites DP, Terr AI (editors). Appleton & Lange, 1990.
Jeske DJ, Capra JD: Immunoglobulins: Structure and function. Chap 7, pp 131–165, in: *Fundamental Immunology.* Paul WE (editor). Raven Press, 1984.

Immunoglobulin Genes

Genes that code for immunoglobulin light and heavy chain molecules undergo rearrangements in the DNA of B cells, which result in the synthesis and expression of the highly diverse group of immunoglobulin molecules. Clonal rearrangements of immunoglobulin genes in B cells are useful for typing the immunologic origin of many leukemias and lymphomas.

Parlsow TG: Immunoglobulin genetics. Chapter 10 in: *Basic & Clinical Immunology,* 7th ed. Stites DP, Terr AI (editors). Appleton & Lange, 1990.

Tests for Immunoglobulins

Immunoglobulin levels can be elevated or reduced in a large number of diseases. In some diseases, particularly gammopathies (see below), increased serum immunoglobulins, especially monoclonal types, are critical for diagnosis. In other diseases such as chronic liver diseases, chronic infection, or idiopathic inflammatory states, polyclonal increases in immunoglobulins are incidental or of unknown significance. If immunodeficiency is suspected in the presence of recurrent bacterial infections, measurement of serum immunoglobulins provides an essential test of B cell and plasma cell function. In acquired immune deficiencies such as AIDS, with many recurrent infections, paradoxic increases in immunoglobulins may occur.

There are various ways of measuring antibody, including the following: (1) quantitative and qualitative determinations of serum immunoglobulins; (2) determination of isohemagglutinin and febrile agglutinin titers; and (3) determination of antibody titers following immunization with tetanus toxoid, diphtheria toxoid, or pertussis vaccines. The first method tests for the presence of serum immunoglobulins but not for the functional adequacy of the immunoglobulins. The second method tests for functional antibodies that are present in the serum of almost all individuals as a consequence of exposure to blood group substances or infection. The third method examines functional antibody activity in the serum after intentional immunization. Commonly used clinical tests of antibody immunity, for many diseases, are protein electrophoresis, immunoelectrophoresis, and quantitative immunoglobulin determinations.

Protein Electrophoresis & Immunoelectrophoresis

Protein electrophoresis is a screening test to semiquantitatively measure various proteins in body fluids, usually serum or urine. Proteins are electrically separated on a strip of cellulose acetate on the basis of charge into albumin, α_1, α_2, β, and γ globulins. The relative concentration of gamma globulins that contains nearly all immunoglobulins is determined with protein stains. This test is useful to screen for diseases with excess or deficiency of immunoglobulins.

Immunoelectrophoresis is used to identify the specific immunoglobulin class in a body fluid. Serum, for example, is separated electrophoretically and then reacted with appropriate antisera directed against IgG, IgA, or IgM. The resulting patterns produced allow identification of abnormal immunoglobulins such as myeloma (M) proteins. This method is also useful in differentiation of monoclonal from polyclonal increases in immunoglobulins. It is only semiquantitative and thus cannot be used to determine immunoglobulin levels precisely, eg, in Waldenström's macroglobulinemia.

Another similar technique called immunofixation electrophoresis has to a large extent replaced immunoelectrophoresis. It has the advantages of more rapid results and slightly higher resolution of low levels of monoclonal immunoglobulin chains. If protein electrophoresis is normal despite suspicion of an M protein, immunoelectrophoresis or immunofixation electrophoresis of both serum and concentrated urine should be performed because of the greater sensitivity of these tests.

Quantitative Immunoglobulin Determinations: Radial Diffusion & Nephelometry Techniques

Quantitative determinations of serum IgG, IgA, and IgM levels can be made using the radial diffusion technique. Circular wells are cut in a gel plate impregnated with a specific antiserum directed against a single human immunoglobulin class. The radius or diameter of the circular precipitin ring is proportionate to the concentration of serum immunoglobulin. The precise immunoglobulin level is determined by comparing the diameter of the unknown serum to that of a standard containing known levels of immunoglobulins.

Determinations of the serum concentrations of IgM, IgG, and IgA can also be made accurately and rapidly by nephelometry. This method employs an instrument to measure the turbidity produced by the interaction of immunoglobulin and anti-immunoglobulin complexes. It is much more rapid than radial diffusion and is useful for measuring a wide spectrum of serum proteins. The measurement of immunoglobulin levels alone does not distinguish monoclonal immunoglobulins, as does the immunoelectrophoresis or immunofixation electrophoresis procedure.

IgD levels have no recognized clinical use, and IgE levels must be measured with more sensitive techniques such as radioimmunoassay or enzyme-linked immunoassay.

DISEASES OF IMMUNOGLOBULIN OVERPRODUCTION (Gammopathies)

The gammopathies include those disease entities in which there is a disproportionate proliferation of a single clone of immunoglobulin-forming cells that produce a homogeneous heavy chain, light chain, or complete molecule. The amino acid sequence of the variable (V) regions is fixed, and only one type (κ or λ) of light chain is produced.

Benign Monoclonal Gammopathy

The diagnosis is made upon finding a homogeneous (monoclonal) immunoglobulin (with either κ or λ chains but not both) in immunoelectrophoresis of the serum of an otherwise normal individual. The incidence of homogeneous immunoglobulins in the serum increases with age and may approach 3% in persons 70 years of age or older. A small percentage of apparently normal persons with a homogeneous serum immunoglobulin will go on to develop multiple myeloma. Parameters that suggest a favorable prognosis in "benign" monoclonal gammopathy include the following: (1) concentration of homogeneous immunoglobulin less than 2 g/dL, (2) no significant increase in the concentration of the homogeneous immunoglobulin from the time of diagnosis, (3) no decrease in the concentration of normal immunoglobulins, (4) absence of a homogeneous light chain in the urine, and (5) normal hematocrit and serum albumin concentration.

Multiple Myeloma

This disease is characterized by the overproduction and spread of neoplastic plasma cells throughout the bone marrow. Rarely, extraosseous plasmacytomas may be found. Anemia, hypercalcemia, increased susceptibility to infection, and bone pain are frequent. Certain diagnosis depends upon the presence of the following: (1) radiographic findings of osteolytic lesions or diffuse osteoporosis, (2) the presence of a homogeneous serum immunoglobulin (myeloma protein) or a single type of light chain in the urine (Bence Jones proteinuria), and (3) finding of an abnormal plasma cell infiltrate in the bone marrow biopsy (see Chapter 10). There is an approximate correlation between the incidence of immunoglobulin type in myeloma and the normal serum concentration of the immunoglobulin involved. That is, IgG {>} IgA {>} IgD {>} IgE. IgM myeloma does not occur for all practical purposes.

Waldenström's Macroglobulinemia

Waldenström's macroglobulinemia is characterized by a proliferation of abnormal lymphoid cells that have morphologic features of both B cells and plasma cells. These cells secrete a homogeneous macroglobulin (IgM) that is easily detected and characterized by immunoelectrophoresis. Monoclonal light chains are present in 10% of cases. Clinical manifestations depend upon the physicochemical characteristics of the macroglobulin. Raynaud's phenomenon and peripheral vascular occlusions are associated with cold-insoluble proteins (cryoglobulins). Retinal hemorrhages, visual impairment, and transient neurologic deficits are common with high-viscosity serum. Bleeding diatheses or hemolytic anemia can occur when the macroglobulin complexes with coagulation factors or binds to the surface of red blood cells.

Amyloidosis

Amyloidosis is manifested by impaired organ function from infiltration of the tissue with insoluble protein fibrils or proteins complexed with polysaccharides. Variations in composition of the fibrils can be largely correlated with the clinical syndromes (Table 14–1).

Amyloid occurs (1) in a primary form or (2) in company with plasmacytosis in bone marrow or lymphoid tissues. These were previously referred to as primary amyloid. The protein fibrils in these entities are composed of immunoglobulin light chains or fragments of light chains, particularly the V region. This form of amyloid has been designated AL.

A nonimmunoglobulin protein (AA) is the major component of amyloid fibrils that form secondary to infection (osteomyelitis, tuberculosis), inflammation, rheumatoid arthritis, Hodgkin's disease, regional enteritis, renal cell carcinoma, leprosy, and intravenous drug abuse. The hereditary systemic amyloidosis associated with familial Mediterranean fever is composed of AA protein. This protein is derived from the acute-phase reactant SAA (serum amyloid-associated). This pattern was previously called secondary amyloidosis.

Symptoms and signs of amyloid infiltration are related to malfunction of the organ involved, eg, nephrotic syndrome, chronic renal failure, cardiomyopathy, cardiac conduction defects, intestinal malabsorption, intestinal obstruction, carpal tunnel syndrome, macroglossia, peripheral neuropathy, end-organ insufficiency of endocrine glands, respiratory failure, obstruction to ventilation, and capillary damage with ecchymosis. Recently, amyloidosis due to deposition of β_2-microglobulin in joints and bones has been de-

Table 14–1. Classification of amyloidosis.[1]

	Clinical Type	**Common Sites of Deposition**	**Chemical Type of Fibril[2]**
Familial	Amyloid polyneuropathy (Portuguese, dominant inheritance)	Peripheral nerves Viscera	AF (prealbumin)
	Familial Mediterranean fever (recessive)	Liver, spleen, kidneys, adrenals	AA
Generalized	Primary	Tongue, heart, gut, skeletal and smooth muscles, nerves, skin, ligaments	AL
	Associated with plasma cell dyscrasia	Liver, spleen, kidneys, heart, adrenals	AL
	Secondary (infection, inflammation, etc)	Any site	AA
	Chronic hemodialysis	Carpal tunnel, bone, joints	AH (β_2-microglobulin)
Localized	Lichen amyloidosis	Skin	AD
	Endocrine-related (eg, thyroid medullary carcinoma, diabetes mellitus, Addison's disease)	Endocrine organ (thyroid)	AE (AE)
Senile		Heart Brain	AS AS

[1] Modified and reproduced, with permission, from Stites DP et al (editors): *Basic & Clinical Immunology,* 7th ed. Appleton & Lange, 1990.
[2] AA = amyloid A; AD = amyloid dermatologic; AE = amyloid endocrine; AF = amyloid familial; AH = amyloid hemodialysis; AL = amyloid light chain; AS = amyloid senile.

scribed in chronic hemodialysis patients. Table 14–1 lists organs characteristically involved with each type of amyloid.

The diagnosis of amyloidosis is based on suspicion, family history, and preexisting long-standing infection or debilitating illness. Microscopic examination of biopsy (eg, gingival, renal, rectal) or surgical specimens is diagnostic. Amyloid binds Congo red dye in tissues and emits apple green fluorescence with ultraviolet light. Fine-needle biopsy of subcutaneous abdominal fat is a simple and reliable method for diagnosing secondary systemic amyloidosis.

Treatment of localized amyloid "tumors" is by surgical excision. There is no effective treatment of systemic amyloidosis, and death usually occurs within 1–3 years. Treatment of the predisposing disease may cause a temporary remission or slow the progress of the disease, but it is unlikely that the established metabolic process is altered. Patients with amyloid due to plasma cell dyscrasia may occasionally respond to treatment with melphalan and prednisone. Colchicine is of use in familial Mediterranean fever. Early and adequate treatment of pyogenic infections may prevent much secondary amyloidosis.

Heavy Chain Disease
(α, γ, μ)

These are rare disorders in which the abnormal serum and urine protein is a part of a homogeneous α, γ, or μ heavy chain. The clinical presentation is more typical of lymphoma than multiple myeloma, and there are no destructive bone lesions. Alpha chain disease is frequently associated with severe diarrhea and infiltration of the lamina propria of the small

intestine with abnormal plasma cells. Mu chain disease is associated with chronic lymphocytic leukemia.

Gertz MA, Kyle RA: Primary systemic amyloidosis: A diagnostic primer. Mayo Clin Proc 1989;64:1505.
Kyle RA, Bayrd EA: *The Monoclonal Gammopathies: Multiple Myeloma and Related Plasma Cell Disorders.* Thomas, 1976.

CELLULAR IMMUNITY

CELLS INVOLVED IN IMMUNITY

Development of T & B Lymphocytes

Lymphocytes interact with antigens via specific receptors and thereby initiate immune responses of vertebrates. In birds, 2 lines of lymphocytes exist: one derived from the thymus and the other from the bursa of Fabricius. The thymus-derived cells are involved in cellular immune responses; the bursa-derived cells are involved in antibody responses. In mammals, T lymphocytes are analogous to the thymus-derived cells in birds and B lymphocytes (bone marrow-derived cells) are analogous to the bursa-derived cells.

Both T and B lymphocytes are derived from precursor or stem cells in the marrow. Precursors of T cells migrate to the thymus, where they develop some of the functional and cell surface characteristics of mature T cells. Clones of autoreactive T cells are eliminated, and mature antigen reactive T cells then migrate to the peripheral lymphoid tissues and enter the pool of long-lived lymphocytes that recirculate from the blood to the lymph.

B cell maturation has antigen-independent or antigen-dependent stages. Antigen-independent maturation includes development from precursor cells in the marrow through the virgin B cell (a cell that has not been exposed to antigen previously) found in the peripheral lymphoid tissues. The production and maturation of virgin B cells are ongoing processes even in adult animals. Antigen-dependent maturation occurs following the interaction of antigen with virgin B cells. The final products of B cell development are circulating long-lived memory B cells and plasma cells that secrete copious amounts of specific antibody. Mature B cells in the periphery are found predominantly in primary follicles and germinal centers of the lymph nodes and spleen.

Subpopulations of T Cells

T lymphocytes are heterogeneous with respect to their cell surface features (Table 14–2) and functional characteristics. At least 4 subpopulations of T cells are now recognized.

A. Helper-Inducer T Cells: These cells help to amplify the production of antibody-forming cells from B lymphocytes after interaction with antigen. Helper T cells also amplify the production of effector T cells that mediate cytotoxicity. The several different functions of T cells may reflect various stages of development rather than unique or separate lineages of these lymphocytes.

B. Cytotoxic or Killer T Cells: These cells are generated after mature T cells interact with certain antigens such as those present on the surface of foreign cells. These cells are responsible for organ graft rejection and for killing of virally infected and some tumor cells.

C. Suppressor T Cells: These cells suppress the formation of antibody-forming cells from B lymphocytes. Suppressor T cells are regarded as regulatory cells that modulate antibody formation. Cell-mediated

immunity (ie, organ graft rejection) is also regulated by suppressor cells.

D. Suppressor-Inducer T Cells: These cells, which have helper cell (not suppressor cell) surface antigens, amplify the development of suppressor T cells.

Identification of T Cell Subpopulations With Monoclonal Antibodies

Monoclonal antibodies to T cell subpopulations are produced by immunizing animals with human T cells and then fusing the spleen cells of the animal with mouse myeloma cells to develop hybridoma cell lines. These hybridoma lines secrete monoclonal antibodies that identify cell surface antigens common to all human T cells (Table 14–2). Lymphocytes stained with fluorescent monoclonal antibodies are enumerated by microscopy or flow cytometry. About 75% of the peripheral blood lymphocytes of normal individuals are T cells; 50% are helper-inducer T cells, and 25% are suppressor or cytotoxic T cells.

Changes in the number or ratio of various T cell subsets occur in a wide variety of clinical conditions. For example, the ratio of helper to suppressor (H/S) cells in healthy individuals is about 1.6–2.2. In many acute viral infections, this ratio falls temporarily both as a result of decrease in helper/inducer cells and of increase in suppressor/cytotoxic cells. In AIDS and related HIV infections, H/S ratios are nearly always reduced—probably irreversibly—by the destructive effects of this lymphotropic virus. Among other clinical applications of the enumeration of these cells are the diagnosis of some immunodeficiencies, phenotyping of leukemias and lymphomas, and monitoring of immunologic changes following organ transplantation.

T Cell Lymphokines

Many T cell functions are mediated by lymphokines, which are humoral factors secreted by lymphocytes or other cells. Lymphokines are secreted when T cells are activated by antigens or other lymphokines. Table 14–3 lists some examples of lymphokines and their functions.

Table 14–2. Surface antigens detected by monoclonal antibodies on T and B cells.

T Cell Antigens			B Cell Antigens
Cluster of Differentiation	Antibody Designations	T Cell Subsets	Ig heavy and light chains DR antigen B cell-specific antigens (CD19, CD20) Fc receptor
CD3	Leu 4, OKT 3, T3	All T cells	
CD2	Leu 5, OKT 11, T11	All T cells with sheep red blood cell receptor	
CD4	Leu 3, OKT 4, T4	Helper-inducer T cells	
CD8	Leu 2, OKT 8, T8	Suppressor or cytotoxic T cells	

Table 14–3. T cell lymphokines.

Lymphokine	Function
Interleukin-1 (IL-1)	Produced by macrophages. Activates T cells. Also causes fever (endogenous pyrogen).
Interleukin-2 (IL-2)	Promotes proliferation of B cells activated by antigens or mitogens.
B cell growth factor (BCGF)	Promotes proliferation of B cells activated by antigens or mitogens.
Gamma interferon	Can inhibit or stimulate T Cells. Inhibits viral replication.

Lymphokines are being used experimentally both to evaluate immune function and to treat disease. Receptors for IL-2 circulate in blood and are a measure of generalized immune stimulation. IL-2 in combination with autologous lymphocytes has been tested as an anticancer treatment in selected patients with limited success.

T Cell Antigen Receptors

T cells interact with several different types of cells during the regulation and mediation of immune responses. These interactions include presentation of antigens to T cells by macrophages or other cells, T cell-induced differentiation of B cells into antibody-secreting cells, and T cell killing of a variety of virus-infected cells. In all of these cell-cell interactions, T cells recognize foreign antigens on the surface of the non-T cell in association with other cell surface antigens that are coded for by the major histocompatibility gene complex of the non-T cell. T cells have cell surface receptors that recognize at least 2 different molecules; one recognition site binds to any single foreign antigen (viral, bacterial, etc), and the other binds to major histocompatibility antigens. An example of this "dual recognition" is observed in the killing of virus-infected target cells by cytolytic T cells. Cytolytic T cells taken from humans immunized to a given virus will kill virus-infected target cells if the target cells carry the same histocompatibility antigens as the immunized host.

These facts raise concerns about host defense against viral infection in bone marrow transplant recipients who do not share the MHC (HLA) antigens of the marrow donors. After marrow transplantation, donor T cells maturing in the host thymus are presumed to recognize foreign antigen in association with host-type histocompatibility antigens. However, most antigen-presenting cells with bear donor-type histocompatibility antigens; this may lead to a severe immunodeficiency state, with a completely mismatched marrow transplant. Fortunately, at the present time, almost all transplant recipients share at least one HLA haplotype with the donor.

The structure of T cell antigen receptors and the genes that encode these glycoproteins have been defined. The antigen recognition structure is a complex of 2 molecules, one containing variable alpha and beta or gamma and delta chains and the other the monomorphic T3 (CD3) molecule. Genes encoding the beta chain have homology to immunoglobulin genes. Clonal rearrangement of T cell receptor genes proceeds during T cell development to generate diversity for antigen recognition in a fashion similar to that of immunoglobulin genes in B cells. T cell receptor gene rearrangements have been used to identify T cell leukemias, lymphomas, and mycosis fungoides, a rare malignant neoplasm of the skin.

Parnes JR: T cell receptors. Chapter 6 in: *Basic & Clinical Immunology*, 7th ed. Stites DP, Terr AI (editors). Appleton & Lange, 1990.

B Lymphocytes

B cells express different classes of surface markers in (Table 14–2). The majority of B cells express both IgM and IgD on the surface and are derived from pre-B cells found mainly in the bone marrow. Pre-B cells contain intracytoplasmic IgM but do not express surface immunoglobulin. Patients with congenital hypogammaglobulinemia frequently show a developmental arrest at the stage of the pre-B cell. The majority of patients with acquired hypogammaglobulinemia have a block of transition from the mature B cell to the plasma cell. Thus, most patients with this disease have normal numbers of circulating mature B cells but reduced numbers of plasma cells.

B cells have been commonly identified by other surface markers in addition to immunoglobulins. These include the receptor for the Fc piece of immunoglobulins, B cell-specific antigens, and surface antigens coded for by the HLA-D genetic region in humans (Table 14–2). All mature B cells bear surface immunoglobulin that is the antigen-specific receptor. Clearly, the major role of B cells is differentiation to antibody-secreting plasma cells. However, B cells may also release lymphokines and function as antigen-presenting cells.

Other Cells Involved in Immune Responses

A. Macrophages: Macrophages are involved in the initial ingestion and processing of particulate antigens before interaction with lymphocytes. They play an important role in T and B lymphocyte cooperation in the induction of antibody responses. In addition, they are effector cells for certain types of tumor immunity.

B. NK (Natural Killer) Cells: These lymphocytic cells, which are indirectly related to the T cell lineage, can kill a wide spectrum of target cells. They are recognized by the presence of specific surface antigens and Fc receptors. Many appear as large granular lymphocytes. Their role in host defense is probably the killing of virally infected cells and tumor cells in the absence of prior sensitization and without MHC restriction.

Broide D: Inflammatory cells: Structure and function. Chapter 12 in: *Basic & Clinical Immunology*, 7th ed. Stites DP, Terr AI (editors). Appleton & Lange, 1990.

Lanier L: Cells of the immune response. Chapter 5 in: *Basic & Clinical Immunology*, 7th ed. Stites DP, Terr AI (editors). Appleton & Lange, 1990.

Schattner A, Duggan DB: Natural killer cells: Toward clinical application. Am J Hematol 1985;18:435.

TESTS FOR CELLULAR IMMUNITY

Techniques for Identification of Human B & T Cells

A. B Cells: Cell surface characteristics usually found on B but not T cells include the following: (1) easily detectable surface immunoglobulin, (2) specific antigens (CD19, CD20), (3) a receptor for the Fc portion of immunoglobulins that have been aggregated or complexed with antigen, and (4) DR antigens (Table 14–2).

Surface immunoglobulin is detected by direct fluorescence staining of live cell suspensions with fluorochrome-conjugated antibodies directed against human immunoglobulin. The Fc receptor is identified by incubating lymphocytes in vitro with fluorochrome-labeled IgG aggregates.

B cell antigens and DR antigens are detected by immunofluorescence with specific monoclonal antibodies.

B. T Cells: T cell markers include surface antigens identified by specific monoclonal antibodies. Monoclonal antisera have been used in both immunofluorescence staining and in vitro cytotoxicity assays to identify T cell subsets (Table 14–2). T cells can also be detected in tissue sections or suspensions using enzyme-labeled antibodies that produce colors on incubation with chromogenic substrates. Approximately 75% of human peripheral blood lymphocytes are T cells, and up to 20% are B cells. The remainder are NK cells.

C. Flow Cytometry: Flow cytometers are instruments that accurately measure the size, density, and multiple colors of immunofluorescent monoclonal antibodies on human lymphocytes. Thousands of cells can be analyzed individually for the presence of all these parameters at once. This method greatly improves the accuracy, speed, and precision of phenotyping human T and B cells in the clinical laboratory.

Procedures for Testing Cell-Mediated Immunity, or T Cell Function

A. Skin Testing: Cell-mediated immunity can be assessed qualitatively by evaluating skin reactivity following intradermal injection of a battery of antigens to which humans are frequently sensitized (ie, streptokinase, streptodornase, purified protein derivative, *Trichophyton, Dermatophyton,* or *Candida*). Intradermal injections of 0.1 mL of recommended test strengths are observed for maximal induration and erythema at 24 and 48 hours. A positive reaction varies in size with particular antigens but is generally at least 10 mm in diameter. Anergy or lack of skin reactivity to all of these substances usually indicates a depression of cell-mediated immunity. Delayed hypersensitivity skin tests depend on complex interactions of T cells, macrophages, and other immunoreactants; thus, failure to respond cannot specifically identify a defect in a particular cell type.

B. In Vitro Stimulation of Peripheral Blood Lymphocytes With Mitogens or Antigens: T lymphocytes are transformed to blast cells upon short-term incubation with mitogens such as phytohemagglutinin or recall antigens in vitro. T cell activation can be determined quantitatively by following the cellular uptake of ^{3}H-thymidine introduced into the culture medium. The in vitro uptake of ^{3}H-thymidine by human peripheral blood lymphocytes indicates T cell function and correlates well with other manifestations of cell-mediated immunity as measured by delayed hypersensitivity skin tests. These functional tests can detect abnormalities in T cells despite normal or slightly reduced cell counts, particularly following bone marrow transplantation or in congenital immunodeficiency diseases. Stimulation of transplant recipients' lymphocytes or donor lymphocytes (the mixed lymphocyte reaction) is critical test for determining histocompatibility, especially in renal and bone marrow transplantation.

APPLICATIONS OF T & B CELL TESTS

Immunodeficiency Diseases

Thymic hypoplasia is associated with a marked decrease in the number of T cells in the peripheral blood. On the other hand, the absence of B cells in the blood is frequently found in X-linked agammaglobulinemia. Marked reduction of both T and B cells occurs in severe combined immunodeficiency disease (SCID). Typing of blood T and B cells can aid in the diagnosis of these diseases in early childhood. Patients with HIV infection and particularly the acquired immunodeficiency syndrome (AIDS) have reduced numbers of T cells and reduced T helper to-suppressor ratios.

Lymphoproliferative Diseases

A marked increase in the number of peripheral blood lymphocytes that bear immunoglobulin of a single heavy chain class and light chain type represents a monoclonal proliferation of cells. Blood lymphocytes from almost all patients with chronic lymphocytic leukemia and non-Hodgkin's lymphoma with blood involvement show this abnormality. On the other hand, lymphocytosis secondary to viral or bacterial infection is associated with a normal percentage of B cells and the usual distribution of immunoglobulin classes on the cell surface.

Lymphocytic leukemias can be classified by phenotyping T and B cells, with implications for prognosis and, sometimes, treatment. Monitoring various T cell subsets is also useful in following patients with organ transplants.

Stites DP: Clinical laboratory methods for detection of cellular immune function. Chapter 19 in: *Basic & Clinical Immunology*, 7th ed. Stites DP, Terr AI (editors). Appleton & Lange, 1990.

IMMUNOLOGIC DEFICIENCY DISEASES

The primary immunologic deficiency diseases include congenital and acquired disorders of humoral immunity (B cell function) or cell-mediated immunity (T cell function). Most of these diseases are rare and—since they are genetically determined—occur almost exclusively in children. A classification of a selected group of immunodeficiency disorders recommended by WHO is shown below:

Infantile X-linked agammaglobulinemia (see below)
Selective immunoglobulin deficiency (see below)
Transient hypogammaglobulinemia of infancy
X-linked immunodeficiency with hyper-IgM
Thymic hypoplasia (pharyngeal pouch syndrome, DiGeorge's syndrome) (see below)
Immunodeficiency with normal serum globulins or hyperimmunoglobulinemia
Immunodeficiency with ataxia-telangiectasia (see below)
Immunodeficiency with thrombocytopenia and eczema (Wiskott-Aldrich syndrome) (see below)
Immunodeficiency with thymoma
Immunodeficiency with generalized hematopoietic hypoplasia

Severe combined immunodeficiency (see below):
  (1) With dysostosis
  (2) With adenosine deaminase deficiency
Variable immunodeficiency (common, largely unclassified) (see below)
Acquired immunodeficiency syndrome (AIDS) (see below)

Ammann AJ, Frank M: Immunodeficiency disorders. Chapters 23–28 in: *Basic & Clinical Immunology*, 7th ed. Stites DP, Terr AI (editors). Appleton & Lange, 1990.
Stiehm ER, Fulginiti VA: *Immunologic Disorders in Infants and Children*, 3rd ed. Saunders, 1988.

INFANTILE X-LINKED AGAMMAGLOBULINEMIA

This hereditary disorder results in a deficit in B cell function with essentially intact T cell function.

Clinical Findings

The diagnosis is based on low IgG levels in serum, an X-linked pattern of heredity, intact cell-mediated immunity, and the absence of plasma cells in biopsy specimens of regional lymph nodes draining the site of recent antigenic stimulation, eg, DPT vaccine.

A. Symptoms and Signs: There are no symptoms during the first 5–6 months of life (probably due to presence of maternal antibody). Thereafter, the infant shows increased susceptibility to pyogenic infections (gram-positive organisms) and *Haemophilus influenzae*, resulting in recurrent furunculosis, pneumonia, and meningitis. There is normal susceptibility to viral exanthematous infections such as rubella, measles, and chickenpox. Other characteristic findings are chronic sinusitis, bronchiectasis, and arthritis of the large joints similar to rheumatoid arthritis.

B. Laboratory Findings: IgG levels in the serum are less than 200 mg/dL, serum IgA and IgM levels are less than 1% of normal, and isohemagglutinins are low or absent. The Schick test is positive, and antitoxin titers do not rise after vaccination with DPT vaccine. The peripheral lymphocyte count and delayed type hypersensitivity skin tests are normal. There are no B lymphocytes but normal or elevated T lymphocytes in the peripheral blood in most cases.

Treatment

Recurrent bacterial infections can be prevented by the administration of gamma globulin for an indefinite period of time. The gamma globulin is usually administered intramuscularly at a dose of 0.2–0.4 mL/kg. Intravenous gamma globulin is also used at a dose of 100–400 mg/kg given over 2–4 hours as often as weekly in severely ill patients. The need for repeated infusions can be determined by monitoring blood levels of IgG. Although the use of appropriate antibiotics has improved the prognosis, it remains poor.

THYMIC HYPOPLASIA
(DiGeorge's Syndrome)

DiGeorge's syndrome is due to failure of embryogenesis of the third and fourth pharyngeal pouches. The mode of transmission and the cause of the morphogeneic failure are unknown. This results in aplasia of the parathyroid and thymus glands. The syndrome presents as a pure T cell functional deficiency with relatively intact B cell function in combination with hypoparathyroidism. Clinical Findings

A. Symptoms and Signs: The major manifestations are neonatal tetany, hypertelorism, and increased susceptibility to viral, fungal, and bacterial infections. Infections are frequently lethal.

B. Laboratory Findings: Serum immunoglobulin levels are usually normal. Antibody responses may be low or normal, depending on the antigen used for immunization. Reactions to delayed hypersensitivity skin tests are absent, lymphocyte counts are low, and functional T cell assays are abnormal. Serum calcium is reduced, phosphorus is elevated, and parathyroid hormone is absent. Biopsy of lymph nodes shows normal germinal center formation but marked deficits in the thymus-dependent or paracortical areas.

Treatment

Transplantation of fetal thymic tissue has been successful in reversing the deficits in cell-mediated immunity and raising the peripheral lymphocyte count to normal. The thymus-dependent areas of the lymph nodes of transplant recipients are also repopulated. Hypoparathyroidism can usually be managed with oral calcium supplemented with vitamin D or its analogues. Spontaneous remissions may occur. The prognosis is primarily related to the severity of associated congenital heart disease.

SEVERE COMBINED
IMMUNODEFICIENCY

Both T and B cell function are markedly decreased in this entity, which is inherited in an autosomal recessive or X-linked pattern. A sporadic appearance in families also occurs. Dysostosis and adenosine deaminase deficiency occur in some cases.

Clinical Findings

A. Symptoms and Signs: Increased susceptibility to infection is noted at 3–6 months of age. Death usually occurs within 2 years. In infancy, there is watery diarrhea, usually associated with *Salmonella* or enteropathic *Escherichia coli* infections. Pulmonary infections, usually with *Pseudomonas* and *Pneumocystis carinii,* are common, as is candidiasis in the mouth and diaper areas. Common viral exanthems such as chickenpox and measles are often lethal.

B. Laboratory Findings: Serum immunoglobulin levels are usually less than 1% of normal, and antibodies do not form in response to vaccinations such as DTP. The peripheral lymphocyte count is less than 2000/μL. Decreased delayed hypersensitivity is manifested by lack of skin reactivity to antigens. Lymph node biopsy shows no lymphocytes, plasma cells, or lymphoid follicles.

Treatment

Passive administration of gamma globulin in doses of 100–400 mg/kg intravenously every 1–4 weeks is temporarily effective. An expert in immunodeficiency disorders should be consulted. Bone marrow transplantation has been successful.

IMMUNODEFICIENCY WITH
THROMBOCYTOPENIA & ECZEMA
(Wiskott-Aldrich Syndrome)

This disorder is characterized by eczema, thrombocytopenia, and recurrent bacterial and viral infections. Inheritance is X-linked, and affected individuals rarely survive more than 10 years. There appears to be a combined T and B cell functional deficit. IgM levels are low and isohemagglutinins absent, but IgG and IgA levels are normal. Cell-mediated immunity is impaired. Treatment is symptomatic for infections and thrombocytopenia. Successful bone marrow transplantation has been achieved.

IMMUNODEFICIENCY WITH
ATAXIA-TELANGIECTASIA

Ataxia-telangiectasia begins in infancy with ataxia and choreoathetoid movements. Telangiectasia of the conjunctiva, face, arms, and eyelids is first noted 5–10 years later. Chronic sinusitis and respiratory infections follow, and death due to intercurrent pulmonary infection or lymphoreticular neoplasm occurs in the second or third decade. Approximately 80% of affected individuals lack serum and secretory IgA. In addition, there is a marked deficit in T cell function associated with a hypoplastic or dysplastic thymus gland. The disease is inherited in an autosomal recessive pattern.

COMMON VARIABLE
IMMUNODEFICIENCY

Onset is in adulthood, with increased susceptibility to pyogenic infections; recurrent sinusitis and pneumonia progressing to bronchiectasis; spruelike syndrome with diarrhea, steatorrhea, malabsorption, and protein-losing enteropathy; and hepatosplenomegaly. Arthritis of the type associated with congenital hypogammaglobulinemia and autoimmune diseases may occur. Serum IgG levels are usually less than 250 mg/dL; serum IgA and IgM levels are subnormal. Lymph node biopsy shows marked reduction in plasma cells. Noncaseating granulomas are frequently found in the spleen, liver, lungs, or skin.

Suppressor T cells inhibit B cells from producing antibody-forming cells in certain cases of adult-onset hypogammaglobulinemia. The absolute B cell count in the peripheral blood in these cases is normal. Therapy at present is similar to that of congenital hypogammaglobulinemia, with 100–400 mg/kg of intravenous gamma globulin at about monthly intervals.

SELECTIVE IMMUNOGLOBULIN DEFICIENCY

Absence of serum IgA with normal levels of IgG and IgM is found in a small percentage of normal individuals. Some cases of IgA deficiency may spontaneously remit. When IgG2 subclass deficiency occurs in combination with IgA deficiency, recurrent infections are common. Occasionally, a spruelike syndrome with steatorrhea has been associated with an isolated IgA deficit. Treatment with commercial gamma globulin is ineffective, since IgA and IgM are not present in this preparation. Frequent infusions of plasma (containing IgA) are hazardous, since anti-IgA antibodies may develop, resulting in systemic anaphylaxis or serum sickness.

ACQUIRED IMMUNODEFICIENCY SYNDROME (AIDS) (See also Chapter 24.)

AIDS is an example of a hitherto unrecognized form of immunodeficiency in which a chronic retroviral infection with HIV—human immunodeficiency virus—in a susceptible host produces severe, life-threatening T cell defects. In addition to reduction of CD4 (T helper cells), there is an increase in CD8 (T suppressor/cytotoxic cells), most of which have a cytotoxic phenotype.

B cell function is altered so that many infected individuals have marked hypergammaglobulinemia, and AIDS patients fail to respond normally to antigens when immunized. Autoantibodies to T cells and circulating immune complexes are present. Most infected individuals progress from health to ARC (AIDS-related complex) to AIDS over several years. The immunologic determinants of the clinical fate of persons infected with HIV are unknown.

In AIDS, immunologic tests reveal a severe deficiency of T lymphocyte function and number, with little alteration in B lymphocyte numbers. Patients are frequently anergic. In vitro tests of peripheral blood T cell function such as proliferative responses to antigens and mitogens are markedly reduced or absent. The absolute lymphocyte count is severely decreased (frequently < 500 cells/μL), and the ratio of helper to suppressor/cytotoxic T cells is considerably lower than normal. The change in the latter ratio is due to a greater reduction in the absolute number of helper T cells in the peripheral blood as compared to suppressor/cytotoxic cells. The immunologic changes that occur in asymptomatic HIV seropositive individuals or those with ARC are usually not as marked as those in AIDS patients.

Gallo RC: The AIDS virus. Sci Am 1987;256:46.

Levy JA: AIDS: Pathogenesis and Treatment. Marcel Dekker, 1988.

What science knows about AIDS. Sci Am (Oct) 1988;259. (Entire issue.)

SECONDARY IMMUNODEFICIENCY

Deficiencies in T cell immunity, antibody immunity, or both have been associated with many diseases. Two examples of altered immunity secondary to underlying disease are discussed below.

Immunodeficiency Associated With Sarcoidosis

The immunodeficiency associated with sarcoidosis is characterized by a partial deficit in T cell function with intact or increased B cell function. Patients with sarcoidosis often are relatively nonreactive to intradermal injections of common antigens. However, complete lack of skin reactivity is infrequent. A positive reaction to purified protein derivative is usually noted during active infection with *Mycobacterium tuberculosis*. Serum immunoglobulin levels are normal or high, and specific antibody formation is generally normal.

Immunodeficiency Associated With Hodgkin's Disease

A moderate to severe deficit in T cell function with intact B cell function is frequently found in Hodgkin's disease. Only 10–20% of patients with Hodgkin's disease show skin reactivity to common antigens, as compared to 70–90% of controls. Many patients show depressed responses to in vitro stimulation of peripheral blood lymphocytes with phytohemagglutinin. Serum immunoglobulins are normal, and specific antibody formation is intact except in agonal cases.

The clinical significance of depressed cell-mediated immunity in Hodgkin's disease is difficult to evaluate, since most patients are treated with potent immunosuppressive agents. Nevertheless, frequent infections with herpes zoster and *Cryptococcus* are probably related to immunodeficiency associated with the underlying disease.

Gotoff SP: The secondary immunodeficiencies. Chapter 20 in: *Immunologic Disorders in Infants and Children,* 3rd ed. Stiehm ER, Fulginiti VA (editors). Saunders, 1988.

AUTOIMMUNITY

Autoimmune diseases cannot be explained by a solitary cause or mechanism. Small amounts of autoantibodies are normally produced and may have physiologic roles in cellular interactions. The major theories regarding the development of autoimmune disease are (1) release of normally sequestered antigens, (2) the presence of abnormal clones, (3) shared antigens between the host and microorganisms, and (4) defects in helper or suppressor T cell function. A genetic susceptibility is also a likely determinant of autoimmune disease. In nearly all autoimmune diseases, multiple mechanisms of autoimmunity are operative and the exact underlying causes are unknown.

Cell-Mediated Autoimmunity

Certain autoimmune diseases are mediated by T cells that have become specifically immunized to autologous tissues. Cytotoxic or killer T cells generated by this aberrant immune response attack and injure specific organs in the absence of serum autoantibodies.

Diminished suppressor T cell activity results in disordered regulation of immune responses and may promote overactivity of other autoreactive mechanisms. The immune damage in nonorganic specific diseases such as systemic lupus erythematosus may be in part due to such a mechanism.

Antibody-Mediated Autoimmunity

Several autoimmune diseases have been shown to be caused by autoantibody in the absence of cell-mediated autoimmunity. The autoimmune hemolytic anemias, idiopathic thrombocytopenia, and Goodpasture's syndrome appear to be mediated solely by autoantibodies directed against autologous cell membrane constituents. In these diseases, antibody attaches to cell membranes, fixes complement, and the ensuing inflammatory reaction severely injures the cells.

The existence of antireceptor antibodies that compete with or mimic various physiologic agonists for cellular receptors is a specific autoimmune mechanism in several diseases. In Graves' disease, antibodies are present that compete with thyroid cells' TSH receptors and thereby stimulate thyroid hormone production. In rare instances of type I diabetes mellitus, anti-insulin receptor antibodies cause insulin resis-

tance in peripheral target tissues. The anti-islet cell antibodies that are usually found in type I diabetes produce insulin deficiency by destroying islet cells in the pancreas. In myasthenia gravis, antibodies to acetylcholine receptors of the myoneural junction block neuromuscular transmission and thereby produce muscle weakness.

Immune Complex Disease

In this group of diseases (systemic lupus erythematosus, rheumatoid arthritis, some drug-induced hemolytic anemias and thrombocytopenias), autologous tissues are injured as "innocent bystanders." Autoantibodies are not directed against cellular components of the target organ but rather against autologous or heterologous antigens in the serum. The resultant antigen-antibody complexes bind nonspecifically to autologous membranes (eg, glomerular basement membrane) and fix complement. Fixation and subsequent activation of complement components produce a local inflammatory response that results in tissue injury.

Steinberg AD: Mechanisms of disordered immune regulation. Chapter 35 in: *Basic & Clinical Immunology,* 7th ed. Stites DP, Terr AI (editors). Appleton & Lange, 1990.

AUTOIMMUNE DISEASES

The diagnosis and treatment of specific autoimmune diseases are described elsewhere in this book. Autoantibodies associated with certain autoimmune diseases are not usually implicated in the pathogenesis of tissue injury but are thought instead to be by-products of the injury (eg, autoimmune thyroiditis and antithyroglobulin antibody).

TESTS FOR AUTOANTIBODIES ASSOCIATED WITH AUTOIMMUNE DISEASES

Assays for autoantibodies are similar to those used for detection of antibodies to foreign antigens. Four commonly used methods are discussed below.

Many of the autoantibodies are not specific for a single disease entity (eg, antinuclear antibody, rheumatoid factor). Tests for the latter autoantibodies are best used as screening procedures in that a negative result makes the diagnosis of certain autoimmune diseases unlikely. For example, a negative antinuclear antibody test makes the diagnosis of systemic lupus erythematosus unlikely, since this antibody is detected in the serum of more than 95% of lupus patients.

Agglutination of Antigen-Coated Red Blood Cells

Red cells (human, sheep, etc) are incubated with

tannic acid or other chemicals so that the cell surface becomes "sticky." The red cells are subsequently incubated with purified specific antigen (eg, thyroglobulin), which is adsorbed to the cell surface. The antigen-coated cells are suspended in an unknown serum, and antibody is detected by red cell agglutination. Antigen-coated latex particles are substituted for red cells in the latex fixation tests.

Enzyme-Linked Immunoassays (ELISA)

Antibodies to various tissue antigens can be readily detected by ELISA tests. Extracted and purified antigens are fixed to a plastic microtiter well or beads. Patient's serum is added, and excess proteins are removed by washing and centrifugation. A second antibody coupled to an enzyme (eg, alkaline phosphatase) is added. The enzyme's substrate is then added, and color forms that is measured in a spectrophotometer. This test can also be adapted to antigen detection by placing the antibody on the plastic surface. ELISA assays are very widely applied in clinical laboratory testing.

Immunofluorescence Microscopy

This technique is most frequently used for detection of antinuclear antibody. Frozen sections of mouse liver or other substrates are cut and placed on glass slides. A patient's serum is placed over the sections and washed away. Fluorescein-conjugated rabbit anti-human immunoglobulin is then applied and washed. Antinuclear antibody specifically binds to the nucleus, and the fluorescein conjugate binds to the human antibody. Fluorescence of the cell nucleus observed by fluorescence microscopy indicates a positive test.

Complement Fixation

Specific antigen, unknown serum, and complement are reacted together. Sheep red blood cells coated with anti-sheep cell antibody are subsequently added to the above reaction mixture for 30 minutes at 37 °C. Lysis of sheep cells indicates that complement is present (attaches to sheep cell surface). Lack of lysis indicates that complement has been consumed by the interaction of antibody in the unknown serum with the specific antigen. Lack of lysis is a positive test for the presence of specific antibody.

Treatment of Autoimmune Diseases

Therapy of autoimmune diseases involves a variety of approaches. Suppression of production of autoantibodies with corticosteroids and cytotoxic agents is often effective. Anti-inflammatory drugs such as aspirin, colchicine, and corticosteroids relieve tissue damage from immune complexes. Plasmapheresis to remove offending autoantibodies and circulating immune complexes, when combined with cytotoxic drugs, has been useful in some diseases. All of these

modalities are directed at symptoms, since the underlying cause of these disorders remains unknown.

Gupta S, Talal N: *Immunology of Rheumatic Diseases.* Plenum, 1985. (Basic and clinical aspects of a variety of autoimmune and rheumatic diseases.)

Morrow J, Isenberg D: *Autoimmune Rheumatic Disease.* Blackwell, 1987. (Only vasculitic and rheumatic diseases.)

IMMUNOGENETICS & TRANSPLANTATION

GENETIC CONTROL OF THE IMMUNE RESPONSE

The ability to mount a specific immune response is under the direct control of genes closely associated on the same chromosome with the structural genes for the major transplantation antigens. The major transplantation antigens are the cell surface glycoproteins (found on most cells of the body), which elicit the strongest transplantation rejection reaction when tissues are exchanged between 2 members of a particular species. In humans, this genetic region has been designated the **human leukocyte antigen (HLA)** complex because these antigens were first detected on peripheral blood lymphocytes. The complex includes antigens HLA-A, -B, -C, -DR and others, each with many alleles.

The HLA region has been localized to chromosome 6, and the order of the different HLA loci is shown in Fig 14–1. Most (98%) of the time, the HLA complex is inherited intact as 2 haplotypes (one from each parent), and within any particular family, therefore, the number of different combinations found will be fairly small; eg, siblings have a 1:4 chance of being HLA-identical. In contrast, the number of antigen combinations among unrelated individuals is huge, resulting in probabilities of fewer than one in several thousand, depending upon the phenotype involved, of finding HLA-compatible individuals in a random donor pool. This is particularly important when compatible donors are needed for allosensitized patients requiring platelet transfusions or organ transplantation. Family members have the highest likelihood of being compatible donors, whereas HLA compatibility between 2 unrelated individuals has a very low probability. HLA-A and -B typing or crossmatching is utilized for selection of compatible donors for platelet transfusions to allosensitized, thrombocytopenic recipients. Typing for these class I antigens as well as for HLA-D antigens is important in determining compatibility for organ transplantation. Typing for HLA markers is of value in studying associa-

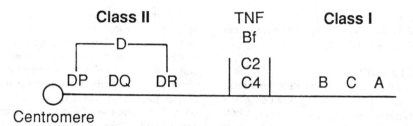

Figure 14–1 Genetic map of the HLA region. The centromere is to the left. Bf, C2, and C4 are genes for components of the complement system. TNF is the tumor necrosis factor gene.

tions between the HLA system and genetic control of disease susceptibility.

In the genetic region determining the major transplantation antigen complex, there are genes determining the ability to mount a specific immune response. These are called immune response, or Ir, genes. Although the exact mechanism of action of Ir genes is not yet known, it is clear that they affect the ability to recognize foreign antigens and to initiate the development of T and B cell immunity to these antigens. Genes with such a strong effect on specific immune responsiveness might be expected to have major effects on resistance or susceptibility to a wide variety of infectious, neoplastic, and autoimmune diseases.

Schwartz BD: The human major histocompatibility HLA complex. Chapter 4 in: *Basic & Clinical Immunology*, 7th ed. Stites DP, Terr AI (editors). Appleton & Lange, 1990.

HLA TYPING

The standard method for detecting HLA-A, -B, and -C antigens is that of lymphocyte microcytotoxicity. Lymphocytes isolated from peripheral blood or lymph nodes are added to each well of a typing tray that has been preloaded with sera containing the appropriate cytotoxic alloantibody. After allowing for the alloantibodies to bind to target lymphocytes, complement is added. Those cells to which antibody has been specifically bound will have complement activated at the cell surface, resulting in cell death or lysis. By addition of a vital dye (eg, eosin, fluorescein diacetate, or trypan blue), viable and nonviable cells can be distinguished. It is thus possible to type for all of the known HLA-A, -B, and -C specificities. At present, the best sources of alloantisera are parous women, 10–30% of whom become sensitized during pregnancy to paternal antigens carried by the fetus. A few antibodies are also provided by individuals allosensitized by other causes, eg, transfusion or transplantation, and a few monoclonal antibodies are also used.

Typing for the class II antigens HLA-DR and -DQ is performed as described above, except that separated B lymphocytes are used as targets rather than unseparated peripheral blood lymphocytes. Antigens of the HLA-D and -DP series are detected by in vitro cellular reactivity. Lymphocytes of one individual will undergo DNA synthesis and proliferation upon encountering lymphocytes from another individual possessing foreign HLA-D antigens. Donor cells are irradiated or treated with mitomycin C to ablate their immune responsiveness. These "stimulator" cells are then mixed with peripheral blood lymphocytes of the recipient (responder) in this mixed leukocyte reaction (MLR) culture. A responder lacking the stimulator's D antigen will respond by brisk DNA synthesis and proliferation that can readily be measured by DNA incorporation of tritiated thymidine. Responders possessing the D antigen of the donor will remain nonreactive.

HLA-DP antigens are identified by an extension of the MLR called primed lymphocyte typing. Following priming stimulation in a first MLR, the responder cells are restimulated in a secondary MLR by a different stimulator cell. If the 2 stimulator cells share the same mismatched DP (or a D) antigen not possessed by the responder, the responder cells will demonstrate a brisk proliferative response.

Although technically demanding and requiring viable lymphoid cells and experienced laboratories, HLA typing is available at most large medical centers or blood banks.

Colombe BW: Histocompatibility testing. Chapter 21 in: *Basic & Clinical Immunology*, 7th ed. Stites DP, Terr AI (editors). Appleton & Lange, 1990.

CLINICAL TRANSPLANTATION

Organ transplants are commonly used in the treatment of many diseases. The main limitation to their more widespread use is the scarcity of donor organs and the expense of these procedures. Failure to achieve completely successful grafts is primarily due to histoincompatibility and lack of totally safe and effective immunosuppressive regimens to halt rejection. Great care in avoiding transmission of infectious agents (eg, HIV, HBV, CMV) from donor to recipient requires extensive pretransplant serologic testing.

Kidney Transplantation

End-stage renal disease is the indication for kidney transplantation. Kidneys from living related donors who are HLA-identical and also red blood cell ABO-matched have 90% survival at 1 year; less identical grafts have a somewhat lower survival rate. Transplants with matched cadaver kidney donors survive nearly as long, especially if the recipient does not contain antibodies to donor antigens. A positive crossmatch by cytotoxicity testing between recipient serum and donor cells is considered a contraindication to that transplant. Donor screening is performed in all cases to avoid transmission of AIDS virus or other infectious agents. Pretreatment of recipients with blood transfusions from the donor appears to extend graft survival even longer. Graft rejection is manifested by diminishing renal function and is treated with immunosuppressive drugs, especially cyclosporine (see below).

Heart Transplantation

The indication for heart transplantation is end-stage cardiac disease clearly refractory to medical treatment. Donors and recipients are matched by excluding anti-HLA antibodies in the recipient, since there is rarely time for HLA typing. Rejection is diagnosed by endomyocardial biopsy and treated with immunosuppressants, particularly cyclosporine. Five-year survival is approximately 40% at selected centers.

Lung Transplantation

Lung transplantation is currently combined with heart transplantation because of the poor results achieved with lung grafts alone. One-year survival may be as high as 70%.

Liver Transplantation

Severe liver dysfunction without serious systemic complications of hepatic failure is the indication for liver transplantation. Children with developmental defects are typical recipients. Recipients are selected on the basis of ABO matching and organ size. HLA typing has not achieved practical results. One-year survival rates approach 70%.

Pancreas & Islet Cell Transplants

The indications for these procedures—largely experimental at present—are pancreatic insufficiency and, in some cases, diabetes mellitus. Clinical results have been disappointing.

Bone Marrow Transplantation

Leukemia, aplastic anemia, and congenital immu-

nologic defects are currently the main indications for marrow transplants. Irradiation and immunosuppressive drugs are used to prepare recipients. Close HLA matching is essential for successful bone marrow transplantation. Graft-versus-host disease caused by attack of donor cells on histocompatible host cells may be fatal. This occurs more commonly in adults, which limits the use of histoincompatible bone marrow transplantation in this age group. Autologous marrow harvested during disease-free periods has been used successfully for marrow reconstitution in selected patients. Infections during the period of emerging immune competence can also present life-threatening problems.

The success rates of bone marrow transplantation are about 70% survival at 1 year in aplastic anemia, 40–75% survival at 1 year in various forms of leukemia, and extremely variable in immunologic deficiency diseases.

Other Organs & Tissues

Transplantations of other organs–skin, cornea, bone, and heart valves–are now routine surgical procedures. Much further research remains to be done on transplantation of other organs–particularly neural tissue.

Garovoy MR et al: Clinical transplantation. Chapter 60 in: *Basic & Clinical Immunology*, 7th ed. Stites DP, Terr AI (editors). Appleton & Lange, 1990.

MECHANISM OF ACTION OF IMMUNOSUPPRESSIVE DRUGS

Therapies that suppress immune or inflammatory responses are used commonly to treat recipients of organ transplants and patients with autoimmune diseases or neoplasms. The most frequently used drugs and their modes of action are briefly summarized below.

(1) Corticosteroids: This group of drugs has potent anti-inflammatory and direct effects on immunocompetent cells. Corticosteroids inhibit cell-mediated immune responses more severely than antibody responses. T helper cells are preferentially reduced owing to redistribution. Neutrophils are increased owing to demargination and bone marrow release. Monocytes and eosinophils are reduced. These cellular changes result in reduced inflammatory responses. Disruption of the interaction between T cells and macrophages appears to be an important mechanism, and corticosteroids have been shown to block the activation of T cells by interleukin-1 (IL-1) derived from macrophages. In addition, corticosteroids inhibit the expression of class II histocompatibility antigens on the macrophage surface, thereby interfering with presentation of antigen to T cells.

(2) Cytotoxic drugs: The most frequently used

cytotoxic drugs are azathioprine and cyclophosphamide. Azathioprine is a derivative of mercaptopurine, an antagonist of purine synthesis. Azathioprine is a phase-specific drug that kills rapidly replicating cells. It inhibits proliferation of both T and B cells as well as macrophages. Cyclophosphamide is an alkylating agent that damages cells by cross-linking DNA. Although this cycle-specific drug is most effective in killing cells going through the mitotic cycle, it can also cause intermitotic cell injury and death. Cyclophosphamide can inhibit both T and B cell immunity as well as inflammation. Azathioprine and cyclophosphamide are effective inhibitors of the production of serum antibodies.

(3) Antimetabolites: The most commonly used antimetabolite is methotrexate, an inhibitor of folic acid synthesis. Methotrexate inhibits rapidly proliferating cells in S phase and suppresses both cell-mediated and humoral immunity as well as inflammation.

(4) Cyclosporine: This cyclic polypeptide derived from a fungus has been used recently as an immunosuppressive drug in organ transplant recipients. Cyclosporine interferes with the secretion of interleukin-2 (IL-2) by T lymphocytes. Since IL-2 is necessary for T cell replication, this drug is a potent inhibitor of T cell proliferation and thereby inhibits T cell-mediated immune responses. Little effect has been shown on direct B cell immune responses or on inflammation. Its toxic effects are primarily on renal and hepatic function.

Many new drugs with potent immunosuppressive actions and reduced toxicities are under development and clinical trials.

Goodwin J: Anti-inflammatory drugs. Chapter 63 in: *Basic & Clinical Immunology,* 7th ed. Stites DP, Terr AI (editors). Appleton & Lange, 1990.
Winkelstein A: Immune suppression. Chapter 61 in: *Basic & Clinical Immunology,* 7th ed. Stites DP, Terr AI (editors). Appleton & Lange, 1990.

ASSOCIATIONS BETWEEN HLA ANTIGENS & SPECIFIC DISEASES

In humans, very striking associations are observed between particular HLA antigens and specific diseases. These facts are important in relating HLA to diseases: HLA antigen frequencies vary substantially among different ethnic groups, and therefore control populations must be carefully selected. Appropriate statistical corrections must be made to compensate for the large number of antigens tested. Accurate clinical definition of disease is necessary to avoid diluting an HLA-disease association by mixing together diseases that are pathogenetically different but clinically similar. If the disease studied has a fatal outcome, then the proper disease phase must be selected to demonstrate associations. Some quantitative measure of strength of association is necessary to compare different HLA-disease relationships.

Table 14–4 is a partial list of HLA-disease associations. Studies have revealed that the strongest association is between HLA-B27 and ankylosing spondylitis, which holds in all ethnic groups but is more striking in Japanese people than in Caucasians studied. Other spondyloarthropathies (eg, Reiter's syndrome, arthritis following *Salmonella* or *Yersinia* infection) are

Table 14–4. HLA and disease associations.

Disease	Antigen	Frequency Patients (%)	Controls (%)	Relative Risk
Ankylosing spondylitis Caucasians	B27	89	4–13	69.1
Japanese	B27	85		207
Reiter's disease	B27	80	9	37
Salmonella arthritis	B27	60–92	8–14	30
Rheumatoid arthritis	DR4	68	25	3.8
Psoriasis vulgaris	Cw6	27	4	8.5
Graves' disease Caucasians	DR3	56	25	3.7
Japanese	Dw12	48	16	5
Diabetes mellitus	DR3 heterozygotes			3
Diabetes mellitus	DR4 heterozygotes			3.6
Diabetes mellitus	DR3/DR4 heterozygotes			33
Acute lymphocytic leukemia	A2	83	44	6
Systemic lupus erythematosus	DR4	73	33	5
Narcolepsy	DR2	100	34	358

also strongly associated with B27, suggesting that despite apparently different causes the pathogeneses of these diseases share some common factor related to the B27 marker. B27 is not specific for all arthritis; eg, rheumatoid arthritis associates not with that antigen but with DR4. Furthermore, disease associations are not restricted to B and DR: eg, psoriasis vulgaris is associated with a C locus antigen and acute lymphocytic leukemia with an A locus antigen. In diabetes mellitus, heterozygote individuals possess both the DR3 and the DR4 antigens and have a relative risk of 33, far greater than expected by simple addition of risks for DR3 plus DR4. It also appears that a single mechanism may associate with different antigens in different ethnic groups. Among Caucasians studied in whom the Dw12 antigen is almost absent, Dw3 is associated with Graves' disease. Among Japanese people where Dw3 is almost completely lacking, Dw12 is associated with Graves' disease.

Sometimes combinations of antigens exhibit disease associations. This suggests either interaction among different genes affecting susceptibility or unusual linkage between the known HLA genes and some nearby gene actually responsible for the disease susceptibility.

Paul WE, Fathman GG, Metzger H (editors): Annu Rev Immunol 1984–present. (Annual entire issue.)

Schwartz BD: The human major histocompatibility HLA complex. Chapter 4 in: *Basic & Clinical Immunology,* 7th ed. Appleton & Lange, 1990.

Stites DP, Terr AI (editors): *Basic & Clinical Immunology,* 7th ed. Appleton & Lange, 1990.

Tiwari JL, Terasaki PI: *HLA and Disease Associations.* Springer, 1985.

Williamson AR, Turner MW: *Essential Immunogenetics.* Blackwell, 1987.

ALLERGIC DISEASES

Allergy is the most common form of immunologic disease. It is defined as an immunologically mediated reaction to a foreign antigen (allergen), causing tissue inflammation and organ dysfunction. The disease can be local or systemic. Because the allergen is foreign—ie, environmental—the skin and respiratory tract are the organs most frequently involved in allergic disease. Allergic reactions may also localize to the vasculature, gastrointestinal tract, or other visceral organs. Anaphylaxis and serum sickness are systemic forms of allergy.

CLASSIFICATION

Allergic diseases can be classified according to (1) the immunologic mechanism involved in pathogenesis, (2) the organ system affected, and (3) the nature and source of the allergen. An immunologic classification is preferred, because it serves as a rational basis for diagnosis and treatment.

Immunologic Mechanisms

The 2 major pathways of immunologically induced inflammation involve the reaction of the allergen with T cells and with B cell products (antibodies). Of the 5 immunoglobulin classes of antibodies (IgG, IgA, IgM, IgD, and IgE) only 3—IgG, IgM, and IgE—are known to be involved in allergy.

A. T Cell-Mediated Allergy (Delayed Hypersensitivity, Cell-Mediated Hypersensitivity): The most common expression of T cell-mediated allergy is allergic contact dermatitis, in which the allergen causes dermal inflammation on direct contact with the skin. The dermatitis appears after a latent period of 1 to several days from the time of contact. Hypersensitivity pneumonitis (extrinsic allergic alveolitis) is a pulmonary allergic disease that has a chronic form in which a T cell-mediated mechanism is prominent.

B. IgE-Mediated Allergy (Immediate Hypersensitivity): IgE antibodies occupy receptor sites on mast cells. Within minutes after exposure to the allergen, vasoactive and inflammatory mediators are activated and released from the mast cell, causing vasodilatation, visceral smooth muscle contraction, and mucous secretory gland stimulation. Other mediators induce a late-phase inflammatory response that appears several hours later. There are 2 clinical subgroups of IgE-mediated allergy: atopy and anaphylaxis.

1. The atopic diseases–Atopy is a clinical term for a group of diseases—allergic rhinitis, allergic asthma, atopic dermatitis, and allergic gastroenteropathy—that occur in certain persons with an inherited tendency to readily develop IgE antibodies to multiple common organic allergens in the air and in foods. The reaction is localized to a susceptible target organ, but more than one of these manifestations may occur in the same allergic individual. There is a strong familial tendency because of complex genetic factors.

2. Anaphylaxis–6Certain allergens—especially drugs, insect venom, and foods—may induce an IgE antibody response that causes a generalized release of mediators from mast cells, resulting in **systemic anaphylaxis.** This disease is characterized by hypotension or shock from generalized vasodilatation, bronchospasm, gastrointestinal and uterine muscle contraction, and urticaria or angioedema. The condition is potentially fatal and is thus a medical emergency. Sensitivities are rarely multiple. The condition affects either nonatopic or atopic persons. **Urticaria and angioedema** are cutaneous forms of anaphylaxis. Like anaphylaxis, they are usually caused by a drug, food, or insect venom, but they are much more common. These disorders are generally benign unless the edematous skin lesions are extensive and cause hypotension or unless angioedema obstructs the larynx or hypopharynx.

C. Immune Complex Allergy: Antibodies of the IgG or IgM isotype can form complexes with the allergen and thereby activate complement to generate mediators of inflammation. Under conditions of high concentrations of both allergen and antibody, the clinical manifestations of disease include the **Arthus reaction,** a localized cutaneous and subcutaneous inflammatory response to injected allergen; **serum sickness,** a systemic disease characterized by fever, arthralgias, and dermatitis; and an acute form of **hypersensitivity pneumonitis** from inhalation of the allergen.

Organ System

Patients present to the physician with symptoms and physical findings that may be either localized or generalized. Knowledge of the organs involved may help to determine the type of allergy and the nature of the allergen (see Table 14–5).

Allergens

Although any exogenous (environmental) material can theoretically be allergenic, certain ones are encountered more frequently than are others. For diag-

nostic purposes, it is convenient to classify them by route of exposure.

A. Inhalants: Pollens, mold spores, animal danders, or other products such as dried saliva, house dust, and insect emanations (especially the house dust mite) are the usual allergens that cause atopic disease. Hypersensitivity pneumonitis (see Chapter 7) has been caused by a long list of airborne organic dusts, microorganisms, and some organic chemicals. Occasionally, the allergens causing contact dermatitis may reach the skin via atmospheric fumes.

B. Ingestants: Foods cause allergic gastroenteropathy and may cause asthma, anaphylaxis, and urticaria or angioedema. Allergic reactions to drugs are most commonly urticaria and anaphylaxis. Drug-induced nonurticarial dermatitis or fixed drug eruptions are suspected to be allergic in origin, though the immunologic mechanism is uncertain. Serum sickness is usually caused by injected foreign protein (eg, antilymphocyte globulin), but mild reactions may occur after administration of oral drugs.

C. Contactants: Plant oils, cosmetics and perfumes, nickel in jewelry or on buckles and undergarment fasteners, hair dyes, topical medications including their additives, and occupational chemicals are the most common causes of allergic contact dermati-

Table 14–5. Allergic diseases classified according to the involved organ or tissue.

Organ or Tissue	Disease	Mechanism			
		T Cell	IgE	Immune Complex	Uncertain
Skin	Allergic contact dermatitis	•			
	Atopic dermatitis		•		
	Urticaria and angioedema		•		
	Arthus reaction			•	
	Generalized drug eruption				•
	Fixed drug eruption				•
Upper respiratory tract	Allergic rhinitis		•		
Bronchi	Asthma		•		
	Allergic bronchopulmonary aspergillosis		•	•	
Alveoli	Hypersensitivity pneumonitis, acute			•	
	Hypersensitivity pneumonitis, chronic	•			
Eyes	Allergic conjunctivitis		•		
GI tract	Allergic gastroenteropathy		•		
Liver	Hepatic drug reaction				•
Kidney	Allergic interstitial nephritis				•
Systemic	Anaphylaxis		•		
	Serum sickness			•	

tis. Occasionally, urticaria may be induced by direct skin contact with the allergen.

D. Injectants: Drugs, Hymenoptera venom, and injected atopic allergens account for most cases of anaphylaxis and acute urticaria or angioedema.

Kaplan AR: *Allergy*. Churchill Livingston, 1985.

Middleton E, Reed C, Ellis E (editors): *Allergy: Principles and Practice*, 3rd ed. Mosby, 1988.

Patterson R (editor): *Allergic Diseases: Diagnosis and Management*, 3rd ed. Lippincott, 1985.

Terr AI: Mechanisms of hypersensitivity. In: *Basic & Clinical Immunology*, 7th ed. Stites, DP, Terr, AI (editors). Appleton & Lange, 1990.

DIAGNOSIS

Virtually all of the diseases caused by allergy can also occur in the absence of an immunologic mechanism. For example, intrinsic asthma is triggered by the nonimmunologic effect of inhaled dusts and fumes, weather changes, stress, etc; irritant contact dermatitis is the result of physical or chemical damage to the skin by chemicals; anaphylactoid reactions are produced nonimmunologically by iodinated radiologic contrast media and some drugs. Therefore, the diagnosis of allergy requires answers to the following 3 questions: (1) What is the nature of the disease? (2) Is the disease caused by allergy? (3) What specific allergens (one or several) are responsible?

A thorough history is essential and must include details of symptomatology and a survey of allergens in the home, at work, associated with hobbies, habits, and medications. Physical examination will reveal evidence of active disease if the patient is examined during a period of allergen exposure. Radiologic or other imaging studies may be necessary to supplement the physical examination. In some cases, physiologic testing such as pulmonary function tests are required to establish the diagnosis of a specific disease, but these procedures do not determine whether there is an allergic cause of that disease.

Tests of Specific Immune Responses

"Allergy tests" show whether or not the patient has been exposed and has developed an immune response to a particular allergen. To confirm a diagnosis of allergic disease, evidence of an immune response (ie, a positive test result) must be correlated with the history before one can conclude that the allergen caused the illness. The type of immune response must be consistent with the nature of the disease; eg, IgE antibody causes allergic rhinitis but not allergic contact dermatitis.

A. IgE Antibody Tests: These can be detected by in vivo (skin tests) or in vitro methods.

1. Skin tests–Epicutaneous or cutaneous exposure to an allergen produces a localized pruritic wheal and erythema which is maximal at 15–20 minutes. It is used most commonly in the diagnosis of allergic respiratory disease (rhinitis and asthma), for which standard sets of allergen extracts are available commercially. These include pollens, fungi, animal danders, dust, and dust mites. The pollen and mold allergens must be appropriate to the patient's geographic area. To avoid a systemic reaction, most allergists perform epicutaneous (prick) testing first, followed by selected intradermal tests to allergens that were negative by prick test but still suspected from the history. Concentrations of extracts for intradermal testing to each allergen are determined by screening in nonallergic subjects. Special allergenic extracts can be prepared for other allergens where indicated. Skin testing for food allergy is appropriate only if the patient has symptoms consistent with IgE-mediated allergy within 2 hours after eating the suspect food. Skin testing to drugs is reliable for protein drugs (eg, heterologous serum, insulin), not for haptenic drugs (low-molecular-weight organic compounds). An important exception is penicillin, which will frequently but not always elicit a positive wheal-and-erythema skin test in patients with anaphylactic allergy to penicillin. Some drugs, notably opiates, cause nonimmunologic release of mast cell mediators and thereby give universal wheal-and-erythema reactions. A negative diluent control test is essential. A positive control with histamine or a histamine liberator—such as morphine—is desirable.

Skin testing is preferred to in vitro methods (discussed below) because it detects the presence of IgE antibody in tissue and shows biologic activity. It is convenient, inexpensive, and provides an immediate result. Any drug with antihistamine effect must be withdrawn prior to testing. Extensive active dermatitis may limit the availability of skin for testing. There is an exceedingly small risk of inducing a systemic reaction when skin testing is conducted properly. Skin testing for anaphylactic reactions to Hymenoptera venom or a drug is performed by serial titration, starting with extremely dilute solutions to avoid a systemic reaction. Some physicians use serial titration of inhalant allergens in testing for atopic diseases.

2. In vitro tests of IgE antibody–IgE antibodies can be detected in serum by radioallergosorbent test (RAST) or enzyme-linked immunosorbent assay (ELISA). Protein allergens are covalently linked to the immunosorbent. Haptenic allergens must first be coupled to a nonallergenic protein carrier such as human serum albumin, which is then linked to the immunosorbent. Many of the usual atopic allergens are available commercially for RAST or ELISA testing.

In vitro tests detect antibody in serum. Since IgE-mediated allergy is caused by IgE antibodies bound to mast cells—not by IgE antibodies in the circulation—in vitro tests generally are less sensitive than skin tests for diagnostic use. They are not affected by antihistamine therapy, but they can give false-positive results in patients with high total serum IgE and false-negative results in patients treated with immunotherapy who have significant allergen-specific IgG antibodies. There is no risk of a systemic reaction. The test is significantly more expensive than skin testing, and results are not immediately available. The RAST or ELISA method is particularly useful for detecting IgE antibodies to certain occupational chemicals or potentially toxic allergens.

The total IgE level in serum is higher on average in atopic patients than it is in nonatopic individuals. There is considerable overlap, so that this measurement is not a satisfactory screening test for atopy.

B. Tests for Immune Complex Allergic Diseases: The IgG antibody may be present in sufficient quantity in serum to be detected by the precipitin-in-gel method. ELISA will detect antibodies present in lesser amounts. Reduced serum levels of C3, C4, or CH_{50} may be evidence of complement activation.

C. Tests for T Cell-Mediated Allergy: Cell-mediated immunity or hypersensitivity is detected by intradermal (tuberculin-type) skin tests which elicit 48-hour inflammatory induration or by patch testing in the diagnosis of allergic contact dermatitis. The patch test is performed by topical application of the suspected contactant allergen. A positive test at 48–72 hours consists of erythema, swelling, and papules. Concentrations of allergens for patch testing must be determined in nonallergic subjects to avoid false-positive irritant responses.

Cell-mediated hypersensitivity can be detected in vitro by exposing peripheral blood mononuclear cells to allergen to detect the release of lymphokines or inhibition of cell migration, but such tests are rarely useful for diagnosis.

Provocation Tests

Occasionally, direct challenge of the affected organ or tissue with the allergen under control conditions is required for a definitive diagnosis. Such challenges can be offered by bronchial, nasal, conjunctival, oral, or cutaneous exposure. This form of testing confirms that the reaction can be caused by the test substance, but a positive test does not prove an immunologic mechanism.

A. Bronchoprovocation Testing: An aerosolized solution of the test allergen is delivered by inhalation through a dosimeter in graded increasing dosages. The response in FEV_1 or FEV_1/FVC is measured by spirometry. Dose-response curves are determined, and the provoking dose producing a 20% fall in FEV 1 (PD_{20}) is determined. This test should be done in a facility where the patient can be monitored for 24 hours after allergen inhalation because of the possibility of a late-phase response. Bronchoprovocation is not necessary in the routine diagnosis of allergic

asthma, but it may be helpful in some cases of occupational asthma.

Provocation testing should not be performed if there is a suspicion that the patient might develop a systemic anaphylactic reaction to the test.

Bronchial provocation field testing can be done by having the patient make serial determinations of peak expiratory flow rate (PEFR) using a portable peak flowmeter during periods of natural exposure to a suspected airborne allergen.

Bronchial provocation with exercise or with inhalation of methacholine, histamine, or cold air is a test for the nonspecific bronchial hyperirritability of asthma. These procedures do not detect allergic sensitivities.

B. Nasal Provocation Testing: This procedure is similar to bronchial provocation except that the allergen is inhaled through the nose and change in nasal airway resistance is measured. The procedure is complicated by the large excursions of nasal airway resistance that occur normally.

C. Conjunctival Provocation: A drop of allergen extract is instilled into one conjunctival sac. An allergic reaction produces itching, conjunctival injection, swelling, and tearing within minutes. The control contralateral eye is not affected. The method is unpleasant and therefore rarely used.

D. Oral Provocation: In most cases of suspected allergy to a food or drug, double-blind placebo-controlled oral challenge is the definitive test. For a positive test, the reported clinical findings must be reproduced. Freeze-dried foods in large opaque capsules provide a sufficient dose of allergen for testing.

AMA Council on Scientific Affairs: In vitro testing for allergy. Report II. JAMA 1987;258:1639.

AMA Council on Scientific Affairs: In vivo diagnostic testing and immunotherapy for allergy. (Two parts.) JAMA 1987;258:1363, 1508.

Terr AI: In vitro tests for immediate hypersensitivity. Ann Rev Med 1988;39:135.

Townley RJ, Hopp RJ: Inhalation methods for the study of airway responsiveness. J Allergy Clin Immunol 1987;80:111.

MANAGEMENT

Allergic disease management requires both symptomatic therapy and allergen-specific treatment. General measures for treating each of the diseases are presented elsewhere in this book. This section will discuss only the management of the allergic causes.

The 3 basic principles of allergy management are: (1) avoidance of the allergen, (2) symptomatic therapy, and (3) immunotherapy.

Avoidance Therapy

Avoidance is the most effective treatment for any allergic condition, and it should always be considered in addition to pharmacologic and immunologic treatment. Avoidance of allergen exposure may or may not reduce the underlying immunologic sensitivity to that allergen. Success requires accurate diagnosis of the causative allergens in each case.

A. Pollens: Remaining indoors in air-conditioned environments will avoid exposure to pollens, but this is not a long-term practical solution.

B. Animal Danders: If the allergy is slight, the patient may benefit from merely keeping the animal out of the bedroom; usually, however, it is necessary to remove the animal from the home altogether.

C. House Dust and Dust Mites: The mattress and pillows should be encased in dust-proof material, and the bedroom floor should be uncarpeted. The room should be dusted frequently. Electronic air purifiers are of unproved effectiveness. Acaricides to eliminate dust mites are under investigation.

D. Foods: Most persons with well-documented food allergy are allergic to one or a small number of foods, so that avoidance is rarely a problem. Persons with peanut anaphylaxis can have a fatal reaction to ingestion of a minute amount of the food. The presence of peanut can be unsuspected in some foods, so that the patient must be vigilant in restaurants or at parties. Soy-based formulas are available for infants with milk allergy.

E. Drugs: It is necessary to avoid all cross-reacting drugs. Allergy to penicillin or to sulfonamides usually encompasses all penicillin or sulfonamide derivatives, respectively. Rarely, a patient exquisitely sensitive to penicillin may react to penicillin in milk products, which then must be avoided.

F. Contactants: Patients with poison ivy or other plant oil allergy must learn to identify and avoid contact with the plant. In California, poison oak allergen is often transmitted to human skin by pets. Nickel-containing jewelry, buckles, etc, can be coated with clear nail polish. Protective clothing and gloves may be necessary for occupational contact dermatitis.

G. Mold Spores: Out of doors, mold spores are unavoidable. Indoor mold contamination can be controlled by repairing leaks and cleaning mold buildup on sinks, shower curtains, pipes, etc.

H. Insect Stings: The sensitive patient should not walk barefoot outdoors, because yellow jackets nest in the ground. Wasp nests and beehives should not be disturbed. Garbage cans should be well covered, and outdoor eating should be avoided.

Drug Therapy

Pharmacotherapy of the immune response and its consequences in allergy is achieved with drugs that alter the inflammatory phase.

A. IgE-Mediated Allergy: Three classes of drugs are useful for IgE-mediated diseases, based on (1) inhibition of release of mediators from mast cells, (2) inhibition of the action of mediators on their target cells, and (3) reversal of the vascular and inflammatory responses in the target tissues.

1. Cromolyn–Numerous studies show that pretreatment with this drug prevents the response to allergen by "stabilizing" the mast cell, though the specific molecular mechanism of action is unknown. Cromolyn is effective only when applied directly to the involved organ, and its action is short-lived. It is therefore available as a bronchial inhaler (Intal), nasal spray (Nasalcrom), and eye drops (Opticrom). Dosage is usually 4 times daily on a continuous maintenance schedule as long as there is exposure to the allergen. Not all patients respond, but the drug has very few side effects and a wide margin of safety. Recently, a high-dose oral form of the drug has been released for use in treating systemic mastocytosis, but its effectiveness in preventing food-induced allergic gastroenteropathy is not known.

2. Anti-mediator drugs–Of the numerous mediators released from mast cells by reaction of allergen with IgE antibody, histamine is the only one that can be effectively blocked pharmacologically. Antihistamine drugs are competitive inhibitors of histamine receptors. Those that inhibit H_1 receptors are used to treat IgE-mediated allergy. There are a number of such drugs on the market (Table 14–6). Their use was limited by side effects, primarily sedation. Terfenadine and astemizole are nonsedating and have prolonged action. Antihistamine therapy is particularly helpful in allergic rhinitis and in urticaria, but it is not effective in all patients. It does not alleviate asthma, though it is not contraindicated in that disease when used to treat a concomitant rhinitis or pruritus. The antipruritic effect of antihistamines may be a useful adjunct in treatment of eczematous diseases. Intramuscular or intravenous antihistamines are used

Table 14–6. H_1 antihistamines.

Chemical Structure	Representative Drugs	Approximate Wholesale Price for 1 Month of Treatment
Ethanolamine	Diphenhydramine	$ 2.40
Ethylenediamine	Pyrilamine	7.20
	Tripelennamine	3.80
Alkylamine	Brompheniramine	7.20
	Chlorpeniramine	2.00
	Triprolidine	5.00
Phenothiazine	Promethazine	1.80
Piperazine	Hydroxyzine	7.00
Piperidine	Astemizole (nonsedating)	36.00
	Azatadine	32.00
	Cyproheptadine	2.40
	Terfenadine (nonsedating)	40.00

in treatment of systemic anaphylaxis but never as the sole method of treatment.

3. Sympathomimetic drugs–Adrenergic agonists are used for both α-adrenergic (vasoconstricting) and β-adrenergic (bronchodilating) properties. Injected epinephrine is initial therapy in anaphylaxis, because it has both effects and acts rapidly. Alpha-adrenergic agonists are used orally as nasal decongestants and conjunctivally as vasoconstrictors in allergic rhinitis and conjunctivitis, respectively. Beta-adrenergic drugs are essential for reversal of acute asthma and for long-term maintenance therapy. These drugs can be given by aerosol, by metered-dose inhaler, or orally. The main side effect is muscle tremor, especially when the drug is taken orally, but tolerance usually develops with continued use.

4. Theophylline–This drug is used as a bronchodilator. Its mechanism of action is unknown, but it may involve inhibition of the bronchodilating effect of endogenous adenosine, liberated during the allergic reaction. If that is true, theophylline could be classified as an anti-mediator drug.

5. Glucocorticoids–These drugs have some therapeutic use in virtually all types of allergic diseases. Effectiveness in allergy is related to the anti-inflammatory and not the immunosuppressive action of these drugs. They are extremely effective, but they do not modify the underlying disease. Their use in allergy treatment requires close attention to side effects and toxicity. Corticosteroid drugs are available in oral, intramuscular, intravenous, intranasal, and bronchial inhalational forms, as eye drops, and in topical formulations for dermatologic use. Short-term systemic burst therapy is indicated for treatment of severe asthma, allergic contact dermatitis, and acute exacerbations of hypersensitivity pneumonitis and allergic bronchopulmonary aspergillosis. Steroid eye drops are for short-term treatment of acute allergic conjunctivitis, and the patient must be monitored for signs of corneal ulceration, keratitis, and glaucoma. Corticosteroid nasal spray is effective and probably safe for long-term use, but epistaxis can occur and nasal septal perforation is a possible complication. Long-term high-dose inhaled corticosteroid therapy for asthma during the inflammatory phase of the disease is currently considered an important aspect of management of the chronic asthmatic, whether allergic or not. Systemic absorption may occur, and oral candidiasis is an unusual but not rare complication that is usually prevented by immediate mouth washing after each application. Topical steroid therapy is the primary treatment of atopic dermatitis. It may be effective in very mild cases of contact dermatitis.

6. Treatment of anaphylaxis–This is a medical emergency that demands immediate recognition and treatment to prevent death or morbidity from respiratory obstruction, circulatory failure, or both.

At the first suspicion of anaphylaxis, aqueous epinephrine 1:1000 in a dose of 0.2–0.5 mL is injected subcutaneously or intramuscularly. Intracardiac injection of 1:10,000 concentration may be necessary for the patient in shock. Repeated injections can be given every 20–30 minutes when necessary.

The definitive therapy of anaphylactic shock is the rapid intravenous infusion of large volumes of fluids—saline, plasma, or colloid solution—to replace loss of intravascular plasma into tissues. Other pressor drugs may be necessary if the patient is refractory to epinephrine.

Airway obstruction may be caused by edema of the larynx and hypopharynx or by bronchospasm. The former is treated by maintenance of an airway with endotracheal intubation or tracheostomy. Bronchospasm responds to subcutaneous epinephrine or terbutaline. Inhalation of selective β_2-adrenergic agonists such as albuterol or terbutaline and intravenous administration of theophylline are also effective, as in asthmatic bronchospasm.

Antihistamines are most useful for alleviating the cutaneous manifestations of urticaria or angioedema and pruritus and for the gastrointestinal and uterine smooth muscle spasms. Corticosteroids will not reverse respiratory obstruction or shock even when given intramuscularly or intravenously, but these drugs may be helpful in moderating later sequelae of the vascular damage.

There may be a clinical "late-phase" IgE response in anaphylaxis, as there is in atopy. Since this begins some hours after exposure to the allergen and subsidence of the immediate-phase response, all patients with anaphylaxis should be monitored for up to 24 hours.

Anaphylaxis in a patient being treated with a beta-blocker drug is a special problem because of refractoriness to epinephrine and selective β -adrenergic agonists. Higher than usual doses of these drugs may be required for the desired effect.

B. Immune Complex Allergic Diseases:

1. Serum sickness–This disease is self-limited, so treatment is usually conservative and symptomatic only. Aspirin will relieve the arthralgias. Antihistamines and topical steroids will control the dermatitis. Corticosteroid therapy is rarely necessary.

2. Allergic bronchopulmonary aspergillosis– Patients with this disease have asthma complicated by periodic episodes of *Aspergillus* pneumonitis. Every effort should be made to prevent the development of bronchiectasis. Attacks characterized by dyspnea, cough, fever, pulmonary infiltrates, and elevated total serum IgE are treated promptly with high-dose systemic steroids. For those patients requiring chronic maintenance steroid therapy, a low dose of systemic corticosteroid is probably more reliable than inhaled beclomethasone.

3. Hypersensitivity pneumonitis–Acute exacerbations are treated with systemic steroids until they resolve fully.

C. T Cell-Mediated Hypersensitivity: Allergic

contact dermatitis is treated with systemic steroids and topical emollients.

Immunotherapy

Treatment of atopy, especially allergic rhinitis, by the repeated long-term injection of allergen has been shown in many controlled clinical trials to be an effective method for reducing or eliminating symptoms and signs of the allergic disorder.

A. Procedure: Based on the clinical evaluation, an aqueous solution of the allergen or allergens responsible for the individual patient's disease is administered repeatedly by subcutaneous injection in increasing doses once or twice a week until a maintenance dose is reached. The maintenance dose is determined individually based on improvement in symptoms and signs of the allergic disease without systemic or excessive local reactions to the injected allergen. Thereafter, the same maintenance dose is injected every 2–4 weeks for several years. It is essential that the patient be monitored closely for correct diagnosis, proper dose, efficacy, and side effects.

B. Immunologic Effects: The term "allergen immunotherapy" is usually used instead of "desensitization," because the immunologic basis for this form of treatment is currently unknown. Nevertheless, certain immunologic changes can be induced by these injections. Circulating levels of IgE antibodies specific to the injected allergens increase slightly during the first few months, then decrease, eventually to substantially lower levels than before treatment. Seasonal rises in IgE antibodies to pollens are blunted or eliminated. IgG "blocking" antibody is produced. Changes in regulatory T cells favoring suppression of IgE antibody production have been reported. All of these effects are allergenically specific.

C. Clinical Effects: Most patients with allergic rhinitis caused by pollen experience progressively less morbidity on natural pollen exposure during successive seasons while on immunotherapy. Some become completely asymptomatic. A few patients derive no benefit. A beneficial response may or may not persist after treatment is stopped. Clinical effects, like the immunologic responses, are specific for the injected allergens only.

D. Adverse Effects: Adverse reactions may be local or systemic. Localized immediate and late-phase skin reactions occur at injection sites. These are not harmful, but the dose must be adjusted to avoid excessively large or prolonged local reactions. Immediate systemic reactions or anaphylaxis are a potential problem for every injection and must be prevented by careful monitoring of dosage. The patient must remain for at least 20 minutes after each injection visit at the treatment facility where drugs and equipment for treating anaphylaxis are available. Late systemic reactions in the form of an exacerbation of the patient's allergic manifestations (rhinitis, asthma, eczema) also calls for reducing the subsequent dosage.

No long-term adverse immunologic or nonimmunologic consequences of aqueous allergen extract immunotherapy are known.

E. Indications: This treatment is recommended for patients with severe allergic rhinitis who respond poorly to drug therapy and whose allergens are not avoidable. It is also used for allergic asthma, though there are few definitive clinical trials in that disease. There is no current evidence for an effect on atopic dermatitis. Inhalant allergens only are used. Food allergy is treated by avoidance.

Immunotherapy of systemic anaphylaxis to Hymenoptera venom has been shown to be extremely effective.

Short-course desensitization for IgE allergy to certain drugs—especially penicillin and insulin—has been successful in many cases. This is usually accomplished by a course of injections of increasing doses over a period of hours rather than the weeks or months as required for atopic disease treatment. Oral, injected, or topical desensitization for contact dermatitis has been attempted without evidence yet that it is efficacious.

Norman PS: Immunotherapy for nasal allergy (Symposium). J Allergy Clin Immunol 1988; 81:992.

Ohman JL: Allergen immunotherapy in asthma: Evidence for efficacy. J Allergy Clin Immunol 1989;84:133.

Terr AI: Desensitization. In: *Basic & Clinical Immunology*, 7th ed. Stites DP, Terr AI (editors). Appleton & Lange, 1990.

Arthritis & Musculoskeletal Disorders

15

David B. Hellmann, MD, & Martin A. Shearn, MD

Examination of the Patient

The diagnosis of a rheumatic disease can often be made in the office or at the bedside by history and physical examination; special attention is paid to signs of articular inflammation (eg, heat, soft tissue swelling, effusion) and the functional status of the joints (eg, range of motion, deformity). Laboratory procedures complete the study, most commonly including sedimentation rate, tests for rheumatoid factor and antinuclear or other antibodies, synovial fluid analysis, and x-rays of affected joints. These studies are important for diagnosis and as a baseline for judging the results of therapy.

Examination of Joint Fluid

Synovial fluid examination (Table 15–1) may provide specific diagnostic information in joint disease.

A. Types of Studies: When performed, the following studies should be included:

1. Gross examination–If fluid is green or purulent, a Gram's stain is indicated. If grossly bloody, consider a bleeding disorder, trauma, or "traumatic tap."

2. Microscopic examination–

a. Cytology–Collect 2–5 mL in a heparinized tube. The red and white cells are counted, using the same equipment and technique as for a standard white count. The diluent, however, should be normal saline solution, since the usual acidified diluent causes the fluid to clot in the pipette. One drop of methylene blue added to the diluent makes the cells distinguishable. Differential counts are performed on thin smears with Wright's stain.

b. Crystals–Compensated polarized light microscopy identifies the existence and type of crystals. The demonstration of urate or calcium pyrophosphate crystals is most important diagnostically.

3. Culture–Collect 1 mL of fluid in a sterile culture tube and perform routine bacterial cultures as well as special studies for gonococci, tubercle bacilli, or fungi when indicated.

4. Glucose–Collect 2–3 mL of fluid in a fluoride tube. Blood glucose should be measured at the time of joint aspiration.

B. Interpretation: (See Table 15–2.) Synovial fluid studies are not diagnostic unless a specific organism is identified in the culture or urate crystals of gout or calcium pyrophosphate crystals of pseudogout are demonstrated. There is considerable overlap in the cytologic and biochemical values obtained in different diseases. These studies do make possible, however, a differentiation according to severity of inflammation. Thus, joint fluids in inflammatory diseases such as infections and rheumatoid arthritis are often turbid, with an elevated white count (usually well above 3000 cells/μL, with over 50% polynucleated forms) and a synovial fluid sugar content that is considerably lower than the blood glucose. In diseases characterized by relatively mild articular inflammation, such as degenerative joint disease or traumatic arthritis, the synovial fluid is usually clear, with a low white cell count (usually below 3000/μL), and the synovial fluid and blood glucose levels are within 10 mg/dL of each other.

AUTOIMMUNE DISEASES (Collagen Diseases, Connective Tissue Diseases)

The autoimmune disorders are a protean group of acquired diseases in which genetic factors appear to play a role. They have in common widespread immunologic and inflammatory alterations of connective tissue.

These illnesses share certain clinical features, and differentiation among them is often difficult because of this. Common findings include synovitis, pleuritis, myocarditis, endocarditis, pericarditis, peritonitis, vasculitis, myositis, skin rash, alterations of connective tissues, and nephritis. Laboratory tests may reveal Coombs-positive hemolytic anemia, thrombocytopenia, leukopenia, immunoglobulin excesses or deficiencies, antinuclear antibodies (which include antibodies to many nuclear constituents, including DNA and extractable nuclear antigen), rheumatoid factors, cryoglobulins, false-positive serologic tests for syphilis, elevated muscle enzymes, and alterations in serum complement.

Table 15–1. Examination of joint fluid.

Measure	Normal	Group I (Noninflammatory)	Group II (Inflammatory)	Group III (Septic)
Volume (mL) (knee)	< 3.5	Often > 3.5	Often > 3.5	Often > 3.5
Clarity	Transparent	Transparent	Translucent-opaque	Opaque
Color	Clear	Yellow	Yellow to opalescent	Yellow to green
WBC (per μL)	< 200	200–3000	3000–50,000	> 50,000[1]
Polymorphonuclear leukocytes (%)	< 25%	< 25%	50% or more	75% or more[1]
Culture	Negative	Negative	Negative	Usually positive
Glucose (mg/dL)	Nearly equal to serum	Nearly equal to serum	> 25, lower than serum	< 25, much lower than serum

[1] Counts are lower with infections caused by organisms of low virulence or if antibiotic therapy has been started.

Although the autoimmune disorders are regarded as acquired diseases, their causes cannot be determined in most instances.

Some of the laboratory alterations that occur in this group of diseases (eg, false-positive serologic tests for syphilis, rheumatoid factor) occur in asymptomatic individuals. These changes may also be demonstrated in certain asymptomatic relatives of patients with connective tissue diseases, in older persons, in patients using certain drugs, and in patients with chronic infectious diseases.

RHEUMATOID ARTHRITIS

Essentials of Diagnosis

- Prodromal systemic symptoms of malaise, fever, weight loss, and morning stiffness.
- Onset usually insidious and in small joints; progression is centripetal and symmetric; deformities common.
- Radiographic findings: juxta-articular osteoporo-

sis, joint erosions, and narrowing of the joint spaces.
- Rheumatoid factor usually present.
- Extra-articular manifestations: subcutaneous nodules, pleural effusion, pericarditis, lymphadenopathy, splenomegaly with leukopenia, and vasculitis.

General Considerations

Rheumatoid arthritis is a chronic systemic inflammatory disease of unknown cause, chiefly affecting synovial membranes of multiple joints. The disease has a wide clinical spectrum with considerable variability in joint and extra-articular manifestations. The prevalence in the general population is 1–2%; female patients outnumber males almost 3:1. The usual age at onset is 20–40 years, although rheumatoid arthritis may begin at any age. Susceptibility to rheumatoid arthritis is genetically determined. Virtually all patients share specific gene products coded in the major histocompatibility complex.

The pathologic findings in the joint include chronic synovitis with pannus formation. The pannus erodes

Table 15–2. Differential diagnosis by joint fluid groups.[1]

Group I (Noninflammatory)	Group II (Inflammatory)	Group III (Purulent)	Hemorrhagic
Degenerative joint disease Trauma[2] Osteochondritis dissecans Osteochondromatosis Neuropathic arthropathy[2] Subsiding or early inflammation Hypertrophic osteoarthropathy[3] Pigmented villonodular synovitis[2]	Rheumatoid arthritis Acute crystal-induced synovitis (gout and pseudogout) Reiter's syndrome Ankylosing spondylitis Psoriatic arthritis Arthritis accompanying ulcerative colitis and regional enteritis Rheumatic fever[3] Systemic lupus erythematosus[3] Progressive systemic sclerosis (scleroderma)[3] Tuberculosis Mycotic infections	Pyogenic bacterial infections	Hemophilia or other hemorrhagic diathesis Trauma with or without fracture Neuropathic arthropathy Pigmented villonodular synovitis Synovioma Hemangioma and other benign neoplasm

[1] Reproduced from Rodnan GP (editor): Primer on the rheumatic diseases, 7th ed. *JAMA* 1973;**244(Suppl):**662.
[2] May be hemorrhagic.
[3] Group I or II.

cartilage, bone, ligaments, and tendons. In the acute phase, effusion and other manifestations of inflammation are common. In the late stage, organization may result in fibrous ankylosis; true bony ankylosis is rare. In both acute and chronic phases, inflammation of soft tissues around the joints may be prominent and is a significant factor in joint damage.

The microscopic findings most characteristic of rheumatoid arthritis are those of the subcutaneous nodule. This is a granuloma with a central zone of fibrinoid necrosis, a surrounding palisade of radially arranged elongated connective tissue cells, and a periphery of chronic granulation tissue. Pathologic alterations indistinguishable from those of the subcutaneous nodule are occasionally seen in the myocardium, pericardium, endocardium, heart valves, visceral pleura, lungs, sclera, dura mater, spleen, and larynx as well as in the synovial membrane, periarticular tissues, and tendons. Nonspecific pericarditis and pleuritis are found in 25–40% of patients at autopsy. Additional nonspecific lesions associated with rheumatoid arthritis include inflammation of small arteries, pulmonary fibrosis, round cell infiltration of skeletal muscle and perineurium, and hyperplasia of lymph nodes. Secondary amyloidosis may also be present.

Clinical Findings

A. Symptoms and Signs: The clinical manifestations of rheumatoid disease are highly variable. The onset of articular signs of inflammation is usually insidious, with prodromal symptoms of malaise, weight loss, and vague periarticular pain or stiffness. Less often, the onset is acute, apparently triggered by a stressful situation such as infection, surgery, trauma, emotional strain, or the postpartum period. There is characteristically symmetric joint swelling with associated stiffness, warmth, tenderness, and pain. Stiffness is prominent in the morning and subsides during the day; its duration is a useful indicator of activity of disease. Stiffness may recur after daytime inactivity and may be much more severe after strenuous activity. Although any joint may be affected in rheumatoid arthritis, the proximal interphalangeal and metacarpophalangeal joints of the fingers as well as the wrists, knees, ankles, and toes are most often involved. Monarticular disease is occasionally seen early. Synovial cysts and rupture of tendons may occur. Entrapment syndromes are not unusual—particularly entrapment of the median nerve at the carpal tunnel of the wrist. Palmar erythema is noted occasionally, as are tiny hemorrhagic infarcts in the nail folds or finger pulps, which are signs of vasculitis. Twenty percent of patients have subcutaneous nodules, most commonly situated over bony prominences but also observed in the bursas and tendon sheaths. A small number of patients have splenomegaly and lymph node enlargement. Low-grade fever, anorexia, weight loss, fatigue, and weakness often persist; chills are rare. After months or years, thickening of the

periarticular tissue, flexion deformities, subluxation, fibrosis, and ankylosis may occur. Atrophy of skin or muscle is common. Dryness of the eyes, mouth, and other mucous membranes is found especially in advanced disease (see Sjögren's Syndrome). Other ocular manifestations include episcleritis and scleromalacia, often due to scleral nodules. Pericarditis and pleural disease, when present, are frequently silent clinically. Aortitis is a rare late complication that can result in aortic regurgitation or rupture and is usually associated with evidence of rheumatoid vasculitis elsewhere in the body.

B. Laboratory Findings: Serum protein abnormalities are often present. Rheumatoid factor, an IgM antibody directed against other globulins, is present in the sera of more than 75% of patients. High titers of rheumatoid factor are commonly associated with severe rheumatoid disease. Titers may also be significantly elevated in a number of diverse conditions, including syphilis, sarcoidosis, infective endocarditis, tuberculosis, leprosy, and parasitic infections; in advanced age; and in asymptomatic relatives of patients with autoimmune diseases. Antinuclear antibodies are demonstrable in 20% of patients, though their titers are lower in rheumatoid arthritis than in systemic lupus erythematosus.

During both the acute and chronic phases, the erythrocyte sedimentation rate and the gamma globulins (most commonly IgM and IgG) are typically elevated. A moderate hypochromic normocytic anemia is common. The white cell count is normal or slightly elevated, but leukopenia may occur, often in the presence of splenomegaly (eg, Felty's syndrome). Joint fluid examination is valuable, reflecting abnormalities that are associated with varying degrees of inflammation. (See Tables 15–1 and 15–2.)

C. Imaging: Often, x-rays taken during the first 6 months are read as normal. The earliest changes occur in the wrists or feet and consist of soft tissue swelling and juxta-articular demineralization. Later, diagnostic changes of uniform joint space narrowing and erosions develop. The erosions are often first evident at the ulnar styloid and at the juxta-articular margin, where the bony surface is not protected by cartilage. Diagnostic changes also occur in the cervical spine, with C1–2 subluxation, but these changes usually take several years to develop.

Differential Diagnosis

The differentiation of rheumatoid arthritis from other diseases of connective tissue can be difficult. However, certain clinical features are helpful. Rheumatic fever is characterized by the migratory nature of the arthritis, an elevated antistreptolysin titer, and a more dramatic and prompt response to aspirin; carditis and erythema marginatum may occur in adults, but chorea and subcutaneous nodules virtually never do. Butterfly rash, discoid lupus erythematosus, photosensitivity, alopecia, high titer to anti-DNA, renal disease, and central nervous system abnormalities point to the diagnosis of systemic lupus erythematosus. Degenerative joint disease (osteoarthritis) is not associated with constitutional manifestations, and the joint pain is characteristically relieved by rest, in contrast to the morning stiffness of rheumatoid arthritis. Signs of articular inflammation, prominent in rheumatoid arthritis, are usually minimal in degenerative joint disease. Osteoarthritis—in contrast to rheumatoid arthritis—spares the wrist and the metacarpophalangeal joints. While in the early years gouty arthritis is almost always intermittent and monarticular, in later years it can become a chronic polyarticular process that mimics rheumatoid arthritis. Gouty tophi can at times resemble rheumatoid nodules. The early history of intermittent monarthritis and the presence of synovial urate crystals are distinctive features of gout. Pyogenic arthritis can be distinguished by chills and fever, demonstration of the causative organism in joint fluid, and the frequent presence of a primary focus elsewhere, eg, gonococcal arthritis. Polymyalgia rheumatica occasionally causes polyarthritis in patients over age 50, but these patients remain rheumatoid factor-negative and have chiefly proximal muscle pain and stiffness. A variety of cancers produce paraneoplastic syndromes, including polyarthritis. One form is hypertrophic pulmonary osteoarthropathy most often produced by lung and gastrointestinal carcinomas, characterized by a rheumatoid-like arthritis associated with clubbing, periosteal new bone formation, and a negative rheumatoid factor. Diffuse swelling of the hands with palmar fasciitis has also been reported with a variety of cancers, especially ovarian carcinoma.

Treatment

A. Basic Program (Conservative Management): The primary objectives of treatment of rheumatoid arthritis are reduction of inflammation and pain, preservation of function, and prevention of deformity. A regimen consisting of education, rest, physical therapy, and nonsteroidal anti-inflammatory agents constitutes the basic program of treatment to which other treatment may be added.

1. Education and emotional factors–Chronic diseases such as rheumatoid arthritis destroy the belief—harbored by most people in good health—that individuals have control over their lives. This feeling of helplessness is often more frightening and disabling than the disease process itself. Therefore, the physician should explain what an autoimmune disease is, what the normal fluctuations of the disease process are like, and how decisions about therapy will be made. Most patients think of "treatment" as a brief course of antibiotic or other drug followed by rapid recovery. The concept of chronic disease control and empiric treatment employing different agents in series must be explained if the patient is to have confidence in the physician.

At some point, the patient's spouse should be invited to the office with the patient for a discussion of the problem and given an opportunity to ask questions. In this way, education of the family serves as a source of the emotional support so critical to the patient's long-term well-being.

2. Systemic rest–The amount of rest required depends upon the severity of the disease. Complete bed rest may be desirable in patients with profound systemic and articular involvement. In mild disease, 2 hours of rest each day may suffice. In general, rest should be continued until significant improvement is sustained for at least 2 weeks; thereafter, the program may be liberalized. However, the increase of physical activity must proceed gradually and with appropriate support for any involved weight-bearing joints.

3. Articular rest–Decrease of articular inflammation may be expedited by articular rest. Relaxation and stretching of the hip and knee muscles, to prevent flexion contractures, can be accomplished by having the patient lie in the prone position for 15 minutes several times daily in addition to nighttime rest. Sitting in a flexed position for prolonged periods is a poor form of joint rest. Appropriate adjustable supports provide rest for inflamed weight-bearing joints, relieve spasm, and may reduce deformities, soft tissue contracture, or instability of the ligaments. The supports must be removable to permit daily range of motion and exercise of the affected extremities (see below). When ambulation is started, care must be taken to avoid weight bearing, which may aggravate flexion deformities. This is accomplished with the aid of crutches or braces until the tendency toward contracture has subsided.

4. Exercise–The management of rheumatoid arthritis is based on the concomitant use of rest and therapeutic exercise in proper balance. Therapeutic exercises are designed to preserve joint motion, muscular strength, and endurance. Initially, passive range of motion and isometric exercises (such as straight leg raising) are best tolerated. As tolerance for exercise increases and the activity of the disease subsides, progressive resistance exercises may be introduced.

5. Heat and cold–These are used primarily for their muscle-relaxing and analgesic effect. Radiant or moist heat is generally most satisfactory. The ambulatory patient will find warm tub baths convenient. Paraffin baths for the hands are inexpensive and help many patients to reduce morning stiffness. Exercise may be better performed after exposure to heat. Some patients derive more relief of joint pain from local application of cold.

6. Nonsteroidal anti-inflammatory drugs (NSAIDs)–

a. Aspirin–Aspirin is an effective anti-inflammatory antipyretic agent and the least expensive of the various drugs available to treat rheumatoid arthritis. It is usually the first drug employed unless there is some contraindication to its use. The proper dose is the amount that provides optimal relief of symptoms without causing toxic reactions. Most adults below the age of 65 can tolerate daily doses of 4–6 g, which result in therapeutic serum salicylate levels of 20–30 mg/dL. After 1 week, the salicylate half-life increases to 15 hours; therefore, the patient need not be given aspirin every 4 hours, as is often recommended. If tinnitus—an early manifestation of toxicity—occurs, the daily dose should be lowered by decrements of 0.6 or 0.9 g until this symptom disappears. Many different preparations of aspirin are now available. Enteric-coated aspirin is recommended because it decreases the high frequency of gastric ulceration seen with chronic use of plain or buffered aspirin. Nonacetylated forms of salicylates, such as salsalate (Disalcid), are probably equally effective at reducing gastric ulceration but are more expensive. Symptoms of gastric irritation may be lessened by the ingestion of salicylates with meals and by taking them with antacid. No salicylate should be used by patients with a history of allergy to aspirin or related products.

b. Other NSAIDs–If aspirin proves ineffective or if intolerable gastrointestinal effects occur, a trial of the newer NSAIDs is indicated. Because of a simpler dosage schedule for most of these agents, compliance may be better. A number of NSAIDs are available, including ibuprofen, fenoprofen, naproxen, tolmetin, sulindac, meclofenamate sodium, piroxicam, flurbiprofen, diclofenac, and ketoprofen. In terms of efficacy for groups of patients, all of the nonsteroidal anti-inflammatory drugs—including aspirin—are equivalent. It is surprising, however, that individual patients may respond to one preparation but not to another.

In terms of toxicity, gastrointestinal side effects are most frequent. All the NSAIDs inhibit gastric prostaglandin E, a local hormone responsible for gastric mucosal cytoprotection. Consequently, these drugs can produce gastric ulceration and bleeding. There is no evidence that any of the newer nonsteroidals produce massive gastrointestinal bleeding any less frequently than does aspirin. But the newer NSAIDs are similar to enteric-coated aspirin in greatly reducing the frequency of gastric symptoms and gastric ulceration seen in patients chronically taking plain aspirin. H_2 blockers and carafate do not reduce the frequency of gastric ulceration. The efficacy of concomitant antacids has not been formally tested.

Only misoprostol, a synthetic analogue of prostaglandin E, reduces the incidence of gastric ulceration. Whether this drug will also decrease the risk of gastrointestinal hemorrhage is not yet known.

NSAIDs can also affect the lower intestinal tract, causing perforation or aggravating inflammatory bowel disease.

The overall rate of bleeding with NSAID use appears to be low: 1:10,000 to 1:6000 users. The frequency of bleeding is increased by chronic use, con-

comitant use of corticosteroids or anticoagulants, the presence of rheumatoid arthritis, a history of peptic ulcer disease or alcoholism, and old age. Thus, though the exact indications for misoprostol have not yet been determined, it should probably be reserved for patients who must take a nonsteroidal drug and have substantial risk factors for gastric bleeding. Misoprostol is an abortifacient and thus is contraindicated in patients who are or might become pregnant.

All of the NSAIDs, including aspirin, can produce renal toxicity, resulting in interstitial nephritis, nephrotic syndrome, reversible renal failure, and aggravation of baseline hypertension. Hyperkalemia due to hyporeninemic hypoaldosteronism may also be seen. The risk of renal toxicity is low but is increased by age over 60, a history of renal disease, congestive heart failure, ascites, and diuretic use.

Indomethacin is probably no more effective than the salicylates in rheumatoid arthritis, and its untoward effects are far greater. Phenylbutazone is not advised for chronic therapy because of its toxicity.

7. Physical therapy–See p 617.

B. Other Anti-inflammatory Drugs: If the patient fails to respond to the basic regimen with a reduction in morning stiffness, fatigue, and joint swelling, additional medications are added.

1. Antimalarials–Hydroxychloroquine sulfate (Plaquenil), is the antimalarial agent most often used against rheumatoid arthritis. It should be reserved for patients with mild disease, since only 25% will respond and in some of those cases only after 3–6 months of therapy. The advantage of hydroxychloroquine is its comparatively low toxicity. A dosage of 200–400 mg/d minimizes the likelihood of toxic reactions. The most important reaction, pigmentary retinitis causing visual loss, is fortunately rare when the dosage is kept low. Biannual ophthalmologic examinations are required when this drug is employed for long-term therapy. Other reactions include neuropathies and myopathies of both skeletal and cardiac muscle, which usually improve when the drug is withdrawn.

2. Gold salts (chrysotherapy)–Gold salts have been the standard second-line treatment for rheumatoid arthritis. There is evidence that these agents may retard the bone erosions associated with rheumatoid arthritis. About 60% of patients may be expected to benefit from gold therapy, although complete remissions are uncommon. Their mode of action is not known.

a. Indications–Disease responding unfavorably to conservative management; erosive disease.

b. Contraindications–Previous gold toxicity; significant renal, hepatic, or hematopoietic dysfunction.

c. Preparations of choice–Intramuscular gold sodium thiomalate or aurothioglucose; oral auranofin.

d. Dosage–Intramuscular gold is given as a 10-mg test dose the first week and a 25-mg dose the second week before reaching the maintenance dose of 50 mg weekly, which is then continued unless toxic reactions appear. If there is no response after 800 mg has been administered, the drug should be discontinued. If the response is good, a total dose of 1 g should be given, followed by a regimen of 50 mg every 2 weeks and, with continued improvement, every 3 and then every 4 weeks for an indefinite period.

The oral dose of auranofin is 3 mg twice daily until benefit or toxicity occurs.

e. Toxic reactions–About 32% of patients (range in various series: 4–55%) experience toxic reactions to gold therapy; the mortality rate is less than 0.4%. The manifestations of toxicity are similar to those of poisoning by other heavy metals (notably arsenic) and include dermatitis (mild to exfoliative, and pruritic), stomatitis, neutropenia, nephritis, and nitritoid reactions (especially to gold thiomalate and presumably due to its vehicle). Auranofin causes side effects less frequently than intramuscular gold, though diarrhea is common. In order to prevent or reduce the severity of toxic reactions, gold should not be given to patients with any of the contraindicating disorders listed above. Periodic urinalyses and complete blood counts should be obtained.

If signs of toxicity appear, the drug should be withdrawn immediately. Severe toxicity may require corticosteroids for control, and failure to respond might then be an indication for the cautious use of penicillamine or dimercaprol (BAL) as chelating agents for the gold. Worsening of articular symptoms after the initial dose is often temporary and is not an indication for withdrawal of the drug. Patients so affected may ultimately respond favorably if treatment is continued.

3. Corticosteroids–Although corticosteroids usually produce an immediate and dramatic anti-inflammatory effect in rheumatoid arthritis, they may not alter the natural progression of the disease; furthermore, clinical manifestations of active disease commonly reappear when the drug is discontinued. The serious problem of untoward reactions resulting from prolonged corticosteroid therapy greatly limits its long-term use. Another disadvantage that might stem from the use of steroids lies in the tendency of the patient and the physician to neglect the less spectacular but proved benefits derived from general supportive treatment, physical therapy, and orthopedic measures.

Corticosteroids may be used on a short-term basis to tide patients over acute disabling episodes, to facilitate other treatment measures (eg, physical therapy), or to manage serious extra-articular manifestations (eg, pericarditis, perforating eye lesions). Corticosteroids may also be indicated for active and progressive disease that does not respond favorably to conservative management and when there are contraindications to or therapeutic failure of gold salts and penicillamine.

The least amount of steroid that will achieve the desired clinical effect should be given, but not more than 10 mg of prednisone or equivalent per day is appropriate for articular disease. Many patients do reasonably well on 5–7.5 mg daily. (The use of 1-mg tablets is to be encouraged.) When the steroids are to be discontinued, they should be phased out gradually on a planned schedule appropriate to the duration of treatment.

Intra-articular corticosteroids may be helpful if one or 2 joints are the chief source of difficulty. Intra-articular hydrocortisone, 25–50 mg, may be given for symptomatic relief, but no more often than 4 times a year.

4. Methotrexate–Many now believe that methotrexate is the treatment of choice for patients with severe rheumatoid arthritis who fail to respond to NSAIDs and gold. Methotrexate is generally well tolerated and often produces a beneficial effect in 2–4 weeks—compared with the 2- to 6-month onset of action for drugs such as gold, penicillamine, and antimalarials. The usual dose is 7.5 mg of methotrexate orally once weekly. The most frequent side effects are gastric irritation and stomatitis. A severe, potentially life-threatening pneumonitis occurs rarely and usually responds to cessation of the drug and institution of corticosteroids. Hepatotoxicity with fibrosis and cirrhosis is another important toxic effect of methotrexate that fortunately appears to be very rare. Diabetes, obesity, and renal disease appear to increase the risk of hepatotoxicity. Liver function tests should be monitored, but because of their insensitivity, periodic liver biopsy is needed. In a patient with no risk factors for hepatotoxicity, liver biopsy should be done after every 2.5–3 g of methotrexate. Cytopenia and infection are other important potential side effects. While methotrexate is an effective medication, its toxicity and potential teratogenic and oncogenic capacities are such that it should only be used by physicians thoroughly familiar with its effects.

5. Azathioprine–This agent, like methotrexate, is an antimetabolite that is effective for severe rheumatoid arthritis not responsive to gold or antimalarials. Its potential for severe toxicity, including immunosuppression complicated by opportunistic infection, restricts its use to physicians experienced with the drug.

6. Penicillamine–Penicillamine may be used in patients with severe rheumatoid arthritis who have continuing rheumatic activity in spite of therapy with the agents discussed above. This agent may prove effective in a number of such patients, although toxicity is substantial. The mechanism of action is not understood. Up to one-half of patients experience some side effects such as oral ulcers, loss of taste, fever, rash, thrombocytopenia, leukopenia, and aplastic anemia. Proteinuria and nephrotic syndrome may occur. Immune complex diseases (eg, myasthenia gravis, systemic lupus erythematosus, polymyositis, Goodpasture's syndrome) appear to be induced by the drug. It should not be used during pregnancy.

If penicillamine is employed, one should start with small doses: 250 mg daily, increasing by 125 mg every 2–3 months up to a maximum of 0.75–1 g/d. Penicillamine is given between meals to enhance absorption. Careful monitoring for toxicity is essential.

C. Experimental Therapy: Cyclophosphamide, chlorambucil, cyclosporine, and total lymph node irradiation have been used with success in experimental studies. Only patients who fail to respond to all other measures should be considered for these treatments, which should be provided by physicians familiar with their toxicities.

D. Surgical Measures: See p 617.

Course & Prognosis

There are 2 general courses that patients with rheumatoid arthritis follow. Of all patients with definite or probable rheumatoid arthritis, 50–75% experience remission within 2 years. These patients are often negative for rheumatoid factor, have good functional status even during disease activity, and are commonly seen in community practices but rarely in academic center practices. Clearly, conservative therapy makes good sense for this patient population.

For the minority of patients who have joint symptoms persisting beyond 2 years, the outcome is not so favorable. In this group, decreased survival is evident. In fact, for patients who have persistent symptoms and poor functional status, the mortality curve resembles that for stage IV Hodgkin's disease or triple-vessel coronary artery disease. Factors that identify those at particular risk of early death from infection, heart disease, or malignancy include poor functional status, more than 30 inflamed joints, extraarticular manifestations (eg, rheumatoid lung disease), and low educational level. These patients, then, need aggressive therapy and probably need it early, since extensive bone damage can occur during the first 2 years. Studies are currently under way to determine whether earlier institution of potent second-line agents such as methotrexate or use of agents in combination will improve the outcome in this unfortunate minority population.

Graham Y, Agrawal NM, Roth SH: Prevention of NSAID-induced gastric ulcer with misoprostol: Multicentre double-blind, placebo-controlled trial. Lancet 1988;2:556. (Misoprostol prevents gastric ulceration associated with NSAID use.)

Paulus HE: The use of combinations of disease-modifying antirheumatic agents in rheumatoid arthritis. Arthritis Rheum 1990;33:113.

Pincus T: Is mortality increased in rheumatoid arthritis? J Musculoskel Med 1988;5:27.

Tugwell P et al: Methotrexate in rheumatoid arthritis. Ann Intern Med 1989;110:581. (Brief review of dosages and toxicities.)

Wilder RL: Treatment of the patient with rheumatoid arthritis refractory to standard therapy. JAMA 1988;259:2446. (Review of options for patients failing gold and nonsteroidals.)

JUVENILE CHRONIC ARTHRITIS

Rheumatoid-like disease with onset before age 17 is referred to as juvenile chronic arthritis. Synovitis that persists for at least 6 weeks is the essential criterion of the diagnosis. Four forms are recognized:

(1) The **polyarticular form** resembles adult rheumatoid arthritis in joint distribution, seropositivity, and prognosis.

(2) The **oligoarticular form** affects chiefly young girls during the peak ages of 2–4, is negative for rheumatoid factor, has a good chance for complete remission, and may be associated with a positive ANA test, which in turn is associated with uveitis. Since the uveitis is often initially silent, all children with the oligoarticular form and a positive ANA test should be examined by an ophthalmologist.

(3) A third form is termed **systemic-onset disease,** or **Still's disease,** characterized by high spiking fevers that may antedate arthritis by months; a characteristic evanescent, salmon-colored morbilliform rash; and—commonly but not always—hepatosplenomegaly, lymphadenopathy, pleuropericarditis, anemia, and leukocytosis.

(4) The fourth form of juvenile chronic arthritis is a juvenile form of **ankylosing spondylitis** characterized initially by inflammatory arthritis involving a few peripheral joints, particularly in a lower extremity, that later extends to the spine.

Systemic-onset disease (Still's disease) can occur in adults and may present initially as fever of undetermined origin. While there is no diagnostic laboratory test, the constellation of signs and symptoms—especially the very characteristic rash—may suggest the diagnosis. The rash is often missed because it is present chiefly during episodes of fever, which characteristically occur during the night.

In many children with polyarticular chronic arthritis, the apophyseal joints of the cervical spine, especially C2–3, are affected. Abnormalities of bony growth and development are related to active disease and may be transient and reversible or, with chronic disease activity, may be irreversible and result in premature closure of epiphyses or ossification centers; micrognathia is one consequence.

The differential diagnosis of juvenile chronic arthritis includes leukemia or lymphoma, inflammatory bowel disease, and chronic infectious disease (eg, Lyme disease; see Chapter 27). Joint fluid examination, culture, serologic tests, and synovial biopsy may be useful in diagnosis.

The treatment of juvenile chronic arthritis must be individualized; in general, the approach to therapy is similar to that for adult rheumatoid arthritis.

Cush JJ et al: Adult-onset Still's disease: Clinical course and outcome. Arthritis Rheum 1987;30:186. (Twenty percent of patients become disabled; polyarticular onset and chronic synovitis are risk factors for poor outcome.)

Leak AM et al: A crossover study of naproxen, diclofenac and tolmetin in seronegative juvenile chronic arthritis. Clin Exp Rheum 1988;6:157. (All 3 medications equally effective.)

Ohta A et al: Adult Still's disease: Review of 228 cases from the literature. J Rheumatol 1987;14:1139. (Recurrence of systemic symptoms is common; one-third develop deforming arthritis with ankylosis.)

SYSTEMIC LUPUS ERYTHEMATOSUS

Essentials of Diagnosis

- Occurs mainly in young women.
- Rash over areas exposed to sunlight.
- Joint symptoms in 90% of patients. Multiple system involvement.
- Depression of hemoglobin, white blood cells, platelets.
- Serologic findings: antinuclear antibody with high titer to native DNA.

General Considerations

Systemic lupus erythematosus is an inflammatory autoimmune disorder that may affect multiple organ systems. Its clinical manifestations are thought to be secondary to the trapping of antigen-antibody complexes in capillaries of visceral structures. The clinical course may vary from a mild episodic disorder to a rapidly fulminating fatal illness.

Systemic lupus erythematosus is not uncommon. Figures from a large representative urban community population indicate a prevalence exceeding one in 2000 persons. About 85% of patients are women. Although the disease may occur at any age, most patients are between ages 10 and 50, with greatest clustering between 20 and 40. Blacks are affected more often than members of other races.

Before making a diagnosis of spontaneous systemic lupus erythematosus, it is imperative to ascertain that the condition has not been induced by a drug. Approximately 25 pharmacologic agents have been implicated as causing a lupus-like syndrome, but only a few cause the disorder with appreciable frequency. Procainamide and hydralazine are the most important and best studied of these drugs. While antinuclear antibody tests and other serologic findings become positive in many persons receiving these agents, in only a few do clinical manifestations occur.

Four features of drug-induced lupus separate it from spontaneously occurring disease: (1) the sex ratio is nearly equal; (2) nephritis and central nervous system features are not ordinarily present; (3) depressed serum complement and antibodies to native DNA are absent; and (4) the clinical features and most laboratory abnormalities must often revert toward normal when the offending drug is withdrawn.

The familial occurrence of systemic lupus erythematosus has been repeatedly documented, and the disorder has involved identical twins in a number of instances. Aggregation of serologic features (positive antinuclear antibody, antibodies to DNA, hypergammaglobulinemia) is seen in asymptomatic family members, and the prevalence of other rheumatic diseases is increased among close relatives of patients. There is increased incidence of HLA-DR2 and -DR3 in lupus. Defective regulation of T cells, B cells, and humoral factors such as complement are all hypothesized to contribute to the pathogenesis of systemic lupus.

The diagnosis of systemic lupus erythematosus should be suspected in patients having a multisystem disease with serologic positivity (eg, antinuclear antibody, serologic test for syphilis). Differential diagnosis includes diseases that may present in a similar manner, such as rheumatoid arthritis, vasculitis, scleroderma, chronic active hepatitis, acute drug reactions, polyarteritis, and drug-induced lupus.

The American Rheumatism Association has proposed that the diagnosis of systemic lupus erythematosus can be made with reasonable probability if 4 of the 11 following criteria are present, serially or simultaneously, during any interval of observation: malar rash; discoid rash; photosensitivity; oral ulcers, nonerosive arthritis; serositis; renal disorder; neurologic disorder; hematologic abnormality (hemolytic anemia, leukopenia, lymphopenia, or thrombocytopenia); immune dysfunction (positive LE preparation, anti-native DNA, anti-Sm, false-positive syphilis serologic tests for more than 6 months); and positive antinuclear antibody.

Clinical Findings

A. Symptoms and Signs: The systemic feature include fever, anorexia, malaise, and weight loss. Most patients have skin lesions at some time; the characteristic "butterfly" rash affects fewer than half of patients. Other cutaneous manifestations are discoid lupus, typical fingertip lesions, periungual erythema, nail fold infarcts, and splinter hemorrhages. Alopecia is common. Mucous membrane lesions tend to occur during periods of exacerbation. Raynaud's phenomenon, present in about 20% of patients, often antedates other features of the disease.

Joint symptoms, with or without active synovitis, occur in over 90% of patients and are often the earliest manifestation. The arthritis is rarely deforming; erosive changes are almost never noted on x-ray study. Subcutaneous nodules are rare.

Ocular manifestations include conjunctivitis, photophobia, transient blindness, and blurring of vision. Cotton-wool spots on the retina (cytoid bodies) represent degeneration of nerve fibers due to occlusion of retinal blood vessels.

Pleurisy, pleural effusion, bronchopneumonia, and pneumonitis are frequent. Restrictive lung disease is often demonstrated.

The pericardium is affected in the majority of patients. Cardiac failure may result from myocarditis and hypertension. Cardiac arrhythmias are common. Atypical verrucous endocarditis of Libman-Sacks is usually clinically silent but occasionally can produce acute or chronic valvular incompetence—most commonly mitral regurgitation—and can serve as a source of thrombotic emboli.

Abdominal pains, ileus, and peritonitis may result from vasculitis; the right colon is especially susceptible. Nonspecific reactive hepatitis or that induced by salicylates may alter liver function.

Neurologic complications of systemic lupus erythematosus include psychosis, organic brain syndrome, seizures, peripheral and cranial neuropathies, transverse myelitis, and strokes. Severe depression and psychosis are sometimes heightened by the administration of large doses of corticosteroids.

Several forms of glomerulonephritis may occur, including mesangial, focal proliferative, diffuse proliferative, and membranous. Some patients may also have interstitial nephritis. With appropriate therapy, the survival rate even for patients with serious renal disease (proliferative glomerulonephritis) is favorable.

Other clinical features include arterial and venous thrombosis, lymphadenopathy, splenomegaly, Hashimoto's thyroiditis, hemolytic anemia, and thrombocytopenic purpura.

B. Laboratory Findings: The LE cell, which is mainly of historical interest, is neither sensitive nor specific for systemic lupus erythematosus. Antinuclear antibody tests are sensitive but not specific for systemic lupus—ie, they are positive in virtually all patients with lupus but are positive also in many patients with nonlupus conditions such as rheumatoid arthritis, various forms of hepatitis, and interstitial lung disease. Antibodies to double-stranded DNA and to Sm are specific for systemic lupus but not sensitive, since they are present in only 60% and 30% of patients, respectively. Depressed serum complement—a finding suggestive of disease activity—often returns toward normal in remission. Anti-native DNA antibody levels also correlate with disease activity; anti-Sm levels do not. Hypergammaglobulinemia, a positive Coombs test reaction, and rheumatoid factor may be demonstrable in the serum.

Three types of antiphospholipid antibodies occur: The first occurs in 10–20% of patients and is responsible for biologic false-positive tests for syphilis. The second is the lupus anticoagulant, which occurs in 7% of patients and, despite its name, is a risk factor for venous and arterial thrombosis and miscarriage. It is most commonly identified by prolongation of the activated partial thromboplastin time, though other phospholipid-dependent coagulation tests, such as Russell's viper venom time, are more sensitive. Anticardiolipin antibodies are the third type of antiphospholipid antibodies, which occur in 25% and may be a risk factor for fetal death in pregnant patients

with lupus. A primary antiphospholipid antibody syndrome is diagnosed in patients who have recurrent venous or arterial occlusions in the presence of antiphospholipid antibodies but without specific features of SLE. Antibody titers to a wide variety of other cellular tissues and organ tissues may be observed.

There is often mild normocytic, normochromic anemia and occasionally autoimmune hemolytic anemia. The sedimentation rate is almost always elevated when the disease is active. Leukopenia and lymphopenia are common; thrombocytopenia occasionally may be severe, resulting in purpura or bleeding.

Liver function tests are often mildly abnormal. Abnormality of urinary sediment is almost always found in association with renal lesions. Showers of red blood cells, with or without casts, and mild proteinuria are frequent during exacerbation of the disease; these usually abate with remission.

Treatment

Many patients with systemic lupus erythematosus have a benign form of the disease requiring only supportive care and need little or no medication. Emotional support, as described for rheumatoid arthritis, is especially important for patients with lupus. Patients with photosensitivity should be cautioned against sun exposure and should apply a protective lotion to the skin while out of doors. Skin lesions often respond to the local administration of corticosteroids. Joint symptoms can usually be alleviated by rest and full dosage with a salicylate or other NSAID. Every drug that may have precipitated the condition should be withdrawn if possible.

Antimalarials (hydroxychloroquine) may be helpful in treating the joint and skin features. When these are used, the dose should not exceed 400 mg/d, and biannual monitoring for retinal changes is necessary. Drug-induced neuropathy and myopathy may be erroneously ascribed to the underlying disease.

Corticosteroids are required for the control of certain serious complications. These include thrombocytopenic purpura, hemolytic anemia, myocarditis, pericarditis, convulsions, and nephritis. Forty to 60 mg of prednisone is often needed initially; however, the lowest dose of corticosteroid that controls the condition should be employed. Central nervous system lupus may require higher doses of corticosteroids than are usually given; however, steroid psychosis may mimic lupus cerebritis, in which case reduced doses are appropriate. In lupus nephritis, sequential studies of serum complement and antibodies to DNA often permit early detection of disease exacerbation and thus prompt increase in corticosteroid therapy. Such studies also allow for lowering the dosage of the drugs and withdrawing them when they are no longer needed. Immunosuppressive agents such as cyclophosphamide, chlorambucil, and azathioprine are used in cases resistant to corticosteroids. The exact role of immunosuppressive agents is controversial.

One study demonstrated that cyclophosphamide improved renal survival in patients with diffuse proliferative glomerulonephritis. Overall patient survival, however, was no better than in the prednisone-treated group. Very close follow-up is needed to watch for potential side effects when immunosuppressants are employed; these agents should be given by physicians experienced in their use. The androgenic steroid danazol may be effective therapy for thrombocytopenia not responsive to corticosteroids. Anticoagulation, most commonly with warfarin (Coumadin), is prescribed for patients who have antiphospholipid antibodies and clotting of the arterial or venous systems. Systemic steroids are not usually given for arthritis, skin rash, leukopenia, or the anemia associated with chronic disease. Positive serologic findings in asymptomatic patients are not an indication for treatment.

Course & Prognosis

The prognosis for patients with systemic lupus appears to be considerably better than older reports implied. From both community settings and university centers, 10-year survival rates exceeding 85% are routine. In most patients, the illness pursues a mild chronic course, occasionally interrupted by disease activity. With time, the number and intensity of exacerbations decrease and the probability of major insult to visceral structures declines. After 5 years of disease, abnormal laboratory findings such as raised sedimentation rates and anti-DNA titers tend to become normal in many patients. However, there are some in whom the disease pursues a virulent course, leading to serious impairment of vital structures such as lung, heart, brain, or kidneys, and the disease may lead to death. With improved control of lupus activity and with increasing use of corticosteroids and immunosuppressive drugs, the mortality and morbidity patterns in lupus have changed. Infections—especially with opportunistic organisms—have become the leading cause of death, followed by active SLE, chiefly due to renal or central nervous system disease. Although such manifestations are more likely to be seen in the early phases of the illness, one must be alert to the possibility of their occurrence at any time. Accelerated atherosclerosis attributed, in part, to corticosteroid use, has been responsible for a rise in late deaths due to myocardial infarction. With more patients living longer, it has become evident that avascular necrosis of bone, affecting most commonly the hips and knees, is responsible for substantial morbidity. Still, it must be emphasized that the outlook for most patients with systemic lupus erythematosus has become increasingly favorable.

Alarcon-Segovia D et al: Antiphospholipid antibodies and the antiphospholipid syndrome in systemic lupus erythematosus: A prospective analysis of 500 consecutive patients. Medicine 1989;68:353. (Anticardiolipin antibodies are associated with venous thrombosis, arterial occlusions, cytopenia, leg ulcers, recurrent fetal loss, and transverse myelitis.)

Asherson RA et al: The "primary" antiphospholipid syndrome: Major clinical and serological features. Medicine 1989;68:366. (Recurrent venous and arterial occlusions in patients with positive ANA tests but no specific features of SLE.)

Balow JE et al: Lupus nephritis. Ann Intern Med 1987;106:79. (Cyclophosphamide improves survival of the kidney but not the patient.)

Galve E et al: Prevalence, morphologic types, and evolution of cardiac valvular disease in systemic lupus erythematosus. N Engl J Med 1988;319:817. (Occurs in 18% of patients.)

Hellmann DB, Petri M, Whiting-O'Keefe Q: Fatal infections in systemic lupus erythematosus: The role of opportunistic organisms. Medicine 1987;66:341. (Infection the leading cause of death.)

Reveille JD et al: Prognosis in systemic lupus erythematosus. Arthritis Rheum 1990;33:37. (Black race, increasing age at onset, and thrombocytopenia associated with worse prognosis.)

PROGRESSIVE SYSTEMIC SCLEROSIS (Scleroderma)

Essentials of Diagnosis

- Diffuse thickening of skin, with telangiectasia and areas of increased pigmentation and depigmentation.
- Raynaud's phenomenon in 90% of patients.
- Systemic features of dysphagia, hypomotility of gastrointestinal tract, pulmonary fibrosis, and cardiac and renal involvement.

General Considerations

Progressive systemic sclerosis is a chronic disorder characterized by diffuse fibrosis of the skin and internal organs. The causes of scleroderma are not known, but autoimmunity, fibroblast disregulation, and occupational exposure have been implicated. Symptoms usually appear in the third to fifth decades, and women are affected 2–3 times as frequently as men.

Scleroderma may be localized or systemic. Localized scleroderma—morphea, linear scleroderma—is not associated with visceral organ involvement and is therefore benign. Two forms of systemic scleroderma are generally recognized: diffuse (20% of patients) and localized (80%). Patients with localized systemic scleroderma frequently have calcinosis cutis, Raynaud's phenomenon, esophageal involvement, sclerodactyly, and telangiectasia (CREST syndrome). Patients with CREST syndrome differ from those with diffuse systemic scleroderma in having skin tightening limited to the hands and face (versus the trunk), a lower risk of renal involvement, a higher risk of pulmonary hypertension, and an overall better prognosis.

Rapid progression of visceral organ disease leading to death within a few years is much more common in diffuse systemic scleroderma than in CREST syndrome.

Clinical Findings

A. Symptoms and Signs: Most frequently, the disease makes its appearance in the skin, although visceral involvement may precede cutaneous alteration. Polyarthralgia and Raynaud's phenomenon (present in 90% of patients) are early manifestations. Subcutaneous edema, fever, and malaise are common. With time the skin becomes thickened and hidebound, with loss of normal folds. Telangiectasia, pigmentation, and depigmentation are characteristic. Ulceration about the fingertips and subcutaneous calcification are seen. Dysphagia due to esophageal dysfunction, which occurs in 90% of patients, results from abnormalities in motility and later from fibrosis. Fibrosis and atrophy of the gastrointestinal tract cause hypomotility, and malabsorption results from bacterial overgrowth. Large-mouthed diverticula occur in the jejunum, ileum, and colon. Diffuse pulmonary fibrosis and pulmonary vascular disease are reflected in low diffusing capacity and decreased lung compliance. Cardiac abnormalities include pericarditis, heart block, myocardial fibrosis, and right heart failure secondary to pulmonary hypertension. Hypertensive uremic syndrome, resulting from obstruction to smaller renal blood vessels, indicates a grave prognosis.

B. Laboratory Findings: Mild anemia is often present, and it is occasionally hemolytic because of mechanical damage to red cells from diseased small vessels. Elevation of the sedimentation rate and hypergammaglobulinemia are also common. Proteinuria and cylindruria appear in association with renal involvement. Antinuclear antibody tests are frequently positive, often with a speckled or nucleolar pattern. Rheumatoid factor and a positive LE preparation may be found. The scleroderma antibody (SCL-70) is found in about 35% of patients with systemic sclerosis and is rare in the CREST syndrome; an anticentromere antibody is seen in 60% of those with CREST syndrome and in 5% of individuals with systemic sclerosis. Though these tests may be useful and of academic interest, their lack of sensitivity and (usually) specificity precludes cost-effective application in diagnosis.

Differential Diagnosis

Eosinophilic fasciitis is a rare disorder presenting with skin changes that appear to be like those in diffuse systemic scleroderma. The inflammatory abnormalities, however, are limited to the fascia rather than the dermis and epidermis. Patients with eosinophilic fasciitis are further distinguished from those with systemic scleroderma by the presence of peripheral blood eosinophilia, the absence of Raynaud's phenomenon, the good response to prednisone, and the increased risk of developing aplastic anemia.

The eosinophilia myalgia syndrome has been recently recognized in some patients who have ingested tryptophan, an essential amino acid that was sold— until removal by the Food and Drug Administration— as an over-the-counter remedy for insomnia and premenstrual symptoms. Weeks to months after beginning ingestion of tryptophan, affected patients developed a syndrome of eosinophilia greater than 1000/ μL, severe generalized myalgias, and cutaneous abnormalities ranging from hives to generalized swelling and induration of the arms and legs similar to that seen in scleroderma or eosinophilic fasciitis. Other common clinical manifestations have included pulmonary symptoms, fever, myopathy, lymphadenopathy, and ascending polyneuropathy. Besides eosinophilia, laboratory features include mild elevations of aldolase with normal creatine kinase levels and, frequently, positive ANA tests. Full-thickness biopsies reveal at times features of scleroderma and at other times evidence of fasciitis or myositis or small vessel vasculitis. Absence of evidence of infection or neoplasm is an important exclusionary feature. While some patients improve after discontinuing tryptophan, others progress and have required corticosteroid therapy, which is not always effective. Deaths have been reported, especially from neurologic involvement. Therefore, anyone with a scleroderma or an eosinophilic fasciitis-like syndrome should be asked about tryptophan use.

Treatment

Treatment is symptomatic and supportive. Severe Raynaud's syndrome may respond to calcium channel blockers. Patients with esophageal disease should take medications in liquid or crushed form. Esophageal reflux can be reduced and scarring prevented by avoiding late-night meals, elevating the head of the bed, and using antacids and H_2 blockers. Omeprazole, the only drug that produces near-complete inhibition of gastric acid production, appears to be remarkably effective for refractory esophagitis. Patients with delayed gastric emptying maintain their weight better if they eat small, frequent meals and remain upright for at least 2 hours after eating. Malabsorption due to bacterial overgrowth responds to antibiotics. The hypertensive crises seen chiefly in diffuse systemic scleroderma can often be treated with angiotensin-converting enzyme inhibitors. The ability of drugs to prevent the development of visceral disease is controversial. The best evidence, however imperfect, suggests that penicillamine may be helpful for patients at high risk of developing early visceral involvement, ie, those with rapidly progressive diffuse systemic scleroderma. Prednisone has little or no role in the treatment of scleroderma.

The prognosis tends to be worse in blacks, in males, and in older patients. In most cases, death results from renal, cardiac, or pulmonary failure.

Barnett AJ, Miller MH, Littlejohn GO: A survival study of patients with scleroderma diagnosed over 30 years

(1953–1983): The value of a simple cutaneous classification in the early stages of the disease. J Rheumatol 1988;15:276. (Ten-year survival, 71% with skin tightness limited to fingers but 21% with diffuse truncal skin involvement.)

Clauw DJ et al: Tryptophan-associated eosinophilic connective-tissue disease. JAMA 1990;263:1502. (Review of seven patients.)

Hertzman P et al: Association of the eosinophilia-myalgia syndrome with the ingestion of tryptophan. N Engl J Med 1990;322:;869. (Detailed description of the original cases.)

Lally EV et al: Progressive systemic sclerosis: Mode of presentation, rapidly progressive disease course, and mortality based on an analysis of 91 patients. Semin Arthritis Rheum 1988;18:1. (Eighteen percent have a rapidly progressive course.)

POLYMYOSITIS-DERMATOMYOSITIS

Essentials of Diagnosis

- Bilateral proximal muscle weakness (all cases).
- Heliotrope suffusion of upper eyelids, characteristic rash, papules over knuckles (many cases).
- Diagnostic tests: elevated CPK and other muscle enzymes, muscle biopsy, electromyogram.
- Increased incidence of malignancy, especially when rash is present and with late age of onset.

General Considerations

Polymyositis is a systemic disorder of unknown cause whose principal manifestation is muscle weakness. It is the most frequent primary myopathy in adults. When skin manifestations are associated with it, the entity is designated dermatomyositis. The true incidence is not known, since milder cases are frequently not diagnosed. The disease may affect persons of any age group, but the peak incidence is in the fifth and sixth decades of life. Women are affected twice as commonly as men.

Clinical Findings

A. Symptoms and Signs: Polymyositis may begin abruptly, although often it is gradual and progressive. The characteristic rash is dusky red and may be seen over the butterfly area of the face, neck, shoulders, and upper chest and back. Periorbital edema and a purplish (heliotrope) suffusion over the upper eyelids are typical signs. Subungual erythema, cuticular telangiectases, and scaly patches over the dorsum of the proximal interphalangeal and metacarpophalangeal joints (Gottron's sign) are highly suggestive. Muscle weakness chiefly involves proximal groups, especially of the extremities. Neck flexor weakness occurs in two-thirds of cases. Pain and tenderness of affected muscles are frequent but not universal, and Raynaud's phenomenon and joint symptoms may be associated. Atrophy and contractures occur late. Associated myocarditis is uncommon. Interstitial pulmonary disease, usually mild, is sometimes associated, and calcinosis may be observed, especially in children. Association with malignant neoplasms, particularly in older patients, is well recognized, but the frequency in several large series appears to be less than 20%. Polymyositis may occur in association with Sjögren's syndrome, systemic lupus erythematosus, or scleroderma.

B. Laboratory Findings: Measurement of serum levels of muscle enzymes, especially creatine phosphokinase and aldolase, is most useful in diagnosis and in assessment of disease activity. Anemia is uncommon. The sedimentation rate is not appreciably elevated in half of the patients. Rheumatoid factor is found in a minority of patients. Antinuclear antibodies are present in 90% of patients, and anti-Jo-1 antibodies are seen in the subset of patients who have associated interstitial lung disease. Chest x-rays are usually normal, though interstitial fibrosis is occasionally seen. Electromyographic abnormalities consisting of polyphasic potentials, fibrillations, and high-frequency action potentials are helpful in establishing the diagnosis. None of the studies are specific.

C. Muscle Biopsy: Biopsy of clinically involved muscle, usually proximal, is the only specific diagnostic study. Findings include necrosis of muscle fibers associated with inflammatory cells, sometimes located near blood vessels. The muscle biopsy may, however, reveal little change in spite of significant muscle weakness owing to the patchy distribution of pathologic abnormalities.

Differential Diagnosis

Most endocrine diseases can be associated with proximal muscle weakness. This is particularly true for hyper- and hypothyroidism, and the latter is associated also with elevations of creatinine phosphokinase. Patients with polymyalgia rheumatica are over the age of 50 and—in contrast to patients with polymyositis—have much more pain than weakness. Disorders of the peripheral and central nervous systems (eg, chronic inflammatory polyneuropathy, multiple sclerosis, myasthenia gravis, Eaton-Lambert disease and amyotrophic lateral sclerosis) can produce weakness but are distinguished by characteristic neurologic signs and electromyographic abnormalities. Many drugs, including corticosteroids, alcohol, clofibrate, penicillamine, tryptophan, and hydroxychloroquine, can produce proximal muscle weakness. Recent reports have indicated that chronic use of colchicine at doses as low as 0.6 mg twice a day in elderly patients with mild to moderate renal insufficiency can produce a mixed neuropathy-myopathy that mimics polymyositis. The weakness and muscle enzyme elevation reverse with cessation of the drug. Lovastatin (Mevacor), a drug increasingly used to treat hypercholesterolemia, also can rarely produce myositis. Polymyositis can occur as a complication of HIV infection and with zidovudine therapy as well.

D. Muscle Biopsy: Biopsy of clinically involved muscle, usually proximal, is the only specific diagnostic study. Findings include necrosis of muscle fibers associated with inflammatory cells, sometimes located near blood vessels. The muscle biopsy may, however, reveal little change in spite of significant muscle weakness owing to the patchy distribution of pathologic abnormalities.

Treatment

Most patients respond to corticosteroids. Often a daily dose of 40–60 mg or more of prednisone is required initially. The dose is then adjusted downward according to the response of sequentially observed serum levels of muscle enzymes. Long-term use of steroids is often needed, and the disease may recur or reemerge when they are withdrawn. Patients with an associated neoplasm have a poor prognosis, although remission may follow treatment of the tumor; steroids may or may not be effective in these patients. In patients resistant or intolerant to corticosteroids, therapy with methotrexate or azathioprine has been advised, but these agents should be used with caution in view of their adverse effects.

Hochberg MC et al: Adult onset polymyositis/dermatomyositis: An analysis of clinical and laboratory features and survival in 76 patients with a review of the literature. Semin Arthritis Rheum 1986;15:168.

Oddis CV, Medsger TA Jr: Relationship between serum creatine kinase level and corticosteroid therapy in polymyositis-dermatomyositis. J Rheumatol 1988;15:807. (After initiation, corticosteroids should be continued until the CPK normalizes, then tapered slowly.)

Plotz PH et al: Current concepts in idiopathic inflammatory myopathies: Polymyositis, dermatomyositis, and related disorders. Ann Intern Med 1989;111:143. (NIH conference and thorough review.)

Takizawa H et al: Interstitial lung disease in dermatomyositis: Clinicopathological study. J Rheumatol 1988;14:102. (Interstitial lung disease occurs more frequently in those with dermatomyositis, polyarthritis, and antibodies to Jo-1.)

OVERLAP (OR MIXED) CONNECTIVE TISSUE DISEASE

Not infrequently, patients have features of more than one rheumatic disease. Special attention has been drawn to patients who have overlapping features of systemic lupus erythematosus, scleroderma, and polymyositis. Initially, these patients were thought to have a distinct entity ("mixed connective tissue disease") defined by a specific autoantibody to ribonuclear protein (RNP). More recent studies suggest that the concept of mixed connective tissue disease is flawed, since with time in many patients the manifestations evolve to one predominant disease, such as scleroderma, and since many patients with antibodies to RNP have clear-cut systemic lupus erythematosus.

Therefore, "overlap connective tissue disease" is the preferred designation for patients having features of different rheumatic diseases.

SJÖGREN'S SYNDROME

Essentials of Diagnosis

- 90% of patients are women; the average age is 50 years.
- Dryness of eyes and dry mouth (sicca components) are the most common features; they occur alone or in association with rheumatoid arthritis or other connective tissue disease.
- Rheumatoid factor and other autoantibodies common.
- Increased incidence of lymphoma.

General Considerations

Sjögren's syndrome, an autoimmune disorder, is the result of chronic dysfunction of exocrine glands in many areas of the body. It is characterized by dryness of the eyes, mouth, and other areas covered by mucous membrane and is frequently associated with a rheumatic disease, most often rheumatoid arthritis. The disorder is predominantly a disease of women, in a ratio of 9:1, with greatest incidence between age 40 and 60 years.

Disorders with which Sjögren's syndrome is frequently associated include rheumatoid arthritis, systemic lupus erythematosus, primary biliary cirrhosis, scleroderma, polymyositis, Hashimoto's thyroiditis, polyarteritis, and interstitial pulmonary fibrosis. When Sjögren's syndrome occurs without rheumatoid arthritis, HLA-DR2 and -DR3 antigens are present with increased frequency.

Clinical Findings

A. Symptoms and Signs: Keratoconjunctivitis sicca results from inadequate tear production caused by lymphocyte and plasma cell infiltration of the lacrimal glands. Symptoms include burning, itching, ropy secretions, and impaired tear production during crying. Parotid enlargement, which may be chronic or relapsing, develops in one-third of patients. Dryness of the mouth (xerostomia) leads to difficulty in speaking and swallowing and to severe dental caries. There may be loss of taste and smell. Desiccation may involve the nose, throat, larynx, bronchi, vagina, and skin.

Systemic manifestations include dysphagia, pancreatitis, pleuritis, neuropsychiatric dysfunction, and vasculitis; they may be related to the associated diseases noted above. Renal tubular acidosis (type I, distal) occurs in 20% of patients. Chronic interstitial nephritis, which may result in impaired renal function, may be seen. A glomerular lesion is rarely observed but may occur secondary to associated cryoglobulinemia.

A spectrum of lymphoproliferation ranging from benign to malignant may be found. Malignant lymphomas and Waldenström's macroglobulinemia occur 44 times more frequently than can be explained by chance alone.

B. Laboratory Findings: Laboratory findings include mild anemia, leukopenia, and eosinophilia. Rheumatoid factor is found in 70% of patients. Heightened levels of gamma globulin, antinuclear antibodies, and antibodies against RNA, salivary gland, lacrimal duct, and thyroid may be noted. Antibodies against cytoplasmic antigens SS-A (or Ro) and SS-B (or La) are found predominantly in Sjögren's syndrome alone, whereas antibodies against salivary ducts and the RANA antigen are found in Sjögren's syndrome in association with rheumatoid arthritis. When SS-A antibodies are present, extraglandular manifestations of Sjögren's syndrome are far more common.

Useful ocular diagnostic tests include the Schirmer test, which measures the quantity of tears secreted. Labial biopsy, a simple procedure, is the only specific diagnostic technique and has minimal risk; if lymphoid foci are seen, the diagnosis is confirmed. Biopsy of the parotid gland should be reserved for patients with atypical presentations such as unilateral gland enlargement.

Treatment & Prognosis

Treatment is symptomatic and supportive. Artificial tears applied frequently will relieve ocular symptoms and avert further desiccation. The mouth should be kept well lubricated. Atropine drugs and decongestants decrease salivary secretions and should be avoided. A program of oral hygiene is essential in order to preserve dentition. If there is an associated rheumatic disease, its treatment is not altered by the presence of Sjögren's syndrome.

The disease is usually benign and may be consistent with a normal life span; it is influenced mainly by the nature of the associated disease.

Fox RI et al: Sjögren's syndrome: Proposed criteria for classification. Arthritis Rheum 1986;29:577. (Four criteria: keratoconjunctivitis sicca, diminished salivary gland flow, positive salivary gland biopsy, and presence of autoantibodies.)

Wise CM, Agudelo CA: Optic neuropathy as an initial manifestation of Sjögren's syndrome. J Rheumatol 1988;15:799. (May antedate Sjögren's.)

VASCULITIS SYNDROMES

The vasculitis syndromes are a heterogeneous group of disorders characterized by the pathologic features of inflammation and necrosis of blood vessels. The cause of most forms of vasculitis is not known. Hepatitis B is strongly associated with some cases of polyarteritis, and other infections have been implicated, eg, the vasculitis that occurs in bacterial endocarditis. Drug reactions—especially to penicillins, sulfonamides, and allopurinol—can produce serum sickness associated with vasculitis. No common pathogenic link has been identified for these disorders, though the deposition of immune complexes in the vascular system occurs in many.

Although vasculitis is seen in multiple disorders, only the major vasculitides will be discussed here.

POLYARTERITIS NODOSA

Essentials of Diagnosis

- Clinical findings depend on arteries involved.
- Affects kidneys, muscles, joints, nerves, heart, gastrointestinal tract in most patients; cutaneous and pulmonary involvement unusual but possible.
- Manifestations of fever, hypertension, abdominal pain, livedo reticularis, mononeuritis multiplex, anemia, hematuria, elevated sedimentation rate.
- Diagnostic confirmation by biopsy or angiogram.

General Considerations

Polyarteritis is characterized by focal or segmental lesions of blood vessels, especially arteries of small to medium size, resulting in a variety of clinical presentations depending upon the specific site of the blood vessel involved. The pathologic hallmark of the disease is acute necrotizing inflammation of the arterial media, with fibrinoid necrosis and extensive inflammatory cell infiltration of all coats of the vessel and surrounding tissue. Aneurysmal dilatations occur; hemorrhage, thrombosis, and fibrosis may lead to occlusion of the lumen. Arterial lesions may be seen in all stages—acute, healing, and healed. Such vascular lesions may involve virtually every organ of the body but are especially prominent in the kidney, heart, liver, gastrointestinal tract, muscle, and testes.

The cause of polyarteritis is unknown. Hepatitis B has been strongly implicated, with 30–50% of patients having serologic evidence of the infection. In addition, immune complexes consisting in part of hepatitis B antigens have been identified in the serum and in the inflamed vessels of some patients. It is not surprising, therefore, that polyarteritis nodosa is more common in intravenous drug abusers and in other groups who have a high prevalence of hepatitis B infection. Yet at least half of patients with polyarteritis have no evidence of hepatitis B infection. Polyarteritis may occur at any age but is more frequent in young adults, and men are affected 3 times as frequently as women.

Clinical Findings

A. Symptoms and Signs: The clinical onset may

be abrupt, often accompanied by fever, chills, and tachycardia. Arthralgia and myositis with muscle tenderness are prominent. A wide variety of cutaneous abnormalities develop. Livedo reticularis is most common; vasculitic involvement causing skin ulcers is less common. Occlusion of retinal vessels results in cotton-wool spots (cytoid bodies). Hypertension occurs in half of patients and renal involvement in more than 80%. The renal lesion is a segmental necrotizing glomerulonephritis with extracapillary proliferation, often with localized intravascular coagulation. Abdominal pain and nausea and vomiting are common. Infarction due to the arteritis compromises the function of major viscera and may lead to cholecystitis, appendicitis, and intestinal obstruction. Cardiac involvement is manifested by pericarditis, myocarditis, and arrhythmias; myocardial infarction secondary to coronary vasculitis also occurs. Multiple asymmetric neuropathies occur as a result of vasculitis of the vasa vasorum. Polyarteritis is an occasional cause of fever of unknown origin.

B. Laboratory Findings: Laboratory findings include proteinuria, hematuria, and cylindruria. Most patients manifest anemia and leukocytosis. Eosinophilia is more frequently encountered in association with pulmonary lesions, which may represent a different disease process (Churg-Strauss vasculitis), though overlap is not universal. The sedimentation rate is almost always elevated. Rheumatoid factor, antinuclear antibody, positive serologic test for syphilis, and increased serum concentration of gamma globulin are neither sensitive nor specific. Serum complement is often normal or elevated.

C. Biopsy and Angiography: Biopsy of symptomatic sites (such as muscle, nerve, or testicle) is sensitive (70%) and specific (97%), with low morbidity and virtually no associated deaths. If these biopsies are negative or if there is no symptomatic site, the patient should undergo visceral angiography to look for characteristic aneurysmal dilatation of the renal, mesenteric, or hepatic arteries. Visceral angiography has sensitivity and specificity similar to those of biopsy of symptomatic sites, but angiography can produce complications such as a rise in creatinine and, rarely, death.

Treatment

Corticosteroids in high doses (up to 60 mg of prednisone daily) may control fever and constitutional symptoms and heal vascular lesions. Immunosuppressive agents, especially cyclophosphamide, appear to improve the survival of patients when given with steroids. These drugs may be required for long periods, and relapses are not infrequent when they are withdrawn.

Prognosis

Without treatment, the 5-year mortality rate is 80%. Corticosteroids alone improve the 5-year survival to 50%. With corticosteroids and immunosuppressive drugs, the 5-year survival has improved to 80–90%.

Albert DA, Rimon D, Silverstein MD: The diagnosis of polyarteritis nodosa. Arthritis Rheum 1988;31:1117. (Best initial strategy: biopsy symptomatic site or perform visceral angiogram.)

Hellmann DB et al: Mononeuritis multiplex: The yield of evaluations for occult rheumatic diseases. Medicine 1988;67:145. (Simultaneous onset of systemic symptoms and mononeuritis multiplex is highly suggestive of polyarteritis.)

POLYMYALGIA RHEUMATICA & GIANT CELL ARTERITIS

Polymyalgia rheumatica, a disorder affecting middle-aged or elderly persons, is rare before age 50. The disease often develops abruptly, with pain and stiffness of the pelvis and shoulder girdle in association with fever, malaise, and weight loss. Anemia and a markedly elevated sedimentation rate are almost always present. The course is generally limited to 1–2 years.

Polymyalgia rheumatica bears a close relationship to giant cell arteritis. The 2 conditions often coexist, but each may occur independently; when they coexist, the clinical manifestations of polymyalgia rheumatica almost always precede those of giant cell arteritis. The importance of diagnosing arteritis lies in the risk of blindness due to obstruction of the ophthalmic arteries; this may occur unless treatment is given. Suggestive symptoms of arteritis include unilateral throbbing headache, scalp sensitivity, visual symptoms, and jaw claudication, but arteritis may be present without local symptoms. Indeed, 40% of patients will have nonclassic presentations with respiratory tract problems (most frequently dry cough), mononeuritis multiplex (most frequently with painful paralysis of a shoulder), or fever of unknown origin.

In the presence of headache and other symptoms suggestive of cranial arteritis, therapy with prednisone, 60 mg daily, is initiated immediately to prevent blindness, and temporal artery biopsy is promptly obtained. How quickly the histologic changes in the temporal artery resolve after initiation of therapy is unclear, but biopsies obtained within 5–7 days after initiation of therapy should be reliable. An adequate biopsy specimen (3–5 cm in length) is essential, because the disease tends to be segmental; bilateral biopsies add 10–20% to the yield. Ten to 15 percent of patients have vasculitis of other major arteries. Prednisone should be continued in a dosage of 60 mg/d for 1–2 months before tapering. When only the symptoms of polymyalgia rheumatic are present, temporal artery biopsy is not necessary. Furthermore, polymyalgia—in the absence of arteritis—responds quickly (1–5 days) and dramatically to smaller doses of prednisone (10–15 mg daily). If such a response does not occur, the diagnosis of polymyalgia rheumatica should be questioned.

In adjusting the dosage of steroid, the erythrocyte sedimentation rate (ESR) is a useful but not absolute guide to disease activity. Blindness rarely occurs when the ESR has reached the normal range. The drug may be discontinued when disease activity ceases, although the disorder may recur and in some patients remains active for years. Chronic infectious disease such as bacterial endocarditis, which have systemic symptoms similar to those of polymyalgia rheumatica, should always be excluded before corticosteroids are started. Multiple myeloma and other malignant disorders should also be considered as causes of anemia and a markedly elevated sedimentation rate.

Machado EBV et al: Trends in incidence and clinical presentation of temporal arteritis in Olmsted County, Minnesota, 1950–1985. Arthritis Rheum 1988;31:745. (Incidence in women has increased; incidence in men and that of classic manifestations has decreased.)

Mehler MF, Rabinowich L: The clinical neuro-ophthalmologic spectrum of temporary arteritis. Am J Med 1988;85:839. (Visual loss, ophthalmoparesis, pupillary autonomic dysfunction, and visual hallucinations.)

WEGENER'S GRANULOMATOSIS

Wegener's granulomatosis is a rare disorder characterized by vasculitis, necrotizing granulomatous lesions of both upper and lower respiratory tract, and glomerulonephritis. Without treatment it is invariably fatal, most patients surviving less than a year after diagnosis. It occurs most commonly in the fourth and fifth decades of life and affects men and women with equal frequency.

Clinical Findings

A. Symptoms and Signs: The disorder presents as a febrile illness with weakness, malaise, and weight loss. Symptoms include those of purulent sinusitis and rhinitis; polyarthralgia may also be present. Dyspnea, cough, chest pain, and hemoptysis may dominate the clinical picture. Ulcerations of the nasal septum are noted in physical examination. X-ray of the chest often reveals nodular pulmonary lesions, frequently cavitating; histologic examination of the lesions shows necrotizing vasculitis with granuloma formation. Although limited forms of Wegener's granulomatosis have been described in which the kidney is spared, severe progressive renal disease usually ensues and results in rapid deterioration of renal function. In such cases the urinary sediment invariably contains red cells, with or without white cells, and red cell casts. Renal biopsy discloses a segmental necrotizing glomerulonephritis with multiple crescents; this is characteristic but not diagnostic. Granulomas are observed in 10%.

B. Laboratory Findings: Laboratory studies show anemia (occasionally microangiopathic), leukocytosis, and a rapid sedimentation rate. Antineutrophil cytoplasmic antibodies appear to be relatively specific and sensitive for this disease (see Nolle reference, below) but have not replaced the need for histologic confirmation.

Treatment

It is essential that the diagnosis be made early, since treatment may be lifesaving; lung tissue is preferred, as findings are more often specific than in tissue from nasal mucosal biopsy. Remissions have been induced in up to 90% of patients treated with cyclophosphamide. Corticosteroids are usually of limited value. The potential role of trimethoprim-sulfamethoxazole in the treatment of Wegener's granulomatosis remains undefined.

Fauci AS et al: Wegener's granulomatosis: Prospective clinical and therapeutic experience with 85 patients for 21 years. Ann Intern Med 1983;98:76.

Nolle B et al: Anticytoplasmic autoantibodies: Their immunodiagnostic value in Wegener granulomatosis. Ann Intern Med. 1989;111:28. (Highly specific (98–99%). Sensitivity was 93–96% for generalized active disease, 60–67% for active regional disease, and 32–40% for disease in remission.)

HENOCH-SCHÖNLEIN PURPURA

This is a form of purpura of unknown cause; the underlying pathologic feature is vasculitis, which principally affects small blood vessels. Although the disease is predominantly seen in children, adults are also affected. Hypersensitivity to aspirin and food and drug additives has been reported. The purpuric skin lesions are typically located on the lower extremities but may also be seen on the hands, arms, and trunk. Localized areas of edema, especially common on the dorsal surfaces of the hands, are frequently observed. Joint symptoms are present in the vast majority of patients, the knees and ankles being most commonly involved. Abdominal pain secondary to vasculitis of the intestinal tract is often associated with gastrointestinal bleeding. Hematuria signals the presence of a renal lesion that is usually reversible, although it occasionally may progress to renal insufficiency. Biopsy of the kidney reveals segmental glomerulonephritis with crescents and mesangial deposition of IgA and, sometimes, IgG. Aside from an elevated sedimentation rate, most laboratory findings are noncontributory; the platelet count is normal or elevated.

The disease is usually self-limited, lasting 1–6 weeks, and subsides without sequelae if renal involvement is not severe. There is no effective treatment, although immunosuppressive drugs have met with some success in the nephropathy of this disorder.

Fogazzi GB et al: Long-term outcome of Schönlein-Henoch nephritis in the adult. Clin Nephrol 1989;31:6. (Eighteen percent develop end-stage renal disease.)

DEGENERATIVE & CRYSTAL-INDUCED ARTHRITIS

DEGENERATIVE JOINT DISEASE (Osteoarthritis)

Essentials of Diagnosis

- A degenerative disorder without systemic manifestations.
- Pain relieved by rest; morning stiffness brief. Articular inflammation minimal.
- X-ray findings: narrowed joint space, osteophytes, increased density of subchondral bone, bony cysts.
- Commonly secondary to other articular disease.

General Considerations

Osteoarthritis is the most common form of joint disease, sparing no age, race, or geographic area. At least 20 million adults in the USA suffer from the effects of this condition at any one time, and 90% of all people will have radiographic features of osteoarthritis in weight-bearing joints by age 40. Symptomatic disease also increases with age.

This arthropathy is characterized by degeneration of cartilage and by hypertrophy of bone at the articular margins. Inflammation is usually minimal. Hereditary and mechanical factors may be variably involved in the pathogenesis.

Degenerative joint disease is traditionally divided into 2 types: (1) primary, which most commonly affects the terminal interphalangeal joints (Heberden's nodes) and less commonly the proximal interphalangeal joints (Bouchard's nodes), the metacarpophalangeal and carpometacarpal joints of the thumb, the hip, the knee, the metatarsophalangeal joint of the big toe, and the cervical and lumbar spine; and (2) secondary, which may occur in any joint as a sequela to articular injury resulting from either intra-articular (including rheumatoid arthritis) or extra-articular causes. The injury may be acute, as in a fracture; or chronic, as that due to occupational overuse of a joint, metabolic disease (eg, hyperparathyroidism, hemochromatosis, ochronosis), or neurologic disorders (tabes dorsalis; see below).

Pathologically, the articular cartilage is first roughened and finally worn away, and spur formation and lipping occur at the edge of the joint surface. The synovial membrane becomes thickened, with hypertrophy of the villous processes; the joint cavity, however, never becomes totally obliterated, and the synovial membrane does not form adhesions. Inflammation is prominent only in occasional patients with acute interphalangeal joint involvement (Heberden's nodes).

Clinical Findings

A. Symptoms and Signs: The onset is insidious. Initially, there is articular stiffness, seldom lasting more than 15 minutes; this develops later into pain on motion of the affected joint and is made worse by prolonged activity and relieved by rest. Deformity may be absent or minimal; however, bony enlargement is occasionally prominent, and flexion contracture or valgus or varus deformity of the knee is not unusual. There is no ankylosis, but limitation of motion of the affected joint or joints is common. Coarse crepitus may often be felt in the joint. Joint effusion and other articular signs of inflammation are mild. There are no systemic manifestations.

B. Laboratory Findings: Elevated sedimentation rate and other laboratory signs of inflammation are not present.

C. Imaging: Radiographs may reveal narrowing of the joint space, sharpened articular margins, osteophyte formation and lipping of marginal bone, and thickened, dense subchondral bone. Bone cysts may also be present.

Differential Diagnosis

Because articular inflammation is minimal and systemic manifestations are absent, degenerative joint disease should seldom be confused with other arthritides. The distribution of joint involvement in the hands also helps distinguish osteoarthritis from rheumatoid arthritis: Osteoarthritis chiefly affects the distal and proximal interphalangeal joints and spares the wrist and metacarpophalangeal joints; rheumatoid arthritis chiefly involves the wrists and metacarpophalangeal joints and spares the distal interphalangeal joints. Furthermore, the joint enlargement is bony-hard and cool in osteoarthritis but spongy and warm in rheumatoid arthritis. Neurogenic arthropathy is easily distinguished by physical examination. Degenerative joint disease may coexist with any other type of joint disease. Furthermore, one must be cautious in attributing all skeletal symptoms to degenerative changes in joints, especially in the spine, where metastatic neoplasia, osteoporosis, multiple myeloma, or other bone disease may coexist.

Treatment

A. General Measures:

1. Rest–Occupational or recreational overuse of an affected joint must be prevented. If weight-bearing joints are involved, activities such as climbing stairs, walking, or prolonged standing should be minimized. Most patients are aware of these limitations by the time they consult a physician.

2. Diet–In obese patients, weight reduction may help diminish stress on the joints.

3. Local heat–Local heat in any form and other forms of physical therapy are often of symptomatic value.

B. Analgesic and Anti-inflammatory Drugs: Salicylates or other nonsteroidal anti-inflammatory drugs (see Chapter 1) are indicated for the relief of pain. High doses of salicylates, as used in more inflammatory arthritides, are unnecessary.

C. Orthopedic Measures: Orthopedic measures to correct developmental anomalies, deformities, disparity in leg length, and severely damaged joint surfaces may be required (see p 617).

D. Surgical Measures: Total hip replacement provides excellent symptomatic and functional improvement when that joint is seriously afflicted, as usually indicated by severely restricted walking and pain at rest, particularly at night. Knee replacement is also an option, though the results are less impressive.

Prognosis

Marked disability is less common than in rheumatoid arthritis, but symptoms may be quite severe and limit activity considerably (especially with involvement of the hips, knees, and cervical spine). Proper treatment may relieve symptoms and improve function.

Felson DT et al: The prevalence of knee osteoarthritis in the elderly: The Framingham osteoarthritis study. Arthritis Rheum 1987;30:914.

Hamerman D: The biology of osteoarthritis. N Engl J Med. 1989;320:1322.

Moskowitz RW: Primary osteoarthritis: Epidemiology, clinical aspects, and general management. Am J Med 1987;83(Suppl 5A):5.

CRYSTAL DEPOSITION ARTHRITIS

1. GOUTY ARTHRITIS

Essentials of Diagnosis

- Acute onset, usually monarticular, often involving the first metatarsophalangeal joint.
- Postinflammatory desquamation and pruritus. Hyperuricemia.
- Identification of urate crystals in joint fluid or tophi.
- Asymptomatic periods between acute attacks. With chronicity, urate deposits in subcutaneous tissue, bone, cartilage, joints, and other tissues.
- Dramatic therapeutic response to NSAIDs or colchicine.

General Considerations

Gout is a metabolic disease of heterogeneous nature, often familial, associated with abnormal amounts of urates in the body and characterized early by a recurring acute arthritis, usually monarticular, and later by chronic deforming arthritis.

Primary gout is a heritable metabolic disease in which hyperuricemia is usually due to overproduction or underexcretion of uric acid—sometimes both. It is rarely due to a specifically determined genetic aberration (eg, Lesch-Nyhan syndrome). Secondary gout, which may have some latent heritable component, is related to acquired causes of hyperuricemia, eg, diuretic use, myeloproliferative disorders, multiple myeloma, hemoglobinopathies, chronic renal disease, and lead poisoning.

About 90% of patients with primary gout are men, usually over 30 years of age. In women the onset is usually postmenopausal. The characteristic histologic lesion is the tophus, a nodular deposit of monosodium urate monohydrate crystals, and an associated foreign body reaction. These may be found in cartilage, subcutaneous and periarticular tissues, tendon, bone, the kidneys, and elsewhere. Urates have been demonstrated in the synovial tissues (and fluid) during acute arthritis; indeed, the acute inflammation of gout is believed to be activated by the phagocytosis by polymorphonuclear cells of urate crystals with the ensuing release from the neutrophils of chemotactic and other substances capable of mediating inflammation. The precise relationship of hyperuricemia to acute gouty arthritis is still obscure, since chronic hyperuricemia is a frequent finding in people who never develop gout or uric acid stones (Table 15–3). Rapid fluctuations in serum urate levels, either increasing or decreasing, are important factors in precipitating acute gout. The mechanism of the late, chronic stage of

Table 15–3. Origin of hyperuricemia.[1]

Primary Hyperuricemia
  A. Increased production of purine:
    1. Idiopathic.
    2. Specific enzyme defects (eg, Lesch-Nyhan syndrome, glycogen storage disease).
  B. Decreased renal clearance of uric acid (idiopathic).

Secondary Hyperuricemia
  A. Increased catabolism and turnover of purine:
    1. Myeloproliferative disorders.
    2. Lymphoproliferative disorders.
    3. Carcinoma and sarcoma (disseminated).
    4. Chronic hemolytic anemias.
    5. Cytotoxic drugs.
    6. Psoriasis.
  B. Decreased renal clearance of uric acid:
    1. Intrinsic kidney disease.
    2. Functional impairment of tubular transport:
      a. Drug-induced (eg, thiazides, probenecid).
      b. Hyperlacticemia (eg, lactic acidosis, alcoholism).
      c. Hyperketoacidemia (eg, diabetic ketoacidosis, starvation).
      d. Diabetes insipidus (vasopressin-resistant).
      e. Bartter's syndrome.

[1] Modified from Rodnan GP: Gout and other crystalline forms of arthritis. *Postgrad Med* (Oct) 1975;**58**:6.

gouty arthritis is better understood. This is characterized pathologically by tophaceous invasion of the articular and periarticular tissues, with structural derangement and secondary degeneration (osteoarthritis).

Uric acid kidney stones are present in 10–20% of patients with gouty arthritis. The term gouty nephropathy (or "gouty nephritis") refers to kidney disease due to sodium urate deposition in the renal interstitium. Uric acid stones are not related to its pathogenesis, and a relationship to renal insufficiency has not been established.

Unless there is a rapid breakdown of cellular nucleic acid following aggressive treatment of leukemia or lymphoma, uric acid-lowering drugs need not be instituted until arthritis, renal calculi, or tophi become apparent. Psoriasis, sarcoidosis, and diuretic drugs are commonly overlooked causes of hyperuricemia and may precipitate attacks in patients with gout. Asymptomatic hyperuricemia should not be treated.

Clinical Findings

A. Symptoms and Signs: The acute arthritis is characterized by its sudden onset, frequently nocturnal, either without apparent precipitating cause or following rapid fluctuations in serum urate levels from food and alcohol excess, surgery, infection, diuretics, chemicals (eg, meglumine diatrizoate, Urografin), or uricosuric drugs. The metatarsophalangeal joint of the great toe is the most susceptible joint, although others, especially those of the feet, ankles, and knees, are commonly affected. Hips and shoulders are rarely involved in gouty arthritis. More than one joint may occasionally be affected during the same attack; in such cases, the distribution of the arthritis is usually asymmetric. As the attack progresses, the pain becomes intense. The involved joints are swollen and exquisitely tender and the overlying skin tense, warm, and dusky red. Fever is common and may reach 39 °C. Local desquamation and pruritus during recovery from the acute arthritis are characteristic of gout but are not always present. Tophi may be found in the external ears, hands, feet, olecranon, and prepatellar bursas. They are usually seen only after several attacks of acute arthritis.

Asymptomatic periods of months or years commonly follow the initial acute attack. Later, gouty arthritis may become chronic, with symptoms of progressive functional loss and disability. Gross deformities, due usually to tophaceous invasion, are seen. Signs of inflammation may be absent or superimposed.

B. Laboratory Findings: The serum uric acid is practically always elevated (> 7.5 mg/dL) unless uricopenic drugs are being given. During an acute attack, the erythrocyte sedimentation rate and white cell count are usually elevated. Examination of the material aspirated from a tophus shows the typical crystals of sodium urate and confirms the diagnosis.

Further confirmation is obtained by identification of sodium urate crystals by compensated polariscopic examination of wet smears prepared from joint fluid aspirates. Such crystals are negatively birefringent and needlelike and may be found free or in neutrophils.

C. Imaging: Early in the disease, radiographs show no changes. Later, punched-out areas in the bone (radiolucent urate tophi) are seen. When these are adjacent to a soft tissue tophus, they are diagnostic of gout.

Differential Diagnosis

Once the diagnosis of acute gouty arthritis is suspected, it is confirmed by the presence of hyperuricemia, dramatic response to NSAIDs or colchicine, local desquamation and pruritus as the edema subsides, and polariscopic examination of joint fluid. Acute gout is often confused with cellulitis. Appropriate bacteriologic studies should exclude acute pyogenic arthritis. Acute chondrocalcinosis (pseudogout) may be distinguished by the identification of calcium pyrophosphate crystals in the joint fluid, usually normal serum uric acid, the x-ray appearance of chondrocalcinosis, and the relative therapeutic ineffectiveness of colchicine.

Chronic tophaceous arthritis may rarely mimic chronic rheumatoid arthritis. In such cases, the diagnosis of gout is suggested by an earlier history of monarthritis and is established by the demonstration of urate crystals in the contents of a suspected tophus. Biopsy may be necessary to distinguish tophi from rheumatoid nodules. An x-ray appearance similar to that of gout may be found in rheumatoid arthritis, sarcoidosis, multiple myeloma, hyperparathyroidism, or Hand-Schüller-Christian disease. Chronic lead intoxication may result in attacks of gouty arthritis and renal insufficiency.

Treatment

A. Acute Attack: The most common mistake in managing gout is starting drug treatment for both the acute arthritis and the hyperuricemia simultaneously. Treatment must be separated by treating the acute arthritis first and hyperuricemia later. Sudden reduction of serum uric acid often precipitates further episodes of gouty arthritis. Treatment of hyperuricemia is more safely started once the acute gouty episode has resolved.

1. Nonsteroidal anti-inflammatory drugs– NSAIDs have become the treatment of choice for acute gout. Traditionally, indomethacin has been the most frequently used agent, but all of the other newer NSAIDs are probably equally effective. Indomethacin is initiated at a dosage of 50 mg every 8 hours and continued until the symptoms have resolved (usually 5–10 days). Active peptic ulcer disease and impaired renal function are contraindications to the use of NSAIDs.

2. Colchicine–Colchicine is also effective for acute gout but is less favored, since 80% of treated patients develop significant abdominal cramping, diarrhea, nausea, or vomiting. Colchicine is thought to work by inhibiting the chemotactic property of leukocytosis and thus interferes with the inflammatory response to urate crystals. Once a full chemotactic response has occurred (after the first 24–48 hours), colchicine loses its effectiveness. The dose is 0.5 or 0.6 mg by mouth every hour until pain is relieved or until nausea or diarrhea appears; the drug is then stopped. The usual total dose required is 4–8 mg. The incidence of gastrointestinal side effects of colchicine can be reduced by intravenous administration in an initial dose of 1–2 mg in 10–20 mL of saline solution. Use of intravenous colchicine, however, should be discouraged because of potential severe toxicity, including local pain, tissue damage from extravasation during injection, bone marrow suppression, and disseminated intravascular coagulation. Single intravenous doses should not exceed 2–3 mg; the total dose should not exceed 4–5 mg; and no additional colchicine should be given by mouth for 1 week. Dosages must be reduced in the presence of renal or hepatic disease or old age. Combined renal and hepatic disease contraindicates the use of intravenous colchicine. Intravenous administration of colchicine is rarely necessary and is inadvisable if the oral route can be used. Oral colchicine should not be used in patients with inflammatory bowel disease.

3. Corticosteroids–Corticosteroids often give dramatic symptomatic relief in acute episodes of gout and will control most attacks if continued long enough. Corticosteroids are best reserved for patients with acute gout who are unable to take oral NSAIDs. If the patient's gout is monarticular, intra-articular administration (eg, triamcinolone, 10–40 mg depending on the size of the joint) is most effective. For polyarticular gout, corticosteroids may be given intravenously (eg, methylprednisolone, 40 mg/d tapered off over 7 days) or orally (eg, prednisone, 40–60 mg/d tapered off over 7 days). It should be recognized that gouty and septic arthritis can coexist, even if rarely. Therefore, joint aspiration and Gram stain of synovial fluid should be performed before corticosteroids are given.

4. Analgesics–At times the pain of an acute attack may be so severe that analgesia is necessary before a more specific drug becomes effective. In these cases, codeine or meperidine may be given. Aspirin should be avoided (see below).

5. Bed rest is important in the management of the acute attack and should be continued for about 24 hours after the acute attack has subsided. Early ambulation may precipitate a recurrence.

6. Physical therapy is of little value during the acute attack, though hot or cold compresses to or elevation of the affected joints makes some patients more comfortable.

B. Management Between Attacks: Treatment during symptom-free periods is intended to minimize urate deposition in tissues, which causes chronic tophaceous arthritis, and to reduce the frequency and severity of recurrences.

1. Diet–It is important to avoid obesity, fasting, excessive alcohol, and dehydration. Rigid diets fail to influence the hyperuricemia or the course of gouty arthritis. Since dietary sources of purines contribute very little to the causation of the disease, restriction of foods high in purine (eg, kidney, liver, sweetbreads, sardines, anchovies, meat extracts) cannot be expected to contribute significantly to the management of the disease. Specific foods or alcoholic beverages that precipitate attacks should be avoided. A high liquid intake and, more importantly, a daily urinary output of 2 L or more will aid urate excretion and minimize urate precipitation in the urinary tract.

2. Avoidance of hyperuricemic medications–Diuretics inhibit renal excretion of uric acid, thereby producing or increasing hyperuricemia. Whenever possible, diuretics should be avoided in patients with gout. Similarly, low doses of aspirin also inhibit renal excretion of uric acid and aggravate hyperuricemia. Nicotinic acid is yet another medication that can produce hyperuricemia.

3. Colchicine–The decision to begin chronic pharmacologic treatment of gout should be based on an estimate of the likelihood of the patient's having another attack. A 43-year-old obese man who has had a single episode of gout and is willing to lose weight and stop taking low-dose aspirin is at low risk of another attack and therefore is unlikely to benefit from chronic medical therapy. In contrast, a 54-year-old man with mild chronic renal failure, a requirement for diuretic use, and a history of multiple attacks of gout is much more likely to benefit from pharmacologic treatment. In general, the higher the uric acid level and the more frequent the attacks of gout, the more likely it is that chronic medical therapy will be beneficial.

Daily colchicine use has 2 indications: (1) Colchicine can be used by itself to prevent future attacks of gout. The drug does not affect the uric acid level but reduces the frequency of attacks. For the person who has mild hyperuricemia and has had several attacks of gouty arthritis, chronic colchicine prophylaxis may be all that is needed to reduce substantially the chance of a future attack. The usual dose is 0.6 mg twice a day. Patients who have coexisting moderate renal insufficiency or heart failure should have the dose reduced to once a day in order to avoid the development of a mixed peripheral neuropathy and myositis that can complicate the use of higher doses. (2) Colchicine prophylaxis is also used when uricosuric drugs or allopurinol (see below) are started, to suppress the acute attacks that can be precipitated by abrupt changes in the serum uric acid level.

4. Reduction of serum uric acid–Indications include frequent acute arthritis not controlled by colchicine prophylaxis, tophaceous deposits, or renal damage. It is emphasized that hyperuricemia with infrequent attacks of arthritis may not require treatment; asymptomatic hyperuricemia should not be treated.

Two classes of agents may be used to lower the serum uric acid—the uricosuric drugs and allopurinol (neither is of value in the treatment of acute gout).

a. Uricosuric drugs–These drugs, by blocking tubular reabsorption of filtered urate and reducing the metabolic pool of urates, prevent the formation of new tophi and reduce the size of those already present. Furthermore, when administered concomitantly with colchicine, they may lessen the frequency of recurrences of acute gout. The indication for uricosuric treatment is the increasing frequency or severity of acute attacks.

The following uricosuric drugs may be employed:

(1) Probenecid 0.5 g daily initially with gradual increase to 1–2 g daily.

(2) Sulfinpyrazone, 100 mg daily initially with gradual increase to 200–400 mg daily. The maintenance dose is determined by observation of the serum uric acid response and the urinary uric acid response. Ideally, one attempts to maintain a normal serum urate level.

Hypersensitivity to either uricosuric drug in the form of fever and rash occurs in 5% of cases; gastrointestinal complaints occur in 10%.

Precautions with uricosuric drugs. It is important to maintain a daily urinary output of 2000 mL or more in order to minimize the precipitation of uric acid in the urinary tract. This can be further prevented by giving alkalinizing agents to maintain a urine pH of above 6.0. If a significant uricosuric effect is not obtained in the presence of overt renal dysfunction, do not increase the dose of the drug beyond the limits stated above. Uricosuric drugs are best avoided in patients with a history of uric acid lithiasis. Avoid using salicylates, since they antagonize the action of uricosuric agents.

b. Allopurinol–The xanthine oxidase inhibitor allopurinol (Zyloprim) promptly lowers plasma urate and urinary uric acid concentrations and facilitates tophus mobilization. The drug is of special value in uric acid overproducers (as defined by urinary excretion of uric acid in excess of 800 mg/d while on a purine-free diet); in tophaceous gout; in patients unresponsive to the uricosuric regimen; and in gouty patients with uric acid renal stones. It should be used cautiously in patients with renal insufficiency and is not indicated in asymptomatic hyperuricemia. The most frequent adverse effect is the precipitation of an acute gouty attack. However, the commonest sign of hypersensitivity to allopurinol (occurring in 5% of cases) is a pruritic rash that may progress to toxic epidermal necrolysis, a potentially fatal complication.

Vasculitis and severe hepatitis are other rare complications.

The daily dose is determined by the serum uric acid response. The initial dose of allopurinol is 100 mg/d for 1 week; the dose is increased if the serum uric acid is still high. A normal serum uric acid level is often obtained with a daily dose of 200–300 mg. Occasionally (and in selected cases) it may be helpful to continue the use of allopurinol with a uricosuric drug. Neither of these drugs is useful in acute gout.

C. Chronic Tophaceous Arthritis: Tophaceous deposits can be made to shrink and disappear altogether with allopurinol therapy. The treatment is essentially the same as that outlined for the intervals between acute attacks. Surgical excision of large tophi offers immediate mechanical improvement in selected deformities but is rarely required.

Prognosis

Without treatment, the acute attack may last from a few days to several weeks, but proper treatment quickly terminates the attack. The intervals between acute attacks vary up to years, but the asymptomatic periods often become shorter if the disease progresses. Chronic tophaceous arthritis occurs after repeated attacks of acute gout, but only after inadequate treatment. Although the deformities may be marked, only a small percentage of patients become bedridden. The younger the patient at the onset of disease, the greater the tendency to a progressive course. Destructive arthropathy is rarely seen in patients whose first attack is after age 50.

Patients with gout have an increased incidence of hypertension, renal disease (eg, nephrosclerosis, tophi, pyelonephritis), diabetes mellitus, hypertriglyceridemia, and atherosclerosis, although these relationships are not well understood.

Kuncl RW et al: Colchicine myopathy and neuropathy. N Engl J Med 1987;316:1562. (Patients developed myopathy [mimicking polymyositis] and neuropathy while taking 0.6 mg twice daily.)

Lawry GV II, Fan PT, Bluestone R: Polyarticular versus monarticular gout: A prospective, comparative analysis of clinical features. Medicine 1988;67:335. (Polyarticular gout develops late in noncompliant patients, often involves the upper extremities, and may be associated with less intense joint inflammation.)

Roberts WN, Liang MH, Stern SH: Colchicine in acute gout: Reassessment of risks and benefits. JAMA 1987;257:1920. (Two percent mortality rate largely due to unguided use of intravenous colchicine.)

Wallace SL, Singer JZ: Review: Systemic toxicity associated with the intravenous administration of colchicine. Guidelines for use. J Rheumatol 1988;15:495.

2. CHONDROCALCINOSIS & PSEUDOGOUT (Calcium Pyrophosphate Dehydrate [CPPD] Deposition Disease)

The term chondrocalcinosis refers to the presence of calcium-containing salts in articular cartilage. It is most often first diagnosed radiologically. It may be familial and is commonly associated with a wide variety of metabolic disorders, eg, hemochromatosis, hyperparathyroidism, ochronosis, diabetes mellitus, hypothyroidism, Wilson's disease, and true gout. Pseudogout, most often seen in persons age 60 or older, is characterized by acute, recurrent and rarely chronic arthritis that usually involves large joints (principally the knees and the wrists) and is almost always accompanied by chondrocalcinosis of the affected joints. Identification of calcium pyrophosphate crystals in joint aspirates is diagnostic of pseudogout. Like the intraarticular urate crystals of gouty synovitis, calcium pyrophosphate crystals are believed to induce the synovitis of pseudogout. They may be seen with the ordinary light microscope but are best visualized under polarized light, in which they exhibit a positive birefringence; like gouty crystals, they may be intracellular or extracellular. X-ray examination shows not only calcification (usually symmetric) of cartilaginous structures but also signs of degenerative joint disease (osteoarthritis). Unlike gout, pseudogout is usually associated with normal serum urate levels and is not dramatically improved by colchicine.

Treatment of chondrocalcinosis is directed at the primary disease, if present. Some of the nonsteroidal anti-inflammatory agents (salicylates, indomethacin, naproxen, and other drugs) are helpful in the treatment of acute episodes of pseudogout. Colchicine may be of benefit. Aspiration of the inflamed joint and intraarticular injection of a hydrocortisone ester is also of value in resistant cases.

McCarty DJ: Arthritis associated with crystals containing calcium. Med Clin North Am 1986;70:437.

SERONEGATIVE SPONDYLOARTHROPATHIES

The diseases included under this heading are noted for onset usually before age 40, inflammatory arthritis of either the spine or the large peripheral joints, uveitis in a significant minority, a strong association with HLA-B27, and the absence of autoantibodies in the serum.

ANKYLOSING SPONDYLITIS

Essentials of Diagnosis

- Chronic low backache in young adults.
- Progressive limitation of back motion and of chest expansion.
- Transient (50%) or permanent (25%) peripheral arthritis.
- Diagnostic x-ray changes in sacroiliac joints.
- Uveitis in 20–25%. Accelerated erythrocyte sedimentation rate and negative serologic tests for rheumatoid factor.
- HLA-B27 usually positive.

General Considerations

Ankylosing spondylitis is a chronic inflammatory disease of the joints of the axial skeleton, manifested clinically by pain and progressive stiffening of the spine. The age at onset is usually in the late teens or early 20s. The incidence is greater in males than in females, and symptoms are more prominent in men, and ascending involvement of the spine is more likely to occur.

Clinical Findings

A. Symptoms and Signs: The onset is usually gradual, with intermittent bouts of back pain that may radiate down the thighs. As the disease advances, symptoms progress in a cephalad direction and back motion becomes limited, with the normal lumbar curve flattened and the thoracic curvature exaggerated. Atrophy of the trunk muscles is common. Chest expansion is often limited as a consequence of costovertebral joint involvement. Radicular symptoms due to the cauda equina syndrome may occur years after onset of the disease. In advanced cases, the entire spine becomes fused, allowing no motion in any direction. Transient acute arthritis of the peripheral joints occurs in about 50% of cases, and permanent changes in the peripheral joints—most commonly the hips, shoulders, and knees—are seen in about 25%.

Spondylitic heart disease, characterized chiefly by atrioventricular conduction defects and aortic insufficiency, occurs in 3–5% of patients with long-standing severe disease. Nongranulomatous anterior uveitis is associated in as many as 25% of cases and may be a presenting feature. Pulmonary fibrosis of the upper lobes, with progression to cavitation and bronchiectasis mimicking tuberculosis, may occur, characteristically long after the onset of skeletal symptoms. Constitutional symptoms similar to those of rheumatoid arthritis are absent in most patients.

B. Laboratory Findings: The erythrocyte sedimentation rate is elevated in 85% of cases, but serologic tests for rheumatoid factor are characteristically negative. There may be leukocytosis and anemia.

HLA-B27 is found in 90% of patients with ankylosing spondylitis, as opposed to 6–8% among normal individuals. These figures are lower in blacks. HLA-

B27 is found with greater than normal frequency in some other rheumatic diseases such as Reiter's syndrome, psoriasis, and inflammatory bowel disease. The incidence of B27 positivity is highest in ankylosing spondylitis. Because of the noted incidence of this antigen in the normal population, it is not an absolutely specific diagnostic test.

Persons with other rheumatic diseases such as rheumatoid arthritis, degenerative joint disease (osteoarthritis), and gout do not show a higher than normal incidence of HLA-B27.

C. Imaging: The earliest radiographic changes are usually in the sacroiliac joints. In the first few months of the disease process, the sacroiliac changes may be detectable only by CT scanning. Later, erosion and sclerosis of these joints are evident on regular radiographs. Later, involvement of the apophyseal joints of the spine, ossification of the annulus fibrosus, calcification of the anterior and lateral spinal ligaments, and squaring and generalized demineralization of the vertebral bodies may occur. The term "bamboo spine" has been used to describe the late radiographic changes.

Additional x-ray findings include periosteal new bone formation on the iliac crest, ischial tuberosities and calcanei, and alterations of the symphysis pubica and sternomanubrial joint similar to those of the sacroiliacs. Radiologic changes in peripheral joints, when present, tend to be asymmetric and lack the demineralization and erosions seen in rheumatoid arthritis.

Differential Diagnosis

Although rheumatoid arthritis may ultimately involve the spine, it does so characteristically in the cervical region, usually sparing the sacroiliac joints. Other features that differentiate ankylosing spondylitis from rheumatoid arthritis are the rare involvement of the small joints of the hands and feet, the absence of subcutaneous nodules, and the negative serologic tests for rheumatoid factor in spondylitis. The history and physical findings of ankylosing spondylitis serve to distinguish this disorder from other causes of low back pain such as disk disease, osteoporosis, soft tissue trauma, and tumors. The single most valuable distinguishing radiologic sign of ankylosing spondylitis is the appearance of the sacroiliac joints, although a similar pattern may be seen in Reiter's syndrome and in the arthritis associated with inflammatory intestinal diseases and psoriasis. In ankylosing hyperostosis (diffuse idiopathic skeletal hyperostosis [DISH], Forestier's disease), there is exuberant osteophyte formation. The osteophytes are thicker and more anterior than the syndesmophytes of ankylosing spondylitis, and the sacroiliac joints are not affected. The x-ray appearance of the sacroiliac joints in spondylitis should be distinguished from that in osteitis condensans ilii. In some geographic areas and in persons with appropriate occupations, brucellosis and fluoride

poisoning may be important in the differential diagnosis.

Treatment

A. Basic Program: In general, treatment is similar to that of rheumatoid arthritis. The importance of postural and breathing exercises should be stressed.

B. Drug Therapy: The nonsteroidal anti-inflammatory agents are employed in the treatment of this disorder. Of these, indomethacin appears to be the most effective, though it is not unreasonable to begin therapy with aspirin. The dosage of indomethacin is usually 25–50 mg 3 times a day, but the least amount should be used that will provide symptomatic improvement. Agents such as naproxen, fenoprofen, tolmetin, sulindac, piroxicam, and other newer NSAIDs are valuable alternatives and may even be used as primary therapy. Indomethacin may produce a variety of untoward reactions, including headache, giddiness, nausea and vomiting, peptic ulcer, renal insufficiency, depression, and psychosis.

C. Physical Therapy: See p 617.

Prognosis

Spontaneous remissions and relapses are common and may occur at any stage. Occasionally, the disease progresses to ankylosis of the entire spine. In general, the functional prognosis is good unless the hips are seriously involved and consequently ankylosed.

Kidd B et al: Disease expression of ankylosing spondylitis in males and females. J Rheumatol 1988;15:1407. (Axial disease more severe in men.)

Nissila M et al: Sulfasalazine in the treatment of ankylosing spondylitis. Arthritis Rheum 1988;31:1111. (Sulfasalazine moderately better than placebo.)

PSORIATIC ARTHRITIS

Essentials of Diagnosis

- Psoriasis precedes onset of arthritis in 80% of cases.
- Arthritis usually asymmetric, with "sausage" appearance of fingers and toes; resembles rheumatoid arthritis; rheumatoid factor is absent from serum.
- Sacroiliac joint involvement common; ankylosing spondylitis may be associated.
- X-ray findings: osteolysis; pencil-in-cup deformity; relative lack of osteoporosis; bony ankylosis; asymmetric sacroiliitis and atypical syndesmophytes.

General Considerations

In 15–20% of patients with psoriasis, arthritis coexists. The patterns or subsets of arthritis that may accompany psoriasis include the following:

(1) Joint disease that resembles rheumatoid arthritis in which polyarthritis is symmetric. Usually, fewer

joints are involved than in rheumatoid arthritis, and rheumatoid factor is absent from the serum.

(2) An oligoarticular form that may lead to considerable destruction of the affected joints.

(3) A pattern of disease in which the distal interphalangeal joints are primarily affected. Early, this may be monarticular, and often the joint involvement is asymmetric. Pitting of the nails and onycholysis are frequently associated.

(4) A severe deforming arthritis (arthritis mutilans) in which osteolysis is severe.

(5) A spondylitic form with sacroiliitis and spinal involvement predominating; 45% of these patients are HLA-B27 positive.

Clinical Findings

A. Symptoms and Signs: Although psoriasis usually precedes the onset of arthritis, in 20–25% of patients the arthritis precedes the skin disease. Arthritis is at least 5 times more common in patients with severe skin disease than in those with only mild skin findings. Occasionally, however, patients may have a single patch of psoriasis (typically hidden in the scalp, gluteal cleft, or umbilicus) and are unaware of it. Thus, a detailed search for cutaneous lesions is essential in patients with arthritis of new onset. Also, the psoriatic lesions may have cleared when arthritis appears—in such cases, the history is most useful. Nail pitting, a residue of previous psoriasis, is sometimes the only clue.

B. Laboratory Findings: Laboratory studies show an elevation of the sedimentation rate, but rheumatoid factor is not present. Uric acid levels may be high, reflecting the active turnover of skin affected by psoriasis. There is a correlation between the extent of psoriatic involvement and the level of uric acid, but gout is no more common than in patients without psoriasis. Desquamation of the skin may also reduce iron stores.

C. Imaging: Radiographic findings are most helpful in distinguishing the disease from other forms of arthritis. There are marginal erosions of bone and irregular destruction of joint and bone, which, in the phalanx, may give the appearance of a sharpened pencil. Fluffy periosteal new bone may be marked, especially at the insertion of muscles and ligaments into bone. Such changes will also be seen along the shafts of metacarpals, metatarsals, and phalanges. Paravertebral ossification occurs, which may be distinguished from ankylosing spondylitis by the absence of ossification in the anterior aspect of the spine.

Treatment

Treatment regimens are symptomatic. Nonsteroidal anti-inflammatory drugs are useful. Antimalarials may exacerbate the psoriasis. Gold therapy is often effective. In resistant cases, methotrexate has been used with some success, but it should be employed only by those fully conversant with its use. Successful treatment of the skin lesions commonly—though not invariably—is accompanied by an improvement in peripheral articular symptoms.

McHugh NJ et al: Psoriatic arthritis: Clinical subgroups and histocompatibility antigens. Ann Rheum Dis 1987;46:184.

Prognosis of psoriatic arthritis. (Editorial.) Lancet 1988; 2:375. (Forty percent have deforming, erosive arthritis; 11% are disabled.)

REITER'S SYNDROME

Reiter's syndrome is a clinical tetrad of unknown cause consisting of urethritis, conjunctivitis (or, less commonly, uveitis), mucocutaneous lesions, and arthritis. It occurs most commonly in young men. It may follow (within days or weeks) infection with *Chlamydia, Campylobacter, Salmonella,* or *Yersinia* and is usually accompanied by a systemic reaction, including fever. The arthritis is most commonly asymmetric and frequently involves the large weight-bearing joints (chiefly the knee and ankle); sacroiliitis or ankylosing spondylitis is observed in at least 20% of patients, especially after frequent recurrences. The mucocutaneous lesions may include balanitis, stomatitis, and keratoderma blenorrhagicum, resembling pustular psoriasis with involvement of the skin and nails. Carditis and aortic regurgitation may occur. While most signs of the disease disappear within days or weeks, the arthritis may persist for several months or even years. The test for HLA-B27 is positive in 80% of white patients, but these percentages are 20–30% lower in blacks. (See Chapter 14 for further discussion of HLA-B27.) Characteristically, the initial attack is self-limited and terminates spontaneously.

Recurrences involving any combination of the clinical manifestations are common and are sometimes followed by permanent sequelae, especially in the joints. X-ray signs of permanent or progressive joint disease may be seen in the sacroiliac as well as the peripheral joints.

Reiter's syndrome must be distinguished from gonococcal arthritis, especially when conjunctivitis has been mild or overlooked. Rheumatoid arthritis, idiopathic ankylosing spondylitis, and psoriatic arthritis must also be considered. Reiter's syndrome appears to be more common in patients infected with HIV and may precede or follow AIDS.

Treatment is symptomatic. Antibiotics are ineffective. As in psoriatic arthritis, the most useful drugs are the NSAIDs.

Granfors K et al: *Salmonella* lipopolysaccharide in synovial cells from patients with reactive arthritis. Lancet 1990;335:685.

Granfors K et al: *Yersinia* antigens in synovial-fluid cells from patients with reactive arthritis. N Engl J Med

1989;320:216. (Synovial fluid from 10 of 15 patients contained *Yersinia* antigens.)

ARTHRITIS & INFLAMMATORY INTESTINAL DISEASES

Arthritis is a common complication of ulcerative colitis, regional enteritis, and Whipple's disease. Occasionally, such joint disease is indistinguishable from rheumatoid arthritis and may represent a coincidence of the 2 disorders. More commonly, however, intestinal arthritis is asymmetric, affects large joints, parallels the course of the bowel disease, and rarely results in residual deformity. Articular symptoms may be prominent enough to cause the patient to overlook intestinal spasm. Ankylosing spondylitis, which may accompany inflammatory bowel disease, is indistinguishable from idiopathic ankylosing spondylitis and usually runs a course separate from bowel disease activity.

The synovitis is pathologically nonspecific. Rheumatoid factor is usually negative and HLA-B27 is often positive, and its presence may predispose to the development of spondylitis. Treatment of intestinal arthritis involves control of intestinal inflammation and use of supportive anti-inflammatory drugs; that of ankylosing spondylitis is the same as for idiopathic ankylosing spondylitis.

About 15% of patients who have jejunoileal bypass surgery for morbid obesity develop an inflammatory symmetric polyarticular disorder. The arthritis is usually acute in onset and nonmigratory and may affect the small as well as the large joints. The sedimentation rate is elevated, and antinuclear antibody and rheumatoid factor tests may be positive. Nonsteroidal anti-inflammatory agents are often effective, although some patients require prednisone.

Danzi JT: Extraintestinal manifestations of idiopathic inflammatory bowel disease. Arch Intern Med 1988; 148:297. (Review of the literature.)
Ratain JS, Hellmann DB: Colitic arthritis and spondylitis. In: *Current Management of Inflammatory Bowel Disease.* Bayless T (editor). Decker, 1989. (Reviews presentations and treatments.)

BEHÇET'S SYNDROME

Named after the Turkish dermatologist who first described it, this disease of unknown cause is characterized by recurrent oral and genital ulcers, uveitis, seronegative arthritis, and central nervous system abnormalities. Other features include ulcerative skin lesions, erythema nodosum, thrombophlebitis, and vasculitis. Arthritis occurs in about two-thirds of patients, most commonly affecting the knees and ankles. Keratitis, uveitis—often with hypopyon (pus in the anterior chamber)—and optic neuritis are observed.

The ocular involvement is often fulminant and may result in blindness. Involvement of the central nervous system often results in serious disability or death. Findings include cranial nerve palsies, convulsions, encephalitis, mental disturbances, and spinal cord lesions. Leukocytosis and a rapid sedimentation rate are common.

The clinical course may be chronic but is often characterized by remissions and exacerbations. Corticosteroids and immunomodulating drugs have been used with beneficial results.

Yazici H et al: A controlled trial of azathioprine in Behçet's syndrome. N Engl J Med 1990; 322:281. (More effective than placebo in preventing uveitis.)

RELAPSING POLYCHONDRITIS

This is a rare disease of unknown cause characterized by inflammatory destructive lesions of cartilaginous structures, principally the ears, nose, trachea, and larynx. It may be associated either with other immunologic disorders such as systemic lupus erythematosus, rheumatoid arthritis, or Hashimoto's thyroiditis or with cancers, especially multiple myeloma. The disease, which is usually episodic, affects males and females equally. The cartilage is painful, swollen, and tender during an attack and subsequently becomes atrophic, resulting in permanent deformity. Biopsy of the involved cartilage shows inflammation, loss of basophilia, and chondrolysis. Noncartilaginous manifestations of the disease include fever, episcleritis, uveitis, deafness, aortic insufficiency, and rarely immune complex-mediated renal disease. In 85% of patients, an arthropathy is seen that tends to be migratory, asymmetric, and seronegative, affecting both large and small joints and the parasternal articulation.

Corticosteroid therapy is often effective. Dapsone may also be effective, sparing the need for chronic high-dose corticosteroid treatment. Involvement of the tracheobronchial tree, leading to its collapse, may cause death if tracheostomy is not done promptly.

Michet CT et al: Relapsing polychondritis: Survival and predictive role of early disease manifestations. Ann Intern Med 1986;104:74. (Below age 51, saddle nose deformity or systemic vasculitis predicted poor outcome. For older patients, anemia predicted worse outcome.)

PALINDROMIC RHEUMATISM

Palindromic rheumatism is a disease of unknown cause characterized by frequent recurring attacks (at irregular intervals) of acutely inflamed joints. Periarticular pain with swelling and transient subcutaneous nodules may also occur. The attacks cease within several hours to several days. The knee and finger joints are most commonly affected, but any peripheral joint may be involved. Systemic manifestations other than fever do not occur. Although hundreds of attacks may take place over a period of years, there is no permanent articular damage. Laboratory findings are usually normal. Palindromic rheumatism must be distinguished from acute gouty arthritis and an atypical, acute onset of rheumatoid arthritis.

Symptomatic treatment is usually all that is required during the attacks. Hydroxychloroquine may be of value in preventing recurrences.

NEUROGENIC ARTHROPATHY
(Charcot's Joint)

Neurogenic arthropathy is joint destruction resulting from loss or diminution of proprioception, pain, and temperature perception. Although traditionally associated with tabes dorsalis, it is more frequently seen in diabetic neuropathy, syringomyelia, spinal cord injury, pernicious anemia, leprosy, and peripheral nerve injury. Prolonged administration of hydrocortisone by the intra-articular route may also cause Charcot's joint. As normal muscle tone and protective reflexes are lost, a marked secondary degenerative joint disease ensues; this results in an enlarged, boggy, painless joint with extensive erosion of cartilage, osteophyte formation, and multiple loose joint bodies. X-ray changes may be degenerative or hypertrophic in the same patient.

Treatment is directed against the primary disease; mechanical devices are used to assist in weight bearing and prevention of further trauma. In some instances, amputation becomes unavoidable.

ARTHRITIS IN SARCOIDOSIS

The frequency of arthritis among patients with sarcoidosis is variously reported between 10% and 35%. It is usually acute in onset, but articular symptoms may appear insidiously and often antedate other manifestations of the disease. Knees and ankles are most commonly involved, but any joint may be affected. Distribution of joint involvement is usually polyarticular and symmetric. The arthritis is commonly self-limiting after several weeks or months; infrequently, the arthritis is recurrent or chronic. Despite its occasional chronicity, the arthritis is rarely associated with joint destruction or significant deformity. Although sarcoid arthritis is often associated with erythema nodosum, the diagnosis is contingent upon the demonstration of other extra-articular manifestations of sarcoidosis and, notably, biopsy evidence of noncaseating granulomas. In chronic arthritis, x-ray shows rather typical changes in the bones of the extremities with intact cortex and cystic changes.

Treatment of arthritis in sarcoidosis is usually symptomatic and supportive. Colchicine may be of value. A short course of corticosteroids may be effective in patients with severe and progressive joint disease.

INFECTIOUS ARTHRITIS*

NONGONOCOCCAL ACUTE BACTERIAL (SEPTIC) ARTHRITIS

Essentials of Diagnosis
- Sudden onset of acute arthritis, usually monarticular, most often in large weight-bearing joints and wrists.
- Chills and fever. Joint fluid findings often diagnostic. Previous joint damage or intravenous drug abuse common risk factors.
- Infection with causative organisms commonly found elsewhere in body.

General Considerations
Nongonococcal acute bacterial arthritis is a disease of an abnormal host. The key risk factors are persistent bacteremia (eg, intravenous drug abuse, endocarditis) and damaged joints (eg, rheumatoid arthritis). *Staphylococcus aureus* is the most common cause of nongonococcal septic arthritis, followed by group A and group B streptococci. Gram-negative septic arthritis, once rare, has become more common, especially in intravenous drug abusers and in other immunocompromised hosts. *Escherichia coli* and *Pseudomonas aeruginosa* are the most common gram-negative isolates in adults.

The widespread use of arthroscopy and prosthetic joint surgery has also increased the frequency of septic arthritis. In the latter conditions, *Staphylococcus epidermidis* is the usual offending organism. Pathologic changes include varying degrees of acute inflammation, with synovitis, effusion, abscess formation in synovial or subchondral tissues, and, if treatment is not adequate, articular destruction.

Clinical Findings
A. Symptoms and Signs: The onset is usually sudden, with acute pain, swelling, and heat of one joint—most frequently the knee. Other commonly affected sites are the hip, wrist, shoulder, and ankle. Unusual sites, such as the sternoclavicular or sacroiliac joint, can be involved in intravenous drug abusers. Chills and fever are common but are absent in up to 20% of patients. Infection of the hip usually does not produce gross swelling but results in groin pain greatly aggravated by walking.

---

* Lyme disease is discussed in Chapter 27.

B. Laboratory Findings: Blood cultures are positive in approximately 50% of patients. The leukocyte count of the synovial fluid may be greater than 100,000/μL, with 90% or more polymorphonuclear cells. Synovial fluid sugar is usually low. Gram stain of the synovial fluid is positive in 75% of staphylococcal infections and in 50% of gram-negative infections.

C. Imaging: Radiographs are usually normal early in the disease, but evidence of demineralization may be present within days of onset. Bony erosions and narrowing of the joint space followed by osteomyelitis and periostitis may be seen within 2 weeks.

Differential Diagnosis

The septic course with chills and fever, the acute systemic reaction, the joint fluid findings, evidence of infection elsewhere in the body, and the response to appropriate antibiotics are diagnostic of bacterial arthritis. Gout and pseudogout are excluded by the failure to find crystals on synovial fluid analysis. Acute rheumatic fever and rheumatoid arthritis commonly involve many joints; Still's disease may mimic septic arthritis, but laboratory evidence of infection is absent. Pyogenic arthritis may be superimposed on other types of joint disease, notably rheumatoid arthritis, and must be excluded (by joint fluid examination) in any apparent acute relapse of the primary disease, particularly when a joint has been needled or one is more strikingly inflamed than the others.

Treatment

Prompt systemic antibiotic therapy of any septic arthritis should be based on the best clinical judgment of the causative organism and the results of smear and culture of joint fluid, blood, urine, or other specific sites of potential infection. If the organism cannot be determined clinically, treatment should be started with bactericidal antibiotics effective against staphylococci, pneumococci, and gram-negative organisms.

Frequent (even daily) local aspiration is indicated when synovial fluid rapidly reaccumulates and causes symptoms. Immediate surgical drainage is reserved for septic arthritis of the hip, because that site is inaccessible to repeated aspiration. For most other joints, surgical drainage is used only if medical therapy fails over 2–4 days to improve the fever and the synovial fluid volume, white blood count, and culture results. Pain can be relieved with local hot compresses and by immobilizing the joint with a splint or traction. Rest, immobilization, and elevation are used at the onset of treatment. Early active motion exercises within the limits of tolerance will hasten recovery.

Prognosis

With prompt antibiotic therapy, functional recovery is usually good. Bony alkalosis and articular destruction commonly occur if treatment is delayed or inadequate.

Cooper C, Cawley MI: Bacterial arthritis in an English health district: A 10-year review. Ann Rheum Dis 1986;45:458.

Goldenberg DL, Reed JI: Bacterial arthritis. N Engl J Med 1985;312:764.

Mozen PH, Zell SC: Sternoclavicular bacterial arthritis. West J Med 1988;148:310.

GONOCOCCAL ARTHRITIS

Essentials of Diagnosis
- Prodromal migratory polyarthralgias.
- Tenosynovitis most common sign.
- Purulent monarthritis in 50%.
- Characteristic skin rash.
- Most common in young women during menses or pregnancy.
- Symptoms of urethritis frequently absent.
- Dramatic response to antibiotics.

General Considerations

Disseminated gonococcal infection is the most common cause of infectious arthritis in large urban areas. In contrast to nongonococcal bacterial arthritis, gonococcal arthritis chiefly occurs in otherwise healthy individuals. Host factors, however, influence the expression of the disease: gonococcal arthritis is 2–3 times more common in women than in men, is especially common during menses and pregnancy, and is rare after age 40. Some of the signs of disseminated gonococcal infection may result from an immunologic reaction to nonviable fragments of the organism's cell wall; this may explain the frequent inability to culture organisms from skin and joint lesions. Recurrent disseminated gonococcal infection should prompt evaluation for a congenital deficiency of complement components, especially C7 and C8.

Clinical Findings

A. Symptoms and Signs: One to 4 days of migratory polyarthralgias involving the wrist, knee, ankle, or elbow is the most common initial course. Thereafter, 2 patterns emerge, one (60% of patients) characterized by tenosynovitis and the other (40%) by purulent monarthritis, most frequently involving the knee. Less than half of patients have fever, and less than one-fourth have any genitourinary symptoms. Most patients will have asymptomatic but highly characteristic skin lesions that usually consist of 2–10 small necrotic pustules distributed over the extremities, especially the palms and soles.

B. Laboratory Findings: The peripheral blood leukocyte count averages 10,400 cells/μL and is elevated in less than one-third of patients. The synovial fluid white blood cell count, however, averages over 50,000 cells/μL. The synovial fluid Gram stain is positive in one-fourth of cases and culture in less than half. Positive blood cultures are seen in 40%

of patients with tenosynovitis and virtually never in patients with suppurative arthritis. Urethral, throat, and rectal cultures should be done in all patients, since they are often positive in the absence of local symptoms. Culturing Neisseria gonorrhoeae is facilitated by rapid transport to the microbiology laboratory, inoculation on chocolate agar, and incubation in carbon dioxide.

C. Imaging: Radiographs are usually normal or show only soft tissue swelling.

Differential Diagnosis

Reiter's syndrome can also produce acute monarthritis in a young person but is distinguished by negative cultures, sacroiliitis, and failure to respond to antibiotics. Lyme disease involving the knee is less acute, does not show positive cultures, and may be preceded by known tick exposure and characteristic rash. The synovial fluid analysis will exclude gout, pseudogout, and nongonococcal bacterial arthritis. Rheumatic fever and sarcoidosis can produce migratory tenosynovitis but have other distinguishing features. Infective endocarditis with septic arthritis can mimic disseminated gonococcal infection.

Treatment

Patients suspected of having gonococcal arthritis should be admitted to the hospital to confirm the diagnosis and to start treatment. While outpatient treatment has been recommended in the past, the rapid rise in gonococci resistant to penicillin makes initial inpatient treatment necessary. Approximately 4–5% of all gonococcal isolates produce a β-lactamase that confers penicillin resistance. An additional 15–20% of gonococcal species have chromosomal mutations that result in relative resistance to penicillin. Therefore, the new recommendations for initial treatment of gonococcal arthritis are to give ceftriaxone, 1 g intravenously daily for 7–10 days. If the diagnosis of gonococcal arthritis and penicillin sensitivity are confirmed, amoxicillin, 500 mg orally 4 times a day, can be given on an outpatient basis to complete a 10- to 14-day course.

Prognosis

Generally, gonococcal arthritis responds dramatically in 24–48 hours after initiation of antibiotics so that daily joint aspirations are rarely needed. Complete recovery is the rule.

Goldenberg DL, Reed JI: Bacterial arthritis. N Engl J Med 1985;312:764.
O'Brien JP et al: Disseminated gonococcal infection: A prospective analysis of 49 patients and a review of pathophysiology and immune mechanisms. Medicine 1983; 62:395.

RHEUMATIC MANIFESTATIONS OF HIV INFECTION

Infection with human immunodeficiency virus (HIV) has been associated with various rheumatic disorders, most commonly Reiter's syndrome or reactive arthritis or arthralgias and more rarely myositis, psoriatic arthritis, Sjögren's syndrome, or vasculitis. It is possible that these disorders stem directly from HIV infection itself or from the many other infections that occur in immunodeficient patients. The rheumatic syndromes can follow or precede by several months the diagnosis of acquired AIDS. Thus, HIV infection must be considered as a possible cause of Reiter's syndrome, and Reiter's syndrome should be considered a possible early manifestation of HIV infection. The lower extremity joints, especially the knees and ankles, are most commonly affected. Often, as in classic Reiter's syndrome, Achilles tendon inflammation (enthesopathy) or knee periarthritis is a prominent and distinguishing feature. Many patients respond to NSAIDs, though a few are unresponsive and develop progressive deformities. The use of immunosuppressive agents, however, is contraindicated in these immunodeficient patients.

Berman A, et al: Rheumatic manifestations of human immunodeficiency virus infection. Am J Med 1988;85:59. (Prospective evaluation of 101 patients: arthralgias in 35, Reiter's syndrome in 10, psoriatic arthritis in 2, myositis in 2, and vasculitis in one.)
Espinoza LR et al: Rheumatic manifestations associated with human immunodeficiency virus infection. Arthritis Rheum 1989;32:1615. (Review of the literature.)

VIRAL ARTHRITIS

Arthritis may be a manifestation of many viral infections. It is generally mild and of short duration, and it terminates spontaneously without lasting ill effects. Mumps arthritis may occur in the absence of parotitis. Rubella arthritis, which occurs more commonly in adults than in children, may appear immediately before, during, or soon after the disappearance of the rash. Its usual polyarticular and symmetric distribution mimics that of rheumatoid arthritis. However, the seronegative tests for rheumatoid factor and the rising rubella titers in convalescent serum help to confirm the diagnosis. Post-rubella vaccination arthritis may have its onset as long as 6 weeks following vaccination and occurs in all age groups.

Polyarthritis may be associated with type B hepatitis and typically occurs before the onset of jaundice; it may occur in anicteric hepatitis as well. Urticaria or other types of skin rash may be present. Indeed, the clinical picture may be indistinguishable from that of serum sickness. Serum transaminase levels are elevated, and hepatitis B surface antigen is most often present. Serum complement levels are usually low during active arthritis and become normal after remission of arthritis. False-positive tests for rheumatoid factor, when present, disappear within several weeks. The arthritis is mild; it rarely lasts more than a few weeks and is self-limiting and without deformity.

Gear AJ et al: Rheumatoid arthritis, juvenile arthritis, iridocyclitis, and the Epstein-Barr virus. Ann Rheum Dis 1986;45:6.
Tingle AJ et al: Rubella-associated arthritis. 1. Comparative study of joint manifestations associated with natural rubella infection and RA 27/3 rubella immunisation. Ann Rheum Dis 1986;45:110.

INFECTIONS OF BONES

Direct microbial contamination of bones results from open fracture, surgical procedures, gunshot wounds, diagnostic needle aspirations, and therapeutic or self-administered drug injections.

Indirect or secondary infections are first noticed in other areas of the body and extend to bones by hematogenous routes.

ACUTE PYOGENIC OSTEOMYELITIS

Essentials of Diagnosis
- Fever and chills associated with pain and tenderness of involved bone.
- Aspiration of involved bone is usually diagnostic.
- Culture of blood or lesion tissue is essential for precise diagnosis.
- Radiographs early in the course are typically negative.

General Considerations
Initial bone infections are indirectly seeded by a single strain of pyogenic bacteria about 95% of the time. About 75% of hematogenous acute infections of bone are due to staphylococci; group A hemolytic streptococci are the next most common pathogens. Vertebral osteomyelitis, due to more indolent organisms, is being encountered with increasing frequency in elderly patients. Infections of bone due to trauma are often polymicrobial.

Salmonellae cause many cases of bacteremia associated with sickle cell disease. Among patients with hemoglobinopathies, osteomyelitis is caused by salmonellae almost 10 times as often as by other pyogenic bacteria. In otherwise healthy patients with salmonellosis, bone lesions are likely to be solitary. In typhoid fever, however, infections of bones occur as a complication in less than 1% of cases. (See Salmonellosis, Chapter 26.)

Bone infection is an uncommon complication of brucellosis, but the clinical picture when it does occur is characteristic. Bone lesions most commonly occur in the lumbar spine or sacroiliac joints.

Clinical Findings
A. Symptoms and Signs: The onset of acute osteomyelitis in adults is less likely to be striking than the sudden and alarming presentation often seen in children. Generalized toxic symptoms of bacteremia may be absent, and vague or evanescent local pain may be the earliest manifestation. Tenderness may be present or absent, depending upon the extent and duration of bone involvement.

B. Laboratory Findings: Aspiration of bone and periosteum to recover organisms for culture is necessary for accurate diagnosis. Blood cultures are frequently positive, particularly when systemic symptoms are prominent, in which case the white count and sedimentation rate are often elevated.

With infections due to *Salmonella* or *Brucella*, significant rising serologic agglutination titers support a tentative diagnosis during the acute stage. Culture of material from the osteoid focus is specific.

C. Imaging: Early findings may include soft tissue swelling, loss of tissue planes, and periarticular demineralization of bone. About 2 weeks after onset of symptoms, erosion of bone and alteration of cancellous bone appear, followed by periostitis. Radionuclide imaging is especially sensitive, becoming positive within 1–2 days after onset of acute osteomyelitis. CT scans and MRI are also more sensitive than conventional radiographs and are particularly helpful in demonstrating the extent of soft tissue involvement. When osteomyelitis involves the vertebrae, it commonly traverses the disk space—a finding that is not observed in tumor.

Differential Diagnosis
Acute hematogenous osteomyelitis should be distinguished from suppurative arthritis, rheumatic fever, and cellulitis. More subacute forms must be differentiated from tuberculous or mycotic infections of bone and Ewing's sarcoma or from metastatic tumor (vertebral osteomyelitis).

Complications
Inadequate treatment of bone infections results in chronicity of infection, and this possibility is increased by delay in diagnosis and treatment. Extension to adjacent bone or joints may complicate acute osteomyelitis. Recurrence of bone infections often results in anemia, weight loss, weakness, and, rarely, amyloidosis or nephrotic syndrome. Pseudoepitheliomatous hyperplasia, squamous cell carcinoma, or fibrosarcoma may occasionally arise in persistently infected tissues.

Treatment

Cultures and antibiotic sensitivity studies should determine the choice of antibiotic agents; the initial selection of drug is based on clinical assessment of the most probable cause. Open or closed drainage of the local lesion is important when prompt clinical response to initial treatment does not occur. Parenteral antibiotic therapy for acute osteomyelitis should be continued for a total of 4–6 weeks. Therapy is extended—often by the oral route—for patients with nosocomial infections and in those with risk factors for a poor response (eg, diabetes). Analgesics, rest, immobilization, and elevation of the part should be used from the beginning of treatment.

Prognosis

If sterility of the lesion is achieved within 2–4 days, a good result can be expected in most cases if there is no compromise of the patient's immune system. However, progression of the disease to a chronic form may occur. It is especially common in the lower extremities and in patients in whom circulation is impaired (eg, diabetics). Surgical saucerization, excision of bone, and debridement of healthy tissues are often necessary.

MYCOTIC INFECTIONS OF BONES & JOINTS

Fungal infections of the skeletal system are usually secondary to a primary infection in another organ, frequently the lungs (see Chapter 30). Although skeletal lesions have a predilection for the cancellous extremities of long bones and the bodies of vertebrae, the predominant lesion—a granuloma with varying degrees of necrosis and abscess formation—does not produce a characteristic clinical picture.

Differentiation from other chronic focal infections depends upon culture studies of synovial fluid or tissue obtained from the local lesion. Serologic tests and skin tests provide presumptive support of the diagnosis.

1. COCCIDIOIDOMYCOSIS

Coccidioidomycosis of bones and joints is usually secondary to primary pulmonary infection. Arthralgia with periarticular swelling, especially in the knees and ankles, occurring as a nonspecific manifestation of systemic coccidioidomycosis, should be distinguished from actual bone or joint infection. Osseous lesions commonly occur in cancellous bone of the vertebrae or near the ends of long bones. These lesions are initially osteolytic and thus may mimic metastatic tumor or myeloma.

The precise diagnosis depends upon recovery of *Coccidioides immitis* from the lesion or histologic examination of tissue obtained by open biopsy. Rising titers of IgA complement-fixing antibodies provide further evidence of the disseminated nature of the disease.

Ketoconazole has become the treatment of choice for bone and joint coccidioidomycosis. It is important to exclude concomitant meningeal infection, for which ketoconazole is ineffective. Chronic infection may require operative excision of infected bone and soft tissue; amputation may be the only solution for stubbornly progressive infections. Immobilization of joints by plaster casts and avoidance of weight bearing provide benefit. Synovectomy, joint debridement, and arthrodesis are reserved for more advanced joint infections.

2. HISTOPLASMOSIS

Focal skeletal or joint involvement in histoplasmosis is rare and generally represents dissemination from a primary focus in the lungs. Skeletal lesions may be single or multiple and are not characteristic.

TUBERCULOSIS OF BONES & JOINTS

Most tuberculous infections in the USA are caused by the human strain of *Mycobacterium tuberculosis* (see Chapter 7). Infection of the musculoskeletal system is caused by hematogenous spread from a primary lesion of the respiratory tract; it may occur shortly after primary infection or may be seen years later as a reactivation disease. Tuberculosis of the thoracic or lumbar spine (Pott's disease) may be associated with an active lesion of the genitourinary tract or may occur as an isolated finding. It is usually a disease of children in Third World nations and of the elderly in the United States. Tuberculous osteomyelitis secondary to cutaneous inoculation has been reported.

Clinical Findings

A. Symptoms and Signs: The onset of symptoms is generally insidious and not accompanied by general manifestations of fever, sweating, toxicity, or prostration. Pain may be mild at onset, is usually worse at night, and may be accompanied by stiffness. As the disease process progresses, limitation of joint motion becomes prominent because of muscle contractures and destruction of the joint. The knee is the most commonly involved peripheral joint. Symptoms of pulmonary tuberculosis may also be present.

Local findings during the early stages may be limited to tenderness, soft tissue swelling, joint effusion, and increase in skin temperature about the involved area. As the disease progresses without treatment, muscle atrophy and deformity become apparent. Abscess formation with spontaneous drainage externally leads to sinus formation. Progressive destruction of bone in the spine may cause a gibbus, especially in the thoracolumbar region.

B. Laboratory Findings: The precise diagnosis rests upon recovery of the acid-fast organism from joint fluid, pus, or tissue specimens. Biopsy of the bony lesion, synovium, or a regional lymph node may demonstrate the characteristic histopathologic picture of caseating necrosis and giant cells.

C. Imaging: There is a latent period between the onset of symptoms and the initial positive radiographic finding. The earliest changes of tuberculous arthritis are those of soft tissue swelling and distention of the capsule by effusion. Subsequently, bone atrophy causes thinning of the trabecular pattern, narrowing of the cortex, and enlargement of the medullary canal. As joint disease progresses, destruction of cartilage, both in the spine and in peripheral joints, is manifested by narrowing of the joint cleft and focal erosion of the articular surface, especially at the margins. Extensive destruction of joint surfaces causes deformity. As healing takes place, osteosclerosis becomes apparent around areas of necrosis and sequestration. Where the lesion is limited to bone, especially in the cancellous portion of the metaphysis, the x-ray picture may be that of single or multilocular cysts surrounded by sclerotic bone. As intraosseous foci expand toward the limiting cortex and erode it, subperiosteal new bone formation takes place. When bony tuberculosis is suspected, a chest film may be helpful in revealing characteristic pulmonary abnormalities even in the absence of symptoms.

Differential Diagnosis

Tuberculosis of the musculoskeletal system must be differentiated from all subacute and chronic infections, rheumatoid arthritis, gout, and, occasionally, osseous dysplasia. In the spine, metastatic tumor may be suggested.

Complications

Destruction of bones or joints may occur in a few weeks or months if adequate treatment is not provided. Deformity due to joint destruction, abscess formation with spread into adjacent soft tissues, and sinus formation are common. Paraplegia is the most serious complication of spinal tuberculosis. As healing of severe joint lesions takes place, spontaneous fibrous or bony ankylosis follows.

Treatment
(See also Chapter 7.)

A. General Measures: General care is especially important when prolonged recumbency is necessary; skillful nursing care must be provided.

B. Chemotherapy: Combinations of antituberculosis agents (eg, isoniazid and rifampin) are recommended. Cure without need for surgical intervention may be effected in most cases, even with extensive disease.

C. Surgical Measures: In acute infections where synovitis is the predominant feature, treatment can be conservative, at least initially: Immobilization by splint or plaster, aspiration, and chemotherapy may suffice to control the infection. This treatment is especially desirable for the management of infections of large joints of the lower extremities in children during the early stage of the infection. Synovectomy may be valuable for less acute hypertrophic lesions that involve tendon sheaths, bursae, or joints.

Alvarez S and McCabe WR: Extrapulmonary tuberculosis revisited: A review of experience at Boston City and other hospitals. Medicine 1984;63:25. (Nineteen percent of extrapulmonary tuberculosis involves spine (50%) or peripheral joints (knee 15%, hips 15%); chest x-ray abnormal in 35%.)

Garrido G et al: A review of peripheral tuberculous arthritis. Semin Arthritis Rheum 1988;18:142. (Ninety percent monarticular, knee most common site; 21% with extra-articular tuberculosis; fever in 10%; normal hematocrit and white blood cell count in 66%.)

PAIN SYNDROMES

CERVICOBRACHIAL PAIN SYNDROMES

A large group of articular and extra-articular disorders is characterized by pain that may involve simultaneously the neck, shoulder girdle, and upper extremity. Diagnostic differentiation is often difficult. Some of these entities and clinical syndromes represent primary disorders of the cervicobrachial region; others are local manifestations of systemic disease. The clinical picture is further complicated when 2 or more of these conditions occur coincidentally.

Clinical Findings

A. Symptoms and Signs: Neck pain may be limited to the posterior neck region or, depending upon the level of the symptomatic joint, may radiate segmentally to the occiput, anterior chest, shoulder girdle, arm, forearm, and hand. It may be intensified by active or passive neck motions. The general distribution of pain and paresthesias corresponds roughly to the involved dermatome in the upper extremity. Radiating pain in the upper extremity is often intensified by hyperextension of the neck and deviation of the head to the involved side. Limitation of cervical movements is the most common objective finding. Neurologic signs depend upon the extent of compression of nerve roots or the spinal cord. Compression of the spinal cord may cause long-tract involvement resulting in paraparesis or paraplegia.

B. Imaging: The radiographic findings depend on

the cause of the pain; many are completely normal. An early finding is loss of the normal anterior convexity of the cervical curve (loss of cervical lordosis). Comparative reduction in height of the involved disk space is a frequent finding. The most common late x-ray finding is osteophyte formation anteriorly, adjacent to the disk; other late changes occur around the apophyseal joint clefts, chiefly in the lower cervical spine. Computer-assisted myelography and MRI are valuable for demonstrating nerve root or spinal cord compression.

Differential Diagnosis & Treatment

The causes of neck pain include acute and chronic cervical strain or sprains, herniated nucleus pulposus, osteoarthritis, ankylosing spondylitis, rheumatoid arthritis, osteomyelitis, neoplasms, spinal stenosis, compression fractures, and functional disorders.

A. Acute or Chronic Cervical Musculotendinous Strain: Cervical strain is generally caused by mechanical postural disorders, overexertion, or injury (eg, whiplash). Acute episodes are associated with pain, decreased cervical spine motion, and paraspinal muscle spasm, resulting in stiffness of the neck and loss of motion. Muscle trigger points can often be localized. Management includes neck and head immobilization by traction, a cervical collar, and administration of analgesics. Gradual return to full activity is encouraged.

Patients with chronic symptoms often have few objective findings. Mechanical stress due to work or recreational activities is often implicated. Chronic pain, especially that radiating into the upper extremity, may require additional treatment such as bracing.

B. Herniated Nucleus Pulposus: Rupture or prolapse of the nucleus pulposus of the cervical disks into the spinal canal causes pain that radiates to the arms at the level of C6–7. When intra-abdominal pressure is increased by coughing, sneezing, or other movements, symptoms are aggravated, and cervical muscle spasm may often occur. Neurologic abnormalities may include decreased reflexes of the deep tendons of the biceps and triceps and decreased sensation and muscle atrophy or weakness in the forearm or hand. Cervical traction, bed rest, and other conservative measures are usually successful. Myelography or electromyography helps delineate lesions that may require surgical treatment (laminectomy, fusion).

C. Arthritic Disorders: Cervical spondylosis (degenerative arthritis) is a collective term describing degenerative changes that occur in the apophyseal joints and intervertebral disk joints, with or without neurologic signs. Osteoarthritis of the articular facets is characterized by progressive thinning of the cartilage, subchondral osteoporosis, and osteophytic proliferation around the joint margins. Degeneration of cervical disks and joints may occur in adolescents but is more common after age 40. Degeneration is progressive and is marked by gradual narrowing of

the disk space, as demonstrated by x-ray. Osteocartilaginous proliferation occurs around the margin of the vertebral body and gives rise to osteophytic ridges that may encroach upon the intervertebral foramens and spinal canal, causing compression of the neurovascular contents. A large anterior osteophyte may occasionally cause dysphagia.

Ankylosing spondylitis is discussed on p 598. Atlantoaxial subluxation may occur in patients with rheumatoid arthritis, regardless of the severity of disease. Inflammation of the synovial structures resulting from erosion and laxity of the transverse ligament can lead to neurologic signs of spinal cord compression. Treatment may vary from use of a cervical collar or more rigid bracing to operative treatment, depending on the degree of subluxation and neurologic progression. Surgical treatment may involve stabilization of the cervical spine.

D. Other Disorders: Osteomyelitis is discussed on p 605 and neoplasms on p 616. Osteoporosis is discussed in Chapter 20.

LOW BACK PAIN

The approach to the patient with nontraumatic low back pain is dictated by several observations. First, low back pain is exceedingly common, experienced at some time by up to 80% of the population. Second, the differential diagnosis of low back pain is broad and includes systemic diseases (eg, metastatic cancer), primary spine disease (eg, disk herniation, degenerative arthritis), and regional diseases (eg, aortic dissection) that refer pain to the low back. Third, a precise diagnosis cannot be made in the majority of cases. The frequent use of the terms "strain," "sprain," or "lumbago" underscores the common imprecision of diagnosis. Even when anatomic defects—such as vertebral osteophytes or a narrowed disk space—are present, clinical disease cannot be assumed since such "defects" are common in asymptomatic patients. Fourth, the great majority of patients will improve in 1–4 weeks with conservative therapy and need no evaluation beyond the initial history and physical examination. The diagnostic challenge, then, is to identify among the many sufferers of low back pain those few patients who require more extensive or urgent evaluation.

In practice this means identifying those patients who have "serious" disease, defined as (1) infection, (2) cancer, (3) inflammatory back disease such as ankylosing spondylitis, (4) important regional disease such as dissecting aortic aneurysm, or (5) significant or rapidly progressing neurologic deficits. If there is no evidence that the patient has any of these 5 problems, conservative therapy is called for.

1. CLINICAL APPROACH TO DIAGNOSIS

General History & Physical Examination

The single most common mistake in evaluating patients with low back pain is to concentrate on the back to the exclusion of a careful general history and physical examination. Yet it is in this very setting that the general history and physical examination are so important in detecting clues or "red flags" suggesting the presence of "serious" back disease. Low back pain is a final common pathway of many processes. The pain of vertebral osteomyelitis is not very different in quality and intensity from the pain due to back strain of the weekend gardener. The physician who concentrates on the back pain symptoms and neglects the general history risks missing the rare patient with low back pain needing further evaluation.

Specifically, the physician should note a history of smoking, weight loss, advanced age, and a history of cancer, all of which are risk factors for vertebral body metastasis. Vertebral body osteomyelitis most frequently occurs in adults with a history of recurrent urinary tract infections and is especially common in diabetics.

A history of peptic ulcer disease and prednisone therapy may be clues suggesting that a patient's refractory back pain is due to a perforated ulcer with retroperitoneal abscess. A history of rheumatic fever or other cardiac valvular lesions should raise concern that new back pain might represent endocarditis with microembolization of the vertebral bodies. Indeed, back pain is a not uncommon manifestation of endocarditis. A history of renal stones or neglected hypertension might indicate another serious cause of referred back pain.

The general physical examination is also of great importance, since elevated temperature or blood pressure, palpable lymph nodes, and abdominal, pelvic, or rectal masses would all be important indications that a patient's back pain has a serious cause.

History of the Back Pain

While most back pain is not distinctive, certain qualities of a patient's pain can indicate a specific diagnosis. Sciatica, characterized by low back pain radiating down the buttock and below the knee, suggest a herniated disk causing nerve root irritation. Other conditions—including sacroiliitis, facet joint degenerative arthritis, spinal stenosis, or irritation of the sciatic nerve from a wallet—can also cause sciatica.

The diagnosis of disk herniation is further suggested by physical examination (see below) and confirmed by imaging techniques. It should be emphasized that disk herniation can be asymptomatic, so that the mere presence of it on a scan does not always signify clinical disease.

Unrelenting low back pain at night, unrelieved by rest or the supine position, should suggest the possibility of malignancy, either vertebral body metastasis or a cauda equina tumor.

Symptoms of large or rapidly evolving **neurologic deficits** identify patients who need urgent evaluation for possible cauda equina tumor, epidural abscess, or, rarely, massive disk herniation. Severe neurologic symptoms with back pain are unusual and should prompt concern. Even with a herniated disk and nerve root impingement, pain is the most prominent symptom; numbness and weakness are less commonly reported and when present are of the magnitude consistent with compression of a single nerve root. Thus, symptoms of bilateral leg weakness (from multiple lumbar nerve root compressions) or of saddle area anesthesia, bowel or bladder incontinence, or impotence (indicating multiple sacral nerve root compressions) indicate an atypically large neurologic deficit requiring urgent evaluation.

Low back pain that **worsens with rest and improves with activity** is characteristic of ankylosing spondylitis or other seronegative spondyloarthropathies, especially when the onset is insidious and begins before age 40. Most degenerative back diseases produce precisely the opposite pattern, with rest alleviating and activity aggravating the pain.

Acute, **writhing** low back pain should suggest referred pain from an abdominal catastrophe such as an aortic dissection.

Low back pain associated with **pseudoclaudication** often indicates spinal stenosis. The typical patient is approximately 60 years old and is bothered less by back pain than by a discomfort occurring in the buttock, thigh, or leg that (like true claudication) is brought on by walking but (unlike claudication) can also be the elicited by prolonged standing. The discomfort is frequently bilateral. Classically, the pain is improved with rest or with flexion of the lumbar spine, which is why patients have less difficulty walking uphill than downhill. Some patients complain less about leg discomfort and more about an exercise-dependent weakness or unsteadiness of the legs—often described as "spaghetti legs" or the gait of a "drunken sailor."

Physical Examination of the Back

Although examination of the back usually does not suggest a specific cause, several physical findings should be sought because they do help identify those few patients who need more than just conservative management.

Neurologic examination of the lower extremities will detect the small deficits produced by disk disease and the large deficits complicating such problems as cauda equina tumors. A positive straight leg raising test indicates nerve root irritation. The examiner performs the test on the supine patient by passively raising the patient's leg. The test is positive if *radicular* pain is produced with the leg raised 60 degrees or less. The test is not specific but is 95% sensitive in patients with herniation at the L4–5 or L5–S1 level (the sites of 95% of disk herniations). It can be falsely negative, especially in patients with herniation above the L4–5 level.

The crossed straight leg sign is less sensitive but much more specific for disk herniation and is positive when raising the contralateral leg reproduces the sciatica.

Detailed examination of the sacral and lumbar nerve roots, especially L5 and S1, are essential for detecting neurologic deficits associated with back pain. Disk herniation produces deficits predictable for the site involved (Table 15–4). Deficits of multiple nerve roots suggest a cauda equina tumor, an epidural abscess, or some other important process that requires urgent evaluation and treatment.

Measurement of spinal motion in the patient with acute pain is rarely of diagnostic utility and usually simply confirms that pain limits motion. An exception to this general rule is that evidence of decreased range of motion in multiple regions of the spine (cervical, thoracic, and lumbar) indicates a diffuse spinal disease such as ankylosing spondylitis. But by the time the patient has such limits, the diagnosis is usually not a mystery.

If the back pain is not severe and does not itself limit motion, Schober's test of lumbar motion is helpful in early diagnosis of ankylosing spondylitis. To perform this test, 2 marks are made, one 10 cm S1 and another 5 cm below. The patient then bends forward as far as possible, and the distraction between the points is measured. Normally, the points distract at least 5 cm. Anything less indicates reduced lumbar motion, which in the absence of severe pain is most commonly due to ankylosing spondylitis or other seronegative spondyloarthropathies.

Palpation of the spine usually does not yield diagnostic information. Point tenderness over a vertebral body is reported to suggest osteomyelitis, but this association appears much tighter in dusty textbooks than in living patients. A step-off noted between the spinous process of adjacent vertebral bodies may indicate spondylolisthesis, but the sensitivity of this evidence is extremely low. Tenderness of the soft tissues

overlying the trochanter is a manifestation of trochanteric bursitis.

Inspection of the spine is not often of value in identifying serious causes of low back pain. The classic posture of ankylosing spondylitis is a late finding. Scoliosis of mild degree is not associated with an increased risk of clinical back disease. Cutaneous neurofibromas can identify the very rare patient who has nerve root encasement.

Examination of the hips should be part of the complete examination. While hip arthritis usually produces groin pain, some patients have buttock or low back symptoms.

Further Examination

If the history and physical examination do not suggest the presence of infection, cancer, inflammatory back disease, major neurologic deficits, or pain referred from abdominal or pelvic disease, further evaluation can be eliminated or deferred while conservative therapy is tried. The great majority of patients will spontaneously improve with conservative care over 1–4 weeks.

Regular radiographs of the lumbosacral spine give 20 times the radiation dose of a chest x-ray and provide limited, albeit important, information. X-rays can provide evidence of vertebral body osteomyelitis, cancer, fractures, or ankylosing spondylitis. Degenerative changes in the lumbar spine are ubiquitous in patients over 40 and do not prove clinical disease. Plain x-rays have very low sensitivity or specificity for disk disease. Thus, plain x-rays are warranted early for patients suspected of having infection, cancer, fractures, or inflammation and in other patients who fail to improve after 2–4 weeks of conservative therapy.

MRI and CT scans provide exquisite anatomic detail but should be reserved for patients in whom the information sought would call for a change in therapy. Clearly, sophisticated imaging is needed urgently in any patient suspected of having an epidural mass or cauda equina tumor. On the other hand, sophisticated imaging is not needed early in the course of a patient suspected of having a routine disk herniation. Since most such patients will improve over 4–6 weeks of conservative therapy, these imaging techniques should be reserved for patients who have failed conservative therapy and who are good surgical candidates. The relative merits of MRI versus CT scanning remain controversial.

Radionuclide bone scanning has limited utility in the evaluation of low back pain. It is most useful for early detection of vertebral body osteomyelitis or metastases. The bone scan is often normal in multiple myeloma.

Blood tests (eg, complete blood count, calcium, alkaline phosphatase, serum protein electrophoresis, sedimentation rate) and urinalysis should be performed early only on patients suspected of having

Table 15–4. Neurologic testing of lumbosacral nerve disorders.

Nerve Root	Motor	Reflex	Sensory Area
L4	Dorsiflexion of foot	Knee jerk	Medial calf
L5	Dorsiflexion of great toe	None	Medial forefoot
S1	Eversion of foot	Ankle jerk	Lateral foot

serious disease. Electrophysiologic testing can be useful in confirming the diagnosis of spinal stenosis.

2. MANAGEMENT

While any management plan must be individualized, key elements of most conservative treatments for back pain include rest, analgesia, and education. Recent studies suggest that 2 days of bed rest is (on average) just as effective as 7 days in achieving relief of acute sciatica, but individual patients vary greatly. Analgesia can usually be provided with nonsteroidal anti-inflammatory drugs, but severe pain may require opiates. Rarely does the need for opiates extend beyond 1–2 weeks, and opiates are contraindicated in the management of chronic low back pain.

Limited evidence supports the use of "muscle relaxants" such as diazepam, cyclobenzaprine, carisoprodol, and methocarbamol. These drugs should also be limited to courses of 1–2 weeks. Their use should be avoided in older patients, who are at risk of falling. All patients should be taught how to protect the back in daily activities—ie, not to lift heavy objects, to use the legs rather than the back when lifting, to use a chair with arm rests, and to arise from bed by first rolling to one side and then using the arms to push to an upright position. Physical therapists are excellent sources for patient education.

The value of corsets or traction is dubious. Back exercises are contraindicated during acute pain but may have some value in preventing recurrences.

Surgical consultation is needed urgently for any patient with a large or evolving neurologic deficit. Surgery for disk disease is indicated when there is documentation of herniation by some imaging procedure, a consistent pain syndrome, and a consistent neurologic deficit that has failed to respond to 4–6 weeks of conservative therapy.

Complaints of a tired and weak back with pain (not necessarily severe) and no objective findings may suggest a psychologic problem. Hysterical back pain may be severe and dramatically exaggerated. A history of domestic or work-related problems and observation of a flat affect with a bizarre reaction to treatment will further suggest the disorder. Treatment may include reassurance and judicious use of mild analgesics and sedatives. Chronicity of complaints is common, and psychiatric referral may be necessary.

The patient with compensatory back or neck pain may be interested in monetary gain, whereas the malingerer seeks a conscious real or imagined secondary gain. Subjective complaints in both types of patients are out of proportion to objective findings. The experienced clinician can often identify the malingerer or the patient with compensatory back or neck pain. These diagnostic impressions should not be conveyed to the patient. It is best to state simply that no organic disorder can be found that explains the patient's symptoms.

Deyo RA et al: Diagnostic imaging procedures for the lumbar spine. Ann Intern Med 1989;111:865. (Relative merits.)

Deyo RA et al: Herniated lumbar intervertebral disk. Ann Intern Med 1990;112:598. (Clinical picture and indications for surgery.)

Frymoyer JW: Back pain and sciatica. N Engl J Med 1988;318:291.

Hall S et al: Lumbar spinal stenosis: Clinical features diagnostic procedures and results of surgical treatment in 68 patients. Ann Intern Med 1985;103:271. (Pseudoclaudication is the most frequent presenting symptom (94%), is frequently bilateral, and is relieved by bending forward.)

Miller GM et al: Magnetic resonance imaging of the spine. Mayo Clin Proc 1989;64:986. (MRI useful, but intraspinal vascular malformations and leptomeningeal metastatic lesions are best seen with myelography.)

THORACIC OUTLET SYNDROMES

Thoracic outlet syndromes include those disorders that result in compression of the neurovascular structures supplying the upper extremity. Among them are cervical rib syndrome, costoclavicular syndrome, scalenus anticus and scalenus medius syndromes, pectoralis minor syndrome, "effort thrombosis" of the axillary and subclavian veins, and the subclavian steal syndrome. Patients often have a history of trauma to the head and neck areas.

Symptoms and signs may arise from intermittent or continuous pressure on elements of the brachial plexus and the subclavian or axillary vessels by a variety of anatomic structures of the shoulder girdle region. The neurovascular bundle can be compressed between the anterior or middle scalene muscles and a normal first thoracic rib or a cervical rib. Descent of the shoulder girdle may continue during adulthood and cause compression. Faulty posture, chronic illness, and occupation may be other predisposing factors. The components of the median nerve that encircle the axillary artery may cause compression and vascular symptoms. Sudden or repetitive strenuous physical activity may initiate "effort thrombosis" of the axillary or subclavian vein.

Pain may radiate from the point of compression to the base of the neck, the axilla, the shoulder girdle region, arm, forearm, and hand. Paresthesias are frequently present and are commonly distributed to the volar aspect of the fourth and fifth digits. Sensory symptoms may be aggravated at night or by prolonged use of the extremities. Weakness and muscle atrophy are the principal motor abnormalities. Vascular symptoms consist of arterial ischemia characterized by pallor of the fingers on elevation of the extremity, sensitivity to cold, and, rarely, gangrene of the digits or venous obstruction marked by edema, cyanosis, and engorgement.

Deep reflexes are usually not altered. When the site of compression is between the upper rib and clavicle, partial obliteration of subclavian artery pulsation may be demonstrated by abduction of the arm to a right angle with the elbow simultaneously flexed and rotated externally at the shoulder so that the entire extremity lies in the coronal plane. Neck or arm position has no effect on the diminished pulse, which remains constant in the subclavian steal syndrome.

Radiographic examination is helpful in differential diagnosis. Chest x-ray will identify patients with cervical rib. MRI with the arms held in different positions is useful in identifying sites of impaired blood flow. Intra-arterial or venous obstruction is confirmed by angiography. Determinations of the conduction velocities of the ulnar and other peripheral nerves of the upper extremity may help to localize the site of their compression.

Thoracic outlet syndrome must be differentiated from symptomatic osteoarthritis of the cervical spine, tumors of the cervical spinal cord or nerve roots, periarthritis of the shoulder, and other cervicobrachial pain syndromes.

Conservative treatment is directed toward relief of compression of the neurovascular bundle. The patient is instructed to avoid physical activities likely to precipitate or aggravate symptoms. Overhead pulley exercises are useful to improve posture. Shoulder bracing, although uncomfortable, provides a constant stimulus to improve posture. When lying down, the shoulder girdle should be bolstered by arranging pillows in an inverted "V" position.

Symptoms may disappear spontaneously or may be relieved by conservative treatment. Operative treatment is more likely to relieve the neurologic rather than the vascular component that causes symptoms.

SCAPULOHUMERAL CALCAREOUS TENDINITIS

Calcareous tendinitis of the shoulder joint is an acute or chronic inflammatory disorder of the capsulotendinous cuff (especially the supraspinatus portion) characterized by deposits of calcium salts among tendon fibers. It is a common cause of acute pain near the lateral aspect of the shoulder joint in men over age 30. The calcium deposit may be restricted to the tendon substance or may rupture into the overlying bursa.

Symptoms consist of pain (at times severe), tenderness to pressure, and restriction of shoulder joint motion.

Radiographic examination confirms the diagnosis and demonstrates the site of the lesion.

Calcareous tendinitis must be differentiated from other cervicobrachial pain syndromes, pyogenic ar-

thritis, osteoarthritis, gout, Pancoast tumors, and tears of the rotator cuff.

The aim of treatment is to relieve pain and restore shoulder joint function. Pain is best treated by injection of the lesion with a local anesthetic with corticosteroid. After treatment, early recovery of shoulder joint function should be fostered by supervised exercises. NSAIDs are also effective. Acute symptoms occasionally subside after spontaneous rupture of the calcium deposit into the subacromial bursa. Chronic symptoms may be treated by analgesics, exercises, and injection of local anesthetics with 20–40 mg of triamcinolone; repeated injections should be avoided. Rarely, calcific deposits may require surgical evacuation.

When x-ray examination shows that a deposit has disappeared, recurrence of that deposit is rare. Symptoms of periarthritis may persist if shoulder joint motion is not completely regained.

Craig EV (editor): The shoulder. Orthopedics 1988;11:37. (Entire issue.)

Petri et al: Randomized, double-blind, placebo-controlled study of the treatment of the painful shoulder. Arthritis Rheum 1987;30:1040. (Both triamcinolone and naproxen are superior to placebo.)

SCAPULOHUMERAL PERIARTHRITIS (Adhesive Capsulitis, Frozen Shoulder)

Periarthritis of the shoulder joint is an inflammatory disorder primarily involving the soft tissues. The condition may be divided into a primary type, in which no obvious cause can be identified, and a secondary type associated with an organic lesion (eg, rheumatoid arthritis, osteoarthritis, fracture or dislocation). The primary type is most common among women after the fourth decade. It may be manifested as inflammation of the articular synovia, the tendons around the joint, the intrinsic ligamentous capsular bands, the paratendinous bursae (especially the subacromial), or the bicipital tendon sheath. Calcareous tendinitis and attritional disease of the rotator cuff, with or without tears, are incidental lesions.

The onset of pain, which is aggravated by extremes of shoulder joint motion, may be acute or insidious. Pain may be most annoying at night and may be intensified by pressure on the involved extremity when the patient sleeps in the lateral decubitus position. Tenderness upon palpation is often noted near the tendinous insertions into the greater tuberosity or over the bicipital groove. Although a sensation of stiffness may be noted only at onset, restriction of shoulder joint motion soon becomes apparent and is likely to progress unless effective treatment is instituted.

Pain can usually be controlled with nonsteroidal anti-inflammatory agents. Passive exercise of the shoulder by an overhead pulley mechanism should be repeated slowly for about 2 minutes 4 times daily. Forceful manipulation of the shoulder joint during this exercise should be avoided. Injection of tender areas with corticosteroids gives transitory relief. Operative treatment should be reserved for the occasional refractory case.

Chard MD, Hazleman BL: Shoulder disorders in the elderly: A hospital study. Ann Rheum Dis 1987;46:684.

EPICONDYLITIS
(Tennis Elbow, Epicondylalgia)

Epicondylitis is a pain syndrome affecting the mid portion of the upper extremity; no single causative lesion has been identified. It has been postulated that chronic strain of the forearm muscles due to repetitive grasping or rotatory motions of the forearm causes microscopic tears and subsequent chronic inflammation of the common extensor or common flexor tendon at or near their respective osseous origins from the epicondyles.

Epicondylitis occurs most frequently in the dominant extremity during middle life. Pain is predominantly on the medial or lateral aspect of the elbow region, may be aggravated by grasping, and may radiate proximally into the arm or distally into the forearm. The point of maximal tenderness to pressure is 1–2 cm distal to the epicondyle but may also be present in the muscle bellies more distally. Resisted dorsiflexion or volar flexion of the wrist may accentuate the pain. X-ray examination generally reveals no significant change.

Treatment is directed toward relief of pain. Most symptoms can be relieved by rest and mild analgesics. An elastic bandage applied about the proximal forearm may ameliorate discomfort when the patient is grasping forcefully. Infiltration of "trigger points" by local anesthetic solutions with corticosteroids may be helpful. Operative treatment is reserved for severe, refractory cases.

FIBROSITIS

Essentials of Diagnosis

- Chronic widespread musculoskeletal pain syndrome with multiple tender points.
- Fatigue, headaches, numbness common.
- Most frequent in women aged 20–50.
- Objective signs of inflammation absent. No specific laboratory or diagnostic test.
- Partially responsive to exercise, amitriptyline.

General Considerations

Fibrositis is one of the most common rheumatic syndromes in ambulatory general medicine. It shares many features with the chronic fatigue syndrome,

namely, an increased frequency among women aged 20–50, absence of objective findings, and absence of diagnostic laboratory tests. While many of the clinical features of the 2 conditions overlap, musculoskeletal pain predominates in fibrositis whereas fatigue dominates the chronic fatigue syndrome.

The cause is unknown, but sleep disorders, hysteria, depression, and viral infections have all been proposed. Subtle histochemical abnormalities in muscle biopsies have been identified and await confirmation. Fibrositis can be a complication of hypothyroidism or rheumatoid arthritis.

Clinical Findings

A. Symptoms and Signs: The typical patient is a premenopausal woman with chronic aching pain and stiffness, frequently involving the entire body but with prominence of pain around the neck, shoulders, low back, and hips. Fatigue, sleep disorders, subjective numbness, chronic headaches, and irritable bowel symptoms are common. The patient feels incapable of performing normal activities, and even minor exertion aggravates pain and increases fatigue. Patients occasionally trace the onset of symptoms to an acute event or viral-like illness. Physical examination is normal except for "trigger points" of pain produced by palpation of various areas such as the trapezius, the medial fat pad of the knee, and the lateral epicondyle of the elbow.

B. Laboratory Findings: There are no laboratory abnormalities in primary fibrositis.

Differential Diagnosis

Fibrositis is a diagnosis of exclusion. A detailed history and physical examination can obviate the need for extensive laboratory testing. Rheumatoid arthritis and systemic lupus erythematosus virtually always present with objective physical findings or abnormalities on routine testing, including the erythrocyte sedimentation rate. Thyroid function tests are useful, since hypothyroidism can produce a secondary fibromyalgia syndrome. Polymyositis usually produces weakness rather than pain. The diagnosis of fibrositis probably should not be made in a patient over age 50 and should never be invoked to explain fever, weight loss, or any other objective signs. Polymyalgia rheumatica produces shoulder and girdle pain, is associated with anemia and an elevated sedimentation rate, and occurs after age 50.

Treatment

Patient education is of paramount importance. Patients can be comforted by the knowledge that they have a recognizable diagnosable syndrome that can be managed by means of specific though imperfect therapies and that the course is not progressive. Placebo-controlled trials have demonstrated modest efficacy of amitriptyline or cyclobenzaprine, 10 mg at bedtime initially and gradually increasing to 40–50 mg depending on efficacy and toxicity. Exercise programs are also beneficial. NSAIDs are generally ineffective. Opiates and corticosteroids are ineffective and should never be used to treat fibrositis.

Prognosis

Most patients have chronic symptoms. With treatment, however, many do eventually resume increased activities. Progressive or objective findings do not develop.

Goldenberg DL: Fibromyalgia syndrome: An emerging but controversial condition. JAMA 1987;257:2782. (Proposes a practical, noninvasive outpatient evaluation and a conservative approach to therapy.)

Wolfe F et al: The American College of Rheumatology 1990 criteria for the classification of fibromyalgia. Arthritis Rheum 1990;33:160. (The combination of widespread musculoskeletal pain and multiple trigger points is 88% sensitive and 81% specific for the diagnosis of fibromyalgia.)

CARPAL TUNNEL SYNDROME

Carpal tunnel syndrome is a common painful disorder caused by compression of the median nerve between the carpal ligament and other structures within the carpal tunnel (entrapment neuropathy). The volume of the contents of the tunnel can be increased by organic lesions such as synovitis of the tendon sheaths or carpal joints, recent or malhealed fractures, tumors, and occasionally congenital anomalies. Even though no anatomic lesion is apparent, flattening or even circumferential constriction of the median nerve may be observed during operative section of the ligament. The disorder may occur in pregnancy and is seen in individuals with a history of repetitive use of the hands, and it may follow injuries of the wrists. A familial type of carpal tunnel syndrome has been reported in which no etiologic factor can be identified.

Carpal tunnel syndrome can also be a feature of many systemic diseases: rheumatoid arthritis and other rheumatic disorders (inflammatory tenosynovitis); myxedema, amyloidosis, sarcoidosis, and leukemia (tissue infiltration); acromegaly; hyperparathyroidism, hypocalcemia, and diabetes mellitus.

Clinical Findings

Pain in the distribution of the median nerve, which may be burning and tingling (acroparesthesia), is the initial symptom. Aching pain may radiate proximally into the forearm and occasionally proximally to the shoulder, neck, and chest. Pain is exacerbated by manual activity, particularly by extremes of volar flexion or dorsiflexion of the wrist. It may be most bothersome at night. Impairment of sensation in the median nerve distribution may not be apparent. Subtle disparity between the affected and opposite sides can be demonstrated by testing for 2-point discrimination

or by requiring the patient to identify different textures of cloth by rubbing them between the tips of the thumb and the index finger. Tinel's or Phalen's sign may be positive. (Tinel's sign is tingling or shocklike pain on volar wrist percussion; Phalen's sign, pain or paresthesia in the distribution of the median nerve when the patient flexes both wrists to 90 degrees with the dorsal aspects of the hands held in apposition for 60 seconds.) Muscle weakness or atrophy, especially of the abductor pollicis brevis, appears later than sensory disturbances. Useful special examinations include electromyography and determinations of segmental sensory and motor conduction delay. Distal median sensory conduction delay may be evident before motor delay.

Differential Diagnosis

This syndrome should be differentiated from other cervicobrachial pain syndromes, from compression syndromes of the median nerve in the forearm or arm, and from mononeuritis multiplex. When left-sided, it may be confused with angina pectoris.

Treatment

Treatment is directed toward relief of pressure on the median nerve. When a primary lesion is discovered, specific treatment should be given. When soft tissue swelling is a cause, elevation of the extremity may relieve symptoms. Splinting of the hand and forearm at night may be beneficial. When nonspecific inflammation of the ulnar bursa is thought to be a cause, injection of corticosteroids into the carpal tunnel may be helpful.

Operative division of the volar carpal ligament gives lasting relief from pain, which usually subsides within a few days. Muscle strength returns gradually, but complete recovery cannot be expected when atrophy is pronounced.

Katz JN et al: The carpal tunnel syndrome: Diagnostic utility of the history and physical examination findings. Ann Intern Med 1990;112:321. (Positive Tinel's sign or Phalen's sign had positive predictive value of approximately 0.50 and negative predictive value of 0.70.)

DUPUYTREN'S CONTRACTURE

This relatively common disorder is characterized by hyperplasia of the palmar fascia and related structures, with nodule formation and contracture of the palmar fascia. The cause is unknown, but the condition has a genetic predisposition and occurs primarily in white men over 50 years of age. The incidence of Dupuytren's contracture is higher among alcoholics and patients with chronic systemic disorders (eg, cirrhosis, diabetes, epilepsy, tuberculosis). The onset may be acute, but slowly progressive chronic disease is more common.

Dupuytren's contracture manifests itself by nodular or cordlike thickening of one or both hands, with the fourth and fifth fingers most commonly affected. The patient may complain of tightness of the involved digits, with inability to satisfactorily extend the fingers, and on occasion there is tenderness. The resulting functional and cosmetic problems may be extremely disabling. Fasciitis involving other areas of the body may lead to plantar fibromatosis (10% of patients) or Peyronie's disease (1–2%).

Periodic examination of patients in early stages of disease is recommended. If the palmar nodule is growing rapidly, injections of triamcinolone into the nodule may be of benefit. Surgical intervention is indicated in patients with significant flexion contractures, depending on the location, but recurrence is not uncommon.

Bradlow A, Mowat AG: Dupuytren's contracture and alcohol. Ann Rheum Dis 1986;45:304.

REFLEX SYMPATHETIC DYSTROPHY

Reflex sympathetic dystrophy is a syndrome of pain and swelling of an extremity accompanied by signs of trophic skin changes in the extremity (eg, skin atrophy, hyperhidrosis) and signs and symptoms of vasomotor instability. Any extremity can be involved, but the disorder most commonly occurs in the hand and is associated with ipsilateral restricted shoulder motion (shoulder-hand syndrome). The swelling in reflex sympathetic dystrophy is diffuse ("catcher's mitt hand") and not restricted to joints. Pain is often described as burning in quality. The shoulder-hand variant of reflex sympathetic dystrophy is common after neck or shoulder injuries or following myocardial infarction. Direct trauma to the hand or foot can also provoke this syndrome. There are no systemic symptoms, and x-rays reveal severe generalized osteopenia. Bone scans also show increased uptake. In a significant minority of cases, symptoms and findings are evident bilaterally.

This syndrome should be differentiated from other cervicobrachial pain syndromes, rheumatoid arthritis, polymyositis, scleroderma, and gout.

In addition to specific treatment of the underlying disorder, treatment is directed toward restoration of function. For most patients, physical therapy is the cornerstone of treatment. Patients who have restricted shoulder motion may benefit from the treatment described for scapulohumeral periarthritis. In resistant cases, prednisone, 30–40 mg/d for 2 weeks and then tapered off over 2 weeks, may be effective.

The prognosis depends in part upon the stage in which the lesions are encountered and the extent and severity of associated organic disease. Early treatment offers the best prognosis for recovery.

BURSITIS

Inflammation of the synovium-like cellular membrane overlying bony prominences may be secondary to trauma, infection, or arthritic conditions. The most common locations are the subdeltoid, olecranon, ischial, and prepatellar bursae. Clinically and anatomically, this syndrome can be differentiated from adjacent inflammatory disorders of tendons, and the attacks may suggest an arthritic process. On occasion, calcific deposits are noted on x-rays of the involved bursae.

Various methods of treatment have been used, including local heat, immobilization, analgesics, nonsteroidal anti-inflammatory agents, and local steroid injections. Infected bursae usually require surgical drainage or aspiration and antibiotic therapy.

Larsson LG, Baum J: The syndromes of bursitis. Bull Rheum Dis 1986;36:1.

JOGGING INJURIES

The beneficial effects on cardiovascular function and the sense of well-being associated with aerobic activity have led to considerable enthusiasm for jogging and running. This has resulted in a large number of musculoskeletal injuries, which are estimated to occur in about 75% of runners. In addition, osteoporosis, hematuria, heat stroke, exercise-induced ectopy, and even death have occurred as consequences of running.

Many of the deleterious effects can be prevented by appropriate precautions, such as stretching exercises, proper footwear, avoidance of overexertion, and prompt attention to injuries. After an injury has healed, a graduated schedule for returning to training is necessary to avoid recurrence. Since injuries occur frequently in long-distance runners, it is most important that these individuals avoid overexertion, and, when early signs of injury appear, reduce the amount of distance run. The psychologic effects of complete inactivation in athletes whose identity is intimately tied to their sport should be recognized and addressed, since severe depression may develop in such circumstances.

Zarins B and Adams M: Knee injuries in sports. N Engl J Med 1988;318:950. (Epidemiology, biomechanics, diagnosis, and treatment of knee injuries in sports.)

TUMORS & TUMORLIKE LESIONS OF BONE

Essentials of Diagnosis

- Persistent pain, swelling, or tenderness of a skeletal part. Pathologic ("spontaneous") fractures.
- Suspicious areas of bony enlargement, deformity, radiodensity, or radiolucency on x-ray.
- Histologic evidence of bone neoplasm on biopsy specimen.

General Considerations

Primary tumors of bone are relatively uncommon in comparison with secondary or metastatic neoplasms. They are, however, of great clinical significance because of the possibility of cancer and because some of them grow rapidly and metastasize widely.

Although tumors of bone have been categorized classically as primary or secondary, there is some disagreement about which tumors are primary to the skeleton. Tumors of mesenchymal origin that reflect skeletal tissues (eg, bone, cartilage, and connective tissue) and tumors developing in bones that are of hematopoietic, nerve, vascular, fat cell, and notochordal origin should be differentiated from secondary malignant tumors that involve bone by direct extension or hematogenous spread. Because of the great variety of bone tumors, it is difficult to establish a satisfactory simple classification of bone neoplasms.

Clinical Findings

Persistent skeletal pain and swelling, with or without limitation of motion of adjacent joints or spontaneous fracture, are indications for prompt clinical, x-ray, laboratory, and possibly biopsy examination. X-rays may reveal the location and extent of the lesion and certain characteristics that may suggest the specific diagnosis. The so-called classic x-ray findings of certain tumors (eg, punched-out areas of the skull in multiple myeloma, "sun ray" appearance of osteogenic sarcoma, and "onion peel" effect of Ewing's sarcoma), although suggestive, are not pathognomonic. Even histologic characteristics of the tumor, when taken alone, cannot provide infallible information about the nature of the process. The age of the patient, the duration of complaints, the site of involvement and the number of bones involved, and the presence or absence of associated systemic disease—as well as the histologic characteristics—must be considered collectively for proper management.

The possibility of benign developmental skeletal abnormalities, metastatic neoplastic disease, infections (eg, osteomyelitis), posttraumatic bone lesions, or metabolic disease of bone must always be kept in mind. If bone tumors occur in or near the joints, they may be confused with the various types of arthritis, especially monarticular arthritis.

Specific Bone Tumors

Tumors arising from osteoblastic connective tissue include osteoid osteoma and osteogenic sarcoma. Osteoid osteomas are benign tumors of children and adolescents that should be surgically removed. Osteogenic sarcomas usually involve the knees or long bones and are treated by resection and chemotherapy, with improving survival in recent years. Fibrosarcomas, which are derived from nonosteoblastic connective tissue, have an outlook similar to that of the osteogenic sarcomas. Tumors derived from cartilage include enchondromas, chondromyxoid fibromas, and chondrosarcomas. Histologic examination is confirmatory in this group, and the outlook with appropriate curettement or surgery is generally good.

Other bone tumors include giant cell tumors (osteoclastomas), chondroblastomas, and Ewing's sarcoma. Of these, chondroblastomas are almost always benign. About 50% of giant cell tumors are benign, while the rest may be frankly malignant or recur after excision. Ewing's sarcoma, which affects children, adolescents, and young adults, has a 50% mortality rate in spite of chemotherapy, irradiation, and surgery.

Treatment

Although prompt action is essential for optimal treatment of certain bone tumors, accurate diagnosis is required because of the great potential for harm that may result either from temporization or from radical or ablative operations or unnecessary irradiation.

Brown KT et al: Computed tomography analysis of bone tumors: Patterns of cortical destruction and soft tissue extension. Skeletal Radiol 1986;15:448.

Sim FH et al: Osteosarcoma: State of the art. Minn Med 1986;69:42.

OTHER DISORDERS OF BONES & JOINTS

OSTEOGENESIS IMPERFECTA (Fragilitas Ossium, Brittle Bones)

Osteogenesis imperfecta is a heritable disorder of connective tissue usually transmitted as an autosomal dominant, although some cases may be autosomal recessive. Two recognized clinical types may occur: osteogenesis imperfecta congenita (fetal type), in which fractures occur in utero and skeletal deformities are apparent at birth; and osteogenesis imperfecta tarda, in which fractures and deformities occur after birth. Fragility of bones is the single most obvious diagnostic criterion. Clearness or blue coloration of the scleras, conduction deafness, and spinal deformities (scoliosis and kyphosis) are often present. Milder cases of the late form may simulate idiopathic juvenile or menopausal osteoporosis. Unfortunately, there is no treatment for the inadequate formation of osteoid.

RHEUMATIC MANIFESTATIONS OF CANCER

Rheumatologic syndromes may be the presenting manifestations for a variety of cancers. Dermatomyositis in adults, for example, is not infrequently associated with cancer. Middle-aged or older patients with polyarthritis that mimics rheumatoid arthritis but is associated with new onset of clubbing and periosteal new bone formation should be suspected of having hypertrophic pulmonary osteoarthropathy, a disorder commonly associated with both malignant diseases (eg, lung and intrathoracic cancers) and nonmalignant ones (eg, cyanotic heart disease, cirrhosis, and lung abscess). Palmar fasciitis is characterized by bilateral palmar swelling and finger contraction and may be the first indication of cancer, particularly ovarian carcinoma. Occasionally, occult cancers produce a polymyalgia rheumatica-like syndrome that uncharacteristically does not respond to low doses of corticosteroids. Palpable purpura due to leukocytoclastic vasculitis may be the presenting complaint in myeloproliferative disorders. Hairy cell leukemia can be associated with medium-sized vessel vasculitis such as polyarteritis nodosa. Acute leukemia can produce joint pains that are disproportionately severe in comparison to the minimal swelling and heat that are present.

AVASCULAR NECROSIS OF BONE

Avascular necrosis of bone is a complication of corticosteroid use, trauma, systemic lupus erythematosus, pancreatitis, alcoholism, gout, sickle cell disease, infiltrative diseases (eg, Gaucher's disease), and caisson disease. The most commonly affected sites are the proximal and distal femoral heads, leading to hip or knee pain. Many patients with hip disease actually first present with referred knee pain. Physical examination will disclose that it is internal rotation of the hip—not movement of the knee—that is painful. Other commonly affected sites include the ankle, shoulder, and elbow. Initially, plain x-rays are often normal; MRI, CT scan, and bone scan are all more sensitive techniques. Treatment involves avoidance of weight bearing on the affected joint for several weeks at least. The merit of surgical core decompression is controversial.

Felson DT and Anderson JJ: Across-study evaluation of association between steroid dose and bolus steroids and avascular necrosis of bone. Lancet 1987;1:901. (Strong correlation between total daily dose and risk of avascular necrosis; no correlation of risk with bolus corticosteroids.)

GENERAL PRINCIPLES IN THE PHYSICAL & SURGICAL MANAGEMENT OF ARTHRITIC JOINTS

Proper physical management of arthritic joints can improve patient comfort and help preserve joint and muscle function and total well-being. In order to obtain optimal results, as well as to conserve financial resources and time, it is important for the physician to be as specific as possible in instructions to the patient or to the occupational and physical therapists conducting treatment.

Exercise

A. Passive Range of Motion: Since someone other than the patient puts the joints through the range of motion once or twice daily, the patient is not directly involved and maintenance of muscle tone is not assisted. Passive exercises should be ordered infrequently and only for specific purposes.

B. Active Range of Motion: This type of exercise requires the patient to actively contract the muscles in order to put joints through the range of motion. The prescribed motions should be repeated 3–10 times once or twice daily. Such active exercise should be encouraged, since it involves the patient, costs no money, protects joint motion, and assists in maintaining muscle tone.

C. Isometric Exercise: With this type of exercise the muscle is contracted but not shortened, while the joint is minimally moved, for 3–10 repetitions several times daily. This maintains or even increases muscle strength and tone; the patient is involved; joint use is minimal; and the cost is nil. Isometric exercise should be used to supplement passive or active range-of-motion exercises.

D. Isotonic Exercise: In isotonic exercise, the muscle is contracted and shortened and the joint is maximally moved and stressed. This type of exercise should seldom be used (see below).

E. Hydrotherapy: The buoyancy of water permits maximum isotonic and isometric exercise with no more stress on joints than active range-of-motion exercises. Although ideal for arthritic patients, its cost often precludes use and it is generally prescribed only for specific short-term goals.

F. Active-Assistive Exercise: The therapist provides direct supervision, physical support, and exercise guidance. Although this is ideal for arthritic patients, cost again often precludes its use except for specific short-term goals. A member of the family may be taught to assist the patient in exercises on a long-term basis.

Any exercise in the arthritic patient may be associated with some pain, but pain lasting for hours after exercise is an indication for a change in the duration or type of exercise.

Heat, Cold, & Massage

A. Heat: Most patients with chronic arthritis find that some form of heat gives temporary muscle relaxation and relief of pain. Generally, moist heat is more effective than electric pads or heat lamps. Tub baths may require bar supports for ease of entry and exit. Paraffin dips may spare the patient the "dishpan hands" caused by water.

B. Cold: Some patients with particularly acute arthritis or acutely injured arthritic joints find that cold (ice pack or bag) relieves pain more effectively than does heat.

C. Massage: While massage is helpful in relaxing muscles and giving psychologic support, it provides only temporary relief, and its cost is usually high.

Splints

Splints may provide joint rest, reduce pain, and prevent contracture, but certain principles should be adhered to.

(1) Night splints of the hands or wrists (or both) should maintain the extremity in the position of optimum function. The elbow and shoulder lose motion so rapidly that other local measures and corticosteroid injections are usually preferable to splints.

(2) The best "splint" for the hip is prone-lying for several hours a day on a firm bed. For the knee, prone-lying may suffice, but splints in maximum tolerated extension are frequently needed. Ankle splints are of the simple right-angle type.

(3) Splints should be applied for the shortest period needed, should be made of lightweight materials for comfort, and should be easily removable for range-of-motion exercises once or twice daily to prevent loss of motion.

(4) Corrective splints, such as those for overcoming knee flexion contractures, should be used under the guidance of a physician familiar with their proper use.

Note: Avoidance of prolonged sitting or knee pillows may decrease the need for splints.

Braces

Unstable joints—particularly the knee and wrist—can be supported, and the pain of weight bearing may be relieved by appropriately prescribed braces.

Assistive Devices

Patient-oriented publications, physical therapists, occupational therapists, and home health nurses can help the patient to obtain appropriate gripping bars, raised toilet seats, long-handled reachers, and other devices to help in coping with daily living.

Joint Protection Program

Physical and occupational therapists can instruct patients in changing their daily habits and their occupational and recreational activities to lesson damage to joints, maintain range of motion, and lessen pain and muscle atrophy.

Delisa JA: Practical use of therapeutic physical modalities. Am Fam Physician (May) 1983;27:129.

Some Orthopedic Procedures for Arthritic Joints

A. Synovectomy: This procedure has been used for over 50 years to attempt to retard joint destruction by invasive synovial pannus of rheumatoid arthritis. However, its prophylactic effect has not been documented, and inflammation of regenerated synovial membrane occurs. Thus, the only indication for synovectomy is intractable pain in an isolated joint, most commonly the knee.

B. Joint Replacement: (See also Total Joint Arthroplasty, below.) Total hip replacement has been highly successful. Infection, the major complication, is uncommon. The long-term effects of replacement of the knee—and more recently the ankle, shoulder, and other joints—have not been fully determined.

C. Arthroplasty: Realignment and reconstruction of the knee, wrist, and small joints of the hand are feasible in a small number of selected patients.

D. Tendon Rupture: This is a fairly common complication in rheumatoid arthritis and requires immediate orthopedic referral. The most common sites are the finger flexors and extensors, the patellar tendon, and the Achilles tendon.

E. Arthrodesis: Arthrodesis (fusion) is being used less now than formerly, but a chronically infected, painful joint may be an indication for this surgical procedure.

F. Total Joint Arthroplasty: In the last 2 decades, remarkable progress has been made in the replacement of severely damaged joints with prosthetic materials. At present, artificial joint replacement is primarily indicated to relieve pain and only secondarily to restore function. Many patients who have minimal pain, therefore, even with marked destruction of the joint on radiographic examination, are not suitable candidates for joint replacement.

Success of the replacement depends upon the amount of physical stress to which the prosthetic components are subjected. Vigorous impact activity, even with the most advanced biomaterials and design, will result in failure of the prosthesis with time. Revision operations are technically more difficult, and the results may not be as good as with the primary procedure. The patient, therefore, must understand the limitations of joint replacement and the consequences of unrestrained joint usage.

1. Total hip arthroplasty–Hip replacement was originally designed for use in patients over 65 years of age with severe osteoarthritis. In these patients— usually less active physically—the prosthesis not only functioned well but outlasted the patients. Severe arthritis that fails to respond to conservative measures remains the principal indication for hip arthroplasty. Hip arthroplasty may also be indicated in younger patients severely disabled by painful hip disease (eg, rheumatoid arthritis), since in such cases it can be assumed that stress on the prosthetic joint will not be great. Contraindications to the operation include active infection and neurotrophic joint disease. Serious complications may occur in about 1% of patients and include thrombophlebitis, pulmonary embolization, sepsis, and dislocation of the joint. Extensive experience has now been accumulated, and the results are generally successful in properly selected patients.

2. Total knee arthroplasty–The indications and contraindications for total knee arthroplasty are similar to those for hip arthroplasty, but experience with the artificial knee is not as extensive. Results are slightly better in osteoarthritis patients than in those with rheumatoid arthritis. Knee arthroplasty is probably not advisable in younger individuals. Complications are similar to those with hip arthroplasty. The failure rate of knee arthroplasty is slightly higher than that of hip arthroplasty.

3. Total arthroplasty–Prostheses are now available for total arthroplasty of every major joint of the extremities, but experience with joints other than the hip and the knee has been limited.

Cornell CN et al: Survivorship analysis of total hip replacements: Results in a series of active patients who were less than fifty-five years old. J Bone Joint Surg (Am) 1986;68:1430.
Scott WN (editor): Symposium on total knee arthroplasty. Orthop Clin North Am 1982;13:1.

REFERENCES

McCarty DJ: *Arthritis and Allied Conditions. A Textbook of Rheumatology,* 11th ed. Lea & Febiger, 1989.
Payan OG, Shearn MA: Nonsteroidal anti-inflammatory drugs; nonopiate analgesics; drugs used in gout. Chapter 35 in: *Basic & Clinical Pharmacology,* 4th ed. Katzung BG (editor). Appleton & Lange, 1989.
Stites DP, Terr AI (editors): *Basic & Clinical Immunology,* 7th ed. Appleton & Lange, 1990.

16

Fluid & Electrolyte Disorders

Marcus A. Krupp, MD

Normally, the body fluids have a specific chemical composition and are distributed in discrete anatomic compartments of relatively fixed volumes. Disease can produce abnormalities in the amounts, distribution, and solute concentrations of the body fluids. Correct diagnosis and treatment of fluid and electrolyte disorders depend upon an understanding of the processes that control volume, distribution, and composition. In addition, the pharmacologic or physiologic action of some components of body fluids must be considered.

BASIC FACTS & TERMS

VOLUME & DISTRIBUTION OF BODY WATER

The volume of body water in a healthy normal individual is quite constant. Body water content varies inversely with obesity. Fat cells contain very little water, and lean tissue is rich in water. Thus, bodies heavy with fat will contain a smaller ratio of water to body weight than lean bodies. After childhood, women usually have a higher ratio of fat to lean tissue. As humans age, they tend to gain proportionately more fat. In the average well-nourished population of the USA, the total body water varies as shown in Table 16–1.

The distribution of water among the body fluid compartments is dependent upon the distribution and content of solute. Membranes and cells restrict movement of solute into and from capillaries, interstitial fluid, and cells. This results in compartmentalization of solute with resultant distribution of water by osmosis to sustain (1) equal osmolal concentrations of solute in compartments and (2) equal concentrations of water in compartments.

Solute concentration is expressed in terms of osmoles. The term osmole (osm) refers to the relationship between molar concentration and osmotic activity of a substance in solution. The osmolality of a substance in solution is calculated by multiplying the molar concentration by the number of particles per mole (mol) provided by ionization. Glucose in solution provides 1 particle per molecule; NaCl in solution—for all practical purposes—totally dissociates into Na^+ and Cl^-, yielding 2 particles per molecule. One mole of glucose in solution thus yields 1 osmole; 1 mole of NaCl, 2 osmoles. The milliunit (mosm) is more convenient. Osmole-per-kilogram-of-water is termed osmolal; osmole-per-liter-of-solution is termed osmolar. The normal osmolality of body fluids is 285–295 mosm/L.

In all problems of altered osmolality, the alteration exists in all body compartments, and the excess or deficit of solute or of water must be calculated on the basis of total body water (TBW).

ELECTROLYTES

In clinical medicine, the measurement of concentrations of electrolyte in body fluids is expressed in milliequivalents per liter of the fluid. Salts in solution dissociate into ions with positive charges (cations) and with negative charges (anions). The numbers of positive and negative charges are equal, ie, a divalent cation (2^+) will be balanced by 2 monovalent anions or 1 divalent anion (2^-).

BODY FLUID COMPARTMENTS
(Table 16–2)

The principal fluid compartments include plasma and interstitial fluid, which comprise the extracellular fluid, and intracellular fluid. Body fluids also are distributed to dense connective tissue, bone, and "transcellular" spaces (gut lumen, cerebrospinal

Table 16–1. Total body water (as percentage of body weight) in relation to age and sex.[1]

Age	Male	Female
10–18	59%	57%
18–40	61%	51%
40–60	55%	47%
Over 60	52%	46%

[1] Modified and reproduced, with permission, from Edelman & Liebman: Anatomy of body water and electrolytes. *Am J Med* 1959;**27**:256.

Table 16–2. Body water distribution in an average normal young adult male.[1]

	mL/kg[2] Body Weight	% of Total Body Water
Total extracellular fluid	270	45
Plasma	45	7.5
Interstitial fluid	120	20
Connective tissue and bone	90	15
Transcellular fluid	15	2.5
Total intracellular fluid	330	55
Total body water	600	100

[1] Modified from Edelman & Liebman: Anatomy of body water and electrolytes. *Am J Med* 1959;**27**:256.

[2] $\dfrac{mL/kg}{10}$ = %, eg, 45 mL/kg = 4.5% body weight.

fluid, intraocular fluid), but these are usually of little clinical significance in body fluid abnormalities except in a few situations (eg, burns, bowel obstruction).

Sodium salts constitute the bulk of osmotically active solute in extracellular water (ECW), whereas potassium salts constitute the bulk of osmotically active solute in intracellular water (ICW). Almost all other solutes present in body water can be considered to be either freely diffusible between ICW and ECW (such as urea) or osmotically inactive (such as intracellular magnesium, which is largely bound to protein) and consequently are not osmotically active in either compartment.

Interstitial fluids are not readily available for assay. One relies on determinations on plasma or serum to assess water and electrolyte derangements in the clinical setting.

PHYSIOLOGY OF WATER & ELECTROLYTE & TREATMENT OF ABNORMAL STATES

In the subsequent discussion, the homeostatic mechanisms and their disturbances are listed under the headings of volume, concentration, and physiologic effects.

WATER VOLUME

The volume of body water is maintained by a balance between intake and excretion. Water as such, in foods and as a product of combustion, is excreted by the kidneys, skin, and lungs. Electrolytes important in maintaining volume and distribution include the cations sodium for extracellular fluid and potassium

and magnesium for intracellular fluid, and the anions chloride and bicarbonate for extracellular fluid and organic phosphate and protein for intracellular fluid.

In response to changes in volume, appropriate feedback mechanisms come into play. The principal elements in regulation are antidiuretic hormone (water); aldosterone and other corticosteroids (sodium and potassium); vascular responses affecting glomerular filtration rate (water and sodium); atrial natriuretic peptide, a hormone from the right atrium (sodium); and renal prostaglandins PGA_2 and PGE_2 (intrarenal circulation and tubule function).

The average adult requires at least 800–1300 mL of water per day to cover obligatory losses. A normal adult on an ordinary diet requires 500 mL of water for renal excretion of solute in a maximally concentrated urine plus additional water to replace that lost via the skin and respiratory tract.

Fluid losses most often include electrolytes as well as water. Sweat, gastrointestinal fluids, urine, and fluid escaping from wounds contain significant quantities of electrolytes. In order to ascertain deficits of water and electrolytes, one must consider the history, change in body weight, clinical state, and appropriate determinations in plasma of concentration of each of the electrolytes, osmolality, protein, and pH. Assessment of renal function is required before repair and maintenance requirements can be determined and prescribed. The capacity of the kidney to excrete a concentrated or a dilute urine sets the limits of water requirement.

1. WATER DEFICIT (Volume Depletion)

Water deficit results in a decrease in volume of both ECW and ICW, with an increase in solute concentration. With decreased blood volume, perfusion of the kidneys and other tissues diminishes and antidiuretic hormone (ADH) release is stimulated, resulting in some conservation of water.

Water deficit results from reduced intake or unusual losses. Reduced intake is likely if the patient is obtunded, unconscious, or disabled or for any reason unable to ingest water because of interference with swallowing or esophageal obstruction. Unusual losses with inadequate replacement include (1) fluid loss via the gastrointestinal tract (vomiting, diarrhea, ileostomy); (2) sequestered fluids (burns, bowel obstruction, peritonitis); or (3) fluid loss due to kidney disorders (diabetes insipidus, osmotic diuresis). Fever or a hot environment increases water loss from the lungs and skin.

Clinical Findings

A. Symptoms and Signs: Early signs are thirst; flushed and loose skin; "dehydrated" appearance, with sunken eyes and dry mucous membranes; hypotension; tachycardia; and oliguria. Later, if dehydration progresses, hallucinations, delirium, and coma may ensue.

B. Laboratory Findings: The decrease in ICW and ECW results in an increase in solute concentration. Serum sodium and protein concentrations are increased. Serum urea nitrogen and, at times, creatinine are elevated, as a result of reduced renal blood flow. Serum osmolality is increased. Urine specific gravity and osmolality are elevated unless the kidney is the primary source of water loss.

Treatment

An essential guideline for treatment is acute change in weight, which is directly related to change in fluid volume.

Water may be provided with or without electrolyte. If water alone is needed, 2.5% or 5% dextrose solution may be given intravenously; the dextrose is rapidly metabolized, leaving free water. Electrolyte (Na^+) is often required to replenish losses and to sustain adequate circulation and urine output; indeed, 0.9% NaCl should be administered first in patients with volume depletion severe enough to cause hypotension even in the presence of mild hypernatremia.

In the presence of normal renal function, 2000–3000 mL of water per day (1500 mL/m^2 of body surface) will provide a liberal maintenance ration. If dehydration is present with increased serum sodium concentration and osmolality, extra water replacement can be estimated on the basis of restoring normal osmolality for the total body fluid volume. The need for intracellular water is reflected in the extracellular fluid with which it is in osmotic equilibrium; therefore, any correction of deviation in osmolality must be considered on the basis of the total volume of body water.

The water requirement is increased in the presence of fever as a result of increased loss via the skin and lungs.

2. WATER EXCESS

Water excess (**dilution syndrome**) produces an expansion of both ECW and ICW, with a corresponding decrease in solute concentration. Both of these effects operate to reduce secretion of antidiuretic hormone (ADH).

Decreased excretion of water can produce an excess of body water, particularly when coupled with increased intake. Decreased renal perfusion results in water retention in the presence of such states as (1) acute or chronic renal failure, (2) nephrotic syndrome, (3) congestive heart failure, or (4) liver disease with ascites. Renal retention of water also occurs in the presence of secretion of vasopressin (ADH) or in the syndrome of inappropriate ADH secretion (SIADH). SIADH is associated with the stress of

surgery or anesthesia; pulmonary disease (pneumonia, lung abscess, tuberculosis, mycoses), central nervous system disease (encephalitis, trauma, tumor, hemorrhage); malignant tumors (small cell carcinoma of the lung, prostate, or pancreas; thymoma); hypothyroidism; and a wide variety of drugs (narcotics, chlorpropamide, barbiturates, clofibrate, indomethacin, cyclophosphamide, vincristine, acetaminophen, psychotropic drugs, and diuretics). (See Hyponatremia, below.)

Clinical Findings

A. Symptoms and Signs: Clinical evidence of water excess depends on the cause. If it occurs acutely or is severe, "water intoxication" is manifested by headache, nausea, vomiting, abdominal cramps, weakness, stupor, convulsions, and coma.

B. Laboratory Findings: The increased volume of body water produces a dilution of solute. Serum Na^+ and protein concentrations are reduced, and serum urea nitrogen concentrations are often low. Plasma osmolality is low. Vasopressin levels are increased.

Treatment

The basic treatment consists of water restriction. If a real deficit of sodium exists as well, saline solutions should be employed. In the presence of severe water intoxication, administration of hypertonic saline solution may be useful to move excess intracellular water to the extracellular space, ie, to increase ECF osmolality and diminish intracellular water volume. Overexpansion of extracellular volume, which may precipitate acute congestive heart failure and pulmonary edema, may be prevented by use of a loop diuretic and replacement of urinary sodium loss with 0.9% sodium chloride supplemented with potassium and magnesium as required.

CONCENTRATION

The total concentration of solute (osmolality) is apparently the same in intracellular and extracellular water. In the intracellular compartment, protein concentration plays a more important osmolal role than in the plasma. The protein content of interstitial fluid is small, and osmolal effects are therefore negligible. The most accessible and best index of osmolality is the measurement of the solute concentration in the plasma or serum by ascertaining the depression of the freezing point or by measurement of vapor pressure. The normal range is 285–295 mosm/L. Serum osmolality can be calculated from the following formula:

$$\text{Osmolaity} = 2(Na^+ \text{ mmol/L}) + \text{Glucose mmol/L} + \text{BUN mmol/L}$$

$$\text{or} = 2(Na^+ \text{ meq/L}) + \frac{\text{Glucose mg/dL}}{18} + \frac{\text{BUN mg/dL}}{2.8}$$

(1 mosm of glucose equals 180 mg/L and 1 mosm of urea nitrogen equals 28 mg/L.)

Measurement of serum sodium by flame photometry may yield an artifactually low result when there is an increased concentration of protein or lipid in the serum. These displace water in which electrolyte is dissolved. Measurement with ion-sensitive electrodes is not so affected.

HYPEROSMOLAL STATES

Hyperosmolal concentrations of solute in body fluids are harmful when increased concentration of solute confined to the extracellular fluid results in loss of water from cells. Hyperosmolality may be asymptomatic or give rise to the manifestations listed below.

Hyperosmolality With Only Transient or No Symptomatic Shift in Water

Urea and alcohol are 2 substances that readily cross cell membranes and can produce hyperosmolality. Urea may be administered acutely in large doses to "draw" water from cells, but the effect is transient, as is the diuresis, and urea soon equilibrates throughout body water. Alcohol quickly equilibrates between intracellular and extracellular water, adding 22 mosm/L for every 1000 mg/L. The hyperosmolality does not produce significant difficulty, but in any condition of stupor or coma in which measured osmolality exceeds that calculated from values of serum Na^+, glucose, and urea nitrogen, alcohol should be considered to explain the discrepancy (osmolal gap). Methanol ingestion is another cause of osmolal gap; it is characterized by severe metabolic acidosis.

Hyperosmolality Associated With Significant Shifts in Water

Increased concentrations of solutes that do not readily enter cells produce a shift of water from the intracellular space to effect a true intracellular dehydration. Sodium and glucose are the solutes commonly involved.

1. HYPERNATREMIA

Hypernatremia almost always follows loss of water in excess of Na^+ (eg, diabetes insipidus or the osmotic diuresis associated with high-protein feedings coupled with inadequate water intake).

Clinical Findings

A. Symptoms and Signs: Usually there is thirst (except if hypothalamic lesions are the cause), weight loss, flushed loose skin, tachycardia and hypotension, and oliguria. Fever, delirium, hyperpnea, and coma may be seen with severe hyperosmolality.

B. Laboratory Findings: Elevated serum Na^+ and osmolality are essential findings. Increased concentrations of serum urea nitrogen reflect decreased renal perfusion. Urine osmolality is elevated.

Treatment

Treatment is directed to correct the cause of the fluid loss and to replace water and, as needed, electrolyte. Water deficit is calculated to restore normal osmolality for total body water. The volume of water required can be determined as follows: Calculate total body water (TBW). (TBW equals 0.5–0.6 of body weight for well-nourished to lean adults.) Then,

$$\text{Volume (in liters) to be replaced} = \text{TBW} \left(\frac{[Na^+] - 140}{140} \right)$$

Initially, dextrose 5% in water may be employed. As correction of water deficit progresses, therapy should continue with 0.45% NaCl with dextrose or, if Na^+ depletion has also been significant, 0.9% saline. Potassium and phosphate may be added as indicated by serum levels. As soon as possible, oral intake should be resumed.

Replacement should be slow (over 24–72 hours) to permit readjustments through diffusion among fluid compartments. Maintenance requirements should be added to each 24-hour replacement ration.

A. Hypernatremia With no Change In Total Body Na^+: This rare occurrence may be associated with a hypothalamic malfunction and requires no treatment besides urging the patient to consume an adequate amount of water.

B. Hypernatremia With an Increase in Total Body Na^+: Accidental intravascular injection of hypertonic saline used for induction of abortion may be responsible. The use of large doses of $NaHCO_3$ in treating cardiac arrest may be a cause, particularly when renal function is impaired. The increase in Na^+ produces expansion of extracellular volume at the expanse of intracellular water, ie, extracellular overload and intracellular dehydration.

Treatment consists of providing water as 5% glucose at a rate that will expand extracellular fluid volume and reduce hyperosmolarity but not induce congestive heart failure. Simultaneously, loop diuretics such as furosemide should be administered intravenously to remove the excess Na^+ and water.

2. HYPERGLYCEMIA (Hyperglycemic Hyperosmolal Syndrome)

Hyperglycemia, usually without ketosis, occurs in patients with non-insulin-dependent diabetes mellitus. When hyperglycemia is severe enough to produce significant hyperosmolality in the extracellular fluid, the loss of water from cells and the loss of total body water consequent to the osmotic diuresis (glycosuria) result in severe dehydration and loss of Na^+, K^+, and phosphate.

Clinical Findings

A. Symptoms and Signs: The common symptoms and signs are obtundation; severe dehydration with loose, dry skin, sunken eyes, and dry mucous membranes; and hypotension with tachycardia and fall in blood pressure that are more severe when the patient is upright. Impaired consciousness and coma are late manifestations.

B. Laboratory Findings: Extreme elevation of serum glucose is seen (usually > 800 mg/dL), as are elevated serum urea nitrogen, creatinine, and, at times, K^+. Serum Na^+ values may be high or low; in either event, the value should be corrected for the shift of water from the cells to the extracellular fluid as follows: For every 100 mg of serum glucose greater than 180 mg/dL, add 1.6 meq to the measured value of Na^+ to obtain the concentration of Na^+ that would exist in the absence of hyperglycemia.

Treatment

Treatment of the hyperosmolal state due to hyperglycemia requires an estimation of the state of total body sodium, for if Na^+ deficit is severe, prompt replacement of both Na^+ and water is essential. The presence of clinical evidence of low blood (plasma) volume is the best immediate indicator of Na^+ deficit. The serum Na^+ level is not a reliable index. Initially, it is essential to expand the extracellular fluid volume until blood pressure and urine volume are stable, employing isotonic saline. Low doses of insulin will reduce hyperglycemia. Once circulation is improved, water losses can be calculated on the basis of the degree of hyperosmolality (see calculation for water replacement for hypernatremia, above) and hyposmolal solutions such as 0.45% saline introduced. Correction of deficit should not be rapid to allow for diffusion and equilibration of water and osmolality. Serum electrolyte and urea nitrogen levels should be monitored closely. Potassium and phosphate may be required, as their concentration falls routinely with correction of blood glucose. If correction with hyposmolal solutions is too rapid, cerebral edema may result.

HYPOSMOLAL STATES

1. HYPONATREMIA WITH DECREASED EXTRACELLULAR FLUID VOLUME

Hyponatremia with decreased extracellular fluid volume is caused by excessive use of diuretics, chronic renal disease, adrenocorticoid deficiency, and fluid sequestration with burns, peritonitis, and pancreatitis.

Clinical Findings

A. Symptoms and Signs: Diminished plasma volume and dehydration occur, with thirst, faintness, and dizziness on standing. There is dry mucosa, loss of skin turgor, tachycardia and orthostatic hypotension, and oliguria. Rarely, shock and coma result.

B. Laboratory Findings: Low serum Na^+ and Cl^- are present. Serum urea and creatinine may be elevated. Serum K^+ may be low or high, depending on the cause.

Treatment

Treatment consists of replacement of volume loss with isotonic saline and treatment of the underlying disorder. Empiric use of corticosteroids is indicated if hypocortisolism is considered in the differential diagnosis.

2. HYPONATREMIA WITH INCREASED EXTRACELLULAR FLUID VOLUME

Hyponatremia with increased extracellular fluid volume occurs when decreased effective circulating blood volume with decreased renal perfusion results in retention of sodium and water. Total body sodium is increased. Secretion of antidiuretic hormone results in a greater retention of water.

Clinical Findings

A. Symptoms and Signs: Edema occurs in congestive heart failure, hepatic cirrhosis, nephrotic syndrome, and hypoproteinemia.

B. Laboratory Findings: Low serum Na^+ is present. Serum urea nitrogen and creatinine may be increased.

Treatment

Diuretics should be given and the underlying disorder treated. Do not attempt to correct hyponatremia with saline solutions.

3. HYPONATREMIA WITHOUT DEHYDRATION OR EDEMA (Normal Extracellular Fluid Volume)

Most commonly, the syndrome of inappropriate secretion of antidiuretic hormone (SIADH) produces retention of water with a dilution of electrolyte. See Water Excess, above, for a list of causes of SIADH.

Clinical Findings

A. Symptoms and Signs: Hyponatremia that occurs acutely produces headache, nausea, vomiting, abdominal cramps, weakness, stupor, coma, and convulsions. Hyponatremia that develops slowly is usually asymptomatic.

B. Laboratory Findings: There is low serum Na^+ and, often, low serum uric acid. There is increased loss in the urine of sodium, urate, and phosphate. Vasopressin concentration in plasma is increased.

Treatment

Water should be restricted to 800 or 500 mL/d until serum Na^+ approaches normal. Demeclocycline (300–600 mg twice daily) is useful in the chronic state. In cases of severe hyponatremia, furosemide or ethacrynic acid may be used to promote diuresis simultaneously with administration of saline 0.9–3% supplemented with K^+ replacement.

Hyponatremia must not be corrected rapidly, but osmotic equilibration must be attained gradually to avoid acute volume overload or central pontine myelinolysis. If hyponatremia (water excess) is life-threatening, rapid correction of serum Na^+ to 120 meq/L can be accomplished, followed by slower correction thereafter.

The cause of SIADH must be treated. Vasopressin antagonists are under development.

4. ARTIFACTUAL HYPONATREMIA

When plasma water per unit volume of plasma is diminished (displaced) by lipids of lipidemia or by protein of hyperproteinemia, sodium concentration will be low when measured by flame photometry. With hyperglycemia, plasma water is increased (shift from cells), and sodium concentration is reduced by 1.6 mmol/L for each 100-mg/dL increase over 180 mg of glucose.

ELECTROLYTES ASSOCIATED WITH PHYSIOLOGIC EFFECTS

Hydrogen ion, K^+, Ca^{2+}, Mg^{2+}, and phosphate ion are included in this category. An abnormality of concentration of any one of these is often accompanied by alteration of concentration and effects of one or more of the others.

HYDROGEN ION CONCENTRATION

The hydrogen ion concentration (H^+) of body fluids is closely regulated with intracellular concentrations of 10^7 mol/L (pH 7.0) and extracellular fluid concentrations of 4 times 10^{-8} mol/L (pH 7.4). These concentrations are maintained at nearly normal levels by buffer substances that remove or release H^+. The capacity of buffers is limited, however, and regulation is accomplished mostly by the lungs and kidneys. The principal buffers include proteins, the oxyhemoglobin-reduced hemoglobin system, primary and secondary phosphate ions, some intracellular phosphate esters, and the carbonic acid-sodium bicarbonate system.

Most of the food used for energy is completely utilized, with production of water, CO_2, and urea. Sulfate and phosphate end products are strong acid anions that must be "neutralized" by cation such as sodium. In the utilization of fat and carbohydrate, intermediate products include the strong acids acetoacetic acid and lactic acid. Buffers provide cation and remove H^+, which is ultimately excreted by the kidneys as acid or as ammonium ion and by the lungs as CO_2 and H_2O, equivalent to carbonic acid. The anions of strong acids with cations such as sodium and ammonium are eliminated by the kidney.

The role of the lung and kidney in removal of H^+ and in regulation of H^+ concentration can be viewed as follows:

$$\frac{[H^+][HCO_3^-]}{[B^+][HCO_3^-]} \rightleftarrows \frac{P_{CO_2}}{HCO_3^-} \quad \frac{\text{lung}}{\text{kidney}}$$

Respiratory control of the partial pressure of CO_2 (P_{CO_2}) in pulmonary alveoli and therefore in the arterial plasma determines the H_2CO_3 concentration in body fluids:

$$CO_2 + H_2O \rightleftarrows H_2CO_3$$

The elimination of CO_2 via the lung in effect removes carbonic acid. The kidney is responsible for $BHCO_3$ concentration in body fluids, which, with H_2CO_3, constitutes one of the buffer systems for regulation of pH.

In kidney tubule cells, carbonic anhydrase catalyzes the conversion of metabolic CO_2 and water to carbonic acid. The carbonic acid serves as a source of H^+ that can be exchanged for Na^+ in the tubular urine so that H^+ is excreted and Na^+ reabsorbed.

Although the pH of urine cannot be lowered below pH 4.5, additional H^+ ion can be excreted by combination with NH_3, generated principally from glutamine within the tubule cell. NH_3 diffuses from the tubule cell into the urine, where it combines with $H^+ \rightarrow NH_4^+$, providing cation for excretion with anions of strong acids with no increase in H^+ concentration (no lowering of pH). These exchanges in the renal tubule involve active transport systems capable of maintaining a gradient in concentration of extracellular fluid H^+ of 4×10^{-8} mol/L (pH 7.4) against a tubular urine H^+ of 32×10^{-6} mol/L (pH 4.5), an 800-fold increase in H^+ concentration.

CLINICAL STATES OF ALTERED H⁺ CONCENTRATION

The clinical term acidosis signifies a decrease in pH (increase in H^+) of extracellular fluid; alkalosis signifies an increase in pH (decrease in H^+) of extracellular fluid. The change in H^+ concentration may be the result of metabolic or respiratory abnormalities.

Note: Mixed metabolic and respiratory abnormalities are frequently encountered.

1. RESPIRATORY ACIDOSIS

Respiratory acidosis follows ventilatory abnormalities resulting in CO_2 retention and elevation of P_{CO_2} in alveoli and arterial blood (hypercapnia), with increased H_2CO_3 and lowered pH. CO_2 retention follows inadequate ventilation during anesthesia, following suppression of the respiratory center by central nervous system disease or drugs, or results from respiratory muscle weakness or paralysis. Structural changes in the lung (emphysema, chronic obstructive disease) or pulmonary circulation and abnormal thoracic structure (kyphoscoliosis) may alter alveolocapillary blood exchange or diminish effective ventilation to prevent CO_2 excretion. In association with impaired CO_2 excretion (Pa_{CO_2}), there usually is impaired O_2 exchange with low alveolar and arterial P_{O_2} (hypoxemia). In the presence of CO_2 retention and the resultant increase in H_2CO_3 concentration, compensatory reabsorption of HCO_3^- by the kidney provides buffer to reduce H^+ concentration, but this protection cannot be accomplished rapidly and is effective only in chronic situations.

The hazard of acute hypercapnia cannot be overemphasized. Buffer protection is severely limited, and renal response is very slow. Thus, an increase in Pa_{CO_2} can quickly produce sharp increases in H^+ concentration (decrease in pH) to levels incompatible with life. Respiratory inadequacy or acute, severe reduction of pulmonary circulation resulting in sudden increase in Pa_{O_2} will usually result in a severe decrease in Pa_{O_2}, compounding the threat to life. It is apparent that periods of hypoventilation constitute a serious and often lethal complication in the immediate postoperative state, following injury of the thoracic cage, in severe illness or shock accompanied by obtunded consciousness, in trauma to the central nervous system, and in the presence of heart failure, cardiac arrhythmias or arrest, and myocardial infarction.

Clinical Findings

A. Symptoms and Signs: With acute onset, there is somnolence, confusion, and asterixis. Coma from CO_2 narcosis ensues. In chronic disease, shortness of breath and cyanosis occur.

B. Laboratory Findings: Arterial blood pH is low; P_{CO_2} is elevated. Serum bicarbonate is elevated but not enough to compensate completely for the hypercapnia. In chronic respiratory acidosis, arterial P_{O_2} is low and polycythemia may be present.

Treatment

Treatment is directed toward improvement of ventilation by maintaining an open airway, use of mechanical aids, treatment with bronchodilators, restoration of circulation, correction of heart failure, and antidotes for anesthetics or drugs suppressing the respiratory center. Tracheal intubation is often required. Close monitoring of arterial blood pH, P_{CO_2}, and P_{O_2} is essential. The respiratory center is readily rendered unresponsive by high Pa_{CO_2} (hypercapnia), and recovery may be slow. In the presence of hypercapnia, relief of hypoxemia with oxygen therapy may deprive the patient of the only remaining stimulus to the respiratory center and produce more severe hypoventilation with resultant CO_2 narcosis. However, hypoxemia also has serious consequences, and it cannot be allowed to exist untreated for fear of CO_2 narcosis. Thus, careful clinical observation is required while judicious amounts of oxygen are given. Endotracheal intubation should be performed if the patient becomes exhausted or if adequate oxygenation cannot be maintained.

2. RESPIRATORY ALKALOSIS

Respiratory alkalosis is a result of hyperventilation, which produces lowered Pa_{CO_2} and elevated pH of extracellular fluid. Anxiety is the usual cause. Hyperventilation may also occur during anesthesia or when mechanical ventilatory devices are incorrectly used. Renal compensation by excretion of HCO_3^- (with Na^+ predominantly) is too slow a response to be effective, and elevation of pH may reach a point at which asterixis, tetany, and increased neuromuscular irritability appear (probably as a result of a decrease in ionized calcium). Respiratory alkalosis often results from the hyperventilation associated with asthma, congestive heart failure, pulmonary embolism, and pneumonia. Chronic hypocapnia is associated with advanced liver disease and pregnancy.

Clinical Findings

A. Symptoms and Signs: In acute cases (hyperventilation), there is light-headedness, anxiety, paresthesias, numbness about the mouth, and a tingling sensation in the hands and feet. Tetany occurs in more severe alkalosis. In chronic cases, asymptomatic findings are those of the primary disease.

B. Laboratory Findings: Arterial blood pH is elevated, and P_{CO_2} is low. Serum bicarbonate is decreased in chronic respiratory alkalosis.

Treatment

Treatment of spontaneous hyperventilation consists

of reducing anxiety by drugs or psychotherapy. Tetany may be alleviated by rebreathing exhaled air, which will increase Pa_{CO_2} and lower blood pH. Regulation of devices used in assisting with ventilation should be guided by measurement of the P_{CO_2} and pH of arterial blood.

3. METABOLIC ACIDOSIS

Metabolic acidosis (lowered blood pH and bicarbonate) occurs with starvation; in uncontrolled diabetes with ketoacidosis and in lactic acidosis; with electrolyte (including bicarbonate) and water loss from diarrhea or enteric fistulas; and with renal insufficiency or tubular defect producing inadequate H^+ excretion. Cation loss (Na^+, K^+, Ca^{2+}) and organic acid anion retention occur with starvation and uncontrolled diabetes mellitus. In the presence of renal insufficiency, phosphate and sulfate are retained and cation (especially Na^+) is lost because of limited H^+ secretion for exchange with cation in the renal tubule. Respiratory compensation for metabolic acidosis by hyperventilation reduces P_{CO_2} and thereby reduces H_2CO_3 concentration in extracellular fluid.

When acidosis is evident, it is important to distinguish between bicarbonate loss and the accumulation or retention of strong acid by calculating the "anion gap," or the amount of anion not identified by the usual serum electrolyte determination (Table 16–3).

$$\text{Anion gap} = [Na^+] - ([HCO_3^-] + [Cl^-]) = 8 - 12 \text{ meq}$$

When bicarbonate is lost (diarrhea, ileostomy, ileal loop bladder, renal tubular acidosis), chloride is usually retained to keep the "gap" normal. When chloride is taken in as NH_4Cl or amino acid-chloride (total parenteral nutrition), bicarbonate is lost and the gap remains normal. An anion gap greater than 12 meq indicates accumulation of organic acids such as acetoacetate, β-hydroxybutyrate, and lactate. In the case of renal insufficiency, an anion gap exists because of retention of phosphate, sulfate, and other ions, but the increased hydrogen ion concentration results from inability to excrete hydrogen ion. A smaller than normal anion gap occurs when there is elevation of monoclonal immunoglobulins (with isoelectric point higher than serum pH), particularly IgG, in plasma cell dyscrasias and lymphoproliferative disorders, or with hypoalbuminemia (about 2.5 meq/g of albumin at normal blood pH).

Clinical Findings

A. Symptoms and Signs: Symptoms include thirst, shortness of breath, weakness, and those of the primary disease (eg, polyuria in diabetic ketoacidosis). Signs include dehydration, tachypnea, restlessness, impaired consciousness, and coma, plus those of the primary disease (eg, fruity breath odor in diabetic ketoacidosis).

Table 16–3. Anion gap.

Normal (8–12 meq)
Loss of HCO_3^-
Diarrhea
Pancreatic fluid loss
Ileostomy (unadapted)
Carbonic anhydrase inhibitors
Chloride retention
Renal tubular acidosis
Ileal loop bladder
Administration of HCl equivalent
NH_4Cl
Arginine and lysine in parenteral nutrition
Increased (>12 meq)
Metabolic anion
Diabetic ketoacidosis
Alcoholic ketoacidosis
Lactic acidosis
Renal insufficiency (PO_4^{3-}, SO_4^{2-})
Starvation
Metabolic alkalosis (increased number of negative charges on protein)
Drug or chemical anion
Salicylate intoxication
Sodium carbenicillin therapy
Methanol (formic acid)
Ethylene glycol (oxalic acid)
Decreased (<8 meq)
Plasma cell dyscrasias
Monoclonal protein (cationic paraprotein) (accompanied by chloride and bicarbonate)
Hypoalbuminemia (decreased unmeasured anion)

B. Laboratory Findings: Blood pH and Pa_{CO_2} and serum HCO_3^- are low. The anion gap may be elevated or normal (see above). Elevated serum urea nitrogen, creatinine, and potassium reflect the degree of renal impairment due to dehydration or renal disease. With diabetic or alcoholic ketoacidosis and with starvation, tests for ketone bodies are positive in urine and serum. Other changes reflect the effects of causes of acidosis.

Treatment

Treatment is directed toward correcting the metabolic defect (eg, insulin for control of diabetes) and replenishment of water and of deficits of Na^+, K^+, HCO_3^-, and other electrolytes. If arterial blood pH is less than 7.1, anion replacement may include bicarbonate, but quantities of bicarbonate should not exceed 50–100 mmol. Renal insufficiency requires careful replacement of water and electrolyte deficit and closely controlled rations of water, sodium, potassium, chloride, and bicarbonate to maintain normal extracellular fluid concentrations; the elevated serum phosphate may be lowered by interfering with phosphate absorption from the gut by oral administration of aluminum hydroxide preparations. In the presence of renal insufficiency, elevated extracellular K^+ concentrations may be reduced by either oral or rectal administration of ion exchange resins that bind K^+ and prevent absorption in the intestine (see Hyperkalemia, below), or by hemodialysis or peritoneal dialysis. (See Diabetic Ketoacidosis in Chapter 21.)

Lactic Acidosis

Lactic acidosis is a serious form of metabolic acidosis characterized by reduced serum bicarbonate concentration, a high anion gap, and usually a normal serum chloride. Two general causes are poor tissue perfusion (anoxia; cardiogenic, septic, or hemorrhagic shock; carbon monoxide poisoning) and metabolic abnormalities (diabetes mellitus, liver disease, renal failure, leukemia; toxicity from phenformin, ethanol, methanol, salicylates, isoniazid; ketoacidosis from any cause). Acidosis usually develops abruptly and is manifested by hyperventilation and often by abdominal pain. Blood chemical changes include low pH (< 7.20) of arterial blood, low bicarbonate, and occasionally high serum phosphate. Arterial blood lactate exceeds 5 mmol/L and may reach 10–15 mmol/L or more. The mortality rate is high (60–70%).

Treatment of severe lactic acidosis is that of the underlying disease: restoring tissue blood flow; correcting hypoxia, ketoacidosis, and liver failure, and removing toxic causative agents. Oxygen, intravenous fluids, avoidance of vasoconstrictors, and general supportive measures are required. The use of bicarbonate is now controversial. Administration of large amounts of bicarbonate may have deleterious effects by reducing cardiac output, blood pressure, perfusion of tissues, and oxygen release from hemoglobin. The metabolism of lactate will yield bicarbonate to restore bicarbonate buffer and pH toward normal. Small doses of sodium bicarbonate (50–100 mmol) may be indicated for severe acidosis with arterial blood pH < 7.20.

4. METABOLIC ALKALOSIS

Metabolic alkalosis results from either acid loss or bicarbonate gain (Table 16–4). In both cases, serum

Table 16–4. Causes of metabolic alkalosis.

Acid loss
  Acid gastric juice (vomiting, suction)
  Chloride excretion with increased reabsorption of HCO_3^- from potent diuretics (furosemide, thiazide, ethacrynic acid)
  Renal acid excretion from excess mineralocorticoid (especially aldosterone)
  K^+ deficiency with H^+ secretion in distal nephron
  Chloride-losing diarrhea (rare)
Bicarbonate gain
  Excessive intake of bicarbonate or precursors (alkalinizing salts). Usually requires some degree of renal insufficiency.
  Milk-alkali syndrome
  Metabolism of acetoacetic acid, β-hydroxybutyric acid, ketones, and lactic acid to bicarbonate
  Abrupt decrease of arterial P_{CO_2} during treatment of chronic hypercapnia (compensated respiratory acidosis)
  Contraction alkalosis (body fluid volume depletion)

bicarbonate is increased, chloride concentration is diminished, and pH is elevated. Moderate or severe metabolic alkalosis (alkalemia) is frequently associated with an increased anion gap because of (1) loss of H^+ and resultant increase in negative charge of plasma proteins, and (2) extracellular fluid volume deficit that results in increased concentration of the plasma proteins.

In defense of plasma pH, a decrease in ventilation permits retention of CO_2 to provide more of the H_2CO_3 fraction of the bicarbonate buffer system. With metabolic alkalosis, K^+ and H^+ are excreted by the kidney, and K^+ depletion commonly results.

Clinical Findings

A. Symptoms and Signs: There are no characteristic symptoms or signs. Weakness and hyporeflexia occur if serum K^+ is markedly low. Tetany and neuromuscular irritability occur rarely.

B. Laboratory Findings: The arterial blood pH and bicarbonate are elevated. The arterial P_{CO_2} is increased. Serum potassium and chloride are decreased. There may be an increased anion gap.

Treatment

Treatment includes restoration of normal body water volume, K^+, Cl^-, and Na^+. The anion should be exclusively Cl^- until correction is achieved. Alkalosis resulting from mineralocorticoid excess is often resistant to treatment, as the kidney is unable to retain Cl^-.

POTASSIUM

Potassium is the major intracellular cation, parallel to that of sodium in extracellular fluid. Potassium plays an important role in muscular contraction, conduction of nerve impulses, enzyme action, and cell membrane function.

Cardiac muscle excitability, conduction, and rhythm are markedly affected by changes in concentration of K^+, Mg^{2+}, and Ca^{2+}, in extracellular fluid. Both an increase and a decrease of extracellular K^+ concentration diminish excitability and conduction rate. Higher than normal concentrations produce a marked depression of conductivity with cardiac arrest in diastole; in the presence of very low concentrations, cardiac arrest occurs in systole. The effects of abnormal K^+ concentrations upon the cell membrane potential of cardiac muscle and upon depolarization and repolarization are manifested in the ECG.

At both extremes of abnormal concentration of K^+ in extracellular fluid, skeletal and smooth muscle contractility is impaired and flaccid paralysis ensues.

Potassium concentration of extracellular fluid is closely regulated between 3.5 and 5 meq/L. Excretion of the 35–100 meq of potassium contained in the daily diet of the average adult is predominantly via the kidney. Loss or retention of K^+ by the kidney depends on many factors; renin-angiotensin-aldosterone effects, blood pH, serum K^+ concentration, glomerular filtration rate, and renal prostaglandins.

1. HYPERKALEMIA

The usual basis for hyperkalemia (K^+ concentration > 5 meq/L) is reduced excretion by the kidney. Table 16–5 lists the common causes.

Clinical Findings

A. Symptoms and Signs: The elevated K^+ concentration interferes with normal neuromuscular function to produce weakness and flaccid paralysis; abdominal distention and diarrhea may occur. As extracellular concentration of K^+ increases, the ECG reflects impaired conduction by peaked T waves of increased amplitude, atrial arrest, widening of the QRS, and biphasic QRS-T complexes. The heart rate may be slow; ventricular fibrillation and cardiac arrest are terminal events.

B. Laboratory Findings: The serum K^+ is elevated. There is evidence of renal impairment (eg, elevated serum urea nitrogen, creatinine, phosphate, and urate; decreased HCO_3^-). With metabolic acidosis, the shift of K^+ from cells into the extracellular fluid produces an increase in serum potassium of approximately 0.6 meq/L per 0.1 unit decrease in pH from 7.4.

Treatment

First confirm that the elevated level of serum or plasma K^+ is genuine (see Table 16–5). Treatment consists of withholding potassium and employing cation exchange resins by mouth or enema. Kayexalate, a sodium cycle sulfonic polystyrene exchange resin, 40–80 g/d in divided doses, is usually effective. In an emergency, insulin plus 10–50% glucose may be employed to deposit K^+ with glycogen in the liver, and Ca_2^+ may be given intravenously as an antagonist ion. Sodium bicarbonate can be given intravenously as an emergency measure in severe hyperkalemia; the increase in blood pH results in a shift of K^+ into cells. Hemodialysis or peritoneal dialysis may be required to remove K^+ in the presence of protracted renal insufficiency. Therapy of the precipitating event proceeds concurrently.

2. HYPOKALEMIA

Hypokalemia is caused by decreased intake or absorption and increased loss (Table 16–6). Potassium deficit may or may not be accompanied by lowered extracellular fluid K^+ concentration (< 3.5 meq/L); however, when hypokalemia is present, total potassium deficit is usually profound. Exceptions to this common circumstance include the hypokalemia of alkalosis and that following administration of insulin.

Clinical Findings

A. Symptoms and Signs: Weakness, paresthesias, and nocturia are frequent complaints. Skeletal muscle weakness, hyporeflexia, and even flaccid paralysis are characteristic. Rhabdomyolysis may occur. Smooth muscle involvement results in paralytic ileus. Impaired ability to concentrate urine and reversal of the diurnal pattern of urine excretion are the typical findings.

B. Laboratory Findings: The serum K^+ is low (< 3.5 meq/L). Depending on the cause, serum Na^+, Ca^{2+}, or Mg^{2+} may be low. The serum HCO_3^- is usually elevated.

Table 16–5. Causes of hyperkalemia.

Diminished excretion
  Renal failure, acute and chronic
  Severe oliguria due to severe dehydration or shock
Increased supply of K^+
  Overtreatment with K^+, orally or parenterally
  Massive release of intracellular K^+ in burns, rhabdomyolysis or crush injury, or severe infection
Endocrine disease
  Adrenocortical insufficiency
  Hyporeninemic-hypoaldosteronism (often with long-term diabetes mellitus)
Physiologic causes
  Metabolic acidosis
Artifacts
  Leakage from erythrocytes if separation of serum from clot is delayed
  Thrombocytosis, with release of K^+ from platelets (plasma K^+ not affected)

Table 16–6. Causes of hypokalemia.

Poor intake
  Starvation, alcoholism
  Prolonged use of intravenous fluids lacking potassium
Reduced absorption
  Malabsorption
  Small bowel bypass; short bowel
Increased loss
  Gastrointestinal: Vomiting, gastrointestinal suction, obstruction, small bowel fistula, diarrhea, villous adenoma, laxative abuse
  Renal: Diuresis (diuretics, osmolar); congenital tubular defects (renal tubular acidosis, Fanconi's syndrome); renal failure; acidosis (especially diabetes); metabolic alkalosis; corticotropin or glucocorticoid excess (Cushing's syndrome); mineralocorticoid excess (aldosterone-renin); licorice abuse; Bartter's syndrome; some antibiotics (amphotericin B, aminoglycosides, sodium load with carbenicillin or ticarcillin); magnesium depletion
  Skin: Burns; excessive sweating
Hypokalemia with no deficit (shift into cells)
  Insulin; beta-adrenergic agonists
  Athletic training; testosterone (anabolic agent) therapy
  Respiratory alkalosis
  Familial periodic paralysis
  Treatment of megaloblastic anemia

The ECG shows decreased amplitude and broadening of T waves, prominent U waves, sagging ST segments, and in more severe deficit, atrioventricular block and finally cardiac arrest. (Hypokalemia increases the likelihood of digitalis toxicity.)

Treatment

Treatment requires replacement of potassium orally or parenterally. If serum Mg^{2+} or Ca^{2+} is low, treatment should include these cations (see below). Because of the toxicity of potassium, it must be administered slowly and cautiously to prevent hyperkalemia. Confirmation of adequate renal function is important when potassium is administered, since the principal route of excretion is via the kidney. KCl in a total dose of 1–3 mmol/kg/d may be given parenterally in glucose or saline solutions (or both) at a rate that will not produce hyperkalemia. Except in an emergency in which serum K^+ is extremely low and cardiac muscle and respiratory muscle activity seriously impaired, the administration of K^+ should be at a rate of 10–20 meq per hour or less. Cl^- is always needed to relieve the hypochloremia of the accompanying metabolic alkalosis. The K^+ depletion of renal tubular acidosis requires K^+ and HCO_3^- replacement. (See Renal Tubular Acidosis.) The hypokalemia of Bartter's syndrome responds to potassium replacement.

CALCIUM

Calcium constitutes about 2% of body weight, but only about 1% of the total body calcium is in solution in body fluid. In the plasma, calcium is present as a nondiffusible complex with protein (33%); as a diffusible but undissociated complex with anions such as citrate, bicarbonate, and phosphate (12%); and as Ca^{2+} (55%). The normal total plasma (or serum) calcium concentration is 2.25–2.6 mmol/L (9–10.3 mg/dL). The serum calcium level is responsive to 2 hormones: parathyroid hormone elevates and calcitonin lowers the concentration. Vitamin D, particularly its active form 1,25-dihydroxycholecalciferol, and serum PO_4^{3-} also influence Ca^{2+} regulation. Bone serves as a reservoir of calcium available to body fluids. Excretion of Ca^{2+} is via the kidney.

Calcium functions as an essential ion for many enzymes. Along with other cations (especially K^+ and Mg^{2+}), calcium exerts an important effect on cell membrane potential and permeability manifested prominently in neuromuscular function. It plays a central role in muscle contraction. At the synapse, the synaptic knobs release acetylcholine. The action potential opens gated Ca^{2+} channels to increase the discharge of acetylcholine commensurate with Ca^{2+} influx.

In cardiac muscle, augmentation of intracellular Ca^{2+} with Ca^{2+} from the extracellular fluid via the slow channels of the muscle cell membrane contributes significantly to contraction. Cardiac muscle responds to elevated Ca^{2+} concentration with increased contractility, ventricular extrasystoles, and idioventricular rhythm. These responses are accentuated in the presence of digitalis. With severe calcium toxicity, cardiac arrest in systole may occur. Low concentration of Ca^{2+} produces diminished contractility of the heart and a lengthening of the QT interval of the ECG by prolonging the ST segment, which may predispose to arrhythmias.

1. HYPERCALCEMIA

Important causes of hypercalcemia are listed in Table 16–7.

Clinical Findings

A. Symptoms and Signs: Anorexia, nausea and vomiting, constipation, polyuria, muscle weakness with hyporeflexia, tremor, lethargy, and confusion are common. Stupor, coma, and azotemia ensue.

B. Laboratory Findings: A significant elevation of serum Ca^{2+} is seen; the level must be interpreted in relation to the serum albumin level (see Hypocalcemia). Serum phosphate may or may not be low, depending on the cause. The ECG shows a shortened QT interval.

Treatment

Treatment consists of control of the primary disease. Symptomatic hypercalcemia is associated with a high mortality rate; treatment must be promptly instituted. Until the primary disease can be brought

Table 16–7. Causes of hypercalcemia.

Increased intake or absorption
  Milk-alkali syndrome
  Vitamin D or vitamin A excess
Endocrine disorders
  Primary hyperparathyroidism (adenoma, hyperplasia, carcinoma)
  Secondary hyperparathyroidism (renal insufficiency, malabsorption)
  Acromegaly
  Adrenal insufficiency
Neoplastic disease
  Tumors producing PTH-like peptides (ovary, kidney, lung)
  Metastases to bone
  Lymphoproliferative disease, including multiple myeloma
  Secretion of prostaglandins and osteolytic factors
Miscellaneous causes
  Thiazide diuretic-induced
  Sarcoidosis
  Paget's disease of bone
  Hypophosphatasia
  Immobilization
  Familial hypocalciuric hypercalcemia
  Complications of renal transplantation
  Iatrogenic

under control, renal excretion of calcium with resultant decrease in serum Ca^{2+} concentration should be promoted. Excretion of Na^+ is accompanied by excretion of Ca^{2+}; therefore, inducing natriuresis by giving Na^+ salts intravenously and by adjunctive use of diuretics is the emergency treatment of choice. Sodium in large quantities (50–80 mmol/h), as chloride or sulfate, with or without diuretics (furosemide), may be required for 12–48 hours. Replacement of water, K^+, and Mg^{2+} is usually necessary. Calcitonin may be a useful adjunct, but tachyphylaxis develops in 24–48 hours. The use of phosphate is hazardous and should be reserved for unusual cases refractory to saline therapy. When elevated Ca^{2+} concentrations result from sarcoidosis or neoplasm, corticosteroids such as prednisone may be effective. Mithramycin is useful if elevated Ca^{2+} is the result of neoplasm metastatic to bone. Recent experience with diphosphonates indicates that they may play a central role in treatment of hypercalcemia; toxicity appears minimal.

2. HYPOCALCEMIA

Important causes of hypocalcemia are listed in Table 16–8.

Clinical Findings

A. Symptoms and Signs: Hypocalcemia affects neuromuscular function to produce muscle cramps and tetany, convulsions, stridor and dyspnea, diplopia, abdominal cramps, and urinary frequency. Chvostek's and Trousseau's signs are usually readily elicited. Cataracts may appear and calcification of basal ganglia of the brain may occur in chronic hypoparathyroidism. Mental retardation and stunted growth are common in childhood. (See Hypoparathyroidism, Chapter 20.)

Table 16–8. Causes of hypocalcemia.

Decreased intake or absorption
  Malabsorption
  Small bowel bypass, short bowel
  Vitamin D deficit (decreased absorption, decreased
    production of 25-hydroxyvitamin D or 1,25-
    dihydroxyvitamin D)
Increased loss
  Chronic renal insufficiency
  Diuretic therapy
Endocrine disease
  Hypoparathyroidism (genetic, acquired; including hypo- and
    hypermagnesemia)
  Pseudohypoparathyroidism
  Calcitonin secretion with medullary carcinoma of the thyroid
Physiologic causes
  Associated with decreased serum albumin
  Decreased end-organ response to vitamin D
  Hyperphosphatemia
  Induced by aminoglycoside antibiotics, mithramycin, loop
    diuretics

B. Laboratory Findings: Serum Ca^{2+} is low. The level of serum Ca^{2+} must be correlated with the simultaneous concentration of serum albumin: When albumin concentration is depressed, serum Ca^{2+} concentration is also depressed in a ratio of 0.8–1 mg of Ca^{2+} to 1 g of albumin. Serum phosphate is usually elevated. Serum Mg^{2+} is commonly low, and hypomagnesemia reduces tissue responsiveness to parathyroid hormone. Other findings are those of the primary disease. The ECG shows a prolonged QT interval.

Treatment

Treatment depends on the primary disease. Treatment of hypoparathyroidism with vitamin D and calcium is discussed in Chapter 20. For tetany due to hypocalcemia, calcium gluconate, 1–2 g, may be given intravenously. A continuous infusion to sustain plasma calcium concentration may be required. Oral medication with the chloride, gluconate, levulinate, lactate, or carbonate salts of calcium will usually control milder symptoms or latent tetany. Vitamin D may be required to ensure adequate absorption of calcium. (See Vitamin D, Chapter 22.) The low serum Ca^{2+} associated with low serum albumin concentration does not require replacement therapy. If serum Mg^{2+} is low, therapy must include replacement of magnesium, which by itself usually will correct hypocalcemia.

MAGNESIUM

About 50% of total body magnesium exists in the insoluble state in bone. Only 5% is present as extracellular cation; the remaining 45% is contained in cells as intracellular cation. The normal plasma concentration is 1.5–2.5 meq/L, with about one-third bound to protein and two-thirds as free cation. Excretion of magnesium ion is via the kidney.

Magnesium is an important activator ion, participating in the function of many enzymes involved in phosphate transfer reactions. Magnesium exerts physiologic effects on the nervous system resembling those of calcium. Magnesium acts directly upon the myoneural junction.

Altered concentration of Mg^{2+} in the plasma usually provokes an associated alteration of Ca^{2+}. Hypermagnesemia suppresses secretion of parathyroid hormone (PTH) with consequent hypocalcemia. Severe and prolonged magnesium depletion impairs secretion of PTH with consequent hypocalcemia. Hypomagnesemia may impair end-organ response to PTH as well.

1. HYPERMAGNESEMIA

Magnesium excess is almost always the result of renal insufficiency and the inability to excrete what has been taken in from food or drugs, especially antacids.

Clinical Findings

A. Symptoms and Signs: Muscle weakness, mental obtundation, and confusion are characteristic manifestations. Weakness, even flaccid paralysis, and fall in blood pressure are evident on examination. There may be respiratory muscle paralysis or cardiac arrest.

B. Laboratory Findings: Serum Mg^{2+} is elevated. In the common setting of renal insufficiency, concentrations of serum creatinine, urea nitrogen, phosphate, and uric acid are elevated; serum K^+ may be elevated. Serum Ca^{2+} is often low. The ECG shows increased PR interval, broadened QRS complexes, and elevated T waves.

Treatment

Treatment is directed toward alleviating renal insufficiency. Calcium acts as an antagonist to Mg^{2+} and may be given intravenously as calcium chloride, 500 mg or more at a rate of 100 mg (4.5 mmol)/min. Hemodialysis or peritoneal dialysis may be indicated.

2. HYPOMAGNESEMIA

Relatively common causes of hypomagnesemia are given in Table 16–9.

Clinical Findings

A. Symptoms and Signs: Common symptoms are weakness, muscle cramps, and tremor. There is marked neuromuscular and central nervous system hyperirritability, with tremors, athetoid movements, jerking, nystagmus, and a positive Babinski response. There may be hypertension, tachycardia, and ventricular arrhythmias. Confusion and disorientation may be prominent.

Table 16–9. Causes of hypomagnesemia.

Diminished absorption or intake
Malabsorption, chronic diarrhea, laxative abuse
Prolonged gastrointestinal suction
Small bowel bypass
Malnutrition
Alcoholism
Parenteral alimentation with inadequate Mg^{2+} content
Increased loss
Diabetic ketoacidosis
Diuretic therapy
Diarrhea
Hyperaldosteronism, Bartter's syndrome
Associated with hypercalciuria
Renal magnesium wasting
Unexplained
Hyperparathyroidism
Postparathyroidectomy
Vitamin D therapy
Induced by aminoglycoside antibiotics, cisplatin

B. Laboratory Findings: The serum Mg^{2+} is low. Hypocalcemia and hypokalemia are often present. The ECG shows a prolonged QT interval particularly due to lengthening of the ST segment.

Treatment

Treatment consists of the use of intravenous fluids containing magnesium as chloride or sulfate, 10–50 mmol/d during the period of severe deficit followed by 5 mmol/d for maintenance. Magnesium sulfate may also be given intramuscularly, 8–33 mmol/d in 4 divided doses. Serum levels must be monitored and dosage adjusted to prevent the concentration from rising above 2.5 mmol/L. K^+ and Ca^{2+} may be required as well. Magnesium oxide, 250–500 mg by mouth 2–4 times daily, is useful for repleting stores in those with chronic hypomagnesemia.

PHOSPHORUS

Eighty percent of the phosphorus in the body is combined with calcium in bones and teeth. Only 10% is incorporated in a variety of organic compounds, and 10% is combined with proteins, lipids, carbohydrates, and other compounds in muscle and blood. Organic phosphate is the principal intracellular anion; inorganic phosphate comprises only a small fraction of intracellular phosphorus.

Phosphate compounds are integral agents in energy transfer and in the metabolism of carbohydrate, protein, and fat. Phosphate serves as the principal urinary buffer (HPO_4^{2-}, $H_2PO_4^-$), constituting most of titratable acidity.

Renal tubular reabsorption of filtered phosphate is reduced (phosphate excretion increased) by parathyroid hormone, expansion of extracellular fluid volume, increased intake of sodium, hypercalcemia, calcitonin, glucocorticoids, and growth hormone.

Phosphorus metabolism and homeostasis are intimately related to calcium metabolism. See sections on calcium metabolism and bone disease.

1. HYPERPHOSPHATEMIA

Causes of hyperphosphatemia are given in Table 16–10. Growing children normally have serum phosphate levels higher than those of adults.

Clinical Findings

A. Symptoms and Signs: The clinical manifestations are those of the underlying disorders (eg, chronic renal failure, hypoparathyroidism).

B. Laboratory Findings: Serum phosphate is increased. Other blood chemistry values are those characteristic of the underlying disease.

Treatment

Treatment is that of the underlying disease and

Table 16–10. Causes of hyperphosphatemia.

Endocrine disease
  Excessive growth hormone (acromegaly)
  Hypoparathyroidism associated with low calcium
  Pseudohypoparathyroidism associated with low calcium
Renal disease
  Chronic renal insufficiency
  Acute renal failure
Catabolic states; tissue destruction
  Stress or injury, rhabdomyolysis (especially if renal insufficiency exists)
  Chemotherapy of malignant disease, particularly lymphoproliferative
Excessive intake or absorption
  Laxatives or enemas containing phosphate
  Hypervitaminosis D

Table 16–11. Causes of phosphate depletion and hypophosphatemia.

Causes of Phosphate Depletion

Diminished supply or absorption
  Starvation
  Parenteral alimentation with inadequate phosphate content
  Malabsorption syndrome, small bowel bypass
  Absorption blocked by aluminum hydroxide or bicarbonate
  Vitamin D-deficient and vitamin D-resistant osteomalacia
Increased loss
  Hyperparathyroidism (primary or secondary)
  Hyperthyroidism
  Renal tubular defects permitting excessive phosphaturia (congenital, induced by monoclonal gammopathy, heavy metal poisoning)
  Hypokalemic nephropathy (potassium depletion)
  Inadequately controlled diabetes mellitus

Causes of Hypophosphatemia

All of the conditions listed above
Intracellular shift of phosphorus
  Administration of glucose, fructose (transient)
  Administration of insulin (transient)
  Anabolic steroids, estrogen, oral contraceptives
  Respiratory alkalosis
  Salicylate poisoning
Electrolyte abnormalities
  Hypercalcemia
  Hypomagnesemia
  Metabolic alkalosis
Causes of clinically significant hypophosphatemia (losses followed by inadequate repletion)
  Diabetes mellitus with acidosis, particularly during aggressive therapy
  Recovery from starvation or prolonged catabolic state
  Total parenteral nutrition with inadequate ration of phosphate
  Chronic alcoholism, particularly during restoration of nutrition; associated with hypomagnesemia (magnesium deficit)
  Respiratory alkalosis
  Recovery from severe burns

of acute onset of hypocalcemia. In acute and chronic renal failure, dialysis will reduce serum phosphate. Absorption of phosphate can be reduced by administration of aluminum hydroxide gel, 30 mL or (as tablets) 4–5 g 3–4 times daily.

2. HYPOPHOSPHATEMIA & PHOSPHORUS DEFICIENCY

Hypophosphatemia may occur in the presence of normal phosphate stores. Serious depletion of body phosphate stores may exist with low, normal, or high concentrations of phosphorus in serum. Leading causes of hypophosphatemia are listed in Table 16–11.

Clinical Findings

A. Symptoms and Signs: Acute, severe hypophosphatemia (0.1–0.2 mg/dL) can lead to acute hemolytic anemia with increased erythrocyte fragility; impaired oxygen delivery to tissues, increased susceptibility to infection from impaired chemotaxis of leukocytes, and platelet dysfunction with petechial hemorrhages. Rhabdomyolysis, encephalopathy (irritability, confusion, dysarthria, convulsive seizures, and coma), and heart failure are uncommon but serious manifestations.

Chronic severe depletion may be manifested by anorexia, pain in muscles and bones, and fractures.

B. Laboratory Findings: In acute symptomatic hypophosphatemia, serum phosphorus is less than 1 mg/dL. Evidence of anemia due to hemolysis may be present (eg, elevated serum lactate dehydrogenase). Rhabdomyolysis results in elevated serum creatine kinase (which contains mostly MM fraction but also some MB fraction) and, often, myoglobin in the urine. Other values vary according to the cause. In chronic depletion, radiographs and biopsies of bones show changes resembling those of osteomalacia.

Treatment

Treatment is best directed toward prophylaxis by including phosphate in repletion and maintenance fluids. For parenteral alimentation, 20 mmol of phosphorus is required for 1000 nonprotein kcal to maintain phosphate balance and to ensure anabolic function. A daily ration for prolonged parenteral fluid maintenance is 20–40 mmol phosphorus. A commercially available KH_2PO_4/K_2HPO_4 mixture (pH 6.5) provides potassium, 4.4 mmol/L, and phosphate, 3 mmol/mL; 5 mL added to each of 2 L of fluid would provide potassium, 44 mmol, and phosphate, 30 mmol (= 930 mg phosphorus). For asymptomatic hypophosphatemia (serum phosphorus 0.7–1 mg/dL), the infusion should provide 9–10 mmol/12 h until the serum phosphorus exceeds 1 mg/dL. A magnesium deficit often coexists and should be treated simultaneously. In administering phosphate-containing solutions, renal function must be assessed and serum calcium must be monitored to guard against production of hypocalcemia. For oral use, phosphate salts are available in skim milk (approximately 33 mmol/L). Tablets or capsules of mixtures of sodium and potassium phosphate may be given to provide 16–32 mmol of phosphorus (0.5–1 g of phosphate) per day.

Contraindications to therapy with phosphate salts include hypoparathyroidism, renal insufficiency, tissue damage and necrosis, and hypercalcemia.

THE APPROACH TO DIAGNOSIS & TREATMENT OF WATER, ELECTROLYTE, & ACID-BASE DISTURBANCES

In the diagnosis and treatment of water and electrolyte derangements, one must rely upon clinical appraisal of the patient, including details of the history, the presenting disease and its complications, recent and abrupt change in weight, the physical examination, and the laboratory data bearing upon altered volume, osmolality, distribution, and physiologic manifestations. Although a thorough knowledge of the physiologic principles of water and electrolyte metabolism and of renal function is essential for sound management, the physician must always consider and be grateful for the homeostatic resources of the patient. If renal function is reasonably good, the range between acceptable lower and upper limits of amounts of water and electrolytes is broad and the achievement of "balance" not difficult. In the presence of renal insufficiency, some endocrinopathies influencing water and electrolyte metabolism, shock, heart failure, hepatic insufficiency, severe gastrointestinal fluid loss, pulmonary insufficiency, and some rarer diseases, the patient is deprived of homeostatic resources, and the physician is called upon to substitute meticulous quantitative therapy.

MAINTENANCE

Most of those who require water and electrolyte intravenously are relatively normal people who cannot take orally what they require for maintenance. Table 16–12 shows that the range of tolerance for water and electrolytes (homeostatic limits) permits reasonable latitude in therapy provided normal renal function exists to accomplish the final regulation of volume and concentration.

An average adult whose entire intake is parenteral would require for maintenance 2500–3000 mL of 5% or 10% dextrose in 0.2% saline solution (34 meq Na+ plus Cl−/L). To each liter, 30 meq of KCl could be added. In 3 L, the total chloride intake would be 192 meq, which is easily tolerated. An alternative would be to eliminate the KCl if parenteral

Table 16–12. Daily maintenance rations for patients requiring parenteral fluids.

	Per m^2 Body Surface	Average Adult (60–100 kg)
Glucose	60–75 g	100–200 g
Na$^+$	50–70 meq	80–120 meq
K$^+$	50–70 meq	80–120 meq
Water	1500 mL	2500 mL

fluids would be required for only 2–3 days. Other solutions available for maintenance therapy contain electrolyte mixtures designed to meet average adult requirements: in one example, each liter contains dextrose, 50 g; Na$^+$, 40 meq; K$^+$, 35 meq; Cl$^-$, 40 meq; HCO$_3$$^-$ equivalent, 20 meq; and PO$_4$$^{3-}$, 15 meq. The daily administration of 2500–3000 mL satisfies the needs listed in Table 16–12.

In situations requiring maintenance or maintenance plus replacement of fluid and electrolyte by parenteral infusion, the total daily ration should be administered continuously over the 24-hour period in order to ensure the best utilization by the patient. Periodic large infusions result in responsive excretion by the kidney. With modern techniques for continuous infusion, around-the-clock administration imposes little discomfort or hardship on the patient.

If parenteral fluids are the only source of water, electrolyte, and calories for longer than a week, more complex fluids containing amino acids, lipid, trace metals, and vitamins should be used under carefully controlled conditions. (See Total Parenteral Nutrition, Chapter 22.)

DEFICITS

To the maintenance ration one must add water and appropriate electrolyte for replacement of losses previously incurred and to replace current losses. The amounts of water and electrolytes are dictated by clinical evaluation of deficits of each, and a further choice of anion would be dictated by the presence of metabolic acidosis or alkalosis and in some instances of respiratory acidosis.

The severity of dehydration (volume depletion) is assessed by means of the history, the magnitude of acute weight loss, and, on physical examination, the loss of elasticity of the skin and subcutaneous tissues, dry mucous membranes, tachycardia and hypotension, lethargy, and weakness. As dehydration becomes more severe, the decrease in plasma volume results in progression of hypotension and shock. An increase in blood urea nitrogen reflects the decreases in glomerular filtration rate associated with low blood volume.

Changes in effective extracellular fluid volume and circulating blood volume accompany the acute redistribution of fluid following burns, bowel obstruction, peritonitis, venous obstruction, and, rarely, lymphatic obstruction.

Treatment consists of replacement of water deficit with appropriate electrolyte according to serum osmolality (Na^+ concentration), blood pH, and serum K^+ concentration. In the presence of hyperosmolality (hypernatremia), electrolyte-free or hypotonic solutions should be employed; if serum Na^+ concentration is normal, repletion can be accomplished with isotonic solutions. If hyposmolality (hyponatremia) exists due to sodium loss, hypertonic (3%) NaCl solutions or hypertonic $NaHCO_3$ solutions may be required, but only if the serum sodium is less than 120 mg/dL. In addition to replacement needs, maintenance requirements must be met, requiring correlation of volume, electrolyte concentration, and rate of administration to effect a normal state.

One should aim for total replacement in 48–72 hours. Time is required for circulation, diffusion, equilibration, renal response, and restoration of normal homeostatic mechanisms; a general rule is to provide daily maintenance needs plus half the deficit in the first 24 hours and a quarter of the deficit daily for 2 days thereafter to complete restitution in 72 hours. To this must be added the equivalent of continuing losses.

SUMMARY OF CLINICAL APPROACH

The following outline summarizes an approach to therapy with water and electrolytes. Listed are factors essential to an assessment of the state of the patient, of the urgency for treatment, and of the choice of the therapeutic agents and the quantities to be administered. This outline has been useful in planning the therapeutic attack and averting the omission of essential elements of treatment.

Problems

1. Maintenance.
2. Repair of deficit plus maintenance.

3. Repair plus replacement of continuing losses plus maintenance.
4. Replacement of continuing losses plus maintenance.

Situations: Acute or Chronic

A. Acute:

1. Respiratory– Pco_2 and pH. Often overlooked. H^+ concentration can change rapidly to life-threatening levels.
2. Organic ion acidosis (lactate, ketones), "anion gap." (Normally, Cl^- plus HCO_3^- plus 12 equals Na^+ in meq/L.)
3. Plasma K^+, Mg^{2+}, Ca^{2+}, and PO_4^{3-} deficit or excess.
4. Hyper- or hyposmolality, often iatrogenic.
5. Explosive gastrointestinal loss; Addison's disease in crisis.
6. Acute renal failure.

B. Chronic:

1. Renal insufficiency.
2. Pulmonary insufficiency.
3. Chronic gastrointestinal disease (gut, liver).
4. Endocrine abnormality, especially myxedema.

Determinants in Establishing Therapy

Sex: Females have proportionately more body fat than males.

Size: Fat or lean; more fat means lower ratios of total body water/kg.

Renal and pulmonary function.

Cause of abnormal state, ie, shock, gastrointestinal obstruction, third space sequestration, diabetes or other endocrine abnormality, malnutrition, drug effect, or therapeutic error. Observations

Weight.

Intake, output, and loss record.

Serum electrolytes, osmolality, urea, creatinine, protein, glucose.

Arterial blood Pco_2, pH, Po_2 as indicated.

Urine specific gravity, osmolality, volume.

REFERENCES

General

Brenner BM, Rector FC Jr (editors): *The Kidney,* 3rd ed. Vol 1. Saunders, 1986.

Knochel JP: Neuromuscular manifestations of electrolyte disorders. Am J Med 1982;72:521.

Maxwell M, Kleeman CR (editors): *Clinical Disorders of Fluid and Electrolyte Metabolism,* 4th ed. McGraw-Hill, 1987.

Mitch WE, Wilcox CS: Disorders of body fluids, sodium and potassium in chronic renal failure. Am J Med 1982;72:536.

Narins RG, Emmett M: Simple and mixed acid-base disorders: A practical approach. Medicine 1980; 59:161.

Narins RG et al: Diagnostic strategies in disorders of fluid, electrolyte and acid-base homeostasis. Am J Med 1982;72:496.

Rose BD: Clinical *Physiology of Acid-Base & Electrolyte Disorders,* 3rd ed. McGraw-Hill, 1989.

Fluid Volume & Sodium

Anderson RJ: Hospital-associated hyponatremia. Kidney Int 1986;29:1237.

Anderson RJ et al: Hyponatremia: A prospective analysis of its epidemiology and the pathogenetic role of vasopressin. Ann Intern Med 1985;102:164.

Ayus JC, Krothapalli RK, Arieff AI: Treatment of symptomatic hyponatremia and its relation to brain damage: A prospective study. N Engl J Med 1987;317:1190.

Berl T: Treating hyponatremia: Damned if we do and damned if we don't. Kidney Int 1990;37:1006.

Cluitmans FHM, Meinders AE: Management of severe hyponatremia: Rapid or slow correction? Am J Med 1990;88:161.

Gardenswartz MH, Berl T: Drug-induced changes in water excretion. Kidney (May) 1981;14:19.

Gennari FJ: Serum osmolality: Uses and limitations. N Engl J Med 1984;310:102.

Jamison RL, Oliver RE: Disorders of urinary concentration and dilution. Am J Med 1982;72:308.

Moran SM et al: The variable hyponatremic response to hyperglycemia. West J Med 1985;142:49.

Narins RG et al: Diagnostic strategies in disorders of fluid, electrolyte and acid-base homeostasis. Am J Med 1982;72:496.

Rose BD: A physiologic approach to solute and water balance in hyponatremia. Kidney (Jan) 1984;17:1.

Schrier RW: Treatment of hyponatremia: Editorial retrospective. N Engl J Med 1985;312:1121.

Spital A, Sterns RD: Paradox of sodium's volume of distribution: Why extracellular solute appears to distribute over total body water. Arch Intern Med 1989;149:1255.

Hydrogen Ion

Bersin RM, Chatterjee K, Arieff AI: Metabolic and hemodynamic consequences of sodium bicarbonate administration in patients with heart disease. Am J Med 1989;87:7.

Cogan MG et al: Metabolic alkalosis. Med Clin North Am 1983;67:903.

Cohen RD, Woods HF: Lactic acidosis revisited. Diabetes 1983;32:181.

Cooper DU et al: Bicarbonate does not improve hemodynamics in critically ill patients who have lactic acidosis. Ann Intern Med 1990;112:492.

Harrington JT: Metabolic alkalosis. (Clinical conference.) Kidney Int 1984;26:88.

Kassirer JP: Life-threatening acid-base disorders. Adv Nephrol 1985;14:67.

Lever E, Jaspan JB: Sodium bicarbonate therapy in severe diabetic ketoacidosis. Am J Med 1983;75:263.

Mizock BA: Controversies in lactic acidosis: Implications in critically ill patients. JAMA 1987;258:497.

Narins RG, Cohen JJ: Bicarbonate therapy for organic acidosis: The case for its continued use. Ann Intern Med 1987;106:615.

Oster JR, Epstein M: Acid-base aspects of ketoacidosis. Am J Nephrol 1984;4:137.

Relman AS: "Blood gases": Arterial or venous? (Editorial.) N Engl J Med 1986;315:188.

Schade DS (editor): Metabolic acidosis. Clin Endocrinol Metab 1983;12:265. (Entire issue.)

Stacpoole PW: Lactic acidosis: The case against bicarbonate therapy. Ann Intern Med 1986;105:276.

Weil MH et al: Difference in acid-base state between venous and arterial blood during cardiopulmonary resuscitation. N Engl J Med 1986;315:153.

Williams HE: Alcoholic hypoglycemia and ketoacidosis. Med Clin North Am 1984;68:33.

Potassium

Cannon-Babb ML, Schwartz AB: Drug-induced hyperkalemia. Hosp Pract 1986;21:99.

Hollenberg NK (editor): Potassium, magnesium and cardiovascular morbidity. Am J Med 1986;80(Suppl 4A):1.

Hollenberg NK, Hollifield JW (editors): Potassium/magnesium depletion: Is your patient at risk of sudden death? Am J Med 1987;82(Suppl 3A):1.

Kaplan NM: Our appropriate concern about hypokalemia. (Editorial.) Am J Med 1984;77:1.

Knochel JP: Etiologies and management of potassium deficiency. Hosp Pract 1987;22:153.

Kurtzman NA: Hypokalemia. Adv Exp Med Biol 1989;252:155.

Narins RG et al: Diagnostic strategies in disorders of fluid, electrolyte and acid-base homeostasis. Am J Med 1982;72:496.

Seldin DW, Giebisch GL (editors): *The Regulation of Potassium Balance.* Raven, 1989.

Williams ME, Rosa RM, Epstein FH: Hyperkalemia. Adv Intern Med 1986;32:265.

Calcium

Alveoli LV, Haddad JG: The vitamin D family revisited. (Editorial.) N Engl J Med 1984;311:47.

Body J-J et al: Dose/response study of aminohydroxypropylidene biphosphonate in tumor-associated hypercalcemia. Am J Med 1987;82:957.

Harinck HIJ et al: Role of bone and kidney in tumor-induced hypercalcemia and its treatment with biphosphonate and sodium chloride. Am J Med 1987;82:1133.

Mundy GR: *Calcium Homeostasis: Hypocalcemia and Hypercalcemia.* Martin Dunitz, 1989.

Mundy GR et al: The hypercalcemia of cancer: Clinical implications and pathogenic mechanisms. N Engl J Med 1984;310:1718.

Ralston SH et al: Comparison of three intravenous biphosphonates in cancer-associated hypercalcemia. Lancet 1989;2:1180.

Sutton RA: Disorders of renal calcium excretion. Kidney Int 1983;23:665.

Zaloga GP et al: Hypocalcemia in critical illness. JAMA 1986;256:1924.

Magnesium

Cronin RE, Knochel JP: Magnesium deficiency. Adv Intern Med 1983;28:509.

Hollenberg NK (editor): Potassium, magnesium and cardiovascular morbidity. Am J Med 1986;80(Suppl 4A):1.

Hollenberg NK, Hollifield JW (editors): Potassium/magnesium depletion: Is your patient at risk of sudden death? Am J Med 1987;82(Suppl 3A):1.

Levine BS, Coburn JW: Magnesium, the mimic/antagonist of calcium. N Engl J Med 1984;310:1253.

Ryzen E, Rude RK: Low intracellular magnesium in

patients with acute pancreatitis and hypocalcemia. West J Med 1990;152:145.

Whang R et al: Frequency of hypomagnesemia in hospitalized patients receiving digitalis. Arch Intern Med 1985;145:655.

Whang R et al: Predictors of clinical hypomagnesemia: Hypokalemia, hypophosphatemia, hyponatremia, and hypocalcemia. Arch Intern Med 1984;144:1794.

Phosphorus

Knochel JP: The clinical status of hypophosphatemia: An update. (Editorial.) N Engl J Med 1985;313:447.

Stoff JS: Phosphate homeostasis and hypophosphatemia. Am J Med 1982;72:489.

Yu GC, Lee DB: Clinical disorders of phosphorus metabolism. West J Med 1987;147:569.

17

Genitourinary Tract

Marcus A. Krupp, MD

NONSPECIFIC MANIFESTATIONS OF GENITOURINARY DISEASES OR DISORDERS

Pain

The localization, pattern of referral, and type of pain are important clues to the diagnosis of genitourinary tract disease.

(1) Pain caused by renal disease is usually felt as a dull ache in the "flanks" or costovertebral angle, often extending along the rib margin toward the umbilicus. Because many renal diseases do not produce sudden distention of the capsules of the kidney, pain is often absent.

(2) Ureteral pain is related to obstruction and is usually acute in onset, severe, and colicky and radiates from the costovertebral angle down the course of the ureter into the scrotum or vulva and the inner thigh. The radiation of the pain may be a clue to the site of obstruction. High ureteral pain is usually referred to the testicle or vulva; midureteral pain to the lower quadrants of the abdomen; and low ureteral pain to the bladder.

(3) Bladder pain accompanies overdistention of the bladder in acute urinary retention with distention of a bladder wall altered by tuberculosis or interstitial cystitis. Relief comes with emptying the bladder. Pain due to bladder infection is usually referred to the distal urethra and accompanies micturition. Pain caused by chronic bladder disease is uncommon.

(4) Acute prostatic inflammation may produce perineal or low mid back pain.

(5) Pain caused by testicular inflammation or trauma is acute and severe and is occasionally referred to the costovertebral angle. Pain associated with infection of the epididymis is similar to that associated with testicular inflammation.

Urinary Symptoms

Infection, inflammation, and obstruction produce symptoms associated with urination.

(1) Frequency, urgency, and nocturia are common when inflammation of the urinary tract is present. Severe infection produces a constant desire to urinate even though the bladder contains only a few milliliters of urine. Frequency and nocturia occur when bladder capacity is diminished by disease or when the bladder cannot be emptied completely, leaving a large volume of residual urine. Nocturia associated with a large urine volume may occur with heart failure, renal insufficiency, mobilization of edema due to any cause, diabetes insipidus, hyperaldosteronism, hypercalcemia, ingestion of large amounts of fluid late in the evening, and diuretics.

(2) Dysuria and burning pain in the urethra on urination are associated with infection of the bladder, prostate, or urethra.

(3) Enuresis may be due to urinary tract disease but is most often caused by functional disorders.

(4) Urinary incontinence may be due to anatomic abnormality, physical stress, the urgency associated with infection or nervous system disease, or the dribbling associated with an overdistended flaccid bladder.

Characteristics of Urine

Urinalysis, an essential part of the examination of all patients, is critical in the study of patients who may have renal disease. Some organic and inorganic materials in solution in the urine are diagnostic of metabolic disease (inherited or acquired) and of renal disease.

(1) Proteinuria (albuminuria): Normally, up to 150 mg of protein is excreted daily in urine. Exercise, febrile illness, or severe dehydration may produce increased proteinuria in persons without renal disease. Rarely, a normal person may have significant proteinuria when in an upright position but none while recumbent (postural or orthostatic proteinuria). Proteinuria in excess of 200–500 mg/d is almost always indicative of renal disease. In most cases of significant proteinuria, increased filtration of protein occurs because of reduction in the density of anionic charges in the glomerular capillary wall, not because of altered epithelial pore size. The "dipstick" test for albumin will usually not detect light-chain globulins (eg, Bence Jones protein) and will be false-positive with highly alkaline urine. Tests with sulfosalicylic acid will be false-positive with sulfisoxazole metabolites, tolbutamide metabolites, acetazolamide, some penicillins (nafcillin, ampicillin, piperacillin), some cephalosporins, levodopa, and tolmetin and with radiographic contrast media.

(2) Urinary sediment provides evidence of renal disease that is not available from other sources, and some elements are characteristic of the type and extent of renal disease. The physician should examine the sediment if renal disease may be present; the highest yield is with a fresh first morning-voided specimen.

(3) Cloudy urine is most frequently due to the urates or phosphates that precipitate out as urine collects in the bladder and is usually of no significance.

(4) Hematuria nearly always means structural genitourinary disease. It may be due to glomerular disease, neoplasms, vascular accidents, infections, anomalies, stones, coagulation defects, or trauma to the urinary tract. When blood appears only during the initial period of voiding, the most likely source is the anterior urethra or prostate. When blood appears during the terminal period of voiding, the most likely source is the posterior urethra, vesical neck, or trigone. Blood mixed in with the total urine volume is from the kidneys, ureters, or bladder. Red blood cells that have come from the glomerulus may be dysmorphic and show a variety of distorted forms and swollen forms. Red cells from elsewhere in the urinary tract are not distorted.

Causes of Hematuria

The causes of hematuria can be summarized as follows:

A. Localized:

1. Urethra and prostate–Trauma, infection.

2. Bladder–Infection, stone, neoplasm, varices (especially of bladder neck with prostatic enlargement), drug reaction (cyclophosphamide), radiation injury, parasite infection (*Schistosoma haematobium*).

3. Ureter–Infection, stone, tumor.

4. Kidney–Glomerular disease, infection, stone, anatomic anomalies (including polycystic disease, arteriovenous malformations), renal vein or artery thrombosis, neoplasms, trauma (including renal biopsy).

B. Systemic:

1. Anticoagulant therapy.

2. Bleeding diathesis–Hemophilia, thrombocytopenia, disseminated intravascular coagulation.

3. Hemolytic disease–Hemoglobinurias, hemolytic-uremic syndrome.

4. Sickle cell disease.

5. Anaphylactoid purpura with renal involvement.

RENAL FUNCTION TESTS

Diagnosis of renal diseases and evaluation of renal function depend on laboratory determinations. As renal function becomes impaired, laboratory observations provide reliable indices of the capacity of the kidney to meet the demands of excretion, reabsorption, and secretion and to fulfill its role in maintaining homeostasis. Useful tests may be categorized according to the physiologic function measured:

(1) Glomerular filtration rate (GFR): Inulin clearance is the reference method for measuring GFR. After a single intravenous injection of ^{51}Cr edetate, ^{99m}technetium diethylenetriamine pentaacetate, or ^{131}I iothalamate, the slope of decreasing concentration in plasma can be determined to give a precise measure of GFR. For routine clinical use, the less precise endogenous creatinine clearance is adequate. Plasma creatinine or urea levels reflect GFR, rising as the filtration rate diminishes. GFR may be estimated from the serum creatinine by the following formula:

$$\text{GFR (mL/min)} = \frac{(140 - \text{Age}) \times \text{Weight (kg)}}{72 \times \text{Serum creatinine (mg/dL)}}$$

The result is for men; for women, multiply the result by 0.85.

Concentrations of serum urea nitrogen and creatinine are used as indicators of adequacy of renal function. Urea nitrogen concentration will vary directly with the quantity of protein in the diet and will increase with increased catabolism following trauma or stressful disease or with decreased renal blood flow (decreased filtration and increased reabsorption). The combination of a high protein load and decreased renal blood flow consequent to bleeding into the upper gastrointestinal tract will result in a transient elevation of serum urea nitrogen. Creatinine is produced at a relatively constant rate independently of diet; total excreted per day is directly related to muscle mass and is therefore diminished in patients who have lost muscle (eg, in the elderly, postpoliomyelitis, with inanition). It is excreted at a fairly constant rate by glomerular filtration; for clinical purposes, tubular secretion is of little consequence except when renal failure is well advanced and tubular secretion produces a significant portion of the total creatinine excreted. Creatinine clearance in the presence of chronic renal failure yields higher values than does inulin clearance. The concentration of serum creatinine increases as renal impairment advances; the concentration exceeds the normal level when creatinine clearance reaches about 50% of normal. Serum creatinine concentration is especially low in patients who have decreased muscle mass. The ratio of concentration of serum urea nitrogen to creatinine is normally about 10:1. Ratios greater than 15:1 occur with prerenal azotemia, postrenal azotemia due to acute obstructive uropathy, and upper gastrointestinal hemorrhage.

(2) Tubular function: Clinical means of assessing tubular function include the ability to produce urine that is more concentrated or less concentrated than the osmolality of plasma and the ability to acidify the urine.

RENAL BIOPSY

Renal biopsy is useful to confirm the diagnosis in instances in which choice of therapy depends on tissue diagnosis. Tissue should be prepared for light and electron microscopy and for immunofluorescent stains. Percutaneous renal biopsy is used to distinguish by structural characteristics the causes of nephrotic syndrome, to determine the presence of generalized disease (amyloidosis, autoimmune diseases), to define the lesion of rapidly progressive glomerulonephritis, and to identify other causes of hematuria and proteinuria. Biopsy is also used to assess rejection response in a transplanted kidney. Absolute contraindications include anatomic presence of only one kidney; severe malfunction of one kidney even though function is adequate in the other; bleeding diathesis; the presence of hemangioma, tumor, or large cysts; perinephric abscess or renal infection; hydronephrosis; and an uncooperative patient. Relative contraindications are the presence of serious hypertension, end-stage chronic renal failure, severe arteriosclerosis, and unusual difficulty in doing a biopsy owing to obesity, anasarca, or inability of the patient to lie flat.

Complications of renal biopsy occur in 5–10% of attempts. The commonest of these is gross hematuria that slowly subsides within 1 or 2 days. Perirenal hemorrhage occurs rarely—and even more rarely, an arteriovenous fistula may be created.

RADIOGRAPHIC EXAMINATION & ULTRASOUND

Renal Radiography

Radiography is an essential resource for the diagnosis and evaluation of renal disease amenable to medical as well as surgical treatment. Kidney size, shape, and position may be critical elements of information. Routine films, tomography, urography, angiography, and CT and MRI scans are sources of anatomic and physiologic data that often are definitive, revealing details of circulation, structure, and calcification available by no other means. Collaboration with the radiologist provides the greatest opportunity for properly performed and interpreted examinations. Radiographic contrast agents are hazardous in the presence of severe dehydration, renal disease, diabetic nephropathy, liver failure, and multiple myeloma.

Scanning With Radionuclides

Use of appropriate radioisotope-tagged compounds (iodohippurate sodium I 131, chlormerodrin Hg 203, technetium 99m Tc pertechnetate), sensitive detectors, and scintillation cameras provides ready assessment of renal blood flow and clearance of the compound, as well as visualization of the size and shape of the kidneys, the site of ureteral obstruction, and the presence of dilated ureters and urinary bladder. The 2 kidneys can be compared as a means of identifying unilateral disease.

Ultrasound (Sonography)

Ultrasound is a noninvasive technique that is free of hazard. Devices utilizing high-frequency sound waves are capable of delineating solid or fluid-filled organs or masses. Kidney size and shape can often be distinguished clearly enough to identify tumors or cysts and anomalies such as horseshoe kidney. Calcification within the kidney and urinary tract can sometimes be best demonstrated in this way. It is a useful guide in performing renal biopsy. Dilated renal calices, the renal pelvis, and the ureters and bladder can be identified. Bladder and prostatic neoplasms can often be demonstrated.

Abuels JG: Proteinuria: Diagnostic principles and procedures. Ann Intern Med 1983;98:186.

Brezis M, Epstein FH: A closer look at radiocontrast-induced nephropathy. (Editorial.) N Engl J Med 1989; 320:179.

Fairley KF, Birch DF: Hematuria: A simple method for detecting glomerular bleeding. Kidney Int 1982;21:105.

Hanglustaine D et al: Detection of glomerular bleeding using a simple staining method for light microscopy. Lancet 1982;2:761.

Morrin PAF: Urinary sediment in the interpretation of proteinuria. (Editorial.) Ann Intern Med 1983;98:254.

Sayer J, McCarthy M, Schmidt JD: Identification and significance of dysmorphic versus isomorphic hematuria. J Urol 1990;143:545.

Smith RF et al: Renal insufficiency in community patients with mild asymptomatic microhematuria. Mayo Clin Proc 1989;64:409.

DISORDERS OF THE KIDNEYS

GLOMERULONEPHRITIS

Clinical manifestations of renal disease are apt to consist only of varying degrees of microscopic hematuria, excretion of characteristic formed elements in the urine, proteinuria, and renal insufficiency and its complications. Alterations in glomerular architecture as observed in tissue examined by light microscopy are also apt to be minimal and difficult to interpret.

Immunologic techniques for demonstrating a variety of antigens, antibodies, and complement fractions have helped toward understanding the origins and pathogenesis of glomerular disease. Electron microscopy has complemented the immunologic methods. Information gleaned from use of these methods has provided a satisfactory basis for diagnosis, treatment, and prognosis.

Briefly, glomerular disease resulting from immunologic reactions may be divided into 2 groups:

(1) Immune complex disease, in which soluble antigen-antibody complexes in the circulation are trapped in the glomeruli. The antigens are not derived from glomerular components; they may be exogenous (bacterial, viral, chemical, including antibiotics and other drugs) or endogenous (circulating native DNA, tumor antigens, thyroglobulin). Factors in the pathogenic potential of the antigen include its origin, quantity, and route of entry and the host's duration of exposure to it. The immune response varies with the capacity of the host to react to antigens.

In the presence of antigen excess and, in some cases, antibody excess, antigen-antibody complexes form in the circulation and are trapped in the glomeruli as they are filtered through capillary walls rendered permeable by the action of vasoactive amines. The antigen-antibody complexes bind components of complement, particularly C3. Activated complement provides factors that attract leukocytes whose lysosomal enzymes incite the injury to the glomerulus.

Light microscopy will show reduced or occluded capillary lumens from proliferating mesangial and endothelial cells and infiltration with polymorphonuclear leukocytes, monocytes, and eosinophils in the mesangium. Bowman's space may be occupied by crescents of accumulated epithelial cells and monocytes. By immunofluorescence methods and by electron microscopy, these complexes appear as lumpy deposits between the epithelial cells and the glomerular basement membrane and in the mesangium. IgG, IgM, occasionally IgA, and C3 have been identified.

(2) Anti-glomerular basement membrane disease, in which antibodies are generated against the glomerular basement membrane of the kidney and often against lung basement membrane, which appears to be antigenically similar to glomerular basement membrane. The autoantibodies may be stimulated by autologous glomerular basement membrane altered in some way or combined with an exogenous agent. The reaction of antibody with glomerular basement membrane is accompanied by activation of complement, the attraction of leukocytes, and the release of lysosomal enzymes. The presence of thrombi in glomerular capillaries is often accompanied by leakage of fibrinogen and precipitation of fibrin in Bowman's space, with subsequent development of epithelial "crescents" in the space.

Immunofluorescence techniques and electron microscopy show the anti-glomerular basement membrane complexes as linear deposits outlining the membrane. IgG and C3 are usually demonstrable.

Classification of Glomerulonephritis

A current classification of glomerulonephritis is based on the immunologic concepts described above. However, the discussions in the following pages are organized according to traditional clinical categories.

I. Immunologic Mechanisms Likely
A. Immune Complex Disease:

Glomerulonephritis clearly poststreptococcal

Glomerulonephritis associated with infectious agents, including staphylococci, pneumococci, infective endocarditis, secondary syphilis, leprosy, malaria, toxoplasmosis, schistosomiasis; viruses of hepatitis (HBAg), measles, varicella; and HIV

Glomerulonephritis associated with other systemic (autoimmune?) disease such as systemic lupus erythematosus, polyarteritis nodosa, scleroderma, anaphylactoid purpura, idiopathic cryoglobulinemia, and tumor antigens (eg, tumors of the colon, bronchus, kidney; melanoma)

Membranous glomerulonephritis, cause unknown

Membranoproliferative glomerulonephritis, cause unknown

Focal glomerulonephritis

Rapidly progressive glomerulonephritis (some cases)

B. Anti-glomerular Basement Membrane Disease:

Goodpasture's syndrome

Rapidly progressive glomerulonephritis (some cases)

II. Immunologic Mechanisms Not Clearly Shown

Lipoid nephrosis (minimal lesion)

Focal glomerulonephritis (some cases)

Focal glomerulosclerosis

Diabetic glomerulosclerosis

Amyloidosis

Hemolytic-uremic syndrome and thrombotic thrombocytopenic purpura

Henoch-Schönlein purpura

Wegener's granulomatosis

Alport's syndrome

Sickle cell disease

1. ACUTE GLOMERULONEPHRITIS

Acute nephritis is often related to an antecedent infection with a group A hemolytic streptococcus or, less frequently, to a variety of other infectious agents. The clinical syndrome of acute nephritis occurs with other renal diseases, including systemic lupus erythematosus, idiopathic mesangiocapillary proliferative (membranoproliferative) glomerulonephritis, Henoch-Schönlein purpura, acute interstitial nephritis, and mixed cryoglobulinemia.

The following description of the clinical presentation of poststreptococcal glomerulonephritis applies in whole or in part to the syndrome of acute glomerulonephritis due to any other cause.

Essentials of Diagnosis

- History of preceding streptococcal or other infection.
- Evidence for systemic vasculitis is present in some cases.
- Malaise, headache, anorexia, low-grade fever.
- Mild generalized edema, mild hypertension, retinal hemorrhages.
- Gross hematuria; protein, red cell casts, granular and hyaline casts, white cells, and renal epithelial cells in urine.
- Evidence of impaired renal function, especially nitrogen retention.

General Considerations

Glomerulonephritis is a disease affecting both kidneys. In most cases, recovery from the acute stage is complete; however, progressive involvement may destroy renal tissue, in which case renal insufficiency results. Poststreptococcal acute glomerulonephritis is most common in children 3–10 years of age, although 5% or more of initial attacks occur in adults over age 50. By far the most common cause is an antecedent infection of the pharynx and tonsils or of the skin with group A β-hemolytic streptococci, certain strains of which are nephritogenic. In children under age 6, pyoderma (impetigo) is the most common antecedent; in older children and young adults, pharyngitis is a common antecedent and skin infection a rare one. Nephritis may follow other infections (see above) and exposure to some drugs, including penicillins, sulfonamides, phenytoin, aminosalicylic acid, and aminoglycoside antibiotics. Rhus dermatitis and reactions to venom or chemical agents may be associated with renal disease clinically indistinguishable from glomerulonephritis.

The pathogenesis of the glomerular lesion has been further elucidated by the use of immunologic techniques (immunofluorescence) and electron microscopy. A likely sequela to infection by nephritogenic strains of β-hemolytic streptococci is injury to the mesangial cells in the intercapillary space. The glomerulus may then become more easily damaged by antigen-antibody complexes developing from the immune response to the streptococcal infection. The C3 component of complement is deposited in association with IgG (rarely IgA or IgM) or alone in a granular pattern on the epithelial side of the basement membrane and occasionally in subendothelial sites as well. Similar immune complex deposits in the glomeruli can often be demonstrated when the origin is other than streptococcal.

Gross examination of the involved kidney shows only punctate hemorrhages throughout the cortex. Microscopically, the primary alteration is in the glomeruli, which show proliferation and swelling of the mesangial and endothelial cells of the capillary tuft. The proliferation of capsular epithelium produces a thickened crescent about the tuft, and in the space between the capsule and the tuft there are collections of leukocytes, red cells, and exudate. Edema of the interstitial tissue and cloudy swelling of the tubule epithelium are common. Immune complexes are demonstrable by means of immunofluorescence techniques. Electron microscopy reveals the dense immune complex deposits as well as altered glomerular structures. As the disease progresses, the kidneys may enlarge. The typical histologic findings in glomerulitis are enlarging crescents that become hyalinized and converted into scar tissue and obstruct the circulation through the glomerulus. Degenerative changes occur in the tubules, with fatty degeneration and necrosis and ultimate scarring of the nephron. Arteriolar thickening and obliteration become prominent.

Clinical Findings

A. Symptoms and Signs: Nephritis begins about 2 weeks after the streptococcal infection or exposure to a drug or other inciting agent. Often the disease is very mild, and there may be no reason to suspect renal involvement unless the urine is examined. In severe cases, the patient develops malaise, headache, mild fever, flank pain, and oliguria. The urine is noted as "bloody," "coffee-colored," or "smoky." Salt and water retention result from the diminished GFR and relatively increased tubular reabsorption. Edema appears in the periorbital areas and may include the extremities and pleural and peritoneal spaces. Increased blood volume is accompanied by increased cardiac output and some increase in arterial peripheral resistance with consequent arterial hypertension. Pulmonary vascular congestion occurs frequently and produces dyspnea. Frank pulmonary edema may ensue.

B. Laboratory Findings: The diagnosis is confirmed by examination of the urine, which may be grossly bloody or coffee-colored (acid hematin) or may show only microscopic hematuria. Red cell morphology provides a clue as to whether the origin of the red cell is glomerular or nonglomerular. Red cells of glomerular origin are dysmorphic and show a variety of distorted forms and swollen forms; red cells of nonglomerular origin are not distorted. Examine the sediment with phase microscopy or with oil immersion in light microscopy after using one of the commercially available sediment stains. The urine contains protein (1+ to 3+) and casts. Hyaline and granular casts are commonly found in large numbers, but the diagnostic sign of glomerulitis, the erythrocyte cast (blood cast), may be rare and require careful search of a centrifuged urinary sediment. The erythrocyte cast resembles a blood clot formed in the lumen of a renal tubule; it is usually of small caliber, intensely orange or red, and under high power with proper lighting may show the mosaic pattern of the packed red cells held together by the clot of fibrin and plasma protein.

With the impairment of renal function and with oliguria, plasma or serum urea nitrogen and creatinine become elevated, the levels varying with the severity of the renal lesion. The sedimentation rate is rapid. Infection of the throat with nephritogenic streptococci is frequently followed by increasing antistreptolysin O (ASO) titers in the serum, whereas high titers are usually not demonstrable following skin infections. Production of antibody against streptococcal deoxyribonuclease B (anti-DNase B) is more regularly observed following both throat and skin infections. Serum complement levels are usually low, as are urinary concentrations of sodium.

These studies are unnecessary in the diagnosis of the typical case. Confirmation is made by examination of the urine, although the history and clinical findings in typical cases leave little doubt. The finding of erythrocytes that are dysmorphic or contained in a cast is proof of their glomerular origin.

Differential Diagnosis

Although considered to be the hallmark of poststreptococcal glomerulonephritis, erythrocyte casts also occur along with other abnormal elements in any disease in which glomerular inflammation is present, ie, polyarteritis nodosa, systemic lupus erythematosus, sarcoidosis, subacute infective endocarditis, IgA nephropathy, Goodpasture's syndrome, Henoch's purpura, and Wegener's granulomatosis.

Complications

In severe cases, signs compatible with cardiac failure appear as a result of salt and water retention; they include cardiac enlargement, tachycardia, S 3 gallop, pulmonary passive congestion, pleural fluid, and peripheral edema. Hypertension may be severe and may contribute to left ventricular failure.

Hypertensive encephalopathy may be striking: severe headache, drowsiness, muscle twitchings and convulsions, vomiting, and at times papilledema and retinal hemorrhage.

Treatment

A. Specific Measures: There is no specific treatment. Residual β-hemolytic streptococci should be eradicated with penicillin or other appropriate antibiotic. Any other etiologic agent should be appropriately treated or removed. Adrenocorticosteroids are of no value and may be contraindicated because they increase protein catabolism, sodium retention, and hypertension. Immunosuppressive and cytotoxic drugs have been ineffective in this form of nephritis. (See Nephrotic Syndrome, below.)

B. General Measures: In uncomplicated cases, treatment is symptomatic and designed to prevent overhydration and hypertension. Hospitalization is indicated if oliguria, nitrogen retention, and hypertension are present. Bed rest is of great importance and should be continued until clinical signs abate. Excretion of protein and formed elements in the urine will increase with resumption of activity, but such increases should not be great. Erythrocytes may be excreted in large numbers for months, and the rate of excretion is not a good criterion for evaluating convalescence.

In the presence of elevated blood urea nitrogen and oliguria, dietary protein restriction is indicated. If severe oliguria is present, no more than 20 g of protein should be given. With subsidence of the acute phase of the disease and in the absence of abnormal nitrogen retention, protein intake may be increased to 0.5–0.6 g/kg/d. Carbohydrates should be given liberally to provide calories and to reduce the catabolism of protein and prevent starvation ketosis. With severe oliguria, hyperkalemia may occur, requiring dialysis.

The degree of oliguria and fluid retention and the severity of circulatory congestion and edema dictate the degree of restriction of salt and water. Loop diuretics are useful in reduction of fluid overload and of accompanying hypertension. Hemodialysis is performed as indicated by the severity of the acute renal insufficiency and for volume overload unresponsive to conservative measures.

If anemia becomes severe and symptomatic, give transfusions of packed red cells.

C. Treatment of Complications:

1. Hypertensive encephalopathy should be treated vigorously. Drowsiness and confusion accompanied by severe headache, nausea, blurred vision, and twitching progress to stupor and coma. A greatly elevated blood pressure (often > 250/150 mm Hg) and evidence of retinal arteriolar spasm with or without papilledema and hemorrhages are characteristic. The goal of therapy is to reduce blood pressure to near normal levels without further impairing renal function. The first-line drugs include nitroprusside, diazoxide, hydralazine, labetalol, and nifedipine.

a. Sodium nitroprusside by intravenous infusion pump at 2–50 μg/kg/min acts promptly but is of brief duration. *Observation in an intensive care unit with intra-arterial blood pressure monitoring is required.*

b. Nifedipine, 10–20 mg sublingually, may be used initially for rapid control under close monitoring.

c. Hydralazine, 5–10 mg intravenously every 15 minutes or 30–50 mg intravenously every 4–6 hours, is slower to act. Propranolol, 1–5 mg intravenously, may be required to reduce tachycardia.

d. Labetalol, an α- and β-adrenergic blocking agent, is given intravenously at a rate of 2 mg/min up to a total of 20 mg. Its effects begin after 5 minutes and last for 3–6 hours. Subsequent infusions of 20–80 mg up to a total of 300 mg may be given. Both this agent, esmolol, and propranolol (as noted above) should be used with caution if at all if cardiac dysfunction is present.

e. Clonidine, minoxidil, or prazosin may be useful for maintenance therapy.

f. Phenytoin may be of value in controlling seizures.

2. Heart failure should be treated as any case of left ventricular failure, ie, with severe restriction of fluid and sodium intake and the use of agents that reduce peripheral resistance (afterload) and venous return (preload) (see Chapter 8). Oxygen helps relieve respiratory distress. Dialysis may be dramatic in relieving symptoms.

Prognosis

Most patients with acute disease recover completely within 1–2 years; 5–20% show progressive renal damage. If oliguria, heart failure, or hypertensive encephalopathy is severe, death may occur during the acute attack.

See references under Chronic Glomerulonephritis, below.

2. CHRONIC GLOMERULONEPHRITIS

If acute glomerulonephritis does not heal within 1–2 years, the vascular and glomerular lesions continue to progress, and tubular changes occur. In the presence of smoldering active nephritis, the patient is usually asymptomatic, and the only evidence of disease is the excretion of abnormal urinary elements.

The urinary excretion of protein, red cells, white cells, epithelial cells, and casts (including erythrocyte casts, granular casts, and hyaline and waxy casts) continues at levels above normal. As renal impairment progresses, signs of renal insufficiency appear (see below).

Treatment

Treat intercurrent infections promptly and vigorously as indicated. Avoid unnecessary vaccinations.

Exacerbations are treated as for the acute attack. A protein intake of 0.5–1 g/kg is permissible as long as renal function is adequate to maintain a normal blood urea nitrogen. A liberal fluid intake is desirable.

Prognosis

Worsening of the urinary findings may occur with infection, trauma, or fatigue. Exacerbations may resemble the acute attack or may be typical of the nephrotic syndrome (see below). Uremia is the usual outcome, but the course is variable, and the patient may live a reasonably normal life for 20–30 years.

Culpepper RM, Andreoli TE: The pathophysiology of the glomerulopathies. Adv Intern Med 1983;28:161.

Glassock RJ: Pathophysiology of acute glomerulonephritis. Hosp Pract (Feb 15) 1988;23:163.

Packham DK et al: Primary glomerulonephritis and pregnancy. Quart J Med (New Series) 1989;266:537. (See editorial comment in Lancet 1989;2:253.)

Wilson CB: Immune aspects of renal diseases. JAMA 1987;258:2957.

3. NEPHROTIC SYNDROME

Essentials of Diagnosis

- Massive edema.
- Proteinuria > 3.5 g/d.
- Hypoalbuminemia < 3 g/dL.
- Hyperlipidemia with cholesterol > 300 mg/dL.
- Free fat, oval fat bodies, fatty casts in urinary sediment.

General Considerations

Glomerular diseases associated with nephrotic syndrome include the following:

(1) Minimal change disease: Lipoid nephrosis accounts for about 20% of cases of nephrotic syndrome in adults.

(2) Membranous glomerulonephritis: About 30% of cases.

(3) Mesangial proliferative glomerulonephritis: About 5% of cases.

(4) Focal glomerular sclerosis: About 10% of cases.

(5) Membranoproliferative glomerulonephritis: About 7% of cases.

(6) Miscellaneous diseases: These include diabetic glomerulopathy, systemic lupus erythematosus, polyarteritis, Wegener's granulomatosis, Henoch-Schönlein purpura, amyloidosis, multiple myeloma, neoplasms (including lymphomas and carcinomas), hepatitis B, syphilis, malaria, reaction to toxins (bee venom, *Rhus* antigen), reaction to drugs, and exposure to heavy metals.

Clinical Findings

A. Symptoms and Signs: Edema may appear insidiously and increase slowly; often it appears suddenly and accumulates rapidly. As fluid collects in the serous cavities, the abdomen becomes protuberant, and the patient may complain of anorexia and become short of breath. Symptoms other than those related to the mechanical effects of edema and serous sac fluid accumulation are not remarkable.

On physical examination of florid cases, massive edema is apparent. Signs of hydrothorax and ascites are common. Pallor is often accentuated by the edema, and striae commonly appear in the stretched skin of the extremities. Hypertension, changes in the retina and retinal vessels, and cardiac and cerebral manifestations of hypertension may be demonstrated more often when autoimmune disease, diabetes mellitus, or renal insufficiency is present.

B. Laboratory Findings: The urine contains large amounts of protein, 4–10 g/24 h or more. The sediment contains casts, including the characteristic fatty and waxy varieties; renal tubule cells, some of which contain lipid droplets (oval fat bodies); and variable numbers of erythrocytes. A mild normochromic anemia is common, but anemia may be more severe if renal damage is great. Nitrogen retention varies with the severity of impairment of renal function. The plasma is often lipemic, and cholesterol and triglycerides are usually elevated. Plasma protein is greatly reduced. The albumin fraction is typically decreased to less than 3 g/dL. Some reduction of gamma globulin occurs in most types of nephrosis, but in inflammatory disease such as systemic lupus erythematosus the protein of the gamma fraction may be greatly elevated. Serum complement may be low in active disease, depending on the cause. The serum electrolyte concentrations are often normal, although the serum sodium may be slightly low; total serum calcium may be low, in keeping with the degree of hypoalbuminemia and decrease in the protein-bound calcium moiety. During edema-forming periods, urinary sodium excretion is very low and urinary aldosterone excretion elevated. If renal insufficiency (see above) is present, the blood and urine findings are usually altered accordingly.

Although renal biopsy has been considered essential to determine the type of lesion, to indicate prognosis, and to guide therapy, response to a trial of therapy has been suggested as a means of avoiding or postponing renal biopsy in many patients.

Differential Diagnosis

Constrictive pericarditis may present with a clinical picture resembling nephrosis. Renal vein thrombosis associated with nephrotic syndrome is probably due to loss of antithrombin III in the urine, which results in increased propensity for intravascular coagulation.

Treatment

There is no specific treatment. Identifiable causative diseases (eg, syphilis, malaria, subacute endocarditis) must be treated and specific antidotes to poisons (eg, heavy metals) given. Bed rest is indicated for patients with severe edema or those who have infections. Hospitalization may be desirable when corticosteroid therapy is initiated. The diet should provide a normal protein ration (0.75–1 g/kg/d), with adequate calories. Sodium intake should be restricted to 0.5–1 g/d. Potassium need not be restricted. If edema, ascites, or pleural effusion becomes disabling, a cautious trial of diuretics is warranted; the physician should watch for reduction of an already diminished plasma volume (postural hypotension, prerenal azotemia, shock).

Adrenocorticosteroids are useful for treatment of the nephrotic syndrome in children and in adults when the underlying disease is the minimal glomerular lesion (lipoid nephrosis), systemic lupus erythematosus, or idiosyncrasy to toxin or venom. In the adult with minimal glomerular lesion, a trial of corticosteroid therapy is justified, although the advantage over no treatment is uncertain and complications of therapy are more frequent. Prednisone, 1 mg/kg/d orally or 2 mg/kg orally as a single morning dose on alternate days for 4–8 weeks, is an adequate trial. Diuresis and diminishing proteinuria are evidence of response to therapy. The dose of prednisone may then be reduced slowly over a period of a month or more. Failure to respond indicates that the cause may not be minimal lesion disease.

For treatment of patients with membranous glomerular lesions, the alternate-day prednisone program (120 mg on alternate mornings) may be employed for up to 8 weeks.

Focal glomerulosclerosis, mesangiocapillary (membranoproliferative) glomerulonephritis, and proliferative glomerulonephritis usually do not respond to steroid alone or to steroid plus immunosuppressive therapy. There is some evidence that immunosuppressive therapy will reduce proteinuria in about 20% of patients, with a third of these having stable renal function after 6 years. Treatment otherwise is symptomatic.

Diuretics are often ineffective, though loop diuretics, thiazides, chlorthalidone, and others may be employed. Spironolactone may be helpful when employed concurrently with other diuretics. Salt-free albumin, dextran, and other oncotic agents are of little help, and their effects are transient.

Caution: Elevation of serum potassium, development of hypertension, and sudden severe increase in edema contraindicate continuation of corticosteroid therapy. Such complications usually arise during the first 2 weeks of continuous therapy.

Immunosuppressive drugs, including alkylating agents, cyclophosphamide, mercaptopurine, azathioprine, cyclosporine, and others, have been employed in the treatment of the nephrotic syndrome. The use of corticosteroids plus immunosuppressive agents is similar to that employed in reversing rejection of homotransplants in humans. Encouraging results have been reported in children. Reports of response to combined therapy have been contradictory for adults with membranous lesions and with systemic lupus erythematosus. Those with minimal lesions refractory to corticosteroid therapy do no better when immunosuppressive agents are added.

Serious side effects related both to corticosteroids and to the cytotoxic agents are common. This form of therapy should be employed only by those experienced in treating the nephrotic syndrome in patients who have proved refractory to well-established treatment regimens.

For renal vein thrombosis, the treatment is directed against progress of thrombus formation and consists of heparin or thrombolytic agents and long-term use of coumarin drugs.

Prognosis

The course and prognosis depend upon the cause of the nephrotic syndrome. In more than half of cases of childhood nephrosis, the disease appears to run a rather benign course when properly treated and to leave insignificant sequelae. Of the others, most develop chronic renal insufficiency. Adults with nephrosis fare less well, particularly when the associated disorder is glomerulonephritis, systemic lupus erythematosus, amyloidosis, or diabetic nephropathy. In those with minimal lesions, remissions, either spontaneous or following corticosteroid therapy, are common. Treatment is more often unsuccessful or only ameliorative when the other glomerular lesions are present.

Glassock RJ et al: The nephrotic syndrome. Page 955 in: *The Kidney,* 3rd ed. Brenner BM, Rector FC (editors). Saunders, 1986.

Levey AS et al: Idiopathic nephrotic syndrome: Puncturing the biopsy myth. Ann Intern Med 1987;107:697.

Relman AS: What have we learned about the treatment of idiopathic membranous nephropathy with steroids? N Engl J Med 1989;320:248.

Schena P, Cameron JS: Treatment of proteinuric idiopathic glomerulonephritides in adults: A retrospective survey. Am J Med 1988;85:315.

Wagoner RD et al: Renal vein thrombosis in idiopathic membranous glomerulopathy and nephrotic syndrome: Incidence and significance. Kidney Int 1983;23:368.

4. IgA NEPHROPATHY

The entity of primary recurrent hematuria (Berger's disease) is now included among the immune complex glomerulopathies in which deposition of IgA with C3 and fibrin-related antigens occurs in a granular pattern in the mesangium of the glomerulus.

Recurrent macroscopic and microscopic hematuria and mild proteinuria are characteristically the only manifestations of renal disease. Prospective studies have shown progression of renal disease, with destruction of glomeruli and loss of renal function, often with hypertension. Exacerbations have been observed with upper respiratory tract disease. Progression is usually slow, extending over 2–3 decades.

Berger's nephropathy has appeared in siblings and identical twins. Males are affected 2–3 times more frequently than females. HLA-DR4 antigen occurs in 49% of patients, an incidence 2.5 times that of the control population.

Diagnosis is made by renal biopsy and demonstration of the mesangial deposits of IgA often accompanied by C3 and by small amounts of IgG. IgA may be deposited in skin capillaries as well. The urine sediment resembles that of any glomerulonephritis, with protein, red cells, and casts, including erythrocyte casts. The paucity of clinical manifestations and slow progress may be determining factors in the diagnosis.

No specific treatment has been advocated for this indolent disease.

Clarkson AR et al: IgA nephropathy. Annu Rev Med 1987;38:157.

D'Amico G: The commonest glomerulonephritis in the world: IgA nephropathy. Q J Med 1987;64:709.

5. ANTI-GLOMERULAR BASEMENT MEMBRANE NEPHRITIS (Goodpasture's Syndrome)

The patient usually gives a history of recent hemoptysis and often of malaise, anorexia, and headache. The clinical syndrome is that of severe acute glomerulonephritis accompanied by diffuse hemorrhagic inflammation of the lungs. Occasionally, acute renal disease with a similar clinical and immunologic pattern may occur without associated lung disease (see next section). The urine shows gross or microscopic hematuria, and laboratory findings of severely suppressed renal function are usually evident. Biopsy shows glomerular crescents, glomerular adhesions, and inflammatory infiltration interstitially. Electron microscopic examination shows an increase in basement membrane material and deposition of fibrin beneath the capillary endothelium. In some cases, circulating antibody against glomerular basement membrane can be identified. IgG and C3 complement can be demonstrated as linear deposits on the basement membranes of the glomeruli and the lung. Anti-glomerular basement membrane antibody also reacts with lung basement membrane.

Only rare cases of survival have been documented. Large doses of corticosteroids in combination with immunosuppressive agents are indicated. In addition, plasmapheresis may be employed to remove circulating antibody. Hemodialysis and nephrectomy with renal transplantation may offer the only hope for rescue. Transplantation should be delayed until circulating antiglomerular antibodies have disappeared.

Johnson JP et al: Therapy of anti-glomerular basement membrane antibody disease: Analysis of prognostic significance of clinical, pathologic, and treatment factors. Medicine 1985;64:219.

6. RAPIDLY PROGRESSIVE GLOMERULONEPHRITIS

Rapid deterioration of renal function in the course of a few weeks to a few months is characteristic of fulminant anti-glomerular basement membrane glomerulonephritis. Other glomerular disorders that can follow the same clinical course include poststreptococcal glomerulonephritis, mesangiocapillary (membranoproliferative) glomerulonephritis, Wegener's granulomatosis, systemic lupus erythematosus, polyarteritis, Henoch-Schönlein purpura, hemolytic-uremic syndrome, thrombotic thrombocytopenic purpura, mixed cryoglobulinemia, and ventriculovenous shunt nephritis. Scleroderma may produce a similar picture.

Oliguria, hematuria and proteinuria, and mild hypertension may be the only signs. Abdominal pain and nausea and vomiting may be prominent.

Exuberant proliferation of epithelial cells of Bowman's capsule with crescent formation is the main feature of renal biopsy. Immunofluorescent stains show either fine linear deposits of IgG and segmental deposits of C3 related to anti-glomerular basement membrane antibody or granular deposits of IgG and IgM accompanied by C3 related to immune complex disease.

Treatment with corticosteroids and immunosuppressive drugs has not been successful. Plasmapheresis may be helpful. Dialysis and transplantation may be necessary.

Spontaneous recovery is rare. Progression of renal failure is the rule.

CHRONIC RENAL INSUFFICIENCY

Essentials of Diagnosis

- Weakness and easy fatigability, headaches, anorexia, nausea and vomiting, pruritus, polyuria, nocturia.
- Hypertension with secondary encephalopathy, retinal damage, heart failure.
- Anemia, azotemia, and acidosis, with elevated serum potassium, phosphate, and sulfate and decreased serum calcium and protein.
- Urine specific gravity low and fixed; mild to moderate proteinuria; few red cells, white cells, and broad renal failure casts.

General Considerations

Chronic renal insufficiency may be a consequence of a variety of diseases involving the kidney parenchyma or obstruction of the excretory tract. Causes of chronic renal failure include the following: (1) primary glomerular disease (immune complex glomerulonephritis), (2) renal vascular disease, (3) metabolic diseases with renal involvement, (4) nephrotoxins, (5) infection, (6) chronic radiation nephritis, (7) interstitial nephritis, (8) chronic obstructive uropathy, (9) congenital anomalies of both kidneys, (10) embolization of glomeruli by cholesterol crystals, and (11) nephropathy of particular geographic distribution.

The pathologic picture varies with the cause of the damage to the kidney. Extensive scarring with decrease in kidney size, hyalinization of glomeruli, and obliteration of some tubules and hypertrophy and dilatation of others produce great distortion of renal architecture. The vascular changes are due to the effects of scar formation and of prolonged hypertension, with thickening of the media, fragmentation of elastic fibers, intimal thickening, and obliteration of the lumens in some areas. In diabetic nephropathy, the typical glomerular lesions of intercapillary sclerosis are often distinct. The vascular lesions of periarteritis or of systemic lupus erythematosus often serve to establish these diagnoses. Obstructive uropathy

presents the classic picture of hydronephrosis with compression and destruction of the renal parenchyma. Polycystic disease, multiple myeloma, amyloid disease, persistent hypercalcemia, and other causes of renal failure usually can be identified by characteristic lesions.

Pathophysiology of Uremia

The clinical findings of the uremic syndrome result from loss of nephrons and decreased renal blood flow and glomerular filtration.

With the loss of nephrons, the burden of solute excretion falls on fewer functional units, with subsequent impaired ability of the kidney to maintain body water, osmolality of body fluids, and electrolyte and acid-base balance. The consequences of nephron loss are, briefly, as follows.

A. Water: Increased solute load per nephron produces an osmotic diuresis with associated impaired ability to excrete concentrated or dilute urine. Dehydration is common and hazardous; water intoxication may occur if fluid intake is excessive.

B. Electrolyte:

1. Both excretion and conservation of electrolyte are inadequate. Reduced filtration and excretion of phosphate, sulfate, and organic acid end products of metabolism result in increased concentration of these anions in body fluids, with displacement of bicarbonate. Furthermore, decreased ability to produce H^+ and NH_4^+ for excretion with anion in the urine contributes to acidosis.

2. Sodium loss due to the impaired reabsorption that accompanies osmotic diuresis contributes to a decrease in extracellular fluid volume. With reduction of plasma volume, renal perfusion declines, with worsening renal failure. Since the kidney cannot respond appropriately, a sudden increase in sodium intake cannot be excreted readily, and edema will usually ensue.

3. Potassium regulation is usually not impaired until oliguria is severe or acidosis becomes prominent.

4. Metabolism of calcium and phosphate is seriously disturbed as a consequence of reduction of glomerular filtration and tubule function, impairment of 1-hydroxylation of the vitamin D metabolite 25-hydroxycholecalciferol to 1,25-dihydroxycholecalciferol, and reduced effect of parathyroid hormone on the skeleton. The ensuing hyperphosphatemia and hypocalcemia elicit the development of secondary hyperparathyroidism. The combination of hyperparathyroidism and impaired vitamin D metabolism results in bone disease (renal osteodystrophy) characterized by osteitis fibrosa, osteomalacia, osteoporosis, osteosclerosis, and, in children, impaired growth. Calcification in soft tissue may occur. Rarely, parathyroid secretion cannot be influenced by therapy, a condition termed tertiary hyperparathyroidism. Pertinent laboratory findings include hyperphosphatemia, hypocalcemia (even when corrected for hypoalbuminemia), hypermagnesemia, and elevated parathyroid hormone levels.

C. Nitrogen Retention: High urea, creatinine, and urate levels are manifestations of reduced clearance. Urea load is related to protein metabolism, while creatinine load is related to muscle mass and is independent of protein intake.

D. Anemia: Depression of red cell production probably results from reduced secretion of erythropoietin by the kidney. Survival time of red cells is shorter than normal. Size and hemoglobin content of red cells are usually normal.

E. Hypertension: With renal ischemia and increasing destruction of the renal parenchyma, hypertension may become evident, with further deterioration of kidney function. The coincidence of malignant hypertension and uremia is particularly ominous.

Clinical Findings

A. Symptoms and Signs: Progressive weakness, easy fatigability, and lethargy are often prominent. Thirst, weight loss, anorexia, gastrointestinal irritability, diarrhea, hiccup, and itching are common complaints. Occasionally, a persistent bad or metallic taste annoys the patient. Symptoms of nervous system involvement include paresthesias and burning sensations associated with peripheral neuropathy, myoclonic jerking, and seizures. Headache, visual difficulties, and symptoms of left heart failure result from hypertension. Cerebral hemorrhage, pulmonary edema, and heart failure are usually late occurrences. Purpura and bleeding from the nose and gastrointestinal tract may be severe. Bone pain and, in children, retarded growth reflect osteodystrophy.

The history should include a review of familial disease and questions regarding previous renal disease, drug ingestion, and symptoms of lower urinary tract obstruction.

Physical examination of the patient reveals pallor, hyperpnea, uremic (sweet uriniferous) breath, dehydration, excoriated skin, and purpura. Hypertension with retinopathy is usually present. Cardiac enlargement, pulmonary edema, and pericarditis may be evident. Evidence of peripheral neuropathy should be sought. Bone deformity and awkwardness of gait are evidence of osteodystrophy.

B. Laboratory Findings: Anemia, azotemia, and acidosis are the principal findings. The anemia is usually normochromic and normocytic, with hemoglobin in the range of 6–9 g/dL. Prolonged bleeding time is attributed to defective platelet function. The urine is usually dilute and contains small amounts of protein; few red, white, and epithelial cells; and a few granular and waxy casts, some of which are large (broad renal failure casts). Serum concentrations of urea nitrogen, creatinine, and often uric acid are greatly elevated. Serum sodium may be slightly lower than normal and serum potassium slightly to markedly elevated; serum calcium is decreased; with bone disease, alkaline phosphatase activity in the serum is increased, and circulating parathyroid hormone is often elevated. Serum magnesium may be elevated. With retention of phosphate, sulfate, and, frequently, chloride, plasma bicarbonate concentration is decreased. (Phosphate and sulfate participate in the "anion gap" of uremia.) Both retention of organic acids and impaired tubular secretion of hydrogen ion plus loss of sodium and bicarbonate buffer are accompanied by a decrease in blood pH.

C. Imaging: Chest radiographs may show evidence of cardiac enlargement, midzone interstitial edema of the lung, frank pulmonary congestion, or pulmonary edema. The size of the kidneys should be determined by ultrasonography, which also may demonstrate evidence of obstructed ureter and bladder outlet. Small kidneys are present in most cases of renal failure; exceptions include amyloid disease, myeloma kidney, obstructive uropathy, and polycystic kidneys. Radiologic evidence of bone disease (osteomalacia and osteitis fibrosa) is commonly present long before overt symptoms and clinical signs appear.

D. Other Findings: Echocardiography is useful in confirming the presence of pericardial effusion. The ECG may reflect left ventricular strain or hypertrophy and changes due to potassium toxicity.

Differential Diagnosis

Chronic renal insufficiency presents symptoms and signs related to the functional disability resulting from a reduction in the number of functioning nephrons rather than to the cause of the renal damage. It is often impossible to distinguish the cause. The presence of large kidneys characteristic of polycystic disease should serve to identify this cause of renal failure. The physician must identify remediable causes of renal insufficiency such as obstruction, infection, persistent hypercalcemia, gout, myeloma, and drug toxicity. Bilaterally small kidneys and the presence of bone disease imply irreversible damage to renal function.

Treatment

Hypertension or heart failure should be treated as indicated with agents that sustain renal function and coronary artery blood flow (see below).

A. Diet and Fluids: Limitation of protein of high biologic value to 0.5 g/kg/d helps to reduce azotemia, acidosis, and hyperkalemia. Trials of mixtures of essential amino acids or of amino acid precursors such as α-keto and α-hydroxy acid analogues are promising approaches to protein replacement.

The diet should include adequate calories and a multivitamin product plus folic acid, 1 mg daily, particularly when protein is severely restricted. Sodium intake need not be restricted and should be tailored to urine losses, which tend to be fixed in amount. Fluid intake should be sufficient to maintain an adequate urine volume, but no attempt should be made to force diuresis. Obligatory water loss may be quite high because of the large solute load (eg, sodium and urea) that must be excreted by a reduced number of nephrons. Intake of up to 2–3 L may be required when creatinine clearance is reduced to 10–20 mL/min. With decreasing clearance, urine volume decreases. Intake must be sufficient to maintain renal function without causing excessive diuresis or water retention. If edema is present, a cautious trial of furosemide or ethacrynic acid is indicated, with careful monitoring of serum electrolytes. Caution: Water restriction for laboratory examination, tests of renal function, or any other reason may lead to serious volume depletion.

B. Electrolyte Replacement:

1. Sodium supplements may be required to restore sodium losses resulting from failure of the kidney to provide NH_4^+ and H^+ for sodium conservation. A mixture of $NaCl$ and $NaHCO_3$ in equal parts, 1–2 g 2–3 times daily with meals, may be required in addition to dietary sources. Weight loss and a decreasing urine volume indicate a need for additional sodium. Hypertension and edema are signs that a trial of sodium restriction is in order.

2. Potassium intake may have to be restricted or supplemented. In severe hyperkalemia, active measures to remove potassium may be required (see discussion in Chapter 16).

3. Serum phosphate levels may be lowered and secondary hyperparathyroidism ameliorated by reducing absorption of phosphate in the gastrointestinal tract with administration of aluminum hydroxide gel, 30 mL, or (as tablets) 4–5 g 3–4 times daily.

C. Bone Disease (Renal Osteodystrophy): In the presence of bone disease, phosphate binders and supplemental calcium are employed as above. In addition, cholecalciferol (vitamin D_3) or, more effectively, its metabolites—ie, calciferol (25-hydroxycholecalciferol) and calcitriol (1,25-dihydroxycholecalciferol)—are useful in correcting osteomalacia and osteitis fibrosa, with some amelioration of myopathy. *Caution:* Close observation is mandatory to prevent hypercalcemia and soft tissue calcification, which may ensue if the dosage is too great. Thorough knowledge of indications and hazards must be obtained before using these potent agents.

Parathyroidectomy may be required if "tertiary" hyperparathyroidism is present or if there is bone pain due to secondary hyperparathyroidism.

D. Anemia; Hemostasis: Iron is of little value unless iron deficit exists. With evidence that transfusion of blood from donors who share at least one HLA-DR antigen with the patient who is potentially a graft recipient is responsible for improved acceptance of renal allografts, there should be no hesitation in giving properly matched blood transfusions to patients whose anemia is symptomatic or if the hematocrit falls to the low 20s.

Recombinant human erythropoietin has proved a safe and effective treatment for patients with end-stage renal disease who are receiving dialysis. When anemia persists after 3 months of adequate hemodialysis or chronic ambulatory peritoneal dialysis, treatment with erythropoietin is warranted. Chronic blood loss, hemolytic disease, infection, cancer, aluminum toxicity, and iron deficiency must be ruled out as causes of anemia. Patients with hemoglobin of less than 8 g/dL who have symptoms attributable to anemia (eg, easy fatigability, angina) should receive erythropoietin. Iron stores must be adequate to achieve the best response and to provide for erythrogenesis (serum ferritin > 100 μg/L). Erythropoietin is given in doses of 100–200 units/kg/wk intravenously or 75–150 units/kg/wk subcutaneously in divided doses (eg, 3 times a week) with close attention to sustaining iron stores (serum transferrin saturation > 20%). Hematocrit of 30% or more is an achievable goal in 95% of patients. Erythropoietin is expensive treatment at present.

Prolonged bleeding time and difficulty with hemostasis can be corrected transiently with cryoprecipitate. Desmopressin acetate (1-deamino-8-D-arginine vasopressin; DDAVP), 0.3 μg/kg body weight diluted in 50–100 mL of saline solution, may be infused intravenously over 30 minutes to shorten the bleeding time for about 4 hours. DDAVP is sometimes used to prevent bleeding during minor surgical procedures.

E. General Measures: Nausea and vomiting may be alleviated with chlorpromazine, 15–25 mg orally or 10–20 mg intramuscularly (or equivalent amounts of related compounds). The barbiturate drugs may be used for sedation as required.

Hypertension is a common manifestation of uremia. An expanded extracellular fluid volume is often responsible for hypertension, and the circumstances can be ameliorated by reduction of extracellular fluid volume by a trial of furosemide or by hemodialysis. Combinations of hydralazine and propranolol may be effective; nifedipine, minoxidil, metoprolol, clonidine, and prazosin are useful drugs. Angiotensin-converting enzyme inhibitors may be of value as antihypertensive agents except in cases of renovascular disease. Very rarely, bilateral nephrectomy may be necessary to rescue the patient from persistent hypertension. (See references for details of management of hypertension in the presence of renal failure.)

F. Approach to Drug Therapy: Because the half-life of many drugs is prolonged in patients with renal failure, the physician must monitor the effects of drugs closely. The dosage of drugs must often be reduced and guided by blood levels (see Bennett reference, below, and Tables 31–4 and 31–7).

G. Chronic Dialysis and Kidney Transplants: These approaches to the treatment of renal insufficiency due to any cause have been under investigation for many years, and encouraging experience has prompted expansion of facilities for scheduled, repeated extracorporeal dialysis. Successful renal transplantation has extended life for patients with chronic renal failure.

Amelioration of complications such as neuropathy, hyperparathyroidism, and anemia can be frequently achieved by dialysis or transplantation.

1. Simplified mechanisms for dialysis with the artificial kidney and ingenious cannulas and arteriovenous fistulas permit periodic dialysis with a minimum of professional supervision in hospital centers and in the patient's home. Patients with creatinine clearances of 0–2 mL/min have been kept alive for 6–10 years in reasonable health and activity by dialysis once or twice a week.

The criteria for selection of patients are now clear. Dialysis is employed when conservative medical treatment is inadequate to forestall overt uremic symptoms—usually when creatinine clearance approaches 5 mL/min and serum creatinine is nearing 10 mg/dL. The goal is to prevent complications of uremia such as anorexia, encephalopathy, pericarditis, and peripheral neuropathy. In anticipation of initiating dialysis, the indications for therapy should be discussed with the patient and preparation for dialysis completed, including placing an arteriovenous shunt or intraperitoneal-space catheter. The route of dialysis, hemodialysis, or continuous ambulatory peritoneal dialysis is selected in consultation with the nephrologist who assumes responsibility for care. Complications of both types of dialysis are many and frequent and should be managed by an experienced nephrologist.

Centers have been established for the treatment of chronic renal insufficiency, and home units are generally available, although considerable skill is required to operate the devices. A recent survey indicates a 1-year survival rate on dialysis of 87%, a 2-year survival rate of 73%, and, in the 20- to 45-year age group, a 6-year survival rate of 60%.

Peritoneal dialysis can be used for temporary or long-term therapy. Chronic ambulatory peritoneal dialysis provides less effective clearance of small molecules (urea, creatinine) than does hemodialysis, but because it is continuous, it is adequate to relieve symptoms of uremia and provides excellent treatment. One to 2 L of dialysate modified to meet the needs of the patient can be exchanged 3–5 times daily. With good technique, the risk of peritonitis is reduced; it can usually be treated successfully with appropriate antibiotics.

Hemofiltration, a variant of dialysis in which a highly permeable membrane is employed, may prove a useful alternative to conventional dialysis.

2. Transplantation of kidneys from one human to another has been technically feasible for many years. Survival of such grafts has been limited by rejection of the foreign organ by the recipient except when donor and recipient were identical twins. Blood typing and leukocyte typing for histocompatibility

antigens have improved the matching of donor and recipient, with an encouraging decrease in the rejection rate. The enhanced survival of cadaver renal grafts in patients who have had 5 or more blood transfusions compared to those who have had none is clear (1-year graft survival > 60% versus 42%). Further experience with immunosuppressive drugs (azathioprine or cyclophosphamide) and adrenal corticosteroids has improved protection of the homologous transplant from rejection for extended periods. The use of cyclosporine to suppress immunity has been impressively effective. The high incidence of nephrotoxicity is a serious complication requiring close monitoring of renal function and reduction of dosage for long-term use. Total lymphoid irradiation (TLI) has resulted in improved tolerance for the graft, permitting reduced dosage of prednisone. The goal with cyclosporine and with TLI is to effect tolerance for the graft in the absence of immunosuppressive drugs. Trials of anti-interleukin-2 receptor antibodies and of prostaglandin E_2 analogues in combination with conventional immunosuppression have been reported to be effective.

When the donor is a parent or an HLA-matched sibling, recipient survival with the first transplant still functional at 2 years is 80% or greater and at 3 years 70%. Cyclosporine has extended survival of the recipient and the transplanted cadaveric kidney, with some reduction of acute rejection episodes.

Beck LH: Kidney function and disease in the elderly. Hosp Pract (Aug 15) 1988;23:75.

Bennett WM et al: Drug Prescribing in Renal Failure: Dosing Guidelines for Adults. American College of Physicians, 1987.

Fraser CL, Arieff AI: Nervous system complications in uremia. Ann Intern Med 1988;109:143.

Gokal R et al: Outcome in patients on continuous ambulatory peritoneal dialysis and haemodialysis: Four-year analysis of a prospective multicentre study. Lancet 1987;2:1105.

Ihle BU et al: The effect of protein restriction on the progression of renal insufficiency. N Engl J Med 1989;321:1773. (Convincing prospective study.)

Keane WF et al: Angiotensin converting enzyme inhibitors and progressive renal insufficiency: Current experience and future directions. Ann Intern Med 1989;111:503.

Langs C et al: Rapid renal failure in acquired immunodeficiency syndrome-associated focal glomerulosclerosis. Arch Intern Med 1990;150:287.

Levin M: The elderly patient with advanced renal failure. Hosp Pract (March 30) 1989;24:35.

Macdougall IC: Treating renal anaemia with recombinant human erythropoietin: Practical guidelines and a clinical algorithm. Br Med J 1990;300:655.

Macdougall IC et al: Long-term cardiorespiratory effects of amelioration of renal anaemia by erythropoietin. Lancet 1990;335:489.

Mallische HH, Faugere M: Renal osteodystrophy. (Editorial.) N Engl J Med 1989;321:317.

Mooradian AD, Morley JE: Endocrine dysfunction in chronic renal failure. Arch Intern Med 1984;144:351.

Selby JV et al: The natural history and epidemiology of

diabetic nephropathy: Implications for prevention and control. JAMA 1990;263:1954.

Tolkoff-Rubin NE, Rubin RH: Uremia and host defenses. (Editorial.) N Engl J Med 1990;322:770.

DISEASES OF THE RENAL TUBULES & INTERSTITIUM

1. ACUTE RENAL FAILURE

Essentials of Diagnosis

- Sudden onset of oliguria; urine volume 20–200 mL/d. (Oliguria may not occur.)
- Proteinuria and hematuria; isosthenuria with a specific gravity of 1.010–1.016.
- Anorexia, nausea and vomiting, lethargy, elevation of blood pressure.
- Progressive increase in serum urea nitrogen, creatinine, potassium, phosphate, sulfate; decrease in sodium, calcium, bicarbonate.
- Spontaneous recovery in a few days to 6 weeks.

General Considerations

Acute intrinsic renal failure is a term applied to a state of sudden cessation of renal function following a variety of insults to normal kidneys. Emphasis has recently been placed on vasomotor constriction of afferent arterioles as the initial lesion—hence the term vasomotor nephropathy. Among the causes of acute renal failure are the following: (1) Toxic agents, eg, carbon tetrachloride, methoxyflurane, sulfonamides, aminoglycoside antibiotics, amphotericin B, mercury bichloride, arsenic, diethylene glycol, and mushroom poisoning. X-ray contrast materials are hazardous in patients with dehydration, renal disease, diabetic nephropathy, liver failure, or multiple myeloma. (2) Traumatic shock due to severe injury, surgical shock, or myocardial infarction, and ischemia associated with surgery on the abdominal aorta (vasomotor nephropathy). (3) Tissue destruction due to crushing injury, rhabdomyolysis, burns, intravascular hemolysis (transurethral resection of the prostate, incompatible blood transfusion). (4) Infectious diseases, eg, leptospirosis, hemorrhagic fever, gram-negative bacteremia with shock, toxic shock syndrome, peritonitis. (5) Disseminated intravascular coagulation. (6) Complications of pregnancy, eg, bilateral cortical necrosis. (7) Immunologic mechanisms induced by methicillin, penicillin, phenytoin, and other drugs.

Renal tubular necrosis is the characteristic pathologic finding. In some instances, after exposure to a specific toxin, the proximal tubule may be primarily damaged; and renal tubule cell disintegration and desquamation with collection of debris in the lumens of the tubules are found uniformly throughout both kidneys. In other cases, tubule cell destruction and basement membrane disruption are scattered throughout both kidneys. In cases due to hemolysis or crushing injury, heme or myoglobin casts may be present, but it is unlikely that such casts produce tubule cell destruction. The spotty distribution of the damage caused by ischemic necrosis is consistent with a great reduction in cortical blood flow in addition to a moderate to marked decrease in total renal blood flow. In bilateral cortical necrosis, ischemic infarcts are distributed throughout both kidneys.

Clinical Findings

The history is critical in identification of the cause. The cardinal sign of acute renal failure is acute reduction of urine output following injury, surgery, a transfusion reaction, or other causes listed above. The daily volume of urine may be reduced to 20–30 mL/d or may be as high as 400–500 mL/d. In some cases, urine volume may always be greater than 600 mL/d. After a few days to 6 weeks of oliguria, the daily urine volume slowly increases. Anorexia, nausea, and lethargy are common symptoms. Other symptoms and signs are related to the causative agent or event.

The course of the disease may be divided into the oliguric and diuretic phases.

A. Oliguric Phase: During the oliguric phase, the urine excretion is greatly reduced. The urine contains protein, red cells, epithelial cells, and characteristic "dirty" brown granular casts; and the specific gravity of the urine is usually 1.010–1.016. The rate of catabolism of protein determines the rate of increase of metabolic end products in body fluids. In the presence of injury, rhabdomyolysis, or fever, the blood urea nitrogen and the serum creatinine, potassium, phosphate, sulfate, and organic acids increase rapidly. Typically, because of dilution and intracellular shifts, the serum sodium concentration drops to 120–130 meq/L. As organic acids and phosphate accumulate, serum bicarbonate concentration decreases. Normochromic anemia is common. With prolonged oliguria, signs of uremia appear, with nausea, vomiting, diarrhea, neuromuscular irritability, convulsions, somnolence, and coma. Hypertension frequently develops and may be associated with retinopathy, left heart failure, and encephalopathy. During this phase of the disease, therapy modifies the clinical picture significantly. Overhydration produces signs of water intoxication, with convulsions, edema, and the serious complication of pulmonary edema. Excess saline administration may produce edema and congestive failure. Failure to restrict potassium intake or to employ agents to remove potassium at the proper time may result in hyperkalemia manifested by neuromuscular depression that progresses to paralysis and interference with the cardiac conduction system, resulting in arrhythmias; death may follow respiratory muscle paralysis or cardiac arrest. With proper treatment, potassium intoxication is almost always reversible, and death should not occur because of it. The oliguric phrase may be very transient or even absent.

B. Diuretic Phase: After a few days to 6 weeks of oliguria, the diuretic phase begins, signifying that the nephrons have recovered to the point that urine excretion is possible. The urine volume usually increases in increments of a few milliliters to 100 mL/d until 300–500 mL/d is excreted, after which the rate of increase in flow is usually more rapid. Rarely, the urine volume increases rapidly during the first day or so of diuresis. Diuresis may be the result of impaired nephron function, with loss of water and electrolytes; but this is uncommon, and true deficits of water, sodium, and potassium seldom occur. More often, diuresis represents an unloading of excess extracellular fluid that has accumulated during the oliguric phase as a result of either overhydration during therapy or unusual metabolic production of water. Diuresis usually occurs when the total nephron function is still insufficient to excrete nitrogenous metabolic products, potassium, and phosphate, and the concentration of these constituents in the serum may continue to rise for several days after urine volumes exceed 1 L/d. Renal function returns slowly toward normal, and blood chemical findings usually become normal.

Differential Diagnosis

Because acute glomerulonephritis, autoimmune disease, acute interstitial nephritis, uric acid nephropathy, myeloma, hepatorenal syndrome, Reye's syndrome, ureteral obstruction due to edema at the ureterovesical junction following ureteral catheterization, ureteral obstruction by neoplasm, bilateral renal artery occlusion due to embolism and, rarely, a ruptured bladder may present with symptoms and signs indistinguishable from those of tubular necrosis, appropriate diagnostic procedures (ultrasound examination of kidneys and bladder, radiograph of abdomen, etc) should be employed as suggested by the history and by physical examination. Functional or prerenal azotemia consequent to shock, severe volume depletion, congestive heart failure, pressor agents, or diuretics must be distinguished to assure appropriate immediate therapy.

In the differentiation between acute renal failure and prerenal azotemia, the ability to excrete creatinine and urea and to conserve sodium are useful criteria (Table 17–1).

The loss of normal capacity to excrete creatinine and to conserve sodium indicates acute renal failure. The clinical setting must be carefully assessed, for in chronic renal insufficiency the ability to conserve sodium is lost, and after administration of diuretics sodium excretion is elevated.

Treatment

A. Specific Measures: Immediate treatment of the cause of oliguria is essential.

Table 17–1. Acute renal failure versus prerenal azotemia.

	Acute Renal Failure	Prerenal Azotemia
Urine osmolality (mosm/L)	<350	>500
Urine/plasma urea	<10	>20
Urine/plasma creatinine	<20	>40
Urine Na (meq/L)	>40	<20
Renal failure index = $\dfrac{U_{Na}}{U/P_{Cr}}$	>1	<1
$FENa^1 = \dfrac{U/P_{Na}}{U/P_{Cr}} \times 100$	>1	<1

[1] Excreted fraction of filtered sodium. See Espinel CH: The FENa test: Use in the differential diagnosis of acute renal failure. *JAMA* 1976;**236**:579; and Miller TR et al: Urinary diagnostic indices in acute renal failure: A prospective study. *Ann Intern Med* 1978;**89**:47.

1. Decreased renal perfusion–Diminished circulating blood volume resulting in decreased renal perfusion (prerenal failure) can be ruled out by infusion of 500–1000 mL of 0.9% NaCl solution and use of a loop diuretic. Treatment in the very early period of acute renal shutdown with mannitol, loop diuretics, or dopamine is controversial.

2. Shock–Vigorous measures to restore normal blood pressure levels are mandatory in order to overcome renal ischemia. *Caution:* When it is apparent that tubular necrosis with oliguria has occurred, the volume of fluid administered must be sharply curtailed.

3. Transfusion reaction–See Chapter 10.

4. Obstruction of ureters–Cystoscopy and catheterization of ureters may be necessary.

5. Heavy metal poisoning—Dimercaprol (BAL) may be of use in mercury or arsenic poisoning, although by the time the renal lesion is apparent it may be too late.

B. General Measures: Conservative medical management often serves adequately for the uncomplicated case. Indications for dialysis include rapidly increasing blood urea nitrogen, serum creatinine, and potassium, and metabolic acidosis often consequent to severe trauma or infection. Overhydration, usually from too vigorous treatment with intravenous solutions, and oliguria lasting 4–5 days are also indications for dialysis. Hemodialysis is more effective, but peritoneal dialysis may be adequate in instances where hemodialysis is not immediately accessible. Aggressive supportive therapy (combating infection, use of hyperalimentation, etc) should accompany treatment by dialysis. Conservative management is summarized below.

1. Oliguric phase–The objectives of therapy are to maintain normal body fluid volume and electrolyte concentration, reduce tissue catabolism to a minimum, and prevent infection until healing occurs.

a. Fluids–Restrict fluids to a basic ration of 400

mL/d for the average adult. Additional fluid may be given to replace unusual losses due to vomiting, diarrhea, sweating, etc. The metabolism of fat, carbohydrate, and protein provides water of combustion; and catabolism of tissues provides intracellular water. These sources must be included in calculations of water balance, thus leaving only a small ration to be provided as "intake" (see ¶ d, below).

b. Diet–In order to limit sources of nitrogen, potassium, phosphate, and sulfate, no protein should be given. Glucose, 100–200 g/d, should be given to prevent ketosis and to reduce protein catabolism. Although fat may be given as butter or emulsion orally or intravenously, it is usually better if the patient fulfills caloric needs from existing fat deposits.

The fluid and glucose may be given orally or intravenously. When administered intravenously as a 20–50% glucose solution, the 400 mL of fluid should be given continuously throughout the 24-hour period through an intravenous catheter threaded into a large vein to reduce the likelihood of thrombosis. Vitamin B complex and vitamin C should be provided.

For patients on dialysis, parenteral hyperalimentation with a mixture of essential amino acids and nonessential amino acids (particularly those partially synthesized in the kidney) supplemented by glucose and lipid for calories prevents excessive catabolism of tissue and enhances recovery.

c. Electrolyte replacement–Electrolyte therapy is not necessary unless it is required to repair clearcut losses, as in vomiting, diarrhea, etc. *Note:* Potassium must not be administered unless proved deficits exist, and then only with caution.

d. Observations–Daily records of fluid intake and output are essential; avoid an indwelling catheter if at all possible. Weight should be recorded daily whenever possible. Because the patient's own tissues are being consumed, weight loss should be about 0.5 kg/d. If weight loss does not occur, too much fluid is being given. Frequent (often daily) measurements of serum electrolytes (especially potassium) and creatinine are essential.

e. Infection–Treat vigorously with appropriate antibiotics in doses adjusted for renal failure.

f. Congestive heart failure–See discussion in Chapter 8.

g. Anemia–A hematocrit of less than 30% is an indication for cautious transfusion with a small volume of packed fresh red blood cells.

h. Hyperkalemia–See discussion in Chapter 16.

i. Uremia–Hemodialysis and peritoneal dialysis are effective, but they require expert management in a well-equipped hospital. With appropriate facilities, dialysis has proved to be of great value if employed "prophylactically" before serum creatinine reaches 7–8 mg/dL.

j. Convulsions and encephalopathy–Seizures are treated as medical emergencies. (See treatment of tonic-clonic seizures, Chapter 18). Hemodialysis

may be instituted if the seizure activity is clearly a result of the renal failure or of treatment (eg, overhydration, administration of bicarbonate).

2. Diuretic phase–Unless water and electrolyte deficits clearly exist, no attempt should be made to "keep up" with the diuresis; collections of excess water and electrolyte are usually being excreted. Fluid and diet intake can be liberalized as diuresis progresses until a normal daily intake is reached. Protein restriction should be continued until blood urea nitrogen and serum creatinine levels are declining. Infection is still a hazard. Diuresis is occasionally accompanied by sodium retention, hypernatremia, and hyperchloremia associated with confusion, neuromuscular irritability, and coma. When this happens, water and glucose must be given in sufficient quantities to correct hypernatremia. Serum electrolytes and blood urea nitrogen or serum creatinine should be measured frequently.

Prognosis

If severe complications of trauma and infection are not present, skillful treatment often will tide the patient over the period of oliguria until spontaneous healing occurs. Death may occur as a result of water intoxication, congestive heart failure, acute pulmonary edema, potassium intoxication, encephalopathy, and infection. With recovery, there often is little residual impairment of renal function.

Better OS, Stein JH: Early management of shock and prophylaxis of acute renal failure in traumatic rhabdomyolysis. N Engl J Med 1990;322:825.

Brenner BM, Lazarus JM (editors): *Acute Renal Failure.* Saunders, 1983.

Schrier RW: Acute renal failure: Pathogenesis, diagnosis, and management. Hosp Pract (March) 1981;16:93.

2. INTERSTITIAL NEPHRITIS

Acute interstitial nephritis may be due to systemic infections from bacteria, viruses, and spirochetes and sensitivity to drugs, including antibiotics (penicillins, cephalosporins, sulfonamides, rifampin, vancomycin), diuretics (thiazides, furosemide), nonsteroidal anti-inflammatory agents, phenindione, allopurinol, cimetidine, and others. Some patients will show other signs of hypersensitivity such as rash, arthralgia, fever, and eosinophilia. Hematuria, proteinuria, and enlargement of the kidneys are commonly demonstrable; eosinophiluria may be observed if urinary sediment is examined after staining with Wright's stain. Occasionally, acute renal failure may occur. Recovery may be complete.

Chronic interstitial nephritis is characterized by focal or diffuse interstitial fibrosis accompanied by infiltration with inflammatory cells ultimately associated with extensive atrophy of renal tubules. It represents a nonspecific reaction to a variety of causes: analgesic abuse, lead and cadmium toxicity, nephrocalcinosis, urate nephropathy, radiation nephritis, sarcoidosis, Balkan nephritis, and some instances of obstructive uropathy. There are cases in which antitubule basement membrane antibodies have been identified by means of immunofluorescence linear staining of IgG and C3. Most patients with antiglomerular basement membrane disease (Goodpasture's syndrome) and some with other forms of rapidly progressive glomerulonephritis will have anti-tubular basement membrane disease as well.

Linton AL, Lindsay RM: Drug-induced acute interstitial nephritis. Kidney 1982;15:1.

Pusey CD et al: Drug-associated acute interstitial nephritis: Clinical and pathological features and the response to high-dose steroid therapy. Q J Med 1983;52:194.

3. DISORDERS RELATED TO NONSTEROIDAL ANTI-INFLAMMATORY DRUGS

The kidney can be adversely affected by nonsteroidal anti-inflammatory drugs (NSAIDs). Renal damage may be structural or functional. Structural changes may produce acute or chronic renal failure, nephrotic syndrome, interstitial nephritis, and renal papillary necrosis. In the United States, about 2% of end-stage renal disease is due to NSAIDs; in Australia, the incidence is estimated to be 20%. Functional changes include abnormal metabolism of water, sodium, and potassium.

Diminished prostaglandin synthesis induced by NSAIDs is the likely cause of the associated kidney disease. The offending drugs include salicylates (acetylated and nonacetylated), oxicams, and the derivatives of indoleacetic acid, propionic acid, anthranilic acid, and pyrazolone.

NSAIDs are particularly dangerous in conditions in which blood volume or effective arterial volume is reduced: congestive heart failure, nephrotic syndrome, diuretic use, and salt depletion. Patients with chronic renal disease may suffer further decrease of kidney function, which may not be reversible.

Papillary necrosis with interstitial nephritis is a serious complication of NSAID use. Associated urinary tract infection, particularly in patients with diabetes mellitus, probably plays a role in the setting of long-term intake of large doses of analgesic drugs.

Water metabolism is regulated in part by renal prostaglandins. NSAIDs inhibit prostaglandin synthesis and thereby reduce excretion of free water, and this may lead to hyponatremia (see Chapter 16). Simultaneous use of thiazides may exaggerate this effect.

Sodium retention is a common side effect of treatment with NSAIDs. Mild to massive edema may occur. Potassium excretion is often reduced; when this occurs in the setting of mild renal insufficiency, hyperkalemia can result. NSAIDs can blunt renin activity and ultimately reduce aldosterone production, which will in turn enhance potassium retention.

Bennett WM, DeBroe ME: Analgesic nephropathy: A preventable renal disease. (Editorial.) N Engl J Med 1989;320:1269.

Carmichael J, Shankel SW: Effects of nonsteroidal anti-inflammatory drugs on prostaglandins and renal function. Am J Med 1985;78:992.

Clive DM, Stoff JS: Renal syndromes associated with nonsteroidal antiinflammatory drugs. N Engl J Med 1984; 310:563.

Dunn MJ: Clinical effects of prostaglandins in renal disease. Hosp Pract (March) 1984;19:99.

Garella S, Matarese RA: Renal effects of prostaglandins and clinical adverse effects of nonsteroidal anti-inflammatory agents. Medicine 1984;63:165.

4. URIC ACID NEPHROPATHY

Crystals of urate produce an interstitial inflammatory reaction. Urate may precipitate out in acid urine in the calices or distally in the ureters to form uric acid stones. Patients with myeloproliferative disease under treatment may develop hyperuricemia and are subject to occlusion of the upper urinary tract by uric acid crystals. Alkalinization of the urine and a liberal fluid intake will help prevent crystal formation. Allopurinol is a useful drug to prevent hyperuricemia and hyperuricosuria.

5. MYELOMA KIDNEY

Features of multiple myeloma that contribute to renal disease include proteinuria (including filtrable Bence Jones protein and κ and λ chains), with precipitation in the tubules leading to accumulation of abnormal proteins in the tubule cells; amyloidosis; hypercalcemia; and, occasionally, increase in viscosity of the blood associated with macroglobulinemia. A Fanconi-like syndrome may develop.

Plugging of tubules, giant cell reaction around tubules, tubular atrophy, and, occasionally, the accumulation of amyloid are evident on examination of renal tissue.

Renal failure may occur acutely or may develop slowly depending on the cause. Radiopaque dyes used for CT scans, angiography, or urograms are likely to produce serious impairment of renal function, particularly in the face of volume depletion. Hemodialysis may rescue the patient during efforts to control the myeloma with chemical agents.

Cohen DJ et al: Acute renal failure in patients with multiple myeloma. Am J Med 1984;76:247.

Kyle RA: Monoclonal gammopathies and the kidney. Annu Rev Med 1989;40:53.

HEREDITARY RENAL DISEASES

Although relatively uncommon in the population at large, hereditary disease must be recognized to permit early diagnosis and treatment in other family members and to prepare the way for genetic counseling.

1. HEREDITARY CHRONIC NEPHRITIS

Evidence of the disease usually appears in childhood, with episodes of hematuria often following an upper respiratory infection. Renal insufficiency, accounting for nearly 5% of patients with end-stage renal disease, commonly develops in males but only rarely in females. Survival beyond age 40 is rare without dialysis or transplant.

In many families, deafness and abnormalities of the eyes accompany the renal disease (Alport's syndrome). Another form of the disease is accompanied by polyneuropathy. Infection of the urinary tract is a common complication.

The anatomic features in some cases resemble proliferative glomerulonephritis; in others, there is thickening of the glomerular basement membrane or podocyte proliferation and thickening of Bowman's capsule. In a few cases, there are fat-filled cells (foam cells) in the interstitial tissue or in the glomeruli.

Laboratory findings are commensurate with existing renal function.

Treatment is symptomatic.

2. CYSTIC DISEASES OF THE KIDNEY

Congenital structural anomalies of the kidney must always be considered in any patient with hypertension, pyelonephritis, or renal insufficiency. The manifestations of structural renal abnormalities are related to the superimposed disease, but management and prognosis are modified by the structural anomaly.

Polycystic Kidneys

Polycystic kidney disease is familial (autosomal dominant) and often involves not only the kidney but the liver and pancreas as well. The incidence of autosomal dominant disease is 1:1000 to 1:400 population.

The formation of cysts in the cortex of the kidney is thought to result from failure of union of the collecting tubules and convoluted tubules of some nephrons. New cysts do not form, but those present enlarge and, by pressure, cause destruction of adjacent tissue. Cysts may be found in the liver and pancreas. The incidence of cerebral vessel (''berry'') aneurysms is higher than normal.

Cases of polycystic disease are discovered during the investigation of hypertension, by diagnostic study in patients presenting with pyelonephritis or hematuria, or by investigating the families of patients with polycystic disease. At times, flank pain due to hemorrhage into a cyst will call attention to a kidney disorder. Otherwise, the symptoms and signs are those commonly seen in hypertension or renal insufficiency. On physical examination the enlarged, irregular kidneys are easily palpable.

The urine may contain leukocytes and red cells. With bleeding into the cysts, there may also be bleeding into the urinary tract. The blood chemical findings reflect the degree of renal insufficiency. Examination by echography or x-ray shows the enlarged kidneys, and urography demonstrates the classic elongated calices and renal pelves stretched over the surface of the cysts.

No specific therapy is available, and surgical interference is contraindicated unless ureteral obstruction is produced by an adjacent cyst. Hypertension, infection, and uremia are treated in the conventional manner; infection in a cyst may be difficult both to localize and to eradicate.

Because persons with polycystic kidneys may live in reasonable comfort with slowly advancing uremia, it is difficult to determine when renal transplantation is in order. Hemodialysis can extend the life of the patient, but recurrent bleeding and continuous pain indicate the need for a transplant, which carries an excellent prognosis.

Although the disease may become symptomatic in childhood or early adult life, it usually is discovered in the fourth or fifth decades. Unless fatal complications of hypertension or urinary tract infections are present, uremia develops very slowly, and patients live longer than with other causes of renal insufficiency.

Cystic Disease of the Renal Medulla

Two syndromes have become more frequent as their diagnostic features have become better known.

Medullary cystic disease is a familial disease (either autosomal dominant or recessive) that may become symptomatic during adolescence. Anemia is usually the initial manifestation, but azotemia, acidosis, and hyperphosphatemia soon become evident. Hypertension may develop. The urine is not remarkable, although there is often an inability to produce a concentrated urine. Many small cysts are scattered through the renal medulla. Renal transplantation is indicated by the usual criteria for the operation.

Sponge kidney is asymptomatic and is discovered by the characteristic appearance of the urogram, often done for other reasons. Enlargement of the papillae and calices and small cavities within the pyramids are demonstrated by the contrast media in the excretory urogram. Many small calculi often occupy the cysts, and infection may be troublesome. Life expectancy is not affected, and only symptomatic therapy for ureteral impaction of a stone or for infection is required.

Acquired Cystic Renal Disease

Patients with end-stage renal disease who have been maintained on hemodialysis will frequently (30–50% of cases) develop cystic degeneration of the end-stage kidneys. The cause is unknown. Although most patients are asymptomatic, hemorrhage into the cysts, rupture, and the development of adenomas or low-grade adenocarcinomas constitute a hazard. CT scan is the preferred diagnostic imaging procedure. Nephrectomy may be necessary.

Gardner KD Jr: Cystic kidneys. Kidney Int 1988;33:610.
Grantham JJ: Polycystic kidney disease: An old problem in a new context. (Editorial.) N Engl J Med 1988;319:44.
Thompson C: Renal disorders. 8. The spectrum of renal cystic diseases. Hosp Pract (April 15) 1988;23:165.

3. ANOMALIES OF FUNCTION OF THE PROXIMAL TUBULE

Defects of Amino Acid Reabsorption

A. Congenital Cystinuria: Cystinuria is an autosomal recessive disease with an incidence ranging from 1:20,000 to 1:1000 in various populations. Increased excretion of cystine results in the formation of cystine calculi in the urinary tract. Ornithine, arginine, and lysine are also excreted in abnormally large quantities. There is also a defect in absorption of these amino acids in the jejunum. Nonopaque stones should be examined chemically to provide a specific diagnosis.

Maintain a high urine volume by giving a large fluid intake. Maintain the urine pH above 7.0 by giving sodium bicarbonate and sodium citrate plus acetazolamide (Diamox) at bedtime to ensure an alkaline night urine. In refractory cases, a low-methionine (cystine precursor) diet may be necessary. Penicillamine has proved useful in some cases.

B. Aminoaciduria: Hereditary defects of renal tubule function or defects of amino acid metabolism are manifested by loss of a variety of amino acids. Failure to thrive and the presence of other tubular deficits suggest the diagnosis.

There is no treatment.

C. Hepatolenticular Degeneration (Wilson's Disease): In this congenital familial disease, aminoaciduria is associated with cirrhosis of the liver and neurologic manifestations.

Multiple Defects of Tubular Function

A. De Toni-Fanconi-Debré Syndrome: Aminoaciduria, phosphaturia, glycosuria, and a variable degree of renal tubular acidosis characterize this syndrome. Osteomalacia is a prominent clinical feature; other clinical and laboratory manifestations are associated with specific tubular defects described above.

The proximal segment of the renal tubule is replaced by a thin tubular structure constituting the swan-neck deformity. The proximal segment also is shortened to less than half the normal length.

Treatment consists of replacing cation deficits (especially potassium), correcting acidosis with bicarbonate or citrate, replacing phosphate loss with isotonic neutral phosphate (mono- and disodium salts) solution, and a liberal calcium intake. Vitamin D is usually helpful, but the dose used must be controlled by monitoring serum calcium and phosphate.

B. Acquired Fanconi Syndrome: Defects in tubular reabsorption resembling those of the Fanconi syndrome can be induced by heavy metal poisoning (cadmium, lead, copper, uranium, mercury), by a degradation product of tetracycline, by cresol poisoning, by galactosemia, by renal tubule damage in myeloma, and by tubulointerstitial disease.

Treatment is directed at the primary cause and at correction of electrolyte abnormalities.

Defects of Phosphorus & Calcium Absorption

A. Vitamin D-Resistant Rickets: Excessive loss of phosphorus and calcium results in rickets or osteomalacia poorly responsive to vitamin D therapy. Treatment consists of giving large doses of vitamin D and dietary phosphorus and calcium supplementation.

B. Pseudohypoparathyroidism: See Chapter 20.

Defects of Glucose Absorption (Renal Glycosuria)

Relative inability to reabsorb glucose means that glycosuria is present when blood glucose levels are normal. Ketosis is not present. The glucose tolerance test response is usually normal. In some instances, renal glycosuria may precede the onset of true diabetes mellitus.

There is no treatment for renal glycosuria.

Defects of Glucose & Phosphate Absorption (Glycosuric Rickets)

The symptoms and signs are those of rickets or osteomalacia, with weakness, pain, or discomfort of the legs and spine, and tetany. The bones become deformed, with bowing of the weight-bearing long bones, kyphoscoliosis, and, in children, signs of rickets. Radiography shows markedly decreased density of the bone, with pseudofracture lines and other deformities. Nephrocalcinosis may occur with excessive phosphaturia, and renal insufficiency may follow. Urinary calcium and phosphorus are increased, and glycosuria is present. Serum glucose is normal, serum calcium normal or low, serum phosphorus low, and serum alkaline phosphatase elevated.

Treatment consists of giving large doses of vitamin D and dietary phosphorus and calcium supplementation.

4. RENAL TUBULAR ACIDOSIS

Both the proximal tubule and the distal tubule can secrete hydrogen ion (H^+) and reclaim bicarbonate (HCO_3^-) from the luminal fluid. Normally, the preponderance of filtered HCO_3^- is reclaimed in the proximal tubule, leaving a smaller demand on the distal segment of the nephron to provide hydrogen for reabsorption of a small amount of HCO_3^- and excretion of metabolic acids.

Proximal Renal Tubular Acidosis (Type II)

The defect in H^+ secretion in the proximal tubule results in a decrease in absorption of filtered bicarbonate, loss of bicarbonate in the urine, and decreased concentration of bicarbonate in extracellular fluid. Secretion of H^+ in the distal tubule is unimpaired.

As plasma bicarbonate concentration diminishes, less bicarbonate is filtered, and ultimately an equilibrium is reached. This sets a limit on bicarbonate loss, and the resultant acidosis is only moderate. Accompanying the limitation of hydrogen ion secretion are increased potassium secretion into the urine and retrieval of Cl^- instead of HCO_3^-. The acidosis is therefore associated with hypokalemia and hyperchloremia. Because Cl^- replaces HCO_3^- in the extracellular fluid, there is no anion gap. Hypercalciuria is moderate, and stone formation is uncommon. Transport of glucose, amino acids, phosphate, and urate may be deficient as well and may result in the Fanconi syndrome (see above).

Proximal renal tubular acidosis may be genetic in origin. It is transiently seen with acetazolamide therapy, use of outdated tetracycline, and exposure to some heavy metals (eg, lead). Proximal renal tubular acidosis may occur when the kidney is involved with medullary cystic disease or multiple myeloma. (See also de Toni-Fanconi-Debré Syndrome, above.)

The pH of the urine is high except if acidosis becomes severe when bicarbonate disappears from the urine and the pH drops to a lower limit of 5.5–5.4.

When treatment is required for the acidosis, it consists of replacement with large amounts of HCO_3^- and replacement of wasted K^+. Bicarbonate in doses of 6–15 mmol/kg/d may be required; some of this should be $KHCO_3$. Shohl's solution, a mixture of sodium citrate and citric acid (1 mL = 1 mmol HCO_3^-), in doses of 20–50 mL 3 times a day, may be substituted for part of the HCO_3^- requirement. A combination of hydrochlorothiazide, to produce slight volume depletion with resultant increased HCO_3^- reabsorption, plus spironolactone, to reduce K^+ excretion, has been employed to ameliorate proximal renal tubular acidosis.

Distal Renal Tubular Acidosis (Type I)

The distal tubule cells, like those of the proximal tubule, generate carbonic acid from CO_2 and H_2O and retrieve the bicarbonate by secreting H^+ to exchange for Na^+ in the tubular fluid. H^+ is excreted with acid anion and buffers in the urine and is also combined with NH_3 to form NH_4^+, an additional cation that accompanies acid anion in the excreted urine.

The defect in distal renal tubular acidosis is either a defect in secretion of H^+ or an inability to transport H^+ against a steep concentration gradient between extracellular fluid and urine in the terminal segments of the nephron (eg, plasma pH 7.4 = 4×10^{-8} molar (H^+) versus urine pH 4.5 = 32×10^{-6} molar [H^+]) or both of these. The defect persists no matter how severe the acidosis, and diagnosis depends on the observation that in the presence of acidosis, the urine pH remains greater than 5.5. Potassium excretion is heightened by failure of H^+ secretion and by activation of the secretion of aldosterone; hypokalemia is often apparent clinically. Hypercalciuria with renal stone and nephrocalcinosis and metabolic bone disease are seen in severe and long-standing cases. There is an incomplete form of distal renal tubular acidosis that is revealed only when it is necessary to excrete a large acid load. To prove that this incomplete form of renal tubular acidosis exists, 0.1 g of NH_4Cl per kilogram is administered orally. Within 6–8 hours, arterial blood pH should be less than 7.35, plasma bicarbonate should be less than 20 mmol/L, and the urine pH should remain greater than 5.5.

Distal renal tubular acidosis may be genetically transmitted. It can occur in association with sickle cell anemia, a variety of autoimmune diseases, chronic interstitial nephritis and urolithiasis, cirrhosis of the liver, diseases in which nephrocalcinosis occurs, and therapy with amphotericin B or analgesics.

Treatment of the acute emergency of severe metabolic acidosis includes vigorous bicarbonate replacement supplemented with adequate K^+. The chronic case requires lifelong therapy with enough $NaHCO_3$, Shohl's solution (a mixture of sodium citrate and citric acid), or potassium citrate (up to 80 meq/d) to neutralize the metabolic acids that must be excreted (50 mmol/d or more) and to correct hypercalciuria. Potassium loss will usually diminish enough so that K^+ replacement is not required, but in some cases, potassium intake may have to be increased.

Appropriate therapy will protect against development of nephrocalcinosis, azotemia, and metabolic bone disease.

Type IV Renal Tubular Acidosis

Recognition of type IV renal tubular acidosis is increasingly common as the clinical manifestations become known. It occurs with hyporeninemic hypoaldosteronism when moderate renal insufficiency is associated with diabetes mellitus; with chronic renal insufficiency from many causes; or as an adverse effect of drugs such as spironolactone (especially with cirrhosis) and nonsteroidal anti-inflammatory agents. It also occurs with normal aldosterone activity when there is chronic renal insufficiency (rarely) or urinary obstruction. The characteristics of type IV renal tubular acidosis include impairment of renal acidification accompanied by reduced renal clearance of potassium, which results in hyperkalemia and acidosis. The disorder is related to lack of aldosterone or inability of aldosterone to stimulate H^+ secretion at the cation exchange portion of the distal tubule.

Treatment with fludrocortisone in doses that do not induce hypervolemia and hypertension (0.1–0.3 mg/d) may correct acidosis and hyperkalemia. Alternatively, reducing potassium intake, use of potassium-binding resins, and use of loop diuretics may correct the hyperkalemia. Acidosis may be corrected by small doses of sodium bicarbonate (2 meq/kg/d).

5. ANOMALIES OF THE DISTAL TUBULE

Excess Potassium Secretion (Potassium "Wastage" Syndrome)

Excessive renal secretion or loss of potassium may occur in 4 situations: (1) chronic renal insufficiency with diminished H^+ secretion; (2) renal tubular acidosis and de Toni-Fanconi syndrome, with cation loss resulting from diminished H^+ and NH_4^+ secretion; (3) aldosteronism and hyperadrenocorticism; and (4) excessive tubular secretion of potassium, the cause of which is unknown. Hypokalemia indicates that the deficit is severe. Muscle weakness, metabolic alkalosis, and polyuria with dilute urine are signs of hypokalemia (see Chapter 16).

Defects of Water Absorption (Renal Diabetes Insipidus)

Nephrogenic diabetes insipidus occurs more frequently in males. Unresponsiveness to antidiuretic hormone is the key to differentiation from pituitary diabetes insipidus.

In addition to congenital refractoriness to antidiuretic hormone, obstructive uropathy, lithium, methoxyflurane, and demeclocycline may also render the tubule refractory. Impaired water reabsorption may be present with sickle cell anemia, medullary cystic disease, hypokalemia, and hypercalcemia.

Symptoms are related to an inability to reabsorb water, with resultant polyuria and polydipsia. The daily urine volume approaches 12 L, and osmolality and specific gravity are low. Atonic bladder and hydronephrosis occur frequently.

Treatment consists primarily of an adequate water intake. Chlorothiazide may ameliorate the diabetes; the mechanism of action is unknown, but the drug may act by increasing isosmotic reabsorption in the proximal segment of the tubule secondary to volume contraction.

6. UNSPECIFIED TUBULAR ABNORMALITIES

Abnormalities

In idiopathic hypercalciuria, decreased reabsorption of calcium predisposes to the formation of renal calculi. Serum calcium and phosphorus are normal. Urine calcium excretion is high; urine phosphorus excretion is low.

Batlle D: Renal tubular acidosis. Med Clin North Am 1983;67:859.

Davidman M, Schmitz P: Renal tubular acidosis: A pathophysiologic approach. Hosp Pract (Jan 30) 1988;23:77.

Rocher LL, Tannen RL: The clinical spectrum of renal tubular acidosis. Annu Rev Med 1986;37:319.

7. CONGENITAL ANOMALIES

Renal Agenesis

Occasionally, one kidney (usually the left) is congenitally absent. The remaining kidney is hypertrophied. Before performing a nephrectomy for any reason, it is mandatory to prove the patient has a second kidney.

Horseshoe Kidney

A band of renal tissue or of fibrous tissue may join the 2 kidneys. Associated abnormalities of the ureterocaliceal system predispose to pyelonephritis, as does hydronephrosis resulting from ureteral obstruction by aberrant vessels.

Ectopic Kidney

The kidney may occupy a site in the pelvis, and the ureter may be shorter than normal. Infection is common in ectopic kidneys compromised by ureteral obstruction or urinary reflux.

Nephroptosis

Unusual mobility of the kidney permits it to move from its normal position to a lower one. The incidence of ureteral occlusion due to movement of a kidney is extremely low.

Anomalies of Renal Calices, Renal Pelvis, & Ureters

Duplication of the ureters is the commonest anomaly. Ureteropelvic junction obstruction, abnormal insertion of ureters into the bladder, and other collecting system anomalies frequently produce stasis of urine with a resulting propensity for recurrent urinary tract infections.

Megaloureter & Hydronephrosis

These anatomic abnormalities may occur congenitally but are more commonly the result of vesicoureteral urinary reflux.

Kissane JM: Congenital malformations. Page 83 in: *Pathology of the Kidney,* 3rd ed. Heptinstall RH (editor). Little, Brown, 1983.

8. RENAL DISEASE INCIDENT TO OTHER DISEASES

Abnormalities of renal function occur with other diseases and may be of therapeutic and prognostic importance. In **sickle cell anemia,** circulatory changes resulting from sickling and aggregation of red cells contribute to decreased concentrating ability, a defect in acidification of urine, hematuria, renal infarction, glomerulopathy, papillary necrosis, and renal failure. With **acute pancreatitis,** acute renal failure may occur in the absence of shock. In **hepatorenal syndrome,** severe renal failure may appear with cirrhosis of the liver and ascites or with severe jaundice of either parenchymatous or obstructive origin. **Acute renal failure in pregnancy** occurs with toxemia, intrauterine hemorrhage, and complications of abortion and in the immediate postpartum period (hemolytic-uremic syndrome).

Acquired immunodeficiency syndrome (AIDS) and AIDS-related complex (ARC) are associated with renal impairment by 3 mechanisms: (1) acute renal failure may be due to sepsis, shock, and respiratory insufficiency and to nephrotoxic drugs used in treatment of AIDS and its complicating infections; (2) use of intravenous drugs and their associated impurities may produce interstitial and glomerular lesions and renal insufficiency; and (3) HIV can produce focal segmental glomerulosclerosis with a particularly rapid progression manifested by proteinuria, microscopic hematuria, and increasingly severe renal failure. The kidneys remain near normal in size; the glomeruli contain mesangial deposits of IgM and C3. Hemodialysis is often useful for treatment of acute renal failure. Patients with glomerulosclerosis who are suitable for dialysis have not survived beyond a year.

Allon M: Renal abnormalities in sickle cell disease. Arch Intern Med 1990;150:501.

Brenner BM, Rector FC Jr: The Kidney, 3rd ed. Saunders, 1986.

Epstein M: The hepatorenal syndrome. Hosp Pract (April 15) 1989;24:65.

Epstein M (editor): The Kidney in Liver Disease, 3rd ed. Williams & Wilkins, 1988.

Langs C et al: Rapid renal failure in acquired immunodefi-
ciency syndrome-associated focal glomerulosclerosis. Arch Intern Med 1990;150:287.

Rao TK, Friedman EA, Nicastri AD: The types of renal disease in the acquired immunodeficiency syndrome. N Engl J Med 1987;316:1062.

INFECTIONS OF THE URINARY TRACT

Ernest Jawetz, MD, PhD

The term urinary tract infection denotes a wide variety of clinical entities in which the common denominator is the presence of a significantly large number of microorganisms in any portion of the urinary tract. Microorganisms may be evident only in the urine (bacteriuria), or there may be evidence of infection of an organ, eg, urethritis, prostatitis, cystitis, pyelonephritis. At any given time, any one of these organs may be asymptomatic or symptomatic. Infection in any part of the urinary tract may spread to any other part of the tract.

Symptomatic urinary tract infection may be acute or chronic. The term relapse implies recurrence of infection with the same organism; the term reinfection implies infection with another organism.

Pathogenesis

Urine secreted by normal kidneys is sterile until it reaches the distal urethra. Bacteria can reach the urinary tract by the ascending route or by hematogenous spread. The latter occurs during bacteremia (eg, with staphylococci) and results in abscess formation in the cortex or the perirenal fat. Far commoner is ascending infection, where bacteria are introduced into the urethra (from fecal flora on the perineum or the vaginal vestibule, or by instrumentation) and travel up the urinary tract to reach the bladder, ureter, or renal pelvis. The most important factor in aiding or perpetuating ascending infection is anatomic or functional obstruction to free urine flow. Free flow, large urine volume, complete emptying of the bladder, and acid pH are important antibacterial defenses.

Age & Sex Distribution of Urinary Tract Infection

In infants, urinary tract infection occurs more frequently in boys than in girls, in keeping with a higher incidence of obstructive anomalies of the urinary tract. After the first year of life, urinary tract infection is more frequent in girls because the female urethra is short and because the vaginal vestibule can become contaminated with fecal flora. In surveys of schoolchildren, only 0.05% of boys have bacteriuria, whereas at least 2% of girls do. In later life, urinary tract infection is rare among men until the age of prostatic hypertrophy (over 40), but there is a regular increase in incidence with age among women. At age 70, about 10% of women have urinary tract infections. In younger women, there is some correlation of the incidence of urinary tract infection with sexual activity and with parity.

Infecting Microorganisms

Virtually any microorganism introduced into the urinary tract may cause urinary tract infection. However, the vast majority of cases of urinary tract infection are caused by aerobic members of the fecal flora, especially *Escherichia* (*E coli* O serotypes 4, 6, and 75 are especially common), *Enterobacter, Klebsiella,* enterococci, *Pseudomonas,* and *Proteus.* Other organisms (eg, *Staphylococcus saprophyticus*) occasionally appear in spontaneous urinary tract infection, but their significance must be assessed as described below. Infections with strict anaerobes are very rare. Viruses may cause immune complex nephritis but—except for adenovirus type 11 in hemorrhagic cystitis of children—do not cause urinary tract infections. Chlamydiae, mycoplasmas, and other organisms causing urethritis, vaginitis, and other genital tract disorders are listed below.

Significant Bacteriuria

The concept of significant bacteriuria is basic to the proper interpretation of urine cultures. Urine secreted by the normal kidney is sterile and remains so while it travels to the bladder. However, the normal urethra has a microbial flora, and any voided urine in normal persons may therefore contain thousands of bacteria per milliliter derived from this normal flora. To differentiate this smaller number of microorganisms from the larger number commonly found in infections of the urinary tract, it is essential to count the number of bacteria in fresh, properly collected specimens by appropriate methods (quantitative culture). In general, acute urinary tract infections are characterized by more than 100,000 bacteria per milliliter. If such numbers are found in 2 consecutive specimens and if the bacteria are of a single type, there is more than a 95% chance that an active infection is present. On the other hand, a significant proportion of acutely dysuric women have pyuria with only 10^3–10^5 bacteria per milliliter at times but respond promptly to antibacterial treatment. In persons who chronically show low-grade bacteriuria, suprapubic aspiration may help in diagnosis.

Pathology

Acute urinary tract infection shows inflammation of any part of the tract and sometimes intense hyperemia or even bleeding of the mucous membranes. The prominent lesion in the kidney is acute inflammation of the interstitial tissue, which may progress to frank suppuration and patchy necrosis. Papillary necrosis (eg, in diabetics) may lead to slough of papillae and ureteral obstruction. Recurrent urinary tract infection may cause only minimal changes or progressively more severe scarring in any part of the tract. Chronic pyelonephritis may lead to widespread fibrosis and scarring of functional cortical and medullary tissue, resulting in renal insufficiency; it appears unlikely that repeated urinary tract infection causes renal insufficiency unless there is concomitant obstruction. Chronic interstitial nephritis may result from bacterial infection or from other causes (eg, hypersensitivity, vasculitis, use of analgesics).

Collection of Urine for Culture

A. Voided Midstream Specimen: This is the optimal method, involving no risk to the patient. The urethral meatus or vaginal vestibule is cleansed, the labia are spread, and the first part of the stream is discarded. The mid part of the stream is aseptically collected in a sterile container.

B. Specimen Obtained by Catheterization: Each urethral catheter insertion carries a 1–2% risk of introducing microorganisms into the bladder and thus initiating urinary tract infection. Results of quantitative culture from a single catheterized urine specimen yielding more than 100,000 bacteria of a single species per milliliter of urine indicate that active urinary tract infection is present. In persons with indwelling urethral catheters, specimens must be obtained by aseptic needle aspiration of urine through the catheter wall, not by disconnecting the closed system.

C. Specimen Obtained by Suprapubic Aspiration: While the bladder is distended, the suprapubic skin is aseptically prepared, and a sterile needle is then thrust into the bladder. This permits aspiration of bladder urine free from urethral contamination. It is especially useful in infants (from whom satisfactory specimens for culture may be difficult to obtain) and in patients with equivocal counts on several occasions. However, this procedure is technically more difficult in adults; it should rarely be necessary.

Examination of Urine

Urine must be cultured or examined microscopically within 1 hour of collection or after no more than 18 hours of refrigeration. Urine is a good culture medium for many microorganisms, and growth can occur at room temperature.

A. Microscopic Examination: A drop of fresh urine or a drop of resuspended sediment from centrifuged fresh urine is placed on a microscope slide, covered with a cover glass, and examined with the high-dry objective under reduced illumination. The prevalence of leukocytes is noted. The presence of more than 10 bacteria (often motile) per field in the unstained specimen suggests a bacteria count of more than 100,000/mL of urine. Smears may also be made from fresh urine, stained with Gram's stain, and examined under the oil immersion objective. Three bacteria or more per field in such stains suggest infection. By immunofluorescence, bacteria in urine are coated with immunoglobulin if they are derived from tissue infection (especially pyelonephritis, prostatitis) but usually are not so coated if the infection is limited to the outflow system (cystitis, urethritis). This procedure is expensive and rarely used in routine cases.

B. Urine Culture: With a calibrated loop, undiluted urine and urine diluted 1:100 are spread on eosin-methylene blue and blood agar plates. After incubation, numbers of colonies are estimated and multiplied by the dilution factor to yield the bacterial count per milliliter. A number of simplified semiquantitative culture methods are available that are readily performed in the physician's office at nominal cost. The dip-slide method and its several variations involve dipping an agar-coated slide or similar device into fresh urine, incubating it, and then comparing the resultant growth with optical density standards.

C. Chemical Tests of Urine: The presence and number of bacteria can also be estimated by various chemical tests that rely on the enzymatic activity of viable bacteria, eg, the reduction of nitrate. These indirect tests are much less reliable than tests employing quantitative estimates of bacterial growth.

D. Identification of Microorganisms: In most cases of acute urinary tract infection, detailed identification of the etiologic organism may not be required. However, in chronic or recurrent urinary tract infection, identification of the organism by standard microbiologic methods is desirable. Antimicrobial drug susceptibility tests are not needed in the first attack of urinary tract infection. Most of these infections are due to coliform organisms and are often treated with sulfonamide, ampicillin, or amoxicillin. In chronic or recurrent urinary tract infection, antimicrobial drug susceptibility tests are needed. It must be kept in mind that many drugs appear in the urine in very high concentration, whereas "standard" tests indicate susceptibility only to levels achieved in blood.

ACUTE URINARY TRACT INFECTION
(Urethritis, Cystitis, Pyelonephritis)

Clinical Findings

A. Lower Tract Involvement (Urethritis, Cystitis):

1. Symptoms and signs–Manifestations include burning pain on urination, often with turbid, foul-smelling, or dark urine; frequency; and suprapubic or lower abdominal discomfort. There are usually no positive physical findings unless the upper tract is involved also.

2. Laboratory findings–Microscopic examination of a properly collected urine specimen usually shows significant bacteriuria and pyuria and occasion-

ally hematuria. Bacteriuria may be confirmed by dip-slide or similar test.

B. Upper Tract Involvement (Pyelonephritis):

1. Symptoms and signs–Findings include headache, malaise, vomiting, chills and fever, costovertebral angle pain and tenderness, and abdominal pain. The absence of upper tract signs does not exclude bacterial invasion of the upper tract, however.

2. Laboratory findings–Significant bacteriuria is often accompanied by proteinuria and pyuria. The bacteria in the urine are often coated with immunoglobulin, as revealed by immunofluorescence. Leukocytosis is common, with a marked shift to the left. Blood culture is only rarely positive.

Differential Diagnosis

Acute urinary tract infection may occasionally present as an "acute abdomen," acute pancreatitis, or pneumonia. In all of these circumstances, the presence of significant bacteriuria usually establishes the diagnosis. On the other hand, dysuria, frequency, nocturia, and lower abdominal pain may be due to traumatic cystitis, the "urethral" or "bladder" syndrome, especially in sexually active women. It may also represent vaginitis ("vaginosis"); urethritis; cervicitis attributable to *Trichomonas*, *Gardnerella*, mixed anaerobes, *Chlamydia*, *Neisseria*, or *Ureaplasma*.

Prevention

Certain women have a high rate of urinary reinfection, sometimes related to sexual activity. In the latter situation, one or 2 doses of an effective antimicrobial (eg, trimethoprim-sulfamethoxazole, nitrofurantoin) taken after intercourse tend to prevent establishment of infection. In other women, recurrences can be greatly reduced if the patient takes trimethoprim-sulfamethoxazole, one tablet 3 times weekly or one-half tablet daily at bedtime for months.

In patients who must have an indwelling catheter postoperatively and in whom closed sterile drainage is established, the onset of bacteriuria is delayed if suitable antimicrobial drugs are given during the first 3 days after insertion. Thereafter, there is no benefit.

Treatment

A. Specific Measures:

1. First attack of urinary tract infection–For uncomplicated acute symptomatic cystitis in nonpregnant women, previously untreated, a single dose of sulfisoxazole, 1 g; amoxicillin, 500 mg; or ciprofloxacin, 500 mg—or 2 tablets of trimethoprim 80 mg plus sulfamethoxazole 400 mg twice in 1 day—is effective treatment in 80–90% of cases. Alternatively, the administration of sulfisoxazole, 4 g/d; ampicillin, 2–4 g/d; cephalexin, 2–4 g/d; or trimethoprim-sulfamethoxazole, 2–4 tablets daily for 1–3 days, may be effective. Acute infection in men or infections suggestive of upper tract involvement should be treated with similar drugs for 7–10 days. If symptoms have not improved and the urine has not cleared as shown by microscopy on day 4 of treatment, culture the urine for possible resistant microorganisms. Follow-up at 2 and 6 weeks after treatment is stopped should show absence of bacteriuria; otherwise, retreat. All men with urinary tract infections should be investigated for obstructive uropathy.

2. Recurrence of urinary tract infection–In this situation, an antimicrobial drug is selected on the basis of antimicrobial susceptibility tests of cultured organisms. The drug is administered for 10–14 days in doses sufficient to maintain high urine levels. Reexamine the urine 2 and 6 weeks after treatment is stopped.

3. Second recurrence, or failure of bacteriuria to be suppressed–Women should be investigated for possible obstruction, reflux, and localization of infection in the upper or lower tract. Men with recurrent urinary tract infection and no obstruction are likely to have a prostatic focus, and a 12- to 20-week trial of trimethoprim-sulfamethoxazole or ampicillin is indicated.

B. General Measures: Forcing fluids may relieve signs and symptoms. Analgesics may be required briefly.

Prognosis

Initial attacks of acute urinary tract infection, in the absence of obstruction, tend to subside with treatment or spontaneously. The symptoms and bacteriuria often disappear. This is not true in recurrent or chronic urinary tract infection. About 20% of pregnant women with asymptomatic bacteriuria in the first trimester develop symptomatic pyelonephritis later in pregnancy and thus may benefit from early treatment.

CHRONIC URINARY TRACT INFECTION
(Cystitis, Pyelonephritis)

Essentials of Diagnosis

- Recurrent episodes of lower or upper tract involvement.
- Absence of symptoms or signs referable to the urinary tract, but persistent asymptomatic bacteriuria.
- Obstruction or other anatomic abnormality in the urinary tract is consistently found in men, occasionally in women.
- Impairment of renal function rare unless obstruction is present.

General Considerations

Chronic or recurrent episodes of urinary tract infection usually produce no permanent harm unless obstruction is present. In these patients, chronic bacterial pyelonephritis may progress to inflammation of in-

terstitial tissue, scarring, atrophy, and, rarely, progressive renal failure. In most patients with these pathologic findings, "chronic pyelonephritis" is in fact not caused by infection but instead represents interstitial nephritis of immunologic or toxic cause. Occasionally, chronic infection is due to a unilateral structural abnormality (eg, ureteral stricture), and nephrectomy may be curative. With bilateral nephritis, chronic suppression of infection may stabilize renal function. Some women have chronic bacteriuria which is asymptomatic; in the absence of anatomic abnormalities, the prognosis for preservation of renal function appears to be good.

Clinical Findings

A. Symptoms and Signs: There are often no positive clinical findings in chronic urinary tract infection except significant bacteriuria. There may be episodes of recurrent acute urinary tract infection with symptoms referable to the lower or to the upper urinary tract. Hypertension and anemia appear only in the late stages of chronic pyelonephritis.

Whenever chronic bacteriuria is discovered, it is mandatory to perform a complete urologic study, including excretory urograms or renal ultrasonography, cystograms, and voiding cystourethrograms, followed by procedures to localize the source of bacteriuria to one or both sides and to the lower or upper tract. Surgical correction of any abnormality (reflux, obstruction, etc) found in these studies must be considered while chronic suppression of bacteriuria is undertaken.

B. Laboratory Findings: The white blood count is usually normal, but significant anemia may be present in early renal failure. Blood urea and serum creatinine are elevated, and creatinine clearance may be reduced. Repeated and meticulous urine culture is crucial as a guide to medical treatment. In addition, methods such as "bladder washout" may be used to distinguish infection of the lower from that of the upper tract. When significant chronic bacteriuria is discovered, an attempt may be made to eradicate or suppress it (see below). If no significant bacteriuria is found in the presence of unexplained hematuria and pyuria, infection by tubercle bacilli, anaerobic bacteria, or fungi must be considered.

Immunofluorescence staining usually shows that bacteria derived from tissue infection are coated with immunoglobulin, eg, in pyelonephritis and prostatitis. Bacteria from the ureter or bladder are not usually stained by this technique.

Treatment

A. Specific Measures: Specific treatment may consist of surgical correction of functional or anatomic abnormalities by the urologist, or it may consist of antimicrobial treatment. The latter usually involves attempts to eradicate the infectious agent by short-term treatment and, if bacteriuria recurs, long-term suppression of the bacteria by administration of urinary antiseptics.

1. If the same organism is isolated from at least 2 sequential urine cultures, antimicrobial drug sensitivity tests should be performed. From the group of drugs to which the organism is susceptible in vitro, the least toxic and least expensive agent is selected (for choice of drugs, see Chapter 31) and administered daily in full systemic doses orally for 4 weeks. The urine is checked after 3 days of treatment and then at weekly intervals to make certain that bacteriuria is suppressed and that a new infection with another organism has not occurred. At the end of treatment, all drug administration is stopped and, 2 and 6 weeks later, the urine is checked again. If bacteriuria is not found, it may be assumed that the particular organism has been eradicated. Repeated examinations for bacteriuria are necessary to confirm absence of recurrent infection.

2. If the foregoing measures fail to eradicate the infection, chronic suppression of bacteriuria is attempted by daily dosage with a urinary antiseptic, eg, nitrofurantoin, methenamine mandelate or hippurate, quinolones, or acidifying agents (see Chapter 31). Urinary pH must be adjusted to the optimum for the drug selected and usually should be held below pH 6.0. The patient can monitor urine pH with indicator paper once a day. After 1 week of treatment and monthly thereafter, the urine must be examined for bacteria. Chronic suppression is continued for 6 months or even longer if the patient can tolerate the drug and superinfection does not occur. If the latter should occur, a specific antimicrobial drug may be selected, by laboratory test, for a 14-day course of treatment, and suppression with another urinary antiseptic may then be continued. At the end of 1 year of suppressive treatment, renal function and bacteriuria are reevaluated.

B. General Measures: Water diuresis may often provide relief from minor discomfort of lower urinary tract symptoms. Water and electrolyte balance must be maintained and renal failure managed as described above. Prevention of infection is all-important, particularly by avoidance of catheterization and instrumentation and by practicing good hygiene. In some women, prophylactic administration of nitrofurantoin, 50–100 mg daily, or trimethoprim-sulfamethoxazole, 2 tablets every other day, may prevent recurrences of infection.

Prolonged drug administration should be avoided in patients with neurogenic bladder or long-term indwelling catheter. Removal of the catheter takes priority over drug treatment.

Prognosis

Probably 10% or fewer of asymptomatic bacteriuria patients develop renal failure attributable to the infection; hypertension is even more rare. Chronic urinary tract infection is eradicated by short-term therapy (2–6 weeks) in about 25–35% of patients. Some of the others have relapses caused by the same organism; some have reinfection caused by other organisms.

Long-term suppression (> 6 months) with urinary antiseptics eradicates bacteriuria in about two-thirds of patients, but some may become reinfected later. Many elderly patients tolerate recurrent urinary tract infection well, and therapy of their asymptomatic bacteriuria is inappropriate. Antimicrobial drugs should be limited to the relief of symptomatic exacerbations.

Komaroff AL: Acute dysuria in women. N Engl J Med 1984;310:368.

Lipsky BA et al: Diagnosis of bacteriuria in men: Specimen collection and culture interpretation. J Infect Dis 1987; 155:847.

Nicolle LE et al: Bacteriuria in elderly institutionalized men. N Engl J Med 1983;309:1420.

Stamm WE: Prevention of urinary tract infections. Am J Med 1984;76:148.

TUBERCULOSIS OF THE GENITOURINARY TRACT

Essentials of Diagnosis

- Fever, easy fatigability, night sweats, or other signs of systemic infection.
- Symptoms or signs of upper or lower urinary tract infection.
- Urine may contain leukocytes and erythrocytes but no visible bacteria.
- Routine urine culture is negative. Special culture of urine for mycobacteria reveals *Mycobacterium tuberculosis.*
- Excretory urogram may show deformed or "motheaten" calices and kidney tissue destruction.
- Cystoscopy may reveal ulcers or granulomas of bladder wall.

General Considerations

Reactivation of foci originating from hematogenous dissemination of tubercle bacilli after primary pulmonary infection is the usual source of tuberculosis of the kidney; rarely does the infection originate in the genital tract. The genital organs may become similarly infected by hematogenous spread or secondary to kidney infection. The prostate, seminal vesicles, epididymides, and, rarely, the testes may be infected. The oviducts are more frequently involved than the ovaries and uterus.

The kidney and ureter may show little gross change. However, caseous nodules in the renal parenchyma and abscess formation with destruction of tissue and fibrosis often produce extensive damage. Calcification in the lesions is common. The ureter and calices are thickened, and stenosis may occur, with total destruction of functioning renal tissue above. The bladder shows mucosal inflammation and submucosal tubercles that become necrotic and form ulcers. Fibrosis of the bladder wall occurs late or upon healing. Tubercles with caseous necrosis and calcification are found in the genital organs. Microscopically, typical tubercles are found, and demonstration of the tubercle bacilli in the lesions is usually easily accomplished.

A search must be made for tuberculosis elsewhere in the body whenever urinary tract tuberculosis is found.

Clinical Findings

A. Symptoms and Signs: Symptoms are not characteristic or specific. Manifestations of chronic infection, with malaise, fever, fatigability, and night sweats, may be present. Tuberculous kidney and ureter infection is usually silent, but bladder infection produces frequency, burning on urination, nocturia, and, occasionally, tenesmus. If bleeding occurs with clot formation, ureteral or vesical colic may occur. Gross hematuria is fairly common. There may be nodular induration of the testes, epididymides, or prostate and thickened seminal vesicles. Occasionally, pain and tenderness occur in the costovertebral angle. A draining sinus may form from any of these sites.

B. Laboratory Findings: The urine contains "pus without bacteria," red cells, and, usually, protein; occasionally, culture for routine bacterial pathogens may also be positive. Culture for tubercle bacilli confirms the diagnosis. If renal damage is extensive, blood urea nitrogen and creatinine are elevated. A mild anemia usually is present, and the sedimentation rate is rapid.

C. Imaging and Cystoscopic Findings: Excretory urograms reveal the moth-eaten appearance of the involved calices or the obliteration of calices, stenosis of calices, abscess cavities, ureteral thickening and stenosis, and the nonfunctioning kidney (autonephrectomy). Calcification of involved tissues is common. Cystoscopic examination is required to determine the extent of bladder wall infection and to provide biopsy material if needed.

Differential Diagnosis

The "sterile" pyuria of chronic interstitial nephritis, chronic nonspecific urethritis, and cystitis may mimic tuberculous infection. If hematuria is prominent, urinary calculi or bladder carcinoma may be suspected.

Treatment

Intensive and prolonged antituberculosis therapy is indicated, employing 2 or 3 drugs simultaneously for 9–18 months (see Chapter 31). In 1991, the drugs of choice are isoniazid, 5–8 mg/kg/d (usually 300 mg/d orally); ethambutol, 15 mg/kg/d as a single oral dose; and rifampin, 10–20 mg/kg/d (usually 600 mg as a single oral dose). Alternative drugs are listed in Chapter 31.

Pyridoxine, 100 mg/d orally, is usually given concurrently with isoniazid to prevent neurotoxic reactions. Surgical procedures are generally limited to situations in which extensive destruction of one kidney makes it unlikely that infection can be eradicated and useful function restored (nephrectomy), obstruction in the tract interferes with proper function, or erosion of a vessel leads to severe bleeding.

Prognosis

The outlook depends largely on the degree of destruction of renal tissue and impairment of renal function. If urinary tract tuberculosis is detected early, prolonged drug treatment can suppress and arrest the infectious process successfully. Structural defects resulting from infection or fibrosis require surgical correction.

Alvarez S, McCabe WR: Extrapulmonary tuberculosis revisited. Medicine 1984;63:25.

American Thoracic Society: Treatment of tuberculosis and other mycobacterial diseases. Am Rev Respir Dis 1983;127:790.

Dutt AK et al: Short-course chemotherapy for extrapulmonary tuberculosis. Ann Intern Med 1986;104:7.

PROSTATITIS

Bacteria may reach the prostate from the bloodstream (eg, tuberculosis) or from the urethra. Prostatitis is thus commonly associated with urethritis (eg, gonococcal, chlamydial, mycoplasmal) or with active bacterial infection of the lower urinary tract. Perineal pain, lumbosacral backache, fever, dysuria, and frequency may be symptoms of acute prostatic infection.

Prostatitis is more often chronic. Symptoms are less impressive, and specific bacterial pathogens are seldom isolated from prostatic secretions.

Clinical Findings

A. Symptoms and Signs: These include perineal pain, fever, dysuria, frequency, and urethral discharge. In acute prostatitis, the prostate feels enlarged, boggy, and very tender; fluctuation occurs only if an abscess has formed. Even gentle palpation of the prostate may express copious purulent discharge.

In chronic prostatitis there may be dull lumbosacral and perineal pain, mild dysuria and frequency, and scanty urethral discharge. Palpation reveals a symmetrically enlarged, boggy, and slightly tender prostate.

B. Laboratory Findings: With acute febrile prostatitis, there is often leukocytosis. The expressed prostatic fluid shows pus cells and bacteria on microscopy and culture. During the acute phase, prostatic palpation may express pus. In acute and chronic prostatitis, the first glass of urine contains a far larger number of white cells than do subsequent urine samples.

Differential Diagnosis

Prostatitis should be differentiated from lower urinary tract infection, although it may form part of it. In the latter case, the infected prostate may serve as a source of recurrent lower urinary tract infections. Perirectal infections may be considered, as well as epididymitis, gonococcal infection, and tuberculosis.

Complications

Epididymitis and cystitis as well as urethritis commonly accompany acute prostatitis. Chronic prostatitis commonly predisposes to recurrent urinary tract infection and occasionally to urethral obstruction and acute urinary retention.

Treatment

A. Specific Measures: For acute prostatitis, initial treatment may consist of sulfamethoxazole, 400 mg, plus trimethoprim, 80 mg, 6–8 tablets daily; tetracycline, 2 g daily by mouth; or ampicillin, 250 mg 6 times daily, until culture of prostatic fluid and susceptibility tests indicate the drug of choice. Treatment for 2 weeks usually abates the acute inflammation, but chronic prostatitis may continue.

Eradication of bacteria in chronically infected prostatic tissue is exceedingly difficult. Antimicrobial drugs diffusing best into prostatic acini must be lipid-soluble and basic (eg, trimethoprim-sulfamethoxazole). Erythromycins are quite active in the prostate but effective mainly against gram-positive organisms, which are rare in urinary tract infections and prostatitis. Conversely, most drugs that are active against gram-negative coliform bacteria (the commonest cause of prostatitis) fail to reach the prostatic acini.

B. General Measures: During the acute phase, the patient should be kept at rest, with good hydration, and kept comfortable by means of analgesics, stool softeners, and sitz baths. Urethral instrumentation and prostatic massage must be avoided. Surgical drainage of an abscess is mandatory.

Chronic prostatitis should be treated by prolonged antimicrobial therapy accompanied by vigorous prostatic massage once weekly to promote drainage. Transurethral prostatectomy offers uncertain benefits.

Prognosis

Although the symptoms of acute prostatitis will usually subside with treatment, the prospects for the eventual elimination of chronic prostatitis are often discouraging.

Krieger JN: Prostatitis syndromes: Pathophysiology, differential diagnosis, and treatment. Sex Transm Dis 1984; 11:100.

URINARY STONES

Urinary stones and calcification in the kidney may be associated with metabolic disease; may be secondary to infection in the urinary tract; may occur in sponge kidney, tuberculosis of the kidney, or papillary necrosis; or may be idiopathic. The incidence of urinary tract calculus is higher in men.

NEPHROCALCINOSIS

Chronic hypercalciuria and hyperphosphaturia may result in precipitation of calcium salts in the renal parenchyma (nephrocalcinosis). The commonest causes are hyperparathyroidism, hypervitaminosis D (particularly with associated high calcium intake), and excess calcium and alkali intake. Chronic interstitial nephritis predisposes to nephrocalcinosis. Other causes include acute osteoporosis following immobilization, sarcoidosis, renal tubular acidosis, the de Toni-Fanconi syndrome, and destruction of bone by metastatic carcinoma.

The symptoms, signs, and laboratory findings are those of the primary disease. The diagnosis is usually established by x-ray demonstration of calcium deposits in the kidney, which appear as minute calcific densities with linear streaks in the region of the renal papillae. True renal stones may be present as well in these patients.

Specific treatment is directed at the primary disorder. Particular attention is directed to treatment of urinary tract infection and renal insufficiency. When renal tubular acidosis or the de Toni-Fanconi defect is present, it is essential to maintain a high fluid intake, to replace cation deficit, and to alkalinize the urine with sodium bicarbonate. See Renal Tubular Acidosis, above.

RENAL STONE

Essentials of Diagnosis

- May be asymptomatic.
- Symptoms of obstruction of calix or ureteropelvic junction, with flank pain and colic.
- Nausea, vomiting, abdominal distention.
- Hematuria.
- Chills and fever and bladder irritability if infection is present.

Etiology

A. Excessive Excretion of Relatively Insoluble Urinary Constituents:

    1. Calcium–

        a. Hypercalciuria with normocalcemia.

(1) Idiopathic hypercalciuria (30–40% of stone formers).

(2) Renal tubular acidosis, type I; distal tubule deficit.

b. Hypercalciuria with hypercalcemia or normocalcemia.

(1) Primary hyperparathyroidism (see Chapter 20). (Five to 7 percent of stone formers.)

(2) High vitamin D intake.

(3) Renal tubular acidosis, type I.

(4) Excessive intake of milk and alkali.

(5) Destructive bone disease due to neoplasm or of metabolic origin (corticosteroid excess, thyrotoxicosis).

(6) Sarcoidosis.

(7) Prolonged immobilization.

2. Oxalate–Over half of urinary stones are composed of calcium oxalate or calcium oxalate mixed with phosphate.

a. Idiopathic (the majority).

b. Congenital or familial oxaluria (rare).

c. Ileal disease; ileal resection or bypass.

d. High oxalate intake (tea, cocoa, spinach, beets, rhubarb, parsley, nuts). Vitamin C is an oxalate precursor.

e. Methoxyflurane anesthesia.

3. Uric acid–

a. Gout–Stones may form spontaneously or as a result of treatment with uricosuric agents.

b. Hyperuricosuria with or without hyperuricemia. Idiopathic or secondary to high purine intake (see ¶C, below).

c. Anticancer therapy with agents that cause rapid destruction of cells, resulting in increased excretion of uric acid.

d. Myeloproliferative disease (leukemia, lymphoma, myeloid metaplasia, etc).

4. Cystine–Hereditary cystinuria.

B. Physical Changes in the Urine:

1. Increased concentration of urine solute as a consequence of low intake of fluid and low urine volume.

2. Urinary pH–

a. Low pH–Organic substances less soluble (uric acid, cystine).

b. High pH–Inorganic salts usually less soluble (calcium phosphate and mixed calcium phosphate-calcium oxalate stones).

c. High pH associated with urinary tract infection with organisms containing urease (especially *Proteus*)–Hydrolysis of urea yields ammonia, which produces an increase in pH. $Mg^+ + NH_4^+ + PO_4^{3+}$ precipitates as magnesium ammonium phosphate (**struvite**) to form stones.

C. Nucleus (Nidus) for Stone Formation:

1. Uricosuria-Crystals of uric acid or sodium hydrogen urate may initiate precipitation of calcium oxalate from solution.

2. Bits of necrotic tissue, blood clots, and clumps of bacteria, particularly in the presence of stasis or infection, may serve as a nucleus for stone formation.

D. Congenital or Acquired Deformities of the Kidneys:

1. Sponge kidney.

2. Horseshoe kidney.

3. Local caliceal obstruction or defect.

General Considerations

The location and size of the stone and the presence or absence of obstruction determine the changes that occur in the kidney and caliceal system. The pathologic changes may be modified by ischemia due to pressure or by infection.

Clinical Findings

A. Symptoms and Signs: Often a stone trapped in a calix or in the renal pelvis is asymptomatic. If a stone produces obstruction in a calix or at the ureteropelvic junction, dull flank pain or even colic may occur. Hematuria and symptoms of accompanying infection may be present. Nausea and vomiting may suggest enteric disease. Flank tenderness and abdominal distention may be the only findings.

B. Laboratory Findings: Urinalysis is the most important laboratory test. In addition to gross or microscopic hematuria, the presence of pyuria suggests associated urinary tract infection. Crystals may provide a lead to the composition of the stone and the underlying metabolic disorder (hypercalciuria, gout, cystinuria, renal tubular acidosis, oxaluria). Chemical analysis of serum with a broad biochemical profile will assist in confirming the metabolic disorder. Always obtain a stone for analysis, and instruct the patient to strain the urine to retrieve any passed calculus for this purpose.

C. Imaging: A plain abdominal radiograph (kidney, ureter, and bladder) will assist in discovering symptomatic and asymptomatic radiopaque stones and related bone lesions (eg, hyperparathyroidism). If the stone has not passed within a day or 2 after the acute onset of symptoms, ultrasonography will usually define renal size and caliceal and ureteral dilatation above the site of obstruction. Radionuclide renography may reveal the presence of persistent obstruction. Excretory and retrograde urograms help to delineate the site and degree of obstruction and to confirm the presence of nonopaque stones (uric acid).

Differential Diagnosis

Renal stone may be confused with acute pyelonephritis, renal tumor, renal tuberculosis, and infarction of the kidney. In occasional cases, the symptoms may mimic those of acute abdomen.

Complications

Infection and hydronephrosis may destroy renal tissue.

Prevention of Further Stone Formation

Prevention of stone formation requires identification of the contributing metabolic defect and of the chemical composition of the stone. Appropriate therapy is directed toward correction or amelioration of the metabolic abnormality and toward favorably altering urine chemistry.

(1) Obtain a stone for analysis whenever possible. It is *essential* for diagnosis and therapy.

(2) Review the family history to identify metabolic causes (cystinuria, gout, hypercalcemia, renal tubular acidosis, hyperoxaluria).

(3) Treat predisposing diseases such as hyperparathyroidism, gout, cystinuria, renal tubular acidosis, infection, sarcoidosis, hypercortisolism, and hyperoxaluria and anatomic defects of the urinary tract.

(4) Instruct the patient to maintain a high fluid intake to produce a dilute urine, ie, urine volume of more than 2000 mL/d with a specific gravity less than 1.015.

(5) Maintain urine pH at a suitable level: (a) Above pH 6.5 for uric acid stones; above 7.5 for cystine stones: Use Shohl's solution (a mixture of sodium citrate and citric acid), 10–30 mL 5 times a day, ie, after each meal, at bedtime, and during the night. (b) Below pH 6.5 for struvite stones: There is no practical long-term therapy that will not produce metabolic acidosis. For a brief trial, one may use ascorbic acid, 3 g/d or more, or methionine, 8–12 g/d.

(6) If hyperuricosuria is present in those who form calcium stones, allopurinol, 100 mg twice a day, plus restriction of intake of purine-containing foods will often reduce stone formation.

(7) If idiopathic hypercalciuria is present, the patient should reduce calcium intake by avoiding milk and milk products, calcium-containing medications, and vitamin D-fortified foods. A high fluid intake is essential. Several regimens are available for chronic prophylaxis: (a) Chronic use of thiazide diuretics (hydrochlorothiazide, 50 mg once or twice daily, or equivalent) plus modest restriction of salt intake will reduce calcium excretion and may enhance excretion of magnesium, which has an inhibitory effect on stone formation. The effectiveness of thiazides tends to diminish, and hypercalciuria may return. (b) Thiazides may not be effective because they reduce citrate excretion in the urine. Citrate inhibits calcium stone formation by complexing with calcium, thus reducing its concentration, and by directly inhibiting crystal growth. The addition of potassium citrate, 10–20 meq 3 times daily by mouth, appears to be effective. (c) Inorganic orthophosphate has proved beneficial when used alone or with thiazides. Combinations of dibasic and monobasic phosphate salts of sodium and potas-

sium provide a mix of neutral pH. Most formulations provide 250 mg of phosphorus per capsule or tablet. Give in divided doses 3 or 4 times a day to provide a total of 1250–1500 mg of phosphorus per day. (d) Cellulose phosphate chelates cations and may be used to reduce intestinal absorption of calcium. When used, it should be accompanied by a low-calcium diet and magnesium supplementation. (e) Magnesium inhibits calcium stone formation. It may be supplied as magnesium oxide in doses that will not produce diarrhea.

(8) If stones consist of **calcium oxalate,** a reduction of oxalate intake is in order. Cocoa, tea, rhubarb, spinach, Swiss chard, beets, parsley, nuts, and excess vitamin C should be avoided. Check for elevated excretion of uric acid or calcium.

(9) Treat patients who are "idiopathic calcium stone formers" according to paragraphs 7 and 8 above.

(10) In the presence of urinary tract infection with urease-containing organisms, suppression of struvite stone formation is difficult. Infection must be eradicated or reduced with appropriate antibiotics.

(11) Prevention of **uric acid stones** by inhibiting the formation of uric acid is possible by blocking the conversion of xanthine to uric acid with the xanthine oxidase inhibitor allopurinol. " . . . xanthine oxidase inhibitor allopurinol, starting with 100 mg/d and increasing as necessary to 200–300 mg/d or even 400–600 mg/d. This will reduce elevated serum uric acid to normal levels and markedly reduce the excretion of uric acid. It is effective even in the presence of renal failure associated with gouty nephropathy, though in such cases the dosage must be reduced commensurate with creatinine clearance. The drug is well tolerated and apparently produces no alteration of renal function. Allopurinol may be used in association with antileukemia and anticancer agents. While the allopurinol effect is developing, treatment should include a high fluid intake and alkalinization of the urine with sodium bicarbonate, 10–12 g/d in divided doses, or Shohl's solution, 50–150 mL/d.

(12) **Cystine stone** formation can be reduced by forcing fluids to produce a urine output of 3–4 L daily and alkalinizing the urine with sodium bicarbonate or sodium citrate and acetazolamide at bedtime. Urine pH should be maintained at 7.5 or higher, at which levels cystine solubility is greatly increased. A low-methionine diet may help, but protein deprivation must be avoided. Patients with severe cystinuria may require penicillamine, which complexes cystine and reduces the total excretion of cystine. There are many side effects of penicillamine that appear to be dose-related.

Treatment

Small stones may be passed. They do no harm if infection is not present. Larger stones may be removed by percutaneous nephrostomy plus mechanical, ultrasonic, or extracorporeal shock-wave lithotripsy to permit easy removal of the debris. Lithotripsy may be employed to shatter stones, fragments of which will be excreted. Indications for percutaneous lithotripsy are being refined, but it is not used for staghorn stones or for multiple stones. Surgical removal may be required. Nephrectomy may be necessary.

Prognosis

If obstruction can be prevented and infection eradicated, the prognosis is good.

URETERAL STONE

Essentials of Diagnosis

- Obstruction of ureter produces severe colic with radiation of pain to regions determined by the position of the stone in the ureter.
- Gastrointestinal symptoms common.
- Urine usually contains fresh red cells.
- May be asymptomatic.
- Exacerbations of infection when obstruction occurs.

General Considerations

Ureteral stones are formed in the kidney but produce symptoms as they pass down the ureter.

Clinical Findings

A. Symptoms and Signs: The pain of ureteral colic is intense. The patient may be in mild shock, with cold, moist skin. There is marked tenderness in the costovertebral angle. Abdominal and back muscle spasm may be present. Referred areas of hyperesthesia may be demonstrated.

B. Laboratory Findings: As for renal stone.

C. Imaging and Instrumental Examination: Radiographs may show the stone lodged in the ureter or at the ureterovesical junction. Nonopaque stones can be demonstrated by radionuclide renography, ultrasonography, or excretory urograms, which reveal the site of obstruction and the dilated ureteropelvic system above it. Because of the danger of infection, cystoscopy and ureteral catheterization should be avoided unless retrograde urography is essential.

Differential Diagnosis

Ureteral stones require differentiation from clots due to hemorrhage, from tumor, and from acute pyelonephritis as well as acute cholecystitis and other causes of acute surgical abdomen.

Prevention

Proceed as for renal stone. Every effort should be made to obtain a stone for analysis.

Treatment

A. Specific Measures: Most stones will pass spontaneously. By a cystoscopic or percutaneous approach, removal of stones may be accomplished with baskets or by ultrasound lithotripsy. Extracorporeal shock-wave lithotripsy is effective in many instances. Surgical ureterolithotomy may be necessary.

B. General Measures: Morphine or other opiates should be given in doses adequate to control pain. Morphine sulfate, 8 mg (or equivalent dosage of other drugs), may be given intravenously and repeated in 5–10 minutes if necessary. Thereafter, subcutaneous administration is usually adequate. Atropine sulfate, 0.8 mg subcutaneously, or methantheline bromide, 0.1 g intravenously, may be used as an antispasmodic.

Prognosis

If obstruction and infection can be treated successfully, the outlook is excellent.

VESICAL STONE

Essentials of Diagnosis

- Bladder irritability, with dysuria, urgency, and frequency.
- Interruption of urinary stream as stone occludes urethra.
- Hematuria and pyuria.
- Benign prostatic hypertrophy is frequently present in men.

General Considerations

Vesical stones occur most commonly when there is residual urine infected with urea-splitting organisms (eg, *Proteus,* staphylococci). Thus, bladder stones are associated with urinary stasis due to bladder neck or urethral obstruction, diverticula, neurogenic bladder, and cystocele. Foreign bodies in the bladder act as foci for stone formation. Ulceration and bladder inflammation predispose to stone formation.

Most vesical stones are composed of magnesium ammonium phosphate (struvite), calcium phosphate, or calcium oxalate. Uric acid stones are common in the presence of an enlarged prostate and uninfected urine.

Clinical Findings

A. Symptoms and Signs: Symptoms of chronic urinary obstruction or stasis and infection are usually present. Dysuria, frequency and urgency, and interruption of the urinary stream (causing pain in the penis) when the stone occludes the urethra are common complaints. Physical findings include prostatic enlargement, evidence of distended (neurogenic) bladder, and cystocele. The stone may be palpable.

B. Laboratory Findings: The urine usually shows signs of infection and contains red cells.

C. Imaging and Cystoscopic Examination:

Radiographic examination shows the calcified stone, and urograms show the bladder abnormalities and upper urinary tract dilatation due to long-standing back pressure. Direct cystoscopic examination may be necessary.

Treatment & Prognosis

Stones can be removed by fragmentation using ultrasound, mechanical, or shock-wave lithotripsy. Surgical lithotomy may be necessary.

Urethral obstruction, cystocele, and other contributing anatomic factors must be eliminated by appropriate surgery.

Infection must be eliminated, usually by administration of an appropriate bactericidal antibiotic for 2–4 weeks to render the urine sterile.

Coe FL, Parks JH: Pathophysiology of kidney stones and strategies for treatment. Hosp Pract (March 15) 1988; 23:185.

Pak CYC et al: Correction of hypocitraturia and prevention of stone formation by combined thiazide and potassium citrate therapy in thiazide-unresponsive hypercalciuric nephrolithiasis. Am J Med 1985;99:284.

Tanagho EA, McAninch JW: *Smith's General Urology,* 12th ed. Appleton & Lange, 1988.

Uribarri J, Oh MS, Carroll HJ: The first kidney stone. Ann Intern Med 1989;111:1006. (Cost-saving advice.)

OBSTRUCTIVE UROPATHY

Obstruction of the urinary tract can result in serious damage to the kidneys; early detection and treatment are required to prevent irreversible function and anatomic damage. The site and degree of obstruction, the duration of obstruction, and the complication of urinary tract infection determine the presenting manifestations.

Etiology & Pathogenesis

Obstructive uropathy is the result of (1) congenital anatomic abnormalities (eg, ureteropelvic, ureterovesical, or urethral stricture); (2) stone, tumor, or clot that obstructs a ureter or the bladder neck; (3) extrinsic tumors, bands, or fibrosis; or (4) neuromuscular disorder related to the spinal cord or peripheral nerve lesions.

Complete obstruction to the flow of urine produces increase in pressure in the ureters and in the renal pelvis, which then become dilated. Renal papillae become flattened, the renal tubules dilate, and glomerular filtration is impeded. Functional impairment of tubule function affects the excretion of solute, the reabsorption of sodium, and the secretion of hydrogen ion. Renal blood flow is reduced. Destruction

of the kidney results within a few weeks. Partial obstruction produces lesser impairment of renal function.

Clinical Findings

A. Symptoms and Signs: The site of obstruction and rapidity of onset determine the presentation. Chronic or low-grade obstruction is usually asymptomatic. Acute and complete obstruction of a ureter will produce pain in the flank or groin associated with distention of the renal capsule or ureteral colic. Acute obstruction of the urethra by an enlarged prostate, postoperative bladder dysfunction, or stone will produce painful distention of the bladder. (See below for discussion of prostatic hyperplasia.) Chronic urethral obstruction may result in a distended bladder with "overflow" dribbling. If a neurologic lesion is the cause of bladder dysfunction, there may be overflow dribbling from a distended bladder, involuntary voiding, and frequency with incomplete emptying of the bladder.

The history and physical examination should be directed at excluding circulatory or intrinsic renal disease as causes of oliguria. The history should focus on recurrent urinary tract infection, symptoms of incomplete lower urinary tract obstruction (nocturia, hesitancy, urgency, incontinence), evidence of diabetes mellitus, use of anticholinergic drugs, stone disease, and neurologic disease. In some patients, the only symptoms may be those of renal failure. The presence of extrinsic tumor, an enlarged prostate, or neurologic disease should be evident on examination. However, the size of the prostate on examination may not correlate with bladder neck obstruction.

B. Laboratory Findings: Bacteriuria and leukocytes in the urine signify accompanying infection. Lower urinary tract obstruction results in elevated BUN and creatinine and, if renal impairment is severe, increased serum K^+, phosphate, and uric acid.

C. Special Examinations: Ultrasound imaging will reveal dilatation of the renal pelvis, ureters, and bladder and help to distinguish unilateral ureteral obstruction from lower tract obstruction. Cystoscopy and retrograde urography may be indicated.

Treatment

Relief of obstruction is urgent. Urethral obstruction can be relieved by catheterization. An indwelling urethral or suprapubic catheter may be required. Operation may be necessary to relieve ureteral obstruction, remove a stone, place nephrostomy tubes or ureteral stents, and relieve urethral obstruction (prostatic resection). Vigorous treatment of infection is imperative. Urologic or surgical consultation should be sought as needed. Treatment of neurogenic bladder is a complex subject that goes beyond the scope of this chapter.

Postobstructive diuresis is usually limited, but

losses may continue beyond elimination of retained fluid and require aggressive replacement of water and electrolyte.

Klahr S: Pathophysiology of obstructive nephropathy. Kidney Int 1983;23:414.

URETERAL OBSTRUCTION

Obstruction of one or both ureters may be due to a variety of acquired diseases, including injury to ureters during pelvic surgery; postirradiation fibrosis; compression by extrinsic neoplastic disease; occlusion of the ureterovesical junction by cancer of the bladder, prostate, uterine cervix, or rectum; endometriosis; chronic infections of the urinary tract; retroperitoneal fibrosis; ureteral stone; chronic vesical outlet obstruction from prostatic hyperplasia or cancer, urethral stricture, or vesical stone.

Although rare, **retroperitoneal fibrosis** warrants further discussion. Chronic inflammatory disease of retroperitoneal tissues over the lower lumbar vertebrae may compress one or both ureters, with consequent dilatation of the ureter and renal pelvis proximal to the site of obstruction. The vena cava and, occasionally, the aorta or other major arteries in the area may be occluded. Rarely, extension upward may extend to the mediastinum.

The reaction occurs in some patients taking methysergide for migraine or beta-blocker drugs (propranolol, atenolol, oxprenolol) for the usual indications. Retroperitoneal fibrosis may accompany sclerosing Hodgkin's disease. Lymphomas and spread of metastatic tumor retroperitoneally may simulate the disease by occluding the ureters and great vessels.

Symptoms and signs include low back pain, abdominal pain, anorexia, weight loss, fever, urinary frequency, and, depending on the degree of renal insufficiency, polyuria or anuria. Occlusion of arteries trapped in the fibrotic reaction can produce claudication and weakness of the legs and impotence. A mass is often palpable over the promontory of the sacrum.

Laboratory findings are those of impaired renal function secondary to chronic obstruction, with elevated blood urea nitrogen and serum creatinine, metabolic acidosis, and anemia (see Chronic Renal Insufficiency). Excretory urograms show medial deviation of the ureters and dilatation of the excretory tract proximal to the obstruction.

Therapy includes abstaining from the offending drug and a trial of corticosteroid. Give prednisone, 30–60 mg/d orally, until evidence of improvement permits reduction to a maintenance dose of 5–15 mg/d. Operation may be required to relieve ureteral obstruction.

TESTICULAR DISEASE

EPIDIDYMITIS

Acute epididymitis is caused by bacterial infection ascending from the urethra or prostate. In older men, it usually follows urinary tract obstruction and infection or instrumentation of the lower genitourinary tract.

Sudden pain in the scrotum, rapid unilateral scrotal enlargement, and marked tenderness of the testes, spermatic cord, and groin are the characteristic manifestations. Secondary orchitis with a swollen, painful testicle may occur. Elevation of the scrotum provides some relief.

Laboratory findings include leukocytosis, pyuria, and bacteriuria. Urine culture will usually demonstrate the organism—frequently *E coli* in men over age 35. A sterile urine culture strongly suggests chlamydial infection, which can be identified in the laboratory. Ultrasound examination often can differentiate a swollen epididymis from testicular tumor.

Bed rest and elevation and support of the scrotum provide symptomatic relief. Nonsteroidal analgesics may be useful. If chlamydial infection is the likely cause, give tetracycline. Appropriate antibiotics should be used for identified bacteria. Trimethoprim-sulfamethoxazole, ampicillin, or a cephalosporin may be employed for men over 35 years of age, in whom *E coli* is the most frequent organism.

Berger RE: Urethritis and epididymitis. Semin Urol 1983; 1:139.

ORCHITIS

Acute orchitis is usually due to mumps and occurs during the years just following adolescence. It is most often unilateral but may be bilateral. Mumps may produce acute oophoritis as well.

Chronic orchitis may be due to syphilis, tuberculosis, leprosy, filariasis, and schistosomiasis haematobia. Destruction of the testis obliterates production of spermatozoa but usually leaves some hormonal cell function.

Meares EM Jr: Nonspecific infections of the urinary tract. In: *Smith's General Urology*, 12th ed. Tanagho EA, McAninch JW (editors). Appleton & Lange, 1988.

TESTICULAR TORSION

Testicular torsion (torsion of the spermatic cord) is most common in adolescent males and young men under age 25. An anomaly of the tunica vaginalis or of the relationship of the epididymis to the testis is usually present.

The characteristic presentation is with a sudden onset of unabating pain in the scrotum, groin, or lower abdomen, made worse by elevation of the scrotum. The testis is swollen, tender, and retracted.

Testicular torsion must be differentiated from epididymitis, orchitis, and trauma to the testis. A technetium 99m Tc pertechnetate scan will demonstrate decreased blood flow with torsion and increased blood flow with epididymitis. Ultrasound examination of the testes may be helpful.

Treatment consists of immediate surgery to remove the infarcted testis. Orchiopexy of the other testis is desirable because of the high incidence of the bilateral anatomic abnormality associated with torsion.

Lee LM, Wright JE, McLoughlin MG: Testicular torsion in the adult. J Urol 1983;130:93.

TUMORS OF THE GENITOURINARY TRACT

ADENOCARCINOMA OF KIDNEY
(Renal Cell Carcinoma, Hypernephroma)

Essentials of Diagnosis
- Gross hematuria with or without flank pain.
- Fever.
- Enlarged kidney may be palpable.

General Considerations

The commonest malignant tumor of the kidney in adults is renal cell carcinoma, which constitutes 6% of all cancers. It rarely occurs before age 35 and more commonly appears after age 50, more commonly in men than in women. This tumor metastasizes early to the lungs, liver, and long bones.

Adenocarcinoma of the kidney apparently arises from renal tubule cells or adenomas. It invades blood vessels early. On microscopic examination, the cells resemble renal tubule cells arranged in cords and varying patterns.

Clinical Findings

A. Symptoms and Signs: Gross hematuria is the most frequent sign. Fever is often the only symptom. A flank mass may be palpable. Pain of renal or ureteral origin may occur with bleeding into the tumor or renal pelvis. Vena caval occlusion may produce characteristic patterns of collateral circulation and edema of the legs.

A hypernephroma may not produce classic symptoms of renal tumor. It may produce symptoms and signs suggesting a wide variety of processes: fever of obscure origin, leukemoid reaction, refractory anemia, erythrocytosis, hypercalcemia, hypoglycemia, peripheral neuropathy, and increased production of gonadotropins and prostaglandins.

B. Laboratory Findings: Polycythemia occasionally develops as a result of increased secretion of erythropoietin by the tumor. Anemia is more commonly found. Hematuria is almost always present, but it may be intermittent or microscopic. Alkaline phosphatase may be elevated in the absence of hepatic metastases. Urinary cytologic examination may aid in diagnosis. The erythrocyte sedimentation rate is increased.

C. Imaging: Ultrasound imaging can define the size and contour of the kidneys. Cysts can often be differentiated from solid tumors. The presence of tumor in the renal vein and vena cava can often be demonstrated. With visualization by real-time ultrasound scan, an experienced operator may perform "thin-needle" biopsy of the renal mass.

Radiographic examination may show an enlarged kidney. Metastatic lesions of bone and lung may be revealed. Excretory or retrograde urograms, as well as angiograms, may be necessary to establish the presence of a renal tumor. CT scans with contrast medium may help differentiate renal cyst or anomaly from tumor, define tumor size and consistency, and document any extension of tumor into the renal vein and vena cava and lymph node and liver metastases. MRI is likely to be the test of choice for diagnosis and staging.

Differential Diagnosis

The differential diagnosis includes hydronephrosis, polycystic kidneys, renal tuberculosis, renal calculi, and renal infarction. The most challenging problem is to distinguish benign renal cyst from carcinoma; aspiration of the lesion may be necessary.

Treatment

Nephrectomy is indicated if no metastases are present. Even when metastases are present, nephrectomy may be indicated for intractable bleeding or pain.

X-ray irradiation of metastases may be of value, although the lesions are usually fairly radioresistant. Isolated single pulmonary metastases can occasionally be removed surgically. At present, chemotherapy is ineffective. Palliation may be achieved with medroxyprogesterone. Trials of alpha interferon and of interleukin-2 plus lymphokine-activated killer cells continue with some promise in spite of significant toxicity.

Prognosis

The course is variable. Some patients may not develop metastases for 10–15 years after removal of the primary tumor. About 35% of patients live more than 5 years.

Garnick MB, Richie JP: Renal neoplasia. Page 1533 in: *The Kidney*, 3rd ed. Brenner B, Rector F (editors). Saunders, 1986.

TUMORS OF THE RENAL PELVIS & URETER

Epithelial tumors of the renal pelvis and ureter are relatively rare. They are usually papillary and tend to metastasize along the urinary tract. Epidermoid tumors are highly malignant and metastasize early. Transitional cell tumors have occurred in cases of interstitial nephritis and papillary necrosis due to phenacetin abuse.

Painless hematuria is the most common complaint. Colic occurs with obstruction due to blood clot or tumor. Tenderness in the flank may be found. Anemia due to blood loss occurs. The urine contains red cells and clots; white cells and bacteria are present when infection is superimposed. Urography should reveal the filling defect in the pelvis or show obstruction and dilatation of the ureter. At cystoscopy, the bleeding from the involved ureter may be seen and satellite tumors identified. Exfoliative cytologic studies should be done.

Radical removal of the kidney, the involved ureter, and the periureteral portion of the bladder should be done unless metastases are extensive.

Irradiation of metastases is usually of little value.

The prognosis depends upon the type of tumor. With anaplastic neoplasms, death usually occurs within 5 years.

TUMORS OF THE BLADDER

Essentials of Diagnosis

- Hematuria, gross or microscopic.
- Malignant cells by urine cytology.
- Suprapubic pain and bladder symptoms associated with infection.
- Visualization of tumor at cystoscopy.

General Considerations

Bladder cancer is the second most common urinary tract tumor. It is 3–4 times more common in men than in women. In men, the tumor occurs almost exclusively in the age group over 50, with a peak occurrence at age 60–70. Use of tobacco, exposure to aniline dyes, and schistosomiasis *(S haematobium)* are risk factors; excessive use of nonsteroidal analgesic drugs (especially phenacetin) may be implicated as well.

Cancers of the bladder may be superficial or invasive, and each type has a different course. The large majority are superficial, confined to the mucosa and submucosa, and rarely metastasize. About 20% of epithelial bladder tumors are invasive, and metastasis occurs frequently. Of the invasive tumors, almost all are transitional cell carcinomas of varying degrees of differentiation. Aggressiveness of the tumors correlates with rapid proliferation and aneuploidy.

Clinical Findings

A. Symptoms and Signs: Hematuria is the commonest symptom and may occur early in the course. Cystitis with frequency, urgency, and dysuria is a frequent complication. With encroachment of the tumor on the bladder neck, the urinary stream is diminished. Suprapubic pain occurs as the tumor extends beyond the bladder. Obstruction of the ureters produces hydronephrosis, frequently accompanied by renal infection, in which case the signs of urinary tract infection may be present. Physical examination is not notable. The bladder tumor may be palpable on bimanual (abdominorectal or abdominovaginal) examination.

B. Laboratory Findings: Anemia is common. The urine contains red cells, white cells, and bacteria. Exfoliative cytology is often confirmatory.

C. Imaging and Instrumental Examination: Excretory urography may reveal ureteral obstruction. Cystograms usually show the tumor. Cystoscopy and biopsy confirm the diagnosis. Ultrasonography, CT scanning, and MRI are helpful in diagnosis and staging.

Differential Diagnosis

Hematuria and pain can be produced by other tumors of the urinary tract, urinary calculi, renal tuberculosis, acute cystitis, or acute nephritis.

Treatment

A. Specific Measures: Tumor staging is required to serve as a guide to selection of treatment. Endoscopic transurethral resection of superficial and submucosal tumors can provide a cure in many cases. Cystectomy with ureterosigmoidostomy or another urinary diversion procedure is required for invasive tumors. Radiation therapy may be useful for more anaplastic tumors. Repeated instillation of either BCG, thiotepa, mitomycin, or doxorubicin may be effective in eradicating superficial and papillary bladder epithelial tumors. For metastatic disease, chemotherapy with methotrexate, vinblastine, cisplatin, and doxorubicin has produced remissions in 40% of patients, with long-term survival in about 20%.

B. General Measures: Urinary tract infection should be controlled with appropriate antibiotics. Anastomosis of ureters to an isolated loop of ileum or sigmoid colon, one end of which is brought to the skin to act as a conduit, is relatively free of renal complications and of alteration of body fluid electrolytes.

Prognosis

Superficial, noninvasive tumors can be satisfactorily controlled with bladder instillations of chemotherapeutic agents with or without transurethral excision. Invasive, aggressive cancer is difficult to treat, readily recurs and is rarely cured by any means. A 50% 5-year absence of overt disease is about the best that can be achieved.

Raghavan D et al: Biology and management of bladder cancer. N Engl J Med 1990;322:1129.

BENIGN PROSTATIC HYPERPLASIA

Essentials of Diagnosis

- Prostatism: hesitancy and straining to initiate micturition, reduced force and caliber of the urinary stream, nocturia.
- Acute urinary retention.
- Enlarged prostate.
- Uremia follows prolonged obstruction.

General Considerations

Hyperplasia of the prostatic lateral and subcervical lobes that are invaded by periurethral glands results in enlargement of the prostate and urethral obstruction.

Clinical Findings

A. Symptoms and Signs: The symptoms of prostatism increase in severity as the degree of urethral obstruction increases. Symptoms may be overlooked or not reported when the progression of obstruction is slow. On rectal examination, the prostate is usually found to be enlarged. The bladder may be seen and palpated as retention of urine increases. Infection commonly occurs with stasis and retention of "residual urine." Hematuria may occur. Uremia may result from prolonged back pressure and severe bilateral hydronephrosis. Determination of blood urea nitrogen may provide the only clue to slowly advancing and relatively asymptomatic obstructive disease. Residual urine can be measured by postvoiding catheterization or estimated by ultrasonography. In the presence of prostatism, ganglionic blocking agents and parasympatholytic drugs used in the treatment of hypertension, as well as tranquilizers, weaken the power of detrusor contraction, thus causing symptoms simulating vesical neck obstruction and in some cases urinary retention.

B. Imaging and Cystoscopic Examination: Ultrasound and excretory urograms reveal the complications of back pressure: ureteral dilatation, hydronephrosis, and postvoiding urinary retention. Cystoscopy will reveal enlargement of the prostate and secondary bladder wall changes such as trabeculation, diverticula, inflammation due to infection, and vesical stone.

Differential Diagnosis

Other causes of urethral obstruction include urethral stricture, vesical stone, bladder tumor, neurogenic bladder, and carcinoma of the prostate.

Treatment

A. Specific Measures: Conservative (nonsurgical) management should be undertaken only in collaboration with a urologist. Acute urinary retention is relieved by catheterization, and catheter drainage is maintained if the degree of obstruction is severe. Surgery is usually necessary. There are various indications for each of the 4 approaches: treatment by transurethral resection or by suprapubic, retropubic, or perineal prostatectomy. Occasionally, partial obstruction may be ameliorated by empirical therapy with trimethoprim-sulfamethoxazole, which relieves the commonly associated chronic prostatitis.

B. General Measures: Treat infection of the urinary tract with appropriate antibiotics. The patient who develops postobstructive diuresis must be sustained with appropriate water and electrolyte replacement.

Prognosis

Surgical resection will relieve symptoms. The surgical mortality rate is low.

Johnson DE, Swanson DA, von Eschenbach AC: Tumors of the genitourinary tract. Pages 330–434 in: *Smith's General Urology,* 12th ed. Tanagho EA, McAninch JW (editors). Appleton & Lange, 1988.

Roos NP et al: Mortality and reoperation after open and transurethral resection of the prostate for benign prostatic hyperplasia. N Engl J Med 1989;320:1120. (An evaluation of alternative surgical interventions.)

Walsh PC: Benign prostatic hyperplasia. In: *Campbell's Urology.* Walsh PC et al (editors). Saunders, 1985.

CARCINOMA OF THE PROSTATE

Essentials of Diagnosis

- Prostatism.
- Hard, irregular prostate.
- Often asymptomatic.
- Elevated serum acid phosphatase signifies extension of cancer beyond capsule.

General Considerations

Carcinoma of the prostate is rare before age 50. It is found more frequently with advancing age and is exceeded only by cancers of the lung and colon as a cause of death in older men. At autopsy, the incidence of asymptomatic carcinoma of the prostate is as high as 60% in men aged 80–90 and 100% in men over 90.

Clinical Findings

A. Symptoms and Signs: The disease is often asymptomatic, even when it has extended beyond the prostate. It may be discovered on physical examination, during examination of tissue obtained in the course of transurethral resection, or at autopsy. Symptoms are those of urethral obstruction (frequency, urgency, difficulty in voiding, urinary retention) or of pain associated with metastases to bone (pelvis, vertebrae, pathologic fracture). On rectal examination, there may be no evidence of tumor. When the lesion is large enough, the prostate is hard, nodular, and irregular; extension of cancer into the seminal vesicles may be evident. Scrotal edema may occur with extension of cancer to regional lymph nodes.

B. Laboratory Findings: Anemia may be present because of replacement of bone marrow by tumor. Serum prostatic acid phosphatase is often elevated when disease extends beyond the prostate and may be used to monitor progress of the disease and response to treatment. Prostate-specific antigen (from the cytoplasm of acinar and ductal epithelium) shows promise as a marker of prostatic cancer but not as a diagnostic tool. Hypercalcemia is a serious complication of bone metastases. Biopsy of the prostate is easily accomplished via a perineal or rectal approach using a core biopsy needle or thin needle directed by sonography or digital examination.

C. Imaging: There is no highly sensitive modality for discovery of carcinoma confined to the prostate. Sonography with a rectal transducer, CT scan, or MRI may identify the lesion, but negative results are not reliable. Sonography is useful for detection of spread to the bladder or seminal vesicles. The presence of metastases to bone is better assessed by radionuclide scan, but a positive scan should be confirmed by x-ray. Radionuclide scans are useful for following the course of the disease in bone, which is typically osteoblastic. Sonography is useful in assessing the presence and severity of lower urinary tract obstruction. Lymphangiography may be employed to determine the presence of metastases in regional lymph nodes but has been reliable in only a few centers; CT scan and MRI may be helpful for this purpose.

Treatment

Grading the cancer and staging its extent are essential for selecting treatment and providing a prognosis. Degree of malignancy is often graded by the Gleason scale (which combines predominant and less characteristic histologic grades to yield an overall score of 2 (well-differentiated) to 10 (poorly differentiated). Staging includes an estimate of the size of the tumor, its confinement within the capsule of the gland (A_1A_2 and B_1B_2), extension beyond the capsule (C_1) and involving the seminal vesicles (C_2), or metastatic disease in regional lymph nodes (D_1) and in bone or other organs (D_2). Surgery may be necessary to assess the presence of disease in regional lymph nodes if imaging procedures are inconclusive.

Treatment for stage A (focal cancer) is usually deferred unless the tumor is highly malignant. For stage A_2 (diffuse cancer within the gland), observation may be in order or treatment as for stage B. For stage B, radical prostatectomy, interstitial irradiation with implantation of ^{125}I seeds, or external beam irradiation may be employed. Stage C is usually treated with external beam irradiation or radical prostatectomy; the latter is losing favor. Stage D is treated with measures designed to reduce androgen secretion. Diethylstilbestrol (DES), 1–3 mg daily, or orchiectomy is most often used. Analogues of luteinizing hormone-releasing hormone (LHRH) used chronically will suppress LH and serum testosterone, and this treatment is associated with fewer side effects than DES. LHRH must be injected, however, and is more expensive than DES. Flutamide, an antiandrogen, may be added to therapy with LHRH in an effort to block all androgen influence. Chemotherapy is reserved for patients who fail to respond to hormone therapy. Palliation for advancing uncontrollable disease requires judicious use of analgesics and irradiation of local lesions. Stage D disease is not treated unless the patient is symptomatic.

Prognosis

Recent 5-year survival rates are as follows: stage A, 85%; stage B, 77%; stage C, 65%; stage D, 29%. These are slightly improved over those of the previous decade.

Donohue JP (editor): Controversies in urologic oncology. (Symposium.) Urol Clin North Am 1987;14:657.) (Entire issue.))

Gibbons RP: Prostate cancer: Chemotherapy. Cancer 1987;60(3 Suppl):586.

Gittes RF: Prostate-specific antigen. (Editorial.) N Engl J Med 1987;317:954.

Huben RP, Murphy GP: Prostate cancer: An update. CA 1986;36:274. (Excellent review.)

Labrie F et al: Benefits of combination therapy with flutamide in patients relapsing after castration. Brit J Urol 1988;61:341.

Stamey TA et al: Prostate-specific antigen as a serum marker for adenocarcinoma of the prostate. N Engl J Med 1987;317:909.

TUMORS OF THE TESTIS
(See also Chapter 20.)

Essentials of Diagnosis

- Painless enlargement of the testis.
- Mass does not transilluminate.
- Evidence of metastases.

General Considerations

The incidence of testicular tumors is about 0.5%

of all types of cancer in males. Tumors occur most frequently between ages 18 and 35 and are often malignant. The incidence of malignancy in an undescended testis is 30–50 times that in the normally positioned gonad. Classification of tumors of the testes is based upon their origin from germinal components or from nongerminal cells. The most common are the germinal tumors: seminomas; embryonal tumors, including embryoma, choriocarcinoma, embryonal carcinoma, teratocarcinoma, and adult teratoma; and the gonadoblastomas of intersexes. Nongerminal tumors include those of interstitial cell, Sertoli cell, and stromal origin. Rarely, lymphomas, leukemias, plasmacytomas, and metastatic carcinoma may involve the testis.

Seminomas, the most common testicular tumors, tend to spread slowly via the lymphatics to the iliac and periaortic nodes and disseminate late. Embryonal tumors invade the spermatic cord and metastasize early, particularly to the lungs. Seminomas are usually radiosensitive; embryonal tumors are usually radioresistant but sensitive to chemotherapy, as is choriocarcinoma also.

Gynecomastia may be associated with testicular tumors. Interstitial cell tumors, which occur at any age and are rarely malignant, are occasionally associated with gynecomastia and with sexual precocity and virilization.

Clinical Findings

A. Symptoms and Signs: Painless enlargement of the testis is typical. The enlarged testis may produce a dragging inguinal pain. The tumor is usually symmetric and firm, and pressure does not produce the typical testicular pain. The tumor does not transilluminate. Attachment to the scrotal skin is rare. Gynecomastia may be present. Virilization may occur in preadolescent boys with Leydig cell tumors. Hydrocele may develop.

Metastases commonly go to regional lymph nodes and then to those of the mediastinum and supraclavicular region. The lungs and the liver are often sites of metastases.

B. Laboratory Findings: Gonadotropins may be present in high concentrations in urine and plasma in cases of choriocarcinoma, and pregnancy tests are positive. Radioimmunoassay for the beta unit of human chorionic gonadotropin is the test of choice for diagnosis and follow-up assessment. Urinary 17-ke-

tosteroids are normal or low in Leydig cell tumors. Estrogens may be elaborated in both Sertoli cell and Leydig cell tumors. Alpha-fetoprotein is a useful tumor marker for diagnosis and assessment of the tumor burden of teratocarcinoma and embryonal carcinoma (derivatives of the extraembryonic primitive yolk sac).

C. Imaging: Tumors of the testicle are easily discerned with ultrasonography. Pulmonary metastases are demonstrated by chest radiographs. CT scans are used in staging to demonstrate intra-abdominal spread and enlarged iliac and periaortic lymph nodes. Displacement of ureters by enlarged lymph nodes can be demonstrated by use of urography or venacavograms.

Differential Diagnosis

Tuberculosis, syphilitic orchitis (gumma of the testicle), hydrocele, spermatocele, and tumors or granulomas of the epididymis may produce similar local manifestations.

Treatment

The testicle should be removed and the lumbar and inguinal nodes examined. Radical resection of iliac and lumbar nodes is usually indicated except for seminoma, which is radiosensitive. Radiation therapy is the treatment of choice following removal of the testis bearing a seminoma. Radiation therapy is employed following radical surgery for other malignant tumors. Chemotherapy is effective against all trophoblastic tumors. Metastatic disease may be curable with combination chemotherapy, including cisplatin, vinblastine, and bleomycin or etoposide plus cisplatin. Other drugs that may be effective in various combinations include vincristine, dactinomycin, doxorubicin, and cyclophosphamide.

Prognosis

Seminomas are least malignant, with 90% 5-year cures. With modern chemotherapeutic regimens, other cell types are increasingly effectively treated, resulting in cures of even widespread metastatic disease.

Einhorn LH: Cancer of the testis: A new paradigm. Hosp Pract (April 15) 1986;21:165. (Staging, therapy, and response to treatment.)
Hainsworth JD, Greco FA: Testicular germ cell neoplasms. Am J Med 1983;75:817.

REFERENCES

Abuelo JG: Renal failure caused by chemicals, foods, plants, animal venoms and misuse of drugs. Arch Intern Med 1990;150:505.

Brenner BM, Lazarus JM (editors): *Acute Renal Failure,* 2nd ed. Churchill Livingstone, 1987.
Brenner BM, Stein JH (editors): *The Kidney in Diabetes*

Mellitus. Churchill Livingstone, 1989.

Brenner BM, Rector FC Jr: *The Kidney*, 3rd ed. Saunders, 1986.

Heptinstall RH: *Pathology of the Kidney*, 3rd ed. Little, Brown, 1983.

Klahr S: Pathophysiology of obstructive nephropathy. Kidney Int 1983;23:414.

Massry SG, Glassock RJ (editors): *Textbook of Nephrology*. Williams & Wilkins, 1983.

Maxwell MH, Kleeman CR, Narins RG (editors): *Clinical Disorders of Fluid and Electrolyte Metabolism*, 4th ed. McGraw-Hill, 1987.

Mitch WE, Klahr S (editors): *Nutrition and the Kidney*. Little, Brown, 1988.

Schrier RW, Gottschalk CW: *Diseases of the Kidney*, 4th ed. Little, Brown, 1988.

Scriver CR et al (editors): *The Metabolic Basis of Inherited Disease*, 6th ed. McGraw-Hill, 1989.

Tanagho EA, McAninch JW: *Smith's General Urology*, 12th ed. Appleton & Lange, 1988.

Williams RD, Donovan JF, Tanagho EA: *Urology*. Pages 825–884 in: *Current Surgical Diagnosis & Treatment*, 8th ed. Way LW (editor). Appleton & Lange, 1988.

Nervous System   18

Michael J. Aminoff, MD, FRCP

HEADACHE

Headache is such a common complaint and can occur for so many different reasons that its proper evaluation may be difficult. Although underlying structural lesions are not present in most patients presenting with headache, it is nevertheless important to bear this possibility in mind. About one-third of patients with brain tumors, for example, present with a primary complaint of headache.

The intensity, quality, and site of pain—and especially the duration of the headache and the presence of associated neurologic symptoms—may provide clues to the underlying cause. The onset of severe headache in a previously well patient is more likely than chronic headache to relate to an intracranial disorder such as subarachnoid hemorrhage or meningitis. Headaches that disturb sleep, exertional headaches, and late-onset paroxysmal headaches are also more suggestive of an underlying structural lesion, as are headaches accompanied by neurologic symptoms such as drowsiness, visual or limb problems, seizures, or altered mental status. Chronic headaches are commonly due to migraine, tension, or depression, but they may be related to intracranial lesions, head injury, cervical spondylosis, dental or ocular disease, temporomandibular joint dysfunction, sinusitis, hypertension, and a wide variety of general medical disorders. Depending on the initial clinical impression, the need for such investigations as CT scan of the head, electroencephalography, and lumbar puncture must be assessed on an individual basis. The diagnosis and treatment of primary neurologic disorders associated with headache are considered separately under these disorders.

Tension Headache

Patients frequently complain of poor concentration and other vague nonspecific symptoms, in addition to constant daily headaches that are often viselike or tight in quality and may be exacerbated by emotional stress, fatigue, noise, or glare. The headaches are usually generalized, may be most intense about the neck or back of the head, and are not associated with focal neurologic symptoms.

When treatment with simple analgesics is not effective, a trial of antimigrainous agents (see Migraine, below) is worthwhile. Techniques to induce relaxation are also useful and include massage, hot baths, and biofeedback. Exploration of underlying causes of chronic anxiety is often rewarding.

Depression Headache

Depression headaches are frequently worse on arising in the morning and may be accompanied by other symptoms of depression. Headaches are occasionally the focus of a somatic delusional system. Tricyclic antidepressant drugs are often helpful, as may be psychiatric consultation.

Migraine

Classic migrainous headache is a lateralized throbbing headache that occurs episodically following its onset in adolescence or early adult life. In many cases, however, the headaches do not conform to this pattern, although their associated features and response to antimigrainous preparations nevertheless suggest that they have a similar basis. In this broader sense, migrainous headaches may be lateralized or generalized, may be dull or throbbing, and are sometimes associated with anorexia, nausea, vomiting, photophobia, and blurring of vision (so-called sick headaches). They usually build up gradually and may last for several hours or longer. They have been related to dilatation and excessive pulsation of branches of the external carotid artery. Focal disturbances of neurologic function may precede or accompany the headaches and have been attributed to constriction of branches of the internal carotid artery. Visual disturbances occur quite commonly and may consist of field defects; of luminous visual hallucinations such as stars, sparks, unformed light flashes (photopsia), geometric patterns, or zigzags of light; or of some combination of field defects and luminous hallucinations (scintillating scotomas). Other focal disturbances such as aphasia or numbness, tingling, clumsiness, or weakness in a circumscribed distribution may also occur.

Patients often give a family history of migraine. Attacks may be triggered by emotional or physical stress, lack or excess of sleep, missed meals, specific foods (eg, chocolate), alcoholic beverages, menstruation, or use of oral contraceptives.

An uncommon variant is so-called basilar artery migraine, in which blindness or visual disturbances throughout both visual fields are initially accompanied or followed by dysarthria, dysequilibrium, tinnitus, and perioral and distal paresthesias and are sometimes followed by transient loss or impairment of consciousness or by a confusional state. This, in turn, is followed by a throbbing (usually occipital) headache, often with nausea and vomiting.

In ophthalmoplegic migraine, lateralized pain—often about the eye—is accompanied by nausea, vomiting, and diplopia due to transient external ophthalmoplegia. The ophthalmoplegia is due to third nerve palsy, sometimes with accompanying sixth nerve involvement, and may outlast the orbital pain by several days or even weeks. The ophthalmic division of the fifth nerve has also been affected in some patients. Ophthalmoplegic migraine is rare; more common causes of a painful ophthalmoplegia are internal carotid artery aneurysms and diabetes.

In rare instances, the neurologic or somatic disturbance accompanying typical migrainous headaches becomes the sole manifestation of an attack (''migraine equivalent''). Very rarely, the patient may be left with a permanent neurologic deficit following a migrainous attack, presumably because of irreversible cerebral ischemic damage.

Management of migraine consists of avoidance of any precipitating factors, together with prophylactic or symptomatic pharmacologic treatment if necessary.

During acute attacks, many patients find it helpful to rest in a quiet, darkened room until symptoms subside. A simple analgesic (eg, aspirin) taken right away often provides relief, but treatment with extracranial vasoconstrictors or other drugs is sometimes necessary. Cafergot, a combination of ergotamine tartrate and caffeine, is often particularly helpful; 1–4 tablets are taken at the onset of headache or warning symptoms, and more are taken after about 20 minutes if symptoms have not begun to subside. Ergonovine maleate, up to 5 tablets (1 mg) taken at the onset of symptoms, may also provide relief. Because of impaired absorption or vomiting during acute attacks,

oral medication sometimes fails to help. Cafergot given rectally as suppositories, ergotamine tartrate given intramuscularly (0.25–0.5 mg), or dihydroergotamine mesylate given either intramuscularly or intravenously (0.5–1 mg) may be useful in such cases. Ergotamine-containing preparations may affect the gravid uterus and thus should be avoided during pregnancy. Mefenamic acid may also help if taken (with food) at the onset of an acute migraine attack.

Prophylactic treatment may be necessary if migrainous headaches occur more frequently than 2 or 3 times a month. Some of the more common drugs used for this purpose are listed in Table 18–1. Their mode of action is unclear and may involve both an effect on extracerebral vasculature and a cerebral effect, eg, by stabilizing serotonergic neurotransmission. Several drugs may have to be tried in turn before the headaches are brought under control. Once a drug has been found to help, it should be continued for several months. If the patient remains headache-free, the dose can then be tapered and the drug eventually withdrawn.

Calcium channel antagonist drugs may decrease the frequency of attacks after an interval of several weeks, but the severity and duration of attacks are not influenced.

Cluster Headache (Migrainous Neuralgia)

Cluster headache affects predominantly middle-aged men. Its cause is unclear but may relate to a vascular headache disorder or a disturbance of serotonergic mechanisms. There is often no family history of headache or migraine. Episodes of severe unilateral periorbital pain occur daily for several weeks and are often accompanied by one or more of the following: ipsilateral nasal congestion, rhinorrhea, lacrimation, redness of the eye, and Horner's syndrome. Episodes usually occur at night, awaken the patient, and last for less than 2 hours. Spontaneous remission

Table 18–1. Prophylactic treatment of migraine.[1]

Drug	Usual Adult Daily Dose (mg)	Common Side Effects
Propranolol	80–240	Fatigue, lassitude, depression, insomnia, nausea, vomiting, constipation.
Amitriptyline	10–150	Sedation, dry mouth, constipation, weight gain, blurred vision, edema, hypotension, urinary retention.
Ergonovine maleate	0.6–2	Nausea, abdominal pain, diarrhea.
Cyproheptadine	12–20	Sedation, dry mouth, epigastric discomfort, gastrointestinal disturbances.
Clonidine	0.2–0.6	Dry mouth, drowsiness, sedation, headache, constipation.
Methysergide	4–8	Nausea, vomiting, diarrhea, abdominal pain, cramps, weight gain, insomnia, edema, peripheral vasoconstriction. Retroperitoneal and pleuropulmonary fibrosis and fibrous thickening of cardiac valves may occur; patients must be closely supervised.

[1] Reproduced, with permission, from Aminoff MJ: Neurologic disorders. In: *Handbook of Medical Treatment,* 17th ed. Watts HD (editor). Jones, 1983.

then occurs, and the patient remains well for weeks or months before another bout of closely spaced attacks occurs. During a bout, many patients report that alcohol triggers an attack; others report that stress, glare, or ingestion of specific foods occasionally precipitates attacks. In occasional patients, typical attacks of pain and associated symptoms recur at intervals without remission. This variant has been referred to as chronic cluster headache.

Examination reveals no abnormality apart from Horner's syndrome that either occurs transiently during an attack or, in long-standing cases, remains as a residual deficit between attacks.

Treatment of an individual attack with oral drugs is generally unsatisfactory, but use of ergotamine tartrate aerosol or inhalation of 100% oxygen (7 L/min for 15 minutes) may be effective. Drugs should be given to prevent further attacks until the ongoing bout is over. Ergotamine tartrate is an effective prophylactic and can be given as rectal suppositories (0.5–1 mg at night or twice daily), by mouth (2 mg daily), or by subcutaneous injection (0.25 mg 3 times daily for 5 days per week). Various prophylactic agents that have been found to be effective in individual patients are propranolol, amitriptyline, cyproheptadine, lithium carbonate (monitored by plasma lithium determination), prednisone (20–40 mg daily or on alternate days for 2 weeks, followed by gradual withdrawal), and methysergide (4–6 mg daily).

Giant Cell (Temporal or Cranial) Arteritis

The superficial temporal, vertebral, ophthalmic, and posterior ciliary arteries are often the most severely affected pathologically. Most patients are elderly. The major symptom is headache, often associated with or preceded by myalgia, malaise, anorexia, weight loss, and other nonspecific complaints. Loss of vision is the most feared manifestation and occurs quite commonly. Clinical examination often reveals tenderness of the scalp and over the temporal arteries. Further details, including approaches to treatment, are given in Chapter 15.

Posttraumatic Headache

A variety of nonspecific symptoms may follow a closed head injury, regardless of whether consciousness is lost. Headache is often a conspicuous feature. Some authorities believe that psychologic factors may be important because there is no correlation of severity of the injury with neurologic signs.

The headache itself usually appears within a day or so following injury, may worsen over the ensuing weeks, and then gradually subsides. It is usually a constant dull ache, with superimposed throbbing that may be localized, lateralized, or generalized. It is sometimes accompanied by nausea, vomiting, or scintillating scotomas.

Dysequilibrium, sometimes with a rotatory component, may also occur and is often enhanced by postural change or head movement. Impaired memory, poor concentration, emotional instability, and increased irritability are other common complaints and occasionally are the sole manifestations of the syndrome. The duration of symptoms relates in part to the severity of the original injury, but even trivial injuries are sometimes followed by symptoms that persist for months.

Special investigations are usually not helpful. The electroencephalogram may show minor nonspecific changes, while the electronystagmogram sometimes suggests either peripheral or central vestibulopathy. CT scans of the head usually show no abnormal findings.

Treatment is difficult, but optimistic encouragement and graduated rehabilitation, depending upon the occupational circumstances, are advised. Headaches often respond to simple analgesics, but severe headaches may necessitate treatment with amitriptyline, propranolol, or ergot derivatives.

Cough Headache

Severe head pain may be produced by coughing (and by straining, sneezing, and laughing) but, fortunately, usually lasts for only a few minutes or less. The pathophysiologic basis of the complaint is not known, and often there is no underlying structural lesion. However, intracranial lesions, usually in the posterior fossa (eg, Arnold-Chiari malformation, basilar impression), are present in about 10% of cases, and brain tumors or other space-occupying lesions may certainly present in this way. Accordingly, CT scanning should be undertaken in all patients and repeated annually for several years, since a small structural lesion may not show up initially.

The disorder is usually self-limited, although it may persist for several years. For unknown reasons, symptoms sometimes clear completely after lumbar puncture. Indomethacin may provide relief.

Headache Due to Other Neurologic Causes

Intracranial mass lesions of all types may cause headache owing to displacement of vascular structures. Posterior fossa tumors often cause occipital pain, and supratentorial lesions lead to bifrontal headache, but such findings are too inconsistent to be of value in attempts at localizing a pathologic process. The headaches are nonspecific in character and may vary in severity from mild to severe. They may be worsened by exertion or postural change and may be associated with nausea and vomiting, but this is true of migraine also. Headaches are also a feature of pseudotumor cerebri (see below). Signs of focal or diffuse cerebral dysfunction or of increased intracranial pressure will indicate the need for further investigation. Similarly, a progressive headache disorder or the new onset of headaches in middle or later life merits investigation if no cause is apparent.

Cerebrovascular disease may be associated with headache, but the mechanism is unclear. Headache may occur with internal carotid artery occlusion or carotid dissection and after carotid endarterectomy. Diagnosis is facilitated by the clinical accompaniments and the circumstances in which the headache developed.

Acute severe headache accompanies subarachnoid hemorrhage and meningeal infections, but the accompanying signs of meningeal irritation and the frequent impairment of consciousness then indicate the need for further investigations. A dramatically severe headache may also occur in association with paroxysmal hypertension in patients with pheochromocytoma.

Dull or throbbing headache is a frequent sequela of lumbar puncture and may last for several days. It is aggravated by the erect posture and alleviated by recumbency. The exact mechanism is unclear, but it is commonly attributed to leakage of cerebrospinal fluid through the dural puncture site. Its incidence may be reduced if a small-diameter needle is used for the spinal tap, and perhaps also if the patient lies prone or supine after the procedure.

Diamond S, Millstein E: Current concepts of migraine therapy. J Clin Pharmacol 1988;28:193.

Lance JW: Headache. Ann Neurol 1981;10:1. (Causes, mechanisms, and treatment.)

Raskin NH: *Headache,* 2nd ed. Churchill Livingstone, 1988. (Emphasis on pathophysiology.)

FACIAL PAIN

Trigeminal Neuralgia

Trigeminal neuralgia ("tic douloureux") is most common in middle and later life. It affects women more frequently than men. The disorder is characterized by momentary episodes of sudden lancinating facial pain that commonly arises near one side of the mouth and then shoots toward the ear, eye, or nostril on that side. The pain may be triggered or precipitated by such factors as touch, movement, drafts, and eating. Indeed, in order to lessen the likelihood of triggering further attacks, many patients try to hold the face still while talking. Spontaneous remissions for several months or longer may occur. As the disorder progresses, however, the episodes of pain become more frequent, remissions become shorter and less common, and a dull ache may persist between the episodes of stabbing pain. Symptoms remain confined to the distribution of the trigeminal nerve (usually the second or third division) on one side only.

The characteristic features of the pain in trigeminal neuralgia usually distinguish it from other causes of facial pain. Neurologic examination shows no abnor-

mality except in a few patients in whom trigeminal neuralgia is symptomatic of some underlying lesion, such as multiple sclerosis or a brain stem neoplasm, in which case the finding will depend on the nature and site of the lesion. Similarly, CT scans and radiologic contrast studies are normal in patients with classic trigeminal neuralgia.

In a young patient presenting with trigeminal neuralgia, multiple sclerosis must be suspected even if there are no other neurologic signs. In such circumstances, findings on evoked potential testing and examination of cerebrospinal fluid may be corroborative. When the facial pain is due to a posterior fossa tumor, CT scanning and MRI generally reveal the lesion.

The drug most helpful for treatment of trigeminal neuralgia is carbamazepine, given in a dose of up to 1200 mg/d, with monitoring by serial blood counts and liver function tests. If carbamazepine is ineffective or cannot be tolerated, phenytoin should be tried. (Doses and side effects of these drugs are shown in Table 18–2.) Baclofen (10–20 mg 3 or 4 times daily) may also be helpful, either alone or in combination with carbamazepine or phenytoin.

In the past, alcohol injection of the affected nerve, rhizotomy, or tractotomy were recommended if pharmacologic treatment was unsuccessful. More recently, however, posterior fossa exploration has frequently revealed some structural cause for the neuralgia (despite normal findings on CT scans or arteriograms), such as an anomalous artery or vein impinging on the trigeminal nerve root. In such cases, simple decompression and separation of the anomalous vessel from the nerve root produce lasting relief of symptoms. In elderly patients with a limited life expectancy, radiofrequency rhizotomy is sometimes preferred because it is easy to perform, has few complications, and provides symptomatic relief for a period of time. Surgical exploration generally reveals no abnormality and is inappropriate in patients with trigeminal neuralgia due to multiple sclerosis.

Atypical Facial Pain

Facial pain without the typical features of trigeminal neuralgia is generally a constant, often burning pain that may have a restricted distribution at its onset but soon spreads to the rest of the face on the affected side and sometimes involves the other side, the neck, or the back of the head as well. The disorder is especially common in middle-aged women, many of them emotionally depressed, but it is not clear whether depression is the cause of or a reaction to the pain. Simple analgesics should be given a trial, as should tricyclic antidepressants, carbamazepine, and phenytoin; the response is often disappointing. Opiate analgesics should be avoided, since addiction is a very real danger in patients with this disorder. Attempts at surgical treatment are not indicated.

Table 18–2. Drug treatment for seizures.[1]

	Usual Adult Daily Dose (mg/kg)	Usual Adult Daily Dose (mg)	Minimum Number of Daily Doses	Time to Steady-State Drug Levels (days)	Optimal Blood Level (per mL)	Selected Side Effects and Idiosyncratic Reactions
Generalized tonic-colonic (grand mal) or partial (focal) seizures						
Phenytoin	4–8	200–400	1	5–10	10–20 µg	Nystagmus, ataxia, dysarthria, sedation, confusion, gingival hyperplasia, hirsutism, megaloblastic anemia, blood dyscrasias, skin rashes, fever, systemic lupus erythematosus, lymphadenopathy, peripheral neuropathy, dyskinesias.
Carbamazepine	5–25	600–1200	2	3–4	4–8 µg	Nystagmus, dysarthria, diplopia, ataxia, drowsiness, nausea, blood dyscrasias, hepatotoxicity.
Phenobarbital	2–5	100–200	1	14–21	10–40 µg	Drowsiness, nystagmus, ataxia, skin rashes, learning difficulties, hyperactivity.
Primidone	5–20	750–1500	3	4–7	5–15 µg	Sedation, nystagmus, ataxia, vertigo, nausea, skin rashes, megaloblastic anemia, irritability.
Valproic acid	10–60		3	2–4	50–100 µg	Nausea, vomiting, diarrhea, drowsiness, alopecia, weight gain, hepatotoxicity, thrombocytopenia, tremor.
Absence (petit mal) seizures						
Ethosuximide	20–35	100–1500	2	5–10	40–100 µg	Nausea, vomiting, anorexia, headache, lethargy, unsteadiness, blood dyscrasias, systemic lupus erythematosus, urticaria, pruritus.
Valproic acid	10–60		3	2–4	50–100 µg	See above.
Clonazepam	0.05–0.2		2	?	20–80 ng	Drowsiness, ataxia, irritability, behavioral changes, exacerbation of tonic-clonic seizures.
Myoclonic seizures						
Valproic acid	10–60		3	2–4	50–100 µg	See above.
Clonazepam	0.05–0.2		2	?	20–80 ng	See above.

[1] Reproduced, with permission, from Aminoff MJ: Neurologic disorders. In: *Handbook of Medical Treatment,* 17th ed. Watts HD (editor). Jones, 1983.

Glossopharyngeal Neuralgia

Glossopharyngeal neuralgia is an uncommon disorder in which pain similar in quality to that in trigeminal neuralgia occurs in the throat, about the tonsillar fossa, and sometimes deep in the ear and at the back of the tongue. The pain may be precipitated by swallowing, chewing, talking, or yawning and is sometimes accompanied by syncope. In most instances, no underlying structural abnormality is present. Carbamazepine is the treatment of choice and should be tried before any surgical procedures are considered.

Postherpetic Neuralgia

About 10% of patients who develop shingles suffer from postherpetic neuralgia. This complication seems especially likely to occur in the elderly and when the first division of the trigeminal nerve is affected. A history of shingles and the presence of cutaneous scarring resulting from shingles aid in the diagnosis. Severe pain with shingles correlates with the intensity of postherpetic symptoms.

The incidence of postherpetic neuralgia may be reduced by the treatment of shingles with steroids but is not influenced by treatment with acyclovir. Management of the established complication is essentially medical. If simple analgesics fail to help, a trial of a tricyclic drug (eg, amitriptyline, up to 100–150 mg/d) in conjunction with a phenothiazine (eg, perphenazine, 2–8 mg/d) is often effective. Other patients respond to carbamazepine (up to 1200 mg/d) or phenytoin (300 mg/d). Application of a cream containing capsaicin (0.025%) to the affected area several times daily may also be helpful.

Facial Pain Due to Other Causes

Facial pain may be caused by temporomandibular joint dysfunction in patients with malocclusion, abnormal bite, or faulty dentures. There may be tenderness of the masticatory muscles, and an association between pain onset and jaw movement is sometimes noted. Treatment consists of correction of the underlying problem.

A relationship of facial pain to chewing or temperature changes may suggest a dental disturbance. The cause is sometimes not obvious, and diagnosis requires careful dental examination and x-rays. Pain on mastication may also occur in giant cell arteritis. Sinusitis and ear infections causing facial pain are usually recognized by the history of respiratory tract infection, fever, and, in some instances, aural discharge. There may be localized tenderness. Radiologic evidence of sinus infection or mastoiditis is confirmatory.

Glaucoma is an important ocular cause of facial pain, usually localized to the periorbital region.

On occasion, pain in the jaw may be the principal manifestation of angina pectoris. Precipitation by exertion and radiation to more typical areas establish the cardiac origin.

Portenoy RK, Duma C, Foley KM: Acute herpetic and postherpetic neuralgia: Clinical review and current management. Ann Neurol 1986;20:651. (Summary of clinical features, pathology, and treatment of herpes and postherpetic neuralgia.)
Sweet WH: The treatment of trigeminal neuralgia (tic douloureux). N Engl J Med 1986;315:174. (A review of therapeutic approaches.)

EPILEPSY

Essentials of Diagnosis

- Recurrent seizures.
- Characteristic electroencephalographic changes accompany seizures.
- Mental status abnormalities or focal neurologic symptoms may persist for hours postictally.

General Considerations

The term epilepsy denotes any disorder characterized by recurrent seizures. A seizure is a transient disturbance of cerebral function due to an abnormal paroxysmal neuronal discharge in the brain. Epilepsy is common, affecting approximately 0.5% of the population in the USA.

Etiology

Epilepsy has several causes. Its most likely cause in individual patients relates to the age at onset.

A. Idiopathic or Constitutional Epilepsy: Seizures usually begin between 5 and 20 years of age but may start later in life. No specific cause can be identified, and there is no other neurologic abnormality.

B. Symptomatic Epilepsy: There are many causes for recurrent seizures.

1. Congenital abnormalities and perinatal injuries may result in seizures presenting in infancy or childhood.

2. Metabolic disorders such as hypocalcemia, hypoglycemia, pyridoxine deficiency, and phenylketonuria are major treatable causes of seizures in newborns or infants. In adults, withdrawal from alcohol or drugs is a common cause of recurrent seizures, and other metabolic disorders such as renal failure and diabetes may also be responsible.

3. Trauma is an important cause of seizures at any age, but especially in young adults. Posttraumatic epilepsy is more likely to develop if the dura mater was penetrated and generally becomes manifest within 2 years following the injury. However, seizures developing in the first week after head injury do not necessarily imply that future attacks will occur. There is suggestive evidence that prophylactic anticonvulsant drug treatment reduces the incidence of posttraumatic epilepsy.

4. Tumors and other space-occupying lesions may lead to seizures at any age, but they are an especially important cause of seizures in middle and later life, when the incidence of neoplastic disease increases. The seizures are commonly the initial symptoms of the tumor and often are partial (focal) in character. They are most likely to occur with structural lesions involving the frontal, parietal, or temporal regions. Tumors must be excluded by appropriate laboratory studies in all patients with onset of seizures after 30 years of age, focal seizures or signs, or a progressive seizure disorder.

5. Vascular diseases become increasingly frequent causes of seizures with advancing age and are the most common cause of seizures with onset at age 60 years or older.

6. Degenerative disorders are a cause of seizures in later life.

7. Infectious diseases must be considered in all age groups as potentially reversible causes of seizures. Seizures may occur with an acute infective or inflammatory illness, such as bacterial meningitis or herpes encephalitis, or in patients with more longstanding or chronic disorders such as neurosyphilis or cerebral cysticercosis. In patients with AIDS, they may result from central nervous system toxoplasmosis, cryptococcal meningitis, secondary viral encephalitis, or other infective complications. Seizures are a common sequela of supratentorial brain abscess, developing most frequently in the first year after treatment.

Classification of Seizures

Seizures can be categorized in various ways, but the descriptive classification proposed by the International League Against Epilepsy is clinically the most useful. Seizures are divided into those that are generalized and those affecting only part of the brain (partial seizures).

A. Partial Seizures: The initial clinical and electroencephalographic manifestations of partial seizures indicate that only a restricted part of one cerebral hemisphere has been activated. The ictal manifestations depend upon the area of the brain involved. Partial seizures are subdivided into simple seizures, in which consciousness is preserved, and complex seizures, in which it is impaired. Partial seizures of either type sometimes become secondarily generalized, leading to a tonic, clonic, or tonic-clonic attack.

1. Simple partial seizures–Simple seizures may be manifested by focal motor symptoms (convulsive jerking) or somatosensory symptoms (eg, paresthesias or tingling) that spread (or "march") to different parts of the limb or body depending upon their cortical representation. In other instances, special sensory symptoms (eg, light flashes or buzzing) indicate involvement of visual, auditory, olfactory, or gustatory regions of the brain, or there may be autonomic symptoms or signs (eg, abnormal epigastric sensations, sweating, flushing, pupillary dilation). When psychic symptoms occur, they are usually accompanied by impairment of consciousness, but the sole manifestations of some seizures are phenomena such as dysphasia, dysmnesic symptoms (eg, déjà vu, jamais vu), affective disturbances, illusions, or structured hallucinations.

2. Complex partial seizures–Impaired consciousness may be preceded, accompanied, or followed by the psychic symptoms mentioned above, and automatisms may occur. Such seizures may also begin with some of the other simple symptoms mentioned above.

B. Generalized Seizures: There are several different varieties of generalized seizures, as outlined below. In some circumstances, seizures cannot be classified because of incomplete information or because they do not fit into any category.

1. Absence (petit mal) seizures–These are characterized by impairment of consciousness, sometimes with mild clonic, tonic, or atonic components (ie, reduction or loss of postural tone), autonomic components (eg, enuresis), or accompanying automatisms. Onset and termination of attacks are abrupt. If attacks occur during conversation, the patient may miss a few words or may break off in mid sentence for a few seconds. The impairment of external awareness is so brief that the patient is unaware of it. Absence seizures almost always begin in childhood and frequently cease by the age of 20 years, although occasionally they are then replaced by other forms of generalized seizure. Electroencephalographically, such attacks are associated with bursts of bilaterally synchronous and symmetric 3-Hz spike-and-wave activity. A normal background in the electroencephalogram and normal or above-normal intelligence imply a good prognosis for the ultimate cessation of these seizures.

2. Atypical absences–There may be more marked changes in tone, or attacks may have a more gradual onset and termination than in typical absences.

3. Myoclonic seizures–Myoclonic seizures consist of single or multiple myoclonic jerks.

4. Tonic-clonic (grand mal) seizures–In these seizures, which are characterized by sudden loss of consciousness, the patient becomes rigid and falls to the ground, and respiration is arrested. This tonic phase, which usually lasts for less than a minute, is followed by a clonic phase in which there is jerking of the body musculature that may last for 2 or 3 minutes and is then followed by a stage of flaccid coma. During the seizure, the tongue or lips may be bitten, urinary or fecal incontinence may occur, and the patient may be injured. Immediately after the seizure, the patient may either recover consciousness, drift into sleep, have a further convulsion without recovery of consciousness between the attacks **(status epilepticus),** or after recovering consciousness have a further convulsion **(serial seizures).** In other cases, patients will behave in an abnormal fashion in the immediate postictal period, without subsequent awareness or memory of events **(postepileptic automatism).** Headache, disorientation, confusion, drowsiness, nausea, soreness of the muscles, or some combination of these symptoms commonly occurs postictally.

5. Tonic, clonic, or atonic seizures–Loss of consciousness may occur with either the tonic or clonic accompaniments described above, especially in children. Atonic seizures **(epileptic drop attacks)** have also been described.

Clinical Findings

A. Symptoms and Signs: Nonspecific changes such as headache, mood alterations, lethargy, and myoclonic jerking alert some patients to an impending seizure hours before it occurs. These prodromal symptoms are distinct from the aura which may precede a generalized seizure by a few seconds or minutes and which is itself a part of the attack, arising locally from a restricted region of the brain.

In most patients, seizures occur unpredictably at any time and without any relationship to posture or ongoing activities. Occasionally, however, they occur at a particular time (eg, during sleep) or in relation to external precipitants such as lack of sleep, missed meals, emotional stress, menstruation, alcohol ingestion (or alcohol withdrawal; see below), or use of certain drugs. Fever and nonspecific infections may also precipitate seizures in known epileptics; in infants and young children, it may be hard to distinguish such attacks from febrile seizures. In a few patients, seizures are provoked by specific stimuli such as flashing lights or a flickering television set **(photosensitive epilepsy),** music, or reading.

Clinical examination between seizures shows no abnormality in patients with idiopathic epilepsy, but in the immediate postictal period, extensor plantar responses may be seen. The presence of lateralized or focal signs postictally suggests that seizures may have a focal origin. In patients with symptomatic epilepsy, the findings on examination will reflect the underlying cause.

B. Imaging: CT or MRI scan is indicated for patients with focal neurologic symptoms or signs, focal seizures, or electroencephalographic findings of a focal disturbance; some physicians routinely order imaging studies for all patients with new-onset seizure disorders. Such studies should certainly be performed in patients with clinical evidence of a progressive disorder and in those presenting with seizures after the age of 30 years, because of the possibility of an underlying neoplasm. A chest radiograph should also be obtained in such patients, since the lungs are a common site for primary or secondary neoplasms.

C. Laboratory and Other Studies: In patients older than 10 years, initial investigations should always include a full blood count, blood glucose determination, liver and renal function tests, and serologic tests for syphilis. The hematologic and biochemical screening tests are important both in excluding various causes of seizures and in providing a baseline for subsequent monitoring of long-term effects of treatment.

Electroencephalography may support the clinical diagnosis of epilepsy (by demonstrating paroxysmal abnormalities containing spikes or sharp waves), may provide a guide to prognosis, and may help classify the seizure disorder. Classification of the disorder is important for determining the most appropriate anticonvulsant drug with which to start treatment. For example, absence (petit mal) and complex partial seizures may be difficult to distinguish clinically, but the electroencephalographic findings and treatment of choice differ in these 2 conditions. Finally, the electroencephalographic findings are important in evaluating candidates for surgical treatment.

Differential Diagnosis

The distinction between the various disorders likely to be confused with generalized seizures is usually made on the basis of the history. The importance of obtaining an eyewitness account of the attacks cannot be overemphasized.

A. Differential Diagnosis of Partial Seizures:
1. Transient ischemic attacks–These attacks are distinguished from seizures by their longer duration, lack of spread, and symptomatology. There is a loss of motor or sensory function (eg, weakness or numbness) with transient ischemic attacks, whereas positive symptomatology (eg, convulsive jerking or paresthesias) characterizes seizures.

2. Rage attacks–Rage attacks are usually situational and lead to goal-directed aggressive behavior.

3. Panic attacks–These may be hard to distinguish from simple or complex partial seizures unless there is evidence of psychopathologic disturbances between attacks and the attacks have a clear relationship to external circumstances.

B. Differential Diagnosis of Generalized Seizures:
1. Orthostatic syncope–Episodes of orthostatic syncope usually occur while the patient is standing or after a sudden change in posture to the erect position, especially in patients with autonomic insufficiency.

2. Cardiac dysrhythmias–Cerebral hypoperfusion due to a disturbance of cardiac rhythm should be suspected in patients with known cardiac or vascular disease or in elderly patients who present with episodic loss of consciousness. Prodromal symptoms are typically absent. A relationship of attacks to physical activity and the finding of a systolic murmur is suggestive of aortic stenosis. Repeated Holter monitoring may be necessary to establish the diagnosis; monitoring initiated by the patient ("event monitor") may be valuable if the disturbances of consciousness are rare.

3. Brain stem ischemia–Loss of consciousness is preceded or accompanied by other brain stem signs. Basilar artery migraine is discussed on p 677 and vertebrobasilar vascular disease on p 690.

4. Pseudoseizures–The term pseudoseizures is used to denote both hysterical conversion reactions and attacks due to malingering when these simulate epileptic seizures. Many patients with pseudoseizures also have true seizures or a family history of epilepsy. Although pseudoseizures tend to occur at times of emotional stress, this may also be the case with true seizures.

Clinically, the attacks superficially resemble tonic-clonic seizures, but there may be obvious preparation before pseudoseizures occur. Moreover, there is usually no tonic phase; instead, there is an asynchronous thrashing of the limbs, which increases if restraints are imposed and which rarely leads to injury. Consciousness may be normal or "lost," but in the latter context the occurrence of goal-directed behavior or of shouting, swearing, etc, indicates that it is feigned. Postictally, there are no changes in behavior or neurologic findings.

Laboratory studies may aid in recognition of pseudoseizures. There are no electrocerebral changes, whereas the electroencephalogram changes during organic seizures accompanied by loss of consciousness. The serum level of prolactin has been found to increase dramatically between 15 and 30 minutes after a tonic-clonic convulsion in most patients, whereas it is unchanged after a pseudoseizure.

Treatment

A. General Measures: For patients with recurrent seizures, drug treatment is prescribed with the goal of preventing further attacks and is usually continued until there have been no seizures for at least 4 years. Epileptic patients should be advised to avoid situations that could be dangerous or life-threatening if further seizures should occur. State legislation may require physicians to report to the state department of motor vehicles any patients with seizures or other episodic disturbances of consciousness.

1. Choice of medication–The drug with which treatment is best initiated depends upon the type of seizures to be treated (Table 18–2). The dose of the selected drug is gradually increased until seizures are controlled, blood levels reach the upper limit of the optimal therapeutic range, or side effects prevent further increases. If seizures continue despite treatment at the maximal tolerated dose, a second drug is added and the dose increased until its blood levels are in the therapeutic range; the first drug is then gradually withdrawn. In treatment of partial and secondarily generalized tonic-clonic seizures, the success rate is higher with carbamazepine or phenytoin than with phenobarbital or primidone. In most patients with seizures of a single type, satisfactory control can be achieved with a single anticonvulsant drug. Treatment with 2 drugs may further reduce seizure frequency or severity, but usually only at the cost of greater toxicity. Treatment with more than 2 drugs is almost always unhelpful unless the patient is having seizures of different types. If the drugs shown in Table 18–2 are ineffective, a number of second-line anticonvulsant drugs can be tried, but these have more frequent and troublesome side effects, which limit their use.

2. Monitoring–Monitoring plasma drug levels has led to major advances in the management of seizure disorders. The same daily dose of a particular drug leads to markedly different blood concentrations in different patients, and this will affect the therapeutic response. Steady-state drug levels in the blood should therefore be measured after treatment is initiated, dosage is changed, or another drug is added to the therapeutic regimen and when seizures are poorly controlled. Dose adjustments are then guided by the laboratory findings. The most common cause of a lower concentration of drug than expected for the prescribed dose is poor patient compliance. Compliance can be improved by limiting to a minimum the number of daily doses. Recurrent seizures or status epilepticus may result if drugs are taken erratically, and in some circumstances noncompliant patients may be better off without any medication.

All anticonvulsant drugs have side effects, and some of these are shown in Table 18–2. A complete blood count should be performed at least annually in all patients, because of the risk of anemia or blood dyscrasia. Treatment with certain drugs may require more frequent monitoring or use of additional screening tests. For example, periodic tests of hepatic function are necessary if valproic acid or carbamazepine is used, and serial blood counts are important with carbamazepine or ethosuximide.

3. Discontinuance of medication–Only when patients have been seizure-free for several (at least 4) years should withdrawal of medication be considered. Unfortunately, there is no way of predicting which patients can be managed successfully without treatment, although seizure recurrence is more likely in patients who initially failed to respond to therapy, those with seizures having focal features or of multiple types, and those with continuing electroencephalographic abnormalities. Dose reduction should be gradual over a period of weeks or months, and drugs should be withdrawn one at a time. If seizures recur, treatment is reinstituted with the same drugs used previously. Seizures are no more difficult to control after a recurrence than before.

B. Special Circumstances:

1. Solitary seizures–In patients who have had only one seizure, investigation should exclude an underlying cause requiring specific treatment. Prophylactic anticonvulsant drug treatment is generally not required unless further attacks occur. The risk of seizure recurrence varies in different series, but in one recent survey it was only 27% over 3 years, with none occurring thereafter. Epilepsy should not be diagnosed on the basis of a solitary seizure. If seizures occur in the context of a transient, nonrecurrent systemic disorder such as acute cerebral anoxia, the diagnosis of epilepsy is inaccurate, and long-term prophylactic anticonvulsant drug treatment is unnecessary.

2. Alcohol withdrawal seizures–One or more generalized tonic-clonic seizures may occur within 48 hours or so of withdrawal from alcohol after a period of high or chronic intake. If the seizures have consistently focal features, the possibility of an associated structural abnormality, often traumatic in origin, must be considered. Treatment with anticonvulsant drugs is generally not required for alcohol withdrawal seizures, since they are self-limited. Status epilepticus may rarely follow alcohol withdrawal and is managed along conventional lines (see below). Further attacks will not occur if the patient abstains from alcohol.

3. Tonic-clonic status epilepticus–Poor compliance with the anticonvulsant drug regimen is the most common cause of tonic-clonic status epilepticus. Other causes include alcohol withdrawal, intracranial infection or neoplasms, metabolic disorders, and drug overdose. The mortality rate may be as high as 20%, and among survivors the incidence of neurologic and mental sequelae may be high. The prognosis relates to the length of time between onset of status epilepticus and the start of effective treatment.

Status epilepticus is a medical emergency. Initial management includes maintenance of the airway and 50% dextrose (25–50 mL) intravenously in case hypoglycemia is responsible. If seizures continue, 10 mg of diazepam is given intravenously over the course of 2 minutes, and the dose is repeated after 10 minutes if necessary. This is usually effective in halting seizures for a brief period but occasionally causes respiratory depression. Regardless of the response to diazepam, phenytoin (15 mg/kg) is given intravenously at a rate of 50 mg/min; this provides initiation of long-term seizure control. The drug is best injected directly but can also be given in saline; it precipitates, however, if injected into glucose-containing solutions. Because arrhythmias may develop during rapid administration of phenytoin, electrocardiographic monitoring is prudent. Hypotension may complicate phenytoin administration, especially if diazepam has also been given.

If seizures continue, phenobarbital is then given in a loading dose of 10–15 mg/kg intravenously by slow or intermittent injection. Respiratory depression and hypotension are common complications and should be anticipated; they may occur also with diazepam alone, though less commonly. If these measures fail, general anesthesia with ventilatory assistance and neuromuscular junction blockade may be required.

Other benzodiazepines than diazepam have been used in the immediate management of status epilepticus. Lorazepam given intravenously is effective but has no particular advantage over diazepam.

After status epilepticus is controlled, an oral drug program for the long-term management of seizures is started, and investigations into the cause of the disorder are pursued.

4. Nonconvulsive status epilepticus–Absence (petit mal) and complex partial status epilepticus are characterized by fluctuating abnormal mental status, confusion, impaired responsiveness, and automatism. Electroencephalography is helpful both in establishing the diagnosis and in distinguishing the 2 varieties. Initial treatment with intravenous diazepam is usually helpful regardless of the type of status epilepticus, but phenytoin, phenobarbital, carbamazepine, and other drugs may also be needed to obtain and maintain control in complex partial status epilepticus.

Berkovic SF et al: Progressive myoclonus epilepsies: Specific causes and diagnosis. N Engl J Med 1986;315:296.

Callaghan N, Garrett A, Goggin T: Withdrawal of anticonvulsant drugs in patients free of seizures for two years: A prospective study. N Engl J Med 1988;318:942. (Factors affecting prognosis.)

Lowenstein DH, Aminoff MJ, Simon RP: Barbiturate anesthesia in the treatment of status epilepticus: Clinical experience with 14 patients. Neurology 1988;38:395. (When standard pharmacologic maneuvers fail.)

Mattson RH et al: Comparison of carbamazepine, phenobarbital, phenytoin, and primidone in partial and secondarily generalized tonic-clonic seizures. N Engl J Med 1985; 313:145.

NEUROLOGIC CAUSES OF SYNCOPE

The term syncope refers to transient loss of consciousness resulting from pancerebral hypoperfusion. The clinical features and certain general causes of syncope are discussed in detail in Chapter 8, and only the neurologic causes are considered here.

Syncope may occur because of orthostatic (postural) hypotension, which occurs in a variety of neurologic contexts when the baroreceptor reflex arc is interrupted. Spinal cord transection and other myelopathies (eg, due to tumor or syringomyelia) above the T6 level may lead to marked postural hypotension, as also do brain stem lesions such as syringobulbia and posterior fossa tumors. Postural hypotension is occasionally found in neurosyphilis (tabes dorsalis) and is a frequent and conspicuous complication of diabetic neuropathy. Other polyneuropathies associated with orthostatic hypotension include Guillain-Barré syndrome, primary amyloidosis, acute porphyric neuropathy, and that associated with carcinoma. An acute or subacute autonomic neuropathy may also develop on an autoimmune basis.

Primary degenerative disorders of the central nervous system may lead to dysautonomia occurring in isolation (primary autonomic failure) or in association with more widespread neurologic abnormalities (multisystem atrophy) that may include parkinsonian, pyramidal, lower motor neuron, and cerebellar deficits.

SENSORY DISTURBANCES

Patients may complain of either lost or abnormal sensations. The term ''numbness'' is often used by patients to denote loss of feeling, but the word also has other meanings and the patient's intention must be clarified. Abnormal spontaneous sensations are generally called paresthesias, and unpleasant or painful sensations produced by a stimulus that is usually painless are called dysesthesias.

Sensory symptoms may be due to disease located anywhere along the peripheral or central sensory pathways. The character, site, mode of onset, spread, and temporal profile of sensory symptoms must be established and any precipitating or relieving factors identified. These features—and the presence of any associated symptoms—help identify the origin of sensory disturbances, as do the physical signs as well. Sensory symptoms or signs may conform to the territory of individual peripheral nerves or nerve roots. Involvement of one side of the body—or of one limb in its entirety—suggests a central lesion. Distal involvement of all 4 extremities suggests polyneuropathy, a cervical cord or brain stem lesion, or—when symptoms are transient—a metabolic disturbance such as hyperventilation syndrome. Short-lived sensory complaints may be indicative of sensory seizures or cerebral ischemic phenomena as well as metabolic disturbances. In patients with cord lesions, there may be a transverse sensory level. ''Dissociated sensory loss'' is characterized by loss of some sensory modalities with preservation of others. Such findings may be encountered in patients with either peripheral or central disease and must therefore be interpreted in the clinical context in which they are found.

The absence of sensory signs in patients with sensory symptoms does not mean that symptoms have a nonorganic basis. Symptoms are often troublesome before signs of sensory dysfunction have had time to develop.

WEAKNESS & PARALYSIS

Loss of muscle power may result from central disease involving the upper or lower motor neurons; from peripheral disease involving the roots, plexus, or peripheral nerves; from disorders of neuromuscular transmission; or from primary disorders of muscle. The clinical findings help to localize the lesion and thus reduce the number of diagnostic possibilities.

Weakness due to upper motor neuron lesions is characterized by selective involvement of certain muscle groups and is associated with spasticity, increased tendon reflexes, and extensor plantar responses. The site of upper motor neuron (pyramidal) involvement may be indicated by the presence of other clinical signs or by the distribution of the motor deficit. Lower motor neuron lesions lead to muscle wasting as well as weakness, with flaccidity and loss of tendon reflexes, but no change in the plantar responses unless the neurons subserving them are directly involved. Fasciculations may be evident over affected muscles. In distinguishing between a root, plexus, or peripheral nerve lesion, the distribution of the motor deficit and of any sensory changes is of particular importance. In patients with disturbances of neuromuscular transmission, weakness is patchy in distribution, often fluctuates over short periods of time, and is not associated with sensory changes. In myopathic disorders, weakness is usually most marked proximally in the limbs, is not associated with sensory loss or sphincter disturbance, and is not accompanied by muscle wasting or loss of tendon reflexes—at least not until an advanced stage.

TRANSIENT ISCHEMIC ATTACKS

Essentials of Diagnosis
- Risk factors for vascular disease often present.
- Focal neurologic deficit of acute onset.
- Clinical deficit resolves completely within 24 hours.

General Considerations
Transient ischemic attacks are characterized by focal ischemic cerebral neurologic deficits that last for less than 24 hours (usually less than 1–2 hours). About 30% of patients with stroke have a history of transient ischemic attacks, and proper treatment of the attacks is an important means of prevention. The incidence of stroke does not relate to either the number or the duration of individual attacks but is increased in patients with hypertension or diabetes.

Etiology
An important cause of transient cerebral ischemia is embolization. In many patients with these attacks, a source is readily apparent in the heart or a major extracranial artery to the head, and emboli sometimes are visible in the retinal arteries. Moreover, an embolic phenomenon explains why separate attacks may affect different parts of the territory supplied by the same major vessel. Cardiac causes of embolic ischemic attacks include rheumatic heart disease, mitral valve disease, cardiac arrhythmia, infective endocarditis, atrial myxoma, and mural thrombi complicating myocardial infarction. Atrial septal defects and patent foramen ovale may permit emboli from the veins to reach the brain (''paradoxical emboli''). An ulcerated plaque on a major artery to the brain may serve as a source of emboli. In the anterior circulation, atherosclerotic changes occur most commonly in the region of the carotid bifurcation extracranially, and these changes may cause a bruit. In some patients with transient ischemic attacks or strokes, an acute or recent hemorrhage is found to have occurred into this atherosclerotic plaque, and this finding may have pathologic significance. Patients with AIDS have an increased risk of developing transient ischemic deficits or strokes.

Other (less common) abnormalities of blood vessels that may cause transient ischemic attacks include fibromuscular dysplasia, which affects particularly the cervical internal carotid artery; inflammatory arterial disorders such as giant cell arteritis, systemic lupus erythematosus, polyarteritis, and granulomatous angiitis; and meningovascular syphilis. Hypotension may cause a reduction of cerebral blood flow if a major extracranial artery to the brain is markedly stenosed, but this is a rare cause of transient ischemic attack.

Hematologic causes of ischemic attacks include polycythemia, sickle cell disease, and hyperviscosity syndromes. Severe anemia may also lead to transient focal neurologic deficits in patients with preexisting cerebral arterial disease.

The **subclavian steal syndrome** may lead to transient vertebrobasilar ischemia. Symptoms develop when there is localized stenosis or occlusion of one subclavian artery proximal to the source of the vertebral artery, so that blood is ''stolen'' from this artery. A bruit in the supraclavicular fossa, unequal radial pulses, and a difference of 20 mm Hg or more between the systolic blood pressures in the arms should suggest the diagnosis in patients with vertebrobasilar transient ischemic attacks.

Clinical Findings
A. Symptoms and Signs: The symptoms of transient ischemic attacks vary markedly among patients; however, the symptoms in a given individual tend to be constant in type. Onset is abrupt and without warning, and recovery usually occurs rapidly, often within a few minutes.

If the ischemia is in the carotid territory, common symptoms are weakness and heaviness of the contralateral arm, leg, or face, singly or in any combination. Numbness or paresthesias may also occur either as the sole manifestation of the attack or in combination with the motor deficit. There may be slowness of movement, dysphasia, or monocular visual loss in the eye contralateral to affected limbs. During an attack, examination may reveal flaccid weakness with pyramidal distribution, sensory changes, hyperreflexia or an extensor plantar response on the affected side, dysphasia, or any combination of these findings. Subsequently, examination reveals no neurologic abnormality, but the presence of a carotid bruit or cardiac abnormality may provide a clue to the cause of symptoms.

Vertebrobasilar ischemic attacks may be characterized by vertigo, ataxia, diplopia, dysarthria, dimness or blurring of vision, perioral numbness and paresthesias, and weakness or sensory complaints on one, both, or alternating sides of the body. These symptoms may occur singly or in any combination. Drop attacks due to bilateral leg weakness, without headache or loss of consciousness, may occur, sometimes in relation to head movements.

The natural history of attacks is variable. Some patients will have a major stroke after only a few attacks, whereas others may have frequent attacks for weeks or months without having a stroke. Attacks may occur intermittently over a long period of time, or they may stop spontaneously. In general, carotid ischemic attacks are more liable than vertebrobasilar ischemic attacks to be followed by stroke.

B. Imaging: CT scan of the head will exclude the possibility of a small cerebral hemorrhage or a cerebral tumor masquerading as a transient ischemic attack. A number of noninvasive techniques, such as ultrasonography, have been developed for studying the cerebral circulation and imaging the major vessels to the head, but they have not replaced arteriography as a means of demonstrating the status of the cerebrovascular system. Accordingly, if findings on CT scan are normal, if there is no cardiac source of embolization, and if age and general condition indicate that the patient is a good operative risk, bilateral carotid arteriography should be undertaken in the further evaluation of carotid ischemic attacks.

C. Laboratory and Other Studies: Clinical and laboratory evaluation must include assessment for hypertension, heart disease, diabetes mellitus, hyperlipidemia, and peripheral vascular disease. It should include complete blood count, fasting blood glucose and serum cholesterol determinations, serologic tests for syphilis, and an ECG and chest x-ray. Echocardiography with bubble contrast is performed if a cardiac source is likely, and blood cultures are obtained if endocarditis is suspected. Holter monitoring is indicated if a transient, paroxysmal disturbance of cardiac rhythm is suspected.

Differential Diagnosis

Focal seizures usually cause abnormal motor or sensory phenomena such as clonic limb movements, paresthesias, or tingling, rather than weakness or loss

of feeling. Symptoms generally spread ("march") up the limb and may lead to a generalized tonic-clonic seizure. The electroencephalogram may help in detecting the epileptogenic source.

Classic migraine is easily recognized by the visual premonitory symptoms, followed by nausea, headache, and photophobia, but less typical cases may be hard to distinguish. The patient's age and medical history (including family history) may be helpful in this regard. Patients with migraine commonly have a history of episodes since adolescence and report that other family members have a similar disorder.

Focal neurologic deficits may occur during periods of hypoglycemia in diabetic patients receiving insulin or oral hypoglycemic agent therapy, and the lack of general hypoglycemic symptoms does not exclude this possibility.

Treatment

When arteriography reveals a surgically accessible lesion on the side appropriate to carotid ischemic attacks and there is relatively little atherosclerosis elsewhere in the cerebrovascular system, operative treatment (carotid thromboendarterectomy) may be appropriate, especially when transient ischemic attacks are of recent onset (< 2 months). When more extensive atherosclerotic disease is angiographically evident in the cerebral circulation, the benefits of surgery are less clear.

In patients with carotid ischemic attacks who are poor operative candidates (and thus have not undergone arteriography) or who are found to have extensive vascular disease, medical treatment should be instituted. Similarly, patients with vertebrobasilar ischemic attacks are treated medically and are not subjected to arteriography unless there is clinical evidence of stenosis or occlusion in the carotid or subclavian arteries.

Medical treatment is aimed at preventing further attacks and stroke. Cigarette smoking should be stopped, and cardiac sources of embolization, hypertension, diabetes, hyperlipidemia, arteritis, or hematologic disorders should be treated appropriately. If anticoagulants are indicated for the treatment of embolism from the heart, they should be started immediately, provided there is no contraindication to their use. There is no advantage in delay, and the common fear of causing hemorrhage into a previously infarcted area is misplaced, since there is a far greater risk of further embolism to the cerebral circulation if treatment is withheld. Treatment is initiated with intravenous heparin while warfarin sodium is introduced.

In patients with presumed or angiographically verified atherosclerotic changes in the extracranial or intracranial cerebrovascular circulation, antithrombotic medication is prescribed. The treatment selected will depend upon the patient's age, the likelihood of compliance in taking the drug, and the ready availability of medical and laboratory services. Some physicians use anticoagulant drugs (eg, warfarin, with temporary heparinization until the dose of warfarin is adequate) unless they are medically contraindicated, continuing them for 3–6 months before they are tapered and ultimately replaced with aspirin or, in women, dipyridamole, which is continued for another year. However, there is no convincing evidence that anticoagulant drugs are of value. Other physicians therefore prefer aspirin, dipyridamole, or both, from the onset.

The evidence supporting a therapeutic role for aspirin and other agents that suppress platelet aggregation is increasing. Platelets adhere to and aggregate around an atherosclerotic plaque and release various substances including thromboxane A_2. One study found that treatment with aspirin significantly reduces the frequency of transient ischemic attacks and the incidence of stroke or death in men. A number of others in which different doses of aspirin were used similarly suggest a beneficial effect and agree that men and women respond differently to treatment. Nevertheless, other investigators have demonstrated therapeutic responses in patients of either sex. The optimal daily dose remains to be established, but 1–4 aspirin tablets (325 mg) is currently recommended. Studies of low-dose aspirin therapy (325 mg or less daily) are in progress. Dipyridamole added to aspirin does not offer any advantage over aspirin alone for stroke prevention, but it may itself have some effect in preventing vascular disease, perhaps by enhancing the production of prostacyclin (which has antithrombotic activities) in the vessel wall.

In recent years, many patients with transient ischemic attacks associated with stenotic lesions of the distal internal carotid or the proximal middle cerebral arteries have undergone surgical extracranial-intracranial arterial anastomosis. However, the indications for such surgery are unclear, and no benefit of surgical treatment could be demonstrated in a large controlled prospective study.

ANA Committee on Health Care Issues: Does carotid endarterectomy decrease stroke and death in patients with transient ischemic attacks? Ann Neurol 1987;22:72.

Engstrom JW, Lowenstein DH, Bredesen DE: Cerebral infarctions and transient neurologic deficits associated with acquired immunodeficiency syndrome. Am J Med 1988;38:677.

Grotta JC: Current medical and surgical therapy for cerebrovascular disease. N Engl J Med 1987;317:1505.

Werdelin L, Juhler M: The course of transient ischemic attacks. Neurology 1988;38:677.

STROKE

Essentials of Diagnosis

- Sudden onset of characteristic neurologic deficit.
- Patient often has history of hypertension, diabetes mellitus, valvular heart disease, or atherosclerosis.

- Distinctive neurologic signs reflect the region of the brain involved.

General Considerations

In the USA, stroke remains the third leading cause of death, despite a general decline in the incidence of stroke in the last 30 years. The precise reasons for this decline are uncertain, but increased awareness of risk factors (hypertension, diabetes, hyperlipidemia, cigarette smoking, cardiac disease, heavy alcohol consumption, family history of stroke) and improved prophylactic measures and surveillance of those at increased risk have been contributory. A previous stroke makes individual patients more susceptible to further strokes.

For years, strokes have been subdivided pathologically into infarcts (thrombotic or embolic) and hemorrhages, and clinical criteria for distinguishing between these possibilities have been emphasized. However, it is often difficult to determine on clinical grounds the pathologic basis for stroke.

1. LACUNAR INFARCTION

Lacunar infarcts are among the most common cerebral vascular lesions. They are small infarcts (usually <5 mm in diameter) that occur in the distribution of short penetrating arterioles in the basal ganglia, pons, cerebellum, anterior limb of the internal capsule, and, less commonly, the deep cerebral white matter. Lacunar infarcts may be associated with poorly controlled hypertension or diabetes and have been found in conjunction with several clinical syndromes, including contralateral pure motor or pure sensory deficit, ipsilateral ataxia with crural paresis, and dysarthria with clumsiness of the hand. The neurologic deficit may progress over 24–36 hours before stabilizing.

Lacunar infarcts are sometimes visible on CT scans as small, punched-out, hypodense areas, but in other patients no abnormality is seen. In some instances, patients with a clinical syndrome suggestive of lacunar infarction are found on CT scanning to have a severe hemispheric infarct.

The prognosis for recovery from the deficit produced by a lacunar infarct is usually good, with partial or complete resolution occurring over the following 4–6 weeks in many instances.

2. CEREBRAL INFARCTION

Thrombotic or embolic occlusion of a major vessel leads to cerebral infarction. Causes include the disorders predisposing to transient ischemic attacks (see above) and atherosclerosis of cerebral arteries. The resulting deficit depends upon the particular vessel involved and the extent of any collateral circulation.

Cerebral ischemia leads to release of excitatory and other neuropeptides that may augment calcium flux into neurons, thereby leading to cell death and increasing the neurologic deficit.

Clinical Findings

A. Symptoms and Signs: Onset is usually abrupt, and there may then be very little progression except that due to brain swelling. Clinical evaluation always includes examination of the heart and auscultation over the subclavian and carotid vessels to determine whether there are any bruits.

1. Obstruction of carotid circulation—Occlusion of the ophthalmic artery is probably symptomless in most cases because of the rich orbital collaterals, but its transient embolic obstruction leads to amaurosis fugax—sudden and brief loss of vision in one eye.

Occlusion of the anterior cerebral artery distal to its junction with the anterior communicating artery causes weakness and cortical sensory loss in the contralateral leg and sometimes mild weakness of the arm, especially proximally. There may be a contralateral grasp reflex, paratonic rigidity, and abulia (lack of initiative) or frank confusion. Urinary incontinence is not uncommon, particularly if behavioral disturbances are conspicuous. Bilateral anterior cerebral infarction is especially likely to cause marked behavioral changes and memory disturbances. Unilateral anterior cerebral artery occlusion proximal to the junction with the anterior communicating artery is generally well tolerated because of the collateral supply from the other side.

Middle cerebral artery occlusion leads to contralateral hemiplegia, hemisensory loss, and homonymous hemianopia (ie, bilaterally symmetric loss of vision in half of the visual fields), with the eyes deviated to the side of the lesion. If the dominant hemisphere is involved, global aphasia is also present. It may be impossible to distinguish this clinically from occlusion of the internal carotid artery. With occlusion of either of these arteries, there may also be considerable swelling of the hemisphere, leading to drowsiness, stupor, and coma in extreme cases. Occlusions of different branches of the middle cerebral artery cause more limited findings. For example, involvement of the anterior main division leads to a predominantly expressive dysphasia and to contralateral paralysis and loss of sensations in the arm, the face, and to a lesser extent, the leg. Posterior branch occlusion produces a receptive (Wernicke's) aphasia and a homonymous visual field defect. With involvement of the nondominant hemisphere, speech and comprehension are preserved, but there may be a confusional state, dressing apraxia, and constructional and spatial deficits.

2. Obstruction of vertebrobasilar circulation—Occlusion of the posterior cerebral artery may lead to a thalamic syndrome in which contralateral hemisensory disturbance occurs, followed by the development of spontaneous pain and hyperpathia. There is often a macular-sparing homonymous hemianopia and sometimes a mild, usually temporary, hemiparesis. Depending on the site of the lesion and the collateral circulation, the severity of these deficits varies and other deficits may also occur, including involuntary movements and alexia. Occlusion of the main artery beyond the origin of its penetrating branches may lead solely to a macular-sparing hemianopia.

Vertebral artery occlusion distally, below the origin of the anterior spinal and posterior inferior cerebellar arteries, may be clinically silent because the circulation is maintained by the other vertebral artery. If the remaining vertebral artery is congenitally small or severely atherosclerotic, however, a deficit similar to that of basilar artery occlusion is seen unless there is good collateral circulation from the anterior circulation through the circle of Willis. When the small paramedian arteries arising from the vertebral artery are occluded, contralateral hemiplegia and sensory deficit occur in association with an ipsilateral cranial nerve palsy at the level of the lesion. An obstruction of the posterior inferior cerebellar artery or an obstruction of the vertebral artery just before it branches to this vessel leads ipsilaterally to spinothalamic sensory loss involving the face, ninth and tenth cranial nerve lesions, limb ataxia and numbness, and Horner's syndrome, combined with contralateral spinothalamic sensory loss involving the limbs.

Occlusion of both vertebral arteries or the basilar artery leads to coma with pinpoint pupils, flaccid quadriplegia and sensory loss, and variable cranial nerve abnormalities. With partial basilar artery occlusion, there may be diplopia, visual loss, vertigo, dysarthria, ataxia, weakness or sensory disturbances in some or all of the limbs, and discrete cranial nerve palsies. In patients with hemiplegia of pontine origin, the eyes are often deviated to the paralyzed side, whereas in patients with a hemispheric lesion, the eyes commonly deviate from the hemiplegic side.

Occlusion of any of the major cerebellar arteries produces vertigo, nausea, vomiting, nystagmus, ipsilateral limb ataxia, and contralateral spinothalamic sensory loss in the limbs. If the superior cerebellar artery is involved, the contralateral spinothalamic loss also involves the face; with occlusion of the anterior inferior cerebellar artery, there is ipsilateral spinothalamic sensory loss involving the face, usually in conjunction with ipsilateral facial weakness and deafness. Massive cerebellar infarction may lead to coma, tonsillar herniation, and death.

3. Coma—Infarction in either the carotid or vertebrobasilar territory may lead to loss of consciousness. For example, an infarct involving one cerebral hemisphere may lead to such swelling that the function of the other hemisphere or the rostral brain stem is disturbed and coma results. Similarly, coma occurs with bilateral brain stem infarction when this involves the reticular formation, and it occurs with brain stem compression after cerebellar infarction.

B. Imaging: Radiography of the chest may reveal cardiomegaly or valvular calcification; the presence of a neoplasm would suggest that the neurologic deficit is due to metastasis rather than stroke. A CT scan of the head is important in excluding cerebral hemorrhage, but it may not permit distinction between a cerebral infarct and tumor.

C. Laboratory and Other Studies: Investigations should include a complete blood count, sedimentation rate, blood glucose determination, and serologic tests for syphilis. Electrocardiography will help exclude a cardiac arrhythmia or recent myocardial infarction that might be serving as a source of embolization. Blood cultures should be performed if endocarditis is suspected, echocardiography if heart disease is suspected, and Holter monitoring if paroxysmal cardiac arrhythmia requires exclusion. Examination of the cerebrospinal fluid is not always necessary but may be helpful if there is diagnostic uncertainty; it should be delayed until after CT scanning.

Treatment

If the neurologic deficit progresses over the following minutes or hours, heparinization may be of value in limiting or arresting further deterioration. Since the signs of progressing stroke may be simulated by an intracerebral hematoma, the latter must be excluded by immediate CT scanning or angiography before the patient is heparinized.

Early management of a completed stroke consists of attention to general supportive measures. During the acute stage, there may be marked brain swelling and edema, with symptoms and signs of increasing intracranial pressure, an increasing neurologic deficit, or herniation syndrome. Corticosteroids have been prescribed in an attempt to reduce vasogenic cerebral edema. Prednisone (up to 100 mg/d) or dexamethasone (16 mg/d) has been used, but the evidence that corticosteroids are of any benefit is conflicting. Dehydrating hyperosmolar agents have also been prescribed in efforts to reduce brain swelling, but there is little evidence of any lasting benefit. Likewise, clinical benefit from treatment with vasodilators such as papaverine is minimal. Neither hypercapnia nor hypocapnia has been shown to have any benefit. Barbiturates are known to decrease neuronal metabolism and energy requirements and have been reported to improve functional recovery in experimental stroke models; their use in humans, however, is experimental. Attempts to lower the blood pressure of hypertensive patients during the acute phase of a stroke should be avoided, since there is loss of cerebral autoregulation and lowering the blood pressure may further compromise ischemic areas.

Anticoagulant drugs have no role in the management of patients with a completed stroke, except when there is a cardiac source of embolization. Treatment is then started with intravenous heparin while warfarin is introduced. If the CT scan shows no evidence of hemorrhage and the cerebrospinal fluid is clear, anticoagulant treatment may be started without delay. Many physicians, however, prefer to wait for about 3–5 days (to reduce any risk of cerebral hemorrhage) before initiating anticoagulant treatment; the CT scan is then repeated and anticoagulant therapy is initiated if it again shows no evidence of hemorrhagic transformation.

Preliminary studies suggest that calcium channel blocking drugs such as nimodipine may reduce the deficit produced by cerebral ischemia and the morbidity and mortality rates from stroke. Multicenter studies are now in progress to study further the effects of these agents in acute cerebral ischemia.

Blockage of glutamate, an excitatory neurotransmitter, reduces the sensitivity of central neurons to ischemia. The N-methyl-D-aspartate (NMDA) type of glutamate receptors are linked to calcium-permeable channels, and studies in animals have shown that specific NMDA-receptor antagonists reduce stroke size, deficits, and the percentage of severely ischemic neurons. The role of this therapeutic approach in humans is currently under study.

The role, if any, of tissue plasminogen activator as a means of providing thrombolytic therapy for acute stroke is also currently the subject of clinical trials.

Physical therapy has an important role in the management of patients with impaired motor function. Passive movements at an early stage will help prevent contractures. As cooperation increases and some recovery begins, active movements will improve strength and coordination. In all cases, early mobilization and active rehabilitation are important. Occupational therapy may improve morale and motor skills, while speech therapy may be beneficial in patients with expressive dysphasia or dysarthria. When there is a severe and persisting motor deficit, a device such as a leg brace, toe spring, frame, or cane may help the patient move about, and the provision of other aids to daily living may improve the quality of life.

Prognosis

The prognosis for survival after cerebral infarction is better than after cerebral or subarachnoid hemorrhage. Loss of consciousness after a cerebral infarct implies a poorer prognosis than otherwise. The extent of the infarct governs the potential for rehabilitation. Patients who have had a cerebral infarct are at risk for further strokes and for myocardial infarcts.

Choi DW: Calcium-mediated neurotoxicity: Relationship to specific channel types and role in ischemic damage. Trends Neurosci 1988;11:465.

Gelmers HJ et al: A controlled trial of nimodipine in acute ischemic stroke. N Engl J Med 1988; 318:203. (May be improved by early therapy.)

Halperin JL, Hart RG: Atrial fibrillation and stroke: New ideas, persisting dilemmas. Stroke 1988;19:937. (Review of prognosis in different patient subgroups and of therapeutic controversies.)

Kochhar A et al: Glutamate antagonist therapy reduces neurologic deficits produced by focal central nervous system ischemia. Arch Neurol 1988; 45:148. (Effect of an NMDA receptor antagonist on cerebral and spinal ischemic models.)

Welin L et al: Analysis of risk factors for stroke in a cohort of men born in 1913. N Engl J Med 1987;317:521.

Yatsu FM et al: Anticoagulation of embolic strokes of cardiac origin: An update. Neurology 1988;38:314.

Zivin JA et al: Tissue plasminogen activator: Reduction of neurologic damage after experimental embolic stroke. Arch Neurol 1988; 45:387. (Studies in animals suggest a therapeutic role.)

3. INTRACEREBRAL HEMORRHAGE

Spontaneous intracerebral hemorrhage in patients with no angiographic evidence of an associated vascular anomaly (eg, aneurysm or angioma) is usually due to hypertension. The pathologic basis for hemorrhage is probably the presence of microaneurysms that are now known to develop on perforating vessels of 100–300 μm in diameter in hypertensive patients. Hypertensive intracerebral hemorrhage occurs most frequently in the basal ganglia and less commonly in the pons, thalamus, cerebellum, and cerebral white matter. Hemorrhage may extend into the ventricular system or subarachnoid space, and signs of meningeal irritation are then found. Hemorrhages usually occur suddenly and without warning, often during activity.

In addition to its association with hypertension, nontraumatic intracerebral hemorrhage may occur with hematologic and bleeding disorders (eg, leukemia, thrombocytopenia, hemophilia, or disseminated intravascular coagulation), anticoagulant therapy, liver disease, cerebral amyloid angiopathy, and primary or secondary brain tumors. Bleeding is primarily into the subarachnoid space when it occurs from an intracranial aneurysm or arteriovenous malformation (see below), but it may be partly intraparenchymal as well. In some cases, no specific cause for cerebral hemorrhage can be identified.

Clinical Findings
A. Symptoms and Signs: With hemorrhage into the cerebral hemisphere, consciousness is initially lost or impaired in about one-half of patients. Vomiting occurs very frequently at the onset of bleeding, and headache is sometimes present. Focal symptoms and signs then develop, depending on the site of the hemorrhage. With hypertensive hemorrhage, there is generally a rapidly evolving neurologic deficit with hemiplegia or hemiparesis. A hemisensory disturbance is also present with more deeply placed lesions. With lesions of the putamen, loss of conjugate lateral

gaze may be conspicuous. With thalamic hemorrhage, there may be a loss of upward gaze, downward or skew deviation of the eyes, lateral gaze palsies, and pupillary inequalities.

Cerebellar hemorrhage may present with sudden onset of nausea and vomiting, disequilibrium, headache, and loss of consciousness that may terminate fatally within 48 hours. Less commonly, the onset is gradual and the course episodic or slowly progressive—clinical features suggesting an expanding cerebellar lesion. In yet other cases, however, the onset and course are intermediate, and examination shows lateral conjugate gaze palsies to the side of the lesion; small reactive pupils; contralateral hemiplegia; peripheral facial weakness; ataxia of gait, limbs, or trunk; periodic respiration; or some combination of these findings.

B. Imaging: CT scanning is important not only in confirming that hemorrhage has occurred but also in determining the size and site of the hematoma. If the patient's condition permits further intervention, cerebral angiography may be undertaken thereafter to determine if an aneurysm or arteriovenous malformation is present (see below).

C. Laboratory and Other Studies: A complete blood count, platelet count, bleeding time, prothrombin and partial thromboplastin times, and liver function tests may reveal a predisposing cause for the hemorrhage. Lumbar puncture is contraindicated because it may precipitate a herniation syndrome in patients with a large hematoma, and CT scanning is superior in detecting intracerebral hemorrhage.

Treatment
Neurologic management is generally conservative and supportive, regardless of whether the patient has a profound deficit with associated brain stem compression, in which case the prognosis is grim, or a more localized deficit not causing increased intracranial pressure or brain stem involvement. In patients with cerebellar hemorrhage, however, prompt surgical evacuation of the hematoma is appropriate, because spontaneous unpredictable deterioration may otherwise lead to a fatal outcome and because operative treatment may lead to complete resolution of the clinical deficit. The treatment of underlying structural lesions or bleeding disorders depends upon their nature.

Caplan L: Intracerebral hemorrhage revisited. (Editorial.) Neurology 1988;38:624.

4. SUBARACHNOID HEMORRHAGE

Between 5% and 10% of strokes are due to subarachnoid hemorrhage. Although hemorrhage is usually from rupture of an aneurysm or arteriovenous malformation, no specific cause can be found in 20% of cases.

Clinical Findings

A. Symptoms and Signs: Subarachnoid hemorrhage has a characteristic clinical picture. Its onset is with sudden headache of a severity never experienced previously by the patient. This may be followed by nausea and vomiting and by a loss or impairment of consciousness that can either be transient or progress inexorably to deepening coma and death. If consciousness is regained, the patient is often confused and irritable and may show other symptoms of an altered mental status. Neurologic examination generally reveals nuchal rigidity and other signs of meningeal irritation, except in deeply comatose patients. A focal neurologic deficit is occasionally present and may suggest the site of the underlying lesion.

B. Imaging: A CT scan should be performed immediately to confirm that hemorrhage has occurred and to search for clues regarding its source. Findings sometimes are normal in patients with suspected hemorrhage, and the cerebrospinal fluid must then be examined before the possibility of subarachnoid hemorrhage is discounted.

Cerebral arteriography may be undertaken to determine the source of bleeding; it is not performed unless or until the patient's condition has stabilized and is good enough so that operative treatment is feasible. In general, bilateral carotid and vertebral arteriography are necessary because aneurysms are often multiple, while arteriovenous malformations may be supplied from several sources.

Treatment

The medical management of patients is important. The measures outlined on p 711 must be applied to comatose patients. Conscious patients are confined to bed, advised against any exertion or straining, treated symptomatically for headache and anxiety, and given laxatives or stool softeners to prevent straining. If there is severe hypertension, the blood pressure can be lowered gradually, but not below a diastolic level of 100 mm Hg. Phenytoin is generally prescribed routinely to prevent seizures. Further comment concerning the specific operative management of arteriovenous malformations and aneurysms follows.

5. INTRACRANIAL ANEURYSM

Saccular aneurysms ("berry" aneurysms) tend to occur at arterial bifurcations, are considerably more common in adults than in children, are frequently multiple (20% of cases), and are usually asymptomatic. They may be associated with polycystic kidney disease and coarctation of the aorta. Most aneurysms are located on the anterior part of the circle of Willis—particularly on the anterior or posterior communicating arteries, at the bifurcation of the middle cerebral artery, and at the bifurcation of the internal carotid artery.

Clinical Findings

A. Symptoms and Signs: Aneurysms may cause a focal neurologic deficit by compressing adjacent structures. However, most are asymptomatic or produce only nonspecific symptoms until they rupture, at which time subarachnoid hemorrhage results. There is often a paucity of focal neurologic signs in patients with subarachnoid hemorrhage, but when present, such signs may relate either to a focal hematoma or to ischemia in the territory of the vessel with the ruptured aneurysm. Hemiplegia or other focal deficit sometimes occurs after a delay of 4–14 days and is due to focal arterial spasm in the vicinity of the ruptured aneurysm. This spasm is of uncertain, probably multifactorial, cause, but it sometimes leads to significant cerebral ischemia or infarction, and it may further aggravate any existing increase in intracranial pressure. Subacute hydrocephalus due to interference with the flow of cerebrospinal fluid may occur after 2 or more weeks, and this leads to a delayed clinical deterioration that is relieved by shunting.

In some patients, "warning leaks" of a small amount of blood from the aneurysm precede the major hemorrhage by a few hours or days. They lead to headaches, sometimes accompanied by nausea and neck stiffness, but the true cause of these symptoms is often not appreciated until massive hemorrhage occurs.

B. Imaging: The CT scan generally confirms that subarachnoid hemorrhage has occurred, but occasionally it is normal. Angiography (bilateral carotid and vertebral studies) generally indicates the size and site of the lesion, sometimes reveals multiple aneurysms, and may show arterial spasm. If subarachnoid hemorrhage is confirmed by lumbar puncture or CT scanning but arteriograms show no abnormality, the examination should be repeated after 2 weeks, because vasospasm may have prevented detection of an aneurysm during the initial study.

C. Laboratory and Other Studies: The cerebrospinal fluid is bloodstained. The electroencephalogram sometimes indicates the side or site of hemorrhage but frequently shows only a diffuse abnormality. Electrocardiographic evidence of arrhythmias or myocardial ischemia has been well described and probably relates to excessive sympathetic activity. Peripheral leukocytosis and transient glycosuria are also common findings.

Treatment

The major aim of treatment is to prevent further hemorrhages. Definitive treatment requires a surgical approach to the aneurysm and ideally consists of clipping of its base. If surgery is not feasible, medical management as outlined above for subarachnoid hemorrhage is continued for about 6 weeks and is followed by gradual mobilization.

Although the operative morbidity and mortality rates are decreased by delaying surgery for at least

10 days after the hemorrhage, the risk of further hemorrhage is greatest within a few days of the first hemorrhage; approximately 20% of patients will have further bleeding within 2 weeks and 40% within 6 months. Attempts have been made to reduce this risk pharmacologically. Since antifibrinolytic drugs prevent lysis of any blood clot that has formed near the site of rupture, aminocaproic acid (Amicar) is often given for the first 2 weeks or so, or until surgery, to reduce the incidence of early recurrence of bleeding. The daily dose is 24–36 g (5 g initially, followed by 1–1.25 g hourly) given intravenously for the first week and then orally, while the streptokinase clot lysis time is monitored. Potential complications include venous thrombosis, pulmonary embolism, and ischemic focal neurologic deficits. Recent studies indicate that this approach may indeed lower the incidence of recurrent bleeding but that it is associated with such an increase in cerebral ischemic complications that the mortality rate and the degree of disability among survivors are unchanged. Thus, early operation (ie, within about 2 days of hemorrhage) is preferred for good operative candidates.

There is currently no specific treatment for cerebral vasospasm, but calcium channel-blocking agents have helped to reduce or reverse experimental vasospasm, and nimodipine has been shown to reduce, in neurologically normal patients, the incidence of ischemic deficits from arterial spasm without producing any side effects. The dose of nimodipine is 60 mg every 4 hours for 21 days.

With regard to unruptured aneurysms, those that are symptomatic merit prompt surgical treatment, whereas small asymptomatic ones discovered incidentally are often followed arteriographically and corrected surgically only if they increase in size to over 5 mm. The natural history of unruptured aneurysms is not clearly defined.

Disney L, Weir B, Petruk K: Effect on management-mortality of a deliberate policy of early operation on supratentorial aneurysms. Neurosurgery 1987;20:695.

Pickard JD et al: Effect of oral nimodipine on cerebral infarction and outcome following subarachnoid haemorrhage. Br Med J 1989;298:636.

6. ARTERIOVENOUS MALFORMATIONS

Arteriovenous malformations are congenital vascular malformations that result from a localized maldevelopment of part of the primitive vascular plexus and consist of abnormal arteriovenous communications without intervening capillaries. They vary in size, ranging from massive lesions that are fed by multiple vessels and involve a large part of the brain to lesions so small that they are hard to identify at arteriography, surgery, or autopsy. In approximately 10% of cases, there is an associated arterial aneurysm, while 1–2% of patients presenting with aneurysms have associated arteriovenous malformations. Clinical presentation may relate to hemorrhage from the malformation or an associated aneurysm or may relate to cerebral ischemia due to diversion of blood by the anomalous arteriovenous shunt or due to venous stagnation. Regional maldevelopment of the brain, compression or distortion of adjacent cerebral tissue by enlarged anomalous vessels, and progressive gliosis due to mechanical and ischemic factors may also be contributory. In addition, communicating or obstructive hydrocephalus may occur and lead to symptoms.

Clinical Findings

A. Symptoms and Signs:

1. Supratentorial lesions–Most cerebral arteriovenous malformations are supratentorial, usually lying in the territory of the middle cerebral artery. Initial symptoms consist of hemorrhage in 30–60% of cases, epilepsy in 20–40%, headache in 5–25%, and miscellaneous complaints (including focal deficits) in 10–15%. Up to 70% of arteriovenous malformations bleed at some point in their natural history, most commonly before the patient reaches the age of 40 years. This tendency to bleed is unrelated to the lesion site or to the patient's sex, but small arteriovenous malformations are more likely to bleed than large ones. Arteriovenous malformations that have bled once are more likely to bleed again. Hemorrhage is commonly intracerebral as well as into the subarachnoid space, and it has a fatal outcome in about 10% of cases. Focal or generalized seizures may accompany or follow hemorrhage, or they may be the initial presentation, especially with frontal or parietal arteriovenous malformations. Headaches are especially likely when the external carotid arteries are involved in the malformation. These sometimes simulate migraine but more commonly are nonspecific in character, with nothing about them to suggest an underlying structural lesion.

In patients presenting with subarachnoid hemorrhage, examination may reveal an abnormal mental status and signs of meningeal irritation. Additional findings may help to localize the lesion and sometimes indicate that intracranial pressure is increased. A cranial bruit always suggests the possibility of a cerebral arteriovenous malformation, but bruits may also be found with aneurysms, meningiomas, acquired arteriovenous fistulas, and arteriovenous malformations involving the scalp, calvarium, or orbit. Bruits are best heard over the ipsilateral eye or mastoid region and are of some help in lateralization but not in localization. Absence of a bruit in no way excludes the possibility of arteriovenous malformation.

2. Infratentorial lesions–Brain stem arteriovenous malformations are often clinically silent, but they may hemorrhage, cause obstructive hydrocephalus, or lead to progressive or relapsing brain stem deficits. Cerebellar arteriovenous malformations may also be clinically inconspicuous but sometimes lead to cerebellar hemorrhage.

B. Imaging: In patients presenting with suspected hemorrhage, CT scanning indicates whether subarachnoid or intracerebral bleeding has recently occurred, helps to localize its source, and may reveal the arteriovenous malformation. If the CT scan shows no evidence of bleeding but subarachnoid hemorrhage is diagnosed clinically, the cerebrospinal fluid should be examined.

When intracranial hemorrhage is confirmed but the source of hemorrhage is not evident on the CT scan, arteriography is necessary to exclude aneurysm or arteriovenous malformation. Even if the findings on CT scan suggest arteriovenous malformation, arteriography is required to establish the nature of the lesion with certainty and to determine its anatomic features so that treatment can be planned. The examination must generally include bilateral opacification of the internal and external carotid arteries and the vertebral arteries. Arteriovenous malformations typically appear as a tangled vascular mass with distended tortuous afferent and efferent vessels, a rapid circulation time, and arteriovenous shunting. Findings on plain radiographs of the skull are often normal unless an intracerebral hematoma is present, in which case there may be changes suggestive of raised intracranial pressure and displacement of a calcified pineal gland.

In patients presenting without hemorrhage, CT scan or MRI usually reveals the underlying abnormality, and MRI frequently also shows evidence of old or recent hemorrhage that may have been asymptomatic. The nature and detailed anatomy of any focal lesion identified by these means is delineated by angiography, especially if operative treatment is under consideration.

C. Laboratory and Other Studies: Electroencephalography is usually indicated in patients presenting with seizures and may show consistently focal or lateralized abnormalities resulting from the underlying cerebral arteriovenous malformation. This should be followed by CT scanning.

Treatment

Surgical treatment to prevent further hemorrhage is justified in patients with arteriovenous malformations that have bled, provided that the lesion is accessible and the patient has a reasonable life expectancy. Surgical treatment is also appropriate if intracranial pressure is increased or if there is cardiac decompensation, as occurs in children, and to prevent further progression of a focal neurologic deficit. In patients presenting solely with seizures, anticonvulsant drug treatment is usually sufficient, and operative treatment is unnecessary unless there are further developments.

Definitive operative treatment consists of excision of the arteriovenous malformation if it is surgically accessible. Arteriovenous malformations that are inoperable because of their location are sometimes treated solely by embolization; although the risk of hemorrhage is not reduced, neurologic deficits may be stabilized or even reversed by this procedure. Two other new techniques for the treatment of intracerebral arteriovenous malformations are injection of a vascular occlusive polymer through a flow-guided microcatheter and permanent occlusion of feeding vessels by positioning detachable balloon catheters in the desired sites and then inflating them with quickly solidifying contrast material. Proton beam therapy may also be useful in the management of inoperable cerebral arteriovenous malformations.

Aminoff MJ: Treatment of unruptured cerebral arteriovenous malformations. Neurology 1987;37:815.
Davis C, Symon L: The management of cerebral arteriovenous malformations. Acta Neurochir 1985;74:4.

7. INTRACRANIAL VENOUS THROMBOSIS

Intracranial venous thrombosis may occur in association with intracranial or maxillofacial infections, hypercoagulable states, polycythemia, sickle cell disease, and cyanotic congenital heart disease and in pregnancy or during the puerperium. It is characterized by headache, focal or generalized convulsions, drowsiness, confusion, increased intracranial pressure, and focal neurologic deficits—and sometimes by evidence of meningeal irritation. The diagnosis is confirmed by CT scanning and MRI or angiography.

Treatment includes anticonvulsant drugs if seizures have occurred and antiedema agents (eg, dexamethasone) to reduce intracranial pressure. The use of anticoagulant drugs is controversial.

Bousser MG et al: Cerebral venous thrombosis: A review of 38 cases. Stroke 1985:16:199.

8. SPINAL CORD VASCULAR DISEASES

Infarction of the Spinal Cord

Infarction of the spinal cord is rare. It occurs only in the territory of the anterior spinal artery because this vessel, which supplies the anterior two-thirds of the cord, is itself supplied by only a limited number of feeders. Infarction usually results from interrupted flow in one or more of these feeders, eg, with aortic dissection, aortography, polyarteritis, or severe hypotension, or after surgical resection of the thoracic aorta. The paired posterior spinal arteries, by contrast, are supplied by numerous arteries at different levels of the cord.

Since the anterior spinal artery receives numerous feeders in the cervical region, infarcts almost always occur more caudally. Clinical presentation is characterized by acute onset of flaccid, areflexive paraplegia that evolves after a few days or weeks into a spastic paraplegia with extensor plantar responses. There is an accompanying dissociated sensory loss, with impairment of appreciation of pain and temperature but preservation of sensations of vibration and position. Treatment is symptomatic.

Epidural or Subdural Hemorrhage

Epidural or subdural hemorrhage may lead to sudden severe back pain followed by an acute compressive myelopathy necessitating urgent myelography and surgical evacuation. It may occur in patients with bleeding disorders or those who are taking anticoagulant drugs, sometimes following trauma or lumbar puncture. Epidural hemorrhage may also be related to a vascular malformation or tumor deposit.

Arteriovenous Malformation of the Spinal Cord

Arteriovenous malformations of the cord are congenital lesions that present with spinal subarachnoid hemorrhage or myeloradiculopathy. Since most of these malformations are located in the thoracolumbar region, they lead to motor and sensory disturbances in the legs and to sphincter disorders. Pain in the legs or back is often severe. Examination reveals an upper, lower, or mixed motor deficit in the legs; sensory deficits are also present and are usually extensive, although occasionally they are confined to radicular distribution. Cervical arteriovenous malformations lead also to symptoms and signs in the arms. Spinal MRI may not detect the arteriovenous malformation, and negative findings do not exclude the diagnosis. In general, the diagnosis is suggested at myelography (performed with the patient prone and supine) when serpiginous filling defects due to enlarged vessels are found. Selective spinal arteriography confirms the diagnosis. Most lesions are extramedullary, are posterior to the cord (lying either intra- or extradurally), and can easily be treated by ligation of feeding vessels and excision of the fistulous anomaly or by embolization procedures. Delay in treatment may lead to increased and irreversible disability or to death from recurrent subarachnoid hemorrhage.

INTRACRANIAL & SPINAL SPACE-OCCUPYING LESIONS

1. PRIMARY INTRACRANIAL TUMORS

Essentials of Diagnosis

- Generalized or focal disturbance of cerebral function, or both.
- Increased intracranial pressure in some patients. Neuroradiologic evidence of space-occupying lesion.

General Considerations

Approximately half of all primary intracranial neoplasms (Table 18–3) are gliomas, and the remainder are meningiomas, pituitary adenomas, neurofibromas, and other tumors. Certain tumors, especially neurofibromas, hemangioblastomas, and retinoblastomas, may have a familial basis, and congenital factors bear on the development of craniopharyngiomas. Tumors may occur at any age, but certain gliomas show particular age predilections (Table 18–3).

Clinical Findings

A. Symptoms and Signs: Intracranial tumors may lead to a generalized disturbance of cerebral function and to symptoms and signs of increased intracranial pressure. In consequence, there may be personality changes, intellectual decline, emotional lability, seizures, headaches, nausea, and malaise. If the pressure is increased in a particular cranial compartment, brain tissue may herniate into a compartment with lower pressure. The most familiar syndrome is herniation of the temporal lobe uncus through the tentorial hiatus, which causes compression of the third cranial nerve, midbrain, and posterior cerebral artery. The earliest sign of this is ipsilateral pupillary dilatation, followed by stupor, coma, decerebrate posturing, and respiratory arrest. Another important herniation syndrome consists of displacement of the cerebellar tonsils through the foramen magnum, which causes medullary compression leading to apnea, circulatory collapse, and death. Other herniation syndromes are less common and of less clear clinical importance.

Intracranial tumors also lead to focal deficits depending on their location.

1. Frontal lobe lesions–Tumors of the frontal lobe often lead to progressive intellectual decline, slowing of mental activity, personality changes, and contralateral grasp reflexes. They may lead to expressive aphasia if the posterior part of the left inferior frontal gyrus is involved. Anosmia may also occur as a consequence of pressure on the olfactory nerve. Precentral lesions may cause focal motor seizures or contralateral pyramidal deficits.

2. Temporal lobe lesions–These lesions may produce a variety of disturbances. Tumors of the uncinate region may be manifested by seizures with olfactory or gustatory hallucinations, motor phenomena such as licking or smacking of the lips, and some impairment of external awareness without actual loss of consciousness. Temporal lobe lesions also lead to depersonalization, emotional changes, behavioral disturbances, sensations of dèjá vu or jamais vu, micropsia or macropsia, visual field defects (crossed upper quadrantanopia), and auditory illusions or hallucinations. Left-sided lesions may lead to dysnomia and receptive aphasia, while right-sided involvement sometimes disturbs the perception of musical notes and melodies.

Table 18–3. Primary intracranial tumors.

Tumor	Clinical Features	Treatment and Prognosis
Glioblastoma multiforme	Presents commonly with nonspecific complaints and increased intracranial pressure. As it grows, focal deficits develop.	Course is rapidly progressive, with poor prognosis. Total surgical removal is usually not possible, and response to radiation therapy is poor.
Astrocytoma	Presentation similar to glioblastoma multiforme but course more protracted, often over several years. Cerebellar astrocytoma, especially in children, may have a more benign course.	Prognosis is variable. By the time of diagnosis, total excision is usually impossible; tumor often is not radiosensitive. In cerebellar astrocytoma, total surgical removal is often possible.
Medulloblastoma	Seen most frequently in children. Generally arises from roof of fourth ventricle and leads to increased intracranial pressure accompanied by brain stem and cerebellar signs. May seed in subarachnoid space.	Treatment consists of surgery combined with radiation therapy and chemotherapy.
Ependymoma	Glioma arising from the ependyma of a ventricle, especially the fourth ventricle; leads early to signs of increased intracranial pressure. Arises also from central canal of cord.	Tumor is not radiosensitive and is best treated surgically if possible.
Oligodendroglioma	Slow-growing. Usually arises in cerebral hemisphere in adults. Calcification may be visible on skull x-ray.	Treatment is surgical, which is usually successful.
Brain stem glioma	Presents during childhood with cranial nerve palsies and then with long-tract signs in the limbs. Signs of increased intracranial pressure occur late.	Tumor is inoperable; treatment is by irradiation and shunt for increased intracranial pressure.
Cerebellar hemangioblastoma	Presents with disequilibrium, ataxia of trunk or limbs, and signs of increased intracranial pressure. Sometimes familial. May be associated with retinal and spinal vascular lesions, polycythemia, and hypernephromas.	Treatment is surgical.
Pineal tumor	Presents with increased intracranial pressure, sometimes associated with impaired upward gaze (Parinaud's syndrome) and other deficits indicative of midbrain lesion.	Ventricular decompression by shunting is followed by surgical approach to tumor; irradiation is indicated if tumor is malignant. Prognosis depends on histopathologic findings and extent of tumor.
Craniopharyngioma	Originates from remnants of Rathke's pouch above the sella, depressing the optic chiasm. May present at any age but usually in childhood, with endocrine dysfunction and bitemporal field defects.	Treatment is surgical, but total removal may not be possible.
Acoustic neurinoma	Ipsilateral hearing loss is most common initial symptom. Subsequent symptoms may include tinnitus, headache, vertigo, facial weakness or numbness, and long-tract signs. (May be familial and bilateral when related to neurofibromatosis.) Most sensitive screening tests are MRI and brain stem auditory evoked potential.	Treatment is excision by translabyrinthine surgery, craniectomy, or a combined approach. Outcome is usually good.
Meningioma	Originates from the dura mater or arachnoid; compresses rather than invades adjacent neural structures. Increasingly common with advancing age. Tumor size varies greatly. Symptoms vary with tumor site—eg, unilateral exophthalmos (sphenoidal ridge); anosmia and optic nerve compression (olfactory groove). Tumor is usually benign and readily detected by CT scanning; may lead to calcification and bone erosion visible on plain x-rays of skull.	Treatment is surgical. Tumor may recur if removal is incomplete.
Primary cerebral lymphoma	Associated with AIDS and other immunodeficient states. Presentation may be with focal deficits or with disturbances of cognition and consciousness. May be indistinguishable from cerebral toxoplasmosis.	Treatment is by whole-brain irradiation; chemotherapy may have an adjunctive role.

3. Parietal lobe lesions–Tumors in this location characteristically cause contralateral disturbances of sensation and may cause sensory seizures, sensory loss or inattention, or some combination of these symptoms. The sensory loss is cortical in type and involves postural sensibility and tactile discrimination, so that the appreciation of shape, size, weight, and texture is impaired. Objects placed in the hand may not be recognized (astereognosis). Extensive parietal lobe lesions may produce contralateral hyperpathia and spontaneous pain (thalamic syndrome). Involvement of the optic radiation leads to a contralateral homonymous field defect that sometimes consists solely of lower quadrantanopia. Lesions of the left angular gyrus cause Gerstmann's syndrome (a combination of alexia, agraphia, acalculia, right-left confusion, and finger agnosia), whereas involvement of the left submarginal gyrus causes ideational apraxia. Anosognosia (the denial, neglect, or rejection of a paralyzed limb) is seen in patients with lesions of the nondominant (right) hemisphere. Constructional apraxia and dressing apraxia may also occur with right-sided lesions.

4. Occipital lobe lesions—Tumors of the occipital lobe characteristically produce crossed homonymous hemianopia or a partial field defect. With left-sided or bilateral lesions, there may be visual agnosia both for objects and for colors, while irritative lesions on either side can cause unformed visual hallucinations. Bilateral occipital lobe involvement causes cortical blindness in which there is preservation of pupillary responses to light and lack of awareness of the defect by the patient. There may also be loss of color perception, prosopagnosia (inability to identify a familiar face), simultagnosia (inability to integrate and interpret a composite scene as opposed to its individual elements), and Balint's syndrome (failure to turn the eyes to a particular point in space, despite preservation of spontaneous and reflex eye movements). The denial of blindness or a field defect constitutes Anton's syndrome.

5. Brain stem and cerebellar lesions—Brain stem lesions lead to cranial nerve palsies, ataxia, incoordination, nystagmus, and pyramidal and sensory deficits in the limbs on one or both sides. Intrinsic brain stem tumors, such as gliomas, tend to produce an increase in intracranial pressure only late in their course. Cerebellar tumors produce marked ataxia of the trunk if the vermis cerebelli is involved and ipsilateral appendicular deficits (ataxia, incoordination and hypotonia of the limbs) if the cerebellar hemispheres are affected.

6. False localizing signs—Tumors may lead to neurologic signs other than by direct compression or infiltration, thereby leading to errors of clinical localization. These false localizing signs include third or sixth nerve palsy produced by herniation syndromes, bilateral extensor plantar responses, and an extensor plantar response occurring ipsilateral to a hemispheric tumor as a result of compression of the opposite cerebral peduncle against the tentorium.

B. Imaging: CT scanning or MRI may detect the lesion and may also define its location, shape, and size; the extent to which normal anatomy is distorted; and the degree of any associated cerebral edema or mass effect. CT scanning is less helpful with tumors in the posterior fossa, but MRI is of particular value there. The characteristic appearance of meningiomas on CT scanning is virtually diagnostic; ie, a lesion in a typical site (parasagittal and sylvian regions, olfactory groove, sphenoidal ridge, tuberculum sellae) that appears as a homogeneous area of increased density in noncontrast CT scans and enhances uniformly with contrast.

Arteriography may show stretching or displacement of normal cerebral vessels by the tumor and the presence of tumor vascularity. The presence of an avascular mass is a nonspecific finding that could be due to tumor, hematoma, abscess, or any space-occupying lesion. In patients with normal hormone levels and an intrasellar mass, angiography is necessary to distinguish with confidence between a pituitary adenoma and an arterial aneurysm.

C. Laboratory and Other Studies: The electroencephalogram provides supporting information concerning cerebral function and may show either a focal disturbance due to the neoplasm or a more diffuse change reflecting altered mental status. Lumbar puncture is rarely necessary; the findings are seldom diagnostic, and the procedure carries the risk of causing a herniation syndrome.

Treatment

Treatment depends on the type and site of the tumor (Table 18–3) and the condition of the patient. Complete surgical removal may be possible if the tumor is extra-axial (eg, meningioma, acoustic neuroma) or is not in a critical or inaccessible region of the brain (eg, cerebellar hemangioblastoma). Surgery also permits the diagnosis to be verified and may be beneficial in reducing intracranial pressure and relieving symptoms even if the neoplasm cannot be completely removed. Clinical deficits are sometimes due in part to obstructive hydrocephalus, in which case simple surgical shunting procedures often produce dramatic benefit. In patients with malignant gliomas, radiation therapy increases median survival rates regardless of any preceding surgery, and its combination with chemotherapy provides additional benefit. Indications for irradiation in the treatment of patients with other primary intracranial neoplasms depend upon tumor type and accessibility and the feasibility of complete surgical removal. Corticosteroids help reduce cerebral edema and are usually started before surgery. Herniation is treated with intravenous dexamethasone and intravenous mannitol (20%). Anticonvulsants are also commonly administered.

Kornblith PL, Walker M: Chemotherapy for malignant gliomas. J Neurosurg 1988;68:1.

Leibel SA, Sheline GE: Radiation therapy for neoplasms of the brain. J Neurosurg 1987;66:1.

2. METASTATIC INTRACRANIAL TUMORS

Cerebral Metastases

Metastatic brain tumors present in the same way as other cerebral neoplasms, ie, with increased intracranial pressure, with focal or diffuse disturbance of cerebral function, or with both of these manifestations. Indeed, in patients with a single cerebral lesion, the metastatic nature of the lesion may only become evident on histopathologic examination. In other patients, there is evidence of widespread metastatic disease, or an isolated cerebral metastasis develops during treatment of the primary neoplasm.

The most common source of intracranial metastasis is carcinoma of the lung; other primary sites are the breast, kidney, and gastrointestinal tract. Most cerebral metastases are located supratentorially. The laboratory and radiologic studies used to evaluate patients with metastases are similar to those described in the preceding section on primary neoplasms. They include MRI and CT scanning performed both with and without contrast material. Lumbar puncture is necessary only in patients with suspected carcinomatous meningitis (see below). In patients with verified cerebral metastasis from an unknown primary, investigation should be guided by symptoms and signs. In women, mammography is regularly indicated; in men, attention should be paid to a possible germ cell origin. Both have therapeutic implications.

In patients with only a single cerebral metastasis who are otherwise well, it may be possible to remove the lesion and then treat with irradiation. Alternatively, irradiation may be selected as the sole means of treatment. In patients with multiple metastases or widespread systemic disease, the long-term outlook is gloomy, and treatment by radiation therapy or chemotherapy is palliative.

Leptomeningeal Metastases (Carcinomatous Meningitis)

The neoplasms metastasizing most commonly to the leptomeninges are carcinoma of the breast, lymphomas, and leukemia. Leptomeningeal metastases lead to multifocal neurologic deficits, which may be associated with infiltration of cranial and spinal nerve roots, direct invasion of the brain or spinal cord, obstructive hydrocephalus, or some combination of these factors.

The diagnosis is confirmed by examination of the cerebrospinal fluid. Findings may include elevated cerebrospinal fluid pressure, pleocytosis, increased protein concentration, and decreased glucose concentration. Cytologic studies may indicate that malignant cells are present; if not, spinal tap should be repeated at least twice to obtain further samples for analysis.

CT scans showing contrast enhancement in the basal cisterns or showing hydrocephalus without any evidence of a mass lesion support the diagnosis. Myelography may show deposits on multiple nerve roots.

Treatment is by irradiation to symptomatic areas, combined with intrathecal methotrexate. The long-term prognosis is poor—only about 10% of patients survive for 1 year.

Henson RA, Urich H: *Cancer and the Nervous System.* Blackwell, 1982.

3. INTRACRANIAL MASS LESIONS IN AIDS PATIENTS

AIDS patients may present with **primary cerebral lymphoma.** This leads to disturbances in cognition or consciousness, focal motor or sensory deficits, aphasia, seizures, and cranial neuropathies. Similar clinical disturbances may result from **cerebral toxoplasmosis,** which is also a common complication in patients with AIDS. Neither CT nor MRI findings distinguish these 2 disorders, and serologic tests for toxoplasmosis are unreliable in AIDS patients. Accordingly, for neurologically stable patients, a trial of treatment with sulfadiazine and pyrimethamine is recommended for 3 weeks; the imaging studies are then repeated, and if any lesion has improved, the antitoxoplasmosis regimen is continued indefinitely. If any lesion does not improve, cerebral biopsy is necessary. Primary cerebral lymphoma is treated with whole-brain irradiation.

Cryptococcal meningitis is also a commonly opportunistic infection in AIDS patients. Clinically, it may resemble cerebral toxoplasmosis or lymphoma, but cranial CT scans are usually normal. The diagnosis is made on the basis of cerebrospinal fluid studies, with positive India ink staining in 75–80% and cryptococcal antigen tests in 95% of cases. Treatment is with amphotericin B and flucytosine.

4. PRIMARY & METASTATIC SPINAL TUMORS

Approximately 10% of spinal tumors are intramedullary. Ependymoma is the most common type of intramedullary tumor; the remainder are other types of glioma. Extramedullary tumors may be extradural or intradural in location. Among the primary extramedullary tumors, neurofibromas and meningiomas are relatively common, are benign, and may be intra- or extradural. Carcinomatous metastases, lymphomatous or leukemic deposits, and myeloma are usually extradural; in the case of metastases, the prostate, breast, lung, and kidney are common primary sites.

Tumors may lead to spinal cord dysfunction by direct compression, by ischemia secondary to arterial or venous obstruction, and, in the case of intramedullary lesions, by invasive infiltration.

Clinical Findings

A. Symptoms and Signs: Symptoms usually develop insidiously. Pain is often conspicuous with extradural lesions; is characteristically aggravated by coughing or straining; may be radicular, localized to the back, or felt diffusely in an extremity; and may be accompanied by motor deficits, paresthesias, or numbness, especially in the legs. When sphincter disturbances occur, they are usually particularly disabling. Pain, however, often precedes specific neurologic symptoms from epidural metastases.

Examination may reveal localized spinal tenderness. A segmental lower motor neuron deficit or dermatomal sensory changes (or both) are sometimes found at the level of the lesion, while an upper motor neuron deficit and sensory disturbance are found below it.

B. Imaging: Findings on plain radiography of the spine may be normal but are commonly abnormal when there are metastatic deposits. CT myelography or MRI may be necessary to identify and localize the site of cord compression. The combination of known tumor elsewhere in the body, back pain, and either abnormal plain films of the spine or neurologic signs of cord compression is an indication to perform these studies on an urgent basis. Some clinicians proceed to myelography based solely on new back pain in a cancer patient. If a complete block is present at lumbar myelography, a cisternal myelogram is performed to determine the upper level of the block and to investigate the possibility of block higher in the cord.

C. Laboratory Findings: The cerebrospinal fluid removed at myelography is often xanthochromic and contains a greatly increased protein concentration with normal cell content and glucose concentration.

Treatment

Intramedullary tumors are treated by decompression and surgical excision (when feasible) and by irradiation. The prognosis depends upon the cause and severity of cord compression before it is relieved.

Treatment of epidural spinal metastases consists of irradiation, irrespective of cell type. Dexamethasone is also given in a high dosage (eg, 25 mg 4 times daily for 3 days, followed by rapid tapering of the dosage, depending on response) to reduce cord swelling and relieve pain. Surgical decompression is reserved for patients with tumors that are unresponsive to irradiation or have previously been irradiated and for cases in which there is some uncertainty about the diagnosis. The long-term outlook is poor, but radiation treatment may at least delay the onset of major disability.

5. BRAIN ABSCESS

Infectious disorders are considered elsewhere in this book, but brief comment will be made here concerning cerebral abscess, which presents as an intracranial space-occupying lesion. Brain abscess may arise as a sequela of disease of the ear or nose, may be a metastatic complication of infection elsewhere in the body, or may result from infection introduced intracranially by trauma or surgical procedures. The most common infective organisms are streptococci, staphylococci, and anaerobes; mixed infections are not uncommon. Headache, drowsiness, inattention, confusion, and seizures are early symptoms, followed by signs of increasing intracranial pressure and then a focal neurologic deficit. There may be little or no evidence of systemic infection.

A CT scan of the head characteristically shows an area of contrast enhancement surrounding a low-density core. Similar abnormalities may, however, be found in patients with metastatic neoplasms. The MRI findings may also be abnormal. Arteriography indicates the presence of a space-occupying lesion, which appears as an avascular mass with displacement of normal cerebral vessels, but this procedure provides no clue to the nature of the lesion.

Treatment consists of intravenous antibiotics, combined with surgical drainage (aspiration or excision) if necessary to reduce the mass effect, or sometimes to establish the diagnosis. Abscesses smaller than 2 cm can often be cured medically. Broad-spectrum antibiotics are used if the infecting organism is unknown. In adults, a common regimen is penicillin G (2 million units every 2 hours intravenously) plus either chloramphenicol (1–2 g intravenously every 6 hours), metronidazole (750 mg intravenously every 6 hours), or both. Nafcillin is added if *Staphylococcus aureus* infection is suspected. Corticosteroids may reduce any associated edema.

NONMETASTATIC NEUROLOGIC COMPLICATIONS OF MALIGNANT DISEASE

A variety of nonmetastatic neurologic complications of malignant disease can be recognized:

(1) Metabolic encephalopathy due to electrolyte abnormalities, infections, drug overdose, or the failure of some vital organ may be reflected by drowsiness, lethargy, restlessness, insomnia, agitation, confusion, stupor, or coma. The mental changes are usually associated with tremor, asterixis, and multifocal myoclonus. The electroencephalogram is generally diffusely slowed. Laboratory studies are necessary to detect the cause of the encephalopathy, which must then be treated appropriately.

(2) Immune suppression resulting from either the malignant disease or its treatment (eg, by chemotherapy) predisposes patients to brain abscess, progressive multifocal leukoencephalopathy, meningitis, herpes zoster infection, and other opportunistic infectious diseases. Moreover, an overt or occult cerebrospinal fluid fistula, as occurs with some tumors, may also increase the risk of infection. CT scanning aids in the early recognition of a brain abscess, but metastatic brain tumors may have a similar appearance. Examination of the cerebrospinal fluid is essential in the evaluation of patients with meningitis but is of no help in the diagnosis of brain abscess. Treatment should be specific for the infective organism.

(3) Cerebrovascular disorders that cause neurologic complications in patients with systemic cancer include nonbacterial thrombotic endocarditis and septic embolization. Cerebral, subarachnoid, or subdural hemorrhages may occur in patients with myelogenous leukemia and may be found in association with metastatic tumors, especially malignant melanoma. Spinal subdural hemorrhage sometimes occurs after lumbar puncture in patients with marked thrombocytopenia.

Disseminated intravascular coagulation occurs most commonly in patients with acute promyelocytic leukemia or with some adenocarcinomas and is characterized by a fluctuating encephalopathy, often with associated seizures, that frequently progresses to coma or death. There may be few accompanying neurologic signs.

Venous sinus thrombosis, which usually presents with convulsions and headaches, may also occur in patients with leukemia or lymphoma. Examination commonly reveals papilledema and focal or diffuse neurologic signs. Treatment is with anticonvulsants and drugs to lower the intracranial pressure. The role of anticoagulants is controversial.

(4) Subacute cerebellar degeneration occurs most commonly in association with carcinoma of the lung. Symptoms may precede those due to the neoplasm itself, which may be undetected for several months or even longer. Typically, there is a pancerebellar syndrome causing dysarthria, nystagmus, and ataxia of the trunk and limbs. Treatment is of the underlying malignant disease.

(5) Encephalopathy, characterized by impaired recent memory, disturbed affect, hallucinations, and seizures, occurs in some patients with carcinomas. The cerebrospinal fluid is often abnormal. EEGs may show diffuse slow-wave activity, especially over the temporal regions. Pathologic changes are most marked in the inferomedian portions of the temporal lobes. There is no specific treatment.

(6) Malignant disease is more commonly associated with sensorimotor polyneuropathy than with pure sensory neuropathy (ie, dorsal root ganglionitis) or autonomic neuropathy.

(7) Dermatomyositis or a myasthenic syndrome may be seen in patients with underlying carcinoma (see Chapter 15).

PSEUDOTUMOR CEREBRI
(Benign Intracranial Hypertension)

Symptoms of pseudotumor cerebri consist of headache, diplopia, and other visual disturbances due to papilledema and abducens nerve dysfunction. Examination reveals the papilledema and some enlargement of the blind spots, but patients otherwise look well. Investigations reveal no evidence of a space-occupying lesion, and the CT scan shows small or normal ventricles. Lumbar puncture confirms the presence

of intracranial hypertension, but the cerebrospinal fluid is normal.

There are many causes of pseudotumor cerebri. Thrombosis of the transverse venous sinus as a noninfectious complication of otitis media or chronic mastoiditis is one cause, and sagittal sinus thrombosis may lead to a clinically similar picture. Other causes include chronic pulmonary disease, endocrine disturbances such as hypoparathyroidism or Addison's disease, vitamin A toxicity, and the use of tetracycline or oral contraceptives. Cases have also followed withdrawal of corticosteroids after long-term use. In many instances, however, no specific cause can be found, and the disorder remits spontaneously after several months.

Untreated pseudotumor cerebri leads to secondary optic atrophy and permanent visual loss. Repeated lumbar puncture to lower the intracranial pressure by removal of cerebrospinal fluid is effective, but pharmacologic approaches to treatment are now more satisfactory. Acetazolamide reduces formation of cerebrospinal fluid and can be used to start treatment; furosemide serves the same function and can be added to the treatment regimen if necessary. Oral corticosteroids have also been used. Obese patients should be advised to lose weight. Treatment is monitored by checking visual acuity, funduscopic appearance, and pressure of the cerebrospinal fluid.

If medical treatment fails to control the intracranial pressure, surgical placement of a lumboperitoneal or other shunt should be undertaken to preserve vision.

In addition to the above measures, any specific cause of pseudotumor cerebri requires appropriate treatment. Thus, hormone therapy should be initiated if there is an underlying endocrine disturbance. Discontinuing the use of tetracycline, oral contraceptives, or vitamin A will allow for resolution of pseudotumor cerebri due to these agents. If corticosteroid withdrawal is responsible, the medication should be reintroduced and then tapered more gradually.

SELECTED NEUROCUTANEOUS DISEASES

Tuberous Sclerosis

Tuberous sclerosis may occur sporadically or on a familial basis with autosomal dominant inheritance. Its pathogenesis is unknown. Neurologic presentation is with seizures and progressive psychomotor retardation beginning in early childhood. The cutaneous abnormality, adenoma sebaceum, becomes manifest usually between 5 and 10 years of age and typically consists of reddened nodules on the face (cheeks, nasolabial folds, sides of the nose, and chin) and sometimes on the forehead and neck. Other typical cutaneous lesions include subungual fibromas, shagreen patches (leathery plaques of subepidermal fibrosis, situated usually on the trunk), and leaf-shaped hypopigmented spots. Associated abnormalities include retinal lesions and tumors, benign rhabdomyomas of the heart, lung cysts, benign tumors in the viscera, and bone cysts.

The disease is slowly progressive and leads to increasing mental deterioration. There is no specific treatment, but anticonvulsant drugs may help in controlling seizures.

Neurofibromatosis

Neurofibromatosis may occur either sporadically or on a familial basis with autosomal dominant inheritance. Two distinct forms are required: Type 1 (**Recklinghausen's disease**) is characterized by multiple hyperpigmented macules and neurofibromas and type 2 by **eighth nerve tumors,** often accompanied by other intracranial or intraspinal tumors. Among familial cases, the gene for type 1 is located on chromosome 17 and that for type 2 on chromosome 22.

Neurologic presentation is usually with symptoms and signs of tumor. Multiple neurofibromas characteristically are present and may involve spinal or cranial nerves, especially the eighth nerve. Examination of the superficial cutaneous nerves usually reveals palpable mobile nodules. In some cases, there is an associated marked overgrowth of subcutaneous tissues (plexiform neuromas), sometimes with an underlying bony abnormality. Associated cutaneous lesions include axillary freckling and patches of cutaneous pigmentation (cafe au lait spots). Malignant degeneration of neurofibromas occasionally occurs and may lead to peripheral sarcomas. Meningiomas, gliomas (especially optic nerve gliomas), bone cysts, pheochromocytomas, scoliosis, and obstructive hydrocephalus may also occur.

It may be possible to correct disfigurement by plastic surgery. Intraspinal or intracranial tumors and tumors of peripheral nerves should be treated surgically if they are producing symptoms.

Barker D et al: Gene for von Recklinghausen neurofibromatosis is in the pericentromeric region of chromosome 17. Science 1987;236:110.

Sturge-Weber Syndrome

Sturge-Weber syndrome consists of a congenital, usually unilateral, cutaneous capillary angioma involving the upper face, leptomeningeal angiomatosis, and, in many patients, choroidal angioma. It has no sex predilection and usually occurs sporadically. The cutaneous angioma sometimes has a more extensive distribution over the head and neck and is often quite disfiguring, especially if there is associated overgrowth of connective tissue. Focal or generalized seizures are the usual neurologic presentation and may commence at any age. There may be contralateral homonymous hemianopia, hemiparesis and hemisensory disturbance, ipsilateral glaucoma or buphthalmos, and mental subnormality. Skull x-rays taken after the first 2 years of life usually reveal gyriform ("tramline") intracranial calcification, especially in the parieto-occipital region, due to mineral deposition in the cortex beneath the intracranial angioma.

Treatment is aimed at controlling seizures pharmacologically. Ophthalmologic advice should be sought concerning the management of choroidal angioma and of increased intraocular pressure.

MOVEMENT DISORDERS

1. BENIGN ESSENTIAL (FAMILIAL) TREMOR

The cause of benign essential tremor is uncertain, but it is sometimes inherited in an autosomal dominant manner. Tremor may begin at any age and is enhanced by emotional stress. The tremor usually involves one or both hands, the head, or the hands and head, while the legs tend to be spared. Examination reveals no other abnormalities. Ingestion of a small quantity of alcohol commonly provides remarkable but short-lived relief by an unknown mechanism.

Although the tremor may become more conspicuous with time, it generally leads to little disability, and treatment is often unnecessary. Occasionally, it interferes with manual skills and leads to impairment of handwriting. Speech may also be affected if the laryngeal muscles are involved. In such circumstances, propranolol may be helpful but will need to be continued indefinitely in daily doses of 60–240 mg. However, intermittent therapy is sometimes useful in patients whose tremor becomes exacerbated in specific predictable situations. It is not clear whether the response to propranolol depends on central or peripheral mechanisms. Primidone may be helpful when propranolol is ineffective, but patients with essential tremor are often very sensitive to it. They are therefore started on 50 mg daily, and the daily dose is increased by 50 mg every 2 weeks depending on the response; a maintenance dose of 125 mg 3 times daily is commonly effective.

Hubble JP, Busenbark KL, Koller WC: Essential tremor. Clin Neuropharmacol 1989;12:453.

2. PARKINSONISM

Essentials of Diagnosis

- Any combination of tremor, rigidity, bradykinesia, progressive postural instability.
- Seborrhea of skin quite common.
- Mild intellectual deterioration is often observed.

General Considerations

Parkinsonism is a relatively common disorder that

occurs in all ethnic groups, with an approximately equal sex distribution. The most common variety, idiopathic Parkinson's disease (paralysis agitans), begins most often between 45 and 65 years of age.

Etiology

Postencephalitic parkinsonism is becoming increasingly rare. Exposure to certain toxins (eg, manganese dust, carbon disulfide) and severe carbon monoxide poisoning may lead to parkinsonism. Typical parkinsonism has occurred in individuals who have taken 1-methyl-4-phenyl-1,2,5,6-tetrahydropyridine (MPTP) for recreational purposes. This compound is converted in the body and selectively destroys dopaminergic neurons in the substantia nigra. Reversible parkinsonism may develop in patients receiving neuroleptic drugs (see Chapter 19) and has also been caused by reserpine and metoclopramide. Only rarely is hemiparkinsonism the presenting feature of a brain tumor or some other progressive space-occupying lesion.

In idiopathic parkinsonism, dopamine depletion due to degeneration of the dopaminergic nigrostriatal system leads to an imbalance of dopamine and acetylcholine, which are neurotransmitters normally present in the corpus striatum. Treatment is directed at redressing this imbalance by blocking the effect of acetylcholine with anticholinergic drugs or by the administration of levodopa, the precursor of dopamine.

Clinical Findings

Tremor, rigidity, bradykinesia, and postural instability are the cardinal features of parkinsonism and may be present in any combination. There may also be a mild decline in intellectual function. The tremor of about 4–6 cycles per second is most conspicuous at rest, is enhanced by emotional stress, and is often less severe during voluntary activity. Although it may ultimately be present in all limbs, the tremor is commonly confined to one limb or to the limbs on one side for months or years before it becomes more generalized. In some patients, tremor is absent.

Rigidity (an increase in resistance to passive movement) is responsible for the characteristically flexed posture seen in many patients, but the most disabling symptoms of parkinsonism are due to bradykinesia, manifested as a slowness of voluntary movement and a reduction in automatic movements such as swinging of the arms while walking. Curiously, however, effective voluntary activity may briefly be regained during an emergency (eg, the patient is able to leap aside to avoid an oncoming motor vehicle).

Clinical diagnosis of the well-developed syndrome is usually simple. The patient has a relatively immobile face with widened palpebral fissures, infrequent blinking, and a certain fixity of facial expression. Seborrhea of the scalp and face is common. There is often mild blepharoclonus, and a tremor may be present about the mouth and lips. Repetitive tapping (about twice per second) over the bridge of the nose produces a sustained blink response (Myerson's sign). Other findings may include saliva drooling from the mouth, perhaps due to impairment of swallowing; soft and poorly modulated voice; a variable rest tremor and rigidity in some or all of the limbs; slowness of voluntary movements; impairment of fine or rapidly alternating movements; and micrographia. There is typically no muscle weakness (provided that sufficient time is allowed for power to be developed) and no alteration in the tendon reflexes or plantar responses. It is difficult for the patient to arise from a sitting position and begin walking. The gait itself is characterized by small shuffling steps and a loss of the normal automatic arm swing; there may be unsteadiness on turning and difficulty in stopping.

Differential Diagnosis

Diagnostic problems may occur in mild cases, especially if tremor is minimal or absent. For example, mild hypokinesia or slight tremor is commonly attributed to old age. Depression, with its associated expressionless face, poorly modulated voice, and reduction in voluntary activity, can be difficult to distinguish from mild parkinsonism, especially since the 2 disorders may coexist; in some cases, a trial of antidepressant drug therapy may be necessary. The family history, the character of the tremor, and lack of other neurologic signs should distinguish essential tremor from parkinsonism. Wilson's disease can be distinguished by its early age at onset, the presence of other abnormal movements, Kayser-Fleischer rings, and chronic hepatitis, and by increased concentrations of copper in the tissues. Huntington's disease presenting with rigidity and bradykinesia may be mistaken for parkinsonism unless the family history and accompanying dementia are recognized. In Shy-Drager syndrome, the clinical features of parkinsonism are accompanied by autonomic insufficiency (leading to postural hypotension, anhidrosis, disturbances of sphincter control, impotence, etc) and more widespread neurologic deficits (pyramidal, lower motor neuron, or cerebellar signs). In progressive supranuclear palsy, bradykinesia and rigidity are accompanied by a supranuclear disorder of eye movements, pseudobulbar palsy, and axial dystonia. Creutzfeldt-Jakob disease may be accompanied by features of parkinsonism, but dementia is usual, myoclonic jerking is common, ataxia and pyramidal signs may be conspicuous, and the electroencephalographic findings are usually characteristic. In patients with tremor, movement may produce an electrocardiographic artifact mimicking atrial flutter.

Treatment

A. Medical Measures: Drug treatment is not required early in the course of parkinsonism, but the nature of the disorder and the availability of medical treatment for use when necessary should be discussed with the patient.

1. Amantadine–Patients with mild symptoms but no disability may be helped by amantadine. This drug improves all of the clinical features of parkinsonism, but its mode of action is unclear. Side effects include restlessness, confusion, depression, skin rashes, edema, nausea, constipation, anorexia, postural hypotension, and disturbances of cardiac rhythm. However, these are relatively uncommon with the usual dose (100 mg twice daily).

2. Anticholinergic drugs–Anticholinergics are more helpful in alleviating tremor and rigidity than bradykinesia. Treatment is started with a small dose (Table 18–4) and gradually increased until benefit occurs or side effects limit further increments. If treatment is ineffective, the drug is gradually withdrawn and another preparation then tried. Ethopropazine is probably the most helpful drug in this group for the relief of tremor.

Common side effects include dryness of the mouth, nausea, constipation, palpitations, cardiac arrhythmias, urinary retention, confusion, agitation, restlessness, drowsiness, mydriasis, increased intraocular pressure, and defective accommodation.

Anticholinergic drugs are contraindicated in patients with prostatic hypertrophy, narrow-angle glaucoma, or obstructive gastrointestinal disease and are often tolerated poorly by the elderly.

3. Levodopa–Levodopa, which is converted in the body to dopamine, improves all of the major features of parkinsonism, including bradykinesia, but does not stop progression of the disorder. The commonest early side effects of levodopa are nausea, vomiting, and hypotension, but cardiac arrhythmias may also occur. Dyskinesias, restlessness, confusion, and other behavioral changes tend to occur somewhat

later and become more common with time. Levodopa-induced dyskinesias may take any conceivable form, including chorea, athetosis, dystonia, tremor, tics, and myoclonus. An even later complication is the "on-off phenomenon," in which abrupt but transient fluctuations in the severity of parkinsonism occur unpredictably but frequently during the day. The "off" period of marked bradykinesia has been shown to relate in some instances to falling plasma levels of levodopa. During the "on" phase, dyskinesias are often conspicuous but mobility is increased.

Carbidopa, which inhibits the enzyme responsible for the breakdown of levodopa to dopamine, does not cross the blood-brain barrier. When levodopa is given in combination with carbidopa, the extracerebral breakdown of levodopa is largely prevented. This reduces the amount of levodopa required daily for beneficial effects, and it lowers the incidence of nausea, vomiting, hypotension, and cardiac irregularities. Such a combination does not prevent the development of the "on-off phenomenon," and the incidence of other side effects (dyskinesias or psychiatric complications) may actually be increased.

Sinemet, a commercially available preparation that contains carbidopa and levodopa in a fixed ratio (1:10 or 1:4), is generally used. Treatment is started with a small dose—eg, one tablet of Sinemet 25/100 (containing 25 mg of carbidopa and 100 mg of levodopa) 3 times daily—and gradually increased depending on the response.

The dyskinesias and behavioral side effects of levodopa are dose-related, but reduction in dose may eliminate any therapeutic benefit. In such circumstances, a drug holiday may be helpful. Levodopa medication is gradually withdrawn over several days and not reinstated for 1–2 weeks. When it is reintroduced, up to two-thirds of patients show improved responsiveness and so derive benefit at a lower daily dose than previously required. The "on-off phenomenon" may also be improved by a drug holiday, but any benefit is usually so transient that a drug holiday is not recommended in this context. There is no way predict which patients will benefit from a drug holiday, and it is a distressing and difficult experience that may necessitate hospitalization. Complications of a drug holiday include depression, decubitus ulcers, aspiration pneumonia, and thromboembolism.

Levodopa therapy is contraindicated in patients with psychotic illness or narrow-angle glaucoma. It should not be given to patients taking monoamine oxidase A inhibitors or within 2 weeks of their withdrawal, because hypertensive crises may result. Levodopa should be avoided in patients with suspected malignant melanomas, which may be activated, and in patients with active peptic ulcers, which may bleed.

4. Bromocriptine–This ergot derivative acts directly on dopamine receptors, and its use in parkinson-

Table 18–4. Some anticholinergic antiparkinsonian drugs.[1]

Drug	Usual Daily Dose (mg)
Benztropine mesylate (Cogentin)	1–6
Biperiden (Akineton)	2–12
Chlorphenoxamine (Phenoxene)	150–400
Cycrimine (Pagitane)	5–20
Ethopropazine (Parsidol)	150–300
Orphenadrine (Disipal, Norflex)	150–400
Procyclidine (Kemadrin)	7.5–30
Trihexyphenidyl (Artane)	6–20

[1] Reproduced, with permission, from Aminoff MJ: Pharmacologic management of parkinsonism and other movement disorders. In: *Basic & Clinical Pharmacology*, 4th ed. Katzung BG (editor). Appleton & Lange, 1989.

ism is associated with a lower incidence of the side effects that occur with long-term levodopa therapy. It was often reserved for patients who had either become refractory to levodopa or developed the "on-off phenomenon." However, it is now best given with a low dose of Sinemet-25/100 (carbidopa 25 mg and levodopa 100 mg), one tablet 3 times daily when dopaminergic therapy is first introduced; the dose of Sinemet is kept constant, while the dose of bromocriptine is gradually increased. The initial dosage of bromocriptine is 1.25 mg twice daily; this is increased by 2.5 mg at 2-week intervals until benefit occurs or side effects limit further increments. The usual daily maintenance dose in patients with parkinsonism is between 10 and 30 mg.

Side effects include anorexia, nausea, vomiting, constipation, postural hypotension, digital vasospasm, cardiac arrhythmias, various dyskinesias and mental disturbances, headache, nasal congestion, erythromelalgia, and pulmonary infiltrates.

Bromocriptine is contraindicated in patients with a history of mental illness or recent myocardial infarction and is probably best avoided in those with peripheral vascular disease or peptic ulcers (bleeding from peptic ulcers has been reported).

A number of other dopamine agonists have been used to treat parkinsonism. Only pergolide has been approved for use in the USA, and it seems to have no particular advantage over bromocriptine.

5. Deprenyl–Deprenyl is a monoamine oxidase B inhibitor that is sometimes used as adjunctive treatment for parkinsonism in patients receiving levodopa. By inhibiting the metabolic breakdown of dopamine, deprenyl has been used to improve fluctuations or declining response to levodopa. In general, however, the response to treatment with it has been disappointing. The drug is taken in a standard dose of 5 mg with breakfast and 5 mg with lunch, and at this dose it does not have the hypertensive effect of the nonselective monoamine oxidase inhibitors. It may, however, increase any adverse effects of levodopa.

It has recently been suggested that treatment with deprenyl may affect the natural history of Parkinson's disease by slowing down its progressive course. Studies to establish this are currently in progress, and preliminary findings have been mixed.

B. General Measures: Physical therapy or speech therapy helps many patients. The quality of life can often be improved by the provision of simple aids to daily living, eg, rails or banisters placed strategically about the home, special table cutlery with large handles, nonslip rubber table mats, and devices to amplify the voice.

C. Surgical Measures: Thalamotomy is generally reserved for the patient who is relatively young, has predominantly unilateral tremor and rigidity that have failed to respond to medication, and has no evidence of diffuse vascular disease. Surgical implan-

tation of adrenal medullary tissue into the caudate nucleus has recently been reported to benefit some patients, but other investigators have failed to substantiate such claims, and the procedure is still being evaluated.

Langston JW: Current theories on the course of Parkinson's disease. J Neurol Neurosurg Psychiatry 1980;13(Special Suppl).

Lees AJ: L-dopa treatment and Parkinson's disease. Q J Med 1986;59:535.

Lindvall O: Transplantation into the human brain: Present status and future possibilities. J Neurol Neurosurg Psychiatry 1989;39(Special Suppl).

Nutt JG: On-off phenomenon: Relation to levodopa pharmacokinetics and pharmacodynamics. Ann Neurol 1987; 22:535. (Pathophysiology of fluctuation in response to levodopa.)

Parkinson Study Group: Effect of deprenyl on the progression of disability in early Parkinson's disease. N Engl J Med 1989;321:1364. (Preliminary report of a multicenter study.)

3. HUNTINGTON'S DISEASE

Essentials of Diagnosis

- Gradual onset and progression of chorea and dementia.
- Family history of the disorder.

General Considerations

Huntington's disease is characterized by chorea and dementia. It is inherited in an autosomal dominant manner and occurs throughout the world, in all ethnic groups, with a prevalence rate of about 5 per 100,000. The gene responsible for the disease has been located on the short arm of chromosome No. 4. Symptoms do not usually develop until after 30 years of age, by which time the patient has usually had children, and so the disease continues from one generation to the next. The cause of Huntington's disease is unknown.

Clinical Findings

Clinical onset is usually between 30 and 50 years of age. The disease is progressive and usually leads to a fatal outcome within 15–20 years. The initial symptoms may consist of either abnormal movements or intellectual changes, but ultimately both occur. The earliest mental changes are often behavioral, with irritability, moodiness, antisocial behavior, or a psychiatric disturbance, but a more obvious dementia subsequently develops. The dyskinesia may initially be no more than an apparent fidgetiness or restlessness, but eventually choreiform movements and some dystonic posturing occur. Progressive rigidity and akinesia (rather than chorea) sometimes occur in association with dementia, especially in cases with childhood onset. CT scanning usually demonstrates cerebral atrophy and atrophy of the caudate nucleus in established cases. MRI and positron emission tomography (PET) have shown reduced glucose utilization in an anatomically normal caudate nucleus.

Chorea developing with no family history of choreoathetosis should not be attributed to Huntington's disease, at least not until other causes of chorea have been excluded clinically and by appropriate laboratory studies. In younger patients, self-limiting Sydenham's chorea develops after group A streptococcal infections on rare occasions. If a patient presents solely with progressive intellectual failure, it may not be possible to distinguish Huntington's disease from other causes of dementia unless there is a characteristic family history or a dyskinesia develops.

Treatment

There is no cure for Huntington's disease, progression cannot be halted, and treatment is purely symptomatic. The reported biochemical changes suggest a relative underactivity of neurons containing gamma-aminobutyric acid (GABA) and acetylcholine or a relative overactivity of dopaminergic neurons. Treatment with drugs blocking dopamine receptors, such as phenothiazines or haloperidol, may control the dyskinesia and any behavioral disturbances. Haloperidol treatment is usually begun with a dose of 1 mg once or twice daily, which is then increased every 3 or 4 days depending on the response. Tetrabenazine, a drug that depletes central monoamines, is widely used in Europe to treat dyskinesia but is not available in the USA. Reserpine is similar in its actions to tetrabenazine and may be helpful; the daily dose is built up gradually to between 2 and 5 mg, depending on the response. Attempts to compensate for the relative GABA deficiency by enhancing central GABA activity or to compensate for the relative cholinergic underactivity by giving choline chloride have not been therapeutically helpful. High levels of somatostatin (a neuropeptide) have recently been reported in certain areas of the brain in patients with Huntington's disease, and the therapeutic response to cysteamine (a selective depleter of somatostatin in the brain) is currently under study.

Offspring should be offered genetic counseling. Their probability of carrying the gene responsible for the disease can be estimated in many instances by identifying a specific DNA marker that is genetically linked to the gene, but this requires analysis of DNA samples from both affected and elderly unaffected family members.

Martin JB, Gusella JF: Huntington's disease: Pathogenesis and management. N Engl J Med 1986;315:1267.

Meissen GJ et al: Predictive testing for Huntington's disease with use of a linked DNA marker. N Engl J Med 1988;318:535.

Myers RH et al: Clinical and neuropathologic assessment of severity in Huntington's disease. Neurology 1988; 38:341.

4. IDIOPATHIC TORSION DYSTONIA

Essentials of Diagnosis

- Dystonic movements and postures.
- Normal birth and developmental history. No other neurologic signs.
- Investigations (including CT scan) reveal no cause of dystonia.

General Considerations

Idiopathic torsion dystonia may occur sporadically or on a hereditary basis, with autosomal dominant, autosomal recessive, and X-linked recessive modes of transmission. It may begin in childhood or later and persists throughout life.

Clinical Findings

The disorder is characterized by the onset of abnormal movements and postures in a patient with a normal birth and developmental history, no relevant past medical illness, and no other neurologic signs. Investigations (including CT scan) reveal no cause for the abnormal movements. Dystonic movements of the head and neck may take the form of torticollis, blepharospasm, facial grimacing, or forced opening or closing of the mouth. The limbs may also adopt abnormal but characteristic postures. The age at onset influences both the clinical findings and the prognosis. With onset in childhood, there is usually a family history of the disorder, symptoms commonly commence in the legs, and progression is likely until there is severe disability from generalized dystonia. In contrast, when onset is later, a positive family history is unlikely, initial symptoms are often in the arms or axial structures, and severe disability does not usually occur, although generalized dystonia may ultimately develop in some patients. If all cases are considered together, about one-third of patients eventually become so severely disabled that they are confined to chair or bed, while another one-third are affected only mildly.

Before a diagnosis of idiopathic torsion dystonia is made, it is imperative to exclude other causes of dystonia. For example, perinatal anoxia, birth trauma, and kernicterus are common causes of dystonia, but abnormal movements usually then develop before the age of 5, the early development of the patient is usually abnormal, and a history of seizures is not unusual. Moreover, examination may reveal signs of mental retardation or pyramidal deficit in addition to the movement disorder. Dystonic posturing may also occur in Wilson's disease, Huntington's disease, or parkinsonism; as a sequela of encephalitis lethargica or previous neuroleptic drug therapy; and in certain other disorders. In these cases, diagnosis is based on the history and accompanying clinical manifestations.

Treatment

Idiopathic torsion dystonia usually responds poorly to drugs. Levodopa, diazepam, baclofen, carbamazepine, amantadine, or anticholinergic medication (in high dosage) is occasionally helpful; if not, a trial of treatment with phenothiazines, haloperidol, or tetrabenazine (not available in the USA) may be worthwhile. However, the doses of these latter drugs that are required for benefit lead usually to mild parkinsonism. Stereotactic thalamotomy is sometimes helpful in patients with predominantly unilateral dystonia, especially when this involves the limbs.

Fahn S: Clinical variants of idiopathic torsion dystonia. J Neurol Neurosurg Psychiatry 1989;96(Special Suppl):1.
Nygaard TG, Marsden CD, Duvoisin RC: Dopa-responsive dystonia. Adv Neurol 1988;50:377.

5. FOCAL TORSION DYSTONIA

A number of the dystonic manifestations that occur in idiopathic torsion dystonia may also occur as isolated phenomena. They are best regarded as focal dystonias that either occur as formes frustes of idiopathic torsion dystonia in patients with a positive family history or represent a focal manifestation of the adult-onset form of that disorder when there is no family history. Medical treatment is generally unsatisfactory. A trial of the drugs used in idiopathic torsion dystonia is worthwhile, however, since a few patients do show some response. In addition, with restricted dystonias such as blepharospasm or torticollis, local injection of botulinum A toxin into the overactive muscles may produce benefit for several weeks or months and can be repeated as needed.

Both blepharospasm and oromandibular dystonia may occur as an isolated focal dystonia. The former is characterized by spontaneous involuntary forced closure of the eyelids for a variable interval. Oromandibular dystonia is manifested by involuntary contraction of the muscles about the mouth causing, for example, involuntary opening or closing of the mouth, roving or protruding tongue movements, and retraction of the platysma.

Spasmodic torticollis, usually with onset between 25 and 50 years of age, is characterized by a tendency for the neck to twist to one side. This initially occurs episodically, but eventually the neck is held to the side. Spontaneous resolution may occur in the first year or so. The disorder is otherwise usually lifelong. Selective section of the spinal accessory nerve and the upper cervical nerve roots is sometimes helpful if medical treatment is unsuccessful. Local injection of botulinum A toxin may provide benefit in some cases.

Writer's cramp is characterized by dystonic posturing of the hand and forearm when the hand is used for writing and sometimes when it is used for other tasks, eg, playing the piano, using a screwdriver or eating utensils. Drug treatment is usually unrewarding, and patients are often best advised to learn to use the other hand for activities requiring manual dexterity.

Gelb DJ, Lowenstein DH, Aminoff MJ: Controlled trial of botulinum toxin injections in the treatment of spasmodic torticollis. Neurology 1989;39:80. (Including evaluation of dose requirements.)
Jankovic J, Schwartz K: Botulinum toxin injections for cervical dystonia. Neurology 1990;40:277.

6. MYOCLONUS

Occasional myoclonic jerks may occur in anyone, especially when drifting into sleep. General or multifocal myoclonus is common in patients with idiopathic epilepsy and is especially prominent in certain hereditary disorders characterized by seizures and progressive intellectual decline, such as the lipid storage diseases. It is also a feature of various rare degenerative disorders, notably Ramsay Hunt syndrome, and is common in subacute sclerosing panencephalitis and Creutzfeldt-Jakob disease. Generalized myoclonic jerking may accompany uremic and other metabolic encephalopathies, result from levodopa therapy, occur in alcohol or drug withdrawal states, or follow anoxic brain damage. It also occurs on a hereditary or sporadic basis as an isolated phenomenon in otherwise healthy subjects.

Segmental myoclonus is a rare manifestation of a focal spinal cord lesion. It may also be the clinical expression of **epilepsia partialis continua,** a disorder in which a repetitive focal epileptic discharge arises in the contralateral sensorimotor cortex, sometimes from an underlying structural lesion. An electroencephalogram is often helpful in clarifying the epileptic nature of the disorder, and CT or MRI scan may reveal the causal lesion.

Myoclonus may respond to certain anticonvulsant drugs, especially valproic acid, or to one of the benzodiazepines, particularly clonazepam. Myoclonus following anoxic brain damage is often responsive to 5-hydroxytryptophan, the precursor of 5-hydroxytryptamine, and sometimes to clonazepam. In patients with segmental myoclonus, a localized lesion should be searched for and treated appropriately.

Berkovic SF et al: Progressive myoclonus epilepsies: Specific causes and diagnosis. N Engl J Med 1986; 315:296.
Kelly JJ, Sharbrough FW, Daube JR: A clinical and electrophysiological evaluation of myoclonus. Neurology 1981;31:581.

7. WILSON'S DISEASE

In this metabolic disorder, abnormal movements and postures of all sorts may occur with or without coexisting signs of liver involvement. It is discussed in detail in Chapter 11.

8. DRUG-INDUCED ABNORMAL MOVEMENTS

Phenothiazines and butyrophenones may produce a wide variety of abnormal movements, including parkinsonism, akathisia (ie, motor restlessness), acute dystonia, chorea, and tardive dyskinesia. These complications are discussed in Chapter 19. Chorea may also develop in patients receiving levodopa, bromocriptine, anticholinergic drugs, phenytoin, carbamazepine, lithium, amphetamines, or oral contraceptives, and it resolves with withdrawal of the offending substance. Similarly, dystonia may be produced by levodopa, bromocriptine, lithium, metoclopramide, or carbamazepine; and parkinsonism by reserpine, tetrabenazine, and metoclopramide. Postural tremor may occur with a variety of drugs, including epinephrine, isoproterenol, theophylline, caffeine, lithium, thyroid hormone, tricyclic antidepressants, and valproic acid.

9. GILLES DE LA TOURETTE'S SYNDROME

Essentials of Diagnosis
- Multiple motor and phonic tics.
- Symptoms begin before age 15 years.
- Chronic lifelong disorder with relapses and remissions.

Clinical Findings
Motor tics are the initial manifestation in 80% of cases and most commonly involve the face, whereas in the remaining 20%, the initial symptoms are phonic tics; all patients ultimately develop a combination of different motor and phonic tics. These are noted first in childhood, generally between the ages of 2 and 15. Motor tics occur especially about the face, head, and shoulders (eg, sniffing, blinking, frowning, shoulder shrugging, head thrusting, etc). Phonic tics commonly consist of grunts, barks, hisses, throat-clearing, coughs, etc, but sometimes also of verbal utterances including coprolalia. There may also be echolalia, echopraxia, and palilalia. Some tics may be self-mutilating in nature, such as severe nail-biting, hair-pulling, or biting of the lips or tongue. The disorder is chronic, but the course may be punctuated by relapses and remissions.

Examination usually reveals no abnormalities other than the multiple tics. Psychiatric disturbances may occur, however, because of the associated cosmetic and social embarrassment. Investigations are unrevealing except that the EEG may show minor nonspecific abnormalities of no diagnostic relevance.

The diagnosis of the disorder is often delayed for years, the tics being interpreted as psychiatric illness or some other form of abnormal movement. Patients are thus often subjected to unnecessary and expensive treatments before the true nature of the disorder is recognized. The ticlike character of the abnormal movements and the absence of other neurologic signs should differentiate this disorder from other movement disorders presenting in childhood. Wilson's disease, however, can simulate the condition and should be excluded.

Treatment
Treatment is symptomatic and may need to be continued indefinitely. Haloperidol is generally regarded as the drug of choice. It is started in a low daily dose (0.25 mg) that is gradually increased (by 0.25 mg every 4 or 5 days) until there is maximum benefit with a minimum of side effects or until side effects limit further increments. A total daily dose of between 2 and 8 mg is usually optimal, but higher doses are sometimes necessary. Treatment with clonazepam or clonidine may also be helpful, and it seems sensible to begin with one of these drugs in order to avoid some of the long-term extrapyramidal side effects of haloperidol. Phenothiazines, such as fluphenazine (2–15 mg daily), have been used, but patients unresponsive to haloperidol are usually unresponsive to these as well.

Pimozide, an oral dopamine-blocking drug related to haloperidol, may be helpful in patients who cannot tolerate or have not responded to haloperidol. Treatment is started with 1 mg daily and the daily dose increased by 1–2 mg every 10 days; the average dose is between 7 and 16 mg daily. The long-term safety of the drug is unclear.

There are a few anecdotal reports that calcium channel blockers may be helpful, but this requires further study.

Regeur L et al: Clinical features and long-term treatment with pimozide in 65 patients with Gilles de la Tourette's syndrome. J Neurol Neurosurg Psychiatry 1986;49:791.
Singer HS, Gammon K, Quaskey S: Haloperidol, fluphenazine, and clonidine in Tourette syndrome: Controversies in treatment. Pediatr Neurosci 1986;12:71.

DEMENTIA

Dementia, the symptom complex of progressive global impairment of intellectual function, is a major medical, social, and economic problem that is worsening as the number of elderly people in the general population increases. It is discussed in Chapter 2, and the only point to be reiterated here is the importance of recognizing early any treatable or reversible causes of dementia, such as normal-pressure hydrocephalus, intracranial mass lesions, vascular disease, hypothyroidism, thiamine or vitamin B_{12} deficiency, Wilson's disease, hepatic or renal failure, neurosyphilis, and the chronic meningitides.

MULTIPLE SCLEROSIS

Essentials of Diagnosis

- Episodic symptoms that may include sensory abnormalities, blurred vision, sphincter disturbances, and weakness with or without spasticity.
- Patient usually under 55 years of age at onset.
- Single pathologic lesion cannot explain clinical findings.
- Multiple foci best demonstrated radiographically by MRI.

General Considerations

This common neurologic disorder of unknown cause has its greatest incidence in young adults. Epidemiologic studies indicate that multiple sclerosis is much more common in persons of western European lineage who live in temperate zones. No population with a high risk for multiple sclerosis exists between latitudes 40° N and 40° S. Genetic, dietary, and climatic factors cannot account for these differences. There may be a familial incidence of the disease, since affected relatives are sometimes reported. The strong association between multiple sclerosis and specific HLA antigens (HLA-DR2) provides support for a theory of genetic predisposition. Many believe that the disease has an immunologic basis. Pathologically, focal—often perivenular—areas of demyelination with reactive gliosis are found scattered in the white matter of brain and spinal cord and in the optic nerves.

Clinical Findings

A. Symptoms and Signs: The common initial presentation is weakness, numbness, tingling, or unsteadiness in a limb; spastic paraparesis; retrobulbar neuritis; diplopia; disequilibrium; or a sphincter disturbance such as urinary urgency or hesitancy. Symptoms may disappear after a few days or weeks, although examination often reveals a residual deficit.

In most patients, there is an interval of months or years after the initial episode before new symptoms develop or the original ones recur. Eventually, however, relapses and usually incomplete remissions lead to increasing disability, with weakness, spasticity, and ataxia of the limbs, impaired vision, and urinary incontinence. The findings on examination at this stage commonly include optic atrophy, nystagmus, dysarthria, and pyramidal, sensory, or cerebellar deficits in some or all of the limbs.

Less commonly, symptoms are steadily progressive from their onset, and disability develops at a relatively early stage. The diagnosis cannot be made with confidence unless the total clinical picture indicates involvement of different parts of the central nervous system at different times.

A number of factors (eg, infection, trauma) may precipitate or trigger exacerbations. Relapses are also more likely during the 2 or 3 months following pregnancy, possibly because of the increased demands and stresses that occur in the postpartum period.

B. Imaging: MRI of the brain or cervical cord is often helpful in demonstrating the presence of a multiplicity of lesions. CT scans are less helpful.

In patients presenting with myelopathy alone and in whom there is no clinical or laboratory evidence of more widespread disease, myelography or MRI may be necessary to exclude a congenital or acquired surgically treatable lesion. The foramen magnum region must be visualized to exclude the possibility of Arnold-Chiari malformation, in which part of the cerebellum and the lower brain stem are displaced into the cervical canal and produce mixed pyramidal and cerebellar deficits in the limbs.

C. Laboratory and Other Studies: A definitive diagnosis can never be based solely on the laboratory findings. If there is clinical evidence of only a single lesion in the central nervous system, multiple sclerosis cannot properly be diagnosed unless it can be shown that other regions are affected subclinically. The electrocerebral responses evoked in the clinical neurophysiology laboratory by monocular visual stimulation with a checkerboard pattern stimulus, by monaural click stimulation, and by electrical stimulation of a sensory or mixed peripheral nerve have been used to detect subclinical involvement of the visual, brain stem auditory, and somatosensory pathways, respectively.

There may be mild lymphocytosis or a slightly increased protein concentration in the cerebrospinal fluid, especially soon after an acute relapse. Elevated IgG in cerebrospinal fluid and discrete bands of IgG, called oligoclonal bands, are present in many patients. The presence of such bands is not specific, however, since they have been found in a variety of inflammatory neurologic disorders and occasionally in patients with vascular or neoplastic disorders of the nervous system.

Treatment

At least partial recovery from acute exacerbations can reasonably be expected, but further relapses may occur without warning, and there is no means of preventing progression of the disorder. Some disability is likely to result eventually, but about half of all patients are without significant disability even 10 years after onset of symptoms.

Recovery from acute relapses may be hastened by treatment with corticosteroids, but the extent of recovery is unchanged. A high dose (eg, prednisone, 60 or 80 mg) is given daily for 1 week, after which medication is tapered over the following 2 or 3 weeks. Long-term treatment with steroids provides no benefit and does not prevent further relapses.

Several recent studies have suggested that intensive immunosuppressive therapy with cyclophosphamide or azathioprine may help to arrest the course of chronic progressive active multiple sclerosis. Further clinical trials are in progress. There is some evidence that plasmapheresis may enhance any beneficial effects of immunosuppression in some patients with chronic progressive multiple sclerosis, at least for a time, but its role in the management of the various clinical forms of multiple sclerosis is uncertain. The findings in a recent trial of systemic interferon therapy suggested some benefit in patients whose disease was characterized by relapses and remissions rather than by steady progression. Further studies to evaluate this form of treatment in selected patients are proceeding. Finally, preliminary studies suggest that Cop 1 (a random polymer-simulating myelin basic protein) may be beneficial in patients with the exacerbating-remitting form of multiple sclerosis, and further evaluation of this approach seems warranted.

Treatment for spasticity (see below) and for neurogenic bladder may be needed in advanced cases. Excessive fatigue must be avoided, and patients should rest during periods of acute relapse.

Bornstein MB et al: A pilot trial of Cop 1 in exacerbating-remitting multiple sclerosis. N Engl J Med 1987;317:408.

Paty DW et al: MRI in the diagnosis of MS: A prospective study with comparison of clinical evaluation, evoked potentials, oligoclonal banding, and CT. Neurology 1988;38:180.

Weiner HL, Hafler DA: Immunotherapy of multiple sclerosis. Ann Neurol 1988;23:211.

SPASTICITY

The term ''spasticity'' is commonly used for an upper motor neuron deficit, but it properly refers to a velocity-dependent increase in resistance to passive movement that affects different muscles to a different extent, is not uniform in degree throughout the range of a particular movement, and is commonly associated with other features of pyramidal deficit. It is often a major complication of stroke, cerebral or spinal injury, static perinatal encephalopathy, and multiple sclerosis.

Physical therapy with appropriate stretching programs is important during rehabilitation after the development of an upper motor neuron lesion and in subsequent management of the patient. The aim is to prevent joint and muscle contractures and perhaps to modulate spasticity.

Drug management is important also, but treatment may increase functional disability when increased extensor tone is providing additional support for patients with weak legs. Dantrolene weakens muscle contraction by interfering with the role of calcium. It may be helpful in the treatment of spasticity but is best avoided in patients with poor respiratory function or severe myocardial disease. Treatment is begun with 25 mg once daily, and the daily dose is built up by 25-mg increments every 3 days, depending on tolerance, to a maximum of 100 mg 4 times daily. The drug should be withdrawn if no benefit has occurred after treatment with the maximum tolerated dose for about 2 weeks. Side effects include diarrhea, nausea, weakness, hepatic dysfunction (that may rarely be fatal, especially in women older than 35), drowsiness, light-headedness, and hallucinations.

Baclofen seems to be the most effective drug for treating spasticity of spinal origin. It is particularly helpful in relieving painful flexor (or extensor) spasms. The maximum recommended daily dose is 80 mg; treatment is started with a dose of 5 or 10 mg twice daily and then built up gradually. Side effects include gastrointestinal disturbances, lassitude, fatigue, sedation, unsteadiness, confusion, and hallucinations. Diazepam may modify spasticity by its action on spinal interneurons and perhaps also by influencing supraspinal centers, but effective doses often cause intolerable drowsiness.

Motor-point blocks by intramuscular phenol have been used to reduce spasticity selectively in one or a few important muscles and may permit return of function in patients with incomplete myelopathies. Intrathecal injection of phenol or absolute alcohol may be helpful in more severe cases, but greater selectivity can be achieved by nerve root or peripheral nerve neurolysis. These procedures should not be undertaken until the spasticity syndrome is fully evolved, ie, only after about 1 year or so, and only if long-term drug treatment either has been unhelpful or carries a significant risk to the patient.

A number of surgical procedures, eg, adductor or heel cord tenotomy, may help in the management of spasticity. Neurectomy may also facilitate patient management. For example, obturator neurectomy is helpful in patients with marked adductor spasms that interfere with personal hygiene or cause gait disturbances. Posterior rhizotomy reduces spasticity, but its effect may be short-lived, whereas anterior rhizotomy produces permanent wasting and weakness in the muscles that are denervated.

Spasticity may be exacerbated by decubitus ulcers, urinary or other infections, and nociceptive stimuli.

MYELOPATHIES IN AIDS

Patients with AIDS may develop a subacute or chronic vacuolar myelopathy leading to paraparesis or quadriparesis, sphincter dysfunction, and sensory disturbances. There is no effective treatment. Myelitis or radiculomyelitis may occur also in AIDS patients as a result of opportunistic viral infections. When extradural lymphomatous deposits cause compressive myelopathy, pain and spinal tenderness are conspicuous, and MRI or myelography reveals the underlying lesion. Treatment is with corticosteroids, radiotherapy, and chemotherapy. Lymphomatous meningitis occurring in AIDS patients has the features described on p 699.

Petito CK et al: Vacuolar myelopathy pathologically resembling subacute combined degeneration in patients with the acquired immunodeficiency syndrome. N Engl J Med 1985;312:874.

SUBACUTE COMBINED DEGENERATION OF THE SPINAL CORD

Subacute combined degeneration of the spinal cord is due to vitamin B_{12} deficiency, such as occurs in pernicious anemia. It is characterized by myelopathy with predominant pyramidal and posterior column deficits, sometimes in association with polyneuropathy, mental changes, or optic neuropathy. Megaloblastic anemia may also occur, but this does not parallel the neurologic disorder, and the former may be obscured if folic acid supplements have been taken. Treatment is with vitamin B_{12}. For pernicious anemia, a convenient therapeutic regimen is 100 mg cyanocobalamin intramuscularly daily for 1 week, then weekly for 1 month, and then monthly for the remainder of the patient's life.

WERNICKE'S ENCEPHALOPATHY

Wernicke's encephalopathy is characterized by confusion, ataxia, and nystagmus leading to ophthalmoplegia (lateral rectus muscle weakness, conjugate gaze palsies); peripheral neuropathy may also be present. It is due to thiamine deficiency and in the USA occurs most commonly in alcoholics. In suspected cases, thiamine (50 mg) is given intravenously immediately and then intramuscularly on a daily basis until a satisfactory diet can be ensured. Intravenous glucose given before thiamine may precipitate the syndrome or worsen the symptoms. The diagnosis is confirmed by the response to treatment, which must not be delayed while laboratory confirmation is obtained.

STUPOR & COMA

The patient who is stuporous is unresponsive except when subjected to repeated vigorous stimuli, while the comatose patient is unarousable and unable to respond to external events or inner needs, although reflex movements and posturing may be present.

Coma is a major complication of serious central nervous system disorders. It can result from seizures, hypothermia, metabolic disturbances, or structural lesions causing bilateral cerebral hemispheric dysfunction or a disturbance of the brain stem reticular activating system. A mass lesion involving one cerebral hemisphere may cause coma by compression of the brain stem.

Assessment & Emergency Measures

The diagnostic workup of the comatose patient must proceed concomitantly with management. Supportive therapy for respiration or blood pressure is initiated if necessary. This is especially true in hypothermia, where all vital signs may be absent; all such patients should be rewarmed before the prognosis is assessed.

The patient can be positioned on one side with the neck partly extended, dentures removed, and secretions cleared by suction; if necessary, the patency of the airways is maintained with an oropharyngeal airway. Blood is drawn for serum glucose, electrolyte, and calcium levels; arterial blood gases; liver and renal function tests; and toxicologic studies if necessary. Dextrose 50% (25 g), naloxone (0.4–1.2 mg), and thiamine (50 mg) to counteract possible hypoglycemia, opiate overdosage, or thiamine deficiency should be given intravenously. The intravenous line is left in place to facilitate further access to the circulation.

After these initial measures, further details are obtained from attendants of the patient's medical history, the circumstances surrounding the onset of coma, and the time course of subsequent events. Abrupt onset of coma suggests subarachnoid hemorrhage, brain stem stroke, or intracerebral hemorrhage, whereas a slower onset and progression occur with other structural or mass lesions. A metabolic cause is likely with a preceding intoxicated state or agitated delirium. On examination, attention is paid to the behavioral response to painful stimuli, the pupils and their response to light, the position of the eyes and their movement in response to passive movement of the head and ice-water caloric stimulation, and the respiratory pattern.

A. Response to Painful Stimuli: Purposive limb withdrawal from painful stimuli implies that sensory pathways from and motor pathways to the stimulated limb are functionally intact, at least in part. Unilateral absence of responses despite application of stimuli to both sides of the body in turn implies a corticospinal lesion; bilateral absence of responsiveness suggests brain stem involvement, bilateral pyramidal tract lesions, or psychogenic unresponsiveness. Inappropriate responses may also occur. Decorticate posturing may occur with lesions of the internal capsule and rostral cerebral peduncle, decerebrate posturing with dysfunction or destruction of the midbrain and rostral pons, and decerebrate posturing in the arms accompanied by flaccidity or slight flexor responses in the legs in patients with extensive brain stem damage extending down to the pons at the trigeminal level.

B. Ocular Findings:

1. Pupils–Hypothalamic disease processes may lead to unilateral Horner's syndrome, while bilateral diencephalic involvement or destructive pontine lesions may lead to small but reactive pupils. Ipsilateral pupillary dilation with no direct or consensual response to light occurs with compression of the third cranial nerve, eg, with uncal herniation. The pupils are slightly smaller than normal but responsive to light in many metabolic encephalopathies; however, they may be fixed and dilated following overdosage with atropine, scopolamine, or glutethimide, and pinpoint (but responsive) with opiates. Pupillary dilatation for several hours following cardiopulmonary arrest implies a poor prognosis.

2. Eye movements–Conjugate deviation of the eyes to the side suggests the presence of an ipsilateral hemispheric lesion or a contralateral pontine lesion. A mesencephalic lesion leads to downward conjugate deviation. Dysconjugate ocular deviation in coma implies a structural brain stem lesion unless there was preexisting strabismus.

The oculomotor responses to passive head turning and to caloric stimulation relate to each other and provide complementary information. In response to brisk rotation of the head from side to side and to flexion and extension of the head, normally conscious patients with open eyes do not exhibit contraversive conjugate eye deviation (doll's-head eye response) unless there is voluntary visual fixation or bilateral frontal pathology. With cortical depression in lightly comatose patients, a brisk doll's-head eye response is seen. With brain stem lesions, this oculocephalic reflex becomes impaired or lost, depending on the site of the lesion.

The oculovestibular reflex is tested by caloric stimulation using irrigation with ice water. In normal subjects, jerk nystagmus is elicited for about 2 or 3 minutes, with the slow component toward the irrigated ear. In unconscious patients with an intact brain stem, the fast component of the nystagmus disappears, so that the eyes tonically deviate toward the irrigated side for 2–3 minutes before returning to their original position. With impairment of brain stem function, the response becomes perverted and finally disappears. In metabolic coma, oculocephalic and oculovestibular reflex responses are preserved, at least initially.

C. Respiratory Patterns: Diseases causing coma may lead to respiratory abnormalities. Cheyne-Stokes respiration may occur with bihemispheric or diencephalic disease or in metabolic disorders. Central neurogenic hyperventilation occurs with lesions of the brain stem tegmentum; apneustic breathing (in which there are prominent end-inspiratory pauses) suggests damage at the pontine level (eg, due to basilar artery occlusion); and atactic breathing (a completely irregular pattern of breathing with deep and shallow breaths occurring randomly) is associated with lesions of the lower pontine tegmentum and medulla.

1. STUPOR & COMA DUE TO STRUCTURAL LESIONS

Supratentorial mass lesions tend to affect brain function in an orderly way. There may initially be signs of hemispheric dysfunction, such as hemiparesis. As coma develops and deepens, cerebral function becomes progressively disturbed, producing a predictable progression of neurologic signs that suggest rostrocaudal deterioration.

Thus, as a supratentorial mass lesion begins to impair the diencephalon, the patient becomes drowsy, then stuporous, and finally comatose. There may be Cheyne-Stokes respiration; small but reactive pupils; doll's-head eye responses with side-to-side head movements but sometimes an impairment of reflex upward gaze with brisk flexion of the head; tonic ipsilateral deviation of the eyes in response to vestibular stimulation with cold water; and initially a positive response to pain but subsequently only decorticate posturing. With further progression, midbrain failure occurs. Motor dysfunction progresses from decorticate to bilateral decerebrate posturing in response to painful stimuli; Cheyne-Stokes respiration is gradually replaced by sustained central hyperventilation; the pupils become middle-sized and fixed; and the oculocephalic and oculovestibular reflex responses become impaired, perverted, or lost. As the pons and then the medulla fail, the pupils remain unresponsive; oculovestibular responses are unobtainable; respiration is rapid and shallow; and painful stimuli may lead only to flexor responses in the legs. Finally, respiration becomes irregular and stops, the pupils often then dilating widely.

In contrast, a subtentorial (ie, brain stem) lesion may lead to an early, sometimes abrupt disturbance of consciousness without any orderly rostrocaudal progression of neurologic signs. Compressive lesions of the brain stem, especially cerebellar hemorrhage, may be clinically indistinguishable from intraparenchymal processes.

A structural lesion is suspected if the findings suggest focality. In such circumstances, a CT scan should be performed before, or instead of, a lumbar puncture in order to avoid any risk of cerebral herniation. Further management is of the causal lesion and is considered separately under the individual disorders.

2. STUPOR & COMA DUE TO METABOLIC DISTURBANCES

Patients with a metabolic cause of coma generally have signs of patchy, diffuse, and symmetric neurologic involvement that cannot be explained by loss of function at any single level or in a sequential manner, although focal or lateralized deficits may occur in hypoglycemia. Moreover, pupillary reactivity is usually preserved, while other brain stem functions are often grossly impaired. Comatose patients with meningitis, encephalitis, or subarachnoid hemorrhage may also exhibit little in the way of focal neurologic signs, however, and clinical evidence of meningeal irritation is sometimes very subtle in comatose patients. Examination of the cerebrospinal fluid in such patients is essential to establish the correct diagnosis.

In patients with coma due to cerebral ischemia and hypoxia, the absence of pupillary light reflexes at the time of initial examination indicates that there is little chance of regaining independence; by contrast, preserved pupillary light responses, the development of spontaneous eye movements (roving, conjugate, or better), and extensor, flexor, or withdrawal responses to pain at this early stage imply a relatively good prognosis.

Treatment of metabolic encephalopathy is of the underlying disturbance and is considered in other chapters. If the cause of the encephalopathy is obscure, all drugs except essential ones may have to be withdrawn in case they are responsible for the altered mental status.

Levy DE et al: Predicting outcome from hypoxic-ischemic coma. JAMA 1985;253:1420.

3. BRAIN DEATH

The definition of brain death is controversial, and diagnostic criteria have been published by many different professional organizations. In order to establish brain death, the irreversibly comatose patient must be shown to have lost all brain stem reflex responses, including the pupillary, corneal, oculovestibular, oculocephalic, oropharyngeal, and respiratory reflexes, and should have been in this condition for at least 6 hours. Spinal reflex movements do not exclude the diagnosis, but ongoing seizure activity or decerebrate or decorticate posturing is not consistent with brain death. The apnea test (presence or absence of spontaneous respiratory activity at a $Paco_2$ of at least 60 mm Hg) serves to determine whether the patient is capable of respiratory activity.

Reversible coma simulating brain death may be seen with hypothermia (temperature <32 °C) and overdosage with central nervous system depressant drugs, and these conditions must be excluded. Certain ancillary tests may assist the determination of brain death but are not essential. An isoelectric electroencephalogram, when the recording is made according to the recommendations of the American Electroencephalographic Society, is especially helpful in confirming the diagnosis. Alternatively, the demonstration of an absent cerebral circulation by intravenous radioisotope cerebral angiography or by 4-vessel contrast cerebral angiography can be confirmatory.

Chatrian GE: Electrophysiologic evaluation of brain death: A critical appraisal. In: *Electrodiagnosis in Clinical Neurology*, 2nd ed. Aminoff MJ (editor). Churchill Livingstone, 1986.

Lynn J: Guidelines for the determination of death: Report of the medical consultants on the diagnosis of death to the President's Commission for the Study of Ethical Problems in Medicine and Biomedical and Behavioral Research. Neurology 1982;32:395.

4. PERSISTENT VEGETATIVE STATE

Patients with severe bilateral hemispheric disease may show some improvement from an initially comatose state, so that, after a variable interval, they appear to be awake but lie motionless and without evidence of awareness or higher mental activity. This persistent vegetative state has been variously referred to as akinetic mutism, apallic state, or coma vigil. Most patients in this persistent vegetative state will die in months or years, but partial recovery has occasionally occurred and in rare instances has been sufficient to permit communication or even independent living.

5. LOCKED-IN SYNDROME (De-efferented State)

Acute destructive lesions (eg, infarction, hemorrhage, demyelination, encephalitis) involving the ventral pons and sparing the tegmentum may lead to a mute, quadriparetic but conscious state in which the patient is capable of blinking and of voluntary eye movement in the vertical plane, with preserved pupillary responses to light. Such a patient can mistakenly be regarded as comatose. Physicians should recognize that "locked-in" individuals are fully aware of their surroundings. Prognosis is variable, but recovery has occasionally been reported, in some cases including resumption of independent daily life, though this may take up to 2 or 3 years.

HEAD INJURY

Trauma is the most common cause of death in young people, and head injury accounts for almost half of these trauma-related deaths. The prognosis following head injury depends upon the site and severity of brain damage. Some guide to prognosis is provided by the mental status, since loss of consciousness for more than 1 or 2 minutes implies a worse prognosis than otherwise. Similarly, the degree of retrograde and posttraumatic amnesia provides an indication of the severity of injury and thus of the prognosis. Absence of skull fracture does not exclude the possibility of severe head injury. During the physical examination, special attention should be given to the level of consciousness and extent of any brain stem dysfunction.

Note: In general, patients who have lost consciousness for 2 minutes or more following head injury should be admitted to the hospital for observation, as should patients with focal neurologic deficits, lethargy, or skull fractures. If patients are not to be detained, responsible family members should be given clear instructions about the need for, and manner of, checking on them at regular (hourly) intervals and for obtaining additional medical help if necessary. Deterioration is an indication for further investigation.

Skull radiographs or CT scans may provide evidence of fractures. Because injury to the spine may have accompanied head trauma, cervical spine radiographs (especially in the lateral projection) should always be obtained in comatose patients and in patients with severe neck pain or a deficit possibly related to cord compression. CT scanning has an important role in demonstrating intracranial hemorrhage and may also provide evidence of cerebral edema and displacement of midline structures.

Cerebral Injuries

These are summarized in Table 18–5 along with comments about treatment.

Scalp Injuries & Skull Fractures

Scalp lacerations and depressed or compound depressed skull fractures should be treated surgically as appropriate. Simple skull fractures require no specific treatment.

The clinical signs of basilar skull fracture include bruising about the orbit (raccoon sign), blood in the external auditory meatus (Battle's sign), and leakage of cerebrospinal fluid (which can be identified by its glucose content) from the ear or nose. Cranial nerve palsies (involving especially the first, second, third, fourth, fifth, seventh, and eighth nerves in any combination) may also occur. If there is any leakage of cerebrospinal fluid, conservative treatment, with elevation of the head, restriction of fluids, and administration of acetazolamide (250 mg 4 times daily), is often helpful; but if the leak continues for more than a few days, lumbar subarachnoid drainage may be necessary. Antibiotics are given if infection occurs, based on culture and sensitivity studies. Only very occasional patients require intracranial repair of the dural defect because of persistence of the leak or recurrent meningitis.

Late Complications of Head Injury

The relationship of chronic subdural hemorrhage to head injury is not always clear. In many elderly persons there is no history of trauma, but in other cases a head injury, often trivial, precedes the onset of symptoms by several weeks. The clinical presentation is usually with mental changes such as slowness, drowsiness, headache, confusion, memory disturbances, personality change, or even dementia. Focal neurologic deficits such as hemiparesis or hemisensory disturbance may also occur but are less common. CT scan is an important means of detecting the hematoma, which is sometimes bilateral. Treatment is by surgical evacuation to prevent cerebral compression and tentorial herniation.

Normal-pressure hydrocephalus may follow head injury, subarachnoid hemorrhage, or meningoencephalitis.

Other late complications of head injury include posttraumatic seizure disorder and posttraumatic headache.

Table 18–5. Acute cerebral sequelae of head injury.

Sequelae	Clinical Features	Pathology
Concussion	Transient loss of consciousness with bradycardia, hypotension, and respiratory arrest for a few seconds followed by retrograde and posttraumatic amnesia. Occasionally followed by transient neurologic deficit.	Bruising on side of impact (coup injury) or contralaterally (contrecoup injury).
Cerebral contusion/ laceration	Loss of consciousness longer than with concussion. May lead to death or severe residual neurologic deficit.	Cerebral contusion, edema, hemorrhage, and necrosis. May have subarachnoid bleeding.
Acute epidural hemorrhage	Headache, confusion, somnolence, seizures, and focal deficits occur several hours after injury and lead to coma, respiratory depression, and death unless treated by surgical evacuation.	Tear in meningeal artery, vein, or dural sinus, leading to hematoma visible on CT scan.
Acute subdural hemorrhage	Similar to epidural hemorrhage, but interval before onset of symptoms is longer. Treatment is by surgical evacuation.	Hematoma from tear in veins from cortex to superior sagittal sinus or from cerebral laceration, visible on CT scan.
Cerebral hemorrhage	Generally develops immediately after injury. Clinically resembles hypertensive hemorrhage. Surgical evacuation is sometimes helpful.	Hematoma, visible on CT scan.

SPINAL TRAUMA

While spinal cord damage may result from whiplash injury, severe injury usually relates to fracture-dislocation causing compression or angular deformity of the cord either cervically or in the lower thoracic and upper lumbar region. Extreme hypotension following injury may also lead to cord infarction.

Total cord transection results in immediate flaccid paralysis and loss of sensation below the level of the lesion. Reflex activity is lost for a variable period, and there is urinary and fecal retention. As reflex function returns over the following days and weeks, spastic paraplegia or quadriplegia develops, with hyperreflexia and extensor plantar responses, but a flaccid atrophic (lower motor neuron) paralysis may be found depending on the segments of the cord that are affected. The bladder and bowels also regain some reflex function, permitting urine and feces to be expelled at intervals. As spasticity increases, flexor or extensor spasms (or both) of the legs become troublesome, especially if the patient develops bed sores or a urinary tract infection. Paraplegia with the legs in flexion or extension may eventually result.

With lesser degrees of injury, patients may be left with mild limb weakness, distal sensory disturbance, or both. Sphincter function may also be impaired, urinary urgency and urgency incontinence being especially common. More particularly, a unilateral cord lesion leads to an ipsilateral motor disturbance with accompanying impairment of proprioception and contralateral loss of pain and temperature appreciation below the lesion (Brown-Séquard syndrome). A central cord syndrome may lead to a lower motor neuron deficit and loss of pain and temperature appreciation, with sparing of posterior column functions. A radicular deficit may occur at the level of the injury—or, if the cauda equina is involved, there may be evidence of disturbed function in several lumbosacral roots.

Treatment of the injury consists of immobilization and—if there is cord compression—decompressive laminectomy and fusion. Anatomic realignment of the spinal cord by traction and other orthopedic procedures is also important. Subsequent care of the residual neurologic deficit—paraplegia or quadriplegia—requires treatment of spasticity and care of the skin, bladder, and bowels.

SYRINGOMYELIA

Destruction or degeneration of gray and white matter adjacent to the central canal of the cervical spinal cord leads to cavitation and accumulation of fluid within the spinal cord. The precise pathogenesis is unclear, but many cases are associated with Arnold-Chiari malformation, in which there is displacement of the cerebellar tonsils, medulla, and fourth ventricle into the spinal canal, sometimes with accompanying meningomyelocele. In such circumstances, the cord cavity connects with and may merely represent a dilated central canal. In other cases, the cause of cavitation is less clear. There is a characteristic clinical picture, with segmental atrophy and areflexia and loss of pain and temperature appreciation in a "cape" distribution owing to the destruction of fibers crossing in front of the central canal. Thoracic kyphoscoliosis is usually present. With progression, involvement of the long motor and sensory tracts occurs as well, so that a pyramidal and sensory deficit develops in the legs. Upward extension of the cavitation (syringobulbia) leads to dysfunction of the lower brain stem and thus to bulbar palsy, nystagmus, and sensory impairment over one or both sides of the face.

Syringomyelia, ie, cord cavitation, may also occur in association with an intramedullary tumor or following severe cord injury, and the cavity then does not communicate with the central canal.

In patients with Arnold-Chiari malformation, there are commonly skeletal abnormalities on plain x-rays of the skull and cervical spine. CT scans show caudal displacement of the fourth ventricle. MRI or positive contrast myelography may demonstrate the malformation itself. Focal cord enlargement is found at myelography or by MRI in patients with cavitation related to past injury or intramedullary neoplasms.

Treatment of Arnold-Chiari malformation with associated syringomyelia is by suboccipital craniectomy and upper cervical laminectomy, with the aim of decompressing the malformation at the foramen magnum. The cord cavity should be drained, and if necessary an outlet for the fourth ventricle can be made. In cavitation associated with intramedullary tumor, treatment is surgical, but radiation therapy may be necessary if complete removal is not possible. Post-traumatic syringomyelia is also treated surgically if it leads to increasing neurologic deficits or to intolerable pain.

MOTOR NEURON DISEASES

This group of disorders is characterized clinically by weakness and variable wasting of affected muscles, without accompanying sensory changes. Certain of these disorders, such as Werdnig-Hoffman disease and Kugelberg-Welander syndrome, occur in infants or children and are not considered further here.

Motor neuron disease in adults generally commences between 30 and 60 years of age. There is degeneration of the anterior horn cells in the spinal cord, the motor nuclei of the lower cranial nerves, and the corticospinal and corticobulbar pathways. The disorder is usually sporadic, but familial cases may occur.

Classification

Five varieties have been distinguished on clinical grounds.

A. Progressive Bulbar Palsy: Bulbar involvement predominates owing to disease processes affecting primarily the motor nuclei of the cranial nerves.

B. Pseudobulbar Palsy: Bulbar involvement predominates in this variety also, but it is due to bilateral corticobulbar disease and thus reflects upper motor neuron dysfunction.

C. Progressive Spinal Muscular Atrophy: This is characterized primarily by a lower motor neuron deficit in the limbs due to degeneration of the anterior horn cells in the spinal cord.

D. Primary Lateral Sclerosis: There is a purely upper motor neuron deficit in the limbs.

E. Amyotrophic Lateral Sclerosis: A mixed upper and lower motor neuron deficit is found in the limbs. This disorder is sometimes associated with dementia, parkinsonism, and other neurologic diseases.

Clinical Findings

A. Symptoms and Signs: Difficulty in swallowing, chewing, coughing, breathing, and talking (dysarthria) occur with bulbar involvement. In progressive bulbar palsy, there is drooping of the palate, a depressed gag reflex, pooling of saliva in the pharynx, a weak cough, and a wasted, fasciculating tongue. In pseudobulbar palsy, the tongue is contracted and spastic and cannot be moved rapidly from side to side. Limb involvement is characterized by motor disturbances (weakness, stiffness, wasting, fasciculations) reflecting lower or upper motor neuron dysfunction; there are no objective changes on sensory examination, though there may be vague sensory complaints. The sphincters are generally spared.

The disorder is progressive and usually fatal within 3–5 years; death usually results from pulmonary infections. Patients with bulbar involvement generally have the poorest prognosis.

B. Laboratory and Other Studies: Electromyography may show changes of chronic partial denervation, with abnormal spontaneous activity in the resting muscle and a reduction in the number of motor units under voluntary control. Motor conduction velocity is usually normal but may be slightly reduced, and sensory conduction studies are also normal. Biopsy of a wasted muscle shows the histologic changes of denervation. The serum creatine phosphokinase may be slightly elevated but never reaches the extremely high values seen in some of the muscular dystrophies. The cerebrospinal fluid is normal.

There have been recent reports of juvenile spinal muscular atrophy due to hexosaminidase deficiency, with abnormal findings on rectal biopsy and reduced hexosaminidase A in serum and leukocytes. Pure motor syndromes resembling motor neuron disease may also occur in association with monoclonal gammopathy or multifocal motor neuropathies due to conduction block. A motor neuronopathy may also develop

in Hodgkin's disease and has a relatively benign prognosis.

Treatment

There is no specific treatment except in patients with gammopathy, in whom plasmapheresis and immunosuppression may lead to improvement. Symptomatic and supportive measures may include prescription of anticholinergic drugs (such as trihexyphenidyl, amitriptyline, or atropine) if drooling is troublesome, braces or a walker to improve mobility, and physical therapy to prevent contractures. Spasticity may be helped by baclofen or diazepam. A semiliquid diet or nasogastric tube feeding may be needed if dysphagia is severe. Gastrostomy or cricopharyngomyotomy is sometimes resorted to in extreme cases of predominant bulbar involvement, and tracheostomy may be necessary if respiratory muscles are severely affected; however, in the terminal stages of these disorders, the aim of treatment should be to keep patients as comfortable as possible.

Mitsumoto H, Hanson MR, Chad DA: Amyotrophic lateral sclerosis: Recent advances in pathogenesis and therapeutic trials. Arch Neurol 1988;45:189.
Parry GJ et al: Gammopathy with proximal motor axonopathy simulating motor neuron disease. Neurology 1986; 36:273.

PERIPHERAL NEUROPATHIES

Peripheral neuropathies can be categorized on the basis of the structure primarily affected. The predominant pathologic feature may be axonal degeneration (axonal or neuronal neuropathies) or paranodal or segmental demyelination. The distinction may be possible on the basis of neurophysiologic findings. Motor and sensory conduction velocity can be measured in accessible segments of peripheral nerves. In axonal neuropathies, conduction velocity is normal or reduced only mildly and needle electromyography provides evidence of denervation in affected muscles. In demyelinating neuropathies, conduction may be slowed considerably in affected fibers, and in more severe cases, conduction is blocked completely, without accompanying electromyographic signs of denervation.

Peripheral neuropathies may also occur as a result of disorders affecting the connective tissues of the nerves or the blood vessels supplying the nerves, but these are much less common than the preceding varieties.

Nerves may be injured or compressed by neighboring anatomic structures at any point along their course. Common **mononeuropathies** of this sort are considered on p 721. They lead to a sensory, motor, or mixed deficit that is restricted to the territory of the affected nerve. A similar clinical disturbance is produced by peripheral nerve tumors, but these are rare except in patients with Recklinghausen's disease. Multiple mononeuropathies suggest a patchy multifocal disease process such as vasculopathy (eg, diabetes, arteritis), an infiltrative process (eg, leprosy, sarcoidosis), radiation damage, or an immunologic disorder (eg, brachial plexopathy). Diffuse **polyneuropathies** lead to a symmetric sensory, motor, or mixed deficit, often most marked distally. They include the hereditary, metabolic, and toxic disorders; idiopathic inflammatory polyneuropathy (Guillain-Barre syndrome); and the peripheral neuropathies that may occur as a nonmetastatic complication of malignant diseases. Involvement of motor fibers leads to flaccid weakness that is most marked distally; dysfunction of sensory fibers causes impaired sensory perception. Tendon reflexes are depressed or absent. Paresthesias, pain, and muscle tenderness may also occur.

1. POLYNEUROPATHIES & MONONEURITIS MULTIPLEX

The cause of polyneuropathy or mononeuritis multiplex is suggested by the history, mode of onset, and predominant clinical manifestations. Laboratory workup includes a complete blood count and sedimentation rate, serum protein electrophoresis, determination of plasma urea and electrolytes, liver and thyroid function tests, tests for rheumatoid factor and antinuclear antibody, a serologic test for syphilis, fasting blood glucose level, urinary heavy metal levels, cerebrospinal fluid examination, and chest radiography. These tests should be ordered selectively, as guided by symptoms and signs. Measurement of nerve conduction velocity is important in confirming the peripheral nerve origin of symptoms and providing a means of following clinical changes, as well as indicating the likely disease process (ie, axonal or demyelinating neuropathy). Cutaneous nerve biopsy may help establish a precise diagnosis (eg, polyarteritis, amyloidosis). In about half of cases, no specific cause can be established; of these, slightly less than half are subsequently found to be heredofamilial.

Treatment is of the underlying cause, when feasible, and is discussed below under the individual disorders. Physical therapy helps prevent contractures, and splints can maintain a weak extremity in a position of useful function. Anesthetic extremities must be protected from injury. To guard against burns, patients should check the temperature of water and hot surfaces with a portion of skin having normal sensation, measure water temperature with a thermometer, and use cold water for washing or lower the temperature setting of their hot-water heaters. Shoes should be examined frequently during the day for grit or foreign objects in order to prevent pressure lesions.

Patients with polyneuropathies or mononeuritis multiplex are subject to additional nerve injury at pressure points and should therefore avoid such behavior as leaning on elbows or sitting with crossed legs for lengthy periods.

Neuropathic pain is sometimes troublesome and may respond to simple analgesics such as aspirin. Narcotics or narcotic substitutes may be necessary for severe hyperpathia or pain induced by minimal stimuli, but their use should be avoided as far as possible. The use of a frame or cradle to reduce contact with bedclothes may be helpful. Many patients experience episodic stabbing pains, which may respond to phenytoin, carbamazepine, or tricyclic antidepressants.

Symptoms of autonomic dysfunction are occasionally troublesome. Postural hypotension is often helped by wearing waist-high elastic stockings and sleeping in a semierect position at night. Fludrocortisone reduces postural hypotension, but doses as high as 1 mg/d are sometimes necessary in diabetics and may lead to recumbent hypertension. Indomethacin (25 or 50 mg 3 times daily) is sometimes helpful. Impotence and diarrhea are difficult to treat; a flaccid neuropathic bladder may respond to parasympathomimetic drugs such as bethanechol chloride, 10–50 mg 3 or 4 times daily.

Inherited Neuropathies

A. Charcot-Marie-Tooth Disease: Several distinct varieties of Charcot-Marie-Tooth disease can be recognized. There is usually an autosomal dominant mode of inheritance, but occasional cases occur on a sporadic, recessive, or X-linked basis. Clinical presentation may be with foot deformities or gait disturbances in childhood or early adult life. Slow progression leads to the typical features of polyneuropathy, with distal weakness and wasting that begin in the legs, a variable amount of distal sensory loss, and depressed or absent tendon reflexes. Tremor is a conspicuous feature in some instances. Pathologic examination reveals segmental demyelination and remyelination of peripheral nerves, an increase in their transverse fascicular area, and hyperplasia of Schwann cells. Electrodiagnostic studies show a marked reduction in motor and sensory conduction velocity (hereditary motor and sensory neuropathy [HMSN] type I).

In other instances (HMSN type II), motor conduction velocity is normal or only slightly reduced, sensory nerve action potentials may be absent, and signs of chronic partial denervation are found in affected muscles electromyographically. The predominant pathologic change is axonal loss rather than segmental demyelination.

A similar disorder may occur in patients with progressive distal spinal muscular atrophy, but there is no sensory loss; electrophysiologic investigation reveals that motor conduction velocity is normal or only slightly reduced, and nerve action potentials are normal.

B. Dejerine-Sottas Disease (HMSN Type III):
Most cases are sporadic or autosomal recessive. The
recessive form has its onset in infancy or childhood
and leads to a progressive motor and sensory polyneuropathy with weakness, ataxia, sensory loss, and depressed or absent tendon reflexes. The peripheral
nerves may be palpably enlarged and are characterized
pathologically by segmental demyelination, Schwann
cell hyperplasia, and thin myelin sheaths. Electrophysiologically, there is slowing of conduction, and
sensory action potentials may be unrecordable.

C. Friedreich's Ataxia: Patients generally present in childhood or early adult life with this autosomal
recessive disorder. The gait becomes atactic, the
hands become clumsy, and other signs of cerebellar
dysfunction develop accompanied by weakness of
the legs and extensor plantar responses. Involvement
of peripheral sensory fibers leads to sensory disturbances in the limbs and depressed tendon reflexes.
There is bilateral pes cavus. Pathologically, there is
a marked loss of cells in the posterior root ganglia
and degeneration of peripheral sensory fibers. In the
central nervous system, changes are conspicuous in
the posterior and lateral columns of the cord. Electrophysiologically, conduction velocity in motor fibers
is normal or only mildly reduced, but sensory action
potentials are small or absent.

D. Refsum's Disease (HMSN Type IV): This
autosomal recessive disorder is due to a disturbance
in phytanic acid metabolism. Clinically, pigmentary
retinal degeneration is accompanied by progressive
sensorimotor polyneuropathy and cerebellar signs.
Auditory dysfunction, cardiomyopathy, and cutaneous manifestations may also occur. Motor and sensory conduction velocity is reduced, often markedly,
and there may be electromyographic evidence of denervation in affected muscles. Dietary restriction of
phytanic acid and its precursors may be helpful therapeutically.

E. Porphyria: Peripheral nerve involvement may
occur during acute attacks in both variegate porphyria
and acute intermittent porphyria. The general clinical
features of these disorders are discussed in Chapter
34. Motor symptoms usually occur first, and weakness
is often most marked proximally and in the upper
limbs rather than the lower. Sensory symptoms and
signs may be proximal or distal in distribution. Autonomic involvement is sometimes pronounced. The
electrophysiologic findings are in keeping with the
results of neuropathologic studies suggesting that
the neuropathy is axonal in type. A high-carbohydrate
diet and, in severe cases, intravenous glucose or levu-
lose may be helpful in treatment. Propranolol may
also be beneficial in acute attacks.

Neuropathies Associated With Systemic & Metabolic Disorders

A. Diabetes Mellitus: In this disorder, involvement of the peripheral nervous system may lead to
symmetric sensory or mixed polyneuropathy, asymmetric motor neuropathy (diabetic amyotrophy), thoracoabdominal radiculopathy, autonomic neuropathy,
or isolated lesions of individual nerves. These may
occur singly or in any combination.

Sensory polyneuropathy, the most common manifestation, may lead to no more than depressed tendon
reflexes and impaired appreciation of vibration in the
legs. When symptomatic, there may be pain, paresthesias, or numbness in the legs, but in severe cases
distal sensory loss occurs in all limbs. Diabetic amyotrophy is characterized by asymmetric weakness and
wasting involving predominantly the proximal muscles of the legs, accompanied by local pain. Thoracoabdominal radiculopathy leads to pain over the trunk.
In patients with autonomic neuropathy, postural hypotension, impaired thermoregulatory sweating, post-
gustatory hyperhidrosis, constipation, flatulence, diarrhea, impotence, urinary retention, and incontinence may occur, and there may be abnormal pupillary
responses. Isolated lesions of individual peripheral
nerves are common and in the limbs tend to occur
at sites of compression or entrapment. Treatment is
symptomatic. Entrapment neuropathies may be helped
by surgical decompression. Treatment of neuropathic
pain is discussed above.

B. Uremia: Uremia may lead to a symmetric sensorimotor polyneuropathy that tends to affect the lower
limbs more than the upper limbs and is more marked
distally than proximally. The diagnosis can be confirmed electrophysiologically, for motor and sensory
conduction velocity is moderately reduced. The neuropathy improves both clinically and electrophysiologically with renal transplantation and to a lesser
extent with chronic dialysis.

C. Alcoholism and Nutritional Deficiency:
Many alcoholics have an axonal distal sensorimotor
polyneuropathy that is frequently accompanied by
painful cramps, muscle tenderness, and painful paresthesias and is often more marked in the legs than
in the arms. Symptoms of autonomic dysfunction
may also be conspicuous. Motor and sensory conduction velocity may be slightly reduced, even in subclinical cases, but gross slowing of conduction is uncommon. A similar distal sensorimotor polyneuropathy
is a well-recognized feature of beriberi (thiamine deficiency). In vitamin B_{12} deficiency, distal sensory
polyneuropathy may develop but is usually overshadowed by central nervous system manifestations
(eg, myelopathy, optic neuropathy, or intellectual
changes).

D. Paraproteinemias: A symmetric sensorimotor polyneuropathy that is gradual in onset, progressive in course, and often accompanied by pain
and dysesthesias in the limbs may occur in patients
(especially men) with multiple myeloma. The neuropathy is of the axonal type in classic lytic myeloma,
but segmental demyelination (primary or secondary)
and axonal loss may occur in sclerotic myeloma and

lead to predominantly motor clinical manifestations. Both demyelinating and axonal neuropathies are also observed in patients with paraproteinemias without myeloma. A small fraction will develop myeloma if serially followed. The demyelinating neuropathy in these patients may be due to the monoclonal protein's reacting to a component of the nerve myelin. The neuropathy of classic multiple myeloma is poorly responsive to therapy. The polyneuropathy of benign monoclonal gammopathy may respond to immunosuppressant drugs and plasmapheresis.

Polyneuropathy may also occur in association with macroglobulinemia and cryoglobulinemia and sometimes responds to plasmapheresis. Entrapment neuropathy, such as carpal tunnel syndrome, is more common than polyneuropathy in patients with (nonhereditary) generalized amyloidosis. With polyneuropathy due to amyloidosis, sensory and autonomic symptoms are especially conspicuous, whereas distal wasting and weakness occur later; there is no specific treatment.

Neuropathies Associated With Infectious & Inflammatory Diseases

A. Leprosy: Leprosy is an important cause of peripheral neuropathy in certain parts of the world. Sensory disturbances are mainly due to involvement of intracutaneous nerves. In tuberculoid leprosy, they develop at the same time and in the same distribution as the skin lesion but may be more extensive if nerve trunks lying beneath the lesion are also involved. In lepromatous leprosy, there is more extensive sensory loss, and this develops earlier and to a greater extent in the coolest regions of the body, such as the dorsal surfaces of the hands and feet, where the bacilli proliferate most actively. Motor deficits result from involvement of superficial nerves where their temperature is lowest, eg, the ulnar nerve in the region proximal to the olecranon groove, the median nerve as it emerges from beneath the forearm flexor muscle to run toward the carpal tunnel, the peroneal nerve at the head of the fibula, and the posterior tibial nerve in the lower part of the leg; patchy facial muscular weakness may also occur owing to involvement of the superficial branches of the seventh cranial nerve.

Motor disturbances in leprosy are suggestive of multiple mononeuropathy, whereas sensory changes resemble those of distal polyneuropathy. Examination, however, relates the distribution of sensory deficits to the temperature of the tissues; in the legs, for example, sparing frequently occurs between the toes and in the popliteal fossae, where the temperature is higher. Treatment is with antileprotic agents (see Chapter 26).

B. AIDS: A variety of neuropathies occur in HIV-infected patients. Patients with AIDS may develop a chronic symmetric sensorimotor axonal **polyneuropathy** associated usually with no abnormal cerebrospinal fluid findings. Treatment is symptomatic, but azidothymidine may be helpful. AIDS patients may also develop progressive **polyradiculopathy** or radiculomyelopathy that leads to leg weakness and urinary retention; sensory loss is less conspicuous than in polyneuropathy. The cerebrospinal fluid may show mononuclear pleocytosis and increased protein and low glucose concentrations. Cytomegalovirus is responsible in at least some cases. The prognosis is generally poor.

An inflammatory **demyelinating polyradiculoneuropathy** sometimes occurs in seropositive patients without AIDS and may follow an acute, subacute, or chronic course. Weakness is usually more conspicuous distally than proximally and tends to overshadow sensory symptoms. Tendon reflexes are depressed or absent. The cerebrospinal fluid shows an increased cell count and protein concentration. Treatment with plasmapheresis has helped some patients. Spontaneous improvement may also occur. Seropositive patients without AIDS may also develop a **mononeuropathy multiplex** that sometimes responds to treatment with plasmapheresis.

C. Sarcoidosis: Sarcoidosis may affect the central nervous system. In addition, cranial nerve palsies (especially facial palsy), multiple mononeuropathy, and, less commonly, symmetric polyneuropathy may all occur, the latter sometimes preferentially affecting either motor or sensory fibers. Improvement may occur with use of corticosteroids.

D. Polyarteritis: Involvement of the vasa nervorum by the vasculitic process may result in infarction of the nerve. Clinically, one encounters an asymmetric sensorimotor polyneuropathy (mononeuritis multiplex) that pursues a waxing and waning course. Steroids and cytotoxic agents—especially cyclophosphamide—may be of benefit in severe cases.

E. Rheumatoid Arthritis: Compressive or entrapment neuropathies, ischemic neuropathies, mild distal sensory polyneuropathy, and severe progressive sensorimotor polyneuropathy can occur in rheumatoid arthritis.

Toxic Neuropathies

Axonal polyneuropathy may follow exposure to industrial agents or pesticides such as acrylamide, organophosphorus compounds, hexacarbon solvents, methyl bromide, and carbon disulfide; metals such as arsenic, thallium, mercury, and lead; and drugs such as phenytoin, perhexiline, isoniazid, nitrofurantoin, vincristine, and pyridoxine in high doses. Detailed occupational, environmental, and medical histories and recognition of clusters of cases are important in suggesting the diagnosis. Treatment is by preventing further exposure to the causal agent. Isoniazid neuropathy is prevented by pyridoxine supplementation.

Diphtheritic neuropathy results from a neurotoxin released by the causative organism and is common in many areas. Palatal weakness may develop 2–4 weeks after infection of the throat, and infection of the skin may similarly be followed by focal weakness of neighboring muscles. Disturbances of accommodation may occur about 4–5 weeks after infection and distal sensorimotor demyelinating polyneuropathy after 1–3 months.

Neuropathies Associated With Malignant Diseases

Both a sensorimotor and a purely sensory polyneuropathy may occur as a nonmetastatic complication of malignant diseases. The sensorimotor polyneuropathy may be mild and occur in the course of known malignant disease; or it may have an acute or subacute onset, lead to severe disability, and occur before there is any clinical evidence of the cancer, occasionally following a remitting course.

Acute Idiopathic Polyneuropathy (Guillain-Barré Syndrome)

This acute or subacute polyradiculoneuropathy sometimes follows infective illness, inoculations, or surgical procedures but often occurs in a previously well person. It probably has an immunologic basis, but the precise mechanism is unclear. The main complaint is of weakness that varies widely in severity in different patients and often has a proximal emphasis and symmetric distribution. It usually begins in the legs, spreading to a variable extent but frequently involving the arms and often one or both sides of the face. The muscles of respiration or deglutition may also be affected. Sensory symptoms are usually less conspicuous than motor ones, but distal paresthesias and dysesthesias are common, and neuropathic or radicular pain is present in many patients. Autonomic disturbances are also common, may be severe, and are sometimes life-threatening; they include tachycardia, cardiac irregularities, hypotension or hypertension, facial flushing, abnormalities of sweating, pulmonary dysfunction, and impaired sphincter control.

The cerebrospinal fluid characteristically contains a high protein concentration with a normal cell content, but these changes may take 2 or 3 weeks to develop. Electrophysiologic studies may reveal marked abnormalities, which do not necessarily parallel the clinical disorder in their temporal course. Pathologic examination has shown that primary demyelination occurs in regions infiltrated with inflammatory cells, and it seems probable that myelin disruption has an autoimmune basis.

When the diagnosis is made, the history and appropriate laboratory studies should exclude the possibility of porphyric, diphtheritic, or toxic (heavy metal, hexacarbon, organophosphate) neuropathies. Poliomyelitis, botulism, and tick paralysis must also be considered. The presence of pyramidal signs, a markedly asymmetric motor deficit, a sharp sensory level, or early sphincter involvement should suggest a focal cord lesion.

Most patients eventually make a good recovery, but this may take many months, and 10–20% patients are left with persisting disability. Treatment with prednisone is ineffective and may actually affect the outcome adversely by prolonging recovery time. Plasmapheresis is of value; it is best performed within the first few days of illness and is best reserved for clinically severe or rapidly progressive cases or those with ventilatory impairment. Patients should be admitted to intensive care units if their forced vital capacity is declining, and intubation should be considered if the forced vital capacity reaches 15 mL/kg, dyspnea becomes evident, or the oxygen saturation declines. Respiratory toilet and chest physical therapy help prevent atelectasis. Marked hypotension may respond to volume replacement or pressor agents. Frequent turning of the patient helps prevent decubitus ulcers, and physical therapy helps prevent contractures. Low-dose heparin to prevent pulmonary embolism should be considered.

Approximately 3% of patients with acute idiopathic polyneuropathy have one or more clinically similar relapses, sometimes several years after the initial illness. Plasma exchange therapy may produce improvement in chronic and relapsing inflammatory polyneuropathy.

Chronic Inflammatory Polyneuropathy

Chronic inflammatory polyneuropathy, an acquired immunologically mediated disorder, is clinically similar to Guillain-Barré syndrome except that it has a relapsing or steadily progressive course over months or years. In the relapsing form, partial recovery may occur after some relapses, but in other instances there is no recovery between exacerbations. Although remission may occur spontaneously with time, the disorder frequently follows a progressive downhill course leading to severe functional disability.

Electrodiagnostic studies show marked slowing of motor and sensory conduction, and focal conduction block. Signs of partial denervation may also be present owing to secondary axonal degeneration. Nerve biopsy may show chronic perivascular inflammatory infiltrates in the endoneurium and epineurium, without accompanying evidence of vasculitis. However, a normal nerve biopsy result or the presence of nonspecific abnormalities does not exclude the diagnosis.

Corticosteroids may be effective in arresting or reversing the downhill course. Treatment is usually begun with prednisone, 60 mg daily, continued for 2–3 months or until a definite response has occurred. If no response has occurred despite 3 months of treatment, a higher dose may be tried. In responsive cases, the dose is gradually tapered, but most patients become corticosteroid-dependent, often requiring prednisone, 20 mg daily on alternate days, on a long-term basis. Patients unresponsive to corticosteroids may benefit instead from treatment with a cytotoxic drug such as azathioprine. There are increasing anecdotal reports of benefit with plasmapheresis.

Hallett M, Tandon D, Berardelli A: Treatment of peripheral neuropathies. J Neurol Neurosurg Psychiatry 1985; 48:1193.
Harati Y: Diabetic peripheral neuropathies. Ann Intern Med 1987;107:546. (Clinical features and pathogenesis.)
Lotti M et al: Occupational peripheral neuropathies. West J Med 1982;137:493.
McKhann GM: Plasmapheresis and acute Guillain-Barré syndrome. (Editorial.) Neurology 1985;35:1096.
McKhann GM, Griffin JW: Plasmapheresis and the Guillain-Barré syndrome. Ann Neurol 1987;22:762.
Parry GJ: Peripheral neuropathies associated with human immunodeficiency virus infection. Ann Neurol 1988; 23(Suppl):S49.

2. MONONEUROPATHIES

An individual nerve may be injured along its course or may be compressed, angulated, or stretched by neighboring anatomic structures, especially at a point where it passes through a narrow space (entrapment neuropathy). The relative contributions of mechanical factors and ischemia to the local damage are not clear. With involvement of a sensory or mixed nerve, pain is commonly felt distal to the lesion. Symptoms never develop with some entrapment neuropathies, resolve rapidly and spontaneously in others, and become progressively more disabling and distressing in yet other cases. The precise neurologic deficit depends on the nerve involved. Percussion of the nerve at the site of the lesion may lead to paresthesias in its distal distribution.

Entrapment neuropathy may be the sole manifestation of subclinical polyneuropathy, and this must be borne in mind and excluded by nerve conduction studies. Such studies are also indispensable for the accurate localization of the focal lesion.

In patients with acute compression neuropathy such as Saturday night palsy, no treatment is necessary. Complete recovery generally occurs, usually within 2 months, presumably because the underlying pathology is demyelination. However, axonal degeneration can occur in severe cases, and recovery then takes longer and may never be complete.

In chronic compressive or entrapment neuropathies, avoidance of aggravating factors and correction of any underlying systemic conditions is important. Local infiltration of the region about the nerve with corticosteroids may be of value; in addition, surgical decompression may help if there is a progressively increasing neurologic deficit or if electrodiagnostic studies show evidence of partial denervation in weak muscles.

Peripheral nerve tumors are uncommon, except in Recklinghausen's disease, but also give rise to mononeuropathy. This may be distinguishable from entrapment neuropathy only by noting the presence of a mass along the course of the nerve and by demonstrating the precise site of the lesion with appropriate electrophysiologic studies. Treatment of symptomatic lesions is by surgical removal if possible.

Carpal Tunnel Syndrome
See Chapter 15.

Pronator Teres or Anterior Interosseous Syndrome
The median nerve gives off its motor branch, the anterior interosseous nerve, below the elbow as it descends between the 2 heads of the pronator teres muscle. A lesion of either nerve may occur in this region, sometimes after trauma or owing to compression from, for example, a fibrous band. With anterior interosseous nerve involvement, there is no sensory loss, and weakness is confined to the pronator quadratus, flexor pollicis longus, and the flexor digitorum profundus to the second and third digits. Weakness is more widespread and sensory changes occur in an appropriate distribution when the median nerve itself is affected. The prognosis is variable. If improvement does not occur spontaneously, decompressive surgery may be helpful.

Ulnar Nerve Lesions
Ulnar nerve lesions are likely to occur in the elbow region as the nerve runs behind the medial epicondyle and descends into the cubital tunnel. In the condylar groove, the ulnar nerve is exposed to pressure or trauma. Moreover, any increase in the carrying angle of the elbow, whether congenital, degenerative, or traumatic, may cause excessive stretching of the nerve when the elbow is flexed. Ulnar nerve lesions may also result from thickening or distortion of the anatomic structures forming the cubital tunnel, and the resulting symptoms may also be aggravated by flexion of the elbow, because the tunnel is then narrowed by tightening of its roof or inward bulging of its floor. A severe lesion at either site causes sensory changes in the medial 1½ digits and along the medial border of the hand. There is weakness of the ulnar-innervated muscles in the forearm and hand. With a cubital tunnel lesion, however, there may be relative sparing of the flexor carpi ulnaris muscle. Electrophysiologic evaluation using nerve stimulation techniques allows more precise localization of the lesion.

If conservative measures are unsuccessful in relieving symptoms and preventing further progression, surgical treatment may be necessary. This consists of nerve transposition if the lesion is in the condylar groove, or a release procedure if it is in the cubital tunnel.

Ulnar nerve lesions may also develop at the wrist or in the palm of the hand, usually owing to repetitive trauma or to compression from ganglia or benign tumors. They can be subdivided depending upon their presumed site. Compressive lesions are treated surgically. If repetitive mechanical trauma is responsible, this is avoided by occupational adjustment or job retraining.

Radial Nerve Lesions

The radial nerve is particularly liable to compression or injury in the axilla (eg, by crutches or by pressure when the arm hangs over the back of a chair). This leads to weakness or paralysis of all the muscles supplied by the nerve, including the triceps. Sensory changes may also occur but are often surprisingly inconspicuous, being marked only in a small area on the back of the hand between the thumb and index finger. Injuries to the radial nerve in the spiral groove occur characteristically during deep sleep, as in intoxicated individuals (Saturday night palsy), and there is then sparing of the triceps muscle, which is supplied more proximally. The nerve may also be injured at or above the elbow; its purely motor posterior interosseous branch, supplying the extensors of the wrist and fingers, may be involved immediately below the elbow, but then there is sparing of the extensor carpi radialis longus, so that the wrist can still be extended. The superficial radial nerve may be compressed by handcuffs or a tight watch strap.

Femoral Neuropathy

The clinical features of femoral nerve palsy consist of weakness and wasting of the quadriceps muscle, with sensory impairment over the anteromedian aspect of the thigh and sometimes also of the leg to the medial malleolus, and a depressed or absent knee jerk. Isolated femoral neuropathy may occur in diabetics or from compression by retroperitoneal neoplasms or hematomas (eg, expanding aortic aneurysm). Femoral neuropathy may also result from pressure from the inguinal ligament when the thighs are markedly flexed and abducted, as in the lithotomy position.

Meralgia Paresthetica

The lateral femoral cutaneous nerve, a sensory nerve arising from the L2 and L3 roots, may be compressed or stretched in obese or diabetic patients and during pregnancy. The nerve usually runs under the outer portion of the inguinal ligament to reach the thigh, but the ligament sometimes splits to enclose it. Hyperextension of the hip or increased lumbar lordosis—such as occurs during pregnancy—leads to nerve compression by the posterior fascicle of the ligament. However, entrapment of the nerve at any point along its course may cause similar symptoms, and several other anatomic variations predispose the nerve to damage when it is stretched. Pain, paresthesia, or numbness occurs about the outer aspect of the thigh, usually unilaterally, and is sometimes relieved by sitting. Examination shows no abnormalities except in severe cases when cutaneous sensation is impaired in the affected area. Symptoms are usually mild and commonly settle spontaneously, so patients can be reassured about the benign nature of the disorder. Hydrocortisone injections about the nerve where it lies medial to the anterosuperior iliac spine often relieve symptoms temporarily, while nerve decompression by transposition may provide more lasting relief.

Sciatic & Common Peroneal Nerve Palsies

Misplaced deep intramuscular injections are probably still the most common cause of sciatic nerve palsy. Trauma to the buttock, hip, or thigh may also be responsible. The resulting clinical deficit depends on whether the whole nerve has been affected or only certain fibers. In general, the peroneal fibers of the sciatic nerve are more susceptible to damage than those destined for the tibial nerve. A sciatic nerve lesion may therefore be difficult to distinguish from peroneal neuropathy unless there is electromyographic evidence of involvement of the short head of the biceps femoris muscle. The common peroneal nerve itself may be compressed or injured in the region of the head and neck of the fibula, eg, by sitting with crossed legs or wearing high boots. There is weakness of dorsiflexion and eversion of the foot, accompanied by numbness or blunted sensation of the anterolateral aspect of the calf and dorsum of the foot.

Tarsal Tunnel Syndrome

The tibial nerve, the other branch of the sciatic, supplies several muscles in the lower extremity, gives origin to the sural nerve, and then continues as the posterior tibial nerve to supply the plantar flexors of the foot and toes. It passes through the tarsal tunnel behind and below the medial malleolus, giving off calcaneal branches and the medial and lateral plantar nerves that supply small muscles of the foot and the skin on the plantar aspect of the foot and toes. Compression of the posterior tibial nerve or its branches between the bony floor and ligamentous roof of the tarsal tunnel leads to pain, paresthesias, and numbness over the bottom of the foot, especially at night, with sparing of the heel. Muscle weakness may be hard to recognize clinically. Compressive lesions of the individual plantar nerves may also occur more distally, with similar clinical features to those of the tarsal tunnel syndrome. Treatment is surgical decompression.

Stewart J: *Focal Peripheral Neuropathies*. Elsevier Science, 1987.

3. BELL'S PALSY

Bell's palsy is an idiopathic facial paresis of lower motor neuron type that has been attributed to an inflammatory reaction involving the facial nerve near the stylomastoid foramen or in the bony facial canal. A relationship of Bell's palsy to reactivation of herpes simplex virus has recently been suggested, but there is little evidence to support this.

The clinical features of Bell's palsy are characteristic. The facial paresis generally comes on abruptly, but it may worsen over the following day or so. Pain about the ear precedes or accompanies the weakness in many cases but usually lasts for only a few days. The face itself feels stiff and pulled to one side. There may be ipsilateral restriction of eye closure and difficulty with eating and fine facial movements. A disturbance of taste is common, owing to involvement of chorda tympani fibers, and hyperacusis due to involvement of fibers to the stapedius occurs occasionally.

The management of Bell's palsy is controversial. Approximately 60% of cases recover completely without treatment, presumably because the lesion is so mild that it leads merely to conduction block. Considerable improvement occurs in most other cases, and only about 10% of all patients are seriously dissatisfied with the final outcome because of permanent disfigurement or other long-term sequelae. Treatment is unnecessary in most cases but is indicated for patients in whom an unsatisfactory outcome can be predicted. The best clinical guide to progress is the severity of the palsy during the first few days after presentation. Patients with clinically complete palsy when first seen are less likely to make a full recovery than those with an incomplete one. A poor prognosis for recovery is also associated with advanced age, hyperacusis, and severe initial pain. Electromyography and nerve excitability or conduction studies provide a guide to prognosis but not early enough to aid in the selection of patients for treatment.

The only medical treatment that may influence the outcome is administration of corticosteroids, but studies supporting this concept have been criticized. Many physicians nevertheless routinely prescribe corticosteroids for patients with Bell's palsy seen within 5 days of onset. The author prescribes them only when the palsy is clinically complete or there is severe pain. Treatment with prednisone, 60 or 80 mg daily in divided doses for 4 or 5 days, followed by tapering of the dose over the next 7–10 days, is a satisfactory regimen. It is helpful to protect the eye with lubricating drops and a patch if eye closure is not possible. There is no evidence that surgical procedures to decompress the facial nerve are of benefit.

Katusic SK et al: Incidence, clinical features, and prognosis in Bell's palsy, Rochester, Minnesota, 1986–1982. Ann Neurol 1986;20:622.

DISCOGENIC NECK & BACK PAIN
(See also Chapter 15.)

1. LOW BACK PAIN

Spinal disease may lead to local pain, root pain, or both. It may also lead to pain that is referred to other parts of the involved dermatomes. Local pain may lead to protective reflex muscle spasm, which in turn causes further pain and may result in abnormal posture and limitation of movement. Radicular pain arises from compression, stretch, or irritation of nerve roots and usually radiates from the back to the territory of the affected root, being exacerbated by coughing, straining, or stretching of the nerve fibers, eg, by straight leg raising. Root disturbances may also lead to paresthesias and numbness in dermatomal (as opposed to peripheral nerve) distribution (Fig 18–1) and to weakness in segmental distribution; reflex changes may accompany involvement of motor or sensory fibers. Only pain due to disk disease is considered here; other causes have been considered in Chapter 15.

Acute Lumbar Intervertebral Disk Prolapse

This cause of low back pain generally involves the L4–5 or the L5–S1 disk and leads to back and radicular (L5 or S1) pain. The L4 root is occasionally affected, but involvement of a higher lumbar root should arouse suspicion of other causes of root compression. There may be accompanying numbness and paresthesias in dermatomal distribution or segmental motor deficit. An L5 radiculopathy causes weakness of dorsiflexion of the foot and toes. With an S1 root lesion, there is weakness of eversion and plantar flexion of the foot and a depressed ankle jerk. A centrally prolapsed disk may lead to bilateral limb disturbances and sphincter involvement. Pelvic and rectal examination and plain x-rays of the spine help to exclude other disorders such as local primary cancers or metastatic deposits. Symptoms are often relieved with simple analgesics, diazepam, and bed rest on a firm mattress. Persisting pain, an increasing neurologic deficit, or any evidence of sphincter dysfunction calls for investigation by CT myelography—or, preferably, by MRI—followed by surgical treatment. The role of percutaneous diskectomy is currently under study as an alternative to operative treatment.

Degenerative Lumbar Osteoarthropathy & Chronic Disk Degeneration

This process leads to local pain, stiffness, and restricted activity. The radiologic findings vary from minor degenerative abnormalities to marked osteophytic spurs, ridges, and other changes. Even minor changes may lead to root or cord dysfunction when there is also a congenitally narrowed spinal canal (spinal stenosis). Pain, sometimes accompanied by weakness or radicular sensory disturbances in the legs, then occurs with activity or with certain postures and

PERIPHERAL NERVE   NERVE ROOT

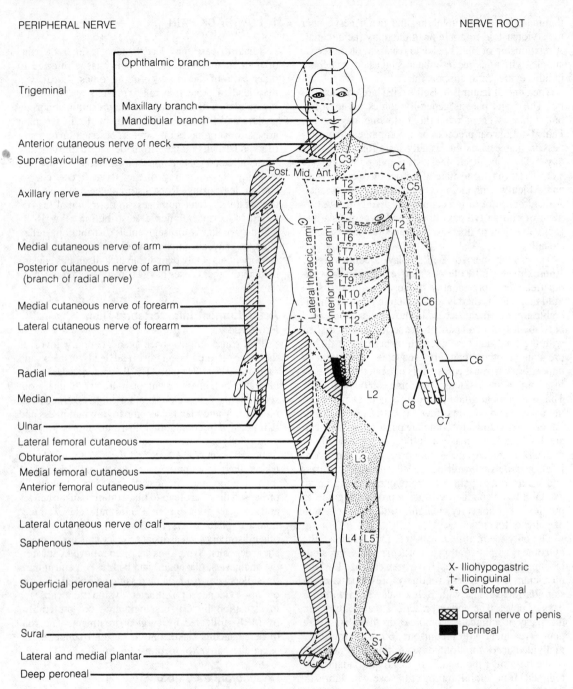

Figure 18–1. Cutaneous innervation. The segmental or radicular (root) distribution is shown on the left side of the body and the peripheral nerve distribution on the right side. **Above:** anterior view; **facing page:** posterior view. (Reproduced, with permission, from Simon RP, Aminoff MJ, Greenberg DA: *Clinical Neurology.* Appleton & Lange, 1989.)

NERVE ROOT   PERIPHERAL NERVE

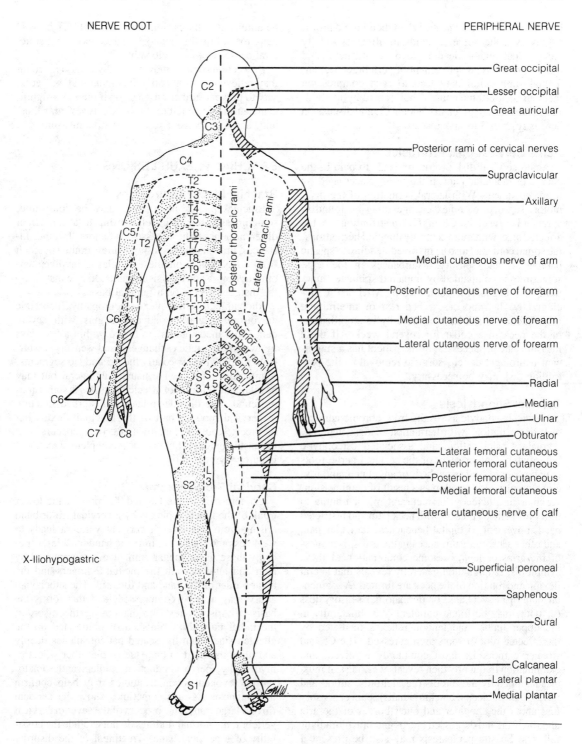

Great occipital
Lesser occipital
Great auricular
Posterior rami of cervical nerves
Supraclavicular
Axillary
Medial cutaneous nerve of arm
Posterior cutaneous nerve of forearm
Medial cutaneous nerve of forearm
Lateral cutaneous nerve of forearm
Radial
Median
Ulnar
Obturator
Lateral femoral cutaneous
Anterior femoral cutaneous
Posterior femoral cutaneous
Medial femoral cutaneous
Lateral cutaneous nerve of calf
Superficial peroneal
Saphenous
Sural
Calcaneal
Lateral plantar
Medial plantar

X-Iliohypogastric

is relieved by rest. This has been referred to as neurogenic claudication; surgical decompression may be helpful in selected cases.

Onik G et al: Automated percutaneous discectomy: A prospective multi-institutional study. Neurosurgery 1990;26:228.

2. NECK PAIN

A variety of congenital abnormalities may involve the cervical spine and lead to neck pain; these include hemivertebrae, fused vertebrae, basilar impression, and instability of the atlantoaxial joint. Traumatic, degenerative, infective, and neoplastic disorders may also lead to pain in the neck. When rheumatoid arthritis involves the spine, it tends to affect especially the cervical region, leading to pain, stiffness, and reduced mobility; displacement of vertebrae or atlantoaxial subluxation may lead to cord compression that can be life-threatening if not treated by fixation. Further details are given in Chapter 15, and discussion here is restricted to disk disease.

Acute Cervical Disk Protrusion

Acute cervical disk protrusion leads to pain in the neck and radicular pain in the arm, exacerbated by head movement. With lateral herniation of the disk, motor, sensory, or reflex changes may be found in a radicular (usually C6 or C7) distribution on the affected side; with more centrally directed herniations, the spinal cord may also be involved, leading to spastic paraparesis and sensory disturbances in the legs, sometimes accompanied by impaired sphincter function. The diagnosis is confirmed by MRI or CT myelography. In mild cases, bed rest or intermittent neck traction may help, followed by immobilization of the neck in a collar for several weeks. If these measures are unsuccessful or the patient has a significant neurologic deficit, surgical removal of the protruding disk may be necessary.

Cervical Spondylosis

Cervical spondylosis results from chronic cervical disk degeneration, with herniation of disk material, secondary calcification, and associated osteophytic outgrowths. One or more of the cervical nerve roots may be compressed, stretched, or angulated; and myelopathy may also develop as a result of compression, vascular insufficiency, or recurrent minor trauma to the cord. Patients present with neck pain and restricted head movement, occipital headaches, radicular pain and other sensory disturbances in the arms, weakness of the arms or legs, or some combination of these symptoms. Examination generally reveals that lateral flexion and rotation of the neck are limited. A segmental pattern of weakness or dermatomal sensory loss (or both) may be found unilaterally or bilaterally in the upper limbs, and tendon reflexes mediated by the affected root or roots are depressed. The C5 and C6 nerve roots are most commonly involved, and examination frequently then reveals weakness of muscles supplied by these roots (eg, deltoids, supra- and infraspinatus, biceps, brachioradialis), pain or sensory loss about the shoulder and outer border of the arm and forearm, and depressed biceps and brachioradialis reflexes. Spastic paraparesis may also be present if there is an associated myelopathy, sometimes accompanied by posterior column or spinothalamic sensory deficits in the legs.

Plain radiographs of the cervical spine show osteophyte formation, narrowing of disk spaces, and encroachment on the intervertebral foramens, but such changes are common in middle-aged persons and may

be unrelated to the presenting complaint. CT or MRI helps to confirm the diagnosis and exclude other structural causes of the myelopathy.

Restriction of neck movements by a cervical collar may relieve pain. Operative treatment may be necessary to prevent further progression if there is a significant neurologic deficit or if root pain is severe, persistent, and unresponsive to conservative measures.

BRACHIAL PLEXUS LESIONS

Brachial Plexus Neuropathy

Brachial plexus neuropathy may be idiopathic, sometimes occurring in relationship to a number of different nonspecific illnesses or factors. In other instances, brachial plexus lesions follow trauma or result from congenital anomalies, neoplastic involvement, or injury by various physical agents. In rare instances, the disorder occurs on a familial basis.

Idiopathic brachial plexus neuropathy (neuralgic amyotrophy) characteristically begins with severe pain about the shoulder, followed within a few days by weakness, reflex changes, and sensory disturbances involving especially the C5 and C6 segments. Symptoms and signs are usually unilateral but may be bilateral. Wasting of affected muscles is sometimes profound. The disorder relates to disturbed function of cervical roots or part of the brachial plexus, but its precise cause is unknown. Recovery occurs over the ensuing months but may be incomplete. Treatment is purely symptomatic.

Cervical Rib Syndrome

Compression of the C8 and T1 roots or the lower trunk of the brachial plexus by a cervical rib or band arising from the seventh cervical vertebra leads to weakness and wasting of intrinsic hand muscles, especially those in the thenar eminence, accompanied by pain and numbness in the medial 2 fingers and the ulnar border of the hand and forearm. The subclavian artery may also be compressed, and this forms the basis of Adson's test for diagnosing the disorder; the radial pulse is diminished or obliterated on the affected side when the seated patient inhales deeply and turns the head to one side or the other. Electromyography, nerve conduction studies, and somatosensory evoked potential studies may help confirm the diagnosis. X-rays sometimes show the cervical rib or a large transverse process of the seventh cervical vertebra, but normal findings do not exclude the possibility of a cervical band. Treatment of the disorder is by surgical excision of the rib or band.

Lumbosacral Plexus Lesions

A lumbosacral plexus lesion may develop in association with diseases such as diabetes, cancer, or bleeding disorders or in relation to injury. It occasionally occurs as an isolated phenomenon similar to idiopathic brachial plexopathy, and pain and weakness then tend to be more conspicuous than sensory symptoms. The distribution of symptoms and signs depends on the level and pattern of neurologic involvement.

Aminoff MJ et al: Relative utility of different electrophysiologic techniques in the evaluation of brachial plexopathies. Neurology 1988;38:546. (Compares utility of different electrodiagnostic studies.)

England JD, Sumner AJ: Neuralgic amyotrophy: An increasingly diverse entity. Muscle Nerve 1987;10:60.

DISORDERS OF NEUROMUSCULAR TRANSMISSION

1. MYASTHENIA GRAVIS

Essentials of Diagnosis

- Fluctuating weakness of commonly used voluntary muscles, producing symptoms such as diplopia, ptosis, and difficulty in swallowing.
- Activity increases weakness of affected muscles.
- Short-acting anticholinesterases transiently improve the weakness.

General Considerations

Myasthenia gravis occurs at all ages, sometimes in association with a thymic tumor or thyrotoxicosis, as well as with rheumatoid arthritis and lupus erythematosus. It is commonest in young women with HLA-DR3; if thymoma is associated, older men are more commonly affected. Onset is usually insidious, but the disorder is sometimes unmasked by a coincidental infection that leads to exacerbation of symptoms. Exacerbations may also occur before the menstrual period or during or shortly after pregnancy. Symptoms are due to a variable degree of block of neuromuscular transmission. This probably has an immunologic basis, and autoantibodies binding to acetylcholine receptors are found in most patients with the disease. These antibodies have a primary role in reducing the number of functioning acetylcholine receptors. Additionally, cellular immune activity against the receptor is found. Clinically, this leads to weakness; initially powerful movements fatigue readily. The external ocular muscles and certain other cranial muscles, including the masticatory, facial, and pharyngeal muscles, are especially likely to be affected, and the respiratory and limb muscles may also be involved.

Clinical Findings

A. Symptoms and Signs: Patients present with ptosis, diplopia, difficulty in chewing or swallowing, respiratory difficulties, limb weakness, or some combination of these problems. Weakness may remain localized to a few muscle groups, especially the ocular muscles, or may become generalized. Symptoms often fluctuate in intensity during the day, and this diurnal variation is superimposed on a tendency to longer-term spontaneous relapses and remissions that may last for weeks. Nevertheless, the disorder follows a slowly progressive course and may have a fatal outcome owing to respiratory complications such as aspiration pneumonia.

Clinical examination confirms the weakness and fatigability of affected muscles. In most cases, the extraocular muscles are involved, and this leads to ocular palsies and ptosis, which are commonly asymmetric. Pupillary responses are normal. The bulbar and limb muscles are often weak, but the pattern of involvement is variable. Sustained activity of affected muscles increases the weakness, which improves after a brief rest. Sensation is normal, and there are usually no reflex changes.

The diagnosis can generally be confirmed by the response to a short-acting anticholinesterase. Edrophonium (Tensilon) can be given intravenously in a dose of 10 mg (1 mL), 2 mg being given initially and the remaining 8 mg about 30 seconds later if the test dose is well tolerated; in myasthenic patients, there is an obvious improvement in strength of weak muscles lasting for about 5 minutes. Alternatively, 1.5 mg of neostigmine can be given intramuscularly, and the response then lasts for about 2 hours; atropine sulfate (0.6 mg) should be available to reverse muscarinic side effects.

B. Imaging: Lateral and anteroposterior x-rays of the chest and CT scans should be obtained to demonstrate a coexisting thymoma, but normal studies do not exclude this possibility.

C. Laboratory and Other Studies: Electrophysiologic demonstration of a decrementing muscle response to repetitive 2- or 3-Hz stimulation of motor nerves indicates a disturbance of neuromuscular transmission. Such an abnormality may even be detected in clinically strong muscles with certain provocative procedures. Needle electromyography of affected muscles shows a marked variation in configuration and size of individual motor unit potentials, and single-fiber electromyography reveals an increased jitter, or variability, in the time interval between 2 muscle fiber action potentials from the same motor unit.

Assay of serum for elevated levels of circulating acetylcholine receptor antibodies is another approach—increasingly used—to the laboratory diagnosis of myasthenia gravis.

Treatment

Medication such as aminoglycosides that may exacerbate myasthenia gravis should be avoided. Anticholinesterase drugs provide symptomatic benefit without influencing the course of the disease. Neostigmine, pyridostigmine, or both can be used, the dose being determined on an individual basis. Overmedication may temporarily increase weakness, which is then unaffected or enhanced by intravenous edrophonium.

Thymectomy usually leads to symptomatic benefit or remission and should be considered in all patients younger than age 60, unless weakness is restricted to the extraocular muscles. If the disease is of recent onset and only slowly progressive, operation is sometimes delayed for a year or so, in the hope that spontaneous remission will occur.

Treatment with corticosteroids is indicated for patients who have responded poorly to anticholinesterase drugs and have already undergone thymectomy. It is introduced with the patient in the hospital, since weakness may initially be aggravated. Once weakness has stabilized after 2–3 weeks or any improvement is sustained, further management can be on an outpatient basis. Alternate-day treatment is usually well tolerated, but if weakness is enhanced on the nontreatment day it may be necessary for medication to be taken daily. The dose of corticosteroids is determined on an individual basis, but an initial high daily dose (eg, prednisone, 60–100 mg) can gradually be tapered to a relatively low maintenance level as improvement occurs; total withdrawal is difficult, however. Treatment with azathioprine may also be effective. The usual dose is 2–3 mg/kg orally daily after a lower initial dose.

In patients with major disability in whom conventional treatment is either unhelpful or contraindicated, plasmapheresis may be beneficial. It may also be useful for stabilizing patients before thymectomy and for managing acute crisis.

Levin KH, Richman DP: Myasthenia gravis. Clin Aspects Autoimm 1989;4:23.

Misulis KE, Fenichel GM: Genetic forms of myasthenic gravis. Pediatr Neurol 1989;5:205.

2. MYASTHENIC SYNDROME (Lambert-Eaton Syndrome)

Myasthenic syndrome may be associated with small-cell carcinoma, sometimes developing before the tumor is diagnosed, and occasionally occurs with certain autoimmune diseases. There is defective release of acetylcholine in response to a nerve impulse, and this leads to weakness especially of the proximal muscles of the limbs. As is not the case in myasthenia gravis, however, power steadily increases with sustained contraction. The diagnosis can be confirmed electrophysiologically, because the muscle response to stimulation of its motor nerve increases remarkably if the nerve is stimulated repetitively at high rates, even in muscles that are not clinically weak.

Treatment with plasmapheresis and immunosuppressive drug therapy (prednisone and azathioprine) may lead to clinical and electrophysiologic improvement, in addition to therapy aimed at tumor when present. Guanidine hydrochloride (25–50 mg/kg/d in divided doses) is occasionally helpful in seriously disabled patients, but adverse effects of the drug include marrow suppression. The response to treatment with anticholinesterase drugs such as pyridostigmine or neostigmine, either alone or in combination with guanidine, is variable.

O'Neill JH et al: The Lambert-Eaton myasthenic syndrome. Brain 1988;111:577. (Review of 50 cases.)

3. BOTULISM

The toxin of *Clostridium botulinum* prevents the release of acetylcholine at neuromuscular junctions and autonomic synapses. Botulism occurs most commonly following the ingestion of contaminated home-canned food and should be suggested by the development of sudden, fluctuating, severe weakness in a previously healthy person. Symptoms begin within 72 hours following ingestion of the toxin and may progress for several days. Typically, there is diplopia, ptosis, facial weakness, dysphagia, and nasal speech, followed by respiratory difficulty and finally by weakness that appears last in the limbs. Blurring of vision (with unreactive dilated pupils) is characteristic, and there may be dryness of the mouth, constipation (paralytic ileus), and postural hypotension. Sensation is preserved, and the tendon reflexes are not affected unless the involved muscles are very weak. If the diagnosis is suspected, the local health authority should be notified and a sample of serum and contaminated food (if available) sent to be assayed for toxin. Support for the diagnosis may be obtained by electrophysiologic studies; with repetitive stimulation of motor nerves at fast rates, the muscle response increases in size progressively.

Patients should be hospitalized in case respiratory assistance becomes necessary. Treatment is with trivalent antitoxin, once it is established that the patient is not allergic to horse serum. Guanidine hydrochloride (25–50 mg/kg/d in divided doses) to facilitate release of acetylcholine from nerve endings sometimes helps to increase muscle strength. Anticholinesterase drugs are of no value. Respiratory assistance and other supportive measures should be provided as necessary. Further details are provided in Chapter 26.

4. DISORDERS ASSOCIATED WITH USE OF AMINOGLYCOSIDES

Aminoglycoside antibiotics, eg, gentamicin, may produce a clinical disturbance similar to botulism by preventing the release of acetylcholine from nerve endings, but symptoms subside rapidly as the responsible drug is eliminated from the body. These antibiotics are particularly dangerous in patients with preexisting disturbances of neuromuscular transmission and are therefore best avoided in patients with myasthenia gravis.

MYOPATHIC DISORDERS

Muscular Dystrophies

These inherited myopathic disorders are characterized by progressive muscle weakness and wasting. They are subdivided by mode of inheritance, age at onset, and clinical features, as shown in Table 18–6. In the Duchenne type, pseudohypertrophy of muscles frequently occurs at some stage; intellectual retardation is common; and there may be skeletal deformities, muscle contractures, and cardiac involvement. The serum creatine phosphokinase level is increased, especially in the Duchenne and Becker varieties, and mildly increased also in limb-girdle dystrophy. Electromyography may help to confirm that weakness is myopathic rather than neurogenic. Similarly, histopathologic examination of a muscle biopsy specimen may help to confirm that weakness is due to a primary disorder of muscle and to distinguish between various muscle diseases.

A genetic defect on the short arm of the X chromosome has recently been identified in Duchenne dystrophy. The affected gene codes for the protein dystrophin, which is markedly reduced or absent from the muscle of patients with the disease. Dystrophin levels are normal in the Becker variety, but the protein is qualitatively altered.

Duchenne muscular dystrophy can now be recognized early in pregnancy in about 95% of women by genetic studies; in late pregnancy, DNA probes can be used on fetal tissue obtained for this purpose by amniocentesis.

There is no specific treatment, but it is important to encourage patients to lead as normal lives as possible. Prolonged bed rest must be avoided, as inactivity often leads to worsening of the underlying muscle disease. Physical therapy and orthopedic procedures may help to counteract deformities or contractures.

Hoffman EP et al: Dystrophin: The protein product of the Duchenne muscular dystrophy locus. Cell 1987; 51:919. (Identification of the primary biochemical defect in Duchenne muscular dystrophy.)

Myotonic Dystrophy

Myotonic dystrophy, a slowly progressive, dominantly inherited disorder, usually manifests itself in the third or fourth decade but occasionally appears early in childhood. Myotonia leads to complaints of muscle stiffness and is evidenced by the marked delay that occurs before affected muscles can relax after a contraction. This can often be demonstrated clinically by delayed relaxation of the hand after sustained grip or by percussion of the belly of a muscle. In addition, there is weakness and wasting of the facial, sternocleidomastoid, and distal limb muscles. Associated clinical features include cataracts, frontal baldness, testicular atrophy, diabetes mellitus, cardiac abnormalities, and intellectual changes. Electromyographic sampling of affected muscles reveals myotonic discharges in addition to changes suggestive of myopathy.

Myotonia can be treated with quinine sulfate (300–400 mg 3 times daily), procainamide (0.5–1 g 4 times daily), or phenytoin (100 mg 3 times daily). More recently, tocainide and mexiletine have been used. In myotonic dystrophy, phenytoin is preferred, since the other drugs may have undesirable effects on cardiac conduction. Neither the weakness nor the course of the disorder is influenced by treatment.

Table 18–6. The muscular dystrophies.

Disorder	Inheritance	Age at Onset (years)	Distribution	Prognosis
Duchenne type	X-linked recessive	1–5	Pelvic, then shoulder girdle; later, limb and respiratory muscles.	Rapid progression. Death within about 15 years after onset.
Becker's	X-linked recessive	5–25	Pelvic, then shoulder girdle.	Slow progression. May have normal life span.
Limb-girdle (Erb's)	Autosomal recessive (may be sporadic or dominant)	10–30	Pelvic or shoulder girdle initially, with later spread to the other.	Variable severity and rate of progression. Possible severe disability in middle life.
Facioscapulo-humeral	Autosomal dominant	Any age	Face and shoulder girdle initially; later, pelvic girdle and legs.	Slow progression. Minor disability. Usually normal life span.
Distal	Autosomal dominant	40–60	Onset distally in extremities; proximal involvement later.	Slow progression.
Ocular	Autosomal dominant (may be recessive)	Any age (usually 5–30)	External ocular muscles. May also be mild weakness of face, neck, and arms.	
Oculopharyngeal	Autosomal dominant	Any age	As in the ocular form but with dysphagia.	

Myotonia Congenita

Myotonia congenita is commonly inherited as a dominant trait. Generalized myotonia without weakness is usually present from birth, but symptoms may not appear until early childhood. Patients complain of muscle stiffness that is enhanced by cold and inactivity and relieved by exercise. Muscle hypertrophy, at times pronounced, is also a feature. A recessive form with later onset is associated with slight weakness and atrophy of distal muscles. Treatment with quinine sulfate, procainamide, tocainide, mexiletine, or phenytoin may help the myotonia, as in myotonic dystrophy.

Polymyositis & Dermatomyositis

See Chapter 15.

Myopathies Associated With Other Disorders

Myopathy may occur in association with chronic hypokalemia, hyper- or hypothyroidism, hyper- or hypoparathyroidism, hyper- or hypoadrenalism, hypopituitarism, and acromegaly and in patients taking corticosteroids, chloroquine, colchicine, clofibrate, emetine, aminocaproic acid, lovastatin, bretylium tosylate, or drugs causing potassium depletion; weakness is mainly proximal, and serum CPK is typically normal. Treatment is of the underlying cause. Myopathy also occurs with chronic alcoholism, whereas acute reversible muscle necrosis may occur shortly after acute alcohol intoxication. Inflammatory myopathy may occur in patients taking penicillamine; myotonia may be induced by diazacholesterol or clofibrate; and preexisting myotonia may be exacerbated or unmasked by depolarizing muscle relaxants (eg, suxamethonium), beta-blockers (eg, propranolol), fenoterol, ritodrine, and, possibly, certain diuretics.

PERIODIC PARALYSIS SYNDROME

Periodic paralysis may have a familial (dominant inheritance) basis. Episodes of flaccid weakness or paralysis occur, sometimes in association with abnormalities of the plasma potassium level. Strength is normal between attacks. The **hypokalemic** variety is characterized by attacks that tend to occur on awakening, after exercise, or after a heavy meal and may last for several days. Patients should avoid excessive exertion. A low-carbohydrate and low-salt diet may help prevent attacks, as may acetazolamide, 250–750 mg/d. An ongoing attack may be aborted by potassium chloride given orally or by intravenous drip, provided the ECG can be monitored and renal function is satisfactory. It is sometimes associated with hyperthyroidism, especially in young Asian men; treatment of the endocrine disorder may then prevent recurrences. In **hyperkalemic** periodic paralysis, attacks also tend to occur after exercise but usually last for less than an hour. They may be terminated by intravenous calcium gluconate (1–2 g) or by intravenous diuretics (furosemide, 20–40 mg), glucose, or glucose and insulin; daily acetazolamide or chlorothiazide may prevent recurrences. **Normokalemic** periodic paralysis is similar clinically to the hyperkalemic variety, but the plasma potassium level remains normal during attacks; treatment is with acetazolamide.

REFERENCES

Adams RD, Victor M: *Principles of Neurology,* 4th ed. McGraw-Hill, 1989.

Aminoff MJ (editor): *Electrodiagnosis in Clinical Neurology,* 2nd ed. Churchill Livingstone, 1986.

Aminoff MJ (editor): *Neurology and General Medicine: The Neurological Aspects of Medical Disorders.* Churchill Livingstone, 1989.

Baraitser M: *The Genetics of Neurological Disorders.* Oxford, 1982.

Dyck PJ et al (editors): *Peripheral Neuropathy,* 2nd ed. Saunders, 1984.

Rosenblum ML et al (editors): *AIDS and the Nervous System.* Raven Press, 1988.

Rowland LP (editor): *Merritt's Textbook of Neurology,* 8th ed. Lea & Febiger, 1989.

Walton JN (editor): *Brain's Diseases of the Nervous System,* 9th ed. Oxford, 1985.

Walton JN (editor): *Disorders of Voluntary Muscle,* 5th ed. Churchill Livingstone, 1988.

Psychiatric Disorders

19

James J. Brophy, MD

Psychiatric disorders are functional impairments that may result from disturbance of one or more of the following interrelated factors: (1) biologic function, (2) psychodynamic adaptation, (3) learned behavior, and (4) social and environmental conditions. Although the clinical situation at a given time determines which area of dysfunction will be emphasized, proper patient care requires an approach that adequately evaluates all factors.

(1) Biologic function: Psychiatric disorders of biologic origin may be secondary to identifiable physical illness or caused by biochemical disturbances of the brain. A wide variety of psychiatric disorders (eg, psychosis, depression, delirium, anxiety), as well as nonspecific symptoms are caused by organic brain disease or by derangement of cerebral metabolism resulting from illness, biochemical aberrations (usually neurotransmitter dysfunction), nutritional deficiencies, or toxic agents.

Neurotransmitter functions have been correlated with the major psychiatric disorders. Cholinergic deficiency is present in some dementias, and adrenergic imbalance is important in some psychoses. Serotonergic mechanisms are involved in affective disorders, aggression, autism, and the anxiety disorders, particularly obsessive compulsive disorders (OCD). Studies of the physiologic interactions that take place along the hypothalamic-pituitary-adrenocortical axis have resulted in a recognized association between depression and endocrine dysfunction. Research in this area is also fundamental to the investigation of psychoimmunologic interactions and biochemical markers in psychiatric disorders.

(2) Psychodynamic maladaptation involves intrapsychic aberrations and is usually treated by a psychotherapeutic approach. There are many forms of psychotherapy: supportive, interpretive, cognitive, persuasive, educative, or some combination of these. Depth, duration, intensity, and frequency of sessions may vary. Various theoretic frameworks may be employed—freudian, jungian, adlerian, sullivanian, kleinian, etc. The "dynamic" approaches have their roots in classic freudian psychoanalytic theory, whereas "experiential" psychotherapy is of more recent origin, including many tenuous offshoots of dubious long-term significance.

(3) Learned behavior is part of the pathogenetic mechanism in all psychiatric disorders. Although a biochemical abnormality may be the matrix of a schizophrenic process, the content of the psychotic material is to a great degree learned and socially relevant. Paranoid delusions reflect current concerns (eg, radar, electronic eavesdropping). In the case of anxiety disorders, many behavioral scientists feel that learned behavior alone is the major consideration. Appropriate parenting or training consists in great part of utilizing proper behavioral practices, rewarding correct behavior, and punishing delinquent behavior. Personality disorders are examples of failure to learn and incorporate patterns of behavior acceptable in societal surroundings.

(4) Social and environmental conditions have always been considered vital factors in the mental balance of the individual. Without the encounter with the environment, there can be no socially recognized illness: the exigencies of everyday life contribute both to the development of a stable personality and to the deviations from the norm. There is a constantly changing ethnic influence that determines which types of behavior will be tolerated or considered deviant as well as variations in the metabolism of drugs. The principal vehicle for modeling and learning in our social structure is the family unit, which has shifted from an extended group with numerous relatives to a smaller nuclear group consisting of one or both parents and their children. This changes when remarriage and perhaps the presence of children of previous unions result in a loose, fluid family unit of stepparents and stepsiblings with variable degrees of bonding. Changes in the family unit have coincided with changes in work patterns of parents and in schooling and work patterns of young adults. The changes are complex and generally have lengthened the period of dependency and increased stresses in the family unit; this, in turn, affects the underlying social fabric, with consequences for each individual.

Barrett JE et al: The prevalence of psychiatric disorders in a primary care practice. Arch Gen Psychiatry 1988; 45:1100. (25% incidence, of which half consists of depression.)

Weiss J: Unconscious mental functioning. Sci Am 1990; 262:103.

PSYCHIATRIC ASSESSMENT

Psychiatric diagnosis rests upon the established principles of a thorough history and examination. All of the forces contributing to the individual's life situation must be identified, and this can only be done if the examination includes the history; mental status; medical conditions (including drugs); and pertinent social, cultural, and environmental factors impinging on the individual.

Interview

The appearance and behavior of the interviewer influences the interviewee. Lateness, obesity, smoking, and use of the patient's first name may all create a negative ambience. The manner in which the history is taken is important not only because it affects success in eliciting pertinent data but also because it may be of therapeutic value in itself. The setting should be quiet, with an appropriate degree of professional decorum at all times, and patients should initially be allowed to talk about their problems in an unstructured way without interruption. The interviewer should minimize writing, unnecessary direct questioning, incoming phone calls, and interpretive comments. Long, rambling discussions may be controlled by subtly interjecting questions relevant to the topic, although the patient's digressions sometimes provide important clues to his or her mental status. The first few minutes are often the most important part of the interview.

The interviewer should be alert for key words or phrases that can be used to help the patient develop the theme of the main difficulty. For example, if the patient says, "Doctor, I hurt, and when we have marital problems, things just get worse"—the words "hurt" and "marital problems" are important clues that need amplification when the physician makes another comment. Nonverbal clues may be as important as words, and one should notice gestures, tones of voice, and facial expressions. Obvious omissions, shying away from painful subjects, and sudden shifts of subject matter give important clues to unconscious as well as conscious sources of difficulty.

Every psychiatric history should cover the following points: (1) complaint, from the patient's viewpoint; (2) the present illness, or the evolution of the complaints; (3) previous disorders and the nature and extent of treatment; (4) the family history—important for genetic aspects and family influences; (5) personal history—childhood development, adolescent adjustment, level of education, and adult coping patterns; (6) sexual history; (7) current life functioning, with attention to vocational, social, educational, and avocational areas; and (8) current medications or other drugs.

It is often essential to obtain additional information from the family. Observing interactions of significant other people with the patient in the context of a family interview may give significant diagnostic information and may even underscore the nature of the problem and suggest a therapeutic approach.

The Mental Status Examination

Observation of the patient and the content of the remarks made during the interview constitute the informal part of the mental status examination, ie, that which is obtained indirectly. The formal mental status examination is performed as noted below and should be particularly detailed when there is any evidence or high risk of cognitive dysfunction.

The mental status examination includes the following: (1) Appearance: Note unusual modes of dress, makeup, etc. (2) Activity and behavior: Gait, gestures, coordination of bodily movements, etc. (3) Affect: Outward manifestation of emotions such as depression, anger, elation, fear, resentment, or lack of emotional response. (4) Mood: Inward feelings, sum of statements, and observable emotional manifestations. (5) Speech: Coherence, spontaneity, articulation, hesitancy in answering, and duration of response. (6) Content of thought: Associations, preoccupations, obsessions, depersonalization, delusions, hallucinations, paranoid ideation, anger, fear, or unusual experiences. (7) Sensorium: (a) orientation to person, place, time, and circumstances; (b) remote and recent memory and recall; (c) calculations, digit retention (forward and backward), serial 7s and 3s; (d) general fund of knowledge (presidents, states, distances, events); (e) abstracting ability, often tested with common proverbs or with analogies and differences (eg, how are a lie and a mistake the same, and how are they different?); (f) ability to identify by naming, reading, and writing specified test names and objects; (g) ideomotor function, which combines understanding and the ability to perform a task (eg, "Show me how to throw a ball"); (h) ability to reproduce geometric constructions (eg, parallelogram, intersecting squares); and (i) right-left differentiation. (8) Judgment regarding commonsense problems such as what to do when one runs out of medicine. (9) Insight into the nature and extent of the current difficulty and its ramifications in the patient's daily life.

The mental status examination is important in establishing a diagnosis and must be *recorded carefully and clearly in the chart*.

Medical Examination

The examination of a psychiatric patient must include a complete medical history and physical examination (with emphasis on the neurologic examination) as well as all necessary laboratory and other special studies. Physical illness may frequently present as psychiatric disease, and vice versa. It is hazardous to assign a "functional" cause to symptoms simply because they arose during an emotional crisis.

Special Diagnostic Aids

Many tests and evaluation procedures are available that can be used to support and clarify initial diagnostic impressions.

A. Psychologic Testing: Psychologic testing by a trained psychologist may measure intelligence and cognitive functioning; provide information about personality, feelings, psychodynamics, and psychopathology; and differentiate psychic problems from organic ones. The place of such tests is similar to that of other tests in medicine—helpful in diagnostic problems but a useless expense when not needed.

1. Objective tests–These tests provide quantitative evaluation compared to standard norms.

a. Intelligence tests–The test most frequently used is the Wechsler Adult Intelligence Scale—Revised (WAIS-R). Intelligence tests often reveal more than IQ. The results, given expert interpretation, can lend objective support to the ultimate psychiatric diagnosis. They provide information regarding different aspects of cognitive functioning, eg, short-term memory, abstract reasoning skills, and judgment.

b. Minnesota Multiphasic Personality Inventory (MMPI)–The MMPI is an empirically based test of personality assessment. The patient's scores are interpreted in comparison with data about others with the same response pattern to assess psychopathologic changes.

c. Bender Gestalt Test–This test is used to elicit evidence of psychomotor dysfunction in persons with organic disorders.

d. Vocational aptitude and interest tests–Several are available and may be used as a source of advice regarding vocational plans.

e. Halstead-Reitan Battery–This test is used when an organic deficit is present but information on location and extent of dysfunction is required.

f. Mini-mental status tests–These tests are short tests easily administered in the office by an assistant to screen for organic brain syndrome or to provide ongoing assessment of the progress of dementia.

2. Projective tests–These tests are unstructured, so that the subject is forced to respond in ways that reflect fantasies and individual modes of adaptation. Conscious and unconscious attitudes (particularly disordered thinking) may be deduced from the subject's responses.

a. Rorschach Psychodiagnostics–This test utilizes 10 inkblots. It requires expert interpretation but can provide important information on psychodynamic themes and aberrations.

b. Thematic Apperception Test (TAT)–This test uses 20 pictures of people in different situations. Interpretation is based on psychoanalytic theory concerning defenses against feelings of anxiety and reflects areas of interpersonal conflicts.

c. Sentence completion tests, draw-a-person tests, etc–These tests are most useful in providing information about the patient's present concerns and conflicts.

3. Miscellaneous tests–Other tests designed for specific purposes include aphasia screening tests, inventories of depression, tests of different types of memory, and neurologic, behavior, and anxiety screening tests.

B. Neurologic Evaluation: Consultation is often necessary and may include specialized tests such as electroencephalography, echoencephalography, brain scanning, CT scanning, positron emission tomography (PET), single photon emission computed tomography (SPECT), magneto-encephalography (MEG), and magnetic resonance imaging (MRI). Brain imaging is useful for detecting structural abnormalities in the patient who presents with a nondefinitive history and examination (eg, dissociative episodes, unusual psychotic episodes not explained by drug abuse). MRI studies (which, unlike CT, can image in all planes and produce a superb gray-white resolution) are particularly useful in delineating temporal lobe lesions, demyelinating disorders, and degenerative diseases (eg, Huntington's disease). PET correlates human behavior with brain chemistry and shows promise in demarcating psychiatric disorders.

C. Amobarbital Interviews: The success of any of the sedative agents in eliciting clinically useful information is quite limited. The suggestive force of giving substances by injection is helpful, as judged from a comparison of amobarbital and saline interviews. The procedure can be helpful in differentiating psychosis from delirium; the former usually improves with amobarbital, whereas the latter worsens. Some cases of conversion disorders or dissociative disorders respond to this approach. Hypnosis can provide similar relief in selected subjects.

D. Biologic Markers: The dexamethasone suppression test (DST) and the thyrotropin-releasing hormone (TRH) test have been used as aids in the diagnosis, treatment, and follow-up of patients with depressive illness. Clinical usefulness of the tests is limited (the DST may be measuring anxiety), but they represent progress in the search for reliable biologic markers.

Formulation of the Diagnosis

A psychiatric diagnosis must be based upon positive evidence accumulated by the above techniques. *It must not be based simply on the exclusion of organic findings.*

A thorough psychiatric evaluation has therapeutic as well as diagnostic value and should be expressed in ways best understood by the patient, family, and other physicians.

Garber HJ et al: Use of magnetic resonance imaging in psychiatry. Am J Psychiatry 1988;145:164. (MRI and PET are major diagnostic advances.)

Kiernan RJ et al: The Neurobehavioral Cognitive Status

Examination: A brief but differentiated approach to cognitive assessment. Ann Intern Med 1987;107:481. (For routine screening.)

TREATMENT APPROACHES

The approaches to treatment of psychiatric patients are, in a broad sense, similar to those in other branches of medicine. For example, the internist treating a patient with heart disease uses not only **medical** measures such as digitalis and pacemakers but also **psychologic** techniques to change attitudes and behaviors, **social** and **environmental** manipulation to mitigate deleterious influences, and **behavioral** techniques to change behavior patterns.

Regardless of the methods employed, treatment must be directed toward an objective, ie, **goal-oriented.** This usually involves (1) obtaining active cooperation on the part of the patient; (2) establishing reasonable goals and modifying the goal downward if failure occurs; (3) emphasizing positive behavior (goals) instead of symptom behavior (problems); (4) delineating the method; and (5) setting a time frame (which can be modified later).

The physician must resist pressures for prescribed treatment and instantaneous results. In almost all cases, psychiatric treatment involves the *active participation* of the significant people in the patient's life. Time must be spent with the patient, but the frequency and duration of appointments are highly variable and should be adjusted to meet both the patient's psychologic needs and financial restrictions. Compliance (collaboration) is the end product of many factors, the most important being clear communication, attention to cost, and simple dosage regimens when drugs are prescribed. *The physician can unwittingly promote chronic illness by prescribing inappropriate medication.* The patient may come to believe that problems respond only to medication, and the more drugs prescribed, the stronger the misconception becomes.

Psychiatric Referrals

All physicians have always treated most psychiatric problems and are in an excellent position to meet their patients' emotional needs in an organized and competent way, referring to psychiatrists for consultation or treatment those patients who represent particularly complex problems. The most pressing problems involve evaluation of suicidal or assaultive potential and diagnostic differentiation in mood disorders and psychoses. The psychiatric problems associated with unusual psychopharmacologic therapy and with medications used in other branches of medicine may require expert pharmacologic consultation. When a psychiatric referral is made, it should be conducted like any

other referral: in an open manner, with full explanation of the problem to the patient and the referral appointment made while the patient is still in the office.

MEDICAL APPROACHES

1. ANTIPSYCHOTIC DRUGS (Neuroleptics, "Major Tranquilizers")

This group of drugs includes **phenothiazines** and **thioxanthenes** (both similar in structure), **butyrophenones, dihydroindolones,** and **dibenzoxazepines.** Table 19–1 lists the drugs in order of increasing milligram potency and decreasing side effects (with the exception of extrapyramidal symptoms). Thus, chlorpromazine has lower milligram potency and causes more severe side effects and fewer extrapyramidal complications than fluphenazine. All are efficacious in reducing symptoms.

The phenothiazines comprise the bulk of the currently used neuroleptic drugs. The only butyrophe-

Table 19–1. Commonly used antipsychotics.

	Chlor-proma-zine Ratio	Usual Daily Oral Dose	Usual Daily Maximum Dose[1]
Phenothiazines			
Chlorpromazine (Thorazine and other trade names)	1:1	100–400 mg	1 g
Thioridazine (Mellaril)	1:1	100–400 mg	600 mg
Mesoridazine (Serentil)	1:2	50–200 mg	400 mg
Perphenazine (Trilafon)[2]	1:10	16–32 mg	64 mg
Trifluoperazine (Stelazine)[2]	1:20	5–15 mg	60 mg
Fluphenazine (Permitil, Prolixin)[2]	1:50	2–10 mg	60 mg
Thioxanthenes			
Chlorprothixene (Taractan)	1:1	100–400 mg	600 mg
Thiothixene[2] (Navane)	1:20	5–10 mg	80 mg
Butyrophenone			
Haloperidol (Haldol)	1:50	2–5 mg	80 mg
Dihydroindolone			
Molindone (Moban)	1:12	30–100 mg	225 mg
Dibenzoxazepine			
Clozapine (Clozaril)	1:1	300–450 mg	900 mg
Loxapine (Loxitane)	1:10	20–60 mg	200 mg

[1] Can be higher in some cases.
[2] Indicates piperazine structure.

none commonly used in psychiatry is haloperidol, which is totally different in structure but very similar in action and side effects to the piperazine phenothiazines such as fluphenazine, perphenazine, and trifluoperazine. These drugs and haloperidol have high potency, a paucity of autonomic side effects and markedly lower arousal levels. Molindone and loxapine, while less potent, are similar in action, side effects, and safety to the piperazine phenothiazines. Clozapine, a dibenzoxazepine derivative, is about 30% effective in the treatment of resistant psychoses. It is helpful in reducing the negative symptoms in chronic schizophrenics and has fewer extrapyramidal effects, though akathisia and tardive dyskinesia have been reported. It has a 1.6% risk of agranulocytosis (higher in persons of Jewish ancestry), and its use must be strictly monitored with weekly blood counts. It also lowers the seizure threshold and has many side effects, including sedation, hypotension, increased liver enzyme levels, hypersalivation, weight gain and changes in both electrocardiogram and electroencephalogram.

None of the antipsychotics produce true physical dependency, and they have a wide safety margins between therapeutic and toxic effects. All decrease adrenergic response and are efficacious in ameliorating psychotic symptoms. Previous response and experience with the drug and its side effects dictate the choice of a drug.

Clinical Indications

The antipsychotics are used to treat all **psychoses,** including the **schizophrenias** and **psychotic ideation in organic brain psychoses, drug-induced psychoses, psychotic depression,** and **mania.** They quickly lower the arousal (activity) level and, perhaps indirectly, gradually improve socialization and thinking. Patients whose behavioral symptoms worsen with use of antipsychotic drugs may have an undiagnosed organic condition.

Symptoms that are ameliorated by these drugs include hyperactivity, hostility, delusions, hallucinations, irritability, and poor sleep. Individuals with acute psychosis and good premorbid function respond quite well. The most common cause of failure in the treatment of acute psychosis is inadequate dosage, and the most common cause of relapse is noncompliance.

Dosage Forms & Patterns

The dosage range is quite broad. For example, haloperidol, 1 mg orally at bedtime, may be sufficient for the elderly person with a mild organic brain syndrome, whereas 60 mg/d may be used in a young schizophrenic patient. For quick response, one may initiate haloperidol, 10 mg intramuscularly, which is absorbed rapidly and achieves an initial 10-fold plasma level advantage over equal oral doses. Psychomotor agitation, racing thoughts, and general arousal are quickly reduced. The dose can be repeated every

3–4 hours; when the patient is less symptomatic, oral doses can replace parenteral administration in most cases.

Various factors play a role in the absorption of oral medications. Of particular importance are previous gastrointestinal surgery and concomitant administration of other drugs, eg, antacids (Table 19–2). There are racial differences in metabolizing these drugs—eg, many Asians require only about half the usual dosage. Bioavailability is influenced by other factors such as smoking or microsomal stimulation with alcohol or barbiturates and enzyme-altering drugs such as carbamazepine or methylphenidate. Plasma drug levels are not of major clinical assistance.

Divided daily doses are not necessary after a maintenance dose has been established, and most patients can then be maintained on a single daily dose, usually taken at bedtime. This is particularly appropriate in a case where the sedative effect of the drug is desired for nighttime sleep, and undesirable sedative effects can be avoided during the day. Costs of medication, nursing time, and patient unreliability are reduced when either a single daily dose or a large bedtime/smaller morning dose schedule is utilized. The maintenance dosage should be the lowest that controls symptoms. This requires adequate follow-up and decreases in dosage when possible. First-episode patients especially should be tapered off medications after about 6 months of stability and carefully monitored; their rate of relapse is lower than that of multiple-episode patients.

Psychiatric patients—particularly paranoid individuals—often neglect to take their medication. In these cases, the enanthate and decanoate (the latter is slightly longer lasting and has fewer extrapyramidal side effects) forms of fluphenazine or the decanoate form of haloperidol may be given by deep subcuta-

Table 19–2. Antipsychotic drug interactions with other drugs.

Drug	Effects
Antacids	Decreased absorption of antipsychotic drugs.
All anticholinergics	Increased anticholinergic effects.
Barbiturates	Central nervous system depression and decreased antipsychotic drug levels.
Carbamazepine	Decreased haloperidol levels.
Cimetidine	Increased chlorpromazine levels.
Cyclic antidepressants	Increased antidepressant blood levels.
Guanadrel	Increased hypotensive effect.
Guanethidine	Decreased hypotensive effect.
Indomethacin	Severe drowsiness (with haloperidol).
Levodopa	Decreased antiparkinson effect.
Methyldopa	Decreased hypotensive effect.
Phenytoin	Increased phenytoin levels.
Propranolol	Increased thioridazine levels.
Thiazide diuretics	Increased hypotensive effect.
Trihexyphenidyl	Decreased antipsychotic levels.

neous injection or intramuscularly to achieve an effect that will usually last 7–28 days. A patient who cannot be depended on to take oral medication (or who overdoses on minimal provocation) will generally agree to come to the physician's office for a "shot." The usual dose of the fluphenazine long-acting preparations is 25 mg (1 mL) every 2 weeks. Dosage and frequency of administration vary from about 100 mg weekly to 12.5 mg monthly. Use the smallest amount as infrequently as possible. A monthly injection of 25 mg of fluphenazine decanoate is equivalent to about 15–20 mg of oral fluphenazine daily.

Intravenous use of haloperidol (the only neuroleptic used in this manner) is reserved for special situations (eg, severely burned patients).

Side Effects

The side effects *decrease* as one goes from the sedating, lower milligram potency drugs such as chlorpromazine to those of higher milligram potency such as fluphenazine and haloperidol (Table 19–1). However, the extrapyramidal effects *increase* as one goes down the list (consider chlorprothixene as similar to chlorpromazine).

The most common anticholinergic side effects include dry mouth (which can lead to ingestion of caloric liquids and weight gain), blurred vision, urinary retention (particularly in elderly men with enlarged prostates), delayed gastric emptying, ileus, and precipitation of acute glaucoma in patients with narrow anterior chamber angles. Other autonomic effects include orthostatic hypotension and sexual dysfunction—problems in achieving erection, ejaculation (including retrograde ejaculation), and orgasm in males (approximately 50% of cases) and females (approximately 30%). Delay in achieving orgasm is often a factor in medication noncompliance. Electrocardiographic changes occur frequently, but clinically significant arrhythmias are much less common. Elderly patients and those with preexisting cardiac disease are at greater risk. For example, thioridazine, which has the fewest extrapyramidal side effects, has the most cardiac effects. One should avoid the concomitant use of thioridazine and sympathomimetic drugs. The most frequently seen electrocardiographic changes include diminution of the T wave amplitude, appearance of prominent U waves, depression of the ST segment, and prolongation of the QT interval. These electrocardiographic findings do not alter treatment.

Metabolic and endocrine effects include weight gain, hyperglycemia, infrequent temperature irregularities (particularly in hot weather), and water intoxication that may be due to inappropriate antidiuretic hormone function. Lactation and menstrual irregularities are common (antipsychotic drugs should be avoided, if possible, in breast cancer patients because of potential trophic effects of elevated prolactin levels on the breast). Both antipsychotic and antidepressant drugs inhibit sperm motility. Bone marrow depression and cholestatic jaundice occur rarely; these are sensitivity reactions, and they usually appear in the first 2 months of treatment. They subside on discontinuance of the drug. There is cross-sensitivity among all of the phenothiazines, and a drug from a different group must be used when allergic reactions occur.

Photosensitivity (including retinal effects) is commonly related to chlorpromazine use. Retinopathy and hyperpigmentation are associated with use of fairly high dosages of thioridazine and chlorpromazine. The appearance of particulate melanin deposits in the lens of the eye is related to the total dose given, and patients on long-term medication should have periodic eye examinations. Teratogenicity has not been causally related to these drugs, but prudence is indicated particularly in the first trimester of pregnancy. The seizure threshold is lowered, but it is safe to use these medications in epileptics controlled by anticonvulsants.

The **neuroleptic malignant syndrome (NMS)** is a catatonialike state with extrapyramidal signs, blood pressure changes, altered consciousness, and hyperpyrexia; it is an uncommon but serious complication of neuroleptic treatment. Muscle rigidity, involuntary movements, confusion, dysarthria, and dysphagia are accompanied by pallor, cardiovascular instability, fever, pulmonary congestion, and diaphoresis and may result in stupor, coma, and death. The cause may be related to a number of factors, including poor dosage control of neuroleptic medication and increased sensitivity of dopamine receptor sites. Lithium in combination with a neuroleptic drug may increase vulnerability, which is already increased in patients with an affective disorder. In most cases, the symptoms develop within the first 2 weeks of antipsychotic drug treatment. The syndrome may occur with small doses of the drugs. Elevated creatine phosphokinase (CPK) and leukocytosis with a shift to the left are present early in about half of cases. Treatment includes bringing down the fever with the usual pharmacologic and cooling methods. Stop dopamine-blocking agents and use a dopamine agonist such as bromocriptine, 2.5–10 mg orally 3 times a day. Amantadine, 100–200 mg orally twice a day, has also been useful. Dantrolene, 50 mg intravenously as needed, is used to alleviate rigidity (do not exceed 10 mg/kg/d). There is ongoing controversy about the efficacy of these 3 agents as well as the use of calcium channel blockers. The syndrome must be differentiated from acute lethal catatonia, malignant hyperthermia, neurotoxic syndromes (including AIDS), and a variety of other conditions such as viral encephalitis, Wilson's disease, central anticholinergic syndrome, and hypertonic states (eg, tetany, strychnine poisoning).

Extrapyramidal symptoms. Akathisia is the most common (about 20%) so-called extrapyramidal symptom. It usually occurs early in treatment (but may persist after neuroleptics are discontinued) and is frequently mistaken for anxiety or exacerbation of psychosis. It is characterized by a subjective desire to be in constant motion followed by an inability to sit or stand still and consequent pacing. It may include feelings of fright, rage, terror, or sexual torment. Insomnia is often present. In all cases, reevaluate the dosage requirement or the type of neuroleptic drug. Antiparkinsonism drugs such as trihexyphenidyl, 2–5 mg orally 3 times daily, or benztropine mesylate, 1–2 mg twice daily, may be helpful. High-potency neuroleptics often require concomitant antiparkinsonism drugs. In resistant cases, propranolol, 30–80 mg/d orally; diazepam, 5 mg 3 times daily; or amantadine, 100 mg orally 3 times daily, may alleviate the symptoms.

Acute dystonias usually occur early, although a tardive occurrence is reported and often includes blepharospasm. Younger patients are at higher risk. The most common signs are bizarre muscle spasms of the head, neck, and tongue. Frequently present are torticollis, oculogyric crises, swallowing or chewing difficulties, and masseter spasms. Laryngospasm is particularly dangerous. Back, arm, or leg muscle spasms are occasionally reported. Diphenhydramine, 50 mg intramuscularly, is effective for the acute crisis; one should then give benztropine mesylate, 2 mg orally twice daily, for several weeks, and then discontinue gradually, since few of the extrapyramidal symptoms require long-term use of the antiparkinsonism drugs (all of which are about equally efficacious)— though trihexyphenidyl tends to be mildly stimulating and benztropine mildly sedating.

Drug-induced parkinsonism is indistinguishable from idiopathic parkinsonism, but it occurs later in treatment than the preceding extrapyramidal symptoms and in some cases appears after neuroleptic withdrawal. The condition includes the typical signs of apathy and reduction of facial and arm movements (akinesia, which can mimic depression), festinating gait, rigidity, loss of postural reflexes, and the pill-rolling tremor. AIDS patients seem particularly vulnerable to extrapyramidal side effects. This extrapyramidal syndrome also responds to the aforementioned antiparkinsonism drugs in the same dosages. After 4–6 weeks, these drugs can often be discontinued with no recurrent symptoms. In any of the extrapyramidal symptoms, amantadine, 100–400 mg daily, may be used instead of the antiparkinsonism drugs if anticholinergic effects are a problem. Benztropine 15 mg is equivalent to atropine 5 mg. (Amantadine is also effective in singultus.) Anticholinergic toxicity is characterized by impaired attention and short-term memory, disorientation, anxiety, visual and auditory hallucinations, and other psychotic ideation. Neuroleptic-induced catatonia is similar to catatonic stupor with rigidity, drooling, urinary incontinence, and cogwheeling. It usually responds slowly to withdrawal of the offending medication and use of antiparkinsonism agents.

Tardive dyskinesia is a syndrome of abnormal involuntary stereotyped movements of the face, mouth, tongue, trunk, and limbs that may occur after months or (usually) years of treatment with neuroleptic agents. The syndrome affects 20–35% of patients who have undergone long-term neuroleptic therapy. *There are no known differences among any of the antipsychotic drugs in the development of this syndrome.*

Early manifestations include fine wormlike movements of the tongue at rest, difficulty in sticking out the tongue, facial tics, increased blink frequency, or jaw movements of recent onset. Later manifestations may include bucco-linguo-masticatory movements, lip smacking, chewing motions, mouth opening and closing, disturbed gag reflex, puffing of the cheeks, disrupted speech, respiratory distress, or choreoathetoid movements of the extremities (the last being more prevalent in younger patients). The symptoms do not necessarily worsen and in rare cases may lessen even though neuroleptic drugs are continued. The dyskinesias do not occur during sleep and can be voluntarily suppressed for short periods. Stress and movements in other parts of the body will often aggravate the condition.

Early signs of dyskinesia must be differentiated from those reversible signs produced by ill-fitting dentures or nonneuroleptic drugs such as levodopa, tricyclic antidepressants (TCAs), antiparkinsonism agents, anticonvulsants, and antihistamines. Other neurologic conditions such as Huntington's chorea can be differentiated by history and examination.

The emphasis should be on prevention. Use the least amount of neuroleptic drug necessary to mute the psychotic symptoms. Detect early manifestations. When these occur, stop anticholinergic drugs and gradually discontinue neuroleptic drugs. Weight loss and cachexia sometimes appear on withdrawal of neuroleptics. In an indeterminate number of cases, the dyskinesias will remit. Keep the patient off the drugs until reemergent psychotic symptoms dictate their resumption, at which point they are restarted in low doses and gradually increased until there is clinical improvement. If the dyskinesic syndrome recurs and it is necessary to continue neuroleptic drugs to control psychotic symptoms, informed consent should be obtained.

Reserpine has occasionally been successfully substituted for the neuroleptic drugs and does not cause dyskinesic syndrome. Benzodiazepines, phosphatidylcholine, clonidine, calcium channel blockers, vitamin E, and propranolol all have had limited usefulness in treating the dyskinetic side effects.

Kalow W: Race and therapeutic drug response. N Engl J Med 1989;320:588. (Differences in metabolism and response.)

Kane JM: The current status of neuroleptic therapy. J Clin Psychiatry 1989;50:322.

Rosebush P, Stewart T: A prospective analysis of 24 episodes of neuroleptic malignant syndrome. Am J Psychiatry 1989;146:717. (Evaluates treatment.)

2. LITHIUM

The use of lithium over the last 4 decades has dramatically affected both diagnosis and treatment in psychiatry. The discovery of lithium's effectiveness in bipolar mood disorders has shown that many of these patients were erroneously diagnosed as having a schizophrenic disorder.

Clinical Indications

As a prophylactic drug for bipolar affective disorder, lithium significantly decreases the frequency and severity of both manic and depressive attacks in about 80% of patients. A positive response is more predictable if the patient has a low frequency of episodes (no more than 2 per year with intervals free of psychopathology). A positive response occurs more frequently in individuals who have blood relatives with a diagnosis of manic or hypomanic attacks. Patients who swing rapidly back and forth between manic and depressive attacks (at least 4 cycles per year) usually respond poorly to lithium prophylaxis initially, but some improve with continued long-term treatment. Carbamazepine has been used with success in this group.

Acute manic or hypomanic symptoms will respond to lithium therapy, but it is common to use neuroleptic drugs to treat the excited or psychotic manic stage (as outlined in the treatment of the psychoses) and then make a decision with the patient and family about the feasibility of long-term prophylactic lithium therapy. The decision is usually based on the severity of the condition. Schizoaffective disorders and some cases of so-called schizophrenia are probably atypical bipolar affective disorder, for which lithium treatment may be effective.

Lithium—either alone or combined with cyclic antidepressants in acute phases—is useful in the prophylaxis of some recurrent unipolar depressions (perhaps undiagnosed bipolar disorder). Its use in the treatment of acute depression is not warranted except in depressions occurring in a bipolar patient who has previously responded to the drug and in cases that have not responded to antidepressant drugs. Most patients with bipolar disease can be managed with lithium alone, though some will require continued or intermittent use of a neuroleptic, antidepressant medication, or carbamazepine. An excellent resource for information pertaining to lithium is the Lithium Information Center, University of Wisconsin, Department of Psychiatry, 600 Highland Avenue, Madison, WI 53792.

Dosage Forms & Patterns

Lithium carbonate (Eskalith, Lithane, Lithobid, Lithonate, Lithotabs) is available in the USA in 300-mg capsules. Tablets (Lithotabs), which can be broken, are used in patients requiring a more exact dosage than a multiple of 300 mg. Side effects can be mitigated by taking the drug with food or by use of Lithobid (slow release). Lithium citrate is available as a syrup for patients in whom compliance is a problem. The dosage is that required to maintain blood levels in the therapeutic range. For acute attacks this ranges from 1 to 1.6 meq/L, whereas the prophylactic dose is usually 0.4–1 meq/L (though levels < 0.6 meq/L may lead to a higher frequency of relapses). Maintenance levels should be kept as low as clinically feasible. The dose required to meet this need will vary in individuals and should be determined by giving a test dose of 600 mg of lithium carbonate after the clinical workup, which should include a medical history and physical examination; complete blood count; T 4, TSH, blood urea nitrogen, creatinine, and electrolyte determinations; urinalysis; and ECG. Twenty-four hours after the administration of the test dose, a blood sample is drawn for lithium determination. (See Table 19–3 for dosage requirements based on a test dose.) The usual practice is to administer lithium in the most convenient way, with a minimum of side effects. There is no evidence that once-a-day dosage is deleterious, but most patients have less nausea when they take the drug in divided doses with meals.

Lithium is readily absorbed, with peak serum levels occurring within 1–3 hours and complete absorption in 8 hours. Half of the total body lithium is excreted in 18–24 hours (95% in the urine). *The blood for the lithium levels should be drawn 12 hours after the last dose.* Serum levels should be measured every 1–3 weeks in the early maintenance stage and thereafter when clinically indicated (at least every 3 months), particularly when there is any condition that may lower sodium levels (eg, diarrhea; dehydration; use of diuretics). Patients receiving lithium should use diuretics with caution and only under close medical supervision. The thiazide diuretics cause increased lithium reabsorption from the proximal renal tubules, resulting in increased serum lithium levels (Table 19–4), and adjustment of lithium intake must be made to compensate for this. Reduce lithium dosage by

Table 19–3. Predicted lithium daily dosage necessary to produce therapeutic levels. (Based on 600-mg test dose.)

24-h Lithium Level (meq/L)	Total Daily Dose (mg)
<0.05	3600
0.05–0.09	2700
0.10–0.14	1800
0.15–0.19	1200
0.20–0.23	900
0.24–0.30	600
>0.30	300

Table 19-4. Lithium interactions with other drugs.

Drug	Effects
Ibuprofen	Increased lithium levels.
Indomethacin	Increased lithium levels.
Iodine	Enhanced goitrogenic effect.
Methyldopa	Rigidity, mutism, fascicular twitching.
Osmotic diuretics (urea, mannitol)	Increased lithium excretion.
Phenylbutazone	Increased lithium levels.
Potassium-sparing diuretics (spironolactone, amiloride, triamterene)	Increased lithium levels.
Sodium bicarbonate	Increased lithium excretion.
Succinylcholine	Increased succinylcholine duration of action.
Theophylline, aminophylline	Increased lithium excretion.
Thiazide diuretics	Increased lithium levels.

25–40% when the patient is receiving 50 mg of hydrochlorothiazide daily. Potassium-sparing diuretics (spironolactone, amiloride, triamterene) may also cause increased serum lithium levels and require careful monitoring of lithium levels. Loop diuretics (furosemide, ethacrynic acid, bumetanide) appear not to alter serum lithium levels.

Side Effects

A. Early Side Effects: Mild gastrointestinal symptoms (take lithium with food), fine tremors (treat with propranolol, 20–60 mg/d orally, only if persistent), slight muscle weakness, and some degree of somnolence are early side effects that are usually transient. Moderate polyuria (reduced renal responsiveness to antidiuretic hormone) and polydipsia (associated with increased plasma renin concentration) are occasionally present. Weight gain (often a result of calories in fluids taken for polydipsia) and leukocytosis are fairly common.

B. Lithium Toxicity: Frank toxicity usually occurs at blood levels above 2 meq/L. This is often a result of sodium loss or kidney disease, since sodium and lithium are reabsorbed at the same loci in the proximal renal tubules. Any sodium loss such as that which occurs with diarrhea, use of diuretics, or excessive perspiration results in increased lithium levels. Symptoms and signs include vomiting and diarrhea, the latter exacerbating the problem since more sodium is lost. Other signs and symptoms, some of which may not be reversible, include tremors, marked muscle weakness, confusion, dysarthria, vertigo, ataxia, hyperreflexia, rigidity, seizures, opisthotonos, and coma. Toxicity is higher in the elderly, who should be maintained on slightly lower serum levels. Lithium overdosage may be accidental or intentional or may occur as a result of poor monitoring. Compliance with lithium therapy is adversely affected by the loss of some hypomanic experiences valued by the patient. These include social extroversion and a sense of heightened enjoyment in many activities such as sex and business dealings, often with increased productivity in the latter (creativity has been positively correlated with affective disorder).

C. Other Side Effects: These include weight gain, goiter (3%; often euthyroid), occasionally hypothyroidism (5%; concomitant administration of lithium and iodide enhances the hypothyroid and goitrogenic effect of either drug), changes in the glucose tolerance test toward a diabeticlike curve, nephrogenic diabetes insipidus, nephrotic syndrome, edema, pseudotumor cerebri (do funduscopy if there are complaints of headache or blurred vision), and leukocytosis. A metallic taste, hair loss, and Raynaud's phenomena have been reported in a small number of cases. Thyroid and kidney function should be checked at 3- to 6-month intervals. Most of these side effects subside when lithium is discontinued; when residual side effects exist, they are usually not serious. Most clinicians treat lithium-induced hypothyroidism (more common in women) with thyroid hormone while continuing lithium therapy. Hypercalcemia and elevated parathyroid hormone levels occur in some patients. Electrocardiographic abnormalities (principally T wave flattening or inversion) may occur during lithium administration but are not of major clinical significance. Sinoatrial block may occur, particularly in the elderly. It is important that other drugs which prolong intraventricular conduction, such as TCAs, be used with caution in conjunction with lithium. Lithium impairs ventilatory function in patients with airway obstruction. Lithium may precipitate or exacerbate psoriasis in some patients. Patients receiving long-term lithium therapy may have cogwheel rigidity and, occasionally, other extrapyramidal signs. Lithium potentiates the parkinsonian effects of haloperidol. A wide variety of neurologic sequelae have been reported; most remit quickly when lithium therapy is discontinued.

The long-term use of lithium has adverse effects on renal function (with interstitial fibrosis, tubular atrophy, and glomerulosclerosis) in some patients that are not always completely reversible. A rise in serum creatinine levels is an indication for in-depth evaluation of renal function. Incontinence has been reported in women, apparently related to changes in bladder cholinergic-adrenergic balance. Lithium increases parathyroid hormone levels, with increased serum calcium and decreased serum phosphate. Long-term lithium therapy has also been associated with a relative lowering of the level of memory and perceptual processing (affecting compliance in some cases). Some impairment of attention and emotional reactivity has also been noted. Lithium-induced delirium with therapeutic lithium levels is an infrequent complication and often persists for several days after serum levels have become negligible. Encephalopathy has occurred in patients on combined lithium/neuroleptic therapy and in those who have cerebrovascular disease, thus requiring careful evaluation of patients who develop neurotoxic signs at subtoxic blood levels.

Lithium exposure in early pregnancy increases the frequency of congenital anomalies, with a marked shift toward major cardiovascular anomalies. *It is advisable for women using lithium either to avoid pregnancy or to not use lithium at all during a planned pregnancy, particularly during the first trimester.* If there has been exposure in the first trimester, especially between the eighth and twelfth weeks, the possibility of teratogenic defect is highest. Bottle-feeding should be considered in mothers using lithium, since concentration in breast milk is one-third to one-half that in serum.

Patients with massive ingestions of lithium or levels above 3 meq/L should be treated with induced emesis and gastric lavage. In normal renal function, osmotic and saline diuresis increases renal lithium clearance. Urinary alkalinization is also helpful, since sodium bicarbonate decreases lithium reabsorption in the proximal tubule, as does acetazolamide also. Aminophylline potentiates the diuretic effect by increasing the glomerular filtration rate of lithium. Drugs affecting the distal loop have no effect on lithium reabsorption. In exceptional cases, hemodialysis and peritoneal dialysis decrease plasma concentration; this gradually shortens recovery time.

Schou M: Lithium prophylaxis: Myths and realities. Am J Psychiatry 1989;146:573. (A practical approach to lithium therapy by the major authority.)

3. ANTIDEPRESSANT DRUGS

The antidepressant drugs are classified into 3 groups; (1) the monoamine oxidase (MAO) inhibitors; (2) the TCAs; and (3) the newer generation drugs, called heterocyclic antidepressants.

Clinical Indications

A. Monoamine Oxidase Inhibitors: The MAO inhibitors have generally been used as second-line drugs (after a failure of tricyclics) because of the dietary and other restrictions (see below and Table 19–5). They should be considered as drugs of first choice in some anxious depressions, atypical depression, panic disorders, and for maintenance therapy of depression in the elderly.

B. Tricyclic Antidepressants (TCAs): The TCAs have been the mainstay of drug therapy for depression for almost 30 years. They have also been used in many other disorders: amitriptyline in chronic pain syndromes; imipramine in panic disorder, enuresis, catalepsy, bulimia, and anorexia nervosa; clomipramine in obsessive compulsive disorder; amoxapine in psychotic depression; and desipramine in reducing craving in cocaine withdrawal.

C. Heterocyclic Antidepressants: The hetero-

Table 19–5. Principal dietary restrictions in MAO use.

1. Cheeses except cream and cottage types and yogurt.
2. Fermented or aged meats or fish such as bologna, pickled herring.
3. Broad bean pods such as Chinese pea pods.
4. Liver of all types.
5. Meat and yeast extracts.
6. Spoiled, dried, or aged fruits, eg, avocados, figs, raisins, bananas.
7. Red wine, sherry, vermouth, cognac, beer, ale.
8. Soy sauce, shrimp paste.

cyclic antidepressants are increasingly being considered front-line drugs in the treatment of depression, particularly when obsessive compulsive disorder is a significant part of the depression or when atypical features predominate.

Dosage Forms & Patterns

Caution: Depressed patients may have suicidal thoughts, and the amount of drug dispensed should be appropriately controlled. The older tricyclics have a narrow therapeutic index, and one advantage of the newer drugs is their wider margin of safety. In all cases of pharmacologic management of depressed states, caution is indicated until the risk of suicide is considered minimal.

A. MAO Inhibitors: MAO inhibitors are administered in gradual stepwise dosage and may be given in the morning or evening, depending upon the effect on sleep. They tend to take effect quickly in a fairly low dosage range (Table 19–6).

B. Tricyclic Antidepressants: TCAs are characterized more by their similarities to each other than by their differences. There is a lag in clinical response for up to several weeks, partly as a result of side effects that prevent rapid increase in dosage and partly because of their neurotransmitter effects. Individuals receiving the same dosages vary markedly in therapeutic drug levels achieved (elderly patients require smaller doses), and determination of plasma drug levels is helpful when clinical response has been disappointing. Nortriptyline is usually effective when plasma levels are between 50 and 150 ng/mL; imipramine at plasma levels of 200–250 ng/mL; and desipramine at plasma levels of about 125 ng/mL. Patients who have had gastric surgery frequently require higher doses to achieve satisfactory plasma levels. Most of the tricyclics can be given in a single dose at bedtime, starting at fairly low doses (eg, desipramine, 50 mg orally) and increasing by 50 mg every several days as tolerated until the therapeutic response is achieved (eg, desipramine, 150–200 mg) or to maximum dose if necessary (eg, desipramine, 300 mg). The most common cause of treatment failure is an inadequate trial. Clomipramine is started at a low dose (25 mg/d orally) and increased slowly in divided doses up to 100 mg/d, held at that level for several days, and then gradually increased as necessary up to 250

Table 19–6. Commonly used antidepressants.

4 = strong effect
1 = weak effect
0 = no effect
— = variable or not established

	Usual Daily Oral Dose (mg)	Usual Daily Maximum Dose (mg)	Sedative Effects	Anticholinergic Effects	Serotonin Reuptake Blockade	Norepinephrine Reuptake Blockade
Monoamine oxidase inhibitors						
Isocarboxazid (Marplan)	10–30	60	—	—	—	—
Phenelzine (Nardil)	45–60	90	—	—	—	—
Tranylcypromine (Parnate)	20–30	50	—	—	—	—
Tricyclic compounds						
Amitriptyline (Elavil)	150–250	300	4	4	4	2
Amoxapine (Asendin)	150–200	400	2	2	1	3
Clomipramine (Anafranil)	100	250	3	4	4	—
Desipramine (Norpramin)	100–250	300	1	1	2	4
Doxepin (Sinequan)	150–200	300	4	2	1	2
Imipramine (Tofranil)	150–200	300	3	3	3	2
Nortriptyline (Pamelor)	100–150	200	2	2	2	3
Protriptyline (Vivactil)	15–40	60	1	2	1	4
Trimipramine (Surmontil)	75–200	200	4	4	1	1
Heterocyclic compounds						
Bupropion (Wellbutrin)	300	450*	0	0	0	†
FluoxetinE (Prozac)	5–40	80	0	0	4	0
Maprotiline (Ludomil)	100–200	300	4	2	1	3
Trazodone (Desyrel)	100–300	600	4	1	2	0

* No single dose should exceed 150 mg.
† Affects dopamine system.

mg/d. Any of the tricyclics should be started at low doses and increased slowly in the treatment of panic disorder.

C. Heterocyclic Antidepressants: Fluoxetine and bupropion are more activating than other heterocyclics and should be given in the morning so as not to interfere with sleep. They may require several weeks to produce a therapeutic response. The half-life of fluoxetine is quite long, and the initial dose (20 mg/d orally) is frequently the therapeutic dose; indeed, the maintenance dose is often 20 mg every other day. Higher doses (40–60 mg/d) are frequently required in the treatment of obsessive compulsive disorder. Bupropion is given early in the day in divided doses and increased very slowly because of concern about the side effect of seizures.

D. Switching and Combination Therapy: Combination therapy with antidepressant drugs is not usually feasible (see Table 19–7), and in switching from one group to another an adequate "washout time" must be allowed. This is critical in certain situations—eg, in switching from a MAO inhibitor to a tricyclic, allow 2–3 weeks between stopping one drug and starting another; in switching from fluoxetine to a MAO inhibitor, allow 4–5 weeks. In switching within groups—eg, from one tricyclic to another (amitriptyline to desipramine, etc)—no washout time is needed, and one can rapidly decrease the dosage of one drug while increasing the other.

However, in any of the 3 groups, one can augment the antidepressant drug if the therapeutic response has been less than satisfactory. Lithium is the most effective augmenting agent. It is added to the regimen and regulated in the usual fashion. Perphenazine, 4–8 mg/d orally, has been used with variable results.

E. Maintenance and Tapering: When clinical relief of symptoms is obtained, medication is continued for several months in the lowest effective maintenance dosage, which is usually about half the dosage required in the acute stage. After about 6 months of effective treatment, the dosage is slowly decreased and, if there is no resurgence of symptoms, discontinued.

Side Effects

A. MAO Inhibitors: The MAO inhibitors commonly cause symptoms of orthostatic hypotension (which may persist) and sympathomimetic effects of tachycardia, sweating, and tremor. Nausea, insomnia (often associated with intense afternoon drowsiness), and sexual dysfunction are common. Central nervous system effects include agitation and toxic psychoses. Dietary limitations (see Table 19–5) and abstinence from drug products containing phenylpropanolamine, phenylephrine, and pseudoephedrine are mandatory, since the reduction of available monoamine oxidase leaves the patient vulnerable to exogenous amines (eg, tyramine in foodstuffs).

Treatment for a resultant hypertensive crisis has been the same as for pheochromocytoma (see Chapter 20), but there have been reports of success with nifedipine, 10 mg sublingually, which normalized blood

Table 19–7. Antidepressant drug interactions with other drugs.

Drug	Effects
Tricyclic and cyclic antidepressants	
Antacids	Decreased absorption of antidepressants.
Anticoagulants	Increased hypoprothrombinemic effect.
Cimetidine	Increased antidepressant blood levels and psychosis.
Clonidine	Decreased antihypertensive effect.
Digitalis	Increased incidence of heart block.
Disulfiram	Increased antidepressant blood levels.
Guanadrel	Decreased antihypertensive effect.
Guanethidine	Decreased antihypertensive effect.
Haloperidol	Increased clomipramine levels.
Insulin	Decreased blood sugar.
Lithium	Increased lithium levels with fluoxetine.
Methyldopa	Decreased antihypertensive effect.
Other anticholinergic drugs	Marked anticholinergic responses.
Phenytoin	Increased blood levels.
Procainamide	Decreased ventricular conduction.
Procarbazine	Hypertensive crisis.
Propranolol	Increased hypotension.
Quinidine	Decreased ventricular conduction.
Rauwolfia derivatives	Increased stimulation.
Sedatives	Increased sedation.
Sympathomimetic drugs	Increased pressor effect.
Monoamine oxidase inhibitors	
Antihistamines	Increased sedation.
Belladonnalike drugs	Increased blood pressure.
Dextromorphan	Same as meperidine.
Guanadrel	Increased blood pressure.
Guanethidine	Decreased blood pressure.
Insulin	Decreased blood sugar.
Levodopa	Increased blood pressure.
Meperidine	Increased mood lability, agitation, seizures.
Methyldopa	Decreased blood pressure.
Reserpine	Increased blood pressure and temperature.
Succinylcholine	Increased neuromuscular blockade.
Sulfonylureas	Decreased blood sugar.
Sympathomimetic drugs	Increased blood pressure.

pressure in 1–5 minutes. The restrictions on the proscribed foodstuffs and sympathomimetic drugs are in effect during treatment and for 1 month after cessation of therapy.

B. Tricyclic Antidepressants: The tricyclics have anticholinergic side effects (amitriptyline 100 mg is equivalent to atropine 5 mg) to varying degrees (see Table 19–6). One must be particularly wary of the effect in elderly men with prostatic hypertrophy.

The anticholinergic effects also predispose to other medical problems such as heat stroke or dental problems such as xerostomia. Orthostatic hypotension is fairly common, may not remit with time, and is a major problem in elderly women with osteoporosis who may suffer a hip fracture after a fall. Cardiac effects of the TCAs are functions of the anticholinergic effect, direct myocardial depression (quinidine effect), and interference with adrenergic neurons. These factors produce altered rate, rhythm, and contractility, particularly in patients with preexisting cardiac disease. Electrocardiographic changes range from benign ST segment and T wave changes and sinus tachycardia to a variety of complex and serious arrhythmias, the latter requiring a change in medication. The seizure threshold may be lowered and is of particular concern in patients with a propensity for seizures (eg, previous head injury, alcohol withdrawal). Loss of libido and erectile, ejaculatory, and orgasmic dysfunction are fairly common and seriously compromise compliance. Delirium, agitation, and mania are infrequent complications.

C. Heterocyclic Antidepressants: These drugs have very little anticholinergic effect. Trazodone tends to be sedating, while fluoxetine and bupropion tend to be activating, with side effects that include headache, nausea, insomnia, nervousness, dyskinesia, and akathisia. Seizures have been a problem with bupropion in the treatment of bulimia. A rare side effect of trazodone has been priapism, which must be treated within 12 hours by injection of epinephrine 1:1000 into the corpus cavernosum. As with most antidepressants, side effects of sexual import are fairly common. Several of the newer drugs are strong serotonin uptake blockers. High doses or combinations of such drugs can cause a "serotonin syndrome" with symptoms of nausea, neuromuscular irritability, hyperthermia, confusion, seizures, and delirium.

Deptula D, Pomara N: Effects of antidepressants on human performance: A review. J Clin Psychopharmacol 1990; 10:105.

Koenig HG, Breitner JCS: Use of antidepressants in medically ill older patients. Psychosomatics 1990;31:22. (Vulnerable population.)

Zisook S: A clinical overview of monoamine oxidase inhibitors. Psychosomatics 1985;26:240. (Still current overview.)

4. SEDATIVE-HYPNOTIC & OTHER ANTIANXIETY DRUGS (Anxiolytic Agents, "Minor Tranquilizers")

The sedatives are a heterogeneous group of drugs that differ in chemical structure but have quite similar pharmacologic and behavioral effects. They are often marketed as "minor tranquilizers" or "antianxiety agents," and all have hypnotic properties when given in adequate dosage. Ethanol is the most commonly used antianxiety drug. The various sedatives differ mainly in milligram potency, dose-response curves, and onset and duration of action. All are general depressants of brain function and decrease anxiety, producing disinhibition and a lowering of passive avoidance in sufficient dosage. To varying degrees, all have the potential for dependency with tolerance and severe withdrawal symptoms. Short-acting drugs may present a greater risk of withdrawal reactions than longer-acting agents. They are addictive and have cross tolerance and cross dependence. Some have anticonvulsant and muscle relaxant properties, although muscle relaxation usually occurs in the ataxic dosage range.

The highly addicting drugs with a narrow margin of safety such as glutethimide, ethchlorvynol, methyprylon, meprobamate, and the barbiturates (with the exception of phenobarbital) should be avoided. Phenobarbital, in addition to its anticonvulsant properties, is a reasonably safe and very cheap sedative but has the disadvantage of enzyme stimulation (not the case with benzodiazepines), which markedly reduces its usefulness if any other medications are being used by the patient. Although its effect on dicumarol is the most widely known, it increases the catabolism of practically all other drugs, including antipsychotics and antidepressants.

The benzodiazepines are the latest in a long line of sedatives that were initially regarded as safe, effective, and not likely to cause dependency. However, like its predecessors, the benzodiazepine group has potential for abuse and complex metabolic actions. When ingested by themselves, these agents are safer than other drugs used in suicide attempts. Despite the fact that the "safer" benzodiazepines are replacing barbiturates for purposes of sedation, there has been no significant reduction in suicides caused by drugs. Furthermore, many attempted suicides involve not only multiple drug use but also alcohol. It is clear that carelessly dispensing drugs for obscure complaints and persistent patient demands is a part of the problem.

Onset of action is a function of rate of absorption (related to lipophilic activity) and varies, with diazepam and clorazepate being the most rapidly absorbed. This characteristic, along with high lipid solubility, may explain the popularity of diazepam. Halazepam and prazepam are the least rapidly absorbed. The length of action of the benzodiazepines varies as a function of the active metabolites they produce. Short-acting benzodiazepines, which do not produce active metabolites, have half-lives of 5–20 hours, and ultra-short-acting ones have half-lives of less than 5 hours. The other benzodiazepines produce active metabolites and have half-lives of 1–8 days. The antihistamines hydroxyzine and diphenhydramine are often prescribed for mild sedation because they are save and produce no dependency.

Buspirone is the only marketed anxiolytic drug that is not a sedative. It is not believed to produce depressant effects or dependence. Abuse potential is thought to be low. Thus, it differs from the sedatives in that motor skills are not impaired and it does not potentiate the effects of alcohol or cause a withdrawal syndrome. Buspirone does not protect from benzodiazepine or alcohol withdrawal. Efficacy is apparently slightly less in patients who have recently been taking benzodiazepines, and there is a 1- to 2-week lag period before the drug takes effect. It is not clear which types of anxiety might respond, but there has been some success in the chronically worried, anxious depressive patient and in some obsessive compulsive patients.

Clinical Indications

The sedatives are used clinically for the treatment of anxiety, which may be the result of many factors, eg, transient situational problems, acute and chronic stresses of life, chronic medical problems, intractable pain exacerbated by apprehension and depression, and problems that people cannot or will not resolve (unhappy marriages, unsatisfactory jobs, etc). In higher doses these drugs act as hypnotics. Whether the indications are anxiety or insomnia, the drugs should be used judiciously. The longer-acting benzodiazepines are used for the treatment of alcohol withdrawal and anxiety symptoms; the shorter-acting drugs are useful as sedatives in sleep and medical procedures such as endoscopy.

Clonazepam, approved in the USA as an oral benzodiazepine antiepileptic agent, has been found to be effective in a variety of other conditions. It has been shown to be effective as an antimanic drug (0.5–16 mg/d orally) and in the treatment of panic attacks (3–6 mg/d orally). Clonazepam is twice as potent and acts twice as long as alprazolam, properties that in many cases make it the preferable drug in panic disorders. It has also been used as an adjunct to antipsychotic drugs in the treatment of agitation in the psychotic patient. Alprazolam is unique in that it is useful in panic disorders and has been used successfully in small doses in the treatment of depression, notably in patients in whom the usual antidepressant drugs are contraindicated (eg, the elderly). Dependency is a major problem, and the antidepressant drugs are preferable in these conditions.

Dosage Forms & Patterns
(Table 19–8)

All of the sedatives may be given orally, and several are available in parenteral form. Short-acting benzodiazepines are absorbed rapidly when given intramuscularly. Disadvantages of intravenous use outweigh advantages in psychiatric disorders. Antacids significantly alter the absorption of clorazepate and prazepam; this is an important consideration, since many anxious individuals suffer from gastrointestinal disturbances and use both types of drugs concomitantly.

Table 19–8. Commonly used antianxiety agents.

	Usual Oral Anxiolytic Dose (mg)	Usual Oral Hypnotic Dose (mg)	Usual Maximum Daily Oral Dose (mg)
Benzodiazepines			
Alprazolam[1] (Xanax)	0.5		4
Chlordiazepoxide (Librium)	5–30	50–100	75–100
Clonazepam (Klonopin)	1.5		10
Clorazepate (Tranxene)	3.25–15	30	60
Diazepam (Valium)	2–10	20–30	40
Flurazepam (Dalmane)		15	60
Halazepam (Paxipam)	20	40–60	160
Lorazepam[1] (Ativan)	2		
Midazolam (Versed)[3]	Use is parenteral preoperative sedation.		
Oxazepam[1] (Serax)	10–30	30–60	90
Prazepam (Centrax)	10		60
Temazepam[1] (Restoril)		15	30
Triazolam[2] (Halcion)		0.125–0.5	1.5
Miscellaneous			
Buspirone (Buspar)	5–10		60
Chloral hydrate (Noctec)[1]	250	500–1000	2000
Hydroxyzine pamoate (Vistaril)	25–50	100	300
Phenobarbital	15–30	90	300

[1] Shorter-acting sedatives.
[2] Ultra-short-acting sedatives.
[3] Ultra-ultra short-acting sedatives.

Food also modifies the absorption of diazepam (and possibly the other benzodiazepines), initially slowing absorption but resulting in higher levels over many hours. In the average case of anxiety, diazepam, 5–10 mg orally every 6–8 hours as needed, is a reasonable starting regimen. Since people vary widely in their response and since the drugs are long-lasting, one must individualize the dosage. Once this is established, an adequate dose early in the course of symptom development will obviate the need for "pill-popping," which contributes to dependency problems. Flurazepam and temazepam are both marketed for management of sleep problems. The latter has a somewhat shorter duration of action but a delayed onset of action in the range of 1–3 hours. Triazolam has achieved popularity as a hypnotic drug because of its very short duration of action. There are problems with dependency and anterograde amnesia, as in the case of all benzodiazepines.

Side Effects

The side effects are mainly behavioral and depend on patient reaction and dosage. As the dosage exceeds the levels necessary for sedation, the side effects include disinhibition, ataxia, dysarthria, nystagmus, and errors of commission. (Machinery should not be operated until the patient is well stabilized, and the patient should be so informed.) Agitation, anxiety, psychosis, confusion, mood lability, and anterograde

amnesia have been reported, particularly with the shorter-acting benzodiazepines.

Overdosage results in respiratory depression, hypotension, shock syndrome, coma, and death. Treatment of overdoses (see Chapter 33) and withdrawal states are medical emergencies. The latter is treated in much the same way as sedative dependency.

A serious side effect of chronic excessive dosage is drug dependency, which may involve tolerance, and physiologic dependency with withdrawal symptoms similar in morbidity and mortality to alcohol withdrawal (withdrawal effects must be distinguished from reemergent anxiety). Abrupt withdrawal of sedative drugs may cause serious and even fatal convulsive seizures. Psychosis, organic manic syndrome, and autonomic dysfunction have also been described. Both duration of action and duration of exposure are major factors; withdrawal symptoms are more severe when the individual has been using the drug for more than 8 months. The symptoms are similar to those of barbiturate withdrawal. They are more gradual in onset in the case of the longer-acting benzodiazepines. They include perceptual distortions, anxiety, faintness, some cardiovascular lability, nightmares, insomnia, and hyperreactivity to external stimuli, with seizures as late as the 12th day of withdrawal. Delirium may be present. Mild withdrawal symptoms may occur even after several weeks of regular usage. Taper dosages every several days for gradual withdrawal (eg, 0.25 mg every 3 days for alprazolam and 5–10 mg every 3 days for diazepam).

The sedatives produce **cumulative** clinical effects with repeated dosage (especially if the patient has not had time to metabolize the previous dose); **additive** effects when given with other classes of sedatives or alcohol (many "accidental" deaths are the result of concomitant use of sedatives and alcohol); and **residual** effects after termination of treatment (particularly in the case of drugs that undergo slow biotransformation). Other side effects are rare, although inhibition of orgasm and hypomania have been reported with the use of alprazolam.

Benzodiazepine interactions with other drugs are listed in Table 19–9.

Table 19–9. Benzodiazepine interactions with other drugs.

Drug	Effects
Antacids	Decreased absorption of benzodiazepines.
Cimetidine	Increased half-life of flurazepam, alprazolam.
Contraceptives	Increased levels of diazepam and triazolam.
Dicumarol	Decreased prothrombin time.
Digoxin	Alprazolam and diazepam raise digoxin level.
Disulfiram	Increased duration of action of sedatives.
Isoniazid	Increased plasma diazepam.
Levodopa	Inhibition of antiparkinsonism effect.
Propoxyphene	Impaired clearance of diazepam.
Rifampin	Decreased plasma diazepam.

Rifkin A: Benzodiazepines for anxiety disorders: Are the concerns justified? Postgrad Med 1990;87:209. (A pertinent question.)

Woods JH, Katz JL, Winger G: Use and abuse of benzodiazepines: Issues relevant to prescribing JAMA 1988; 260:3476. (Dependency a major concern.)

5. OTHER DRUGS USED IN PSYCHIATRIC DISORDERS

Carbamazepine (Tegretol), an anticonvulsive drug, has been used with increasing frequency in the treatment of bipolar patients who cannot be satisfactorily treated with lithium (nonresponsive or side effects). It has also been used in the treatment of resistant depressions and alcohol withdrawal and in patients with behavioral dyscontrol. It suppresses some phases of kindling and has been used to treat residual symptoms in previous stimulant abusers (eg, impulse control problems). The patients most responsive are those bipolars who tend not to respond to lithium (eg, lack of family history, rapid cycling, severe mania). Dose-related side effects include sedation and ataxia. Dosages start at 400–600 mg orally daily and are increased slowly. Skin rashes and a mild reduction in white count are common. Hyponatremia and water intoxication occur rarely. Congenital anomalies have been reported along with growth deficiency and developmental delay. Nonsteroidal anti-inflammatory drugs (except aspirin); the antibiotics erythromycin, troleandomycin, and isoniazid; the calcium channel blockers verapamil and diltiazem (but not nifedipine); and cimetidine all increase carbamazepine levels. Carbamazepine can be effective in conjunction with lithium, though there have been reports of reversible neurotoxicity with the combination. Carbamazepine stimulates liver enzymes and so tends to decrease levels of haloperidol and oral contraceptives. Cases of fetal malformation have been reported. Hepatic and hematologic status should be monitored in patients taking carbamazepine.

Valproic acid has been used successfully in rapid-cycling bipolar patients refractory to other treatments. It is usually added to the other regimen—lithium, carbamazepine, or neuroleptic drug. It increases liver enzyme activity, causes tremor, increases appetite and weight gain, and may result in fetal malformation.

Calcium channel blockers are increasingly being used in psychiatric conditions. This has come about with the realization that a number of drugs used in psychiatry (eg, lithium, antidepressants, neuroleptics, and carbamazepine) have calcium channel-blocking activity. Mania has been the principal disorder studied to date. There is also preliminary evidence that these drugs may be useful in the treatment of tardive dyskinesia and panic attacks.

Beta-blockers such as atenolol and propranolol have been used to mute the peripheral symptoms of anxiety without significantly affecting motor performance. They block symptoms mediated by sympathetic stimulation (eg, palpitations, tremulousness) but not noradrenergic symptoms (eg, diarrhea, muscle tension). Contrary to current belief, they do not generally cause depression as a side effect.

6. OTHER ORGANIC THERAPIES

Electroconvulsive therapy (ECT) causes a central nervous system seizure (peripheral convulsion is not necessary) by means of electric current. The key objective is to exceed the seizure threshold, which can be accomplished by a variety of means. Electrical stimulation is more reliable and simpler than the use of chemical convulsants such as hexafluorodiethyl ether (flurothyl). The mechanism of action is not known, but it is thought to involve major neurotransmitter responses at the cell membrane. Current insufficient to cause a seizure produces no therapeutic benefit.

Electroconvulsive therapy is the most effective (about 70%) treatment of severe depression, particularly with delusions and agitation commonly seen in the involutional period. It is indicated when medical conditions preclude the use of antidepressants or in cases of nonresponsiveness to these medications. Comparative controlled studies of electroconvulsive therapy in severe depression show that it is more effective than chemotherapy. It is also effective in the manic disorders and psychoses during pregnancy (when drugs may be contraindicated). It has not been shown to be helpful in chronic schizophrenic disorders, and it is generally not used in acute schizophrenic episodes unless drugs are not effective and it is urgent that the psychosis be controlled (eg, a catatonic stupor complicating an acute medical condition).

Before electroconvulsive therapy is administered, a history and physical examination are performed, along with indicated laboratory tests. Lateral spine films and an electroencephalogram (EEG) are frequently done, particularly in elderly patients. Occasionally, the EEG will reveal a clinically silent intracranial lesion that may be a factor in the depression and is a contraindication to electroconvulsive therapy. The patient should not eat or drink for at least 8 hours before treatment. Medications that heighten the seizure threshold (eg, sedatives, clonidine) should be discontinued several days prior to electroconvulsive therapy. Lithium may aggravate the central nervous system side effects, including memory loss. Dentures are removed prior to electroconvulsive therapy. An empty bladder is desirable because of incontinence resulting from the seizure. Atropine sulfate, 0.6–1 mg intramuscularly, is given for its vagolytic effect. A short-acting drug such as methohexital, 40–70 mg, is given carefully intravenously (extravasation is very irritating to tissues) to cause unconsciousness. Succinylcholine, 30–60 mg intravenously, will produce a flaccid paralysis, and the anesthesiologist can then ventilate the patient with 100% oxygen from the onset of unconsciousness until spontaneous respiration resumes. Succinylcholine is contraindicated if the patient is using echothiophate iodide for glaucoma, since the latter is absorbed in amounts sufficient to interfere with the hydrolysis of succinylcholine and can thus precipitate prolonged apnea. Chronic renal dialysis, excessive supported ventilation, and congenital pseudocholinesterase deficiency may also result in prolonged apnea.

Placement of electrodes may be bitemporal or unilateral on the nondominant side. The latter is considered to produce less impairment of memory, although it may be slightly less effective and require more than the usual 9–12 treatments. Patients with a history of manic symptoms respond better to bitemporal electroconvulsive therapy. Electroconvulsive therapy may be performed every few days (3 per week is usual), or all of the treatments may be given in 1–3 sessions under electrocardiographic monitoring of seizure activity (multiple-monitored electroconvulsive therapy).

A seizure usually lasts 5–20 seconds, with a brief postictal state. The patient can resume activity in about 1 hour. The most common side effects are memory disturbance and headache. Memory loss or confusion is usually related to number and frequency of electroconvulsive therapy treatments and proper oxygenation during treatment. Some memory loss is occasionally permanent, but most memory faculties return to full capacity within several weeks. There have been reports that lithium administration concurrent with electroconvulsive therapy resulted in greater memory loss. Before anesthesia was used, spinal compression fractures and severe anticipatory anxiety were common.

Increased intracranial pressure is a positive contraindication. Other problems such as cardiac disorders, aneurysms, bronchopulmonary disease, and venous thrombosis are relative contraindications and must be evaluated in light of the severity of the medical problem versus the need for electroconvulsive therapy. Serious complications arising from electroconvulsive therapy occur in less than one in 1000 cases. Most of these problems are cardiovascular or respiratory in nature (eg, aspiration of gastric contents). Poor patient understanding and lack of acceptance of the technique by the public are the biggest obstacles to the use of electroconvulsive therapy.

Psychosurgery has a limited place in selected cases of severe, unremitting anxiety and depression, obsessional neuroses, and, to a lesser degree, some of the schizophrenias. The stereotactic techniques now being used, including modified bifrontal tractotomy, are great improvements over the crude methods of the past. In the controversial area of **megavitamin treatment** for the schizophrenic patient, the overall

therapeutic efficacy of nicotinic acid or nicotinamide as the sole or adjuvant medication is no better than that of an inactive placebo. **Acupuncture** and **electrosleep** are of unproved usefulness for any psychiatric conditions.

Phototherapy is used in seasonal affective disorder. It consists of exposure (at a 3-foot distance) to a light source of 2500 lux for 2 hours daily in the morning.

Hussain ES, Freeman HL, Jones RA: A cohort study of psychosurgery cases from a defined population. J Neurol Neurosurg Psychiatry 1988;51:345. (Procedures and indications.)

Reiter S et al: Effects of verapamil on tardive dyskinesia and psychosis in schizophrenic patients. J Clin Psychiatry 1989;50:26. (Preliminary results.)

Scott AI: Which depressed patient will respond to electroconvulsive therapy? The search for biological predictors of recovery. Br J Psychiatry 1989;154:8.

7. HOSPITALIZATION

The need for hospital care may range from admission to a medical bed in a general hospital for an acute situational stress reaction to admission to a psychiatric ward when the patient is in acute psychosis. The trend over recent years has been to admit patients to general hospitals in the community, treat patients aggressively, and discharge them promptly to the next appropriate level of treatment—day hospital, halfway house, outpatient therapy, etc. Involuntary hospitalization should be objectively determined on the basis of patient and society welfare. Sixty percent of admissions are readmissions. The total "in residence" population (hospital plus residential) is about the same as the hospital total of 25 years ago. This does not include the homeless mentally ill, a population that would have been institutionalized in past years.

Hospital care may be indicated when patients are too sick to care for themselves or when they present serious threats to themselves or others; when observation and diagnostic procedures are necessary; or when specific kinds of treatment such as electroconvulsive therapy, complex medication trials, or hospital environment (milieu) are required. Symptoms correlating best with hospitalization are self-neglect, violent or bizarre behavior, paranoid ideation or delusions, marked intellectual impairment, and poor judgment.

The disadvantages of psychiatric hospitalization include decreased self-confidence as a result of needing hospitalization; the stigma of being a "psychiatric patient"; possible increased dependency and regression; and the expense. Generally, there is no advantage to prolonged hospital stays for most psychiatric disorders.

Drake RE, Wallach MA: Mental patients' attitudes toward hospitalization: A neglected aspect of hospital tenure.

Am J Psychiatry 1988;145:29. (Often ignored, and should be a major consideration in the decision to hospitalize.)

PSYCHOLOGIC APPROACHES

Psychotherapy attempts to make sense of the chaotic aspects of a person's life and, secondarily, to change the patient's attitudes and behaviors. There are over 100 different types of psychotherapy, and all are reported to give similar results. Harm as well as good can be done by psychotherapy. Bad results can usually be shown to be due to the inexperience, poor judgment, or inflexibility of the therapist.

Dynamic psychotherapy. The basic concepts of dynamic psychotherapy rest in the role of the unconscious with libidinal drives and conflicts that remain out of awareness and in the importance of determinism, which emphasizes that each psychic event is determined by the ones that preceded it. The ideologic framework is not a critical factor. The variables that correlate highly with improvement are support by the therapist and identification with the therapist (both being functions of the patient-therapist relationship), improved self-esteem, and appropriate use of defense mechanisms.

The defense mechanisms of particular importance are **repression** (barring from consciousness), **reaction formation** (substituting a pleasant thought for a painful one), **isolation** (separating original memory from affective response), **denial** (refusing to deal with obvious reality issues), **projection** (attributing a wish or impulse to some other person), **rationalization** (substituting acceptable reason for unacceptable reason), and **undoing** (neutralizing objectionable thoughts).

The focus is rooted in the subjective past, and the mode of change is to make the unconscious conscious, ie, to achieve insight with an understanding of the early past and its connection with conflicts. To achieve reduction of the conflicts, the therapist in a dyadic relationship uses free associations, interpretations, and analysis of both resistance and transference of feelings (a repetition of the past that is inappropriate to the present) onto the therapist. The process is long-term—in classic psychoanalysis, with major psychic reorganization, daily sessions; in later modifications, weekly or twice weekly meetings with the focus on insight and change of behavior.

Experiential psychotherapy. This includes gestalt therapy, client-centered psychotherapy, cognitive therapy, existential analysis, and structural analysis. Experiential therapy evolved from the concepts of fragmentation of the self, existential despair, and the lack of unity with one's own experiences. The focus of therapy is on the present. The mode of change is in the immediate experiencing of one's emotions. The past is not significant in the therapeutic process. The therapist uses intense interactions in a comfortable setting that stimulates self-expression. The sharing is an important element in the encounter to ameliorate the feelings of isolation and alienation and emphasize the possibility of unlimited psychic growth. The goals in this short-term process (weekly meetings for weeks or months) are self-determination; integration of new perceptions, thinking patterns, and self-awareness; rational thinking; creativity; and self-affirmation within a setting of adult, humanistic, peer-oriented relationships.

Cognitive therapy. Corrects faulty impressions (upon which the person acts) and counteracts learned behavior such as helplessness (eg, "Everybody must love me," or "If I make a mistake, I am no good"). The therapist challenges the patient's negative self-image, negative interpretations, and negative views of the future. Daily logs often help the patient see the incongruity between established conceptions and reality and help substitute more reality-oriented and positive cognitions.

Supportive psychotherapy. It usually denotes a positive relationship with the patient, strengthening of existing defenses, enhancing self-esteem (remoralization), and an emphasis on the here and now. The goals are primarily alleviation of symptoms and termination of therapy when this has been accomplished. There is little effort to make substantial changes in the personality structure. Emphasis is on maintaining morale and hope in the future, recognizing responses to stress, and identifying and practicing new ways of coping with stress. Success in all forms of disorders (medical and psychiatric) has been correlated with assumption of responsibility by the patient, a positive approach with a will to live, confidence in the treating professional, and supportive family and friends. Termination should occur within the framework of therapist availability in the event of future needs.

Group therapy. The decision for group versus individual therapy is usually based on the patient's need to improve interpersonal relationships, and the group setting may provide the "laboratory" for improvisation and practice of new behaviors that can then be generalized to everyday activities. Therapy groups are usually composed of individuals who have no outside connection with one another, but groups may be made up of couples or families.

The various schools of therapy often purport to be unique, more effective, or of more lasting value than others. In reality, they have many similarities and common derivations, with about the same results. The attitude of the patient, the cultural variations, and the skill of the therapist rather than the ideology are usually the major factors in producing change.

Beitman BD, Goldfried MR, Norcross JC: The movement toward integrating the psychotherapies: An overview. Am J Psychiatry 1989;146:138.

Ursano RJ, Hales RE: A review of brief individual psychotherapies. Am J Psychiatry 1986;143:1507. (Still relevant.)

SOCIAL APPROACHES

In contrast to psychologic techniques, which deal principally with intrapsychic phenomena and interpersonal problems, the social approaches to psychiatric treatment attempt to modify attitudes and behavior by altering the **environmental** factors contributing to the patient's maladaptation. The scope of the attempt may range from provision of a therapeutic milieu—eg, in a day hospital or residential community—to minor alterations in school procedures or daily family activities. The family, friends, and neighbors provide the major social support in the large majority of cases. Various psychologic and behavioral techniques are used within social approaches.

Part-Time Hospitalization

The patient either participates in the hospital milieu during the day (day hospitals—going home at night), or stays the night (night hospitals—going to work or school during the day), or spends several hours a day in the hospital for up to 5 or 6 days a week. This is a cost-effective alternative to full hospitalization.

Self-Help Communities

These are usually sponsored by nongovernmental agencies for the purpose of helping people with a particular type of difficulty. The individual lives-in full-time for varying periods and usually continues to be affiliated with the group after leaving. Examples of self-help communities include halfway houses, lodge societies (autonomous financial and social entities) across the USA, residences for alcoholics, Salvation Army, and church-sponsored agencies. They are often a bridge between hospitalization and independent living.

Substitute Homes

Substitute homes provide shelter and treatment-related programs for longer periods of time. Examples of "substitute" homes are foster homes, usually for children; board-and-care homes, primarily for people who are disabled and unlikely to return to productive function; residential treatment centers, taking a number of children and offering fairly intensive treatment programs; and shelters for young people—often in the process of withdrawing from drugs.

Nonresidential Self-Help Organizations

The following are examples of organizations usually administered by people who have survived similar problems and have banded together to help others cope with the same problem: Alcoholics Anonymous (and Al-Anon, to help families of alcoholics); Recovery Inc., organized and run by people who have had an emotional problem that required hospitalization; Schizophrenics Anonymous; Gamblers Anonymous;

Overeaters Anonymous; colostomy clubs; mastectomy clubs; the Epilepsy Society; Body Positive, for AIDS victims; the Alzheimer's Disease and Related Disorders Association; the American Heart Association's Stroke Clubs of America; burn recovery groups; other groups organized to help people deal with practical and psychologic problems of a particular illness; and friendship centers that assist people in their efforts to find specific kinds of help. At times, the best support for a patient is contact with another patient who has conquered a similar problem.

A national self-help clearinghouse at the City University of New York, 33 West 42nd St., New York, NY 10036, maintains up-to-date listings of mutual aid organizations in the USA.

Special Professional & Paraprofessional Organizations

Examples of special organizations of this type are Homemaker Service, made up of individuals who come into the home to help the partially disabled maintain the household; Visiting Nurse Associations, which usually provide more than medical assistance; adult protective services for the elderly; genetic counseling services; family service agencies, for marriage counseling and family problems; crisis centers, eg, "free clinics" and county-sponsored satellite clinics; and church-sponsored agencies. Religion (personal beliefs) and churches (organized groups) play major roles in psychosocial adjustment.

Stress Reduction Techniques

Social and environmental factors are major aids in lowering stress and should be part of the activities of daily living. Both active recreation (sports, physical exercise, participant hobbies) and passive pursuits (reading, music, painting) are necessary for a balanced life and alleviation of stress. Family structure and dynamics must be evaluated, and there will be occasions (eg, adult children living at home, presence of in-laws) when a social restructuring is in order.

Galanter M: Zealous self-help groups as adjuncts to psychiatric treatment: A study of Recovery Inc. Am J Psychiatry 1988;145:1248. (A typical self-help group.)

BEHAVIORAL APPROACHES

Behavior therapy has its foundations in theories of the learning process. The role of the behavior therapist is that of a teacher who attempts to bring about change in the patient's maladaptation. The specific problem (target behavior) and the factors that play a role in precipitating or perpetuating the problem must first be identified. An attempt can then be made to alter those factors that perpetuate unwanted behavior.

The emphasis of behavior therapy is on "here and

now'' and *direct* change. The goal is to "unlearn" those destructive or unproductive types of behavior that result from faulty learning and to enhance the individual's repertoire of useful social and adaptive skills. Great emphasis is placed on identifying and then ablating whatever is maintaining the maladaptive behavior.

Whereas **conditioning** is understood by some to be synonymous with a specific type of learning (eg, Pavlov's dogs), behavior therapy is much broader. It includes the relationship with the therapist, utilizes verbal techniques, although to a lesser degree than other therapies, and interprets "behavior" in a broad sense that includes thoughts and feelings.

Many of the techniques of behavior therapy require a cooperative effort on the part of a number of people who must all understand and be consistent in their responses to specified behaviors. Thus, a cooperative social setting such as a milieu ward or the patient's own home and family is important in implementing many of the following techniques.

Techniques of Behavior Therapy

A. Modeling: Much learning occurs by imitation. From the earliest years of childhood, the individual's behavior is modeled after parents, teachers, peers, employers, public personalities, historical figures, etc ("significant others"). The therapist makes a conscious effort to serve as a model of particular kinds of behavior that are significant to and attainable by the patient. This device is particularly useful in treating patients with low self-esteem.

B. Operant Conditioning: Operant conditioning is the deliberate implementation of a system of rewards to encourage repetition of specific desired behaviors. A voluntary behavior is singled out for a specific reward every time the behavior is used. The objective is to develop a habit in the use of that behavior. Like modeling, operant conditioning is a common procedure in families, and the child soon learns that "good" behavior is rewarded.

C. Aversive Conditioning: Aversive conditioning is the opposite of operant conditioning but is a less potent shaper of behavior. Undesirable behavior (eg, alcohol ingestion) is paired with an unpleasant consequence (eg, vomiting induced by apomorphine, mild electric or sound shock), whereas satisfactory alternative responses are operantly encouraged. The most common conditions treated by this technique have been enuresis, smoking, alcoholism, and sexual arousal disorders.

D. Extinction: Extinction is the process of refusing to reinforce behavior on the theory that behavior cannot be sustained without some sort of reinforcement. Temper tantrums and noxious behavior, usually contrived to gain attention of any sort, are "extinguished" in this way.

E. Desensitization: Familiarity lessens anxiety and reduces the tendency to avoid exposure to the feared object, person, or situation. The subject is repeatedly exposed to the feared stimulus (eg, looking at a picture of an elevator when the fear has been riding in elevators) at such a low level of intensity that the fear response is minimal. Exposures are then gradually increased (eg, walking past a real elevator) until the subject is able to tolerate the real experience with markedly reduced fear. This technique has been most effective in the treatment of phobias and a variety of situations (such as frigidity or impotence) that engender fears of failure, disapproval, and embarrassment.

F. Emotive Imagery: Deliberate evocation of mental images that arouse certain feelings can be used as a way of warding off painful emotions resulting from stress-inducing circumstances. Noxious imagery can be used in aversive conditioning and "pleasant thoughts" in operant training. A graded exposure to the thoughts results in gradually lower anxiety levels.

G. Flooding: Flooding (implosion) consists of overwhelming the individual, in a safe setting, with anxiety-producing stimuli. The anxiety responses gradually lessen (law of diminishing returns) until extinction occurs. In some ways, flooding is a desensitization technique without the graded approach. It has been used in treatment of patients with such behavior problems as compulsive hoarding.

H. Role Playing: In the role-playing technique, patients can practice various types of behaviors in anxiety-producing but "safe" situations. For example, the therapist may assume the role of an angry friend and the patient uses different ways of handling the situation. Role reversal—where the therapist and the patient change roles—then gives the patient a chance to experience the other's feelings and attitudes. Assertiveness training for inhibited individuals is a variant to help people learn to be more spontaneous.

I. Relaxation Techniques: These include muscle relaxation, self-hypnosis, and biofeedback procedures. The names are descriptive. Biofeedback requires some equipment to measure and signal physiologic change. It is particularly helpful in such somatic disorders as migraine headache and hyperactive bowel syndrome (see Somatoform Disorders). Relaxation, meditation, and hypnosis share some common features and are valuable ancillary modalities in effecting change and modifying symptoms.

COMMON PSYCHIATRIC DISORDERS

STRESS & ADJUSTMENT DISORDERS (Situational Disorders)

Stress exists when the adaptive capacity of the individual is overwhelmed by events. The event may be an insignificant one objectively considered, and even favorable changes (eg, promotion and transfer) requiring adaptive behavior can produce stress. For each individual, stress is subjectively defined, and the response to stress is a function of each person's personality and physiologic endowment.

Classification & Clinical Findings

Opinion differs about what events are most apt to produce stress reactions. The Holmes/Rahe studies of psychosocial factors provide some insights into the stress-inducing potential of marriage, family relationships, work and social relationships, financial problems, illness and injury, etc. The causes of stress are different at different ages—eg, in young adulthood, the sources of stress are found in the marriage or parent-child relationship, the employment relationship, and the struggle to achieve financial stability; in the middle years, the focus shifts to changing spousal relationships, problems with aging parents, and problems associated with having young adult offspring who themselves are encountering stressful situations; in old age, the principal concerns are apt to be retirement, loss of physical capacity, major personal losses, and thoughts of death.

An individual may react to stress by becoming anxious or depressed, by developing a physical symptom, by running away, by having a drink or starting an affair, or in limitless other ways. Common subjective responses are fear (of repetition of the stress-inducing event), rage (at frustration), guilt (over aggressive impulses), and shame (over helplessness). Acute stress may be manifested by restlessness, irritability, fatigue, increased startle reaction, and a feeling of tension. Inability to concentrate, sleep disturbances (insomnia, bad dreams), and somatic preoccupations often lead to self-medication, most commonly with alcohol or other central nervous system depressants. Maladaptive behavior to stress is called adjustment disorder, with the major symptom specified (eg, "adjustment disorder with depressed mood").

Posttraumatic stress disorder (PTSD) is a syndrome with symptoms of **reexperiencing** the traumatic event (eg, rape, military combat), along with decreased responsiveness to and **avoidance** of current events, and **physiologic arousal,** which includes startle reactions, intrusive thoughts, illusions, overgener-alized associations, sleep problems, nightmares, difficulties in concentration, and hyperalertness. The symptoms may be precipitated or exacerbated by distant events that are a reminder of the original stress. Symptoms frequently arise after a long latency period (eg, child abuse can result in later posttraumatic stress syndrome). The sooner the symptoms arise after the initial trauma and the sooner therapy is initiated, the better the prognosis. The therapeutic approach is to facilitate the normal recovery that was blocked at the time of the traum. Therapy at that time should be brief, simple (catharsis and working through of the traumatic experience), and expectant (of quick recovery and a rapid return to work).

Differential Diagnosis

Adjustment disorders must be distinguished from anxiety disorders, affective disorders, and personality disorders exacerbated by stress and from structural somatic disorders with psychic overlay.

Treatment

A. Behavioral: Stress reduction techniques include immediate symptom reduction (eg, rebreathing in a bag for hyperventilation) or early recognition and removal from a stress source before full-blown symptoms appear. It is often helpful for the patient to keep a daily log of stress precipitators, responses, and alleviators. Relaxation and exercise techniques are also helpful in reducing the reaction to stressful events. Specific behavioral techniques such as desensitization are indirectly helpful in anxiety reduction of stress reactions.

B. Social: The stress reactions of life crisis problems are—more than any other category—a function of psychosocial upheaval, and patients frequently present with somatic symptoms. While it is not easy for the patient to make necessary changes (or they would have been made long ago), it is important for the therapist to establish the framework of the problem, since the patient's denial system may obscure the issues. Clarifying the problem allows the patient to begin viewing it within the proper context and facilitates the sometimes difficult decisions the patient eventually must make (eg, change of job or relocation of adult dependent offspring).

C. Psychologic: Prolonged in-depth psychotherapy is seldom necessary in cases of isolated stress response or adjustment disorder. Supportive psychotherapy (see above) with an emphasis on the here and now and strengthening of existing defenses, is a helpful approach while time and the patient's own resiliency allow a restoration to the previous level of function. Posttraumatic stress syndromes respond to catharsis and dynamic psychotherapy oriented toward acceptance of the event. Marital problems are a major area of concern, and it is important that the physician have available a dependable referral source when marriage counseling is indicated. In posttraumatic stress disorder, group psychotherapy and individual counseling are both helpful.

D. Medical: Judicious use of sedatives (eg, lorazepam, 1–2 mg orally daily) for a limited time and as part of an overall treatment plan can provide relief from acute anxiety symptoms. Problems arise when the situation becomes chronic through inappropriate treatment or when the treatment approach supports the development of chronicity (see Sedative-Hypnotic Drugs, above).

While treatment of posttraumatic stress disorder is difficult, antidepressant drugs in full dosage help in decreasing panic, startle response, and depression. Beta-blockers are used to lessen the peripheral symptoms of anxiety (eg, tremor, palpitations).

Prognosis

Return to satisfactory function after a short period is part of the clinical picture of this syndrome. Resolution may be delayed if others' responses to the patient's difficulties are thoughtlessly harmful or if the secondary gains outweigh the advantages of recovery.

Goldberg J et al: A twin study of the effects of the Vietnam war on posttraumatic stress disorder. JAMA 1990; 263:1227.

Helzer JE, Robins LN, McEvoy L: Post-traumatic stress disorder in the general population. N Engl J Med 1987;317:1630. (The incidence and prevalence are greater than supposed, and the patient presents in the primary physician's office.)

ANXIETY DISORDERS & DISSOCIATIVE DISORDERS (Neuroses)

Essentials of Diagnosis

- Overt anxiety or an overt manifestation of a defense mechanism (such as a phobia) or both.
- Not limited to an adjustment disorder.
- Somatic symptoms referable to the autonomic nervous system or to a specific organ system (eg, dyspnea, palpitations, paresthesias).
- Not a result of physical disorders, psychiatric conditions (eg, schizophrenia), or drugs (eg, caffeine).

General Considerations

Stress, fear, and anxiety all tend to be interactive. The principal components of anxiety are **psychologic** (tension, fears, difficulty in concentration, apprehension) and **somatic** (tachycardia, hyperventilation, palpitations, tremor, sweating). Other organ systems (eg, gastrointestinal) may be involved in multiple-system complaints. Fatigue and sleep disturbances are common. Sympathomimetic symptoms of anxiety are both a response to a central nervous system state and a reinforcement of further anxiety. Anxiety can become self-generating, since the symptoms reinforce the reaction, causing it to spiral.

The resultant anxiety is handled in different ways. Anxiety may be free-floating, resulting in acute anxiety attacks, occasionally becoming chronic. When one or several defense mechanisms (see above) are functioning, the consequences are well-known problems such as phobias, conversion reactions, dissociative states, obsessions, and compulsions. *Lack of structure is frequently a contributing factor,* as noted in those people who have "Sunday neuroses." They do well during the week with a planned work schedule but cannot tolerate the unstructured weekend. Planned-time activities tend to bind anxiety, and many people have increased difficulties when this is lost, as in retirement.

Some believe that various manifestations of anxiety are not a result of unconscious conflicts but are "habits"—persistent patterns of nonadaptive behavior acquired by learning. The "habits," being nonadaptive, are unsatisfactory ways of dealing with life problems—hence the resultant anxiety. Help is sought only when the anxiety becomes too painful. *Exogenous factors such as stimulants (eg, caffeine, cocaine) must be considered as causative or contributing factors.*

Clinical Findings

A. Generalized Anxiety Disorder: This is the most common of the clinically significant anxiety disorders. Initial manifestations appear at age 20–35 years, and there is a slight predominance in women. The disabling anxiety symptoms of apprehension, worry, irritability, hypervigilance (preparation for threat), and somatic complaints are long-lasting and persist for at least 1 month. Symptoms include cardiac (eg, tachycardia, increased blood pressure), gastrointestinal (eg, increased acidity, epigastric pain), and neurologic (eg, headache, syncope) systems. Some of the origins or exacerbating causes of the anxiety may be identified in life situations.

B. Panic Disorder: This is characterized by short-lived, recurrent, unpredictable episodes of intense anxiety (with or without agoraphobia) accompanied by marked physiologic manifestations. Distressing symptoms such as dyspnea, tachycardia, palpitations, headaches, dizziness, paresthesias, choking, smothering feelings, nausea, and bloating are associated with feelings of impending doom (alarm response). Recurrent sleep panic attacks (not nightmares) occur in about 30% of panic disorders. Anticipatory anxiety develops in all these patients and further constricts their daily lives. Panic disorder tends to be familial, with onset under age 25; it affects 3–5% of the population, is related to temporal lobe dysfunction, and there is a 2:1 prevalence in women. The premenstrual period is one of heightened vulnerability. Stimulants can induce the symptoms. Patients frequently undergo emergency medical evaluations (eg, for "heart attacks" or "hypoglycemia") before the correct diagnosis is made. Gastrointestinal symptoms are especially common, occurring in about one-third of cases. Myocardial infarction, pheochromocytoma, thyroid disease, and various recreational drug reactions can mimic panic disorder. Lactate infusion with reemergence of the symptoms is corroborative evidence of panic disorder. Mitral valve prolapse may be present but is not necessarily a significant factor. "Air hunger" and tetany due to **hyperventilation syndrome** are promptly relieved when rebreathing is induced by placing an airtight bag over the patient's nose and mouth. Patients with recurrent panic disorder often become **demoralized, hypochondriacal, agoraphobic,** and **depressed.** About one-fourth have obsessive compulsive features. Alcohol abuse (about 20%) results from self-treatment and is not infrequently combined with dependence on sedatives. Suicide attempts are a significant complication.

C. Phobic Disorder: Phobic ideation can be considered a mechanism of "displacement" in which the patients transfers feelings of anxiety from their true object to one that can be avoided. However, since phobias are ineffective defense mechanisms, there tends to be an increase in their scope, intensity, and number. Social phobias are global or specific; in the former, all social situations are poorly tolerated, while the latter group includes performance anxiety or well-delineated phobias. Agoraphobia (fear of open places and public areas) is frequently associated with severe panic attacks. Patients often develop the syndrome in early adult life, making a normal life-style difficult.

D. Obsessive Compulsive Disorder: In the obsessive compulsive reaction, the irrational idea or the impulse persistently intrudes into awareness. Obsessions (constantly recurring thoughts such as fears of hitting somebody) and compulsions (repetitive actions such as washing hands many times prior to peeling a potato) are recognized by the individual as absurd and are resisted, but anxiety is alleviated only by ritualistic performance or mechanical impulse or entertainment of the idea. The primary underlying concern of the patient is to not lose control. These patients are usually predictable, orderly, conscientious, and intelligent, traits that are seen in many compulsive behaviors such as anorexia and compulsive running. There is an overlapping of obsessive compulsive disorder and tics, including trichotillomania (hair-pulling), and major depression occurs in two-thirds of these patients during their lifetimes. The 2–3% incidence in the USA is a much higher incidence than was previously recognized. Male:female ratios are similar, with the highest rates occurring in the young, divorced, separated, and unemployed. There are many case reports linking obsessive compulsive disorder to previous neurologic insults (eg, encephalitis). In these patients, neurologic abnormalities of fine motor coordination and involuntary movements are common. Under extreme stress, these patients sometimes exhibit paranoid and delusional behaviors,

often associated with depression, and can mimic schizophrenia.

E. Dissociative Disorder: Fugue, amnesia, somnambulism, and multiple personality are the usual dissociative states. The reaction is precipitated by emotional crisis, and although the primary gain is anxiety reduction, the secondary gain is a temporary solution of the crisis. Mechanisms include repression and isolation as well as particularly limited concentration such as seen in hypnotic states. This condition is similar in many ways to symptoms seen in patients with temporal lobe dysfunction.

Treatment

A. Medical: In all cases, underlying medical disorders must be ruled out (eg, cardiovascular, endocrine, respiratory, and neurologic disorders and substance-related syndromes, both intoxication and withdrawal states). These and other disorders can coexist with panic disorder. Benzodiazepines and buspirone are the anxiolytics of choice in most cases of generalized anxiety. Other classes of drugs, such as antipsychotics, and the older sedatives, such as the barbiturates, have no advantages over the benzodiazepines and numerous disadvantages (diverse side effects and more dependency problems, respectively). Beta-blockers such as propranolol may help reduce peripheral somatic symptoms. Ethanol is the most frequently self-administered drug, but it has no role in the treatment of anxiety.

Panic attacks may be treated in several ways. TCAs and MAO inhibitors (imipramine, 100–300 mg/d orally) (adequate blood levels will require dosages similar to those used in the treatment of depression, or phenelzine, 30–60 mg/d orally) are effective against the panic attacks. Fluoxetine also is effective, particularly if obsessive compulsive disorder is present with the panic disorder. Because of overresponsiveness to the tricyclics, starting doses should be low and very gradually increased. Clonazepam (1–8 mg/d orally) is effective as an alternative to antidepressants. Alprazolam (0.5–8 mg/d orally) is also effective but causes significant dependency problems. Because of chronicity of the disorders and the problem of dependency with benzodiazepine drugs, it is generally desirable to use antidepressant drugs as the principal pharmacologic approach. Nonresponse may indicate the presence of limbic overstimulation and warrant a trial of carbamazepine. Antidepressants have been used in conjunction with propranolol (40–160 mg/d orally) in resistant cases. Phobic disorder may be part of the panic disorder and is treated within that framework. Global social phobias may be treated with MAO inhibitors in the same dosage as used for depression, while specific phobias such as performance anxiety may respond to moderate doses of β-blockers.

Obsessive compulsive disorders respond to serotonergic drugs in about 60% of cases. Clomipramine has proved effectiveness in doses equivalent to those used for depression and has produced remission in cases of trichotillomania. Fluoxetine has been widely used in this disorder but in doses higher than those used in depression (up to 60–80 mg/d).

B. Behavioral: Behavioral approaches are widely used in various anxiety disorders. Any of the behavioral techniques (see above) can be used beneficially in altering the contingencies (precipitating factors or rewards) supporting any anxiety-provoking behavior. Relaxation techniques can sometimes be helpful in reducing anxiety. Desensitization, by exposing the patient to graded doses of a phobic object or situation, is an effective technique and one that the patient can practice outside the therapy session. Emotive imagery, wherein the patient imagines the anxiety-provoking situation while at the same time learning to relax, helps to decrease the anxiety when the patient faces the real life situation. Physiologic symptoms in panic attacks respond well to relaxation training.

C. Psychologic: Cognitive approaches have been effective in treatment of panic disorders when erroneous beliefs need correction. Other individual approaches such as reality therapy and transactional analysis are helpful when problems with interpersonal relationships are a major factor. Group therapy is the treatment of choice when the anxiety is clearly a function of the patient's difficulties in dealing with others, and if these other people are part of the family it is appropriate to include them and initiate family or couples therapy. The analysis of early life origins of the condition is not fruitful.

D. Social: Social modification may require measures such as family counseling to aid acceptance of the patient's symptoms. Any help in maintaining the social structure is anxiety-alleviating, and work, school, and social activities should be maintained. School and vocational counseling may be provided by professionals, who often need help from the physician in defining the patient's limitations.

Prognosis

Anxiety disorders are usually of long standing and may be quite difficult to treat. All can be relieved to varying degrees with medications and behavioral techniques. The prognosis is much better if one can break the commonly observed anxiety-panic-phobia-depression cycle with a combination of the therapeutic interventions discussed above.

Dobrovsky SL et al: Anxiety and mood disorders: New developments and their clinical applications. J Clin Psychiatry 1990;51(Suppl):1. (Overview of current treatments.)

Hollander E et al: Signs of central nervous system dysfunction in obsessive-compulsive disorder. Arch Gen Psychiatry 1990;47:27. (Importance in genesis of this disorder.)

Stein MB, Shea CA, Uhde TW: Social phobic symptoms in patients with panic disorders: Practical and theoretical implications. Am J Psychiatry 1989;146:235. (Common in office practice.)

Weissman MM et al: Suicidal ideation and suicide attempts in panic disorder and attacks. N Engl J Med 1989; 321:1209. (A significant suicide problem.)

SOMATOFORM DISORDERS (Psychophysiologic Disorders, Psychosomatic Disorders)

Essentials of Diagnosis

- Physical symptoms may involve one or more organ systems and are not intentional.
- Subjective complaints exceed objective findings.
- Correlations of symptom development and psychosocial stresses.
- Matrix of biogenetic and developmental patterns.

General Considerations

A major source of diagnostic confusion in medicine has been to assume cause-and-effect relationships when parallel events have been observed. This post hoc ergo propter hoc reasoning has been particularly vexing in many situations where the individual exhibits psychosocial distress that could well be secondary to a chronic illness but has been assumed to be primary and causative. An example is the person with a chronic bowel disease who becomes querulous and demanding. Is this a result of problems of coping with a chronic disease, or is it a personality pattern that causes the gastrointestinal problem?

People react differently to illness. Emotional stress often exacerbates or precipitates an acute illness—or an acute illness, such as an opioid peptide-secreting tumor, may produce psychiatric symptoms as a result of the endogenous opiates. Vulnerability in one or more organ systems and exposure to family members with somatization problems play a major role in the development of particular symptoms, and the "functional" versus "organic" dichotomy is a hindrance to good treatment.

In any patient presenting with a condition judged to be somatoform, depression must be considered in the diagnosis.

Clinical Findings

A. Conversion Disorder: "Conversion" (formerly "hysterical conversion") of psychic conflict into physical symptoms in parts of the body innervated by the sensorimotor system (eg, paralysis, aphonia) is a disorder that is more common in unsophisticated individuals and certain cultures. The defense mechanisms utilized in this condition are repression (a barring from consciousness) and isolation (a splitting of the affect from the idea). The somatic manifestation that takes the place of anxiety is typically paralysis, and in some instances the organ dysfunction may have symbolic meaning (eg, arm paralysis in marked anger). Hysterical seizures ("pseudoseizures") are usually difficult to differentiate from intoxication states or panic attacks. Retention of consciousness, random flailing with asynchronous movements of the right and left sides, and resistance to having the nose and mouth pinched closed *during the attack* all point toward a hysterical event. Electroencephalography during the attack is the most helpful diagnostic aid in excluding seizure states. Serum prolactin levels rise abruptly in the postictal state but not in pseudoseizures. There is usually a history of other conversion situations. La belle indiffearence is not a significant characteristic (as commonly believed). Important criteria in diagnosis include a history of conversion or somatization disorder, modeling, a serious precipitating emotional event, associated psychopathology (eg, schizophrenia, personality disorders), a temporal correlation between the precipitating event and the symptom, and a temporary "solving of the problem" by the conversion. *It is important to differentiate physical disorders with unusual presentations (eg, multiple sclerosis).*

B. Somatization Disorder (Briquet's Syndrome, Hysteria): This is characterized by multiple physical complaints referable to several organ systems. Anxiety, panic disorder, and depression are often present, and **major depression** is an important consideration in the differential diagnosis. There is a significant relationship (20%) to a lifetime history of panic-agoraphobia-depression. It usually occurs before age 30 and is more common in women. Polysurgery is often a feature of the history. Preoccupation with medical and surgical therapy becomes a lifestyle that excludes most other activities. The symptoms are a reflection of adaptive patterns, coping techniques, and reactivity of the particular organ system. There is often evidence of long-standing somatic symptoms (particularly dysmenorrhea, a lump in the throat, vomiting, shortness of breath, burning in the sex organs, painful extremities, and amnesia), often with a history of similar organ system involvement in other family members. Multiple symptoms that constantly change and inability of more than 3 doctors to make a diagnosis are strong clues to the problem.

C. Psychogenic Pain Disorder: This involves a long history of complaints of severe pain not consonant with anatomic and clinical signs. This diagnosis must not be one of exclusion and should be made only after extended evaluation has established a clear correlation of psychogenic factors with exacerbations and remissions of complaints.

D. Hypochondriasis: This is a fear of disease and preoccupation with the body, with perceptual amplification and heightened responsiveness. A process of social learning is usually involved, frequently with a role model who was a member of the family and may be a part of the underlying psychodynamic etiology. It is common in panic disorders.

E. Factitious Disorders: These disorders, in which symptom production is intentional, are not somatoform conditions. They are characterized by self-

induced symptoms or false physical and laboratory findings for the purpose of deceiving physicians or other hospital personnel. The deceptions may involve self-mutilation, fever, hemorrhage, hypoglycemia, seizures, and an almost endless variety of manifestations—often presented in an exaggerated and dramatic fashion (Munchausen's syndrome). "Proxy Munchausen" is the term used when a parent creates an illness in a child so that treatment can be given to satisfy a somatization disorder in the parent. The duplicity may be either simple or extremely complex and difficult to recognize. The patients are frequently connected in some way with the health professions, they are often migratory, and their motivation in complex cases is usually unclear.

Complications

A poor doctor-patient relationship, with iatrogenic disorders and "doctor shopping," are the principal problems. Sedative and analgesic dependency is the most common iatrogenic complication.

Treatment

A. Medical: Medical support with careful attention to building a therapeutic doctor-patient relationship is the mainstay of treatment. *It must be accepted that the patient's distress is real. Every problem not found to have an organic basis is not necessarily a mental disease.* Diligent attempts should be made to relate symptoms to adverse developments in the patient's life. It may be useful to have the patient keep a meticulous diary, paying particular attention to various pertinent factors evident in the history. Regular, frequent, short appointments may be helpful. Drugs (not infrequently abused) should not be prescribed to replace appointments. One doctor should be the primary physician, and consultants should be used mainly for evaluation. An emphatic, realistic, optimistic approach must be maintained in the face of the expected ups and downs. Ongoing reevaluation is necessary, since somatization can coexist with a concurrent physical illness.

B. Psychologic: Psychologic approaches can be used by the primary physician when it is clear that the patient is ready to make some changes in lifestyle in order to achieve symptomatic relief. This is often best approached on a here-and-now basis and oriented toward pragmatic changes rather than an exploration of early experiences that the patient frequently fails to relate to current distress. Group therapy with other individuals who have similar problems is sometimes of value to improve coping, allow ventilation, and focus on interpersonal adjustment. Hypnosis and amobarbital interviews used early are helpful in resolving conversion disorders. If the primary physician has been working with the patient on psychologic problems related to the physical illness, the groundwork is often laid for successful psychiatric referral.

C. Behavioral: Behavioral therapy is probably best exemplified by the current efforts in biofeedback techniques. In biofeedback, the particular abnormality (eg, increased peristalsis) must be recognized and monitored by the patient and therapist (eg, by an electronic stethoscope to amplify the sounds). This is immediate feedback, and after learning to recognize it the patient can then learn to identify any change thus produced (eg, a decrease in bowel sounds) and so become a conscious originator of the feedback instead of a passive recipient. Relief of the symptom operantly conditions the patient to utilize the maneuver that relieves symptoms (eg, relaxation causing a decrease in bowel sounds). With emphasis on this type of learning, the patient is able to identify symptoms early and initiate the countermaneuvers, thus decreasing the symptomatic problem. Migraine and tension headaches have been particularly responsive to biofeedback methods.

D. Social: Social endeavors include family, work, and other interpersonal activity. Family members should come for some appointments with the patient so that they can learn how best to live with the patient. This is particularly important in treatment of the somatization and psychogenic pain disorders. Ileostomy clubs and similar mutual aid groups provide a climate for encouraging the patient to accept and live with the problem. Ongoing communication with the employer may be necessary to encourage long-term continued interest in the employee. Employers can become just as discouraged as physicians in dealing with employees who have chronic problems.

Prognosis

The prognosis is much better if the primary physician is able to intervene early before the situation has deteriorated. After the problem has crystallized into chronicity, it is very difficult to effect change.

Lipowski ZJ: Somatization: The concept and its clinical application. Am J Psychiatry 1988;145:1358.

CHRONIC PAIN DISORDERS

Essentials of Diagnosis

- Chronic complaints of pain.
- Symptoms frequently exceed signs.
- Minimal relief with standard treatment.
- History of many physicians.
- Frequent use of many nonspecific medications.

General Considerations

A problem in the management of pain is the lack of distinction between acute and chronic pain syndromes. Most physicians are adept at dealing with acute pain problems but have difficulty handling the patient with chronic pain. This type of patient frequently takes too many medications, stays in bed a

great deal, has had many physicians, has lost skills, and experiences little joy in either work or play. All relationships suffer (including those with physicians), and life becomes a constant search for succor. The search results in complex physician-patient relationships that usually include many drug trials, particularly sedatives. Treatment failures provoke angry responses and depression from both the physician and the patient, and the pain syndrome is exacerbated. When frustration becomes too great, a new physician is found, and the cycle is repeated. The longer the existence of the pain, the more important the psychologic factors of anxiety and depression, which are often a consequence rather than a cause of chronic pain. As with all other conditions, it is counterproductive to speculate about whether the pain is "real." It is real to the patient, and acceptance of the problem underlines a mutual endeavor to alleviate the disturbance.

Clinical Findings

Components of the chronic pain syndrome consist of anatomic changes, chronic anxiety and depression, anger, and changed life-style. Usually, the anatomic problem is irreversible, since it has already been subjected to many interventions with increasingly unsatisfactory results.

Chronic anxiety and depression produce heightened irritability and overreaction to stimuli. A marked decrease in pain threshold is apparent. This pattern develops into a hypochondriacal preoccupation with the body and a constant need for reassurance. The pressure on the doctor becomes wearing and often leads to covert rejection devices, such as not being available or making referrals to other physicians. This is perceived by the patient, who then intensifies the effort to get help, and the typical cycle is under way. Anxiety and depression are seldom discussed, almost as if there is a tacit agreement not to deal with these issues.

Changes in life-style involve some of the so-called pain games. These usually take the form of a family script in which the patient accepts the role of being sick, and this role then becomes the focus of most family interactions and may become important in maintaining the family, so that neither the patient nor the family wants the patient's role to change. Demands for attention and efforts to control the behavior of others revolve around the central issue of control of other people (including physicians). Cultural factors frequently play a role in the behavior of the patient and how the significant people around the patient cope with the problem. Some cultures encourage demonstrative behavior, while others value the stoic role. The physician's recognition of this fact is important, since overt dramatization of the discomfort is sometimes helpful in alleviating the problem.

Another secondary gain that frequently maintains the patient in the sick role is financial compensation or other benefits ("green poultice"). Frequently, such systems are structured so that they reinforce the maintenance of sickness and discourage any attempts to give up the role. Physicians unwittingly reinforce this role because of the very nature of the practice of medicine, which is to respond to complaints of illness. Helpful suggestions are often met with responses like "Yes, but. . . ." Medications then become the principal approach, and drug dependency problems may develop.

Treatment

A. Behavioral: The cornerstone of a unified approach to chronic pain syndromes is a comprehensive behavioral program. This is necessary to identify and eliminate pain reinforcers, to decrease drug use, and to use effectively those positive reinforcers that shift the focus from the pain. *It is critical that the patient be made a partner in the effort to alleviate pain.* (Avoid the concept of cure.) The patient should agree to discuss the pain only with the physician and not with family members; this tends to stabilize the patient's personal life, since the family is usually tired of the subject. At the beginning of treatment, the patient should be assigned self-help tasks graded up to maximal activity, as a means of positive reinforcement. The tasks should not exceed capability. The patient can also be asked to keep a self-rating chart to log accomplishments, so that progress can be measured and remembered. Instruct the patient to record degrees of pain on a self-rating scale in relation to various situations and mental attitudes so that similar circumstances can be avoided or modified.

Avoid negative reinforcers such as sympathy and attention to pain. Emphasize a positive response to productive activities, which remove the focus of attention from the pain. Activity is also desensitizing, since the patient learns to tolerate increasing activity levels.

Biofeedback techniques (see Somatoform Disorders, above) and hypnosis have been successful in ameliorating some pain syndromes. Hypnosis tends to be most effective in those patients with a high level of denial, who are more responsive to suggestion. Hypnosis can be used to lessen anxiety, alter perception of the length of time that pain is experienced, and encourage relaxation.

B. Medical: A *single physician* in charge of the multiple treatment approach is the highest priority. Consultations as indicated and technical procedures done by others are appropriate, but the care of the patient should remain in the hands of the primary physician. Referrals should not be allowed to raise the patient's hopes unrealistically or to become a way for the physician to reject the case. The attitude of the doctor should be one of honesty, interest, and hopefulness—not for a cure but for control of pain and improved function. If the patient is heavily addicted to narcotics, detoxification should be the first treatment goal.

If analgesics or sedatives are prescribed, they should not be given on an "as-needed" schedule. A fixed schedule lessens the conditioning effects of these drugs. TCAs (eg, amitriptyline) in doses smaller than those used in depression may be helpful.

In addition to medications, a variety of alternative strategies may be offered, including physical therapy (including daily application of heat or cold) and acupuncture.

C. Social: *Involvement of family members and other significant persons in the patient's life should be an early priority.* The best efforts of both patient and therapists can be unwittingly sabotaged by other persons who may feel that they are "helping" the patient. They frequently tend to reinforce the negative aspects of the pain syndrome. The patient becomes more dependent and less active, and the pain syndrome becomes an immutable way of life. The more destructive "pain games" described by many experts in chronic pain syndromes are results of well-meaning but misguided efforts of family members. Ongoing therapy with the family can be helpful in the early identification and elimination of these behavior patterns.

Alteration of behavior in others (including employers and friends) requires repetition of instructions and fairly frequent contact. The tendency is to slip back into behavior patterns that impede progress. Group instruction by a nurse or physician's assistant is valuable and is enhanced by interchanges of people in the group. Repetition and group interaction tend to fix the instructions.

D. Psychologic: In addition to group therapy with family members and others, groups of patients can be helpful if properly led. The major goal, whether of individual or group therapy, is to gain patient *involvement.* A group can be a powerful instrument for achieving this goal, with the development of group loyalties and cooperation. People will frequently make efforts with group encouragement that they would never make alone. Individual therapy should be directed toward strengthening existing defenses and improving self-esteem. The rapport between patient and physician, as in all psychotherapeutic efforts, is the major factor in therapeutic success.

Dworkin SF, VonKorff M, LeResche L: Multiple pains and psychiatric disturbance. Arch Gen Psychiatry 1990;47:239. (Significant linkage.)

PSYCHOSEXUAL DISORDERS

The stages of sexual activity include **excitement** (arousal), **plateau, orgasm,** and **resolution.** The precipitating excitement or arousal is psychologically determined. Arousal response leading to plateau is a physiologic and psychologic phenomenon of vasocongestion, a parasympathetic reaction causing erection in the male and labial/clitoral congestion in the female. The orgasmic response includes emission in the male and clonic contractions of the analogous striated perineal muscles of both male and female. Resolution is a gradual return to normal physiologic status.

While the arousal stimuli—vasocongestive and orgasmic responses—constitute a single response in a well-adjusted person, they can be considered as separate stages that can produce different syndromes responding to different treatment procedures.

Clinical Findings

There are 3 major groups of sexual disorders.

A. Paraphilias (Sexual Arousal Disorders): In these conditions, formerly called "deviations" or "variations," the excitement stage of sexual activity is associated with sexual objects or orientations different from those usually associated with adult heterosexual stimulation. The stimulus may be a woman's shoe, a child, animals, instruments of torture, or incidents of aggression. The pattern of sexual stimulation is usually one that has early psychologic roots. Poor experiences with heterosexual activity frequently reinforce this pattern over time.

Exhibitionism is the impulsive behavior of exposing the genitalia in order to achieve sexual excitation. It is a childhood sexual behavior carried into adult life.

Transvestism is the wearing of clothes and the enactment of a role of the opposite sex for the purpose of sexual excitation. Such fetishistic cross-dressing can be part of masturbation foreplay. Transvestism in homosexuality and transsexualism is not done to cause sexual excitement but is a function of the homosexual preference or gender disorder.

Voyeurism involves the achievement of sexual arousal by secretly watching the activities of the opposite sex, usually in various stages of undress or sexual activity. In both exhibitionism and voyeurism, excitation leads to masturbation as a *replacement* for heterosexual activity.

Pedophilia is the use of a child of either sex to achieve sexual arousal and, in many cases, gratification. Contact is frequently oral, with either participant being dominant, but pedophilia includes intercourse of any type. Adults of both sexes engage in this behavior, but because of social and cultural factors it is more commonly identified with males. The pedophile has difficulty in adult sexual relationships, and males who perform this act are frequently impotent.

Incest involves a sexual relationship with a person in the immediate family, most frequently a child. In many ways it is similar to pedophilia (intrafamilial pedophilia). Incestuous feelings are fairly common, but cultural mores are usually sufficiently strong to act as a barrier to the expression of sexual feelings.

Bestiality is the attainment of sexual gratification by intercourse with an animal. The intercourse may involve penetration or simply contact with the human genitalia by the tongue of the animal. The practice is more common in rural or isolated areas and is frequently a substitute for human sexual contact rather than an expression of preference.

Sadism is the attainment of sexual arousal by inflicting pain upon the sexual object, and **masochism** is the attainment of sexual excitation by enduring pain. Much sexual activity has aggressive components (eg, biting, scratching). Forced sexual acquiescence (eg, rape) is considered to be primarily an act of aggression.

Bondage is the achievement of erotic pleasure by being humiliated, enslaved, physically bound, and restrained. It is life-threatening, since neck binding or partial asphyxiation usually forms part of the ritual.

Necrophilia is sexual intercourse with a dead body or the use of parts of a dead body for sexual excitation, often with masturbation.

B. Gender Identity Variations: *Core gender identity* reflects a biologic self-image—the conviction that "I am a male" or "I am a female." While this is a fixed self-image, *gender role identity* is a dynamic, changing self-representation. Variances of core gender identity are rare, while those of gender role identity are common. The major gender variation is transsexualism.

Transsexualism (a core gender identity problem) is an attempt to deny and reverse biologic sex by maintaining sexual identity with the opposite gender. Transsexuals do not alternate between gender roles; rather, they assume a fixed role of attitudes, feelings, fantasies, and choices consonant with those of the opposite sex, all of which clearly date back to early development. For example, male transsexuals in early childhood behave, talk, and fantasize as if they were girls. They do not grow out of feminine patterns, they do not work in professions traditionally considered to be masculine, and they have no interest in their own penises either as evidence of maleness or as organs for erotic behavior. The desire for sex change starts early and may culminate in assumption of a feminine life-style, hormonal treatment, and use of surgical procedures, including castration and vaginoplasty.

Homosexuality is no longer considered to be a classifiable sexual disorder. Problems arise in this group when the individual has difficulty accepting the sexual orientation or is under stress in a society that is intolerant.

C. Psychosexual Dysfunction: This category includes a large group of vasocongestive and orgasmic disorders. Often, they involve problems of sexual adaptation, education, and technique that are often initially discussed with, diagnosed by, and treated by the family physician.

There are 2 conditions common in the male: impotence and ejaculation disturbances.

Impotence (erectile dysfunction) is inability to

achieve or maintain an erection firm enough for satisfactory intercourse; patients sometimes use the term to mean premature ejaculation. Careful questioning is necessary, since causes of this vasocongestive disorder can be psychologic, physiologic, or both. After onset of the problem, a history of occasional erections—especially nocturnal penile tumescence, which may be evaluated by a simple monitoring device, or a sleep study in the sleep laboratory—is evidence that the dysfunction is psychologic in origin, with the caveat that decreased nocturnal penile tumescence occurs in some depressed patients. **Psychologic impotence** is caused by interpersonal or intrapsychic factors (eg, marital disharmony, depression). **Organic factors** (which usually develop gradually) include arteriosclerosis, hypertension, diabetes mellitus, drug abuse (alcohol, nicotine, narcotics, stimulants), pharmacologic agents (anticholinergic drugs, antihypertensive medication, antihistamines, disulfiram, all psychotherapeutic drugs, narcotics, estrogens), organ system failure (circulatory, cardiorespiratory, renal), surgical complications (prostatectomy, vascular and back surgery), trauma (disk and spinal cord injuries), endocrine disturbances (pituitary, thyroid, adrenal), zinc deficiency, neurologic disorders (multiple sclerosis, tumors, peripheral neuropathies, injuries) (eg, trauma from bicycle or motorcycle seats), pernicious anemia, syphilis), urologic problems (phimosis, Peyronie's disease, priapism), and primary developmental abnormalities (Klinefelter's syndrome).

Ejaculation disturbances include premature ejaculation, inability to ejaculate, and retrograde ejaculation. (One may ejaculate even though impotent.) Ejaculation is usually connected with orgasm, and ejaculatory control is an acquired behavior that is minimal in adolescence and increases with experience. Pathogenic factors are those that interfere with learning control, most frequently sexual ignorance. Intrapsychic factors (anxiety, guilt, depression) and interpersonal maladaptation (marital problems, unresponsiveness of mate, power struggles) are also common. Organic causes include interference with sympathetic nerve distribution (often due to surgery or trauma) and the effects of pharmacologic agents on sympathetic tone. Postcoital cephalalgia is common and may be a variant of migraine.

In females, the 2 most common forms of sexual dysfunction are vaginismus and frigidity.

Vaginismus is a conditioned response in which a spasm of the perineal muscles occurs if there is any stimulation of the area. The desire is to avoid penetration. Sexual responsiveness and vasocongestion may be present, and orgasm can result from clitoral stimulation.

Frigidity is a complex condition in which there is a general lack of sexual responsiveness. The woman has difficulty in experiencing erotic sensation and does not have the vasocongestive response. Sexual activity varies from active avoidance of sex to an occasional orgasm. Orgasmic dysfunction—in which a woman has a vasocongestive response but varying degrees of difficulty in reaching orgasm—is sometimes differentiated from frigidity. Causes for the dysfunctions include poor sexual techniques, early traumatic sexual experiences, interpersonal disharmony (marital struggles, use of sex as a means of control), and intrapsychic problems (anxiety, fear, guilt). Organic causes include any conditions that might cause pain in intercourse, pelvic pathology, mechanical obstruction, and neurologic deficits.

Disorders of sexual desire refer to reduction or absence of sexual desire in either sex and may be a function of organic or psychologic difficulties (eg, anxiety, phobic avoidance). Any chronic illness can sap desire, but cerebral problems such as partial complex seizures, panhypopituitarism, Cushing's syndrome, and parkinsonism frequently cause a decrease in sexual drive. Hormonal variations, including use of antiandrogen compounds such as cyproterone acetate, and chronic renal failure contribute to deterioration in sexual activity. Alcohol, sedatives, narcotics, marihuana, and some medications may affect sexual drive and performance.

Treatment

A. Paraphilias and Gender Identity Disorders:

1. Psychologic–Sexual arousal disorders involving variant sexual activity (paraphilia), particularly those of a more superficial nature (eg, voyeurism) and those of recent onset, are responsive to psychotherapy in a moderate percentage of cases. The prognosis is much better if the motivation comes from the individual rather than the legal system; unfortunately, however, court intervention is frequently the only stimulus to treatment, because the condition persists and is reinforced until conflict with the law occurs. Therapies frequently focus on barriers to normal arousal response; the expectation is that the variant behavior will decrease as normal behavior increases.

2. Behavioral–Aversive and operant conditioning techniques have been tried frequently in gender role disorders but have been only occasionally successful. In some cases, the sexual arousal disorders improve with modeling, role-playing, and conditioning procedures. Emotive imagery is occasionally helpful in lessening anxiety in fetish problems.

3. Social–Although they do not produce a change in sexual arousal patterns or gender role, self-help groups have facilitated adjustment to an often hostile society. Attention to the family is particularly important in helping persons in such groups to accept their situation and alleviate their guilt about the role they think they had in creating the problem.

4. Medical–Medroxyprogesterone acetate, a suppressor of libidinal drive, is used to mute disruptive sexual behavior in males of all ages. Onset of action is usually within 3 weeks, and the effects are generally reversible. After careful evaluation, some transsexuals are treated with hormones and genital surgery.

B. Psychosexual Dysfunction:

1. Medical–Identification of a contributory reversible cause is most important. Even if the condition is not reversible, identification of the specific cause helps the patient to accept the condition. Marital disharmony, with its exacerbating effects, may thus be avoided. Of all the sexual dysfunctions, impotence is the condition most likely to have an organic basis. As part of the evaluation, vascular factors can be assessed in the office by injections of papaverine and phentolamine to produce an erection. Ultrasound examination is helpful in detecting arterial abnormalities. Yohimbine, 18 mg orally daily, has had modest effectiveness in both organic and psychogenic impotence. When the condition is irreversible, penile implants may be considered. Revascularization surgery has been done in patients with impotence due to circulatory problems.

2. Behavioral–Syndromes resulting from conditioned responses have been treated by conditioning techniques, with excellent results. Vaginismus responds well to desensitization with graduated Hegar dilators along with relaxation techniques. Masters and Johnson have used behavioral approaches in all of the sexual dysfunctions, with concomitant supportive psychotherapy and with improvement of the communication patterns of the couple.

3. Psychologic–The use of psychotherapy by itself is best suited for those cases in which interpersonal difficulties or intrapsychic problems predominate. Anxiety and guilt about parental injunctions against sex constitute the most frequent psychopathology contributing to sexual dysfunction. Even in these cases, however, a combined behavioral-psychologic approach usually produces results most quickly.

4. Social–The proximity of other people (eg, a mother-in-law) in a household is frequently an inhibiting factor in sexual relationships. In such cases, some social engineering may alleviate the problem.

Fuller AK: Child molestation and pedophilia. JAMA 1989;261:602.

Gitlin MJ, Pasnau RO: Psychiatric syndromes linked to reproductive function in women. Am J Psychiatry 1989;146:1413.

Krane RJ, Goldstein I, Saenz I: Impotence. N Engl J Med 1989;321:1648.

Segraves RT: Effects of psychotropic drugs on human erection and ejaculation. Arch Gen Psychiatry 1989; 46:275. (Drugs are a common cause of erectile problems, and a result is treatment noncompliance.)

PERSONALITY DISORDERS

Essentials of Diagnosis

- Long history dating back to childhood.
- Recurrent maladaptive behavior.
- Low self-esteem and lack of confidence.
- Minimal introspective ability.
- Major difficulties with interpersonal relationships or society.
- Depression with anxiety when maladaptive behavior fails.

General Considerations

Personality—a hypothetical construct—is the result of a genetic substrate and the prolonged interaction of an individual with personal drives and with outside influences (parent-child interactions, peer influences, random events), the sum being the enduring and unique patterns of behavior which are adopted in order to cope with the environment and which characterize one as an individual. The personality structure, or character, is an integral part of self-image and is important to one's sense of identity.

The classification of subtypes depends upon the predominant symptoms and their severity. The most severe disorders—those that bring the patient into greatest conflict with society—tend to be classified as antisocial (psychopathic) or borderline.

Classification & Clinical Findings

Paranoid: Defensive, oversensitive, secretive, suspicious, hyperalert, with limited emotional response.

Schizoid: Shy, introverted, withdrawn, avoids close relationships.

Compulsive: Perfectionist, egocentric, indecisive, with rigid thought patterns and need for control.

Histrionic (hysterical): Dependent, immature, seductive, histrionic, egocentric, vain, emotionally labile (a mnemonic device describing these traits is *dishevel*).

Schizotypal: Superstitious, socially isolated, suspicious, with limited interpersonal ability and odd speech.

Narcissistic: Exhibitionist, grandiose, preoccupied with power, lacks interest in others, with excessive demands for attention.

Avoidant: Fears rejection, hyperreacts to rejection and failure, with poor social endeavors and low self-esteem.

Dependent: Passive, overaccepting, unable to make decisions, lacks confidence, with poor self-esteem.

Passive-aggressive: Stubborn, procrastinating, argumentative, sulking, helpless, clinging, negative to authority figures.

Antisocial: Selfish, callous, promiscuous, impulsive, unable to learn from experience, has legal problems.

Borderline: Impulsive; has unstable and intense interpersonal relationships; is suffused with anger, fear, and guilt; lacks self-control and self-fulfillment; has identity problems and affective instability; is suicidal (a serious problem—up to 80% of hospitalized borderline patients make an attempt at some time during treatment, and the incidence of completed suicide is as high as 5%); aggressive behavior, feelings of emptiness, and occasional psychotic decompensation. This group has a high drug abuse rate, which plays a role in symptomatology. There is extensive overlap with other diagnostic categories, particularly mood disorders.

Differential Diagnosis

Patients with personality disorders tend to show anxiety and depression when pathologic techniques fail, and their symptoms can be similar to those occurring with anxiety disorders. Occasionally, the more severe cases may decompensate into psychosis under stress and mimic other psychotic disorders.

Treatment

A. Social: Social and therapeutic environments such as day hospitals, halfway houses, and self-help communities utilize peer pressures to modify the self-destructive behavior. The patient with a personality disorder often has failed to profit from experience, and difficulties with authority impair the learning experience. The use of peer relationships and the repetition possible in a structured setting of a helpful community enhances the educational opportunities and increases learning. When one's companions note every flaw in one's character and insist that it be corrected immediately, a powerful learning environment is being created. When problems are detected early, both the school and the home can serve as foci of intensified social pressure to change the behavior, particularly with the use of behavioral techniques.

B. Behavioral: The behavioral techniques used are principally operant and aversive conditioning. The former simply emphasizes the recognition of acceptable behavior and reinforcement of this with praise or other tangible rewards. Aversive responses usually mean punishment, although this can range from a mild rebuke to some specific punitive responses such as verbal abuse or deprivation of privileges. Extinction plays a role in that an attempt is made not to respond to inappropriate behavior, and the lack of response eventually causes the person to abandon that type of behavior. Pouting and tantrums, for example, diminish quickly when such behavior elicits no reaction.

C. Psychologic: Psychologic intervention is most usefully accomplished in group settings. Group therapy is helpful when specific interpersonal behavior needs to be improved (eg, schizoid and inadequate types, in which involvement with people is markedly impaired). This mode of treatment also has a place with so-called acting-out patients, ie, those who frequently act in an impulsive and inappropriate way. The peer pressure in the group tends to impose restraints on rash behavior. The group also quickly identifies the patient's types of behavior and helps

to improve the validity of the patient's self-assessment, so that the antecedents of the unacceptable behavior can be effectively handled, thus decreasing its frequency. Individual therapy should initially be supportive, ie, helping the patient to restabilize and mobilize defenses. If the individual has the ability to observe his or her own behavior, a longer-term and more introspective therapy may be warranted. The therapist must be able to handle countertransference feelings (which are frequently negative), maintain appropriate boundaries in the relationship (no physical contacts, however well-meaning), and refrain from premature confrontations and interpretations.

D. Medical: Hospitalization is rarely indicated except in the case of serious suicidal danger. In most cases, treatment can be accomplished in the day treatment center or self-help community. Antipsychotics may be required for short periods in conditions that have temporarily decompensated into transient psychoses (eg, haloperidol, 2–5 mg orally every 3–4 hours until the patient has quieted down and is regaining contact with reality). In most cases, these drugs are required only for several days and can be discontinued after the patient has regained a previously established level of adjustment. Carbamazepine, 800 mg orally daily in divided doses, decreases the severity of behavioral dyscontrol. Antidepressants have improved anxiety, depression, and sensitivity to rejection in some borderline patients.

Prognosis

Antisocial and borderline categories generally have a guarded prognosis, whereas persons with mild schizoid or passive-aggressive tendencies have a good prognosis with appropriate treatment.

Cowdry RW, Gardner DL: Pharmacotherapy of borderline personality disorders. Arch Gen Psychiatry 1988;45:111.
Zanarini MC, Gunderson JG, Frankenberg FR: Cognitive features of borderline personality disorder. Am J Psychiatry 1990;147:57. (Recognition is difficult but necessary for early treatment.)

SCHIZOPHRENIC & OTHER PSYCHOTIC DISORDERS

Essentials of Diagnosis (Schizophrenia)
- Social withdrawal, usually slowly progressive, often with deterioration in personal care.
- Loss of ego boundaries, with inability to perceive oneself as a separate entity.
- Loose thought associations, often with slowed thinking or overinclusive and rapid shifting from topic to topic.
- Autism with absorption in inner thoughts and frequent sexual or religious preoccupations.

- Auditory hallucinations, often of a derogatory nature.
- Delusions, frequently of a grandiose or persecutory nature.
- Symptoms of at least 6 months' duration.

Frequent additional signs:
- Flat affect and rapidly alternating mood shifts irrespective of circumstances.
- Hypersensitivity to environmental stimuli, with a feeling of enhanced sensory awareness.
- Variability or changeable behavior incongruent with the external environment.
- Concrete thinking with inability to abstract; inappropriate symbolism.
- Impaired concentration worsened by hallucinations and delusions.
- Depersonalization, wherein one behaves like a detached observer of one's own actions.

General Considerations

The schizophrenic disorders are a group of syndromes manifested by massive disruption of thinking, mood, and overall behavior, as well as poor filtering of stimuli. According to *DSM-III-R* criteria, the onset of illness occurs before age 45; signs must be continuous for at least 6 months; the illness is not preceded by a full depressive or manic syndrome; and symptoms are not due to mental retardation or organic mental disorder. The characterization and nomenclature of the disorders are quite arbitrary and are influenced by sociocultural factors and schools of psychiatric thought.

It is currently believed that the schizophrenic disorders are of multifactorial cause, with genetic, environmental, neuroendocrine, and pathophysiologic components. At present, there is no laboratory method to confirm the diagnosis of schizophrenia. There may or may not be a history of a major disruption in the individual's life (failures, losses, physical illness) before gross psychotic deterioration is evident. Females tend to have a benign course. History obtained from others may indicate a long-standing "strange" premorbid personality.

"Other psychotic disorders" are conditions that are similar to schizophrenic illness in their acute symptoms but have a less pervasive influence over the long term. The individual usually attains higher levels of functioning. The acute psychotic episodes tend to be less disruptive of the person's life-style, with a fairly quick return to previous levels of functioning.

Classifications

A. Schizophrenic Disorders: Schizophrenic disorders are subdivided on the basis of certain prominent phenomena that are frequently present. **Disorganized (hebephrenic) schizophrenia** is characterized by marked incoherence and an incongruous or silly affect. **Catatonic schizophrenia** is distinguished by a marked psychomotor disturbance of either excitement (purposeless and stereotyped) or rigidity with mutism. Infrequently, there may be rapid alternation between excitement and stupor (see under catatonic syndrome, below). **Paranoid schizophrenia** includes marked persecutory or grandiose delusions often consonant with hallucinations of similar content. **Undifferentiated schizophrenia** denotes a category in which symptoms are not specific enough to warrant inclusion of the illness in the other subtypes. **Residual schizophrenia** is a classification that includes persons who have clearly had an episode warranting a diagnosis of schizophrenia but who at present have no overt psychotic symptoms, although they show milder signs such as social withdrawal, flat affect, and eccentric behaviors.

B. Paranoid (Delusional) Disorders: Paranoid disorders are psychoses in which the predominant symptoms are persistent persecutory delusions, with minimal impairment in daily function (the schizophrenic disorders show significant impairment). Intellectual and occupational activities are little affected, whereas social and marital functioning tend to be markedly involved. Hallucinations are not usually present. Many of these patients are misdiagnosed as paranoid schizophrenics. The category includes such states as paranoia, shared paranoid disorder (folie à deux), and paranoid state, the last being characterized by its transitory nature, whereas the others are more chronic.

C. Schizoaffective Disorders: Schizoaffective disorders are those cases that fail to fit comfortably either in the schizophrenic or in the affective categories. They are usually cases with affective symptoms that precede or develop concurrently with psychotic manifestations.

D. Schizophreniform Disorders: Schizophreniform disorders are similar in their symptoms to the schizophrenic disorders except that the duration of the illness is less than 6 months but more than 1 week.

E. Brief Reactive Psychotic Disorders: These disorders last less than 1 week. They are the result of psychologic stress. The shorter duration is significant and correlates with a more acute onset and resolution as well as a much better prognosis.

Clinical Findings (Schizophrenia)

The signs and symptoms vary markedly among individuals as well as in the same person at different times. **Appearance** may be bizarre, although the usual finding is a mild to moderate unkempt blandness. **Motor activity** is generally reduced, although extremes ranging from catatonic stupor to frenzied excitement occur. **Social behavior** is characterized by marked withdrawal, coupled with disturbed interpersonal relationships and a reduced ability to experience pleasure. Dependency and a poor self-image are common. **Verbal utterances** are variable, the language being concrete yet symbolic, with unassociated rambling statements (at times interspersed with mutism) during an acute episode. Neologisms (made-up words or phrases), echolalia (repetition of words spoken by others), and verbigeration (repetition of senseless words or phrases) are occasionally present. **Affect** is usually flattened and shallow, with occasional inappropriateness. **Depression** is ubiquitous but may be less apparent during the acute psychotic episode and become more obvious during recovery. Depression is sometimes confused with akinetic side effects of antipsychotic drugs.

Thought content may vary from a paucity of ideas to a rich complex of delusional fantasy with archaic thinking. One frequently notes after a period of conversation that little if any information has actually been conveyed. Incoming stimuli produce varied responses. In some cases a simple question may trigger explosive outbursts, whereas at other times there may be no overt response whatsoever (catatonia). When paranoid ideation is present, the patient is often irritable and less cooperative. Delusions (false beliefs) are characteristic of paranoid thinking, and they usually take the form of a preoccupation with the supposedly threatening behavior exhibited by other individuals. This ideation may cause the patient to adopt active countermeasures such as locking doors and windows, taking up weapons, covering the ceiling with aluminum foil to counteract radar waves, and other bizarre efforts. Somatic delusions revolve around issues of bodily decay or infestation. **Perceptual distortions** usually include auditory hallucinations—visual hallucinations are more commonly associated with organic mental states—and may include illusions (distortions of reality) such as figures changing in size or lights varying in intensity. Cenesthetic hallucinations (eg, burning sensation in the brain, feeling blood flowing in blood vessels) are fairly common. Lack of humor, feelings of dread, depersonalization (a feeling of being apart from the self), and fears of annihilation may be present. Any of the above symptoms generates higher anxiety levels, with heightened arousal and occasional panic, as the individual fails to cope.

Ventricular enlargement in the brain, as seen on the CT scan, has been correlated with a chronic course, severe cognitive impairment, and nonresponsiveness to neuroleptic medications.

The development of the acute episode in schizophrenia frequently is the end product of a gradual decompensation. Frustration and anxiety appear early, followed by depression and alienation, along with decreased effectiveness in day-to-day coping. This often leads to feelings of panic and increasing disorganization, with loss of the ability to test and evaluate the reality of perceptions. The stage of so-called psychotic resolution includes delusions, autistic preoccupations, and psychotic insight, with acceptance of the decompensated state. The schizophrenic process

is frequently complicated by the use of alcohol and other recreational drugs. Polydipsia and polyuria with secondary hyponatremia may produce water intoxication—characterized by symptoms of confusion, lethargy, psychosis, seizures, and occasionally death—in any psychiatric disorder, but most commonly schizophrenia. Possible pathogenetic factors include a hypothalamic defect, inappropriate ADH secretion (rule out lung, duodenal, or pancreatic cancer; pituitary or hypothalamic tumor), neuroleptic medications (anticholinergic effects, withdrawal of medication, stimulation of hypothalamic thirst center, effect on ADH), smoking (nicotine and SIADH), psychotic thought processes (delusional beliefs), and other medications (eg, diuretics, antidepressants, lithium, alcohol). Other causes must be ruled out (eg, diabetes mellitus, diabetes insipidus, renal disease).

Differential Diagnosis

First and foremost should be a reconsideration of the diagnosis of schizophrenia in any person who has been so diagnosed in the past, particularly when the clinical course has been atypical. A number of these patients have been found to actually have atypical episodic affective disorders that have responded well to lithium. Manic episodes often mimic schizophrenia. Also, many individuals have been diagnosed as schizophrenic because of inadequacies in psychiatric nomenclature. Thus, persons with brief reactive psychoses, paranoid disorders, and schizophreniform disorders were often inappropriately diagnosed as having schizophrenia. Toxic reactions to drugs have also been incorrectly diagnosed as schizophrenia in many instances.

Psychotic depressions, psychotic organic mental states, and any illness with psychotic ideation tend to be confused with schizophrenia, partly because of the regrettable tendency to use the terms interchangeably. Adolescent phases of growth and counterculture behaviors constitute another area of diagnostic confusion. It is particularly important to avoid a misdiagnosis in these groups, because of the long-term implications arising from having such a serious diagnosis made in a formative stage of life.

Medical disorders such as thyroid dysfunction, adrenal and pituitary disorders, and practically all of the organic mental states in the early stages must be ruled out. **Complex partial seizures,** especially when psychosensory phenomena are present, are an important differential consideration. Toxic drug states arising from prescription, over-the-counter, and street drugs may mimic all of the psychotic disorders. The chronic use of amphetamines, cocaine, and other stimulants frequently produces a psychosis that is almost identical to the acute paranoid schizophrenic episode. Stimulants (including caffeine) and marihuana (antagonizes neuroleptics) may precipitate acute psychiatric symptoms in the schizophrenic. The presence of formication and stereotypy suggests the possibility of stimulant abuse. Phencyclidine (see below) has become a very common street drug, and in many cases a reaction to it is difficult to distinguish from other psychotic disorders. Cerebellar signs, excessive salivation, dilated pupils, and increased deep tendon reflexes should alert the physician to the possibility of a toxic psychosis. Industrial chemicals (both organic and metallic), degenerative disorders, and metabolic deficiencies must be considered in the differential diagnosis.

Catatonic syndrome, frequently assumed to exist solely as a component of schizophrenic disorders, is actually the end product of a number of illnesses, including various organic conditions. Neoplasms, viral and bacterial encephalopathies, central nervous system hemorrhage, metabolic derangements such as diabetic ketoacidosis, sedative withdrawal, and hepatic and renal malfunction have all been implicated. It is particularly important to realize that drug toxicity (eg, overdoses of antipsychotic medications such as fluphenazine or haloperidol) can cause catatonic syndrome, which may be misdiagnosed as a catatonic schizophrenic disorder and inappropriately treated with more antipsychotic medication.

Treatment

A. Medical: Hospitalization is often necessary, particularly when the patient's behavior shows gross disorganization. The presence of competent family members lessens the need for hospitalization, and each case should be judged individually. The major considerations are to prevent self-inflicted harm or harm to others and to provide the patient's basic needs. A full medical evaluation and CT scanning or MRI should be considered in first episodes of schizophreniform disorder and other psychotic episodes of unknown cause.

Antipsychotic medications (see Antipsychotic Drugs) are the treatment of choice. They block the response to stimulation. The relapse rate can be reduced by 50% with proper maintenance neuroleptic therapy. So-called **positive symptoms** such as hallucinations and delusions respond best, while **negative symptoms** such as withdrawal, psychomotor retardation, and poor interpersonal relationships may show little improvement. Trihexyphenidyl has been helpful in alleviating negative symptoms independently of its action on extrapyramidal side effects. Antidepressant drugs may be used in conjunction with neuroleptics if significant depression is present. Resistant cases may require concomitant use of lithium. The addition of a benzodiazepine drug to the neuroleptic regimen may prove helpful in treating the agitated or catatonic psychotic patient who has not responded to neuroleptics alone; the benzodiazepine may make possible maintenance with a lower neuroleptic dose. Treatment-resistant schizophrenics may be candidates for a trial of clozapine (30% improvement rate).

B. Social: Environmental considerations are most

important in the individual with a chronic illness, who usually has a history of repeated hospitalizations, a continued low level of functioning, and symptoms that never completely remit. This type of patient has usually never lived up to basic potential and frequently has been rejected by family members. The work record has frequently been poor, with a disability pension being the usual means of financial support. In these cases, board and care homes experienced in caring for psychiatric patients are most important. There is frequently an inverse relationship between stability of the living situation and the amounts of required antipsychotic drugs, since the most salutary environment is one that reduces stimuli.

Nonresidential self-help groups such as Recovery, Inc. should be utilized whenever possible. They provide a setting for sharing, learning, and mutual support and are frequently the only social involvement with which this type of patient is comfortable. Work agencies (eg, Goodwill Industries, Inc.) and vocational rehabilitation departments provide assessment, training, and job opportunities at a level commensurate with the person's clinical condition.

C. Psychologic: The need for psychotherapy varies markedly depending on the patient's current status and history. In a person with a single psychotic episode and a previously good level of adjustment, supportive psychotherapy may be helpful in assisting the patient to reintegrate the experience, gain some insight into antecedent problems, and become a more self-observant individual who can recognize early signs of stress. Insight-oriented psychotherapy is often counterproductive in this type of disorder. More importantly, family therapy should be given concomitantly to help alleviate the patient's stress and to assist relatives in coping with the patient.

D. Behavioral: Behavioral techniques (see above) are most frequently used in therapeutic settings such as day treatment centers, but there is no reason why they cannot be incorporated into family situations or any therapeutic setting. Many behavioral techniques are used unwittingly (eg, positive reinforcement—whether it be a word of praise or an approving nod—after some positive behavior), and with some careful thought, this approach can be a most powerful instrument for helping a person learn behaviors that will facilitate social acceptance. The family or board and care situation is the most important place for practice of such techniques, since so much of the patient's time is spent in such settings.

Prognosis

In any psychosis, the prognosis for alleviation of positive symptoms with medication is excellent in the large majority of patients. Negative symptoms are much more difficult to treat and are the principal reason schizophrenic patients do not achieve optimal function. Unavailability of structured work situations and lack of family therapy are 2 other reasons why the prognosis is so guarded in such a large percentage of schizophrenic patients. Psychosis connected with a history of serious drug abuse has a poor prognosis because of the central nervous system damage, usually from multiple drug abuse and the indirect factors (sepsis, infections, anoxia).

Frank AF, Gunderson JG: The role of the therapeutic alliance in the treatment of schizophrenia. Arch Gen Psychiatry 1990;47:228. (Always underestimated.)

Goldman MB, Luchins DJ, Robertson GL: Mechanisms of altered water metabolism in psychotic patients with polydipsia and hyponatremia. N Engl J Med 1988; 318:397. (A problem in about 20% of schizophrenic patients.)

Kramer MS et al: Antidepressants in "depressed" schizophrenic in-patients. Arch Gen Psychiatry 1989;46:922. (Always controversial.)

MOOD DISORDERS
(Depression & Mania)

Essentials of Diagnosis

Present in most depressions:
- Lowered mood, varying from mild sadness to intense feelings of guilt, worthlessness, and hopelessness.
- Difficulty in thinking, including inability to concentrate, ruminations, and lack of decisiveness.
- Loss of interest, with diminished involvement in work and recreation.
- Somatic complaints such as headache; disrupted, lessened, or excessive sleep; loss of energy; change in appetite; decreased sexual drive.
- Anxiety.

Present in some severe depressions:
- Psychomotor retardation or agitation.
- Delusions of a hypochondriacal or persecutory nature.
- Withdrawal from activities.
- Physical symptoms of major severity, eg, anorexia, insomnia, reduced sexual drive, weight loss, and various somatic complaints.
- Suicidal ideation.

General Considerations

Depression, like anxiety (with which it is associated), is ubiquitous and is a reality of everyday life. It may be the final expression of (1) genetic factors (neurotransmitter dysfunction), (2) developmental problems (personality defects, childhood events), or (3) psychosocial stresses (divorce, job loss). It frequently presents in the form of somatic complaints with negative medical workup. It can be a normal reaction to a wide variety of events and must be evaluated as such. When the depression is appropriate to a life event and is not of major magnitude, specific treatment is not necessary. The whole issue of depression is further confused by the fact that the word is used as an expression of a mood, a symptom, a syndrome, or a disease.

Clinical Findings

In general, there are 3 major groups of depressions, with similar symptoms in each group.

A. Reactive to Psychosocial Factors: Depression may occur in reaction to some outside (exogenous) adverse life situation, usually loss of a person by death (grief reaction), divorce, etc; financial reversal (crisis); or loss of an established role, such as being needed. Anger is frequently associated with the loss, and this in turn often produces a feeling of guilt. Adjectives such as reactive and neurotic (implying anxiety, which is often present in these depressions) are often used in this group of depressions. They are properly classified as adjustment disorders with depressed mood. The symptoms range from mild sadness, anxiety, irritability, worry, lack of concentration, discouragement, and somatic complaints to the more severe symptoms of the next group.

B. Depressive Disorders: The subclassifications include major depressive episodes and dysthymia.

1. A major depressive episode (endogenous unipolar disorder, involutional melancholia) is a period of serious mood depression that occurs relatively independently of the patient's life situations or events. Many consider a physiologic or metabolic aberration to be causative. Complaints vary widely but most frequently include a loss of interest and pleasure (anhedonia), withdrawal from activities, and feelings of guilt. Also included are inability to concentrate, some cognitive function, anxiety, chronic fatigue, feelings of worthlessness, somatic complaints (unidentifiable somatic complaints frequently indicate depression), and loss of sexual drive. Diurnal variation with improvement as the day progresses is common. Vegetative signs that frequently occur are insomnia, anorexia with weight loss, and constipation. Occasionally, severe agitation and psychotic ideation (paranoid thinking, somatic delusions) are present. Paranoid symptoms may range from general suspiciousness to ideas of reference with delusions. The somatic delusions frequently revolve around feelings of impending annihilation or hypochondriacal beliefs (eg, that the body is rotting away with cancer). Hallucinations are uncommon. Major depressive disorders may occur at any time from childhood through adult life. The incidence is somewhat higher in women, and there is a greater chance of occurrence during the involutional period with symptoms of severe agitation, somatic complaints, insomnia, an obsessive preoccupation with personal inadequacies, and feelings of guilt. Atypical depression is a subtype that is characterized by hypersomnia, overeating, lethargy, and rejection sensitivity. Postnatal depression may be linked to the major affective disorders, as is seasonal affective depression (SAD), a dysfunction of circadian rhythms that occurs more commonly in the winter and is believed to be due to decreased exposure to full-spectrum light. A questionnaire called the Seasonal Pattern Assessment Questionnaire (SPAQ) has been developed at NIMH to distinguish this disorder. Common symptoms include carbohydrate craving, hyperphagia, and hypersomnia.

2. Dysthymia is a chronic depressive disturbance. Sadness, loss of interest, and withdrawal from activities over a period of 2 or more years with a relatively persistent course is necessary for this diagnosis. Generally, the symptoms are milder but longer-lasting than those in a major depressive episode.

C. Bipolar Disorders: Bipolar disorders (manic and depressive episodes) and individual manic episodes usually occur earlier (late teens or early adult life) than major depressive episodes.

1. A manic episode is a mood change characterized by elation with hyperactivity, overinvolvement in life activities, low irritability threshold, flight of ideas, easy distractibility, and little need for sleep. The overenthusiastic quality of the mood and the expansive behavior initially attract others, but the irritability, mood lability, aggressive behavior, and grandiosity usually lead to marked interpersonal difficulties. Activities may occur that are later regretted, eg, excessive spending, resignation from a job, a hasty marriage, sexual acting out, and exhibitionistic behavior, with alienation of friends and family. Atypical manic episodes can include gross delusions, paranoid ideation of severe proportions, and auditory hallucinations usually related to some grandiose perception. The episodes begin abruptly (sometimes precipitated by life stresses) and may last from several days to months. Spring and summer tend to be the peak periods. Generally, the manic episodes are of shorter duration than the depressive episodes. In almost all cases, the manic episode is part of a broader bipolar (manic-depressive) disorder. Manic patients differ from schizophrenics in that the former use more effective interpersonal maneuvers, are more sensitive to the social maneuvers of others, and are more able to utilize weakness and vulnerability in others to their own advantage. Creativity has been positively correlated with mood disorders, but the best work done is between episodes of mania and depression.

2. Cyclothymic disorders are chronic mood disturbances with episodes of depression and hypomania. The symptoms must have at least a 2-year duration and are milder than those in a depressive or manic episode. Occasionally, the symptoms will escalate into a full-blown manic or depressive episode, in which case it would be classified as a bipolar disorder.

D. Secondary to Illness and Drugs: (All are classified as organic mood disorders.) Any illness, severe or mild, can cause significant depression. Conditions such as rheumatoid arthritis, multiple sclerosis, and chronic heart disease are particularly likely to be associated with depression, as are all other chronic illnesses. Hormonal variations clearly play a role in some depressions. Varying degrees of depression occur at various times in schizophrenic disorders, central nervous system disease (including cerebral dysrhythmias), and organic mental states. **Alcohol dependency** frequently coexists with serious depression.

The classic model of drug-induced depression occurs with the use of reserpine, both in a clinical and a neurochemical sense. Corticosteroids and oral contraceptives are commonly associated with affective changes. Antihypertensive medications such as methyldopa, guanethidine, clonidine, and propranolol have been associated with the development of depressive syndromes, as have digitalis and antiparkinsonism drugs. Infrequently, disulfiram and anticholinesterase drugs may be associated with symptoms of depression. All stimulant use results in a depressive syndrome when the drug is withdrawn. Alcohol, sedatives, opiates, and most of the psychedelic drugs are depressants and, paradoxically, are often used in self-treatment of depression. Limbic kindling may be one of the mechanisms by which the drugs of abuse cause central dysrhythmias and secondary depression.

Differential Diagnosis

Since depression may be a part of any illness—either reactively or as a secondary symptom—careful attention must be given to personal life adjustment problems, the role of medications (eg, reserpine, steroids, levodopa). Schizophrenia, partial complex seizures, brain syndromes, and anxiety disorders must be differentiated. Subtle thyroid dysfunction must be ruled out (check antithyroid antibodies).

Complications

The longer the depression continues, the more crystallized it becomes—particularly when there is an element of secondary reinforcement. The most important complication is **suicide,** which always includes some elements of aggression. Suicide rates vary from 4 per 100,000 in Greece to 12 per 100,000 in the USA to 45 per 100,000 in Hungary. Males tend toward successful suicide, particularly in older age groups, whereas women make more attempts with lower mortality rates. An increased suicide rate is being observed in the younger population, ages 15–35. Patients with cancer, respiratory illnesses, AIDS, and those being maintained on hemodialysis have higher suicide rates.

There are 4 major groups of people who make suicide attempts:

(1) Those who are overwhelmed by problems in living. By far the greatest number fall into this category. There is often great ambivalence; they don't really want to die, but they don't want to go on as before either.

(2) Those who are clearly attempting to control others. This is the blatant attempt in the presence of a significant other person in order to hurt or control that person.

(3) Those with severe depressions *(high-risk group)*. This group includes both exogenous (eg, AIDS, which has a suicide rate 60 times that of the general population) and endogenous conditions. It also includes those who may not be diagnosed as having depression but who are overwhelmed by a serious stressful situation (eg, the man charged with child molestation who hangs himself in his cell). Anxiety, panic, and fear are major findings in suicidal behavior. A patient may seem to make a dramatic improvement, but the lifting of depression may be due to the patient's decision to commit suicide.

(4) Those with psychotic illness *(high-risk group)*. These individuals tend not to verbalize their concerns, are unpredictable, and are often successful but comprise a small percentage of the total. Borderline personality disorders are included in this group.

The immediate goal of psychiatric evaluation is to assess the current suicidal risk and the need for hospitalization versus outpatient management. The intent is less likely to be truly suicidal, for example, if small amounts of poison or drugs were ingested or scratching of wrists was superficial; if the act was performed in the presence of others or with early notification of others; or if the attempt was arranged so that early detection would be anticipated. Alcohol, hopelessness, delusional thoughts, and complete or nearly complete loss of interest in life or ability to experience pleasure are all positively correlated with suicide attempts. Other risk factors are previous attempts, a family history of suicide, medical or psychiatric illness (eg, anxiety, depression, psychosis), male sex, older age, contemplation of violent methods, and drug use (including long-term sedative or alcohol use), which contributes to impulsiveness or mood swings. Successful treatment cannot be achieved if the patient continues to abuse drugs.

The patient's current mood status is best evaluated by direct evaluation of plans and concerns about the future, personal reactions to the attempt, and thoughts about the reactions of others. The patient's immediate resources should be assessed—people who can be significantly involved (most important), family support, job situation, financial resources, etc.

If hospitalization is not indicated, the physician must formulate and institute a treatment plan or make an adequate referral. Medication should be dispensed in small amounts to at-risk patients. Guns and drugs should be removed from the patient's household. Driving should be interdicted until the patient improves. The problem is often worsened by the long-term complications of the suicidal attempt, eg, brain damage due to hypoxia; peripheral neuropathies caused by staying for long periods in one position, causing nerve compressions; and medical or surgical problems such as esophageal strictures and tendon dysfunctions.

The reasons for self-mutilation, most commonly wrist cutting (but also autocastration, autoamputation,

and autoenucleation, which are associated with psychoses), may be very different from the reasons for a suicide attempt. The initial treatment plan, however, should presume suicidal ideation, and conservative treatment should be initiated as for attempted suicide.

Sleep disturbances in the depressions are discussed below.

Treatment

A. Medical: Depression associated with reactive disorders usually does not call for drug therapy and can be managed by psychotherapy and the passage of time. In severe cases—particularly when vegetative signs are present or impending—antidepressant drug therapy (see Antidepressant Drugs) is often effective. Drug selection depends on previous response if that information is available. In a patient presenting for the first time, one chooses either a serotonergic or adrenergic enhancing drug (see Table 19–6) and gives a full trial of the medication. If the depression is atypical, an MAO inhibitor or heterocyclic antidepressant (eg, fluoxetine, or bupropion) is indicated. In the event of nonresponse, the initial drug is discontinued and a drug from the neurotransmitter class not chosen initially is then given a trial. In either case, augmentation with lithium is accepted practice. With continued nonresponse, a drug from a group not previously used (eg, after failure with a tricyclic and an MAO inhibitor, a heterocyclic antidepressant) may be tried with or without lithium. Electroconvulsive therapy is usually reserved for involutional depression and cases that have not responded to pharmacotherapy.

If psychotic ideation is present—usually paranoia or somatic delusions—antipsychotic drugs should be given initially (eg, trifluoperazine, 10–20 mg/d orally) and the dosage increased every 2–3 days until symptoms abate. If depression persists as the psychosis comes under control, it may be necessary to add an antidepressant drug later.

Hospitalization is necessary if suicide is a realistic possibility or if symptoms are incapacitating. Suicide precautions should be instituted. In patients who do not respond to medications—particularly those with involutional melancholia or those who are considered at risk of suicide—hospitalization is mandatory and should not be withheld out of concern for cost to the family or the presumed social stigma of psychiatric detention.

Electroconvulsive therapy has consistently been more effective than the antidepressant groups of drugs, particularly for involutional depressions (see Other Organic Therapies, above). It is also effective in mania. Convenience, expense, and public opinion have been major limiting factors in the use of electroconvulsive therapy. It should be considered in those who are considered significant suicide risks and in those who fail to respond to adequate trials of medication.

Stimulants have little, if any, place in the treatment of depression. Their uses are in the treatment of apathy in geriatric cases, depression in severe medical illness when antidepressants or electroconvulsive therapy is not feasible, and attention deficit disorders. Atypical depression is treated with fluoxetine or MAO inhibitors. Progesterone has shown promise in the treatment of postnatal depression. Full-spectrum light therapy for 1–2 hours daily in the morning has been successful in depression related to seasonal affective disorder (SAD).

Manic episodes are treated with haloperidol, 5–10 mg orally or intramuscularly every 2–3 hours until symptoms subside. A decision must then be made about the need for long-term lithium maintenance. The dosage of haloperidol is gradually reduced after lithium is started (see Lithium, above).

If lithium alone does not control symptoms, a neuroleptic may be added. The addition of L-tryptophan or clonazepam may obviate the need for a neuroleptic. If lithium is contraindicated or if problems develop with lithium (eg, kidney dysfunction), clonazepam alone (0.5–16 mg/d orally) may be effective in acute episodes but is questionable for long-term prophylaxis. Carbamazepine, 800–1600 mg/d orally, is also an effective substitute. Valproic acid in initial studies has been shown to be comparable in effectiveness to carbamazepine. Calcium channel blockers are increasingly being used in the treatment of mania in patients for whom lithium or carbamazepine is either ineffective or contraindicated (eg, verapamil is safer than lithium or carbamazepine during pregnancy, though it decreases uterine contractility and must be discontinued before delivery).

B. Psychologic: It is seldom possible to engage an individual in penetrating psychotherapeutic endeavors during the acute stage of a severe depression. While medications may be taking effect, a supportive approach to strengthen existing defenses and appropriate consideration of the patient's continuing need to function at work, to engage in recreational activities, etc, are necessary as the severity of the depression lessens. If the patient is not seriously depressed, it is often quite appropriate to initiate intensive psychotherapeutic efforts, since flux periods are a good time to effect change. A catharsis of repressed anger and guilt may be beneficial. Therapy during or just after the acute stage may focus on coping techniques, with some practice of alternative choices. When lack of self-confidence and identity problems are factors in the depression, individual psychotherapy can be oriented to ways of improving self-esteem, increasing assertiveness, and lessening dependency. It is usually helpful to involve the spouse or other significant family members early in treatment.

C. Social: Flexible use of appropriate social services can be of major importance in the treatment of depression. Since alcohol is often associated with depression, early involvement in alcohol treatment programs such as Alcoholics Anonymous can be important to future success (see Alcohol Dependency and Abuse, below). The *structuring* of daily activities during severe depression is often quite difficult for the patient, and loneliness is often a major factor. The help of family, employer, or friends is often necessary to mobilize the patient who experiences no joy in daily activities and tends to remain uninvolved and to deteriorate. Insistence on sharing activities will help involve the patient in simple but important daily functions. In some severe cases, the use of day treatment centers or support groups of a specific type (eg, mastectomy groups) is indicated. It is not unusual for a patient to have multiple legal, financial, and vocational problems requiring legal and vocational rehabilitation.

D. Behavioral: When depression is a function of self-defeating coping techniques such as passivity, the role-playing approach can be useful. Behavioral techniques, including desensitization, may be used in problems such as phobias where depression is a by-product. When depression is a regularly used interpersonal style, behavioral counseling to family members or others can help in extinguishing the behavior in the patient.

Prognosis

Reactive depressions are usually time-limited, and the prognosis with treatment is good if suicide or a pathologic pattern of adjustment does not intervene. Major affective disorders frequently respond well to a full trial of drug treatment.

Elkin IE et al: National Institute of Mental Health treatment of depression collaborative research program: General effectiveness of treatments. Arch Gen Psychiatry 1989; 46:971.

Gold PW, Goodwin FK, Chrousos GP: Clinical and biochemical manifestations of depression: Relation to the neurobiology of stress. (2 parts.) N Engl J Med 1988; 319:348, 413. (Correlative psychophysiology.)

Karasu TB: Toward a clinical model of psychotherapy for depression. 2. An integrative and selective treatment approach. Am J Psychiatry 1990;147:269.

SLEEP DISORDERS

Sleep consists of 2 distinct states as shown by electroencephalographic studies: REM (rapid eye movement) sleep, also called dream sleep, D state sleep, paradoxic sleep; and NREM (non-REM) sleep, also called S state sleep, which is divided into stages 1, 2, 3, and 4 recognizable by different electroencephalographic patterns. Stages 3 and 4 are "delta" sleep. Dreaming occurs mostly in REM and to a lesser extent in NREM sleep.

Sleep is a cyclic phenomenon, with 4–5 REM periods during the night accounting for about one-fourth of the total night's sleep (1½–2 hours). The first REM period occurs about 80–120 minutes after onset of sleep and lasts about 10 minutes. Later REM periods are longer (15–40 minutes) and occur mostly in the last several hours of sleep. Most stage 4 (deepest) sleep occurs in the first several hours.

Age-related changes in normal sleep include an unchanging percentage of REM sleep and a marked decrease in stage 3 and stage 4 sleep, with an increase in wakeful periods during the night. These normal changes, early bedtimes, and daytime naps play a role in the increased complaints of insomnia in older people. Variations in sleep patterns may be due to circumstances (eg, "jet lag") or to idiosyncratic patterns ("night owls") in persons who perhaps because of different "biologic rhythms" habitually go to bed late and sleep late in the morning. Creative facilities and rapidity of response to unfamiliar situations are impaired by loss of sleep. There are also rare individuals who have chronic difficulty in adapting to a 24-hour sleep-wake cycle (desynchronization sleep disorder), which can be resynchronized by altering exposure to light.

The 3 major sleep disorders are discussed below.

Dyssomnias (Insomnia)

Patients may complain of difficulty getting to sleep or staying asleep, intermittent wakefulness during the night, early morning awakening, or combinations of any of these. Transient episodes are usually of little significance. Stress, caffeine, physical discomfort, daytime napping, and early bedtimes are common factors.

A. Clinical Conditions: Psychiatric disorders are often associated with persistent insomnia. **Depression** is usually associated with fragmented sleep, decreased total sleep time, earlier onset of REM sleep, a shift of REM activity to the first half of the night, and a loss of slow wave sleep—all of which are nonspecific findings. In **manic disorders,** sleeplessness is a cardinal feature and an important early sign of impending mania in bipolar cases. Total sleep time is decreased, with shortened REM latency and increased REM activity. Sleep-related panic attacks occur in the transition from stage 2 to stage 3 sleep in some patients with a longer REM latency in the sleep pattern preceding the attacks.

Abuse of alcohol may cause or be secondary to the sleep disturbance. There is a tendency to use alcohol as a means of getting to sleep without realizing that it disrupts the normal sleep cycle. Chronic alcohol abuse increases stage 1 and decreases REM sleep (most drugs delay or block REM sleep), with symptoms persisting for many months after the individual has stopped drinking. Acute alcohol or other sedative withdrawal causes delayed onset of sleep and REM rebound with intermittent awakening during the night.

Heavy smoking (more than a pack a day) causes difficulty falling asleep—apparently independently of the often associated increase in coffee drinking. Excess intake near bedtime of caffeine, cocaine, and other stimulants (eg, over-the-counter cold remedies) causes decreased total sleep time—mostly NREM sleep—with some increased sleep latency.

Sedative-hypnotics—specifically, the benzodiazepines, which are the prescription drugs of choice to promote sleep—tend to increase total sleep time, decrease sleep latency, and decrease nocturnal awakening, with variable effects on NREM sleep. Withdrawal causes just the opposite effects and results in continued use of the drug for the purpose of preventing withdrawal symptoms. Antidepressants decrease REM sleep (with marked rebound on withdrawal in the form of nightmares) and have varying effects on NREM sleep. The effect on REM sleep correlates with reports that REM sleep deprivation parallels improvement in some depressions.

Persistent insomnias are also related to a wide variety of medical conditions, particularly delirium, pain, respiratory distress syndromes, uremia, asthma, and hypothyroidism. Adequate analgesia and proper treatment of medical disorders will reduce symptoms and decrease the need for sedatives.

B. Treatment: In transient insomnias, deemphasis and reassurance are sufficient treatment. The patient should be given commonsense advice about consistent bedtimes, room temperature (cool is best), late snacks (a small amount of food or liquid), daily exercise, avoidance of noxious habits (too much coffee, alcohol, cigarettes), and daytime naps (including dozing at the TV set). Patients in acute distress because of sleepless nights may require a short course of benzodiazepine (eg, temazepam, 15 mg at bedtime). Antihistamines such as diphenhydramine or hydroxyzine are acceptable milder substitutes for benzodiazepines or chloral hydrate. Antidepressive and antipsychotic drugs with sedative effects (eg, trazodone, thioridazine) may be selected when dyssomnia is a symptom of the underlying condition requiring these types of medication.

Hypersomnias (Disorders of Excessive Sleepiness)

The hypersomnias are a more severe problem than insomnia.

A. Clinical Conditions:

1. Sleep apnea–This disorder is characterized by cessation of breathing for at least 30 episodes (each lasting 10 seconds) during the night. There are 2 types: obstructive and central. The obstructive type is discussed in Chapter 7. Central sleep apnea is due to failure during sleep of the respiratory drive mechanism. Obese middle-aged and older men with hypertension are most often affected. Both types may occur simultaneously. Symptoms include snoring, restless sleep, and excessive daytime sleepiness, which may be associated with headaches and depression. Cardiac arrhythmias (particularly bradycardia) and blood gas irregularities occur during episodes. The patients tend to have poor judgment and a history of work-related problems. Definitive diagnostic evaluation may include thyroid evaluation and otolaryngologic examination; polysomnography in the hospital to record sleep, heart rate, and respiratory movement; and oxygen saturation studies. Moderate alcohol intake at bedtime has produced sleep apnea episodes (10–12 nightly) in healthy men.

2. Narcolepsy–Narcolepsy consists of a tetrad of symptoms: (1) Sudden, brief (about 15 minutes) sleep attacks that may occur during any type of activity; (2) cataplexy—sudden loss of muscle tone involving specific small muscle groups or generalized muscle weakness that may cause the person to slump to the floor, unable to move, often associated with emotional reactions and sometimes confused with seizure disorder; (3) sleep paralysis—a generalized flaccidity of muscles with full consciousness in the transition zone between sleep and waking; and (4) hypnagogic hallucinations, visual or auditory, which may precede sleep or occur during the sleep attack. The attacks are characterized by an abrupt transition into REM sleep—a necessary criterion for diagnosis. The disorder begins in early adult life, affects both sexes equally, and usually levels off in severity at about 30 years of age.

3. Kleine-Levin syndrome–This syndrome, which occurs mostly in young males, is characterized by hypersomnic attacks 3–4 times a year lasting up to 2 days, with hyperphagia, hypersexuality, irritability, and confusion on awakening. It has often been associated with antecedent neurologic insults. It usually remits after age 40.

4. Nocturnal myoclonus–Periodic lower leg movements during sleep with subsequent daytime sleepiness, anxiety, depression, and cognitive impairment.

B. Treatment: Treatment of sleep attacks may include medical measures such as weight reduction, administration during sleep of low-flow oxygen by nasal prongs, and tongue restraining devices. Surgical treatment is discussed in Chapter 7. Diaphragmatic pacing has been helpful for central sleep apnea. Trials with protriptyline have improved daytime somnolence and nocturnal oxygenation, with no significant change, however, in the number of apneic episodes.

Narcolepsy is managed by daily administration of a stimulant such as amphetamine sulfate, 10 mg in the morning, with increased dosage as necessary. Imipramine, 75–100 mg daily, has been effective in treatment of cataplexy but not narcolepsy.

Nocturnal myoclonus is treated with clonazepam with variable results. There is no treatment for Kleine-Levin syndrome.

Parasomnias (Abnormal Behaviors During Sleep)

These disorders are fairly common in children and less so in adults.

A. Clinical Presentations: Sleep terror (pavor nocturnus) is an abrupt, terrifying arousal from sleep, usually in preadolescent boys. Symptoms are fear, sweating, tachycardia, and confusion for several minutes, with amnesia for the event. **Nightmares** occur during REM sleep; sleep terrors in stage 3 or stage 4 sleep. **Sleepwalking (somnambulism)** includes ambulation or other intricate behaviors while still asleep, with amnesia for the event. It affects mostly children aged 6–12 years, and episodes occur during stage 3 or stage 4 sleep in the first third of the night. Sleepwalking in elderly people is a feature of organic brain syndrome. Idiosyncratic reactions to drugs (eg, marihuana, alcohol) and medical conditions (eg, partial complex seizures) may be causative factors in adults.

Enuresis is involuntary micturition during sleep in a person who usually has voluntary control. Like other parasomnias, it is more common in children, usually in the 3–4 hours after bedtime, but is not limited to a specific stage of sleep. Confusion during the episode and amnesia for the event are common.

B. Treatment: Treatment for sleep terrors is with benzodiazepines (eg, diazepam, 5–20 mg at bedtime), since it will suppress stage 3 and stage 4 sleep. Somnambulism responds to the same treatment for the same reason, but simple safety measures should not be neglected. Enuresis may respond to imipramine, 50–100 mg at bedtime. Behavioral approaches (eg, bells that ring when the pad gets wet) have also been successful.

Ford DE, Kamerow DB: Epidemiologic study of sleep disturbances and psychiatric disorders. JAMA 1989; 262: 1479.

Moran MG, Thompson TL, Nies AS: Sleep disorders in the elderly. Am J Psychiatry 1988;145:1369.

DISORDERS OF AGGRESSION

Acts performed with the deliberate intent of causing physical harm to persons or property have a wide variety of causative factors. Aggression and violence are symptoms rather than diseases, and most frequently they are *not* associated with an underlying medical condition. Clinicians are unable to predict dangerous behavior with greater than chance accuracy. In terms of demographic characteristics, the perpetrator of an act of aggression is often a male under age 25, a member of a minority group, a person in socially and economically deprived circumstances, and a resident of an inner-city area. Depression, paranoia, temporal lobe dysfunction, and organic mental states may be associated.

Those who commit acts of aggression fall into 2 general types. The more common is a person with a pattern of physically aggressive behavior from an early age, with a poor capacity for peer relationships; truancy; and a family member (usually the father) who has a history of brutality, psychosis, or antisocial behavior. The less common type is the overcontrolled, chronically frustrated person who seethes inside until some event precipitates a violent overreaction. Some clues to the dangerous patient include statements that they feel powerless, feel humiliated, have headaches, or feel that they are "going to explode" or have "something terribly wrong with my body." *In both types, disinhibiting drugs (most commonly alcohol) play a role in the aggressive outburst.*

In the USA, 50% of all violent deaths are alcohol-related. The ingestion of even small amounts of alcohol can result in pathologic intoxication that resembles an acute organic mental condition. Amphetamines, crack cocaine, or other stimulants are frequently associated with aggressive behavior. Phencyclidine is a drug commonly associated with violent behavior that is occasionally of a bizarre nature. Impulse control disorders are characterized by physical abuse, usually of wife or children, pathologic intoxication, impulsive sexual activities, and automobile misuse.

Wife beating and rape are much more widespread than heretofore recognized. Awareness of the problem is to some degree due to increasing recognition of the rights of women and the understanding by women that they do not have to accept abuse. Acceptance of this kind of aggression inevitably leads to more, with the ultimate aggression being murder—20–50% of murders in the USA occur within the family. Police are called in more domestic disputes than *all other criminal incidents combined.* Children who are a part of such relationships inevitably become victims. The majority of abused children come from this type of household.

Features of individuals who have been subjected to chronic physical or sexual abuse are as follows: trouble expressing anger, staying angry longer, general passivity in relationships, feeling "marked for life" with accompanying feeling of deserving to be victimized, lack of trust, and dissociation of affect from experiences. The physician should be suspicious about the origin of any injuries not fully explained, particularly if such incidents recur.

Treatment

A. Psychologic: Management of any violent individual includes appropriate psychologic maneuvers. Move slowly, talk slowly with clarity and reassurance, and evaluate the situation. Strive to create a setting that is minimally disturbing and eliminate people or things threatening to the violent individual. Do not threaten or abuse and do not touch or crowd the person. Allow no weapons in the area. Proximity to a door is comforting to both the patient and the exam-

iner. Use a negotiator whom the violent person can relate to comfortably. Food and drink are helpful in defusing the situation (as are cigarettes for those who smoke). Honesty is important. Make no false promises, bolster the patient's self-esteem, and continue to engage the subject verbally until the situation is under control. This type of individual does better with strong external controls to replace the lack of inner controls over the long term. Close probationary supervision and court-mandated restrictions can be most helpful. There should be a major effort to help the individual avoid drug use (eg, Alcoholics Anonymous). Victims of abuse are essentially treated as any victim of trauma and, not infrequently, have evidence of posttraumatic stress disorder.

B. Pharmacologic: Pharmacologic means are often necessary whether or not psychologic approaches have been successful. This is particularly true in the agitated or psychotic patient. The drug of choice in psychotic aggressive states is haloperidol, 10 mg intramuscularly every hour until symptoms are alleviated. Benzodiazepine sedatives (eg, diazepam, 5 mg orally or intravenously every several hours) can be used for mild to moderate agitation, but an antipsychotic drug is preferred for management of the seriously violent and psychotic patient. Chronic aggressive states, particularly in retardation and brain damage (rule out causative organic conditions and medications such as anticholinergic drugs) have been ameliorated with propranolol, 40–240 mg/d orally, or pindolol, 5 mg twice daily orally (pindolol causes less bradycardia and hypotension). Anticonvulsant medication has produced variable results, carbamazepine appearing to be the most effective drug.

C. Physical: Physical management is necessary if psychologic and pharmacologic means are not sufficient. It requires the active and visible presence of an adequate number of personnel to reinforce the idea that the situation is under control despite the patient's lack of inner controls. Such an approach often precludes the need for actual physical restraint. When adequate personnel are not available, however, 2 people shielded by a mattress (single-bed size) can usually corner and subdue the patient without injury to anyone. Seclusion rooms and restraints should be used only when necessary (ambulatory restraints are an alternative), and the patient must then be observed at frequent intervals. Design of corridors and seclusion rooms is important. Narrow corridors, small spaces, and crowded areas exacerbate the potential for violence in an anxious patient.

D. Other: The treatment of victims (eg, beaten wives) is a frustrating experience, chiefly because of the woman's reluctance to leave the situation. Reasons for staying vary, but common themes include the fear of more violence because of leaving; the hope that the situation may ameliorate (in spite of steady worsening); and the financial aspects of the situation, which are seldom to the woman's advantage. Concerns for the children often finally compel the woman to seek help. An early step is to get the woman into a therapeutic situation that provides the support of others in similar straits. Al-Anon is frequently a valuable asset and quite appropriate when alcohol is one of the factors in the abuse of the woman. The group can support the victim while she gathers strength to consider alternatives without being paralyzed by fear. Many cities now offer temporary emergency centers and counseling. "Rescue" attempts by physicians and other well-meaning individuals are often unsuccessful and discourage the would-be helper from ever again dealing with such problems. Use the available resources, attend to any medical or psychiatric problems, and maintain a compassionate interest.

Jacobson A: Physical and sexual assault histories among psychiatric outpatients. Am J Psychiatry 1989;146:755. (They are often interrelated.)

SUBSTANCE USE DISORDERS
(Drug Dependency, Drug Abuse)

The term "drug dependency" is used in a broad sense here to include both addictions and habituations. It involves the triad of compulsive drug use referred to as drug addiction, which includes (1) a **psychologic craving** or dependence and the behavior included in the procurement of the drug ("hustle"); (2) **physiologic dependence,** with withdrawal symptoms on discontinuance of the drug; and (3) **tolerance,** ie, the need to increase the dose to obtain the desired effects. Drug dependency is a function of the amount of drug used and the duration of usage. The amount needed to produce dependency varies with the nature of the drug and the idiosyncratic nature of the user. The frequency of use is usually daily, and the duration is inevitably greater than 2–3 weeks. Polydrug abuse is very common. Transgenerational continuity of drug abuse is also common. A large percentage of drug abusers present themselves for something other than treatment (eg, avoiding legal consequences, obtaining more drugs).

There is accumulating evidence that an impairment syndrome exists in many former (and current) drug users. It is believed that drug use has damaged neurotransmitter receptor sites and that the consequent imbalance produces symptoms that may mimic other psychiatric illnesses. "Kindling"—repeated stimulation of the brain—renders the individual more susceptible to focal brain activity with minimal stimulation. Stimulants and depressants can produce kindling, leading to relatively spontaneous effects no longer dependent on the original stimulus. These effects may

be manifested as mood swings, panic, and occasionally overt seizure activity. The imbalance also results in an individual who simply does not produce: poor job retention, marriage problems, poor planning, and generally erratic behavior. Early recognition is important, mainly to establish realistic treatment programs that are chiefly symptom-directed.

The physician faces 3 problems with substance abuse: (1) the prescribing of substances such as sedatives, stimulants, or narcotics that might produce dependency; (2) the treatment of individuals who have already abused drugs, most commonly alcohol; and (3) the detection of illicit drug use in patients presenting with psychiatric symptoms. The usefulness of urinalysis for detection of drugs varies markedly with different drugs and under different circumstances (pharmacokinetics is a major factor). Water-soluble drugs (eg, alcohol, stimulants, opioids) are eliminated in a day or so. Lipophilic substances (eg, phencyclidine, tetrahydrocannabinol) appear in the urine over longer periods of time: several days in most cases, 1–2 months in chronic marihuana users. Sedative drug determinations are quite variable, amount of drug and duration of use being important determinants. False-positives can be a problem related to ingestion of some legitimate drugs or foods (eg, phenytoin for barbiturates, phenylpropanolamine for amphetamines, chlorpromazine for opiates) and some foods (eg, poppy seeds for opiates, coca leaf tea for cocaine). Manipulations can alter the legitimacy of the testing. Dilution, either in vivo or in vitro, can be detected by checking urine specific gravity. Addition of ammonia, vinegar, or salt may invalidate the test, but odor and pH determinations are simple. Hair analysis can determine drug use over longer periods.

ALCOHOL DEPENDENCY & ABUSE
(Alcoholism)

Essentials of Diagnosis
Major criteria:
- Physiologic dependence as manifested by evidence of withdrawal when intake is interrupted.
- Laboratory tests.
- Tolerance to the effects of alcohol.
- Evidence of alcohol-associated illnesses, such as alcoholic liver disease, cerebellar degeneration.
- Continued drinking despite strong medical and social contraindications and life disruptions.
- Impairment in social and occupational functioning.
- Depression.
- Blackouts.
Other signs:
- Alcohol stigmas: Alcohol odor on breath, alcoholic facies, flushed face, scleral injection, tremor, ecchymoses, peripheral neuropathy.
- Surreptitious drinking.
- Unexplained work absences.

● Frequent accidents, falls, or injuries of vague origin; in smokers, cigarette burns on hands or chest.

General Considerations

Alcoholism is a syndrome consisting of 2 phases: problem drinking and alcohol addiction. Problem drinking is the repetitive use of alcohol, often to alleviate anxiety or solve other emotional problems. Alcohol addiction is a true addiction similar to that which occurs following the repeated use of other sedative-hypnotics. Concurrent dependence on sedative-hypnotics is very common. There is a high incidence among homeless individuals. Alcohol and other drug abuse patients have a much higher prevalence of lifetime psychiatric disorders. Adoption and twin studies indicate some genetic influence. *Depression is often present and should be evaluated carefully.* The majority of suicides and intrafamily homicides involve alcohol, and it is a major factor in rapes and assaults.

Clinical Findings

A. Acute Intoxication: The signs of alcoholic intoxication are the same as those of overdosage with any other central nervous system depressant: drowsiness, errors of commission, disinhibition, dysarthria, ataxia, and nystagmus. For a 70-kg person, an ounce of whiskey, a glass of wine, or a 12-oz bottle of beer raises the level of alcohol in the blood by 25 mg/dL. Blood levels below 50 mg/dL rarely cause significant motor dysfunction. Intoxication as manifested by ataxia, dysarthria, and nausea and vomiting indicates a blood level above 150 mg/dL, and lethal blood levels range from 350 to 900 mg/dL. In severe cases, overdosage is marked by respiratory depression, stupor, seizures, shock syndrome, coma, and death. Serious overdoses are frequently due to a combination of alcohol with other sedatives.

B. Withdrawal: There is a wide spectrum of manifestations of alcoholic withdrawal, ranging from anxiety, decreased cognition, and tremulousness through increasing irritability and hyperreactivity to full-blown **delirium tremens.** The latter is an acute organic psychosis that is usually manifest within 24–72 hours after the last drink (but may occur up to 7–10 days later). It is characterized by mental confusion, tremor, sensory hyperacuity, visual hallucinations (often of snakes, bugs, etc), autonomic hyperactivity, diaphoresis, dehydration, electrolyte disturbances (hypokalemia, hypomagnesemia), seizures, and cardiovascular abnormalities. The acute withdrawal syndrome is often completely unexpected and occurs when the patient has been hospitalized for some unrelated problem and presents as a diagnostic problem. *Suspect alcohol withdrawal in every unexplained delirium.* Seizures occur early (the first 24 hours) and are more prevalent in persons who have a history of withdrawal syndromes. The mortality rate from delirium tremens has steadily decreased with early diagnosis and improved treatment.

C. Alcoholic (Organic) Hallucinosis: This syndrome occurs either during heavy drinking or on withdrawal and is characterized by a paranoid psychosis without the tremulousness, confusion, and clouded sensorium seen in withdrawal syndromes. The patient appears normal except for the auditory hallucinations, which are frequently persecutory and may cause the patient to behave aggressively and in a paranoid fashion.

D. Chronic Alcoholic Brain Syndromes: These encephalopathies are characterized by increasing erratic behavior, memory and recall problems, and emotional instability—the usual signs of organic brain syndrome due to any cause (see Organic Mental Disorders, below). Early recognition and treatment of alcoholic with intravenous thiamine and B complex vitamins, particularly thiamine, can minimize damage.

Differential Diagnosis

The differential diagnosis of problem drinking is essentially between primary alcoholism (when no other major psychiatric diagnosis exists) and secondary alcoholism, when alcohol is used as self-medication for major underlying psychiatric problems such as schizophrenia or affective disorder. The differentiation is important, since the latter group requires treatment for the specific psychiatric problem.

The differential diagnosis of alcoholic withdrawal includes other sedative abuse. Acute alcoholic hallucinosis must be differentiated from other acute paranoid states such as amphetamine psychosis or acute paranoid schizophrenia. An accurate history is the most important differentiating factor. The history and laboratory test results are the most important features in differentiating chronic organic brain syndromes due to alcohol from those due to other causes. The form of the brain syndrome is of little help—eg, chronic brain syndromes from lupus erythematosus may be associated with confabulation similar to that resulting from long-standing alcoholism.

Complications

The medical, economic, and psychosocial problems of alcoholism are staggering. The central and peripheral nervous system complications include chronic brain syndromes, cerebellar degeneration, cardiovascular disorders, and peripheral neuropathies. The effects on the liver result not only in cirrhosis with its direct complications such as liver failure and esophageal varicosities but also in the systemic effects of altered metabolism and the immune system, changes in hormone levels, cardiovascular disease, an increased incidence of cancer, protein abnormalities, and coagulation defects.

Fetal alcohol syndrome includes one or more of the following developmental defects in the offspring of alcoholic women: (1) low birth weight and small size with failure to catch up in size or weight; (2) mental retardation, with an average IQ in the 60s;

and (3) a variety of birth defects, with a large percentage of facial and cardiac abnormalities. The fetuses are very quiet in utero, and there is an increased frequency of breech presentations. There is a higher incidence of delayed postnatal growth and behavior development. The risk factors are appreciably higher the more alcohol ingested by the mother each day. Cigarette and marihuana smoking can produce similar effects on the fetus.

Treatment of Problem Drinking

A. Psychologic: The most important consideration for the physician is to suspect the problem early and take a nonjudgmental attitude, though this does not mean a passive one. The problem of **denial** must be met, preferably with significant family members at the first meeting. This means dealing from the beginning with any enabling behavior of the spouse or other significant people. This is particularly true when the problem has become a "chronic rescue operation." There must be an emphasis on the things that can be done. This approach emphasizes the fact that the physician cares and strikes a positive and hopeful note early in treatment. Valuable time should not be wasted trying to find out why the patient drinks; come to grips early with the immediate problem of how to stop the drinking. Total abstinence (not "controlled drinking") should be the primary goal.

B. Social: Get the patient into Alcoholics Anonymous (AA) and the spouse into Al-Anon. Success is usually proportionate to the utilization of AA, religious counseling, and other resources. The patient should be seen frequently for short periods and charged an appropriate fee.

Do not underestimate the importance of religion, particularly since the alcoholic is often a dependent person who needs a great deal of support. Early enlistment of the help of a concerned religious adviser can often provide the turning point for a personal conversion to sobriety.

One of the most important considerations is the job; it is usually lost or in jeopardy. The business community has become painfully aware of the problem, with the result that about 70% of the Fortune 500 companies offer programs to their employees to help with the problem of alcoholism. In the latter case, some specific recommendations to employers can be offered: (1) Avoid placement in jobs where the alcoholic must be alone, eg, traveling buyer or sales executive. (2) Use supervision but not surveillance. (3) Keep competition with others to a minimum. (4) Avoid positions that require quick decision making on important matters (high stress situations).

C. Medical: Hospitalization is not usually necessary or even desirable at this stage, which is not an acute one. It is sometimes used to dramatize a situation and force the patient to face the problem of alcoholism, but generally it should be used on medical indications.

Because of the many medical complications of alcoholism, a complete physical examination with appropriate laboratory tests is mandatory, with special attention to the liver and nervous system. Two tests of major importance are γ-glutamyl transferase (findings above 30 mU/mL are suggestive of heavy drinking) and mean corpuscular volume (> 95 fL in males and > 100 fL in females). If both these findings are elevated, there is a high probability of a serious drinking problem. HDL cholesterol elevations combined with elevated γ-glutamyl transferase concentrations also can predictably help to identify heavy drinkers. *Use of sedatives as a replacement for alcohol is not desirable.* Usually the result is a concomitant use of sedatives and alcohol and a worsening of the problem. Lithium is not helpful in the treatment of primary alcoholism.

Disulfiram blocks the metabolism of alcohol with acetaldehyde buildup, with the result that unpleasant symptoms of headaches, flushing, and nausea occur within 30 minutes after exposure and may progress to more serious signs and symptoms, including hypertension, shock, and coma. Disulfiram is helpful in deterrence, particularly binge drinking. There should be no surreptitious use of the drug. The patient should have full knowledge of the consequences of using alcohol with the drug (including elixirs and sunscreens with alcohol). Cardiac disease and psychoses are contraindications to the use of disulfiram. Side effects without concomitant alcohol use include impotence, liver damage (obtain hepatic baseline studies), drowsiness, and fetal anomalies in pregnant women. The initial dose is 500 mg orally daily (after abstention from alcohol for 12 hours), reduced to 250 mg daily after a week. Disulfiram impairs elimination of caffeine and interacts with phenytoin, sedatives, and narcotics. A disulfiram regimen need not interfere with other treatment approaches such as AA.

D. Behavioral: Conditioning approaches have been used in many settings in the treatment of alcoholism, most commonly as a type of aversion therapy. For example, the patient is given a drink of whiskey and then a shot of apomorphine, and proceeds to vomit. In this way a strong association is built up between the vomiting and the drinking. Although this kind of treatment has been successful in some cases, many people do not retain the learned aversive response.

Treatment of Withdrawal & Hallucinosis

A. Medical:

1. Alcoholic hallucinosis—Alcoholic hallucinosis, which can occur either during or on cessation of a prolonged drinking period, is not a typical withdrawal syndrome and is handled differently. Since the symptoms are primarily those of a psychosis in the presence of a clear sensorium, they are handled like any other psychosis: hospitalization (when indicated) and adequate amounts of antipsychotic drugs. Haloperidol, 5 mg orally twice a day for the first day or so, usually ameliorates symptoms quickly, and the drug can be decreased and discontinued over several days as the patient improves. It then becomes necessary to deal with the chronic alcohol abuse, which has been discussed.

2. Withdrawal symptoms–Withdrawal symptoms, ranging from a mild syndrome to the severe state usually called delirium tremens, are a medical problem with a significant morbidity and mortality rate. They usually occur (onset 12 hours, peak intensity 48–72 hours after cessation of alcohol intake) when an intake of at least 7–8 pints of beer or 1 pint of spirits daily for several months has been stopped. The patient should be hospitalized and given adequate central nervous system depressants to counteract the excitability resulting from the sudden cessation of alcohol. Monitoring of vital signs and fluids and electrolyte levels is essential for the severely ill patient. Antipsychotic drugs such as chlorpromazine should *not* be used. The choice of the specific sedative is less important than using *adequate* doses to bring the patient to a level of moderate sedation, and this will vary from person to person. Mild to moderate dependency requires "drying out"—a short course of oral benzodiazepines on an outpatient basis with *no alcohol intake*. In severe withdrawal, hospitalize and use diazepam orally in a dosage of 5–10 mg every 1–4 hours depending on the clinical need. After stabilization, the amount of diazepam required to maintain a sedated state may be given orally every 8–12 hours. If restlessness, tremulousness, and other signs of withdrawal persist, the dosage is increased until moderate sedation occurs. The dosage is then gradually reduced by 20% every 24 hours until withdrawal is complete. This usually requires a week or so of treatment. Clonidine, 5 μg/kg orally every 2 hours, suppresses cardiovascular signs of withdrawal and also has some anxiolytic effect. Carbamazepine, 400–800 mg daily orally, compares favorably with benzodiazepines for alcohol withdrawal..

Meticulous examination for other medical problems is necessary. Alcoholics commonly have liver disease and associated clotting problems and are also prone to injury—and the combination all too frequently leads to undiagnosed subdural hematoma.

Anticonvulsant drugs are not needed unless there is a history of seizures. In these situations, phenytoin can be given in a loading dose—500 mg orally and, several hours later, another 500 mg orally (ie, 1 g over 4–6 hours). This drug is then continued in a dosage of 300 mg daily, which is checked by serum drug level.

A general diet should be given, and vitamins in high doses: thiamine, 100 mg 3 times a day; pyridoxine, 100 mg/d; folic acid, 5 mg 3 times a day; and ascorbic acid, 100 mg twice a day. Intravenous glucose solutions should not be given prior to the vita-

mins. Concurrent administration is satisfactory, and hydration should be meticulously assessed on an ongoing basis.

Chronic brain syndromes secondary to a long history of alcohol intake are not responsive to any specific measures. Attention to the social and environmental care of this type of patient is paramount.

B. Psychologic and Behavioral: The comments in the section on problem drinking apply here also; these methods of treatment become the primary consideration after the successful treatment of withdrawal or alcoholic hallucinosis. Psychologic and social measures should be initiated in the hospital shortly before discharge. This increases the possibility of continued posthospitalization treatment.

Chainess ME, Simon RP, Greenberg DA: Ethanol and the nervous system. N Engl J Med 1989;321:442.

Moore RD et al: Prevalence, detection, and treatment of alcoholism in hospitalized patients. JAMA 1989;261: 403.

OTHER DRUG & SUBSTANCE DEPENDENCIES

Opiates

The terms "opiates" and "narcotics" are used interchangeably and include a group of drugs with actions that mimic those of morphine. The group includes natural derivatives of opium, synthetic surrogates, and a number of polypeptides, some of which have been discovered to be natural neurotransmitters. The principal narcotic of abuse is heroin (metabolized to morphine), which is not used as a legitimate medication. A large percentage of heroin addicts are infected with HIV because of nonsterile needles. The other common narcotics are prescription drugs and differ in milligram potency, duration of action, and agonist and antagonist capabilities (see Chapter 1). All of the narcotic analgesics can be reversed by the narcotic antagonist naloxone.

The clinical signs of mild narcotic intoxication include needle tracks; changes in mood, with feelings of euphoria; drowsiness; nausea with occasional emesis; and miosis. The incidence of snorting and inhaling heroin ("smoking") is increasing, particularly among cocaine users. This coincides with a decrease in the availability of methaqualone (no longer on the market) and other sedatives used to temper the cocaine "high." Combined cocaine and heroin smoking has increased, with associated increases in dependency and morbidity. Overdosage causes respiratory depression, peripheral vasodilatation, pinpoint pupils, pulmonary edema, coma, and death.

Dependency is a major concern when continued use of narcotics occurs, although withdrawal causes only moderate morbidity (about the severity of a bout with the "flu"). Addicts sometimes consider themselves more addicted than they really are and may not require a withdrawal program. Grades of withdrawal are categorized from 0–4: grade 0 includes craving and anxiety; grade 1, yawning, lacrimation, rhinorrhea, and perspiration; grade 2, previous symptoms plus mydriasis, piloerection, anorexia, tremors, and hot and cold flashes with generalized aching; grades 3 and 4, increased intensity of previous symptoms and signs, with increased temperature, blood pressure, pulse, and respiratory rate and depth. In withdrawal from the most severe addiction, vomiting, diarrhea, weight loss, hemoconcentration, and spontaneous ejaculation or orgasm commonly occur.

Treatment for overdosage (or suspected overdosage) is naloxone (Narcan), 0.4 mg intravenously. If an overdose has been taken, the results are dramatic and occur within 2 minutes. Since the length of action of naloxone is much shorter than that of the narcotics, the patient must be under close observation. Hospitalization, supportive care, naloxone administration, and observation for withdrawal from other drugs should be maintained for as long as necessary. Complications of heroin administration include infections (eg, pneumonia, septic emboli, hepatitis), traumatic insults (eg, arterial spasm due to drug injection, gangrene), and pulmonary edema (50% of patients).

Treatment for withdrawal begins if grade 2 signs develop. If a withdrawal program is necessary, use methadone, 10 mg orally (use parenteral administration if the patient is vomiting), and observe. If signs (piloerection, mydriasis, cardiovascular changes) persist for more than 4–6 hours, give another 10 mg; continue to administer methadone at 4- to 6-hour intervals until signs are not present (rarely more than 40 mg of methadone in 24 hours). Divide the total amount of drug required over the first 24-hour period by 2 and give this dose every 12 hours. Each day, reduce the total 24-hour dose by 5–10 mg. Thus, a moderately addicted patient initially requiring 30–40 mg of methadone could be withdrawn over a 4- to 8-day period. Clonidine, 0.1 mg in several divided doses over a 10- to 14-day period, is an alternative to methadone detoxification; it is not necessary to taper the dose. Clonidine is helpful in alleviating cardiovascular symptoms but does not significantly relieve anxiety, insomnia, or generalized aching.

Methadone maintenance programs are of some value in chronic recidivism. Under carefully controlled supervision, the narcotic addict is maintained on fairly high doses of methadone (40–120 mg/d) that satisfy craving and block the effects of heroin to a great degree. Methadyl acetate is longer lasting and is replacing methadone in some programs. Abrupt withdrawal from methadyl acetate does not result in more severe withdrawal problems than gradual withdrawal.

Narcotic antagonists (eg, naltrexone) can also be used successfully for treatment of the patient who has been free of opioids for 7–10 days. Naltrexone blocks the narcotic "high" of heroin when 50 mg is given orally every 24 hours initially for several days and then 100 mg is given every 48–72 hours. Liver disorders are a major contraindication. Compliance tends to be poor, partly because of the dysphoria that can persist long after opioid discontinuance.

Sedatives (Anxiolytics)
See p 742.

Psychedelics
About 6000 species of plants have psychoactive properties. All of the common psychedelics (LSD, mescaline, psilocybin, dimethyltryptamine, and other derivatives of phenylalanine and tryptophan) produce similar behavioral and physiologic effects. An initial feeling of tension is followed by emotional release such as crying or laughing (1–2 hours). Later, perceptual distortions occur, with visual illusions and hallucinations, and occasionally there is fear of ego disintegration (2–3 hours). Major changes in time sense and mood lability then occur (3–4 hours). A feeling of detachment and a sense of destiny and control occur (4–6 hours). Of course, reactions vary among individuals, and some of the current street drugs produce markedly different time frames. Occasionally, the acute episode is terrifying (a "bad trip") which may include panic, depression, confusion, or psychotic symptoms. Preexisting emotional problems, the attitude of the user, and the setting where the drug is used affect the experience.

Treatment of the acute episode primarily involves protection of the individual from erratic behavior that may lead to injury or death. A structured environment is usually sufficient until the drug is metabolized. In severe cases, antipsychotic drugs with minimal side effects (eg, haloperidol, 5 mg intramuscularly) may be given every several hours until the individual has regained control. In cases where "flashbacks" occur (mental imagery from a "bad trip" that is later triggered by mild stimuli such as marihuana, alcohol, or psychic trauma), a short course of an antipsychotic drug (eg, trifluoperazine, 5 mg orally) for several days is usually sufficient. An occasional patient may have "flashbacks" for much longer periods and require small doses of neuroleptic drugs over the longer term.

Phencyclidine
Phencyclidine (PCP, angel dust, peace pill, hog), developed as an anesthetic agent, first appeared as a street drug deceptively sold as tetrahydrocannabinol (THC). Because it is simple to produce and mimics to some degree the traditional psychedelic drugs, it has become a common deceptive substitute for LSD, THC, and mescaline. It is available in crystals, capsules, and tablets to be inhaled, injected, swallowed, or smoked (it is commonly sprinkled on marihuana).

Absorption after smoking is rapid, with onset of symptoms in several minutes and peak symptoms in 15–30 minutes. Mild intoxication produces a euphoria accompanied by a feeling of numbness. Moderate intoxication (5–10 mg) results in disorientation, detachment from surroundings, distortion of body image, combativeness, unusual feats of strength, and loss of ability to integrate sensory input, especially touch and proprioception. Physical symptoms include dizziness, ataxia, dysarthria, nystagmus, retracted upper eyelid with blank stare, hyperreflexia, and tachycardia. There are increases in blood pressure, respiration, muscle tone, and urine production. Usage in the first trimester of pregnancy is associated with an increase in spontaneous abortion and congenital defects. Severe intoxication (20 mg or more) produces an increase in degree of moderate symptoms, with the addition of seizures, deepening coma, hypertensive crisis, and severe psychotic ideation. The drug is particularly long lasting (several days to several weeks) owing to high lipid solubility, gastroenteric recycling, and the production of active metabolites. Overdosage may be directly fatal, with the major causes of death being hypertensive crisis, respiratory arrest, and convulsions. Acute rhabdomyolysis has been reported and can result in myoglobinuric renal failure.

Differential diagnosis involves the whole spectrum of street drugs, since in some ways phencyclidine mimics sedatives, psychedelics, and marihuana in its effects. Blood and urine testing can detect the acute problem.

Treatment is discussed in Chapter 33.

Marihuana

Cannabis sativa, a hemp plant, is the source of marihuana. The parts of the plant vary in potency. The resinous exudate of the flowering tops of the female plant (hashish, charas) is the most potent, followed by the dried leaves and flowering shoots of the female plant (bhang) and the resinous mass from small leaves of inflorescence (ganja). The least potent parts are the lower branches and the leaves of the female plant and all parts of the male plant. Mercury may be a contaminant in marihuana grown in volcanic soil. The drug is usually inhaled by smoking. Effects occur in 10–20 minutes and last 2–3 hours. "Joints" of good quality contain about 500 mg of marihuana (which contains approximately 5–15 mg of tetrahydrocannabinol with a half-life of 7 days). Marihuana soaked in formaldehyde and dried ("AMP") has produced unusual effects, including autonomic discharge and severe, transient cognitive impairment.

With moderate dosage, marihuana produces 2 phases: mild euphoria followed by sleepiness. In the acute state, the user has an altered time perception, less inhibited emotions, impaired immediate memory, and conjunctival injection. High doses produce transient psychotomimetic effects. No specific treatment is necessary except in the case of the occasional "bad trip," in which case the person is treated in the same way as for psychedelic usage. Marihuana frequently aggravates existing mental illness and slows the learning process in children.

Studies of long-term effects have conclusively shown abnormalities in the pulmonary tree. Laryngitis and rhinitis are related to prolonged use, along with chronic obstructive pulmonary disease. Electrocardiographic abnormalities are common, but no long-term cardiac disease has been linked to marihuana use. Chronic usage has resulted in depression of plasma testosterone levels and reduced sperm counts. Abnormal menstruation and failure to ovulate have occurred in some female users. Sudden withdrawal produces insomnia, nausea, myalgia, and irritability. Psychologic effects of chronic marihuana usage are still unclear. Urine testing is reliable if samples are carefully collected and tested. Detection periods span 4–6 days in acute users and 20–50 days in chronic users.

Stimulants

The abuse of stimulants has increased markedly since World War II, partly because of the proliferation of drugs marketed for weight reduction. The **amphetamines,** including methedrine ("speed")—the latest variant is a "smokable" form called "ice," which gives an intense and fairly long-lasting high—methylphenidate, and phenmetrazine, are under prescription control, but street availability remains high. Moderate usage of any of the stimulants produces hyperactivity, a sense of enhanced physical and mental capacity, and sympathomimetic effects. The clinical picture of acute stimulant intoxication includes sweating, tachycardia, elevated blood pressure, mydriasis, hyperactivity, and an acute brain syndrome with confusion and disorientation. Tolerance develops quickly and, as the dosage is increased, paranoid ideation (with delusions of parasitosis), stereotypy, bruxism, and full-blown psychoses occur, often with aggressive responses. Stimulant withdrawal is characterized by depression with symptoms of hyperphagia and hypersomnia.

People who have used stimulants chronically (eg, anorexigenics) occasionally become sensitized ("kindling") to future use of stimulants. In these individuals, even small amounts of mild stimulants such as caffeine can cause symptoms of paranoia and auditory hallucinations.

Cocaine is a stimulant, not a narcotic. It is a product of the coca plant. The derivatives include seeds, leaves, coca paste, cocaine hydrochloride, and the free base of cocaine. Coca paste is a crude extract that contains 40–80% cocaine sulfate and other impurities. Cocaine hydrochloride is the salt and the most commonly used form. Free base, a purer (and stronger) derivative called "crack" is prepared by simple extraction from cocaine hydrochloride.

There are various modes of use. Coca leaf chewing involves toasting the leaves and chewing with alkaline material (eg, the ash of other burned leaves) to enhance buccal absorption. One achieves a mild high, with onset in 5–10 minutes and lasting for about an hour. Intranasal use is simply snorting cocaine through a straw. Absorption is slowed somewhat by vasoconstriction (which may eventually cause tissue necrosis and septal perforation); the onset of action is in 2–3 minutes, with a moderate high (euphoria, excitement, increased energy) lasting about 30 minutes. The purity of the cocaine is a major determinant of the high. Intravenous use of cocaine hydrochloride or free-base cocaine is effective in 30 seconds and produces a short-lasting, fairly intense high of about 15 minutes' duration. Smoking free-base cocaine (volatilized cocaine because of the lower boiling point) acts in seconds and results in an intense high lasting several minutes. The intensity of the reaction is related to the marked lipid solubility of the free-base form and produces by far the most severe medical and psychiatric symptoms.

Cardiovascular collapse, arrhythmias, myocardial infarction, and transient ischemic effects have been reported. Seizures, strokes, hyperthermia, and lung damage may occur, and there are several obstetric complications, including spontaneous abortion, abruptio placentae, teratogenic effects, delayed fetal growth, and prematurity. Cocaine can cause mood swings and delirium, and chronic use can cause the same problems as other stimulants (see above).

Physicians should be alert to cocaine use in patients presenting with unexplained nasal bleeding, headaches, fatigue, insomnia, anxiety, depression, and chronic hoarseness. Sudden withdrawal of the drug is not life-threatening but usually produces craving, sleep disturbances, hyperphagia, lassitude, and severe depression (sometimes with suicidal ideation) lasting days to weeks.

Treatment is imprecise and difficult. Since the high is related to blockage of dopamine reuptake, the dopamine agonist bromocriptine, 1.5 mg orally 3 times a day, alleviates some of the symptoms of craving associated with acute cocaine withdrawal. Other dopamine agonists such as apomorphine, levodopa, and amantadine are under study for this purpose. There is preliminary evidence that carbamazepine in the usual doses reduces craving in withdrawal (probably owing to its effect on kindling), and desipramine in moderate doses has been useful in helping maintain abstinence in the early stages of treatment. Treatment of psychosis is the same as that of any psychosis: antipsychotic drugs in dosages sufficient to alleviate the symptoms. These approaches should be used in conjunction with a structured program, most often based on the AA model. Hospitalization may be required if the self-harm or violence toward others is a perceived threat (usually indicated by paranoid delusions).

Caffeine

The most popular mind-affecting drugs are caffeine, nicotine, and alcohol. Some 10 billion pounds of coffee (the richest source of caffeine) are consumed yearly throughout the world. Tea, cocoa, and cola drinks also contribute to an intake of caffeine that is often astoundingly high in a large number of people. Low and moderate doses (30–200 mg/d) tend to improve some aspects of performance (eg, vigilance). The approximate content of caffeine in a (180-mL) cup of beverage is as follows: brewed coffee, 80–140 mg; instant coffee, 60–100 mg; decaffeinated coffee, 1–6 mg; leaf tea, 30–80 mg; tea bags, 25–75 mg; instant tea, 30–60 mg; cocoa, 10–50 mg; and 12-oz cola drinks, 30–65 mg. A 2-oz chocolate candy bar has about 20 mg. Caffeine-containing analgesics usually contain approximately 30 mg per unit. Symptoms of caffeinism (usually associated with ingestion of over 500 mg/d) include anxiety, agitation, restlessness, insomnia, a feeling of being "wired," and somatic symptoms referable to the heart and gastrointestinal tract. *It is common for a case of caffeinism to present as an anxiety disorder.* It is also common for caffeine and other stimulants to precipitate severe symptoms in compensated schizophrenic and manic-depressive patients. Chronically depressed patients often use caffeine drinks as self-medication. This diagnostic clue may help distinguish some major affective disorders. Withdrawal from caffeine (> 500 mg/d) can produce headaches, irritability, and occasional nausea.

Nicotine

Nicotine is generally taken via snuff, chewing, or smoking tobacco products. While the percentage of people in the USA who smoke tobacco has decreased to about one-third of the population, the use of snuff or chewing tobacco has increased, and tobacco smoking in the rest of the world remains highly prevalent. Nicotine enhances alertness, with later muscular relaxation. It is highly addicting, with abstinence symptoms that include irritability, headache, and lethargy. Withdrawal symptoms may continue for 4–6 weeks, and craving may continue for many months.

Treatment involves some medical approaches such as substitution therapy with nicotine-containing chewing gum (Nicorette), one piece for each cigarette habitually smoked in a 24-hour period, gradually reduced. Clonidine, 0.1–0.4 mg/d orally, reduces symptoms but is still controversial. Many treatment programs combine the above medications with a behavioral approach that can include aversive conditioning or flooding.

Miscellaneous Drugs & Solvents

The principal over-the-counter drugs (OTC) of concern are phenylpropanolamine and an assortment of antihistaminic agents. Frequently, these drugs are sold in combination as cold remedies (eg, Dristan, Triaminic). Not infrequently, a mild analgesic is added to the preparation. Most appetite suppressant drugs are combinations of phenylpropanolamine and caffeine (fenfluramine is an exception); these drugs are also heavily marketed as "stay-awake" drugs. Practically all of the so-called sleep aids are now antihistamines. Scopolamine and bromides have generally been removed from the over-the-counter market.

The major problem in the use of all these drugs relates to phenylpropanolamine, which has all the side effects of any stimulant, including precipitation of anxiety states, increased pressor effect, auditory and visual hallucinations, paranoid ideation, and, occasionally, delirium. Aggressiveness and some loss of impulse control have been reported. Sleep disturbances are common even with reasonably small doses.

Antihistamines usually produce some central nervous system depression—thus their use as over-the-counter sedatives. Drowsiness may be a problem. Antihistamine intoxication can produce excitement. The mixture of antihistamines with alcohol usually exacerbates the central nervous system effects.

The abuse of laxatives sometimes can lead to electrolyte disturbances that may contribute to the manifestations of an organic brain syndrome. The greatest use of laxatives tends to be in the elderly, who are most vulnerable to physiologic changes.

Steroids are being abused by people who wish to increase muscle mass for cosmetic reasons or for greater strength. In addition to the medical problems, there are significant mood swings associated with such abuse.

Amyl nitrite, a drug useful in angina pectoris, has been used in recent years as an "orgasm expander." The changes in time perception caused by the drug prompted its nonmedical use, and popular lore concerning the effects of inhalation just prior to orgasm has led to increased use. Tolerance develops readily, but there are no known withdrawal symptoms. Abstinence for several days reestablishes the previous level of responsiveness. Long-term effects are unknown.

Sniffing of solvents and inhaling of gases (including aerosols) produce a form of inebriation similar to that of the volatile anesthetics. Agents include gasoline, toluene, petroleum ether, lighter fluids, cleaning fluids, paint thinners, solvents for "Scotch Gard," glue, typewriter correction fluids, and nail polish. Typical intoxication states include euphoria, slurred speech, hallucinations, and confusion, and with high doses, acute manifestations are unconsciousness and cardiorespiratory depression or failure; chronic exposure produces a variety of symptoms related to the liver, kidney, or bone marrow. Lead encephalopathy can be associated with sniffing leaded gasoline. In addition, studies of workers chronically exposed to jet fuel showed significant increases in neurasthenic symptoms, including fatigue, anxiety, mood changes, memory difficulties, and somatic complaints. These same problems have been noted in long-term solvent abuse.

The so-called designer drugs are synthetic substitutes for commonly used recreational drugs and are produced in small, clandestine laboratories. The most common designer drugs have been methyl analogues of fentanyl and have been used as heroin substitutes. MDMA, an amphetamine derivative sometimes called "ecstasy," is also a designer drug with high abuse potential and a potential for causing irreversible neurotoxicity. Manufacture and use of these substances are a vexing problem for law enforcement, since the newest drugs have not yet reached an illegal status and there are no tests developed for detection. Furthermore, they present problems for physicians faced with symptoms from a totally unknown cause.

Benowitz NL: Pharmacologic aspects of cigarette smoking and nicotine addiction. N Engl J Med 1988;319:1318.

Gawin FH et al: Desipramine facilitation of initial cocaine abstinence. Arch Gen Psychiatry 1989;46:117. (Relapse rate in cocaine addiction is very high.)

Pollack MH, Brotman AW, Rosenbaum JF: Cocaine abuse and treatment. Compr Psychiatry 1989;30:31.

Schwartz RH: Urine testing in the detection of drugs of abuse. Arch Intern Med 1988;148:2407.

Tzu-Chin W et al: Pulmonary hazards of smoking marijuana as compared with tobacco. N Engl J Med 1988;318:347. (A serious problem about which there is no controversy.)

Westermeyer J: The psychiatrist and solvent-inhalant abuse: Recognition, assessment, and treatment. Am J Psychiatry 1987;144:903. (An often overlooked type of drug abuse.)

Zuckerman B et al: Effects of maternal marijuana and cocaine use on fetal growth. N Engl J Med 1989;320:762.

ORGANIC MENTAL DISORDERS
(Organic Brain Syndrome [OBS])

Essentials of Diagnosis

- Transient or permanent brain dysfunction.
- Cognitive impairment to varying degrees: may include disorientation; impaired recall and recent memory; distorted perception, often with psychotic ideation.
- Emotional disorders frequently present: depression, anxiety, irritability.
- Behavioral disturbances may include problems of impulse control, sexual acting out, aggression, exhibitionism.

General Considerations

The organic problem may be a primary brain disease or a secondary manifestation of some general disorder. All of the brain syndromes show some degree of cognitive impairment depending on the site of involvement, the rate of onset and progression, and the duration of the underlying brain lesion. Emotional disturbances are often inversely proportionate to the severity of the cognitive disorder. The behavioral disturbances tend to be more common with chronicity, more directly related to the underlying personality, and not necessarily correlated with cognitive dysfunction.

Etiology

A. Intoxication: Alcohol, sedatives, bromides, anticholinergic drugs, antidepressants, analgesics (eg, pentazocine), pollutants, psychedelic drugs, salicylates (chronic use), solvents, a wide variety of over-the-counter and prescribed drugs, and household, agricultural, and industrial chemicals.

B. Drug Withdrawal: Withdrawal from alcohol, sedative-hypnotics, corticosteroids.

C. Long-Term Effects of Alcohol: Wernicke-Korsakoff syndrome.

D. Infections: Septicemia; meningitis and encephalitis due to bacterial, viral, fungal, parasitic or tuberculous organisms or to central nervous system syphilis; acute and chronic infections due to the entire range of microbiologic pathogens.

E. Endocrine Disorders: Thyrotoxicosis, hypothyroidism, adrenocortical dysfunction (including Addison's disease and Cushing's syndrome), pheochromocytoma, insulinoma, hypoglycemia from insulin overdose, hyperparathyroidism, hypoparathyroidism, panhypopituitarism, diabetic ketoacidosis.

F. Respiratory Disorders: Hypoxia, hypocapnia, any imbalance in respiratory exchange.

G. Metabolic Disturbances: Fluid and electrolyte disturbances (especially hyponatremia), acid-base disorders, hepatic disease (hepatic encephalopathy, leukodystrophies, Wilson's disease), renal failure, porphyria.

H. Nutritional Deficiencies: Deficiency of vitamin B_1 (beriberi), vitamin B_{12} (pernicious anemia), nicotinic acid (pellagra); protein-calorie malnutrition.

I. Trauma: Subdural hematoma, subarachnoid hemorrhage, intracerebral bleeding, concussion syndrome.

J. Cardiovascular Disorders: Cardiac infarctions, arrhythmias, cerebrovascular spasms, hypertensive encephalopathy, hemorrhages, embolisms, occlusions.

K. Neoplasms: Primary or metastatic lesions of the central nervous system, cancer-induced hypercalcemia.

L. Idiopathic Epilepsy: Ictal and interictal dysfunction.

M. Collagen and Immunologic Disorders: Systemic lupus erythematosus, acquired immunodeficiency syndrome (AIDS), Sjodgren's syndrome.

N. Degenerative Diseases: Alzheimer's disease, Pick's disease, multiple sclerosis, parkinsonism, Huntington's chorea, amyotrophic lateral sclerosis, normal pressure hydrocephalus.

O. Miscellaneous: Tourette's syndrome.

Clinical Findings

The manifestations are many and varied and include problems with orientation, short or fluctuating attention span, loss of recent memory and recall, impaired judgment, emotional lability, lack of initiative, impaired impulse control, inability to reason through problems, depression (worse in mild to moderate types), confabulation (not limited to alcohol organic brain syndrome), constriction of intellectual functions, visual and auditory hallucinations, and delusions. Physical findings will naturally vary according to the cause. The EEG is often abnormal.

A. Delirium: Delirium (acute confusional state) is a transient global disorder of attention, with clouding of consciousness, usually a result of systemic problems (eg, drugs, hypoxemia). Onset is usually rapid. The mental status fluctuates (impairment is usually least in the morning), with varying inability to concentrate, maintain attention, and sustain purposeful behavior. (''Sundowning''—mild to moderate delirium at night—is more common in patients with preexisting dementia and may be precipitated by drugs and sensory deprivation.) There is a marked deficit of short-term memory and recall. Anxiety and irritability are common. Amnesia is retrograde (impaired recall of past memories) and anterograde (inability to recall events after the onset of the delirium). Orientation problems follow the inability to retain information. Perceptual disturbances (often visual hallucinations) and psychomotor restlessness with insomnia are common. Autonomic changes include tachycardia, dilated pupils, and sweating. The average duration is about 1 week, with full recovery in most cases. Delirium can coexist with dementia.

B. Dementia: (See also Chapter 2.) Dementia is characterized by chronicity and deterioration of selective mental functions. Onset is insidious in most cases. Dementia is usually progressive, more common in the elderly (occurring in about 50% of people over age 55), and rarely reversible even if underlying disease can be corrected. Dementia can be classified as cortical or subcortical.

There are 3 types of cortical dementia: (1) primary degenerative dementia, accounting for about 50–60% of cases; (2) atherosclerotic (multi-infarct) dementia, 15–20% of cases; and (3) mixtures of the first 2 types or dementia due to miscellaneous causes, 15–20% of cases (see also Chapter 2). Examples of primary degenerative dementia are Alzheimer's dementia (most common) and Pick, Parkinson, Creutzfeldt-Jakob, and Huntington dementias (less common).

Dementia of the Alzheimer type (DAT) has in many cases a genetic link and is characterized by initial short-term memory loss (both anterograde and retrograde), gradual loss of expressive and comprehensive language (aphasia of a word finding type occurs early), constructional apraxia, visuoperceptual defects, a decreased sense of smell, problem-solving difficulties, and personality changes, including thought disorder (usually paranoid) and increased irritability. There is enormous diversity in symptoms and momentum of the disease. Sudden onset, seizures, gait disturbance, or focal neurologic signs tend to rule out the diagnosis.

Subcortical forms include degeneration of subcortical structures (eg, parkinsonism, HIV infection) and are less likely to be associated with aphasia, agnosia, or loss of higher associative functions but more likely to produce major problems in retrieval of information (very poor on recall but much better at recognition of items), major attention deficits, early arithmetic difficulties, some constructional apraxia, and personality changes in which depression—which imposes an increased suicidal risk— is a major feature (this adversely affects neuropsychologic testing). In both types, loss of impulse control (sexual and language) is common. The tenuous level of functioning makes the individual most susceptible to minor physical and psychologic stresses. The course depends on the underlying cause, and the general trend is steady deterioration.

Pseudodementia is a term applied to depressed patients who appear to be demented. It is occasionally used to include other reversible conditions that mimic dementia (eg, mass lesions, effects of medication). Electroencephalographic sleep data help in differentiating dementia from depression.

C. Amnestic Syndrome: This is a memory disturbance without delirium or dementia. It is usually associated with thiamine deficiency and chronic alcohol use (eg, Korsakoff's syndrome). It impairs selective areas of cognitive functioning. The onset is usually sudden, but the course is usually chronic.

D. Organic Hallucinosis: This condition is characterized by persistent or recurrent hallucinations (usually auditory) without the other symptoms usually found in delirium or dementia. Alcohol or hallucinogens are often the cause. There does not have to be any other mental disorder, and there may be complete spontaneous resolution.

E. Organic Personality Syndrome: This syndrome is characterized by emotional lability and loss of impulse control along with a general change in personality. Cognitive functions are preserved. Social inappropriateness is common. Loss of interest and lack of concern with the consequences of one's actions are often present. The course depends on the underlying cause (eg, frontal lobe contusion may resolve completely).

Differential Diagnosis

Patients with nonorganic ("functional") psychoses usually remain oriented; the onset is usually gradual; hallucinations are usually auditory rather than visual; and intellectual functions are relatively intact, with good memory and a normal EEG and no demonstrable organic disease.

Complications

Chronicity is sometimes a function of early nonreversal, eg, subdural hematoma, low-pressure hydrocephalus. Prompt correction of reversible causes improves recovery of mental function. Accidents secondary to impulsive behavior and poor judgment are a major consideration. Secondary depression and impulsive behavior not infrequently lead to suicide attempts. Drugs, particularly sedatives, may worsen thinking abilities and contribute to the overall problems.

Treatment
(See also Chapter 2.)

A. Medical: Provide a pleasant, comfortable, nonthreatening, and physically safe environment with adequate nursing or attendant services. *Establish the diagnosis and correct underlying medical problems* (electrolyte abnormalities, abnormal thyroid function, etc). Discontinue drugs that may be contributing to the problem (eg, cimetidine, lidocaine, anticholinergic drugs, central nervous system depressants). Do not overlook any possibility of reversible organic disease. Avoid analgesic drugs. Give antipsychotics in small doses at first (eg, haloperidol, 2 mg orally at bedtime) and increase according to the need to reduce psychotic ideation or excessive irritability. Aggressiveness and rage states in central nervous system lesions can be reduced with beta-blockers in moderate doses. Since the serotonergic system has been implicated in arousal conditions, drugs that affect serotonin have been studied and found to be of some benefit in aggression and agitation. Included in this group are lithium, trazodone, and clonazepam. Dopamine blockers (eg, the neuroleptic drugs such as haloperidol) have been used for many years to attenuate aggression, and newer ones such as pimozide show promise for these conditions as well as for the treatment of the motor and phonic tics of Tourette's syndrome. Emotional lability in some cases responds to small doses of imipramine, 25 mg 3 times daily; and depression, which often occurs early in the course of Alzheimer type dementia, responds to the usual doses of antidepressant drugs, preferably those with the least anticholinergic side effects.

Cerebral vasodilators were originally used on the assumption that cerebral arteriosclerosis and ischemia were the principal causes of the dementias. Although there is a slight reduction of blood flow in primary degenerative dementia (probably as a result of the basic disorder), there is no evidence that this is a major factor in this group of disorders or that vasodilators are of value. Ergotoxine alkaloids (Hydergine) have been studied, with mixed results; improvement in ambulatory self-care and depressed mood has been noted, but there has been no improvement of cognitive functioning on any standardized tests. Hyperbaric oxygen treatment has not produced significant improvement. Drugs having a stimulatory effect, such as methylphenidate, may cause affective improvement without a change in cognitive function. The affective improvement can benefit the patient and family by providing some improvement in the quality of life. Numerous investigational drugs have been used, but the responses have been variable and inconsistent.

Failing sensory functions should be supported as necessary, with hearing aids, cataract surgery, etc.

B. Social: Substitute home care, board care, or convalescent home care may be most useful when the family is unable to care for the patient. The setting should include familiar people and objects, lights at night, and a simple schedule. Family counseling may help the family to cope with problems that may occur and may help keep the patient at home as long as possible. Volunteer services, including homemakers, visiting nurses, and adult protective services may be helpful in maintaining the patient at home.

C. Behavioral: Behavioral techniques include operant responses that can be used to induce positive behaviors, eg, paying attention to the patient who is trying to communicate appropriately, and extinction by ignoring inappropriate responses. Alzheimer's patients can learn skills and retain them but do not recall the circumstances in which they were learned.

D. Psychologic: Formal psychologic therapies are not usually helpful and may make things worse by taxing the patient's limited cognitive resources.

Prognosis

The prognosis is good in acute (reversible) cases, fair in moderate cases, and poor in deteriorated states.

Dickson LR, Ranseen JD: An update on selected organic mental syndromes. Hosp Community Psychiatry 1990; 41:290. (Overview of AIDS dementia complex, cocaine abuse, cerebrovascular accident, traumatic brain injury.)

Lipowski ZJ: Delirium (acute confusional states). JAMA 1987;258:1789. (Review article by the leading expert in the field.)

GERIATRIC PSYCHIATRIC DISORDERS
(See also Chapter 2.)

Essentials of Diagnosis

- Some degree of organic brain syndrome often present.
- Depression, paranoid ideation, and easy irritability are common.
- High frequency of medical problems.
- Patient is frequently worsened by a wide variety of medications.
- Loneliness and fear of death are often factors.
- Vague somatic complaints common.

General Considerations

There are 3 basic factors in the process of aging: biologic, sociologic, and psychologic.

The complex **biologic** changes depend on inherited characteristics (the best guarantee of long life is to have long-lived parents), nutrition, declining sensory functions such as hearing or vision, disease, trauma, and life-style. A definite correlation between hearing loss and paranoid ideation exists in the elderly. (See Organic Brain Syndrome, above.) As a person ages, the central nervous system and immune system become less hardy, and relatively minor disorders or combinations of disorders may cause deficits in cognition and affective response. Hypochondriasis is frequently a mechanism of compensating for decreased function. (eg, preoccupation with bowel function).

The **sociologic** factors derive from stresses connected with occupation, family, and community. Any or all of these areas may be disrupted in a general phenomenon of "disengagement" and lack of intimacy that older people experience as friends die, the children move away, and the surroundings become less familiar. Retirement commonly precipitates a major disruption in a well-established life structure. This is particularly stressful in the person whose compulsive devotion to a job has precluded other interests, so that sudden loss of this outlet leaves a void that is not easily filled.

The **psychologic** withdrawal of the elderly person is frequently related to a loss of self-esteem, which is based on the economic insecurity of older age with its congruent loss of independence, the realization of decreasing physical and mental ability, loneliness, and the fear of approaching death. The process of aging is often poorly accepted, and the real or imagined loss of physical attractiveness may have a traumatic impact that the plastic surgeon can only soften for a time. In a culture that stresses physical and sexual attractiveness, it is difficult for most people to accept the change.

Clinical Findings & Complications

The most common psychiatric syndrome in the elderly is organic brain syndrome of varying degree (see Chapter 2). Psychotic ideation (usually paranoid) may coexist with the organic brain syndrome. Frequently, in milder cases, the individual is aware of the deficiency in sensorium and becomes depressed about actual or threatened loss of function. Depression becomes the most obvious symptom. Unless the examination is done with great care, organic brain syndrome is missed, and the patient is treated for the secondary symptom of depression without evaluation of the organic problem.

Overt depression is often related to life exigencies (80% of people over age 65 have some kind of medical problem). Alcoholism is present in approximately 15% of older patients presenting with psychiatric symptoms. The incidence of suicide is higher in elderly people—loneliness, age, and medical problems being directly related. Depression in the absence of a brain syndrome is frequently manifested in the elderly as a somatic complaint without the overt signs of depression (see Affective Disorders, above). Anxiety is often associated with organic illness. In organic brain syndrome, anxiety heightens preexisting confusion.

Abuse of the elderly—both physical neglect (passive) and physical injury (active)—demands early recognition. Bruises, welts, fractures, and debilitation should alert the physician. The battered elderly are probably just as numerous as battered children, but less reported, and require the same diligence in physician recognition.

Polypharmacy (with both prescription and over-the-counter drugs) is a major cause of accidents and illness in the elderly. Cognitive impairment increases as the number of drugs used increases; sedatives are one of the major culprits (eg, overuse in sleep problems). The increased and varied complaints are often an attempt to compensate and divert attention from decreased mental function.

Treatment

A. Social: Socialization, a structured schedule of activities, familiar surroundings, continued achievement, and avoidance of loneliness (probably the most important factor) are some of the major considerations in prevention and amelioration of the psychiatric problems of older age. Whenever possible, the patient should remain in a familiar setting or return to one for as long as possible. An inexorable downhill trend frequently follows dislocation, with the accompanying disengagement from adaptable activities. The patient can be supported in the primary environment by various agencies that can help avoid a premature change of habits. For patients with disabilities that make it difficult to cope with the problems of living alone, homemaker services can assist in continuing the day-to-day activities of the household; visiting nurses can administer medications and monitor the physical condition of the patient; and geriatric social groups can help maintain socialization and human contacts. In the hospital or nursing home, attention to the kinds of people placed in the same room is most important. Attention to the proper mixture of active and inactive people can help relieve the loneliness that so often pervades such placement.

B. Medical: Treatment of any reversible components of an organic brain syndrome is obviously the major medical consideration. One commonly overlooked factor is self-medication, frequently with over-the-counter drugs that further impair the patient's already precarious functioning. Common culprits are antihistamines and anticholinergic drugs.

Any signs of psychosis, such as paranoid ideation and delusions, respond very well to *small amounts* of antipsychotics. Trifluoperazine, 2–5 mg orally once a day, or fluphenazine, 1–2 mg orally daily, will usually decrease psychotic ideation markedly. Associated agitation is usually ameliorated. The use of long-acting fluphenazine for acute paranoid ideation or agitation is appropriate if it is used initially in low dosage (12.5 mg) every 2–3 weeks with close attention to the possibility of extrapyramidal side effects, which are more frequent in the geriatric population.

Judicious use of antipsychotics can often maintain the older person in the home environment and delay the traumatic dislocation that usually worsens the patient's condition. Do not use drugs that cause significant orthostatic hypotension (resulting in dizziness, falls, fractures). Long-acting benzodiazepines, TCAs, and antipsychotic drugs double the possibility of hip fracture in this population. Because of sensitivity to anticholinergic effects, avoid nonpiperazine phenothiazines and unnecessary antiparkinsonism drugs. Sedatives frequently have a worsening effect and should generally be avoided. All psychoactive drugs have a higher incidence of side effects and are metabolized and excreted more slowly in the elderly.

Antidepressants (in one-half to one-third the doses given to young adults) are used when indicated for depression. Monoamine oxidase inhibitors have been particularly valuable in maintenance therapy. Low doses of amitriptyline have been effective in pathologic laughing and weeping, which occur in neurologic conditions such as multiple sclerosis. Infrequently, a stimulant in small doses (eg, methylphenidate, 5–10 mg orally daily) can be used to treat apathy. The stimulant may help increase the patient's energy for social involvement and help the patient to maintain life activities.

When sedatives are to be used, consider triazolam, 0.125 mg orally daily, which has an ultra-short half-life. Sedatives can worsen memory and confusional states in people who are already impaired. The appropriate use of wine and beer for mild sedative effects is quite rewarding in the hospital and other care facilities as well as at home.

C. Behavioral: The impaired cognitive abilities of the geriatric patient necessitate simple behavioral techniques. Positive responses to appropriate behavior encourage the patient to repeat desirable kinds of behavior, and frequent repetition offsets to some degree the defects in recent memory and recall. It also results in participation—a most important element, since there is a tendency in the older population to withdraw, thus increasing isolation and functional decline.

One must be careful not to reinforce and encourage obstreperous behavior by responding to it; in this way, extinction or at least gradual reduction of inappropriate behavior will occur. At the same time, the obstreperous behavior often represents a nondirective response to frustration and inability to function, and a structured program of activity is necessary.

D. Psychologic: Patients may require help in adjusting to changing roles and commitments and in finding new goals and viewpoints. The older person steadily loses an important commodity—the future—and may attempt to compensate for this by preoccupation with the past. Involvement with the present and psychotherapy on a here-and-now basis can help make the adjustment easier.

Blazer D: Depression in the elderly. N Engl J Med 1989;320:164. (A significant problem with or without brain syndrome.)

Lipowski ZJ: Geriatrics: Delirium in the elderly patient. N Engl J Med 1989;320:578.

Montamat SC, Cusack BJ, Vestal RE: Current concepts—Geriatrics: Management of drug therapy in the elderly. N Engl J Med 1989;321:303.

DEATH & DYING

As Thomas Browne said, "The long habit of living indisposeth us for dying." It is only when death comes close to us that we really begin to respond to the possibility of our own death.

Death means different things to different people. For some it may represent an escape from unbearable suffering or other difficulties; for others, entrance into a new transcendental life. Death may come as a narcissistic attempt to find lasting fame or importance in martyrdom or heroic adventure, or it may be an atonement for real or imagined guilt or a means of extorting from others posthumously the affection that was not forthcoming during life.

Often the process is more shattering to those whose charge it is to maintain life, and there is a good deal of question about the so-called agony of death. Some observers, including Sir William Osler, take the view that there is no such thing, and the experiences of people who have been resuscitated from cardiac standstill seem to substantiate his view. They describe a sensation of detachment, a final peaceful "letting go"; and one is at times impressed with the fact that the dying patient resents any interference with the process by physicians and nurses.

How each individual responds to imminent death is a function not only of what death means to that person but also of the mechanisms used to deal with problems—and these are usually the same as those used throughout life. Patients frequently worry more about *how* they will die than about death itself. Responses frequently seen in the dying patient include denial, anger, bargaining, depression, and acceptance—stages that are seen in many people as they go through any significant flux or loss. Seldom are these stages seen in isolation, and the complexity of the process contributes to the juxtaposition of the stages and the noted lability of mood and attitude in the dying patient.

An ill person may at first deny any concern with dying and then later admit to a fear of going to sleep because of the possibility of not waking up. This is often demonstrated by a need to keep the light on and to call frequently during the night with minor complaints. Some find it necessary to deny impending death to the end. Their families and doctors will often join in the conspiracy of denial, either out of sympathy or for their own reasons. It is important not to force the patient to realize the truth but to allow the opportunity, *when the patient is ready*, to discuss and deal with the problem of impending death. Frank discussion can mitigate the terror some patients feel. For many it is a comfort to be actively involved in the process of dying, sharing in the anticipation of death, and making whatever plans may be important. Alleviation of pain is a primary concern of many patients. The physician should not be concerned about addiction to narcotics when treating a dying patient.

The reactions of the family are often a combination of pain, anger, sadness, and depression. They react to each other and to the personnel caring for the patient. The problem to be resolved with the survivors is the guilt feelings they may have—that they continue to exist while the other person has died. Also to be reconciled are the vague sense of being responsible for the death and the subconscious refusal to believe that the person is really dead. The staff must be careful not to alienate the family, because this can result in less than optimum care. Some emotional investment in the patient by the staff is proper and inevitable, but it must be handled with insight and professional restraint. An insecure staff member may respond to a patient's death as if it were a professional failure. If the emotional investment is too little, the staff member may seem to be aloof and insensitive, while overconcern may lead to depression and despair, further impairing the person's capacity to serve as a source of support for the family in a time of distress.

The physician and staff must be aware of their own anxieties; maintain an appropriate level of involvement (a change of physicians may be necessary when this is impossible); allow for free and ongoing communication between patient, physician, and family; and share as a group—staff and family—the impending and unavoidable loss.

Smedra NG et al: Withholding and withdrawal of life support from the critically ill. N Engl J Med 1990;322:309.

PSYCHIATRIC PROBLEMS ASSOCIATED WITH MEDICAL & SURGICAL DISORDERS

Essentials of Diagnosis

Acute problems:

- Psychotic organic brain syndrome secondary to the medical or surgical problem, or compounded by effect of treatment.
- Acute anxiety, often related to ignorance and fear of the immediate problem as well as uncertainty about the future.
- Anxiety as an intrinsic aspect of the medical problem (eg, hyperthyroidism).

Intermediate problems:

- Depression as a function of the illness or acceptance of the illness, often associated with realistic or fantasied hopelessness about the future.
- Behavioral problems, often related to denial of illness and, in extreme cases, causing the patient to leave the hospital against medical advice.

Recuperative problems:

- Decreasing cooperation as the patient sees improvement and is not compelled to follow orders closely.
- Readjustment problems with family, job, and society.

General Considerations

A. Acute Problems:

1. "Intensive care unit psychosis" is a type of delirium that is frequently accompanied by psychotic ideation. It is an expression of organic (frequently including a preexisting organic brain syndrome), psychologic, and environmental factors. Some factors include sleep deprivation, sedative and analgesic medications, alcohol withdrawal, metabolic fluctuations (particularly hypoxemia and hyponatremia), fear, and overstimulation. It is important to consider and recognize the problem early when it is more easily treated. (See Organic Mental Disorders, above.)

2. Pre- and postsurgical anxiety states are common—and commonly ignored. Presurgical anxiety is ubiquitous and is principally a fear of death (note the high number of surgical patients who make out their wills). Patients may be fearful of anesthesia (improved by the preoperative anesthesia interview), the mysterious operating room, and the disease processes that might be uncovered by the surgeon. Such fears frequently cause people to delay examinations that might result in earlier surgery and a greater incidence of cure.

The opposite of this is **surgery proneness,** the quest for surgery to escape from overwhelming life stresses. Polysurgery patients are not easily catego-

rized. Dynamic motivations include narcissism, unconscious guilt, a masochistic need to suffer, an attempt to deal with another family member's illness, and psychogenic pain. More apparent reasons may include an attempt to get relief from pain and a lifestyle that has become almost exclusively medically oriented, with all of the risks entailed in such an endeavor.

Postsurgical anxiety states are usually related to pain, procedures, and loss of body image. Acute pain problems are quite different from chronic pain disorders (see Chronic Pain Disorders, above); the former are readily handled with *adequate* analgesic medication. The alteration in body image is particularly difficult for mastectomy patients. Any procedure that results in a stoma has the attendant ramifications of odor, excretion bag, and concern about intimate relationships with others.

3. Iatrogenic problems usually pertain to medications, complications of diagnostic and treatment procedures, and impersonal and unsympathetic staff behavior. Polypharmacy is often a factor. Patients with unsolved diagnostic problems are at higher risk. They are desirous of relief, and the quest engenders more diagnostic procedures with a higher incidence of complications. The upset patient and family may be very demanding. Negative responses or a lack of attention by the staff to excessive demands may result in complications that escape the attention of the staff. Experience teaches medical personnel to appreciate that obstreperous behavior or excessive demands usually result from anxiety. Such behavior is best handled with calm and measured responses.

B. Intermediate Problems:

1. Prolonged hospitalization presents unique problems in certain hospital services, eg, burn units, orthopedic services, and tuberculosis wards. The acute problems of the severely burned patient are discussed in Chapter 32. The problems often are behavioral difficulties related to length of hospitalization and necessary procedures. For example, in burn units, pain is a major problem in addition to anxiety about procedures. Debridement and grafting seem neverending to the patient, who is angry about and becoming resistant to immobilization and apparent lack of progress. This is especially true for people who have led an unencumbered life-style. Disputes with staff are common and often concern pain medication or ward privileges. Some patients regress to infantile behavior and dependency. Staff members must agree about their approach to the patient in order to ensure the smooth functioning of the unit.

2. Depression frequently intervenes during this period. It can contribute to irritability and overt anger. Severe depression can lead to anorexia, which further complicates healing and metabolic balance. It is during this period that the issue of disfigurement arises. Relief at survival gives way to concern about future function and appearance.

C. Recuperative Problems:

1. Anxiety about return to the outside world can cause regression to a dependent position. Complications increase, and staff forbearance again is tested. Anxiety at this stage usually is handled more easily than previous behavior problems.

2. Posthospital adjustment is related to the severity of the deficits and the use of outpatient facilities (eg, physical therapy, rehabilitation programs, psychiatric outpatient treatment). In a broad sense, the issue of "survivorship"—attention to the quality of life in someone who had or has a major illness. Some patients may experience posttraumatic stress symptoms. Lack of appropriate follow-up can contribute to depression in the patient, who may feel that he or she is making poor progress and may have thoughts of "giving up." Reintegration into work, educational, and social endeavors may be painfully slow. Life is simply much more difficult when one is disfigured, disabled, or disfranchised.

Clinical Findings

The symptoms that occur in these patients are similar to those discussed in previous sections of this chapter, eg, organic brain syndrome, anxiety, and depression. Behavior problems may include lack of cooperation, increased complaints, demands for medication, sexual approaches to nurses, threats to leave the hospital, and actual signing out against medical recommendations. The underlying personality structure of the individual is a major factor in coping styles (eg, compulsive increases indecision, hysterical increases dramatic behavior).

Differential Diagnosis

Organic brain syndrome must always be ruled out, since it often presents with symptoms resembling anxiety, depression, or psychosis. Personality disorders existing prior to hospitalization often underlie the various behavior problems, but particularly the management problems.

Complications

Prolongation of hospitalization causes increased expense, deterioration of patient-staff relationships, and increased probabilities of iatrogenic and legal problems. The possibility of increasing posthospital treatment problems is enhanced.

Treatment

A. Medical: The most important consideration by far is to have *one* physician in charge, a physician whom the patient trusts and who is able to oversee multiple treatment approaches (see Somatoform Disorders, above). In the acute problems, attention must be paid to metabolic imbalance, alcohol withdrawal, and previous drug use—prescribed, recreational, or over-the-counter. Adequate sleep and analgesia are important in the prevention of delirium.

Most physicians are attuned to the early detection of the surgery-prone patient. Plastic and orthopedic surgeons are at particular risk. Appropriate consultations may help detect some problems and mitigate future ones.

Postsurgical anxiety states can be alleviated by personal attention from the surgeon. Anxiety is not so effectively lessened by ancillary medical personnel, whom the patient perceives as lesser authorities, until after the physician has reassured the patient. Inappropriate use of "as needed" analgesia places an unfair burden on the nurse. "Patient-controlled analgesia" can improve pain control, decrease anxiety, and minimize side effects.

Depression should be recognized early. If severe, it may be treated by antidepressant medications (see Antidepressant Drugs, above). High levels of anxiety can be lowered with *judicious* use of anxiolytic agents. Unnecessary medications tend to reinforce the patient's impression that there must be a serious illness or medication would not be required.

B. Psychologic: Prepare the patient for what is to come. This includes the types of units where the patient will be quartered, the procedures that will be performed, and any disfigurements that will result from surgery. Often because of anxiety, a great number of patients do not really listen to these explanations and are greatly surprised after surgery. Explanations with other family members present *on several occasions* may be necessary, since repetition gives the patient time to digest the information and ask further questions. The nursing staff can be helpful, since patients frequently confide a lack of understanding to a nurse but are reluctant to do so to the physician.

Denial of illness is frequently a block to acceptance of treatment. This, too, should be handled with family members present (to help the patient face the reality of the situation) in a series of short interviews (for reinforcement). Dependency problems resulting from long hospitalization are best handled by focusing on the changes to come as the patient makes the transition to the outside world. Key figures are teachers, vocational counselors, and physical therapists. Challenges should be realistic and practical and handled in small steps.

Depression is usually related to the loss of familiar hospital supports, and the outpatient therapists and counselors help to lessen the impact of the loss. Some of the impact can be alleviated by anticipating, with the patient and family, the signal features of the common depression to help prevent the patient from assuming a permanent sick role (invalidism).

Suicide is always a concern when a patient is faced with despair. An honest, compassionate, and supportive approach will help sustain the patient during this trying period.

C. Behavioral: Prior desensitization can significantly allay anxiety about medical procedures. A "dry run" can be done to reinforce the oral description.

Cooperation during acute problem periods can be enhanced by the use of appropriate reinforcers such as a favorite nurse or *helpful* family member. People who are positive reinforcers are even more helpful during the intermediate phases when the patient becomes resistant to the seemingly endless procedures (eg, debridement of burned areas).

Specific situations (eg, psychologic dependency on the respirator) can be corrected by weaning with appropriate reinforcers (eg, a loved one allowed in the room whenever the patient is disconnected from the respirator). Behavioral approaches should be done in a positive and optimistic way for maximal reinforcement.

D. Social: A change in environment requires adaptation. Because of the illness, admission and hospitalization may be more easily handled than discharge. Reintegration into society can be difficult. In some cases, the family is a negative influence. A predischarge evaluation must be made to determine whether the family will be able to cope with the physical or mental changes in the patient. Working with the family while the patient is in the acute stage may presage a successful transition later on.

A positive work situation is critical to the restoration of self-esteem. In many cases, the previous form of employment is no longer available. Vocational counseling can provide new career directions. It should be started in the hospital as early as possible and may include the occupational therapists.

Development of a new social life can be facilitated by various self-help organizations (eg, the stoma club). Sharing problems with others in similar circumstances eases the return to a social life which may be quite different from that prior to the illness.

Prognosis

The prognosis is good in all patients who have reversible medical and surgical conditions. It is guarded when there is serious functional loss that impairs vocational, educational, or societal possibilities—especially in the case of progressive and ultimately life-threatening illness.

White PF: Use of patient-controlled analgesia for management of acute pain. JAMA 1988;259:243. (An improved approach.)

REFERENCES

Abrams R: *Electroconvulsive Therapy*. Oxford Univ Press, 1988.

Drugs that cause psychiatric symptoms. Med Lett Drugs Ther 1989;31:113. (Excellent compendium.)

Grilly DM: *Drugs and Human Behavior*. Allyn & Bacon, 1989.

Robins LN, Barrett JE (editors): *The Validity of Psychiatric Diagnoses*. Raven Press, 1989.

Siegel RK: *Intoxication: Life in Pursuit of Artificial Paradise*. Dutton, 1989.

Schuckit M: *Drug and Alcohol Abuse: A Clinical Diagnosis and Treatment*, 3rd ed. Plenum Press, 1989.

Zonderman AB, Costa PT, McCrae RR: Depression as a risk for cancer morbidity and mortality in a nationally representative sample. JAMA 1989;262:1191. (Challenges some established myths.)

Endocrine Disorders

20

Carlos A. Camargo, MD

Concepts of the endocrine system, the mechanisms of action of hormones, the complex interrelationships among hormones in maintaining our internal milieu, and the diagnosis and therapy of disorders of the endocrine glands continue to undergo radical changes. The line separating a hormone from other information-carrying molecules is becoming a tenuous one. This chapter, however, deals with the classically accepted hormonal systems.

It is now clear that all hormones regulate intracellular mechanisms responsible for the production of cellular proteins and that the induction or activation of these proteins is responsible for the effects of the hormones. Many hormones have predecessors without biologic activity and that these "prohormones" must be transformed into active moieties. These changes may take place inside the endocrine gland itself (eg, many pituitary hormones), in other tissues peripheral in location such as liver or kidney (eg, vitamin D transformations), or inside the target organ cell (eg, testosterone-dihydrotestosterone transformation in prostatic cells). It is also possible for a hormone to exert most of its actions via a mediator formed in another organ (eg, growth hormone → IGF-I).

Hormones attach to cells via specific receptors found either on the surface of the cells (most peptide hormones) or inside the cell (steroid and thyroid hormones). The importance of these receptors in modern concepts of endocrine function cannot be overemphasized. Our understanding of disease processes in endocrinology is currently being greatly enhanced by knowledge of the dynamic aspects of hormone receptors, their modulation and control, and endocrine abnormalities.

Muldoon TG, Evans AC Jr: Hormones and their receptors. Arch Intern Med 1988;148:961.

COMMON PRESENTING COMPLAINTS

Delayed Growth

Normal growth is a complex process resulting from the interplay of multiple hormonal, metabolic, nutri-

tional, genetic, and environmental factors. Normal growth requires, among other things, a normal chromosomal complement; normal cardiovascular, renal, and gastrointestinal systems; adequate diet and exercise; and the absence of harmful drugs or toxins. The possible causes of growth failure are multiple, and determination of the cause requires comprehensive evaluation of the entire patient, not just of the endocrine status.

Bone diseases such as rickets as well as nutritional, metabolic, emotional, and chronic cardiorespiratory, gastrointestinal, hematologic, or renal disorders may delay growth. A common cause of short stature in girls is Turner's syndrome: look for sexual infantilism, webbing of the neck, and other signs of this chromosomal disorder. There are many variants of Turner's syndrome without somatic anomalies. Chromosomal analysis is often required for diagnosis.

Hormonal abnormalities to be considered include the following:

A. Juvenile Hypothyroidism: Thyroid deficiency in children may be subtle and difficult to recognize clinically. It should be suspected whenever a growth chart shows arrest in a previously normally growing child. The most common cause is Hashimoto's thyroiditis. Skeletal maturation is delayed. Low serum thyroxine and elevated TSH levels confirm the diagnosis.

B. Glucocorticoid Excess: Cushing's syndrome, whether naturally occurring or due to exogenous glucocorticoid administration, in childhood or adolescence is always associated with growth retardation. Look for red or violaceous striae, centripetal obesity, and easy bruisability. If the diagnosis is in doubt, perform a screening test such as the overnight dexamethasone suppression test. If the results reveal an abnormality, a complete evaluation is indicated.

C. Gonadal Steroid Excess: Precocious puberty and pseudoprecocious puberty, of whatever origin, are associated with early rapid growth and premature epiphyseal closure, resulting in short final stature. Look for signs of masculinization or feminization. If gonadal steroid excess is suspected, a complete workup is indicated.

D. Hypopituitarism: Any disease of the hypothalamus or the pituitary, with the exception of pituitary growth hormone-secreting tumors, is capable of impairing growth. Ask in detail about a history of headaches, visual disturbances, or polyuria. Remember that craniopharyngiomas are common in childhood and adolescence. Modern imaging techniques (CT scan, MRI) will detect pituitary and hypothalamic disease in the early stages. If pituitary disease is suspected, a complete endocrine evaluation is in order.

E. Monotropic Lack of Growth Hormone: This syndrome is a common cause of dwarfism. It is often "idiopathic" in that no specific cause such as neoplasia, infection, vascular disease, or anatomic abnormality is ever found. A hypothalamic defect may be found. Many of these patients are able to synthesize growth hormone when growth hormone-releasing factor is administered.

F. Other Syndromes Affecting Growth: In addition to the disorders mentioned, there are a myriad of rare syndromes, most of them heritable, in which deficient growth is one feature. These include genetic syndromes causing deafness or facial or limb anomalies, mental retardation, or retinitis pigmentosa.

Excessive Growth

Excessive growth may be a familial or ethnic characteristic or a physiologic event (eg, the growth spurt of puberty) as well as a sign of endocrine disease. If precocious genital development occurs, consider true precocity due to pituitary or hypothalamic disorders, or pseudoprecocious puberty due to excess of adrenal, ovarian, or testicular hormones (often due to tumors). These patients, if not treated rapidly, will eventually be of short stature as a result of premature closure of their epiphyses. The administration of a synthetic luteinizing hormone-releasing hormone (LHRH, GnRH) analogue has recently been shown to be effective in suppressing gonadotropin secretion in cases of true precocious puberty. Pituitary tumors secreting excess growth hormone cause gigantism if present before puberty and acromegaly if growth hormone excess occurs after closure of the epiphyseal plates of long bones. A few cases of nonpituitary "cerebral gigantism" have been described. Marfan's syndrome should also be considered. Klinefelter's syndrome and its variants can also be associated with tall stature. Individuals with XYY genotype are often tall and may exhibit mental retardation and antisocial behavior. Purely hypogonadal individuals tend to be tall, with eunuchoid proportions (span exceeds height; excessive length of floor-to-pubis segment of body).

Obesity

Although obesity is a common presenting "endocrine" complaint, the overwhelming majority of cases are due to excessive food intake or physical inactivity, or both. There is some experimental evidence favoring the concept that there may be slightly different rates of thermogenesis in obese and nonobese individuals, but the matter remains controversial. Recent studies

of twins separated soon after birth have emphasized the importance of genetic factors in obesity. Likewise, separated twin studies indicate that there is an important genetic predisposition to obesity. It is clear, however, that obesity is *always* the result of a positive energy balance and will not occur if "excess" calories are not ingested. This is true for *all* types of obesity.

Endocrine causes of obesity are uncommon. A rapid onset of massive obesity associated with lethargy or polyuria suggests a hypothalamic lesion. Some cases of obesity are associated with delayed puberty. Hypothyroidism is usually *not* associated with marked obesity. In Cushing's disease or syndrome, there is roundness of the face with a characteristic "buffalo hump" and trunk obesity with thin extremities. Striae are common with any type of obesity. They are wider (> 10 mm) and more violaceous in Cushing's syndrome. Amenorrhea, hypertension, and glucose intolerance are commonly associated with obesity and often improve after adequate weight loss. Insulin-secreting adenomas are often associated with weight gain, but these are quite rare. Rare causes of obesity include Prader-Willi syndrome (with mental retardation, hypotonia, and hypogonadism) and Laurence-Moon-Biedl syndrome (with retinitis pigmentosa, polydactyly, and hypogonadism). In most instances, the obese patient requires increased activity and reduction in caloric intake, and all such patients require sympathetic understanding and reinforcement of motivation.

Wasting & Weakness

Nonendocrine causes such as occult cancer, depression, anorexia nervosa, dietary fanaticism, gastrointestinal malabsorption, etc, should always be considered first. Hypopituitarism is only rarely associated with cachexia. Diabetes mellitus, thyrotoxicosis, pheochromocytoma, and Addison's disease are often accompanied by progressive weight loss.

Abnormal Skin Pigmentation or Color

Increased skin pigmentation is often present in conditions associated with ACTH excess such as Addison's disease. It may be very marked after bilateral adrenalectomy for Cushing's disease (Nelson's syndrome). Pregnancy and, less frequently, the ingestion of oral contraceptives may be associated with spotty brown pigmentation, especially over the face (chloasma). Nonendocrine conditions such as sprue, chronic iron deposition, chronic ingestion of chlorpromazine, arsenic poisoning, etc, may also be associated with hyperpigmentation, which is common also in severe malnutrition.

Vitiligo is frequent in Addison's disease and is often associated with autoimmune endocrinopathies.

Hypertrichosis & Hirsutism

Hypertrichosis and hirsutism are disorders involving increased growth of body hair. It is important to distinguish between the two.

A. Hypertrichosis: Hypertrichosis is a disorder in which there is a generalized increase in body hair, including areas that are *not* androgen-sensitive, such as the arms and legs, the forehead, and the eyebrows. The disorder occurs in both men and women. Hypertrichosis is seen rarely in patients with porphyria cutanea tarda, sometimes in patients with anorexia nervosa, and in patients taking phenytoin, diazoxide, or minoxidil. There is no known endocrine abnormality underlying hypertrichosis in these cases.

B. Hirsutism: In hirsutism, excess androgen causes **vellus hair** follicles, which produce fine, short, nonpigmented hairs, to become **terminal hair** follicles, which produce coarse, long, pigmented hairs. This occurs only in areas of the body sensitive to the effects of androgens (mainly testosterone), eg, the face, chest, and lower abdomen. This disorder occurs only in women. In diagnosing hirsutism, racial, familial, and individual differences must be taken into account (eg, Native American women have much less body hair than southern European or eastern Mediterranean women). If the increased hair growth began at puberty and is not progressing, if there are no signs of virilization, and if menstruation is regular, the process is probably benign.

Laboratory evaluation of hirsutism may include levels of serum testosterone, androstenedione (peripheral conversion of which accounts for 40–60% of circulating testosterone levels), LH, FSH, and prolactin.

1. Idiopathic and familial hirsutism–These are the most common forms of hirsutism. In the idiopathic form (hirsutism for which no metabolic cause can be found), there may be increased skin sensitivity to androgens. Familial or genetic hirsutism is evident in certain family or ethnic groups in which women tend to have a greater proportion of terminal facial or body hair (eg, eastern Mediterranean peoples). Localized treatment such as electrolysis, depilatory agents, bleaching compounds, and shaving are usually effective.

2. True hirsutism–True hirsutism is always caused by a relative or absolute excess of androgen, which may be of adrenal or ovarian origin, or both. This excess cannot always be demonstrated by laboratory tests; the free, non-protein-bound fraction of plasma testosterone is the most sensitive test. Adrenal disorders such as Cushing's syndrome are easily ruled out on the basis of the history, physical examination, and dexamethasone suppression test. Late-onset congenital adrenal hyperplasia (deficiency of 21-hydroxylase or 11β-hydroxylase) can be diagnosed by measuring the steroid precursors immediately before the enzymatic block (17-hydroxyprogesterone and 11-deoxycortisol, respectively). ACTH stimulation is sometimes necessary to demonstrate the defect. Obesity may cause a previously asymptomatic defect to become apparent. 11-Hydroxylase deficiency is often associated with hypertension and hypokalemia. Satisfactory results are obtained with adrenal suppression (dexamethasone, 0.5–0.75 mg/d at bedtime).

Other systemic agents used for symptomatic therapy of hirsutism are androgen antagonists such as cimetidine, spironolactone, and, in Europe, cyproterone acetate. Results are variable and experience inconclusive.

3. Ovarian abnormalities–Other common causes of hirsutism are ovarian abnormalities such as polycystic ovary syndrome. This syndrome is accompanied by menstrual irregularities or amenorrhea, increased free plasma testosterone, decreased sex steroid-binding globulin, a high LH to FSH ratio ($>$ 2), and multiple ovarian cysts. The hirsutism often responds to chronic ovarian suppression with an oral contraceptive agent.

4. Ovarian and adrenal tumors– Androgen-secreting ovarian and adrenal tumors are rare causes of hirsutism, but the possibility should always be taken into account. A sudden onset of hirsutism is suggestive, as well as signs of increased muscle mass, frontal balding, deepening of the voice, enlargement of the clitoris, and amenorrhea. The plasma testosterone is usually markedly elevated ($>$ 150 ng/dL). Urinary 17-ketosteroids are usually also markedly elevated in adrenal tumors causing hirsutism. Plasma levels of dehydroepiandrosterone (DHEA) sulfate are almost always high in adrenal tumors and normal in ovarian tumors. Pelvic and adrenal CT scan and ovarian ultrasound often localize the tumor. Surgical removal of the neoplasm is often curative, but the patient should be warned that it may be years before the hair pattern returns to normal.

5. Hyperprolactinemia–A rare cause of hirsutism is hyperprolactinemia, which can result in excessive production of adrenal androgens. If a prolactinoma is demonstrated, surgical resection or bromocriptine therapy is in order.

Rittmaster RS, Loriaux DL: Hirsutism. Ann Intern Med 1987;106:95.

Change in Appetite

Polyphagia (associated with polydipsia and polyuria) is classically found in uncontrolled diabetes mellitus. However, excessive eating is usually not an endocrine problem but a compulsive personality trait. Only rarely is it due to a hypothalamic lesion, in which case it is associated with somnolence and other signs of the hypothalamic disease, eg, hypogonadism. Excessive appetite with weight loss is observed in thyrotoxicosis; polyphagia with weight gain may rarely indicate acromegaly or hypoglycemia due to an insulin-secreting islet cell adenoma.

Anorexia and nausea associated with weight loss and diarrhea may occur at the onset of addisonian crisis or uncontrolled diabetic acidosis. Weight loss due to anorexia plus increased metabolic rate is often seen in patients with pheochromocytoma. Anorexia and nausea with constipation are found with any state of hypercalcemia, eg, hyperparathyroidism.

Polyuria & Polydipsia

Polyuria, often associated with polydipsia, is commonly of nonendocrine origin, resulting from a habit of drinking excessive water (psychogenic). However, if it is severe and of sudden onset, it suggests diabetes mellitus or diabetes insipidus. Diabetes insipidus may develop insidiously or may appear suddenly after head trauma or brain surgery. Lithium and demeclocycline may induce polyuria by interfering with the renal action of ADH.

Polyuria and polydipsia are frequently seen in any state of hypercalcemia, such as hyperparathyroidism, and are also part of the syndrome of hypokalemic nephropathy, such as can occur in disorders of mineralocorticoid excess. Polyuria may occur in renal tubular disorders, such as renal tubular acidosis and Fanconi's syndrome, as well as in a multitude of renal diseases associated with damage to the medullary interstitium that is responsible for establishing the osmotic gradient required for concentration of urine.

Gynecomastia

Gynecomastia, or breast enlargement in men, is fairly common. It is a physiologic phenomenon during puberty, when at least half of males experience enlargement of one or both breasts. Pubertal hypertrophy is characterized by a tender discoid enlargement of breast tissue 2–3 cm in diameter beneath the areola; it usually subsides spontaneously within a year. Gynecomastia is also common among elderly men, particularly when there is associated weight gain; however, the exact incidence in men who are not suffering from hepatic, renal, or cardiac disease or are not taking drugs causing breast enlargement has not been ascertained. Gynecomastia can be the first sign of a serious disorder such as a testicular tumor, and medical evaluation is always indicated when breast enlargement occurs. Carcinoma of the male breast is an extremely rare cause of gynecomastia. It is more common, however, in patients with Klinefelter's syndrome.

The causes of gynecomastia are multiple and diverse (Table 20–1). A search for a common mechanism has not been successful. A number of researchers believe that in many cases (but not all), an altered androgen/estrogen ratio causes changes in cellular elements in breast tissue. This could be due to the following mechanisms: (1) A decrease in production of androgen (all cases of male hypogonadism; see Table 20–13). (2) An increase in estrogen formation (adrenal or testicular tumors, excessive gonadotropin secretion, hyperthyroidism, hepatic disease). (3) A decrease in sensitivity of breast tissue to androgens (hereditary states of androgen resistance such as Reif-

Table 20–1. Causes of gynecomastia.

Physiologic causes	Drugs (cont'd)
Neonatal period	Methyldopa
Puberty	Metoclopramide
Aging	Penicillamine
Drugs	Phenothiazines
Alcohol	Reserpine
Alkylating agents	Spironolactone
Amphetamines	Testosterone
Busulfan	Tricyclic antidepressants
Chorionic gonadotropin	**Endocrine diseases**
Cimetidine	Male hypogonadism
Clomiphene	Hyperthyroidism
Cyclophosphamide	Androgen resistance syn-
Diazepam	dromes
Diethylstilbestrol	**Systemic diseases**
Digitalis	Chronic liver disease
Estrogens	Chronic renal disease
Ethionamide	Refeeding after starvation
Heroin	**Neoplasias**
Hydroxyzine	Testicular tumors
Isoniazid	Adrenal tumors
Ketoconazole	Bronchogenic carcinoma
Marihuana	Carcinoma of the breast
Meprobamate	Hepatoma (rare)
Methadone	**Idiopathic**

enstein's syndrome, complications of drugs such as cimetidine or spironolactone).

It is theoretically possible that increased tissue sensitivity to estrogens may also cause gynecomastia. This mechanism has been postulated by some to account for idiopathic gynecomastia.

Many drugs induce gynecomastia by a variety of mechanisms. Estrogens or drugs having estrogenic effects (diethylstilbestrol, marihuana, digitalis, possibly heroin) are one group. Other drugs cause liver damage, which in turn can result in hyperestrogenemia (alcohol, isoniazid). A few drugs cause damage to the testicle or block the synthesis of testosterone by Leydig cells, with resulting hypotestosteronemia (cyclophosphamide, spironolactone, ketoconazole). Others (phenothiazines) induce hyperprolactinemia, with a resulting decrease in gonadotropin and testosterone secretion. It is paradoxic that testosterone itself can produce gynecomastia when given parenterally as testosterone esters over the long term. This is due to increased peripheral conversion of testosterone by aromatases to estradiol. Undoubtedly, some drugs produce gynecomastia by a combination of mechanisms. The mechanism of action has not yet been found in some drugs (busulfan, penicillamine, diazepam).

The history and physical examination will often clarify the cause of gynecomastia. An adolescent with slight gynecomastia or a patient with prostatic carcinoma taking diethylstilbestrol needs no further study. Careful examination of the testes is mandatory to look for a testicular tumor. The small, firm testes of Klinefelter's syndrome are characteristic. Eunuchoid features, signs of liver disease, or the enlarged thyroid of Graves' disease are also helpful.

Laboratory investigation of unclear cases should include the following:

(1) A chest x-ray to search for metastatic or primary lung tumors.

(2) Measurements of plasma levels of the beta subunit of human chorionic gonadotropin (hCG). High levels may lead to finding a choriocarcinoma or other hCG-secreting tumors.

(3) Measurements of plasma testosterone and luteinizing hormone (LH) are valuable in the diagnosis of primary or secondary hypogonadism. A high testosterone level may be seen in hyperthyroidism (due to increased sex steroid-binding protein). High testosterone levels *plus* high LH levels should alert the physician to the possibility of androgen resistance.

(4) Serum estradiol is often measured but is usually normal. Many estrogens and substances with estrogen activity are *not* detected by the estradiol radioimmunoassay. Other laboratory tests such as serum prolactin, thyroid function, and chromosomal analysis should not be performed indiscriminately but can be valuable when clinically indicated.

The treatment of gynecomastia is that of the underlying condition. It can be surgically corrected if aesthetic or psychologic considerations so indicate.

Abnormal Lactation

Lactation may rarely be seen as part of the syndrome of pseudocyesis. It is frequently present in acromegaly and, more rarely, in thyrotoxicosis and myxedema. A common cause of the galactorrhea-amenorrhea syndrome is a prolactin-secreting tumor of the pituitary gland. The level of serum prolactin is usually above 100 ng/mL in these patients (see Clinical Disorders of Prolactin Secretion). CT scan or MRI allows visualization of small pituitary adenomas. Galactorrhea may also occur after pituitary stalk section. It can occur after thoracotomy or other injuries to the chest wall as well as after breast surgery. Abnormal lactation occurs rarely with estrogen-secreting adrenal tumors and quite rarely with corpus luteum cysts and choriocarcinoma. Many drugs (phenothiazines, antihypertensive agents such as reserpine and methyldopa, estrogen-containing medications such as oral contraceptives, etc) may produce lactation. Serum prolactin levels are high in many patients with galactorrhea, and they can be used to evaluate the response to therapy.

If the serum prolactin is normal, the condition is usually benign (idiopathic galactorrhea); it is interesting to note that galactorrhea ceases in many of these patients with bromocriptine therapy.

Precocious Puberty
(in Both Sexes)

Precocious puberty is often a normal variant or a familial trait, but it may indicate serious organic disease. One must differentiate true precocity (caused by release of pituitary gonadotropins) from pseudopre-

cocity. At times there is only premature breast development ("thelarche") or only premature appearance of pubic and axillary hair ("adrenarche") with normal subsequent menarche. Hypothalamic lesions, encephalitis, hydrocephalus, and certain tumors (eg, hamartoma of the tuber cinereum, pineal tumors) may cause true sexual precocity. Precocious puberty also occurs in girls who have associated fibrous dysplasia of bone and pigment spots (McCune-Albright syndrome). Adrenal hyperplasia or tumor and gonadal tumors usually cause pseudoprecocious puberty with virilization or feminization. Hepatomas, chorioepitheliomas, and pineal germinomas may produce human chorionic gonadotropin (hCG) and may rarely cause isosexual precocity in males. Reversible precocity with lactation and pituitary enlargement may be seen in juvenile hypothyroidism. The cause must be detected early, since untreated children with precocious puberty will eventually be short or even dwarfed as a result of premature closure of the epiphyses, and because many of the tumors responsible for precocious puberty are potentially malignant.

Sexual Infantilism
& Delayed Puberty

It is often difficult to differentiate between simple functional delay of puberty (often a familial trait) and organic causes for such delays. Any type of gonadal or genetic defect may manifest itself primarily by failure of normal sexual development (see Diseases of the Testes, and Diseases of the Ovaries). Many patients grow to eunuchoid proportions, with span exceeding height. Hypothalamic lesions may be responsible, especially if familial and associated with loss of sense of smell (Kallmann's syndrome). Other causes include craniopharyngioma, pituitary tumors, defective testes or ovaries, Turner's syndrome, and Klinefelter's syndrome). The serum gonadotropins are very helpful in determining the site of disease. If high, they point to the gonad as the defective organ. Chromosomal disorders should be ruled out by chromosomal analysis. It should be remembered that systemic disorders such as malnutrition or chronic renal, cardiac, or gastrointestinal disease may also be associated with delayed puberty.

Impotence & Lack
of Libido in Males

Erectile impotence is a frequent, complex problem. Psychogenic factors are less important in causing impotence than formerly believed and endocrine, vascular, and neurologic abnormalities are more important. Hypogonadism of whatever origin (Table 20–13) is associated with lack of libido and consequent erectile dysfunction. These can also be the first clinical manifestations of a hyperprolactinemic disorder (Table 20–4). Other endocrine causes of impotence include hyperthyroidism, Addison's disease, and acromegaly.

Diabetes mellitus is a very common cause; as many as 50% of males seen in outpatient diabetic clinics suffer from erectile dysfunction. In the past, this was thought to be due to autonomic neuropathy. Arteriosclerotic disease leading to decrease of penile blood flow is a more frequent cause. Vascular disease is also a frequent factor in impotence in elderly men. Any debilitating systemic disorder (eg, heart failure, renal insufficiency, infections, cancer) can cause impotence at any age.

A history of drug use is extremely important. Many pharmacologic agents are known to cause impotence through a variety of mechanisms; some interfere directly with the neural erectile reflex, and a few induce hyperprolactinemia or interfere with testosterone action (Table 20–2). For many drugs, the mechanism is not known. All drugs that are associated with impotence are variable in effect, with some patients developing severe impotence with a given dose and others retaining normal erectile function with double that dose. The reasons for this are not known. If the cause is in doubt, the suspected offending agent should be discontinued and the patient's response evaluated.

Techniques such as monitoring of nocturnal penile tumescence, Doppler penile blood flow analysis, and bulbocavernosus reflex timing have been helpful in distinguishing "organic" from "psychogenic" impotence. Overlap does occur, however, and organic impotence can cause psychologic problems (fear of failure, performance anxiety) that persist even after the underlying disorder has been treated.

Treatment will vary with the cause. Testosterone administration is helpful in hypogonadal states. Bromocriptine is useful in hyperprolactinemic syndromes. Revascularization procedures can be effective in selected cases when performed by expert technicians. A variety of penile prostheses are now available for surgical implantation in patients not responsive to medical or psychologic therapy. Several psychologic therapeutic approaches can be tried for patients found to have no evidence of organic disease. Several mechanical devices to help produce and maintain erection are now available. The rate of success is variable. Intrapenile injections of papaverine and other vasoactive agents have also been used to induce erections of long duration. Priapism has been a serious complication.

Table 20–2. Drugs causing impotence.

Alcohol	Methadone
Atropine	Methyldopa
Barbiturates	Monoamine oxidase inhibitors
Chlordiazepoxide	Phenothiazines
Cimetidine	Phenoxybenzamine
Clonidine	Propranolol
Diazepam	Reserpine
Ethionamide	Spironolactone
Guanethidine	Thiazides
Marihuana	Tricyclic antidepressants

Cryptorchidism

Failure of descent of the testes is a common but poorly understood phenomenon. Not infrequently, spontaneous descent takes place at the time of puberty. Cryptorchid testes may be intra-abdominal or located anywhere in the inguinal canal. Cryptorchidism may be an isolated defect or associated with other congenital anomalies.

There is no agreement about when hormonal therapy should be instituted. If the testes are present, gonadotropic hormone will bring them down unless a hernia or blockage of the passageway prevents their descent. hCG, 1000 units 3 times per week for 3 weeks, is usually sufficient. If this fails, surgical orchiopexy is indicated. Early surgical repair is advisable because intra-abdominal testes may later fail to produce sperm normally and because the incidence of malignancy in intra-abdominal testes is high.

A new approach to cryptorchidism is therapy with gonadorelin (gonadotropin-releasing hormone). The use of synthetic gonadorelin in a nasal spray for 4 weeks has resulted in successful descent of the testes in a significant proportion of cases.

Bone & Joint Pains & Pathologic Fractures

If the onset is at an early age and if there is a family history of similar disorders, consider osteogenesis imperfecta (blue scleras may be present). Bowing of the bone and pseudofractures suggest rickets or osteomalacia, due either to intestinal or, more commonly, renal tubular disorders. Always consider hyperparathyroidism, specifically if bone pain, bone cysts, and fractures are associated with renal stones. Back pain in postmenopausal women suggests osteoporosis. In cases of osteopenia of unknown cause, hyperthyroidism and Cushing's syndrome should always be considered. Rickets and osteomalacia are accompanied by pain in the extremities. Bone pain may occur also as a result of metastatic tumors, multiple myeloma, and Paget's disease. Dual-photon bone densitometry has been helpful in the diagnosis and follow-up of bone demineralization disorders.

Renal Colic; Gravel & Stone Formation

A metabolic cause must be sought for recurrent stone formation in adults and for kidney stones in children. If there is a family history, cystinuria and uric acid stones must be considered, as well as renal tubular acidosis with nephrocalcinosis. About 5% of stones are due to hyperparathyroidism, which must be ruled out in every instance of calcium stones by obtaining a parathyroid hormone assay if the serum calcium is elevated. Hypercalciuria may also be present. Other causes of stone formation include vitamin D intoxication and sarcoidosis as well as diseases characterized by rapid bone breakdown such as Cushing's syndrome, bone cancer, etc. Uric acid stones may occur in patients with gouty arthritis, but often they occur simply because the urinary pH is very acid; they are also observed after any type of intensive therapy for leukemia or lymphoma. Idiopathic hypercalciuria is the most common metabolic cause of recurrent calcium stones in males. Primary hyperoxaluria is a rare cause of severe renal calcification and may be associated with deposition of oxalate in soft tissues (oxalosis). Oxalate stones are seen frequently in patients with intestinal disorders (eg, ileitis, shunt procedures for obesity). At times, stones form in a structurally abnormal kidney (eg, medullary sponge kidney). Metabolic causes of renal stones must be corrected early before renal damage due to infection and obstruction occurs, since this may not be reversed upon removal of the initiating factor. The keys to proper diagnosis are chemical stone analysis and blood and urine tests for calcium, phosphate, and uric acid.

Tetany & Muscle Cramps

Mild tetany with paresthesias and muscle cramps is usually due to hyperventilation with alkalosis resulting from an anxiety state. If tetany occurs in children, rule out idiopathic hypoparathyroidism or pseudohypoparathyroidism. Look for calcification in the lens, poor teeth, and x-ray evidence of basal ganglia calcification. Hypoparathyroidism occurs in the postthyroidectomy patient. Tetany may be the presenting complaint of osteomalacia or rickets or of acute pancreatitis. Severe vomiting can produce systemic alkalosis and tetany. Neonatal tetany may rarely indicate maternal hyperparathyroidism. Severe hypocalcemic tetany will occasionally produce convulsions and must be differentiated from "idiopathic" epilepsy. Classic signs of tetany are Chvostek's sign and Trousseau's phenomenon. Leg cramps may occur in some diabetic patients. Muscle cramps are also frequent in hypothyroidism. Magnesium deficiency must be considered in tetany unresponsive to calcium.

Mental Changes

Disturbances of mentation are often subtle and may be difficult to recognize, but they may be important indications of underlying endocrine disorders. Nervousness, flushing, and excitability are characteristic of the menopause, hyperthyroidism, and anxiety states. Prolonged hypothyroidism in infancy is associated with severe mental deficits. In adults, it is accompanied by mental slowness, depression, and lethargy. Occasionally it may be manifested by delusional psychosis ("myxedema madness"). Prolonged hypocalcemia from untreated hypoparathyroidism may be associated with intellectual deterioration. Convulsions with abnormal electroencephalographic findings may occur in hypocalcemic tetany or in hypoglycemia. Islet cell tumors may cause confusion, abnormal speech, and behavior or personality changes as well as sudden loss of consciousness, somnolence and prolonged lethargy, or coma. Frank psychosis can occur

but is rare. Diabetic acidosis may progress gradually into coma. Hypercalcemia leads to somnolence and lethargy, with marked weakness. Mental confusion may occur in hypopituitarism or Addison's disease. Confusion, lethargy, and nausea may be the presenting symptoms of water intoxication due to inappropriate or excessive secretion of antidiuretic hormone. Insomnia, mood changes, anxiety, and even frank psychosis can be associated with Cushing's syndrome. Rapid changes in glucocorticoid status (either a sudden increase or a sudden decrease) may be associated with acute psychosis. Mental deficiency may be associated with abnormal excretion of amino acids in the urine (eg, phenylketonuria) and with chromosomal abnormalities.

DISEASES OF THE HYPOTHALAMUS & PITUITARY GLAND

The function of the pituitary gland is controlled by regulating hormones (factors) produced by the hypothalamus. These releasing and release-inhibiting hormones are, for the most part, relatively simple polypeptides, many of which have been identified and synthesized (Table 20–3). A clinical disorder may be due to lack or excess of a pituitary hormone or, more commonly, to lack of releasing or inhibiting factor of the hypothalamus. Isolated or multiple defects may occur. Accurate radioimmunoassays and stimulation tests have made it possible to classify accurately the location of the defect. Clinical use of

Table 20–3. The pituitary hormones and their hypothalamic regulatory factors (hormones).[1]

Hormones	Regulatory Factors (Hormones)
Growth hormone (somatotropin, STH)	Somatotropin-releasing factor (SRF, GH-RH, GH-RF); somatotropin release-inhibiting hormone (SIF, somatostatin)
Corticotropin (ACTH)	Corticotropin-releasing factor (CRF or CRH)
Thyrotropin (TSH)	Thyrotropin-releasing hormone (TRF, TRH)
Follicle-stimulating hormone (FSH)	FSH and LH share a common hypothalamic peptide, gonadotropin-releasing hormone or gonadorelin (FSH-RH, LH-RH, LH-RF, LRH, GnRH)
Luteinizing hormone (LH)	
Prolactin	Prolactin-releasing factor (PRF); prolactin inhibitory factor (PIF) or dopamine

[1] Modified from Schally AV et al: Hypothalamic regulatory hormones. *Science* 1973;**179**:341.

synthetic hypothalamic factors and their agonist or antagonist analogues is a new and promising development (eg, use of GnRH and analogues in cryptorchidism, delayed puberty, induction of ovulation, management of precocious puberty). A fascinating feature of at least one of the hypothalamic peptides (GnRH) is the opposite effects produced when it is given by constant infusion versus pulsatile administration; the latter mode stimulates and the former inhibits gonadotropin secretion. Hypothalamic disease may be caused by infiltrative or inflammatory diseases (sarcoidosis, histiocytosis X, tuberculosis), by tumors, or by trauma. The symptomatology can be neurologic (somnolence, hyperphagia, thermal regulation disorders), endocrine, or visual. Tumors of the pituitary gland are recognized with increased frequency thanks to new methods of visualization of soft structures within the sella turcica (CT scans and MRI). Some are hormonally inactive or only secrete subunits of gonadotropins. Others have been found to secrete excessive ACTH, growth hormone, prolactin, thyrotropin, LH, and FSH. A certain degree of overlap in function has been noted, eg, pituitary enlargement and lactation in juvenile myxedema reversed by the administration of thyroid hormone. Prolactin assays may be most important for the early diagnosis of hypothalamic or pituitary lesions.

Chakeres DW, Curtin A, Ford G: Magnetic resonance imaging of pituitary and parasellar abnormalities. Radiol Clin North Am 1989;27:265.

Gillies G, Grossman A: The CRFs and their control: Chemistry, physiology and clinical implications. Clin Endocrinol Metab 1985;14:821.

Jordan RM, Kohler PO: Recent advances in diagnosis and treatment of pituitary tumors. Adv Intern Med 1987; 32:299.

Lechan RM: Neuroendocrinology of pituitary hormone regulation. Endocrinol Metab Clin North Am 1987;16:475.

Molitch ME (editor): Pituitary tumors. (Symposium.) Endocrinol Metab Clin North Am 1987;16:475.

Molitch ME, Russell EJ: The pituitary "incidentaloma." Ann Intern Med 1990;112:925.

Whitcomb RW, Crowley WF Jr: Diagnosis and treatment of isolated gonadotropin-releasing hormone in men. J Clin Endocrinol Metabl 1990;70:3.

PANHYPOPITUITARISM

Essentials of Diagnosis

- Sexual dysfunction; weakness; easy fatigability; lack of resistance to stress, cold, and fasting; axillary and pubic hair loss.
- Low blood pressure; may have visual field defects.
- Low or low normal: T_4, TSH, FSH, LH, testosterone, urinary 17-ketosteroids and hydroxycorticosteroids, growth hormone. Prolactin may be elevated.
- CT scan or MRI may reveal a pituitary lesion.

General Considerations

Hypopituitarism is a relatively rare disorder in which inactivity of the pituitary gland leads to insufficiency in the target organs. All or several of the tropic hormones may be involved. Isolated defects, eg, of the gonadotropins, are not rare. There is also great variation in the severity of the lesions, from those merely involving pathways (hypothalamic lesions) to almost complete destruction of the gland itself. Causes of this disorder include circulatory collapse due to hemorrhage following delivery and subsequent pituitary necrosis (Sheehan's syndrome), granulomas, hemochromatosis, cysts and tumors (chromophobe adenomas and craniopharyngiomas are most common), surgical hypophysectomy, external irradiation to the skull, trauma, metastatic disease, and aneurysms involving the sella turcica.

The pituitary tumor may be part of the syndrome of multiple endocrine adenomatosis (type I), with concomitant involvement of the parathyroid glands and pancreatic islets. Isolated or partial deficiencies of anterior pituitary hormones (eg, FSH, LH, TSH) or their releasing hormones may also occur.

Clinical Findings

These vary with the degree of pituitary destruction, and are related to the lack of hormones from the "target" endocrine glands.

A. Symptoms and Signs: Weakness; lack of resistance to cold, to infections, and to fasting; and sexual dysfunction (lack of development of secondary sex characteristics, or regression of function) are the most common symptoms. In expanding lesions of the sella, interference with the visual tracts may produce temporal hemianopia or other visual field defects. Short stature is the rule if the onset is during the growth period. Amenorrhea and galactorrhea may be the first indications of a pituitary tumor. In men, impotence is usually an early complaint.

In both sexes there is sparseness or loss of axillary and pubic hair, and there may be thinning of the eyebrows and of the head hair.

The skin is often dry, with lack of sweating, and the patient appears pale. Pigmentation is lacking even after exposure to sunlight. Fine wrinkles are seen, and the facies presents a "sleepy" appearance.

The heart is small and the blood pressure low. Orthostatic hypotension is often present. Visual field defects (bitemporal hemianopia) may be present if an enlarging pituitary mass compresses the optic chiasm.

B. Laboratory Findings: The fasting blood glucose may be low. Dilutional hyponatremia is often present if hypocortisolism exists, due to impaired free water clearance, because of inappropriate secretion of vasopressin. Hyperkalemia does not occur, since aldosterone production, which is mainly controlled by the renin-angiotensin system, is not affected. Mild anemia may be present. Systematic analysis of pituitary hormones should be done: Serum growth hormone, measured by radioimmunoassay, is low and does not increase in response to insulin hypoglycemia, arginine infusion, or levodopa. The insulin tolerance test (use only 0.05 unit/kg intravenously) shows marked insulin sensitivity and may be dangerous in these patients, since severe hypoglycemia reactions may occur. The T_4 level is low, and the TSH is not elevated (as in primary myxedema). Urinary 17-ketosteroids and 17-hydroxycorticosteroids and plasma cortisol are low but rise slowly after corticotropin administration. Corticotropin may have to be given for several days to demonstrate an adrenal response. Serum ACTH is low. Plasma levels of sex steroids (testosterone and estradiol) are low, and so are the serum gonadotropins. TSH response to repeated intravenous infusions of thyrotropin-releasing hormone (TRH) may be of help in differentiating hypothalamic from pituitary lesions. Elevated prolactin levels are found in patients with prolactinomas and in cases of hypothalamic disease.

The demonstration of a low level of a hormone secreted by a target gland in the presence of a low level of a trophic hormone is strongly suggestive of hypothalamic or pituitary disease (low plasma cortisol *and* ACTH, T_4 *and* TSH, estradiol or testosterone *and* LH).

C. Imaging: Radiographs of the skull may show a lesion. Craniopharyngiomas are often calcified and may be seen in a plain film. CT scan is helpful in ascertaining the degree of suprasellar extension of a tumor, the presence of cysts, "empty sella," etc. Magnetic resonance imaging (MRI) provides even better detail.

Differential Diagnosis

Anorexia nervosa may occasionally simulate hypopituitarism. In fact, severe malnutrition may give rise to functional hypopituitarism. Cachexia is rare in hypopituitarism. Loss of axillary and pubic hair is rare in anorexia nervosa. The 17-ketosteroids are low normal or not as low as in hypopituitarism; plasma and urinary cortisol are normal or high and may respond rapidly to corticotropin stimulation; the gonadotropins are usually present at low levels. Thyroid function tests are not abnormal in anorexia nervosa except for low T_3. Pituitary growth hormone assays show high levels in anorexia nervosa and very low levels in hypopituitarism.

Primary adrenal or thyroid insufficiency is easily differentiated from pituitary insufficiency, since serum ACTH or TSH is invariably elevated in the former conditions.

Enlargement of the sella may require CT scans or MRI to rule out "empty sella syndrome," where minimal endocrine abnormalities are present and radiation or surgery is not indicated.

Hypoglycemia after fasting may occasionally cause confusion with hyperinsulinism.

The mental changes of hypopituitarism may be mistaken for a primary psychosis.

Complications

In addition to those of the primary lesion (eg, tumor), complications may develop at any time as a result of the patient's inability to cope with minor stressful situations. This may lead to high fever, shock, coma, and death. Sensitivity to thyroid may precipitate an adrenal crisis if thyroid hormone is administered without glucocorticoid treatment. Rarely, acute hemorrhage may occur in large pituitary tumors with rapid loss of vision, headache, and evidence of acute pituitary failure (pituitary apoplexy) requiring emergency decompression of the sella.

Treatment

The pituitary lesion, if a tumor, is treated by surgical removal, x-ray irradiation, or both. Removal is usually via a transsphenoidal approach, which in expert hands is an effective and safe surgical procedure. Craniotomy is rarely necessary. Endocrine substitution therapy must be used before, during, and often permanently after such procedures.

Recently, new therapeutic vistas have been opened by the development of purified pituitary hormones and of hypothalamic releasing hormones or their analogues. The mainstay of substitution therapy for pituitary insufficiency remains the replacement of the end-organ deficiencies (adrenal, thyroid, and gonad). This must be continued throughout life. Almost complete replacement therapy can be carried out with corticosteroids, thyroid hormone, and sex steroids. In adults, growth hormone replacement therapy does not seem necessary for metabolic normalcy.

A. Corticosteroids: Give hydrocortisone tablets, 15–25 mg/d orally in divided doses. Most patients do well with 15 mg in the morning and 5–10 mg in the late afternoon. A mineralocorticoid is rarely needed, since the adrenal conserves the capacity to secrete aldosterone. Additional amounts of rapid-acting corticosteroids must be given during states of stress, eg, during infection, trauma, or surgical procedures.

B. Thyroid: Thyroid (and insulin) should rarely, if ever, be used in panhypopituitarism unless the patient is receiving corticosteroids. Because of lack of adrenal function, patients may be exceedingly sensitive to these drugs. Levothyroxine is the drug of choice. The usual maintenance dose is 0.125 mg daily (range, 0.1–0.175 mg daily).

C. Sex Hormones:

1. If gonadal failure is present, appropriate sex steroid replacement should be instituted. For males, testosterone enanthate, cypionate, or any other long-acting ester is given intramuscularly every 2 weeks (200–400 mg/dose). Because of hepatic complications, the long-term use of oral androgens is not recommended.

2. Estrogens are extremely important in the female to prevent osteoporosis and to maintain secondary sex characteristics. The most frequently used oral agents are conjugated estrogens (eg, Premarin) and ethinyl estradiol. Give 0.625–1.25 mg of Premarin daily or 0.02–0.05 mg of ethinyl estradiol. Three weeks of estrogen therapy are usually followed by 5–10 days of a progestational agent such as medroxyprogesterone acetate, 10 mg daily. If the patient is unwilling to take 2 different kinds of pills every month, a "low-dose" (30 μg of ethinyl estradiol) combination estrogen-progestin oral contraceptive preparation may be used, but not in women over 40 or in those who smoke. (See Table 13–5.)

3. Chorionic gonadotropic hormone (hCG) in combination with human pituitary FSH or postmenopausal urinary gonadotropin may be used in an attempt to produce fertility.

4. Clomiphene citrate and GnRH are sometimes useful in hypothalamic hypogonadism.

Note: Sex hormones, especially estrogens, should be employed cautiously in young patients with panhypopituitarism, or the epiphyses will close before maximum growth is achieved. Most androgens also share this property—especially when given in large doses.

D. Human Growth Hormone: This hormone is by far the most effective agent for increasing height. Previously used preparations were obtained from human pituitary glands collected at autopsy. They have been withdrawn from the market because of demonstrated transmission of Creutzfeldt-Jakob disease to recipients. New methods of production of hGH (human growth hormone) using recombinant DNA techniques have ensured increased availability and safety of this hormone. The very high cost, however, remains a problem. It has been used to increase the stature of some children who do *not* have clear-cut growth hormone deficiency and even in perfectly normal children who were within 2 SD of the mean for height. This use is experimental and not recommended.

E. Other Drugs: Bromocriptine has been used successfully in the treatment of pituitary lesions producing lactation and amenorrhea, especially in prolactinomas. It is given orally in divided doses. Most patients respond very well to 5–10 mg daily. This treatment often induces marked regression in tumor size in addition to dramatic decreases of serum prolactin levels, with resumption of menses and ovulation. Unfortunately, cessation of therapy is almost always associated with regrowth of tumor. (See Disorders of Prolactin Secretion.)

Prognosis

This depends on the primary cause. If it is due to postpartum necrosis (Sheehan's syndrome), partial or even complete recovery may occur. Functional hypopituitarism due to starvation and similar causes may also be corrected.

If the gland has been destroyed, the problem is to replace target organ hormones, since chronic replacement with pituitary tropic hormones is not yet feasible. With appropriate therapy, a patient with hypopituitarism can expect a normal life span. Major improvements in pituitary surgical techniques in the last decade have resulted in safe and satisfactory removal of many pituitary tumors. Unfortunately, the rate of postsurgical recurrence is significant.

Brook CED et al: Clinical features and investigation of growth hormone deficiency. Clin Endocrinol Metab 1986;15:479.

Hickstein D, Chandler WF, Marshall JC: The spectrum of pituitary adenoma hemorrhage. West J Med 1986; 144:435.

Oelkers W: Hyponatremia and inappropriate secretion of vasopressin (antidiuretic hormone) in patients with hypopituitarism. N Engl J Med 1989;321:492.

ACROMEGALY & GIGANTISM

Essentials of Diagnosis

- Excessive growth of hands (increased glove size), feet (increased shoe size), jaw (protrusion of lower jaw), and internal organs; or gigantism before closure of epiphyses.
- Amenorrhea, headaches, visual field loss, sweating, weakness.
- Increased heel pad.
- Elevated serum inorganic phosphorus; T_4 normal; glycosuria.
- Elevated serum growth hormone with failure to suppress after glucose.
- Elevated insulinlike growth factor I.
- Imaging: Sellar enlargement and terminal phalangeal "tufting" on radiographs. CT or MRI demonstration of pituitary tumor.

General Considerations

Growth hormone seems to exert its peripheral effects through the release of several somatomedins produced in the liver and other tissues, the most important of which is known as insulinlike growth factor I (IGF-I).

An excessive amount of growth hormone is most often produced by a benign pituitary adenoma. Recent studies indicate that many growth hormone-secreting tumors have genetic mutations resulting in loss of regulation by GHRH. This dysregulation of growth hormone results in acromegaly. The disease may be associated with adenomas elsewhere, such as in the parathyroids or pancreas (multiple endocrine neoplasia type I). Acromegaly may also rarely occur as a result of secretion of ectopic growth hormone-releasing hormone (GHRH) by tumors such as bronchial and intestinal carcinoids, hypothalamic gangliocytomas, pancreatic islet cell adenomas, and lung carcinomas. If the onset is before closure of the epiphyses, gigantism will result. If the epiphyses have already closed at onset, only overgrowth of soft tissues and terminal skeletal structures (acromegaly) results. At times the disease is transient ("fugitive acromegaly") and followed by pituitary insufficiency.

Clinical Findings

A. Symptoms and Signs: Crowding of other hormone-producing cells, especially those concerned with gonadotropic hormones, causes amenorrhea and loss of libido. Production of excessive growth hormone causes doughy enlargement of the hands with spadelike fingers, large feet, jaw, face, tongue, and internal organs, wide spacing of the teeth, and an oily, tough, "furrowed" skin and scalp with multiple fleshy tumors (mollusca). Hoarse voice is common. Sleep apnea may occur. At times, acanthosis nigricans is present. Pressure of the pituitary tumor causes headache, bitemporal hemianopia, lethargy, and diplopia. In long-standing cases, secondary hormonal changes take place, including diabetes mellitus, goiter, and abnormal lactation. Less commonly, these may be the presenting picture in acromegaly. Excessive sweating may be the most reliable clinical sign of activity of the disease.

B. Laboratory Findings: Serum inorganic phosphorus is often elevated (> 4 mg/dL) during the active phase of acromegaly. Serum gonadotropins are normal or low. Glycosuria and hyperglycemia may be present, and there is resistance to insulin. Hypercalciuria is common. The T_4 is normal or low. 17-Ketosteroids and hydroxycorticosteroids may be high or low, depending upon the stage of the disease. In the active phase of the disease, serum levels of growth hormone are almost always elevated above 7 ng/mL. Administration of glucose fails to suppress the serum level of growth hormone (as it does in normal individuals). Intravenous infusion of TRH or LRH often results in stimulation of growth hormone secretion, whereas in normal individuals there is no such effect. The plasma levels of immunoreactive IGF-I have been reported to correlate closely with disease activity. Serum prolactin is often elevated. This may be due to simultaneous secretion of prolactin by the growth hormone-secreting tumor, to the presence of a small prolactinoma, or to interference with delivery of hypothalamic prolactin inhibitory factor (PIF) to the normal prolactin-secreting cells of the anterior pituitary.

C. Imaging: Radiography of the skull may show a large sella with destroyed clinoids, but a sella of usual size does not rule out the diagnosis. The frontal sinuses may be large. One may also demonstrate thickening of the skull and long bones, with typical overgrowth of vertebral bodies and severe spur formation. Dorsal kyphosis is common. Typical "tufting" of the terminal phalanges of the fingers and toes occurs, with increase in size of the sesamoid bone. A lateral view of the feet shows increased thickness of the heel pad. Modern techniques of CT and MRI scanning can demonstrate even small pituitary tumors.

Differential Diagnosis

Growth hormone excess is to be considered if there is rapid growth or resumption of growth once stopped (eg, change in shoe size or ring size). Consider the diagnosis also in unexplained amenorrhea or insulin-resistant diabetes mellitus. Physiologic spurts of growth and increase in tissue size from exercise, weight gain, or certain occupations enter into the differential diagnosis. The syndrome of cerebral gigantism with mental retardation and ventricular dilatation but normal growth hormone levels resembles acromegalic gigantism. Myxedema and, rarely, pachydermoperiostosis may resemble acromegaly. Serial photographs are of help in differentiating familial nonendocrine gigantism and facial enlargement. Other conditions causing visceromegaly must be considered.

Complications

Complications include pressure of the tumor on surrounding structures, rupture of the tumor into the brain or sinuses, the appearance of glucose intolerance or frank diabetes mellitus, cardiac enlargement, and cardiac failure. The carpal tunnel syndrome, due to compression of the median nerve at the wrist, may cause disability of the hand. Arthritis of hips, knees and spine can be troublesome. Cord compression due to large intervertebral disks may be seen. Weakness due to myopathy often affects the limbs. Visual field defects may be severe and progressive. Acute loss of vision may occur if the tumor undergoes spontaneous hemorrhage and necrosis (pituitary apoplexy).

Treatment

Pituitary surgery is the treatment of choice. Transsphenoidal microsurgery has removed the hyperfunctioning tissue while preserving anterior pituitary function in most patients. Pituitary irradiation is useful if surgical therapy fails to return the elevated growth hormone levels to normal. Periodic reassessment of pituitary function after these procedures is advisable. In the "burnt out" case, hormonal replacement as for hypopituitarism may be required. Reports of medical treatment with bromocriptine have been disappointing. Large doses are often necessary (30–40 mg/d), and normalization of growth hormone secretion is not often achieved. A somatostatin analogue, octreotide, has been described as effective in lowering growth hormone concentration and rapidly improving clinical symptoms in a small series of patients with acromegaly.

Prognosis

Prognosis depends upon the age at onset and, more particularly, the age at which therapy is begun. Menstrual function may be restored. Severe headaches may persist even after treatment. Secondary tissue and skeletal changes do not respond completely to removal of the tumor. The diabetes may be permanent in spite of adequate pituitary ablation. The patient may succumb to the cardiovascular complications. The tumor may "burn out," causing symptoms of hypopituitarism, or it may appear as an "empty" sella.

Barkan AL: Acromegaly: Diagnosis and therapy. Endocrinol Metab Clin North Am 1989;18:277.

Gorden P et al: NIH conference: Somatostatin and somatostatin analogue (SMS 201–995) in treatment of hormone-secreting tumors of the pituitary and gastrointestinal tract and nonneoplastic diseases of the gut. Ann Intern Med 1989;110:35.

Landis CA et al: GTPase inhibiting mutations activate the alpha chain of Gs and stimulate adenylyl cyclase in human pituitary tumours. Nature 1989;340:692.

Melmed S et al: Acromegaly. N Engl J Med 1990;322:966.

Sano T et al: Growth hormone-releasing hormone-producing tumors: Clinical, biochemical and morphological manifestations. Endocr Rev 1988;9:357.

CLINICAL DISORDERS OF PROLACTIN SECRETION

Essentials of Diagnosis

- Women: Menstrual cycle disturbances (oligomenorrhea, amenorrhea).
- Men: Decreased libido and erectile impotence.
- Elevated serum prolactin.
- CT scan or MRI often demonstrates pituitary adenoma.

Normal Physiology

Prolactin is a peptide hormone with a molecular weight of 21,000 which is secreted by the pituitary and in the mammalian species has as its main role that of inducing lactation. The hormone is hypersecreted during pregnancy, and the levels in plasma increasingly rise until the time of delivery. Under the combined effect of prolactin, increased estrogen, and progesterone, further breast development takes place, with eventual formation of milk in the acini. After parturition, the sudden withdrawal of estrogen caused by the expulsion of the placenta results in the onset of lactation. Estrogens play a synergistic role along with prolactin to promote the differentiation and development of the breast, but they antagonize prolactin in inhibiting the actual secretion of milk. The presence of prolactin is absolutely essential for lactation. During the puerperal period, the act of suckling constitutes a powerful stimulus for the continued production of prolactin. Lactation will cease if prolactin secretion is interrupted by prolactin-lowering drugs or by pituitary destruction. Prolactin is an unusual hormone in terms of control of secretion in that it is under a predominantly inhibitory control. Thus, section of the pituitary stalk will result in marked increases in prolactin secretion. Also, a pituitary transplanted to another anatomic site will abundantly secrete prolactin. There is mounting evidence that the prolactin inhibitory factor (PIF) is dopamine and that the control of prolactin secretion is primarily modulated by secretion of PIF. A prolactin-stimulating factor also exists, but its physiologic role is less clear. Prolactin, like other peptide hormones, is secreted episodically, and its concentration in blood is not stable (0–20 ng/mL).

Elevated serum prolactin is found in association with multiple physiologic and pathologic causes (Table 20–4). It should be remembered that exercise and stress frequently raise prolactin concentration. Estrogens increase serum prolactin levels slowly by increasing the number of prolactin-secreting cells in the anterior pituitary gland. Many drugs inhibit prolactin inhibitory factor, thereby raising the production of prolactin.

Clinical Consequences of Prolactin Excess

In women, prolactin excess produces (1) disturbances of pituitary ovarian function with anovulatory cycles, oligomenorrhea, or (frequently) amenorrhea; (2) galactorrhea (less common); and (3) hirsutism (rare). (See p 788.)

In men, excess prolactin is associated with (1) impotence and decreased libido (very common), (2) hypogonadism (less common), and (3) galactorrhea (very rare). (See p 791.)

Of all women with secondary amenorrhea, about one-fourth have elevated prolactin levels. In men, increased prolactin concentrations are usually not associated with galactorrhea, because the male breast tissue has not been primed by estrogens and progesterone.

Most women with hyperprolactinemia have amen-

Table 20–4. Causes of hyperprolactinemia.

Physiologic Causes	Pharmacologic Causes	Pathologic Causes
Sleep (REM phase)	Phenothiazines	Pituitary stalk section
Exercise	Tricyclic antidepressants	Hypothalamic disease
Stress (trauma, surgery)	Reserpine	Prolactin-secreting tumors
Pregnancy	Methyldopa	Nelson's syndrome
Puerperium	Amphetamines	Acromegaly
Suckling	Anesthetic agents	Hypothyroidism
	Estrogens	Renal failure
	Metoclopramide	Chronic chest wall stimulation (post-thoracotomy; post-mastectomy; herpes zoster, etc)
	Amoxepin	Pseudocyesis
	Verapamil	Spinal cord lesions
	MAO inhibitors	

orrhea or manifestations of a short luteal phase. The combination of amenorrhea and galactorrhea is characteristic of hyperprolactinemic syndromes, but studies indicate that amenorrhea is much more common than galactorrhea. Hyperprolactinemic women also tend to have decreased bone density and are therefore at increased risk to develop clinical osteoporosis if left untreated. Finally, about 25% of women with hyperprolactinemia have increased acne, seborrhea, or hirsutism as manifestations of increased androgenic activity, probably of adrenal origin.

The most important cause of high serum prolactin is a pituitary tumor. As many as 65% of all pituitary tumors may be associated with hyperprolactinemia. The tumors may be small (microadenomas) or produce clear-cut enlargement of the sella (macroadenomas). A great number of tests have been devised to separate a prolactin-secreting tumor from other causes of hyperprolactinemia. All of them are unreliable. The actual level of serum prolactin is useful, however. In patients with proved pituitary tumors, plasma levels of prolactin are almost always over 100 ng/mL. Levels greater than 250 ng/mL are, in the absence of renal failure, almost diagnostic of prolactinoma. Macroadenomas tend to cause higher levels of serum prolactin than microadenomas and are more frequently associated with decreased secretion of gonadotropins (LH and FSH). CT scan of the pituitary often demonstrates small prolactinomas. Differentiation from normal variants, however, is not always possible. Magnetic resonance imaging (MRI) may prove superior to CT scan for evaluation of pituitary disease.

Treatment

The treatment of a hyperprolactinemic state obviously depends upon the cause. If the problem is due to administration of exogenous estrogens, discontinuance of these drugs will produce improvement after a period of several months. Discontinuance of psychotropic agents usually results in a much faster recovery and resumption of menses. If hyperprolactinemia is due to hypothyroidism, administration of thyroid hormone will rapidly correct the situation. The treatment of prolactinomas remains controversial. In expert hands, transsphenoidal removal of a microadenoma results in prompt normalization of serum prolactin, resumption of menses, etc. The recurrence rate, however, is approximately 20% after 5 years. Macroadenomas, on the other hand, respond to surgical resection less favorably: fewer than 30% of cases result in "cures," and surgical morbidity and mortality are higher. Bromocriptine, a drug that binds to the pituitary dopamine receptor, thus inhibiting both spontaneous as well as TRH-provoked secretion from the gland, is useful in the medical therapy of hyperprolactinemic syndromes. In doses of 2.5–10 mg/d, it promptly reduces the levels of circulating prolactin, with rapid resumption of menses and cessation of galactorrhea. Always start with a small dose (eg,

1.25 mg/d) given at bedtime to minimize problems of nausea, dizziness, and orthostatic hypotension. Gradually increase the dose as necessary to bring prolactin levels down to normal. The exact role of bromocriptine in the treatment of prolactin-secreting pituitary tumors is debatable at present, with many endocrinologists favoring medical over surgical therapy. The choice of surgery or bromocriptine as primary therapy requires awareness of the skill and experience of the surgeon in this type of procedure. Dramatic reductions in size of prolactinomas can occur during bromocriptine administration. Intratumoral hemorrhages have also been reported. Unfortunately, discontinuance of therapy usually results in reappearance of hyperprolactinemia and galactorrhea-amenorrhea, even after many years of therapy. Since the patient's fertility is usually promptly restored with bromocriptine therapy, many pregnancies have resulted, with no clear evidence that the drug is teratogenic. Pregnancy, however, with its concomitant hypersecretion of estrogens, may result in marked increase in pituitary tumor size, with danger of sudden development of visual disturbances. This seldom occurs, however, in patients with microadenomas.

Hartog M, Hull MG: Hyperprolactinaemia. Br Med J 1988;297:701.

Vance ML, Thorner MO: Prolactinomas. Endocrinol Metab Clin North Am 1987;16:731.

Yousem DM et al: Pituitary adenomas: Possible role of bromocriptine in intratumoral hemorrhage. Radiology 1989;170:239.

DIABETES INSIPIDUS

Essentials of Diagnosis

- Polydipsia (4–20 L/d); excessive polyuria.
- Urine specific gravity < 1.006.
- Inability to concentrate urine on fluid restriction.
- Hyperosmolality of plasma.
- Vasopressin reduces urine output (except in nephrogenic diabetes insipidus).

General Considerations

Diabetes insipidus is an uncommon disease characterized by an increase in thirst and the passage of large quantities of urine of a low specific gravity. The urine is otherwise normal. The disease may occur acutely, eg, after head trauma or surgical procedures near the pituitary region, or may be chronic and insidious in onset. It is due to decreased or absent vasopressin secretion or, more rarely, unresponsiveness of the kidney to vasopressin (nephrogenic diabetes insipidus).

The causes may be classified as follows:

A. Due to Deficiency of Vasopressin:

1. Primary diabetes insipidus, due to a defect inherent in the gland itself (no organic lesion), may be familial, occurring as a dominant trait; or, more commonly, sporadic or "idiopathic."

2. Secondary diabetes insipidus is due to destruction of the functional unit by surgical or accidental trauma, infection (eg, encephalitis, tuberculosis, syphilis), primary tumor or metastatic tumors from the breast or lung (common), and histiocytosis X (eosinophilic granuloma or Hand-Schüller-Christian disease).

B. "Nephrogenic" Diabetes Insipidus: This disorder is due to a defect in the kidney tubules that interferes with water reabsorption and occurs as an X-linked recessive trait. The polyuria is unresponsive to vasopressin. In fact, these patients have normal secretion of vasopressin. Serum levels of ADH are normal or high. Adults with familial nephrogenic diabetes insipidus often have hyperuricemia. Acquired forms of vasopressin-resistant diabetes insipidus are seen in some patients with pyelonephritis, renal amyloidosis, potassium depletion, Sjögren's syndrome, sickle cell anemia, or chronic hypercalcemia. Certain drugs (eg, demeclocycline, lithium) may induce nephrogenic diabetes insipidus.

Clinical Findings

A. Symptoms and Signs: The outstanding signs and symptoms of the disease are intense thirst, especially with a craving for ice water, and polyuria, the volume of ingested fluid varying from 4 to 20 L daily, with correspondingly large urine volumes. Restriction of fluids causes marked weight loss, dehydration, headache, irritability, fatigue, muscular pains, hypothermia, tachycardia, and shock.

B. Laboratory Findings: Polyuria of over 6 L daily with a specific gravity below 1.006 is suggestive of diabetes insipidus. Random serum osmolality is usually above 290 mosm/kg in diabetes insipidus and below 280 mosm/kg in psychogenic polydipsia. Simple water deprivation with measurement of urine osmolality may be diagnostic. Special tests have been devised to distinguish true diabetes insipidus from psychogenic polydipsia. The latter will often respond (with reduction in urine flow and increase in urinary specific gravity) to administration of hypertonic (3%) saline solution; true diabetes insipidus does not. Hypertonic saline infusions may be dangerous to patients with abnormal cardiovascular status. Although a positive response tends to rule out true diabetes insipidus, a negative result must be followed by careful prolonged dehydration and measurement of both urine and plasma osmolality and body weight under hospital conditions. Plasma osmolality is normally maintained in the range of 285–290 mosm/kg associated with ADH concentrations of 1–3 μU/mL. Impaired ability to either synthesize or release ADH results in diminished ability of the kidney to conserve water. Patients with severe diabetes insipidus minimally concentrate urine following dehydration. After administration of 5 units of vasopressin, urine osmolality promptly rises

if the problem is central diabetes insipidus. Patients with milder degrees may fail to release ADH in response to hypertonicity but retain the ability to release hormone following nonosmotic stimuli. Some patients respond to an osmotic stimulus only when the plasma osmolality exceeds normal levels ("high set osmoreceptor"). The presence of intact thirst perception results in polydipsia and polyuria. Failure to respond to vasopressin (Pitressin) indicates "nephrogenic" diabetes insipidus, acquired or congenital. Radioimmunoassay for arginine vasopressin has facilitated the differential diagnosis of diabetes insipidus and psychogenic polydipsia. The plasma levels of vasopressin should always be correlated with the simultaneously obtained plasma and urine osmolalities. The high levels of plasma vasopressin in nephrogenic diabetes insipidus are characteristic.

If true primary diabetes insipidus seems likely on the basis of these tests, CT scan and MRI of the pituitary hypothalamic area are indicated. Search also for associated bone lesions of histiocytosis, and consider a primary tumor in the lung or breast. In nephrogenic diabetes insipidus, one must exclude chronic hypokalemia or hypercalcemia, sickle cells disease or trait, pyelonephritis, and hydronephrosis as well as demeclocycline and lithium administration.

Differential Diagnosis

The most important differentiation is from the "psychogenic" water-drinking habit (see above). This may be difficult, since patients with long-standing polydipsia develop a true defect in renal concentrating ability. The baseline serum osmolality is helpful, since subjects with psychogenic polydipsia tend to have low values, whereas the serum osmolality is normal or high in patients with diabetes insipidus. Serum sodium concentrations parallel serum osmolalities. Polydipsia and polyuria may also be seen in diabetes mellitus, renal insufficiency, hypokalemia (eg, in primary hyperaldosteronism), and in hypercalcemic states such as hyperparathyroidism.

Complications

If water is not readily available, the excessive output of urine will lead to severe dehydration, which rarely proceeds to a state of shock. Insomnia and dysphagia may occur. All the complications of the primary disease may eventually become evident. In patients who also have a disturbed thirst mechanism and who are receiving effective antidiuretic therapy, there is a danger of induced water intoxication. In untreated subjects, the passage of large volumes of urine for many years may be associated with dilatation of the ureters and urinary bladder.

Treatment

A. Specific Measures: Aqueous vasopressin injection is rarely used in continuous treatment because of its short duration of action (1–4 hours). A synthetic analogue of arginine vasopressin (desmopressin acetate [DDAVP]) is longer-acting and has become the treatment of choice. It is given intranasally in a dose of 5–10 μg once or twice daily. It has displaced old preparations such as vasopressin tannate in oil.

B. Other Measures: Mild cases require no treatment other than adequate fluid intake. Hydrochlorothiazide, 50–100 mg/d (with potassium chloride), is the only effective therapy available for nephrogenic diabetes insipidus. Chlorpropamide (Diabinese) has been found to enhance the activity of ADH upon the renal tubule and is useful in patients with partial diabetes insipidus, who still maintain a residual secretion of vasopressin. It has no effect in the nephrogenic type. After an initial dose of 250 mg twice daily, many patients can be maintained on 125–250 mg daily. Side effects include nausea, skin allergy, hypoglycemia, and a disulfiramlike reaction to alcohol.

Other drugs with antidiuretic activity are clofibrate and carbamazepine. They induce release of ADH and may be used in combination with chlorpropamide for selected patients with partial vasopressin deficiency. They have no effect on nephrogenic diabetes insipidus.

Solute restriction (low-sodium, no-excess-protein diet) may be of additional help. Psychotherapy is required for most patients with compulsive water drinking.

C. X-Ray Therapy: This may be used in the treatment of some cases due to tumor (eg, eosinophilic granuloma).

Prognosis

Diabetes insipidus may be latent, especially if there is associated lack of anterior pituitary function; and may be transient, eg, following head trauma. In most patients, the condition is permanent. With adequate therapy, all symptoms disappear and the patient can live a normal life. The ultimate prognosis is essentially that of the underlying disorder. In cases associated with organic brain disease, the prognosis is often poor. Surgical correction of the primary brain lesion rarely alters the diabetes insipidus.

If the disease is due to an eosinophilic granuloma of the skull, amelioration or even complete cure may be effected with x-ray therapy.

The prognosis of the ''nephrogenic'' type is only fair, since intercurrent infections are common, especially in infants affected with the disease. The acquired forms of this type may be reversible—eg, if urinary tract infection or obstruction is alleviated.

Illowsky BP, Birch DG: Polydipsia and hyponatremia in psychiatric patients. Am J Psychiatry 1988;145:675.

Richardson DWW, Robinson AG: Drugs twenty years later: Desmopressin. Ann Intern Med 1985;103:228. (Drug of choice for central diabetes insipidus.)

Robertson GL: Differential diagnosis of polyuria. Annu Rev Med 1988;39:425.

Seckl J, Dunger D: Postoperative diabetes insipidus. (Editorial.) Br Med J 1989;298:2.

INAPPROPRIATE SECRETION OF ANTIDIURETIC HORMONE

This syndrome, which is essentially water intoxication, may be mild and may only be manifested as asymptomatic hyponatremia, or it may be accompanied by irritability, lethargy, confusion, and seizures. It may lead to coma and death if not recognized. Laboratory findings include hyponatremia (which usually suggests the diagnosis) and hypo-osmolality of the serum, continued renal excretion of sodium, formation of hyperosmolar urine, and expanded fluid volume. Adrenal and renal function are normal. Plasma arginine vasopressin levels are elevated or high normal but are inappropriate for plasma osmolality. Serum amino acid levels are typically low.

The disorder is commonly caused by small-cell carcinoma of the lung, but it may also be present in patients with malignant tumors of the pancreas, prostate, and other organs. It is also seen in pulmonary tuberculosis, porphyria, acute leukemia, acute myocardial infarction, and central nervous system disorders. It can also occur in hypopituitarism and is often found in patients with AIDS and acute infections. It may be induced by chlorpropamide, vincristine, cyclophosphamide, and potassium-depleting diuretics.

Treatment is best accomplished by water restriction, which succeeds if the syndrome is recognized early. In severe cases of hyponatremia, when rapid correction is required, the use of furosemide diuresis with electrolyte replacement may be tried. If serum sodium concentration is extremely low (< 115 meq/L), judicious use of hypertonic saline may be necessary at the initiation of therapy. Lithium carbonate has been found to be effective in this syndrome, but lithium intoxication may occur. Demeclocycline is a safer drug to correct antidiuresis if water restriction is not sufficient. A search for the primary cause of the disorder must always be undertaken (see Chapter 16).

Kinzie BJ: Management of the syndrome of inappropriate secretion of antidiuretic hormone. Clin Pharm 1987; 6:625.

Robertson GL: Syndrome of inappropriate antidiuresis. N Engl J Med 1989;321:538.

Sterns RH: Treatment of hyponatremia: First, do no harm. Am J Med 1990;88:557.

DISEASES OF THE THYROID GLAND

Thyroid hormone affects cellular oxidative processes throughout the body. Tyrosine and inorganic iodine combine to form monoiodotyrosine and diiodotyrosine, which further combine to form thyroxine (T_4) and triiodothyronine (T_3), which are stored in the thyroid follicles linked to thyroglobulin.

Under the influence of TSH, T_4 and T_3 are released from the gland as the need arises. Most of the circulating T_3, however, results from extrathyroidal metabolism of T_4. Circulating thyroxine is bound to plasma proteins, primarily thyroxine-binding globulins (TBG) but also to prealbumin and albumin. T_3 is bound to TBG and to albumin. Only the free, unbound fractions of T_4 and T_3 are metabolically active and regulate TSH release. High levels of estrogen (eg, in pregnancy or in women taking oral contraceptives) increase the thyroxine-binding globulin levels and thus also the total level of T_4. The binding can be inhibited by certain compounds, eg, phenytoin and high doses of aspirin, which lower the T_4.

The requirements for iodine are minimal (about 50–200 μg/d), but if a true deficiency arises or if the demand for iodine is increased (eg, during puberty), hormone production will be insufficient and circulating levels will be low. This leads to increase in pituitary TSH output, and thyroid hyperplasia follows.

The peripheral metabolism of the thyroid hormones, especially by the liver, and its alteration in disease states are significant. Most circulating T_3 derives from peripheral conversion of T_4, which is also metabolized to a biologically inactive compound, reverse T_3. In many acute and chronic nonthyroidal illnesses, starvation, etc, the proportion of T_3 formed decreases and that of reverse T_3 increases. Serum concentrations of free T_4 are usually normal, less frequently low (patients with more serious disease), and rarely elevated. Euthyroid hyperthyroxinemia is especially common in acute psychiatric illness and in hyperemesis gravidarum; the mechanisms are unclear.

Thyroid disorders may occur with or without diffuse or nodular enlargement of the gland (goiter). Symptoms may be due to pressure alone or to hyperfunction or hypofunction. A strong genetic predisposition to thyroid disease has been recognized.

Since thyroid hormone affects all vital processes of the body, the time of onset of a deficiency state is most important in mental and physical development. Prolonged insufficiency that is present since infancy (cretinism) causes irreversible changes. Milder degrees of hypofunction, especially in adults, may go unrecognized or may masquerade as symptoms of disease of another system, eg, menorrhagia. Diagnosis will then depend to a large extent upon laboratory aids, especially the finding of an elevated TSH level.

In any age group, whenever an isolated thyroid nodule is felt that is not associated with hyperfunction—and especially if there is any change in size of the nodule—the possibility of neoplasm must be considered.

Kaplan MM, Larsen PR (editors): Thyroid disease. (Symposium.) Med Clin North Am 1985;69(5):September. [Entire issue.]

Thomas R, Reid RL: Thyroid disease and reproductive dysfunction: A review. Obstet Gynecol 1987:70:789.

Wall JR (editor): Autoimmune thyroid disease. (Symposium.) Endocrinol Metab Clin North Am 1987;16:229.

TESTS OF THYROID FUNCTION (Tables 20–5 and 20–6)

The tests most widely used in clinical practice are T_4 and "free" T_4 radioimmunoassays. When the latter is not available, the resin uptake of T_3 and determination of free thyroxine index (FTI) are useful. The TSH (RIA) assay has been of great help in diagnosis.

1. THYROID HORMONES IN SERUM

T_4 (RIA)

Normal: 5–12 μg/dL.

This test measures thyroxine by radioimmunoassay. It is affected by states of altered thyroxine binding.

"Free" Thyroxine Determination (FT$_4$)

Normal: 0.8–2.3 ng/dL.

This test measures the metabolically effective fraction of circulating T_4. If properly performed, it is the best measurement of thyroid hormones, since it is not affected by binding problems, chronic illness, etc.

Radioactive T_3 Uptake of Resin

Normal (varies with methods): 25–35%.

In general, this test parallels the T_4 (high in hyperthyroidism, low in hypothyroidism). It is an indirect measure of the interaction of thyroid hormone with protein binding sites and is of value in certain patients, eg, pregnant women or patients taking estrogens, since estrogens increase thyroxine binding and raise the total serum T_4 while T_3 uptake is low. In conditions accompanied by decreased thyroxine binding (malnutrition, nephrotic syndrome, congenital deficiency of TBG, etc), the total T_4 is low but the T_3 resin uptake is high.

Free Thyroxine Index (FTI)

The normal range varies in different laboratories.

The product of T_4 and resin T_3 uptake ($T_4 \times T_3$ uptake) usually (not always) corrects for abnormalities of thyroxine binding. If a free T_4 determination is available, this calculation is unnecessary.

Thyroxine-Binding Globulin (TBG-RIA)

Normal: 2–4.8 mg/dL.

This is a direct and specific test for the most impor-

Table 20–5. Typical results of some blood thyroid function tests in various conditions.[1]
(N = Normal range. ↑ = Elevated. ↓ = Decreased. V = Variable.)

Note: The more direct tests are subject to technical variables. They should be used when the more standard tests do not give decisive information, since many drugs cause interference with these thyroid tests.

	T_4 (RIA)	T_3 Resin	Free T_4 Index	T_3 Serum	RAI (^{123}I) Uptake	Other Useful Tests and Comments
Hyperthyroidism	↑	↑	↑	↑	↑	TSH ↓
Hypothyroidism	↓	↓	↓	↓	↓	TSH ↑ in primary myxedema, ↓ in pituitary myxedema
Euthyroid, or hypothyroid therapy with: T_4	N	N	N	V	↓	TSH ↓ with 0.1–0.2 mg T_4
T_3[2]	↓	↓	↓		↓	TSH ↓ with 50 μg T_3
Desiccated thyroid[3]	N	N	N		↓	TSH ↓ with 120–200 mg
Euthyroid following[4] Radiographic contrast dyes	N	N	N or ↑	N	↓	Effects may persist for 2 weeks to years
Pregnancy Hyperthyroid	↑	N or ↑	↑	↑	↑	Effects persist for 6–10 weeks after termination
Euthyroid	↑	↓	N	↑	↑	
Hypothyroid	N or ↓	↓	↓	↓	↓	
Birth control pills	↑	↓	N	↑	N	TSH normal
Nephrotic syndrome[5]	↓	↑	N	N	N	Low TP and TBG
Phenytoin, high doses of salicylates, testosterone	↓	↑	N	↓	N	TSH normal
Iodine deficiency	N	N	N	N	↑	^{123}I ↓ by T_4 or T_3
Iodide ingestion	N	N	N	N	↓	

[1] Modified and reproduced, with permission, from Leeper RD: *Current Concepts* 1972;**1**:1. Courtesy of the Upjohn Co., Kalamazoo, Mich.
[2] T_3 causes decreased measurements of serum thyroxine because T_4 secretion is depressed or absent. T_3 resin uptake is decreased because of decreased saturation of TBG with T_4.
[3] Assuming normal T_3:T_4 ratio. Different batches of thyroid extract may vary.
[4] Free T_4 index may be increased if measurement for serum T_4 is elevated by contamination.
[5] TBG is lost in this disease, which accounts for decreased serum thyroxine.

tant thyroid-binding protein and is not affected by alterations in other serum proteins.

T_3 by Radioimmunoassay

Normal: 80–200 ng/mL.

This test is of value in the diagnosis of thyrotoxicosis with normal T_4 values (T_3 thyrotoxicosis) and in some cases of toxic nodular goiter. It decreases rapidly in states of malnutrition, chronic illnesses, weight reduction diets, etc.

2. IN VIVO UPTAKE OF THYROID GLAND

Radioiodine (^{123}I) Uptake of Thyroid Gland

Normal: 5–35% in 24 hours. The normal range has been markedly lowered (by 4–20%) in the USA because of increase of dietary intake of iodine (primarily due to the addition of sodium iodate to bread).

A. Elevated: Thyrotoxicosis, hypofunctioning large goiter, iodine lack; at times, chronic thyroiditis.

B. Low: Administration of iodides or iodine in any form (drugs, radiology contrast dyes, etc), T_4, antithyroid drugs, thyroiditis, hypothyroidism, and iodine contrast dye exposure.

A scintiscan over the gland outlines areas of increased and decreased activity. If the uptake of ^{123}I is blocked, technetium (^{99m}Tc) may be used to obtain a scintiscan. Suppression of uptake after administration of 100 μg of T_3 daily for several days will determine if the area in the gland is autonomous or TSH-dependent.

3. MISCELLANEOUS TESTS OF THYROID FUNCTION

Achilles Tendon Reflex

The relaxation time is often prolonged in hypothyroidism but also in diabetes, old age, peripheral vascular disease, etc. It is rapid in hyperthyroidism. Although it lacks specificity for diagnosis, this test may be of value in following response to therapy.

Table 20–6. Appropriate use of thyroid tests.

Purpose	Test	Comment
For screening	Free-T_4	Excellent test.
	T_4 (RIA)	Varies with TBG.
	T_3 resin uptake	Varies with TBG.
	Free thyroxine index	Useful combination.
For hypo-thyroidism	Serum TSH	Primary vs secondary hypothyroidism. "Feed-back" with T_4 and T_3.
	TRH stimulation	Differentiates pituitary and hypothalamic disorders.
	Antithyroglobulin and antimicrosomal antibodies	Elevated in Hashimoto's thyroiditis.
For hyper-thyroidism	Serum TSH	Usually suppressed.
	T_3 (RIA)	Elevated.
	^{123}I uptake and scan	Increased diffuse vs "hot" areas.
	Suppression test (100 μg T_3 for 7 days)	Autonomy. For atypical Graves' disease with normal uptake.
	TRH stimulation	No response; safer than suppression test.
	Antithyroglobulin and antimicrosomal	Elevated in Graves' disease.
	TSH displacing immunoglobulin (TD)	Positive in Graves' disease (not always).
For nodules	^{123}I uptake and scan	"Warm" vs "cold."
	^{99m}Tc scan	Vascular vs avascular.
	Echo scan	Solid vs cystic. Pure cysts are not malignant.
	Thyroglobulin (TG)	High in metastatic, papillary, or follicular carcinomas.
	Calcitonin	High in medullary carcinoma.
	Thin-needle aspiration	Best diagnostic method for thyroid cancer.

Thyrotropin Immunoassay & Response to TRH

Normal: TSH-RIA less than 8 μU/mL (varies with laboratory); TRH response: doubling of TSH within 40 minutes after administration of 400 μg intravenously.

Radioimmunoassay of serum TSH is the most sensitive test for the early detection of primary hypothyroidism. TSH elevations may occur in subclinical hypothyroidism (eg, after destructive thyroid treatment), in iodine deficiency goiter, and in some dyshormonogenic goiters. It may also be elevated in rare cases of resistance to the action of thyroid hormone (Refetoff syndrome). After adequate T_4 replacement,

patients with myxedema should have undetectable or low TSH levels. A normal TSH response to TRH rules out pituitary hypothyroidism. A prolonged and exaggerated rise in TSH after administration of thyrotropin-releasing hormone (TRH) in patients with borderline elevations of TSH may provide further evidence of primary thyroid failure. Patients with hyperthyroidism fail to respond to TRH, and a normal response virtually excludes hyperthyroidism.

"Ultrasensitive" assays for TSH have been developed that separate the normal range from the "suppressed" values found in hyperthyroidism. These may be of help in the diagnosis of mild hyperthyroidism and will render obsolete the use of TRH stimulation tests for this purpose. These new assays may provide the best cost-effective screening test for thyroid dysfunction (hypo- or hyperthyroidism).

Thyroid Antibodies

Antibodies against several thyroid constituents (antithyroglobulin and antimicrosomal) are most commonly found in Hashimoto's thyroiditis but are also found in most patients with Graves' disease, a few patients with goiters or thyroid carcinomas, and in about 5–10% of normal subjects. In the latter, the titers tend to be low, and they increase with age. Thyroid-specific stimulating autoantibodies such as LATS (long-acting thyroid stimulator) are found in Graves' disease. A generic test for these thyroid-stimulating immunoglobulins (TSI) measures their displacement of TSH in thyroid cell membranes. TSI titers are elevated in approximately 80% of patients with Graves' disease. These titers—and those of antithyroglobulin and antimicrosomal antibodies—often decrease during pregnancy and during treatment of Graves' disease with propylthiouracil. TSI titers have been used with variable results to predict the rate of relapse of Graves' disease after chronic thiourea therapy and to predict neonatal hyperthyroidism. Other antibodies include thyroid growth-promoting antibodies, blocking antibodies, etc. Most of these factors can be measured only in research laboratories.

Serum Thyroglobulin

The level of serum thyroglobulin rises in autoimmune thyroid disease, thyroid injury or inflammation, and thyroid cancer. Levels are of little value in diagnosing or distinguishing among these conditions, but they provide a useful marker in thyroid cancer to indicate recurrence of disease and the need for further studies and therapy.

Ultrasound

This simple technique has been used to determine if thyroid lesions are solid or cystic. Cysts are less likely to be malignant, since thyroid carcinomas rarely undergo cystic degeneration. One should remember, however, that most solid lesions are also benign.

Fine-Needle Aspiration

Aspiration of thyroid tissue with a fine-gauge (21–26) needle has been shown to be helpful in the diagnosis of thyroid disorders, especially nodular lesions. Reading by an experienced cytopathologist is mandatory. This technique has recently become the preferred approach to the diagnosis of thyroid masses.

Calcitonin Assay

Elevated in medullary carcinoma.

de los Santos ET, Mazzaferri EL: Sensitive thyroid-stimulating hormone assays: Clinical applications and limitations. Compr Ther 1988;14:26.
Gavin LA: The diagnostic dilemmas of hyperthyroxinemias and hypothyroxinemias. Adv Intern Med 1987;33:185.
Ross DS: New sensitive immunoradiometric assays for thyrotropin. (Editorial.) Ann Intern Med 1986;104:718.
Tani EM, Skoog L. Lowhagen T: Clinical utility of fine-needle aspiration cytology of the thyroid. Annu Rev Med 1988;39:255.

SIMPLE & NODULAR GOITER

Essentials of Diagnosis

- Enlarged thyroid gland, often nodular.
- No symptoms except those associated with compression by large gland.
- T_4 and serum cholesterol normal; radioactive iodine uptake normal or elevated.
- TSH may be elevated.

General Considerations

Simple goiter in many parts of the world is due to iodine lack and occurs in endemic areas away from the seacoast. Deficiency of iodine leads to functional overactivity and hyperplasia of the gland, which becomes filled with colloid poor in iodine. If the deficiency is corrected, the enlargement may subside. In long-standing cases, the goiter persists and is often nodular. In the USA, the ingestion of iodine is now so high (due to iodates in bread and other iodine sources in the diet) that iodine deficiency due to lack of ingestion is extremely rare. Iodine excess can also cause goiter (excessive chronic ingestion of seaweed in Hokkaido, Japan; chronic treatment with saturated solution of potassium iodide or Lugol's solution). Unknown factors other than iodine lack play a role in the genesis of goiter. Simple goiter may occur transiently in persons living in iodine-deficiency areas when there is greater demand for thyroid hormone, eg, with the onset of puberty or during pregnancy. Rarely, goiter may occur in spite of adequate iodine intake when there is interference with formation of thyroid hormones, eg, due to excess intake of certain goitrogenic vegetables (rutabagas, turnips), exposure to thiocyanate, or congenital lack of enzyme systems involved in thyroxine biosynthesis. Goitrogens occurring in contaminated water supplies have been de-

scribed. Thyroid growth-stimulating immunoglobulins have been demonstrated in the serum of patients with goiters previously thought not to be autoimmune. A suggestion has been made that IGF-I (insulinlike growth factor I) may play a role in the pathogenesis of certain goiters. Goiter is more easily prevented than cured; it is rarer since the introduction of iodized salt. Simple goiters may show chronic thyroiditis on biopsy.

Clinical Findings

A. Symptoms and Signs: The gland is visibly enlarged and palpable. There may be no symptoms, or symptoms may occur as a result of compression of the structures in the thoracic outlet: wheezing, dysphagia, respiratory embarrassment. Large goiters with intrathoracic extension may intermittently block the thoracic outlet: raising of the arms above the neck may result in facial congestion, jugular venous distention, and dizziness (Pemberton's sign). Most patients with large multinodular goiters are euthyroid. A few may be hypothyroid. Exposure to large amounts of iodine may produce thyrotoxicosis, but this can also occur spontaneously if nodular autonomy has taken place (Plummer's disease).

B. Laboratory Findings: The T_4 is usually normal. The TSH levels may be elevated. The radioiodine uptake of the gland may be normal or high. The uptake over nodules usually shows them to be low in activity (in contrast to toxic nodular goiters).

With special techniques it is possible to demonstrate enzymatic defects in thyroid hormone production or abnormal circulating compounds in a number of patients with goiters, especially the familial types. Antimicrosomal and antithyroglobulin antibody titers are usually not elevated.

C. Ultrasound Examination: Echography provides information about the structure of the thyroid rapidly and safely: presence of single or multiple nodules, intrathoracic extension of goiters, etc. It should be remembered that demonstration of the cystic nature of a mass does not rule out malignancy.

D. CT Scan and MR Imaging: These techniques are useful in the presence of large goiters to demonstrate tracheal compression, impingement upon neighboring structures, etc.

Differential Diagnosis

It may be difficult, by examination alone, to differentiate simple goiter from toxic diffuse or nodular goiter, especially in a patient with a great many nervous symptoms. A history of residence in an endemic area, a family history of goiter, or onset during stressful periods of life (eg, puberty or pregnancy) will often help. Thyroid function tests are usually normal in simple goiter. High titers of antithyroid antibodies point to the presence of autoimmune thyroid disease (Hashimoto's thyroiditis or Graves' disease). If the lesion is nodular, and especially if only a single nodule is present, neoplasm must be considered. Fine-needle aspiration of the nodule is the most useful technique to distinguish neoplasia from other causes of nodule formation.

Prevention

With a dietary intake of 100–200 μg of iodine daily, simple goiter due to iodine deficiency should not occur. During times of stress (puberty, pregnancy, and lactation), the upper limits of this dose may be necessary. This amount is provided in 1–2 g of iodized salt daily. Parenteral administration of iodinated oil has been introduced in certain areas of the world for goiter prophylaxis.

Treatment

A. Specific Measures:

1. Thyroid–Levothyroxine, 0.1 mg or more, is of value in most cases. The goiter will stop growing and often will decrease in size. As a guide to therapy, T_4 should be maintained in the high normal range, suppressing TSH levels. Since long-standing simple goiters may contain autonomous nodules, it is prudent to watch the patient carefully for possible hyperthyroidism.

2. Iodine therapy–If the enlargement is discovered early and occurs in an area of known endemic iodine deficiency, it may disappear completely with adequate iodine administration. One daily drop of saturated solution of potassium iodide in one-half glass of water is sufficient. Continue therapy until the gland returns to normal size, and then place the patient on a maintenance dosage or use iodized table salt.

B. Indications for Surgery:

1. Signs of pressure–If signs of local pressure are present that are not helped by medical treatment, the gland should be removed surgically. If the patient's age or poor health makes surgical therapy too hazardous, radioactive iodine in large doses (20–100 mCi) is an alternative.

2. Potential cancer–Surgery should be considered for any thyroid gland with a single "cold" (low ^{123}I or ^{99m}Tc uptake) noncystic nodule, since these characteristics increase the likelihood of its being malignant. If the nodule has grown rapidly, is associated with lymphadenopathy, or is attached to surrounding tissues, malignancy is much more likely. Fine-needle aspiration of the nodule is very helpful to decide whether or not surgery is necessary. In a patient with a history of neck radiation during childhood or adolescence, thyroid cancer is common, and surgical removal of a cold nodule is recommended even if aspiration biopsy is negative for malignancy.

Prognosis

Simple goiter may disappear spontaneously or may become large, causing compression of vital structures. Multinodular goiters of long standing, especially in people over 50 years of age, may become toxic. This often happens after ingestion of large amounts of iodine such as administration of radiologic contrast agents (jodbasedow phenomenon). Whether they ever become malignant is not established.

Botazzo GF, Doniach D: Autoimmune thyroid disease. Annu Rev Med 1986;37:353.

Kay TW et al: Treatment of nontoxic multinodular goiter with radioactive iodine. Am J Med 1988;84:19.

Lever EG et al: Inherited disorders of thyroid metabolism. Endocr Rev 1983;4:213.

Mazzaferri EL, de los Santos ET, Rofagha-Keyhani S: Solitary thyroid nodule: Diagnosis and management. Med Clin North Am 1988;72:1177.

HYPOTHYROIDISM

In view of the profound influence exerted on all tissues of the body by thyroid hormone, lack of the hormone may affect virtually all body functions. The degree of severity ranges from mild and unrecognized hypothyroid states to striking myxedema.

A state of hypothyroidism may be due to primary disease of the thyroid gland itself or lack of pituitary TSH or hypothalamic TRH. A true end-organ insensitivity to normal amounts of circulating hormone has been rarely observed. Although gross forms of hypothyroidism, ie, myxedema and cretinism, are readily recognized on clinical grounds alone, the far more common mild forms often escape detection without adequate laboratory facilities.

1. CRETINISM & JUVENILE HYPOTHYROIDISM

Essentials of Diagnosis

- Dwarfism; mental retardation; dry, yellow, cold skin; "pot belly" with umbilical hernia.
- T_4 low; serum cholesterol elevated. Delayed bone age; "stippling" of epiphyses.
- TSH elevated.

General Considerations

The causes of cretinism and juvenile hypothyroidism are as follows:

A. Congenital (Cretinism):

1. Thyroid gland absent or rudimentary (embryogenic defect; most cases of sporadic cretinism).

2. Thyroid gland present but defective in hormone secretion, goitrous, or secondarily atrophied. Due to extrinsic factor (deficient iodine, goitrogenic substances, in most cases of endemic cretinism); or due to maternal factors (some cases of congenital goiter). Many cases are familial, and enzymatic defects in thyroid hormone synthesis may be demonstrated.

B. Acquired (Juvenile Hypothyroidism): Atrophy of the gland or defective function may be due to unknown causes, thyroiditis, or operative removal (lingual thyroid or toxic goiter) or secondary to pituitary deficiency.

Clinical Findings

A. Symptoms and Signs: Dwarfism may be seen, with delayed skeletal maturation; apathy; physical and mental torpor; dry skin with coarse, dry, brittle hair; constipation; slow teething; poor appetite; large tongue; "pot belly" with umbilical hernia; deep voice; cold extremities and cold sensitivity; and true myxedema of subcutaneous and other tissues. A yellow skin due to carotenemia is not infrequent. The thyroid gland is usually not palpable, but a large goiter may be present that may be diffusely enlarged or nodular. Sexual development is retarded, but maturation eventually occurs. Deafness is occasionally associated with congenital goiter (Pendred's syndrome).

B. Laboratory Findings: Total serum T_4 and free T_4 are markedly decreased. Serum cholesterol is frequently elevated. Radioactive iodine uptake is very low in athyroid individuals, but it may be high in cases of congenital iodine organification defects. Other congenital errors of thyroid hormone biosynthesis may be demonstrated by special techniques. Some patients show circulating autoantibodies to thyroid constituents. TSH by radioimmunoassay is invariably elevated; this may be the best screening test.

C. Imaging: Delayed skeletal maturation is a constant finding, often with "stippling" of the epiphyses (especially of the femoral head), with flattening; widening of the cortices of the long bones, absence of the cranial sinuses, and delayed dentition may also be noted.

Differential Diagnosis

It is important to measure serum TSH to differentiate primary hypothyroidism from pituitary failure. Cretinism is sometimes confused with Down's syndrome, although retarded skeletal development is rare in mongoloid infants. In children and adolescents, any unexplained decrease in the rate of growth should alert the physician to the possibility of early hypothyroidism. All causes of stunted growth and skeletal development must be considered as well.

Treatment

See Myxedema, below.

Prognosis

The progress and outcome of the disease depend largely upon the duration of thyroid deficiency and the adequacy and persistence of treatment. Since mental development is at stake, it is of utmost importance to start treatment early.

The prognosis for full mental and physical maturation is much better if the onset of disease occurs later in life. Congenital cretins often have variable degrees of intellectual impairment. With implementation of large-scale thyroid screening programs at birth, appropriate therapy is being instituted much earlier than before, and it is expected that most cretins will have a reasonably normal mental development.

By and large, the response to thyroid therapy is gratifying, but therapy usually must be maintained throughout life.

Eastman CJ, Phillips DI: Endemic goitre and iodine deficiency disorders: Aetiology, epidemiology and treatment. Clin Endocrinol Metab 1988;2:719.

LaFranchi S: Diagnosis and treatment of hypothyroidism in children. Compr Ther 1987;13:20.

Larsen PR: Maternal thyroxine and congenital hypothyroidism. N Engl J Med 1989;321:44.

2. ADULT HYPOTHYROIDISM & MYXEDEMA

Essentials of Diagnosis

- Weakness, fatigue, cold intolerance, constipation, menorrhagia, hoarseness.
- Dry, cold, yellow, puffy skin; scant eyebrows; thick tongue; bradycardia; delayed return of deep tendon reflexes.
- Anemia (often macrocytic).
- T_4 and radioiodine uptake low.
- TSH elevated in primary myxedema.

General Considerations

Primary thyroid deficiency is much more common than secondary hypofunction due to pituitary insufficiency. Primary myxedema occurs after thyroidectomy, eradication of thyroid by radioactive iodine, ingestion of goitrogens (eg, thiocyanates, rutabagas, lithium carbonate), or chronic thyroiditis. The widely used antiarrhythmic agent amiodarone has induced goiter, hypothyroidism, and hyperthyroidism in many patients as a consequence of its high iodine content. Thyroid deficiency can also occur after external x-ray irradiation of the neck (as in patients with lymphoma). Most cases, however, are due to atrophy of the gland from unknown causes, probably due to an autoimmune mechanism. This may also involve other endocrine glands, eg, adrenals, in the same patient (Schmidt's syndrome).

Secondary hypothyroidism may follow destructive lesions of the pituitary gland, eg, chromophobe adenoma or postpartum necrosis (Sheehan's syndrome). It is frequently accompanied by associated disorders of the adrenals and gonads. Since thyroid hormone is necessary for all glandular functions, severe primary myxedema may lead to secondary hypofunction of the pituitary, adrenals, and other glands, making diagnosis difficult.

Clinical Findings

These may vary from the rather rare full-blown myxedema to mild states of hypothyroidism, which are far more common and may escape detection unless a high index of suspicion is maintained.

A. Symptoms and Signs:

1. Early–The principal symptoms are weakness, fatigue, muscle cramps, cold intolerance, constipation, lethargy, constipation, dryness of skin, headache, and menorrhagia. Physical findings may be few or absent. Outstanding are thin, brittle nails; thinning of hair, which may be coarse; and pallor, with poor turgor of the mucosa. Delayed return of deep tendon reflexes is often found.

2. Late–The principal symptoms are slow speech, absence of sweating, modest weight gain, constipation, peripheral edema, pallor, hoarseness, decreased sense of taste and smell, muscle cramps, aches and pains, dyspnea, and deafness. Some women have amenorrhea; others have menorrhagia. Galactorrhea may also be present. Physical findings include puffiness of the face and eyelids, typical carotenemic skin color, thinning of the outer halves of the eyebrows, thickening of the tongue, hard pitting edema, and effusions into the pleural, peritoneal, and pericardial cavities, as well as into joints. Cardiac enlargement ("myxedema heart") is often due to pericardial effusion. The heart rate is slow; the blood pressure is more often normal than low, and even diastolic hypertension that reverses with treatment may be found. Hypothermia may be present. Pituitary enlargement due to hyperplasia of TSH-secreting cells, which may be reversible following thyroid therapy, may be seen in long-standing hypothyroidism. True obesity is relatively unusual in hypothyroidism.

B. Laboratory Findings: The T_4 is under 3.5 μg/dL; the free T_4 is less than 0.8 ng/dL. Radioiodine uptake is decreased ($< 10\%$ in 24 hours), but this test is not always reliable—especially in early or mild cases. The radioactive T_3 resin uptake is usually low. TSH is invariably elevated in primary hypothyroidism. Plasma cholesterol is elevated in primary and, less commonly, in secondary hypothyroidism. Anemia is often present; it may be macrocytic, due in some cases to associated pernicious anemia, or hypochromic microcytic, due to iron deficiency in women with menorrhagia. Serum creatine phosphokinase (CPK) is often elevated. Plasma cortisol is normal unless the patient has associated autoimmune Addison's disease or the hypothyroidism is secondary to pituitary disease with associated adrenal insufficiency. Serum prolactin is elevated in some patients with primary hypothyroidism, presumably due to hypersecretion of hypothalamic thyrotropin-releasing hormone (TRH). Antithyroid antibody titers (antimicrosomal and antithyroglobulin) are high in patients with Hashimoto's thyroiditis and idiopathic primary myxedema.

Differential Diagnosis

Hypothyroidism must be considered in many states of neurasthenia, unexplained menstrual disorders or weight gain, and anemia. Myxedema enters into the differential diagnosis of unexplained heart failure that does not respond to digitalis or diuretics, and unexplained ascites. The protein content of myxedematous effusions is high. The thick tongue may be confused with that seen in primary amyloidosis. Pernicious anemia may be suggested by the pallor and the macrocytic type of anemia seen in myxedema, and the 2 disorders may even coexist. Some cases of primary psychosis and structural diseases of the brain have been confused with myxedema. Some cases of primary psychosis and structural diseases of the brain have been confused with myxedema.

Complications

Complications are mostly cardiac in nature, occurring as a result of advanced coronary artery disease and congestive failure, which may be precipitated by too vigorous thyroid therapy. There is an increased susceptibility to infection. Megacolon has been described in long-standing hypothyroidism. Organic psychoses with paranoid delusions may occur ("myxedema madness"). Rarely, adrenal crisis may be precipitated by thyroid therapy of pituitary or primary myxedema. Hypothyroidism is a rare cause of infertility, which may respond to thyroid medication. Pregnancy in a woman with untreated hypothyroidism often results in miscarriage. On the other hand, if the hypothyroidism is due to autoimmune disease, it may improve during pregnancy. Sellar enlargement and even well-defined TSH-secreting tumors may develop in untreated cases. These tumors decrease in size after replacement therapy is instituted.

A rare complication of severe hypothyroidism is deep stupor, at times progressing to **myxedema coma,** with severe hypothermia, hypoventilation, hypoxia, hypercapnia, and hypotension. Water intoxication and severe hyponatremia are common. Convulsions and abnormal central nervous system signs may occur. Myxedema coma is often induced by an underlying infection; cardiac, respiratory, or central nervous system illness; cold exposure; or drug use. It is most often seen in elderly women. The mortality rate is high. Myxedematous patients are unusually sensitive to opiates and may die from average doses.

Refractory hyponatremia is often seen in severe myxedema. Inappropriate secretion of antidiuretic hormone has been observed in some patients, but a defect in distal tubular reabsorption of sodium and water has been demonstrated in many others.

Treatment

A. Specific Therapy: Levothyroxine is the drug of choice. Other thyroid preparations are still available (Table 20–7), but their use is to be discouraged. Levo-

Table 20–7. Equivalency of thyroid preparations.

Desiccated Thyroid	Approximate Equivalent In		
	Levothyroxine Sodium (Levothroid, Synthroid, Etc)	Liothyronine Sodium (T₃, Cytomel)	Liotrix (Euthroid, Thyrolar)
60 mg	0.05 mg	12.5 μg	Code: ½
65 mg	0.1 mg	25 μg	1
130 mg	0.2 mg	50 μg	2
200 mg	0.3 mg	75 μg	3

thyroxine is easily available, inexpensive, and well standardized and is converted in the body to T_3, the most active thyroid hormone, in an enzymatically regulated manner that best meets the metabolic needs of the patient.

1. When treating patients with severe myxedema or myxedema heart disease, or elderly patients with hypothyroidism with other associated heart disease, begin with small doses of levothyroxine, 25–50 μg daily for 1 week, and increase the dose every week by 25 μg daily up to a total of 100–150 μg daily. This dosage should be continued until signs of hypothyroidism have vanished and the TSH normalizes.

2. Patients with early hypothyroidism may be started with larger doses, 50–100 μg daily, increasing by 25 μg every week until the TSH normalizes.

3. Maintenance—Each patient's dose must be adjusted to obtain the optimal effect. Most patients require 100–150 μg daily for maintenance. Optimal dosage can be estimated by following the free T_4 and TSH levels.

4. Myxedema coma is a medical emergency with a high mortality rate. Levothyroxine sodium, 100–300 μg intravenously as a slow (5- to 10-minute) injection and repeated once in a dose of 100 μg in 12 hours, with the addition of hydrocortisone, 100 mg as an initial bolus, followed by 25–50 mg every 8 hours, may be lifesaving. The patient must not be warmed, adequate pulmonary ventilation must be provided, and fluid and electrolyte replacement must be carefully monitored. Infection is often present and must be vigorously treated. Since assisted mechanical ventilation is almost always necessary to correct the hypercapnia and since patients require very close supervision of state of consciousness, blood pressure, cardiac rhythm, temperature, etc, hospitalization in a well-equipped intensive care unit is strongly recommended.

5. There are special situations where the daily maintenance dose of thyroxine may have to be altered: Slightly higher doses may be necessary during pregnancy or in patients taking drugs that increase thyroxine clearance, such as phenytoin or carbamazepine. Conversely, lower doses are required in subjects with decreased thyroxine clearance (the elderly) or when thyroxine-binding globulin is markedly reduced. At all times, the best guide to therapy of primary hypothyroidism is the level of plasma TSH.

B. Needless Use of Thyroid: The use of thyroid medication as nonspecific stimulating therapy is mentioned only to be condemned. It has been shown that the doses usually employed merely suppress the activity of the patient's own gland. Larger doses given to euthyroid individuals to induce weight loss are irrational and dangerous.

"Metabolic insufficiency" is a questionable entity. The use of thyroid in cases of amenorrhea or infertility is indicated only if the patient is proved to be hypothyroid.

Prognosis

The patient may succumb to the complications of the disease if treatment is withheld too long, eg, myxedema coma. With early treatment, striking transformations take place both in appearance and mental function. Return to a normal state is usually the rule, but relapses will occur if treatment is interrupted. On the whole, response to thyroid treatment is most satisfactory. Chronic maintenance therapy with unduly large doses of thyroid hormone may lead to subtle but important side effects (eg, bone demineralization) and is to be avoided.

Amino N: Autoimmunity and hypothyroidism. Clin Endocrinol Metab 1988;2:591.

Becker C: Hypothyroidism and atherosclerotic heart disease: Pathogenesis, medical management, and the role of coronary artery bypass surgery. Endocr Rev 1985; 6:432.

Camargo CA: Hypothyroidism and goiter during pregnancy. In: *Endocrine Disorders in Pregnancy.* Brody SA, Ueland K (editors). Appleton & Lange, 1989.

Fish LH et al: Replacement dose, metabolism, and bioavailability of levothyroxine in the treatment of hypothyroidism: Role of triiodothyronine in pituitary feedback in humans. N Engl J Med 1987;316:764.

Lazarus JH, Hall R (editors): Hypothyroidism and goitre. (Symposium.) Clin Endocrinol Metab 1988;2:53.

Utiger RD: Therapy of hypothyroidism: When are changes needed? N Engl J Med 1990;323:126.

HYPERTHYROIDISM
(Thyrotoxicosis)

Essentials of Diagnosis

- Weakness, sweating, weight loss, nervousness, loose stools, heat intolerance.
- Tachycardia; warm, thin, soft, moist skin; exophthalmos; stare; tremor.
- Goiter, bruit. T_4, radio-T_3 resin uptake, and radioiodine uptake elevated.
- Failure of suppression by T_3 administration.

General Considerations

The term "thyrotoxicosis" denotes a series of clinical disorders associated with increased circulating levels of free thyroxine or triiodothyronine. By far the most common form of thyrotoxicosis is that associated with diffuse enlargement of the thyroid, hyperactivity of the gland, and the presence of antibodies against different fractions of the thyroid gland. This autoimmune thyroid disorder is called **Graves' disease** (or Basedow's disease in Europe and Latin America). It is much more common in women than in men (8:1), and its onset is usually between the ages of 20 and 40. It may be accompanied by a poorly understood infiltrative ophthalmopathy (Graves' exophthalmos) and, less commonly, by infiltrative dermopathy (pretibial myxedema). It may also be associated with other systemic autoimmune disorders such as pernicious anemia, myasthenia gravis, diabetes mellitus, etc. It has a familial tendency, and histocompatibility studies have shown an association with group HLA-B8 and HLA-DRW3 in white subjects. Current thinking about the pathogenesis of the hyperthyroidism of Graves' disease involves the formation of autoantibodies that bind to the TSH receptor in thyroid cell membranes and stimulate the gland to hyperfunction. These thyroid-stimulating immunoglobulins (TSI) are demonstrable by special techniques in the plasma of most (but not all) patients with Graves' disease. Recent studies suggest that many other antibodies are generated in Graves' disease and even in some forms of thyrotoxicosis that have been traditionally thought to be nonautoimmune.

Other causes of hyperthyroidism include the following:

(1) Plummer's disease, or autonomous toxic adenoma of the thyroid, which may be single or multiple. This is not accompanied by infiltrative ophthalmopathy or dermopathy. Antithyroid antibodies are usually not present in the plasma, and tests for TSI are negative.

(2) Jodbasedow disease, or iodine-induced hyperthyroidism, which may occur in patients with multinodular goiters after intake of large amounts of iodine, especially in the form of radiographic contrast materials.

(3) Thyrotoxicosis factitia, which is due to ingestion of excessive amounts of exogenous thyroid hormone. An unusual variant has been recently reported, with epidemics of thyrotoxicosis due to consumption of ground beef contaminated with bovine thyroid gland.

(4) Struma ovarii (hydatidiform mole), which causes rare cases of clinical hyperthyroidism, although asymptomatic elevation of T_4 may be seen in chorionic tumors, presumably due to ectopic production of a TSH-like material.

(5) TSH-secreting tumor of the pituitary, which is an extremely rare cause of hyperthyroidism. Much more commonly, these tumors are the consequence of long-standing hypothyroidism.

(6) Thyroiditis, which may be associated with transient hyperthyroidism during the initial phase.

Clinical Findings

A. Symptoms and Signs: Restlessness, nervousness, irritability; easy fatigability, especially toward the latter part of the day; and unexplained weight loss in spite of ravenous appetite are often the early features. There is usually excessive sweating and heat intolerance, and quick movements with incoordination varying from fine tremulousness to gross tremor. Less commonly, patients' primary complaints are difficulty in focusing their eyes, pressure from the goiter, diarrhea, or rapid, irregular heart action.

The patient is quick in all motions, including speech. The skin is warm and moist and the hands tremble. A diffuse or nodular goiter may be seen or felt with a thrill or bruit over it. The eyes appear bright, there may be a stare, at times periorbital edema, and commonly lid lag, lack of accommodation, exophthalmos, and even diplopia. The hair and skin are thin and of silky texture. Vitiligo may also occur. Spider angiomas and gynecomastia are common. Cardiovascular manifestations vary from tachycardia, especially during sleep, to paroxysmal atrial fibrillation and congestive failure of the "high-output" type. Mitral valve prolapse occurs much more frequently than in the general population. At times, a harsh pulmonary systolic murmur is heard (Means' murmur). Lymphadenopathy and splenomegaly may be present. Proximal muscle weakness and osteoporosis are common features, especially in long-standing thyrotoxicosis. Rarely, one finds nausea, vomiting, and even fever and jaundice (in which case the prognosis is poor). Mental changes are common, varying from mild exhilaration to delirium and exhaustion progressing to severe depression.

Associated with severe or malignant exophthalmos is at times a localized, bilateral, hard, nonpitting, symmetric swelling ("pretibial myxedema") over the tibia and dorsum of the feet (infiltrative dermopathy). At times there is clubbing and swelling of the fingers (acropachy). It often subsides spontaneously. Onycholysis (separation of nails from the nail bed) may also occur.

Thyroid "storm," rarely seen today, is an extreme form of thyrotoxicosis that may occur after stress, thyroid surgery, or radioactive iodine administration and is manifested by marked delirium, severe tachycardia, vomiting, diarrhea, dehydration, and in many cases, very high fever. The mortality rate is high.

B. Laboratory Findings: The T_4 level and radioiodine and T_3 resin uptakes are increased. On rare occasions, the T_4 level may be normal but the serum T_3 elevated ("T_3 thyrotoxicosis"). Free T_4 is elevated and TSH suppressed. The radioiodine uptake is elevated. In toxic nodular goiter, a high radioiodine uptake in the nodule is diagnostic if combined with elevated T_4 or T_3 and low TSH levels. Postprandial glycosuria is occasionally found. Lymphocytosis is common. Urinary and, at times, serum calcium and phosphate are elevated. Serum alkaline phosphatase may be elevated. In patients with Graves' disease, thyroid-stimulating immunoglobulins (TSI) are often present in serum and tests for antithyroid antibodies (antimicrosomal and antithyroglobulin) are also positive.

C. Imaging: Skeletal changes may include diffuse demineralization or, at times, resorptive changes (osteitis). Hypertrophic osteoarthropathy with proliferation of periosteal bone may be present, especially in the hands (acropachy). CT or MRI scans of the orbit show swelling of the extraocular muscles in cases of Graves' ophthalmopathy.

D. Electrocardiographic Findings: Electrocardiography may show tachycardia, atrial fibrillation, and P and T wave changes.

Differential Diagnosis

Hyperthyroidism may be confused with anxiety neurosis or mania, but in the latter the thyroid is not enlarged and thyroid function tests are normal. Subacute thyroiditis may present with toxic symptoms, and the gland is usually quite tender. The thyroid antibody tests may be positive; T_4 may be elevated, but radioiodine uptake is very low. Exogenous thyroid administration will present the same laboratory features as thyroiditis. A rare pituitary tumor may produce the picture of thyrotoxicosis with high levels of TSH.

Some states of hypermetabolism without thyrotoxicosis, notably severe anemia, leukemia, polycythemia, and cancer, rarely cause confusion. Pheochromocytoma is often associated with hypermetabolism, tachycardia, weight loss, and profuse sweating. Acromegaly may also produce tachycardia, sweating, and thyroid enlargement. Appropriate laboratory tests will easily distinguish these entities.

Cardiac disease (eg, atrial fibrillation, failure) refractory to treatment with digitalis, quinidine, or diuretics suggests the possibility of underlying hyperthyroidism. Other causes of ophthalmoplegia (eg, myasthenia gravis) and exophthalmos (eg, orbital tu-

mor) must be considered. Thyrotoxicosis must also be considered in the differential diagnosis of muscle weakness and osteoporosis. Hypercalciuria and bone demineralization may resemble hyperparathyroidism. The two diseases may be present in the same patient. Diabetes mellitus and Addison's disease may coexist with thyrotoxicosis.

Complications

The ocular and cardiac complications of long-standing thyrotoxicosis are most serious. Severe malnutrition and wasting with cachexia may become irreversible. If jaundice is present, the mortality rate increases. Episodes of periodic paralysis induced by exercise or heavy carbohydrate ingestion and accompanied by hypokalemia may complicate thyrotoxicosis in Oriental men. Thyroid "storm" (see above) is rarely seen but may be fatal. Hypercalcemia and nephrocalcinosis may occur. Decreased libido, impotence, decreased sperm count, and gynecomastia are often found in men with Graves' disease. Complications of treatment for goiter include drug reactions following iodine and thiouracil treatment, hypoparathyroidism and laryngeal palsy after surgical treatment, and progressive exophthalmos. The exophthalmos may progress, despite adequate therapy, to the point of corneal ulceration and destruction of the globe unless orbital decompression is done.

Treatment

Treatment is aimed at halting excessive secretion of the thyroid hormone. Three methods are available: medical therapy (thioureas, iodine, propranolol), subtotal thyroidectomy, and radioactive iodine ablation of the gland. The method of choice is still being debated and varies with different patients. The most widely accepted method in the past has been subtotal thyroidectomy after adequate preparation. There is a greater tendency toward trying long-term medical treatment with antithyroid drugs to achieve remission of the disease and to use radioactive iodine therapy rather than surgical thyroidectomy for thyroid ablation except for large multinodular glands. The age of the patient and reproductive history and wishes are important considerations. Children and young adults who have not yet had children are better treated with antithyroid drugs rather than with radioactive iodine. If medical therapy fails or the gland is very large, subtotal thyroidectomy should be considered, subject to the availability of a skilled and experienced thyroid surgeon. It should be pointed out that even among experts, there is wide divergence of opinion as to the best "definitive" treatment of Graves' disease, especially in the young.

A. Subtotal Thyroidectomy: Adequate preparation is of the utmost importance. One or 2 drugs are generally necessary for adequate preparation: one of the thiouracil group of drugs alone, or, preferably, a thiouracil plus iodine. The sympatholytic agent propranolol has been used successfully as the sole agent before surgery. This drug, however, does not return the patient to a normal metabolic rate, and most experts prefer to render the patient euthyroid prior to surgery.

1. Preoperative use of thiouracil and similar drugs–Several thiouracil drugs are available: propylthiouracil, methimazole, and carbimazole. The modes of action are probably identical. These agents block the intrathyroidal synthesis of hormone. Propylthiouracil has also been shown to impede the peripheral conversion of T_4 to T_3, and carbimazole has been described as decreasing autoimmune response in Graves' disease.

Propylthiouracil has been most widely used and appears to be the least toxic. It is the thiouracil preparation most often used in the USA. The T_4 invariably falls, the rate of fall depending upon the total quantity of previously manufactured hormone available from the gland. (More hormone is present if iodine has been given previously.) The average time required for the T_4 to return to normal is about 4–6 weeks. If the drug dose is not tapered, the T_4 will continue to fall until the patient becomes myxedematous.

Preparation is usually continued and surgery deferred until the T_4 and T_3 uptake are normal. There is no need to rush surgery and no danger of "escape" as with iodine. In severe cases, 100–200 mg 4 times daily (spaced as close to every 6 hours as possible) is generally adequate. Larger doses (eg, for patients with very large glands) are occasionally necessary. In milder cases, 100 mg 3 times daily is sufficient.

There are 2 hazards in the use of propylthiouracil: (1) Agranulocytosis may develop, usually during the first 10 weeks of therapy; patients should be instructed to watch for fever, or sore throat and to notify their physicians immediately if any of these occurs, so that blood count and examination can be performed. If the white count falls below $3000/\mu L$ or if less than 45% granulocytes are present, therapy should be discontinued. Other reactions are drug fever, rash, and jaundice. Rash is common (about 5% of patients); it is usually self-limited and responds to antihistaminic drugs. (2) The gland may remain hyperplastic and highly vascular, rendering surgical removal more difficult. For this reason, combined therapy, using propylthiouracil and iodine, is the method of choice in preparing patients for thyroidectomy (see below).

Methimazole (Tapazole) has a mode of action similar to that of the thiouracils, though it does not alter the T_4 to T_3 conversion. The average dose is 5–10 mg every 8–12 hours, though a single dose often suffices for patients with mild disease. Drug rash and agranulocytosis may also occur.

Carbimazole (not available in the USA but commonly used in Europe) is rapidly converted to methimazole and is similar in action. The average dose is 10–15 mg every 8 hours. Toxic side effects are slightly more common with this drug.

2. Preoperative use of iodine–Iodine is given in daily doses of 5–10 drops of strong iodine solution (Lugol's solution) or saturated solution of potassium iodide along with a thiourea in preparation for surgery. It should not be used as a single agent, since (1) a few patients may not respond, especially those who have received iodine recently; (2) sensitivity to iodides may be present; (3) after 10–14 days of therapy, the gland may "escape" and the patient may develop a more severe hyperthyroidism than before; and (4) it is generally impossible to reduce the T_4 to normal with iodine alone.

3. Combined propylthiouracil-iodine therapy–The advantage of this method is that one obtains the complete inhibition of thyroid secretion with the involuting effect of iodine.

Propylthiouracil followed by iodine appears at present to be the preoperative method of choice. Begin therapy with propylthiouracil; about 10–21 days before surgery is contemplated (when all thyroid tests have returned to normal or low normal range), begin the iodine and *continue* for 1 week after surgery.

4. Propranolol–This drug may be used alone for the preoperative preparation of the patient in doses of 80–240 mg daily. It is the most rapid way of reversing some of the seemingly catecholamine-mediated toxic manifestations of the disease, and less time is necessary to prepare the patient for thyroidectomy. It has been suggested as the treatment of choice for thyrotoxicosis in pregnancy. Since it does not reverse the hypermetabolic state itself, escape and even thyroid storm may occur in patients so prepared. It should not be used in patients with bronchial asthma, and it should be employed with extreme caution if congestive heart failure seems likely to develop.

B. Continuous Propylthiouracil Therapy (Medical Treatment): Control of hyperthyroidism with propylthiouracil alone is often the preferred treatment, especially in young people, who are not good candidates for ^{131}I therapy. The advantage is that it avoids the risks and postoperative complications of surgery, eg, laryngeal palsy, hypoparathyroidism. The disadvantages are the possibility of toxic reactions and the need to watch for signs of hypothyroidism.

Begin with 100–200 mg every 6–8 hours and continue until the T_4 and T_3 uptake are normal and all signs and symptoms of the disease have subsided; then place the patient on a maintenance dose of 50–150 mg daily, observing the thyroid function tests periodically to avoid hypothyroidism.

An alternative method is to continue with doses of 50–200 mg every 6–8 hours until the patient becomes hypothyroid and then maintain the T_4 at normal levels with thyroid hormone.

The optimal duration of therapy and the recurrence

rate with medical therapy have not been agreed upon. At present it would seem that of the patients kept on propylthiouracil between 18 and 24 months, about 20–40% will remain euthyroid as the drug is tapered off and discontinued. Patients with large thyroid glands that fail to decrease in size with medical therapy have a greater chance of recurrence of thyrotoxicosis after cessation of therapy. In some laboratories, decreasing levels of thyroid-stimulating immunoglobulins (TSI) have been helpful in predicting successful outcome of medical therapy. Those having recurrences after cessation of treatment may be treated again with propylthiouracil, radioiodine, or surgery. Since the natural history of untreated Graves' disease often includes eventual development of hypothyroidism, all such patients should have reevaluation of thyroid status at regular intervals.

C. Radioactive Iodine (^{131}I): The administration of radioiodine has proved to be an excellent method for destruction of overfunctioning thyroid tissue (either diffuse or toxic nodular goiter). The rationale of treatment is that the radioiodine, being concentrated in the thyroid, will destroy the cells that concentrate it. Objections to radioiodine therapy include the possibility of carcinogenesis and the possibility of damage to the genetic pool of the individual treated, but all studies to date have failed to show evidence of these effects. Nevertheless, the use of radioiodine is generally limited to older age groups (25 or above); however, the age level is not absolute, and some children may be best treated with radioiodine. Since fetal radiation is harmful, *do not use this drug in pregnant women.* In the majority of patients, it is preferable to render the subject euthyroid with propylthiouracil before ^{131}I ablation. The drug is discontinued 3–5 days before administration of radioiodine. There is a high incidence of hypothyroidism several years after this form of treatment, even when small doses are given. Several studies have shown, however, that hypothyroidism also occurs quite frequently years after surgical or medical treatment of Graves' disease and that eventual hypothyroidism may be part of the natural history of this condition. Prolonged follow-up, preferably with T_4 and TSH measurements, is therefore mandatory. There is a greater tendency toward higher-dosage radioiodine ablation of the toxic gland, with subsequent permanent replacement therapy with thyroid hormone. If smaller doses are used initially, re-treatment may be required and myxedema may still occur several years later.

D. General Measures:

1. The patient with hyperthyroidism should not engage in strenuous activities. In severe cases, bed rest may be necessary. Most cases are treated with thioureas or radioiodine on an ambulatory basis.

2. Hyperthyroid patients are often in negative nitrogen and calcium balance and need a well-balanced and nutritious diet.

3. Many of the symptoms of hyperthyroidism

respond to adrenergic blockade. Propranolol has been very useful to ameliorate tachycardia, palpitations, tremor, and nervousness. Atrial fibrillation may convert to sinus rhythm. Propranolol also decreases the frequency of periodic hypokalemic paralysis in Oriental men with thyrotoxicosis and ameliorates other neuromuscular manifestations such as thyrotoxic myopathy.

E. Treatment of Complications:

1. Exophthalmos–The exact cause of exophthalmos in Graves' disease is still not known. It has been shown that exophthalmos is due to edema and cellular infiltration of the orbital muscles, possibly because of an autoimmune reaction that may be facilitated by lymphatic channel communication between the thyroid gland and the ocular orbits. The onset and severity of this ocular complication bear no relationship to the hypermetabolic state. Treatment of hypothyroidism does not necessarily help this condition and may possibly even aggravate it, leading to malignant exophthalmos. It has been suggested that this is because the thyroid secretion exerts an inhibitory effect on the anterior pituitary, and removal of the gland allows the anterior pituitary to secrete more hormones and aggravate the condition. However, since the pituitary TSH levels are *always* low in thyrotoxicosis due to Graves' disease, it is doubtful that thyroid therapy is of use unless the patient is becoming hypothyroid.

a. Dark glasses, protection from dust, eye shields, tarsorrhaphy, and other measures may be necessary to protect the eyes. Elevation of the head of the bed at night, diuretics, and local use of methylcellulose solution (1%) to prevent drying of the protruding eyes are helpful. Ophthalmologic consultation should be requested.

b. Glucocorticoid therapy in large doses (60–100 mg of prednisone daily) has proved helpful in some cases. The inflammatory reaction in the periorbital tissues is reduced, and symptoms such as lacrimation, chemosis, and photophobia may rapidly improve. Ocular protrusion is less responsive. Unfortunately, relapse occurs frequently when the drug is discontinued, and the severe side effects of high-dose glucocorticoid therapy preclude prolonged therapy. A recent study indicates that a course of prednisone following ^{131}I therapy for Graves' disease prevents exacerbation of ophthalmopathy.

c. Because of the persistent belief that the ophthalmopathy is an immune phenomenon, many modifiers of the immune response have been used, such as azathioprine, cyclophosphamide, and cyclosporine. Results have been erratic and not reproducible.

d. Surgery for malignant exophthalmos– In severe progressive cases, where corneal edema or ulceration, limitation of extraocular muscle movements, and failing vision occur, orbital decompression may be necessary to save the eyesight.

e. X-ray radiation of the retro-orbital area, with

careful shielding of the lens, may be helpful and should be considered in severe cases.

2. Cardiac complications–

a. Some degree of tachycardia is almost always found if normal rhythm is present in thyrotoxicosis. This requires only the treatment of the thyrotoxicosis. Severe tachycardia responds promptly to propranolol therapy.

b. Congestive failure tends to occur in long-standing thyrotoxicosis, especially in the older age groups. Treatment is the same as for congestive failure due to any cause.

c. Atrial fibrillation may occur in association with thyrotoxicosis. Ventricular response rates remain rapid despite digitalis. Many cases revert to normal rhythm soon after toxicity is removed. However, if fibrillation persists after euthyroidism is achieved, electrical conversion is necessary after appropriate anticoagulation therapy to prevent embolism.

3. "Crisis" or "storm"–Therapy of thyroid storm is multifactorial. Treat aggressively any precipitating illness (infection, ketoacidosis, etc). Give large doses of antithyroid drugs, by nasogastric tube if necessary. Propylthiouracil, 1000–1500 mg daily in divided doses, is of crucial importance. Administer iodine to block release of thyroid hormone from glandular stores (SSKI, 5 drops every 6 hours, or sodium iodide, 500 mg intravenously every 12 hours. Give large doses of adrenergic blocking agents, eg, propranolol (60–120 mg every 6 hours) to block adrenergic-mediated effects of thyroid hormone and to decrease synthesis of T_3 from T_4. Intravenous propranolol may be necessary, with careful monitoring of cardiac rhythm and function. Large doses of glucocorticoids (hydrocortisone sodium succinate, 300 mg/d) have traditionally been used in these patients, who are at risk of developing adrenal insufficiency. Glucocorticoids may inhibit the peripheral transformation of T_4 to T_3 and should be of help.

General supportive therapy, best carried out in an intensive care unit, includes antipyretic therapy, oxygen, sedation, glucose infusions, multivitamins, and careful monitoring of the state of hydration, electrolyte balance, etc.

4. Hyperthyroidism and pregnancy–Since hyperthyroidism is a condition preferentially affecting women during their reproductive years, it is not surprising that the 2 entities often coincide in the same subject. Diagnosis may be difficult, since normal pregnancy may be accompanied by tachycardia, warm skin, heat intolerance, increased sweating, and a palpable thyroid. Laboratory tests are helpful: although the T_4 is elevated in all pregnant women, values over 15 mg/dL are encountered only in hyperthyroidism. The T_3 resin uptake, which is low in normal pregnancy because of high TBG concentration, is "normal" in thyrotoxic subjects. The free T_4 is clearly elevated. Pregnancy often has a beneficial effect upon the thyrotoxicosis of Graves' disease, with decreasing antibody

titers and decreasing free T_4 levels as the pregnancy advances. Pregnant women with hyperthyroidism are best treated with propylthiouracil in the smallest dose consistent with "high normal" thyroid function. The drug *does* cross the placenta and rarely may induce TSH hypersecretion and thyroid enlargement in the fetus. Thyroid hormone administration to the mother *does not* prevent hypothyroidism in the fetus, since T_4 and T_3 do not freely cross the placenta. Fetal hypothyroidism is rare, however, since the mother's hyperthyroidism is often controlled with small (50–150 mg/d) daily doses of propylthiouracil. If hyperthyroidism is severe, surgery may be necessary, better done during the second trimester.

Rarely, the child may be born with transient thyrotoxicosis due to placental passage of maternal thyroid stimulators. This neonatal thyrotoxicosis resolves spontaneously in 3–12 weeks. Rarely, hyperthyroidism may persist because of the presence of active Graves' disease in the infant.

A question often arises about whether a mother taking thioureas should breast feed her baby. Recent studies indicate that only minimal amounts of propylthiouracil are transferred to the maternal milk and that breast feeding is safe. Apparently this is less true for methimazole, which appears in higher concentrations in the milk.

5. Dermopathy–Severe pretibial myxedema, an uncommon complication of Graves' disease, responds well to local glucocorticoid therapy.

Prognosis

Graves' disease is a cyclic entity and may subside spontaneously and may even result in spontaneous hypothyroidism. More commonly, however, it progresses, especially with recurrent psychic trauma and other types of stress. The ocular, cardiac, and psychic complications often are more serious than the chronic wasting of tissues and may become irreversible even after treatment. Permanent hypoparathyroidism and vocal cord palsy are risks of surgical thyroidectomy. With any form of therapy, unless radical thyroidectomy or large dosage ^{131}I therapy is used, recurrences are common. With adequate treatment and long-term follow-up, the results are good. It is perhaps wiser to speak of induced remission rather than cure. Post-treatment hypothyroidism is common. It may occur several years after radioactive iodine therapy or subtotal thyroidectomy. Use of ^{131}I to treat Graves' disease has not resulted in any demonstrable increase of thyroid cancer, leukemia, or other cancers.

Patients with jaundice and fever have a less favorable prognosis, and so do those with thyroid storm. Malignant exophthalmos also has a poor prognosis, even with optimal therapy.

Bahn RS et al: Diagnostic evaluation of Graves' ophthalmopathy. Endocrinol Metab Clin North Am 1988;17:527.
Bartalena L et al: Use of corticosteroids to prevent progres-

sion of Graves' ophthalmopathy after radioiodine therapy for hyperthyroidism. N Engl J Med 1989;321:1349.

Becker DV: Choice of therapy for Graves' hyperthyroidism. (Editorial.) N Engl J Med 1984;311:464.

Burrow GN: The management of thyrotoxicosis in pregnancy. (Current Concepts.) N Engl J Med 1985;313:562.

Cooper DS: Antithyroid drugs. N Engl J Med 1984; 311:1353.

Dunn JT: Choice of therapy in young adults with hyperthyroidism of Graves' disease. Ann Intern Med 1984; 100:891.

Fradkin JE, Wolff J: Iodide-induced thyrotoxicosis. Medicine 1983;62:1.

Gruebeck-Loebenstein B et al: Immunological features of non-immunogenic hyperthyroidism. J Clin Endocrinol Metab 1985;60:150.

Roth RH, McAuliffe MJ: Hyperthyroidism and thyroid storm. Emerg Med Clin North Am 1989;7:873.

Smith LH, Rapoport B: The ophthalmopathy of Graves' disease. West J Med 1985;142:532.

Utiger RD: Treatment of Graves' ophthalmopathy. N Engl J Med 1989;321:1403.

Weetman AP, McGregor AM: Autoimmune thyroid disease: Developments in our understanding. Endocr Rev 1984; 5:309.

THYROID CANCER

Essentials of Diagnosis

- Painless swelling in region of thyroid, or thyroid nodule not responding to suppression.
- Normal thyroid function tests.
- Past history of irradiation to neck may be present.
- Positive thyroid needle aspiration.

General Considerations
(Table 20–8)

Although carcinoma of the thyroid is rarely associated with functional abnormalities, it enters into the differential diagnosis of all types of thyroid lesions. It is common in all age groups but especially in patients who have received radiation therapy in childhood or infancy to the face, neck, or upper mediastinum. The cell type determines to a large extent the type of therapy required and the prognosis for survival. The most common varieties are papillary and follicular carcinomas, which are usually associated with prolonged survival. The anaplastic tumor is rare and carries a very bad prognosis. Finally, the medullary carcinoma of the thyroid originates in the parafollicular cells derived from the last branchial pouch, contains amyloid deposits, and secretes calcitonin. It is familial and often associated with pheochromocytomas (multiple endocrine neoplasia type II) and with the syndrome of multiple mucosal neuromas (multiple endocrine neoplasia type III). Other tumors of the thyroid, much less common than those mentioned above, include lymphomas, primary sarcomas, and teratomas.

Clinical Findings

A. Symptoms and Signs: The principal signs of thyroid cancer are a painless nodule, a hard nodule in an enlarged thyroid gland, so-called lateral aberrant thyroid tissue, or palpable lymph nodes with thyroid enlargement. Signs of pressure or invasion of surrounding tissues are present in anaplastic or longstanding tumors with recurrent laryngeal nerve palsy, fixation of nodule to neighboring structures, etc.

B. Laboratory Findings: With very few exceptions, all thyroid function tests are normal unless the disease is associated with thyroiditis. The scintiscan usually shows a "cold" nodule. Serum thyroid autoantibodies are sometimes found. Thyroglobulin levels are high in metastatic papillary and follicular tumors. In medullary carcinoma, the calcitonin levels are elevated, especially after a calcium infusion. Calcitonin assay is a reliable clue to silent medullary carcinoma, especially in the familial syndrome, although an occasional extrathyroidal tumor (eg, lung) may also produce calcitonin. The best way to deter-

Table 20–8. Some characteristics of thyroid cancer.

	Papillary	Follicular	Medullary	Anaplastic
Incidence[1] (%)	61	18	6	15
Average age[1]	42	50	50	57
Females[1] (%)	70	72	56	56
Deaths due to thyroid cancer[1,2] (%)	6	24	33	98
Invasion: Juxtanodal	+++++	+	++++++	+++
Blood vessels	+	+++	+++	+++++
Distant sites	+	+++	++	++++
Resemblance to normal thyroid	+	+++	+	±
^{123}I uptake	+	++++	0	0
Degree of malignancy	+	++ to +++	+++	++++++++

[1] Data based upon 885 cases analyzed by Woolner et al; figures have been rounded to the nearest digit. (After Woolner.)
[2] Some patients have been followed up to 32 years after diagnosis.

mine the nature of a thyroid nodule is fine-needle aspiration biopsy. It requires the services of an experienced cytopathologist.

C. Imaging: Extensive bone and soft tissue metastases (some of which may take up radioiodine) may be demonstrable on radiographs or radioisotope scans. Calcified areas may be seen in medullary carcinoma (primary tumor or metastases).

Differential Diagnosis
(Table 20–9)

Nonmalignant enlargements of the thyroid gland are far more common than carcinoma. Echography may be helpful in differentiating cystic and solid nodules. Purely cystic lesions are very frequently benign. The incidence of malignancy is much greater in single than in multinodular lesions, and far greater in nonfunctioning than in functioning nodules. The differentiation from chronic thyroiditis is at times most difficult, and the 2 lesions may occur together. Any nonfunctioning lesion in the region of the thyroid that increases rapidly must be considered carcinoma until proved otherwise. Thyroid therapy has been traditionally used to differentiate benign from malignant nodules, the benign ones being expected to decrease in

Table 20–9. Differential diagnosis of thyroid nodules.[1]

Clinical Evidence	Low Index of Suspicion	High Index of Suspicion
History	Familial history of goiter Residence in area of endemic goiter	Previous therapeutic irradiation of head, neck, or chest Hoarseness
Physical characteristics	Older women Soft nodule Multinodular goiter	Children, young adults; men Solitary, firm nodule Vocal cord paralysis Enlarged lymph nodes Distant metastatic lesions
Serum factors	High titer of antithyroid antibody	Elevated serum calcitonin High serum thyroglobulin
Scanning techniques Uptake of ^{123}I Echo scan Thermography Roentgenogram Technetium flow	"Hot" nodule Cystic lesion Cold Shell-like calcification Avascular	"Cold" nodule Solid lesion Warm Punctate calcification Vascular
Thyroxine therapy	Regression after 0.2 mg/d for 6 months or more	Increase in size

[1] Reproduced, with permission, from Greenspan FS: Thyroid nodules and thyroid cancer. *West J Med* 1974;121:359.

size, though this often does not happen. Percutaneous needle aspiration biopsy has been extremely useful in diagnosis and is the diagnostic procedure of choice to separate benign from malignant lesions prior to surgery. If there is a history of neck radiation in childhood or adolescence, excision of the suspected thyroid nodule is mandatory.

Complications

The complications vary with the type of carcinoma. Papillary tumors invade local structures, such as lymph nodes; follicular tumors metastasize through the bloodstream; anaplastic carcinomas are highly aggressive, both locally and systemically. Medullary carcinomas may be complicated by the coexistence of pheochromocytomas. The complications of radical neck surgery often include permanent hypoparathyroidism, and, less commonly, vocal cord palsy; permanent hypothyroidism is expected and should always be treated.

Treatment

Surgical removal is the treatment of choice for most thyroid carcinomas. The appropriate extent of surgical removal is debatable, some surgeons favoring lobectomy and others near-total thyroidectomy. ^{131}I has been used by most as an adjunct to surgical therapy, especially for follicular carcinoma. Complete ablation of the thyroid with ^{131}I after thyroidectomy is advocated by many. The patient is rendered hypothyroid by withdrawing thyroid hormone for 4–6 weeks until the TSH is significantly elevated to maximize the iodine uptake by thyroid tissue. At this time, a tracer dose of radioiodine is given, uptake determination and scan are done, and the ablative dose of ^{131}I is calculated and given subsequently. This allows visualization and therapy of thyroid tissue left in place after surgery and even of metastases that could not be visualized prior to thyroidectomy. Following this procedure, the patient is placed on suppressive doses of T_4 indefinitely. Some repeat the cycle of stopping therapy, rendering the patient hypothyroid, and scanning and treating—if residual uptake is present— every 6–12 months until all thyroid tissue, benign or malignant, has disappeared. There is a risk of hematologic malignancy with multiple ^{131}I therapy at the large doses used. The risk of leukemia increases significantly after a cumulative dose greater than 300 mCi. The protracted course of most thyroid cancers, with or without therapy, has made it difficult to establish a consensus for optimal therapy. Thyroxine administration to suppress TSH to undetectable levels is mandatory for papillary and follicular cancers. External irradiation may be useful for local as well as distant metastases. Postoperative hypoparathyroidism must be treated in the usual manner.

Prognosis

The prognosis is directly related to the cell type.

The anaplastic carcinomas advance rapidly in spite of early diagnosis and treatment, while papillary and follicular tumors—in spite of frequent bouts of recurrence—are rarely fatal. Early detection and removal of medullary carcinomas by finding elevated calcitonin levels may lead to a better prognosis. In general, the prognosis is less favorable in elderly patients.

Crile G et al: The advantages of subtotal thyroidectomy and suppression of TSH in the primary treatment of papillary carcinoma of the thyroid. Cancer 1985;55:2691.

DeGroot LJ: Radiation and thyroid disease. Clin Endocrinol Metab 1988;2:777.

Franklyn JA, Sheppard MC: Thyroid nodules and thyroid cancer: Diagnostic aspects. Clin Endocrinol Metab 1988:2:761.

Griffin JE: Management of thyroid nodules. Am J Med Sci 1988;296:336.

Kramer JB, Wells SA Jr: Thyroid carcinoma. Adv Surg 1989;22:195.

Mazzaferri EI, Young RL: Papillary thyroid carcinoma: A 10-year follow-up report of the impact of therapy in 576 patients. Am J Med 1981;70:511. (A classic paper in thyroid carcinoma.)

THYROIDITIS

Essentials of Diagnosis

- Swelling of thyroid gland, causing pressure symptoms in acute and subacute forms; painless enlargement in chronic form.
- Thyroid function tests variable; discrepancy in T_4 and radioiodine uptake common.
- Serologic autoantibody tests often positive.

General Considerations

Thyroiditis has been more frequently diagnosed in recent years, since special serologic tests for thyroid autoantibodies became available. This heterogeneous group can be divided into 2 groups: (1) due to a specific cause (usually infection), and (2) due to unknown, often autoimmune factors. The second is the more common form.

Clinical Findings

A. Symptoms and Signs:

1. Thyroiditis due to specific infections–A rare disorder causing severe pain, tenderness, redness, and fluctuation in the region of the thyroid gland and due to pyogenic organisms, usually in the course of systemic infection.

2. Nonspecific (?autoimmune) thyroiditis–

a. Subacute nonsuppurative thyroiditis–This disorder—also called de Quervain's thyroiditis, granulomatous thyroiditis, giant cell thyroiditis—is an acute, usually painful enlargement of the thyroid gland, with dysphagia. The pain radiates to the ears. The manifestations may persist for weeks or months and may be associated with signs of thyrotoxicosis and malaise. Young and middle-aged women are most commonly affected. Viral infection has been suggested as the cause. The erythrocyte sedimentation rate is markedly elevated, which helps differentiate this form of thyroiditis from others. Aspiration biopsy shows characteristic giant multinucleated cells.

b. Lymphocytic subacute thyroiditis–This form of thyroiditis—also called lymphocytic thyroiditis with hyperthyroidism, and silent subacute thyroiditis—is characterized by a silent (painless) swelling of the thyroid and associated with symptoms and signs of hyperthyroidism. It is being increasingly recognized in the USA. The clinical manifestations are similar to those of moderate Graves' disease, and the differential diagnosis is not simple. Both may present with symmetric, painless, modest enlargement of the thyroid, tremor, weight loss, stare, lid lag, etc, as well as elevated levels of serum T_4. Antibody titers (antithyroglobulin and antithyroid microsomal) are higher in Graves' disease. The ^{123}I uptake is low in this form of thyroiditis and high in Graves' disease. The hyperthyroid symptoms abate spontaneously, and normalcy is restored within a few months. The transient hyperthyroid state is due to leakage of preformed thyroid hormone from the inflamed gland and not to hyperactivity of the thyroid cells. These patients, therefore, should not receive propylthiouracil. Propranolol is useful for symptomatic control of the hyperthyroid phase. The etiology of this entity is unknown.

c. Postpartum thyroiditis is a form of autoimmune thyroiditis occurring soon after parturition and accompanied by transient hyperthyroidism followed by hypothyroidism. It has been described in women with thyroid autoimmune disease who had suppression of antibody titers during pregnancy and a rebound of immune activity after delivery.

d. Hashimoto's thyroiditis–Hashimoto's thyroiditis—also called struma lymphomatosa, lymphadenoid goiter, and chronic lymphocytic thyroiditis—is the most common form of thyroiditis and probably the most common thyroid disorder. Evidence for an autoimmune cause is uniformly present. Onset of enlargement of the thyroid gland is insidious, with few pressure symptoms. The gland is firm, symmetrically enlarged, lobulated, and nontender to palpation. Thyroid antibody titers (antithyroglobulin and antimicrosomal) are very high. The condition is more frequent in women and has a familial clustering. It occurs at all ages. Signs of thyroid dysfunction seldom appear, but rarely the disease may progress to myxedema or even present as thyrotoxicosis ("hashitoxicosis"), which may be transient.

e. Riedel's thyroiditis–Riedel's thyroiditis is also called chronic fibrous thyroiditis, Riedel's struma, woody thyroiditis, ligneous thyroiditis, and invasive thyroiditis. It is the rarest form of thyroiditis and is found most frequently in middle-aged women. Enlargement is often asymmetric; the gland is stony hard and adherent to the neck structures, causing signs of compression and invasion, including dysphagia, dyspnea, and hoarseness. It may be part of a systemic fibrosis syndrome with retroperitoneal, mediastinal, and biliary tract sclerosis.

B. Laboratory Findings: The T_4 and T_3 resin uptake are usually markedly elevated in acute and subacute thyroiditis and normal or low in the chronic forms. Radioiodine uptake is characteristically very low in the initial, hyperthyroid phase of subacute thyroiditis; it may be high with an uneven scan in chronic thyroiditis, with enlargement of the gland, and low in Riedel's struma. Leukocytosis, elevation of the sedimentation rate, and increase in serum globulins are common in acute and subacute (de Quervain) forms. Thyroid autoantibodies are most commonly demonstrable in Hashimoto's thyroiditis but are also found in the other types. The serum TSH level is elevated if inadequate amounts of thyroid hormone is elaborated by the thyroid gland.

Complications

In the suppurative forms of thyroiditis, any of the complications of infection may occur; the subacute and chronic forms of the disease are complicated by the effects of pressure on the neck structures: dyspnea and, in Riedel's struma, vocal cord palsy. Hashimoto's thyroiditis may lead to hypothyroidism. Carcinoma or lymphoma may be associated with chronic thyroiditis and must be considered in the diagnosis of uneven painless enlargements that continue in spite of treatment. Hashimoto's thyroiditis may be associated with Addison's disease, hypoparathyroidism, diabetes, pernicious anemia, biliary cirrhosis, vitiligo, and other autoimmune conditions. Mitral valve prolapse is also much more frequent in patients with Hashimoto's thyroiditis than in normal persons. The reason for this is unknown.

Differential Diagnosis

Thyroiditis must be considered in the differential diagnosis of all types of goiters, especially if enlargement is rapid. In the acute or subacute stages it may simulate primary hyperthyroidism, and only a careful evaluation of several of the laboratory findings will point to the correct diagnosis. The very low radioiodine uptake in subacute thyroiditis with elevated T_4 and T_3 uptake and a rapid sedimentation rate is of the greatest help. Chronic thyroiditis, especially if the enlargement is uneven and if there is pressure on surrounding structures, may resemble carcinoma, and both disorders may be present in the same gland. The subacute and suppurative forms of thyroiditis may resemble any infectious process in or near the neck structures; and the presence of malaise, leukocytosis, and a high sedimentation rate is confusing. Because of referred ear pain, patients with subacute thyroiditis may be misdiagnosed as having otitis. The thyroid autoantibody tests have been of help in the diagnosis of chronic lymphocytic (Hashimoto's) thyroiditis, but the tests are not specific and may also be positive in patients with goiters, carcinoma, and thyrotoxicosis, though the titers are often higher in Hashimoto's thyroiditis. Biopsy may be required for diagnosis.

Treatment

A. Suppurative Thyroiditis: Antibiotics, and surgical drainage when fluctuation is marked.

B. Subacute Thyroiditis:

1. De Quervain's thyroiditis– All treatment is empiric and must be maintained for several weeks, since the recurrence rate is high. The drug of choice is aspirin, which relieves pain and inflammation. Severe cases may require a brief course of prednisone therapy: 10 mg 3 times a day for 1 or 2 weeks is effective, but symptoms and signs may recur after the drug is tapered off.

2. Silent lymphocytic thyroiditis with hyperthyroidism does not require the use of anti-inflammatory agents. The symptoms of hyperthyroidism may be treated with propranolol. If hypothyroidism develops later, thyroid replacement therapy is indicated.

C. Hashimoto's Thyroiditis: Levothyroxine should be given in the usual doses (0.1–0.15 mg daily) if hypothyroidism or large goiter is present. If the thyroid gland is only minimally enlarged and the patient is euthyroid (with *normal* TSH levels), regular observation is in order, since hypothyroidism may develop in later years.

D. Riedel's Struma: Partial thyroidectomy is often required to relieve pressure; adhesions to surrounding structures make this a difficult operation.

Prognosis

The course of this group of diseases is quite variable. Spontaneous remissions and exacerbations are common in the subacute form, and therapy is nonspecific. The disease process may smolder for months. Hashimoto's thyroiditis may be associated with other autoimmune disorders (diabetes mellitus, Addison's disease, pernicious anemia, etc), with all the complications of those diseases. In general, however, patients with Hashimoto's thyroiditis have an excellent prognosis, since the condition either remains stable for years or progresses slowly to hypothyroidism, which is easily treated. Rarely, lymphoma of the thyroid may complicate Hashimoto's thyroiditis.

Hamburger JI: The various presentations of thyroiditis: Diagnostic considerations. Ann Intern Med 1986;104:219.

Jansson R, Dahlberg PA, Karlsson FA: Postpartum thyroiditis. Clin Endocrinol Metab 1988;2:619.

Schwaegerle SM, Bauer TW, Esselstyn CB Jr: Riedel's thyroiditis. Am J Clin Pathol 1988;90:715.

THE PARATHYROIDS

Parathyroid gland secretion is most important in maintenance of calcium homeostasis. Parathyroid hormone (PTH) is a polypeptide hormone composed of 84 amino acids with a molecular weight of 9500. Together with calcitonin (CT), secreted by the parafollicular cells of the thyroid gland, and 1,25-dihydroxycholecalciferol, the active form of vitamin D, parathyroid hormone is responsible for maintenance of calcium, phosphate, and magnesium balance, the integrity and normal mineralization of the teeth and skeleton, and maintenance of normal neuromuscular excitability.

The main physiologic effects of PTH are as follows: (1) It increases the osteoclastic activity in bone, with increased delivery of calcium and phosphorus to the extracellular compartment and the circulation; (2) it increases the renal tubular reabsorption of calcium in the glomerular filtrate; (3) it inhibits the net absorption of phosphate and bicarbonate by the renal tubule; and (4) it stimulates the synthesis of 1,25-dihydroxycholecalciferol by the kidney. All of these steps result in a net increase in the amount of ionized calcium circulating in plasma.

Calcitonin (CT) is a weak hormone whose main function is to antagonize the effect of PTH on bone. Neither excess nor deficiency of this hormone seems to result in chronic derangement of calcium homeostasis.

Vitamin D is a hormone with a complex set of actions and mechanism of synthesis. Cholecalciferol (vitamin D_3) is synthesized in the skin, under the influence of ultraviolet radiation, from 7-dehydrocholesterol. Two sequential hydroxylations, are necessary for full biologic activity: The first one takes place in the liver—to 25-hydroxycholecalciferol—and the second one in the kidney, resulting in the formation of the most potent biologic metabolite of vitamin D, 1,25-dihydroxycholecalciferol $(1,25[OH]_2D_3)$. The main action of vitamin D is the acceleration of calcium and phosphate absorption in the intestine. Deficiency or excess of vitamin D results in profound disturbances of calcium and phosphate homeostasis and, in the case of deficiency, of skeletal formation and maturation. Other actions of vitamin D are now under intense scrutiny, and it is possible that this hormone plays a significant role in cell communication and differentiation, especially in immunologically important cell lines.

HYPOPARATHYROIDISM & PSEUDOHYPOPARATHYROIDISM

Essentials of Diagnosis

- Tetany, carpopedal spasms, tingling of lips and hands, muscle and abdominal cramps, psychologic changes.
- Positive Chvostek's sign and Trousseau's phenomenon; defective nails and teeth; cataracts.
- Serum calcium low; serum phosphate high; alkaline phosphatase normal; urine calcium excretion reduced.
- Basal ganglia calcification on x-ray of skull.

General Considerations

Hypoparathyroidism is most commonly seen following thyroidectomy or surgery for primary hyperparathyroidism. Very rarely, it follows x-ray irradiation to the neck or radioactive iodine administration. Transient hypoparathyroidism occurs in a significant number of patients after thyroidectomy. After surgical removal of parathyroid tissue for primary hyperparathyroidism, a profound hypocalcemia may occur as a result of accelerated remineralization of the skeleton (hungry bone syndrome).

Parathyroid deficiency in the absence of surgical or radiation injury is referred to as **idiopathic hypoparathyroidism.** It is often associated with candidiasis, may be familial or sporadic, and may be accompanied by other endocrine deficiencies, presumably on an autoimmune basis. It usually begins in childhood. Patients may later develop diabetes mellitus, pernicious anemia, thyroid immune disease, or most often, Addison's disease. Candidiasis usually occurs first, before the age of 8; hypoparathyroidism becomes apparent a few years later; and Addison's disease or other endocrinopathies are last to appear. This syndrome is called **polyglandular autoimmune syndrome type I** and also **MEDAC (multiple endocrine deficiency, autoimmune, candidiasis) syndrome.**

Occasionally, idiopathic hypoparathyroidism occurs in an adult with no family history or other manifestations of disease. The cause of these sporadic cases is unknown.

Functional hypoparathyroidism may also occur as a result of magnesium deficiency (malabsorption, chronic alcoholism), which prevents the secretion of PTH. Correction of hypomagnesemia results in rapid disappearance of the condition.

Finally, a few rare cases of hypoparathyroidism due to destruction of the parathyroid glands by metastatic malignant tissue (carcinoma of the breast) have been reported. Hemochromatosis may also occasionally cause hypoparathyroidism.

Pseudohypoparathyroidism is a genetic defect associated with short stature, round face, obesity, bone abnormalities including short metacarpals and metatarsals, and ectopic bone formation. The parathyroids are present and often hyperplastic, but there is resistance to the hormone action. It appears to be a heterogeneous group of disorders, with several different subgroups having been identified. The classic cases present with clinical and chemical evidence of hypoparathyroidism (increased neuromuscular irritability, cataracts, basal ganglia calcification, hypocalcemia, hyperphosphatemia, etc) and elevated serum PTH. Most patients with the phenotypic abnormalities just described have tissue resistance to PTH and to other hormones that act by stimulating cAMP (glucagon, vasopressin, TSH). A recent important discovery was the gene mutation responsible for the defect in a subgroup of patients with this condition (also known as Albright's hereditary osteodystrophy). Patients without hypocalcemia but sharing the phenotypic abnormalities are described as having **pseudopseudohypoparathyroidism.**

Clinical Findings

A. Symptoms and Signs: Acute hypoparathyroidism causes tetany, with muscle cramps, irritability, carpopedal spasm, and convulsions; stridor, wheezing, dyspnea; tingling of the circumoral area, hands, and feet is almost always present. Symptoms of the chronic disease are lethargy, personality changes, anxiety state, blurring of vision due to cataracts, and mental retardation.

Chvostek's sign (facial muscle contraction on tapping the facial nerve in front of the tragus) is positive, and Trousseau's phenomenon (carpal spasm after application of a cuff) is present. Cataracts may occur; the nails may be thin and brittle; the skin dry and scaly, at times with fungus infection (candidiasis) and loss of hair (eyebrows); deep tendon reflexes may be hyperactive. Papilledema and elevated cerebrospinal fluid pressure are occasionally seen. Teeth may be defective if the onset of the disease occurs in childhood. Branchial anomalies (eg, cleft palate) may be found. In pseudohypoparathyroidism, the fingers and toes are short, especially the fourth finger, where a dimple instead of a knuckle is seen on making a fist, due to a short fourth metacarpal bone.

B. Laboratory Findings: Serum calcium is low, serum phosphate high, urinary phosphate low (tubular reabsorption of phosphate above 95%), urinary calcium low to absent, and alkaline phosphatase normal. Alkaline phosphatase may be elevated in pseudohypoparathyroidism. Creatinine clearance is normal. Parathyroid hormone levels are low or absent in idiopathic or postsurgical hypoparathyroidism but normal or even markedly elevated in pseudohypoparathyroidism. Administration of parathyroid hormone results in phosphaturia and increase of urinary cAMP in patients with hypoparathyroidism, whereas most patients with pseudohypoparathyroidism do not show a response.

C. Imaging: Radiographs or CT scans of the skull may show basal ganglia calcifications; the bones may be denser than normal. In pseudohypoparathyroidism, short metacarpals and ectopic bone may be seen and bones may be demineralized.

D. Other Examinations: Slit-lamp examination may show early posterior lenticular cataract formation. The ECG shows prolonged QT intervals and T wave abnormalities.

Complications

Acute tetany with stridor, especially if associated with vocal cord palsy, may lead to respiratory obstruction requiring tracheostomy. The complications of chronic hypoparathyroidism depend largely upon the duration of the disease and the age at onset. If it starts early in childhood, there may be stunting of growth, malformation of the teeth, and retardation of mental development. There may be associated sprue syndrome, pernicious anemia, and Addison's disease, probably on the basis of an autoimmune mechanism. In pseudohypoparathyroidism, tissue resistance to the action of other hormones (TSH, glucagon, vasopressin) may be present. In long-standing cases, cataract formation and calcification of the basal ganglia are seen. Occasionally, parkinsonian symptoms develop. Ossification of the paravertebral ligaments may occur with nerve root compression; surgical decompression may be required. Seizures are common in untreated patients. Overtreatment with vitamin D and calcium may produce impairment of renal function and nephrocalcinosis.

Differential Diagnosis

The symptoms of hypocalcemic tetany may be confused with or mistaken for tetany due to respiratory alkalosis, in which the serum calcium is normal. Symptoms of anxiety are common in both instances, and fainting is not uncommon in the hyperventilation syndrome. The typical blood and urine findings should differentiate the 2 disorders. Other causes of hypocalcemia include the vitamin D deficiency syndromes, where serum phosphate is low instead of high. Acute pancreatitis is easily recognizable by the acute onset, abdominal symptoms, elevated serum and urinary amylase, etc. In the "hungry bone syndrome," previously mentioned, serum phosphate is low and alkaline phosphatase is elevated. Confusion might arise with the tetany due to magnesium deficiency or in chronic renal failure, in which retention of phosphorus will produce a high serum phosphorus with low serum calcium, but the differentiation should be obvious on clinical grounds (eg, uremia).

At times hypoparathyroidism is misdiagnosed as idiopathic epilepsy, choreoathetosis, or brain tumor (on the basis of brain calcifications, convulsions, choked disks) or, more rarely, as "asthma" (on the basis of stridor and dyspnea). Hypocalcemia, of course, does not occur in any of these conditions. Other causes of cataracts and basal ganglia calcification also enter into the differential diagnosis.

Treatment

A. Emergency Treatment for Acute Attack (Hypoparathyroid Tetany): This usually occurs after surgery and requires immediate treatment.

1. Be sure an adequate airway is present.

2. Calcium gluconate, 10–20 mL of 10% solution intravenously, may be given *slowly* until tetany ceases. Ten to 50 mL of 10% calcium gluconate may be added to 1 L of 5% glucose in water or saline and administered by slow intravenous drip. The rate should be so adjusted that the serum calcium is raised above 7 mg/dL and maintained between 8 and 9 mg/dL. Careful monitoring of serum calcium is important to avoid hypercalcemia.

3. Oral calcium–Calcium salts should be given orally as soon as possible to supply 1–2 g of calcium daily. Calcium carbonate (40% calcium) is effective and is the calcium salt of choice. Tablets containing 250 mg of calcium are well tolerated; the dosage is 4–8 tablets per day. Other calcium preparations, such as calcium lactate or gluconate, have lower calcium content and are more expensive.

4. Vitamin D preparations–(Table 20–10.) Therapy should be started as soon as oral calcium is begun. The choice of agent is not easy, since multiple factors such as availability, duration of action, and cost must be considered. Vitamin D_2 (ergocalciferol) has been used successfully for many years in the chronic treatment of hypoparathyroidism. The usual daily dose ranges from 50,000 to 100,000 units/d. It is a slow-acting preparation, and if toxicity develops hypercalcemia may persist for weeks after the drug is discontinued. Dihydrotachysterol is faster in onset of action and is 3 times more potent than ergocalciferol. The usual daily maintenance dose is 0.125–1 mg/d. It is more expensive than vitamin D_2. The active metabolite of vitamin D, 1,25-dihydroxycholecalciferol (calcitriol), has a very rapid onset of action, and if toxicity develops it is not long-lasting. Because of its very high cost, it has been used primarily in the treatment of acute hypocalcemia in doses ranging from 1–4 µg/d rather than for prolonged, chronic therapy.

5. Magnesium–If hypomagnesemia is present (chronic alcoholism, malnutrition, drugs such as cisplatin, etc), it must be corrected in order to treat the resulting hypocalcemia. Acutely, $MgSO_4$ is given intravenously, 1–2 g every 6 hours. Chronic magnesium replacement requires magnesium oxide tablets (600 mg), 1 or 2 per day.

B. Maintenance Treatment: The goal should be to maintain the serum calcium in the low normal range (8.5–9 mg/dL). This will minimize the hypercalciuria that would otherwise occur and provides a safety margin against overdosage and hypercalcemia, which may produce permanent damage to renal function. Calcium supplementation (1–2 g/d) is continued, and a vitamin D preparation, as previously outlined, is given. Monitoring of serum calcium at regular intervals (every 3 months at a minimum) is mandatory.

Caution: Phenothiazine drugs should be administered with caution in hypoparathyroid patients, since they may precipitate extrapyramidal symptoms. Furosemide should be avoided, since it may enhance hypocalcemia.

Prognosis

The outlook is fair if prompt diagnosis is made and treatment instituted. Some changes (eg, in the electroencephalogram) are reversible by appropriate treatment, but the dental changes, cataracts, and brain calcifications are permanent. Periodic blood chemical evaluation is required, since changes in calcium levels may call for modification of the treatment schedule. Sudden appearance of hypercalcemia, especially in children, may be due to Addison's disease.

Hosking DJ, Kerr D: Mechanisms of parathyroid hormone resistance in pseudohypoparathyroidism. Clin Sci 1988; 74:561.

Mallette LE et al: Synthetic human parathyroid hormone-(1–34) for the study of pseudohypoparathyroidism. J Clin Endocrinol Metab 1988;67:964.

Patten JL et al: Mutation in the gene encoding the stimulatory G protein of adenylate cyclase in Albright's hereditary osteodystrophy. N Engl J Med 1990;322:1412.

Zaloga GP, Chernow B: Hypocalcemia in critical illness. JAMA 1986;256:1924.

Table 20–10. Vitamin D preparations used in the treatment of hypoparathyroidism.[1]

	Potency[2]	How Supplied	Daily Dose (Range)	Time Required for Toxic Effects to Subside
Ergocalciferol (ergosterol, vitamin D_2)	40,000 USP units/mg.	Capsules of 25,000 and 50,000 units; solution, 500,000 units/mL.	25,000–200,000 units	6–18 weeks.
Dihydrotachysterol (Hytakerol)	120,000 USP units/mg.	Tablets of 0.125, 0.2, and 0.4 mg.	0.2–1 mg.	1–3 weeks.
Calcifediol (Calderol)	. . .	Capsules of 20 and 50 µg.	20–200 µg.	3–6 weeks.
Calcitriol (Rocaltrol)	. . .	Capsules of 0.25 and 0.5 µg.	0.25–5 µg.	½–2 weeks.

[1] Reproduced, with permission, from Greenspan FS, Forsham PH (editors): *Basic & Clinical Endocrinology,* 2nd ed. Lange, 1986.
[2] Number of units of vitamin D provided by 1 mg of the preparation.

HYPERPARATHYROIDISM

Essentials of Diagnosis

- Renal stones, nephrocalcinosis, polyuria, polydipsia, hypertension, uremia, intractable peptic ulcer, constipation.
- Bone pain, cystic lesions, and, rarely, pathologic fractures.
- Serum and urine calcium elevated; urine phosphate high with low to normal serum phosphate; alkaline phosphatase normal to elevated.
- Hypercalcemia is often the only abnormality present (found in routine screening).
- X-ray: subperiosteal resorption, loss of lamina dura of teeth, renal parenchymal calcification or stones, bone cysts, chondrocalcinosis.
- Elevated parathyroid hormone.

General Considerations

Primary hyperparathyroidism is an increasingly recognized disorder. Surveys suggest that hyperfunction of the parathyroids, often as asymptomatic hypercalcemia, may be present in 0.1% of patients examined. It should always be suspected in obscure bone and renal disease, especially if nephrocalcinosis or calculi are present. At least 5% of renal stones are associated with this disease. It is more frequent in persons over the age of 50 and more common in women than in men. It may be hereditary in a minority of cases.

The disease is due to hypersecretion of parathyroid hormone either by hyperplastic glands or by a parathyroid adenoma or carcinoma (the latter is very rare). The pathologic classification of parathyroid adenoma versus hyperplasia is difficult when examining an isolated gland. Even the separation between a "normal" gland and an abnormal one (adenoma or hyperplasia) may be difficult, since there are few absolute criteria. The findings at surgery are very important: how many glands were identified, what was their size, etc. In most published series, a simple "adenoma" was more frequently found than hyperplasia of all glands.

Multiple neoplasms, often familial, of the pancreas, pituitary, thyroid, and adrenal glands may be associated with primary hyperparathyroidism due to tumor or, more commonly, due to hyperplasia of the parathyroids (multiple endocrine adenomatosis types I, IIa, and IIb; see Table 20–14).

Secondary hyperparathyroidism is almost always associated with hyperplasia of all 4 glands, but on rare occasions an autonomous tumor may arise in hyperplastic glands ("tertiary hyperparathyroidism"). It is most commonly seen in chronic renal disease but is also found in chronic vitamin D deficiency states.

Hyperparathyroidism causes excessive excretion of calcium and phosphate by the kidneys; this can result in either calculus formation within the urinary tract or, less commonly, diffuse parenchymal calcification (nephrocalcinosis). Chronic bone resorption induced by excessive PTH in the circulation may produce diffuse demineralization, pathologic fractures, or cystic bone lesions throughout the skeleton ("osteitis fibrosa cystica").

Clinical Findings

A. Symptoms and Signs: The manifestations of hyperparathyroidism may be divided into those referable to (1) skeletal involvement, (2) renal and urinary tract damage, and (3) hypercalcemia per se. Since the adenomas are small and deeply located, they are almost never palpable. In many patients, the disease is discovered when they are entirely asymptomatic as the result of a blood "multipanel" screening test that reveals unsuspected hypercalcemia. Others complain only of nonspecific symptoms such as fatigue, lack of energy, or mild "aches and pains."

1. Skeletal manifestations–These may vary from simple back pain, joint pains, painful shins, and similar complaints, to actual pathologic fractures of the spine, ribs, or long bones, with loss of height and progressive kyphosis. At times an epulis of the jaw (actually a "brown tumor") may be the telltale sign of osteitis fibrosa.

2. Urinary tract manifestations–Polyuria and polydipsia may be present and are due to hypercalcemia. Stones containing calcium oxalate or phosphate may be passed. Nephrocalcinosis and renal failure may eventually occur.

3. Manifestations of hypercalcemia–Mild hypercalcemia is often asymptomatic. In more severe cases, thirst, anorexia, and nausea and vomiting are outstanding symptoms. Often one finds a history of peptic ulcer, with obstruction or even hemorrhage. There may be stubborn constipation, asthenia, anemia, and weight loss. Hypertension is commonly found. Some patients present primarily with neuromuscular disorders such as muscle weakness, easy fatigability, or paresthesias. Depression and psychosis may occur. Intense pruritus may accompany severe hypercalcemia. Calcium may precipitate in the corneas ("band keratopathy"). In secondary (renal) hyperparathyroidism, calcium also precipitates in the soft tissues, especially around the joints. Recurrent pancreatitis occurs in some patients.

B. Laboratory Findings: The hallmark of primary hyperparathyroidism is hypercalcemia (serum calcium > 10.2 mg/dL). In hyperproteinemic states, the total serum calcium may be elevated but the ionized fraction is normal, whereas in primary hyperparathyroidism the ionized calcium is always elevated. The serum phosphate is often low (< 2.5 mg/dL). The urine calcium excretion may be high or normal, but it is usually low for the degree of hypercalcemia. There is an excessive loss of phosphate in the urine in the presence of low to low normal serum phosphate (low tubular reabsorption of phosphate [below 80–90%]). The alkaline phosphatase is elevated only if bone disease is present. The plasma chloride and uric acid levels may be elevated. (In secondary hyperparathyroidism, the serum phosphate is high as a result of renal failure.) Elevated levels of parathyroid hormone confirm the diagnosis. Multiple radioimmunoassays are available. The best recognizes the intact molecule at 2 different sites—the N-terminal and the C-terminal ends—with 2 different antibodies. This assay, known as *imunoradiometric assay* (IRMA), is totally specific, highly sensitive, and makes it easy to differentiate primary hyperparathyroidism from other causes of hypercalcemia.

The localization of parathyroid tumors by selective radioimmunoassay for parathyroid hormone via venous catheter is rarely done—only after an unsuccessful prior neck exploration.

C. Imaging: Since the gland or glands affected are rarely larger than 1.5 cm in diameter (and often *much* smaller), imaging techniques are often unsuccessful and are usually not necessary. In experienced hands, ultrasonography may be helpful. CT scan reveals only the rare large neck or mediastinal adenoma. Angiographic studies may be of great help in unusual, complicated cases but only if special expertise is available. Bone x-rays may show diffuse demineralization, subperiosteal resorption of bone (especially in the radial aspects of the fingers), and often loss of the lamina dura of the teeth. There may be cysts throughout the skeleton, mottling of the skull ("salt-and-pepper appearance"), or pathologic fractures. Articular cartilage calcification (chondrocalcinosis) is sometimes found. One may find calculi in the urinary tract or diffuse stippled calcifications in the region of the kidneys (nephrocalcinosis). Soft tissue calcifications around the joints and in the blood vessels may be seen in renal osteitis.

Complications

Although the striking complications are those associated with skeletal damage (eg, pathologic fractures), the serious ones are those referable to renal damage. Urinary tract infection due to stone and obstruction may lead to renal failure and uremia. If the serum calcium level rises rapidly, clouding of sensorium, renal failure, and rapid precipitation of calcium throughout the soft tissues may occur. Peptic ulcer and pancreatitis may be intractable before surgery. Insulinomas or gastrinomas may be associated, as well as pituitary tumors (multiple endocrine neoplasia type I). Pseudogout may complicate hyperparathyroidism both before and after surgical removal of tumors. Subcutaneous, soft tissue, and extensive vascular calcification—as well as dermal necrosis—may occur in secondary hyperparathyroidism due to renal insufficiency.

Differential Diagnosis

High serum calcium associated with high PTH is highly indicative of primary hyperparathyroidism. It is important, however, to consider all other possible causes of hypercalcemia. A complete history and physical examination are sufficient to exclude some of the causes. Other hypercalcemic syndromes include the following:

(1) Vitamin D intoxication: Usually the history alone is sufficient to exclude this cause. Patients may take large amounts of vitamin D for unclear reasons, and a check of all medications is important. Serum levels of 25-hydroxycholecalciferol are helpful to confirm the diagnosis. A brief course of glucocorticoid therapy may be necessary if hypercalcemia is significant.

(2) Sarcoidosis and other granulomatous disorders: The demonstration that macrophages and perhaps other cells present in granulomatous tissue have the ability to synthesize 1,25-dihydroxycholecalciferol has greatly clarified our understanding of the calcium abnormality in these disorders, which include tuberculosis, berylliosis, histoplasmosis, coccidioidomycosis, and even foreign-body granuloma formation. Increased intestinal calcium absorption and hypercalciuria are more common than hypercalcemia. Serum levels of 1,25-dihydroxycholecalciferol are elevated.

(3) Hyperthyroidism: Increased calcium turnover is a feature of thyrotoxicosis. Mild hypercalcemia may also be present.

(4) Adrenal insufficiency: Hypercalcemia is common in untreated Addison's disease. The mechanism is unclear, but a partial explanation relates to the hyperproteinemia often found in a dehydrated, hemoconcentrated addisonian patient, so that it is the total rather than the ionized calcium that is elevated.

(5) Milk-alkali syndrome: The history of peptic ulcer and prolonged therapy with milk or antacids such as sodium bicarbonate or calcium carbonate is of paramount importance. Hypercalcemia is rapidly reversible following discontinuance of such therapy. If it persists, the possibility of associated hyperparathyroidism should be strongly considered.

(6) Multiple myeloma: This bone marrow cancer is a common cause of hypercalcemia in the older population. Many other hematologic cancers such as monocytic leukemia, T cell leukemia and lymphoma, Burkitt's lymphoma, etc, have also been associated with hypercalcemia. An osteoclastic activating factor (OAF) has been identified in the genesis of hypercalcemia. Other local osteolytic tissue factors are being actively investigated at present. Blood analyses, serum protein electrophoresis and immunoelectrophoresis and bone marrow biopsy usually make the diagnosis without difficulty.

(7) Hypercalcemia of cancer: Many malignant tumors (breast, lung, pancreas, uterus, hypernephroma, etc) can produce severe hypercalcemia. In some cases (breast carcinoma especially), bony metastases are clearly present and the diagnosis presents little difficulty. In many others, no metastases to bone can be demonstrated. Recent investigations have demonstrated the secretion of a polypeptide substance by the tumor that has effects on bone resorption similar to those of parathyroid hormone. This peptide has been isolated and sequenced. It has homology with PTH in amino acids 1–13 only. It has been named parathyroid hormone-related peptide (PTH-RP), and its gene locus has been identified in the short arm of chromosome 12 (the PTH gene is in the short arm of chromosome 11). A radioimmunoassay is now commercially available and has proved useful to separate the humoral hypercalcemia of malignancy (HHM) from other forms of hypercalcemia. The clinical features of the hypercalcemia of cancer can closely simulate hyperparathyroidism. Serum phosphate is often low, but the plasma level of PTH by IRMA is *low*. The search for the occult cancer may, on occasion, be quite difficult.

(8) Familial hypocalciuric hypercalcemia: It is important to rule out this benign condition in subjects with mild hypercalcemia because it can be easily mistaken for mild hyperparathyroidism. It is an autosomal dominant inherited disorder characterized by severe hypocalciuria (usually < 50 mg/24 h), variable hypermagnesemia, and normal or minimally elevated levels of PTH. These patients do not normalize their hypercalcemia after subtotal parathyroid removal and should not be subjected to surgery. The condition has an excellent prognosis and is easily diagnosed with family history and urinary calcium clearance determination.

Other causes of hypercalcemia, usually easily diagnosed, include bone fractures or Paget's disease with immobilization, acute renal failure, and vitamin A intoxication. Modest hypercalcemia is also occasionally seen in patients taking thiazide diuretics.

Treatment

A. Surgical Measures: The mainstay of therapy for primary hyperparathyroidism is surgical removal of the excess parathyroid tissue. Removal of a parathyroid adenoma usually results in surgical cure. However, multiple tumors may occasionally be present; the tumor may be in the thyroid gland or in an ectopic site, eg, the mediastinum. Hyperplasia of all glands requires removal of 3 glands and subtotal resection of the fourth before cure is likely. Success is related to the experience and expertise of the surgeon. After surgery, the patient may, in the course of several hours or days, develop tetany (usually transient) as a result of rapid fall of blood calcium even though the calcium level may fall only to the normal or low normal range. *Caution:* Be certain that an adequate airway is present. Therapy is as for hypoparathyroid tetany (see p 820). Prolonged hypocalcemia due to recalcification of the "hungry" skeleton may require large amounts of calcium and vitamin D. Additional magnesium salts may be required postoperatively. Not every patient with hyperparathyroidism,

however, requires surgical treatment. Patients with mild hypercalcemia (< 11 mg/dL) may be followed medically unless they show evidence of deterioration of renal function, bone demineralization, significant hypertension, etc. (See Table 20–11.)

B. Fluids: A large fluid intake is necessary so that a diluted urine will be excreted to minimize the formation of calcium-containing renal stones.

C. Treatment of Hypercalcemia: If symptomatic and severe, hypercalcemia requires hospitalization and intensive hydration with intravenous saline. Loop diuretics such as furosemide are helpful for inducing calcium excretion and lowering the serum calcium. If used initially, however, furosemide may further dehydrate the patient and worsen the hypercalcemia. It should be used, therefore, only *after* circulatory volume has been restored by saline administration. Thiazide diuretics should *never* be used, since they decrease calcium excretion and worsen the hypercalcemia. In subjects in renal failure, hemodialysis may be necessary.

Agents that inhibit bone resorption include mithramycin, which effectively reduces the hypercalcemia due to hyperparathyroidism or cancer, but this drug is toxic. Calcitonin combined with glucocorticoids has been used in the treatment of hypercalcemia, but its value is uncertain. Glucocorticoid therapy is very useful in cases of vitamin D intoxication, sarcoidosis, and hematologic disorders associated with hypercalcemia. Intravenous etidronate (a diphospho-

Table 20–11. Categories of treatment for patients with primary hyperparathyroidism.[1]

Criteria	Preferred Treatment
1. One or more of the following: Serum calcium > 11 mg/dL. 　Osteitis fibrosa cystica. 　Progressive osteopenia. 　Metabolically active nephrolithiasis. 　Intractable peptic ulcer. 　Pancreatitis. 　Serious psychiatric disease. 　Severe hypertension.	Surgical removal of parathyroid lesion.
2. Unsuccessful surgery, or recurrence with manifestations noted in category 1.	Surgical removal of parathyroid lesion; preoperative localization may be indicated.
3. Serum calcium <11 mg/dL. Abnormal serum iPTH. Absence of manifestations noted in category 1.	Surgical removal of parathyroid lesion or medical management (see text).
4. Surgery contraindicated.	Medical management for hypercalcemia and prevention of nephrolithiasis (see text).

[1] Reproduced, with permission, from Greenspan FS, Forsham PH (editors): *Basic & Clinical Endocrinology*, 2nd ed. Lange, 1986.

nate) has been used successfully to reverse the hypercalcemia of cancer with minimal side effects. Another drug recently advocated for severe hypercalcemia is gallium nitrate, but experience with it is limited. The patient with hypercalcemia is very sensitive to the toxic effects of digitalis. Propranolol may be useful in preventing the adverse cardiac effects of hypercalcemia.

D. Medical Treatment of Mild Hyperparathyroidism: Since this disorder is more frequently recognized by routine chemical screening procedures, a number of patients with relatively mild hypercalcemia (< 11 mg/dL) and few symptoms are encountered. They are best managed by forcing fluids; avoiding immobilization and thiazides; adding phosphate preparations if renal function is good; and giving estrogenic hormones if postmenopausal. Careful follow-up is necessary, with attention paid to evaluation of renal function (creatinine clearance) and monitoring of skeletal mineralization with dual photon bone densitometry. If the patient cannot be followed periodically or becomes symptomatic—eg, passes a stone or shows progressive bone disease—neck exploration must be considered.

Prognosis

The disease is usually a chronic progressive one unless treated successfully by surgical removal of the abnormal parathyroid glands. There are at times unexplained exacerbations and partial remissions. Completely asymptomatic patients with mild hypercalcemia may be followed by means of serial calcium determinations and treated medically as outlined above.

Spontaneous cure due to necrosis of the tumor has been reported but is exceedingly rare. The prognosis is directly related to the degree of renal impairment. The bones, in spite of severe cyst formation, deformity, and fracture, will heal completely if a tumor is successfully removed, but this may take several years. Significant renal damage, however, may progress even after removal of an adenoma, and life expectancy is reduced. In carcinoma of the parathyroid (rare), the prognosis is not necessarily hopeless. The presence of pancreatitis increases the mortality rate. If hypercalcemia is severe, the patient may suddenly die in cardiac arrest or may develop acute renal failure. However, early diagnosis and treatment of this disease in an increasing number of patients have led to dramatic recovery. Prolonged postoperative follow-up must be stressed to ensure that the state of hyperparathyroidism has been reversed.

The distressing bone disease of secondary hyperparathyroidism due to renal failure (renal osteodystrophy) can be partially prevented and treated by careful monitoring of the phosphate and parathyroid hormone levels. Resistance to vitamin D can now be overcome by the newer biologically active derivatives, eg, 1,25-dihydroxycholecalciferol and 1 α-hy-

droxycholecalciferol. "Tertiary hyperparathyroidism," ie, hypercalcemia following correction of renal failure, is uncommon in patients so managed, and parathyroidectomy is rarely required nowadays for this disorder.

Some patients with chronic renal failure have severe osteodystrophy and hypercalcemia due to chronic aluminum intoxication rather than to autonomous hyperparathyroidism (pseudohyperparathyroidism).

Bilezikian JP: Parathyroid hormone-related peptide in sickness and in health. N Engl J Med 1990;322:1151.
Breslau NA: Update on secondary forms of hyperparathyroidism. Am J Med Sci 1987;294:120.
Canfield RE (editor): Etidronate disodium: A new therapy for hypercalcemia of malignancy. (Proceedings of a symposium.) Am J Med 1987;82(2A):1.
Chapman I et al: Primary hyperparathyroidism: Pathogenesis, diagnosis, and management. Compr Ther 1988; 14:65.
Higgins CB, Auffermann W: MR imaging of thyroid and parathyroid glands: A review of current status. AJR 1988;151:1095.
Marons R: Laboratory diagnosis of hyperparathyroidism. Endocrinol Metab Clin North Am 1989;18:647.
Schaiff RA, Hall TG, Bar RS: Medical treatment of hypercalcemia. Clin Pharm 1989;8:108.
Stewart AF et al: Humoral hypercalcemia of malignancy. Ann Intern Med 1988;108:454.

METABOLIC BONE DISEASE*

OSTEOPOROSIS

Essentials of Diagnosis

- Asymptomatic to severe backache.
- Spontaneous fractures and collapse of vertebrae without spinal cord compression, often discovered "accidentally" on radiography; loss of height.
- Serum calcium, phosphorus, and alkaline phosphatase normal.
- Demineralization, especially of spine and pelvis.

General Considerations

Osteoporosis is the most common metabolic bone disease in the USA and is a major public health problem. As a result of osteoporosis, hundreds of thousands of fractures take place every year. The morbidity and (indirect) mortality rates are very high. Since the usual form of the disease is clinically evident in middle life and beyond and since women are more frequently affected than men, it is often termed "postmenopausal" or "senile" osteoporosis. It is charac-

---

* The causes of osteomalacia are summarized in Table 20–12.

Table 20–12. Causes of osteomalacia.[1]

Vitamin D deficiency
Inadequate sunlight exposure without dietary supplementation.
  House- or institution-bound people.
  Atmospheric smog.
  Chronic residence in far northern and far southern latitudes.
  Excessive covering of body with clothing.
Gastrointestinal disease that interrupts the normal enterohepatic recycling of vitamin D and its metabolites, resulting in their fecal loss.
  Chronic steatorrhea (pancreatic).
  Malabsorption (gluten-sensitive enteropathy).
  Surgical resection of large parts of intestine.
  Biliary fistula formation.
Impaired synthesis of $1,25(OH)_2D_3$ by the kidney.
  Nephron loss as in chronic kidney disease (see section on renal hyperparathyroidism).
  Functional impairment of $1,25(OH)_2D_3$ hydroxylase (eg, hypoparathyroidism).
  Congenital absence of $1,25(OH)_2D_3$ hydroxylase (vitamin D-dependent rickets type I).
  Suppression of $1,25(OH)_2D_3$ production by endogenously produced substances (cancer).
Target cell resistance to $1,25(OH)_2D_3$-absent or diminished number of $1,25(OH)_2D_3$ receptors, vitamin D-dependent rickets type II.

Phosphate deficiency
Dietary.
  Low intake of phosphate.
  Excessive aluminum hydroxide ingestion (phosphate binders).
Impaired renal tubular reabsorption of phosphate.
  Other acquired and hereditary renal tubular disorders associated with renal phosphate loss (Fanconi's syndrome).
  Tumor-associated hypophosphatemia.
  X-linked hypophosphatemia.
  Adult-onset hypophosphatemia.

Systemic acidosis
Chronic renal failure.
Distal renal tubular acidosis.
Ureterosigmoidoscopy.
Chronic acetazolamide and ammonium chloride administration.

Drug-induced osteomalacia
Excessive alcohol intake.
Excessive diphosphonate administration.
Excessive fluoride administration.
Anticonvulsant administration (enhanced vitamin D metabolism).
Aluminum, lead, cadmium excess.
Outdated tetracyclines.

Primary mineralization defects
Hypophosphatasia.
Osteopetrosis.
Fibrogenesis imperfecta ossium.

[1] Modified and reproduced, with permission, from Greenspan FS, Forsham PH (editors): *Basic & Clinical Endocrinology*, 2nd ed. Lange, 1986.

terized by an absolute decrease in the amount of bone present to a level below which it is capable of maintaining the structural integrity of the skeleton. The rate of bone formation is often normal, whereas the rate of bone resorption is increased. There is a greater loss of trabecular bone than compact bone, accounting for the primary features of the disease, ie, crush fractures of vertebrae, fractures of the neck of the femur, and fractures of the distal end of the radius. Whatever bone is present is normally mineralized. Osteoporosis may be produced secondarily by a number of disorders (see below), but more commonly it is primary and of unknown cause. The inheritance of low skeletal mass in young adult life (especially in white females), loss of sex hormones at the time of the menopause, the effects of aging, lack of activity, inadequate dietary calcium intake, impaired intestinal calcium absorption, a high phosphate intake, acid ash diet, inappropriate secretion of parathyroid hormone or calcitonin, or some combination of these factors have been considered as possible contributing causes. In some patients, no obvious contributing factor is identified.

Etiology

A. Principal Associations:

1. Lack of estrogens (postmenopausal, physiologic, or postoophorectomy osteoporosis). (Females are deprived of estrogens relatively early in life. About 30% of women over 60 years of age have clinical osteoporosis. Some degree of osteoporosis is almost always present in advanced age.)

2. Lack of activity, eg, immobilization as in paraplegia or rheumatoid arthritis. (Osteoblasts depend upon strains and stresses for proper function.) While a moderate amount of physical activity is of benefit both to prevent and treat osteoporosis, excessive athletic activity, which leads to weight loss and amenorrhea, causes bone loss.

3. Malabsorption, at times with intestinal lactase deficiency or after gastrectomy, may be an important factor in elderly patients with osteoporosis.

4. Deficient 1,25-dihydroxyvitamin D production may be a cause of some types.

B. Less Common Associations:

1. Developmental disturbances (eg, osteogenesis imperfecta).

2. Nutritional disturbances (eg, anorexia nervosa, protein starvation or excess, ascorbic acid deficiency).

3. Chronic calcium deficiency due to inadequate intake or renal loss may cause osteoporosis.

4. Endocrine diseases—Lack of androgens (congenital or acquired hypogonadism), hypopituitarism and hyperprolactinemia (secondary gonadal failure), acromegaly (mechanism unknown; possibly due to hypogonadism), thyrotoxicosis (not constant; causes excessive turnover of skeletal tissue), excessive exogenous or endogenous ACTH or corticosteroids causing increased bone resorption (eg, Cushing's disease), and long-standing uncontrolled diabetes mellitus (rare).

5. Bone marrow disorders–The presence of abnormal cells in the bone marrow, such as in myeloma or leukemia, may stimulate osteoclastic activity and cause osteoporosis. This is in addition to the active replacement of the marrow with tumor cells. A bone marrow factor may also play an etiologic role in senile osteoporosis.

6. Prolonged use of heparin may lead to osteoporosis. Tobacco smoking may be an important factor.

7. Chronic alcoholism.

Clinical Findings

A. Symptoms and Signs: Osteoporosis may first be discovered on x-ray examination. It may present as backache of varying degrees of severity or as a spontaneous fracture or collapse of a vertebra. Loss of height is common.

B. Laboratory Findings: Serum calcium, phosphate, and alkaline phosphatase are normal. The alkaline phosphatase may be slightly elevated in osteogenesis imperfecta and also in other forms of osteoporosis if there has been a recent fracture.

C. Imaging: The principal areas of demineralization are the spine and pelvis, especially in the femoral neck and head; demineralization is less marked in the skull and extremities. Compression of vertebrae is common. The lamina dura is preserved. The increasing availability of instruments for quantitating bone mineral mass with low radiation exposure (especially dual photon absorptiometry) makes screening for premature bone loss feasible in high-risk individuals and allows assessment of response to therapy.

Differential Diagnosis

It is important not to confuse this condition with other metabolic bone diseases, especially osteomalacia and hyperparathyroidism; or with the diffuse demineralization sometimes seen in myeloma and metastatic bone disease. Bone scintiscans and biopsy may be required, since these conditions may coexist in the postmenopausal patient.

Treatment

A. Specific Measures: Specific treatment varies with the cause; combined hormone therapy is usually used, although its effectiveness may be in preventing bone loss rather than increasing bone mass.

1. Postmenopausal–Estrogens appear to decrease bone resorption. Before beginning estrogen therapy in a postmenopausal woman, perform a careful pelvic examination to rule out neoplasm or other abnormality and warn the patient that vaginal bleeding may occur. Administer estrogen daily except for the last 5–7 calendar days of each month, and then repeat the cycle. Any of the following may be used: (1) Estradiol (Estrace), 1–2 mg orally. (2) Ethinyl estra-

diol, 0.02–0.05 mg orally daily as tolerated. (3) Estrone sulfate and conjugated estrogenic substances (Amnestrogen, Premarin, etc) are well tolerated and widely used. The dosage is 0.625–1.25 mg orally daily. The long-acting injectable estrogen preparations may be useful. The addition of a progestin, eg, medroxyprogesterone acetate (Provera), 10 mg daily for the last week to 10 days of each estrogen cycle, reduces the risk of endometrial carcinoma. See discussion of menopause (Chapter 13) for dangers of estrogen therapy.

2. Sodium fluoride increases the mineral density of cancellous bone but decreases that of cortical bone and induces increased bone fragility.

3. Calcitonin (Calcimar) has been approved by the FDA for the treatment of osteoporosis in doses of 100 IU/d. It must be used parenterally and has limited efficacy.

4. Diphosphonates–These agents inhibit osteoclastic-induced bone resorption. Etidronate is available in the USA, and recent studies demonstrate the efficacy of long-term cyclical therapy with this agent in reducing the rate of vertebral fractures and increasing vertebral bone mineral density. Daily administration of 400 mg of etidronate for 2 weeks every 3 months is safe and inexpensive. Whether additional benefit is obtained by estrogen supplementation is not known.

B. General Measures: The diet should be adequate in protein, calcium (milk and milk products are desirable except in lactose intolerance), and vitamin D. Increased calcium intake by use of supplementary calcium salts (eg, calcium carbonate), up to 1–2 g calcium per day, is advisable. Additional vitamin D (2000–5000 units/d) may be needed if there is associated malabsorption or osteomalacia. The importance of exercise in preventing bone loss cannot be overemphasized. Thiazides may be useful if hypercalciuria is present. Patients should be kept active; bedridden patients should be given active or passive exercises. The spine must be adequately supported (eg, with a Taylor brace or corset), but rigid or excessive immobilization must be avoided. Elderly patients must be protected from falling. Alcohol should be avoided.

Prognosis

The prognosis is good for postmenopausal osteoporosis if estrogen therapy is started early and maintained for years. Spinal involvement is not reversible on x-ray, but progression of the disease is often halted. In general, osteoporosis is a crippling rather than a killing disease, and the prognosis is essentially that of the underlying disorder (eg, Cushing's syndrome). The idiopathic variety does not respond appreciably to any form of therapy except possibly fluoride. Careful periodic records of the patient's height will indicate if the disease has become stabilized. Periodic measurements of bone mass in a given individual, using modern techniques (eg, bone densitometry), may alert the physician to a progressive bone loss before clinical or x-ray evidence of osteoporosis occurs. Measures to prevent progressive loss of bone mass may be more effective than treatment of the clinical disease, which at present is costing several billions of dollars in medical care annually in the USA alone.

Barzel US: Estrogens in the prevention and treatment of postmenopausal osteoporosis: A review. Am J Med 1988;85:847.

Bikle DD: Effects of alcohol abuse on bone. Compr Ther 1988;14:16.

Eastell R, Riggs BL: Calcium homeostasis and osteoporosis, Endocrinol Metab Clin North Am 1987;16:829.

Eastell R, Riggs BL: Diagnostic evaluation of osteoporosis. Endocrinol Metab Clin North Am 1988;17:547.

Hodgson SF: Corticosteroid-induced osteoporosis. Endocrinol Metab Clin North Am 1990;19:95.

Lukert BP, Raisz LG: Glucocorticoid induced osteoporosis: Diagnosis and management. Ann Intern Med 1990; 112:352.

Martin TJ (editor): Metabolic bone disease. (Symposium.) Clin Endocrinol Metab 1988;2:1.

Parfitt AM: Use of calciferol and its metabolites and analogues in osteoporosis. Drugs 1988;36:513.

Raisz LG: Local and systemic factors in the pathogenesis of osteoporosis. N Engl J Med 1988;318:818.

Riggs BL: A new option for treating osteoporosis. N Engl J Med 1990;323:124. (Editorial on diphosphonates.)

Riggs BL et al: Effect of fluoride treatment on the fracture rate in postmenopausal women with osteoporosis. N Engl J Med 1990;322:802.

Ryan WG: Prevention and treatment of osteoporosis. Compr Ther 1987;13:51.

Stevenson JC: Pathogenesis, prevention, and treatment of osteoporosis. Obstet Gynecol 1990;75(No. 4 Suppl):36S.

Watts NB et al: Intermittent cyclical etidronate treatment of postmenopausal osteoporosis. N Engl J Med 1990; 323:73.

NONMETABOLIC BONE DISEASE

POLYOSTOTIC FIBROUS DYSPLASIA

Polyostotic fibrous dysplasia is a rare disease that is frequently mistaken for osteitis fibrosa generalisata due to hyperparathyroidism, since both are manifested by bone cysts and fractures. Polyostotic fibrous dysplasia is not a metabolic disorder of bone but a congenital dysplasia in which bone and cartilage do not form but remain as fibrous tissue.

McCune-Albright syndrome is polyostotic fibrous dysplasia with "brown spots" having ragged margins along with a variety of endocrinopathies, including precocious puberty. Precocious puberty occurs more frequently in girls. Other endocrine disorders include

gigantism and acromegaly, hyperthyroidism, hypogonadism, Cushing's syndrome due to adrenal adenoma, and a rare syndrome of hypophosphatemic osteomalacia. The reason for the occurrence of these endocrine abnormalities in this disease is unknown.

The manifestations are painless swelling of the involved bone beginning in childhood (usually the skull, upper end of femur, tibia, metatarsals, metacarpals, phalanges, ribs, and pelvis), either singly or in multiple distribution, with cysts or hyperostotic lesions and at times with brown pigmentation of the overlying skin. Skull involvement may give a "leonine" appearance. Involvement is segmental and may be unilateral. Precocious puberty in girls may be due to estrogen-secreting ovarian cysts, in which case serum gonadotropins are low, or to hypothalamic disease, with true precocious puberty.

Radiographs reveal rarefaction and expansion of the affected bones, at times with cystic changes, or hyperostosis (especially of base of the skull). Fractures and deformities may also be visible, eg, "shepherd's crook" deformity of the hip.

The bone cysts and fractures should, by their distribution and skin pigmentation, be distinguished from those of hyperparathyroidism and neurofibromatosis. All other types of bone cyst and tumor must be considered also. The hyperostotic lesions of the skull must be distinguished from those of Paget's disease. Biopsy of bone may be required to settle the diagnosis.

There is no treatment for this disease except for surgical correction of bone fractures and deformities. The endocrine problems must be individualized and treated independently as they occur.

Most lesions heal, and the progression is slow. On rare occasions, sarcomatous transformation of bone occurs.

Harris RI: Polyostotic fibrous dysplasia with acromegaly. Am J Med 1985;78:539.

PAGET'S DISEASE
(Osteitis Deformans)

Essentials of Diagnosis

- Often asymptomatic.
- Bone pain may be the first symptom.
- Kyphosis, bowed tibias, large head, waddling gait, and frequent fractures that vary with location of process.
- Serum calcium and phosphate normal; alkaline phosphatase elevated; urinary hydroxyproline elevated.
- Dense, expanded bones on x-ray.

General Considerations

Paget's disease is a nonmetabolic bone disease of unknown etiology. A possible viral etiology has recently been suggested. It causes excessive bone destruction and repair—with associated deformities, since the repair takes place in an unorganized fashion. Up to 3% of persons over age 50 will show isolated lesions, but clinically important disease is much less common. There is a strong familial incidence of Paget's disease. A rare form occurs in young people ("juvenile Paget's disease").

Clinical Findings

A. Symptoms and Signs: Often mild or asymptomatic. Deep "bone pain" is usually the first symptom. The bones become soft, leading to bowed tibias, kyphosis, and frequent fractures with slight trauma. The head becomes larger, and headaches are a prominent symptom. Increased vascularity over the involved bones causes increased warmth.

B. Laboratory Findings: The blood calcium and phosphorus are normal, but the alkaline phosphatase is markedly elevated. Urinary hydroxyproline and calcium are elevated in active disease.

C. Imaging: On radiographs the involved bones are expanded and denser than normal. Multiple fissure fractures may be seen in the long bones. The initial lesion may be destructive and radiolucent, especially in the skull ("osteoporosis circumscripta"). Technetium pyrophosphate bone scans are helpful in delineating activity of bone lesions even before any radiologic changes are apparent.

Differential Diagnosis

Differentiate from primary bone lesions such as osteogenic sarcoma, multiple myeloma, and fibrous dysplasia and from secondary bone lesions such as metastatic carcinoma and osteitis fibrosa cystica. If serum calcium is elevated, hyperparathyroidism may be present in some patients as well.

Complications

Fractures are frequent and occur with minimal trauma. If immobilization takes place and there is an excessive calcium intake, hypercalcemia and kidney stones may develop. Involvement of the bones in the auditory apparatus may cause hearing loss, vertigo, and tinnitus. Vertebral collapse may lead to spinal cord compression. Osteosarcoma may develop in long-standing lesions. Sarcomatous change is suggested by marked increase in bone pain, sudden rise in alkaline phosphatase, and appearance of a new lytic lesion. The increased vascularity, acting like multiple arteriovenous fistulas, may give rise to high-output cardiac failure. Rheumatic manifestations and hyperuricemia with acute and chronic joint pain often complicate this disease, especially in joints near involved bone.

Treatment

Asymptomatic patients require no treatment.

Three therapeutic agents have been introduced to reduce excessive bone resorption, with consequent fall of serum alkaline phosphatase and urinary hydroxyproline. They should be reserved for active and progressive disease. The calcitonins (porcine, human, and salmon) act by reducing osteoclastic activity. **Synthetic salmon calcitonin (Calcimar)** is given in doses of 50–100 IU subcutaneously daily or 3 times weekly for several months to years. Aside from local sensitivity reactions, systemic side effects—eg, flushing, nausea—are rare. It is expensive, and antibody formation is common. Escape from treatment (return of abnormal laboratory features or symptoms even though treatment is maintained) commonly occurs. **Synthetic human calcitonin (Cibacalcin)** has been recently released in the USA for the treatment of active Paget's disease. It is of use in patients who fail to respond to salmon calcitonin or have developed resistance due to antibodies. It is more expensive than other forms of therapy and causes side effects, including nausea and flushing, in as many as 20% of patients. The dose is 0.5 mg/d subcutaneously. The **diphosphonates** inhibit osteoclast-mediated bone resorption. Etidronate disodium (Didronel) is available in 200 and 400 mg tablets. The safest dose is 5 mg/kg daily for 90–180 days. In severe disease, 10 mg/kg/d may be used for 90 days, with rest periods before another course is given. Etidronate disodium is effective orally with minor side effects (eg, diarrhea), but it must never be used for periods longer than 6 months in order to avoid adverse effects on bone mineralization with increased susceptibility to fractures. Newer diphosphonates (eg, ADP; 3-amino-1-hydroxypropylidene-1,1-bisphosphonate) do not impair bone mineralization but are not yet available in the USA. **Mithramycin,** an antitumor agent, rapidly suppresses osteoclastic activity and has been effective in severe cases. Because of renal, hepatic, and bone marrow toxicity, however, it should be used only in the most serious cases. Patients may respond to one agent after they have escaped from the beneficial effects of another. Combined or sequential therapy using several agents is under investigation. The choice of the best agent and the duration of treatment must be individualized.

Prognosis

The prognosis in general is good, but sarcomatous changes (in 1–3%) or renal complications secondary to hypercalciuria (in 10%) alter the prognosis unfavorably. In general, the prognosis is worse the earlier in life the disease starts. Fractures usually heal well. In the severe forms, marked deformity, intractable pain, and cardiac failure are found. The recently introduced therapeutic agents may improve the prognosis significantly, but osteogenic sarcoma is unresponsive to any form of therapy, including mithramycin.

Merkow RL, Lane JM: Paget's disease of bone. Endocrinol Metab Clin North Am 1990;19:177.

DISEASES OF
THE ADRENAL CORTEX

Total destruction of both adrenal cortices is not compatible with human life. The adrenal cortex regulates a variety of metabolic processes by means of secretion of some 30 steroid hormones, of which 2, cortisol and aldosterone, are of paramount importance.

The secretion of cortisol is regulated by ACTH and that of aldosterone primarily by the renin-angiotensin system. ACTH is under the control of the hypothalamic corticotropin-releasing hormone (CRH). The plasma free cortisol level, in turn, is one of the factors that regulates ACTH secretion. Aldosterone secretion, in contrast, is principally controlled by volume receptors that activate renin release, leading to the production of angiotensin II, which stimulates the zona glomerulosa of the adrenal to release aldosterone. Aldosterone secretion is also influenced by ACTH and by the plasma potassium concentration. Clinical syndromes of adrenal insufficiency or excess may thus be due to primary lesions of the adrenal glands themselves or may be secondary to pituitary disorders.

(1) Catabolic (glucocorticoids): Cortisol and related steroids, the "stress hormones" of the adrenal cortex, are vital for survival. These steroids have a general "catabolic" action, increasing protein breakdown, inducing hyperaminoacidemia, and causing a negative nitrogen balance. They increase gluconeogenesis and have an "anti-insulin" effect. They also possess significant anti-inflammatory properties and alter the body's immune response.

(2) Electrolyte-regulating (mineralocorticoids): The principal hormone in this group is aldosterone. Its primary role is in retaining sodium and excreting potassium and thus "regulating" the extracellular fluid compartment and the blood pressure. It has minor effects on carbohydrate metabolism.

(3) Anabolic (sex steroids): Androstenedione and related C_{19} steroids are protein builders; they are also virilizing and androgenic and represent the principal source of androgens in the female.

Improved chemical and radioimmunoassays of various hormones, stimulation and suppression tests, and refined radiologic procedures have facilitated accurate diagnosis of adrenal disorders.

ADRENOCORTICAL HYPOFUNCTION
(Adrenocortical Insufficiency)

1. ACUTE ADRENAL INSUFFICIENCY
(Adrenal Crisis)

Essentials of Diagnosis

- Weakness, abdominal pain, high fever, confusion, nausea and vomiting.
- Low blood pressure, dehydration.
- Skin pigmentation may be increased.
- Serum potassium high, sodium low, blood urea nitrogen high.
- Corticosteroids low in blood and urine.

General Considerations

Acute adrenal insufficiency is an emergency caused by sudden marked deprivation or insufficient supply of adrenocortical hormones. Crisis may occur in the course of chronic insufficiency in a known addisonian patient, or it may be the presenting manifestation of adrenal insufficiency. Acute adrenal crisis is more commonly seen in diseases of the cortex itself than in disorders of the pituitary gland causing secondary adrenocortical hypofunction.

Adrenal crisis may occur in the following situations: (1) Following stress, eg, trauma, surgery, infection, or prolonged fasting in a patient with latent insufficiency. (2) Following sudden withdrawal of adrenocortical hormone after replacement in a patient with chronic insufficiency or in a patient with temporary insufficiency due to suppression by exogenous glucocorticoids. (3) Following bilateral adrenalectomy or removal of a functioning adrenal tumor that had suppressed the other adrenal. (4) Following sudden destruction of the pituitary gland (pituitary necrosis), or when thyroid or insulin is given to a patient with panhypopituitarism. (5) Following injury to both adrenals by trauma, hemorrhage, anticoagulant therapy, thrombosis, infection, or, rarely, metastatic carcinoma. In overwhelming sepsis, massive bilateral adrenal hemorrhage may occur (Waterhouse-Friderichsen syndrome).

Clinical Findings

A. Symptoms and Signs: The patient complains of headache, lassitude, nausea and vomiting, abdominal pain, and often diarrhea. Confusion or coma may be present. Fever may be 40.6 °C (105 °F) or more. The blood pressure is low. Other signs may include cyanosis, petechiae (especially with meningococcemia), dehydration, abnormal skin pigmentation with sparse axillary hair, and lymphadenopathy.

B. Laboratory Findings: A high eosinophil count is often found in adrenal failure, but it is not specific. The blood glucose and serum sodium levels are low. Serum potassium and blood urea nitrogen are high. Hypercalcemia may be present. Blood culture may be positive if bacterial infection is the precipitating cause. Urinary and blood cortisol levels are very low. Plasma ACTH is markedly elevated if the patient has primary adrenal disease (generally > 200 pg/mL).

C. Electrocardiographic Findings: The ECG may show decreased voltage.

Differential Diagnosis

This condition must be differentiated from other causes of coma and confusion, such as diabetic coma, cerebrovascular accident, and acute poisoning, and from other causes of high fever. The high serum potassium is not specific, but it should alert the physician to the possibility of adrenal insufficiency. The blood glucose is usually low, but the condition may coexist with diabetes mellitus, in which case the blood sugar is high, which may be misleading. Eosinophilia and lymphocytosis, which are usually absent in other emergencies, are characteristic. A low plasma cortisol in the presence of severe systemic illness is diagnostic of adrenal failure. If the diagnosis is suspected, draw blood sample for cortisol and treat with hydrocortisone, 100–300 mg intravenously, and saline *immediately*, without waiting for the results of laboratory tests.

Treatment

A. Acute Phase: Institute appropriate antishock measures (see Chapter 9), especially intravenous fluids and plasma, vasopressor drugs, and oxygen. Do not give narcotics or sedatives.

Give hydrocortisone phosphate or hydrocortisone sodium succinate, 100 mg intravenously immediately, and continue intravenous infusions of 50–100 mg every 6 hours for the first day. Give the same amount every 8 hours on the second day and then gradually reduce the dosage every 8 hours.

Since bacterial infection is frequently the precipitating factor of acute adrenal crisis, it is wise to administer empirical wide-spectrum antibiotics while waiting for the results of initial cultures. Hypoglycemia should be vigorously treated while serum electrolytes, urea nitrogen, and creatinine are monitored.

B. Convalescent Phase: When the patient is able to take food by mouth, give oral hydrocortisone, 10–20 mg every 6 hours, and reduce dosage to maintenance levels as needed. Mineralocorticoid therapy is not needed when large amounts of hydrocortisone are being given, but as the dose is reduced it is necessary to add fludrocortisone acetate, 0.05–0.1 mg daily.

C. Complications During Treatment: Excessive use of intravenous fluids and corticosteroids may cause generalized edema with hypertension; flaccid paralysis due to potassium depletion and psychotic reactions may occur. Monitor blood pressure and ECGs throughout treatment.

Prognosis

Before replacement therapy and antibiotics became available, acute adrenal crisis was often rapidly fatal. Even today, if treatment is not early and vigorous, death may occur. Once the crisis has passed, the patient must be investigated to assess the degree of permanent adrenal insufficiency and to establish the cause if possible.

2. CHRONIC ADRENOCORTICAL INSUFFICIENCY (Addison's Disease)

Essentials of Diagnosis

- Weakness, easy fatigability, anorexia; frequent episodes of nausea and vomiting.
- Sparse axillary hair; increased skin pigmentation of creases, pressure areas, and nipples.
- Hypotension, small heart.
- Serum sodium and chloride are low. Serum potassium and blood urea nitrogen are elevated. Eosinophilia and lymphocytosis are present.
- Plasma cortisol levels are low to absent and fail to rise after administration of corticotropin. Urinary 17-ketosteroids and 17-hydroxycorticosteroids are low.
- Plasma ACTH level elevated.

General Considerations

Addison's disease is a rare disorder due to progressive destruction of the adrenal cortices. It is characterized by chronic deficiency of hormones concerned with gluconeogenesis and mineral metabolism and causes often striking skin pigmentation. Volume and sodium depletion and potassium excess are characteristic of primary adrenal failure. In contrast, if chronic adrenal insufficiency is secondary to pituitary failure (atrophy, necrosis, tumor), mineralocorticoid production (controlled by the renin-angiotensin system) persists and hyperkalemia is not present. Furthermore, since ACTH is not elevated, skin pigmentary changes are not encountered. Isolated aldosterone lack has been described, with persistent hyperkalemia, salt wasting, and acidosis. The majority of these patients have hypoaldosteronism on the basis of reduced renin production or release. This syndrome is commonly seen in patients with chronic renal disease and especially in elderly diabetics.

The term Addison's disease should be reserved for adrenal insufficiency due to adrenocortical disease. Tuberculosis of the adrenals is no longer the most common cause, accounting today for less than one-third of cases. Idiopathic atrophy accounts for most of the other cases. There may be associated thyroiditis, hypoparathyroidism, hypogonadism, diabetes mellitus, pernicious anemia, and candidiasis. An autoimmune mechanism has been established for these and other causes of idiopathic atrophy.

Rare causes include metastatic carcinoma (especially of the breast or lung), coccidioidomycosis, and histoplasmosis of the adrenal gland (more frequent in patients with AIDS), syphilitic gummas, scleroderma, amyloid disease, and hemochromatosis. Bilateral adrenal hemorrhage may occur in patients taking anticoagulants, in patients in shock, or during open heart surgery, resulting in Addison's disease. Familial adrenoleukodystrophy (with demyelinating disorder) is due to accumulation of very long fatty acids and is being recognized with increasing frequency.

Clinical Findings

A. Symptoms and Signs: The symptoms are weakness and fatigability, weight loss, anorexia, nausea and vomiting, and, less frequently, diarrhea and nervous and mental irritability. Pigmentary changes consist of diffuse tanning over nonexposed as well as exposed parts or multiple freckles; or accentuation of pigment over pressure points and over the nipples, buttocks, perineum and recent scars. Dark brown spots may appear on the mucous membranes of the mouth. Some patients have associated vitiligo. Other findings include hypotension with small heart, hyperplasia of lymphoid tissues, stiffness and calcification of the cartilages of the ear, and scant to absent axillary and pubic hair (especially in women).

B. Laboratory Findings: The white count shows moderate neutropenia (about 5000/μL), lymphocytosis (35–50%), and a total eosinophil count over 300/μL. Serum potassium and urea nitrogen are elevated; serum sodium is low. Fasting blood glucose is low. Hypercalcemia may be present.

Low plasma cortisol (< 5 mg/dL) at 8 AM is diagnostic, especially if accompanied by simultaneous elevation of the plasma ACTH level (usually > 200 pg/mL). Urinary 17-hydroxysteroids, 17-ketosteroids, and free cortisol are low. A good screening test is the cosyntropin (Cortrosyn) stimulation test: Plasma cortisol samples are obtained in the basal state and 45 minutes after intramuscular injection of 0.25 mg of cosyntropin (Cortrosyn). If the plasma cortisol does not rise by at least 10 μg/dL and reach at least 18 μg/dL, the diagnosis of primary or secondary adrenal insufficiency is likely.

C. Imaging: Adrenal calcification on x-ray may be found in about 10% of cases, most frequently in granulomatous diseases such as tuberculosis and coccidioidomycosis.

Differential Diagnosis

Addison's disease should be considered in any patient with hypotension and hyperkalemia. Unexplained weight loss, weakness, and anorexia may be mistaken for occult cancer. Nausea, vomiting, diarrhea, and abdominal pain may be misdiagnosed as intrinsic gastrointestinal disease. The hyperpigmentation may be confused with that due to ethnic or racial causes. Hemochromatosis also enters the differential diagnosis of skin hyperpigmentation, but it should be remembered that it may be a cause of Addison's disease, especially if the patient also has diabetes or cardiac arrhythmias.

Complications

Any of the complications of the underlying disease (eg, tuberculosis) are more likely to occur, and the patient is susceptible to intercurrent infections that may precipitate crisis. Diabetes mellitus and, rarely, thyrotoxicosis, as well as Hashimoto's thyroiditis, hypoparathyroidism, pernicious anemia, and ovarian failure of autoimmune origin may be associated with idiopathic adrenal failure.

The dangers of overzealous treatment as well as inadequate replacement must be guarded against. Psychosis, gastric irritation, and low-potassium syndrome may occur with excessive corticosteroid treatment. Corticosteroid treatment may impair the patient's resistance to tuberculosis, which may spread. Excessive mineralocorticoid administration leads to hypertension, edema, and muscular weakness.

Treatment

A. Specific Therapy: Replacement therapy should include a combination of glucocorticoids and mineralocorticoids. In mild cases, hydrocortisone alone may be adequate.

1. Hydrocortisone is the drug of choice. Most addisonian patients are well maintained on 15–25 mg of hydrocortisone orally daily in 2 divided doses, two-thirds in the morning and one-third in the late afternoon or early evening. On this dosage, most of the metabolic abnormalities are corrected. Many patients, however, do not obtain sufficient salt-retaining effect and require desoxycorticosterone or fludrocortisone supplementation or extra dietary salt.

2. Fludrocortisone acetate has a potent sodium-retaining effect. The dosage is 0.05–0.1 mg orally daily or every other day. If postural hypotension, hyperkalemia, or weight loss occurs, raise the dose. If weight gain, edema, hypokalemia, or hypertension ensues, lower the dose.

B. General Measures: If replacement therapy is adequate, most patients need no special diets or precautions. Treat all infections immediately and vigorously, and raise the dose of cortisone appropriately. The dose of glucocorticoid should also be raised in case of trauma, surgery, complicated diagnostic procedures, or other forms of stress. Patients are well advised to carry at all times a card or bracelet giving information about their disease and their need for hydrocortisone.

Prognosis

With adequate replacement therapy, the life expectancy of patients with Addison's disease is markedly prolonged. Active tuberculosis responds to specific chemotherapy. Withdrawal of treatment or increased demands due to infection, trauma, surgery, or other types of stress may precipitate crisis with a sudden fatal outcome unless large doses of parenteral corticosteroids are employed. Pregnancy may be followed by exacerbation of the disease. With appropriate therapy, however, a fully active life is now possible for most patients.

Burke CW: Adrenocortical insufficiency. Clin Endocrinol Metab 1985;14:947.

Sadeghi-Nejad A, Senior B: Adrenomyeloneuropathy presenting as Addison's disease in childhood. N Engl J Med 1990;322:13.

ADRENOCORTICAL OVERACTIVITY

Hyperadrenalism is caused either by bilateral hyperplasia or by adenoma or, more rarely, carcinoma of one adrenal. The clinical picture will vary with the type of secretion produced, but in general, 3 clinical disorders can be differentiated: (1) Cushing's syndrome, in which the glucocorticoids predominate; (2) the adrenogenital syndrome, in which the adrenal androgens predominate (feminizing tumors are rare); and (3) hyperaldosteronism, with mineralocorticoid excess. The clinical picture is most apt to be mixed in cases of malignant tumor and in bilateral hyperplasia. All syndromes of adrenal overactivity are far more common in females than in males.

1. CUSHING'S SYNDROME (Hypercortisolism)

Essentials of Diagnosis

- Centripetal obesity, easy bruisability, psychosis, hirsutism, purple striae.
- Osteoporosis, hypertension.
- Hyperglycemia, glycosuria, low serum potassium and chloride, low total eosinophils, and lymphocytopenia.
- Elevated serum cortisol and urinary 17-hydroxysteroids. Abnormal suppression by exogenous dexamethasone.

General Considerations

The term Cushing's syndrome refers to hypercortisolism due to any cause. The primary lesion may be in the pituitary or the hypothalamus, with resultant hypersecretion of ACTH and anatomic or functional bilateral adrenal hyperplasia. It has been speculated that ACTH hypersecretion by the pituitary may be the result of autonomous ACTH-secreting adenoma or of increased release of corticotropin-releasing factor by the hypothalamus. This is the most common form of the disorder (about 70%) and is usually referred to as Cushing's disease. Hypercortisolism may also be due to an autonomous adrenal tumor (adenoma or carcinoma) or to ectopic secretion of ACTH by a nonpituitary neoplasm.

Hypercortisolism due to a tumor of one adrenal is usually associated with atrophy of the contralateral gland. Carcinoma of the adrenal (5%) is always unilateral and often metastasizes late. A mixed picture with virilization is often present.

Administration of corticotropin causes adrenal hyperplasia; administration of glucocorticoid causes adrenal atrophy associated with most features of Cushing's syndrome. These effects are partially reversible when medication is withdrawn.

Certain extra-adrenal malignant tumors (eg, small-cell carcinoma of the lung) may secrete ACTH or, more rarely, corticotropin-releasing factor and produce severe Cushing's syndrome with bilateral adrenal hyperplasia. Severe hypokalemia and hyperpigmentation are commonly found in this group.

Clinical Findings

A. Symptoms and Signs: Cushing's syndrome causes "moon face" and "buffalo hump," obesity with protuberant abdomen, and thin extremities; a plethoric appearance; oligomenorrhea or amenorrhea (or impotence in the male); weakness, backache, headache; hypertension; mild acne and superficial skin infections; chloasma-like pigmentation (especially on the face), hirsutism (mostly of the lanugo hair over the face and upper trunk, arms, and legs), purple striae (especially around the thighs, breasts, and abdomen), and easy bruisability (eg, hematoma formation following venipuncture). Mental symptoms may range from increased lability of mood to frank psychosis.

B. Laboratory Findings: Glucose tolerance is impaired, often with glycosuria. The patient is resistant to the action of insulin. Urinary 17-hydroxycorticosteroids and plasma cortisol are high. The usual diurnal variation in plasma cortisol levels is absent in Cushing's syndrome. Urinary free cortisol is always elevated. Urinary 17-ketosteroids are often low or normal in Cushing's syndrome due to adenoma; normal or high if the disorder is due to hyperplasia; and very high if due to carcinoma. Total eosinophils are low ($< 50/\mu L$), lymphocytes are under 20%, and red and white blood cell counts are elevated. Serum bicarbonate is high, and serum Cl^+ and K^- are low in some cases, especially those associated with ectopic production of ACTH by extra-adrenal tumors.

C. Imaging: Osteoporosis of the skull, spine, and ribs is common. Nephrolithiasis may be present. CT scan or MRI easily demonstrates adrenal tumors if present. Bilateral adrenal hyperplasia can also be visualized. Since the pituitary adenomas causing Cushing's disease are usually very small, they are always missed by conventional radiographic techniques, but many can be demonstrated by CT or MRI scans of the pituitary. Adrenal angiography or ^{131}I-19-iodocholesterol scanning may demonstrate small adrenal tumors or hyperplastic glands.

Diagnostic Tests

A. Dexamethasone Suppression Tests: Administering dexamethasone in low doses (0.5 mg every 6 hours for 2 days) separates patients with all forms of Cushing's syndrome from those who do not have the disorder. (A common problem is to decide whether an obese, hypertensive, slightly hirsute woman does or does not have hypercortisolism.) In patients with Cushing's syndrome, the 24-hour urinary 17-hydroxycorticosteroids are not reduced to less than 3.5 mg in the second day of dexamethasone administration as they are in normals.

Once it is clear that the patient has hypercortisolism, one proceeds to the high-dose dexamethasone suppression test (2 mg every 6 hours for 2 days). In patients with Cushing's *disease* (pituitary hypersecretion of ACTH), the urinary 17-hydroxycorticosteroids are lowered to less than 50% of the baseline value. This does not occur in those with adrenal tumors or ectopic ACTH production—with the exception of patients with bronchial carcinoids (secreting ACTH), who may show suppression.

A faster, less accurate screening test for Cushing's syndrome is administration of 1 mg of dexamethasone at midnight. In most normal subjects, plasma cortisol levels are suppressed the following morning to less than 5 μg/dL. Patients with Cushing's syndrome do not suppress to this value and should have additional workup.

B. ACTH Stimulation Test: The administration of ACTH causes marked hypersecretion of plasma cortisol and urinary 17-hydroxycorticosteroids and 17-ketosteroids in Cushing's disease and often also in cases due to adrenal adenoma; but ACTH does not stimulate secretion in cases due to adrenal carcinoma or ectopic ACTH.

C. Metyrapone (Metopirone) Stimulation Test: Failure of 11-deoxycortisol (compound S) to rise after a 4-hour infusion or after an oral dose of metyrapone 500 mg every hour for 6 doses indicates that the hypercortisolism is due to adrenal tumor or ectopic ACTH secretion.

D. Direct Assay of Plasma ACTH: The new assay for ACTH, utilizing a double antibody technique for 2-site recognition of the ACTH molecule (immunoradiometric assay [IRMA]), is both sensitive and specific. The increased sensitivity and reliability of measurement for ACTH will make some of the other tests for Cushing's syndrome unnecessary.

The plasma ACTH is suppressed in cases of autonomous secretion of cortisol by an adrenal tumor (adenoma or carcinoma). It is high normal or elevated in patients with Cushing's disease and usually very high in those with ACTH-secreting ectopic tumors producing Cushing's syndrome and in Nelson's syndrome (see below).

E. The Urinary Free Cortisol Test: This test is very useful for the diagnosis of Cushing's syndrome, since, unlike the 17-hydroxycorticosteroids, free cortisol excretion is not affected by drugs, obesity, hyperthyroidism, etc. Patients with hypercortisolism have values greater than 130 μg/24 h.

F. Corticotropin-Releasing Hormone Test: This new stimulation test is not yet generally available. It has proved useful in the differential diagnosis of hypercortisolism—and especially in the clarification of the mechanism of the hypercortisolism of depression, which is associated with decreased response of the pituitary to corticotropin-releasing hormone, whereas patients with Cushing's disease have plasma ACTH hyperresponsiveness to the same stimulus.

Differential Diagnosis

A frequent problem is differentiating true Cushing's syndrome from obesity associated with diabetes mellitus, especially if there is hirsutism and amenorrhea. The distribution of fat, the presence or absence of muscle atrophy in the extremities, and the color and width of the striae often help but are not infallible signs. Dexamethasone suppression tests are very helpful to clarify the diagnosis. Cushing's syndrome must be differentiated from the adrenogenital syndrome (see below), since the latter is amenable to medical treatment. Exogenous administration of corticosteroids must be kept in mind. Hypercortisolism secondary to alcoholism has been reported (pseudo-Cushing's syndrome).

In rare cases, the outstanding manifestation of Cushing's disease or syndrome may be only diabetes, osteoporosis, hypertension, or psychosis. Adrenal disease must be ruled out in patients with these disorders, especially in insulin-resistant diabetes mellitus, since early treatment may be curative. The overnight dexamethasone suppression test and the 24-hour urinary free cortisol determination are useful for determining whether hypercortisolism is present.

Complications

The patient may suffer from any of the complications of hypertension, including congestive failure, cerebrovascular accidents, and coronary attacks, or of diabetes. Susceptibility to infections, especially of the skin and urinary tract, is increased. Compression fractures of the osteoporotic spine and aseptic necrosis of the femoral head may cause marked disability. Nephrolithiasis may occur. Intractable peptic ulcer may be present. Most serious, perhaps, are the psychotic complications not infrequently observed in this disease. Pituitary enlargement (due to ACTH-secreting adenomas) and deepening skin pigmentation have been observed following adrenalectomy for hyperplasia (Nelson's syndrome), causing, at times, visual field abnormalities.

Treatment

A. Specific Measures: Primary treatment of a malignant tumor producing Cushing's syndrome by ectopic secretion of ACTH is often not possible but is obviously the treatment of choice when feasible.

1. Surgical treatment–Adrenal tumors are removed surgically. For Cushing's disease, the preferred initial therapy is transsphenoidal surgical removal of the ACTH-secreting pituitary adenoma. An experienced neurosurgeon is required. Although the "cure" rate is reported to be over 75% with this procedure, recurrences of disease in subsequent years have occurred with disturbing frequency. In selected cases, pituitary irradiation may be used, and there are a few patients who may respond well to pharmacologic inhibition of ACTH secretion. If all these measures prove unsuccessful to correct the hypercortisolism, total adrenalectomy may be necessary. Adequate preoperative medication and care are of utmost importance. The patient should receive all general measures listed below, plus adequate hormonal supplementation.

If bilateral adrenalectomy is contemplated, give high doses of hydrocortisone sodium succinate (Solu-Cortef) in divided doses intramuscularly or intravenously, on the day of surgery; continue the intramuscular dosage for 1–2 days after surgery, then gradually decrease the dose and maintain on oral hydrocortisone as for Addison's disease. Because of the danger of precipitating heart failure, care must be taken to avoid excessive fluids and sodium.

In cases of unilateral tumor, the patient is prepared as for total adrenalectomy. After surgery, cortisol must be provided. Treatment with cortisol may have to be continued for weeks or months, since the contralateral gland has undergone atrophy because of ACTH suppression and may be slow to recover function.

A less frequent form of Cushing's syndrome is bilateral nodular adrenal hyperplasia. These patients have low or undetectable serum ACTH, do not suppress well with dexamethasone, and appear to have autonomous secretion of cortisol. Bilateral adrenalectomy is the treatment of choice.

An unusual form of Cushing's syndrome is known as **Carney complex,** a familial genetic disorder manifested by pigmented bilateral adrenal nodules, pigmented skin lesions, testicular and pituitary tumors, multiple myxomas, and schwannomas. Treatment consists of surgical removal of adrenal nodules.

2. X-ray therapy to the pituitary has been the treatment of choice in children with Cushing's disease. Transsphenoidal microadenomectomy is now preferred. Partial destruction of the pituitary by other means (proton beam, yttrium implant, cryotherapy)

has been attempted. Hypophysectomy may be required for large adenomas.

3. Adrenocortical inhibitors–Chemical treatment by means of adrenocortical inhibitors has been largely unsuccessful. Mitotane has limited use in inoperable carcinomas and occasionally in Cushing's disease. Metyrapone and aminoglutethimide have been used to reduce adrenocortical overactivity, but the results are erratic. The antifungal agent ketoconazole decreases steroid biosynthesis by the adrenal and has proved useful to decrease hypercortisolism, but experience is limited.

B. General Measures: A high-protein diet should be given, although dietary attempts to correct the negative nitrogen balance are never successful. Potassium chloride administration may replace losses before and after surgery.

Insulin is usually unnecessary, as the diabetes is mild; however, if the hyperglycemia is severe, it should be given in spite of the insulin resistance usually present.

Prognosis

The best prognosis for total recovery is for patients in whom a benign adrenal adenoma has been removed and who have survived the postadrenalectomy state of adrenal insufficiency. Cushing's disease has a more guarded prognosis. Fewer than 50% of patients with Cushing's *disease* respond to pituitary irradiation alone. Microsurgery of the pituitary, involving removal of small adenomas, has markedly improved the prognosis of this condition. If extensive hypophysectomy is necessary to remove the ACTH-secreting tumor, panhypopituitarism supervenes. Diabetes insipidus, transient or permanent, may also ensue. The more extensive the surgical procedure, the more frequent will be the rate of postoperative complications. Bilateral adrenalectomy cures the hypercortisolism but is associated with high morbidity. Furthermore, it may be followed by severe hyperpigmentation and rapid growth of ACTH-secreting pituitary tumors (Nelson's syndrome) with visual complications and sometimes malignant transformation.

Complete adrenalectomy necessitates chronic replacement therapy with glucocorticoid and mineralocorticoid hormones. A small number of patients with Cushing's disease treated with bilateral adrenalectomy have a subsequent recurrence of hypercortisolism. It is postulated that a small piece of adrenal tissue, either ectopic tissue or tissue left inadvertently by the surgeon, undergoes hyperplasia in response to the very high ACTH levels that are found after adrenalectomy.

Hypercortisolism due to ectopic ACTH-secreting malignant extra-adrenal tumors has a poor prognosis, since tumors are frequently advanced and inoperable at the time of diagnosis.

Findling JW: Cushing's syndromes: An enlarged clinical spectrum. N Engl J Med 1989;321:1677.

Hermus AR et al: Transition from pituitary-dependent to adrenal-dependent Cushing's syndrome. N Engl J Med 1988;318:966.

Kaye TB, Crapo L: The Cushing's syndrome: An update on diagnostic tests. Ann Intern Med 1990;112:434.

Krakoff LR: Glucocorticoid excess syndromes causing hypertension. Cardiol Clin 1988;5:537.

Schteingart D: Cushing's syndrome. Endocrinol Metab Clin North Am 1989;18:311.

2. THE ADRENOGENITAL SYNDROME: PREPUBERTAL

Adrenal virilizing syndromes in infancy or childhood are of great interest to the pediatrician and may be due to excessive production of androgens by a tumor (benign or malignant) or, more commonly, to congenital adrenal hyperplasia.

Congenital Adrenal Hyperplasia

The term congenital adrenal hyperplasia refers to a complex series of rare but well-studied enzymatic errors of metabolism, with deficient levels of different enzymes involved in the synthesis of cortisol. By far the most common forms are 21- and 11β-hydroxylase deficiencies, both characterized by excessive formation of adrenal androgens under the ACTH drive induced by hypocortisolism. This excess of androgens results in masculinization in the female (ranging from mild hirsutism and clitoral hypertrophy to frank pseudohermaphroditism) and in premature virilization in the male. In both entities, there is a variable degree of clinical hypocortisolism. In untreated 11β-hydroxylase deficiency, there is hypertension due to excessive formation of desoxycorticosterone, a metabolic precursor with potent mineralocorticoid activity. Hypertension never occurs in untreated 21-hydroxylase deficiency; on the contrary, a salt-losing form with clear-cut mineralocorticoid deficiency is present in approximately 50% of cases. In both enzymatic deficiencies, one finds high ACTH levels, plasma androgens, urinary pregnanetriol, and 17-ketosteroids. Specific diagnosis is made by demonstrating elevated plasma levels of the metabolic precursor immediately before the enzymatic block: 11-deoxycortisol in 11β-hydroxylase deficiency and 17-hydroxyprogesterone in 21-hydroxylase deficiency.

The fundamental step in the treatment of congenital adrenal hyperplasia is the administration of enough glucocorticoid to suppress ACTH and reverse the metabolic abnormalities. A mineralocorticoid is required in the salt-losing form. Plastic surgery may be necessary in females with ambiguous genitalia. It should be performed early in life.

Hughes IA: Management of congenital adrenal hyperplasia. Arch Dis Child 1988;63:1399.

White PC, New MI, Dupont B: Congenital adrenal hyperplasia. (2 parts.) N Engl J Med 1987;316:1519, 1580.

3. ADRENOGENITAL SYNDROME & VIRILIZING DISEASES OF WOMEN

Essentials of Diagnosis

- Menstrual disorders and hirsutism.
- Regression or reversal of primary and secondary sex characteristics, with balding, hoarse voice, acne, and enlargement of the clitoris.
- Occasionally a palpable pelvic tumor.
- Urinary 17-ketosteroids elevated in adrenal disorders, variable in others.
- Plasma testosterone often elevated.

General Considerations

The diagnosis of virilizing disorders in women is more difficult than in young girls, since sources of abnormal androgens other than the adrenal exist, principally the ovaries. Modest androgen excess from whatever source will cause increases in sexual hair (chin, upper lip, abdomen, and chest) and increased activity of sebaceous glands, with acne and menstrual irregularities or amenorrhea. If androgen excess is pronounced, defeminization (decrease in breast size, loss of feminine adipose tissue) and virilization (frontal balding, muscularity, clitoridean hypertrophy, and deepening of the voice) occurs.

Syndromes of androgen excess in previously menstruating and normal-appearing adult women may be caused by the following disorders:

(1) Ovarian disorders: Stein-Leventhal syndrome (large polycystic ovaries most common), theca luteinization (thecosis ovarii), Sertoli-Leydig cell tumors (arrhenoblastoma), hilar cell tumor or hyperplasia, adrenal cell rests, dysgerminoma (rare).

(2) Adrenal disorders: Congenital adrenal hyperplasia (late form of 21- and 11β-hydroxylase deficiencies), virilizing adrenal adenoma, adrenal carcinoma, Cushing's syndrome.

(3) Miscellaneous causes: Exposure to exogenous androgens (anabolic agents, testosterone, 19-norprogestins).

Clinical Findings

A. Symptoms and Signs: Symptoms include scant menstrual periods or amenorrhea, acne and roughening of the skin, odorous perspiration, and hoarseness or deepening of the voice. Hirsutism is present over the face, body, and extremities, with thinning or balding of head hair. Musculature is increased and feminine contours are lost. The breasts and genitalia are atrophied, the clitoris and larynx enlarged. A tumor may rarely be palpable on pelvic examination (arrhenoblastoma, polycystic ovaries).

B. Laboratory Findings: Urinary 17-ketosteroids are elevated in almost all cases of adrenal overproduction of androgens (whether adrenal tumors or hyperplasia). High levels are seen in adrenal tumors. Elevated serum dehydroepiandrosterone sulfate levels suggest an adrenal lesion. Plasma 11-deoxycortisol (compound S) and 17-hydroxyprogesterone assays help rule out the most common forms of congenital adrenal hyperplasia (see above).

Ovarian lesions are more likely to produce testosterone, which can be markedly elevated in plasma. If very high (> 250 mg/dL) and with low LH and FSH, an ovarian tumor is likely and should be actively looked for. In polycystic ovary syndrome, the plasma testosterone is usually only moderately elevated although the free, non-protein-bound fraction is higher. The serum LH is high, and the LH:FSH ratio is usually greater than 2.0.

C. Imaging: Ultrasonography is an accurate and noninvasive procedure to demonstrate ovarian enlargement or the presence of cysts or solid tumors. CT scan or MRI may reveal an adrenal tumor.

D. Special Examinations: Laparoscopy is often helpful.

Differential Diagnosis

Since hirsutism may be the only sign of adrenal tumor, all of the disorders characterized by excessive hair have to be considered in the differential diagnosis. From the practical standpoint, however, the diagnosis commonly depends upon whether one is dealing simply with racial, familial, or idiopathic hirsutism, where an unusual end-organ sensitivity to endogenous androgen exists; or whether excessive amounts of male hormone are being produced. Most cases of idiopathic hirsutism are due to an ovarian abnormality in testosterone and androstenedione production. The dexamethasone test is not reliable in differentiating between adrenal and ovarian sources of excess androgen. In general, if hirsutism is associated with enlargement of the clitoris, deepening of the voice, frontal baldness, development of heavy musculature, or breast atrophy and amenorrhea and if the onset is rapid, one can assume that a tumor of the adrenal or ovary is present. CT or MRI visualizes even small adrenal tumors, and ultrasound diagnoses even small ovarian tumors or cysts, so that blind exploratory surgery is rarely necessary. Although virilization is not the rule with Cushing's syndrome, a mixed picture is at times seen in malignant adrenal tumors and, more rarely, in adrenal hyperplasia.

Complications

Aside from the known high incidence of malignancy in tumors causing virilization, the interference with femininity and consequent infertility may be irreversible. Diabetes and obesity may be complicating features. At times, mental disorders accompany states of defeminization.

Treatment

Treatment varies with the cause of the androgen excess. When ovarian or adrenal tumors are present, surgical removal is the treatment of choice. Polycystic ovary syndrome is best treated with an estrogen-progestin preparation to suppress the excessive ovarian production of androgens. Rarely, bilateral partial resection of the ovaries may be necessary.

It has become clear that in addition to the classic presentations there are many cases of mild adrenal enzymatic deficiencies that may not be manifested clinically until adult life. "Late-onset" adrenal hyperplasia is now being recognized as a cause of hirsutism or menstrual abnormalities in many women. The most common variant is due to 21-hydroxylase deficiency. Treatment with corticosteroids has proved valuable in reducing the activity of the glands (by suppressing endogenous ACTH). In adults, the drug of choice is dexamethasone, 0.5–1.5 mg daily orally in divided doses; use the smallest dose that keeps the 17-ketosteroid, pregnanetriol, and 17-hydroxyprogesterone levels within the normal range.

In cases of idiopathic hirsutism, where the origin of the offending androgen is not clear (probably of combined ovarian-adrenal origin), drugs such as spironolactone, which interferes with the cellular action of testosterone, have been used with variable results. Other antiandrogens such as cyproterone acetate have been found useful for virilizing disorders in Europe but are not available in the USA.

Prognosis

The outlook is favorable if a malignant tumor is removed early, since metastasis often occurs late.

The ultimate fate of the virilized woman depends not only upon the underlying cause (ie, tumor or hyperplasia) but more particularly upon the age at onset of the virilizing influence and its duration. If virilization is of long standing, restoration of normal femininity or loss of hirsutism is unlikely even though the causative lesion is successfully removed.

Many cases of simple hirsutism in females are not due to a readily demonstrable endocrine disease but to hereditary or racial factors and cannot be treated effectively with systemic medications or surgery. Bleaching, shaving, and electrolysis are the treatments of choice.

Barnes R, Rosenfield RL: The polycystic ovary syndrome: Pathogenesis and treatment. Ann Intern Med 1989; 110:386.

Rittmaster RS, Loriaux DL: Hirsutism. Ann Intern Med 1987;106:95.

PRIMARY HYPERALDOSTERONISM

Essentials of Diagnosis

- Hypertension, polyuria, polydipsia, muscular weakness.
- Hypokalemia, hypernatremia, alkalosis.
- Elevated plasma and urine aldosterone levels and low plasma renin level.

General Considerations

Primary hyperaldosteronism is a relatively rare disorder caused by aldosterone excess. It accounts for less than 2% of cases of hypertension. It is more common in females. The 2 main types of primary hyperaldosteronism are those due to unilateral adrenocortical adenoma (Conn's syndrome) and those due to bilateral cortical hyperplasia. Edema is rarely seen in primary hyperaldosteronism, but secondary hyperaldosteronism is often found in edematous states such as cardiac failure and hepatic cirrhosis.

Clinical Findings

A. Symptoms and Signs: Hypertension, muscular weakness (at times with paralysis simulating periodic paralysis), paresthesias with frank tetanic manifestations, headache, polyuria (especially nocturnal), and polydipsia are the outstanding complaints. Edema is rarely present. On the other hand, some patients have only diastolic hypertension, without other signs or symptoms. Hypertension is typically moderate. Malignant hypertension is rare.

B. Laboratory Findings: Low serum potassium, hypernatremia, and alkalosis are characteristic. Urinary and plasma aldosterone levels are markedly elevated, and plasma renin levels are low.

A good screening test in a patient with hypertension in whom primary aldosteronism is suspected is the determination of plasma renin after sodium depletion (diet or diuretic) and after several hours of being in the upright position. These stimuli normally increase renin production. In primary aldosteronism, the renin level characteristically remains low.

A high-sodium diet, saline infusion, or desoxycorticosterone acetate administration fails to suppress the elevated aldosterone levels.

C. Electrocardiographic Findings: Electrocardiographic changes are those of prolonged hypertension and hypokalemia.

D. Imaging: Cardiac hypertrophy due to hypertension is present. CT scan or MRI frequently allows visualization of unilateral adenoma or bilateral hyperplasia. Adrenal arteriography is rarely necessary today for visualization of adrenal adenomas. Adrenal vein catheterization for measurement of aldosterone and cortisol is sometimes necessary to confirm unilateral disease. [131]I iodocholesterol scanning can be used for the same purpose (dexamethasone is used to suppress ACTH-mediated steroid production).

Differential Diagnosis

This important reversible cause of hypertension must be considered in the differential diagnosis in any patient who shows muscular weakness and tetanic manifestations; and in the differential diagnosis of periodic paralysis, potassium- and sodium-losing nephritis, nephrogenic diabetes insipidus, and hypokalemia (be certain the patient has not been receiving diuretic agents). Excessive ingestion of licorice or laxatives may simulate hyperaldosteronism. The oral contraceptives may raise aldosterone secretion in some patients. Unilateral renal vascular disease producing secondary hyperaldosteronism with severe hypertension must be ruled out. Plasma renin activity is low in primary hyperaldosteronism and elevated in renal vascular disease. Excessive secretion of desoxycorticosterone and corticosterone may produce a similar clinical picture. Low renin levels are found in about 25% of cases of essential hypertension. Their response to diuretics and their prognosis are better than those of patients with hypertension associated with high renin levels. Excess of an as yet unidentified mineralocorticoid is thought by some to be responsible. Aldosteronism due to a malignant ovarian tumor has been reported.

It is important to differentiate primary aldosteronism due to an adenoma and that due to bilateral nodular hyperplasia, since the hypertension can be cured or greatly ameliorated by removal of the adenoma, whereas it usually does not respond after bilateral adrenalectomy in patients with hyperplasia. Subjects with adenoma tend to have lower serum potassiums, higher aldosterone levels, and lower renal vein renins. Postural studies are useful. Aldosterone and renin activity are determined with the patient in the recumbent position and again a few hours later after ambulation. In adenoma, the plasma aldosterone and renin levels do not change. In bilateral hyperplasia, both levels rise, reflecting the incomplete suppression of renin and its increase by assumption of the upright posture. In doubtful cases, adrenal vein catheterization may yield the diagnosis.

Complications

All of the complications of chronic hypertension are encountered in primary hyperaldosteronism. Progressive renal damage is less reversible than hypertension.

Treatment

Conn's syndrome (unilateral adrenal adenoma secreting aldosterone) is treated by surgical removal of the lesion. Bilateral adrenal hyperplasia is best treated with spironolactone. Bilateral adrenalectomy corrects the hypokalemia but not the hypertension and should *not* be performed. Antihypertensive agents may also be necessary. A rare type of hyperplasia responds well to dexamethasone suppression.

Prognosis

The hypertension is reversible in about two-thirds of cases but persists or returns in spite of surgery in the remainder.

The prognosis is much improved by early diagnosis with chemical tests and scanning procedures.

Bravo EL: Clinical aspects of endocrine hypertension. Med Clin North Am 1987;71:907.

Young WF Jr et al: Primary aldosteronism: Diagnosis and treatment. Mayo Clin Proc 1990;65:96.

DISEASES OF THE ADRENAL MEDULLA

PHEOCHROMOCYTOMA

Essentials of Diagnosis

- "Spells" or "attacks" of headache, visual blurring, severe sweats, vasomotor changes in a young adult, weight loss.
- Hypertension, often paroxysmal ("spells") but frequently sustained.
- Postural tachycardia and hypotension; cardiac enlargement.
- Hypermetabolism with normal T_4. Elevation of plasma and urinary catecholamines or their metabolites.

General Considerations

Pheochromocytoma is a rare disease characterized by paroxysmal or sustained hypertension due to a tumor of pheochrome tissue, located in either or both adrenals or anywhere along the sympathetic nervous chain, and rarely in such aberrant locations as the thorax, bladder, or brain. In about 10% of cases, the tumor involves both adrenal glands. Most tumors are sporadic; only 10–15% are familial. Bilateral adrenal tumors tend to occur more frequently in familial cases.

The following familial syndromes have been identified:

(1) Familial pheochromocytoma without other abnormalities.

(2) Pheochromocytoma associated with islet cell tumors of the pancreas.

(3) Pheochromocytoma associated with calcitonin-secreting medullary carcinoma of the thyroid and hyperparathyroidism (multiple endocrine neoplasia type II).

(4) Pheochromocytoma in association with medullary carcinoma of the thyroid and the syndrome of multiple mucosal neuromas, without hyperparathyroidism (multiple endocrine neoplasia type III).

(5) Pheochromocytoma with neurofibromatosis (Recklinghausen's disease).

(6) Pheochromocytoma with Hippel-Lindau disease (hemangioblastomas of retina, cerebellum, and other parts of the nervous system).

Clinical Findings

A. Symptoms and Signs: Pheochromocytoma is manifested by attacks of severe headache, palpitations, tachycardia, profuse sweating, vasomotor changes (including facial pallor), precordial or abdominal pain, increasing nervousness and irritability, increased appetite, and loss of weight. Anginal attacks may occur. Physical findings include hypertension, either in attacks or sustained, with cardiac enlargement; postural tachycardia (change of more than 20 beats/min) and postural hypotension; mild elevation of basal body temperature. Retinal hemorrhage or papilledema occurs occasionally.

B. Laboratory Findings: Hypermetabolism is present; T_4 and free T_4 are normal; and glycosuria or hyperglycemia (or both) may be present. Blood volume is usually contracted.

C. Special Tests: Pharmacologic provocative and suppressive tests that evaluate the rise or fall in blood pressure have become obsolete and are not recommended.

1. Assay of urinary catecholamines on a 24-hour urine specimen–and the simpler tests for 3-methoxy-4-hydroxymandelic acid (vanillylmandelic acid, VMA), or total metanephrines—are now generally available. Urinary catecholamines are usually elevated. One should remember that stress, catecholamine-containing topical nasal medications, many bronchodilators, and methyldopa will also produce abnormally high values. Since VMA determinations can also be affected by a number of drugs, avoidance of drug taking during the urine collection is desirable. Antihypertensive agents such as thiazides, clonidine, and ganglionic blockers do not elevate VMA, metanephrines, or catecholamines.

Most patients with pheochromocytoma have clear-cut elevations of urinary catecholamines (normal range up to 130 μg/24 h) and VMA (normal range, 2–7 mg/24 h). Occasionally there are patients with large tumors who have normal excretion of catecholamines but high VMA, presumably due to intratumoral metabolism of the catecholamines. Conversely, a very small, actively catecholamine-releasing tumor may be associated with normal VMA and very high urinary catecholamines. In any patient with pheochromocytoma, the secretion of catecholamines may be sporadic and intermittent.

2. Direct assay of epinephrine and norepinephrine in blood and urine during or following an attack is the most reliable test for pheochromocytoma associated with paroxysmal hypertension. High epinephrine levels favor tumor localization within the adrenal gland. Proper collection of specimens is essential. Determination of blood catecholamines via a venous catheter—a research procedure—will help localize ectopic lesions and paragangliomas.

3. Imaging–CT scan and MRI have been shown to be very accurate in the diagnosis of these tumors.

Differential Diagnosis

Pheochromocytoma should always be suspected in any patient with labile hypertension, especially if some of the other features such as hypermetabolism or glycosuria are present in a young person. Because of such symptoms as tachycardia, tremor, palpitation, and hypermetabolism, pheochromocytoma may be confused with thyrotoxicosis. It should be considered in patients with unexplained acute anginal attacks. About 10% are mistakenly treated for diabetes mellitus because of hyperglycemia and glycosuria. Pheochromocytoma may also be misdiagnosed as essential hypertension, myocarditis, glomerulonephritis or other renal lesions, toxemia of pregnancy, eclampsia, and psychoneurosis. It rarely masquerades as gastrointestinal hemorrhage and abdominal disorders of an emergency nature. Catecholamine determination has made the diagnosis much more accurate.

Complications

All of the complications of severe hypertension may be encountered. Hypertensive crises with sudden blindness or cerebrovascular accidents are not uncommon. These may be precipitated by sudden movement, by manipulation during or after pregnancy, by emotional stress or trauma, or during surgical removal of the tumor. Cardiomyopathy may develop. Occasionally, the initial manifestation of pheochromocytoma may be hypotension or even shock.

After removal of the tumor, a state of severe hypotension and shock (resistant to epinephrine and norepinephrine) may ensue with precipitation of renal failure or myocardial infarction. These complications can be avoided by judicious preoperative and operative use of catecholamine-blocking agents such as phentolamine and phenoxybenzamine and by the use of blood or plasma to restore blood volume. Hypotension and shock may occur from spontaneous infarction or hemorrhage of the tumor; emergency surgical removal of the tumor is necessary in these cases.

On rare occasions, a patient dies as a result of the complications of diagnostic tests or during surgery. No patient with suspected pheochromocytoma should be subjected either to an invasive diagnostic procedure or to surgery unless there has been adequate alpha blockade with phenoxybenzamine.

Cholelithiasis is often associated.

Treatment

Surgical removal of the tumor or tumors is the treatment of choice. This may require exploration of the entire sympathetic chain as well as both adrenals. Administration of α-adrenergic blocking drugs and blood or plasma before and during surgery has made this type of surgery a great deal safer in recent years. Give phenoxybenzamine, 10 mg orally every 12 hours, and increase the dose gradually until hypertension is controlled. The usual maintenance dose is 40–120 mg daily. Do not increase the dose further when postural hypotension and nasal stuffiness become manifest.

After appropriate α-adrenergic receptor blockade

with phenoxybenzamine, the beta-blocker propranolol can be employed to control tachycardia and other arrhythmias. Maintain adrenergic blockade for a minimum of 10 days or until optimal cardiac status is established. Monitor the ECG until it becomes stable. (It may take a week or even months to correct electrocardiographic changes in patients with catecholamine myocarditis, and it is prudent to defer surgery until then in such cases.) An experienced anesthesiologist should always be present at surgery to prevent (and control if unavoidable) sudden changes in blood pressure, cardiac arrhythmias, etc.

Since there may be multiple tumors, it is essential to recheck urinary catecholamine levels postoperatively (1–2 weeks after surgery).

Long-term treatment with phentolamine is not successful. Oral phenoxybenzamine (Dibenzyline) has been successfully used as chronic treatment in inoperable carcinoma.

Metyrosine (Demser) is a competitive blocker in the synthesis of catecholamines. It is useful in the medical management of malignant or inoperable tumors. The initial dosage is 250 mg 4 times daily, increased daily by increments of 250–500 mg to a maximum of 4 g/d.

Prognosis

The prognosis depends upon how early the diagnosis is made. If the tumor is successfully removed before irreparable damage to the cardiovascular system has occurred, a complete cure is usually achieved. Complete cure (or improvement) may follow removal of a tumor that has been present for many years. Rarely, hypertension persists or returns in spite of successful surgery. Only a small percentage of tumors are malignant.

Before the advent of blocking agents, the surgical mortality rate was as high as 30%, but this has rapidly decreased. The importance of a team approach—endocrinologist, experienced anesthesiologist, and surgeon—cannot be overemphasized. In good hands, the surgical mortality rate is less than 3%.

If after removal of a tumor a satisfactory fall of blood pressure does not occur, always consider the presence of another tumor.

It has been estimated that in the USA alone about 800 deaths a year may be due to unrecognized pheochromocytoma.

Benowitz NL: Pheochromocytoma. Adv Intern Med 1990; 35:195.

DISEASES OF THE PANCREATIC ISLET CELLS*

ISLET CELL FUNCTIONING PANCREATIC TUMORS

The pancreatic islet is composed of several types of cells, each with distinct chemical and microscopic features: the A cells (20%) secrete glucagon, the B cells (70%) secrete insulin, and the D cells (5%) secrete somatostatin or gastrin. F cells secrete "human pancreatic polypeptide." Each cell may give rise to benign or malignant neoplasms that are often multiple and usually present with a clinical syndrome related to hypersecretion of a native or ectopic hormonal product. Diagnosis of the tumor depends principally on specific assay of the hormone produced. In malignant insulinoma, an increase in plasma proinsulin—and, in the Zollinger-Ellison syndrome, the prohormone "big" gastrin—may be the most specific finding. The exact hormone responsible for the "pancreatic cholera" syndrome remains unknown, but a biologically active substance called vasoactive intestinal peptide (VIP) is often found both in the plasma and in the tumors of patients with this condition. Glucagon-secreting A cell tumors are rare; patients present with diabetes, anemia, weight loss, hypoaminoacidemia, and a chronic generalized skin rash (migratory necrolytic erythema). Somatostatinomas are very rare and are associated with weight loss, diabetes, malabsorption, and hypochlorhydria.

In addition to the native hormones, aberrant or ectopic hormones are often secreted by islet cell tumors, including ACTH, melanocyte-stimulating hormone, serotonin, and chorionic gonadotropin, with a variety of clinical syndromes. Islet cell tumors may be part of the syndrome of multiple endocrine adenomatosis type I (with pituitary and parathyroid adenomas).

Direct resection of the tumor (or tumors), which often spreads locally, is the primary form of therapy for all types of islet cell neoplasm except Zollinger-Ellison syndrome, where treatment choices include blockade of acid secretion by the gastric mucosa with H_2 blocking agents or removal of the end organ (total gastrectomy). A new class of "acid pump" inhibitors (omeprazole) may become the therapy of choice for Zollinger-Ellison syndrome. Palliation of functioning malignant disease often requires both antihormonal and anticancer chemotherapy. The use of streptozocin, doxorubicin, and asparaginase, especially for malignant insulinoma, has produced some encouraging

results, although these drugs are quite toxic. Recently, a somatostatin analogue has been used in the therapy of islet cell tumor. This therapy is still experimental.

Prognosis in these neoplasms is variable. Long-term survival in spite of widespread metastases has been reported. Earlier diagnosis by hormonal assay may lead to earlier detection and a higher cure rate.

Mignon M, Bonfile S: Diagnosis and treatment of Zollinger-Ellison syndrome. Clin Gastroenterol 1988;2:677.

Rossi P et al: Endocrine tumors of the pancreas. Radiol Clin North Am 1989;27:129.

Solcia E et al: The gastroenteropancreatic endocrine system and related tumors. Gastroenterol Clin North Am 1989; 18:671.

DISEASES OF THE TESTES

MALE HYPOGONADISM

Male hypogonadism may be classified according to time of onset, ie, prepubertal or postpubertal. It may also be classified as primary or secondary, depending on whether the lesion is in the testes (hypergonadotropic) or in the hypothalamic-pituitary area (hypogonadotropic).

The etiologic diagnosis of hypogonadism (eg, primary or secondary) is based on a careful history and physical examination and is confirmed by laboratory tests (Table 20–13).

1. PREPUBERTAL HYPOGONADISM

The diagnosis of secondary hypogonadism cannot usually be made in boys under age 16 or 17, since it is difficult to differentiate from "physiologic" delay of puberty.

Prepubertal hypogonadism is most commonly due to a specific gonadotropic deficiency of the pituitary.

Table 20–13. Causes of hypogonadism.

Primary Hypogonadism (Hypergonadotropic)	Secondary Hypogonadism (Hypogonadotropic)
Klinefelter's syndrome	Kallmann's syndrome
Anorchia	Pituitary tumors
Surgical or accidental castration	Craniopharyngiomas
Viral infections (mumps)	Hypothalamic lesions
Tuberculosis	Hemochromatosis
Leprosy	Prader-Willi syndrome
Myotonic dystrophy	Laurence-Moon-Biedl syndrome
Ionizing radiation injury	
Chemotherapeutic agents	

---

* Diabetes mellitus and the hypoglycemic states are discussed in Chapter 21.

It may be familial and associated with anosmia (Kallmann's syndrome) or hyposmia. It may also occur as a result of destructive lesions near the pituitary region (eg, suprasellar cyst) or, more rarely, as a result of destruction or malformation of the testes (prepubertal castration). Rare causes include Prader-Willi syndrome (obesity, hypogonadism, mental retardation, and hypotonia associated with deletions of chromosome 15), Laurence-Moon-Biedl syndrome (obesity, hypogonadism, polydactyly, retinitis pigmentosa), and Alstrom's syndrome (hypogonadism, nerve deafness, obesity, and retinitis pigmentosa).

In cases associated with a complete pituitary defect, the patient is of short stature or fails to grow and mature. Otherwise, the patient is strikingly tall due to overgrowth of the long bones due to delay in closure of epiphyseal plates. The external genitalia are underdeveloped, the voice is high-pitched, the beard does not grow, and the patient lacks libido and potency. In adult life he presents a youthful appearance, with obesity (often in girdle distribution), disproportionately long extremities (span exceeds height), lack of temporal recession of the hairline, and a small Adam's apple. Gynecomastia is occasionally seen (but apparent gynecomastia may be merely fat). The skin is fine-grained, wrinkled, and sallow, especially on the face. There is no acne or sebum production. The penis is small and the prostate undeveloped. Pubic and axillary hair are scant. The testes may be absent from the scrotum (cryptorchidism) or may be in the scrotum but very small. Rarely, and for unknown reasons, they may be entirely absent (anorchia).

Bone age is retarded. Anemia may be present. Urinary 17-ketosteroids are low or normal in testicular failure, very low or absent in primary pituitary failure. Serum FSH and LH are low in cases of hypothalamic or pituitary origin and elevated in patients with primary testicular failure. Serum testosterone is subnormal and is an excellent index of Leydig cell function.

The response to chorionic gonadotropin injections in cases due to pituitary failure will be maturation, elevation of plasma testosterone, and, occasionally, descent of cryptorchid testes. In primary testicular failure, no such response occurs.

Testosterone therapy can produce adequate secondary sexual characteristics in hypogonadal patients but will not induce spermatogenesis. To induce spermatogenesis in patients with *secondary* hypogonadism, a combination of an FSH preparation, eg, human menopausal gonadotropin (hMG [Pergonal]), with human chorionic gonadotropin (hCG) is usually required. This treatment is expensive. Spermatogenesis can occasionally be achieved with the use of hCG alone. Patients with hypogonadism must be placed on testosterone and maintained for life on adequate doses. Long-acting testosterone preparations such as enanthate or cypionate, 200–300 mg intramuscularly every 2–4 weeks, are employed. These doses are well tolerated, although gynecomastia may occur with prolonged therapy. It is due to conversion of testosterone to estradiol by peripheral aromatases. The use of oral synthetic androgenic preparations is less desirable, since they have a significant hepatotoxicity, especially when used for long periods of time. Recently, transdermal testosterone preparations have become available and appear to be well tolerated. Reports demonstrating a dramatic response of FSH and LH to LH-releasing factor (GnRH, LHRH) seem to locate the defect in isolated hypogonadotropic hypogonadism to the hypothalamus and offer renewed hope for future treatment. Pulsatile LHRH infusion to induce both puberty and spermatogenesis has been described.

Castro-Maguna M et al: Genetic forms of male hypogonadism. Urology 1990;35:195.
Sitruk-Ware R: Transdermal delivery of steroids. Contraception 1989;39:1.
Wu FC: Male hypogonadism: Current concepts and trends. Clin Obstet Gynecol 1985;12:531.

2. KLINEFELTER'S SYNDROME

The most common primary developmental abnormality causing hypogonadism is Klinefelter's syndrome (seminiferous tubule dysgenesis). It afflicts one out of every 400–500 males. It is caused by the presence of one or more supernumerary X chromosomes and is usually recognized at or shortly after puberty. It is at times familial. Most commonly, there is only failure of the tubules with permanent sterility. The secretory function of the Leydig cells ranges from normal to definite failure. An abnormality in the LH feedback control as well as a disorder in steroidogenesis has been demonstrated in Klinefelter's syndrome.

The clinical findings are swelling of the breasts (gynecomastia), sterility, lack of libido and potency (rare), and at times lack of development of body hair, and female escutcheon. Excessive growth of long bones is present. There may be associated mental retardation. The testes are usually small (< 2 cm in longest diameter) and firm. The penis and prostate are usually normal. The ejaculate usually contains no spermatozoa, although an occasional case of spermatogenesis in a patient with a mosaic variant has been described. Urinary 17-ketosteroids are low normal or normal. Serum testosterone is usually low to normal. LH and FSH levels are invariably elevated. Serum estradiol is higher than normal. Testicular biopsy shows sclerosis of the tubules, nests of Leydig cells, and no spermatozoa. The cell karyotype is most commonly 47,XXY, with a chromatin-positive buccal smear. Mosaicism may have clinical features ranging from normal to the classic picture just described here. Chromosomal analysis is necessary to diagnose the condition. In mosaics with a normal 46,XY cell line, spermatogenesis may be present.

All causes of gynecomastia must be differentiated from Klinefelter's syndrome. Testicular size, plasma FSH, and, if necessary, chromosomal analysis will settle the diagnosis.

Testosterone replacement should be given if secondary sexual characteristics have failed to appear or if impotence and low blood testosterone develop later in life. There is no treatment for the infertility. If gynecomastia is disfiguring, plastic surgical removal is indicated.

Hsueh WA et al: Endocrine features of Klinefelter's syndrome. Medicine 1978;57:447.
Klinefelter HF: Klinefelter's syndrome: Historical background and development. South Med J 1986;79:1089.

3. POSTPUBERTAL HYPOGONADISM

Any pituitary lesion (eg, tumor, infection, necrosis) may lead to lack of gonadotropin; often, hypogonadism is an early sign. The testes may be damaged by trauma, x-ray irradiation, infection, or in other ways. Viral (mumps) and bacterial (gonorrhea, leprosy) orchitis usually affects only the seminiferous tubules and spermatogenesis, leaving Leydig cell function intact. Occasionally, low plasma testosterone and high LH are seen. Many drugs can affect testicular function—cyclophosphamide rapidly causes azoospermia, ketoconazole inhibits testosterone biosynthesis, and hepatic and renal failure are often associated with low testosterone levels. Myotonic dystrophy should be considered if myotonia, frontal baldness, and diabetes are present. States of malnutrition, anemia, and similar disorders may lead to functional gonadal underactivity. The hormonal aging process is also associated with decreased gonadal function: at age 80 years, 70% of men have low plasma free testosterone levels.

The symptoms of acquired adult hypogonadism are varying degrees of loss of libido and potency; retardation of hair growth, especially of the face; vasomotor symptoms (flushing, dizziness, chills); lack of aggressiveness and interest; sterility; and muscular aches and back pain. Atrophy or hypoplasia of external genitalia and prostate is rare. The skin of the face is thin and finely wrinkled, and the beard is scant. Girdle type obesity and kyphosis of the spine are present.

Urinary and plasma testosterone levels are low. Urinary and serum FSH or LH are low in cases due to pituitary lesions and elevated in primary testicular failure. Serum prolactin is often elevated in hypothalamic or pituitary lesions, especially in pituitary tumors. In fact, the first manifestation of a prolactin-secreting pituitary tumor in a male may be impotence. The sperm count is low, or spermatozoa may be absent.

True adult hypogonadism must be differentiated from the far more commonly seen psychogenic lack of libido and potency. Measurement of plasma testosterone is useful in this regard. Confusion may also arise in men who are obese and have a sparse beard and small genitalia but normal sperm counts and urinary FSH ("fertile eunuchs"). These patients may represent examples of end-organ unresponsiveness or isolated lack of LH. The usual form of male infertility is "spermatogenic arrest." The disorder can only be diagnosed by testicular biopsy. Most of these patients have normal gonadotropin levels and are not benefited by therapy.

Acquired male hypogonadism is treated with androgens. Oral methyltestosterone or fluoxymesterone is effective, but these synthetic oral preparations are not recommended for chronic therapy because of their hepatotoxicity. They may cause peliosis hepatis and even hepatic tumors. It is preferable to use the long-acting injectable preparations of testosterone (cypionate, enanthate). The dose used is 200–400 mg every 3 weeks. Recently, preparations of testosterone for transdermal use (scrotal skin) have become available. They appear to be effective and well tolerated. Treatment of long-standing hypogonadism with androgens may precipitate anxiety and acute emotional problems that often require concomitant psychotherapy. Watch for acute urinary retention in older patients. In cases of hypogonadism due to hyperprolactinemia, excellent results may be achieved by administration of bromocriptine or, more permanently, with removal of a pituitary prolactin-secreting tumor.

In cases of *secondary* hypogonadism, it is possible to restore spermatogenesis in many patients with parenteral gonadotropin therapy (see previous section for details).

Prognosis of Hypogonadism

If hypogonadism is due to a pituitary lesion, the prognosis is that of the primary disease (eg, tumor, necrosis). The prognosis for restoration of virility is good if testosterone is given. The sooner administration is started, the fewer stigmas of eunuchoidism remain (unless therapy is discontinued).

The prognosis for fertility is dismal for the overwhelming majority of patients with primary testicular failure (primary hypogonadism). In many subjects with gonadotropin deficiency, it is possible to induce spermatogenesis. It is only feasible in instances where the testicular elements are present but are unstimulated due to lack of pituitary tropic hormones.

Cryptorchidism should be corrected early, since the incidence of malignant testicular tumors is higher in ectopic testicles and the chance of ultimate fertility is lessened in long-standing cases, even after orchiopexy. The advantages of medical therapy with human chorionic gonadotropin or (recently) with gonadotropin-releasing hormone versus surgical orchiopexy are still controversial.

Colodny AH: Undescended testes: Is surgery necessary? (Editorial.) N Engl J Med 1986;314:511.

Griffin JE: Diagnosis and management of male infertility. Ann Intern Med 1987;32:259.

Melman A: Evaluation and management of erectile dysfunction. Surg Clin North Am 1988;68:965.

Krane RJ et al: Impotence. N Engl J Med 1989;321:1648.

Snyder PJ: Clinical use of androgens. Annu Rev Med 1984;35:207.

MALE HYPERGONADISM & TESTICULAR TUMORS IN ADULTS*
(See also Chapter 17.)

In adults, almost all lesions causing male hypergonadism are functioning testicular tumors, which quite frequently are malignant. An unusual form of hypergonadism in recent years has been androgen abuse by athletes in an attempt to enhance athletic performance. Significant toxic effects (gynecomastia, infertility, marked decrease in high-density lipoproteins, etc) have been noted.

Many or most testicular neoplasms are functioning. The majority originate in germ cells and may secrete human chorionic gonadotropin. Leydig and Sertoli cell tumors secrete androgens or estrogens (or both). Germ cell tumors are highly malignant, whereas many non-germ cell tumors are benign. They are at times quite small and are clinically recognized because of their hormonal effects or because of the presence of metastases. The sudden appearance of gynecomastia in an otherwise healthy male should raise the possibility of testicular tumor. hCG levels in blood are often high and serve as a marker of disease activity. Ultrasonography is helpful in early diagnosis. In general, once hormonal manifestations have become pronounced, cure by surgical removal is unlikely. Some tumors are bilateral, eg, interstitial cell tumors. Often, a mixed picture is present.

The incidence of cancer in cryptorchidism is high.

Treatment

If the diagnosis is made early, surgical removal may be curative; radiotherapy is very useful in radiosensitive types. Great advances in the chemotherapy of testicular tumors have taken place in recent years, and many patients are cured of the disease.

The serum concentration of the beta subunit of human chorionic gonadotropin (hCG) is elevated in choriocarcinomas and, less commonly, in other testicular tumors. The response to therapy can be monitored in such cases by following the level of this glycoprotein.

Ozols RF, Williams SD: Testicular cancer. Curr Probl Cancer 1989;3:285

Peckham M: Testicular cancer. Acta Oncol 1988;27:439.

Sternberg CN, Bosl GJ: Advances in testicular cancer: Role of chemotherapy. Prog Clin Biol Res 1988; 277:79.

Wilson JD: Androgen abuse by athletes. Endocr Rev 1988;9:181.

DISEASES OF THE OVARIES
(See also Chapter 13.)

FEMALE HYPOGONADISM*

The outstanding symptom of female hypogonadism is amenorrhea (see below). Partial deficiencies, principally corpus luteum failure, may occur; these do not always cause amenorrhea but more often produce anovulatory periods or metrorrhagia.

Estrogenic failure has far-reaching effects, especially if it begins early in life (eg, Turner's syndrome).

Primary pituitary disorders are much less common causes of hypogonadism in the female than primary ovarian disorders and are often associated with other signs of pituitary failure.

Ovarian failure starting in early life will lead to delayed closure of the epiphyses and retarded bone age, often resulting in tall stature with long extremities. On the other hand, in ovarian agenesis due to chromosomal disorder, dwarfism is the rule (see below). In adult ovarian failure, changes are more subtle, with some regression of secondary sex characteristics, including breast atrophy, diminished vaginal secretions, changes in vaginal epithelium, etc. Vasomotor instability with "hot flushes" is a typical sign of estrogen secretory failure. In estrogenic deficiency of long standing in any age group, osteoporosis, especially of the spine, is almost always found, since estrogen protects bone against excessive resorption.

A relatively rare form of ovarian failure is seen in states of androgen excess originating in the adrenal cortex or ovary, when estrogens, though present in the body, are suppressed by the presence of large amounts of androgens.

1. AMENORRHEA

Since regular menstruation depends upon normal function of the entire physiologic axis extending from the hypothalamus and pituitary to the ovary and the uterine lining, it is not surprising that menstrual disorders are among the most common presenting complaints of endocrine disease in women. Correct diagnosis depends upon proper evaluation of each component of the axis, and nonendocrine factors must also be considered.

If menstruation is defined as shedding of endometrium which has been stimulated by estrogen or by estrogen and progesterone which are subsequently withdrawn, it is obvious that amenorrhea can occur either when hormones are deficient or lacking (the hypohormonal or ahormonal type) or when these hormones, though present in adequate amounts, are never withdrawn (the continuous hormonal type).

Primary amenorrhea implies that menses have never been established. This diagnosis is not usually made before the age of about 16. Secondary amenorrhea means that menses once established have ceased (temporarily or permanently).

The most common type of hypohormonal amenorrhea is the menopause, or physiologic failure of ovarian function. The most common example of continuous hormonal amenorrhea is that due to pregnancy, when cyclic withdrawal is prevented by the placental secretions. These 2 conditions should always be considered before extensive diagnostic studies are undertaken.

The principal diagnostic aids that are used in the study of amenorrhea are as follows: (1) vaginal smear for estrogen effect; (2) endometrial biopsy; (3) "medical D&C" (see below); (4) basal body temperature determination; (5) urine determinations of 17-ketosteroids, FSH, pregnanediol, and pregnanetriol; (6) culdoscopy and gynecography; (7) chromosomal studies; (8) pelvic exploratory operation or laparoscopy and gonadal biopsy; (9) radioimmunoassays of FSH, LH, and prolactin, which are now available for specific diagnosis of certain types of amenorrhea; (10) plasma testosterone assay; (11) x-ray studies of the hypothalamic and pituitary areas; and (12) in young females, bone age.

Primary Amenorrhea

Because of the frequency with which "delayed puberty" is found in otherwise normal females, the diagnosis of primary amenorrhea usually is not made until the patient is clearly beyond the age at which normal menarche occurs. In the USA, the mean age at menarche is 12 ½ years. If menses have not started by age 16, primary amenorrhea is definitely present, and the cause should be investigated.

Most cases of primary amenorrhea are of the hypohormonal or ahormonal type. Exact diagnosis is essential to rule out an organic lesion along the hypothalamic-pituitary-gonadal axis. The chromosomal sex pattern must be determined in many cases. Laparoscopy or pelvic exploration may be required to establish the diagnosis. In large series, the most common cause has always been Turner's syndrome.

The causes are as follows:

(1) Hypothalamic causes: Constitutional delay in onset, severe malnutrition, serious organic illness, lack of LHRH (GnRH).

(2) Pituitary causes (with low or absent FSH): Suprasellar cyst, pituitary tumors (eosinophilic adenomas, chromophobe adenomas, basophilic adenomas, craniopharyngiomas, etc), isolated lack of pituitary gonadotropins.

(3) Ovarian causes (with high FSH): Ovarian dysgenesis with XO karyotype (Turner's syndrome), mosaic variants, mixed gonadal dysgenesis (XO-XY karyotype), pure gonadal dysgenesis, etc. Rarely, "resistant ovaries" syndrome.

(4) Uterine causes: Malformations, congenital müllerian dysgenesis, imperforate hymen, hermaphroditism, unresponsive or atrophic endometrium.

(5) Miscellaneous causes: All forms of male pseudohermaphroditism (enzymatic defects in testosterone synthesis, androgen resistance syndromes), androgen excess syndromes (adrenal or ovarian tumors, adrenal enzymatic defects with excess androgen formation, such as 21- or 11β-hydroxylase deficiencies, polycystic ovaries).

Since primary amenorrhea is only a manifestation of multiple and often complex underlying defects, treatment must be individualized according to the specific cause.

Secondary Amenorrhea

Temporary cessation of menses is extremely common and usually does not require extensive endocrine investigation. In the childbearing age, pregnancy must be ruled out. In women beyond the childbearing age, menopause should be considered first. States of emotional stress, malnutrition, anemia, and similar disorders may be associated with temporary amenorrhea and correction of the primary disorder will usually also reestablish menses. Some women fail to menstruate regularly for prolonged intervals after stopping oral contraceptive pills. Lactation may be associated with amenorrhea, either physiologically or for abnormally prolonged periods after delivery. An increasing number of small prolactin-secreting pituitary tumors causing secondary amenorrhea and often lactation have been discovered by means of prolactin assays and pituitary imaging studies.

By the use of the "medical D&C," ie, the administration of progesterone with subsequent withdrawal, these amenorrheas can be arbitrarily divided into amenorrhea with negative D&C and amenorrhea with positive D&C. The former (with the exception of pregnancy) show an atrophic or hypoestrin type of endometrium; the latter show an endometrium of the proliferative type but lacking progesterone.

(1) Secondary amenorrhea with negative medical D&C may be due to the following causes: premature ovarian failure, pituitary tumor, or pituitary infarction (Sheehan's syndrome). The measurement of serum FSH and LH is extremely helpful in separating ovarian causes (high gonadotropins) from hypothalamic-pituitary origin (low gonadotropins). Serum prolactin levels must be measured. Less common causes include

virilizing syndromes such as arrhenoblastoma, Cushing's disease, Addison's disease, and miscellaneous causes such as anorexia nervosa, profound myxedema, and scarring of the uterine cavity with synechia formation (Asherman's syndrome).

(2) Secondary amenorrhea with positive medical D&C may be due to polycystic ovary syndrome, estrogen medication, estrogenic granulosa cell tumors (rare), or hyperthyroidism. A common cause is "psychogenic amenorrhea" related to emotional trauma (divorce, going to college, stressful new job, etc). Menses usually return in a few months without any specific therapy. Tonic elevation of serum LH with normal FSH is helpful in the diagnosis of polycystic ovary syndrome. Amenorrhea or oligomenorrhea is also often found in athletes (long-distance runners, dedicated ballet dancers, etc). Depletion of body fat due to strenuous exercise may play a role in the pathogenesis of this problem.

Some degree of overlap in these 2 groups is sometimes found.

The aim of therapy is not only to reestablish menses (although this is valuable for psychologic reasons) but also to attempt to establish the cause (eg, pituitary tumor) of the amenorrhea and to restore reproductive function.

Treatment depends upon the underlying disease. It is not necessary to treat all cases, especially temporary amenorrhea or irregular menses in unmarried girls or women. These cases usually are corrected spontaneously after marriage or the first pregnancy.

In patients whose response to progesterone is normal, the administration of this hormone during the last 5–10 days of each month, orally or parenterally, will correct the amenorrhea.

In patients who are unresponsive to progesterone and whose urinary gonadotropin levels are low, treatment of a pituitary lesion may restore menstruation; gonadotropins would appear to be of value, and human pituitary FSH has been used with some success experimentally. This, or gonadotropins from postmenopausal urine (menotropins, hMG), has given good results in secondary amenorrhea. Clomiphene citrate (Clomid) has been extensively and often successfully tried for the treatment of these patients. However, if pregnancy is not desirable, estrogen alone or in combination with progesterone is more commonly used. If gonadotropin levels are high, gonadotropins are of no value; treat with estrogens alone or with estrogens and progesterone. A commonly used schedule is the oral administration of 1.2 mg of conjugated estrogens from days 1 to 20 of each month and 10 mg of medroxyprogesterone daily during days 21 to 25. Corticosteroids may restore menstruation in virilizing disorders that are due to enzymatic abnormalities in cortisol biosynthesis. Wedge resection of the ovaries often restores regular menstruation in the polycystic ovary syndrome. The use of LHRH (GnRH) is under investigation at present and appears promising. In patients with the galactorrhea-amenorrhea syndromes associated with elevated prolactin levels, restoration of ovulatory menses has been achieved with the ergot derivative bromocriptine (bromoergocryptine). Transsphenoidal resection of small prolactin-producing pituitary adenomas likewise has resulted in restoration of fertility.

General measures include dietary management as required to correct overweight or underweight; psychotherapy in cases due to emotional disturbance; and correction of anemia and any other metabolic abnormality that may be present (eg, mild hypothyroidism).

Hypothalamic Amenorrhea

Secondary hypothalamic amenorrhea, due to emotional or psychogenic causes, is far more common in young women than amenorrhea due to organic causes (except for pregnancy). It is probably mediated by a hypothalamic block of the release of pituitary gonadotropic hormones, especially LH. Pituitary FSH is still produced and is found in normal or low levels in the urine. Since some LH is necessary in the production of estrogen as well as FSH, a state of hypoestrinism with an atrophic endometrium will eventually result.

A history of psychic trauma just preceding the onset of amenorrhea can usually be obtained. The urinary FSH level is normal or low normal, and the 17-ketosteroid level is low normal. Plasma LH is low. Vaginal smear and endometrial biopsy show mild hypoestrin effects. The response to progesterone (medical D&C) is variable. The endometrium responds to cyclic administration of estrogens.

Menses often return spontaneously, after weight gain, or after several induced "cycles." Psychotherapy may be of value. Clomiphene citrate (Clomid) may be tried to reestablish menses. If amenorrhea persists for years, signs of estrogen deficiency will appear and must be treated.

It is most important to recognize this syndrome and not to mistake it for an organic type of amenorrhea with a very different prognosis.

Tan SL: Recent advances in the management of patients with amenorrhea. Clin Obstet Gynecol 1985;12:725.
Veldhuis JD: Management of amenorrhea. Hosp Pract 1988;23(Suppl 11A):40.

2. TURNER'S SYNDROME (Primary Ovarian Agenesis, Gonadal Dysgenesis)

Turner's syndrome is a chromosomal disorder associated with congenital absence of the ovaries and with short stature and other phenotypic anomalies. It represents the most common cause of primary amenorrhea. Patients with the classic syndrome lack one of the two X chromosomes.

The principal features include bilateral streak gonads, genital hypoplasia with infantile uterus, vagina, and breasts and primary amenorrhea; scant axillary and pubic hair; short stature, usually between 122 and 142 cm (48 and 56 inches); increased carrying angle of arms; webbing of neck (quite common); stocky "shield" chest with widely spaced nipples; cardiovascular disorders, especially coarctation of the aorta, congenital valve defects; osteoporosis and other skeletal anomalies (short fourth metacarpals, exostosis of tibia, etc) with increasing age; and prematurely senile appearance. Nevi are common. Lymphedema of hands and feet is seen in infants. There is an increased incidence of autoimmune thyroiditis and diabetes.

Serum FSH and LH are high. Bone age is retarded. Chromosomal analysis shows a 45,X pattern. Mosaicism is common; most frequent is the 45,X, 46,XX chromosomal pattern.

The principal disorder to be differentiated is pituitary dwarfism. In this disorder, urinary and serum FSH is low or absent, and other signs of pituitary failure are present. In Noonan's syndrome, a rare inherited disorder, the female patient has many similar phenotypic characteristics (short stature, shield chest, short neck), but cardiac lesions are in the right side of the heart (pulmonary stenosis is common), the ovaries are normal, the chromosomal pattern is 46,XX, and the serum FSH and LH are not elevated.

With administration of estrogens, some increase in height can be achieved, but this is almost never enough to increase stature significantly; androgens may also promote growth, especially fluoxymesterone in low doses. Some cases respond to administration of growth hormone.

Without treatment, growth will eventually cease, since the epiphyses will close spontaneously (though late). The administration of estrogen will develop the breasts and uterus and lead to anovulatory menses upon cyclic withdrawal. Administration of an oral progestogen such as medroxyprogesterone acetate (Provera) for the last 5–10 days of each cycle is recommended. Fertility can never be achieved.

The associated congenital cardiovascular anomalies may cause early death or may require surgical correction (eg, coarctation). Webbing of the neck can be corrected by plastic surgery.

Similar syndromes with different chromosomal patterns exist. "Pure gonadal dysgenesis" has only "streak" gonads and sexual infantilism, with normal stature and normal 46,XX chromosomal pattern. "Mixed" or "atypical" gonadal dysgenesis has a "streak" gonad on one side and an abnormal gonad, prone to neoplasm, on the other side, making prophylactic removal a desirable procedure. It is very often associated with XY mosaicism.

FEMALE HYPERGONADISM

Excesses of ovarian hormones are often encountered during the normal reproductive life of women and most frequently give rise to irregular or excessive menstrual bleeding and, more rarely, to amenorrhea. Excesses before the age of puberty or after the menopause, however, should be thoroughly investigated, since the possibility of malignant lesions is great. Several ovarian tumors may secrete estrogens. Other extraovarian sources of estrogens are malignant tumors of the adrenals. Since these tumors usually produce excesses of androgens as well, their hyperestrogenic effects are rarely detectable clinically in the female. Another cause of hyperestrogenism is the ingestion or other use of hormones (eg, in face or vaginal creams).

POLYCYSTIC OVARY SYNDROME

This term is used to denote a heterogeneous group of disorders all characterized by bilateral polycystic ovaries but with variable incidence and degree of hirsutism, amenorrhea, and obesity. Patients may have only mild hirsutism or may present with signs and symptoms of virilization. Some women have normal menses; in others, anovulatory cycles and infertility are present. An occasional patient presents with primary amenorrhea. Conditions found to be associated with this syndrome include adrenal defects in the synthesis of cortisol, central nervous system lesions, thyroid diseases, and adrenal and ovarian tumors. In most cases, however, no associated disorder is found, and the exact mechanism of the syndrome remains unclear.

The eponym **Stein-Leventhal syndrome** is usually reserved for patients who have amenorrhea, hirsutism, and obesity associated with polycystic ovaries without other associated endocrine disease.

Patients with polycystic ovary syndrome usually have normal or elevated estrogen levels; frequently show a tonic elevation of serum LH; and often have elevated levels of plasma testosterone. Gonadal steroid-binding globulin levels in plasma are decreased, so that the free (active) fraction of testosterone is elevated even if the level of total testosterone is normal.

Urinary 17-ketosteroids are usually normal or modestly elevated. FSH is normal or low. Administration of progesterone results in withdrawal bleeding. The hirsutism has been shown to be related to abnormal production of testosterone and related compounds by the ovaries and possibly also by the adrenals. Glucose intolerance and elevated serum insulin levels (associated with peripheral insulin resistance) are often found, even in subjects who are not obese. Hereditary factors may be involved. Pelvic sonography is helpful in demonstrating bilateral enlargement of the ovaries.

At operation, the enlarged ovaries are found to have many follicles on the surface and are surrounded by a thick capsule ("oyster ovaries").

Therapy must be individualized depending on the severity of the disorder, the presenting complaint, and any associated endocrine disease. Excess hair usually responds to oral contraceptive steroids. Glucocorticoid suppression (with small doses of dexamethasone at bedtime) is sometimes helpful. Combined adrenal and ovarian suppression has been reported to have additional beneficial effect. The dopamine agonist bromocriptine has been reported to improve the menstrual abnormalities and hirsutism of polycystic ovary syndrome. Experience is lacking for this use of the drug. If the patient wants to maintain fertility, several procedures are available. Wedge resection often restores ovulatory periods and fertility, but hirsutism is not helped by this procedure unless large doses of estrogens are also used. Recently, ovulation followed by pregnancy has been produced by human pituitary or urinary FSH and also by clomiphene. There is danger of rapid enlargement of the ovaries due to cyst formation and rupture if the dosage is not carefully controlled. Multiple pregnancies may occur.

Barnes R, Rosenfield RL: The polycystic ovary syndrome: Pathogenesis and treatment. Ann Intern Med 1989; 110:386.

DISORDERS OF PLURIGLANDULAR INVOLVEMENT

Involvement of multiple endocrine glands in the same patient is becoming recognized with increasing frequency. Many of these disorders are familial, although sporadic cases are also seen. The syndromes may consist of excessive hormone formation, usually due to the presence of hormone-secreting tumors, or they may consist of failure of multiple endocrine glands.

DISORDERS OF HORMONE EXCESS

Several familial syndromes with multiple gland involvement have been described. The most common one is multiple endocrine neoplasia (or adenomatosis) type I (MEN I or MEA I; see Table 20–14). In this condition, tumors of the pituitary gland, the parathyroid gland, and the pancreatic islets occur in the same patient, although not necessarily at the same time. The disorder is inherited as an autosomal dominant, but there is considerable phenotypic variability. Some

Table 20–14. Multiple endocrine gland neoplasia or adenomatosis (MEN).[1]

	Tissue Affected	Clinical Presentation
Type I (MEN I)	Parathyroid	Adenoma or hyperplasia
	Pancreas	Adenoma (often multiple) of islet cells, gastrinoma
	Pituitary	Adenoma (acromegaly, prolactinoma)
	Adrenal	Adenoma (cortical)
	Miscellaneous	Lipomas, thyroid tumors (other than medullary carcinoma)
Type II or IIa (MEN II)	Thyroid	Medullary carcinoma or C cell hyperplasia
	Adrenal	Pheochromocytomas
	Parathyroid	Hyperplasia or adenoma
Type III or IIb (MEN III)	Thyroid	Medullary carcinoma or C cell hyperplasia
	Adrenal	Pheochromocytomas (adenoma or hyperplasia)
	Neural tissue	Ganglioneuromas
	Somatic manifestations	Marfanoid habitus, thick lips, "blubbery tongue," megacolon

[1] Modified after Deftos LJ: Calcitonin in clinical medicine. *Adv Intern Med* 1978;23:159.

individuals in the same family express the abnormality as children, whereas in others the clinical manifestations may not appear until late in adult life. The clinical manifestations of this syndrome are extremely variable, since the glandular tumors may secrete a variety of different hormones. The most common finding is hypercalcemia due to primary hyperparathyroidism. Either hyperplasia or adenoma of the parathyroid glands may be found. The clinical manifestations and laboratory findings are identical to those found in spontaneously occurring primary hyperparathyroidism. The pituitary gland tumors may secrete **prolactin** (galactorrhea-amenorrhea syndrome) or **growth hormone** (producing gigantism or acromegaly). The tumors of the pancreatic islets may produce **insulin,** giving all of the clinical manifestations found in a spontaneously occurring insulinoma, or **gastrin,** giving rise to gastric acid hypersecretion (Zollinger-Ellison syndrome). Elevation of serum gastrin (measured by radioimmunoassay) is characteristic of Zollinger-Ellison syndrome and is associated with increased hydrochloric acid secretion. Tumors of the pancreatic islets have also been described as secreting additional peptide hormones such as substance P, secretin, vasoactive intestinal peptide (VIP), glucagon, and others. The glucagon-producing tumors are associated with a typical skin rash (migratory necrolytic erythema), with diabetes mellitus, and with very low levels of amino acids in plasma.

A separate disorder of familial hypersecretion of hormones is the so-called multiple endocrine neoplasia type II (MEN II or MEA II), or Sipple's syndrome.

In this syndrome, one finds pheochromocytomas (often bilateral) associated with medullary carcinoma of the thyroid, a tumor that originates in the C cells of the thyroid. These cells are the remnants of the ultimobranchial body found in lower species, and they secrete calcitonin. The baseline levels of calcitonin in blood are often markedly elevated and are helpful in the diagnosis of these tumors as well as in monitoring the response to therapy. In members of affected families, one can demonstrate the presence of small calcitonin-producing tumors by stimulatory tests such as calcium infusion or pentagastrin administration that result in markedly elevated levels of calcitonin. In patients with MEA II, one may also find hypercalcemia, which is often due to parathyroid hyperplasia.

A few families have been described with the so-called MEA type III syndrome, which consists of pheochromocytomas and medullary carcinomas of the thyroid associated with multiple mucosal neuromas and a peculiar phenotypic appearance: bumpy lips, enlarged tongue, visible corneal nerves, marfan-like habitus, muscular hypotonia, etc.

Case reports of "overlap" between MEA I and MEA II have been published in the last few years, but the significance is not clear. A more meaningful association may be that of pheochromocytoma and islet cell tumors of the pancreas.

Although many theories have been proposed to explain the existence of these syndromes, none are consistent with the facts known at present (see references at end of next section).

Thakker RV, Ponder BA: Multiple endocrine neoplasia. Clin Endocrinol Metab 1988;2:1031.

DISORDERS OF MULTIPLE ENDOCRINE DEFICIENCIES

It has long been known that primary adrenal insufficiency and primary thyroid failure could occur simultaneously in the same patient for unclear reasons (Schmidt's syndrome). It has been demonstrated that many of these patients have an autoimmune disorder, with formation of antibodies against cellular fractions of many endocrine glands. In addition to adrenal and thyroid failure, patients with these syndromes may have failure of the gonads, of the pituitary gland, of the insulin-secreting cells of the pancreatic islets, etc. There is often an association with pernicious anemia and with vitiligo and nontropical sprue as well as other autoimmune disorders. This syndrome has also been designated **polyglandular autoimmune syndrome type II** to differentiate it from **polyglandular autoimmune syndrome type I,** which is characterized by the appearance of mucocutaneous candidiasis (often in childhood), associated or followed by hypoparathyroidism and adrenal insufficiency. The

type I condition occurs in siblings, without involvement of other generations in the family. It is also known as autoimmune polyendocrinopathy-candidiasis-ectodermal dystrophy (APECED).

The basic mechanisms for the formation of autoantibodies are not clear at present. Although a familial tendency is often seen, many patients present with a sporadic disorder. An increased association of certain HLA antigens has been described in afflicted individuals with the type II disorder. No treatment other than hormone replacement is known at present.

A very rare syndrome involving endocrine systems is the POEMS syndrome, consisting of *p*olyneuropathy, *o*rganomegaly, *e*ndocrinopathy, *m*-protein, and *s*kin changes. The endocrine involvement includes diabetes mellitus, primary hypogonadism, and hyperpigmentation. The disorder is associated with sclerotic bone lesions, hepatosplenomegaly, and lymph node enlargement. The bone lesions contain plasma cells, and it is postulated that pathogenic immunoglobulins are produced there since radiation of the affected bone has resulted in resolution of the endocrine abnormalities.

Ahonen P et al: Clinical variations of autoimmune polyendrocrinopathy-candidiasis-ectodermal dystrophy (APECED) in a series of 68 patients. N Engl J Med 1990;322:1829.
McGregor AM: Immunoendocrine interactions and autoimmunity. N Engl J Med 1990;322:1739.

CLINICAL USE OF CORTICOTROPIN (ACTH) & THE CORTICOSTEROIDS

Both pituitary adrenocorticotropin (ACTH), acting by adrenal stimulation, and the C-11-oxygenated adrenal steroids (corticosteroids) have been shown to have profound modifying effects on many pathologic processes, especially those associated with immunologic problems and inflammation. These effects cannot be entirely explained at present on the basis of the known metabolic and immunologic activities of these compounds.

These agents do not appear to "cure." Their action is primarily anti-inflammatory and appears to be related to multiple effects upon blood vessels, leukocytes, macrophages, fibroblasts, cell membrane permeability, etc, rather than to one discrete, all-encompassing effect. They suppress the inflammatory process but do not deal with the underlying cause of the disease process. When they are discontinued, the disease often recurs.

Even though there is no support for the claim that a patient or a disease process may be responsive to one and not to another of these classes of drugs, there is no reason to use ACTH given its parenteral route of administration and lack of predictability of its corticosteroid response. Both ACTH and the corticosteroids cause varying degrees of pituitary suppression, while the corticosteroids lead to adrenal atrophy after prolonged use as well. They should not be stopped suddenly, and during periods of stress (eg, surgery, trauma), additional amounts of rapidly acting steroids must be provided. Many patients become dependent on corticosteroids, and withdrawal is difficult.

The systemic and topical efficacies of the corticosteroids are compared in Table 20–15.

Toxicity & Side Reactions

These agents are potentially dangerous, but with proper precautions most of these dangers can be avoided (see below). Corticosteroids are generally contraindicated during early pregnancy, except in the adrenogenital syndromes.

A. Hyperglycemia and glycosuria (diabetogenic effect) is of major significance in the early or potential diabetic.

B. Marked retention of sodium and water, with subsequent edema, increased blood volume, and hypertension, is minimized by the use of the newer agents.

C. Negative nitrogen and calcium balance may occur, with loss of body protein and consequent osteoporosis.

D. Potassium loss may lead to hypokalemic alkalosis.

E. Hirsutism and acne are cosmetic problems that may be of greater concern to females. Amenorrhea may occur.

F. Cushing's features or facies may develop with prolonged administration.

G. Peptic ulcer may be produced or aggravated.

Table 20–15. Systemic versus topical activity of corticosteroids. (Hydrocortisone = 1 in potency.)

	Systemic Activity	Topical Activity
Prednisolone	4–5	1–2
Fluprednisolone	8–10	10
Triamcinolone	5	1
Triamcinolone acetonide	5	40
Dexamethasone	30	10
Betamethasone	30	5–10
Betamethasone valerate		50–150
Methylprednisolone	5	5
Fluocinolone acetonide		40–100
Flurandrenolone acetonide		20–50
Fluorometholone	1–2	40

H. Resistance to infectious agents is lowered.

I. Impotence and decreased libido associated with decreased serum testosterone have been recently described.

Techniques Employed to Correct or Minimize Dangers

(1) Always reduce the dosage as soon as consistent with the clinical response. Intermittent alternate-day use may be a preferable and safer method of treatment. This method works well with prednisone or prednisolone but not with longer-acting drugs such as dexamethasone.

(2) During the first 2 weeks of therapy, blood pressure and weight should be carefully observed. Take an initial complete blood count and sedimentation rate and repeat as indicated. Serum potassium, bicarbonate, and chloride should be checked occasionally if large doses of these hormones are to be given over a period of more than several days. Blood and urine glucose should be followed as well.

(3) All patients should be on high-protein diets (100 g or more of protein daily) with adequate calcium intake.

(4) If edema develops, place the patient on a low-sodium diet (200–400 mg of sodium daily). Diuretics may be employed when strict sodium restriction is impossible.

(5) Potassium chloride, as 10% or 20% solution, effervescent tablets, or powder, 3–15 g daily in divided doses, should be administered if prolonged use or high dosage is employed.

(6) In cases of long-continued administration, anabolic preparations may be used to counteract the negative protein, calcium, and potassium balance. Unfortunately, the distressing osteoporosis cannot be prevented.

(7) Do not stop either ACTH or corticosteroids abruptly, since sudden withdrawal may cause a severe "rebound" of the disease process or a malignant necrotizing vasculitis. Also remember that glucocorticoids cause atrophy of the adrenal cortex through endogenous ACTH inhibition; sudden withdrawal may lead to symptoms of adrenal insufficiency.

(8) When treating mild disorders, giving corticosteroids during the daytime only or on alternate days causes less suppression of endogenous ACTH. When discontinuing therapy, withdraw evening dose first.

Contraindications & Special Precautions

A. Stress in Patients Receiving Maintenance Corticosteroids: Patients receiving corticosteroids, especially the oral preparations (or even ACTH), must be carefully watched because suppression of endogenous ACTH interferes with the normal response to stressful situations (eg, surgery or infections). Patients should be warned of this danger and should carry identification cards showing what drug they are taking, the dosage, and the reason for taking it. Whenever such a situation occurs or is about to occur, the dosage of cortisone or hydrocortisone should be increased or parenteral corticosteroids given (or both). If oral cortisone or hydrocortisone can be administered, it must be administered in larger doses at least every 6 hours.

B. Heart Disease: These agents should be used with caution in patients with cardiac disease or hypertension. Blood pressure may be increased by sodium retention or by increases in plasma renin substrate. The increase in extracellular fluid may lead to cardiac decompensation. Always begin with small doses and place the patient on a low-sodium diet.

C. Predisposition to Psychosis: These drugs cause a sense of well-being and euphoria in most persons, but in predisposed patients, an acute psychotic reaction may occur. (Insomnia may be the presenting symptom.) In these cases the drug should be stopped or the dosage reduced, and the patient should be carefully observed and protected. Persons have committed suicide under the influence of these drugs.

D. Effect on Peptic Ulcer: Active peptic ulcer is a contraindication to the use of these drugs because of the danger of perforation or hemorrhage. These agents also tend to activate ulcers and should be used only in emergency situations or with optimal antiulcer therapy in patients who have a history of peptic ulcer. Acute pancreatitis has been reported as well.

E. Tuberculosis: Active or recently healed tuberculosis is a contraindication to the use of these drugs unless intensive antituberculosis therapy is also carried out. A chest x-ray should be taken before and periodically during prolonged treatment with corticosteroids.

F. Infectious Diseases: Because these drugs tend to lower resistance and therefore to promote dissemination of infections, they must be used with caution, even when appropriate antibiotics are being given, in any acute or chronic infection.

G. Myopathy: A peculiar steroid myopathy has been reported, especially with the substituted steroids. Proximal muscle weakness without atrophy and with normal serum creatine kinase is relatively common and not correlated with dose or duration of therapy.

H. Fatty Liver: Fatty liver and fat embolism may occur.

I. Diagnostic Errors: Administration of these drugs may interfere with certain immune mechanisms that are of diagnostic value, eg, in skin tests and agglutination tests; they produce leukocytosis and lymphopenia, which may be confusing. The potent substituted corticosteroids (eg, dexamethasone) will suppress the urinary ketosteroids and hydroxycorticosteroid values. The signs and symptoms of infection may be masked by corticosteroid therapy. These drugs may also interfere with normal pain perception (eg, joint pain), which may lead to Charcot-like disintegration of the weight-bearing joints after local or systemic corticosteroid therapy.

J. Withdrawal of Corticosteroids: Prolonged use of these agents leads to combined pituitary-adrenal gland suppression that may last for as long as 1 year after stopping the drug. In the presence of infection, trauma, surgery, or other forms of stress, the patient may have signs of adrenal insufficiency unless given supplemental hydrocortisone.

Always withdraw corticosteroids slowly to minimize both flare-ups of the original disease and to prevent "steroid withdrawal reactions" (arthralgias, aches and pains, fatigue, nausea, fine desquamation of skin with a "chalky" appearance, etc).

REFERENCES

DeGroot LJ et al: *Endocrinology,* 2nd ed. 3 vols. Grune & Stratton, 1989.

Felig P et al (editors): *Endocrinology and Metabolism,* 2nd ed. McGraw-Hill, 1987.

Ingbar SH, Braverman LE (editors): *The Thyroid: A Fundamental and Clinical Text,* 5th ed. Lippincott, 1986.

McKusik VA: *Mendelian Inheritance in Man: Catalogue of Autosomal Dominant, Autosomal Recessive, and X-linked Phenotypes,* 8th ed. Johns Hopkins Univ Press, 1988.

Scriver CR et al (editors): *The Metabolic Basis of Inherited Disease,* 6th ed. McGraw-Hill, 1989.

Speroff L et al: *Clinical Gynecologic Endocrinology and Infertility,* 4th ed. Williams & Wilkins, 1988.

Wilson JD, Foster DW (editors): *Williams' Textbook of Endocrinology,* 7th ed. Saunders, 1985.

Yen SSC, Jaffe RB (editors): *Reproductive Endocrinology,* 2nd ed. Saunders, 1986. *The causes of osteomalacia are summarized in Table 20–12.

21

Diabetes Mellitus, Hypoglycemia, & Lipoprotein Disorders

John H. Karam, MD

DIABETES MELLITUS

Essentials of Diagnosis

Type I diabetes, or insulin-dependent diabetes mellitus (IDDM):

- Presence of symptoms such as polyuria, polydipsia, and rapid weight loss associated with unequivocal hyperglycemia.
- Plasma glucose of 140 mg/dL or higher after an overnight fast, documented on more than one occasion.
- Ketonemia, ketonuria, or both.

Type II diabetes, or non-insulin-dependent diabetes mellitus (NIDDM):

- Comprises more than 90% of the diabetic population.
- Symptoms include polyuria and polydipsia; catabolic features such as ketonuria and weight loss generally are uncommon at time of diagnosis. Candidal vaginitis in women may be an initial manifestation. Many patients have few or no symptoms.
- Plasma glucose of 140 mg/dL or higher after an overnight fast on more than one occasion. After 75 g oral glucose, diagnostic values are 200 mg/dL or more 2 hours after the oral glucose and at least once between 0 and 2 hours.
- Glycosylated hemoglobin levels above the upper range of normal suggest the diagnosis of incipient type II diabetes.

Classification & Pathogenesis

Diabetes mellitus represents a syndrome with disordered metabolism and inappropriate hyperglycemia due to either an absolute deficiency of insulin secretion or a reduction in its biologic effectiveness or both. It is classified into 2 major types in which age at onset is not a criterion (Table 21–1).

A. Type I: Insulin-Dependent Diabetes Mellitus (IDDM): This severe form is associated with ketosis in the untreated state. It occurs most commonly in juveniles but occasionally in adults, especially the nonobese and those who are elderly when hyperglycemia first appears. It is a catabolic disorder in which circulating insulin is virtually absent, plasma glucagon is elevated, and the pancreatic B cells fail to respond to all insulinogenic stimuli. Exogenous insulin is therefore required to reverse the catabolic state, prevent ketosis, reduce the hyperglucagonemia, and bring the elevated blood glucose level down.

The highest prevalence of type I diabetes is in Scandinavia, where it comprises as many as 20% of the total number of patients with diabetes. This decreases in prevalence to 13% in southern Europe and 8% in the USA, while in Japan and China less than 1% of patients with diabetes have type I diabetes.

Certain human leukocyte antigens (HLA) are strongly associated with the development of type I diabetes. About 95% of type I patients possess either HLA-DR3 or HLA-DR4, compared to 45–50% of Caucasian controls. HLA-DQ genes are even more specific markers of IDDM susceptibility, since a particular variety (HLA-DQw3.2) is invariably found in the DR4 patients with IDDM, while a "protective" gene (HLA-DQw3.1) is prevalent in the DR4 controls. Moreover, HLA-DR2, which is generally protective against IDDM, seems to be so only because it is often linked to protective DQ genes. In addition, circulating islet cell antibodies have been detected in as many as 85% of patients tested in the first few weeks of their diabetes, and when sensitive immunoassays are used, the majority of these patients also have detectable anti-insulin antibodies prior to receiving insulin therapy.

Because of these immune characteristics, type I diabetes is felt to result from an infectious or toxic environmental insult to pancreatic B cells of persons whose immune system is genetically predisposed to develop a vigorous autoimmune response against altered pancreatic B cell antigens. Extrinsic factors that affect B cell function include damage caused by viruses such as mumps or coxsackie B4 virus, by toxic chemical agents, or by destructive cytotoxins and antibodies released from sensitized immunocytes. An underlying genetic defect on chromosome 11 relating to B cell replication or function may predispose to

Table 21–1. Clinical classification of idiopathic diabetes mellitus syndromes.

Type	Ketosis	Islet Cell Antibodies	HLA Association	Treatment
(I) Insulin-dependent (IDDM)	Present	Present at onset	Positive	Insulin (mixtures of rapid- and intermediate-acting, at least twice daily) and diet
(II) Non-insulin-dependent (NIDDM) (a) Nonobese	Absent	Absent	Negative	(1) Eucaloric diet alone (2) Diet plus insulin or sulfonylureas
(b) Obese				(1) Weight reduction (2) Hypocaloric diet, plus sulfonylureas or insulin for symptomatic control only

development of B cell failure after viral infection; alternatively, specific HLA genes may increase susceptibility to a diabetogenic virus or be linked to certain immune response genes that predispose patients to a destructive autoimmune response against their own islet cells (autoaggression). A recent study showing amelioration of hyperglycemia in patients given cyclosporine shortly after onset of type I diabetes lends further support to the pathogenetic role of autoimmunity.

B. Type II: Non-Insulin-Dependent Diabetes Mellitus (NIDDM): This represents a heterogeneous group comprising milder forms of diabetes that occur predominantly in adults but occasionally in juveniles. More than 90% of all diabetics in the USA are included under this classification. Circulating endogenous insulin is sufficient to prevent ketoacidosis but is inadequate in the face of increased needs owing to tissue insensitivity. Type II diabetes is defined in essentially negative terms: It is a *non* ketotic form of diabetes that is *not* linked to HLA markers on the sixth chromosome; it has *no* islet cell antibodies; and it is *not* dependent on exogenous insulin therapy to sustain life, thereby being termed "*non*-insulin-dependent diabetes mellitus" (NIDDM). In most cases of this type of diabetes, the cause is unknown.

An element of tissue insensitivity to insulin has been noted in most NIDDM patients irrespective of weight and has been attributed to several interrelated factors. These include a primary (and as yet undefined) genetic factor, which is aggravated in time by additional enhancers of insulin resistance such as aging and abdominal-visceral obesity. In addition, there is an accompanying deficiency in the response of pancreatic B cells to glucose. Both the tissue resistance to insulin and the impaired B cell response to glucose appear to be further aggravated by increased hyperglycemia, and both defects are ameliorated by treatment that reduces the hyperglycemia toward normal. Attempts to identify a genetic marker for NIDDM have as yet been unsuccessful. However, most epidemiologic data indicate strong genetic influences, since in monozygotic twins over 40 years of age, concordance is uniform within a year whenever one twin develops NIDDM.

Two subgroups of patients with type II diabetes are currently distinguished by the absence or presence of obesity. The degree and prevalence of obesity varies among different racial groups. While obesity occurs in less than 30% of Chinese and Japanese patients with NIDDM, it is found in 75–80% of North Americans, Europeans, or Africans with NIDDM and approaches 100% of patients with NIDDM among Pima Indians or Pacific Islanders from Nauru or Samoa.

1. Nonobese NIDDM patients–These patients generally show an absent or blunted early phase of insulin release in response to glucose; however, it may often be elicited in response to other insulinogenic stimuli such as acute intravenous administration of sulfonylureas, glucagon, or secretin. Among this heterogeneous subgroup may be certain unrecognized patients with a milder expression of type I diabetes who initially retain enough B cell function to avoid ketosis but later develop increasing dependency on insulin therapy. Also included within this subgroup are those with diabetes characterized as "maturity-onset diabetes of the young," whose strongly positive family history of a mild form of diabetes suggests an autosomal dominant transmission.

The hyperglycemia in this subgroup of patients often responds to oral hypoglycemic agents or, at times, to dietary therapy alone. Occasionally, insulin therapy is required to achieve satisfactory glycemic control even though it is not needed to prevent ketoacidosis.

Although residual insulin resistance may persist after therapeutic correction of the hyperglycemia in some cases, it does not seem to be clinically relevant to the treatment of nonobese NIDDM patients, who generally respond to appropriate therapeutic supplements of insulin in the absence of rare associated conditions such as lipoatrophy or acanthosis nigricans.

2. Obese NIDDM patients–This form of diabetes is secondary to extrapancreatic factors that produce insensitivity to endogenous insulin. It is characterized by nonketotic mild diabetes, mainly in adults but occasionally also in children. The primary problem is a "target organ" disorder resulting in ineffective insulin action (Table 21–2) that can secondarily influ-

Table 21–2. Factors reducing response to insulin.

Prereceptor inhibitors: Anti-insulin antibodies
Receptor inhibitors:
  Insulin receptor antibodies
  "Down regulation" of receptors by hyperinsulinism:
    Primary hyperinsulinism (B cell adenoma)
    Hyperinsulinism secondary to a postreceptor defect (obesity, Cushing's syndrome, acromegaly, pregnancy) or prolonged glycemia (diabetes mellitus, post-glucose tolerance test)
Postreceptor influences:
  Poor responsiveness of principal target organs; obesity; hepatic disease; muscle inactivity; sustained hyperglycemia
  Hormonal excess: glucocorticoids, growth hormone, oral contraceptive agents, progesterone, human chorionic somatomammotropin, catecholamines, thyroxine

ence pancreatic B cell function. Hyperplasia of pancreatic B cells is often present and probably accounts for the fasting hyperinsulinism and exaggerated insulin responses to glucose and other stimuli seen in the milder forms of this disorder. In more severe cases, secondary (but potentially reversible) failure of B cell secretion may result after exposure to prolonged fasting hyperglycemia. This phenomenon has been called "desensitization" of the pancreatic B cell. It is selective for glucose, and the B cell recovers sensitivity to glucose stimulation once the sustained hyperglycemia is corrected by any form of therapy, including diet, sulfonylureas, and insulin. Obesity is common in this type of diabetes and is generally associated with abdominal distribution of fat, producing an abnormally high waist-to-hip ratio. Refined radiographic techniques of assessing abdominal fat distribution with CT scans have documented that a "visceral" obesity, due to accumulation of fat in the omental and mesenteric regions, correlates with insulin resistance, whereas fat predominantly in subcutaneous tissues of the abdomen has little if any association with insulin insensitivity. In obese patients, insulin insensitivity is positively correlated with the presence of distended adipocytes, but liver and muscle cells also resist the deposition of additional glycogen and triglycerides in their storage depots.

A major cause of the observed resistance to insulin in target tissues of obese patients is believed to be a postreceptor defect in insulin action. This is associated with overdistended storage depots, and there is a reduced ability to clear nutrients from the circulation after meals. A resulting hyperinsulinism can further enhance insulin resistance by down-regulation of insulin receptors. Moreover, when hyperglycemia develops, a specific glucose transporter protein within insulin target tissue also becomes down-regulated after continuous activation. This contributes to further defects in postreceptor insulin action, thereby aggravating the hyperglycemia.

When overfeeding is corrected so that storage depots become less saturated, the cycle is interrupted. There is improvement in insulin sensitivity, which is further restored toward normal by a reduction of both the hyperinsulinism and the hyperglycemia.

Epidemiologic Considerations

An estimated 7 million people in the USA are known to have diabetes, of which 560,000 have the insulin-dependent type. Use of the current "therapeutic" classification has been widely accepted throughout the world, but its deficiencies are apparent in many individual cases. For example, a 23-year-old nonobese woman whose mild diabetes is presently responding adequately to diet alone and who shows a low-normal C-peptide response to stimuli had presented with severe diabetes with ketosis and required insulin for several weeks following diagnosis. In addition, she has an associated autoimmune disorder, myasthenia gravis. From an etiologic standpoint, she probably has type I diabetes, but her present clinical status is "non-insulin-dependent." The National Diabetes Data Group is reviewing the present classification system so that such cases may be incorporated. Most persons with adult-onset diabetes are obese and thus may well represent a type of diabetes in which tissue insensitivity to insulin is a fundamental pathologic feature.

Clinical Findings

The principal clinical features of the 2 major types of diabetes mellitus are listed for comparison in Table 21–3.

Patients with type I diabetes (IDDM) present with a characteristic symptom complex, as outlined below. An absolute deficiency of insulin results in excessive accumulation of circulating glucose and fatty acids, with consequent hyperosmolality and hyperketonemia. The severity of the insulin deficiency and the acuteness with which the catabolic state develops determine the intensity of the osmotic and ketotic excess.

Patients with type II diabetes (NIDDM) may or may not present with characteristic signs and symptoms. The presence of obesity or a strongly positive family history for mild diabetes suggests a high risk for the development of type II diabetes.

A. Symptoms:

1. Type I diabetes (IDDM)–Increased urination is a consequence of osmotic diuresis secondary to

Table 21–3. Clinical features of diabetes at diagnosis.

	Diabetes Type I (IDDM)	Diabetes Type II (NIDDM)
Polyuria and thirst	+ +	+
Weakness or fatigue	+ +	+
Polyphagia with weight loss	+ +	−
Recurrent blurred vision	+	+ +
Vulvovaginitis or pruritus	+	+ +
Peripheral neuropathy	+	+ +
Nocturnal enuresis	+ +	−
Often asymptomatic	−	+ +

sustained hyperglycemia. This results in a loss of glucose as well as free water and electrolytes in the urine. Enuresis may signal the onset of diabetes in very young children. Thirst is a consequence of the hyperosmolar state, as is blurred vision, which often develops as the lenses and retinas are exposed to hyperosmolar fluids.

Weight loss despite normal or increased appetite is a common feature of IDDM when it develops subacutely over a period of weeks. The weight loss is initially due to depletion of water, glycogen, and triglyceride stores; thereafter, reduced muscle mass occurs as amino acids are diverted to form glucose and ketone bodies.

Lowered plasma volume produces dizziness and weakness due to postural hypotension when sitting or standing. Total body potassium loss and the general catabolism of muscle protein contribute to the weakness.

Paresthesias may be present at the time of diagnosis of type I diabetes, particularly when the onset is subacute. They reflect a temporary dysfunction of peripheral sensory nerves, which clears as insulin replacement restores glycemic levels closer to normal, suggesting neurotoxicity from sustained hyperglycemia.

When insulin deficiency is absolute and of acute onset, the above symptoms progress in an accelerated manner. Ketoacidosis exacerbates the dehydration and hyperosmolality by producing anorexia and nausea and vomiting, thus interfering with oral fluid replacement. As serum osmolality exceeds 320–330 mosm/L (normal, 285–295 mosm/L), impaired consciousness ensues; increased osmolality has a better correlation with progression to coma and subsequent outcome than does lowered pH. With progression of acidosis, deep breathing with a rapid ventilatory rate (Kussmaul respiration) occurs in an attempt to eliminate carbon dioxide. With worsening acidosis and increasing osmolality, the cardiovascular system may be unable to maintain compensatory vasoconstriction; severe circulatory collapse may result.

2. Type II diabetes (NIDDM)–Most patients with type II diabetes have an insidious onset of hyperglycemia and may be relatively asymptomatic initially. This is particularly true in obese patients, whose diabetes may be detected only after glycosuria or hyperglycemia is noted during routine laboratory studies. Occasionally, NIDDM patients may present with evidence of neuropathic or cardiovascular complications because of underlying occult disease present for some time prior to diagnosis. Chronic skin infections are common. Generalized pruritus and symptoms of vaginitis are frequently the initial complaints of women with NIDDM. Diabetes should be suspected in women with chronic candidal vulvovaginitis as well as in those who have delivered large babies (> 9 lb, or 4.1 kg) or have had polyhydramnios, preeclampsia, or unexplained fetal losses.

B. Signs:

1. Type I diabetes (IDDM)–The patient's level of consciousness can vary depending on the degree of hyperosmolality. When insulin deficiency develops relatively slowly and sufficient water intake is maintained, patients remain relatively alert and physical findings may be minimal. When vomiting occurs in response to worsening ketoacidosis, dehydration progresses and compensatory mechanisms become inadequate to keep serum osmolality below 320–330 mosm/L. Under these circumstances, stupor or even coma may occur. The fruity breath odor of acetone further suggests the diagnosis of diabetic ketoacidosis.

Postural hypotension indicates a depleted plasma volume; hypotension in the recumbent position is a serious prognostic sign. Loss of subcutaneous fat and muscle wasting are features of more slowly developing insulin deficiency. In occasional patients with slow, insidious onset of insulin deficiency, subcutaneous fat may be considerably depleted. An enlarged liver, eruptive xanthomas on the flexor surface of the limbs and on the buttocks, and lipemia retinalis indicate that chronic insulin deficiency has resulted in chylomicronemia, with circulating triglycerides elevated usually to over 2000 mg/dL.

2. Type II diabetes (NIDDM)–Nonobese patients with this mild form of diabetes often have no characteristic physical findings at the time of diagnosis. Obese diabetics may have any variety of fat distribution; however, diabetes seems to be more often associated in both men and women with localization of fat deposits on the upper segment of the body (particularly the abdomen, chest, neck, and face) and relatively less fat on the appendages, which may be quite muscular. Standardized tables of waist-to-hip ratio indicate that ratios of "greater than 0.9" in men and "greater than 0.8" in women are associated with an increased risk of diabetes in obese subjects. Mild hypertension may be present in obese diabetics. In women, candidal vaginitis with a reddened, inflamed vulvar area and a profuse whitish discharge may herald the presence of diabetes.

C. Laboratory Findings:

1. Urinalysis–

a. Glucosuria–A specific and convenient method to detect glucosuria is the paper strip impregnated with glucose oxidase and a chromogen system (Clinistix, Diastix, TesTape), which is sensitive to as little as 0.1% glucose in urine. Diastix can be directly applied to the urinary stream, and differing color responses of the indicator strip reflect glucose concentration.

Certain common therapeutic agents interfere with this determination. When taken in large doses, ascorbic acid, salicylates, methyldopa (Aldomet), and levodopa can give false-negative results, since these powerful reducing agents interfere with the color reaction and thus prevent accurate estimation of glucose in the urine of diabetics. A normal renal threshold for glucose as well as reliable bladder emptying is essential for interpretation.

b. Ketonuria–Qualitative detection of ketone bodies can be accomplished by nitroprusside tests (Acetest or Ketostix). Although these tests do not detect β-hydroxybutyric acid, which lacks a ketone group, the semiquantitative estimation of ketonuria thus obtained is nonetheless usually adequate for clinical purposes.

2. Blood testing procedures–

a. Glucose tolerance test–

(1) Methodology and normal fasting glucose: Plasma or serum from venous blood samples may be used and has the advantage over whole blood of providing values for glucose that are independent of hematocrit and that reflect the glucose concentration to which body tissues are exposed. For these reasons, and because plasma and serum are more readily measured on automated equipment, plasma and serum glucose measurements are rapidly replacing the whole blood glucose determinations used heretofore in most laboratories. Fluoride anticoagulant in the collecting tube prevents enzymatic glycolysis by blood corpuscles and prevents pseudohypoglycemia, seen in states of extreme leukocytosis. If serum is used, samples should be refrigerated and separated within 1 hour after collection.

(2) Criteria for laboratory confirmation of diabetes mellitus: If the fasting plasma glucose level is over 140 mg/dL on more than one occasion, further evaluation of the patient with a glucose challenge is unnecessary. However, when fasting plasma glucose is less than 140 mg/dL in suspected cases, a standardized oral glucose tolerance test may be done (see Table 21–4).

For proper evaluation of the test, the subjects should be normally active and free from acute illness. Medications that may impair glucose tolerance include diuretics, contraceptive drugs, glucocorticoids, nicotinic acid, and phenytoin.

Because of difficulties in interpreting oral glucose tolerance tests and the lack of standards related to aging, these tests are generally being replaced by documentation of fasting hyperglycemia as a means of diagnosing diabetes mellitus.

Since fasting plasma glucose is known to increase with aging, physicians should be more tolerant of slight abnormalities of fasting glucose values in elderly people (over 70 years of age) and not deprive patients of occasional sugar-containing snacks when symptoms are not evident. However, an occasional elderly patient may benefit from the diagnosis of mild diabetes in that macular edema may be detected earlier and laser treatment initiated before vision deteriorates permanently.

b. Glycosylated hemoglobin (hemoglobin A₁) **b. Glycosylated hemoglobin (hemoglobin A_1) measurements**–Glycosylated hemoglobin is abnormally high in diabetics with chronic hyperglycemia and reflects their metabolic control. It is produced by nonenzymatic condensation of glucose molecules with free amino groups on the globin component of hemoglobin. The higher the prevailing ambient levels of blood glucose, the higher will be the level of glycosylated hemoglobin. The major form of glycohemoglobin is termed hemoglobin A_{1c}, which normally comprises only 4–6% of the total hemoglobin. The remaining glycohemoglobins (2–4% of the total) consist of phosphorylated glucose or fructose and are termed hemoglobin A_{1a} and hemoglobin A_{1b}. Most laboratories measure the sum of these 3 glycohemoglobins and report it as hemoglobin A_1.

Since glycohemoglobins circulate within red blood cells whose life span lasts up to 120 days, they generally reflect the state of glycemia over the preceding 8–12 weeks, thereby providing an improved method of assessing diabetic control. When glycohemoglobins are measured in a reliable laboratory, they are extremely useful in monitoring the progress of patients. Measurements should be made in patients with either type of diabetes mellitus at 3- to 4-month intervals. In patients monitoring their own blood glucose levels, glycohemoglobin values provide a valuable

Table 21–4. National Diabetes Data Group criteria for evaluating standard oral glucose tolerance test.[1]

	Normal Glucose Tolerance	Impaired Glucose Tolerance	Diabetes Mellitus[2]
Fasting plasma glucose (mg/dL)	< 115	116–139	> 140
Points between 0 and 120 minutes (mg/dL)	< 200	< 200	200 at least once
Two hours post glucose load (mg/dL)	< 140	> 140 but < 200	> 200

[1] Give 75 g of glucose dissolved in 300 mL of water for adults (1.75 g/kg ideal body weight for children) after an overnight fast in subjects who have been receiving at least 150–200 g of carbohydrate daily for 3 days before the test.
[2] A fasting plasma glucose greater than 140 mg/dL is diagnostic of diabetes. However, if the plasma glucose is less than 140 mg/dL, both of the lower columns must be fulfilled to make the diagnosis of diabetes mellitus.

check on the accuracy of monitoring. In patients who do not monitor their own blood glucose levels, glycohemoglobin values are essential for adjusting therapy. Attempts to use glycohemoglobin methods for diabetes screening have been controversial. Sensitivity in detecting known diabetes cases by hemoglobin A_{1c} measurements is only 85%, indicating that diabetes cannot be excluded by a normal value. On the other hand, elevated hemoglobin A_{1c} assays are quite specific (91%) in identifying the presence of diabetes mellitus.

Occasionally, fluctuations in hemoglobin A_1 are due to an acutely generated, reversible, intermediary (aldimine-linked) product that can falsely elevate glycohemoglobins when measured with "short-cut" chromatographic methods. This can be eliminated by using more intricate methods or by dialysis of the hemolysate before chromatography. When hemoglobin variants are present, such as negatively charged hemoglobin F, acetylated hemoglobin from high-dose aspirin therapy, or carbamylated hemoglobin produced by the complexing of urea with hemoglobin in uremia, falsely *high* "hemoglobin A_1" values are obtained with commonly used chromatographic methods. In the presence of positively charged hemoglobin variants such as hemoglobin S or C, or when the life span of red blood cells is reduced by increased hemolysis or hemorrhage, falsely *low* values for "hemoglobin A_1" result.

Serum fructosamine is formed by nonenzymatic glycosylation of serum proteins (predominantly albumin). Since serum albumin has a much shorter half-life than hemoglobin, serum fructosamine generally reflects the state of glycemic control for only the preceding 2 weeks. When abnormal hemoglobins or hemolytic states affect the interpretation of glycohemoglobin or when a narrower time frame is required, such as for ascertaining glycemic control at the time of conception in a diabetic woman who has recently become pregnant, serum fructosamine assays offer some advantage.

c. Self-monitoring of blood glucose–Capillary blood glucose measurements performed by patients themselves, as outpatients, are extremely useful, particularly in IDDM patients in whom "tight" metabolic control is attempted. A portable battery-operated Glucometer II (Ames Co.) or Glucosan II (Lifescan, Inc.) provides a digital readout of the intensity of color developed when glucose oxidase paper strips are exposed to a drop of capillary blood for up to 60 seconds. Similar diagnostic strips made by Biodynamics Corp. (Chemstrip-bG) have 2 chromogen indicators that permit *visual* estimation of the glucose concentration when compared to a series of color standards. The Chemstrip-bG can also be read by a reflectance meter (Accu-chek II). Newer glucometers—One Touch (Lifescan, Inc) or ExacTech (Baxter Corp)—automatically time the reaction as soon as a drop of blood is applied to the previously inserted test strip. This

relieves patients of the need to wipe off the strip after an exact interval of time and eliminates technical errors from improper blotting or timing. To eliminate the expense of test strips, Eli Lilly Co. has introduced the direct 30/30 meter, which provides 30 days of unlimited testing using a disposable 30-day cartridge that requires no strips. In self-monitoring of blood glucose, patients must prick their finger with a small lancet (Monolet, Ames Co.), which can be facilitated by a small plastic trigger device such as an Autolet (Ames Co.), Autoclix (Bio-Dynamics), or Penlet (Lifescan, Inc.).

The accuracy of data obtained by glucose monitoring requires careful education and training of the patient in sampling and measuring procedures as well as in proper calibration of the instruments. Bedside glucose monitoring in a hospital setting requires rigorous quality control programs and certification of personnel to avoid serious errors. When this is not feasible, glucose testing at the bedside is best done by technicians from the central laboratory.

3. Capillary morphometry (biopsy of the quadriceps muscle)–The basement membrane of capillaries from skeletal muscle tissue of the quadriceps area is abnormally thickened in cases of overt spontaneous diabetes in adults with fasting hyperglycemia of 140 mg/dL or more. Capillary morphometry appears to be less useful in diabetic children, being normal in as many as 60% of those below age 18.

Whether basement membrane thickening in diabetics can result from hyperglycemia alone with no genetic component appears to have been resolved by documented observation of thickened capillary basement membranes in the muscle of patients with acquired chronic hyperglycemia after ingestion of a diabetogenic toxin (Vacor rodenticide) during attempted suicide. While this finding establishes that glucose toxicity can produce abnormally thick membranes, it is still possible that the degree of abnormal thickening may depend on varying genetic susceptibility among diabetic patients. Moreover, it remains unclear whether a thickened capillary basement membrane of skeletal muscle has clinical significance, since it has not been possible to demonstrate a correlation between this marker and clinically evident renal dysfunction or renal mesangial changes associated with progressive diabetic nephropathy.

Differential Diagnosis

A. Hyperglycemia Secondary to Other Causes: (Table 21–5.) Secondary hyperglycemia has been associated with various disorders of insulin target tissues (liver, muscle, and adipose tissue).

Other secondary causes of carbohydrate intolerance include endocrine disorders—often specific endocrine tumors—associated with excess production of growth hormone, glucocorticoids, catecholamines, glucagon, or somatostatin. In the first 4 situations, peripheral

Table 21–5. Secondary causes of hyperglycemia.

Hyperglycemia due to tissue insensitivity to insulin
  Hormonal tumors (acromegaly, Cushing's syndrome, gluca-
    gonoma, pheochromocytoma)
  Pharmacologic agents (glucocorticoids, sympathomimetic
    drugs, nicotinic acid)
  Liver disease (cirrhosis, hemochromatosis)
  Muscle disorders (myotonic dystrophy)
  Adipose tissue disorders (lipoatrophy, lipodystrophy, truncal
    obesity)
  Insulin receptor disorders (acanthosis nigricans syndromes,
    leprechaunism)
Hyperglycemia due to reduced insulin secretion
  Hormonal tumors (somatostatinoma, pheochromocytoma)
  Pancreatic disorders (pancreatitis, hemosiderosis from ex-
    cess transfusions, idiopathic hemochromatosis)
  Pharmacologic agents (thiazide diuretics, phenytoin, pen-
    tamidine, Vacor rodenticide)

responsiveness to insulin is impaired. With excess of glucocorticoids, catecholamines, or glucagon, increased hepatic output of glucose is a contributory factor; in the case of catecholamines, decreased insulin release is an additional factor in producing carbohydrate intolerance, and with excess somatostatin production it is the major factor.

A rare syndrome of extreme insulin resistance associated with acanthosis nigricans is divided into 2 major groups on the basis of clinical and laboratory manifestations: Group A consists of younger women with androgenic features (hirsutism, amenorrhea, polycystic ovaries) in whom insulin receptors are deficient in number and often are structurally abnormal. Group B consists of older people, mostly women, in whom immunologic disease is suspected (high erythrocyte sedimentation rate, anti-DNA antibodies, and a circulating immunoglobulin that binds to insulin receptors, reducing their affinity to insulin).

Medications such as thiazide diuretics, phenytoin, and high-dose glucocorticoids can produce hyperglycemia that is reversible once the drugs are discontinued. Chronic pancreatitis reduces the number of functioning B cells and can result in a metabolic derangement very similar to that of genetic diabetes mellitus except that a concomitant reduction in pancreatic A cells may reduce glucagon secretion so that relatively lower doses of insulin replacement are needed. Insulin-dependent diabetes is occasionally associated with Addison's disease and autoimmune thyroiditis (Schmidt's syndrome). This occurs particularly in women and probably represents an autoimmune disorder in which there are circulating antibodies to adrenocortical and thyroid tissue, thyroglobulin, and gastric parietal cells.

B. Nondiabetic Glycosuria: Nondiabetic glycosuria (renal glycosuria) is a benign, asymptomatic condition wherein glucose appears in the urine despite a normal amount of glucose in the blood, either basally or during a glucose tolerance test. Its cause may vary from an autosomally transmitted genetic disorder to

one associated with dysfunction of the proximal renal tubule (Fanconi's syndrome, chronic renal failure), or it may merely be a consequence of the increased load of glucose presented to the tubules by the elevated glomerular filtration rate during pregnancy. As many as 50% of pregnant women normally have demonstrable sugar in the urine, especially during the third and fourth months. This sugar is practically always glucose except during the late weeks of pregnancy, when lactose may be present.

Treatment

A. Goals of Treatment of Diabetes: Diabetes mellitus is a chronic disease that requires ongoing medical care and education both to prevent acute illness and to reduce the risk of long-term complications. Therapy directed toward these goals should not be too restrictive to the patient's quality of life. At present, there is conflicting evidence about whether microangiopathy is related to the existence and duration of hyperglycemia or whether it reflects a separate, coexisting genetic disorder. Until this conflict is resolved, the therapeutic objective is to attempt to restore known metabolic derangements to normal in the hope that this approach will impede if not prevent the progression of microvascular disease.

B. Treatment Regimens:

1. Diet–A well-balanced, nutritious diet remains a fundamental element of therapy. However, in more than half of cases, diabetic patients fail to follow their diet. In prescribing a diet, it is important to relate dietary objectives to the type of diabetes. In obese patients with mild hyperglycemia, the major goal of diet therapy is weight reduction by caloric restriction. Thus, there is less need for exchange lists, emphasis on timing of meals, or periodic snacks, all of which are so essential in the treatment of insulin-requiring nonobese diabetics. This type of patient represents the most frequent challenge for the physician. Weight reduction is an elusive goal that can only be achieved by close supervision and education of the obese patient. See Chapter 22 for dietary management of obesity.

a. ADA diet–Exchange lists for meal planning can be obtained from the American Diabetes Association and its affiliate associations or from the American Dietetic Association, 430 North Michigan Avenue, Chicago 60611. The ADA diet stresses the major goal of caloric restriction as a means of achieving or maintaining ideal weight. A prudent diet is recommended, which includes restriction of fat intake to 35% or less of the total calories and suggests that saturated fat be reduced to only one-third of this by substituting poultry, veal, and fish for red meats as a major protein source. At the same time, cholesterol is restricted to less than 300 mg daily. Carbohydrates may be consumed liberally (as much as 50–60% of total calories) as long as refined and simple sugars are avoided as snacks. Dietary sucrose need not aggravate postprandial hyperglycemia in diabetic patients if consumed as part of a mixed meal and in exchange for other carbohydrate components of the meal. Unrefined carbohydrates with a fiber content sufficient to provide 15–20 g of fiber daily are recommended for both type I and type II diabetic patients.

b. Dietary fiber–Plant components such as cellulose, gum, and pectin are indigestible by humans and are termed dietary "fiber." Insoluble fibers such as cellulose or hemicellulose, as found in bran, tend to increase intestinal transit and may have beneficial effects on colonic function. In contrast, soluble fibers such as gums and pectins, as found in beans, oatmeal, or apple skin, tend to retard nutrient absorption rates so that glucose absorption is slower and hyperglycemia is diminished. Although the ADA diet does not include insoluble fiber supplements such as added bran, it recommends food such as oatmeal, cereals, and beans with relatively high soluble fiber content as staple components of the diet in diabetics. High soluble fiber content in the diet may also have a favorable effect on blood cholesterol levels.

c. Artificial sweeteners–The nonnutritive sweetener saccharin continues to be available in certain foods and beverages despite recent warnings by the FDA about its potential long-term carcinogenicity to the bladder. A restriction on the use of saccharin in children and pregnant women is recommended; however, in patients with diabetes or obesity, physicians should determine on an individual basis its comparative benefit versus risk.

Nutritive sweeteners such as sorbitol and fructose have recently increased in popularity. Except for acute diarrhea induced by ingestion of large amounts of sorbitol-containing foods, their relative risk has yet to be established. Fructose represents a "natural" sugar substance that is a highly effective sweetener which induces only slight increases in plasma glucose levels.

Aspartame (NutraSweet) has proved to be a popular sweetener for diabetic patients. It consists of 2 amino acids (aspartic acid and phenylalanine) that combine to produce a nutritive sweetener 180 times as sweet as sucrose. A major limitation is that it cannot be used in baking or cooking because of its lability to heat.

2. Oral hypoglycemic drugs–Only the sulfonylureas remain in use as oral hypoglycemic drugs in the USA. Some discussion of the biguanides is included here because these drugs are still used overseas.

a. Sulfonylureas–(Table 21–6.) Slight modifications of the basic structure produce agents that have similar qualitative actions but differ widely in potency. The mechanism of action of the sulfonylureas when they are acutely administered is due to their insulinotropic effect on pancreatic B cells. However, it remains unclear whether this well-documented *acute* action requires additional extrapancreatic effects such

Table 21–6. Sulfonylureas.

	Tablet Size (mg)	Daily Dose	Duration of Action (hours)
Tolbutamide (Orinase)[1]	250, 500	0.25–2 g in divided doses	6–12
Tolazamide (Tolinase)[1]	100, 250, 500	0.1–1 g as single dose or in divided doses	10–14
Acetohexamide (Dymelor)[1,2]	250, 500	0.25–1.5 g as single dose or in divided doses	12–24
Chlorpropamide (Diabinese)[1,2]	100, 250	0.1–0.5 g as single dose	Up to 60
Glyburide (Diaβeta, Micronase)	1.25, 2.5, 5	1.25–20 mg	10–24
Glipizide (Glucotrol)	5, 10	5–30 mg	10–20

[1] Generic form available.
[2] There has been a decline in use of these formulation. In the case of chlorpropamide, this is due to its numerous side effects (see text).

as an increase in insulin binding to receptors to explain more adequately the hypoglycemic effect of sulfonylureas during chronic administration.

Sulfonylureas are presently not indicated in the juvenile type ketosis-prone insulin-dependent diabetic, since these drugs seem to depend on functioning pancreatic B cells. There is little, if any, potentiation of insulin effectiveness on long-term glycemic control when sulfonylureas are added in IDDM patients.

The sulfonylureas seem most appropriate for use in the nonobese insulinopenic mild maturity-onset diabetic in whom acute administration improves the early phase of insulin release that is refractory to acute glucose stimulation. In obese mild diabetics and others with peripheral insensitivity to levels of circulating insulin, primary emphasis should be on weight reduction. When hyperglycemia in obese diabetics has been more severe, with consequent impairment of pancreatic B cell function, sulfonylureas may improve glycemic control until concurrent measures such as diet, exercise, and weight reduction can sustain the improvement without the need for oral drugs.

(1) Tolbutamide (Orinase) is supplied in tablets of 250 and 500 mg. It is rapidly oxidized in the liver to an inactive form, and its approximate duration of effect is relatively short (6–10 hours). Tolbutamide is probably best administered in divided doses (eg, 500 mg before each meal and at bedtime); however, some patients require only 1 or 2 tablets daily. Because of its short duration of action, which is independent of renal function, tolbutamide is probably the safest agent to use in elderly patients, in whom hypoglycemia would be a particularly serious risk. Prolonged hypoglycemia has been reported rarely, mostly in patients receiving certain antibacterial sulfonamides (sulfisoxazole, sulfaphenzole), an anticoagulant (dicumarol), or phenylbutazone for arthralgias. These drugs apparently compete with sulfonylureas for oxidative enzyme systems in the liver, resulting in maintenance of high levels of unmetabolized, active sulfonylureas in the circulation.

(2) Chlorpropamide (Diabinese) is supplied in tablets of 100 and 250 mg. This drug, with a half-life of 32 hours, is slowly metabolized, with approximately 20–30% excreted unchanged in the urine. Since the metabolites retain hypoglycemic activity, elimination of the biologic effect is almost completely dependent on renal excretion, so that its use is contraindicated in patients with renal insufficiency. The average maintenance dose is 250 mg daily, given as a single dose in the morning. Chlorpropamide is a potent agent, and prolonged hypoglycemic reactions are more common than with tolbutamide, particularly in elderly patients, in whom chlorpropamide therapy should be monitored with special care. Doses in excess of 500 mg daily increase the risk of cholestatic jaundice. A flush may occur when alcohol is ingested by patients taking chlorpropamide, appearing within 8 minutes of ingesting the alcohol and lasting for 10–12 minutes; it is believed to be dose-related.

Hyponatremia is a complication of chlorpropamide therapy in some patients, apparently because chlorpropamide both stimulates vasopressin secretion and potentiates its action at the renal tubule. The antidiuretic effect of chlorpropamide is relatively unique, since 3 other sulfonylureas (acetohexamide, tolazamide, and glyburide) facilitate water excretion in humans. Since other sulfonylureas have now become available with comparable potency but without the disadvantage of causing water retention or alcohol flushing, there is less need to prescribe chlorpropamide in managing patients with NIDDM.

(3) Tolazamide (Tolinase) is supplied in tablets of 100, 250, and 500 mg. It is comparable to chlorpropamide in potency but has a shorter duration of action and does not cause water retention. Tolazamide is more slowly absorbed than the other sulfonylureas, with effects on blood glucose not appearing for several hours. Its duration of action may last up to 20 hours, with maximal hypoglycemic effect occurring between the fourth and 14th hours. Tolazamide is metabolized to several compounds that retain hypoglycemic effects. If more than 500 mg/d is required, the dose should be divided and given twice daily. Doses larger than 1000 mg daily do not improve the degree of glycemic control.

(4) Acetohexamide (Dymelor) is supplied in tablets of 250 and 500 mg. Its duration of action is about 10–16 hours, being intermediate in action between tolbutamide and chlorpropamide. A dose of 0.25–1.5 g is given daily in one or 2 doses. Liver metabolism is rapid, but the metabolite produced remains active.

(5) Second-generation sulfonylureas (glyburide and glipizide): Glyburide and glipizide are 100-fold more potent than tolbutamide. These drugs should be used with caution in patients with cardiovascular disease or in elderly patients, in whom hypoglycemia would be especially dangerous.

Diabetic patients who have not responded to tolbutamide or even tolazamide may respond to the more potent first-generation sulfonylurea chlorpropamide or to either of the second-generation sulfonylureas. Unfortunately, substantial glycemic benefit has not always resulted when a maximum therapeutic dose of chlorpropamide has been replaced with that of a second-generation drug in NIDDM patients whose glucose control has been unsatisfactory.

(a) Glyburide (glibenclamide; Diaβeta, Micronase): Glyburide is available in 1.25-, 2.5-, and 5-mg tablets. The usual starting dose is 2.5 mg/d, and the average maintenance dose is 5–10 mg/d given as a single morning dose; maintenance doses higher than 20 mg/d are not recommended. Glyburide is metabolized in the liver into products with such low hypoglycemic activity that they are considered clinically unimportant. Although assays specific for the unmetabolized compound suggest a plasma half-life of only 1–2 hours, the biologic effects of glyburide are clearly persistent 24 hours after a single morning dose in diabetic patients.

Glyburide has few adverse effects other than its potential for causing hypoglycemia. Flushing has rarely been reported after ethanol ingestion. It does not cause water retention, as chlorpropamide does, but rather slightly enhances free water clearance. Glyburide is absolutely contraindicated in the presence of hepatic impairment and probably should not be used in patients with renal insufficiency, in elderly patients, or in those who would be put at serious risk from an episode of hypoglycemia.

(b) Glipizide (Glucotrol): Glipizide is available in 5- and 10-mg tablets. For maximum effect in reducing postprandial hyperglycemia, this agent should be ingested 30 minutes before meals, since rapid absorption is delayed when the drug is taken with food. The recommended starting dose is 5 mg/d with up to 15 mg/d given as a single daily dose before breakfast. When higher daily doses are required, they should be divided and given before meals. The maximum recommended dose is 40 mg/d.

At least 90% of glipizide is metabolized in the liver to inactive products, and 10% is excreted unchanged in the urine. Glipizide therapy is therefore contraindicated in patients with hepatic or renal impairment, who would therefore be at high risk for hypoglycemia, but because of its lower potency it is preferable to glyburide in elderly patients.

b. Biguanides–These compounds were introduced in the 1950s for the management of non-insulin-dependent diabetes mellitus. Phenformin (DBI, Meltrol-50) was available in the USA until 1977, when it was discontinued because of its association with lactic acidosis. While it is still prescribed in some areas overseas to a limited extent, it has generally been replaced by other biguanides such as buformin and particularly metformin. Only metformin is discussed here.

Metformin (1,1-dimethylbiguanide hydrochloride) was introduced in France in 1957 as an oral agent for therapy of type II diabetes, either alone or in conjunction with sulfonylureas. It is awaiting FDA approval in the USA pending the outcome of multicenter clinical trials. It is marketed in many parts of the world under the brand name Glucophage and is also known as Diabefagos and Haurymellin.

(1) Clinical pharmacology: The exact mechanism of action of metformin remains unclear. It reduces both the fasting level of blood glucose and the degree of postprandial hyperglycemia in patients with type II diabetes but has no effect on fasting blood glucose in normal subjects. Metformin does not stimulate insulin action, particularly in reducing hepatic gluconeogenesis. Other proposed mechanisms include a slowing down of gastrointestinal absorption of glucose and increased glucose uptake by skeletal muscle, which have been reported in some but not all clinical studies.

Metformin has a half-life of 1½–3 hours, is not bound to plasma proteins, and is not metabolized in humans, being excreted unchanged by the kidneys.

(2) Indications and dosage: Metformin may be used as an adjunct to diet for the control of hyperglycemia and its associated symptomatology in patients with type II diabetes, particularly those who are obese or are not responding optimally to maximal doses of sulfonylureas. A side benefit of metformin therapy is its tendency to improve hyperglycemia and hypertriglyceridemia in obese diabetics without the weight gain associated with insulin or sulfonylurea therapy. Metformin is not indicated for patients with type I diabetes and is contraindicated in diabetics with renal or hepatic insufficiency, alcoholism, or a propensity to develop hypoxia (eg, disease associated with cardiorespiratory insufficiency).

Metformin is dispensed as 500-mg or 850-mg tablets, and the dosage range is from 500 mg to a maximum of 2.5 g daily, with the lowest possible effective dose being recommended. It is important that metformin be taken in divided doses—and with meals—to reduce minor gastrointestinal upsets. A common schedule would be one 500-mg tablet 3 times a day with meals or one 850-mg tablet twice daily at breakfast and dinner.

(3) Adverse reactions: The most frequent side effects of metformin are gastrointestinal symptoms (anorexia, nausea, vomiting, abdominal discomfort, diarrhea), which occur in up to 20% of patients. These effects are dose-related, tend to occur at onset of therapy, and often are transient. However, in 3–5% of patients, therapy may have to be discontinued because of persistent diarrheal discomfort.

Hypoglycemia does not occur with therapeutic doses of metformin, which permits its description as a "euglycemic" or "antihyperglycemic" drug rather than an oral hypoglycemic agent. Dermatologic or hematologic toxicity is rare.

Lactic acidosis has been reported as a side effect but is uncommon with metformin in contrast to phenformin, and almost all reported cases have involved subjects with associated risk factors that should have contraindicated its use (renal, hepatic, or cardiorespiratory insufficiency, alcoholism, advanced age).

c. Safety of the oral hypoglycemic agents– The University Group Diabetes Program (UGDP) reported that the number of deaths due to cardiovascular disease in diabetic patients treated with tolbutamide or the no longer used phenformin was excessive compared to either insulin-treated patients or those receiving placebos. Controversy persists about the validity of the conclusions reached by the UGDP because of the heterogeneity of the population studied, with its preponderance of obese subjects, and certain features of the experimental design such as the use of a fixed dose of oral drug. At present a warning label is inserted in each package of sulfonylureas, but there is no restriction to recommending their use by the American Diabetes Association.

Idiosyncratic reactions to sulfonylureas are rare, with skin rashes or hematologic toxicity (transient leukopenia, thrombocytopenia) occurring in less than 0.1% of patients.

3. Insulin–Insulin is indicated for type I (IDDM) diabetics as well as for nonobese type II diabetics with insulinopenia whose hyperglycemia does not respond to diet therapy either alone or combined with oral hypoglycemic drugs.

With the development of highly purified human insulin preparations, immunogenicity has been markedly reduced, thereby decreasing the incidence of therapeutic complications such as insulin allergy, immune insulin resistance, and localized lipoatrophy at the injection site. However, the problem of achieving optimal insulin delivery remains unsolved with the present state of technology. It has not been possible to reproduce the physiologic patterns of intraportal insulin secretion with subcutaneous injections of soluble or longer-acting insulin suspensions. Even so, with the help of appropriate modifications of diet and exercise and careful monitoring of capillary blood glucose levels at home, it has often been possible to achieve acceptable control of blood glucose by using portable insulin infusion pumps or variable mixtures of short- and longer-acting insulins injected at least twice daily.

a. Characteristics of available insulin preparations–Commercial insulin preparations differ with respect to the animal species from which they are obtained, their purity and solubility, and the time of onset and duration of their biologic action. In the fall of 1989, more than 40 different formulations of insulin were available in the USA.

(1) Species of insulin: Because the supply of pork insulin has been too limited to satisfy the insulin requirements of all diabetic patients, most commercial insulins contain the slightly more antigenic beef insulin, which differs by 3 amino acids from human insulin (in contrast to the single amino acid distinguishing pork and human insulins). Standard preparations of Iletin I (Eli Lilly) are mixtures containing 70% beef and 30% pork insulin. However, a limited supply of monospecies pork or beef insulin (Iletin II) has been available for use in certain patients with insulin allergy or immune insulin resistance. The production of highly purified insulins by Danish manufacturers has resulted in a substantial increase in the availability of porcine insulin. Human insulin is now produced by recombinant DNA techniques (biosynthetic human insulin) or by enzymatic conversion of pork insulin to human insulin structure (semisynthetic human insulin), in which alanine, the terminal amino acid on the beta chain of pork insulin, is replaced by threonine. Human insulin prepared by the recombinant DNA method has been introduced for clinical use as Humulin (Eli Lilly) and dispensed as either Regular, NPH, or Lente Humulin. Human insulin prepared by enzymatic conversion of pork insulin or by recombinant DNA methods is marketed by Novo Nordisk. Novolin R (formerly Actrapid Human), a zinc suspension of human insulin, Novolin L (formerly Monotard Human), and an isophane suspension of human, Novolin N, are also products of Novo Nordisk. The R, L, and N refer to the particular formulation (regular, lente, and NPH, respectively). The cost of human insulin is approximately 1¼ times the cost of standard beef or pork insulin but slightly less than the cost of purified pork or beef insulin. Since human insulin tends to be slightly more hydrophilic than beef insulin, it was not until July 1987 that Eli Lilly was able to produce an ultralente formulation of human insulin with the required degree of insolubility characteristic of beef insulin products.

(2) Purity of insulin: Recent improvements in purification techniques for insulins extracted from animal pancreas have reduced or eliminated contaminating insulin precursors which had molecular weights greater than that of insulin and which were biologically inactive yet capable of inducing anti-insulin antibodies. The degree of purification in which proinsulin contamination is greater than 10 but less than 25 ppm characterizes the main form of insulin produced commercially in the USA by Eli Lilly as Iletin I. When proinsulin content is reduced to less than 10 ppm, manufacturers are entitled by FDA regulations to label the insulin as "purified." Such highly purified insulins are presently marketed in the USA by Eli Lilly and Novo Nordisk. The Eli Lilly product is called Iletin II to identify this highly purified insulin, and it presently is available only as a monospecies pork or beef insulin. All human insulins are also highly purified.

The more purified insulins that have recently become available seem to preserve their potency quite well, so that refrigeration is recommended but not crucial. During travel, reserve supplies of insulin can thus be readily transported for weeks without losing potency if protected from extremes of heat or cold.

(3) Concentration of insulin: At present, most insulins are available in a concentration of 100 units/mL (U100), and all are dispensed in 10–mL vials. To accommodate children and occasional adults who may require small quantities, a U40 insulin continues to be available. However, with the popularity of "low-dose" (0.5- or 0.3-mL) disposable insulin syringes, there is less need for U40 insulin, since U100 can now be measured with acceptable accuracy in doses as low as 1–2 units. For use in rare cases of severe insulin resistance in which large quantities of insulin are required, a limited supply of U500 regular porcine insulin (Iletin II) is available from Eli Lilly.

b. Insulin preparations–(Table 21–7.) Three principal types of insulins are available: (1) short-acting, with rapid onset of action; (2) intermediate-acting; and (3) long-acting, with slow onset of action (Fig 21–1). Short-acting insulin (unmodified insulin) is a crystalline zinc insulin provided in soluble form and thus is dispensed as a clear solution. All other commercial insulins have been specially modified to retain more prolonged action and are dispensed as turbid suspensions at neutral pH with either protamine in phosphate buffer (protamine zinc insulin and NPH) or varying concentrations of zinc in acetate buffer (ultralente and semilente). The use of protamine zinc insulin and semilente preparations is currently decreasing, and almost no indications for their use exist.

(1) Regular insulin is a short-acting soluble crystalline zinc insulin whose effect appears within 15 minutes after subcutaneous injection and lasts 5–7 hours when usual quantities are administered. It is the only type of insulin that can be administered intravenously. It is particularly useful in the treatment of diabetic ketoacidosis and when the insulin requirement is changing rapidly, such as after surgery or during acute infections.

Two preparations of regular insulin are used for insulin infusion pumps since they contain a phosphate buffer that prevents aggregation in the tubing. These are Velosulin (Novo Nordisk) and a specially prepared Humulin BR (Eli Lilly) which is only recommended for pump use.

(2) Lente insulin is a mixture of 30% semilente (an amorphous precipitate of insulin with zinc ions) with 70% ultralente insulin (an insoluble crystal of zinc and insulin). Its onset of action is delayed for up to 2 hours (Fig 21–1), and because its duration of action often is less than 24 hours (with a range

Table 21–7. Insulin preparations available in the USA.[1]

Preparation	Special Source	Concentration
SHORT-ACTING INSULINS		
Standard[2]		
Regular (Novo Nordisk)	Pork	U100
Regular Iletin I (Lilly)	Beef and pork	U100
Semilente (Novo Nordisk)	Beef	U40, U100
Semilente Iletin I (Lilly)	Beef and pork	U40, U100
"Purified"[3]		
Regular (Novo Nordisk)[4]	Pork or human	U100
Regular Humulin (Lilly)	Human	U100
Regular Iletin II (Lilly)	Pork or beef	U100, U500[6]
Semilente (Novo Nordisk)	Pork	U100
Velosulin (Nordisk)	Pork or human	U100
Humulin BR (Lilly)[5]	Human	U100
INTERMEDIATE-ACTING INSULINS		
Standard[2]		
Isophane NPH (Novo Nordisk)	Beef	U100
Lente (Novo Nordisk)	Beef	U100
Lente Iletin I (Lilly)	Beef and pork	U40, U100
NPH Iletin I (Lilly)	Beef and pork	U40, U100
"Purified"[3]		
Insulatard NPH (Nordisk)	Pork or human	U100
Lente Humulin (Lilly)	Human	U100
Lente Iletin II (Lilly)	Pork of beef	U100
Lente (Novo Nordisk)[5]	Pork or human	U100
NPH Humulin (Lilly)	Human	U100
NPH Iletin II (Lilly)	Pork or beef	U100
NPH (Novo Nordisk)	Pork or human	U100
PREMIXED INSULINS		
(70% NPH, 30% REGULAR)		
Mixtard (Nordisk)	Pork	U100
Novolin 70/30 (Novo Nordisk)	Human	U100
Humulin 70/30 (Lilly)	Human	U100
LONG-ACTING INSULINS		
Standard[2]		
PZI Iletin I (Lilly)	Beef and pork	U40, U100
Ultralente (Novo Nordisk)	Beef	U100
Ultralente Iletin I (Lilly)	Beef and pork	U40, U100
"Purified"[3]		
PZI Iletin II (Lilly)	Pork or beef	U100
Ultralente (Novo Nordisk)	Beef	U100
Ultralente Humulin (Lilly)	Human	U100

Modified from Katzung BG: *Clinical Pharmacology '90*. Appleton & Lange, 1990.

[1] These agents are all available without prescription. Wholesale prices for all preparations are similar.

[2] Greater than 10 but less than 25 ppm proinsulin.

[3] Less than 10 ppm proinsulin.

[4] Novo Nordisk human insulins are termed Novolin R, L, and N.

[5] Humulin BR (Buffered Regular) is recommended to be used only in pumps. Its phosphate buffer precludes its being mixed with lente insulin.

[6] U500 available only as pork insulin.

of 18–24 hours), most patients require at least 2 injections daily to maintain a sustained insulin effect. Lente insulin has its peak effect in most patients between 8 and 12 hours, but individual variations in peak response time must be considered when interpreting unusual or unexpected patterns of glycemic responses in individual patients. While lente insulin is the most widely used of the lente series, particularly in conjunction with regular insulin, there has recently been a resurgence of the use of ultralente in combination with multiple injections of regular insulin as a means of attempting optimal control in IDDM patients. Ultralente has a very slow onset of action with a prolonged duration (Fig 21–1), and its administration once or twice daily has been advocated to provide a basal level of insulin comparable to that achieved by basal endogenous secretion or the overnight infusion rate programmed into insulin pumps.

(3) NPH (neutral protamine Hagedorn or isophane) insulin is an intermediate-acting insulin

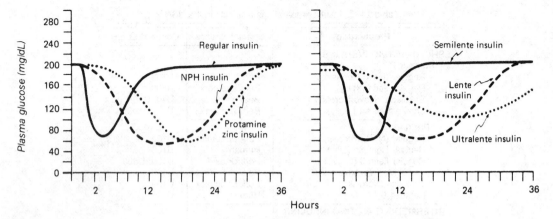

Figure 21–1. Extent and duration of action of various types of insulin (in a fasting diabetic). Duration of action is extended considerably when the dose of a given insulin formulation increases above the average therapeutic doses depicted here.

whose onset of action is delayed by combining 2 parts soluble crystalline zinc with 1 part protamine zinc insulin. This produces equivalent amounts of insulin and protamine, so that neither is present in an uncomplexed form ("isophane").

The onset and duration of action of NPH insulin are comparable to those of lente insulin (Fig 21–1); it is usually mixed with regular insulin and given at least twice daily for insulin replacement in IDDM patients.

(4) Mixtures of insulin: Since intermediate insulins require several hours to reach adequate therapeutic levels, their use in IDDM patients requires supplements of regular insulin preprandially. Recent reports caution that insulin mixtures containing increased proportions of lente to regular insulins may retard the rapid action of admixed regular insulin. The excess zinc in lente insulin may bind the soluble insulin and partially blunt its action, particularly when a relatively small proportion of regular insulin is mixed with lente (eg, 1 part regular to 1½ or more parts lente). NPH preparations that do not contain excess protamine do not delay absorption of admixed regular insulin. They are therefore preferable to lente when mixtures of intermediate and regular insulins are prescribed. For convenience, regular or NPH insulin may be mixed together in the same syringe and injected subcutaneously in split dosage before breakfast and supper. It is recommended that the regular insulin be withdrawn first, then the NPH insulin. No attempt should be made to mix the insulins in the syringe, and the injection is preferably given immediately after loading the syringe. Stable premixed insulins (70% NPH and 30% regular) are available as a convenience to patients who have difficulty mixing insulin because of visual problems or impairment of manual dexterity.

Occasional vials of NPH insulin have tended to show unusual clumping of their contents or "frosting" of the container, with considerable loss of bioactivity.

This instability is a rare phenomenon which may not be restricted to NPH human insulin and might occur less frequently if NPH human insulin were refrigerated when not in use.

c. Methods of insulin administration–

(1) Insulin syringes and needles: Plastic disposable syringes with needles attached are available in 1-mL, 0.5-mL, and 0.3-mL sizes. In cases where very low insulin doses are prescribed, as in young children, the specially calibrated 0.5-mL and 0.3-mL disposable syringes facilitate accurate measurement of U100 insulin in doses up to 50 or 30 units, respectively. The "low-dose" syringes have become increasingly popular, because diabetics generally should not take more than 30–50 units of insulin in a single injection, except in rare instances of extreme insulin resistance. Several recent reports have indicated that "disposable" syringes may be reused until blunting of the needle occurs (usually after 3–5 injections). Sterility adequate to avoid infection with reuse appears to be maintained by refrigerating syringes between uses. One concern, however, arises from a recent report that flecks of silicone may become suspended in insulin bottles in which disposable syringes have repeatedly been reused; the silicone flecks seem to reduce the activity of the insulin.

(2) Site of injection: Any part of the body covered by loose skin can be used, such as the abdomen, thighs, upper arms, flanks, and upper buttocks. Rotation of sites continues to be recommended to avoid delayed absorption when fibrosis or lipohypertrophy occurs from repeated use of a single site. However, considerable variability of absorption rates from different sites, particularly with exercise, may contribute to the instability of glycemic control in certain IDDM patients if injection sites are rotated too frequently in different areas of the body. Consequently, it is best to limit injection sites to a single region of the body and rotate sites within that region. The abdomen is recommended for subcutaneous injections, since regular insulin has been shown to absorb more rapidly from that site than from other subcutaneous sites.

(3) Insulin delivery systems: Efforts to administer soluble insulin by "closed-loop" systems (glucose-controlled insulin infusion system) have been successful for acute situations such as diabetic ketoacidosis or for administering insulin to diabetics during surgery. However, chronic use is precluded by the need for continually aspirating blood to reach an external glucose sensor and the large size of the computerized pump system.

Current research into smaller "open-loop" means of insulin delivery (insulin reservoir and pump programmed to deliver regular insulin at a calculated rate without a glucose sensor) has developed several relatively small pumps for subcutaneous, intravenous, or intraperitoneal infusion. With improving methods for patients' self-monitoring of blood glucose, these pump systems have become more useful for managing diabetics. However, at present, conventional methods of insulin administration with multiple subcutaneous injections of soluble, rapid-acting insulin and a single injection of long-acting insulin usually can provide as effective glycemic control in most cases as the more expensive open-loop systems if frequent self-monitoring of blood glucose is practiced.

To facilitate these multiple injection regimens, portable pen-sized injectors have been introduced which contain cartridges of U100 regular human insulin and retractable needles (NovoPen, NovolinPen, Insuject). These injectors eliminate the need for patients to carry an insulin bottle and syringes during the day while adhering to a regimen of multiple injections of regular insulin supplementing a single injection of long-acting insulin.

C. General Considerations in Treatment of Diabetes: Patients with diabetes can have a full and satisfying life. However, "free" diets and unrestricted activity are still not advised for insulin-requiring diabetics. Until new methods of insulin replacement are developed that provide more normal patterns of insulin delivery in response to metabolic demands, multiple feedings will continue to be recommended, and certain occupations potentially hazardous to the patient or others will continue to be prohibited.

Exercise increases the effectiveness of insulin, and moderate exercise is an excellent means of improving utilization of fat and carbohydrate in diabetic patients. A judicious balance of the size and frequency of meals with moderate regular exercise can often stabilize the insulin dosage in diabetics who tend to slip out of control easily. Strenuous exercise could precipitate hypoglycemia in an unprepared patient, and diabetics must therefore be taught to reduce their insulin dosage in anticipation of strenuous activity or to take supplemental carbohydrate. Injection of insulin into a site farthest away from the muscles most involved in exercise may help ameliorate exercise-induced hy-

poglycemia, since insulin injected in the proximity of exercising muscle may be more rapidly mobilized.

All diabetic patients must receive adequate instruction on personal hygiene, especially with regard to care of the feet (see below), skin, and teeth. All infections—but especially pyogenic infections with fever and toxemia—provoke the release of high levels of insulin antagonists such as catecholamines or glucagon and thus bring about a marked increase in insulin requirements. Supplemental regular insulin is often required to correct hyperglycemia during infection.

Psychologic factors are of great importance in the control of diabetes, particularly when the disease is difficult to stabilize. One reason the diabetic may be particularly sensitive to emotional upset is that A cells of diabetics are hyperresponsive to physiologic levels of epinephrine, producing excessive levels of glucagon with consequent hyperglycemia.

Counseling should be directed at avoiding extremes of compulsive rigidity or self-destructive neglect and is especially important for adolescents.

Steps in the Management of the Diabetic Patient

A. Diagnostic Examination: Any features of the clinical picture that suggest end-organ insensitivity to insulin, such as obesity, must be identified. The family history should document not only the incidence of diabetes in other members of the family but also the age at onset, whether it was associated with obesity, and whether insulin was required. Other factors that increase cardiac risk, such as smoking history, presence of hypertension or hyperlipidemia, or oral contraceptive pill use, should be recorded.

Laboratory diagnosis should document fasting plasma glucose levels above 140 mg/dL or postprandial values consistently above 200 mg/dL and whether ketonuria accompanies the glycosuria. A glycohemoglobin measurement is useful for assessing the effectiveness of future therapy. Some flexibility of clinical judgment is appropriate when diagnosing diabetes mellitus in the elderly patient with borderline hyperglycemia.

Baseline values include fasting plasma triglycerides, total cholesterol and HDL cholesterol, electrocardiography, renal function studies, peripheral pulses, and neurologic, podiatric, and ophthalmologic examinations to help guide future assessments.

B. Patient Education: Since diabetes is a lifelong disorder, education of the patient is probably the most important obligation of the physician who provides initial care. The best persons to manage a disease that is affected so markedly by daily fluctuations in environmental stress, exercise, diet, and infections are the patients themselves and their families. The "teaching curriculum" should include explanations by the physician of the nature of diabetes and its potential acute and chronic hazards and how they can be recognized early and prevented or treated.

INSTRUCTIONS IN THE CARE OF THE FEET
FOR PERSONS WITH DIABETES MELLITUS OR VASCULAR DISTURBANCES

Hygiene of the Feet

(1) Wash feet daily with mild soap and lukewarm water. Dry thoroughly between the toes by pressure. Do not rub vigorously, as this is apt to break the delicate skin.

(2) When feet are thoroughly dry, rub well with vegetable oil to keep them soft, prevent excess friction, remove scales, and prevent dryness. Care must be taken to prevent foot tenderness.

(3) If the feet become too soft and tender, rub them with alcohol about once a week.

(4) When rubbing the feet, always rub upward from the tips of the toes. If varicose veins are present, massage the feet very gently; never massage the legs.

(5) If the toenails are brittle and dry, soften them by soaking for one-half hour each night in lukewarm water containing 1 tbsp of powdered sodium borate (borax) per quart. Follow this by rubbing around the nails with vegetable oil. Clean around the nails with an orangewood stick. If the nails become too long, file them with an emery board. File them straight across and no shorter than the underlying soft tissues to the toe. Never cut the corners of the nails. (The podiatrist should be informed if a patient has diabetes.)

(6) Wear low-heeled shoes of soft leather that fit the shape of the feet correctly. The shoes should have wide toes that will cause no pressure, fit close in the arch, and grip the heels snugly. Wear new shoes one-half hour only on the first day and increase by 1 hour each day following. Wear thick, warm, loose stockings.

Treatment of Corns & Calluses

(1) Corns and calluses are due to friction and pressure, most often from improperly fitted shoes and stockings. Wear shoes that fit properly and cause no friction or pressure.

(2) To remove excess calluses or corns, soak the feet in lukewarm (not hot) water, using a mild soap, for about 10 minutes and then rub off the excess tissue with a towel or file. Do not tear it off. Under no circumstances must the skin become irritated.

(3) Do not cut corns or calluses. If they need attention it is safer to see a podiatrist.

(4) Prevent callus formation under the ball of the foot (a) by exercise, such as curling and stretching the toes several times a day; (b) by finishing each step on the toes and not on the ball of the foot; and (c) by wearing shoes that are not too short and that do not have high heels.

Aids in Treatment of Impaired Circulation (Cold Feet)

(1) Never use tobacco in any form. Tobacco contracts blood vessels and so reduces circulation.

(2) Keep warm. Wear warm stockings and other clothing. Cold contracts blood vessels and reduces circulation.

(3) Do not wear circular garters, which compress blood vessels and reduce blood flow.

(4) Do not sit with the legs crossed. This may compress the leg arteries and shut off the blood supply to the feet.

(5) If the weight of the bedclothes is uncomfortable, place a pillow under the covers at the foot of the bed.

(6) Do not apply any medication to the feet without directions from a physician. Some medicines are too strong for feet with poor circulation.

(7) Do not apply heat in the form of hot water, hot water bottles, or heating pads without a physician's consent. Even moderate heat can injure the skin if circulation is poor.

(8) If the feet are moist or the patient has a tendency to develop athlete's foot, a prophylactic dusting powder should be used on the feet and in shoes and stockings daily. Change shoes and stockings at least daily or oftener.

Treatment of Abrasions of the Skin

(1) Proper first-aid treatment is of the utmost importance even in apparently minor injuries. Consult a physician immediately for any redness, blistering, pain, or swelling. Any break in the skin may become ulcerous or gangrenous unless properly treated by a physican.

(2) Dermatophytosis (athlete's foot), which begins with peeling and itching between the toes or discoloration or thickening of the toenails, should be treated immediately by a physician or podiatrist.

(3) Avoid strong irritating antiseptics such as tincture of iodine.

(4) As soon as possible after any injury, cover the area with sterile gauze, which may be purchaed at drugstores. Only fine paper tape or cellulose tape (Scotch Tape) should be used on the skin if adhesive retention of the gauze is required.

(5) Elevate and, as much as possible until recovery, avoid using the foot.

The importance of regular tests for glucose on either capillary blood or double-voided urine specimens should be stressed and instructions on proper testing and recording of data provided. Moreover, patients should be provided with algorithms they can use to adjust the timing and quantity of their insulin dose, food, and exercise in response to recorded blood glucose values for optimal blood glucose control. The targets for blood glucose control should be elevated appropriately in elderly patients since they have the greatest risk if subjected to hypoglycemia and the least long-term benefit from more rigid glycemic control. Advice on personal hygiene, including detailed instructions on foot care, as well as individual instruction on diet and specific hypoglycemic therapy, should be provided. Patients should be told about community agencies, such as Diabetes Association chapters, that can serve as a continuing source of instruction. Finally, vigorous efforts should be made to persuade new diabetics who smoke to give up the habit, since large vessel peripheral vascular disease and debilitating retinopathy are less common in nonsmoking diabetic patients.

C. Self-Monitoring of Blood Glucose: Monitoring of blood glucose by patients has allowed greater flexibility in management while achieving improved glycemic control. It involves educating the patient to perform 3 essential steps: (1) The obtaining of a drop of capillary blood from the fingertip by means of a specially designed lancet. Automatic spring-loaded devices facilitate finger-pricking and ensure an adequate blood sample. (2) Application of the sample to the test strip and removal at the proper time. (3) Accurate quantitation of the color developed (either visually or with a colorimeter).

Self-monitoring of blood glucose is particularly useful in brittle diabetics, those attempting "ideal" glycemic control such as during pregnancy, patients who have little or no early warning of hypoglycemic attacks, and those with dysfunctional bladders from diabetic neuropathy or altered renal thresholds for glucose. Self-monitoring of blood glucose is recommended for all insulin-treated diabetic patients. The expert consensus on self-monitoring is that its proper use is to develop a data base as an aid in making day-to-day decisions about therapy as well as to determine when emergency situations arise. It is particularly valuable as an educational and training tool to enhance understanding of diabetes by patients and their families. The usefulness of self-monitoring depends on the accuracy of the results obtained. Patients must be taught proper techniques, cautioned to calibrate instruments each day despite the expense of strips, to keep proper records, and, particularly, how to respond to unacceptably high or low blood glucose levels with appropriate therapeutic maneuvers. Self-monitoring has proved to be an effective and safe clinical tool that can improve glycemic control in compliant patients.

D. Initial Therapy: Treatment must be individualized on the basis of the type of diabetes and specific needs of each patient. However, certain general principles of management can be outlined for hyperglycemic states of different types.

1. The obese NIDDM patient–The most common type of diabetic patient is obese, is non-insulin-dependent, and has hyperglycemia because of insensitivity to normal or elevated circulating levels of insulin.

a. Weight reduction–Treatment is directed toward achieving weight reduction, and prescribing a diet is only one means to this end. Behavior modification to achieve adherence to the diet, as well as increased physical activity to expend energy, is also required. Cure can be achieved by reducing adipose stores, with consequent restoration of tissue sensitivity to insulin. The presence of diabetes with its added risk factors may motivate the obese diabetic to greater efforts to lose weight. (See also Chapter 22.)

b. Hypoglycemic agents–No hypoglycemic agents, including insulin as well as oral hypoglycemic drugs, are indicated for long-term use in the obese patient with mild diabetes. The weight reduction program can be upset by real or imagined hypoglycemic reactions when insulin therapy is used and weight gain is a frequent complication. It is also possible that administration of insulin to an obese patient who already has excessive circulating levels may have the ill effects of maintaining insulin insensitivity of receptor sites as well as interfering with catabolic mechanisms during caloric deprivation. The obese diabetic who has been previously treated with conventional beef-pork insulin—often in interrupted fashion—and who requires high doses both to offset excess caloric intake and to overcome tissue insensitivity may develop immune insulin resistance. This not only increases the requirements for exogenous insulin but also impairs the effectiveness of endogenous insulin and may even precipitate ketosis.

Oral sulfonylureas have a role in the management of obese patients with diabetes causing nocturia, blurred vision, or candidal vulvovaginitis. Insulin injections may be required if a trial of sulfonylurea therapy does not ameliorate symptoms. In such cases, short-term therapy (weeks or months) with either sulfonylureas or insulin may be indicated to abate symptoms until simultaneous caloric restriction leading to weight reduction can occur.

Combining sulfonylureas with insulin replacement has not been effective in reducing insulin requirements or improving glycemic control in IDDM patients who have no residual pancreatic B cell function. On the other hand, NIDDM patients do show modest glycemic improvement with a combined sulfonylurea-insulin regimen, but one that generally can be achieved with insulin therapy alone. At present, there is no overall consensus for using combined sulfonylurea therapy with insulin in NIDDM. One regimen has been proposed that adds a bedtime intermediate-acting insulin to reduce excessive nocturnal hepatic glucose output in NIDDM patients doing poorly on maximal doses of sulfonylureas, but until more data are available to validate this approach, most diabetologists recommend stopping the sulfonylureas in these circumstances and changing over to insulin therapy alone. It is only in the case of NIDDM patients requiring excessive amounts of insulin—exceeding 100 units/d—that it is considered a reasonable option to add sulfonylureas to improve glycemic control rather than prescribing higher insulin doses.

2. The nonobese patient–In the nonobese diabetic, mild to severe hyperglycemia is usually due to refractoriness of B cells to glucose stimulation. Treatment depends on whether insulinopenia is mild (NIDDM or mild IDDM in partial remission) or severe, with ketoacidosis (IDDM).

a. Diet therapy–If hyperglycemia is mild, normal metabolic control can occasionally be restored by means of multiple feedings of a diet limited in simple sugars and with a caloric content sufficient to maintain ideal weight. Restriction of saturated fats and cholesterol is also strongly advised.

b. Oral hypoglycemic agents–When diet therapy is not sufficient to correct hyperglycemia, a trial of sulfonylureas is often successful in reducing the glycohemoglobin concentration below 9.5%. Once the dosage of one of the more potent sulfonylureas reaches the upper recommended limit in a compliant patient without maintaining blood glucose below 200 mg/dL during the day, insulin therapy is indicated.

c. Treatment of IDDM with insulin–(Table 21–8.) The patient requiring insulin therapy should be initially regulated under conditions of optimal diet and normal daily activities. In patients with IDDM, information and counseling should be provided about the advantages of taking multiple injections of insulin in conjunction with self blood glucose monitoring. If tight control is attempted, urine glucose measurements are not sufficient, and at least 3 measurements of capillary blood glucose are required daily to avoid frequent hypoglycemic reactions. A single injection of long-acting insulin is not recommended in patients with IDDM for the reasons given in Table 21–8, which describes the advantages and disadvantages of various insulin regimens in this type of diabetes.

(1) Conventional split-dose insulin mixtures: A typical initial dose schedule in a 70-kg patient taking 2200 kcal divided into 6 or 7 feedings might be 10 units of regular and 15 units of NPH insulin in the morning and 5 units of regular and 5 units of

Table 21–8. Advantages and disadvantages of various insulin regimens in treatment of type I diabetes.

	Single Injection of NPH or Lente	Conventional Split Dose of Mixture (Regular and NPH Twice Daily)	Three Injections (Mixture of Regular and NPH in AM; Regular at Dinner; NPH at Bedtime)	Four Injections (Regular Before Meals and NPH, Lente, or Ultralente at Bedtime) or Subcutaneous Infusion of Regular Insulin With Pump
Advantages	Convenience only	Relatively convenient. Controls postprandial glycemia at breakfast and dinner.	Controls postprandial glycemia at breakfast and dinner. Can prevent prebreakfast hyperglycemia with less risk of nocturnal hypoglycemia. Less variability of absorption of NPH, since lower doses are injected to last overnight.	Controls postprandial glycemia. Allows flexibility of meal schedules and quantity. Less variability of absorption of small doses of insulins given more frequently. Tight glycemic control is possible with least risk of hypoglycemia.
Disadvantages	Poor glycemic control or nocturnal hypoglycemia. Requires frequent feedings to avoid hypoglycemia if acceptable control attempted. Inflexible feeding schedules. Variability of absorption of large doses predisposes to hypoglycemia, which is common. Because of these disadvantages, this regimen is not recommended.	Prebreakfast hyperglycemia is common. Increased risk of nocturnal hypoglycemia in attempt to control prebreakfast hyperglycemia. Variability of absorption due to relatively large NPH doses to last overnight.	Less convenient. Lunch schedule is relatively inflexible as to time and quantity to avoid hypoglycemia from morning NPH. Dinner schedule cannot be delayed without extra feedings.	Relatively inconvenient. Pumps are expensive and are generally less convenient than multiple injections and add risk of skin infections and pump failures.

NPH insulin in the evening. The morning capillary blood glucose gives a measure of the effectiveness of NPH insulin administered the previous evening; the noon blood glucose reflects the effects of the morning regular insulin; and the 5:00 PM and 9:00 PM sugars represent the effects of the morning NPH and evening regular insulins, respectively. A properly educated patient should be taught to adjust insulin dosage by observing the pattern of glycemia and correlating it with the approximate duration of action and the time of peak effect after injection of the various insulin preparations (Fig 21–1). Adjustments to correct patterns of hyperglycemia should be made gradually and preferably not more often than every 3 days.

(2) Intensive insulin therapy: In cases where conventional split doses of insulin mixtures cannot maintain near normalization of blood glucose without hypoglycemia, particularly at night, multiple injections of insulin may be required. An increasingly popular regimen consists of reducing or omitting the evening dose of intermediate insulin and adding a portion of it at bedtime. For example, 10 units of regular insulin mixed with 10 units of NPH insulin in the morning, 8–10 units of regular insulin before the evening meal, and 6 units of NPH insulin at bedtime might be more efficacious than the conventional split-dose regimen mentioned above.

In cases where hypoglycemia occurs unexpectedly and at inconsistent times day or night, variable or delayed insulin absorption from large subcutaneous depots containing regular and NPH insulin may be a contributing factor. Reducing the size and changing the character of the depots by administering small doses of regular insulin more frequently (eg, 4 times a day), with one injection of a long-acting insulin (eg, ultralente insulin) at bedtime has often been most helpful in reducing the frequency and severity of hypoglycemia in patients attempting near normalization of blood glucose. This regimen has become more convenient with the advent of pen-injectors and gives greater flexibility regarding meal patterns and diet

than conventional therapy with split-dose insulin mixtures. Certain patients do not accept multiple injections of regular insulin but often prefer continuous subcutaneous infusions with portable open-loop insulin pumps, which require subcutaneous needle insertion only every 48 hours.

(3) Management of early morning hyperglycemia in IDDM: (Table 21–9.) One of the more difficult therapeutic problems in managing patients with IDDM is determining the proper adjustment of insulin dose when the prebreakfast blood glucose level is high.

(a) Somogyi effect: Patients with IDDM may develop nocturnal hypoglycemia, which may in turn stimulate a surge of counterregulatory hormones (Somogyi effect) to produce high blood glucose levels by 7:00 AM.

Clinicians have often observed that by reducing inappropriately high doses of administered insulin, hyperglycemia on the following morning may improve substantially. This "Somogyi effect" remains a factor to be considered as contributing to early morning hyperglycemia in patients treated with relatively high doses of insulin. Prescribing a lower dose of intermediate-acting insulin before dinner or at bedtime is a reasonable therapeutic option, particularly when nocturnal hypoglycemia is suspected.

(b) Waning of circulating insulin levels: A possibly more common cause of prebreakfast hyperglycemia is the waning of circulating insulin levels. This would suggest that *more*, rather than less, intermediate insulin should be given the evening before. The Somogyi effect and the waning of insulin levels are not mutually exclusive; if they occur together, more severe hyperglycemia develops.

(c) Dawn phenomenon: The recently described dawn phenomenon is found in as many as 75% of IDDM patients and occurs in most NIDDM and normal subjects as well. It is characterized by reduced tissue sensitivity to insulin developing between 5:00 AM and 8:00 AM. Recent evidence suggests that this phenomenon is evoked by spikes of growth hormone

Table 21–9. Prebreakfast hyperglycemia: Classification by blood glucose and insulin levels.

	Blood Glucose (mg/dL)			Free Immunoreactive Insulin (μU/mL)		
	10:00 PM	3:00 AM	7:00 AM	10:00 PM	3:00 AM	7:00 AM
Somogyi effect	90	40	200	High	Slightly high	Normal
Dawn phenomenon	110	110	150	Normal	Normal	Normal
Waning of insulin dose plus dawn phenomenon	110	190	220	Normal	Low	Low
Waning of insulin dose plus dawn phenomenon plus Somogyi effect	110	40	380	High	Normal	Low

released hours before, at the onset of sleep. When the dawn phenomenon occurs alone, it may produce only mild hyperglycemia in the early morning, but when it is associated with either the Somogyi effect or the waning phenomenon, or both, the hyperglycemia may be more severe. Table 21–9 shows that diagnosis of the cause of prebreakfast hyperglycemia can be facilitated by the self-monitoring of blood glucose at 3:00 AM in addition to the usual bedtime and 7:00 AM measurements. This is required for only a few nights until the diagnosis is established and appropriate adjustment of bedtime insulin dose or nighttime feeding is achieved.

(d) Therapy of prebreakfast hyperglycemia: When a particular pattern emerges from monitoring blood glucose levels overnight, appropriate therapeutic measures can be taken. The Somogyi effect can be treated by reducing the dose of intermediate insulin, giving a portion of it at bedtime, or supplying more food at bedtime. When the dawn phenomenon alone is present, the dosage of intermediate insulin can be divided between dinnertime and bedtime, or when insulin pumps are used, the basal infusion rate can be increased (eg, from 0.8 unit/h to 1 unit/h from 6:00 AM until breakfast). With waning insulin levels, either increasing the evening dose or shifting it from dinnertime to bedtime, or both, can be effective.

d. Treatment of NIDDM with insulin–When sulfonylureas fail and NIDDM patients require insulin to control their hyperglycemia, various insulin regimens may be effective. Although a single morning injection of insulin is not recommended in type I diabetes (see Table 21–8), in some patients with type II diabetes enough residual insulin secretion persists to allow a single morning injection of 25–30 units of NPH or lente insulin to replace their deficient insulin secretion. If prebreakfast hyperglycemia persists on this regimen, a number of alternatives are available. A convenient regimen includes split doses of a fixed 70:30 mixture of NPH:regular insulin, which can be started as 20 units before breakfast and 15 units before dinner and increased appropriately depending on target blood glucoses at 7:00 AM and 5:00 PM . When more than 50 units a day are required without achieving proper control, these patients may benefit from 3 or 4 injection regimens as described for IDDM in Table 21–8.

e. Acceptable levels of glycemic control: Limited data are available concerning the level of glucose control needed to avoid diabetic complications. Postprandial blood glucose levels below 200 mg/dL have been advocated by retrospective analysis of 2 populations of NIDDM patients. A reasonable aim of therapy is to approach normal glycemic excursions without provoking severe or frequent hypoglycemia. What has been considered "acceptable" control includes blood glucose levels of 80–130 mg/dL before meals and after an overnight fast and levels no higher than 180 mg/dL 1 hour after meals and 150 mg/dL

2 hours after meals. Glycohemoglobin levels should be no higher than 1% or 2% above the upper limit of the normal range. In elderly patients, criteria for optimal control should be adjusted upward, with glycohemoglobins 2–3% above the upper limits of normal and preprandial blood glucose levels below 200 mg/dL being acceptable. A long-term multicenter clinical trial sponsored by the National Institute of Health is now in progress to evaluate the benefits of achieving these goals of glycemic control in diabetic patients with IDDM. No data are available on the benefits of glycemic control in patients with NIDDM.

Indications for Purified Insulins

Human insulin or purified pork insulins are indicated when insulin of conventional purity has been associated with allergy, immune resistance, or lipoatrophy. Also, they are preferable in any patient undergoing insulin therapy for the first time, since they reduce or eliminate the risk of occurrence of these rare immune complications. Moreover, absent or very low levels of anti-insulin antibodies enhance recovery from insulin-induced hypoglycemia and facilitate the measurement of therapeutic levels of circulating insulin as a guide for optimal management. In patients with NIDDM whose therapy with insulin is to be for a limited time (eg, in gestational diabetes or during acute infections or surgery), human insulin or purified insulin reduces the risks of immunologic sensitization to future exposures to insulin.

Complications of Insulin Therapy

A. Hypoglycemia: Hypoglycemic reactions, the most common complication of insulin therapy, may result from delay in taking a meal or unusual physical exertion. With more IDDM patients attempting "tight" control, this complication has become even more frequent. In older diabetics, in those taking only longer-acting insulins, and often in those attempting to maintain euglycemia on infusion pumps, autonomic counterregulatory responses are less readily elicited, and the manifestations are mainly from impaired function of the central nervous system, ie, mental confusion, bizarre behavior, and ultimately coma. Even focal neurologic deficits mimicking stroke may be observed. More rapid development of hypoglycemia from the effects of regular insulin causes signs of autonomic hyperactivity, both sympathetic (tachycardia, palpitations, sweating, tremulousness) and parasympathetic (nausea, hunger), that may progress to coma and convulsions. Except for sweating, most of the sympathetic symptoms of hypoglycemia are blunted in patients receiving beta-blocking agents for angina or hypertension. Though not absolutely contraindicated, these drugs must be used with great caution in insulin-requiring diabetics.

Since autonomic responses correlate strongly with

"awareness" of hypoglycemia, many poorly controlled diabetics—whose nervous systems have adapted to chronic hyperglycemia—may trigger adrenergic alarms at levels of blood glucose above the usual hypoglycemic range. Conversely, IDDM patients overtreated with insulin may be unaware of critically low levels of blood glucose because of an adaptive blunting of their alarm systems owing to chronic hypoglycemia.

For unexplained reasons, patients with IDDM lose their glucagon responses to hypoglycemia (but not to amino acids in protein-containing meals) within a year or so after developing diabetes. These patients then rely predominantly on the sympathetic nervous system to counterregulate hypoglycemia and are at special risk in later years when aging or autonomic neuropathy blunts their sympathetic responses.

Because of the potential danger of insulin reactions, the diabetic patient should carry packets of table sugar or a candy roll at all times for use at the onset of hypoglycemic symptoms. Recently, tablets containing 3 g of glucose have become available (dextrosol). The educated patient soon learns to take the amount of glucose needed and avoids the excess that may occur with eating candy or drinking orange juice, causing very high hyperglycemia. An ampule of glucagon (1 mg) should be provided to every diabetic receiving insulin therapy, and family or friends should be instructed how to inject it in the event that the patient is unconscious or refuses food. An identification bracelet, necklace, or card in the wallet or purse should be carried by every diabetic receiving hypoglycemic drug therapy.

All of the manifestations of hypoglycemia are rapidly relieved by glucose administration. If more severe hypoglycemia has produced unconsciousness or stupor, the treatment is 50 mL of 50% glucose solution by rapid intravenous infusion. If intravenous therapy is not available, 1 mg of glucagon injected intramuscularly will usually restore the patient to consciousness within 15 minutes to permit ingestion of sugar. If the patient is stuporous and glucagon is not available, small amounts of honey or syrup can be inserted within the buccal pouch, but, in general, oral feeding is contraindicated in unconscious patients. Rectal administration of syrup or honey (30 mL per 500 mL of warm water) has been effective.

B. Immunopathology of Insulin Therapy: At least 5 molecular classes of insulin antibodies are produced during the course of insulin therapy in diabetes, including IgA, IgD, IgE, IgG, and IgM.

1. Insulin allergy–Insulin allergy, or immediate-type hypersensitivity, is a rare condition in which local or systemic urticaria is due to histamine release from tissue mast cells sensitized by adherence of anti-insulin IgE antibodies. In severe cases, anaphylaxis results. A subcutaneous nodule appearing several hours later at the site of insulin injection and lasting for up to 24 hours has been attributed to an IgG-mediated complement-binding Arthus reaction. When only human insulin has been used from the onset of insulin therapy, insulin allergy is exceedingly rare. When allergy to beef or, more rarely, pork insulin is present, a species change (eg, to human insulin) may correct the problem, although in many cases cross-reaction between human and animal insulins results in persistent allergic responses. Antihistamines, corticosteroids, and even desensitization may be required, especially for systemic hypersensitivity.

2. Immune insulin resistance–All insulin-treated patients develop a low titer of circulating IgG anti-insulin antibodies that neutralize to a small extent the action of insulin. In some diabetic patients, principally those with some degree of tissue insensitivity to insulin (such as in the obese) and with a history of interrupted exposure to therapy with beef insulin, a high titer of circulating IgG anti-insulin antibodies develops. This results in extremely high insulin requirements—often more than 200 units daily. This is often a self-limited condition and may clear spontaneously after several months. However, in cases where the circulating antibody is specifically more reactive with beef insulin—a more potent immunogen in humans than pork insulin—changing the patient to a less antigenic insulin (pork or human) may make possible a dramatic reduction in insulin dosage or at least may shorten the duration of immune resistance. In some adults, the foreign insulin can be completely discontinued and the patient maintained on diet along with oral sulfonylureas. This is possible only when the circulating antibodies do not effectively neutralize endogenous (human) insulin.

C. Lipodystrophy at Injection Sites: Atrophy of subcutaneous fatty tissue leading to disfiguring excavations and depressed areas may rarely occur at the site of injection. This complication results from an immune reaction, and it has become rarer with the development of pure insulin preparations. Injection of these preparations directly into the atrophic area often results in restoration of normal contours. Lipohypertrophy, on the other hand, is a consequence of the pharmacologic effects of insulin being deposited in the same location repeatedly. It can occur with purified insulins and is best treated with localized liposuction of the hypertrophic areas by an experienced plastic surgeon. Rotation of injection sites will prevent lipohypertrophy.

Chronic Complications of Diabetes

Late clinical manifestations of diabetes mellitus include a number of pathologic changes that involve small and large blood vessels, cranial and peripheral nerves, the skin, and the lens of the eye. These lesions lead to hypertension, renal failure, blindness, autonomic and peripheral neuropathy, amputations of the lower extremities, myocardial infarction, and cerebrovascular accidents. The cause of these late manifestations is not well understood, but they correlate with the duration of the diabetic state. In patients with type I diabetes, end-stage renal disease is a major cause of death, whereas patients with type II diabetes are more likely to have macrovascular diseases leading to myocardial infarction and stroke as the main causes of death.

A. Ocular Complications:

1. Diabetic cataracts–Premature cataracts occur in diabetic patients. These opacities resemble those found in elderly patients with "senile" cataracts but occur at a younger age and seem to correlate with both the duration of diabetes and the severity of chronic hyperglycemia. Nonenzymatic glycosylation of lens protein is twice as high in diabetic patients as in age-matched nondiabetic persons and may contribute to the premature occurrence of cataracts.

2. Diabetic retinopathy–Three main categories exist: background, or "simple," retinopathy, consisting of microaneurysms, hemorrhages, exudates, and retinal edema; proliferative retinopathy with arteriolar ischemia manifested as cotton-wool spots (small infarcted areas of retina); and proliferative, or "malignant," retinopathy, consisting of newly formed vessels. Proliferative retinopathy is a leading cause of blindness in the USA, particularly since it increases the risk of retinal detachment. After 10 years of diabetes, half of all patients have retinopathy, and this proportion increases to more than 80% after 15 years of diabetes. Annual consultation with an ophthalmologist should be arranged for patients who have had type I diabetes for more than 5 years and for *all* patients with type II diabetes. Extensive "scatter" xenon or argon photocoagulation and focal treatment of new vessels reduce severe visual loss in those cases in which proliferative retinopathy is associated with *recent* vitreous hemorrhages or in which extensive new vessels are located on or near the optic disk. Macular edema, which is more common than proliferative retinopathy in patients with type II diabetes (about 6% prevalence), has also responded to this therapy with improvement in visual acuity. Avoiding tobacco use and correction of associated hypertension are important therapeutic measures in the management of diabetic retinopathy.

3. Glaucoma–Glaucoma occurs in approximately 6% persons with diabetes. It is generally responsive to the usual therapy for open-angle disease. Neovascularization of the iris in diabetics can predispose to closed-angle glaucoma, but this is relatively uncommon except after cataract extraction, when growth of new vessels has been known to progress rapidly, involving the angle of the iris and obstructing outflow

B. Diabetic Nephropathy:

As many as 4000 cases of end-stage renal disease occur each year among diabetic people in the United States. This is about one-fourth of all patients being treated for end-stage renal disease and represents a considerable national health expense.

Patients developing diabetes before the age of 20 years have a 50% chance of having diabetic nephropathy after 20 years—in contrast to those with diabetes occurring after the age of 40 years, who have only a 4% incidence of diabetic renal disease after 20 years.

Diabetic nephropathy is initially manifested by proteinuria; subsequently, as kidney function declines, urea and creatinine accumulate in the blood.

1. Microalbuminuria–New methods of detecting small amounts of urinary albumin have permitted detection of microgram concentrations—in contrast to the less sensitive dipstick strips, whose minimal detection limit is 0.3–0.5%. Conventional 24-hour urine collections, in addition to being inconvenient for patients, also show wide variability of albumin excretion, since several factors such as sustained erect posture, dietary protein, and exercise tend to increase albumin excretion rates. For these reasons, most laboratories prefer to screen patients with a timed overnight urine collection beginning at bedtime, when the urine is discarded and the time noted. Normal subjects excrete less than 15 μg/min during overnight urine collections; values of 20 μg/min or higher are considered to represent abnormal microalbuminuria.

Subsequent renal failure can be predicted by urinary albumin excretion rates exceeding 30 μg/min. Increased microalbuminuria correlates with increased levels of blood pressure, and this may explain why increased proteinuria in diabetic patients is associated with an increase in cardiovascular deaths even in the absence of renal failure. Careful glycemic control as well as a low-protein diet (0.6 g/kg/d) may reduce both the hyperfiltration and the elevated microalbuminuria in patients in the early stages of diabetes and those with incipient diabetic nephropathy. Antihypertensive therapy also decreases microalbuminuria, and clinical trials with inhibitors of angiotensin I converting enzyme (eg, enalapril, 20 mg/d) show a documented reduction of microalbuminuria in diabetic patients even in the absence of hypertension.

2. Progressive diabetic nephropathy–Progressive diabetic nephropathy consists of proteinuria of varying severity occasionally leading to nephrotic syndrome with hypoalbuminemia, edema, and an increase in circulating betalipoproteins as well as progressive azotemia. In contrast to all other renal disorders, the proteinuria associated with diabetic nephropathy does not diminish with progressive renal failure (patients continue to excrete 10–11 g daily as creatinine clearance diminishes). As renal failure progresses, there is an elevation in the renal threshold at which glycosuria appears.

Hypertension develops with progressive renal involvement, and coronary and cerebral atherosclerosis seems to be accelerated. Approximately two-thirds of adult patients with diabetes have hypertension.

Once diabetic nephropathy has progressed to the stage of hypertension, proteinuria, or early renal failure, glycemic control is not beneficial in influencing its course. In this circumstance, antihypertensive medications, including ACE inhibitors, and restriction of dietary protein to 0.6 g/kg body weight per day are recommended.

When the serum creatinine reaches 3 mg/dL, consultation with a nephrologist or a diabetologist experienced in the treatment of diabetic nephropathy is recommended. When the serum creatinine reaches 5 mg/dL, consultation with personnel at a center where renal transplantation is performed is indicated.

Dialysis has been of limited value in the treatment of renal failure due to diabetic nephropathy. At present, experience in renal transplantation—especially from related donors—is more promising and is the treatment of choice in cases where there are no contraindications such as severe cardiovascular disease.

C. Gangrene of the Feet: The incidence of gangrene of the feet in diabetics is 20 times the incidence in matched controls. The factors responsible for its development are ischemia, peripheral neuropathy, and secondary infection. Occlusive vascular disease involves both microangiopathy and atherosclerosis of large and medium-sized arteries. Cigarette smoking should be avoided, and prevention of foot disease should be emphasized, since treatment is difficult once ulceration and gangrene have developed. Patients should be instructed to inspect their feet daily for reddened areas, blisters, abrasions, or lacerations, particularly when the foot is insensitive. Physicians should inspect the feet of diabetic patients at each visit and instruct patients as necessary on filing calluses with an emery board, cutting toenails straight across, not walking barefoot, and avoiding tight shoes. When an uncomplicated neuropathic ulcer is present and blood flow is not impaired, consultation with a podiatrist or orthopedist is recommended. If blood supply is diminished or absent, patients with foot ulcers should be referred to an appropriate specialist (vascular or orthopedic surgeon). Special custom-built shoes are usually required to redistribute weight evenly over an insensitive foot, particularly when it has been deformed by surgery or asymptomatic fractures (Charcot's joint). Amputation of the lower extremities is sometimes required.

Beta blockers are relatively contraindicated in patients with ischemic foot ulcers, because these drugs reduce peripheral blood flow.

D. Diabetic Neuropathy: Peripheral and autonomic neuropathy, the 2 most common chronic complications of diabetes, are poorly understood. Peripheral neuropathy is generally bilateral, symmetric, and associated with dulled perception of vibration, pain, and temperature, particularly in the lower extremities. At times, discomfort of the lower extremities can be incapacitating. Both motor and sensory nerve conduction are delayed in peripheral nerves, and ankle jerks may be absent.

Contrasting with this axonal neuropathic process is ischemic neuropathy resulting from small vessel disease of the vasa nervorum. Femoral and cranial nerves are commonly involved, and motor abnormalities predominate. These can result in sudden onset of diplopia due to ophthalmoplegia or in acute pain and weakness of thigh muscles (diabetic amyotrophy). Spontaneous resolution of these ischemic neuropathies generally occurs in 6–12 weeks.

Amitriptyline, 50–75 mg at bedtime, has been recommended for pain associated with diabetic neuropathy. Dramatic relief has often resulted within 48–72 hours. This rapid response is in contrast to the 2 or 3 weeks required for an antidepressive effect. Patients often attribute benefit to their having a full night's sleep after amitriptyline compared to many previously sleepless nights occasioned by neuropathic pain. Mild to moderate morning drowsiness is a side effect that generally improves with time or can be lessened by giving the medication several hours before bedtime. This drug should not be continued if improvement has not occurred after 5 days of therapy. Other drugs used include carbamazepine and phenytoin, both of questionable benefit for leg pain. There has also been recent interest in use of the antiarrhythmic drug mexiletine for this purpose.

With autonomic neuropathy, there is evidence of postural hypotension, decreased cardiovascular response to Valsalva's maneuver, gastroparesis, alternating bouts of diarrhea (particularly nocturnal) and constipation, inability to empty the bladder, and impotence. Gastroparesis should be considered in insulin-dependent diabetic patients who develop unexpected fluctuations and variability in their blood glucose levels after meals. Impotence due to neuropathy differs from psychogenic impotence in that the latter may be intermittent (erections occur under special circumstances), whereas diabetic impotence is usually persistent; aortoiliac occlusive disease may contribute to this problem.

Local injection of papaverine into the corpus cavernosum produces a penile erection if blood supply is competent. This helps differentiate erectile disabilities due to neuropathic causes from those that do not respond to papaverine because of vasculopathy.

There is no consistently effective treatment for diabetic autonomic neuropathy. Metoclopramide has been of some help in treating diabetic gastroparesis over the short term, but its effectiveness seems to diminish over time. It is a dopamine antagonist that has central antiemetic effects as well as a cholinergic action to facilitate gastric emptying. It can be given intravenously (10–20 mg) or orally (20 mg of liquid metoclopramide) before breakfast and dinner. Drowsiness is a common adverse effect, and tardive dyskinesia can be a particularly troublesome side effect. Diarrhea associated with autonomic neuropathy has occasionally responded to broad-spectrum antibiotic therapy, though it often undergoes spontaneous remission. Bethanechol (Urecholine) has occasionally improved emptying of the atonic urinary bladder. Impotence is usually permanent, and a penile prosthesis should be considered as a therapeutic option in selected cases. Mineralocorticoid therapy and pressure suits have reportedly been of some help in patients with orthostatic hypotension occurring as a result of loss of postural reflexes.

E. Skin and Mucous Membrane Complications: Chronic pyogenic infections of the skin may occur, especially in poorly controlled diabetic patients. Eruptive xanthomas can result from hypertriglyceridemia, associated with poor glycemic control. An unusual lesion termed **necrobiosis lipoidica diabeticorum** is usually located over the anterior surfaces of the legs or the dorsal surfaces of the ankles. They are oval or irregularly shaped plaques with demarcated borders and a glistering yellow surface and occur in women 2–4 times more frequently than in men.

"Shin spots" are not uncommon in adult diabetics. They are brownish, rounded, painless atrophic lesions of the skin in the pretibial area. Candidal infection can produce erythema and edema of intertriginous areas below the breasts, in the axillas, and between the fingers. It causes vulvovaginitis in most chronically uncontrolled diabetic women with persistent glucosuria and is a frequent cause of pruritus.

While antifungal creams containing nystatin offer immediate relief of vulvovaginitis, recurrence is frequent unless glucosuria is reduced.

F. Special Situations:

1. Insulin replacement during surgery–During major surgery and in the immediate recovery period in patients with insulin-requiring diabetes, 5% dextrose in physiologic saline should be infused intravenously at a rate of 100–200 mL/h with regular human insulin (25 units/250 mL normal saline) infused into the intravenous tubing at a rate of 1–3 units/h. The patient's blood glucose should be monitored every hour initially and the rates of insulin or dextrose adjusted to maintain blood glucose values between 120 and 190 mg/dL.

2. Pregnancy and the diabetic patient–Several features distinguish the management of diabetics during pregnancy from the general therapy of diabetes. These include the following: (1) Oral hypoglycemic agents are contraindicated. (2) Weight reduction is not advised, since fetal nutrition can be adversely affected. (3) Intensive insulin therapy with frequent self-monitoring of blood glucose is generally recommended to improve the likelihood of having healthy normal babies. Every effort should be made, utilizing multiple injections of insulin or a continuous infusion of insulin by pump, to maintain near-normalization of fasting and preprandial blood glucose values while avoiding hypoglycemia. Glycohemoglobin should be maintained in the normal range.

Since many diabetic pregnancies persist beyond the expected term—or because the infants are usually large and hydramnios may be present—it has been suggested that pregnancy be terminated early (at 37–38 weeks), especially if glycemic control during pregnancy has been inadequate (eg, glycohemoglobin > 10%). There is a present trend away from elective cesarean section and toward induction of labor.

See Chapter 13 for further details.

Prognosis

The effect of diabetic control on the development of complications remains an unresolved controversy. The observation that most diabetic patients receiving standard treatment regimens often have elevated levels of hemoglobin A_{1c} indicates the ineffectiveness of present conventional therapeutic methods for controlling hyperglycemia. Until pancreatic islet transplants or improved insulin delivery systems are available, this important question of control affecting complications may not be resolved. Korean patients who developed chronic hyperglycemia after accidental ingestion of Vacor, a rodenticide with potent toxicity for pancreatic B cells, were examined 6–7 years after the onset of their acquired diabetes. More than half of them showed thickened muscle capillary basement membranes, while 44% showed retinopathy and 28% had proteinuria. These findings suggest that hyperglycemia associated with insulin deficiency can itself be responsible for microvascular changes in diabetic patients. Intervention trials in small groups of IDDM patients with background or proliferative retinopathy have shown that despite 1 year of "tight" glycemic control with insulin pumps, worsening of the retinopathy continued. Moreover, there was no difference in the progression of diabetic retinopathy during a 2-year follow-up in IDDM patients achieving normal glycohemoglobins after successful pancreatic transplantation compared to a matched group with elevated glycohemoglobins in whom an attempted pancreas transplant was unsuccessful. A large-scale prevention trial involving 25 centers in the USA is under way to determine if "tight" glycemic control in IDDM can delay or prevent the *onset* of microvascular disease. Until these questions are resolved, the prognosis remains uncertain.

The period between 10 and 20 years after onset of diabetes seems to be a critical one. If the patient survives this period without fulminating complications, there is a strong likelihood that reasonably good health will continue. In addition to poorly understood factors relating to differences in individual susceptibility to development of long-term complications of hyperglycemia, it is clear that the diabetic patient's intelligence, motivation, and awareness of the potential complications of the disease contribute significantly to the ultimate outcome.

Alberti KG, Gries FA: Management of non-insulin-dependent diabetes mellitus in Europe: A consensus view. Diabetic Med 1988;5:275.

American Diabetes Association Committee on Professional Practice: Standards of medical care for patients with diabetes mellitus. Diabetes Care 1989;12:365.

Bailey CJ: Metformin revisited: Its actions and indications for use. Diabetic Medicine 1988;5:315.

Bailey TS, Mezitis NHE: Combination therapy with insulin and sulfonylureas for type II diabetes. Diabetes Care 1990;13:687.

Bantle JP: The dietary treatment of diabetes mellitus. Med Clin North Am 1988;72:1285.

Bennett PH: The diagnosis of diabetes: New international classification and diagnostic criteria. Annu Rev Med 1983;34:295.

DCCT Research group: Diabetes control and complications trial (DCCT): Update. Diabetes Care 1990;13:427.

DeFronzo RA: The triumvirate: Beta-cell, muscle, liver: A collusion responsible for NIDDM. Diabetes 1988; 37:667.

Feingold KR et al: Muscle capillary basement membrane width in patients with Vacor-induced diabetes mellitus. J Clin Invest 1986;78:102.

Fujioka S et al: Contribution of intra-abdominal fat accumulation to the impairment of glucose and lipid metabolism in human obesity. Metabolism 1987;36:54.

Gerich JE: Glucose counterregulation and its impact on diabetes mellitus. Diabetes 1988;37:1608.

Gerich JE: Oral hypoglycemic agents. N Engl J Med 1989; 321:1231.

Godine JE: The relationship between metabolic control and vascular complications of diabetes mellitus. Med Clin North Am 1988;72:1271.

Herold KC, Rubenstein AH: Immunosuppression for insulin-dependent diabetes. N Engl J Med 1988; 318:701.

Horton ES: Exercise and diabetes mellitus. Med Clin North Am 1988;72:1301.

Jackson RA et al: Mechanism of metformin action in non-insulin-dependent diabetes. Diabetes 1987;36:632.

Kennedy WR et al: Effects of pancreatic transplantation on diabetic neuropathy. N Engl J Med 1990;322:1031.

Lebovitz HE (editor): Physician's Guide to Non-Insulin-Dependent (Type II) Diabetes: Diagnosis and Treatment, 2nd ed. American Diabetes Association, 1988.

Merimee TJ: Diabetic retinopathy: A synthesis of perspectives. N Engl J Med 1990;322:978.

Nathan DM: Modern management of insulin-dependent diabetes mellitus. Med Clin North Am 1988;72:1365.

Ogbonnaya KI, Arem R: Diabetic diarrhea. Arch Intern Med 1990;150:262.

Parfrey PS et al: Contrast material-induced renal failure in patients with diabetes mellitus, renal insufficiency, or both: A prospective controlled study. N Engl J Med 1989;320:143.

Pecoraro RE, Reiber GE, Burgess EM: Pathways to diabetic limb amputation: Basis for prevention. Diabetes Care 1990;13:513.

Reaven GM: Role of insulin resistance in human disease. Diabetes 1988;37:1595.

Reddi AS, Camerini-Davalos RA: Diabetic nephropathy. Arch Intern Med 1990;150:31.

Schade DS: Surgery and diabetes. Med Clin North Am 1988;72:1531.

Singer DE et al: Tests of glycemia in diabetes mellitus: Their use in establishing a diagnosis and in treatment. Ann Intern Med 1989;110:125.

Stephenson JM, Schernthaner G: Dawn phenomenon and Somogyi effect in IDDM. Diabetes Care 1989;12:245.

The Working Group of Hypertension in Diabetes: Statement on hypertension in diabetes mellitus. (Two parts.) Arch Intern Med 1987;147:830, 1165.

Wu MS et al: Effect of metformin on carbohydrate and lipoprotein metabolism in NIDDM patients. Diabetes Care 1990;13:1.

Zinman B: The physiologic replacement of insulin: an elusive goal. N Engl J Med 1989;321:363.

DIABETIC COMA

Coma may be due to a variety of causes not directly related to diabetes. Certain causes directly related to diabetes require differentiation: (1) Hypoglycemic coma resulting from excessive doses of insulin or oral hypoglycemic agents. (2) Hyperglycemic coma associated with either severe insulin deficiency (diabetic ketoacidosis) or mild to moderate insulin deficiency (hyperglycemic nonketotic hyperosmolar coma). (3) Lactic acidosis associated with diabetes, particularly in diabetics stricken with severe infections or with cardiovascular collapse.

DIABETIC KETOACIDOSIS

Diabetic ketoacidosis may be the initial manifestation of type I diabetes or may result from increased insulin requirements in type I diabetes patients during the course of infection, trauma, myocardial infarction, or surgery. Type II diabetics may develop ketoacidosis under severe stress such as sepsis. Recently, diabetic ketoacidosis has been found to be one of the more common serious complications of insulin pump therapy, occurring in approximately one per 80 patient-months of treatment. Many patients who monitor capillary blood glucose regularly ignore urine ketone measurements, which would signal the possibility of insulin leakage or pump failure before serious illness develops. Poor compliance is one of the most common causes of diabetic ketoacidosis, particularly when episodes are recurrent.

Clinical Findings

A. Symptoms and Signs: The appearance of diabetic ketoacidotic coma is usually preceded by a day or more of polyuria and polydipsia associated with marked fatigue, nausea and vomiting, and, finally, mental stupor that can progress to coma. On physical examination, evidence of dehydration in a stuporous patient with rapid deep breathing and a "fruity" breath odor of acetone would strongly suggest the diagnosis. Hypotension with tachycardia indicates profound fluid and electrolyte depletion. Abdominal pain and even tenderness may be present in the absence of abdominal disease. Conversely, cholecystitis or pancreatitis may occur with minimal symptoms and signs.

B. Laboratory Findings: (Table 21–10.) Glycosuria of 4+ and strong ketonuria with hyperglycemia, ketonemia, low arterial blood pH, and low plasma bicarbonate are typical of diabetic ketoacidosis. Serum potassium is often elevated despite total body potassium depletion resulting from protracted polyuria or vomiting. Elevation of serum amylase is common but often represents salivary as well as pancreatic amylase. Thus, in this setting, serum amylase is not a good marker for acute pancreatitis. Multichannel chemical analysis of serum creatinine (SMA-6) is falsely elevated by nonspecific chromogenicity of keto acids and glucose. Most laboratories can correct for these interfering substances on request. Leukocytosis as high as 25,000/ mL with a leftward shift may occur with or without associated infection.

Complications

The 2 major metabolic aberrations of diabetic ketoacidosis are hyperglycemia and ketoacidemia, both due to insulin lack associated with hyperglucagonemia.

A. Hyperglycemia: Hyperglycemia results from increased hepatic production of glucose as well as diminished glucose uptake by peripheral tissues. Hepatic glucose output is a consequence of increased gluconeogenesis resulting from insulinopenia as well as from an associated hyperglucagonemia. Hyperglycemia produces an osmotic overload in the kidney, causing diuresis, with a critical loss of electrolytes and a disproportionate loss of free water in the urine with intracellular dehydration. When serum hyperosmolality exceeds 320–330 mosm/L, central nervous system depression or coma may ensue.

B. Ketoacidemia: Ketoacidemia represents the effect of insulin lack at multiple enzyme loci. Insulin lack associated with elevated levels of growth hormone and glucagon contributes to an increase in lipolysis from adipose tissue and in hepatic ketogenesis. In addition, there is evidence that reduced ketolysis by insulin-deficient peripheral tissues contributes to the ketoacidemia. The only true "keto" acid present is acetoacetic acid, which, along with its by-product acetone, is measured by nitroprusside reagents (Acetest and Ketostix). The sensitivity for acetone, however, is poor, requiring over 10 mmol, which is seldom reached in the plasma of ketoacidotic subjects—although this detectable concentration is readily achieved in urine. Thus, in the plasma of ketotic patients, only acetoacetate is measured by these reagents. The more prevalent β-hydroxybutyric acid has no ketone group and is therefore not detected by conventional nitroprusside tests. This takes on special importance in the presence of circulatory collapse during diabetic ketoacidosis, wherein an increase in lactic acid can shift the redox state to increase β-hydroxybutyric acid at the expense of the readily detectable acetoacetic acid. Bedside diagnostic reagents would then be unreliable, suggesting no ketonemia in cases where β-hydroxybutyric acid is a major factor in producing the acidosis.

Treatment

A. Prevention: Education of diabetic patients to recognize the early symptoms and signs of ketoacidosis has done a great deal to prevent severe acidosis. Urine ketones should be measured in patients with signs of infection or in insulin pump-treated patients when capillary blood glucose is unexpectedly and persistently high. When heavy ketonuria and glycosuria persist on several successive examinations, supplemental regular insulin should be administered and liquid foods such as lightly salted tomato juice and broth should be ingested to replenish fluids and

Table 21–10. Laboratory diagnosis of coma in diabetic patients.

	Urine		Plasma		
	Glucose	Acetone	Glucose	Bicarbonate	Acetone
Related to diabetes					
Hypoglycemia	0[1]	0 or +	Low	Normal	0
Diabetic ketoacidosis	+ + + +	+ + + +	High	Low	+ + + +
Nonketotic hyperglycemic coma	+ + + +	0	High	Normal or slightly low	0
Lactic acidosis	0 or +	0 or +	Normal or low or high	Low	0 or +
Unrelated to diabetes					
Alcohol or other toxic drugs	0 or +	0 or +	May be low	Normal or low[2]	0 or +
Cerebrovascular accident or head trauma	+ or 0	0	Often high	Normal	0
Uremia	0 or +	0	High or normal	Low	0 or +

[1] Leftover urine in bladder might still contain glucose from earlier hyperglycemia.
[2] Alcohol can elevate plasma lactate as well as keto acids to reduce pH.

electrolytes. The patient should be instructed to contact the physician if ketonuria persists, and especially if vomiting develops or if appropriate adjustment of the infusion rate on an insulin pump does not correct the hyperglycemia and ketonuria. In juvenile-onset diabetics, particularly in the teen years, recurrent episodes of severe ketoacidosis often indicate poor compliance with the insulin regimen, and these patients will require intensive family counseling.

B. Emergency Measures: If ketosis is severe, the patient should be placed in the hospital for correction of the hyperosmolality as well as the ketoacidemia.

1. Therapeutic flow sheet–One of the most important steps in initiating therapy is to start a flow sheet listing vital signs and the time sequence of diagnostic laboratory values in relation to therapeutic maneuvers. Indices of the metabolic defects include urine glucose and ketones as well as arterial pH, plasma glucose, acetone, bicarbonate, serum urea nitrogen, and electrolytes. Serum osmolality should be estimated and tabulated during the course of therapy.

A convenient method of estimating serum osmolality is as follows (normal values in humans are 280–300 mosm/L:

$$mosm/L = 2[Na^+] + \frac{Glucose\ (mg/dL)}{18} + \frac{BUN\ (mg/dL)}{2.8}$$

These calculated estimates are usually 10–20 meq/L lower than values recorded by standard cryoscopic techniques in patients with diabetic coma. One physician should be responsible for maintaining this therapeutic flow sheet and prescribing therapy. An indwelling catheter is required in all comatose patients but should be avoided if possible in a fully cooperative diabetic because of the risk of introducing bladder infection. Fluid intake and output should be recorded. Gastric intubation is recommended in the comatose patient to correct the commonly associated gastric dilatation that may lead to vomiting and aspiration. The patient should not receive sedatives or narcotics.

2. Insulin replacement–Only regular insulin should be used initially in all cases of severe ketoacidosis, and it should be given immediately after the diagnosis is established. Regular insulin can be given in a loading dose of 0.3 unit/kg as an intravenous bolus followed by 0.1 unit/kg/h, continuously infused or given hourly as an intramuscular injection; this is sufficient to replace the insulin deficit in most patients. Replacement of insulin deficiency helps correct the acidosis by reducing the flux of fatty acids to the liver, reducing ketone production by the liver, and also improving removal of ketones from the blood. Insulin treatment reduces the hyperosmolality by reducing the hyperglycemia. It accomplishes this by increasing removal of glucose through peripheral

utilization as well as by decreasing production of glucose by the liver. This latter effect is accomplished by direct inhibition of gluconeogenesis and glycogenolysis, as well as by lowered amino acid flux from muscle to liver and reduced hyperglucagonemia.

The insulin dose should be "piggy-backed" into the fluid line so the rate of fluid replacement can be changed without altering the insulin delivery rate. For optimal effects, continuous low-dose insulin infusions should always be preceded by a rapid intravenous loading dose of regular insulin, 0.3 unit/kg, to prime the tissue insulin receptors. If the plasma glucose level fails to fall at least 10% in the first hour, a repeat loading dose is recommended. The availability of instruments for rapid and accurate glucose analysis (Beckman or Yellow Springs glucose analyzer) has contributed much to achieving optimal insulin replacement. Rarely, a patient with immune insulin resistance is encountered, and this requires doubling the insulin dose every 2–4 hours if hyperglycemia does not improve after the first 2 doses of insulin. One must be alert to the danger of anaphylactic shock when very high doses of insulin are administered intravenously to patients whose insulin resistance is due to very high titers of anti-insulin antibodies. Sudden saturation of anti-insulin IgG blocking antibodies can result in discharge of most cells containing anti-insulin IgE antibodies.

3. Fluid and electrolyte replacement–In most patients, the fluid deficit is 4–5 L. Initially, normal saline solution is the solution of choice to help reexpand the contracted vascular volume. The use of sodium bicarbonate has been questioned because of the following potentially harmful consequences: (1) Hypokalemia from rapid potassium shifts into cells. (2) Tissue anoxia from reduced dissociation of oxygen from hemoglobin when acidosis is rapidly reversed. (3) Cerebral acidosis resulting from a reduction of cerebrospinal fluid pH. However, these considerations are relatively less important in certain clinical settings, and 1–2 ampules of sodium bicarbonate (44 meq per 50-mL ampule) added to a bottle of *hypotonic* saline solution may be administered whenever the blood pH is 7.0 or less or blood bicarbonate is below 9 meq/L. Once the pH reaches 7.2, no further bicarbonate should be given, since it aggravates rebound metabolic alkalosis as ketones are metabolized. Alkalosis causes potassium shifts that increase the risk of cardiac arrhythmias. In the first hour, at least 1 L of normal saline should be infused, and fluid should be given thereafter at a rate of 300–500 mL/h with careful monitoring of serum potassium. If the blood glucose is above 500 mg/dL, 0.45% saline solution may be used after the first hour, since the water deficit exceeds the sodium loss in uncontrolled diabetes with osmotic diuresis. When blood glucose falls to 250 mg/dL or less, 5% glucose solutions should be used to maintain blood glucose between 200 and 300 mg/

dL while insulin therapy is continued in order to clear the ketonemia. Glucose administration has the dual advantage of preventing hypoglycemia and furthermore of reducing the likelihood of cerebral edema, which could result from too rapid a decline in hyperglycemia.

4. Potassium and phosphate replacement– Total body potassium loss from polyuria as well as from vomiting may be as high as several hundred milliequivalents. However, because of shifts from cells due to the acidosis, serum potassium is usually normal or high until after the first few hours of treatment, when acidosis improves and serum potassium returns into cells. Potassium in doses of 20–30 meq/h should be infused within 3–4 hours after beginning therapy, or sooner if initial serum potassium is inappropriately low. Potassium replacement should be deferred if serum potassium remains above 5.8 meq/L, as in cases of renal insufficiency. An ECG can be of help in monitoring the patient and reflecting the state of potassium balance at the time, but it should not replace accurate laboratory measurements.

Foods high in potassium content can be prescribed when the patient has recovered sufficiently to take food orally. (Tomato juice and grapefruit juice contain 14 meq of potassium per 240 mL and a medium-sized banana 10 meq.)

Because severe hypophosphatemia also develops during insulin therapy of diabetic ketoacidosis, a small amount of phosphate can be replaced as the potassium salt. The potassium need is several times that of phosphate and should be replaced separately, since replacing phosphorus ions too rapidly (while meeting potassium requirements) can precipitate a drop in serum calcium in the tissues and induce tetany.

A significant therapeutic benefit of phosphate replacement has not been documented. However, certain potential advantages have been suggested. Treatment of hypophosphatemia helps to restore the buffering capacity of the plasma, thereby facilitating renal excretion of hydrogen; and it corrects the impaired oxygen dissociation from hemoglobin by regenerating 2,3-diphosphoglycerate. To minimize the risk of inducing tetany from an overload of phosphate replacement, an average deficit of 40–50 mmol phosphate in adults with diabetic ketoacidosis should be replaced by intravenous infusion *at a rate not to exceed 3 mmol/h.*

A stock solution available from Abbott Laboratories provides a mixture of 1.12 g KH_2PO_4 and 1.18 g K_2HPO_4 in a 5-mL single-dose vial representing 22 meq potassium and 15 mmol phosphate (27 meq). Five milliliters of this stock solution in 2 L of either 0.45% saline or 5% dextrose in water, infused at 400 mL/h, will replace the phosphate at the optimal rate of 3 mmol/h and will provide 4.4 meq of potassium per hour. If serum phosphate remains below 2.5 mg/dL, a repeat 5-hour infusion of potassium phosphate at a rate of 3 mmol/h would be reasonable.

5. Treatment of associated infection–Antibiotics are prescribed as indicated. Cholecystitis and pyelonephritis may be particularly severe in these patients.

Prognosis

The frequency of deaths due to diabetic ketoacidosis has been dramatically reduced by improved therapy of young diabetics, but this complication remains a significant risk in the aged and in patients in profound coma in whom treatment has been delayed. Acute myocardial infarction and infarction of the bowel following prolonged hypotension worsen the outlook. A serious prognostic sign is renal failure, and prior kidney dysfunction worsens the prognosis considerably because the kidney plays a key role in compensating for massive pH and electrolyte abnormalities. Cerebral edema has been reported to occur rarely as metabolic deficits return to normal. This is best prevented by avoiding sudden reversal of marked hyperglycemia. Maintaining glycemic levels of 200–300 mg/dL for the initial 24 hours after correction of severe hyperglycemia reduces this risk.

NONKETOTIC HYPERGLYCEMIC COMA

This second most common form of hyperglycemic coma is characterized by severe hyperglycemia in the absence of significant ketosis, with hyperosmolality and dehydration. It occurs in patients with mild or occult diabetes, and most patients are at least middle-aged to elderly. Underlying renal insufficiency or congestive heart failure is common, and the presence of either worsens the prognosis. A precipitating event such as infection, myocardial infarction, stroke, or recent operation is often present. Certain drugs such as phenytoin, diazoxide, glucocorticoids, and diuretics have been implicated in its pathogenesis, as have procedures associated with glucose loading such as peritoneal dialysis.

Pathogenesis

A partial or relative insulin deficiency may initiate the syndrome by reducing glucose utilization of muscle, fat, and liver while inducing hyperglucagonemia and increasing hepatic glucose output. With massive glycosuria, obligatory water loss ensues. If a patient is unable to maintain adequate fluid intake because of an associated acute or chronic illness or has suffered excessive fluid loss, marked dehydration results. As plasma volume contracts, renal insufficiency develops, and the resultant limitation of renal glucose loss leads to increasingly higher blood glucose concentrations. Severe hyperosmolality develops that causes mental confusion and finally coma. It is not clear why ketosis is virtually absent under these conditions of insulin insufficiency, although reduced levels of although reduced levels of growth hormone may be associated along with portal vein insulin concentrations sufficient to restrain ketogenesis.

Clinical Findings

A. Symptoms and Signs: Onset may be insidious over a period of days or weeks, with weakness, polyuria, and polydipsia. The lack of features of ketoacidosis may retard recognition of the syndrome and delay therapy until dehydration becomes more profound than in ketoacidosis. Reduced intake of fluid is not an uncommon historical feature, due to either inappropriate lack of thirst, nausea, or inaccessibility of fluids to elderly, bedridden patients. Lethargy and confusion develop, progressing to convulsions and deep coma. Physical examination confirms the presence of profound dehydration in a lethargic or comatose patient without Kussmaul respirations.

B. Laboratory Findings: Severe hyperglycemia is present, with blood glucose values ranging from 800 to 2400 mg/dL. In mild cases, where dehydration is less severe, dilutional hyponatremia as well as urinary sodium losses may reduce serum sodium to 120–125 meq/L, which protects to some extent against extreme hyperosmolality. However, as dehydration progresses, serum sodium can exceed 140 meq/L, producing serum osmolality readings of 330–440 mosm/kg. Ketosis and acidosis are usually absent or mild. Prerenal azotemia is the rule, with serum urea nitrogen elevations over 100 mg/dL being typical.

Treatment

A. Saline: Fluid replacement is of paramount importance in treating nonketotic hyperglycemic coma. If hypovolemia is present, fluid therapy should be initiated with isotonic saline. In all other cases, hypotonic (0.45%) saline appears to be preferable as the initial replacement solution because the body fluids of these patients are markedly hyperosmolar. As much as 4–6 L of fluid may be required in the first 8–10 hours. Careful monitoring of the patient is required for proper sodium and water replacement. Once blood glucose reaches 250 mg/dL, fluid replacement should include 5% dextrose in either water, 0.45% saline solution, or 0.9% saline solution. The rate of dextrose infusion should be adjusted to maintain glycemic levels of 250–300 mg/dL in order to reduce the risk of cerebral edema. An important end point of fluid therapy is to restore urine output to 50 mL/h or more.

B. Potassium: With the absence of acidosis, there may be no initial hyperkalemia unless associated renal failure is present. This results in less severe total potassium depletion than in diabetic ketoacidosis, and less potassium replacement is therefore needed. However, because initial serum potassium is usually not elevated and because it declines rapidly as a result of the sensitivity of the nonketotic patient to insulin, it has been recommended that potassium replacement be initiated earlier than in ketotic patients, assuming that no renal insufficiency or oliguria is present. Potassium chloride (10 meq/L) can be added to the initial bottle of fluids administered if the patient's serum potassium is not elevated.

C. Phosphate: When hypophosphatemia develops during insulin therapy, phosphate replacement can be given as described for ketoacidotic patients (at 3 mmol/h).

D. Insulin: Less insulin may be required to reduce the hyperglycemia in nonketotic patients as compared to those with diabetic ketoacidotic coma. In fact, fluid replacement alone can reduce hyperglycemia considerably. An initial dose of only 15 units intravenously and 15 units subcutaneously of regular insulin is usually quite effective, and in most cases subsequent doses need not be greater than 10–25 units subcutaneously every 4 hours.

Prognosis

The overall mortality rate of hyperglycemic, hyperosmolar, nonketotic coma is more than 10 times that of diabetic ketoacidosis, chiefly because of its higher incidence in older patients, who may have compromised cardiovascular systems or associated major illnesses. (When patients are matched for age, the prognoses of these 2 hyperglycemic emergencies are reasonably comparable.) When prompt therapy is instituted, the mortality rate can be reduced from nearly 50% to that related to the severity of coexistent disorders.

LACTIC ACIDOSIS

Lactic acidosis is characterized by accumulation of excess lactic acid in the blood. Normally, the principal sources of this acid are the erythrocytes (which lack enzymes for aerobic oxidation), skeletal muscle, skin, and brain. Conversion to glucose and oxidation principally by the liver but also by the kidneys represent the chief pathways for its removal. Overproduction of lactic acid (tissue hypoxia), deficient removal (hepatic failure), or both (circulatory collapse) can cause accumulation. Lactic acidosis is not uncommon in any severely ill patient suffering from cardiac decompensation, respiratory or hepatic failure, septicemia, or infarction of bowel or extremities. With the discontinuance of phenformin therapy in the USA, lactic acidosis in patients with diabetes mellitus has become uncommon, but it still must be considered in the acidotic diabetic, especially if the patient is seriously ill.

Clinical Findings

A. Symptoms and Signs: The main clinical features of lactic acidosis are marked hyperventilation and mental confusion leading to stupor and coma. When lactic acidosis is secondary to tissue hypoxia or vascular collapse, the clinical presentation is variable, being that of the prevailing catastrophic illness. However, in the idiopathic, or spontaneous, variety, the onset is rapid (usually over a few hours), blood pressure is normal, peripheral circulation is good, and there is no cyanosis.

B. Laboratory Findings: Plasma bicarbonate and blood pH are quite low, indicating the presence of severe metabolic acidosis. Ketones are usually absent from plasma and urine or at least not prominent. The first clue may be a high anion gap (serum sodium minus the sum of chloride and bicarbonate anions [in meq/L] should be no greater than 15). A higher value indicates the existence of an abnormal compartment of anions. If this cannot be clinically explained by an excess of keto acids (diabetes), inorganic acids (uremia), or anions from drug overdosage (salicylates, methyl alcohol, ethylene glycol), then lactic acidosis is probably the correct diagnosis. (See Chapter 16 also.) In the absence of azotemia, hyperphosphatemia may be a clue to the presence of lactic acidosis. The diagnosis is confirmed by demonstrating, in a sample of blood that is promptly chilled and separated, a plasma lactic acid concentration of 7 mmol/L or higher (values as high as 30 mmol/L have been reported). Normal plasma values average 1 mmol/L, with a normal lactate/pyruvate ratio of 10:1. This ratio is greatly exceeded in lactic acidosis.*

Treatment

Aggressive treatment of the precipitating cause of lactic acidosis is the main component of therapy. Empiric antibiotic coverage should be given after culture samples are obtained in any patient in whom the cause of the lactic acidosis is not apparent.

Alkalinization with intravenous sodium bicarbonate to keep the pH above 7.2 has been recommended in the emergency treatment of severe lactic acidosis. Massive doses may be required (as much as 2000 meq in 24 hours has been used); however, there is no evidence that the mortality rate is favorably affected by administering bicarbonate, and the matter is at present controversial. Hemodialysis may be useful in cases where large sodium loads are poorly tolerated. Dichloroacetate, an anion that facilitates pyruvate removal by activating pyruvate dehydrogenase, reverses certain types of lactic acidosis in animals and may prove useful in treating some types of lactic acidosis in humans.

Prognosis

The mortality rate of spontaneous lactic acidosis approaches 80%. The prognosis in most cases is that of the primary disorder that produced the lactic acidosis.

Cooper DJ et al: Bicarbonate does not improve hemodynamics in critically ill patients who have lactic acidosis. Ann Intern Med 1990;112:492.

Foster DW, McGarry JD: The metabolic derangements and treatment of diabetic ketoacidosis. N Engl J Med 1983; 309:159.

Fulop M: The treatment of severely uncontrolled diabetes mellitus. Adv Intern Med 1984;29:327.

Kitabachi AE, Murphy MB: Diabetic ketoacidosis and hyperosmolar hyperglycemic nonketotic coma. Med Clin North Am 1988;72:1545.

Kitabachi AE, Rumbak M: The management of diabetic emergencies. Hosp Pract (June 15) 1989;24:129.

Morris LR, Murphy MB, Kitabchi AE: Bicarbonate therapy in severe ketoacidosis. Ann Intern Med 1986;105:836.

Narins RG, Cohen JJ: Bicarbonate therapy for organic acidosis: The case for its continued use. Ann Intern Med 1987;106:615.

Rosenbloom AL: Intracerebral crises during treatment of diabetic ketoacidosis. Diabetes Care 1990;13:22.

Stacpoole PW et al: Dichloroacetate in the treatment of lactic acidosis. Ann Intern Med 1988;108:58.

Wachtel TJ, Silliman RA, Lamberton P: Predisposing factors for the diabetic hyperosmolar state. Arch Intern Med 1987;147:499.

THE HYPOGLYCEMIC STATES

Spontaneous hypoglycemia in adults is of 2 principal types: fasting and postprandial. Fasting hypoglycemia is often subacute or chronic and usually presents with neuroglycopenia as its principal manifestation; postprandial hypoglycemia is relatively acute and is often heralded by symptoms of adrenergic discharge (sweating, palpitations, anxiety, tremulousness).

Differential Diagnosis
(See Table 21–11.)

Fasting hypoglycemia may occur in certain endocrine disorders, such as hypopituitarism, Addison's disease, or myxedema; in disorders related to liver malfunction, such as acute alcoholism or liver failure; and in instances of renal failure, particularly in patients requiring dialysis. These conditions are usually obvious, with hypoglycemia being only a secondary feature. When fasting hypoglycemia is a primary manifestation developing in adults without apparent endocrine disorders or inborn metabolic diseases from childhood, the principal diagnostic possibilities include (1) hyperinsulinism, due to either pancreatic B cell tumors or surreptitious administration of insulin (or sulfonylureas); and (2) hypoglycemia due to noninsulin-producing extrapancreatic tumors.

---

* In collecting samples, it is essential to rapidly chill and separate the blood in order to remove red cells, whose continued glycolysis at room temperature is a common source of error in reports of high plasma lactate. Frozen plasma remains stable for subsequent assay.

Table 21–11. Common causes of hypoglycemia.[1]

Fasting hypoglycemia
Hyperinsulinism
  Pancreatic B cell tumor
  Surreptitious administration of insulin or sulfonylureas
Extrapancreatic tumors
Postprandial (reactive) hypoglycemia
Early hypoglycemia (alimentary)
  Postgastrectomy
  Functional (increased vagal tone)
Late hypoglycemia (occult diabetes)
  Delayed insulin release due to B cell dysfunction
Counterregulatory deficiency
Idiopathic
Alcohol hypoglycemia
Immunopathologic hypoglycemia
Idiopathic anti-insulin antibodies (which release their bound insulin)
Antibodies to insulin receptors (which act as agonists)
Pentamidine-induced hypoglycemia

[1] In the absence of clinically obvious endocrine or hepatic disorders.

Postprandial (reactive) hypoglycemia may be classified as early (within 2–3 hours after a meal) or late (3–5 hours after eating). Early, or alimentary, hypoglycemia occurs when there is a rapid discharge of ingested carbohydrate into the small bowel followed by rapid glucose absorption and hyperinsulinism. It may be seen after gastrointestinal surgery and is particularly associated with the dumping syndrome after gastrectomy. In some cases, it is functional and may represent overactivity of the parasympathetic nervous system mediated via the vagus nerve. Rarely, it results from defective counterregulatory responses such as deficiencies of growth hormone, glucagon, cortisol, or autonomic responses.

Alcohol hypoglycemia is due to hepatic glycogen depletion combined with alcohol-mediated inhibition of gluconeogenesis. At presentation, blood ethanol may be below levels usually associated with legal standards relating to being "under the influence."

Immunopathologic hypoglycemia is an extremely rare condition in which anti-insulin antibodies or antibodies to insulin receptors develop spontaneously. In the former case, the mechanism is unclear, but it may relate to increasing dissociation of insulin from circulating pools of bound insulin. When antibodies to insulin receptors are found, most patients do not have hypoglycemia but rather severe insulin-resistant diabetes and acanthosis nigricans. However, during the course of the disease in these patients, certain anti-insulin receptor antibodies with agonist activity mimicking insulin action predominate, producing severe hypoglycemia.

Factitious hypoglycemia is self-induced hypoglycemia due to surreptitious administration of insulin or sulfonylureas.

HYPOGLYCEMIA DUE TO PANCREATIC B CELL TUMORS

Fasting hypoglycemia in an otherwise healthy adult is most commonly due to an adenoma of the islets of Langerhans. Ninety percent of such tumors are single and benign, but multiple adenomas can occur as well as malignant tumors with functional metastases. Beta cell hyperplasia as a cause of fasting hypoglycemia is rare and not well documented in adults. Adenomas may be familial, and multiple adenomas have been found in conjunction with tumors of the parathyroids and pituitary (Werner's syndrome; multiple endocrine neoplasia type I).

Clinical Findings
A. Symptoms and Signs: The signs and symptoms are those of subacute or chronic hypoglycemia, which may progress to permanent and irreversible brain damage. Delayed diagnosis has often resulted in prolonged psychiatric care or treatment for psychomotor epilepsy before the true diagnosis was established. In long-standing cases, obesity can result as a consequence of overeating to relieve symptoms.

Whipple's triad is characteristic of hypoglycemia regardless of the cause. It consists of (1) a history of hypoglycemic symptoms, (2) an associated fasting blood glucose of 40 mg/dL or less,* and (3) immediate recovery upon administration of glucose. The hypoglycemic symptoms in insulinoma often develop in the early morning or after missing a meal. Occasionally, they occur after exercise. They typically begin with evidence of central nervous system glucose lack and can include blurred vision or diplopia, headache, feelings of detachment, slurred speech, and weakness. Personality and mental changes vary from anxiety to psychotic behavior, and neurologic deterioration can result in convulsions or coma. Sweating and palpitations may not occur.

B. Laboratory Findings: Beta cell adenomas do not reduce secretion in the presence of hypoglycemia, and the critical diagnostic test is to demonstrate inappropriately elevated serum insulin levels at a time when hypoglycemia is present. A reliable serum insulin level of 8 μU/mL or more in the presence of blood glucose values below 40 mg/dL is diagnostic of inappropriate hyperinsulinism. Other causes of hyperinsulinemic hypoglycemia must be considered, including factitious administration of insulin or sulfonylureas. An elevated circulating proinsulin level is characteristic of most B cell adenomas and does not occur in factitious hyperinsulinism.

C. Diagnostic Tests:
1. Prolonged fasting under hospital supervision until hypoglycemia is documented is probably the most dependable means of establishing the diagnosis,

* Plasma glucose values are generally 10–15% higher than blood glucose values.

especially in men. In patients with insulinoma, the blood glucose levels often drop below 40 mg/dL after an overnight fast. In normal male subjects, the blood glucose does not fall below 55–60 mg/dL during a 3-day fast. In contrast, in premenopausal women who have fasted for only 24 hours, the plasma glucose may fall normally to such an extent that it can reach values as low as 35 mg/dL. After 36 hours of fasting, premenopausal normal women occasionally achieve such low levels of glucose that clinical evaluation of this test for insulinoma becomes quite difficult. In these cases, however, the women are not symptomatic, presumably owing to the development of sufficient ketonemia to supply energy needs to the brain. Insulinoma patients, on the other hand, become symptomatic when plasma glucose drops to subnormal levels, since inappropriate insulin secretion restricts ketone formation. Moreover, the demonstration of a nonsuppressed insulin level ($\geq$ 8 units/mL) in the presence of hypoglycemia and of an *increasing* ratio of insulin to glucose (ie, glucose falls more rapidly than does insulin) suggests the diagnosis of insulinoma, since normal females show a falling insulin-to-glucose ratio during a fast. If hypoglycemia does not develop in a male patient after fasting for up to 72 hours—and particularly when this prolonged fast is terminated with a period of moderate exercise—insulinoma must be considered an unlikely diagnosis.

2. Failure to suppress C peptide during insulin-induced hypoglycemia is the basis of another diagnostic test for insulinoma. This small peptide connecting A and B chains of insulin is released in equimolar quantities with endogenous insulin and thus reflects endogenous insulin secretion, which cannot be directly monitored during insulin infusion. Whereas normal persons suppress their C peptide levels to 50% or more during hypoglycemia induced by 0.1 unit of insulin per kilogram body weight per hour, absence of suppression suggests the presence of an autonomous insulin-secreting tumor.

3. Proinsulin determinations–In contrast to normal subjects, whose proinsulin concentration is less than 20% of the total immunoreactive insulin, patients with insulinoma have elevated levels of proinsulin representing 30–90% of total immunoreactive insulin. New assays for human proinsulin incorporating specific monoclonal antibodies offer considerable potential for the evaluation of patients with suspected insulinoma.

4. Stimulation tests with pancreatic B cell secretagogues such as tolbutamide, glucagon, or leucine are generally not needed in most cases if basal insulin is found to be nonsuppressible and therefore inappropriately elevated during fasting hypoglycemia. However, in occasional patients with a relatively fixed level of circulating insulin that is only barely inappropriate, stimulation may be helpful, bearing in mind that false-negative results can occur if the tumor is poorly differentiated and agranular.

Intravenous glucagon (1 mg over 1 minute) can be useful in patients with "borderline" fasting inappropriate hyperinsulinism. A rise above baseline of 200 μU/mL or more at 5 and 10 minutes strongly suggests insulinoma, although poorly differentiated tumors may not respond. Glucagon has the advantage over tolbutamide of correcting rather than provoking hypoglycemia during stimulation testing and is diagnostic in 60–70% of patients with insulinoma.

D. Preoperative Localization of B Cell Tumors: Pancreatic arteriography has been disappointing, with an accuracy rate of only 20% and a false-positive rate of about 5%. CT scan and MRI are not helpful in the preoperative localization of insulinoma because they do not distinguish small tumors within the pancreas. However, intraoperative ultrasound is proving to be a valuable means of localizing small tumors within the pancreas not palpable at laparotomy.

Percutaneous transhepatic pancreatic vein catheterization with insulin assay is useful for localizing small insulinomas. It offers promise in helping localize small B cell tumors, particularly in the head of the pancreas, where they may be difficult to see or palpate at the time of surgery. It may also detect multiple tumors or islet cell hyperplasia preoperatively. This technique is not widely available.

Treatment

A. Surgical Measures: Resection is the treatment of choice, preferably by a surgeon with previous experience in removing islet cell tumors. Diazoxide, 300–400 mg/d orally with 25–50 mg hydrochlorothiazide, inhibits insulin release from tumors and is useful in the interval prior to surgery for prevention of hypoglycemic episodes. However, because effective doses are tolerated poorly over the long term, diazoxide is not considered a desirable alternative to surgical excision. Blood glucose should be monitored throughout surgery, and 10% dextrose in water should be infused at a rate of 100 mL/h or faster. In cases where the diagnosis has been established but no adenoma is located, subtotal pancreatectomy is usually indicated, including the entire body and tail of the pancreas. Total pancreatectomy is seldom required now in view of the efficacy of long-term medical therapy with diazoxide in most patients with insulinomas. Intraoperative utilization of the "closed loop" artificial pancreas permits monitoring of plasma glucose and infusion of dextrose. This not only protects against hypoglycemia but also may aid in determining whether all insulin-secreting tumors have been removed, at which time the dextrose infusion stops and blood glucose rises.

B. Diet and Medical Therapy: In patients with inoperable functioning islet cell carcinoma or in patients in whom subtotal removal of the pancreas has failed to produce cure, reliance on frequent feedings is necessary. Since most tumors are not responsive to glucose, carbohydrate feedings every 2–3 hours are usually effective in preventing hypoglycemia, although obesity may become a problem. Glucagon should be available for emergency use as indicated in the discussion of treatment of diabetes. Diazoxide, 300–600 mg daily orally, has been useful with concomitant thiazide diuretic therapy to control concomitant sodium retention. When patients are unable to tolerate diazoxide because of gastrointestinal upset, hirsutism, or edema, the calcium channel blocker verapamil may be beneficial in view of its inhibitory effect on insulin release from insulinoma cells. Recently, a potent long-acting synthetic octapeptide analogue of somatostatin (octreotide, Sandoz) has been used to inhibit release of hormones from a number of endocrine tumors, including inoperable insulinomas. When hypoglycemia persists after attempted surgical removal of the insulinoma and if diazoxide or verapamil is poorly tolerated or ineffective, a trial of 50 μg of octreotide (Sandostatin) injected subcutaneously twice daily may control the hypoglycemic episodes in conjunction with multiple small feedings. Streptozocin is useful in decreasing insulin secretion in islet cell carcinomas, and effective doses have been achieved without the undue renal toxicity that characterized early experience.

Prognosis

When insulinoma is diagnosed early and cured surgically, complete recovery is likely, although brain damage following severe hypoglycemia is not reversible. A significant increase in survival rate has been shown in streptozocin-treated patients with islet cell carcinoma, with reduction in tumor mass as well as decreased hyperinsulinism.

HYPOGLYCEMIA DUE TO EXTRAPANCREATIC TUMORS

These rare causes of hypoglycemia include mesenchymal tumors such as retroperitoneal sarcomas, hepatomas, adrenocortical carcinomas, and miscellaneous epithelial type tumors. The tumors are frequently large and readily palpated or visualized on urograms.

Laboratory diagnosis depends upon fasting hypoglycemia associated with serum insulin levels that are generally below 8 μU/mL. The mechanism of these tumors' hypoglycemic effect remains obscure. Although they do not release immunoreactive insulin, it has been suggested that they may produce certain insulinlike substances similar to the somatomedins or growth factors that may bind to the insulin receptor.

The prognosis for these tumors is generally poor, and surgical removal should be attempted when feasible. Dietary management of the hypoglycemia is the mainstay of medical treatment, since diazoxide is usually ineffective.

POSTPRANDIAL HYPOGLYCEMIA (Reactive Hypoglycemia)

Postgastrectomy Alimentary Hypoglycemia

Reactive hypoglycemia following gastrectomy is a consequence of hyperinsulinism resulting from rapid gastric emptying of ingested food. Symptoms result from adrenergic hyperactivity in response to the hypoglycemia. Treatment consists of more frequent feedings with smaller portions of less rapidly assimilated carbohydrate and more slowly absorbed fat and protein.

Functional Alimentary Hypoglycemia

This syndrome is classified as functional when no postsurgical explanation exists for the presence of early alimentary type reactive hypoglycemia. It is most often associated with chronic fatigue, anxiety, irritability, weakness, poor concentration, decreased libido, headaches, hunger after meals, and tremulousness. However, most patients with these symptoms do not have hypoglycemia. (See Chronic Fatigue Syndrome in Chapter 1.)

Indiscriminate use and overinterpretation of glucose tolerance tests have led to an unfortunate tendency to overdiagnose functional hypoglycemia. As many as one-third or more of *normal* subjects have hypoglycemia reaching nadirs as low as 40–50 mg/dL with or without symptoms during a 4-hour glucose tolerance test. Accordingly, to increase diagnostic reliability, hypoglycemia should preferably be documented during a spontaneous symptomatic episode accompanying routine daily activity, with clinical improvement following feeding.

In patients with documented postprandial hypoglycemia on a functional basis, there is no harm and occasional benefit in reducing the proportion of carbohydrate in the diet while increasing the frequency and reducing the size of meals. Support and mild sedation should be the mainstays of therapy, with dietary manipulation only an adjunct.

Late Hypoglycemia (Occult Diabetes)

This condition is characterized by a delay in early insulin release from pancreatic B cells, resulting in initial exaggeration of hyperglycemia during a glucose tolerance test. In response to this hyperglycemia, an exaggerated insulin release produces a late hypoglycemia 4–5 hours after ingestion of glucose. These patients are usually quite different from those with early hypoglycemia, often being obese and frequently having a family history of diabetes mellitus.

In obese patients, treatment is directed at weight reduction to achieve ideal weight. Like all patients with postprandial hypoglycemia, regardless of cause, these patients often respond to reduced carbohydrate intake with multiple, spaced, small feedings high in protein. They should be considered potential diabetics and advised to have periodic medical evaluations.

ALCOHOL HYPOGLYCEMIA

Fasting Hypoglycemia After Ethanol

During the postabsorptive state, normal plasma glucose is maintained by hepatic glucose output derived from both glycogenolysis and gluconeogenesis. With prolonged starvation, glycogen reserves become depleted within 18–24 hours and hepatic glucose output becomes totally dependent on gluconeogenesis. Under these circumstances, a blood concentration of ethanol as low as 45 mg/dL (considerably below the California legal "under the influence" level for drivers of 80 mg/dL) can induce profound hypoglycemia by blocking gluconeogenesis. Neuroglycopenia in a patient whose breath smells of alcohol may be mistaken for alcoholic stupor. Prevention consists of adequate food intake during ethanol ingestion. Therapy consists of glucose administration to replenish glycogen stores until gluconeogenesis resumes.

Postethanol Reactive Hypoglycemia

When sugar-containing soft drinks are used as mixers to dilute alcohol in beverages (gin and tonic, rum and cola), there seems to be a greater insulin release than when the soft drink alone is ingested and a tendency for more of a late hypoglycemic overswing to occur 3–4 hours later. Prevention would consist of avoiding sugar mixers while ingesting alcohol or ensuring supplementary food intake to provide sustained absorption.

FACTITIOUS HYPOGLYCEMIA

Factitious hypoglycemia may be difficult to document. A suspicion of self-induced hypoglycemia is supported when the patient is associated with the health professions or has access to insulin or sulfonylurea drugs taken by a diabetic member of the family. The triad of hypoglycemia, high immunoreactive insulin, and suppressed plasma C peptide immunoreactivity is pathognomonic of exogenous insulin administration. Demonstration of circulating antibodies supports this diagnosis in suspected cases. When sulfonylureas are suspected as a cause of factitious hypoglycemia, a chemical test of the plasma to detect the presence of these drugs may be required to distinguish laboratory findings from those of insulinoma.

IMMUNOPATHOLOGIC HYPOGLYCEMIA

This rare cause of hypoglycemia, documented in isolated case reports, may occur as 2 distinct disorders: one associated with spontaneous development of circulating anti-insulin antibodies and another associated with antibodies to insulin receptors, in which the antibodies apparently have agonist capabilities.

PENTAMIDINE-INDUCED HYPOGLYCEMIA

With the increased prevalence of pulmonary infection by *Pneumocystis carinii* in patients with acquired immune deficiency syndrome, pentamidine given intravenously or by aerosol is being used more frequently and in 10–20% of patients produce symptomatic hypoglycemia. This apparently is due to lytic destruction of pancreatic B cells, causing acute hyperinsulinemia and hypoglycemia, followed later by insulinopenia and hyperglycemia which occasionally is persistent. Intravenous glucose should be administered during pentamidine administration and for the period immediately following to prevent or ameliorate hypoglycemic symptoms. Following a complete course of therapy with pentamidine, fasting blood glucose or a subsequent glycohemoglobin should be monitored to assess the extent of pancreatic B cell recovery or residual damage.

Axelrod L, Ron D: Insulinlike growth factor II and the riddle of tumor-induced hypoglycemia. N Engl J Med 1988;319:1477.

Campbell PJ, Gerich JE: Mechanisms for prevention, development, and reversal of hypoglycemia. Adv Intern Med 1988;33:205.

Cohen RM, Camus F: Update on insulinomas or the case of the missing (Pro) insulinoma. Diabetes Care 1988; 11:506.

Daughaday WH et al: Synthesis and secretion if insulinlike growth factor II by a leiomyosarcoma with associated hypoglycemia. N Engl J Med 1988;319:1434.

Fischer KF, Lees JA, Newman JH: Hypoglycemia in hospitalized patients: Causes and outcomes. N Engl J Med 1986;315:1245.

Grunberger G et al: Factitious hypoglycemia due to surreptitious administration of insulin: Diagnosis, treatment, and long-term follow-up. Ann Intern Med 1988;108:252.

Kvols LK et al: Treatment of metastatic islet cell carcinoma with a somatostatin analogue (SMS 201–995). Ann Intern Med 1987;107:162.

Palardy J et al: Blood glucose measurements during symptomatic episodes in patients with suspected postprandial hypoglycemia. N Engl J Med 1989;321:1421.

Rifkin MD, Weiss SM: Intraoperative sonographic identification of nonpalpable pancreatic masses. J Ultrasound Med 1984;3:409.

Waskin H et al: Risk factors for hypoglycemia associated with pentamidine therapy for Pneumocystis pneumonia. JAMA 1988;260:345.

Williams HE: Alcoholic hypoglycemia and ketoacidosis. Med Clin North Am 1984;68:33.

DISTURBANCES OF LIPID METABOLISM

The principal circulating lipids in humans are of 4 types: (1) triglycerides, (2) free cholesterol, (3) cholesteryl esters, and (4) phospholipids. These are transported as spherical macromolecular complexes termed **lipoproteins,** wherein an inner core of hydrophobic lipids (triglycerides and cholesteryl esters) is encased by a membrane of unimolecular thickness consisting of various proteins (apolipoproteins, or simply apoproteins) in association with hydrophilic lipids (free cholesterol and phospholipids).

Classification of Lipoproteins

Specific differences among the various lipoprotein classes depend on the amount each class contains of each of the 4 lipids (this affects their size and density) and on the nature of the apoprotein in their membrane. These differences allow for classification of lipoproteins on the basis of ultracentrifugal density, with those containing mostly triglyceride being termed **very low density lipoproteins (VLDL)** and those containing mostly cholesterol called **low-density lipoproteins (LDL);** when the total lipid content is slightly less than the weight of protein in the membrane, the density is **high (HDL).**

When classified on the basis of their mobility on paper electrophoresis, LDL are termed betalipoproteins; VLDL, prebetalipoproteins; and HDL, alphalipoproteins. These 3 classes of lipoproteins are normally present in fasting sera. Chylomicrons constitute a fourth class, normally present only after ingestion of fat. These are of such low density that they float even without centrifugation, and because of their large size and proportionately low protein content, they fail to migrate on paper electrophoresis.

Metabolism of Lipoproteins

Chylomicrons, which carry ingested fat, and VLDL, which contain triglyceride converted from endogenous fatty acids and ingested carbohydrate, are transported in plasma to fat depots, where they are cleared by an enzyme, lipoprotein lipase, attached to capillary endothelium. The normal end products of both chylomicrons and VLDL are "remnant" particles of very low density that contain different B apoproteins in their membranes. The B apoprotein of chylomicron remnants (B-48) is smaller than that of VLDL remnants (B-100), and studies of apoprotein metabolism indicate that chylomicron remnants are completely metabolized by the liver, while VLDL remnants are further hydrolyzed by hepatic lipase and either removed by the liver or converted to LDL and then returned to the circulation. Low-density lipoproteins are responsible for transporting cholesteryl esters to peripheral tissues where the transported cholesterol can be used for membrane synthesis, thus sparing these tissues in their endogenous production of cholesterol. High-density lipoproteins contribute to lipid transport by transferring apoprotein C-II to VLDL particles and chylomicrons, which activates lipoprotein lipase; they also participate in the removal of cholesterol either from aging cell membranes or from tissue deposits by providing apoprotein A-I, which activates a circulating enzyme, lecithin-cholesterol acyltransferase (LCAT). This produces cholesteryl esters that are subsequently removed by the HDL and either recycled via remnant lipoproteins and LDL for resynthesis of cell membrane or taken to the liver for excretion as biliary cholesterol or bile salts.

Diagnostic Evaluation of Hypercholesterolemia

In most adult patients, a fasting serum cholesterol measurement is indicated. In those at high risk, such as relatives of patients with a strongly positive family history of myocardial infarction, children as well as other adult members of the family should be screened. If the total serum cholesterol is above 200 mg/dL, a further assessment by measuring a repeat serum cholesterol along with an HDL cholesterol and a serum triglyceride measurement would permit indirect estimation of the LDL cholesterol concentration based on the following approach: After an overnight fast, total serum cholesterol is generally composed of the cholesterol contained within 3 major lipoprotein particles: LDL, HDL, and VLDL. HDL cholesterol can readily be measured in most clinical laboratories using a simple modification of the same assay used to quantitate the total serum cholesterol. The VLDL cholesterol must be indirectly estimated as follows: In the average-sized VLDL particle, there is a ratio of 5:1 (by weight) of triglyceride to cholesterol. Thus, it is possible to estimate the VLDL cholesterol content by taking one-fifth of the serum triglyceride value. This estimate is inapplicable in 2 situations: chylomicrons have higher ratios (8:10) of triglyceride to cholesterol, and in the rare type III disorder, remnant particles have a lower ratio of 1:1 or 2:1.

As long as fasting serum triglyceride levels are below 600–800 mg/dL (lower than would be expected from chylomicronemia) and there are no clinical suggestions of dysbetalipoproteinemia (type III), the following equation provides an indirect estimate of LDL cholesterol (LDL_c):

$$LDL_c = \text{Total cholesterol} - \left(HDL_c + \frac{\text{Serum triglyceride}}{5}\right)$$

Values of LDL cholesterol above 160 mg/dL in adults would generally increase risk factors to a degree that would justify a recommendation for a modified diet initially and, if this is not effective, consideration of a subsequent trial of drug therapy—assuming that

Table 21-12. Risk factors for coronary heart disease (CHD) other than LDL cholesterol.

Male sex
Family history of CHD before age 55 years
Cigarette smoking
Hypertension
Diabetes mellitus
Severe obesity (> 30% above ideal weight)
Peripheral vascular disease
HDL cholesterol below 35 mg/dL
Lipoprotein(a) above 30 mg/dL

secondary causes of LDL elevation are not identified. In elderly people with reduced life expectancy, pharmacologic therapy is seldom indicated for hypercholesterolemia.

In persons with coronary heart disease or at least 2 positive risk factors for it (including male sex), a value of 130 mg/dL or higher for LDL cholesterol would qualify them for a therapeutic regimen. Table 21-12 lists the important risk factors.

When fasting levels of triglycerides are moderately elevated in the serum in association with an elevated serum cholesterol to give a triglyceride:cholesterol ratio of 1:1 or 2:1, the most probable diagnosis statistically is the mixed hyperlipidemic disorder familial combined hyperlipidemia, characterized by elevation of both LDL and VLDL, rather than the rare type III disorder characterized by increased numbers of remnant particles. Although certain clinical features such as distinctive planar xanthomas may identify the patient with dysbetalipoproteinemia (type III), for a definite laboratory diagnosis, analytic ultracentrifugation with fractionation of the various lipoproteins is helpful in distinguishing these 2 disorders. Similarly, genetic analysis of DNA for the presence of

alleles for apoprotein E_2 is informative or diagnostic. Differentiating these 2 causes of hypertriglyceridemia may be important, since the triglyceride-containing remnant in type III disease is perhaps more atherogenic than the larger VLDL particle and is a better responder to pharmacologic therapy (eg, to estrogens in postmenopausal women as well as to either clofibrate or gemfibrozil in lipemic patients).

Lipoprotein Disorders

An excess or deficiency of certain lipoproteins can result from primary genetic disorders or may be secondary to acquired metabolic dysfunction. Until more information becomes available to permit classification on the basis of cause, the use of electrophoresis to define various phenotypes has been accepted by WHO. These phenotypes, together with their acquired (secondary) counterparts, include the main types of hyperlipidemia seen clinically (Table 21-13). These "types" should not be considered disease entities but may be useful for determining the most rational therapy.

A. Primary Hyperlipoproteinemias:

1. Type I hyperlipoproteinemia (hyperchylomicronemia)—This is the rarest form of familial hyperlipoproteinemia and is characterized by massive chylomicronemia when a patient is on a normal diet and complete disappearance of the chylomicronemia a few days after fat is eliminated from the diet. Postheparin lipolytic activity is absent in the serum in most cases, indicating that this autosomal recessive defect is a deficiency of lipoprotein lipase. However, several families have been reported to have a deficiency of C-II apoprotein, which interferes with normal activation of lipoprotein lipase and in the case of homozygotes results in marked hyperchylomicro-

Table 21-13. More common causes of primary hyperlipidemia.

Type[1]	Lipoprotein Abnormalities and Defect	Appearance of Serum[2]	Cholesterol Elevation[3]	Triglyceride Elevation[3]	Clinical Presentation	Rule Out
IIA	Hyperbetalipoproteinemia (lack of a cell surface receptor involved in degrading LDL). Common.	Clear	Usually 300–600 but may be higher	None	Xanthelasma, tendon xanthomas, accelerated atherosclerosis; detectable in childhood.	Hypothyroidism, nephrotic syndrome, hepatic obstruction.
IIB	Familial combined lipidemia (both LDL and VLDL elevation). Quite common.	Turbid	Usually 250–600	Usually 200–600	Relatively common. Severe forms are like IIA; milder forms associated with obesity or diabetes.	Same as IIA.
IV	Hyperprebetalipoproteinemia (delay in clearance or overproduction of VLDL). Common.	Turbid	300–800	200–5000	Most common, usually in adults. Eruptive xanthomas; accelerated vascular disease, mild glucose intolerance, hyperuricemia.	Nephrotic syndrome, hypothyroidism, glycogen storage disease; oral contraceptives.

[1] Types I, III, and V are omitted from the table because of their clinical rarity. See text.
[2] Refrigerated serum overnight at 4 °C.
[3] mg/dL. Normal cholesterol, 150–250 mg/dL; triglycerides, <150 mg/dL.

nemia. Lipemia retinalis is seen when serum triglycerides exceed 2500 mg/dL. Total serum cholesterol is often quite high, since it accounts for as much as 10% of the weight of chylomicron particles; however, LDL cholesterol is subnormal. Spurious hyponatremia may result from displacement of plasma water by high fat content during routine blood sampling. Pancreatitis is the major hazard, and patients with this disorder may not have accelerated atherosclerosis despite hypercholesterolemia. The diagnosis is suspected in children with recurrent abdominal pain, especially when hepatosplenomegaly is present. Eruptive xanthomas and creamy serum that separates into a creamy supernate and a clear infranate confirm the diagnosis.

Treatment consists of a fat-restricted diet (10–20 g daily), and the response is usually good.

2. Type IIA (hyperbetalipoproteinemia; familial hypercholesterolemia)–This disorder in homozygotes is due to absence of normal LDL receptors and their replacement by defective ones, which results in impaired clearance of betalipoproteins; in heterozygotes, half of the LDL receptors are defective, causing partial impairment of betalipoprotein clearance. This receptor defect also prevents normal feedback inhibition of cholesterol synthesis by cholesterol released after internalization of betalipoproteins. It is one of the commonest of familial hyperlipoproteinemias and is transmitted as an autosomal dominant, at least in the severe variety. The major clinical manifestations of familial hypercholesterolemia include an accelerated atherosclerosis, early myocardial infarction, and the presence of tendon xanthomas and xanthelasma. The diagnosis is based on hypercholesterolemia in the presence of clear serum after overnight incubation at 4° C. Total serum cholesterol is elevated, with a normal serum triglyceride and normal HDL cholesterol level—indicating that LDL cholesterol accounts for the elevated serum cholesterol. Dietary restriction of saturated fat and cholesterol is seldom of help in severe cases but should be advised, along with intense efforts to correct any reversible risk factors for macrovascular disease (smoking, hypertension, obesity). Vigorous measures, including oral administration of combinations of bile acid-binding resins with either nicotinic acid or with inhibitors of hydroxymethyl glutaryl-coenzyme A reductase (lovastatin), have recently been shown to restore serum cholesterol to normal in highly compliant patients. Jejunoileal bypass surgery has produced discouraging results. Chronic plasma-exchange therapy is expensive and inconvenient but can lower cholesterol and reduce the size of xanthomas. Milder forms of hypercholesterolemia whose genetics are as yet unclear may phenotypically resemble familial hypercholesterolemia but are much more responsive to dietary treatment.

3. Type IIB (mixed hyperbeta- and hyperprebetalipoproteinemia)–This disorder has been termed familial combined hyperlipidemia (FCHL) or

multiple type hyperlipoproteinemia, since affected individuals and their relatives tend to change their lipid profiles from an excess of either VLDL or LDL particles alone to a combination of both, or even at times to a normal lipid phenotype. Generally, however, an excess of Apo B-100 lipoproteins can be detected even when serum cholesterol values are normal; this is due to increased numbers of smaller and denser LDL particles that are enriched with Apo B-100 and relatively depleted in cholesterol content. An overproduction of Apo B-100, along with an increased sensitivity to dietary indiscretion, has been invoked to explain the genesis of this disorder. It aggregates in families, has features of autosomally dominant transmission, and is associated with a high risk for coronary artery disease. When the combined pattern is present in affected members, both the triglyceride/cholesterol ratio and the electrophoretic pattern are indistinguishable from those of type III disease, as is the character of serum turbidity after overnight incubation at 4 °C. Ultracentrifugal analysis confirms the diagnosis by showing both an LDL and a VLDL elevation, whereas in type III, a ''floating beta'' particle is obtained. Patients with multiple type hyperlipoproteinemia are at high risk for coronary artery disease, and this condition accounts for the vast majority of patients with myocardial infarction who also have hyperlipidemia. A prudent diet designed to achieve or maintain normal weight, avoidance of smoking, and correction of hypertension are essential recommendations for all affected individuals. Drug therapy is advocated in patients manifesting only hypertriglyceridemia if a family history of coronary artery disease is present, and it is indicated in patients with elevated LDL cholesterol that has not responded to diet therapy. Combined treatment with nicotinic acid and a bile acid-binding resin has generally been effective in FCHL, though maintaining compliance with this regimen may be difficult.

4. Type III (hyper-''remnant''-lipoproteinemia; dysbetalipoproteinemia)–This rare disorder results from absence of the apoprotein E-3, which normally activates hepatic lipase to clear chylomicron remnants and transforms VLDL remnants to LDL. In its place is an abnormal isoform (E-2) that binds poorly to hepatic lipase. This results in accumulation of lipoprotein remnants of intermediate density (IDL), which have flotation characteristics on ultracentrifugation in the lower range of VLDL but have the electrophoretic mobility of betalipoproteins (beta-VLDL), hence the name dysbetalipoproteinemia. Although hypercholesterolemia is present, the excess cholesterol is in the IDL fraction and the LDL cholesterol concentration is generally low due to impaired removal of VLDL remnants. In this circumstance, attempts to estimate lipoprotein cholesterol content derived from an equation using standard clinical laboratory lipid measurements incorrectly indicate an increase in LDL cholesterol. Therefore, when hypertriglyceridemia accompanies hypercholesterolemia, the possibility of dysbetalipoproteinemia may require direct quantitation of lipoprotein cholesterol fractions rather than a calculated estimate.

The genetic mode of transmission of dysbetalipoproteinemia suggests a mendelian-recessive trait; however, its expression as hyperlipidemia seems to require precipitating factors such as obesity or hypothyroidism. It occurs predominantly in adults and is rare in premenopausal women, since estrogens seem to reduce accumulation of the "remnant" particles. Patients are often obese and may have tuberous xanthomas, xanthelasma, and accelerated atherosclerosis. Planar xanthomas on the palms have been considered diagnostic. Treatment is especially gratifying in type III disease. Reduction to ideal weight in the obese patient and maintenance on a low-cholesterol diet may produce dramatic improvement, and total correction of hyperlipoproteinemia may result, especially in response to the addition of clofibrate, 1 g twice daily, to the dietary regimen. Estrogen therapy after menopause can also produce a dramatic increase in removal of these remnant particles, even though it does not affect the abnormal apoprotein E distribution.

5. Type IV (hyperprebetalipoproteinemia)– This type of lipemia is endogenous in contrast to type I hyperlipoproteinemia and represents a failure in removal of prebetalipoproteins (VLDL) produced by the liver, either in normal amounts or excessively.

Since carbohydrate intake induces production of this triglyceride-enriched lipoprotein from esterification of endogenous fatty acids, this disorder has been termed carbohydrate-induced hyperlipemia. It is common in adults and often associated with caloric excess, obesity, and hyperuricemia. Serum triglyceride levels above 500 mg/dL after an overnight fast are considered abnormally high, while those between 250 and 500 mg/dL are "borderline." Very high triglyceride levels exceeding 1000 mg/dL occasionally occur and indicate associated chylomicronemia. This results from exacerbating factors such as poorly controlled diabetes or alcohol ingestion being superimposed on this disorder, or it may occur when drugs such as estrogens or high-dose glucocorticoids are prescribed for affected persons. Eruptive xanthomas may accompany triglyceride levels above 1000 mg/dL. Treatment is directed at weight reduction in the obese, avoiding high carbohydrate or alcohol intake and caloric excess. Whether hypertriglyceridemia represents a significant coronary risk factor is still controversial. While small elevations of serum triglycerides may not increase cardiac risk when cholesterol is normal, moderate elevations exceeding 250 mg/dL have been reported to increase coronary risk in young subjects. Moreover, since patients with marked hypertriglyceridemia (> 100 mg/dL) are at risk for pancreatitis, pharmacologic therapy should be prescribed if they have not responded adequately to dietary measures. Nicotinic acid is an effective and inexpensive drug

that most lipid specialists favor to lower triglycerides. However, patient acceptance must be encouraged by physicians, since the drug has side effects of flushing and because it requires multiple doses per day. Gemfibrozil, while more expensive, is more readily tolerated and has proved to be quite effective in reducing triglyceride levels.

6. Type V (mixed lipemia)– This is a rare disorder wherein excessive prebetalipoproteins and chylomicrons are both present. Onset is usually in early adult life and is characterized by recurrent abdominal pain, pancreatitis, hepatosplenomegaly, eruptive xanthomas, and glucose intolerance. The disorder is markedly aggravated by alcohol excess.

Therapy is similar to that for type IV except that fat restriction is necessary as in type I.

7. Hyperlipoprotein(a)– Lipoprotein antigen, or Lp(a), is a recently characterized variant of LDL that is strongly correlated with the risk of coronary heart disease. This lipoprotein contains a unique large apoprotein consisting of an apo-B component linked to a second protein, apo(a), which is closely related to plasminogen in structure. The medial level of Lp(a) is 5–10 mg/dL, but 20% of people have elevated levels of 30–80 mg/dL, particularly if they have a history of myocardial infarction or a parental history of premature coronary artery disease. Elevated levels of Lp(a) increase coronary risk, and this risk is additive when LDL levels are also increased.

B. Secondary Hyperlipoproteinemias: In all cases of hyperlipoproteinemia, secondary forms should be ruled out before a diagnosis of primary genetic hyperlipoproteinemia is made. In uncontrolled diabetes mellitus, circulating levels of lipoprotein are often elevated along with glucose. Since lipoprotein lipase is an insulin-dependent enzyme, elevated levels of both chylomicrons and VLDL result from diabetes in which insulin levels are low (insulinopenic diabetes) or ineffective (insulin-insensitive diabetes). Replacement of deficient insulin or restriction of caloric intake to restore effectiveness of endogenous insulin in obese diabetics facilitates clearance of these lipoproteins. In addition, when lipemia is resolving after insulin replacement in insulin-deficient diabetics, an increase of betalipoproteins inevitably follows clearance of the larger triglyceride-carrying particles because of the much longer half-life of the betalipoproteins. Hyperbetalipoproteinemia is commonly a consequence of hypothyroidism or mild forms of nephrotic syndrome.

Hyperprebetalipoproteinemia and mixed lipemia can result from hypopituitarism, lipodystrophy, renal failure with azotemia, severe hypothyroidism, hypergammaglobulin disorders, or advanced nephrotic syndrome (with serum albumin below 2 g/dL). These lipemic manifestations are seen in genetically predisposed persons with mild diabetes mellitus or hyperestrogenemia (as in pregnancy or with oral contraceptive therapy) or in those who use alcohol excessively.

Dysbetalipoproteinemia can become apparent during hypothyroidism and revert to a latent state with thyroid replacement.

Antihypertensive therapy and serum lipids. Antihypertensive agents such as thiazide diuretics and β-adrenergic blockers have an adverse effect on serum lipids, tending to slightly raise serum levels of LDL cholesterol and triglycerides while at the same time lowering HDL cholesterol. Sensitivity differs among individuals; however, long-term adverse effects are generally minimal with lower doses of diuretics. Prazosin and clonidine lower serum LDL cholesterol and triglycerides while raising levels of HDL cholesterol. Angiotensin-converting enzyme inhibitors, calcium channel blockers, and captopril have no demonstrable effects on serum lipids.

Relationship of Lipoproteins to Atheroma (Fig 21–2)

Studies suggest that the arterial wall intima is permeable to small molecular complexes in inverse proportion to their size. Elastin, a component of arterial wall, has a demonstrable affinity for apoprotein B, which is present on all lipoproteins except HDL. Accordingly, small lipoproteins such as HDL, LDL, and certain of the smaller VLDL and remnants may enter through defects and tears in the intimal walls of arteries, where all except HDL adhere to elastin, which retards their exit and allows their accumulation. This would explain why chylomicrons, owing to their large size, are not considered atherogenic in type I disorders despite severe hypercholesterolemia and why hypertension, aging, and hyperlipidemia, either individually or (especially) in combination, could exaggerate normal atherogenic processes.

In addition to atheroma, thrombogenic factors contribute to cardiac risk. Hypertriglyceridemia and smoking may increase platelet aggregation and predispose to clotting as well as contribute to atherogenesis. For these reasons, avoiding tobacco, correcting hypertension, and lowering excessive serum triglyceride and LDL cholesterol levels are recommended for reduction of cardiac risk.

A number of recent studies have documented a consistent negative correlation between plasma concentration of HDL cholesterol and clinically evident atherosclerosis. In its transit through the wall of the artery, HDL may incorporate cholesteryl esters into its central core for recycling onto cell membranes or for transport to excretory systems in the liver. The presumed role of HDL in clearing cholesterol from tissues may account for the observed increase in risk of atherosclerosis when HDL levels are relatively low, as in obesity, diabetes, and hyperlipidemic disorders and in males, especially when physically inactive. Conversely, in persons with a lower than normal risk of atherosclerosis, such as chronic alcoholics, women of childbearing age, and marathon runners, there is a high level of HDL. The "scavenger" role of HDL in clearing cholesterol from tissues could slow down atherogenesis and thereby contribute to the apparent protective effect of high plasma HDL in relation to atherosclerosis.

Treatment

Treatment of the secondary hyperlipoproteinemias consists, where possible, of treatment of the primary disorder, eg, hypothyroidism, nephrotic syndrome, diabetes mellitus, obstructive jaundice, or estrogen excess due to use of oral contraceptives. In primary hyperlipoproteinemia, no one diet is effective in all the lipid transport disorders. Similarly, none of the pharmacologic agents are universally effective. An understanding of lipid transport mechanisms and drug actions has improved the therapeutic approach to the hyperlipidemic patient. Flow sheets recommended by an NIH expert panel are depicted in Figs 21–3 and 21–4 for classification and therapy based on elevated LDL cholesterol and the presence of coronary artery risk factors. See Chapter 1 for a discussion of the general approach to diagnosis and management of hypercholesterolemia, particularly in elderly individuals.

A. Diet Therapy: When chylomicrons are elevated, total fat intake should be reduced (including polyunsaturated fats) and alcohol avoided. In all other hyperlipidemias, certain general principles apply: Calories are restricted to achieve or maintain ideal body weight and daily cholesterol intake is limited to 300 mg, which results in an increase in high-affinity LDL receptors on cell membranes. Reduction of total fat in the diet to less than 30% is recommended, with less than 10% saturated, approximately 10% polyunsaturated, and 10–12% monounsaturated (eg, olive oil). Unsaturated fats improve palatability when saturated fats must be restricted and may have a beneficial role in reducing platelet factors that promote an in-

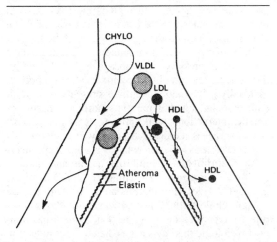

Figure 21–2. Lipoproteins and atheromas.

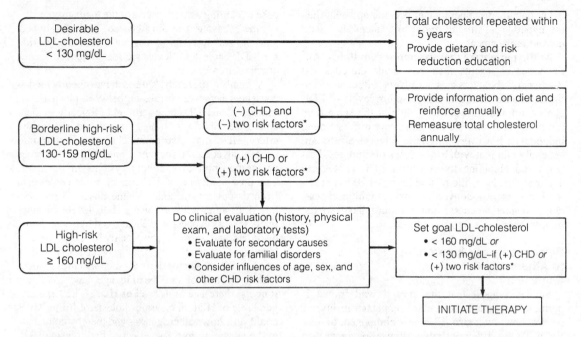

Figure 21–3. Management algorithm based on low-density lipoprotein (LDL) cholesterol. Clinical judgment should determine whether elderly patients whose benefit/risk ratio may be low should receive pharmacologic therapy. Asterisk means that one risk factor may be male sex (Table 21–12). CHD = coronary heart disease. (Modified from Report of the National Cholesterol Education Program Expert Panel on Detection, Evaluation, and Treatment of High Blood Cholesterol in Adults. Arch Int Med 1988;148:36.)

creased coagulability of blood. Alcohol is restricted when triglycerides are elevated but is permitted in moderation when the lipid elevation is predominantly in the LDL fraction.

Epidemiologic studies from the Netherlands indicate that over a 20-year follow-up period, mortality rates from coronary heart disease were more than 50% lower among those who consumed at least 30 g of fish per day than in those who did not eat fish. Moreover, a specific triglyceride-lowering effect has been produced by dietary fish oils containing highly unsaturated fatty acids of the omega-3 family (in which the first of 5 or 6 double bonds begins at the third carbon from the methyl terminal). Application of these principles of diet to the general population as a means of reducing the risk of atherosclerosis remains a controversial subject, particularly since hyperglycemia may be aggravated by large quantities of omega-3 fatty acids in diabetic patients.

B. Hypolipidemic Drugs: Several major classes of drugs are currently in use (Table 21–14):

1. Nicotinic acid–Nicotinic acid reduces lipolysis and diminishes production of VLDL and is equally effective at lowering LDL. The dosage is 100 mg 3 times daily initially, gradually building up to a level of 3–7 g daily taken with meals. Cutaneous flushing and pruritus, as well as gastrointestinal upsets and hyperuricemia, are major side effects, but the flushing is transient and readily tolerated if dosage increments are introduced gradually and the patient is warned

to anticipate it. Aspirin may also help to alleviate flushing. Nicotinic acid decreases the hepatic production of VLDL and is particularly useful in primary hyperbetalipoproteinemia when combined with resins that bind bile acids, but it may be effective in all types of primary hyperlipoproteinemia except type I. Nicotinic acid is less useful in treating lipid abnormalities in diabetic patients because of its tendency to aggravate hyperglycemia by interfering with the action of insulin.

2. Clofibrate–Clofibrate has many known effects in the body and both decreases the synthesis of VLDL and increases its catabolism. It is most effective in type III remnant excess but is of occasional value also in disorders with increased VLDL (IIB, IV, V). In cases of hyperbetalipoproteinemia, its effects have been less impressive. The dosage is 1.5–2 g daily. Side effects are few, but myositis has been reported, especially if hypoalbuminemia is present, as in lipidemia associated with nephrotic syndrome. Pharmacokinetic interactions with anticoagulants may occur. A major risk is increased frequency of cholelithiasis and a possible association with gastrointestinal cancer.

3. Gemfibrozil–Gemfibrozil is an analogue of clofibrate. It is primarily and highly effective in lowering triglycerides, and there is an associated increase in HDL cholesterol. When patients with elevated serum triglycerides have not responded to usual nonpharmacologic therapy such as diet, weight reduction (in case of obesity), avoiding ethanol, and normaliza-

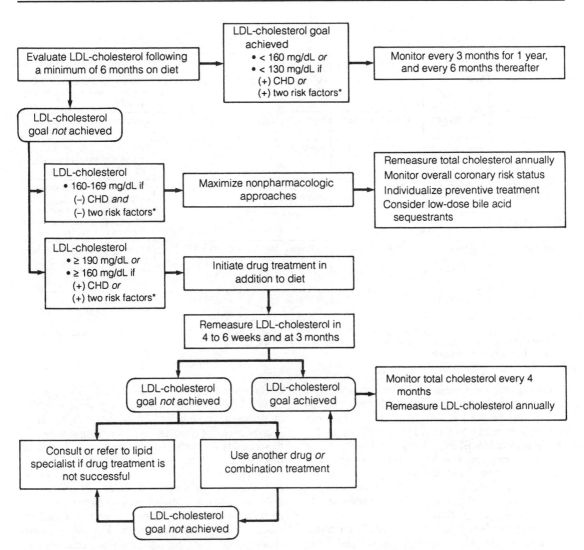

Figure 21–4. Indications for drug therapy of elevated LDL cholesterol. Clinical judgment should determine whether elderly patients whose benefit/risk ratio may be low should receive pharmacologic therapy. Asterisk means that one risk factor may be male sex (Table 21–12). CHD = coronary heart disease. (Modified from Report of the National Cholesterol Education Program Expert Panel on Detection, Evaluation, and Treatment of High Blood Cholesterol in Adults. Arch Int Med 1988;148:36.)

tion of glycemia in diabetics, gemfibrozil in a dose of 1200 mg/d (one 600-mg tablet before breakfast and dinner) is a reasonable choice for initial therapy. It is less useful in lowering LDL cholesterol levels in cases of hypercholesterolemia. Results of the Helsinki study suggest that gemfibrozil reduced the incidence of coronary heart disease by 34% in 4081 asymptomatic men without causing serious adverse effects. It lowered LDL cholesterol by 10% and serum triglycerides by 43%. Its side effects (similar to those of clofibrate) include gastrointestinal symptoms, occasional abnormalities in liver function, an increase in biliary lithogenicity, and potentiation of the effects of oral anticoagulants.

4. Resins to absorb bile acids (cholesty-

ramine, colestipol)–Cholestyramine is an insoluble resin that absorbs bile acids and is thus able to increase cholesterol catabolism and enhance LDL removal. It is not very palatable, and 16 –32 g/d is required in 2–4 divided doses, preferably in orange juice or applesauce. Flavored ''candy bar'' cholestyramine resins are also available and contain 4 g per bar (Cholybar). Gastrointestinal side effects, especially constipation, are common. Similar doses of colestipol are as effective as cholestyramine while being more palatable. VLDL excess is not helped and may be aggravated by these agents due to their tendency to increase VLDL production by the liver, thereby modestly raising serum triglyceride levels. They are the drugs of choice in treating types IIA and IIB, particularly when

Table 21–14. Summary of the major hypolipidemic drugs.[1]

Drugs	Reduce CHD Risk[2]	Long-Term Safety	Maintaining Adherence	LDL Cholesterol Lowering	Special Precautions
Nicotinic acid	Yes	Yes	Requires considerable education	15–30%	Test for hyperuricemia, hypoglycemia, and liver function abnormalities.
Clofibrate	Not proved	Not established	Relatively easy	Minimal	Myositis (when albumin is <2 g/dL). Lithogenic.
Gemfibrozil	Yes	Yes	Relatively easy	8–15%	Gemfibrozil is lithogenic and should not be used in patients with gallbladder disease.
Cholestyramine, colestipol	Yes	Yes	Requires considerable education	15–30%	Can alter absorption of other drugs and can raise triglyceride levels; should not be used in patients with hypertriglyceridemia.
Probucol	Not proved	Not established	Relatively easy	10–15%	Lowers HDL cholesterol; significance of this has not been established; prolongs QT interval.
Lovastatin	Not proved	Not established	Very easy	25–45%	Monitor for liver function and muscle enzyme abnormalities.

[1] Modified from Cleeman JI: Report of the National Cholesterol Education Program expert panel on detection, evaluation, and treatment of high blood cholesterol in adults. *Arch Intern Med* 1988;**148**:36.
[2] CHD = coronary heart disease.

combined with nicotinic acid. In patients with type IIA hypercholesterolemia, combined therapy with colestipol and nicotinic acid resulted in complete and sustained normalization of LDL levels. Recently, psyllium (Metamucil) in a dosage of 1 tsp 3 times daily has been found to have cholesterol-lowering effects (see Anderson et al reference). Therefore, it can be very useful as an adjunct to resin therapy, since it abates the gritty texture of resins while correcting their constipating effects.

5. Probucol–Probucol is reported to modestly lower serum cholesterol levels by as yet undefined mechanisms, but its major effect may be to protect blood vessels from the harmful effects of hypercholesterolemia. Probucol is an antioxidant that has the unique feature among lipid-lowering drugs of also reducing tissue deposition of LDL, which appears to be an oxidation-dependent phenomenon. Rabbits with LDL receptor deficiency are protected from atherosclerosis by probucol despite very high serum LDL cholesterol levels, and patients with hypercholesterolemia showed regression of xanthoma during probucol therapy. Probucol in doses of 500 mg twice daily is generally well tolerated, but cardiotoxicity in animals, a prolonged QT interval in humans, and a reduction of HDL cholesterol levels in addition to LDL cholesterol levels make further trials necessary before the benefit-to-risk ratio can be properly assessed.

6. HMG-CoA reductase inhibitors–The most effective therapy at present for lowering elevated LDL cholesterol levels includes drugs that competitively inhibit HMG-CoA reductase, the rate-limiting enzyme in cholesterol biosynthesis. Reduction in biosynthesis

of cholesterol induces increased numbers of high-affinity LDL receptors on cell membranes, resulting in increased clearance of LDL from serum. In homozygous cases of familial hyperbetalipoproteinemia, these agents are ineffective owing to the absence of functioning LDL receptors. However, in heterozygotes, clinical trials have shown lovastatin (Mevacor) to be extremely effective in lowering LDL cholesterol as much as 40% in conjunction with diet and as much as 65% when combined with other drugs such as nicotinic acid or bile sequestrants. The recommended starting dose is 20 mg once daily with the evening meal; this can be raised at monthly intervals to a maximum of 80 mg/d divided into 2 doses. Side effects are surprisingly minimal, with only myositis reported in approximately 0.5% and subclinical serum transaminase elevations in 1.5%. However, its long-term safety cannot be ascertained until patients have been followed over longer periods of therapy.

Anderson JW et al: Cholesterol-lowering effects of psyllium hydrophilic mucilloid for hypercholesterolemic men. Arch Intern Med 1988;148:292.

Cleeman JI: Report of the National Cholesterol Education Program Expert Panel on detection, evaluation, and treatment of high blood cholesterol in adults. Arch Intern Med 1988;148:36.

Denke MA, Grundy SM: Hypercholesterolemia in elderly persons: Resolving the treatment dilemma. Ann Intern Med 1990;112:780.

Frick MH et al: Helsinki Heart Study: Primary-prevention trial with gemfibrozil in middle-aged men with dyslipidemia. Safety of treatment, changes in risk factors, and incidence of coronary heart disease. N Engl J Med 1987;317:1237.

Garber AM, Sox HC Jr, Littenberg B: Screening asymptomatic adults for cardiac risk factors: The serum cholesterol level. Ann Intern Med 1989;110:622.

Garg A, Grundy SM: Lovastatin for lowering cholesterol levels in non-insulin-dependent diabetes mellitus. N Engl J Med 1988;318:81.

Garg A, Grundy SM: Management of dyslipidemia in NIDDM. Diabetes Care 1990;13:153.

Gordon DJ, Rifkind BM: High-density lipoprotein: The clinical implications of recent studies. N Engl J Med 1989;321:1311.

Havel RJ, Yamada N, Shames DM: Role of apolipoprotein E in lipoprotein metabolism. Am Heart J 1987; 113:470.

Kane JP, Malloy MJ: When to treat hyperlipidemia. Adv Intern Med 1988;33:143.

Malloy MJ et al: Complementarity of colestipol, niacin, and lovastatin in treatment of severe familial hypercholesterolemia. Ann Intern Med 1987;107:616.

O'Connor P, Feely J, Shepherd J: Lipid lowering drugs. Br Med J 1990;300:667.

Rohlfing JJ, Brunzell JD: The effects of diuretics and adrenergic-blocking agents on plasma lipids. West J Med 1986; 145:210.

Seed M et al: Relation of serum lipoprotein(a) concentration and apolipoprotein(a) phenotype to coronary heart disease in patients with familial hypercholesterolemia. N Engl J Med 1990;322:1494.

Steinberg D et al: Beyond cholesterol: Modifications of low-density lipoprotein that increase its atherogenicity. N Engl J Med 1989;320:915.

Taylor WC et al: Cholesterol reduction and life expectancy: A model incorporating multiple risk factors. Ann Intern Med 1987;106:605.

Tobert JA: Efficacy and long-term adverse effect pattern of lovastatin. Am J Cardiol 1988;62:28.

22

Nutrition

Robert B. Baron, MD

NUTRITIONAL REQUIREMENTS

Approximately 40 nutrients are required by the human body. Nutrients are considered essential if they cannot be synthesized by the body and if a deficiency causes recognizable abnormalities that disappear when the deficit is corrected. Required nutrients include the essential amino acids, water-soluble vitamins, fat-soluble vitamins, minerals, and the essential fatty acids. The body also requires an adequate energy substrate, a small amount of metabolizable carbohydrate, indigestible carbohydrate (fiber), additional nitrogen, and water.

Most of the required nutrients are harmful when consumed in excessive amounts. Thus, a range of acceptable intake levels can be established for most of them.

Nutritional requirements are most commonly expressed as the average daily amounts of nutrients a population group should consume. Requirements for any given individual cannot be stated, because of the great range of biologic variability. In the USA, the most widely used estimates of nutritional requirements are the Recommended Dietary Allowances (RDAs) developed by a subcommittee of the Food and Nutrition Board of the National Academy of Sciences. RDAs have been established for energy and protein; the water-soluble vitamins thiamine, riboflavin, niacin, vitamin B_6, folic acid, vitamin B_{12}, and vitamin C; the fat-soluble vitamins A, D, and K; and the minerals calcium, phosphorus, magnesium, iron, zinc, iodine, and selenium (Table 22–1).

The RDA Subcommittee has also established "estimated safe and adequate intakes" for 7 additional nutrients. These include the vitamins pantothenic acid and biotin and the trace elements copper, chromium, fluoride, manganese, and molybdenum. Minimal requirements for the electrolytes sodium, potassium, and chloride are also given by the RDA Subcommittee.

The RDAs exceed the actual requirements of most individuals in the population because they are stated as 2 standard deviations above the estimated mean requirement. Therefore, a dietary intake of less than the RDA of a specific nutrient is not necessarily inadequate for a given individual—it increases the *risk* of an inadequate intake. For most clinical situations, two-thirds of the RDA is considered an adequate nutritional intake.

The RDAs for energy are treated in a different manner. Because energy needs vary so greatly among individuals, the RDA Committee sets forth estimates of the average needs of the population rather than recommended intakes for individuals. About half of the population will require more energy than the RDA and half will require less.

Nutritional requirements vary not only from one individual to the next but from one day to the next in any given subject. They differ also with age, sex, and body size and during pregnancy and lactation. Different RDAs have been developed for different age and sex groups. Requirements vary also with such clinical circumstances as premature birth, aging, metabolic disorders, infections, chronic illness, medications, extremes of climate and physical activity, and the route of ingestion. The RDAs do not cover such situations—they are intended only for healthy populations.

ENERGY

The human body requires energy to support normal functions and physical activity, growth, and repair of damaged tissues. Energy is provided by oxidation of dietary protein, fat, carbohydrate, and alcohol. Oxidation of 1 g of each provides 4 kcal of energy from protein and carbohydrate, 9 kcal from fat, and 7 kcal from alcohol.

In healthy individuals, energy expenditure is primarily determined by 3 factors: basal energy expenditure (BEE), diet-induced thermogenesis (DIT), and physical activity.

The BEE is the amount of energy required to maintain basic physiologic functions. It is measured under a defined set of circumstances. The subject must be in a warm room, awake, and at rest and must not have eaten for 12 hours. In healthy persons, the BEE (in kcal/24h) can be estimated by the Harris-Benedict equation, which will correctly predict measured BEE in 90% ± 10% of healthy subjects. In clinical practice, patients rarely meet the strict criteria for basal status. Energy expenditure measured in individuals at

Table 22–1. Recommended daily dietary allowances for adults (revised 1989).[1]

		Weight		Height				Fat-Soluble Vitamins				Water-Soluble Vitamins							Minerals						
Category	Age (years) or Condition	(kg)	(lb)	(cm)	(in)	Protein (g)	Vita-min A (µg RE)	Vita-min D (µg)	Vita-min E (mg α-TE)	Vita-min K (µg)	Vita-min C (mg)	Thia-mine (mg)	Ribo-flavin (mg)	Niacin (mg NE)	Vita-min B6 (mg)	Folate (µg)	Vitamin B12 (µg)	Cal-cium (mg)	Phos-phorus (mg)	Mag-nesium (mg)	Iron (mg)	Zinc (mg)	Iodine (µg)	Sele-nium (µg)
Males	15–18	66	145	176	69	59	1,000	10	10	65	60	1.5	1.8	20	2.0	200	2.0	1,200	1,200	400	12	15	150	50
	19–24	72	160	177	70	58	1,000	10	10	70	60	1.5	1.7	19	2.0	200	2.0	1,200	1,200	350	10	15	150	70
	25–50	79	174	176	70	63	1,000	5	10	80	60	1.5	1.7	19	2.0	200	2.0	800	800	350	10	15	150	70
	51+	77	170	173	68	63	1,000	5	10	80	60	1.2	1.4	15	2.0	200	2.0	800	800	350	10	15	150	70
Females	15–18	55	120	163	64	44	800	10	8	55	60	1.1	1.3	15	1.5	180	2.0	1,200	1,200	300	15	12	150	50
	19–24	58	128	164	65	46	800	10	8	60	60	1.1	1.3	15	1.6	180	2.0	1,200	1,200	280	15	12	150	55
	25–50	63	138	163	64	50	800	5	8	65	60	1.1	1.3	15	1.6	180	2.0	800	800	280	15	12	150	55
	51+	65	143	160	63	50	800	5	8	65	60	1.0	1.2	13	1.6	180	2.0	800	800	280	10	12	150	55
Pregnant						60	800	10	10	65	70	1.5	1.6	17	2.2	400	2.2	1,200	1,200	320	30	15	175	65
Lactating	1st 6 months					65	1,300	10	12	65	95	1.6	1.8	20	2.1	280	2.6	1,200	1,200	355	15	19	200	75
	2nd 6 months					62	1,200	10	11	65	90	1.6	1.7	20	2.1	260	2.6	1,200	1,200	340	15	16	200	75

[1] From: National Research Council: *Recommended Dietary Allowances*, 10th ed. National Academy of Sciences, 1989.

Table 22–2. Average energy calories expended per hour by adults at selected weights engaged in various activities.[1]

Activity	54 kg (120 lb)	64 kg (140 lb)	73 kg (160 lb)	82 kg (180 lb)	91 kg (200 lb)	100 kg (220 lb)
Sleeping: Reclining	50	58	69	78	86	99
Very light: Sitting	73	83	103	115	127	150
Light: Walking on level, shopping, light housekeeping	143	166	200	225	250	290
Moderate: Cycling, dancing, skiing, tennis	226	262	307	345	382	430
Heavy: Walking uphill, shoveling, swimming, playing basketball or football	440	512	598	670	746	840

Note: Range of rate of expenditure of calories per minute of activity (for a 70-kg man or a 58-kg woman): Sleeping, 0.9–1.2; very light, 1.5–2.5; light, 2–4.9; moderate, 5–7.4; heavy, 6–12.
[1] Data from: *Recommended Dietary Allowances,* 9th ed. National Academy of Sciences—National Research Council, 1980. Adapted from McArdle WD, Katch FI, Katch VL: *Exercise Physiology: Energy, Nutrition and Human Performance.* Lea & Febiger, 1981.

rest without food for 2 hours is the resting metabolic expenditure (RME) and is about 10% greater than BEE.

Diet-induced thermogenesis (DIT) is the amount of energy expended during and following the ingestion of food. The precise cause of this increase in energy expenditure is still uncertain. DIT averages approximately 10% of the BEE.

Physical activity has a major impact on energy expenditure. The average energy expenditure per hour by adults engaged in typical activities is shown in Table 22–2.

Daily recommended energy intakes for healthy individuals are shown in Table 22–3.

PROTEIN

Protein is required for growth and for maintenance of body structure and function. Although the nutri-

Table 22–3. Median heights and weights and recommended energy intake (REE).[1]

Category	Age (years) or Condition	Weight (kg)	Weight (lb)	Height (cm)	Height (in)	REE (kcal/d)	Multiples of REE	Per kg	Per day[3]
Infants	0.0–0.5	6	13	60	24	320		108	650
	0.5–1.0	9	20	71	28	500		98	850
Children	1–3	13	29	90	35	740		102	1300
	4–6	20	44	112	44	950		90	1800
	7–10	28	62	132	52	1330		70	2000
Males	11–14	45	99	157	62	1440	1.70	55	2500
	15–18	66	145	176	69	1760	1.67	45	3000
	19–24	72	160	177	70	1780	1.67	40	2900
	25–50	79	174	176	70	1800	1.60	37	2900
	51+	77	170	173	68	1530	1.50	30	2300
Females	11–14	46	101	157	62	1310	1.67	47	2200
	15–18	55	120	163	64	1370	1.60	40	2200
	19–24	58	128	164	65	1350	1.60	38	2200
	25–50	63	138	163	64	1380	1.55	36	2200
	51+	65	143	160	63	1280	1.50	30	1900
Pregnant	1st trimester								+0
	2nd trimester								+300
	3rd trimester								+300
Lactating	1st 6 months								+500
	2nd 6 months								+500

Average Energy Allowance[2] (kcal) spans the last three columns (Multiples of REE, Per kg, Per day[3]).

[1] From: National Reserach Council: *Recommended Dietary Allowances,* 19th ed. National Academy of Sciences, 1989.
[2] In the range of light to moderate activity, the coefficient of variation is ±20%.
[3] Figure is rounded.

tional requirement is commonly stated in grams of protein, the true requirement is for 9 **essential amino acids** plus additional nitrogen for protein synthesis. The essential amino acids are leucine, isoleucine, lysine, methionine, phenylalanine, threonine, tryptophan, valine, and histidine.

Adequate protein must be consumed each day to replace essential amino acids lost through protein turnover. On a protein-free diet, the average male loses 3.8 g of nitrogen per day—equivalent to 24 g of protein. Allowing for differences in protein quality and utilization and for individual variability, the RDA for protein is 56 g/d for men and 45 g/d for women.

Amino acids are required by the body in a specific pattern very similar to that found in egg protein. Proteins that most closely resemble this pattern are commonly referred to as "high-quality" (milk, eggs, other animal proteins), while others with lower amounts of one or more amino acids are considered to be of "lower quality" (seeds, grains, other vegetable proteins). Actually, the amino acid composition of various food proteins represents a continuum of quality. Proteins of "lower quality" can be ingested with other "low-quality" proteins to provide amounts of deficient amino acids sufficient to make up a protein intake of high quality.

Protein and energy requirements are closely related. Diets that provide insufficient energy will require additional protein to maintain nitrogen equilibrium.

CARBOHYDRATE

As long as adequate energy and protein are provided in the diet, there is no specific requirement for dietary carbohydrate. A small amount of carbohydrate—approximately 100 g/d—is necessary to prevent ketosis. In practice, however, most dietary energy should be provided by carbohydrate. In the USA, the average diet contains 45% of calories as carbohydrate. Current recommendations are to increase carbohydrate intakes to 55–60% of total calories in the diet.

Dietary carbohydrates include simple sugars, complex carbohydrates (starches), and undigestible carbohydrates (dietary fiber). Although simple sugars and complex carbohydrates provide equal amounts of calories, the bulk of dietary carbohydrates should be derived from starches. Sugars—particularly sucrose—are concentrated sources of calories without other sources of essential nutrients. Sucrose consumption is also thought to be an important factor in the development of tooth decay. Complex carbohydrates, when unrefined, provide carbohydrate calories and vitamins, minerals, and dietary fiber.

Dietary fiber is that portion of plant foods that cannot be digested by the human intestine. Fiber increases the bulk of the stool and facilitates excretion. Epidemiologic evidence suggests that diets high in dietary fiber are associated with a lower incidence of digestive and cardiovascular diseases. The more insoluble fibers, such as those found in wheat bran, have the greatest impact on colonic function. Soluble fibers such as those found in legumes, oats, and fruit result in lower blood sugar levels in diabetics and lower blood cholesterol.

FAT

Dietary fat is the most concentrated source of food energy. Like energy from dietary carbohydrate, energy derived from fat can support protein synthesis. Dietary fat also provides the essential fatty acid linoleic acid. Other than the need for adequate quantities of linoleic acid, there is no specific requirement for dietary fat as long as the diet provides adequate nutrients oxidizable for energy. Although the average American diet contains 40% of calories as fat, current recommendations are to limit dietary fat to 30% or less of total calories. Diets containing as little as 5–10% of total calories as fat appear to be safe and well tolerated.

Dietary fats are composed chiefly of fatty acids and dietary cholesterol. Fatty acids contain either no double bonds (saturated), one double bond (monounsaturated), or more than one double bond (polyunsaturated). Typical American diets contain predominantly saturated fatty acids. Current recommendations are to equalize the intake of saturated, monounsaturated, and polyunsaturated fatty acids. Saturated fatty acids are associated with increased dietary cholesterol, while polyunsaturated fatty acids lower serum cholesterol. Monounsaturated fatty acids, which were previously thought to have no significant effect on serum cholesterol, have recently been shown to lower it. Saturated fats are solid at room temperature and in general are derived from animal foods; unsaturated fats are liquid at room temperature and in general are derived from plant foods.

The polyunsaturated fatty acid **linoleic acid** is an essential nutrient, required by the body for the synthesis of arachidonic acid, the major precursor of prostaglandins. Deficiencies of linoleic acid result in dermatitis, hair loss, and impaired wound healing. For individuals with average energy requirements, approximately 5 g of linoleic acid per day—1–2% of total calories—is required to prevent essential fatty acid deficiency. The polyunsaturated fatty acid **linolenic acid** is also an essential fatty acid in some mammalian species, but its role in human nutrition is less clear. Most foods that contain linoleic acid also contain linolenic acid. If there is a human requirement for linolenic acid, it would be met by diets that provide adequate linoleic acid.

Cholesterol is a major constituent of cell membranes. It is synthesized easily by the body and is not an essential nutrient. Diets that contain large amounts of cholesterol partially inhibit endogenous cholesterol synthesis but result in a net increase in serum cholesterol concentrations because of suppression of synthesis of low-density lipoprotein receptors. Average American diets contain approximately 450 mg/d of cholesterol. Current recommendations are to limit dietary cholesterol to 300 mg or less per day.

VITAMINS

Vitamins are a heterogeneous group of organic molecules required by the body for a variety of essential metabolic functions. They are grouped as **water-soluble vitamins:** thiamine, riboflavin, niacin, vitamin B_6 (pyridoxine), vitamin B_{12} (cobalamin), folacin, pantothenic acid, biotin, and vitamin C (ascorbic acid); and **fat-soluble vitamins:** A, D, E, and K. Disorders of vitamin metabolism are discussed on pp. 908-912.

MINERALS

The body also requires a number of inorganic minerals, commonly grouped as the **major minerals** calcium, magnesium, and phosphorus; the **electrolytes** sodium, potassium, and chloride; and the **trace elements** iron, zinc, copper, manganese, molybdenum, fluoride, iodine, cobalt, chromium, and selenium. Important characteristics of major and electrolytes summarized in Table 22–4.

DRUG-NUTRIENT INTERACTIONS

Many commonly used medications can have important effects on nutritional requirements. Chronic therapy with a variety of drugs can induce nutrient deficiencies by appetite suppression, intestinal malabsorption, and alterations in nutrient metabolism. The effects of selected drugs on nutrient absorption and metabolism are summarized in Table 22–5.

DIETARY RECOMMENDATIONS

Prior to 1977, the emphasis in nutrition education and diet planning was to ensure that the RDAs were met by diets that contained a wide variety of foods. The most important dietary education tool used for this purpose was *The Four Food Groups,* published by the United States Department of Agriculture and the National Dairy Council. According to this model, 2 servings per day from both the milk group and the meat group and 4 servings per day from both the fruit and vegetable group and the cereal group would meet the minimal nutritional requirements for most individuals.

Although this model does ensure that the RDAs are met by a variety of foods, it does not guarantee that the individual foods selected are of high quality. The effects of food processing on the nutrient density of food, the balance of macronutrients (percentages of fat, carbohydrate, and protein), and the character

Table 22–4. Essential macrominerals: Summary of major characteristics.[1]

Elements	Functions	Deficiency Disease or Symptoms	Toxicity Disease or Symptoms
Calcium	Constituent of bones, teeth; regulation of nerve, muscle function.	Children: rickets. Adults: osteomalacia. May contribute to osteoporosis.	Occurs with excess absorption due to hypervitaminosis D or hypercalcemia due to hyperparathyroidism, or idiopathic hypercalcemia.
Phosphorus	Constituent of bones, teeth, ATP, phosphorylated metabolic intermediates. Nucleic acids.	Children: rickets. Adults: osteomalacia.	Low serum $Ca^{2+}:P_i$ ratio stimulates secondary hyperparathyroidism; may lead to bone loss.
Sodium	Principal cation in extracellular fluid. Regulates plasma volume, acid-base balance, nerve and muscle function, Na^+/K^+-ATPase.	Unknown on normal diet; secondary to injury or illness.	Hypertension (in susceptible individuals).
Potassium	Principal cation in intracellular fluid; nerve and muscle function, Na^+/K^+-ATPase.	Occurs secondary to illness, injury, or diuretic therapy; muscular weakness, paralysis, mental confusion.	Cardiac arrest, small bowel ulcers.
Chloride	Fluid and electrolyte balance; gastric fluid.	Infants fed salt-free formula. Secondary to vomiting, diuretic therapy, renal disease.	
Magnesium	Constituent of bones, teeth; enzyme cofactor (kinases, etc).	Secondary to malabsorption or diarrhea, alcoholism.	Depressed deep tendon reflexes and respiration.

[1] Reproduced, with permission, from Murray RK et al: *Harper's Biochemistry,* 21st ed. Appleton & Lange, 1988.
[2] Excess mineral intake produces toxic symptoms. Unless otherwise specified, symptoms include nonspecific nausea, diarrhea, and irritability.

Table 22–5. Effect of drugs on nutrient absorption and metabolism.[1]

Drug	Effect
Analgesics and anti-inflammatories	
Salicylates	Decreases serum ascorbic acid; increases urinary loss of ascorbic acid, potassium, and amino acids.
Sulfasalazine	Impairs folate absorption and antagonizes folate supplementation.
Antacids	
Aluminum antacids	Decrease absorption of phosphate and vitamin A.
Others	Alkaline destruction of thiamine; some decrease absorption of vitamin A, iron; steatorrhea.
Anticonvulsants	
Phenobarbital	Decreases serum folate; increases vitamin D and vitamin K turnover and may cause deficiency.
Phenytoin	Decreases serum folate; increases vitamin D and vitamin K and may cause deficiency.
Primidone	Decreases serum folate and vitamins B_6, B_{12}; decreases calcium absorption; increases vitamin D and vitamin K turnover and may cause deficiency.
Antimicrobials	
Neomycin	Binds bile acids and decreases absorption of fat, carotene; vitamins A, D, K, B_{12}; potassium, sodium, calcium, nitrogen.
Amphotericin B	Decreases serum magnesium and potassium.
Aminosalicyclic acid	Increases absorption of folate, vitamin B_{12}, iron, cholesterol, fat.
Chloramphenicol	Increases need for vitamins B_2, B_6, B_{12}; increases serum iron.
Penicillin	Hypokalemia; renal potassium wasting.
Tetracycline	Calcium, iron, magnesium inhibit drug absorption; decreases vitamin K synthesis.
Cycloserine	May decrease absorption of calcium, magnesium; may decrease serum folate and vitamins B_6, B_{12}; decreases protein synthesis.
Isoniazid	Vitamin B_6 antagonist; may cause deficiency.
Sulfonamides	Decrease absorption of folate; decrease serum folate, iron.
Nitrofurantoin	Decreases serum folate.
Pyrimethamine	Decreases serum B_{12} and folate.
Antimitotics	
Methotrexate	Decreases absorption of folate, vitamin B_{12}, and fat.
Colchicine	Decreases absorption of vitamin B_{12}, carotene, fat, sodium, potassium, cholesterol, lactose, nitrogen.
Cathartics	
Phenolphthalein	Malabsorption, hypokalemia; deficiency of vitamin D, calcium.
Mineral oil	Malabsorption; decreased absorption of vitamins A, D, K.
Diuretics	Some cause hypokalemia, hypomagnesemia; may increase urinary excretion of vitamins B_1, B_6; calcium, magnesium, potassium.
Hypocholesterolemics	
Cholestyramine	Binds bile acids; decreases absorption of fat, carotene; vitamins A, D, K, B_{12}; folate, iron.
Clofibrate	Decreases absorption of carotene, vitamin B_{12}, iron, glucose.
Hypotensives	
Hydralazine	Vitamin B_6 deficiency.
Captopril	May cause hyponatremia, hyperkalemia; decreased taste acuity.
Oral contraceptives	Vitamin B_6, folate deficiency; may increase the need for other nutrients.

of macronutrients (simple versus complex carbohydrate; saturated versus unsaturated fat) are omitted.

Since 1977, literally dozens of governmental, professional, and public health agencies and associations have published dietary recommendations that attempt to deal with these issues. Although attention has been directed to the differences between these reports, most agree on the basic principles of eating a wide variety of foods; increasing the consumption of foods containing complex carbohydrates; restricting the intake of sugar, fat (particularly saturated fat), cholesterol, salt, and alcohol; and maintaining an ideal body weight.

The 2 most important recent publications are *The Surgeon General's Report on Nutrition and Health* (1988) and the National Research Council's *Diet and Health* (1989). Although both reports reflect similar

Table 22–6. Summary of dietary recommendations published by the Surgeon General and the National Research Council.

	Surgeon General's *Report on Nutrition and Health* (1988)	National Research Council's *Diet and Health* (1989)
Fats and cholesterol	Reduce consumption (especially saturated fat) and cholesterol.	Reduce total fat intake to 30% or less of calories and cholesterol to less than 300 mg/d.
Energy and weight control	Achieve and maintain desirable body weight.	Balance food intake and physical activity to maintain appropriate body weight.
Complex carbohydrates and fiber	Increase consumption of whole grains, cereals, vegetables (including dried beans and peas), and fruits.	Eat 5 servings or more per day of a combination of vegetables and fruits. Also increase intake of starches and other complex carbohydrates by eating 6 servings per day of bread, cereals, and legumes. Increase carbohydrates to >55% of total calories.
Sodium	Reduce intake by choosing low-sodium foods and limiting added salt.	Limit salt (sodium chloride) to 6 < g.
Alcohol	Take in moderation (no more than 2 drinks per day).	Intake not recommended. For those who drink alcohol, limit consumption to 1 oz of pure alcohol per day.
Protein	Not specifically discussed.	Maintain protein intake at moderate levels (0.8–1.6 g/kg body weight per day).
Dietary supplements	Not specifically discussed.	Avoid taking dietary supplements in excess of the RDA in any one day.
Fluoride	Include in community water systems.	Maintain an optimal intake of fluoride, particularly during years of tooth formation and growth.
Sugars	Those vulnerable to dental caries, especially children, should limit consumption.	Maintain current intake.
Calcium	Adolescent girls and adult women should increase consumption.	Maintain adequate calcium intake.
Iron	Children, adolescents, and women of childbearing age should be sure to consume good sources of iron.	Not specifically discussed.

basic goals, the Surgeon General's report makes primarily qualitative recommendations while the National Research Council makes specific quantitative recommendations. These reports are contrasted in Table 22–6.

National Research Council: *Diet and Health: Implications for Reducing Chronic Disease Risk.* National Academy Press, 1989.

National Research Council: *Recommended Dietary Allowances,* 10th ed. National Academy Press, 1989.

US Department of Health and Human Services: *The Surgeon General's Report on Nutrition and Health.* DHHS (PHS) Publication No. 88–50210. US Government Printing Office, 1988.

ASSESSMENT OF NUTRITIONAL STATUS

The prevention and treatment of nutritional problems require the identification of patients at risk for the development of malnutrition and the identification of patients who already show symptoms and signs of malnutrition. Unfortunately, no single biochemical test or clinical technique is sufficiently accurate to serve as a reliable test for malnutrition. Current techniques of nutritional assessment utilize a combination of methods, including evaluation of dietary intake, anthropometric measurements, clinical examination, and laboratory tests. Some patients require serial measurements and close observation to confirm the diagnosis of malnutrition.

DIETARY HISTORY

Virtually all patients undergoing a complete history and physical examination should be asked screening dietary questions to help identify those high-risk patients who require further evaluation. Of particular importance are the regularity and availability of meals; who does the shopping and food preparation; recent changes in appetite, intake, or body weight; use of special diets or dietary supplements; use of alcohol, drugs, or medications; food preferences and food allergies; and the presence of illnesses that affect nutritional intakes, losses, or requirements. Elderly and adolescent patients, pregnant or lactating women, and the poor and socially isolated are at particular risk for nutritional problems.

Further quantification of dietary intake can be performed using a variety of techniques. **Twenty-four-hour diet recalls** can be performed quickly and easily and provide rough estimates of nutrient intakes. Patients are asked to describe their dietary intake over the preceding 24 hours, including snacks, beverages, and alcohol. Questions should be asked also about food preparation. Intake can then be rapidly assessed by determining the numbers of servings ingested from each food group and by evaluating the quality of food within each group. Problems with this technique include inaccurate reporting by patients, difficulties in estimating serving sizes, and the usual problems of generalizing from inadequate data: in this case, a single day's intake. These problems can be partially solved by showing the patient serving-size models and by repeating the procedure several times on different occasions.

More accurate quantitative information can be obtained by asking patients to complete a **3- to 5-day diet record.** Nutrient composition can then be analyzed with the aid of standard handbooks or computer software. Although this technique is prospective and less likely to be invalidated by memory lapses, omissions are still common as well as the usual difficulties in estimating serving sizes. Furthermore, 3–5 days may not be truly representative of long-term intakes because of random and seasonal variations and changes in eating behavior induced by record keeping.

ANTHROPOMETRICS

Anthropometric measurement is a method of assessing nutritional status by estimating body composition, particularly fat stores and skeletal muscle. The most commonly used measurements are those of height and weight, the triceps skin fold, and the mid arm muscle circumference. Because of great individual variation, the latter have limited applicability.

Evaluation of body weight is the most useful anthropometric technique. Body weight in relationship to height should be checked against reference tables of "desirable weights" (Table 22–7) and expressed as **relative weight:** Relative weights in excess of 120% are defined as obesity. Recent change in body weight is a better index of undernutrition than low relative weight. Changes in body weight are best expressed as the percentage of usually weight lost per unit of time. A loss of 10% or more of usual weight within a period of 1–2 months is generally considered to be predictive of a poor clinical outcome.

LABORATORY TESTS

Serum albumin is the most important test for the diagnosis of protein-calorie undernutrition. Most patients with severe protein depletion will have abnormally low serum albumin levels. Unfortunately, many nonnutritional conditions can also cause low levels of serum albumin—particularly liver disease and se-

Table 22–7. Reference height and body weight ranges for adult males and females.[1,2]

Height, Men and Women		Weight, lb (kg)					
		Men			Women		
in	cm	Small Frame	Medium Frame	Large Frame	Small Frame	Medium Frame	Large Frame
58	147	. . .	. . .	. . .	102–111 (46–50)	109–121 (49–55)	118–131 (54–59)
59	150	. . .	. . .	. . .	103–113 (47–51)	111–123 (50–56)	120–134 (54–61)
60	152	. . .	. . .	. . .	104–115 (47–52)	113–126 (51–57)	122–137 (55–62)
61	155	. . .	. . .	. . .	106–118 (48–54)	115–129 (52–59)	125–140 (57–64)
62	158	128–134 (58–61)	131–141 (59–64)	138–150 (63–68)	108–121 (49–55)	118–132 (54–60)	128–143 (58–65)
63	160	130–136 (59–62)	133–143 (60–65)	140–153 (64–69)	111–124 (50–56)	121–135 (55–61)	131–147 (59–67)
64	163	132–138 (60–63)	135–145 (61–66)	142–156 (64–71)	114–127 (52–58)	124–138 (56–63)	134–151 (61–68)
65	165	134–140 (61–64)	137–148 (62–67)	144–160 (65–73)	117–130 (53–59)	127–141 (58–64)	137–155 (62–70)
66	168	136–142 (62–65)	139–151 (63–68)	146–164 (66–74)	120–133 (54–60)	130–144 (59–65)	140–159 (64–72)
67	170	138–145 (63–66)	142–154 (64–69)	149–168 (68–76)	123–136 (56–62)	133–147 (60–67)	143–163 (65–74)
68	173	140–148 (64–67)	145–157 (66–71)	152–172 (69–78)	126–139 (57–63)	136–150 (62–68)	146–167 (66–76)
69	175	142–151 (64–68)	148–160 (67–73)	155–176 (70–80)	129–142 (59–64)	139–153 (63–69)	149–170 (68–77)
70	178	144–154 (65–69)	151–163 (68–74)	158–180 (72–82)	132–145 (60–66)	142–156 (64–71)	152–173 (69–78)
71	181	146–157 (66–71)	154–166 (70–75)	161–184 (73–83)	135–148 (61–67)	145–159 (66–72)	155–176 (70–80)
72	183	149–160 (68–73)	157–170 (71–77)	164–188 (74–85)	138–151 (63–68)	148–162 (67–73)	158–179 (71–81)
73	185	152–164 (69–74)	160–174 (73–79)	168–192 (76–87)	. . .	. . .	. . .
74	188	155–168 (70–76)	164–178 (74–81)	172–197 (78–89)	. . .	. . .	. . .
75	190	158–172 (72–78)	167–182 (76–83)	176–202 (80–92)	. . .	. . .	. . .
76	193	162–176 (73–80)	171–187 (78–85)	181–207 (82–94)	. . .	. . .	. . .

[1] From: Metropolitan Life Foundation: 1983 Metropolitan height and weight tables. *Stat Bull Metropol Life Insur Co* 1983;**64**:2.
[2] Ages 25 through 59, for 5 lb of indoor clothing for men and 3 lb of indoor clothing for women, and 1-in heels for both.

vere illness in general. Other serum proteins with shorter half-lives (transferrin, prealbumin, etc) may more accurately reflect short-term changes in nutritional status but suffer from similar shortcomings.

Qualitative and quantitative tests of cellular immunity are also abnormal in many patients with protein-calorie undernutrition. Measurements of the **total lymphocyte count** and **delayed hypersensitivity reactions** to common skin test antigens are commonly used but are also nonspecific; ie, abnormalities may be due to nonnutritional factors.

Thus, the use of laboratory tests to diagnose protein-calorie malnutrition is limited by confounding factors that make the tests unreliable for differentiating malnutrition from nonnutritional health disorders. The judicious interpretation of these tests, however—particularly the serum albumin—may help to confirm the diagnosis of protein-calorie undernutrition in selected patients. Despite their uncertain diagnostic utility, these tests are useful prognostic indicators. Patients with abnormal nutritional assessment parameters have a markedly increased risk of poor clinical outcomes. Combining the tests into quantitative indices further improves their prognostic validity.

CLINICAL EXAMINATION

Clinical evaluation is the most important aspect of the assessment of nutritional status. A **nutritionally focused history and physical examination** should be performed on each patient at risk for nutritional problems. The history emphasizes recent reduction in dietary intake, weight loss, and evaluation of the patient's functional status. The physical examination focuses on muscle wasting, fat stores, volume status, and signs of micronutrient deficiencies (Table 22–8). This type of clinical assessment has recently been demonstrated to be more accurate than techniques relying primarily on laboratory tests or anthropometry.

Despite these techniques, it is often difficult to confirm a diagnosis of malnutrition. Continued close observation is often necessary. Monitoring dietary intakes during hospitalization can be quite helpful. **Calorie counts** by registered dietitians can be used to estimate energy and protein intakes for comparison with estimated requirements. Serial measurements of body weight and serial clinical assessments should also be performed.

Table 22–8. Clinical signs that may be due to nutrient deficiency.

Clinical Sign	Nutrient	Clinical Sign	Nutrient
Hair		**Mouth (cont'd)**	
Transverse depigmentation	Protein, copper	Atrophic lingual papillae	Niacin, iron, riboflavin, folate, vitamin B_{12}
Easily pluckable	Protein	Hypogeusia	Zinc, vitamin A
Sparse and thin	Protein, zinc, biotin	Tongue fissuring	Niacin
Skin		**Neck**	
Dry, scaling	Zinc, vitamin A, essential fatty acids	Goiter	Iodine
Flaky paint dermatitis	Protein, niacin, riboflavin	**Chest**	
Follicular hyperkeratosis	Vitamins A and C	Thoracic rosary	Vitamin D
Perifollicular petechiae	Vitamin C	**Heart**	
Petechiae, purpura	Vitamins C and K	High-output failure	Thiamine
Pigmentation, desquamation	Niacin	Decreased output	Protein-calorie
Nasolabial seborrhea	Niacin, riboflavin, pyridoxine	**Abdomen**	
Pallor	Iron, folate, vitamin B_{12}, copper	Hepatosplenomegaly	Protein-calorie
		Distention	Protein-calorie
Scrotal/vulvar dermatoses	Riboflavin	Diarrhea	Niacin, folate, vitamin B_{12}
Subcutaneous fat loss	Calorie	**Extremities**	
Nails		Muscle tenderness, pain	Thiamine, vitamin C
Spooning	Iron	Muscle wasting	Protein-calorie
Transverse lines, ridging	Protein-calorie	Edema	Protein, thiamine
Head		Bone tenderness	Vitamin D, vitamin C, calcium, phosphorus
Temporal muscle wasting	Protein-calorie		
Parotid enlargement	Protein	**Neurologic**	
Eyes		Hyporeflexia	Thiamine
Night blindness	Vitamin A, zinc	Decreased position and vibratory sense	Vitamin B_{12}, thiamine
Corneal vascularization	Riboflavin		
Xerosis, Bitot spots, keratomalacia	Vitamin A	Paresthesias	Vitamin B_{12}, thiamine, niacin
		Confabulation, disorientation	Thiamine
Conjunctival inflammation	Riboflavin	Dementia	Niacin
Mouth		Ophthalmoplegia	Thiamine, phosphorus
Glossitis (scarlet, raw)	Niacin, pyridoxine, riboflavin, vitamin B_{12}, folate	Tetany	Calcium, magnesium
		Other	
Bleeding gums	Vitamin C, riboflavin	Delayed wound healing	Zinc, protein-calorie, vitamin C
Cheilosis	Riboflavin		
Angular stomatitis	Riboflavin, iron		

Detsky AS et al: What is subjective global assessment of nutritional status? JPEN 1987;11:8.

NUTRITIONAL DISORDERS

PROTEIN-CALORIE UNDERNUTRITION

Protein-calorie undernutrition occurs as a result of a relative or absolute deficiency of calories and protein. For most developing nations, protein-calorie undernutrition remains the most important nutritional problem and among the most significant of all health problems. Classically, protein-calorie undernutrition has been described as 2 distinct syndromes. **Kwashiorkor,** caused by a deficiency of protein in the presence of adequate calories, is typically seen in weaning infants at the birth of a sibling in areas where foods containing protein are insufficiently abundant. **Marasmus,** caused by combined protein and calorie deficiency, is most commonly seen where adequate quantities of food are not available.

In industrialized societies, protein-calorie undernutrition is most commonly seen among hospitalized medical and surgical patients. As many as 20% of all patients admitted to hospital have significant protein-calorie undernutrition. In these patients, protein-calorie undernutrition is caused either by decreased intake of calories and protein, increased nutrient losses, or increased nutrient requirements dictated by the underlying illness. For example, diminished oral intake may result from poor dentition or various gastrointestinal disorders. Loss of nutrients results from malabsorption and diarrhea as well as from glycosuria. Requirements are increased by fever, surgery, neoplasia, and burns. Few patients are sick enough to require acute hospitalization without manifesting some of these risk factors.

Pathophysiology

Protein-calorie undernutrition results in important pathophysiologic changes that can affect virtually every organ system. The most obvious results are loss of body weight, adipose stores, and skeletal muscle mass. Weight losses of 5–10% are usually tolerated without significant loss of physiologic function; losses of 35–40% of body weight usually result in death. Loss of protein from skeletal muscle and internal organs is usually proportionate to weight loss. Protein mass is lost from the liver, gastrointestinal tract, kidneys, and heart.

As protein-calorie undernutrition progresses, organ dysfunction may develop. Hepatic synthesis of serum proteins decreases, and depressed levels of circulating proteins may be observed. Cardiac output and contractility are decreased, and the ECG may show decreased voltage and a rightward axis shift. Autopsies of patients who die with severe undernutrition show myofibrillar atrophy and interstitial edema of the heart.

The lungs are affected primarily by weakness and atrophy of the muscles of respiration. Vital capacity and tidal volume are depressed, and mucociliary clearance is abnormal. The gastrointestinal tract is most importantly affected by mucosal atrophy and loss of villi of small intestine, resulting in a decrease in absorptive capacity. Intestinal disaccharidase deficiency and mild pancreatic insufficiency can also develop and result in malabsorption.

Changes in immunologic function are among the most important changes seen in protein-calorie undernutrition. The total lymphocyte count is commonly decreased, primarily because of a reduction in circulating T cells. T cell function is also depressed. Changes in B cell function are more variable. Other aspects of immunologic function are also affected, including total complement activity, granulocyte function, and anatomic barriers to infection. Virtually every phase of wound healing is also affected.

Clinical Findings

Patients with severe protein-calorie malnutrition—particularly children in developing countries—often exhibit signs of the classic syndromes of kwashiorkor and marasmus. The child with severe kwashiorkor will have marked edema, ascites, and muscle wasting. Lethargy, irritability, anorexia, and growth failure are common. The blood pressure and pulse are depressed, and the temperature may be low. The skin shows a "flaky paint" dermatitis, with dry, hyperpigmented lesions. The hair is sparse, dry, and depigmented. Cheilosis, stomatitis, and conjunctivitis are usually present. The liver is commonly enlarged. Laboratory manifestations include hypoalbuminemia, anemia (usually normochromic normocytic unless other deficiencies are present), and a decreased total lymphocyte count. Liver enzymes are most commonly normal, and BUN and the serum creatinine, cholesterol, potassium, magnesium, and calcium are usually low.

Patients with marasmus also exhibit growth retardation and muscle wasting. In contrast to kwashiorkor, there is no edema or ascites or specific dermatitis. Subcutaneous fat is usually absent and the skin dry and loose, giving the child a "skin and bones" appearance. Weakness and irritability are common, but there is usually less lethargy than with kwashiorkor. The appetite may be normal or increased. Blood pressure, pulse, and temperature are depressed. Laboratory values are more likely to be normal than in kwashiorkor—particularly serum albumin and other serum protein levels.

Most patients with protein-calorie undernutrition do not manifest the classic syndromes of kwashiorkor and marasmus but have intermediate syndromes. Similarly, most hospitalized patients in industrialized nations have less characteristic signs of malnutrition. In these instances, the features of malnutrition are often obscured by the underlying disease. Detection of hospitalized patients with protein-calorie undernutrition requires identification of high-risk patients, application of current techniques of nutritional assessment, and close observation of every patient's nutritional status during the course of hospitalization.

The diagnosis of protein-calorie undernutrition is particularly difficult in 2 further circumstances. Patients with significant obesity often appear to be overnourished because of their excess adipose stores. Rapid weight loss, however—particularly when due to illness—commonly results in depletion of skeletal and visceral protein and can lead to the pathophysiologic abnormalities described above despite the external appearance of obesity. In such patients, significant weight loss and depletion of serum proteins may be the only clues to protein depletion. Acutely ill patients—particularly those who are "hypermetabolic" and unable to eat—may develop visceral protein depletion rapidly without manifesting significant weight loss or other signs of undernutrition. In these patients, signs of hypermetabolism and decreased levels of serum protein may be the only clues to the diagnosis of undernutrition.

Treatment

The treatment of severe protein-calorie undernutrition is a slow process requiring great care. Initial efforts should be directed at correcting fluid and electrolyte abnormalities and any significant acute infections. Of particular concern is depletion of potassium, magnesium, and calcium and acid-base abnormalities. The second phase of treatment is directed at repletion of protein, energy, and micronutrients. Treatment should be started with modest quantities of protein and calories calculated according to the patient's actual body weight. Adult patients can initially be given 0.8 g of protein and 30 kcal per kilogram. Concomitant administration of vitamins and minerals is necessary. Either the enteral or parenteral route can be used, although the former is preferable. Enteral fat and lactose are usually withheld initially. Patients with less severe protein-calorie undernutrition can be given calories and protein simultaneously with the correction of fluid and electrolyte abnormalities. Similar quantities of protein and calories are recommended for initial treatment.

All patients initially treated for protein-calorie undernutrition require close follow-up. Both calories and protein can be advanced as tolerated. Adult patients can be advanced to 1.5 g/kg/d of protein and 40 kcal/kg/d.

Patients who are refed too rapidly can develop a number of untoward clinical sequelae. During refeeding, circulating potassium, magnesium, phosphorus, and glucose move intracellularly and can result in

low serum levels of each. The administration of water and sodium in combination with carbohydrate refeeding can overload hearts with depressed cardiac function and result in congestive heart failure. Enteral refeeding can result in malabsorption and diarrhea due to abnormalities in the gastrointestinal tract.

Refeeding edema is a benign condition that must be differentiated from congestive heart failure. Changes in renal sodium reabsorption and poor skin and blood vessel integrity result in the development of edema in dependent areas without other signs of congestive heart failure. Treatment is with reassurance, elevation of the dependent area, and modest sodium restriction. Diuretics are usually ineffective in this situation, may aggravate electrolyte deficiencies, and should not be used.

The prevention and early detection of protein-calorie malnutrition in hospitalized patients require constant awareness of that possibility by the physicians and others responsible for their care. Each patient admitted to the hospital should be screened for risk factors. Patients at risk require formal assessment of nutritional status and close observation of dietary intake, body weight, and nutritional requirements during the hospital stay.

The prevention of protein-calorie malnutrition in the developing world is, of course, a more complex problem. Most important is the redistribution of food and food-related resources from industrialized nations to the still developing ones. Poverty—not overpopulation or world food shortages—is the primary cause of most of the world's undernutrition.

The distribution of infant formula to the developing world to replace traditional breast-feeding practices has had a deleterious effect in many nations and should be discouraged.

Baron RB: Malnutrition in hospitalized patients: Diagnosis and treatment. West J Med 1986;144:63.
Baron RB: Protein-calorie undernutrition. Chap 214, pp 1212–1215, in: *Cecil Textbook of Medicine*, 18th ed. Wyngaarden JB, Smith LH (editors). Saunders, 1988.
Keys A et al: *The Biology of Human Starvation.* Univ of Minnesota Press, 1950.

OBESITY

Obesity is one of the most common disorders in medical practice and among the most frustrating and difficult to manage. Little progress has been made in obesity treatment in the last 25 years, yet major changes have occurred in our understanding of its causes and its implications for health.

Definition & Measurement

Obesity is defined as an excess of adipose tissue. The exact criterion for how much is too much is controversial. Accurate quantification of body fat requires sophisticated techniques not usually available in clinical practice. In most situations, physical examination is sufficient to detect excess body fat. Two methods commonly used for more quantitative evaluation are relative weight (RW) and body mass index (BMI).

Relative weight (RW) is the measured body weight divided by the "desirable weight." Desirable weight is defined as the midpoint value recommended for a "medium-frame" person in the 1983 Metropolitan Life Insurance Tables (Table 22–7). This technique does not differentiate between patients with excess fat or "excess" muscle.

The **body mass index (BMI),** more accurately reflects the presence of excess adipose tissue. BMI is calculated by dividing measured body weight in kilograms by the height in meters squared. The "normal" BMI is 20–25 kg/m^2.

The National Institutes of Health currently define obesity as a relative weight over 120% (BMI $>$ 27.5 kg/m^2): Mild obesity is a relative weight of 120–140% (BMI 27.5–30 kg/m^2); moderate obesity is a relative weight of 140–200% (BMI 30–40 kg/m^2); and severe or "morbid" obesity is a relative weight over 200% (BMI $>$ 40 kg/m^2). Other factors besides total weight, however, are also important. Recent data suggest that excess fat around the waist and flank is a greater health hazard than fat in the thighs and buttocks. Obese patients with high waist-hip ratios ($>$ 1.0 in men; $>$ 0.8 in women) have a significantly greater risk of diabetes mellitus, stroke, coronary artery disease, and early death than equally obese patients with lower waist-hip ratios. Further differentiation of the location of excess fat suggests that visceral fat is more metabolically active and hazardous to health than subcutaneous fat.

Age is also an important factor. As age increases, moderate increases in body weight are not associated with increased mortality rates. New weight tables accounting for the effect of age have recently been developed.

About 25% of people in the USA have relative weights in excess of 120%. Blacks—particularly black women—are more apt to be obese than whites, and the poor are more obese than the rich regardless of race.

Health Consequences of Obesity

Obesity is associated with significant increases in both morbidity and mortality. A great many disorders occur with greater frequency in obese people. The most important and common of these are hypertension, type II diabetes mellitus, hyperlipidemia, coronary artery disease, degenerative joint disease, and psychosocial disability; but certain cancers (colon, rectum, and prostate in men; uterus, biliary tract, breast, and ovary in women), thromboembolic disorders, digestive tract diseases (gallstones, reflux esophagitis), and skin disorders are also more prevalent in the obese. Surgical and obstetric risks are greater as well. Obese patients also have a greater risk of pulmonary functional impairment, endocrine abnormalities, proteinuria, and increased hemoglobin concentration.

The death rate increases in proportion to the degree of obesity: Relative weights of 130% are associated with an excess mortality rate of 35% and relative weights of 150% a greater than 2-fold excess death rate. Patients with "morbid" obesity (relative weight $>$ 200%) have as much as a 10-fold increase in death rate.

Etiology

Until recently, obesity was considered to be the direct result of a sedentary life-style plus chronic ingestion of excess calories. Obese people were *blamed* for being obese—by their friends and families, their employers, their physicians, and even by themselves. Although these factors are undoubtedly the principal cause of obesity in many cases, there is now evidence that many other factors are also involved. In laboratory animals, for example, a variety of hypothalamic abnormalities can lead to obesity. Genetic factors are also important. A recent study of 540 adopted children demonstrated a close relationship between their body mass index and that of their biologic parents. No such relationship was found between the children and their adoptive parents. Twin studies have also demonstrated substantial genetic influences on body mass index and little influence from the childhood environment. Many metabolic abnormalities have recently been described in obese patients that may also be the cause—rather than the effect—of obesity.

Further research will probably permit classification of obese patients into subgroups according to different etiologic features. Given our imperfect understanding of the causes of obesity, it is essential not to hold the patients personally responsible for their condition.

Medical Evaluation of the Obese Patient

The history and physical examination are the most important parts of the evaluation of obese patients. Historical information should be obtained about age at onset, recent weight changes, family history of obesity, occupational history, eating and exercise behavior, cigarette and alcohol use, previous weight loss experience, and psychosocial factors. Particular attention should be directed at use of laxatives, diuretics, hormones, nutritional supplements, and over-the-counter medications.

Physical examination should assess the degree and distribution of body fat, overall nutritional status, and signs of secondary causes of obesity.

Less than 1% of obese patients have an identifiable secondary cause of obesity. Hypothyroidism and Cushing's syndrome are important examples that can usually be diagnosed by physical examination in patients with unexplained recent weight gain. Such patients with physical findings suggesting hypothyroidism or Cushing's syndrome may require further endocrinologic evaluation, including serum TSH determination and dexamethasone suppression testing (see Chapter 20).

All obese patients should be evaluated for medical consequences of their obesity. Fasting levels of glucose, cholesterol, and triglycerides should be measured.

Treatment

There is no single effective method of treatment for obesity. Using conventional techniques, only 20% of patients will lose 20 lb and maintain the loss for over 2 years; 5% will maintain a 40-lb loss. Continued close provider-patient contact appears to more important for success of treatment than the specific features of any given treatment regimen. Careful patient selection will improve success rates and lessen frustration of both patients and therapists. Only sufficiently motivated patients should enter treatment programs. Specific attempts to identify motivated patients—eg, requesting a 3-day diet record—are often useful.

Most successful programs employ a multidisciplinary approach to weight loss, with hypocaloric diets, behavior modification or other strategies to change eating behavior, aerobic exercise, and social support. Emphasis must be on *maintenance* of weight loss.

Dietary instructions should incorporate the same principles that apply to healthy people who are not obese, ie, a low-fat, high-complex carbohydrate, high-fiber diet. This is achieved by emphasizing intake of a wide variety of predominantly "unprocessed" foods. Special attention is usually paid to limiting foods that provide large amounts of calories without other nutrients, ie, fat, sucrose, and alcohol. There is no special advantage to diets that restrict carbohydrates, advocate large amounts of protein or fats, or recommend ingestion of foods one at a time.

Long-term changes in eating behavior are required to maintain weight loss. Although formal **behavior modification** programs are available to which patients can be referred, the clinician caring for obese patients can teach a number of useful behavioral techniques. The most important technique is to emphasize planning and record keeping. Patients can be taught to plan menus and exercise sessions and to record their actual behavior. Record keeping not only aids in behavioral change; the availability of records also helps the health care provider to make specific suggestions for problem solving. Patients can be taught to recognize "eating cues" (emotional, situational, etc) and how to avoid or control them. Reward systems and refundable financial contracts are also useful for many patients.

Exercise offers a number of advantages to patients trying to lose weight and keep it off. Aerobic exercise directly increases the daily energy expenditure and is particularly useful for long-term weight maintenance. Exercise will also preserve lean body mass and partially prevent the decrease in basal energy expenditure seen with semistarvation.

Social support is essential for a successful weight loss program. Continued close contact with the therapist, family and peer group involvement, etc, are useful techniques for reinforcing behavioral change and preventing social isolation.

Patients with severe obesity may require more aggressive treatment regimens. **Very low calorie diets** (400–500 kcal/d) result in rapid weight loss and marked improvement in obesity-related metabolic complications. Side effects such as fatigue, orthostatic hypotension, cold intolerance, and fluid and electrolyte disorders are common and require regular supervision by a physician. Other less common complications include gout, gallbladder disease, and cardiac arrhythmias. Patients are commonly maintained on such programs for 4–6 months and lose an average of 2–4 pounds a week. Long-term weight maintenance is less predictable and requires concurrent behavior modification and exercise.

Medications for obesity are widely available over the counter and with prescription. The most commonly used medications are phenylpropanolamine, phentermine, mazindol, fenfluramine, and the antidepressant fluoxitene. Controversy exists concerning the efficacy of these agents and specific indications for their use. Although many studies show a short-term benefit, there is little evidence of long-term weight loss.

Although it is generally considered to be the last resort for the treatment of obesity, more than 100,000 obese patients have had **surgical therapy.** Few controlled trials exist, and the development of rational indications for surgery has been difficult. Most surgeons require relative weights greater than 200% before they will proceed. Gastric operations, such as the vertical-banded gastroplasty and gastric bypass procedures, are now the operations of choice. Although both types of procedures result in significant weight loss, direct comparisons tend to favor gastric bypass. The perioperative mortality rate averages less than 1% but ranges from nil to 4% at different centers. When reversals, revisions, and patients lost to follow-up are considered, failure rates approach 50%. Jejunoileal bypass operations have been abandoned by most surgeons owing to unacceptable long-term complications.

Bray GA, Gray DS: Obesity: 1. Pathogenesis. 2. Treatment. West J Med 1988;149:429, 555. (An excellent comprehensive 2-part review.)

Stunkard AJ et al: The body mass index of twins who have been reared apart. N Engl J Med 1990;322:1483.

Wadden TA, Van Itallie TB, Blackburn GL: Responsible and irresponsible use of very-low-calorie diets in the treatment of obesity. JAMA 1990;263:83.

EATING DISORDERS

ANOREXIA NERVOSA

Anorexia nervosa characteristically begins in the years between adolescence and young adulthood. Over 95% of patients are females, most commonly from the middle and upper socioeconomic strata. The diagnosis is based on the loss of 25% or more of body weight, a distorted body image, and fear of weight gain or of loss of control over food intake. Other medical or psychiatric illnesses that can account for anorexia and weight loss must be excluded.

The prevalence of anorexia nervosa is estimated to be about one per 100,000 in the population at large, but in Caucasian adolescent girls from middle and upper class families the rate may be as high as 1:200. Many other adolescent girls have features of the disorder without the severe weight loss.

The cause of anorexia nervosa is not known. Although multiple endocrinologic abnormalities exist in these patients, most authorities believe they are secondary to malnutrition and not primary disorders. Most authors favor a primary psychiatric origin, but no single psychiatric hypothesis satisfactorily explains all cases. The patient characteristically comes from a family whose members are highly goal- and achievement-oriented. Interpersonal relationships may be inadequate or destructive. The parents are usually overly directive and concerned with slimness and physical fitness, and much of the family conversation centers around dietary matters. One theory holds that the patient's refusal to eat is an attempt to regain control of her body in defiance of parental control. The patient's unwillingness to inhabit an "adult body" may also represent a rejection of adult responsibilities and the implications of adult interpersonal relationships. Patients are commonly perfectionistic in behavior and exhibit obsessional personality characteristics. Marked depression or anxiety may be present.

Clinical Findings

A. Symptoms and Signs: Clinically, patients with anorexia nervosa may exhibit severe emaciation and may complain of cold intolerance or constipation. Amenorrhea is almost always present. Bradycardia, hypotension, and hypothermia may be present in severe cases. Examination demonstrates loss of body fat, dry and scaly skin, and increased lanugo body hair. Parotid enlargement and edema may also be present.

B. Laboratory Findings: Laboratory findings are variable but may include anemia, leukopenia, electrolyte abnormalities, and elevations of BUN and serum creatinine. Serum cholesterol levels are often increased. Endocrine abnormalities included depressed levels of luteinizing and follicle-stimulating hormones and impaired response of LH to luteinizing hormone-releasing hormone.

Diagnosis & Differential Diagnosis

The diagnosis of anorexia nervosa can be difficult, since many common social and cultural factors promote and maintain anorexic behavior. Diagnosis depends upon identification of the common behavioral features and exclusion of medical disorders that would account for weight loss.

Behavioral features required for the diagnosis include intense fear of becoming obese, disturbance of body image, weight loss of at least 25%, and refusal to maintain body weight over a minimal normal weight.

The differential diagnosis includes endocrine and metabolic disorders such as panhypopituitarism, Addison's disease, hyperthyroidism, and diabetes mellitus; gastrointestinal disorders such as Crohn's disease and celiac sprue; chronic infections and cancers such as tuberculosis and lymphoma; and rare central nervous system disorders such as hypothalamic tumors.

Treatment

The goal of treatment is restoration of normal body weight and resolution of psychologic difficulties. Hospitalization is usually necessary for frank anorexia nervosa. Treatment programs conducted by experienced teams are successful in about two-thirds of cases, restoring normal weight and menstruation. One-half continue to experience difficulties with eating behavior and psychiatric problems. Occasional patients with anorexia develop obesity after treatment. Two to 6% of patients die from the complications of the disorder or commit suicide.

Various treatment methods have been used without clear evidence of superiority of one over another. Supportive care by physicians and nurses is probably the most important feature of therapy. Structured behavioral therapy, intensive psychotherapy, and family therapy may be tried. A variety of medications including tricyclic antidepressants and lithium carbonate are effective in some cases. Patients with severe malnutrition must be hemodynamically stabilized and may require enteral or parenteral feeding. Forced feedings should be reserved for life-threatening situations, since the goal of treatment is to reestablish normal eating behavior.

Garfinkel PE, Garner DM, Goldbloom DS: Eating disorders: Implications for the 1990s. Can J Psychiatry 1987; 32:624.

Health and Public Policy Committee, American College of Physicians: Eating disorders: Anorexia nervosa and bulimia. Ann Intern Med 1986;105:790.

Heroz DB, Copeland PM: Eating disorders. N Engl J Med 1985;313:295.

BULIMIA & BULIMAREXIA

Bulimia is the episodic uncontrolled ingestion of large quantities of food. When combined with purging, either by self-induced vomiting or abuse of diuretics or cathartics, the disorder is called bulimarexia, or the binge-purge syndrome.

Like anorexia, bulimia and bulimarexia are predominantly disorders of young, white middle- and upper-class women. It is more difficult to detect than anorexia, and some studies have estimated the prevalence to be as high as 19% in college-age women.

Patients with bulimia typically consume large quantities of easily ingested high-calorie foods, usually in secrecy. Some patients may have several such episodes a day for a few days; others report regular and persistent patterns of binge eating. Binging is usually followed by vomiting, cathartics, or diuretics and is usually accompanied by feelings of guilt or depression. Periods of binging may be followed by intervals of self-imposed starvation. Body weights may fluctuate but generally are within 20% of desirable weights.

Some patients with bulimia also have a cryptic form of anorexia nervosa with significant weight losses and amenorrhea. Family and psychologic issues are generally similar to those encountered among patients with anorexia nervosa. Bulimics, however, have a higher incidence of premorbid obesity, greater use of cathartics and diuretics, and more impulsive or antisocial behaviors. Weights are closer to normal, and menstruation is usually preserved.

Depending on the type and severity of abnormal behavior, a variety of medical complications can occur. Gastric dilatation and pancreatitis have been reported after binges. Vomiting can result in poor dentition, pharyngitis, esophagitis, aspiration, and electrolyte abnormalities. Cathartic and diuretic abuse also commonly result in electrolyte abnormalities or dehydration. Constipation and hemorrhoids are common.

Treatment of bulimia and bulimarexia requires supportive care and psychotherapy. Individual, group, family, and behavioral therapy have all been utilized with modest success. Antidepressants may be helpful in some patients. Although death from bulimia is rare, the long-term psychiatric prognosis in severe bulimia is worse than the prognosis in anorexia nervosa, which suggests that the underlying psychiatric disorder may be more severe.

Fitzgerald BA, Wright JH, Atala KD: Bulimia nervosa: Uncovering a secret disorder. Postgrad Med (Aug) 1988;84:119. (Early recognition results in improved outcome.)
See also references under Anorexia Nervosa, above.

DISORDERS OF VITAMIN METABOLISM

Deficiencies of single vitamins are rarely encountered in current clinical practice, even in developing countries. Deficiencies of multiple vitamins are more commonly seen along with protein-calorie undernutrition. Although any cause of protein-calorie undernutrition can result in concurrent vitamin deficiency, most such instances are associated with malabsorption, alcoholism, medications, hemodialysis, total parenteral nutrition, food faddism, or inborn errors of metabolism.

Vitamin deficiency syndromes develop gradually. Symptoms are commonly nonspecific, and the physical examination is rarely helpful in early diagnosis. Most characteristic physical findings, such as the perifollicular hemorrhages associated with vitamin C deficiency, are seen late in the course of the syndrome. Other characteristic physical findings, such as glossitis and cheilosis, are seen with deficiencies of many B vitamins. Such abnormalities strongly suggest the presence of a nutritional deficiency but do not indicate which nutrient is deficient.

Despite the relative ease of meeting the recommended daily allowances with a mixed diet, many adults in the USA take vitamin supplements. In fact, syndromes of vitamin excess may be more common than deficiency syndromes, particularly those due to excess of vitamins A, D, and B_6. Most claims for significant health benefits of such supplements, particularly those taken in megadoses, remain unsubstantiated.

Some vitamins can be used efficaciously as drugs. Derivatives of vitamin A are used to treat cystic acne and, more recently, skin wrinkles. Niacin is an effective medication for hyperlipidemia. Vitamin-responsive inborn errors of metabolism also commonly require pharmacologic doses of vitamins.

Council on Scientific Affairs: Vitamin preparations as dietary supplements and as therapeutic agents. JAMA 1987;257:1929.
Suter PM, Russell RM: Vitamin requirements of the elderly. Am J Clin Nutr 1987;45:501.

WATER-SOLUBLE VITAMINS

1. THIAMINE

The primary role of thiamine is as precursor of thiamine pyrophosphate, a coenzyme required for several important biochemical reactions necessary for carbohydrate oxidation. Thiamine is also thought to have an independent role in nerve conduction in peripheral nerves. The recommended daily allowances of thiamine are listed in Table 22–1.

Thiamine Deficiency

A. Clinical Findings: Most thiamine deficiency in the USA is due to alcoholism. Chronic alcoholics have poor dietary intakes of thiamine and impaired thiamine absorption, metabolism, and storage. Thiamine deficiency is also associated with malabsorption, dialysis, and other causes of chronic protein-calorie undernutrition. Thiamine deficiency can be precipitated in marginally replete patients with intravenous dextrose solutions. A number of thiamine-responsive inborn errors of metabolism have also been described.

Early manifestations of thiamine deficiency include anorexia, muscle cramps, paresthesias, and irritability. Advanced deficiency affects chiefly the cardiovascular system (''wet beriberi'') or the nervous system (''dry beriberi''). Wet beriberi occurs if severe physical exertion and high carbohydrate intakes accompany thiamine deficiency, whereas dry beriberi is seen with inactivity and low-calorie intake.

Beriberi heart disease is characterized by marked peripheral vasodilatation resulting in classic high-output heart failure with dyspnea, tachycardia, cardiomegaly, and pulmonary and peripheral edema, with warm extremities mimicking cellulitis.

Involvement of the nervous system can include both the peripheral and the central nervous systems. Peripheral nerve involvement is typically a symmetric motor and sensory neuropathy with pain, paresthesias, and loss of reflexes. The legs are usually affected more than the arms. Central nervous system involvement results in Wernicke-Korsakoff syndrome. Wernicke's encephalopathy consists of nystagmus progressing to ophthalmoplegia, truncal ataxia, and confusion. Korsakoff's syndrome is characterized by amnesia, confabulation, and impaired learning.

B. Diagnosis: A variety of biochemical tests are available to assess thiamine deficiency. In most instances, however, the clinical response to empirical thiamine therapy is used to support a diagnosis of thiamine deficiency. The most commonly used and widely available biochemical tests are measurement of erythrocyte transketolase activity and urinary thiamine excretion. A transketolase activity coefficient greater than 15–20% suggests thiamine deficiency.

C. Treatment: Suspected thiamine deficiency should be treated promptly with large parenteral doses of thiamine. Fifty to 100 mg/d are typically administered for the first few days, followed by daily oral doses of 5–10 mg/d. All patients should simultaneously receive therapeutic doses of other water-soluble vitamins. Although treatment results in complete resolution in one-half of patients (one-fourth immediately and another one-fourth over days), the other half obtain only partial resolution or no benefit.

Thiamine Toxicity

Although extremely large doses of thiamine can be administered either orally or parenterally without significant toxicity, prolonged injections of large doses can result in an anaphylactoid reaction.

2. RIBOFLAVIN

Riboflavin—as the coenzymes flavin mononucleotide and flavin adenine dinucleotide—participates in a variety of important oxidation-reduction reactions and is an essential component of a number of other enzymes. The recommended daily allowances of riboflavin are listed in Table 22–1.

Riboflavin Deficiency

A. Clinical Findings: Riboflavin deficiency almost always occurs in combination with deficiencies of other vitamins. Dietary inadequacy, interactions with a variety of medications, alcoholism, and other causes of protein-calorie undernutrition are the most common causes of riboflavin deficiency. A number of riboflavin-responsive inborn errors of metabolism have been described.

Manifestations of riboflavin deficiency include mouth soreness, cheilosis, angular stomatitis, glossitis, seborrheic dermatitis, weakness, corneal vascularization, and anemia.

B. Diagnosis: Riboflavin deficiency is usually treated empirically when the diagnosis is clinically suspected. Deficiency can be confirmed by measuring the riboflavin-dependent enzyme erythrocyte glutathione reductase. Activity coefficients greater than 1.2–1.3 are suggestive of riboflavin deficiency. Urinary riboflavin excretion and serum levels of plasma and red cell flavins can also be measured.

C. Treatment: Riboflavin deficiency is easily treated with riboflavin-containing foods or oral preparations of the vitamin. Administration of 10–15 mg/d until clinical findings are resolved is usually adequate. Riboflavin can also be given parenterally, but it is poorly soluble in aqueous solutions.

Riboflavin Toxicity

There is no known toxicity of riboflavin.

3. NIACIN

Niacin is a generic term for nicotinic acid and other derivatives with similar nutritional activity. Unlike most other vitamins, niacin can be synthesized by the human body from the essential amino acid tryptophan. Niacin is an essential component of the coenzymes nicotinamide adenine dinucleotide (NAD) and nicotinamide adenine dinucleotide phosphate (NADP), which are involved in many oxidation-reduction reactions. The recommended daily allowances of niacin are listed in Table 22–1; major food sources are protein foods containing tryptophan and numerous cereals, vegetables, and dairy products.

Niacin can also be used therapeutically for the treatment of hypercholesterolemia and hypertriglyceridemia. Daily doses of 3–6 g can result in significant reductions in levels of low-density lipoproteins (LDL) and very low density lipoproteins (VLDL) and in elevation of high-density lipoproteins (HDL). Niacinamide does not exhibit the lipid-lowering effects of nicotinic acid.

Niacin Deficiency

A. Clinical Findings: Historically, niacin deficiency occurred when corn, which is relatively deficient in both tryptophan and niacin, was the major source of calories. Currently, niacin deficiency is more commonly due to alcoholism and nutrient-drug interactions. Niacin deficiency can also occur in inborn errors of metabolism.

As with other B vitamins, the early manifestations of niacin deficiency are nonspecific. Common complaints include anorexia, weakness, irritability, mouth soreness, glossitis, stomatitis, and weight loss. More advanced deficiency results in the classic triad of pellagra: dermatitis, diarrhea, and dementia. The characteristic dermatitis is symmetric, involving sun-exposed areas. Skin lesions are dark, dry, and scaling. The dementia begins with insomnia, irritability, and apathy and progresses to confusion, memory loss, hallucinations, and psychosis. The diarrhea can be severe and may result in malabsorption due to atrophy of the intestinal villi. Advanced pellagra can result in death.

B. Diagnosis: In advanced cases, the diagnosis of pellagra can be made on clinical grounds. In early cases, diagnosis requires a high index of suspicion and attempts at confirmation of niacin deficiency. Niacin metabolites, particularly N-methylnicotinamide, can be measured in the urine. Low levels suggest niacin deficiency but may also be found in patients with generalized undernutrition. Serum and red cell levels of NAD and NADP are also low but are similarly nonspecific.

C. Treatment: Pellagra can be effectively treated with oral niacin, usually given as nicotinamide. Doses ranging from 10 to 150 mg/d have been used without difficulty.

Niacin Toxicity

At the high doses of niacin used to treat hyperlipidemia, side effects are common. These include cutaneous flushing and gastric irritation. Elevation of liver enzymes, hyperglycemia, and gout are less common untoward effects.

Canner PL et al: Fifteen-year mortality in Coronary Drug Project patients: Long-term benefit with niacin. J Am Coll Cardiol 1986;8:1245.

4. PYRIDOXINE

"Pyridoxine" is actually a group of closely related substances involved in intermediary metabolism. These include pyridoxine itself, pyridoxal, pyridoxamine, and their 5-phosphate esters. As the major coenzyme involved in the metabolism of amino acids, pyridoxal 5-phosphate is the most important. Pyridoxal phosphate is also required for the synthesis of heme. The recommended daily allowances of pyridoxine are listed in Table 22–1.

Pyridoxine Deficiency

A. Clinical Findings: Pyridoxine deficiency most commonly occurs as a result of interactions with medications—especially isoniazid, cycloserine, penicillamine, and oral contraceptives—and of alcoholism. A number of inborn errors of metabolism and other pyridoxine-responsive syndromes, particularly pyridoxine-responsive anemia, are not clearly due to vitamin deficiency but commonly respond to high doses of the vitamin.

Manifestations of pyridoxine deficiency result in a clinical syndrome similar to that seen with deficiencies of other B vitamins, including mouth soreness, glossitis, cheilosis, weakness, and irritability. Severe deficiency can result in peripheral neuropathy, anemia, and seizures.

B. Diagnosis: The diagnosis of pyridoxine deficiency can be confirmed by measurement of pyridoxal phosphate in blood. Normal levels are greater than 50 ng/mL.

C. Treatment: Pyridoxine deficiency can be effectively treated with oral pyridoxine supplements. Doses of 10–20 mg/d are usually adequate, though some patients taking medications that interfere with pyridoxine metabolism may need doses as high as 100 mg/d. Inborn errors of metabolism and the pyridoxine-responsive syndromes often require up to 500 mg/d.

Pyridoxine should be routinely prescribed for patients receiving medications that interfere with pyridoxine metabolism to prevent pyridoxine deficiency. This is particularly true for elderly patients, the urban poor, and alcoholics, who are more likely to have diets marginally adequate in pyridoxine.

Large doses of pyridoxine have also been advocated for treatment of premenstrual syndrome and carpal tunnel syndrome. No significant clinical benefits have been consistently demonstrated.

Pyridoxine Toxicity

A sensory neuropathy, at times irreversible, occurs in patients receiving large doses of pyridoxine. Although most patients have taken 2 g or more per day, some patients have taken only 200 mg/d.

5. VITAMIN B$_{12}$ & FOLIC ACID

Vitamin B$_{12}$ (cobalamin) and folic acid are discussed in Chapter 10. The recommended daily allowances of vitamin B$_{12}$ and folic acid are listed in Table 22–1. Vitamin B$_{12}$ is abundant in meat and dairy products; fresh vegetables supply ample folic acid.

6. VITAMIN C
(Ascorbic Acid)

Vitamin C is a potent antioxidant involved in many oxidation-reduction reactions and is also required for the synthesis of collagen. It increases the absorption of nonheme iron and is involved in tyrosine metabolism, wound healing, and drug metabolism. With the exception of collagen synthesis, the exact mechanism of action for most of these functions is poorly understood. The recommended daily allowances of vitamin C are listed in Table 22–1; major food sources are fresh fruits and vegetables.

Vitamin C Deficiency
A. Clinical Findings: Most cases of vitamin C deficiency seen in the USA are due to dietary inadequacy, most commonly in the urban poor, the elderly, and chronic alcoholics. Infants 6–12 months of age whose diets are not supplemented with vitamin C or vitamin C-containing foods are also at high risk.

Early manifestations of vitamin C deficiency are nonspecific and include malaise and weakness. In more advanced stages, the typical features of scurvy develop. Manifestations may include perifollicular hemorrhages, perifollicular hyperkeratotic papules, petechiae and purpura, splinter hemorrhages, bleeding gums, joint hemorrhages, and subperiosteal hemorrhages. Anemia is common, and wound healing is impaired. The late stages of scurvy are characterized by edema, oliguria, neuropathy, intracerebral hemorrhage, and death.

B. Diagnosis: The diagnosis of advanced scurvy can be made clinically on the basis of the characteristic skin lesions and other manifestations. The diagnosis can be confirmed with decreased plasma levels, typically below 0.1 mg/dL. Platelet ascorbic acid levels can also be measured.

C. Treatment: Adult scurvy can be treated with 100–300 mg of ascorbic acid per day. Improvement typically occurs, even in advanced cases, within days.

A number of inborn errors of metabolism, including osteogenesis imperfecta and Chédiak-Higashi syndrome, may respond to similar doses of vitamin C. Certain types of Ehlers-Danlos syndrome may improve with larger doses of vitamin C.

Vitamin C in extremely large doses has also been enthusiastically advocated for prevention and treatment of the common cold and cancer. When evaluated in randomized blinded trials, no significant benefit has been consistently demonstrated in either of these conditions.

Vitamin C Toxicity
Although generally extremely safe, very large doses of vitamin C can have side effects. Most common are gastric irritation, flatulence, or diarrhea. Oxalate kidney stones are of theoretic concern because ascorbic acid is metabolized to oxalate, but stone formation has not been frequently reported. Vitamin C can also confuse common diagnostic tests by causing false-negative tests for stool occult blood and both false-negative and false-positive tests for urine glucose.

FAT-SOLUBLE VITAMINS

1. VITAMIN A

Vitamin A (retinol) is a high-molecular-weight alcohol either ingested preformed or synthesized from plant carotenoids, particularly β-carotene. Isomers and derivatives of retinol are commonly called retinoids. Vitamin A is essential for normal retinal function and plays an important but still not fully understood role in cell growth and differentiation, particularly of epithelial cells. Epidemiologic biochemical evidence suggests that this role may be important for prevention of certain cancers. The recommended daily allowances of vitamin A are listed in Table 22–1; the principal food sources are highly pigmented vegetables.

Vitamin A Deficiency
A. Clinical Findings: Vitamin A deficiency is one of the most common vitamin deficiency syndromes, particularly in developing countries. In many such regions, vitamin A deficiency is the most common cause of blindness. In the USA, vitamin A deficiency is usually due to fat malabsorption syndromes and alcoholism and to laxative abuse with mineral oil and occurs most commonly in the elderly and the urban poor.

Night blindness is the earliest symptom of vitamin A deficiency. Dryness of the conjunctiva (xerosis) and the development of small white patches on the sclera (Bitot's spots) are early signs. Ulceration and necrosis of the cornea (keratomalacia), perforation, endophthalmitis, and blindness are late manifestations. Xerosis and hyperkeratinization of the skin and loss of taste may also occur.

B. Diagnosis: Abnormalities of dark adaptation are strongly suggestive of vitamin A deficiency. Serum levels below the normal range of 30–65 mg/dL are commonly seen in advanced deficiency.

C. Treatment: Night blindness and other signs of early deficiency can be effectively treated with 30,000 IU of vitamin A daily for 1 week. Advanced deficiency with corneal damage calls for administration of 20,000 IU/kg for at least 5 days.

Vitamin A Toxicity

Excess intake of β-carotenes (hypercarotenosis) results in staining of the skin a yellow-orange color but is otherwise benign. Skin changes are most marked on the palms and soles, while the scleras remain white, clearly distinguishing hypercarotenosis from jaundice. Hypercarotenosis is usually due to excess consumption of carrots, usually as carrot juice.

Excessive vitamin A (hypervitaminosis A), on the other hand, can be quite toxic. Chronic toxicity usually occurs after ingestion of daily doses of over 50,000 IU/d for more than 3 months. Early manifestations include dry, scaly skin, hair loss, mouth sores, painful hyperostoses, anorexia, and vomiting. More serious findings include increased intracranial pressure, with papilledema, headaches, and decreased cognition; and hepatomegaly, occasionally progressing to cirrhosis. Acute toxicity can result from ingestion of massive doses of vitamin A, such as in drug overdoses or consumption of polar bear liver. Manifestations include nausea, vomiting, abdominal pain, headache, papilledema, and lethargy.

The diagnosis can be confirmed by elevations of serum vitamin A levels. The only treatment is withdrawal of vitamin A from the diet. Most symptoms and signs improve rapidly.

2. VITAMIN D

Vitamin D is discussed in Chapter 20. The recommended daily allowances of vitamin D are listed in Table 22–1; a major food source is fortified milk, but sunlight on the skin is a prime resource as well.

3. VITAMIN E

Vitamin E activity is derived from at least 8 naturally occurring tocopherols, the most potent of which is α-tocopherol. Although the exact function and mechanism of action of vitamin E in humans are unclear, it is commonly thought to function as an antioxidant, protecting membranes and other cellular structures from attack by free radicals. Dietary selenium and other antioxidants work in conjunction with vitamin E and may partially spare its requirement and reverse signs of vitamin E deficiency in animals. The recommended daily allowances of vitamin E are listed in Table 22–1; the major food source is vegetable seed oil.

Vitamin E Deficiency

A. Clinical Findings: Clinical deficiency of vitamin E is most commonly due to severe malabsorption, the genetic disorder abetalipoproteinemia, and, in children with chronic cholestatic liver disease, biliary atresia or cystic fibrosis. Manifestations of deficiency include areflexia, disturbances of gait, decreased proprioception and vibration, and ophthalmoplegia. In premature infants, hemolytic anemia, intraventricular hemorrhage, and thrombocytosis have been reported.

B. Diagnosis: Plasma vitamin E levels can be measured; normal levels are 0.5–0.7 mg/dL or higher. Since vitamin E is normally transported in lipoproteins, the serum level should be interpreted in relation to circulating lipids.

C. Treatment: The optimum therapeutic dose of vitamin E has not been clearly defined. Twenty-five units of vitamin E can be administered to premature infants to treat hemolytic anemia and to prevent intraventricular hemorrhage. Larger doses, often administered parenterally, can be used to improve the neurologic complications seen in abetalipoproteinemia and cholestatic liver disease.

Vitamin E Toxicity

Vitamin E is the least toxic of the fat-soluble vitamins. Large doses, 20–80 times the recommended daily requirement, have been taken for extended periods of time without apparent harm, although nausea, flatulence, and diarrhea have been reported. Large doses of vitamin E can increase the vitamin K requirement and can result in bleeding in patients taking oral anticoagulants.

4. VITAMIN K

Vitamin K is discussed in Chapter 10. The recommended daily allowances of vitamin K are listed in Table 22–1; it is synthesized by intestinal bacteria.

DIET THERAPY

Specific therapeutic diets can be designed to facilitate the medical management of most common illnesses. In most cases, consultation with a registered dietitian is necessary in order to design and implement major dietary changes. Physicians should be familiar with the indications for special diets and their basic composition to facilitate patient referrals and to maximize patient compliance.

Diet therapy is a difficult process, and not all patients are able to cooperate fully. Before starting specific dietary changes, one should assess the patient's motivation for change in eating habits. Patients who are not adequately motivated or who for other reasons are unable to change their diets should not be started on diet therapy, since embarking on a course that can only fail will interfere with other aspects of the therapeutic relationship between doctor and patient. Requesting the patient to record dietary intake for 3–5 days may provide useful insight into the patient's motivation.

Prescribed diets should take into account personal food preferences, cultural habits, and eating behavior. Changes should be introduced gradually. Close follow-up and a close patient-therapist relationship are necessary for sustained dietary change.

Therapeutic diets can be divided into 3 groups: (1) diets that alter the consistency of food; (2) diets that restrict or otherwise modify dietary components; and (3) diets that supplement dietary components.

DIETS THAT ALTER CONSISTENCY

Clear Liquid Diet

This diet provides adequate water, up to 1000 kcal as simple sugar, and some electrolytes. It is fiber-free and requires minimal digestion or intestinal motility.

A clear liquid diet is useful for patients with resolving postoperative ileus, acute gastroenteritis, partial intestinal obstruction, and as preparation for diagnostic gastrointestinal procedures. It is commonly used as the first diet for patients who have been taking nothing by mouth for long periods. Because of the low calorie and minimal protein content of the clear liquid diet, it should be used only for short periods.

Full Liquid Diet

The full liquid diet provides adequate water and can be designed to provide adequate calories and protein. Vitamins and minerals—especially folic acid, iron, and vitamin B_6—may be inadequate and should be provided in the form of supplements. Dairy products, soups, eggs, and soft cereals are used to supplement clear liquids. Commercial oral supplements can also be incorporated into the diet or used alone.

This diet is low in residue and can be used in many instances instead of the clear liquid diet described above—especially in patients with difficulty in chewing or swallowing, with partial obstructions, or in preparation for some diagnostic procedures. Full liquid diets are commonly used following clear liquid diets to "advance" diets in patients who have been taking nothing by mouth for long periods.

Mechanical Soft Diet

This diet includes foods permitted in the liquid diets as well as foods containing easily digested protein and carbohydrates. Eggs, cottage cheese, ground meat, crackers, refined cereals and grains, skinless potatoes and starches, cooked skinless fruits and vegetables, and cakes and cookies are included.

The diet is low in residue. It can be designed to meet all other nutritional requirements. It is most commonly used for patients who have difficulty with chewing and swallowing or with partial intestinal obstruction. Mechanical soft diets that restrict spices and seasonings—the bland diet—have traditionally been used for patients with peptic disease. There is no evidence that such diets are useful, and they should no longer be prescribed.

DIETS THAT RESTRICT NUTRIENTS

Diets can be designed to restrict (or eliminate) virtually any nutrient or food component (see Table 22–9). The most commonly used restricted diets are those that limit sodium, fat, and protein. Other restrictive diets include gluten restriction in sprue, potassium and phosphate reduction in renal insufficiency, and various elimination diets for food allergies.

Sodium-Restricted Diets

Low-sodium diets are useful in the management of hypertension and in conditions in which sodium retention and edema are prominent features, particularly congestive heart failure, chronic liver disease, and chronic renal failure. Sodium restriction is beneficial with or without diuretic therapy. When used in conjunction with diuretics, sodium restriction allows lower dosage of the diuretic medication and may prevent side effects. Potassium excretion, in particular, is directly related to distal renal tubule sodium delivery, and sodium restriction will decrease diuretic-related potassium losses.

Typical American diets contain about 4–6 g (175–260 meq) of sodium per day. Typical sodium-restricted diets contain 2000 mg (88 meq), 1000 mg (44 meq), and 500 mg (22 meq) of sodium per day. Diets containing intermediate quantities of sodium can also be designed.

Dietary sodium includes sodium naturally occurring in foods, sodium added during food processing, and sodium added by the consumer during cooking and at the table. About a third of current dietary intake is derived from each. Diets that allow 2000 mg of sodium daily are easiest to design and implement. Such diets generally eliminate added salt, most processed foods, and selected foods with particularly high sodium content. Patients who follow such diets for 2–3 months lose their craving for salty foods and can often continue to restrict their sodium intake indefinitely. Many patients with mild hypertension will achieve significant reductions in blood pressure (approximately 5 mm Hg diastolic) with this degree of sodium restriction. Other patients require more severe sodium restriction (approximately 1000 mg of sodium per day) for reduction in blood pressure, and other may actually have increased blood pressure with sodium restriction.

Diets allowing 1000 mg and 500 mg of sodium require, in addition to the restrictions outlined above, restrict more commonly eaten foods. Special "low-sodium'' products are now available to facilitate such diets. These diets are difficult for most people to follow and are generally reserved for hospitalized patients and highly motivated outpatients—most commonly those with severe liver disease and ascites.

Fat-Restricted Diets

Traditional fat-restricted diets are useful in the treatment of fat malabsorption syndromes. Such diets will improve the symptoms of diarrhea with steatorrhea independently of the primary physiologic abnormality by limiting the quantity of fatty acids that reach the colon. The degree of fat restriction necessary to control symptoms must be individualized. Patients with severe malabsorption can be limited to 40–60 g of fat per day. Diets containing 60–80 g of fat per day can be designed for patients with less severe abnormalities.

In general, fat-restricted diets require broiling, baking, or boiling meat and fish; discarding the skin of poultry and fish and using those foods as the main protein source; using nonfat dairy products; and avoiding desserts, sauces, and gravies.

Low-Cholesterol, Low-Saturated Fat Diets

Fat-restricted diets that specifically restrict saturated fats and dietary cholesterol are the mainstay of dietary treatment of hyperlipidemia (see Chapter 21). Similar diets are recommended also for diabetes

(Chapter 21) and for the prevention of coronary artery disease (Chapter 8). Current recommendations for the prevention of cancer by dietary modification also include fat restriction.

The aim of these diets is to restrict total fat to 30% of calories and to achieve a normal body weight by caloric restriction. Saturated fat and dietary cholesterol are further restricted. In the first phase of treatment (''step 1''), saturated fat is restricted to 10% of total calories and dietary cholesterol to 300 mg/d. ''Step 2'' consists of further reduction of saturated fat to 7% of total calories and dietary cholesterol to 200 mg/d. In both cases, up to 10% of calories is derived from polyunsaturated fats and 10–15% is monounsaturated. In both diets also, 50–60% of calories is from carbohydrates, particularly complex carbohydrates high in dietary fiber. Ideally, the ''step 1'' diet can lead to a decrease in serum cholesterol of 15–20% and the ''step 2'' diet a further 5% reduction.

Protein-Restricted Diets

Protein-restricted diets are most commonly used in patients with hepatic encephalopathy due to chronic liver disease and in patients with renal failure to ameliorate the progression of early disease and to decrease symptoms of uremia in more severe disease. Patients with selected inborn errors of amino acid metabolism and other abnormalities resulting in hyperammonemia also require protein restriction.

Protein restriction is intended to limit the production of nitrogenous waste products. Energy intake must be adequate to facilitate the efficient use of dietary protein. Proteins must be of high biologic value and be provided in sufficient quantity to meet minimal requirements. For most patients, the diet should contain at least 0.5 g/kg/d of protein. Patients with encephalopathy who fail to respond to this degree of restriction are unlikely to respond to more severe restriction.

Table 22–9. Diets that restrict nutrients.

	Common Indication
Sodium-restricted	Hypertension, congestive heart failure, chronic liver disease, chronic renal failure
Fat-restricted	Malabsorption syndromes
Fat- and cholesterol-restricted	Hyperlipidemia, diabetes
Protein-restricted	Hepatic encephalopathy, chronic renal failure
Calorie-restricted	Obesity, diabetes (type II)
Lactose-restricted	Lactose intolerance
Potassium-restricted	Chronic renal failure
Gluten-restricted	Celiac sprue
Phosphate-restricted	Chronic renal failure
Copper-restricted	Wilson's disease
Oxalate-restricted	Hyperoxaluria
Elimination diets	Food allergies
Salicylate-restricted	Chronic urticaria
Tyramine-restricted	Monoamine oxidase inhibitor use
Amino acid-restricted	Amino acid disorders, eg, phenylketonuria

DIETS THAT SUPPLEMENT NUTRIENTS

High-Fiber Diet

Dietary fiber is a diverse group of plant constituents that are resistant to digestion by the human digestive tract. Typical American diets contain about 5–10 g of dietary fiber per day. Epidemiologic evidence has suggested that populations consuming greater quantities of fiber have a lower incidence of certain gastrointestinal disorders, including diverticulitis and colon cancer. Most authorities currently recommend higher intakes of dietary fiber for health maintenance.

Diets high in dietary fiber (20–35 g/d) are also commonly used in management of a variety of gastrointestinal disorders, particularly the irritable bowel syndrome and recurrent diverticulitis. Diets high in fiber may also be useful to reduce blood sugar in patients with diabetes and to reduce cholesterol levels in patients with hypercholesterolemia. Such diets include greater intakes of fresh fruits and vegetables, whole grains, legumes and seeds, and bran products. For some patients, the addition of psyllium seed (2 tsp per day) or natural bran (½ cup per day) may be preferable.

High-Potassium Diets

Potassium-supplemented diets are used most commonly to compensate for potassium losses caused by diuretics. Although potassium losses can be partially prevented by using lower doses of diuretics, concurrent sodium restriction, and potassium-sparing diuretics, some patients require additional potassium to prevent hypokalemia. Epidemiologic and experimental evidence suggests that high-potassium diets may also have a direct antihypertensive effect. Typical American diets contain about 3 g (80 meq) of potassium per day. High-potassium diets commonly contain 4.5–7 g (120–180 meq) of potassium per day.

Most fruits, vegetables, and their juices contain high concentrations of potassium. Supplemental potassium can also be provided with potassium-containing salt substitutes or as potassium chloride in solution or capsules, but this is rarely necessary if the above measures are followed to prevent potassium losses and supplement dietary potassium.

High-Calcium Diets

Additional intakes of dietary calcium have recently been recommended for the prevention of postmenopausal osteoporosis, the prevention and treatment of hypertension, and the prevention of colon cancer. Although the evidence in each case is preliminary, most authorities currently recommend intakes of 1 g of calcium per day for most adults and 1.5 g/d for postmenopausal women. Current USA intakes are approximately 700 mg/d.

Low-fat and nonfat dairy products are the mainstay of supplemental calcium intakes. Patients with lactose intolerance who cannot tolerate liquid dairy products may be able to tolerate nonliquid products such as cheese and yogurt. Leafy green vegetables and canned fish with bones also contain high concentrations of calcium, although the latter is also very high in sodium.

American Dietetic Association: Health implications of dietary fiber. J Am Diet Assoc 1988;88:216.

Baron RB: Management of hypercholesterolemia: A primary care perspective. West J Med 1989;150:562. (Practical suggestions for implementing diet therapy.)

Expert Panel Report of the National Cholesterol Education Program (NCEP): Detection, evaluation, and treatment of high blood cholesterol in adults. Arch Intern Med 1988;148:36.

Kaplan N: Nondrug treatment of hypertension. Ann Intern Med 1985;102:359.

NUTRITIONAL SUPPORT

Nutritional support is the provision of nutrients to patients who cannot meet their nutritional requirements by eating standard diets. Nutrients may be delivered enterally, using oral nutritional supplements, nasogastric and nasoduodenal feeding tubes, and tube enterostomies; or parenterally, using lines or catheters placed in peripheral or central veins, respectively. Current nutritional support techniques permit adequate nutrient delivery to virtually any patient. Nutrition support should only be utilized, however, if it is likely to improve the patient's clinical outcome. The financial costs and risks of side effects must be balanced against the potential advantages of improved nutritional status in each clinical situation.

INDICATIONS FOR NUTRITIONAL SUPPORT

The precise indications for nutritional support remain controversial. Most authorities agree that nutritional support is indicated for at least 4 groups of adult patients: (1) those with inadequate bowel syndromes; (2) those with severe prolonged hypercatabolic states (eg, due to extensive burns, multiple trauma, mechanical ventilation); (3) those requiring prolonged therapeutic bowel rest; and (4) those with severe protein-calorie undernutrition with a treatable disease who have sustained a loss of over 25% of body weight.

It has been difficult to prove the efficacy of nutritional support in the treatment of most other conditions. Over 100 randomized controlled clinical trials have been conducted in an attempt to address this question. In most cases it has not been possible to show a clear advantage of treatment by means of nutritional support over treatment without such support. Unfortunately, most of these studies have design flaws and do not disprove the effectiveness of nutritional support.

The American Society for Parenteral and Enteral Nutrition (ASPEN) has published recommendations for the rational use of nutritional support. These are shown in Table 22–10. The recommendations emphasize the need to individualize the decision to begin nutritional support, carefully weighing the risks and costs against the benefit to each patient. They also demonstrate the need to identify high-risk malnourished patients by nutritional assessment.

Table 22–10. Indications and contraindications for nutritional support.[1]

1. Normally nourished patients who are eating sufficiently—no additional therapy.
2. Normally nourished patients who are not eating sufficiently for a period of less than 5–7 days—no further therapy. For a period of over 5–7 days, enteral and/or parenteral nutrition support to meet requirements should be considered.
3. Malnourished patients who are eating sufficiently—no further therapy.
4. Malnourished patients who are not eating sufficiently—enteral and/or parenteral nutrition support to meet requirements should be considered.
5. Selected patients who are hypermetabolic may require specialized nutrition therapy before 5–7 days.

[1] Reprinted from: *Standards for Nutrition Support: Hospitalized Patients.* American Society for Parenteral and Enteral Nutrition (ASPEN), 1984.

NUTRITIONAL SUPPORT METHODS

Selection of the most appropriate nutritional support method involves consideration of gastrointestinal function, the anticipated duration of nutritional support, and the ability of each method to meet the patient's nutritional requirements. The method chosen should meet the patient's nutritional needs with the lowest risk and lowest cost possible. For most patients, enteral feeding is safer and cheaper and offers significant physiologic advantages. An algorithm for selection of the most appropriate nutritional support method is presented in Fig 22–1.

Prior to initiating specialized enteral nutritional support, efforts should be made to supplement food intake. Careful attention to patient preferences, timing of meals, diagnostic procedures and use of medica-

tions, and the use of foods brought to the hospital by family and friends can often significantly increase oral intake. Patients unable to eat enough at regular mealtimes to meet their nutritional requirements can be given **oral supplements** as snacks or to replace low-calorie beverages. Supplements of differing nutritional composition are available for the purpose of individualizing the diet in accordance with specific clinical requirements. Fiber and lactose content, caloric density, protein level, and amino acid profiles can all be modified as necessary.

Patients unable to take adequate oral nutrients who have functioning gastrointestinal tracts and who meet the criteria for nutritional support are candidates for **tube feedings.** Small-bore feeding tubes are placed via the nose into the stomach or duodenum. Patients able to sit up in bed who can protect their airways can be fed into the stomach. Because of the increased risk of aspiration, patients who cannot adequately protect their airways should be fed nasoduodenally. Feeding tubes can be passed into the duodenum by leaving an extra length of tubing and placing the patient in the right decubitus position. Metoclopramide, 10 mg intravenously, can be given 20 minutes prior to insertion and continued every 6 hours thereafter to facilitate passage through the pylorus. Occasionally patients will require fluoroscopy or endoscopic guidance to insert the tube distal to the pylorus. Placement of nasogastric and, particularly, nasoduodenal tubes should be confirmed radiographically before delivery of feeding solutions.

Feeding tubes can also be placed directly into the gastrointestinal tract using **tube enterostomies.** Most tube enterostomies are placed in patients who require long-term enteral nutritional support. The most common application is the surgical placement of gastrostomies and jejunostomies. Gastrostomies have the ad-

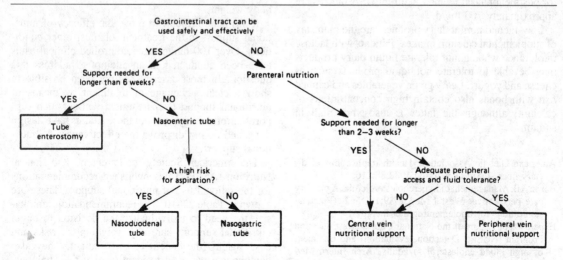

Figure 22–1. Nutritional support method decision tree.

vantage of allowing bolus feedings, while jejunostomies require continuous infusions. Gastrostomies—like nasogastric feeding—should only be used in patients at low risk for aspiration. Gastrostomies can also be placed percutaneously with the aid of endoscopy. These tubes can then be advanced to jejunostomies. Tube enterostomies can also be used in patients with unrelievable obstructions.

Patients who require nutritional support but whose gastrointestinal tracts are nonfunctional should receive **parenteral nutritional support.** Most patients receive parenteral feedings via a central vein—most commonly the subclavian vein. Peripheral veins can be used in some patients, but because of the high osmolality of parenteral solutions this is rarely tolerated for long periods.

Peripheral vein nutritional support is most commonly used in patients with nonfunctioning gastrointestinal tracts who require immediate support but whose clinical status is expected to improve within 1–2 weeks, allowing enteral feeding. Peripheral vein nutritional support is administered via standard intravenous lines. Solutions should always include lipid and dextrose in combination with amino acids to provide adequate nonprotein calories. Serious side effects are infrequent, but there is a high incidence of phlebitis and infiltration of intravenous lines.

Central vein nutritional support is most commonly delivered via intravenous catheters placed percutaneously using aseptic technique. Proper placement in the superior vena cava is documented radiographically before the solution is allowed to start running. Catheters must be carefully maintained by experienced nursing personnel and not used for anything other than nutritional support.

NUTRITIONAL REQUIREMENTS

Each patient's nutritional requirements should be determined independently of the method chosen. In most situations, solutions of equal nutrient value can be designed for delivery via enteral and parenteral routes, but differences in absorption must be considered. A complete nutritional support solution must contain water, energy, amino acids, electrolytes, vitamins, and minerals.

Water

For most patients, water requirements can be calculated by allowing 1500 mL for the first 20 kg of body weight plus 20 mL for every kilogram over 20. Additional losses should be replaced as they occur. For average-sized adult patients, fluid needs are about 30–35 mL/kg, or approximately 1 mL/kg of energy required (see below).

Energy

Energy requirements can be estimated by one of

3 methods: (1) by using standard equations to calculate basal energy expenditure (BEE) plus additional calories for activity and illness; (2) by applying a simple calculation based on calories per kilogram of body weight; or (3) by measuring energy expenditure with indirect calorimetry.

Basal energy expenditure (BEE) can be calculated by the Harris-Benedict equation (see p 1690). For undernourished patients, actual body weight should be used; and for obese patients, ideal body weight should be used. For most patients, an additional 20–50% of BEE is administered as nonprotein calories to accommodate energy expenditures during activity or relating to the illness. Occasional patients are noted to have energy expenditures greater than 150% of BEE.

Energy requirements can be estimated also by multiplying actual body weight in kilograms (for obese patients, ideal body weight) by 30–35 kcal.

Both of these methods provide imprecise estimates of actual energy expenditures. Studies using indirect calorimetry have demonstrated that as many as 30–40% of patients will have measured expenditures 10% above or below estimated values. For accurate determination of energy expenditure, indirect calorimetry should be used. Unfortunately, calorimeters are available in only a few medical centers. This means that patients must be closely monitored and regularly reassessed to determine whether estimates are close enough for clinical purposes.

Protein

Protein and energy requirements are closely related. If adequate calories are provided, most patients can be given 0.8–1.2 g of protein per kilogram per day. Patients undergoing moderate to severe stress should receive up to 1.5 g/kg/d. As in the case of energy requirements, actual weights should be used for normal and underweight patients and ideal weights for patients with significant obesity.

Patients who are receiving protein without adequate calories will catabolize protein for energy rather than utilizing it for protein synthesis. Thus, when energy intake is low, excess protein is needed for nitrogen balance. If both energy and protein intakes are low, extra energy will have a more significant positive effect on nitrogen balance than extra protein.

Electrolytes & Minerals

Requirements for sodium, potassium, and chloride vary widely. Most patients require 45–145 meq/d of each. The actual requirement in individual patients will depend on the patient's cardiovascular, renal, endocrine, and gastrointestinal status as well as measurements of serum concentration.

Patients receiving enteral nutritional support should receive adequate vitamins and minerals according to the recommended daily allowances (Table 22–1). Most premixed enteral solutions provide adequate vitamins and minerals as long as adequate calories are administered.

Patients receiving parenteral nutritional support require smaller amounts of minerals: calcium, 10–15 meq/d; phosphorus, 15–20 meq per 1000 nonprotein calories; and magnesium, 16–24 meq/d. Most patients receiving nutritional support do not require supplemental iron because body stores are adequate. Iron nutrition should be monitored closely by following the hemoglobin concentration, MCV, and iron studies. Parenteral administration of iron is associated with a number of adverse effects and should be reserved for iron-deficient patients unable to take oral iron.

Patients receiving parenteral nutritional support should be given the trace elements zinc (about 5 mg/d) and copper (about 2 mg/d). Patients with diarrhea will require additional zinc to replace fecal losses. Additional trace elements—especially chromium, manganese, and selenium—are provided to patients receiving long-term parenteral nutrition.

Parenteral vitamins are provided daily. Standardized multivitamin solutions are currently available to provide adequate quantities of vitamins A, B_{12}, C, D, E, thiamine, riboflavin, niacin, pantothenic acid, pyridoxine, folic acid, and biotin. Vitamin K is not given routinely but administered when the prothrombin time becomes abnormal.

Essential Fatty Acids

Patients receiving nutritional support should be given 2–4% of their total nonprotein calories as linoleic acid to prevent essential fatty acid deficiency. Most prepared enteral solutions contain adequate linoleic acid. Patients receiving parenteral nutrition should be given 500 mL of intravenous fat (emulsified soybean or safflower oil) about 2–3 times a week. Intravenous fat can also be used as an energy source in place of dextrose.

ENTERAL NUTRITIONAL SUPPORT SOLUTIONS

Most patients who require enteral nutritional support can be given commercially prepared enteral solutions (Table 22–11). Nutritionally complete solutions have been designed to provide adequate proportions of water, energy, protein, and micronutrients. Nutritionally incomplete solutions are also available to provide specific macronutrients (eg, protein, carbohydrate, and fat) to supplement complete solutions for patients with unusual requirements or to design solutions that are not available commercially.

Nutritionally complete solutions are characterized as follows: (1) by osmolality (isotonic or hypertonic), (2) by lactose content (present or absent), (3) by the molecular form of the protein component (intact proteins; peptides or amino acids), (4) by the quantity

Table 22–11. Enteral solutions.

Complete
  Blenderized (eg, Compleat, Compleat-Modified, Vitaneed)
  Whole protein, lactose-containing (eg, Meritene, Sustagen)
  Whole protein, lactose-free, low-residue:
    1 kcal/mL (eg, Ensure, Entrition, Isocal, Osmolite)
    1.5 kcal/mL (eg, Ensure Plus, Sustacal HC)
    2 kcal/mL (eg, Isocal HCN, Magnacal, TwoCal HN)
    High-nitrogen: > 16% total calories from protein (eg, Ensure HN, Isotein HN, Sustacal)
  Whole protein, lactose-free, high-residue:
    1 kcal/mL (eg, Enrich)
  Defined (elemental) formulas (eg, Vital, Vivonex)
  "Disease-specific" formulas:
    Renal failure: with essential amino acids (eg, Amin-Aid, Travasorb Renal)
    Malabsorption: with medium-chain triglycerides (eg, Portagen, Travasorb MCT)
    Respiratory failure: with > 50% calories from fat (eg, Pulmocare)
    Hepatic encephalopathy: with high amounts of branched-chain amino acids (eg, Hepatic-Aid II, Travasorb Hepatic)
Incomplete (modular)
  Protein (eg, Nutrisource Protein, Promed, Propac)
  Carbohydrate (eg, Nutrisource Carbohydrate, Polycose, Sumacal)
  Fat (eg, MCT Oil, Microlipid, Nutrisource Lipid)
  Vitamins (eg, Nutrisource Vitamins)
  Minerals (eg, Nutrisource Minerals)

of protein and calories provided, and (5) by fiber content (present or absent). For most patients, isotonic solutions containing no lactose or fiber are preferable. Such solutions generally contain relatively higher quantities of fat and intact protein. Most commercial isotonic solutions contain 1000 kcal and about 37–45 g of protein per liter.

Solutions containing hydrolyzed proteins or crystalline amino acids and with no significant fat content are called elemental solutions, since macronutrients are provided in their most "elemental" form. These solutions have been designed for patients with malabsorption, particularly pancreatic insufficiency and limited fat absorption. Elemental diets are extremely hypertonic and often result in more severe diarrhea. Their use should be limited to patients who cannot tolerate isotonic solutions.

Although formulas have been designed for specific clinical situations—solutions containing primarily essential amino acids (for renal failure), medium-chain triglycerides (for fat malabsorption), more fat (for respiratory failure and CO_2 retention), and more branched-chain amino acids (for hepatic encephalopathy and severe trauma)—they have not been shown to be superior to standard formulas for most patients.

Enteral solutions should be administered via continuous infusion, preferably with an infusion pump. Feedings should be started at full strength at about 25–33% of the estimated final infusion rate. Feedings can be advanced by similar amounts every 12 hours as tolerated.

Complications of Enteral Nutritional Support

Minor complications of tube feedings occur in 10–15% of patients. Gastrointestinal complications include diarrhea (most common), inadequate gastric emptying, emesis, esophagitis, and occasionally gastrointestinal bleeding. Diarrhea associated with tube feeding may be due to intolerance to the osmotic load or to one of the macronutrients (eg, fat, lactose) in the solution. Patients being fed in this way may also have diarrhea from other causes (as side effect of antibiotics or other drugs; associated with infection, etc), and these possibilities should always be investigated in appropriate circumstances.

Mechanical complications of tube feedings are potentially the most serious. Of particular importance are aspiration and aspiration pneumonia. All patients receiving nasogastric tube feedings are at risk for these life-threatening complications. Limiting nasogastric feedings to those patients who can adequately protect their airway and careful monitoring of patients being fed by tube should limit these serious complications to 1–2% of cases. Minor mechanical complications are common and include tube obstruction and dislodgment.

Metabolic complications during enteral nutritional support are common but in most cases easily managed. The most important problem is hypernatremic dehydration, most commonly seen in elderly patients unable to respond to thirst. Abnormalities of potassium, glucose, and acid-base balance may also occur.

PARENTERAL NUTRITIONAL SUPPORT SOLUTIONS

Parenteral nutritional support solutions can be designed to deliver adequate nutrients to virtually any patient. The basic parenteral solution is composed of dextrose, amino acids, and water. Electrolytes, minerals, trace elements, vitamins, and medications can also be added. Most commercial solutions contain the monohydrate form of dextrose that provides 3.4 kcal/g. Crystalline amino acids are available in a variety of concentrations, so that a broad range of solutions can be made up that will contain specific amounts of dextrose and amino acids as required.

Typical solutions for central vein nutritional support contain 25–35% dextrose and 2.75–4.25% amino acids depending upon the patient's estimated nutrient and water requirements. These solutions typically have osmolalities in excess of 1800 mosm/L and require infusion into a central vein.

Solutions with lower osmolalities can also be designed for infusion into peripheral veins. Typical solutions for peripheral infusion contain 5–10% dextrose and 2.75–4.25% amino acids. These solutions have osmolalities between 800 and 1200 mosm/L and result in a high incidence of thrombophlebitis and line infiltration. These solutions will provide adequate protein for most patients but inadequate energy. Additional energy must be provided in the form of emulsified soybean or safflower oil. Such intravenous fat solutions are currently available in 10% and 25% solutions providing 1.1 and 2.2 kcal/mL, respectively. Intravenous fat solutions are isosmotic and well tolerated by peripheral veins. Typical patients are given 500 mL of a 10% or 20% solution each day. As much as 60% of total nonprotein calories can be administered in this manner.

Intravenous fat can also be provided to patients receiving central vein nutritional support. In this instance, dextrose concentrations should be decreased to provide a fixed concentration of energy. Intravenous fat has been shown to be equivalent to intravenous dextrose in providing energy to "spare protein." Intravenous fat is associated with less glucose intolerance, less production of carbon dioxide, and less fatty infiltration of the liver and has been increasingly utilized in patients with hyperglycemia, respiratory failure, and liver disease. Intravenous fat has also been increasingly used in patients with large estimated energy requirements. Recent studies suggest that the maximum glucose utilization rate is approximately 5–7 mg/min/kg. Patients who require additional calories can be given them as fat to prevent excess administration of dextrose. Intravenous fat can also be used to prevent essential fatty acid deficiency. The optimal ratio of carbohydrate and fat in parenteral nutritional support has not been determined.

Infusion of parenteral solutions should be started slowly to prevent hyperglycemia and other metabolic complications. Typical solutions are given initially at a rate of 50 mL/h and advanced by about the same amount every 24 hours.

COMPLICATIONS OF PARENTERAL NUTRITIONAL SUPPORT

Complications of central vein nutritional support occur in up to 50% of patients. Although most are minor and easily managed, about 5% of patients will develop significant complications. Complications of central vein nutritional support can be divided into catheter-related complications and metabolic complications.

Catheter-related complications can occur during insertion or while the catheter is in place. Pneumothorax, hemothorax, arterial laceration, air emboli, and brachial plexus injury can occur during catheter placement. The incidence of these complications is inversely related to the experience of the physician performing the procedure but will occur in at least 1–2% of cases even in major medical centers. Each catheter placement should be documented by chest radiograph prior to initiation of nutritional support.

Catheter thrombosis and catheter-related sepsis are

Table 22–12. Metabolic complications of parenteral nutritional support.

Complication	Common Causes	Possible Solutions
Hyperglycemia	Too rapid infusion of dextrose, "stress," gluco-corticoids.	Decrease glucose infusion. Insulin. Replacement of dextrose with fat.
Hyperosmolar non-ketotic dehydration	Severe, unde-tected hyper-glycemia.	Insulin, hydration, potassium.
Hyperchloremic metabolic acidosis	High chloride ad-ministration.	Decrease chloride.
Azotemia	Excessive protein administration.	Decrease amino acid concentration.
Hyperphosphatemia, hypokalemia, hypomagnesemia	Extracellular to intracellular shift-ing with refeeding.	Increase solution concentration.
Liver enzyme abnormalities	Lipid trapping in hepatocytes, fatty liver.	Decreased dextrose.
Acalculous chole-cystitis	Biliary stasis.	Oral fat.
Zinc deficiency	Diarrhea, small bowel fistulas.	Increase concentration.
Copper deficiency	Biliary fistulas.	Increase concentration.

the most important complications of indwelling catheters. Patients with indwelling central vein catheters who develop signs of sepsis without an apparent source should have their lines removed immediately, the tip cultured, and antibiotics begun empirically. Patients with less significant fevers without an apparent source should have their lines removed and cultured and be observed without antibiotics. Catheter-related sepsis occurs in 2–3% of patients even if maximal efforts are made to prevent infection.

Metabolic complications of central vein nutritional support occur in over 50% of patients (Table 22–12). Most are minor and easily managed, and termination of support is seldom necessary.

PATIENT MONITORING DURING NUTRITIONAL SUPPORT

Every patient receiving enteral or parenteral nutritional support should be followed closely. Formal nutritional support teams composed of a physician, a nurse, a dietitian, and a pharmacist have been shown to decrease the rate of complications.

Patients should be monitored both for the adequacy of treatment and to prevent complications or detect them early when they occur. Because estimates of nutritional requirements are imprecise, frequent reassessment is necessary. Daily intakes should be recorded and compared with estimated requirements. Body weight, hydration status, and overall clinical status should be followed. Patients who do not appear to be responding as anticipated can be evaluated for nitrogen balance by means of the following equation:

$$\text{Nitrogen balance} = \frac{\text{24-hour protein intake (g)}}{6.25} - \left(\frac{\text{24-hour urinary}}{\text{nitrogen (g)}} + 4 \right)$$

Patients with positive nitrogen balances can be continued on their current regimens; patients with negative balances should receive moderate increases in calorie and protein intake and then be reassessed.

Feeding tubes and catheters should be examined often to avoid mechanical and infectious complications.

Monitoring for metabolic complications should include urine glucose determination every 6 hours and daily measurements of electrolytes; serum glucose, phosphorus, magnesium, calcium, and creatinine; and BUN until the patient is stabilized. Once the patient is stabilized, electrolytes, phosphorus, calcium, magnesium, and glucose should be checked at least twice weekly. Red blood cell folate, zinc, and copper should be checked at least once a month.

American Society of Parenteral and Enteral Nutrition Board of Directors: Guidelines for the use of enteral nutrition in the adult patient. JPEN 1987;11:435.

American Society of Parenteral and Enteral Nutrition Board of Directors: Guidelines for use of home total parenteral nutrition. JPEN 1987;11:342.

American Society of Parenteral and Enteral Nutrition Board of Directors: Guidelines for use of total parenteral nutrition in the hospitalized adult patient. JPEN 1986;10:441.

Baron RB: Nutrition support of the critically ill obese patient. Top Clin Nutr (Apr) 1986;1:71.

Cerra FB: Hypermetabolism, organ failure, and metabolic support. Surgery 1987;101:1.

Detsky AS et al: Perioperative parenteral nutrition: A meta-analysis. Ann Intern Med 1987;107:195.

Murphy LM, Lipman TO: Central venous catheter care in parenteral nutrition: A review. JPEN 1987;11:190.

Task Force on Nutrition Support in AIDS: Guidelines for nutrition support in AIDS. Nutrition 1989;5:39.

REFERENCES

Alpers DH, Clouse RE, Stenson WF: *Manual of Nutritional Therapeutics*, 2nd ed. Little, Brown, 1988.

National Research Council: *Recommended Dietary Allowances*, 10th ed. National Academy of Science, 1989.

Kinney JM et al: *Nutrition and Metabolism in Patient Care.* Saunders, 1988.

Pennington JAT, Church HN: *Bowes and Church's Food Values of Portions Commonly Used,* 14th ed. Lippincott, 1985.

Rombeau JL, Caldwell MD: *Enteral Nutrition,* 2nd ed. Saunders, 1990.

Rombeau JL, Caldwell MD: Parenteral Nutrition. Saunders, 1986.

Shils ME, Young VR: *Modern Nutrition in Health and Disease,* 7th ed. Lea & Febiger, 1988.

Wyngaarden JB, Smith LH: Nutritional diseases. Part XV of: *Cecil Textbook of Medicine,* 18th ed. Wyngaarden JB, Smith LH (editors). Saunders, 1988.

23

Introduction to Infectious Diseases

Richard A. Jacobs, MD, PhD, Ernest Jawetz, MD, PhD, & Moses Grossman, MD

Most infections are confined to specific organ systems. In a book organized as this one is—principally by organ system—many of the important infectious disease entities are discussed in chapters devoted to specific anatomic areas. In this chapter are discussed some important general problems in infectious diseases that are not covered elsewhere.

FEVER OF UNKNOWN ORIGIN (FUO)

To fulfill the criteria of FUO, a patient must have an illness of at least 3 weeks' duration, fevers over 38.3 °C (101 °F), and must remain undiagnosed after 1 week of study in the hospital. The intervals specified are arbitrary ones intended to exclude patients with prolonged but self-limited viral illnesses and to allow time for the usual radiographic, serologic, and cultural studies to be performed. However, because of concerns over costs of hospitalization and the availability of most screening tests on an outpatient basis, the criteria often are not adhered to.

Etiologic Considerations

Certain general principles about FUO are helpful to keep in mind in the diagnostic approach to these patients.

A. Common Causes: Most cases represent unusual manifestations of common diseases and not rare or exotic diseases—ie, tuberculosis, endocarditis, and gallbladder disease are more common causes of FUO than Whipple's disease or familial Mediterranean fever.

B. Age of Patient: In adults, infections (30–40% of cases) and cancer (20–35% of cases) account for the majority of FUOs. In children, infections (30–50% of cases) are the most common cause of FUO and usually occur at age less than 6 years. Viral illnesses and occult urinary tract infections are leading infectious causes in children. Unlike adults, children rarely have cancer as a cause of FUO (5–10% of cases). Autoimmune disorders occur with equal frequency in adults and children (10–20% of cases), but the diseases differ. Juvenile rheumatoid arthritis is particularly common in children, whereas systemic lupus erythematosus, Wegener's granulomatosis, and polyarteritis nodosa are more common in adults.

C. Duration of Fever: The cause of FUO changes dramatically in patients who have been febrile for a prolonged period of time—ie, 6 months or longer. Infection, cancer, and autoimmune disorders combined account for only 20% of FUOs in these patients. Instead, other entities such as granulomatous diseases (granulomatous hepatitis, Crohn's disease, ulcerative colitis) and factitious fever become important causes. Up to 27% of patients who say they have been febrile for 6 months or longer actually have no true fever or underlying disease. Instead, the usual normal circadian variation in temperature (temperature 1–2 °F higher in the afternoon than in the morning) is interpreted as abnormal.

D. Immunologic Status: In the neutropenic patient, fungal infections and occult bacterial infection are important and common causes of FUO. In the patient taking immunosuppressive medications (particularly organ transplant patients), cytomegalovirus infections are a frequent cause of fever.

E. Classification of Causes of FUO: Most patients with FUO will fit into one of 5 categories.

1. Patients with infection–Both systemic and localized infections can cause FUO. Tuberculosis and endocarditis are the most common systemic infections, but mycoses, viral diseases (particularly infection with Epstein-Barr virus and cytomegalovirus), toxoplasmosis, brucellosis, salmonellosis, malaria, and many other less common infections have been implicated. Primary infection with human immunodeficiency virus (HIV) or opportunistic infections associated with the acquired immunodeficiency syndrome (AIDS), particularly mycobacterial infections, can also present at FUO. The most common form of localized infection causing FUO is an obscure abscess. Liver, spleen, kidney, brain, and bone are organs in which abscess may be difficult to find. A collection of pus may form in the peritoneal cavity or in the subdiaphragmatic, subhepatic, paracolic, or other areas. Cholangitis, urinary tract infection, dental abscess, or a collection of pus in a paranasal sinus may cause prolonged fever.

2. Patients with neoplasms–Many cancers can present as FUO. The most common are lymphoma and leukemia. Primary and metastatic tumors of the liver also are frequently associated with fever, as in renal cell carcinomas. Chronic lymphocytic leukemia and multiple myeloma are rarely associated with fever, and the presence of fever in patients with these diseases should prompt a careful search for infection.

3. Patients with autoimmune disorders– Still's disease, systemic lupus erythematosus, and polyarteritis nodosa are the more common autoimmune causes of FUO.

4. Patients with miscellaneous causes–Many other diseases have been associated with FUO but less commonly than the foregoing types of illness. Examples include temporal arteritis, sarcoidosis, Whipple's disease, familial Mediterranean fever, recurrent pulmonary emboli, alcoholic hepatitis, drug fever, factitious fever, and others.

5. Patients with undiagnosed FUO–Despite extensive evaluation, in 10–15% of patients the diagnosis remains elusive. In about three-fourths of these patients, the fever abates spontaneously and the clinician never knows the cause; in the remainder, more classic manifestations of the underlying disease appear over time, and the diagnosis then becomes apparent.

Approach to Diagnosis of FUO

Because the evaluation of a patient with FUO is so costly and time-consuming, it is imperative to document the presence of fever. This is done most reliably by observing the patient while the temperature is being taken to make certain that fever is not factitious (self-induced). Associated findings that usually accompany fever include tachycardia, chills, and piloerection. A thorough history—including family, occupational, social (sexual preference, use of intravenous drugs), and travel histories—may give clues to the underlying diagnosis. Detailed and repeated physical examination may reveal subtle, evanescent clinical findings that are the key to diagnosis.

In addition to "routine" laboratory studies, blood cultures should always be obtained, preferably when the patient is off antibiotics. Serologic studies may be diagnostic for certain immunologic diseases but are less useful in diagnosing infectious causes of FUO. A single elevated titer rarely allows one to make a diagnosis of infection; instead, one must demonstrate a 4-fold rise or fall in titer to confirm a specific infectious cause.

Almost all patients with FUO should have a chest radiograph, sinus films, upper gastrointestinal series with small bowel follow-through, barium enema, proctosigmoidoscopy, and some evaluation of gallbladder function. The usefulness of radionuclide studies has not been extensively studied in FUO. Theoretically, a gallium scan would be more helpful than an indium-labeled white blood cell scan, because gallium is useful for detecting infection and neoplasm whereas the indium scan is useful only for detecting infection. Both studies are limited by a high rate of

false positivity. Indium-labeled immunoglobulin is another radionuclide study that may prove to be useful in detecting infection and neoplasm and is presently under investigation.

CT scan of the abdomen and pelvis can be quite useful in evaluating patients with FUO. When positive, the findings on CT scan are usually confirmed and often lead to a specific diagnosis. It is important to realize that a negative CT scan is not quite as useful; even with a negative CT scan, more invasive procedures such as exploratory laparotomy may lead to the diagnosis. The role of magnetic resonance imaging (MRI) in the diagnosis of FUO has not been evaluated.

Invasive procedures are often required for diagnosis. Any abnormal finding should be aggressively evaluated: headache calls for lumbar puncture to rule out meningitis; skin from an area of rash should be biopsied to look for cutaneous manifestations of collagen vascular disease or infection; and enlarged lymph nodes should be aspirated or biopsied and examined for cytologic features to rule out neoplasm and sent for culture and infection. Bone marrow aspiration with biopsy is a relatively low-yield procedure, but the risk is low and the procedure should be done if other less invasive tests have not yielded a diagnosis. Liver biopsy will yield a specific diagnosis in 10–15% of patients with FUO. One should consider this procedure in any patient with abnormal liver function tests even if the liver is normal in size on physical examination. The role of exploratory laparotomy is debatable. Studies on usefulness of laparatomy in the diagnosis of FUO have not been done since the advent of CT scanning and MRI. One should consider laparotomy in the deteriorating patient if the diagnosis is elusive despite extensive evaluation.

Therapeutic Trials

Therapeutic trials are indicated if a diagnosis is strongly suspected—eg, it is reasonable to give antituberculous drugs if one suspects tuberculosis, or tetracycline if brucellosis is suspected. However, if there is no clinical response in several weeks, it is imperative to stop therapy and reevaluate the situation. Empiric use of steroids should be discouraged; these agents can suppress fever if given in high enough doses, but they can also exacerbate many infections, and infection remains a leading cause of FUO. Suppression of fever with low doses of nonsteroidal antiinflammatory agents (eg, naproxen, 250 mg twice daily) has been reported to be specific for fever associated with malignancy, but published data are limited.

Chang JC: Neoplastic fever: A proposal for diagnosis. Arch Intern Med 1989;149:1728.

Dinarello CA, Cannon JG, Wolff SM: New concepts on the pathogenesis of fever. Rev Infect Dis 1988;10:168.

Larson EB et al: Fever of undetermined origin: Diagnosis

and follow-up of 105 cases, 1970–1980. Medicine 1982;61:269.

Quinn MJ et al: Computed tomography of the abdomen in evaluation of patients with fever of unknown origin. Radiology 1980;136:407.

INFECTIONS IN THE IMMUNOCOMPROMISED PATIENT

A description of the cellular basis of immune responses, the role of various host responses in maintaining health and the methods used for detection of deficiencies in the immune system can be found in Chapter 14. Immunodeficiency may be congenital but more often is due to suppression of the immune system by diseases or drugs. Deficiencies of polymorphonuclear cells, T lymphocytes, or B lymphocytes tend to predispose the host to infection with different agents. Thus, polymorphonuclear cell deficiency predisposes particularly to infection with gram-negative enteric bacteria, staphylococci, and fungi; B lymphocyte deficiency and hypogammaglobulinemia to infection with extracellular encapsulated organisms, eg, pneumococci or *Haemophilus* sp; and T lymphocyte deficiency to infection with intracellular bacteria (eg, mycobacteria, *Listeria, Legionella*), fungi (*Candida, Cryptococcus, Aspergillus,* etc), protozoa (*Pneumocystis carinii,* etc), and viruses (cytomegalovirus, herpes simplex, etc).

Many opportunistic organisms (ie, organisms that rarely produce invasive infections in an uncompromised host) do not produce disease except in the immunodeficient host. Such hosts are often infected with several opportunists simultaneously.

Infections caused by common organisms may present uncommon clinical manifestations. Determination of the specific infecting agents is essential for effective treatment.

Immunodeficient Hosts

Patients deficient in normal immune defenses fall into several groups:

(1) Congenital defects of cellular or humoral immunity or a combination of both, eg, Wiskott-Aldrich syndrome. These are usually children.

(2) Patients with cancer, particularly lymphoreticular cancer.

(3) Patients receiving immunosuppressive therapy. These include patients with neoplastic disease and transplant recipients who are receiving corticosteroids, other immunosuppressive drugs, or radiation treatment. Patients receiving high-dose corticosteroid therapy for other diseases (asthma, temporal arteritis, systemic lupus erythematosus, etc) also fall into this group.

(4) Patients who have very few polymorphonuclear cells ($< 500/\mu L$) or those whose polymorphonuclear cells do not function normally with respect to phagocytosis or the intracellular killing of microorganisms (eg, chronic granulomatous disease).

(5) A larger group of patients who are not classically immunodeficient but whose host defenses are seriously compromised by prior splenectomy, debilitating illness, diabetes mellitus, surgical or other invasive procedures (eg, intravenous drug abuse or intravenous hyperalimentation), burns, or broad-spectrum antimicrobial therapy.

(6) Patients with variants of the acquired immunodeficiency syndrome (AIDS). (See Chapter 24.) This profound disturbance in T lymphocyte subpopulations produces extreme susceptibility to opportunistic infections and to rapidly disseminating Kaposi's sarcoma and other neoplasms, with an exceedingly high death rate.

Infectious Agents

A. Bacteria: Any bacterium pathogenic for humans can infect an immunosuppressed host. Furthermore, noninvasive and nonpathogenic organisms (opportunists such as *Staphylococcus epidermidis,* diphtheroids, *Propionibacterium acnes*) may also cause disease in such cases. Examples include gram-negative bacteria—particularly *Pseudomonas, Serratia, Proteus, Providencia*—and *Nocardia.* Many come from the hospital environment and are resistant to antimicrobial drugs. Mycobacteria—both *Mycobacterium tuberculosis* and atypical organisms—must be considered.

B. Fungi: *Candida, Aspergillus, Cryptococcus, Mucor,* and others can all cause disease in immunosuppressed hosts. Candidiasis is the most common and is often found in patients receiving intensive antimicrobial therapy.

C. Viruses: Cytomegalovirus is the most common, but varicella-zoster and herpes simplex viruses are also important.

D. Protozoa: *Pneumocystis carinii* is an important cause of pneumonia in many immunodeficient patients. This diagnosis must be made early, because reasonably effective therapy is available. *Toxoplasma gondii* is also important and is susceptible to therapy.

Cryptosporidium may cause chronic, severe diarrhea.

Approach to Diagnosis

A systematic approach is necessary, including the following steps:

(1) Review carefully the patient's current immune status, previous antimicrobial therapy, and all previous culture reports.

(2) Obtain pertinent cultures for bacteria, fungi, yeasts, and viruses.

(3) Consider which of the serologic tests for fungal, viral, and protozoal diseases are pertinent.

(4) Consider special diagnostic procedures. The cause of pulmonary infiltrates can be easily determined with simple techniques in some situations—

eg, induced sputum yields a diagnosis of *Pneumocystis carinii* pneumonia in 50–80% of AIDS patients with this infection. In other situations, more invasive procedures (bronchoalveolar lavage, transbronchial biopsy, or even open lung biopsy) may be required. Other procedures such as skin, liver, or bone marrow biopsy may be helpful in establishing a diagnosis.

(5) Consider whether the infection (eg, candidiasis) is superficial or systemic. Therapeutic considerations are quite different in each case.

Because infections in the immunocompromised patient can be rapidly progressive and life-threatening, diagnostic procedures must be done promptly, and empiric therapy is often instituted before a specific diagnostic agent has been isolated.

Approach to Treatment

Caution: It is essential to avoid aggravating the patient's other problems and to avoid gross alterations of the host's normal microbial flora.

Take measures to improve host defenses, correct electrolyte imbalance, offer adequate caloric intake, etc. Improve the patient's immune status whenever possible. This includes temporary decrease in immunosuppressive drug dosage in transplant patients and modification of chemotherapy in cancer patients. It is important in the prevention of nosocomial infections to minimize the use of venous and Foley catheters and central lines. Their continuing use must be evaluated regularly, and—if their colonization by microbes is suspected—they must be replaced and appropriate cultures performed.

Injection of immune globulin USP (human gamma globulin) at regular intervals can compensate for certain B cell deficiencies. Granulocyte transfusions are only rarely able to tide the patient over a prolonged period of neutropenia.

Antimicrobial drug therapy should be rationally chosen in order to be specific and bactericidal for the infecting agent. Combinations of antimicrobial drugs may be necessary, since multiple infectious agents may be involved.

Empiric therapy is often instituted in the immunosuppressed patient. The antibiotic or combination of antibiotics used first depends on the type of immunocompromise and the site of infection. For example, in the febrile neutropenic patient, one is concerned primarily about bacterial and fungal infections. A commonly used regimen would be an antipseudomonal penicillin (ticarcillin, mezlocillin, pipericillin) or third-generation cephalosporin (cefotaxime, ceftizoxime, or ceftazidime) in combination with tobramycin (see Chapter 31 for dosing information). If the patient fails to respond in 3 days, amphotericin B is usually added. In the organ transplant patient with interstitial infiltrates, one is concerned mainly about *Pneumocystis carinii* or *Legionella* spp, so that empiric treatment with intravenous erythromycin and trimethoprim-sulfamethoxazole would be reasonable.

If the patient fails to respond to empiric treatment, one must often decide between empiric addition of more antimicrobial agents or doing invasive procedures outlined above to make a specific diagnosis. By making a specific diagnosis, therapy can be specific and "polypharmacy" with multiple potentially toxic agents avoided.

Anaissie EG et al: Randomized trial of beta-lactam regimens in febrile neutropenic patients. Am J Med 1988;84:581.

Press DW et al: Hickman catheter infections in patients with malignancies. Medicine 1984;63:189.

Schimpf SC, Klastersky J, Goya H (editors): Therapy for immunocompromised patients. Am J Med 1986;80(Suppl 5C):1. (Entire issue.)

Wheeler RR et al: Esophagitis in the immunocompromised host. Rev Infect Dis 1987;9:88.

Young LS: Empirical antimicrobial therapy in the neutropenic host. N Engl J Med 1986;315:580.

NOSOCOMIAL INFECTIONS

Nosocomial infections are by definition those acquired in the course of hospitalization. At present in the USA, 3–7% of patients who enter the hospital free from infection acquire a nosocomial infection. Generally, patients acquire hospital infections with common organisms because of their own increased susceptibility to infection or because of procedures carried out in the hospital.

Nosocomial infections can be attributed principally to the following aspects of contemporary medical care:

(1) Many hospitalized patients (especially in tertiary care hospitals, which have the highest nosocomial infection rate) are compromised because of deficiencies in their immunologic responses or impaired host defenses (skin ulcers, aspiration tendencies, etc). These may be congenital but commonly are acquired as a result of the administration of drugs for the treatment of cancer, for the maintenance of transplants, or for the suppression of autoimmune processes. The very young and the elderly are particularly susceptible to infection.

(2) Many aspects of medical care now require the use of invasive techniques for diagnosis, monitoring, and therapy. Examples are the indwelling urinary catheter; intravascular lines used for measurements, infusions of fluids or drugs, or parenteral alimentation; drainage tubes; and shunts.

(3) Materials administered in the intensive care unit may themselves be vectors of infection: common examples are contaminated intravenous solutions or their containers; respirators and humidifiers that may introduce microorganisms into particularly susceptible lungs; and plastic tubing that may carry infectious agents into the body.

(4) The widespread use of antimicrobial drugs contributes to the selection of drug-resistant microor-

ganisms both in the individual patient and in the hospital environment. Thus, nosocomial infections are often attributable to members of the endogenous human microflora or free-living microorganisms that happen to be particularly resistant to antimicrobial drugs, presenting difficult management problems. Such organisms often are not established human "pathogens" but can be classed as "opportunists."

The principal anatomic sites of hospital-acquired infection are the urinary tract, surgical wounds, the respiratory tract, and skin sites where indwelling needles or tubes penetrate. Most notorious among nosocomial infections are those due to gram-negative enteric bacteria, staphylococci, or mycotic organisms that develop in patients with granulocyte counts below 500/μL as a result of cancer chemotherapy or organ transplant. In such patients, bloodstream invasion often occurs without a well-defined portal of entry. Patients with markedly depressed cell-mediated immunity may also develop viral infections in the hospital, eg, varicella-zoster, cytomegalovirus, hepatitis, and others. They are likewise open to opportunists like *Legionella*, *Nocardia*, and other bacteria and protozoa, eg, *P carinii*.

In general, organisms that cause nosocomial infections tend to be multidrug-resistant and are often not sensitive to antibiotics used to treat community-acquired infections. For example, *Staphylococcus aureus* strains that cause hospital infections may be resistant to nafcillin and cephalosporins; *Staphylococcus epidermidis*—a frequent pathogen in patients with foreign bodies (shunts, hyperalimentation catheters, prosthetic heart valves, etc)—similarly may be resistant to nafcillin and sensitive only to vancomycin; and gram-negative organisms that cause nosocomial infections may be unusual (*Enterobacter* spp, *Acinetobacter* spp, *Pseudomonas*) and sensitive only to aminoglycosides. For these reasons, it is often necessary to institute empiric therapy with drugs such as vancomycin and tobramycin (or amikacin) until a specific agent is isolated and sensitivities are known, at which time the least toxic and least costly active drug can be used. The bacteriology and sensitivity patterns of nosocomial infections are quite variable, and one needs to be aware of local patterns to best treat these patients.

Prevention is of paramount importance in controlling nosocomial infections. Foley catheters, intravenous lines, hemodynamic monitoring devices, hyperalimentation lines, and similar such "invasive" devices should only be used when critical to patient care and, when used, should be discontinued at the earliest possible time. Attentive nursing care (positioning to prevent decubitus ulcers, wound care, elevating the head during tube feedings to prevent aspiration) is critical in preventing nosocomial infections. In addition, careful monitoring of high-risk areas (intensive care units, neonatal units, surgical floors, hemodialysis and transplant units, etc) by skilled personnel—hospital epidemiologists—to detect increases in infection rates early is a key factor in prevention of these types of infections.

Garibaldi RA et al: Infections among patients in nursing homes. N Engl J Med 1981;305:731.
Haley RW et al: The efficacy of infection surveillance and control programs in preventing nosocomial infections. Am J Epidemiol 1985;121:183.
McGowan JE Jr: Antimicrobial resistance in hospital organisms and its relation to antibiotic use. Rev Infect Dis 1983;5:1033.

INFECTIONS OF THE CENTRAL NERVOUS SYSTEM

Infections of the central nervous system can be caused by almost any infectious agent but most commonly are due to bacteria, mycobacteria, fungi, spirochetes, and viruses. Certain symptoms and signs are more or less common to all types of central nervous system infection: headache, fever, sensorial disturbances, neck and back stiffness, positive Kernig and Brudzinski signs, and cerebrospinal fluid abnormalities. In patients presenting with these manifestations, the possibility of central nervous system infection must be considered.

Such an infection constitutes a *medical emergency*. Immediate diagnostic steps must be instituted to establish the specific cause. Normally, these include the history, physical examination, blood count, blood culture, lumbar puncture with careful study and culture of the cerebrospinal fluid, and a chest film. The cerebrospinal fluid must be examined for cell count, glucose, and protein, and a smear must be stained for bacteria (and acid-fast organisms when appropriate) and cultured for pyogenic organisms and for mycobacteria and fungi when indicated. Counterimmunoelectrophoresis and latex agglutination can detect antigens of encapsulated organisms. These tests are particularly helpful for diagnosis when the patient has already received antibiotics, so that cultures are likely to be negative. In bacterial meningitis, prompt therapy is essential to prevent death and minimize serious sequelae.

If a space-occupying lesion (brain abscess, subdural empyema) is suspected, its presence should be confirmed by CT scan, which ideally should precede lumbar puncture.

Etiologic Classification

Central nervous system infections can be divided into several categories that usually can be readily distinguished from each other by cerebrospinal fluid examination as the first step toward etiologic diagnosis (Table 23–1).

A. Purulent Meningitis: Patients with bacterial meningitis usually present acutely within hours or 1–2 days after onset of symptoms. The organisms responsible depend primarily on the age of the patient as summarized in Table 23–2. The diagnosis usually based on the gram-stained smear (positive in 60–80%) or culture (positive in over 90%).

B. Granulomatous Meningitis: Patients with granulomatous meningitis present less acutely with a history of symptoms lasting weeks to months. The most common pathogens are *Mycobacterium tuberculosis,* atypical mycobacteria, fungi (*Cryptococcus, Coccidioides, Histoplasma,* etc.), and *Treponema pallidum* (meningovascular syphilis). The diagnosis is made by culture or in some cases by serologic tests (cryptococcosis, coccidioidomycosis, syphilis).

C. Aseptic Meningitis: Aseptic meningitis—a much more benign and self-limited syndrome—is caused principally by viruses, especially mumps virus, the enterovirus group (including coxsackieviruses and echoviruses), and herpesviruses. Infectious mononucleosis may be accompanied by aseptic meningitis. Leptospiral infection is usually placed in the aseptic group because of the lymphocytic cellular response and its relatively benign course. This type of meningitis also occurs during secondary syphilis and stage 2 Lyme disease.

D. Encephalitis: Due to herpesviruses, arboviruses, and many other viruses. Produces disturbances of the sensorium, seizures, and many other manifestations. Cerebrospinal fluid may be entirely normal or may show some lymphocytes.

E. Partially Treated Bacterial Meningitis: Bacterial meningitis following partly effective antimicrobial therapy may present with the same course and some of the same cerebrospinal fluid findings as aseptic meningitis.

F. "Neighborhood" Reaction: As noted in Table 23–1, this term denotes a purulent infectious process in close proximity to the central nervous system that spills some of the products of the inflammatory

process—white blood cells or protein—into the cerebrospinal fluid. Such an infection might be a brain abscess, osteomyelitis of the vertebrae, epidural abscess, subdural empyema, bacterial sinusitis, etc.

G. Noninfectious Meningeal Irritation: Meningismus, presenting with the classic signs of meningeal irritation with totally normal cerebrospinal fluid findings, may occur in the presence of other infections such as pneumonia, shigellosis, etc. Carcinomatous meningitis, sarcoidosis, systemic lupus erythematosus, and chemical meningitis can also produce signs and symptoms of meningeal irritation with associated cerebrospinal fluid pleocytosis, increased protein, and low or normal glucose.

H. Brain Abscess: Brain abscess presents as a space-occupying lesion; symptoms may include vomiting, fever, and neurologic manifestations. If brain abscess is suspected, a CT scan should precede lumbar puncture.

I. Amebic Meningoencephalitis: These infections are caused by free-living amebas and present as 2 distinct syndromes. The diagnosis is confirmed by culture or identification of the organism on biopsy specimens. No effective therapy is available.

1. Primary amebic meningoencephalitis is caused by *Naegleria fowleri* and is an acute fulminant disease characterized by signs of meningeal irritation that rapidly progresses to encephalitis.

2. Granulomatous amebic encephalitis is caused by *Acanthamoeba* species. It is an indolent disease characterized by headache, nausea, vomiting, cranial neuropathies, seizures, and hemiparesis.

Treatment

Treatment consists of supporting circulation, ventilation, the airway, and other life-support functions that may be compromised by infection and resulting disturbance of the central nervous system. Increased

Table 23–1. Typical cerebrospinal fluid findings in various central nervous system diseases.

Diagnosis	Cells/µL	Glucose (mg/dL)	Protein (mg/dL)	Opening Pressure
Normal[1]	0–5 lymphocytes	45–85	15–45	70–180 mm H$_2$O
Purulent meningitis (bacterial)[2] (community-acquired)	200–20,000 polymorphonuclear neutrophils	Low (<45)	High (>50)	++++
Granulomatous meningitis (mycobacterial, fungal)[2,3]	100–1000, mostly lymphocytes	Low (<45)	High (>50)	+++
Aseptic meningitis, viral or meningoencephalitis[3,4]	100–1000, mostly lymphocytes	Normal	Moderately high (>50)	Normal to +
Spirochetal meningitis[3]	25–2000, mostly lymphocytes	Normal or low	High (>50)	+
"Neighborhood" reaction[5]	Variably increased	Normal	Normal or high	Variable

[1] Cerebrospinal fluid glucose must be considered in relation to blood glucose level. Normally, cerebrospinal fluid glucose is 20–30 mg/dL lower than blood glucose, or 50–70% of the normal value of blood glucose.
[2] Organisms in smear of culture of cerebrospinal fluid; counterimmunoelectrophoresis or latex agglutination may be diagnostic.
[3] Polymorphonuclear neutrophils may predominate early.
[4] Viral isolation from cerebrospinal fluid early; antibody titer rise in paired specimens of serum.
[5] May occur in mastoiditis, brain abscess, epidural abscess, sinusitis, septic thrombus, brain tumor. Cerebrospinal fluid culture results usually negative.

intracranial pressure due to brain edema often requires therapeutic attention. Hyperventilation, mannitol, and even drainage of cerebrospinal fluid through placement of ventricular catheters have been employed to control cerebral edema and increased intracranial pressure. Dexamethasone may also decrease cerebral edema and may be useful in preventing some long-term sequelae (hearing loss) of bacterial meningitis. In the case of purulent meningitis proper, antimicrobial treatment is imperative. Since the identity of the causative microorganism may remain unknown or doubtful for a few days, initial antibiotic treatment as listed in Table 23–2 should be directed against the microorganisms most common for each age group.

The usual duration of therapy for most bacterial meningitides is 10–14 days. Meningitis caused by gram-negative bacilli should be treated longer (ie, for 3 weeks). The role of adjunctive therapy with corticosteroids or nonsteroidal anti-inflammatory drugs is under investigation, and these agents cannot be recommended at this time.

Therapy of other types of meningitis is discussed elsewhere in this book (fungal meningitis, Chapter 30; syphilis and Lyme borreliosis, Chapter 27; tuberculous meningitis, Chapter 26).

Lebel MH et al: Dexamethasone therapy for bacterial meningitis: Results of 2 double-blind, placebo-controlled trials. N Engl J Med 1988;319:964.

Ma P et al: *Naegleria* and *Acanthamoeba* infections: Review. Rev Infect Dis 1990;12:490.

Schaad UB et al: A comparison of ceftriaxone and cefuroxime for the treatment of bacterial meningitis in children. N Engl J Med 1990;322:141.

Shapiro ED: Prophylaxis for bacterial meningitis. Med Clin North Am 1985;69:269.

Tunkel AR, Wispelway B, Schald M: Bacterial meningitis: Recent advances in pathophysiology and treatment. Ann Intern Med 1990;112:610.

ANIMAL & HUMAN BITE WOUNDS

About 1% of emergency room visits in urban areas are for treatment of animal and human bites. Dog

Table 23–2. Initial antimicrobial therapy for purulent meningitis of unknown cause.

Age Group	Common Microorganisms	Standard Therapy
0–4 weeks	*Escherichia coli*, group B *Streptococcus*, *Listeria monocytogenes*	Ampicillin[1] + a third-generation cephalosporin[2] or ampicillin + an aminoglycoside[3]
4–12 weeks	*E coli*, group B *Streptococcus*, *L monocytogenes*, *Haemophilus influenzae*, *Streptococcus pneumoniae*	Ampicillin + third-generation cephalosporin
3 months to 18 years	*H influenzae*, *Neisseria meningitidis*, *S pneumoniae*	Third-generation cephalosporin or ampicillin + chloramphenicol[4]
18–60 years	*S pneumoniae*, *N meningitidis*	Penicillin G[5] or ampicillin
Over 60 years	*S pneumoniae*, *N meningitidis*, *L monocytogenes*, gram-negative bacilli	Ampicillin + third-generation cephalosporin
Postsurgical or posttraumatic	*Staphylococcus aureus*, *S pneumoniae*, gram-negative bacilli	Third-generation cephalosporin with or without nafcillin[6]

[1] Ampicillin dose in neonates (< 7 days old) is 50 mg/kg IV every 12 hours; for infants > 7 days, children, and adults, 50–100 mg/kg IV every 6 hours.
[2] Third-generation cephalosporins are cefotaxime, ceftizoxime, and ceftriaxone. The dosage of cefotaxime and ceftizoxime in neonates (0–1 week of age) is 50 mg/kg every 12 hours; in infants 1–4 weeks of age, 50 mg/kg IV every 8 hours; in infants > 1 month of age (including adults), 50 mg/kg IV every 6 hours. The dosage of ceftriaxone (including adults) is 50 mg/kg IV every 12 hours over 4 weeks.
[3] The aminoglycosides are gentamicin and tobramycin. The dosage for infants < 7 days old is 2.5 mg/kg IV every 12 hours; ages 1 week to 10 years, 2.5 mg/kg every 8 hours; > 10 years, 1.7 mg/kg IV every 8 hours adjusted for renal failure.
[4] Chloramphenicol dosage is 100 mg/kg/d IV in divided doses in children, 50 mg/kg/d IV in divided doses in adults.
[5] Penicillin G dosage is 3–4 million units IV every 4 hours.
[6] Nafcillin dosage is 2 g IV every 4 hours.

bites occur most commonly in the summer months, and most occur in children. Biting animals are usually known by their victims, and most biting incidents are provoked (ie, bites occur while playing with the animal or after surprising the animal or waking it abruptly from sleep). Failure to elicit a history of provocation is important, because an unprovoked attack raises the possibility that the animal is rabid. Human bites are usually inflicted by children while playing or fighting; in adults, bites are associated with alcohol use and closed-fist injuries that occur during fights.

The animal inflicting the bite, the location of the bite, and the type of injury inflicted are all important determinants of whether these injuries become infected. Cat bites are more likely to become infected than human bites—between 30% and 50% of all cat bites subsequently become infected. Infections following human bites are variable: Those inflicted by children rarely become infected, because they are superficial; and bites by adults become infected in 15–20% of cases, with a particularly high rate of infection in closed-fist injuries. Dog bites, for unclear reasons, become infected only 5% of the time. Bites of the head, face, and neck are less likely to become infected than bites on the extremities. Puncture wounds become infected more frequently than lacerations, probably because the latter are easier to irrigate and debride.

The bacteriology of bite infections depends upon the biting animal and when the infection occurs after the biting incident. Early infections (within 24 hours after the bite) following dog and cat bites are most frequently caused by *Pasteurella multocida*. These infections are characterized by rapid onset and progression, fevers, chills, cellulitis, and local adenopathy. Early infections following human bites are usually caused by mixed aerobic and anaerobic mouth flora and can produce a rapidly progressive necrotizing infection. Late infections (longer than 24 hours after the bite) are caused mainly by staphylococci and streptococci, but innumerable organisms have been implicated in these infections. *Capnocytophaga canimorsus* (formerly called a DF2 organism), a gram-negative organism that is part of canine oral flora; *Eikenella corrodens,* another gram-negative organism that can be part of human mouth flora; *Haemophilus* spp, *Pseudomonas* spp, and other gram-negative organisms have all been implicated in bite infections.

The possibility of AIDS transmission from a bite by an HIV-infected person is exceedingly remote. There have been no documented cases of HIV transmission by this route.

Treatment

A. Local Care: Vigorous cleansing and irrigation of the wound as well as debridement of necrotic material are the most important factors in decreasing the incidence of infections.

B. Suturing: If wounds require closure for cosmetic or mechanical reasons, suturing can be done. However, one should never suture a wound that is already infected, and wounds of the hand should generally not be sutured since a closed-space infection of the hand can result in loss of function.

C. Prophylactic Antibiotics: Prophylaxis is indicated in high-risk bites, eg, cat bites in any location (dicloxacillin, 0.5 g orally 4 times a day for 3–5 days) and hand bites by any animal or by humans (penicillin V, 0.5 g orally 4 times a day for 3–5 days). Other regimens that have not been adequately studied but may be effective based on bacteriologic findings include an oral cephalosporin or amoxicillin/clavulanic acid (Augmentin).

D. Antibiotics: For wounds that are infected, antibiotics are clearly indicated. How they are given (orally or intravenously) and the need for hospitalization are clinical decisions that depend on the assessment of each individual patient. In general, *P multocida* is best treated with penicillin or a tetracycline. Response to therapy is slow, and therapy should be continued for at least 2–3 weeks. Human bites frequently require admission to the hospital and intravenous therapy with either penicillin or clindamycin. Because the bacteriology of these infections is so variable, one should always culture infected wounds and adjust therapy appropriately, especially if the patient is not responding to initial empiric treatment.

E. Tetanus and Rabies: All patients must be evaluated for the need for tetanus (see Chapter 26) and rabies (see Chapter 25) prophylaxis.

Brook I: Microbiology of human and animal bite wounds in children. Pediatr Inf Dis J 1987;6:29.

Brown CG: Dog bites: The controversy continues. Am J Emerg Med 1985;3:83.

Elliott DL: Pet-associated illness. N Engl J Med 1985;313:985.

SEXUALLY TRANSMITTED DISEASES

Some infectious diseases are transmitted most commonly—or most efficiently—by sexual contact. The frequency of some of these infections (eg, gonorrhea) has increased markedly in recent years as a result of changing patterns of sexual behavior. Others (eg, herpetic and chlamydial genital infections) are only now beginning to be appreciated as important systemic infections with a primarily sexual mode of transmission. Rectal and pharyngeal infections caused by these microorganisms are common as a result of varied sexual practices.

Most of the infectious agents that cause sexually transmitted diseases are fairly easily inactivated when exposed to a harsh environment. They are thus particularly suited to transmission by contact with mucous membranes. They may be bacteria (eg, gonococci), spirochetes (syphilis), chlamydiae (nongonococcal urethritis, cervicitis), viruses (eg, herpes simplex, hepatitis B virus, cytomegalovirus, AIDS virus), or protozoa (eg, *Trichomonas*). In most infections caused by these agents, early lesions occur on genitalia or other sexually exposed mucous membranes; however, wide dissemination may occur, and involvement of nongenital tissues and organs may mimic many noninfectious disorders. All sexually transmitted diseases have subclinical or latent phases that may play an important role in long-term persistence of the infection or in its transmission from infected (but largely asymptomatic) persons to other contacts. Laboratory examinations are of particular importance in the diagnosis of such asymptomatic patients. Simultaneous infection by several different agents is common, and any person with a sexually transmitted disease should be tested for syphilis. If the test is negative, a repeat study should be done in 3 months, since seroconversion can be delayed.

For each patient, there are one or more sexual contacts who require diagnosis and treatment. As a rule, sexual partners should be treated simultaneously to avoid prompt reinfection. Finding a sexually transmitted disease in a child strongly suggests sexual abuse, and the case should be reported to the authorities. The commonest sexually transmitted diseases are gonorrhea,* syphilis,* condyloma acuminatum, chlamydial genital infections, cytomegalovirus and herpesvirus genital infections, *Trichomonas* vaginitis, chancroid,* granuloma inguinale,* scabies, and lice. However, shigellosis,* hepatitis,* amebiasis,* giardiasis, cryptosporidiasis, salmonellosis,* and campylobacteriosis may also be transmitted by sexual (oral-anal) contact, especially in homosexual males. Homosexual or heterosexual contact is the most prevalent method of transmission of HIV and AIDS* (see Chapter 24).

The risk of developing a sexually transmitted disease following a sexual assault is unknown. Victims should be evaluated within 24 hours of the assault, and cultures for *Neisseria gonorrhoeae* and *Chlamydia trachomatis* should be obtained as well as a blood sample for serologic testing for syphilis. (An additional sample should be stored for future testing for HIV and hepatitis B if needed.) Follow-up serologic testing for syphilis should be performed in 3 months. If infection is found, it should be treated. Use of presumptive therapy is controversial, some workers feeling that all patients should receive it and others that it should be limited to those in whom follow-up cannot be ensured or that it should be given only to those who request it. If therapy is given, a reasonable regimen would be ceftriaxone, 250 mg intramuscularly, following by doxycycline, 100 mg orally twice daily for 7 days.

Clinical and epidemiologic details and methods of diagnosis and treatment are discussed for each infection separately elsewhere in this book (see Index).

Centers for Disease Control: Sexually transmitted diseases: Treatment guidelines. MMWR 1989;38:38.

Holmes KK et al: *Sexually Transmitted Diseases*. McGraw-Hill, 1984.

INFECTIONS IN DRUG ADDICTS

The abuse of parenterally administered narcotic drugs has increased enormously. There are an estimated 300,000 or more narcotic addicts in the USA, mostly in or near large urban centers. Consequently, many physicians and hospitals serving such urban and suburban populations are faced with the diagnosis and treatment of problems that are closely related to drug abuse. Infections are a large part of these problems.

Common Infections That Occur With Greater Frequency in Drug Users

(1) Skin infections are associated with poor hygiene and multiple needle punctures, commonly due to *S aureus*.

(2) Hepatitis is nearly universal among habitual drug users and is transmissible both by the parenteral and by the fecal-oral route. Many addicts experience hepatitis more than once.

(3) Aspiration pneumonia and its complications (lung abscess, empyema, brain abscess) result from altered consciousness associated with drug abuse. Mixed aerobic and anaerobic mouth flora are usually involved.

(4) Pulmonary septic emboli may originate from venous thrombi or right-sided endocarditis.

(5) Sexually transmitted diseases are not directly related to drug abuse but, for social reasons, occur with greater frequency in population groups that are also involved in drug abuse.

(6) AIDS has a high incidence among intravenous drug abusers and their sexual contacts and the offspring of infected women (see Chapter 24).

(7) Infective endocarditis (see below).

Infections Rare in USA Except in Drug Users

(1) Tetanus: Drug users now form a majority of cases of tetanus in the USA, especially in unimmunized female addicts who inject drugs subcutaneously ("skin-popping").

(2) Malaria: Needle transmission occurs from addicts who acquired the infection in malaria-endemic areas outside the USA.

(3) Melioidosis: This chronic pulmonary infection caused by *Pseudomonas pseudomallei* is occasionally seen in debilitated drug users.

---

* Reportable to public health authorities.

Osteomyelitis

Osteomyelitis involving vertebral bodies, sternoclavicular joints, and other sites usually results from hematogenous distribution of injected organisms or septic venous thrombi. Pain and fever precede roentgenologic changes by several weeks. While staphylococci, often methicillin-resistant, are common organisms, *Serratia, Pseudomonas,* and other organisms rarely encountered in "spontaneous" bone or joint disease are found in addicts who use drugs intravenously.

Infective Endocarditis

The organisms that cause infective endocarditis in those who use drugs intravenously are most commonly *S aureus, Candida* (especially *Candida parapsilosis*), *Streptococcus faecalis,* and gram-negative bacteria (especially *Pseudomonas* and *Serratia marcescens*).

Involvement of the right side of the heart is somewhat more frequent than involvement of the left side, and infection of more than one valve is not infrequent. Right-sided involvement, especially in the absence of murmurs, is often suggested by manifest pulmonary emboli. The diagnosis must be established by blood culture. Until the etiologic organism is known, treatment must be directed against the most probable organisms. One commonly used regimen includes ampicillin (6–9 g/d), nafcillin (9–12 g/d), and either gentamicin or tobramycin (4.5–6 mg/kg/d). In the penicillin-allergic patient or if methicillin-resistant *S aureus* is a concern, vancomycin (20–30 mg/kg/d in 2 or 3 divided doses) can be used with an aminoglycoside.

Chandrasekar PH, Narula AP: Bone and joint infections in intravenous drug abusers. Rev Infect Dis 1986;8:904.

Levine DP et al: Bacteremia in narcotic addicts: Infective endocarditis. Rev Infect Dis 1986;8:374.

Scheidegger C, Zimmerli W: Infectious complications in drug addicts: Seven-year review of 269 hospitalized narcotics abusers in Switzerland. Rev Infect Dis 1989; 11:486.

BACTERIAL ENDOCARDITIS

Discussions of the pathogenesis, clinical findings, complications, and prevention of endocarditis can be found in Chapter 8. Antimicrobial therapy of bacterial endocarditis is discussed in this section.

Approximately 90% of cases of native valve endocarditis are due to viridans streptococci (60%), *S aureus* (20%), and enterococci (5–10%). Gram-negative organisms and fungi account for a small percentage.

The bacteriology of native valve endocarditis in intravenous drug users differs from that of other patients. *S aureus* accounts for 60% or more of all cases and for 80–90% of cases in which the tricuspid valve is infected. Enterococci and streptococci comprise the balance in about equal proportion. Gram-negative aerobic bacilli, fungi, and unusual organisms that rarely infect others may cause endocarditis in intravenous drug users.

The bacteriology of prosthetic valve endocarditis also is distinctive. Early infections (ie, those occurring within 2 months after valve implantation) are commonly caused by staphylococci—both coagulase-positive and coagulase-negative—gram-negative organisms, and fungi. Late prosthetic valve endocarditis resembles native valve endocarditis, with the majority of infections caused by streptococci, though coagulase-negative staphylococci still cause a significant proportion of cases.

Diagnosis

Blood culture is the single most important test in diagnosis of endocarditis. Blood cultures are positive in 95% or more of cases. For patients with suspected endocarditis, 3 blood cultures should be obtained at different times; in 95–99% of cases, one or more of the 3 cultures will be positive.

Prior antimicrobial therapy is the most common cause of culture-negative endocarditis. To recover the causative organism in patients who have been treated previously, more than 3 blood cultures obtained over 24–48 hours are recommended before starting antimicrobials unless the patient is acutely ill.

Echocardiography may provide useful adjunctive information to identify the specific valve or valves that are infected. The sensitivity of echocardiography is between 30% and 75%; therefore, it cannot reliably rule out endocarditis but may confirm a clinical suspicion. Transesophageal echocardiography is a new technique that is useful in identification of valve ring abscess and may also be more sensitive than 2-dimensional and M-mode echocardiography.

Treatment

Empiric regimens for endocarditis while culture results are pending should include agents active against staphylococci, streptococci, and enterococci. Nafcillin or oxacillin, 1.5 g every 4 hours, plus penicillin, 4 million units every 4 hours, plus gentamicin, 1 mg/kg every 8 hours, is such a regimen. Vancomycin, 1 g every 12 hours, may be used instead of the penicillins in the penicillin-allergic patient.

A. Streptococci: For penicillin-susceptible viridans group streptococcal endocarditis (ie, MIC ≤ 0.1 μg/mL), penicillin G, 3 million units (400,000 units/kg for children) intravenously every 4 hours for 4 weeks, is recommended. The duration of therapy can be shortened to 2 weeks if streptomycin, 500 mg intramuscularly every 12 hours, or gentamicin, 1 mg/kg every 8 hours, is added to the regimen. For infections due to nutritionally deficient streptococci which tend to persist or recur after 2 weeks of combination therapy, total duration of therapy should be 4 weeks, with addition of gentamicin for the first 2 weeks.

For the penicillin-allergic patient, either cefazolin, 1 g every 8 hours for 4 weeks, or vancomycin, 1 g every 12 hours for 4 weeks, may be used. Two-week regimens including aminoglycosides have not been proved to be effective except with penicillin. Anecdotal reports and animal studies suggest that ceftriaxone as a single daily dose of 2–4 g for 4 weeks may be effective, but more study is needed before this regimen can be recommended.

For viridans streptococci with a penicillin MIC greater than 0.1 μg/mL, gentamicin, 1 mg/kg, should be included in the 4-week penicillin regimen for at least 2 weeks, though some authorities recommend a total duration of 4 weeks. This regimen is recommended also for prosthetic valve infection.

B. Enterococci: For enterococcal endocarditis, the relapse rate is unacceptably high when penicillin is used alone; either streptomycin or gentamicin must be included in the regimen. Because aminoglycoside resistance occurs in enterococci, susceptibility to it should be documented. Gentamicin is probably the aminoglycoside of choice, because streptomycin resistance is more common than gentamicin resistance and the nephrotoxicity of gentamicin is generally more easily managed than the vestibular toxicity of streptomycin. Penicillin, 4 million units every 4 hours (or vancomycin, 1 g every 12 hours in penicillin-allergic patients), plus gentamicin, 1 mg/kg every 8 hours for at least 4 weeks, is recommended. Patients who have had symptoms of endocarditis for 3 months or longer may be more prone to relapse and should be treated for 6 weeks with the combination.

C. Staphylococci: For methicillin-susceptible *S aureus,* nafcillin or oxacillin, 1.5 g every 4 hours for 4 weeks, is the preferred therapy. For penicillin-allergic patients, cephalothin, 2 g every 4 hours, cefazolin 1 g every 6 hours, or vancomycin, 1 g every 12 hours, may be used. For methicillin-resistant strains, vancomycin is the only agent of proved effectiveness.

The role of aminoglycoside combination regimens for *S aureus* endocarditis remains unclear, but they may be useful in shortening the duration of bacteremia. In selected patients with tricuspid valve endocarditis (with or without pulmonary involvement) who do not have serious extrapulmonary sites of infection, the total duration of therapy can be shortened from 4 weeks to 2 weeks.

Because coagulase-negative staphylococci—a common cause of prosthetic valve endocarditis—are routinely resistant to methicillin, β-lactam antibiotics should not be used for this infection until the isolate is known to be susceptible. A combination of vancomycin for 6 weeks, rifampin, 300 mg twice daily for 6 weeks, and gentamicin, 1 mg/kg every 8 hours for the first 2 weeks, is the regimen of choice.

Bisno AL et al: Antimicrobial treatment of infective endocarditis due to viridans streptococci, enterococci, and staphylococci. JAMA 1989;261:1471. (Consensus statement.)

Chambers HF, Miller RT, Newman MG: Right-sided *Staphylococcus aureus* endocarditis in intravenous drug abusers: Two-week combination therapy. Ann Intern Med 1988;109:619. (Nafcillin plus tobramycin for 2 weeks.)

"FOOD POISONING" & ACUTE GASTROENTERITIS

Food poisoning is a nonspecific term often applied to the syndrome of acute anorexia, nausea, vomiting, or diarrhea that is attributed to food intake, particularly if it afflicts groups of people and is not accompanied by fever. The actual cause of such acute gastrointestinal upsets might be emotional stress, viral or bacterial infections, food intolerance, inorganic (eg sodium nitrite) or organic (eg, mushroom, shellfish) poisons, or drugs (eg, antimicrobials). More specifically, food poisoning may refer to toxins produced by bacteria growing in food (staphylococci, clostridia, *Bacillus cereus*) or to acute food infections with short incubation periods and a mild course (*Salmonella enterocolitis* or to infection with enterotoxigenic *Escherichia coli,* shigellae, or vibrios (*Vibrio cholerae,* El Tor vibrios, marine vibrios including *Vibrio parahaemolyticus, Vibrio vulnificus*). *Campylobacter jejuni* and *Yersinia enterocolitica* may produce similar clinical enterocolitis and can be identified only by special stool culture methods. Adenoviruses, rotaviruses, and Norwalk-type viruses may produce a similar syndrome. *E coli* O157:H7 is an infrequent cause of hemorrhagic colitis. Some prominent features of some of these "food poisonings" are listed in Table 23–3. In general, the diagnosis must be suspected when groups of people who have shared a meal develop acute vomiting or diarrhea. Food and stools must be secured for bacteriologic and toxicologic examination. In febrile patients, blood cultures are indicated.

Treatment usually consists of replacement of fluids and electrolytes and, very rarely, management of hypovolemic shock and respiratory embarrassment. If botulism is suspected, polyvalent antitoxin must be administered. Antimicrobial drugs are not indicated unless a specific microbial agent producing progressive systemic involvement can be identified.

Blacklow NR, Cukor G: Viral gastroenteritis. N Engl J Med 1981;304:397.

Blaser MJ, Reller LB: *Campylobacter* enteritis. N Engl J Med 1981;305:1444.

Fekety R: Recent advances in management of bacterial diarrheas. Rev Infect Dis 1983;5:246.

Spika JS et al: Chloramphenicol-resistant *Salmonella newport* traced through hamburger to dairy farms. N Engl J Med 1987;316:565.

Table 23-3. Acute bacterial diarrheas and "food poisoning."

Organism	Incubation Period (Hours)	Vomiting	Diarrhea	Fever	Epidemiology	Pathogenesis	Clinical Features
Staphylococcus	1–8, rarely up to 18	+++	+	–	Staphylococci grow in meats, dairy, bakery products and produce enterotoxin.	Enterotoxin acts on receptors in gut that transmit impulse to medullary centers.	Abrupt onset, intense vomiting for up to 24 hours, regular recovery in 24–48 hours. Occurs in persons eating the same food. No treatment usually necessary except to restore fluids and electrolytes.
Bacillus cereus	1–8, rarely up to 18	+++	++	–	Reheated fried rice causes vomiting or diarrhea.	Enterotoxins formed in food or in gut from growth of B cereus.	After 1–6 hours, mainly vomiting. After 8–16 hours, mainly diarrhea. Both self-limited to less than 1 day.
Clostridium perfringens	8–16	±	+++	–	Clostridia grow in rewarmed meat dishes and produce enterotoxin.	Enterotoxin produced in food and in gut causes hypersecretion in small intestine.	Abrupt onset of profuse diarrhea; vomiting occasionally. Recovery usual without treatment in 1–4 days. Many clostridia in cultures of food and feces of patients.
Clostridium botulinum	24–96	±	Rare	–	Clostridia grow in anaerobic foods and produce toxin.	Toxin absorbed from gut blocks acetylcholine at neuromuscular junction.	Diplopia, dysphagia, dysphonia, respiratory embarrassment. Treatment requires clear airway, ventilation, and intravenous polyvalent antitoxin (see p 984). Toxin present in food and serum. Mortality rate high.
Escherichia coli (some strains)	24–72	±	++	–	Organisms grow in gut and produce toxin. May also invade superficial epithelium.	Toxin causes hypersecretion in small intestine.	Usually abrupt onset of diarrhea; vomiting rare. A serious infection in neonates. In adults, "traveler's diarrhea" is usually self-limited in 1–3 days. Use diphenoxylate (Lomotil) but no antimicrobials.
Vibrio para-haemolyticus	6–96	+	++	±	Organisms grow in seafood and in gut and produce toxin, or invade.	Hypersecretion in small intestine; stools may be bloody.	Abrupt onset of diarrhea in groups consuming the same food, especially crabs and other seafood. Recovery is usually complete in 1–3 days. Food and stool cultures are positive.
Vibrio cholerae (mild cases)	24–72	+	+++	–	Organisms grow in gut and produce toxin.	Toxin causes hypersecretion in small intestine. Infective dose: 10^7–10^9 organisms.	Abrupt onset of liquid diarrhea in endemic area. Needs prompt replacement of fluids and electrolytes (see p 993) IV or orally. Tetracyclines shorten excretion of vibrios. Stool cultures positive.
Shigella spp (mild cases)	24–72	±	++	+	Organisms grow in superficial gut epithelium and gut lumen and produce toxin.	Organisms invade epithelial cells; blood, mucus, and PMNs in stools. Infective dose: 10^2–10^3 organisms.	Abrupt onset of diarrhea, often with blood and pus in stools, cramps, tenesmus, and lethargy. Stool cultures are positive. In severe cases, give trimethoprim-sulfamethoxazole, ampicillin, or chloramphenicol. Do not give opiates. Restore fluids. Often mild and self-limited.
Salmonella spp	8–48	±	++	+	Organisms grow in gut. Do not produce toxin.	Superficial infection of gut, little invasion. Infective dose: 10^5 organisms.	Gradual or abrupt onset of diarrhea and low-grade fever. No antimicrobials unless systemic dissemination is suspected. Stool cultures are positive. Prolonged carriage is frequent.
Clostridium difficile	?	–	+++	+	Associated with antimicrobial drugs, eg, clindamycin.	Toxin causes epithelial necrosis in colon; pseudomembranous colitis.	Especially after abdominal surgery; abrupt bloody diarrhea, and fever. Toxin in stool. Oral vancomycin useful in therapy.
Campylobacter jejuni	2–10 days	–	+++	+	Organism grows in jejunum and ileum.	Invasion and toxin production uncertain.	Fever, diarrhea; PMNs and fresh blood in stool, especially in children. Usually self-limited. Special media needed for culture at 43 °C. Erythromycin in severe cases with invasion. Usual recovery in 5–8 days.
Yersinia entero-colitica	?	±	++	+	Fecal-oral transmission (occasionally). Food-borne. ?In pets.	Gastroenteritis or mesenteric adenitis. Occasional bacteremia. Toxin produced.	Severe abdominal pain, diarrhea, fever; PMNs and blood in stool; polyarthritis, erythema nodosum in children. If severe, give tetracycline or gentamicin. Keep stool at 4 °C before culture.

Terranova W, Blake PA: *Bacillus cereus* food poisoning. N Engl J Med 1978;298:143.

Walker RI et al: Pathophysiology of *Campylobacter* enteritis. Microbiol Rev 1986;50:81.

TRAVELER'S DIARRHEA

Whenever a person travels from one country to another, particularly if the change involves a marked difference in climate, social conditions, or sanitation standards and facilities, diarrhea is likely to develop within 2–10 days. There may be up to 10 or even more loose stools per day, often accompanied by abdominal cramps, nausea, occasionally vomiting, and, rarely, fever. The stools do not usually contain mucus or blood, and aside from weakness, dehydration, and occasionally acidosis, there are no systemic manifestations of infection. The illness usually subsides spontaneously within 1–5 days; rarely, it lasts 2–3 weeks.

Stool cultures rarely reveal salmonellae or shigellae. Contributory causes may at times include unusual food and drink, change in living habits, occasional viral infections (enteroviruses or rotaviruses), and change in bowel flora. A significant number of cases of traveler's diarrhea are caused by acquisition of strains of *Escherichia coli* that produce an enterotoxin.

Other less common pathogens are *Salmonella, Shigella, Campylobacter,* and *Entamoeba.* In patients with fever and bloody diarrhea, stool culture may be indicated, though the illness usually has resolved by the time the patient seeks medical attention. Chronic watery diarrhea may be due to amebiasis or giardiasis or, rarely, tropical sprue.

For most individuals, the affliction is short-lived, and symptomatic therapy with opiates or diphenoxylate with atropine (Lomotil) is all that is required. Antimicrobial drugs generally are not indicated. Avoidance of fresh foods and water sources that are likely to be contaminated is recommended for travelers to developing countries, where infectious diarrheal illnesses are endemic. For prophylaxis, bismuth subsalicylate is effective. Numerous antimicrobial regimens also are effective, such as norfloxacin, 400 mg, ciprofloxacin, 500 mg, or trimethoprim-sulfamethoxazole, 160/800 mg, once daily. Tetracyclines also are effective, but photosensitization with these drugs makes them less desirable. Because not all travelers will have diarrhea and because most episodes are brief and self-limited, an alternative approach is to provide the traveler with a 5-day supply of antimicrobials to be taken if significant diarrhea occurs during the trip.

DuPont HL, Ericsson CD, Johnson PC: Chemotherapy and chemoprophylaxis of travelers' diarrhea. Ann Intern Med 1985;102:260.

DuPont HL et al: Prevention of travelers' diarrhea by the tablet formulation of bismuth subsalicylate. JAMA 1987;257:1347.

Gorbach SL, Edelman R: Travelers' diarrhea (NIH Consensus Development Conference). Rev Infect Dis 1986; 255:S227.

Mathewson JJ et al: A newly recognized cause of travelers' diarrhea: Enteroadherent *Escherichia coli.* J Infect Dis 1985;151:471.

ACTIVE IMMUNIZATION AGAINST INFECTIOUS DISEASES

RECOMMENDED IMMUNIZATION OF CHILDREN

Every individual—child or adult—should maintain an adequate defense against infectious disease by immunization. The recommended schedules and dosages change often, so that one should always consult the manufacturers' package inserts.

The schedule for active immunizations in children is presented in Table 23–4.

RECOMMENDED IMMUNIZATION OF ADULTS

Several vaccines are recommended for adults depending upon previous vaccination status and the risks of exposure to certain diseases.

Tetanus-Diphtheria Toxoid

Everyone should receive a primary series of immunizations against tetanus and diphtheria once (Table 23–4). Thereafter, routine booster doses of tetanus-diphtheria toxoid for adults (Td) should be given every 10 years. Adults who have not previously been immunized should receive 2 doses of Td 1–2 months apart, followed by a booster dose 6–12 months later. Adults partially immunized in childhood with DTP need only a total of 3 doses of tetanus and diphtheria toxoid (ie, if one dose was given in childhood, give 2 doses of Td; if 2 doses were given, only one dose of Td is needed to complete primary immunization). If booster doses are given too frequently, an Arthus reaction as well as severe local pain and swelling can occur. Pertussis vaccine, which is combined with tetanus-diphtheria toxoid for use in children under 7 years of age (DPT), should *not* be used in adults.

Measles

Adults born before during or 1957 are considered immune to measles. Adults born after 1956 or later who were not immunized after age 1 year and who do not have a physician-documented history or labora-

Table 23–4. Recommended schedule of active immunization of children.

Age	Product Administered[1]
2 months	DTP-1,[2] OPV-1[3]
4 months	DTP-2, OPV-2
6 months	DTP-3
15 months[4]	MMR-1,[5] DTP-4, OPV-3
18 months	Hb CV[6]
4–6 years	DTP-5, OPV-4, MMR-2
14–16 years and every 10 years thereafter	Td[7]

(Adapted from: General recommendations on immunization: Guidelines from the Immunization Practices Advisory Committee. Ann Intern Med 1989;111:133.)

[1] Package insert should be consulted for doses, storage, and handling. Preparations from different manufacturers may vary, and individual manufacturers may change their products from time to time.

[2] DTP = diphtheria and tetanus toxoids and pertussis vaccine, absorbed. DTP can be used up to the seventh birthday.

[3] OPV = live oral poliovirus vaccine, trivalent (contains poliovirus types 1, 2, and 3).

[4] At least 6 months should have elapsed since DTP-3; or, if fewer than 3 doses of DTP have been given, at least 6 weeks should have elapsed since the last DTP or OPV. MMR should not be delayed to allow for MMR, DTP-4, and OPV-3 to be given simultaneously. Giving MMR at 15 months and DTP-4 and OPV-3 at 18 months is acceptable.

[5] MMR = measles, mumps, rubella virus vaccine, live. In high-risk areas (5 or more cases of measles in preschool children in each of the last 5 years, or a county with a recent outbreak among unvaccinated children of preschool age), initial vaccination with MMR should be at 12 months of age.

[6] Haemophilus influenzae b polysaccharide antigen conjugated to a protein carrier. The conjugated vaccine is preferred over the polysaccharide vaccine. If the conjugate is not available, the polysaccharide vaccine can be given at 24 months or older. Children less than 5 years of age who have been previously vaccinated with polysaccharide vaccine between ages 18 and 23 months should be revaccinated with the conjugated vaccine.

[7] Td = tetanus and diphtheria toxoids, absorbed. For use in persons older than 7 years. Contains the same amount of tetanus as DTP but less diphtheria toxoid.

tory evidence of previous infection should receive 2 doses of vaccine at least 1 month apart. Persons born between 1963 and 1967—during which time inactivated measles vaccine was the only product available—should also be revaccinated with 2 doses of live attenuated vaccine separated by at least 1 month. Persons vaccinated before their first birthday should also be revaccinated. Because outbreaks of measles have occurred in young adults who have received a single dose of measles vaccine, revaccination is recommended, particularly before going to college, entering a health care profession, or embarking on foreign travel.

About 5–15% of unimmunized individuals will develop fever and about 5% a mild rash 5–12 days after vaccination. Fever and rash are self-limiting, lasting only 2–3 days. Local swelling and induration

is particularly common in individuals previously vaccinated with inactivated vaccine. Pregnant women and persons with a history of anaphylaxis to eggs or egg products should not be vaccinated. Milder allergic reactions to eggs are not a contraindication to vaccination.

Rubella

The major purpose of rubella vaccination is to prevent transmission to the fetus. Immunization is recommended for all adults but particularly for women of childbearing age who have not previously been immunized. In addition, both male and female hospital workers who may be exposed to patients with rubella or who might have contact with pregnant patients should be immunized. A single immunization is given.

Adverse effects are usually mild. Up to 40% of unvaccinated adults (usually women) experience joint pain. Joint symptoms begin 1–3 weeks after vaccination and are self-limited, lasting 3–10 days. Frank arthritis is rare. Although vaccination of pregnant women is *not* recommended, available data suggest that with the RA27/3 vaccine strain (the one presently available), the congenital rubella syndrome does not occur in the offspring of those inadvertently vaccinated during pregnancy or within 3 months before conception.

Mumps

Most adults who have been exposed to mumps are immune even if they did not have clinically recognized disease. Thus, this vaccine is not often used though it is recommended for all adults—particularly males—who are susceptible.

Influenza

Influenza vaccination is recommended yearly. Those at greatest risk for severe complications of influenza should have priority in vaccination programs: (1) adults with chronic cardiopulmonary disease severe enough to require either regular medical follow-up or hospitalization in the last year, and (2) residents of nursing homes and other chronic care facilities. Others who would benefit from vaccination include medical personnel who have extensive contact with high-risk patients; healthy adults over age 65; and adults with chronic metabolic or renal disease, those with anemia, and those receiving immunosuppressive drugs. Vaccination is recommended also for otherwise healthy adults who provide essential community services.

Local reactions (erythema and tenderness) at the site of injection are common, but fevers, chills, and malaise (which lasts in any case only 2–3 days) are rare. Like measles, mumps, and yellow fever vaccines, influenza vaccine is prepared using embryonated chicken eggs, and persons with a history of anaphylaxis to eggs should not be vaccinated.

Pneumococcal Pneumonia

Pneumococcal vaccine contains purified polysaccharide from 23 of the most common strains of *Streptococcus pneumoniae*, which cause 90% of bacteremic episodes in the USA. Although the efficacy of pneumococcal vaccine has been questioned, it is presently recommended for patients at increased risk for developing severe pneumococcal disease, especially asplenic patients and those with sickle cell disease. It is also recommended for adults who are at increased risk of developing pneumococcal disease, including those with chronic illnesses (eg, cardiopulmonary disease, alcoholism, cirrhosis, cerebrospinal fluid leaks), those who are immunocompromised (eg, patients with Hodgkin's disease, lymphoma, chronic renal failure, nephrotic syndrome, and asymptomatic or symptomatic HIV infection), and those taking immunosuppressive medications. In addition, it is recommended for all individuals over 65 years of age. A single dose of vaccine usually confers lifelong immunity. Revaccination every 5–6 years should be considered only in those at highest risk of fatal pneumococcal infection (eg, asplenic patients) and those known to have a rapid decline in antibody titers (eg, nephrotic syndrome, transplant recipients, renal failure). Revaccination should also be considered for high-risk individuals previously immunized with the older 14-valent vaccine. Since immunocompetent patients respond best to the vaccine, it should be given before splenectomy or starting chemotherapy if that can be anticipated.

Mild reactions (erythema and tenderness) occur in up to 50% of recipients, but systemic reactions are uncommon. The incidence of adverse reactions with revaccination is unknown but is probably related to the interval between vaccinations. Early reports suggested frequent adverse reactions when revaccination occurred within 1–2 years. Subsequent reports have indicated few adverse reactions when revaccination occurs 5 or more years later.

Hepatitis B

Hepatitis B vaccine is given on 3 separate occasions—the first 2 doses 1 month apart and the last dose 5 months after the second one. It is recommended for all individuals at increased risk of developing hepatitis B for social reasons (intravenous drug users, male homosexuals), family reasons (household and sexual contacts of hepatitis B carriers), or occupational reasons (those with frequent exposure to blood and blood products, hemodialysis patients and staff, house officers, morticians). Although most often used for preexposure prophylaxis, the vaccine is also given as postexposure prophylaxis along with hepatitis B immunoglobulin following needle stick injury or mucous membrane exposure to blood from an individual who is HBAg-positive. It is also given along with hepatitis B immunoglobulin to infants of mothers who are HBAg-positive. Immunity wanes with time, but recommendations for revaccination have not been established. Adverse reactions are minor and limited to local soreness.

RECOMMENDED IMMUNIZATIONS FOR TRAVELERS

Individuals traveling to other countries frequently require immunizations in addition to those listed above and may benefit from chemoprophylaxis against various diseases. Every traveler must fulfill the immunization requirements of the health authorities of different countries. These are listed in *Health Information for International Travel*, published by the Centers for Disease Control. An updated version is published yearly and is available from the Superintendent of Documents, United States Government Printing Office, Washington DC 20402.

When individuals request information and vaccinations for travel from a physician, their entire immunization history should be reviewed and updated, including those immunizations listed above that are not specifically required for travel.

Various vaccines can be given simultaneously at different sites. Some, such as cholera, plague, and typhoid vaccine, which cause significant discomfort, are best given at different times. In general, live attenuated vaccines (measles, mumps, rubella, yellow fever, and oral poliovaccine) should not be given to immunosuppressed individuals or household members of immunosuppressed people or to pregnant women. Immunoglobulin should not be given for 3 months before or at least 2 weeks after live virus vaccines, because it may attenuate the antibody response.

Chemoprophylaxis of malaria is discussed in Chapter 28.

Cholera

Because the incidence of cholera among travelers is very low and because the vaccine is only marginally effective, the World Health Organization does not routinely require immunization even when traveling to and from endemic areas. Certain countries, however, still require vaccination for travel (Middle Eastern countries, Asian countries, occasionally others).

Cholera vaccine contains a suspension of killed vibrios, including prevalent antigenic types. Two injections are given intramuscularly 2–6 weeks apart, followed by booster injections every 6 months during periods of possible exposure. Protection depends largely on booster doses. The WHO certificate is valid for 6 months only.

Hepatitis A

No active immunization is available. Temporary passive immunity may be induced by the intramuscular injection of immune globulin, 0.02 mL/kg every 2–3 months or 0.1 mL/kg every 6 months. Immune globulin is recommended for all parts of the world where environmental sanitation is poor and the risk of exposure to hepatitis A is high because of contaminated food and water supplies and contact with infected persons.

Hepatitis B

This vaccine is not ordinarily recommended for travelers other than medical personnel who will be handling body fluids of individuals in highly endemic areas (southeast Asia and sub-Saharan Africa). The dosing schedule is as outlined above.

Meningococcal Meningitis

If travel is contemplated to an area where meningococcal meningitis is epidemic or highly endemic (Nepal, sub-Saharan Africa, New Delhi), polysaccharide vaccines from types A, C, W-135, and Y may be indicated. Follow manufacturer's dosage recommendations.

Plague

Plague vaccine is a suspension of killed plague bacilli that is given intramuscularly, 3 injections 4 or more weeks apart. A single booster injection 6 months later is desirable. Vaccination is generally recommended only for travelers who will have exposure to rodents or rabbits in rural areas where plague is endemic. (Some areas in South America, southeast Asia, occasionally others.)

Poliomyelitis

Adult travelers to tropical or developing countries who have not previously been immunized against poliomyelitis should receive a primary series of 3 doses of inactivated enhanced-potency poliovaccine (IPV), as follows: 2 doses 4–8 weeks apart and then a third dose 6–12 months after the second. Because of the risk of vaccine-associated paralytic poliomyelitis, live attenuated oral poliovaccine (OPV) should not be routinely used to vaccinate adults. It may be used if protection is needed within 4 weeks of travel, in which case a single dose of OPV is given and primary immunization is then completed with either IPV or OPV. Travelers who have previously been fully immunized with OPV or IPV should receive a booster dose with either OPV or IPV.

Rabies

For travelers to areas where rabies is common in domestic animals (eg, India, Mexico), preexposure prophylaxis with human diploid cell vaccine should be considered. It usually consists of 3 injections given 1 week apart, with a booster 3 weeks later.

Typhoid

Typhoid vaccine is a suspension of killed *Salmo-*

nella typhi that provides only moderate short-term protection. Two doses are given 4 weeks or more apart. A single booster dose is given every 3 years if exposure is a probability. (Many countries.)

Paratyphoid vaccines are ineffective and are not recommended at present.

Yellow Fever

The live attenuated yellow fever virus vaccine is administered once subcutaneously. The WHO certificate requires registration of the manufacturer and the batch number of the vaccine. Vaccination is available in the USA only at approved centers. Vaccination must be repeated at intervals of 10 years or less. (Africa, South America.) Because it is a live attenuated vaccine prepared in embryonated eggs, the yellow fever vaccine should not be given to immunosuppressed individuals or those with a history of anaphylaxis to eggs. Pregnancy is a relative contraindication to vaccination.

Japanese B Encephalitis

This disease is a mosquito-borne viral encephalitis that affects primarily children and older adults (65 years and older) and occurs primarily from June to September. It is prevalent in India and Asia. The vaccine is an inactivated viral preparation given 3 times at weekly intervals. Vaccination is recommended for those traveling to endemic areas in the summer months who will be exposed for 3 weeks or more.

HYPERSENSITIVITY TESTS & DESENSITIZATION

Before injecting antitoxin, materials derived from animal sources, or drugs (eg, penicillin) to which a patient has had a severe reaction in the past, test for hypersensitivity. If the test described below is negative, desensitization is not necessary, and a full dose of the material may be given. If the test is positive, alternative drugs should be strongly considered. If that is not feasible, desensitization is necessary.

Intradermal Test for Hypersensitivity

Penicillin is the drug that most frequently serves as an indication for sensitivity testing and desensitization. Skin testing requires 2 preparations: PPL (penicilloyl-polylysine) and a freshly prepared solution of penicillin G in a concentration of 10,000 units per milliliter. A "pinprick" test is performed with each solution at different sites by placing a small drop of solution on the skin and making small indentations of the skin with a needle. If there is no reaction within 10 minutes, 0.01–0.02 mL is injected intradermally, raising a small bleb. Development of a wheal greater than 5 mm in diameter is considered a positive test and an indication for desensitization. If the test is negative, the drug can be administered with the precautions listed below.

Desensitization

A. Precautions:

1. The desensitization procedure is not innocuous—deaths from anaphylaxis have been reported. If extreme hypersensitivity is suspected, it is advisable to use an alternative structurally unrelated drug and to reserve desensitization for situations when treatment cannot be withheld and no alternative drug is available.

2. An antihistaminic drug should be administered before desensitization is begun in order to lessen any reaction that should occur. An airway device must be available.

3. Epinephrine, 1 mL of 1:1000 solution, must be ready for immediate administration.

B. Desensitization Method:
Several methods of desensitization have been described for penicillin, including use of both oral and intravenous preparations. All methods start with very small doses of drug and gradually increase the dose until therapeutic doses are achieved. For penicillin, 1 unit of drug is given intravenously and the patient observed for 15–30 minutes. If there is no reaction, some recommend doubling the dose while others recommend increasing it 10-fold every 15–30 minutes until therapeutic doses are reached.

For recommendations on skin testing and desensitization for other preparations (botulism antitoxin, diphtheria antitoxin, etc), one should consult the manufacturers' package inserts.

Treatment of Reactions

A. Mild Reactions: If a mild reaction occurs, drop back to the next lower dose and continue with desensitization. If a severe reaction occurs, administer epinephrine (see below) and discontinue the drug unless treatment is urgently needed. If desensitization is imperative, continue slowly, increasing the dosage of the drug more gradually.

B. Severe Reactions: If manifestations of a severe reaction appear, give 0.5–1 mL of 1:1000 epinephrine into an intravenous drip of 5% dextrose in water at once. The symptoms include urticaria, angioneurotic edema, dyspnea, coughing, choking, and shock. Observe the patient closely and repeat epinephrine as necessary.

Corticosteroids may be used (eg, hydrocortisone, 100 mg intravenously), but their effort begins only after 18 hours.

Borish L, Tamir R, Rosenwasser L: Intravenous desensitization to beta-lactam antibiotics. J Allergy Clin Immunol 1987;30:314.

Penicillin Allergy. Med Lett Drugs Ther 1980;30:79.

Wendel GD et al: Penicillin allergy and desensitization in serious infections during pregnancy. N Engl J Med 1985;312:1229.

REFERENCES

Feigin RD, Cherry JD: *Textbook of Pediatric Infectious Diseases,* 2nd ed. Saunders, 1987.

Jawetz E et al: *Review of Medical Microbiology,* 18th ed. Appleton & Lange, 1989.

Mandell GL, Douglas RG Jr, Bennett JE: *Principles and Practice of Infectious Disease,* 2nd ed. Wiley, 1985.

AIDS & Related Conditions

24

Harry Hollander, MD, & Mitchell H. Katz, MD

Essentials of Diagnosis

- Risk factors: sexual contact with an infected person, parenteral exposure to infected blood by transfusion or needle sharing, perinatal exposure.
- Prominent systemic complaints such as sweats, diarrhea, weight loss, and wasting.
- Opportunistic infections due to diminished cellular immunity—often life-threatening.
- Aggressive cancers, particularly Kaposi's sarcoma and extranodal lymphoma.
- Neurologic manifestations, including dementia, aseptic meningitis, and neuropathy.

General Considerations

When AIDS was first recognized in the USA in 1981, cases were identified by finding severe opportunistic infections such as *Pneumocystis carinii* pneumonia that indicated profound defects in cellular immunity in the absence of other causes of immunodeficiency. When the syndrome was found to be caused by the human immunodeficiency virus (HIV), it became obvious that severe opportunistic infections and unusual neoplasms were at one end of a spectrum of disease, while healthy seropositive individuals were at the other end.

The 1987 Centers for Disease Control (CDC) classification of HIV disease defines a variety of definitively or presumptively diagnosed opportunistic infections (eg, *P carinii* pneumonia) and neoplasms (eg, Kaposi's sarcoma) as evidence of AIDS. The CDC criteria also specify AIDS diagnoses based upon documented weight loss, diarrhea, or dementia in a patient with positive HIV serology. In general, the term "AIDS-related complex" (ARC) was used to denote those HIV-infected patients who were symptomatic but did not fit the CDC definition of AIDS. This group of patients is heterogeneous, with varying clinical problems and prognoses. Therefore, the use of the term "ARC" should be avoided. Because the CDC's definition is for surveillance purposes and does not stratify patients by severity of illness, other classification systems have been developed.

Epidemiology

The modes of transmission of HIV are similar to those of hepatitis B, in particular with respect to sexual, parenteral, and vertical transmission. The risk of sexual transmission varies with particular sexual practices; anal intercourse is the riskiest. The risk of sustaining HIV infection from a needle stick with infected blood is approximately 1:200, which is significantly less than the risk of contracting hepatitis B from a contaminated needle stick. Between 30 and 50 percent of children born to HIV-infected mothers contract HIV-infection. The HIV virus has not been shown to be transmitted by respiratory droplet spread, by vectors such as mosquitoes, or by casual nonsexual contact.

In the USA, 80% of AIDS cases are reported in gay or bisexual men, and 16% are intravenous drug users, the majority of whom live in major metropolitan areas. The remainder of cases occur in infants of infected mothers, heterosexual contacts of infected individuals, and recipients of contaminated blood or blood products. Bidirectional heterosexual spread occurs occasionally in the USA but is the most common route of transmission in Africa. The reasons for this difference may relate to cofactors such as general health status and the presence of genital ulcers.

Current estimates are that about 1 million Americans are infected with HIV. Estimates of the number of people who will develop AIDS in the 1990's have been scaled down from prior estimates, based on recent AIDS incidence data. It is estimated that in 1991 there will between 127,000 and 153,000 people alive with AIDS, with more than 50,000 new cases per year. Among risk groups, the most rapid percentage increases are anticipated among inner city intravenous drug users and heterosexuals, especially blacks and Latinos. HIV infection will continue to spread outward from major metropolitan areas to suburban and rural parts of the country. Because blood donor screening is universally practiced in the USA, the number of new AIDS cases due to transfusion has already peaked and is expected to decline further. The current risk of contracting HIV from a screened unit of blood is 1:100,000. Since 1983, transmission of HIV to at-risk gay men in San Francisco has dramatically fallen to less than 1% per year. This development offers hope that education about risk behavior modification will interrupt the spread of infection in other at-risk populations.

Etiology

The syndromes described below are due to infection with human retroviruses known as human immunodeficiency viruses (HIV, formerly HTLV-III or LAV). Retroviruses depend upon a unique enzyme, reverse transcriptase (RNA-directed DNA-polymerase), to replicate within host cells. The other major pathogenic human retrovirus, HTLV-I, is associated with lymphoma, while HIV is not directly oncogenic. The genome of HIV viruses contains genes for 3 basic structural proteins and at least 5 other regulatory proteins; *gag* codes for group antigen proteins, *pol* codes for polymerase, and *env* codes for the external envelope protein. The greatest variability in strains of HIV occurs in the viral envelope. Since neutralizing activity is found in antibodies directed against the envelope, this variability presents problems for vaccine development.

In addition to the classic AIDS virus (HIV-I), a group of related viruses, HIV-II, have been isolated in West African patients. HIV-II has the same genetic organization as HIV-I, but there are significant differences in the envelope glycoproteins. Some infected individuals exhibit AIDS-like illnesses, but most West Africans infected with HIV-II are currently asymptomatic. HIV-II has been found in several people in the USA. Thus, this variant may be less pathogenic or have a longer period of latency preceding disease.

Pathogenesis

The hallmark of symptomatic HIV infection is immunodeficiency. The virus can infect all cells expressing the T4 CD4 antigen, which serves as a receptor for HIV. Once it enters a cell, HIV can replicate and cause cell fusion or death by unknown mechanisms. In many cases, a latent state is established, with integration of the HIV genome into the cell's genome. The cell principally infected is the CD4 (helper-inducer) lymphocyte, which directs many other cells in the immune network. With increasing duration of infection, the number of CD4 lymphocytes falls. Some of the immunologic defects, however, are explained not by *quantitative* abnormalities of lymphocyte subsets but by *qualitative* defects in CD4 responsiveness induced by HIV.

Other cells in the immune network that are infected by HIV include B lymphocytes and macrophages. The defect in B cells is partly due to disordered CD4 lymphocyte function. However, HIV can also alter B cell function directly. These direct and indirect effects can lead to generalized hypergammaglobulinemia and can also depress B cell responses to new antigen challenges. Because of these defects, the immunodeficiency of HIV is mixed. Elements of humoral and cellular immunodeficiency are present, especially in children.

The role of macrophage-monocyte infection in immunodeficiency is not as clear. It is possible that macrophage dysfunction plays a role in some of the clinical manifestations of the disease, such as *P carinii* pneumonia. Macrophages also act as a reservoir for HIV and serve to disseminate it to other organ systems (eg, the central nervous system).

Apart from the immunologic effects of HIV, the virus can also directly cause a variety of neurologic effects. Rare glial cells and oligodendrocytes express CD4 antigen and thus may be permissive of infection by HIV. However, these cells are rarely infected, whereas multinucleated giant cells of macrophage origin are more commonly seen in brain specimens of infected individuals. The envelope of HIV is homologous with neuroleukins; the neuropathologic features may be partly dependent upon inhibition of neurologic growth factors by the virus. Other mechanisms may also be important.

Pathology

Most histopathologic changes in HIV infection are caused by secondary opportunistic infections or neoplasms rather than direct effects of HIV infection. Several pathologic findings, however, are unique to HIV. The lymph nodes may demonstrate different pathologic changes at different stages of clinical disease. Early, a pattern of benign but florid follicular hyperplasia is seen. Immunologic staining reveals a profound decrease in CD4 lymphocytes in the paracortical areas of the lymph nodes, consistent with the depressed CD4 lymphocyte count in peripheral blood. Later, as immunodeficiency progresses, involution and atrophy of formerly hyperplastic lymph nodes often take place. Pulmonary involvement by HIV may result in a lymphocytic interstitial pneumonitis seen in lung biopsies. Whether this pathologic pattern represents direct HIV infection or is an autoimmune response to infection is unclear. This pathologic pattern is common in childhood HIV infection and is being recognized more commonly in adults. It has a variable clinical course.

Pathologic involvement of the nervous system is frequent in infected individuals. Over 90% of patients dying of AIDS have abnormal brain histopathologic findings, with diffuse involvement of the cerebrum and cerebellum. Findings include focal subcortical demyelination and, less commonly, the presence of multinucleated giant cells. A vacuolar myelopathy resembling that due to vitamin B_{12} deficiency may also be seen.

Finally, a variety of pathologic changes have been observed in peripheral nerves, ranging from demyelinating neuropathy, which resembles Guillain-Barré syndrome, to an axonal sensory neuropathy with little surrounding inflammatory response. Thus, HIV does leave some pathologic footprints in several organ systems. Far more common, however, is secondary disease due to immunodeficiency.

Pathophysiology

Clinically, the syndromes caused by HIV infection are usually explicable by one of 3 known mechanisms. Some HIV-associated manifestations, however, are not explained by any of these proposed mechanisms.

A. Immunodeficiency: Immunodeficiency is a direct result of the effects of HIV upon immune cells. A spectrum of infections and neoplasms is seen, as in other congenital or acquired immunodeficiency states. Two remarkable features of HIV immunodeficiency are the low incidence of infections such as listeriosis and aspergillosis and the frequent occurrence of Kaposi's sarcoma. This latter complication has been seen primarily in gay or bisexual men, and its incidence has steadily declined through the first 10 years of the epidemic. This epidemiologic fact and other basic science advances suggest that Kaposi's sarcoma is not a true neoplasm but a multicentric hyperplasia of endothelial elements stimulated by an unidentified sexually transmitted or behaviorally related cofactor.

B. Autoimmunity: Autoimmunity can occur as a result of disordered cellular immune function or B lymphocyte dysfunction. Examples of both lymphocytic infiltration of organs (eg, lymphocytic interstitial pneumonitis) and autoantibody production (eg, immunologic thrombocytopenia) occur. These phenomena may be the only clinically apparent disease or may coexist with obvious immunodeficiency.

C. Neurologic Dysfunction: Little is known about the mechanisms of neurologic dysfunction, since relatively few neural cells are infected and the inflammatory response is minimal. Possibilities include homology with and blockade of neurologic growth factors, other toxic effects of viral products, or release of neurotoxic compounds from infected macrophages.

Clinical Findings

A. Symptoms and Signs: Many individuals with HIV infection remain asymptomatic for years, with a mean time of approximately 10 years between exposure and development of AIDS. When symptoms occur, they may be remarkably protean and nonspecific. Systemic complaints such as weight loss, fevers, and night sweats are common. Ear, nose, and throat complaints include sinus fullness and drainage, painful swallowing, mouth lesions (candidal plaques, leukoplakia), and periodontal irritation. Cough or shortness of breath raises a suspicion of HIV-related pulmonary disease. Gastrointestinal complaints include changes in bowel function, especially diarrhea. Central nervous system symptoms include depression, changes in personality, difficulty in concentrating, and frank confusion. Tingling, numbness, and weakness suggest peripheral neuropathy. Cutaneous complaints are common and include dry skin, new rashes, and nail changes. Since virtually all of these findings may be seen with other diseases, a combination of complaints is more suggestive of HIV infection than any one symptom.

Physical examination may be entirely normal. Ab-

normal findings range from completely nonspecific to highly specific for HIV infection. Those that are predictive of HIV infection include hairy leukoplakia of the tongue and disseminated Kaposi's sarcoma. Kaposi's lesions may appear anywhere; careful examination of the eyelids, conjunctiva, pinnae, palate, and toe webs is mandatory to locate potentially occult lesions. Hairy leukoplakia is commonly seen as a white lesion on the lateral aspect of the tongue. It may be flat or slightly raised, is usually corrugated, and has vertical parallel lines with fine or thick ("hairy") projections. A funduscopic finding of cytomegalovirus retinitis (perivascular hemorrhages and fluffy exudates) and the presence of oral candidiasis are both suggestive if no other cause of these conditions is found. Other less specific findings include evidence of recent weight loss, folliculitis, seborrheic dermatitis, onycholysis, retinal cotton-wool spots, oral aphthous ulcerations, and generalized lymphadenopathy. Neuropsychiatric findings may include depression, emotional lability, psychomotor slowing, abnormalities of pursuit eye movements, focal deficits, decreased vibratory sensation, and depressed or accentuated reflexes.

B. Laboratory Findings: Laboratory findings may include anemia, leukopenia (particularly lymphopenia) and thrombocytopenia in any combination, polyclonal hypergammaglobulinemia, and hypocholesterolemia. Cutaneous anergy is frequent early in the course and becomes universal as the disease progresses. More specific for HIV infection are abnormalities of T lymphocyte subsets. While an increased number and percentage of suppressor cells occur in other viral infections or medical conditions, the progressive decrease in helper CD4 lymphocytes is typical of HIV infection.

Specific tests for HIV include antibody and antigen detection and direct viral culture. Screening serology is done either by enzyme immunoassay (EIA) or immunofluorescent assay (IFA). Positive specimens are then confirmed by a different method (eg, Western blot). False-positive screening tests may occur as normal biologic variants or in association with other disease states, such as connective tissue disease. These are usually detected by negative confirmatory tests. The specificity of positive results by 2 different methods approaches 100%, even in low-risk populations. Similarly, the sensitivity of screening serologic tests is now over 99.5%. Newer molecular biology techniques (polymerase chain reaction) show a small incidence of individuals ($< 1\%$) who are infected with HIV for up to 36 months without generating an antibody response. However, the vast majority will develop antibodies detectable by screening serologic tests within several months of infection. Core protein antigen may be detectable before a serologic response occurs, and antigenemia may also reappear in the course of the disease as immunosuppression progresses. The reappearance of core (p24) antigen in asymptomatic individuals has correlated with an increased risk of disease progression. Since culture techniques are costly and labor-intensive and require specialized biocontainment facilities, they are of little clinical usefulness.

Tests that determine evidence of macrophage-monocyte stimulation may provide additional useful prognostic information in infected individuals. Beta$_2$-microglobulin, for example, is a cell surface protein that tends to rise in a high percentage of cases over the course of HIV disease. Asymptomatic individuals with elevated serum β_2-microglobulin concentrations may have a 2- to 3-fold increased incidence of disease progression. However, this test must be interpreted cautiously, since autoimmune processes, malignant tumors, and other infections are also associated with elevated values. Neopterin is another monocyte product that has been used in some studies as a predictive marker. Neopterin determination is not yet generally available in clinical laboratories.

Differential Diagnosis

HIV infection may mimic a variety of other medical illnesses. Specific differential diagnosis depends upon the mode of presentation. In patients presenting with constitutional symptoms such as weight loss and fevers, differential considerations include cancer, chronic infections such as tuberculosis and endocarditis, and endocrinologic diseases such as hyperthyroidism. When pulmonary processes dominate the presentation, acute and chronic lung infections must be considered as well as other causes of diffuse interstitial pulmonary infiltrates. When neurologic disease is the mode of presentation, conditions that cause mental status changes or neuropathy—eg, alcoholism, liver disease, renal dysfunction, thyroid disease, and vitamin deficiency—should be considered. If a patient presents with headache and a cerebrospinal fluid pleocytosis, other causes of chronic meningitis enter the differential. When diarrhea is a prominent complaint, infectious enterocolitis, antibiotic-associated colitis, inflammatory bowel disease, and malabsorptive symptoms must be considered.

Complications & Sequelae

The complications of HIV-related infections and neoplasms affect virtually every organ. The general approach to the HIV-infected person with symptoms is to evaluate the organ systems involved, aiming to diagnose treatable conditions rapidly.

A. Systemic Complaints: Fever, night sweats, and weight loss are common symptoms in HIV-infected patients and may occur without a complicating opportunistic infection. Patients with persistent fever and no localizing symptoms should nonetheless be carefully examined, and evaluated with a chest radiograph (*P carinii* pneumonia can present without respiratory symptoms), bacterial blood cultures if the fever is greater than 38.5 °C, serum cryptococcal antigen,

and mycobacterial cultures of the blood. If these studies are normal, patients should be observed closely. Antipyretics are useful because HIV-infected patients have a propensity for high fevers and subsequent dehydration. Generally, nonsteroidal anti-inflammatory agents are more effective than aspirin or acetaminophen in the relief of fever.

Weight loss is a particularly distressing complication of long-standing HIV infection. The mechanism of HIV-related cachexia is not well understood. Frequent episodes of anorexia, nausea, vomiting, and diarrhea all contribute to weight loss among AIDS patients. Depression and adrenal insufficiency are 2 potentially treatable causes of weight loss. For some patients with poor appetite, the progestational agent megestrol acetate (80 mg 4 times a day) can increase appetite and lead to subsequent weight gain. Effective fever control decreases the metabolic rate. Many patients will benefit from the use of high-caloric food supplementation. Selected patients with otherwise good functional status and weight loss due to unrelenting nausea, vomiting, or diarrhea may benefit from total parenteral nutrition.

B. Pulmonary Disease: The lungs are a frequently involved site of disease. *P carinii* pneumonia is the most common opportunistic infection, affecting 75% of patients. *P carinii* pneumonia may be difficult to diagnose because the symptoms—fever, cough, and shortness of breath—are nonspecific. Furthermore, the severity of symptoms ranges from fever and no respiratory symptoms through mild cough or dyspnea to frank respiratory distress.

The cornerstone of diagnosis is the chest radiograph. Diffuse or perihilar infiltrates are most characteristic, but only two-thirds of patients with *P carinii* pneumonia have this finding. Normal chest radiographs are seen in 5–10% of patients with *P carinii* pneumonia, while the remainder have atypical infiltrates. Apical infiltrates are commonly seen among patients with *P carinii* pneumonia who have been receiving aerosolized pentamidine prophylaxis, presumably because the drug is not well distributed in the upper zones. Isolated elevations of lactate dehydrogenase concentrations are consistent with a diagnosis of *P carinii* pneumonia.

Definitive diagnosis can be obtained by Wright-Giemsa stain of induced sputum in 50–80% of cases at centers with experience performing this test. A negative sputum induction does not, however, rule out the disease. Therefore, the next step for patients suspected of having *P carinii* pneumonia should be bronchoalveolar lavage. This technique establishes the diagnosis in over 95% of cases. The use of fluorescent antibodies for staining sputum samples may increase the sensitivity of sputum examination, decreasing the need for bronchoscopy.

In patients with symptoms suggestive of *P carinii* pneumonia but with negative or atypical chest radiographs and negative sputum examinations, other diagnostic tests may provide additional information in deciding whether to proceed to bronchoalveolar lavage. These tests include pulmonary function tests such as carbon monoxide diffusing capacity, lung gallium scanning, and exercise oximetry. In addition, a CD4 count above 250 cells μL within 2 months after evaluation of respiratory symptoms makes a diagnosis of *P carinii* pneumonia unlikely.

Other infectious causes of pulmonary disease in AIDS patients include bacterial, mycobacterial, and viral pneumonias. An increased incidence of pneumococcal pneumonia with septicemia and *Haemophilus influenzae* pneumonia has been reported. *Mycobacterium tuberculosis* is thought to result from reactivation of prior infection; atypical infiltrates and disseminated disease occur more commonly than among immunocompetent hosts. Atypical mycobacteria can cause pulmonary disease in AIDS patients with or without preexisting lung disease and responds variably to treatment. Isolation of cytomegalovirus from bronchoalveolar lavage fluid occurs commonly in AIDS patients but does not establish a definitive diagnosis. Diagnosis of cytomegalovirus pneumonia requires biopsy; response to treatment is poor.

Noninfectious causes of lung disease include Kaposi's sarcoma, non-Hodgkin's lymphoma, and interstitial pneumonitis. In patients with known Kaposi's sarcoma, pulmonary involvement complicates the course in approximately one-third of cases. Non-Hodgkin's lymphoma may involve the lung as the sole site of disease but more commonly involves other organs as well, especially the brain, liver, and gastrointestinal tract. Both of these processes may show nodular or diffuse parenchymal involvement, pleural effusions, and mediastinal adenopathy on chest radiographs.

Nonspecific interstitial pneumonitis may mimic *P carinii* pneumonia. Typically, these patients present with several months of mild cough and dyspnea; chest radiographs show interstitial infiltrates. Many patients with this entity undergo transbronchial biopsies in an attempt to diagnose *P carinii* pneumonia. Instead, the tissue shows interstitial inflammation ranging from an intense lymphocytic infiltration (consistent with lymphoid interstitial pneumonitis) to a mild mononuclear inflammation. Corticosteroids may be helpful in some cases.

C. Central Nervous System Disease: Central nervous system disease in HIV-infected patients can be divided into intracerebral space-occupying lesions, encephalopathy, meningitis, and spinal cord processes.

Toxoplasmosis is the most common space-occupying lesion in HIV-infected patients. Patients may present with headache, focal neurologic deficits, seizures, or altered mental status. The diagnosis is usually made presumptively based on the characteristic appearance of cerebral imaging studies. Typically, toxoplasmosis appears as multiple lesions, contrast-enhancing on CT scan, with a predilection for the basal ganglia.

Single lesions are atypical of toxoplasmosis. When a single lesion has been detected by CT scanning, MRI scanning—because of its greater sensitivity—may reveal multiple lesions. If a patient has a single lesion on MRI and is neurologically stable, clinicians may either pursue an immediate tissue diagnosis or a 2-week empiric trial of toxoplasmosis therapy. Biopsy is then performed if the lesion does not diminish in size. Serologic testing for toxoplasmosis is not helpful in confirming the diagnosis, since most HIV-infected patients will have detectable titers. Conversely, 15% of patients with toxoplasmosis have negative titers by enzyme immunoassay or immunofluorescence assays.

Non-Hodgkin's lymphoma is the second most common space-occupying lesion in HIV-infected patients. Symptoms are similar to those with toxoplasmosis. While imaging techniques cannot distinguish these 2 diseases with certainty, lymphoma more often is solitary. Other less common lesions should be suspected if there is preceding bacteremia, fungemia, or intravenous drug use. These include bacterial abscesses, cryptococcomas, tuberculomas, and *Nocardia* lesions.

Because techniques for stereotactic brain biopsy have improved, this procedure plays an increasing role in diagnosing cerebral lesions. Biopsy should be strongly considered if lesions are solitary or do not respond to toxoplasmosis treatment, especially if they are easily accessible. Diagnosis of lymphoma is important because patients who have not had a prior opportunistic infection are likely to benefit from treatment (radiation therapy).

AIDS dementia complex (HIV encephalopathy) is the most common cause of mental status changes in HIV-infected patients. The diagnosis is one of exclusion based on a brain imaging study and spinal fluid analysis which exclude other pathogens. Neuropsychiatric testing is helpful in distinguishing patients with dementia from those with depression. Patients with AIDS dementia complex typically have difficulty with cognitive tasks and exhibit diminished motor speed. Although the mechanism by which HIV causes neurologic dysfunction is not known, many patients improve with AZT. Metabolic abnormalities may also cause changes in mental status: hypoglycemia, hyponatremia, hypoxia, and drug overdose are important considerations in this population. Other less common infectious causes of encephalopathy include progressive multifocal leukoencephalopathy, cytomegalovirus, and herpes simplex encephalitis.

Cryptococcal meningitis typically presents with fever and headache. Less than 20% of patients have meningismus. Diagnosis is based on a positive latex agglutination test or positive culture of spinal fluid for *Cryptococcus*. Seventy to ninety percent of patients with cryptococcal meningitis have a positive serum agglutination test for *Cryptococcus* (CRAG). Thus, a negative serum CRAG test makes a diagnosis of cryptococcal meningitis unlikely and can be useful in the initial evaluation of a patient with headache, fever, and normal mental status. HIV meningitis, characterized by lymphocytic pleocytosis of the spinal fluid with negative culture, is common early in HIV infection and may mimic cryptococcal meningitis in its clinical presentation.

Spinal cord function may also be impaired in HIV-infected individuals. HIV myelopathy presents with leg weakness and incontinence. Spastic paraparesis and sensory ataxia are seen on neurologic examination. Myelopathy is usually a late manifestation of HIV disease, and most patients will have concomitant HIV encephalopathy. Pathologic evaluation of the spinal cord reveals vacuolation of white matter. Because HIV myelopathy is a diagnosis of exclusion, symptoms suggestive of myelopathy should be evaluated by lumbar puncture to rule out cytomegalovirus polyradiculopathy (described below) and an MRI or CT scan to exclude epidural lymphoma.

D. Peripheral Nervous System: Peripheral nervous system syndromes include inflammatory polyneuropathies, sensory neuropathies, and mononeuropathies.

An inflammatory demyelinating polyneuropathy similar to Guillain-Barré syndrome occurs in HIV-infected patients, usually prior to frank immunodeficiency. The syndrome in many cases improves with plasmapheresis, supporting an autoimmune basis of the disease. Cytomegalovirus can cause an ascending polyradiculopathy characterized by lower extremity weakness and a neutrophilic pleocytosis on spinal fluid analysis with a negative bacterial culture. Transverse myelitis can be seen with herpes zoster or cytomegalovirus.

About 30% of patients with advanced HIV disease develop sensory neuropathies. Affected patients typically complain of numbness, tingling, and pain in their lower extremities. Symptoms are disproportionate to findings on gross sensory and motor evaluation. In contrast to inflammatory demyelinating polyneuropathy, sensory neuropathies occur late in HIV-disease progression and are due to axonal loss. Evaluation should rule out other causes of sensory neuropathy such as alcoholism, thyroid disease, vitamin B_{12} deficiency, and syphilis. Severe sensory neuropathy is a contraindication to initiation of 2 of the experimental antiviral drugs, the dideoxynucleosides ddI and ddC. Occasionally, sensory neuropathies improve with AZT therapy, but more commonly treatment is symptomatic with amitriptyline.

E. Myopathy: Myopathies are increasingly noted in HIV-infected patients. Proximal muscle weakness is typical, and patients may have varying degrees of muscle tenderness. The most important clinical distinction is between myopathy due to the primary effect of HIV and that due to AZT. Patients with symptomatic myopathy, especially with creatine kinase levels greater than 1000 IU/L, should have their dose of AZT decreased or stopped and be considered for experimental antiviral therapy (ddI). A muscle biopsy can distinguish HIV myopathy from AZT myopathy and should be considered in patients for whom continuation of AZT is essential.

F. Retinitis: Complaints of visual changes must be evaluated immediately in HIV-infected patients. Cytomegalovirus retinitis is the most common retinal infection in AIDS patients and can be rapidly progressive. In contrast, cotton wool spots, which are also common in HIV-infected people, are benign, remit spontaneously, and appear as small indistinct white spots without exudation or hemorrhage. This distinction may be difficult at times for the nonspecialist, and patients with visual changes should be seen by an ophthalmologist. Other rare retinal processes include toxoplasmosis and other herpesvirus infections.

G. Oral Lesions: The findings of oral candidiasis and hairy leukoplakia are significant for several reasons. First, these lesions are almost pathognomonic for HIV infection. Second, several studies have indicated that patients with these lesions have a high rate of progression to AIDS, though it is not known whether this increased risk is independent of other parameters of immune function, such as the CD4 count.

Hairy leukoplakia is caused by the Epstein-Barr virus. The lesion is not usually troubling to patients and sometimes recedes with acyclovir or AZT treatment. Oral candidiasis can be bothersome to patients, many of whom report an unpleasant taste or mouth dryness. There are 2 types of oral candidiasis: pseudomembranous (removable white plaques) and erythematous (red friable plaques). Treatment is with topical agents such as clotrimazole troches (one 4 or 5 times a day). Patients with candidiasis that does not respond to topical antifungals can be treated with oral ketoconazole (200 mg once a day). Angular cheilitis—fissures at the sides of the mouth—is usually due to *Candida* as well and can be treated topically with ketoconazole cream.

Gingival disease is common in HIV-infected patients and is thought to be due to an overgrowth of microorganisms. It usually responds to professional dental cleaning and chlorhexidine rinses. Some HIV-infected patients will develop a particularly aggressive gingivitis or periodontitis; these patients should be started on antibiotics that cover anaerobic oral flora (eg, metronidazole, 250 mg 4 times a day for 4 or 5 days) and referred to oral surgeons with experience with these entities.

Other lesions seen in the mouths of HIV-infected patients include Kaposi's sarcoma (usually on the hard palate), recurrent aphthous ulcers (best treated with topical steroids), and warts.

H. Gastrointestinal Manifestations: Esophageal candidiasis is a common AIDS infection. Typically, patients complain of substernal pain or burning, worse with swallowing. Nausea may also occur. In a patient with these characteristic symptoms and oral candidiasis, empiric antifungal treatment is begun. Patients who can take oral medications should be started on ketoconazole (200 mg twice a day). Patients who do not improve with ketoconazole may be given fluconazole (200 mg daily). Further evaluation to identify other causes of esophagitis (herpes simplex, cytomegalovirus) is reserved for patients who do not improve with treatment or those without visible oral candidiasis.

Autopsy studies have demonstrated that the liver is a frequent site of infections and neoplasms in HIV-infected patients. However, many of these infections are not clinically symptomatic. Clinicians may note elevations of alkaline phosphatase and transaminases on routine chemistry panels. Mycobacterial disease, cytomegalovirus, and lymphoma cause liver disease and can present with varying degrees of nausea, vomiting, and right upper quadrant abdominal pain. Sulfonamide drugs and ketoconazole have also been associated with hepatitis. HIV-infected patients with chronic active hepatitis tend to have less severe bouts of hepatitis because of the concomitant immunodeficiency. Percutaneous liver biopsy may be helpful in diagnosing liver disease, but frequently the cause can be determined by other tests (eg, blood culture, biopsy of a more accessible site). Moreover, because the majority of hepatic infections do not respond well to treatment (eg, *M avium-intracellulare*), the procedure should be reserved for people with persistent symptoms and laboratory abnormalities in whom no other cause for illness can be determined.

Biliary disease is common in AIDS patients. Cholecystitis presents with similar manifestations as seen in immunocompetent hosts but is more likely to be acalculous. Sclerosing cholangitis and papillary stenosis have also been increasingly reported in HIV-infected patients. Typically, the syndrome presents with severe nausea, vomiting, and right upper quadrant pain. Liver function tests generally show alkaline phosphatase elevations disproportionate to elevation of the transaminases. Although dilated ducts can be seen on ultrasound, the diagnosis is made by endoscopic retrograde cholangiopancreatography, which reveals intraluminal irregularities of the proximal intrahepatic ducts with "pruning" of the terminal ductal branches. Stenosis of the distal common bile duct at the papilla is commonly seen with this syndrome. Cytomegalovirus and *Cryptosporidium* are thought to play inciting roles in this syndrome. Initial reports of symptomatic improvement with performance of sphincterotomies were encouraging, but enthusiasm for the procedure has waned because many patients had recurrence of symptoms.

Entercolitis is a common problem in HIV-infected individuals. Organisms known to cause enterocolitis include bacteria *(Campylobacter, Salmonella, Shigella),* viruses (cytomegalovirus, adenovirus), and protozoans *(Cryptosporidium, E histolytica, Giardia).* Several of the organisms causing enterocolitis in HIV-infected individuals also cause diarrhea in immunocompetent hosts. However, HIV-infected patients tend to have more severe symptoms, including high fevers and severe abdominal pain that can mimic acute abdominal catastrophes. Bacteremia and concomitant biliary involvement are also more common with enterocolitis in HIV-infected patients. Relapses of enterocolitis following adequate therapy have been reported with both *Salmonella* and *Shigella* infections.

Because of the wide range of agents known to cause enterocolitis, a stool culture and multiple stool examinations for ova and parasites (including modified acid-fast staining for *Cryptosporidium*) should be performed. Those patients who have *Cryptosporidium* on one stool with improvement in symptoms in less than 1 month should not be considered to have AIDS, as *Cryptosporidium* is a cause of self-limited diarrhea in HIV-negative hosts. More commonly, HIV-infected patients with *Cryptosporidium* have persistent enterocolitis with profuse watery diarrhea.

Patients with a negative stool examination and persistent symptoms should be evaluated with sigmoidoscopy and biopsy. Patients whose symptoms last longer than 1 month with no identified cause of diarrhea are considered to have a presumptive diagnosis of AIDS. A primary effect of the HIV virus on the colonic epithelium may be the cause, and some patients will improve with AZT therapy.

Two other important gastrointestinal abnormalities in HIV-infected patients are gastropathy and malabsorption. It has been documented that some HIV-infected patients do not produce normal levels of stomach acid and therefore are unable to absorb drugs such as ketoconazole that require an acid medium. This decreased acid production may explain, in part, the susceptibility of HIV-infected patients to *Campylobacter* and *Shigella,* both of which are sensitive to acid concentration.

A malabsorption syndrome occurs commonly in HIV-infected patients. It can be due to infection of the small bowel with *M avium-intracellure* or *Cryptosporidium.* In other cases, biopsy of the small bowel reveals no pathogens but histologic changes consistent with Whipple's disease.

I. Skin: HIV-infected patients commonly develop skin manifestations that can be grouped into viral, bacterial, fungal, neoplastic, and nonspecific dermatitides.

Herpes simplex infections occur more frequently, tend to be more severe, and are more likely to disseminate than in AIDS patients than in immunocompetent hosts. Because of the risk of progressive local disease, all herpes simplex attacks should be treated with acyclovir. To avoid the complications of attacks, many clinicians recommend chronic acyclovir administration for HIV-infected patients with a history of recurrent herpes. However, the finding of acyclovir resistance among some herpes strains cultured from HIV-infected patients raises concern about this practice.

Herpes zoster is a common manifestation of HIV-infection. As with herpes simplex infections, patients with zoster should be treated with acyclovir to prevent dissemination (800 mg orally 4 or 5 times per day). Vesicular lesions should be cultured if there is any question about their origin, since herpes simplex responds to much lower doses of acyclovir. Disseminated zoster and cases with ocular involvement should be treated with intravenous rather than oral acyclovir.

Molluscum contagiosum is seen in HIV-infected patients, as in other immunocompromised patients. Lesions have a propensity for spreading widely over the patient's skin and should be treated with topical liquid nitrogen.

Staphylococcus is the most common bacterial cause of skin disease in HIV-infected patients; it usually presents as folliculitis, superficial abscesses (furuncles), or bullous impetigo. Because dissemination with sepsis has been reported, attempts should be made to aggressively treat these lesions. Folliculitis is initially treated with topical clindamycin, and patients may benefit from regular washing with an antibacterial soap such as chlorhexidine (Hibiclens). Abscesses often require incision and drainage. Patients may need systemic antibiotics for severe folliculitis.

The majority of fungal rashes afflicting AIDS patients are due to dermatophytes and *Candida*. These are particularly common in the inguinal region but may occur anywhere on the body. Fungal rashes generally respond well to topical clotrimazole or ketoconazole.

Kaposi's sarcoma lesions are red or purple, flat or raised papules that generally do not blanch. About 40% of patients with dermatologic Kaposi's sarcoma will develop visceral disease (eg, gastrointestinal, pulmonary). Aggressive cutaneous and visceral Kaposi's sarcoma frequently requires systemic chemotherapy. Other dermatologic malignancies seen disproportionately among HIV-infected persons include basal cell and squamous cell carcinomas. The latter have been associated with anal condylomas, suggesting that papillomavirus may play a role in carcinogenesis.

Seborrheic dermatitis is more common in HIV-infected patients. Scrapings of seborrhea have revealed *Pityrosporum ovale,* implying that the seborrhea is caused by this fungus. Consistent with the isolation of this fungus is the clinical finding that seborrhea responds well to topical clotrimazole as well as hydrocortisone cream.

Xerosis presents in HIV-infected patients with severe pruritus. The patient may have no rash, or nonspecific excoriations from scratching. Treatment is with emollients and antipruritic lotions.

Psoriasis can be very severe in HIV-infected pa-

tients. Because of the underlying immunodeficiency, methotrexate should be avoided.

Treatment

Treatment of common HIV infections and malignancies is detailed in Table 24–1. In general, AIDS patients require protracted therapy, including lifelong therapy for toxoplasmosis, cryptococcosis, and cytomegalovirus retinitis. The emergence of resistance is more common for some infections of HIV-infected people (eg, acyclovir-resistant herpes simplex) than among immunocompetent individuals. In addition, HIV-infected patients have an increased incidence of side effects to standard drugs. For example, the incidence of side effects with trimethoprim-sulfamethoxazole is about 80% in this population.

The development of drugs that suppress the HIV infection itself rather than its complications has been an important development. Zidovudine (AZT) is the first approved—and the most thoroughly studied—antiviral drug for HIV infection. It has been proved to decrease symptoms and prolong the life of patients with AIDS or severe symptomatic disease. Recently, AZT has been shown to slow the progression to severe disease among patients with mild symptoms as well as asymptomatic patients with CD4 counts below 500 cells per microliter.

Side effects seen with AZT are listed in Table 24–2. Approximately 40% of patients will experience subjective side effects that generally remit within 6 weeks. The common dose-limiting side effects of AZT are anemia and neutropenia. Although the anemia is usually macrocytic, it does not respond to vitamin B_{12} or folic acid supplementation. Both the anemia and the neutropenia generally respond to dose reductions and interruptions.

The dosing of AZT is controversial. The initial trials of AZT utilized 1500 mg/d. More recent studies in AIDS patients have shown that a dose of 200 mg 3 times a day results in fewer side effects and improved survival compared to 200 mg 6 times a day. Similarly, studies in asymptomatic HIV-infected individuals indicate that over the first year of therapy, 100 mg 5 times a day is as efficacious as 300 mg 5 times a day. While lower doses appear to be preferable over the short term, there is some concern about whether these lower doses will be as effective as higher doses in preventing neurologic disease in HIV-infected patients. The cost of AZT (at a dose of 500 mg/d) is approximately $225.00 a month.

In monitoring patients receiving AZT, complete blood counts—with platelet and differential counts—should be done every 2 weeks for the first month of therapy and then every 1–3 months depending on the clinical situation. Liver function tests and creatine phosphokinase levels should be checked every 3 months. AZT can be taken concomitantly with other medicines except probenecid, which prolongs the serum half-life of AZT. In the initial AZT trial, aceta-

Table 24–1. Treatment of AIDS-related opportunistic infections and malignancies.[1]

Infection	Treatment	Complications
P carinii infection	Trimethoprim-sulfamethoxazole, 15 mg/kg (based on trimethoprim component) orally or IV	Nausea, neutropenia, anemia, hepatitis, drug rash, Stevens-Johnson syndrome
	Pentamidine, 3–4 mg/kg IV	Hypotension, hypoglycemia, anemia, neutropenia, pancreatitis, hepatitis.
	Trimethoprim, 300 mg 3 times daily, with dapsone, 100 mg daily	Nausea, rash, hemolytic anemia in G6PD-deficient patients. Methemoglobinemia (weekly levels should be < 10% of total hemoglobin).
	Primaquine, 15–30 mg daily, and clindamycin, 300–600 mg every 6 hours (not well established)	Hemolytic anemia in G6PD-deficient patients. Methemoglobinemia, neutropenia, colitis.
	Trimetrexate[2] (given with folinic acid)	Leukopenia, rash, mucositis
	Aerosolized pentamidine[2]	Bronchospasm
M avium complex infection	No proven effective therapy. Combination drug regimens in use: Clofazimine, 100 mg daily, plus	Abdominal pain, discoloration of skin
	Rifampin, 600 mg daily, plus	Rash, hepatitis
	Amikacin, 1 mg/kg IV twice daily for 2–4 weeks	Nephrotoxicity, ototoxicity
Toxoplasmosis	Pyrimethamine, 100–200 mg orally as loading dose, followed by 25–75 mg/d, combined with sulfadiazine, 4–8 g daily in 4 divided doses, and folinic acid, 5 mg 3 times a week. Clindamycin, 600–1200 mg every 8 hours, may be an alternative in patients allergic to sulfonamides.	Leukopenia, rash
Lymphoma	Combination chemotherapy (eg, modified CHOP, M-BACOD, with or without GM-CSF). Central nervous system disease: radiation treatment with dexamethasone for edema.	Nausea, vomiting, anemia, leukopenia, cardiotoxicity (with doxorubicin)
Cryptococcal meningitis	Amphotericin B, 0.6 mg/kg/d, to a total dose of about 1.5 g. Maintenance therapy is with amphotericin B, 1 mg/kg/wk, or with fluconazole, 200–400 mg daily. (Initiation of therapy with fluconazole is not well established.)	For amphotericin B, fever, anemia, and azotemia. For fluconazole, hepatitis.
Cytomegalovirus infection	Ganciclovir, 10 mg/kg/d in 2 divided doses for 10 days, followed by 6 mg/kg 5 days a week indefinitely. Decrease dose for renal impairment). Foscarnet.[2]	Neutropenia
Esophageal candidiasis	Ketoconazole, 200 mg twice a day.	Hepatitis, adrenal insufficiency
	Fluconazole, 100–200 mg daily	Hepatitis
Herpes simplex infection	Acyclovir, 200 mg 5 times daily for 7–10 days; or acyclovir, 5 mg/kg IV every 8 hours for severe cases. Foscarnet.[2]	Resistant herpes simplex with chronic therapy
Herpes zoster	Acyclovir, 800 mg 4–5 times daily for 7–10 days. Intravenous therapy at 15 mg/kg for ocular involvement, disseminated disease.	See above
Kaposi's sarcoma Limited cutaneous disease	Observation, intralesional vinblastine (Velban)	Local blistering
Extensive/aggressive cutaneous disease	Systemic chemotherapy (eg, alternating weekly vinca alkaloids). Alpha interferon (for patients with CD4 > 400 cells/μL and no constitutional symptoms). Radiation (amelioration of edema).	Bone marrow suppression, peripheral neuritis, flulike syndrome
Visceral disease (eg, pulmonary)	Combination chemotherapy	Bone marrow suppression

[1] For treatment of *Mycobacterium tuberculosis* infection: see Chapter 7.
[2] Experimental drugs or unapproved indications.

Table 24–2. AZT side effects.

Subjective[1]
  Malaise
  Headache
  Nausea
  Vomiting
  Insomnia
Long-term
  Anemia (macrocytic typical, normocytic rare)
  Neutropenia
  Myopathy
  Hepatitis (rare)
  Hyperpigmentation of skin and nail beds.

[1] Usually resolve within 6 weeks.

Table 24–3. Approach to antiretroviral therapy.

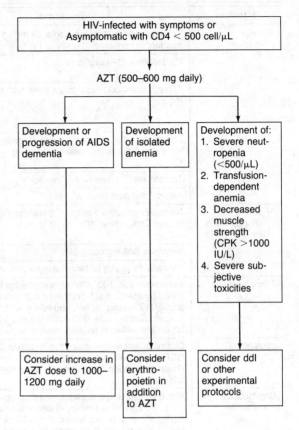

minophen use was associated with an increased incidence of neutropenia. However, this association has been disproved. Therefore, acetaminophen can be used in patients with contraindications to aspirin or nonsteroidal anti-inflammatory agents. Because of the synergistic bone marrow toxicity with some antibiotics, it may be prudent to withhold AZT while treating patients for serious opportunistic infections such as *P carinii* pneumonia. Long-term administration of AZT with ganciclovir can pose a difficult problem, since patients receiving this combination are prone to neutropenia.

The demonstration of in vitro resistance to AZT in patients who had been treated for longer than 6 months, has raised new questions about AZT, especially its use in early infection. This finding must be interpreted cautiously, since the resistance was quantitative, and patients in whom resistance was demonstrated were doing well clinically. Nonetheless, development of resistance is consistent with experience with other antimicrobial agents and with the clinical observation that in many AIDS patients, the benefits of AZT do not last beyond 18 months. The effects of earlier use and lower doses of AZT on emergence of resistance are unknown.

Concern about AZT resistance is also tempered by the finding that resistant isolates were not resistant to other related dideoxynucleosides (eg, ddI, ddC). Among other antiviral drugs, ddI has undergone the most testing. It appears to have fewer hematologic toxicities than AZT, but its efficacy is unknown. Side effects with ddI include a dose-related, reversible, painful peripheral neuropathy, pancreatitis, and diarrhea (due to the buffering agent mixed with the drug). Ultimately, combinations of antiviral drugs will probably be used to minimize side effects, diminish resistance, and maximize efficacy. Immunomodulating drugs such as interferons or interleukin-2 in combination with antiviral drugs are also under study. Hematopoietic stimulating factors such as erythropoietin and granulocyte colony stimulating factor may have a role in diminishing side effects with antiviral drugs. An approach to currently available antiretroviral therapy is outlined in Table 24–3.

Prevention

A. Primary Prevention: In spite of intensive research on vaccine development, no vaccine is available now. Thus, prevention of HIV infection depends upon effective screening of blood products, precautions regarding sexual practices, and infection control practices in the health care setting. Although HIV may be found in virtually all body fluids, the principal mode of sexual transmission involves the exchange of semen or blood. Homosexual or heterosexual anal intercourse remains the sexual practice with highest risk. Condoms appear to be effective in bidirectionally preventing viral transmission. Use of bleach to clean needles appears to inactivate HIV. In the hospital, concerns about nosocomial infection have led to the recommendation for universal body fluid precautions. This involves the rigorous use of gloves when handling any body fluid and the addition of gown, mask, and goggles for procedures that may result in splash or droplet spread.

B. Secondary Prevention: The percentage of HIV-infected persons who will ultimately progress to AIDS is not known. However, cohort studies of individuals with documented dates of seroconversion demonstrate that approximately 50% of untreated seropositive persons develop AIDS within 10 years.

The risk of developing AIDS is inversely correlated with the CD4 count; over 80% of patients with a CD4 count below 200 cells/μL develop AIDS within 3 years.

However, there is increasing evidence that medical intervention can slow the progression of disease among healthy HIV-infected people. Recommended interventions for health care maintenance of HIV-infected individuals are listed in Table 24–4.

Patients should have monitoring of clinical status and laboratory parameters, including a CD4 lymphocyte count, on a 3- to 6-month basis. Patients with values between 200 and 350/μL should have the more frequent counts. Because the CD4 count is one of the best predictors of progression of disease, it is the main criterion for administration of AZT and *P carinii* prophylaxis. Unfortunately, counts are laboratory-dependent, vary diurnally within the same individual (lower in the morning), and are frequently lower with concomitant viral infections. Thus, comparison counts should be performed at the same laboratory and at the same time of day. The trend of CD4 counts is much more helpful clinically than any single count.

Because of the increased occurrence of tuberculosis among HIV-infected patients, all such individuals should undergo PPD testing. Although anergy is common among AIDS patients, the likelihood of a false-negative result is much lower when the test is done early in infection. Those with positive tests (> 5 mm of induration) need a chest x-ray. Patients with an infiltrate in any location, especially if accompanied by mediastinal adenopathy, should have sputum sent for acid-fast staining. Those patients with a positive PPD but negative evaluations for active disease should receive isoniazid (300 mg daily) for 9 months to a year regardless of their age.

HIV-infected patients are at increased risk of reactivation of syphilis and progression to tertiary syphilis despite standard treatment. Because the only widely available tests for syphilis are serologic and because HIV-infected individuals are known to have disordered antibody production, there is concern about the interpretation of these titers. This concern has been fueled by a report of an HIV-infected patient with secondary syphilis and negative syphilis serologic testing. In addition, persistence of treponemes in the spinal fluid after one dose of benzathine penicillin has been demonstrated in HIV-infected patients with primary and secondary syphilis. Therefore, the CDC has recommended an aggressive diagnostic approach to HIV-infected patients with reactive RPR or VDRL tests of greater than 1 year or unknown duration. All such patients should have a lumbar puncture with cerebrospinal fluid cell count and CSF-VDRL. Those with a normal cerebrospinal fluid evaluation are treated as having late latent syphilis (benzathine penicillin G, 2.4 million units intramuscularly weekly for 3 weeks) with follow-up titers. Those with a pleocytosis or a positive CSF-VDRL test are treated as having neurosyphilis (aqueous penicillin G, 2–4 million units intravenously every 4 hours; or procaine penicillin G, 2.4 million units intramuscularly daily, with probenecid, 500 mg 4 times daily, for 10 days.) Some clinicians take a less aggressive approach to patients who have low titers (less than 1:8), a history of having been treated for syphilis, and a normal neurologic examination. Close follow-up of titers is mandatory if such a course is taken.

The efficacy of pneumococcal and influenza vaccines is debated, but since they are safe, HIV-infected individuals should receive them. Patients without evidence of hepatitis surface antibody should receive hepatitis vaccination if they are practicing unsafe sex or actively using intravenous drugs. Live vaccines, such as yellow fever vaccine, should be avoided.

Patients with CD4 counts below 200–250 cells should be provided prophylaxis for *P carinii* pneumonia, especially if they have systemic symptoms of fever, weight loss, fatigue, or signs of hairy leukoplakia or candidiasis. Three regimens for prophylaxis are aerosolized pentamidine, trimethoprim-sulfamethoxazole, and dapsone (see Table 24–5). Aerosolized pentamidine has the advantage of minimal systemic side effects. Its disadvantages are expense (approximately $160.00 per monthly treatment) and decreased effectiveness in the apical and peripheral areas of the lung. Several cases of extrapulmonary *P carinii* infections in patients receiving aerosolized pentamidine have also been reported. Trimethoprim-sulfamethoxazole is inexpensive and widely available. However, the side effects include anemia and neutropenia, which can be especially problematic in patients receiving AZT. Dapsone is undergoing study as a potential prophylactic agent. The use of prophylaxis for other AIDS infections, including toxoplasmosis and cytomegalovirus retinitis, is also under study.

Table 24–4. Health care maintenance of HIV-infected individuals.

For all HIV-infected individuals
  CD4 counts every 3–6 months.
  PPD with anergy controls.
  INH for those with positive PPD and normal chest x-ray.
  RPR or VDRL.
  Pneumococcal vaccine; influenza vaccine in season.
  Hepatitis vaccine for those HBsAb-negative and at risk.
For HIV-infected individuals with CD4 < 500 cells
  AZT.
For HIV-infected individuals with CD4 < 200 cells
  P carinii prophylaxis.

Course & Prognosis

The rate of progression to symptomatic disease is reviewed above. Once clinical findings develop, outcome varies. With improvements in therapy, some

Table 24–5. *P carinii* prophylaxis.

Drug	Dose	Side Effects	Limitations
Aerosolized pentamidine	300 mg monthly	Bronchospasm (pretreat with bronchodilators)	Apical *P carinii* pneumonia, extrapulmonary *P carinii* infections
Trimethoprim-sulfamethoxazole	One double-strength tablet daily	Anemia, neutropenia, hepatitis, rash, Stevens-Johnson syndrome	Incidence of side effects is high, especially among patients receiving AZT
Dapsone	50–100 mg daily	Anemia, neutropenia, hepatitis, methemoglobinemia	Efficacy not well established. G6PD level should be normal. Monitor methemoglobin level.

cohorts of patients are living longer after the diagnosis of AIDS. In San Francisco, mean survival after a first bout of *Pneumocystis* pneumonia is 18–24 months. This is increased from approximately 12 months at the start of the epidemic. However, survival after diagnosis of HIV-related lymphomas still averages less than 6 months.

REFERENCES

Centers for Disease Control: Estimates of HIV prevalence and projected AIDS cases. MMWR 1990;39:110. (Projections of the AIDS epidemic in the 1990's.)

Chaisson RE et al: Tuberculosis in patients with the acquired immunodeficiency syndrome. Am Rev Respir Dis. 1987;136:570-574. (Comparison of HIV-positive and HIV-negative patients.)

Chuck SL, Sande MA: Infections with *Cryptococcus neoformans* in the acquired immunodeficiency syndrome. N Engl J Med. 1989;321:794. (Review of 106 patients.)

Hook EW: Syphilis and HIV infection. J Infect Dis. 1989;160:530.

McArthur JC: Neurologic manifestations of AIDS. Medicine 1987;66:407. (Review of 186 patients.)

Masur H et al: *Pneumocystis* pneumonia: From bench to clinic. Ann Intern Med. 1989; 111:813.

Phair JP, Wolinsy S: Diagnosis of infection with the human immunodeficiency virus. J Infect Dis. 1989;159:320. (ELISA and Western Blot tests and discussion of indications for other HIV tests, including p24 antigen, polymerase chain reaction, and viral cultures.)

Yarchoan R et al: Clinical pharmacology of 3'-azido-2',3'-dideoxythymidine (zidovudine) and related dideoxynucleosides. N Engl J Med. 1989;321:726. (Pharmacology of AZT and new antiviral therapy such as ddI and ddC.)

Infectious Diseases: Viral & Rickettsial

25

Moses Grossman, MD, Ernest Jawetz, MD, PhD, & Lawrence M. Tierney, Jr., MD

VIRAL DISEASES

DIAGNOSIS OF VIRAL INFECTIONS

Some viral illnesses present a clear-cut clinical syndrome (chickenpox, measles, mumps) that identifies the virus involved. Though specific identification of most viruses is technically possible, laboratory assistance is required only for confirmation in atypical cases or for the differential diagnosis of similar syndromes. In some instances, the clinical picture has a number of features that are suggestive of viral infection in general but could be caused by any one of a number of viruses. Such a "viral" picture is seen in aseptic meningitis. The viruses involved in aseptic meningitis include mumps and several enteroviruses; the specific viral diagnosis can only be made with laboratory assistance. In the case of the respiratory tract, viral infections also have certain features in common—widespread involvement of the respiratory epithelium with redness and clear nasal secretion, absence of a purulent response—and, if pneumonia is present, it is more apt to be interstitial pneumonia.

Sometimes the statistical predilection of one of the respiratory viruses for an anatomic site allows one to make an "educated guess." For example, respiratory syncytial virus is the most common cause of bronchiolitis, and parainfluenza virus is the most common cause of croup.

At times, accurate diagnosis is of such import to the patient (rubella during pregnancy) or the community (hepatitis) that rapid laboratory confirmation of the suspected diagnosis is essential. In most cases, however, specific identification is not needed for patient management purposes.

Laboratory Considerations

There are 3 basic laboratory techniques for making a viral diagnosis:

A. Isolation and Identification of the Virus: This requires prompt transport (best on wet ice) to the laboratory and inoculation of the appropriate speci-

men into a suitable cell culture or into a live animal. A variety of techniques are then utilized to determine the presence and nature of the particular virus. At times this can be done very simply (eg, in the case of herpes simplex); at times it may be laborious, time-consuming, and expensive (eg, in the case of coxsackievirus). The isolation of virus from a specimen that is normally free of virus (eg, cerebrospinal fluid, lung biopsy) or from a pathologic lesion (herpes or varicella vesicle) has great diagnostic significance. However, finding a virus in the nasopharynx or in the stool may denote carriage rather than disease; in this case, additional evidence of a rise in antibody titer will be necessary before a specific diagnosis can be made.

B. Microscopic Methods: This entails the microscopic examination of cells, body fluids, or aspirates to demonstrate either the presence of the virus or specific cytologic changes peculiar to one virus or a group of viruses (eg, multinucleate giant cells at the base of herpesvirus lesions; rotavirus structures seen in electron micrographs of diarrheal stools). Immunofluorescence methods, especially when employing monoclonal antibodies, can rapidly identify some virus antigens (rabies, varicella, herpes simplex, respiratory syncytial, etc) in desquamated or scraped cells rather than in exudates or transudates.

C. Serologic Methods: During viral illnesses, specific antibodies develop. The timing of rise in titer and persistence of antibodies varies. A 4-fold rise in antibody titer during the course of the illness is usually considered significant evidence of disease. Since a single serum titer is not particularly helpful, many laboratories will not do the test until paired sera (taken 2–3 weeks apart) are available. It is not practical to do serologic tests for a large number of viruses in any patient. Thus, the use of this method requires a specific suspicion of which virus might be involved.

HERPESVIRUSES OF HUMANS

This large group of DNA viruses shares common features that are important in the general clinical patterns manifested in humans. The better-defined clinical pictures are described under the specific disease entities. The most important herpesviruses in human disease states are herpes simplex type 1, herpes simplex type 2, varicella-zoster, cytomegalovirus, and EB-infectious mononucleosis virus.

Each virus tends to produce subclinical primary infection more often than clinically manifest illness. Each tends to persist in a latent state (evidenced only by persistent immunologic reactivity) for the rest of the person's life. Reactivation producing a clinical recurrence of disease may follow a known or unrecognized triggering mechanism. In herpes simplex and varicella-zoster, the virus is latent in sensory ganglia, and reactivation is followed by the appearance of lesions in the distal sensory nerve distribution. As a result of the suppression of cell-mediated immunity by disease, drugs, or radiation, reactivation of virus may lead to widespread disseminated lesions on and within affected organs and the central nervous system. Severe or even fatal illness may also occur in the newborn or the immunodeficient child.

Herpesviruses can infect the fetus and induce serious congenital malformations. They have also been linked to neoplasia (eg, cervical carcinoma, Burkitt's lymphoma), but the relationship remains uncertain. Herpesvirus infections that involve epithelial surfaces may lead to prolonged shedding of virus and its spread to contacts of the infected person.

Several drugs can inhibit replication of herpesviruses. Of these, idoxuridine and trifluridine are effective topically in human herpetic keratitis, but they are too toxic for systemic use. Acyclovir, 15 mg/kg/d, has been used intravenously in disseminated herpes simplex or herpetic encephalitis. The latter should be diagnosed by brain biopsy with immunofluorescent stain and culture of virus. If the diagnosis is made very early before onset of coma, the mortality rate can be significantly reduced. However, many of the survivors are not neurologically normal. Because of the need for rapid treatment and the difficulty of brain biopsy, many suspected cases of herpetic encephalitis receive drug therapy prior to the establishment of the diagnosis.

Acyclovir, 15 mg/kg/d intravenously, is clearly beneficial in symptomatic primary genital infections (particularly in females) and in disseminating herpetic mucocutaneous lesions of immunosuppressed patients or newborns. It can limit varicella lesions in immunocompromised patients if used early. Oral acyclovir (200 mg 5 times daily) can be effective systemically in such patients and can also be used to reduce the frequency and severity of recurrent herpetic lesions.

Topical acyclovir (5%) applied to primary genital herpetic lesions can reduce viral shedding and local pain and shorten healing time, but it has little effect on recurrent lesions. It helps in treating mucocutaneous lesions in immunocompromised patients (see Chapter 31). No drug currently available affects the recurrence rate of herpetic lesions following a course of treatment.

Corey L, Spear PG: Infections with herpes simplex viruses. (2 parts.) N Engl J Med 1986;314:686, 749.
Mertz GJ et al: Long-term acyclovir suppression of frequently recurring genital herpes, simplex virus infection. JAMA 1988;260:201.
Straus SE et al: Acyclovir suppression of frequently recurring genital herpes. JAMA 1988;260:2227.

MEASLES
(Rubeola)

Essentials of Diagnosis

- Prodrome of fever, coryza, cough, conjunctivitis, photophobia, Koplik's spots.
- Rash: brick-red, irregular, maculopapular; onset 3 days after onset of prodrome; face to trunk to extremities.
- Leukopenia. Exposure 10–14 days previously.

General Considerations

Measles is an acute systemic viral (paramyxovirus) infection transmitted by inhalation of infective droplets. Its highest incidence is in young children. One attack confers permanent immunity. Communicability is greatest during the preeruptive stage but continues as long as the rash remains. Sporadic recent outbreaks of the disease in adults have led to changes in recombinations concerning prevention (see below).

Clinical Findings

A. Symptoms and Signs: (Table 25–1.) Fever is often as high as 40–40.6 °C (104–105 °F). It persists through the prodrome and rash (about 7 days) but may remit briefly at the onset of rash. Malaise may be marked. Coryza resembles that seen with upper respiratory infections (nasal obstruction, sneezing, and sore throat). Cough is persistent and nonproductive. There is conjunctivitis, with redness, swelling, photophobia, and discharge.

Koplik's spots are pathognomonic of measles. They appear about 2 days before the rash and last 1–4 days as tiny "table salt crystals" on the dull red mucous membranes of the cheeks and often on inner conjunctival folds and vaginal mucous membranes. The pharynx is red, and a yellowish exudate may appear on the tonsils. The tongue is coated in the center; the tip and margins are red. Moderate generalized lymphadenopathy is common. Splenomegaly occurs occasionally.

The rash usually appears first on the face and behind the ears 4 days after the onset of symptoms. The initial lesions are pinhead-sized papules which coalesce to form the brick-red, irregular, blotchy maculopapular rash and which may further coalesce in severe cases to form an almost uniform erythema on

Table 25–1. Diagnostic features of some acute exanthems.

Disease	Prodromal Signs and Symptoms	Nature of Eruption	Other Diagnostic Features	Laboratory Tests
Measles (rubeola)	3–4 days of fever, coryza, conjunctivitis, and cough.	Maculopapular, brick-red; begins on head and neck; spreads downward. In 5–6 days rash brownish, desquamating. See atypical measles.	Koplik's spots on buccal mucosa.	White blood count low. Virus isolation in cell culture. Antibody tests by hemagglutination inhibition or neutralization.
Atypical measles	Same as measles.	Maculopapular centripetal rash, becoming confluent.	History of measles vaccination.	Measles antibody present in past, with titer rise during illness.
Rubella (German measles)	Little or no prodrome.	Maculopapular, pink; begins on head and neck, spreads downward, fades in 3 days. No desquamation.	Lymphadenopathy, postauricular or occipital.	White blood count normal or low. Serologic tests for immunity and definitive diagnosis (hemagglutination inhibition).
Chickenpox (varicella)	0–1 day of fever, anorexia, headache.	Rapid evolution of macules to papules, vesicles, crusts; all stages simultaneously present; lesions superficial, distribution centripetal.	Lesions on scalp and mucous membranes.	Specialized complement fixation and virus neutralization in cell culture. Fluorescent antibody test of smear of lesions.
Scarlet fever	½–2 days of malaise, sore throat, fever, vomiting.	Generalized, punctate, red; prominent on neck, in axilla, groin, skinfolds; circumoral pallor; fine desquamation involves hands and feet.	Strawberry tongue, exudative tonsillitis.	Group A hemolytic streptococci cultures from throat; antistreptolysin O titer rise.
Exanthem subitum	3–4 days of high fever.	As fever falls by crisis, pink maculopapules appear on chest and trunk; fade in 1–3 days.		White blood count low.
Erythema infectiosum	None. Usually in epidemics.	Red, flushed cheeks; circumoral pallor; maculopapules on extremities.	"Slapped face" appearance.	White blood count normal.
Meningococcemia	Hours of fever, vomiting.	Maculopapules, petechiae, purpura.	Meningeal signs, toxicity, shock.	Cultures of blood. Cerebrospinal fluid. High white blood count.
Rocky Mt. spotted fever	3–4 days of fever, chills, severe headaches.	Maculopapules, petechiae, initial distribution centripetal (extremities to trunk).	History of tick bite.	Agglutination (OX19, OX2), complement fixation.
Typhus fevers	3–4 days of fever, chills, severe headaches.	Maculopapules, petechiae, initial distribution centrifugal (trunk to extremities).	Endemic area, lice.	Agglutination (OX19), complement fixation.
Infectious mononucleosis	Fever, adenopathy, sore throat.	Maculopapular rash resembling rubella, rarely papulovesicular.	Splenomegaly, tonsillar exudate.	Atypical lymphocytes in blood smears; heterophil agglutination. Monospot test.
Enterovirus infections	1–2 days of fever, malaise.	Maculopapular rash resembling rubella, rarely papulovesicular or petechial.	Aseptic meningitis.	Virus isolation from stool or cerebrospinal fluid; complement fixation titer rise.
Drug eruptions	Occasionally fever.	Maculopapular rash resembling rubella, rarely papulovesicular.		Eosinophilia.
Eczema herpeticum	None.	Vesiculopustular lesions in area of eczema.		Herpes simplex virus isolated in cell culture. Multinucleate giant cells in smear of lesion.
Kawasaki disease	Fever, adenopathy, conjunctivitis.	Cracked lips, strawberry tongue, maculopapular polymorphous rash, peeling skin on fingers and toes.	Edema of extremities. Angiitis of coronary arteries.	Thrombocytosis, electrocardiographic changes.

some areas of the body. By the second day, the rash begins to coalesce on the face as it appears on the trunk. On the third day, the rash is confluent on the trunk, begins to appear on the extremities, and begins to fade on the face. Thereafter, it fades in the order of its appearance. Hyperpigmentation remains in fair-skinned individuals and severe cases. Slight desquamation may follow.

Atypical measles is a syndrome occurring in adolescents or adults who have received inactivated measles vaccine or who received live measles vaccine before age 12 months and as a result have developed hypersensitivity rather than protective immunity. When they are infected with wild measles virus, such individuals may develop a severe illness with high fever, unusual rashes (papular, hemorrhagic) without Koplik's spots, headache and arthralgias, and interstitial infiltrates, occasionally with pleural effusions. There is a substantial mortality rate.

B. Laboratory Findings: Leukopenia is usually present unless secondary bacterial complications exist. Febrile proteinuria is present. Virus can be recovered from nasopharyngeal washings and from blood. A 4-fold rise in serum antibody supports the diagnosis.

Complications

A. Central Nervous System Complications: Encephalitis occurs in approximately 1:2000 to 1:1000 cases. Its onset is usually 3–7 days after the rash. Vomiting, convulsions, coma, and a variety of severe neurologic signs and symptoms develop. Treatment is symptomatic and supportive. There is an appreciable mortality rate, and many patients are left with permanent sequelae. Subacute sclerosing panencephalitis is a very late form of central nervous system complication, the measles virus acting as a "slow virus" to produce this degenerative central nervous system disease years after the initial infection.

B. Respiratory Tract Disease: Early in the course of the disease, bronchopneumonia or bronchiolitis due to the measles virus may occur and result in serious difficulties with ventilation.

C. Secondary Bacterial Infections: Immediately following measles, secondary bacterial infection—particularly cervical adenitis, otitis media, and pneumonia—occurs in about 15% of patients.

D. Tuberculosis: Measles produces temporary anergy to the tuberculin skin test; there may be exacerbations in patients with tuberculosis.

Prevention

In the United States, most children receive their first vaccine dose at 15 months and a second at age 4–6 years prior to entry into school (see Table 23–4). In high-risk areas and in counties with large inner city populations—or if there have been recent cases among unvaccinated preschool children—the first dose may be administered at 12 months. Students beyond high school and medical staff starting employment must have the above vaccination schedule documented—or must have serologic evidence of immunity—if they were born after 1957. For individuals born during or before 1957, herd immunity can be assumed.

Outbreak control is similar. If outbreaks are occurring in preschool children under 1 year of age, initial vaccination may be given at 6 months, with repeat at 15 months. When outbreaks take place in day care centers, K–12 institutions, or colleges and universities, revaccination is indicated for all students and their siblings born during or after 1957 who do not have documentation of immunity as defined above. If outbreaks occur in medical facilities, revaccination is indicated for all medical workers born in 1957 or after who have direct patient contact and no evidence of immunity. Susceptible personnel who have been exposed should be isolated from patient contact from the fifth to the 21st day after exposure irrespective of whether they have been vaccinated or have received immune globulin; if they should develop measles,

they should be isolated from patient contact until 7 days after the rash develops.

When susceptible individuals are exposed to measles, the live virus vaccine can prevent disease if given within 24 hours of exposure. This is rarely feasible in a household. Later, gamma globulin (0.25 mL/kg [0.1 mL/lb] body weight) can be injected for prevention of clinical illness. This must be followed by active immunization 3 months later.

Treatment

A. General Measures: Isolate the patient for the week following onset of rash and keep at bed rest until afebrile. Give aspirin, saline eye sponges, vasoconstrictor nose drops, and a sedative cough mixture as necessary.

B. Treatment of Complications: Secondary bacterial infections are treated with appropriate antimicrobial drugs. Postmeasles encephalitis can only be treated symptomatically.

Prognosis

The mortality rate of measles in children in the USA is 0.2%, but it may be as high as 10% in children in underdeveloped areas. Deaths are due principally to encephalitis (15% mortality rate) and bacterial pneumonia.

ACIP: Measles prevention. MMWR 1989;24:11.

Bloch AB et al: Health impact of measles vaccination in the United States. Pediatrics 1985;76:524.

Markowitz LE et al: Pattern of transmission in measles outbreak in the United States, 1985–86. N Engl J Med 1989;320:75.

ERYTHEMA INFECTIOSUM (Fifth Disease)

This acute, communicable viral illness is common, mainly in children 4–10 years old, and occurs in focal and community-wide outbreaks. It is caused by a human parvovirus (HPV—a 20-nm DNA virus). The initial manifestation of illness is a distinctive fiery red appearance of the cheeks ("slapped cheeks"), with circumoral pallor. A few days later, there is a red, lacy, maculopapular rash on the trunk that may wax and wane for several days. Malaise, headache, and pruritus occur, but fever is rare. At the time of the rash, there may be arthralgia, synovitis, and arthritis, particularly in females. The arthritis is symmetric and involves mainly the hands, wrists, and knees. It usually resolves in 4 weeks but may last for months. HPV is also implicated in aplastic crisis, especially in sickle cell disease, and may cause disturbances in pregnancy.

The diagnosis is clinical (Table 25–1) but may be confirmed by an elevated titer of IgM anti-HPV antibodies in serum. Scarlet fever is the main differential diagnosis. The prognosis is excellent. Besides arthritis, which is common in some outbreaks, encephalitis has been described as a rare complication. Treatment is symptomatic.

Centers for Disease Control: Risks associated with human parvovirus B19 infection. MMWR 1989;38:81.

RUBELLA
(German Measles)

Essentials of Diagnosis

- No prodrome; mild symptoms (fever, malaise, coryza) coinciding with eruption.
- Posterior cervical and postauricular lymphadenopathy.
- Fine maculopapular rash of 3 days' duration; face to trunk to extremities.
- Leukopenia. Exposure 14–21 days previously.
- Arthralgia, particularly in young women.

General Considerations

Rubella is a systemic viral disease transmitted by inhalation of infective droplets. It is only moderately communicable. One attack usually confers permanent immunity. The incubation period is 14–21 days (average, 16 days). The disease is transmissible for 1 week before the rash appears.

The clinical picture of rubella is difficult to distinguish from other viral illnesses such as infectious mononucleosis, echovirus infections, and coxsackievirus infections. Definitive diagnosis can only be made by isolating the virus or by serologic means.

The principal importance of rubella lies in the devastating effect this virus has on the fetus in utero, producing teratogenic effects and a continuing congenital infection.

Clinical Findings

A. Symptoms and Signs: (Table 25–1.) Fever and malaise, usually mild, accompanied by tender suboccipital adenitis, may precede the eruption by 1 week. Mild coryza may be present. Joint pain (polyarthritis) occurs in about 25% of adult cases. These symptoms usually subside within 7 days but may persist for weeks.

Posterior cervical and postauricular lymphadenopathy is very common. Erythema of the palate and throat, sometimes blotchy, may be noted. A fine, pink maculopapular rash appears on the face, trunk, and extremities in rapid progression (2–3 days) and fades quickly, usually lasting 1 day in each area. Rubella without rash may be at least as common as the exanthematous disease. Diagnosis can be suspected when there is epidemiologic evidence of the disease in the community but requires laboratory confirmation.

B. Laboratory Findings: Leukopenia may be present early and may be followed by an increase in plasma cells. Virus isolation and serologic tests of immunity (rubella virus hemagglutination inhibition and fluorescent antibody tests) are available. Definitive diagnosis is based on a 4-fold rise in the antibody titer.

Complications

A. Complications in Pregnancy: It is important to know whether rubella antibodies are present at the beginning of pregnancy.

If a pregnant woman is exposed to a possible case of rubella, an immediate hemagglutination-inhibiting rubella antibody level should be obtained. If antibodies are found, there is no reason for concern. If no antibodies are found, careful clinical and serologic follow-up is essential. If the occurrence of rubella in the expectant mother can be confirmed, therapeutic abortion may be considered. Judgment in this regard is tempered by personal, religious, legal, and other considerations. The risk to the fetus is highest in the first trimester but continues into the second.

B. Congenital Rubella: An infant acquiring the infection in utero may be normal at birth but more likely will have a wide variety of manifestations, including growth retardation, maculopapular rash, thrombocytopenia, cataracts, deafness, congenital heart defects, organomegaly, and many other manifestations. Viral excretion in the throat and urine persists for many months despite high antibody levels. The diagnosis is confirmed by isolation of the virus. A specific test for IgM rubella antibody is useful for making this diagnosis in the newborn. Treatment is directed to the many anomalies.

Prevention

Live attenuated rubella virus vaccine (eg, RA 27/3) should be given to all infants and to girls before the menarche. When adult women are immunized, they must not be pregnant, and the absence of antibodies should be established. (In the USA, about 80% of 20-year-old women are immune to rubella.) Birth control must be practiced for at least 3 months after the use of this live vaccine. Arthritis may follow administration of rubella vaccine and is often more severe than that which occurs with the disease.

Treatment

Give aspirin or acetaminophen as required for symptomatic relief. Encephalitis and thrombocytopenic purpura can only be treated symptomatically.

Prognosis

Rubella (other than the congenital form) is a mild illness and rarely lasts more than 3–4 days. Congenital rubella, on the other hand, has a high mortality rate, and the congenital defects associated with it require many years of medical and surgical management.

Centers for Disease Control: Rubella and congenital rubella syndrome: United States 1985–88. MMWR 1989;38:173.

CYTOMEGALOVIRUS DISEASE

The vast majority of cytomegalovirus infections are clinically inapparent. The virus (human herpesvirus 5) can be cultured from the salivary glands of 10–25% of healthy individuals, from the cervix of 10% of healthy women, and from the urine of 1% of all newborns. Cytomegalovirus infection occurs in 85–95% of homosexual men and is sexually transmitted. In immunocompromised persons, including AIDS patients, cytomegalovirus infection is often a serious illness (see Chapter 24), and its virtually ubiquitous presence in that disorder poses many clinical problems.

Clinical Findings

A. Classification: Three important clinical entities are recognized.

1. Perinatal disease–Intrauterine infection results in serious disease, with jaundice, hepatosplenomegaly, thrombocytopenia, and purpura. Of congenitally infected children, more than 15% develop a hearing deficit and up to 30% have mental retardation. Infection acquired soon after birth is asymptomatic but may induce neurologic deficits later.

2. Acute acquired cytomegalovirus disease– The clinical picture is that of infectious mononucleosis with fever, malaise, muscle and joint pains, generalized lymphadenopathy, and an enlarged liver. Pharyngitis and respiratory symptoms are not pronounced. Laboratory findings include atypical lymphocytes and abnormal liver function tests. In contrast to Epstein-Barr herpesvirus infection, the heterophil antibody test is negative. This disease may occur after massive blood transfusions, including those given to infants.

3. Disease in the immunosuppressed host– In immunocompromised persons, cytomegalovirus can cause an opportunistic severe pneumonia. Cytomegalovirus infection itself can result in immunosuppression and may provide a favorable environment for spread of other opportunistic pathogens (eg, *Pneumocystis carinii* pneumonia, disseminated herpes simplex lesions).

B. Laboratory Findings: (In addition to those listed above.) Cytomegalovirus can be grown in cell culture from urine, cervical secretions, semen, saliva, blood, and other tissues. Serologic tests are used to determine the incidence of infection in various groups. A significant titer rise is the only indication of recent infection.

Treatment

Control fever, pain, and convulsions with appropriate drugs. The antiviral drug ganciclovir (DHPG) has yielded some benefits, though at the cost of signifi-

cant toxicity (see Chapter 31). Hyperimmune cytomegalovirus globulin given intravenously to bone marrow transplant recipients may have some prophylactic value.

Onorato IM et al: Epidemiology of cytomegaloviral infection: Recommendations for prevention and control. Rev Infect Dis 1985;7:479.

Preiksaitis JK, Brown L, McKenzie M: The risk of cytomegalovirus infection in seronegative transfusion recipients not receiving exogenous immunosuppression. J Infect Dis 1988;157:523.

Stagno S, Whitley RJ: Herpesvirus infections of pregnancy: Cytomegalovirus infections. N Engl J Med 1985; 313:1270.

VARICELLA (Chickenpox) & HERPES ZOSTER (Shingles)

Essentials of Diagnosis

- Fever and malaise just before or with eruption.
- Rash: pruritic, centripetal, papular, changing to vesicular, pustular, and finally crusting.
- Leukopenia.
- Exposure 14–20 days previously.

General Considerations

Varicella is a viral (human herpesvirus 3) disease spread by inhalations of infective droplets or contact with lesions. Most cases occur in children. One attack confers permanent immunity. The incubation period of varicella is 10–20 days (average, 14 days).

Herpes zoster is caused by the varicella virus in persons who experienced chickenpox with the initial varicella infection.

Clinical Findings

A. Varicella:

1. Symptoms and signs–(Table 25–1.) Fever and malaise are usually mild in children and more severe in adults. Itching is characteristic of the eruption. Vesicular lesions, quickly rupturing to form small ulcers, may appear first in the oropharynx. The rash is most prominent on the face, scalp, and trunk but to a lesser extent commonly involves the extremities (centripetal). Maculopapules change in a few hours to vesicles that quickly become pustular and eventually form crusts. New lesions may erupt for 1–5 days, so that all stages of the eruption are generally present simultaneously. The crusts usually slough in 7–14 days. The vesicles and pustules are superficial and elliptic and have slightly serrated borders.

The distribution and evolution of varicella distinguish it from herpes zoster.

2. Laboratory findings–Leukopenia is common. Multinucleated giant cells may be found in scrapings of the base of the vesicles. Virus isolation is possible.

B. Herpes Zoster: This syndrome is caused by

the same virus as varicella. Usually a single, unilateral dermatome is involved. Pain, sometimes very severe, may precede the appearance of the skin lesions. The lesions follow the distribution of a nerve root. Thoracic and lumbar roots are most common, but cervical roots and the trigeminal nerve may be involved. The skin lesions are similar to those of chickenpox and develop in the same way from maculopapules to vesicles to pustules. When the trigeminal nerve is involved, a lesion on the tip of the nose implies ophthalmic division disease, mandating systemic therapy (see below). Complete resolution of lesions may take 2–6 weeks. Antibody levels are higher and more persistent in zoster than they are in varicella.

Complications

Secondary bacterial infection of the lesions is common and may produce a pitted scar. Cellulitis, erysipelas, and surgical scarlet fever may occur.

Pneumonia of the interstitial type occurs more often in adults and may lead to adult respiratory distress syndrome (ARDS) and sometimes death.

Encephalitis occurs infrequently. It tends to be characterized by ataxia and nystagmus. Most patients recover without sequelae.

Varicella in immunosuppressed patients (eg, those receiving antileukemia drugs or kidney transplants) is often very severe and may be fatal. Chickenpox contracted during the first or second trimester of pregnancy carries a small risk of a distinctive pattern of congenital malformations in the fetus. If a mother develops varicella within 5 days of delivery, the newborn is at great risk of severe disease and should receive varicella-zoster immune globulin (VZIG).

In immunosuppressed patients, herpes zoster may disseminate, producing skin lesions beyond the dermatome, visceral lesions, and encephalitis. This is a serious, sometimes fatal complication.

Prevention

VZIG is effective in preventing chickenpox in exposed susceptible immunosuppressed individuals, but it has no place in therapy. A live attenuated vaccine for immunocompromised susceptible children appears to be safe and effective.

VZIG may be obtained by calling the nearest regional Red Cross Blood Center or the Centers for Disease Control, Atlanta; day phone (404) 329–3311 or (404) 329–2888.

Treatment

A. General Measures: Isolate the patient until primary crusts have disappeared, and keep at bed rest until afebrile. Hospital patients with varicella-zoster should be placed in isolation rooms, and personnel entering the room should wear gowns, gloves, and masks. Keep the skin clean by means of frequent tub baths or showers when afebrile. Calamine lotion locally and antihistaminics may relieve pruritus. If

antipyretics are necessary, acetaminophen rather than aspirin should be given to avoid risk of Reye's syndrome.

B. Treatment of Complications: Secondary bacterial infection of local lesions may be treated with bacitracin-neomycin ointment; if lesions are extensive, appropriate antimicrobial therapy may be indicated. Antiviral therapy with high-dose acyclovir should be started early for varicella or zoster in immunocompromised individuals. It should also be instituted for severe disease (pneumonitis, corneal involvement by zoster) in immunocompetent persons (see Chapter 31). Steroids (eg, prednisone, 40 mg orally daily for 10 days and then tapered to zero) tend to reduce the incidence of postherpetic neuralgia in the elderly and are not likely to have deleterious effects. While acyclovir tends to accelerate healing of lesions, it has little effect on postherpetic pain.

Prognosis

The total duration from onset of symptoms to disappearance of crusts rarely exceeds 2 weeks. Fatalities are rare except in immunosuppressed patients.

Plotkin SA: Hell's fire and varicella-vaccine safety. N Engl J Med 1988;318:573.
Straus SE et al: Varicella-zoster virus infections: Biology, natural history, treatment, and prevention. (NIH Conference.) Ann Intern Med 1988;108:221.

VARIOLA
(Smallpox, Variola Major)

Smallpox was a highly contagious viral (poxvirus) disease characterized by severe headache, fever, and prostration and accompanied by a centrifugal rash developing from macules to papules to vesicles to pustules.

Immunization with vaccinia virus culminating in a worldwide effort by WHO has apparently succeeded in eradicating smallpox from the world as of 1979.

VACCINIA

The efficacy of vaccination was the essential factor in the eradication of smallpox. Since the world has been declared free of smallpox, civilian vaccination is now indicated only for laboratory workers working with smallpox virus or closely related viruses. Vaccination is still practiced among military forces. Smallpox vaccination is no longer required for international travel.

Any form of immunosuppression is an absolute contraindication to smallpox vaccination. Eczema in the patient or family member (including a past history of eczema), other forms of dermatitis, and burns also contraindicate vaccination. Smallpox vaccine should never be used "therapeutically."

Complications range from minor rashes to life-threatening complications such as postvaccinal encephalitis, vaccinia necrosum, and eczema vaccinatum. Vaccinia can be transmitted from military personnel and their families to contacts. Assistance with the management of such complications may be obtained through the Centers for Disease Control.

US Public Health Service Advisory Committee on Immunization Practices: Smallpox vaccine. MMWR 1985; 34:341.

MUMPS
(Epidemic Parotitis)

Essentials of Diagnosis

- Painful, swollen salivary glands, usually parotid.
- Orchitis, meningoencephalitis, pancreatitis.
- Cerebrospinal fluid lymphocytic pleocytosis in meningoencephalitis.
- Exposure 14–21 days previously.

General Considerations

Mumps is a viral (paramyxovirus) disease spread by respiratory droplets that usually produces inflammation of the salivary glands and, less commonly, orchitis, meningoencephalitis, pancreatitis, and oophoritis. Most patients are children. The incubation period is 14–21 days (average, 18 days). Infectivity precedes the symptoms by about 1 day, is maximal for 3 days, and then declines until the swelling is gone.

Clinical Findings

A. Symptoms and Signs: Fever and malaise are variable but are often minimal in young children. High fever usually accompanies orchitis or meningoencephalitis. Pain and swelling of one or both (75%) of the parotid or other salivary glands occur, usually in succession 1–3 days apart. Occasionally, one gland subsides completely (usually in 7 days or less) before others become involved. Orchitis occurs in 25% of men. Headache and lethargy suggest meningoencephalitis. Upper abdominal pain and nausea and vomiting suggest pancreatitis. Lower abdominal pain in females suggests oophoritis.

Tender parotid swelling is the commonest physical finding. Edema is occasionally marked. Swelling and tenderness of the submaxillary and sublingual glands are variable. The orifice of Stensen's duct may be reddened and swollen. Neck stiffness and other signs of meningeal irritation suggest meningoencephalitis. Testicular swelling and tenderness (unilateral in 75%) denote orchitis. Epigastric tenderness suggests pancreatitis. Lower abdominal tenderness and ovarian enlargement may be noted in mumps oophoritis, but the diagnosis is often difficult. Salivary gland involvement must be differentiated from lymph node involvement in the anterior cervical space.

B. Laboratory Findings: Relative lymphocytosis may be present, but the blood picture is not typical. Serum amylase is commonly elevated with or without pancreatitis. Lymphocytic pleocytosis of the cerebrospinal fluid is present in meningoencephalitis, which may be asymptomatic. The diagnosis is confirmed by isolating mumps virus from saliva or demonstrating a 4-fold rise in complement-fixing antibodies in paired sera.

Differential Diagnosis

Swelling of the parotid gland may be due to calculi in the parotid ducts, and a reaction to iodides may produce such swelling. Other causes include starch ingestion, sarcoidosis, cirrhosis, diabetes, and bulimia. Parotitis may also be produced by pyogenic organisms, particularly in debilitated individuals. Swelling of the parotid gland must be differentiated from inflammation of the lymph nodes that are located more posteriorly and inferiorly than the parotid gland.

Complications

The "complications" of mumps are simply other manifestations of the disease less common than inflammation of the salivary glands. These usually follow the parotitis but may precede it or occur without salivary gland involvement: meningoencephalitis (30%), orchitis (occurs mainly after puberty in 25% of infected men), pancreatitis, oophoritis, thyroiditis, neuritis, myocarditis, and nephritis.

Aseptic meningitis is common during the course of mumps and may occur without salivary gland involvement. This is a very benign self-limited illness. Occasionally, however, encephalitis develops. This is associated with cerebral edema, serious neurologic manifestations, and sometimes death. Deafness may develop (rarely) as a result of eighth nerve neuritis.

Prevention

Mumps live virus vaccine is safe and highly effective. It is recommended for routine immunization for children over age 1 year, either alone or in combination with other virus vaccines. It should not be given to immunocompromised individuals. Its use has markedly decreased the incidence of mumps in the USA. The mumps skin test is less reliable in determining immunity than are serum neutralization titers.

Treatment

A. General Measures: Isolate the patient until swelling subsides and keep at bed rest during the febrile period. Give aspirin or codeine for analgesia as required and alkaline aromatic mouthwashes.

B. Treatment of Complications:

1. Meningoencephalitis–The treatment of aseptic meningitis is purely symptomatic. The management of encephalitis requires attention to cerebral edema, the airway, and maintenance of vital functions.

2. Orchitis–Suspend the scrotum in a suspensory or toweling "bridge" and apply ice bags. Incision of the tunica may be necessary in severe cases. Give codeine or morphine as necessary for pain. Pain can also be relieved by injection of the spermatic cord at the external inguinal ring with 10–20 mL of 1% procaine solution. Reduce inflammatory reaction with hydrocortisone sodium succinate, 100 mg intravenously, followed by 20 mg orally every 6 hours for 2–3 days.

3. Pancreatitis–Symptomatic relief only and parenteral fluids if necessary.

4. Oophoritis–Symptomatic treatment only.

Prognosis

The entire course of the infection rarely exceeds 2 weeks. Fatalities (due to encephalitis) are very rare.

Orchitis often makes the patient very uncomfortable but very rarely results in sterility.

Centers for Disease Control: Mumps: United States, 1985–1988. MMWR 1988;38:101.

POLIOMYELITIS

Essentials of Diagnosis

- Muscle weakness, headache, stiff neck, fever, nausea and vomiting, sore throat.
- Lower motor neuron lesion (flaccid paralysis) with decreased deep tendon reflexes and muscle wasting.
- Cerebrospinal fluid shows excess cells. Lymphocytes predominate; rarely more than 500/μL.

General Considerations

Poliomyelitis virus (enterovirus) is present in throat washings and stools. Infection is most commonly acquired by the fecal-oral route. Since the introduction of effective vaccine, poliomyelitis has become a rare disease in developed areas of the world.

Three antigenically distinct types of poliomyelitis virus (I, II, and III) are recognized, with no cross-immunity between them.

The incubation period is 5–35 days (usually 7–14 days). Infectivity is maximal during the first week, but virus is excreted in stools for several weeks.

Clinical Findings

A. Symptoms and Signs:

1. Abortive poliomyelitis–The symptoms are fever, headache, vomiting, diarrhea, constipation, and sore throat.

2. Nonparalytic poliomyelitis–Headache, neck, back, and extremity pain; fever, vomiting, abdominal pain, lethargy, and irritability are present.

Muscle spasm is always present in the extensors of the neck and back and often in hamstring and other muscles. The muscles may be tender to palpation.

3. Paralytic poliomyelitis–Paralysis may occur at any time during the febrile period. Tremors, muscle weakness, constipation, and ileus may appear. Paralytic poliomyelitis may be divided into 2 forms, which may coexist: (1) spinal poliomyelitis, with weakness of the muscles supplied by the spinal nerves; and (2) bulbar poliomyelitis, with weakness of the muscles supplied by the cranial nerves and variable "encephalitis" symptoms. Bulbar symptoms include diplopia (uncommon), facial weakness, dysphagia, dysphonia, nasal voice, weakness of the sternocleidomastoid and trapezius muscles, difficulty in chewing, inability to swallow or expel saliva, and regurgitation of fluids through the nose. The most life-threatening aspect of bulbar poliomyelitis is respiratory paralysis.

Paralysis of the shoulder girdle often precedes intercostal and diaphragmatic paralysis, which leads to diminished chest expansion and decreased vital capacity. Cyanosis and stridor may appear later as a result of hypoxia. Paralysis may quickly become maximal or may progress over a period of several days until the temperature becomes normal.

Deep tendon reflexes are diminished or lost, often asymmetrically, in areas of involvement.

In bulbar poliomyelitis there may be loss of gag reflex, loss of movement of palate and pharyngeal muscles, pooling of secretions in the oropharynx, deviation of tongue, and loss of movement of the vocal cords.

Lethargy or coma may be due to encephalitis or hypoxia, most often caused by hypoventilation.

Hypertension, hypotension, and tachycardia may occur. Convulsions are rare.

B. Laboratory Findings: The white blood cell count may be normal or mildly elevated. Cerebrospinal fluid pressure and protein are normal or slightly increased; glucose is not decreased; cells usually number fewer than 500/μL (predominantly lymphocytes; polymorphonuclear cells may be elevated at first). Cerebrospinal fluid is normal in 5% of patients. The virus may be recovered from throat washings (early) and stools (early and late). Neutralizing and complement-fixing antibodies appear during the first or second week of illness.

Differential Diagnosis

Nonparalytic poliomyelitis is very difficult to distinguish from other forms of aseptic meningitis due to other enteroviruses. The distinction is made by laboratory means. Acute infectious polyneuritis (Guillain-Barré) and paralysis from a tick bite may initially resemble poliomyelitis. In Guillain-Barré syndrome (see Chapter 18), the weakness is more symmetric, and the cerebrospinal fluid has a high protein content but normal cell count.

Complications

Urinary tract infection, atelectasis, pneumonia, myocarditis, and pulmonary edema may occur.

Prevention

Oral live trivalent virus vaccine (Sabin) is easily administered, safe, and very effective in providing local gastrointestinal immunity as well as a good level of circulating antibody. It is essential for primary immunization of all infants. Routine immunization of adults in the USA is not recommended because of the low incidence of the disease. However, adults who are exposed to poliomyelitis or plan to travel to endemic areas and who have not received polio immunization within the past decade should be given inactivated poliomyelitis vaccine (Salk). This vaccine should also be given to immunodeficient or immunosuppressed individuals and members of their households.

Treatment

Cranial nerve involvement must be detected promptly. Maintain comfortable but changing positions in a "polio bed": firm mattress, foot board, sponge rubber pads or rolls, sandbags, and light splints. Fecal impaction and urinary retention (especially with paraplegia) must be managed. In cases of respiratory paralysis or weakness, intensive care is needed.

To prevent future deformity, active exercise is avoided during fever but passive range-of-motion exercises are carried out, as well as frequent changes in position. As soon as the fever has subsided, early mobilization and active exercise under skilled direction are begun.

Prognosis

During the febrile period, paralysis may develop or progress. Mild weakness of small muscles is more likely to regress than severe weakness of large muscles. Bulbar poliomyelitis carries the highest mortality rate (up to 50%). New muscle weakness may develop and progress slowly years after recovery from acute paralytic poliomyelitis. While it presents with signs of chronic and new denervation, it is not infectious activity but caused by increasing dysfunction of surviving motor neurons.

Dalakas MC et al: A long-term follow-up of patients with post-poliomyelitis neuromuscular symptoms. N Engl J Med 1986;314:959.

Nikowane BM et al: Vaccine-associated paralytic poliomyelitis. JAMA 1987;257:1335.

ENCEPHALITIS

Essentials of Diagnosis

- Fever, malaise, stiff neck, sore throat, and nausea and vomiting, progressing to stupor, coma, and convulsions.
- Signs of an upper motor neuron lesion (exaggerated deep tendon reflexes, absent superficial reflexes, pathologic reflexes, spastic paralysis).
- Cerebrospinal fluid protein and pressure often increased, with lymphocytic pleocytosis.

General Considerations

A. Viral Encephalitis: While arboviruses (Table 25–2) are the principal causes, many other viruses may produce encephalitis. Herpes simplex produces "mass-like" lesions in the temporal lobes. Rabies virus invariably produces encephalitis; mumps virus, poliovirus, and other enteroviruses can cause aseptic meningitis or meningoencephalitis.

B. Encephalitis Accompanying Exanthematous Diseases of Childhood: This may occur in the course of measles, varicella, infectious mononucleosis, and rubella.

C. Encephalitis Following Vaccination: Encephalitis of the demyelinating type may follow use of certain immunizing agents. These include vaccines against smallpox, rabies, and pertussis.

D. Toxic Encephalitis: Toxic encephalitis due to drugs, poisons, or bacterial toxins (*Shigella dysenteriae* type 1) may be clinically indistinguishable from infectious encephalitis.

E. Reye's Syndrome: See p 966.

Clinical Findings

A. Symptoms and Signs: The symptoms are

Table 25–2. Arbovirus (arthropod-borne) encephalitis.[1]

Disease	Geographic Distribution	Vector; Reservoir	Comment
California encephalitis	Throughout USA	Mosquitoes; small mammals	Mainly in children
Eastern (equine) encephalitis	Eastern part of North, Central, and South America	Mosquitoes; birds, small rodents	Often occurs in horses in the area
St. Louis encephalitis	Western and central USA, Florida	Mosquitoes; birds (including domestic fowl)	
Venezuelan encephalitis	South America	Mosquitoes	Rare in USA
Western (equine) encephalitis	Throughout western hemisphere	Mosquitoes; birds	Often occurs in horses in the area; particularly affects young children

[1] Seasonal incidence varies with the mosquito season in different areas. It is mainly summer and fall (May through October).

fever, malaise, sore throat, nausea and vomiting, lethargy, stupor, coma, and convulsions. Signs include stiff neck, signs of meningeal irritation, tremors, convulsions, cranial nerve palsies, paralysis of extremities, exaggerated deep reflexes, absent superficial reflexes, and pathologic reflexes.

B. Laboratory Findings: The white blood cell count is variable. Cerebrospinal fluid pressure and protein content are often increased; glucose is normal; lymphocytic pleocytosis may be present (polymorphonuclears may predominate early in some forms). The virus may sometimes be isolated from blood or, rarely, from cerebrospinal fluid. Serologic tests of blood may be diagnostic in a few specific types of encephalitis. A CT scan of the brain may reveal the temporal lobe lesions indicative of herpesvirus but is more important in excluding mass lesions.

Differential Diagnosis

Mild forms of encephalitis must be differentiated from aseptic meningitis, lymphocytic choriomeningitis, and nonparalytic poliomyelitis; severe forms from cerebrovascular accidents, brain tumors, brain abscess, and poisoning.

Complications

Bronchial pneumonia, urinary retention and infection, and decubitus ulcers may occur. Late sequelae are mental deterioration, parkinsonism, and epilepsy.

Prevention

Effective measures include vigorous mosquito control and active immunization against childhood infectious diseases. Special inactivated virus vaccines have been prepared for high-risk persons.

Treatment

Although specific therapy for the majority of causative entities is not available, vigorous supportive measures can be helpful. Such measures include reduction of intracranial pressure (by the use of mannitol and glucocorticoids), the control of convulsions, maintenance of the airway, administration of oxygen, and attention to adequate nutrition during periods of prolonged coma.

Prevention or early treatment of decubiti, pneumonia, and urinary tract infections is important. Give anticonvulsants as needed.

Acyclovir is an effective drug in a dosage of 15 mg/kg/d intravenously for herpes simplex encephalitis if administered early in the disease before onset of coma. It has no effect on other viral encephalitides (see Chapter 31).

Prognosis

The prognosis should always be guarded, especially in younger children. Sequelae may become apparent late in the course of what appears to be a successful recovery.

Arvin AM et al: Management of the patient with herpes simplex encephalitis. Pediatr Infect Dis 1987;6:2.

LYMPHOCYTIC CHORIOMENINGITIS

Essentials of Diagnosis

- "Influenzalike" prodrome of fever, chills, malaise, and cough, followed by meningitis with associated stiff neck.
- Kernig's sign, headache, nausea, vomiting, and lethargy.
- Cerebrospinal fluid: slight increase of protein, lymphocytic pleocytosis (500–1000/μL).
- Complement-fixing antibodies within 2 weeks.

General Considerations

Lymphocytic choriomeningitis is a viral (arenavirus) infection of the central nervous system. The reservoir of infection is the infected house mouse, although naturally infected guinea pigs, monkeys, dogs, and swine have been observed. Pet hamsters may be a source of infection. The virus is shed by the infected animal via oronasal secretions, urine, and feces, with transmission to humans probably through contaminated food and dust. The incubation period is probably 8–13 days to the appearance of systemic manifestations and 15–21 days to the appearance of meningeal symptoms. The disease is not communicable from person to person. Complications are rare.

This disease is principally confined to the eastern seaboard and northeastern states of the USA.

Clinical Findings

A. Symptoms and Signs: The prodromal illness is characterized by fever, chills, headache, myalgia, cough, and vomiting; the meningeal phase by headache, nausea and vomiting, and lethargy. Signs of pneumonia are occasionally present during the prodromal phase. During the meningeal phase there may be neck and back stiffness and a positive Kernig sign (meningeal irritation). Severe meningoencephalitis may disturb deep tendon reflexes and may cause paralysis and anesthesia of the skin.

The prodrome may terminate in complete recovery, or meningeal symptoms may appear after a few days of remission.

B. Laboratory Findings: Leukocytosis may be present. Cerebrospinal fluid lymphocytic pleocytosis (total count is often 500–3000/μL) may occur, with slight increase in protein and normal glucose. Complement-fixing antibodies appear during or after the second week. The virus may be recovered from the blood and cerebrospinal fluid by mouse inoculation.

Differential Diagnosis

The influenzalike prodrome and latent period help distinguish this from other aseptic meningitides, meningismus, and bacterial and granulomatous meningitis. A history of exposure to mice is an important diagnostic clue.

Treatment

Treat as for encephalitis.

Prognosis

Fatality is rare. The illness usually lasts 1–2 weeks, although convalescence may be prolonged.

DENGUE
(Breakbone Fever, Dandy Fever)

Essentials of Diagnosis

- Sudden onset of high fever, chills, severe aching, headache, sore throat, prostration, and depression.
- Biphasic fever curve: initial phase, 3–4 days; remission, few hours to 2 days; second phase, 1–2 days.
- Rash: maculopapular, scarlatiniform, morbilliform, or petechial; on extremities to torso, occurring during remission or second phase.
- Leukopenia.

General Considerations

Dengue is a viral (group B arbovirus, togavirus) disease transmitted by the bite of the *Aedes* mosquito. It may be caused by one of several serotypes widely distributed between latitudes 25 °N and 25 °S (eg, Thailand, India, Philippines; Caribbean, including Puerto Rico and Cuba; Central America; Africa). It occurs only in the active mosquito season (warm weather). The incubation period is 3–15 days (usually 5–8 days).

Clinical Findings

A. Symptoms and Signs: Dengue begins with a sudden onset of high fever, chilliness, and severe aching (''breakbone'') of the head, back, and extremities, accompanied by sore throat, prostration, and depression. There may be conjunctival redness and flushing or blotching of the skin. The initial febrile phase lasts 3–4 days, typically but not inevitably followed by a remission of a few hours to 2 days. The skin eruption appears in 80% of cases during the remission or during the second febrile phase, which lasts 1–2 days and is accompanied by similar but usually milder symptoms than in the first phase. The rash may be scarlatiniform, morbilliform, maculopapular, or petechial. It appears first on the dorsum of the hands and feet and spreads to the arms, legs, trunk, and neck but rarely to the face. The rash lasts 2 hours to several days and may be followed by desquamation. Petechial rashes and gastrointestinal hemorrhages occur in a high proportion of cases (mosquito-borne hemorrhagic fever) in southeast Asia. These probably involve an immunologic reaction (immune complex disease).

Before the rash appears, it is difficult to distinguish dengue from malaria, yellow fever, or influenza. With the appearance of the eruption, which resembles rubella, the diagnosis is usually clear.

B. Laboratory Findings: Leukopenia is characteristic. Thrombocytopenia occurs in the hemorrhagic form of the disease. Virus may be recovered from the blood during the acute phase. Serologic diagnosis must consider the several viruses that can produce this clinical syndrome.

Complications

Depression, pneumonia, iritis, orchitis, and oophoritis are rare complications. Shock occurs in hemorrhagic dengue.

Prevention

Available prophylactic measures include control of mosquitoes by screening and insect repellents. An effective vaccine has been developed but has not been produced commercially.

Treatment

Treat shock by expanding circulating blood volume. Give salicylates as required for discomfort. Permit gradual restoration of activity during prolonged convalescence.

Prognosis

Fatalities are rare. Convalescence is slow.

Centers for Disease Control: Dengue and dengue hemorrhagic fever in the Americas, 1986. MMWR 1988; 37:129.

COLORADO TICK FEVER

Essentials of Diagnosis

- Fever, chills, myalgia, headache, prostration.
- Leukopenia.
- Second attack of fever after remission lasting 2–3 days.
- Onset 3–6 days following tick bite.

General Considerations

Colorado tick fever is an acute viral (orbivirus) infection transmitted by *Dermacentor andersoni* bites. The disease is limited to the western USA and is most prevalent during the tick season (March to August). The incubation period is 3–6 days.

Clinical Findings

A. Symptoms and Signs: The onset of fever (to 38.9–40.6 °C [102–105 °F]) is abrupt, sometimes with chills. Severe myalgia, headache, photophobia, anorexia, nausea and vomiting, and generalized weakness are prominent symptoms. Abnormal physical findings are limited to an occasional faint rash. Fever continues for 3 days, followed by a remission of 2–3 days and then by a full recrudescence lasting 3–4 days. In an occasional case there may be 2 or 3 bouts of fever.

Influenza, Rocky Mountain spotted fever, and other acute leukopenic fevers must be differentiated.

B. Laboratory Findings: Leukopenia (2000–3000/μL) with a shift to the left occurs. Viremia may be demonstrated by inoculation of blood into mice or by fluorescent antibody staining of the patient's red cells (with adsorbed virus). Complement-fixing antibodies appear during the third week after onset of the disease.

Complications

Aseptic meningitis or encephalitis occurs rarely. Asthenia may follow, but fatalities are very rare.

Treatment

No specific treatment is available. Aspirin or codeine may be given for pain.

Prognosis

The disease is self-limited and benign.

HEMORRHAGIC FEVERS

This is a diverse group of illnesses resulting from virus infections and perhaps immunologic responses to them. The common clinical features include high fever; hemorrhagic diathesis with petechiae or purpura; and bleeding from the nose, gastrointestinal tract, and genitourinary tract, with thrombocytopenia, leukopenia, and marked toxicity, often leading to shock and death. The viruses may be tick-borne (eg, Omsk hemorrhagic fever, Russia; Kyasanur Forest hemorrhagic fever, India), mosquito-borne (eg, Chikungunya hemorrhagic fever, yellow fever, dengue), or zoonotic (often derived from rodents, eg, Junin hemorrhagic fever, Argentina; Machupo hemorrhagic fever, Bolivia; Lassa hemorrhagic fever, West Africa). This last (zoonotic) group includes Marburg hemorrhagic fever (from contact with African vervet monkeys) and Ebola hemorrhagic fever in central Africa.

Persons who present with symptoms compatible with those of hemorrhagic fever and who have traveled from a possible endemic area should be strictly isolated for diagnosis and symptomatic treatment. Conclusive diagnosis may be made by growing the virus from blood obtained early in the disease or by showing a significant specific antibody titer rise. Isolation is particularly important, because some of these infections are highly transmissible to close contacts, including medical personnel, and carry a mortality rate of 50–70%.

For most of these entities, no specific treatment is available. Lassa fever can be effectively treated with intravenous ribavirin if started early (see Chapter 31). It is more important to differentiate hemorrhagic fever from such easily treated entities as meningococcemia and Rocky Mountain spotted fever.

Centers for Disease Control: Management of patients with suspected viral hemorrhagic fever. MMWR 1988;37:53.

RABIES

Essentials of Diagnosis

- Paresthesia, hydrophobia, rage alternating with calm.
- Convulsions, paralysis, thick tenacious saliva.
- History of animal bite.

General Considerations

Rabies is a viral (rhabdovirus) encephalitis transmitted by infected saliva that gains entry into the body by a bite or an open wound. Bats, skunks, foxes, and raccoons are widely infected. Dogs and cats are infected in some countries. Rodents are unlikely to have rabies. The virus gains entry into the salivary glands of dogs 5–7 days before their death from rabies, thus limiting their period of infectivity. The incubation period may range from 10 days to 2 years but is usually 3–7 weeks. The virus travels in the nerves to the brain, multiplies there, and then migrates along the efferent nerves to the salivary glands.

Rabies is almost uniformly fatal. The most common clinical problem confronting the physician is the management of a patient bitten by an animal (see Prevention).

Clinical Findings

A. Symptoms and Signs: There is usually a history of animal bite. Pain appears at the site of the bite, followed by tingling. The skin is quite sensitive to changes of temperature, especially air currents. Attempts at drinking cause extremely painful laryngeal spasm, so that the patient refuses to drink (hydrophobia). The patient is restless and behaves in a peculiar manner. Muscle spasm, laryngospasm, and extreme excitability are present. Convulsions occur, and blowing on the back of the patient's neck will often precipitate a convulsion. Large amounts of thick tenacious saliva are present.

B. Laboratory Findings: Biting animals who are apparently well should be kept under observation. Sick or dead animals should be examined for rabies. The diagnosis of rabies in the brain of a rabid animal may be made rapidly by the fluorescent antibody technique.

Prevention

Since the disease is almost always fatal, prevention is the only available approach. Immunization of household dogs and cats and active immunization of persons with an unusual degree of exposure (eg, veterinarians) are important. However, the most important common decisions concern handling animal bites.

A. Local Treatment of Animal Bites and Scratches: Thorough and repeated flushing and cleansing of wounds with soap and water are important. If rabies immune globulin or antiserum is to be used, a portion should be infiltrated locally around the wound (see below). Wounds caused by animal bites should not be sutured.

B. The Biting Animal: A dog or cat should be captured, confined, and observed by a veterinarian for 7–10 days. A wild animal, if captured, should be sacrificed and the head shipped on ice to the nearest laboratory qualified to examine the brain for rabies. When the animal cannot be examined, skunks, bats, coyotes, foxes, and raccoons should be presumed to be rabid. The rabies potential of bites by other animals must be evaluated individually.

C. Postexposure Immunization: The physician must reach a decision based on the recommendations of the USPHS Advisory Committee but should also be influenced by the circumstances of the bite, the extent and location of the wound, the presence of rabies in the region, the type of animal responsible for the bite, etc. (Consultation is provided by state health departments.) Treatment includes both passive antibody and vaccine. The optimal form of passive immunization is human rabies immune globulin (20 IU/kg). Up to 50% of the globulin should be used to infiltrate the wound; the rest is administered intramuscularly. If the human gamma globulin is not available, equine rabies antiserum (40 IU/kg) can be used after appropriate tests for horse serum sensitivity. As of 1989 in the USA, the inactivated human diploid cell rabies vaccine is licensed. It is given as 5 injections intramuscularly on days 0, 3, 7, 14, and 28 after exposure. The vaccine effectively produces a regular antibody response. Allergic reactions are rare. The vaccine is commercially available or can be obtained through state health departments.

In other countries, inactivated duck embryo vaccine or mouse brain vaccine may be available, but the method of administration is much more complex, the rate of allergic reactions is higher—particularly ascending paralysis—and the efficacy is less.

Preexposure prophylaxis with 3 injections of diploid cell vaccine is recommended for persons at high risk of exposure (veterinarians, animal handlers, etc). Simultaneous chloroquine prophylaxis for malaria may diminish the antibody response.

Treatment

This very severe illness with an almost universally fatal outcome requires skillful intensive care with attention to the airway, maintenance of oxygenation, and control of seizures.

Prognosis

Once the symptoms have appeared, death almost inevitably occurs after 2–3 days as a result of cardiac or respiratory failure or generalized paralysis.

Centers for Disease Control: Rabies surveillance, United States, 1987. MMWR 1988;37:554.

Warrell DA, Warrell MJ: Human rabies and its prevention: An overview. Rev Infect Dis 1988;10(Suppl 4):S726.

YELLOW FEVER

Essentials of Diagnosis

- Sudden onset of severe headache, aching in legs, and tachycardia. Later, bradycardia, hypotension, jaundice, hemorrhagic tendency (''coffee-ground'' vomitus).
- Proteinuria, leukopenia, bilirubinemia, bilirubinuria.
- Endemic area.

General Considerations

Yellow fever is a viral (group B arbovirus, togavirus) infection transmitted by the *Aedes* and jungle mosquitoes. It is endemic to Africa and South America (tropical or subtropical), but epidemics have extended far into the temperate zone during warm seasons. The mosquito transmits the infection by first biting an individual having the disease and then biting a susceptible individual after the virus has multiplied within the mosquito's body. The incubation period in humans is 3–6 days.

Clinical Findings

A. Symptoms and Signs:

1. Mild form–Symptoms are malaise, headache, fever, retro-orbital pain, nausea, vomiting, and photophobia. Bradycardia may be present.

2. Severe form–Symptoms are the same as in the mild form, with sudden onset and then severe pains throughout the body, extreme prostration, bleeding into the skin and from the mucous membranes (''coffee-ground'' vomitus), oliguria, and jaundice. Signs include tachycardia, erythematous face, and conjunctival redness during the congestive phase, followed by a period of calm (on about the third day) with a normal temperature and then a return of fever, bradycardia, hypotension, jaundice, hemorrhages (gastrointestinal tract, bladder, nose, mouth, subcutaneous), and later delirium. The short course and mildness of the icterus distinguish yellow fever from leptospirosis. The mild form is difficult to distinguish from infectious hepatitis.

B. Laboratory Findings: Leukopenia occurs, although it may not be present at the onset. Proteinuria is present, sometimes as high as 5–6 g/L, and disappears completely with recovery. With jaundice there are bilirubinuria and bilirubinemia. The virus may be isolated from the blood by intracerebral mouse inoculation (first 3 days). Antibodies appear during and after the second week.

Differential Diagnosis

It may be difficult to distinguish yellow fever from leptospirosis and other forms of jaundice on clinical evidence alone.

Prevention

Transmission is prevented through mosquito control. Live virus vaccine is highly effective and should be provided for persons living in or traveling to endemic areas. (See Chapter 23.)

Treatment

Treatment consists of giving a liquid diet, limiting food to high-carbohydrate, high-protein liquids as tolerated; intravenous glucose and saline as required; analgesics and sedatives as required; and saline enemas for obstipation.

Prognosis

The mortality rate is high in the severe form, with death occurring most commonly between the sixth and the ninth days. In survivors, the temperature returns to normal by the seventh or eighth day. The prognosis in any individual case should be guarded at the onset, since sudden changes for the worse are common. Hiccup, copious black vomitus, melena, and anuria are unfavorable signs.

Monath TP: Yellow fever: A medically neglected disease. Rev Infect Dis 1987;9:165.

MISCELLANEOUS RESPIRATORY INFECTIONS

Infections of the respiratory tract are perhaps the most common human ailments. While they are a source of discomfort, disability, and loss of time for most average adults, they are a substantial cause of morbidity and serious illness in young children and in the elderly. Specific associations of certain groups of viruses with certain disease syndromes have been established. Many of these viral infections run their natural course in older children and in adults without specific treatment and without great risk of bacterial complications. In young infants and in the elderly, or in persons with impaired respiratory tract reserves, bacterial superinfection increases morbidity and mortality rates.

The Common Cold

See Chapter 6.

Croup
(Laryngotracheobronchitis)

This is most commonly a parainfluenza virus infection of small children, with anatomic localization in the subglottal area. It produces hoarseness, a "seal bark" cough, and signs of upper airway obstruction with inspiratory stridor, xiphoid and suprasternal retraction, but no pain on swallowing. It must be differentiated from epiglottitis due to *H influenzae*. Treatment includes hydration, steam inhalation (hot or cold), and alertness to the possibility of complete airway obstruction. Should that emergency occur, intubation or tracheostomy is lifesaving.

Epiglottitis

This is a medical emergency requiring urgent attention to the airway. It occurs most commonly in children 1–6 years old, who develop a swollen, "cherry-red" epiglottis and airway obstruction with fever, pain on swallowing, and a "croupy" cough. Lateral neck x-ray can help to demonstrate swelling of the epiglottis. Direct laryngoscopy may precipitate obstruction and must therefore be performed only in a setting where immediate intubation can be done expertly. Epiglottitis sometimes occurs in adults with pale erythematous swelling of the supraglottic region. In adults, laryngoscopy is less likely to precipitate an airway crisis, and for that reason immediate intubation is not critical.

Treatment consists of airway maintenance, antimicrobials (either ampicillin plus chloramphenicol, or cefuroxime) and close observation.

Bronchiolitis

This viral infection is caused most often by respiratory syncytial virus in children under 2 years of age. It results in a "ball valve" obstruction to expiration at the level of the bronchiole, resembling bronchial asthma in pathophysiology. Clinical signs include low-grade fever, severe tachypnea (up to 100 respirations per minute), an expiratory wheeze, overinflation of lungs, depressed diaphragm, decreased air exchange, and greatly increased work of breathing. Foreign body aspiration and bronchial asthma may have to be considered in differential diagnosis.

Treatment consists of hydration, humidification of inspired air, and—with rising blood P_{CO_2}—the possible need for ventilatory support. In infants, the clinical course of respiratory syncytial viral infections can be favorably modified by use of aerosolized ribavirin.

INFLUENZA

Essentials of Diagnosis

- Abrupt onset with fever, chills, malaise, cough, coryza, and muscle aches.
- Aching, fever, and prostration out of proportion to catarrhal symptoms.
- Leukopenia.
- Cases usually in epidemic pattern, not sporadic.

General Considerations

Influenza (orthomyxovirus) is transmitted by the respiratory route. Although sporadic cases occur, epidemics and pandemics appear at varying intervals, usually in the fall or winter. Antigenic types A and B produce clinically indistinguishable infections, whereas type C is usually a minor illness. The incubation period is 1–4 days.

It is difficult to diagnose influenza in the absence of a classic epidemic. The disease resembles many other mild febrile illnesses but is always accompanied by a cough.

Clinical Findings

A. Symptoms and Signs: The onset is usually abrupt, with fever, chills, malaise, muscular aching, substernal soreness, headache, nasal stuffiness, and occasionally nausea. Fever lasts 1–7 days (usually 3–5). Coryza, nonproductive cough, and sore throat are present. Signs include mild pharyngeal injection, flushed face, and conjunctival redness.

B. Laboratory Findings: Leukopenia is common. Proteinuria may be present. The virus may be isolated from the throat washings by inoculation of embryonated eggs or cell cultures. Complement-fixing and hemagglutination-inhibiting antibodies appear during the second week.

Complications

Influenza causes necrosis of the respiratory epithelium, which predisposes to secondary bacterial infections. Frequent complications are acute sinusitis, otitis media, purulent bronchitis, and pneumonia.

Pneumonia is commonly due to bacterial infection with pneumococci or staphylococci and rarely to the influenza virus itself. The circulatory system is not usually involved, but pericarditis, myocarditis, and thrombophlebitis sometimes occur.

Reye's syndrome is a rare and severe complication of influenza and other viral diseases (eg, varicella, coxsackievirus, echovirus), particularly in young children. It consists of rapid development of hepatic failure and encephalopathy, and there is a 30% fatality rate. The pathogenesis is unknown; aspirin may be a risk factor. Hypoglycemia, elevation of serum transaminases and blood ammonia, prolonged prothrombin time, and change in mental status all occur within 2–3 weeks after onset of the virus infection. Histologically, the periphery of liver lobules shows striking fatty infiltration and glycogen depletion. Treatment is supportive and directed to the management of cerebral edema.

Prevention

Polyvalent influenza virus vaccine given twice (1–2 weeks apart) exerts moderate temporary protection. Partial immunity lasts a few months to 1 year. Partial immunity lasts a few months to 1 year. Antigenic configuration of the vaccine changes yearly. Vaccination is recommended every year for persons with chronic respiratory insufficiency, cardiac disease, or other debilitating illness. Effective chemoprophylaxis

for epidemiologically or virologically confirmed influenza A consists of amantadine hydrochloride, 200 mg/d orally. This markedly reduces the incidence of infection in individuals exposed to influenza A if begun immediately and continued for 10 days.

Treatment

Many patients with influenza prefer to rest in bed. Analgesics and a sedative cough mixture may be used. Antibiotics should be reserved for treatment of bacterial complications. If antipyretics are needed, acetaminophen rather than aspirin should be used, especially in children. Ribavirin by aerosol has helped severely ill patients with influenza A or B.

Prognosis

The duration of the uncomplicated illness is 1–7 days, and the prognosis is excellent. Purulent bronchitis and bronchiectasis may result in chronic pulmonary disease and fibrosis that persist throughout life. Most fatalities are due to bacterial pneumonia. Pneumococcal pneumonia is most common, but staphylococcal pneumonia is most serious. In recent epidemics, the mortality rate has been low except in debilitated persons—especially those with severe heart disease.

If the fever persists for more than 4 days, if the cough becomes productive, or if the white blood cell count rises to about 12,000/μL, secondary bacterial infection should be ruled out or verified and treated.

INFECTIOUS MONONUCLEOSIS (EB Virus Infection)

Essentials of Diagnosis

- Fever, sore throat, malaise, lymphadenopathy.
- Frequently splenomegaly, occasionally maculopapular rash.
- Positive heterophil agglutination test (Monospot).
- "Atypical" large lymphocytes in blood smear; lymphocytosis.
- Hepatitis frequent, and occasionally myocarditis, neuritis, encephalitis.

General Considerations

Infectious mononucleosis is an acute infectious disease due to the Epstein-Barr (EB) herpesvirus (human herpesvirus 4). It is universal in distribution and may occur at any age but usually occurs between the ages of 10 and 35, either in an epidemic form or as sporadic cases. Its mode of transmission is probably by saliva. The incubation period is probably 5–15 days.

Clinical Findings

A. Symptoms and Signs: Symptoms are varied but typically include fever; discrete, nonsuppurative, slightly painful, enlarged lymph nodes, especially those of the posterior cervical chain; and, in approximately half of cases, splenomegaly. Sore throat is often present, and toxic symptoms (malaise, anorexia, and myalgia) occur frequently in the early phase of the illness. A maculopapular or occasionally petechial rash occurs in less than 50% of cases. Exudative pharyngitis, tonsillitis, or gingivitis may occur.

Common manifestations of infectious mononucleosis are hepatitis with hepatomegaly, nausea, anorexia, and jaundice; central nervous system involvement with headache, neck stiffness, photophobia, pains of neuritis, and occasionally even Guillain-Barré syndrome; pulmonary involvement with chest pain, dyspnea, and cough; and myocardial involvement with tachycardia and arrhythmias.

The varying symptoms of infectious mononucleosis—especially sore throat, hepatitis, rash, and lymphadenopathy—raise difficult problems in differential diagnosis.

B. Laboratory Findings: Initially, there is a granulocytopenia followed within 1 week by a lymphocytic leukocytosis. Many lymphocytes are atypical, ie, are larger than normal adult lymphocytes, stain more darkly, and frequently show vacuolated, foamy cytoplasm and dark chromatin in the nucleus. Hemolytic anemia secondary to anti-i antibodies is occasionally encountered, as is thrombocytopenia (at times severe).

The mononucleosis spot test and the heterophil (sheep cell agglutination) test usually become positive in infectious mononucleosis before the fourth week after onset of the illness. Titer rises in antibodies directed at several EB virus antigens can be detected by immunofluorescence. During acute illness, there is always a rise in antibody to EB virus capsid antigen (VCA). A false-positive VDRL or RPR test occurs in 10% of cases.

In central nervous system involvement, the cerebrospinal fluid may show increase of pressure, abnormal lymphocytes, and protein.

With myocardial involvement, the electrocardiographic studies may show abnormal T waves and prolonged PR intervals.

Liver function tests are commonly abnormal.

Differential Diagnosis

Causes of pharyngitis with exudate include diphtheria and adenovirus, herpes simplex, gonococcal, and streptococcal infections. Cytomegalovirus infection may be indistinguishable from infectious mononucleosis due to EB virus, but the heterophil antibody and Monospot tests are negative. The same applies to toxoplasmosis and rubella.

Complications

These usually consist of secondary throat infections, often streptococcal, and (rarely) rupture of the spleen or hypersplenism. Very rarely, there may be a variety of neurologic involvements, eg, myelitis.

EB virus infections rarely may result in the production of B cell lymphomas. A special case, Burkitt's lymphoma of the jaw in African children, regularly shows the presence of EB viral antigens. The etiologic role of EB virus in this neoplasm is not established. While Burkitt's lymphoma in Africa responds to radiation therapy or anticancer chemotherapy, the effect of antiviral drugs is unknown. The rare cases of Burkitt's lymphoma in the USA are much more invasive, respond poorly to therapy, and are not regularly associated with EB virus. EB virus has also been associated with nasopharyngeal carcinoma in some populations, but again, the role of the virus is unclear.

There is no credible evidence that chronic fatigue syndrome is caused by chronic EBV infection. This disorder is discussed in Chapter 1.

Treatment

A. General Measures: No specific treatment is available. The patient requires support and reassurance because of the frequent feeling of lassitude and the duration of symptoms. Symptomatic relief can be afforded by the administration of aspirin, and hot saline or 30% glucose throat irrigations or gargles 3 or 4 times daily. In severely ill patients, when an enlargement of lymphoid tissues is so marked as to threaten to obstruct the airway, a 5-day course of corticosteroids (eg, prednisolone, 50 mg/d for 3 days, then less) may be beneficial if the diagnosis is well-established.

B. Treatment of Complications: Hepatitis, myocarditis, and encephalitis are treated symptomatically. Rupture of the spleen requires emergency splenectomy. In order to avoid this complication, it is best to avoid frequent deep palpation of the spleen or vigorous activity.

Prognosis

In uncomplicated cases, fever disappears in 10 days and lymphadenopathy and splenomegaly in 4 weeks. The debility sometimes lingers for 2–3 months.

Death is uncommon; when it does occur it is usually due to splenic rupture or hypersplenic phenomena (severe hemolytic anemia, thrombocytopenic purpura) or to encephalitis.

COXSACKIEVIRUS INFECTIONS

Coxsackievirus infections cause several clinical syndromes. As with other enteroviruses, infections are most common during the summer. Two groups, A and B, are defined by their differing behavior after injection into suckling mice. There are more than 50 serotypes.

Clinical Findings

A. Symptoms and Signs: The clinical syndromes associated with coxsackievirus infection may be described briefly as follows:

1. Summer grippe (coxsackie A and B)–A febrile illness, principally of children, which lasts 1–4 days; minor symptoms and respiratory tract infection are often present.

2. Herpangina (coxsackie A2, 4, 5, 6, 7, 10)– Sudden onset of fever, which may be as high as 40.6 °C (105 °F), sometimes with febrile convulsions; headache, myalgia, vomiting; and sore throat, characterized early by petechiae or papules on the soft palate that become shallow ulcers in about 3 days and then heal.

3. Epidemic pleurodynia (coxsackie B1, 2, 3, 4, 5)–Sudden onset of recurrent pain in the area of diaphragmatic attachment (lower chest or upper abdomen); fever is often present during attacks of pain; headache, sore throat, malaise, nausea; tenderness, hyperesthesia, and muscle swelling of the involved area; orchitis, pleurisy, and aseptic meningitis may occur. Relapse may occur after recovery.

4. Aseptic meningitis (coxsackie A2, 4, 7, 9, 10, 16; B viruses)–Fever, headache, nausea, vomiting, stiff neck, drowsiness, cerebrospinal fluid lymphocytosis without chemical abnormalities; rarely, muscle paralysis. See also Viral Meningitis.

5. Acute nonspecific pericarditis (coxsackie B types)–Sudden onset of anterior chest pain, often worse with inspiration and in the supine position; fever, myalgia, headache; pericardial friction rub appears early; pericardial effusion with paradoxic pulse, increased venous pressure, and increase in heart size may appear; electrocardiographic and x-ray evidence of pericarditis is often present. One or more relapses may occur.

6. Myocarditis (coxsackie B3, 4, and others)– Heart failure in the neonatal period may be the result of myocarditis associated with infection acquired in utero. Adult heart disease may be caused by coxsackievirus group B.

7. Hand, foot, and mouth disease–Coxsackievirus type A16 and several other types produce an illness characterized by stomatitis and a vesicular rash on the hands and feet. This may take an epidemic form.

B. Laboratory Findings: Routine laboratory studies show no characteristic abnormalities. Neutralizing antibodies appear during convalescence. The virus may be isolated from throat washings or stools inoculated into suckling mice.

Treatment & Prognosis

Treatment is symptomatic. With the exception of myocarditis, all of the syndromes caused by coxsackieviruses are benign and self-limited.

Melnick JL: Enteroviruses: Polioviruses, coxsackieviruses, echoviruses, and newer enteroviruses. Pages 739–794 in: *Virology*. Fields BN et al (editors). Raven Press, 1985.

ECHOVIRUS INFECTIONS

Echoviruses are enteroviruses that produce several clinical syndromes, particularly in children. Infection is most common during the summer.

Over 20 serotypes have been demonstrated. Types 4, 6, and 9 cause aseptic meningitis, which may be associated with rubelliform rash. Types 9 and 16 cause an exanthematous illness (Boston exanthem) characterized by a sudden onset of fever, nausea, and sore throat, and a rubelliform rash over the face and trunk that persists 1–10 days. Orchitis may occur. Type 18 causes epidemic diarrhea, characterized by a sudden onset of fever and diarrhea in infants. Types 18 and 20 cause common respiratory disease (see Chapter 6). Myocarditis has also been reported.

As is true of the other enterovirus infections also, the diagnosis is best established by correlation of the clinical, epidemiologic, and laboratory evidence. The virus produces cytopathic effects in tissue culture and can be recovered from the feces, throat washings, blood, and cerebrospinal fluid. A 4-fold rise in antibody titer signifies systemic infection.

Treatment is purely symptomatic. The prognosis is excellent, although occasional mild paralysis has been reported following central nervous system infection.

ADENOVIRUS INFECTIONS

Adenoviruses (there are more than 30 antigenic types) produce a variety of clinical syndromes. These infections are self-limited and most common among military recruits, although sporadic cases occur in civilian populations. The incubation period is 4–9 days.

There are 5 clinical types of adenovirus infection:

(1) The common cold: Many infections produce rhinitis, pharyngitis, and mild malaise without fever and are indistinguishable from other infections that produce the common cold syndrome.

(2) Acute undifferentiated respiratory disease, nonstreptococcal exudative pharyngitis: Fever lasts 2–12 days and is accompanied by malaise and myalgia. Sore throat is often manifested by diffuse injection, a patchy exudate, and cervical lymphadenopathy. Cough is sometimes accompanied by rales and x-ray evidence of pneumonitis (primary atypical pneumonia). Conjunctivitis is often present.

(3) Pharyngoconjunctival fever: Fever and malaise, conjunctivitis (often unilateral), and mild pharyngitis.

(4) Epidemic keratoconjunctivitis: In adults, an iatrogenic infection with unilateral conjunctival redness, pain, tearing, and an enlarged preauricular lymph node. Keratitis leads to subepithelial opacities (especially with types 8, 19, or 37).

(5) Acute hemorrhagic cystitis in children: (Often associated with type 11.)

Vaccines are not available for general use. Live oral vaccines containing attenuated type 4 and type 7 have been used in military personnel.

Treatment is symptomatic.

INFECTIONS WITH SLOW VIRUSES

Several animal diseases (scrapie, visna) are caused by viruses that are definitely communicable but replicate in the host very slowly—for months without producing symptoms. Eventually, they produce progressive disease and death. At least 4 human degenerative diseases are believed to be caused by similar "slow" viruses.

Kuru and **Creutzfeldt-Jakob disease** are spongiform encephalopathies. The virus can be transmitted by brain or eye tissue, and perhaps by other forms of contact, to humans, chimpanzees, and monkeys. After many weeks or months, the diseases pursue an inexorable downhill course and end in death. Kuru is characterized by cerebellar ataxia, tremors, dysarthria, and emotional lability; Creutzfeldt-Jakob disease by progressive dementia, myoclonic fasciculations, ataxia, and somnolence. Little is known about the characteristics of the causative viruses. There is no specific treatment, and prevention is limited to avoidance of specific risks (contamination by affected brain tissue, transplant of cornea from patient).

Subacute sclerosing panencephalitis (SSPE) is a slowly progressive demyelinating disorder of the central nervous system, ending in death. Altered measles viruses have been grown from brain tissue, and the cerebrospinal fluid antibody to measles is high.

Progressive multifocal leukoencephalopathy (PML) is an extremely rare progressive demyelinating neurologic disease that occurs particularly in persons immunosuppressed by drugs or disease (eg, HIV infection). Certain papovaviruses (eg, JC virus) have been grown from brain tissue of patients with PML, but no etiologic relationship can be assumed.

It is possible that other degenerative central nervous system diseases in humans (eg, multiple sclerosis) may be caused by "slow" viruses.

Brown P et al: Diagnosis of Creutzfeld-Jakob disease by Western blot identification of marker protein in human brain tissue. N Engl J Med 1986;314:547.

RICKETTSIAL DISEASES (Rickettsioses)

The rickettsioses are a group of febrile diseases caused by infection with rickettsiae. Rickettsiae are small obligate intracellular bacteria that are parasites of arthropods. In arthropods, rickettsiae grow in the cells lining the gut, often without harming the host. Human infection results either from the bite of the specific arthropod or from contamination with its feces. In humans, rickettsiae grow principally in endothelial cells of small blood vessels, producing vasculitis, necrosis of cells, thrombosis of vessels, skin rashes, and organ dysfunctions.

Different rickettsiae and their vectors are endemic in different parts of the world, but 2 or more types may coexist in the same geographic area. A summary of epidemiologic features is given in Table 25–3. The clinical picture is variable but usually includes a prodromal stage followed by fever, rash, and prostration. Isolation of rickettsiae from the patient is cumbersome and difficult and can be undertaken only by specialized laboratories. Laboratory diagnosis relies on the development of nonspecific antibodies to certain *Proteus* strains (Weil-Felix reaction) and of specific antibodies detected by complement fixation or immunofluorescence tests.

Prevention & Treatment

Preventive measures are directed at control of the vector, specific immunization when available, and (occasionally) drug chemoprophylaxis. All rickettsiae can be inhibited by tetracyclines or chloramphenicol. All early clinical infections respond in some degree to treatment with these drugs. Treatment usually consists of giving either tetracycline hydrochloride or chloramphenicol, 0.5 g orally every 4–6 hours for 4–10 days (50 mg/kg/d). In seriously ill patients, initial treatment may consist of 1 g of tetracycline or chloramphenicol intravenously. Supportive measures may include parenteral fluids, sedation, oxygen, and skin care. The vector (louse, tick, mite) must be removed from patients.

EPIDEMIC LOUSE-BORNE TYPHUS

Essentials of Diagnosis

- Prodrome of headache, then chills and fever.
- Severe, intractable headaches, prostration, persisting high fever.
- Maculopapular rash appears on the fourth to seventh days on the trunk and in the axillas, spreading to the rest of the body but sparing the face, palms, and soles.
- Laboratory confirmation by *Proteus* OX19 agglutination and specific serologic tests.

General Considerations

Epidemic louse-borne typhus is due to infection with *Rickettsia prowazekii*, a parasite of the body louse that ultimately kills the louse. Transmission is favored by crowded living conditions, famine, war, or any circumstances that predispose to heavy infesta-

Table 25–3. Rickettsial diseases.[1]

Disease	Rickettsia	Geographic Area of Prevalence	Insect Vector	Mammalian Reservoir	Weil-Felix Agglutination		
					OX19	OX2	OXK
Typhus group							
Epidemic typhus	Rickettsia prowazekii	South America, Africa, Asia, North America (?)[2]	Louse	Humans	++	±	−
Murine typhus	Rickettsia typhi	Worldwide; small foci	Flea	Rodents	++	−	−
Scrub typhus	Rickettsia tsutsugamushi	Southeast Asia, Japan	Mite[3]	Rodents	−	−	++
Spotted fever group							
Rocky Mountain spotted fever (RMSF)	Rickettsia rickettsii	Western Hemisphere	Tick[3]	Rodents, dogs	+	+	−
Fièvre boutonneuse Kenya tick typhus South African tick fever Indian tick typhus	Rickettsia conorii	Africa, India, Mediterranean countries	Tick[3]	Rodents, dogs	+	+	−
Queensland tick typhus	Rickettsia australis	Australia	Tick[3]	Rodents, marsupials	+	+	−
North Asian tick typhus	Rickettsia sibirica	Siberia, Mongolia	Tick[3]	Rodents	+	+	−
Rickettsialpox	Rickettsia akari	USA, Korea, USSR	Mite[3]	Mice	−	−	−
RMSF-like	Rickettsia canada	North America	Tick[3]	Rodents	?	?	−
Other							
Q fever	Coxiella burnetii	Worldwide	None[4]	Cattle, sheep, goats	−	−	−
Trench fever	Rochalimaea quintana	Rare	Louse	Humans	?	?	?

[1] Reproduced, with permission, from Jawetz E et al: *Review of Medical Microbiology*, 18th ed. Appleton & Lange, 1989.
[2] Contact with flying squirrels or their ectoparasites.
[3] Also serve as arthropod reservoir by maintaining rickettsiae through transovarian transmission.
[4] Human infection results from inhalation of dust.

tion with lice. When the louse sucks the blood of a person infected with *R prowazekii*, the organism becomes established in the gut of the louse and grows there. When the louse is transmitted to another person (through contact or clothing) and has a blood meal, it defecates simultaneously, and the infected feces are rubbed into the itching bite wound. Dry, infectious louse feces may also enter the respiratory tract and result in human infection. A deloused and bathed typhus patient is no longer infectious for other humans.

In a person who recovers from clinical or subclinical typhus infection, *R prowazekii* may survive in lymphoid tissues. Years later, there may be a recrudescence of disease (Brill's disease) without exposure to infected lice.

Recently, mild and atypical cases of *R prowazekii* have rarely occurred in the USA after contact with flying squirrels or their ectoparasites.

Clinical Findings

A. Symptoms and Signs: (Table 25–1.) Prodromal malaise, cough, headache, and chest pain begin after an incubation period of 10–14 days. There is then an abrupt onset of chills, high fever, and prostration, with "influenzal symptoms" progressing to de-

lirium and stupor. The headache is intractably severe, and the fever is unremitting for many days.

Other findings consist of conjunctivitis, flushed face, rales at the lung bases, and often splenomegaly. A macular rash (that soon becomes papular) appears first in the axillas and then over the trunk, spreading to the extremities but rarely involving the face, palms, or soles. In severely ill patients, the rash becomes hemorrhagic, and hypotension becomes marked. There may be renal insufficiency, stupor, and delirium. In spontaneous recovery, improvement begins 13–16 days after onset with rapid drop of fever.

B. Laboratory Findings: The white blood cell count is variable. Proteinuria and hematuria commonly occur. Serum obtained 5–12 days after onset of symptoms usually shows agglutinating antibodies for *Proteus* OX19 (rarely also OX2)—*R prowazekii* shares antigens with these *Proteus* strains—and specific antibodies for *R prowazekii* antigens demonstrated by complement fixation, microagglutination, or immunofluorescence. In primary rickettsial infection, early antibodies are IgM; in recrudescence (Brill's disease), early antibodies are predominantly IgG, and the Weil-Felix test is negative.

C. Imaging: Radiographs of the chest may show patchy consolidation.

Differential Diagnosis

The prodromal symptoms and the early febrile stage are not specific enough to permit diagnosis in nonepidemic situations. The rash is usually sufficiently distinctive for diagnosis, but it may be missing in 5–10% of cases and may be difficult to observe in dark-skinned persons. A variety of other acute febrile diseases may have to be considered.

Brill's disease (recrudescent epidemic typhus) has a more gradual onset than primary *R prowazekii* infection, fever and rash are of shorter duration, and the disease is milder and rarely fatal.

Complications

Pneumonia, vasculitis with major vessel obstruction and gangrene, circulatory collapse, myocarditis, and uremia may occur.

Prevention

Prevention consists of louse control with insecticides, particularly by applying chemicals to clothing or treating it with heat, and frequent bathing. Immunization with vaccines consisting of inactivated egg-grown *R prowazekii* gives some protection This vaccine was not available in the USA or Canada in 1989. An improved cell culture vaccine is being developed.

Treatment

See p 969.

Prognosis

The prognosis depends greatly upon age and immunization status. In children under age 10, the disease is usually mild. The mortality rate is 10% in the second and third decades but may reach 60% in the sixth decade. Effective vaccination can convert a potentially serious disease into a mild one.

Duma RJ et al: Epidemic typhus in the United States associated with flying squirrels. JAMA 1981;245:2318.

ENDEMIC FLEA-BORNE TYPHUS (Murine Typhus)

Rickettsia typhi (R mooseri) is transmitted from rat to rat through the rat flea (rarely, the rat louse). Humans acquire the infection (eg, in Central America, Texas) when bitten by an infected flea, which releases infected feces while sucking blood.

Flea typhus resembles recrudescent epidemic typhus in that it has a gradual onset and the fever and rash are of shorter duration (6–13 days) and the symptoms less severe than in louse-borne typhus. The rash is maculopapular and concentrated on the trunk and fades fairly rapidly. Pneumonia or gangrene is rare. Fatalities are rare and limited to the elderly.

Complement-fixing or immunofluorescent antibodies can be detected in the patient's serum with specific *R typhi* antigens. There is a rising titer of agglutinating antibodies to *Proteus* OX19.

Preventive measures are directed at control of rats and their ectoparasites. Insecticides are first applied to rat runs, nests, and colonies, and the rats are then poisoned or trapped. Finally, buildings must be made ratproof. Antibiotic treatment need not be intensive because of the mildness of the natural disease. An experimental vaccine was fairly effective, but it is not commercially available now.

Taylor JP, Betz TG, Rawlings JA: Epidemiology of murine typhus in Texas: 1980 through 1984. JAMA 1986; 255:2173.

SPOTTED FEVERS (Tick Typhus)

Tick-borne rickettsial infections occur in many different regions of the world and have been given regional or local names, eg, Rocky Mountain spotted fever in North America, Queensland tick typhus in Australia, boutonneuse fever in North Africa, Kenya tick typhus, etc. The causative agents are all antigenically related to *Rickettsia rickettsii*, and all are transmitted by hard (ixodid) ticks and have cycles in nature that involve dogs, rodents, or other animals. There is some similarity in the epidemiology and clinical presentation of spotted fevers and Lyme disease (see Chapter 27). Rickettsiae are often transmitted from one generation of ticks to the next (transovarian transmission) without passage through a vertebrate host. Patients infected with spotted fevers usually develop antibodies to *Proteus* OX19 and OX2 in low titer, in addition to specific rickettsial antibodies, detected best by immunofluorescence, microagglutination, or complement fixation.

Control of spotted fevers involves prevention of tick bites, specific immunization when available, and antibiotic treatment of patients.

1. ROCKY MOUNTAIN SPOTTED FEVER

Essentials of Diagnosis

- Exposure to tick bite in endemic area.
- "Influenzal" prodrome followed by chills, fever, severe headache, widespread aches and pains, restlessness, and prostration; occasionally, delirium and coma.
- Red macular rash appears between the second and sixth days of fever, first on the wrists and ankles and then spreading centrally; it may become petechial.
- Laboratory confirmation by agglutination of *Proteus* OX19 and OX2 and by specific antibodies with complement fixation and immunofluorescence.

General Considerations

The causative agent, *R rickettsii*, is transmitted to humans by the bite of the wood tick, *Dermacentor andersoni*, in the western USA and by the bite of the dog tick, *Dermacentor variabilis*, in the eastern USA. Other hard ticks transmit the organism in the southern USA and in Central and South America and are responsible for transmitting it among rodents, dogs, porcupines, and other animals. Most human cases occur in late spring and summer. In the USA, most cases occur in the eastern third of the country, with nearly 1000 reported per year.

Clinical Findings

A. Symptoms and Signs: Three to 10 days after the bite of an infectious tick, anorexia, malaise, nausea, headache, and sore throat occur. These progress, with chills, fever, myalgia, aches in bones, joints, and muscles, abdominal pain, nausea and vomiting, restlessness, insomnia, and irritability. Cough and pneumonitis may develop. Delirium, lethargy, stupor, and coma may appear. The face is flushed and the conjunctivas infected. Between days 2 and 6 of fever, a rash appears first on the wrists and ankles, spreading centrally to the arms, legs, and trunk. The rash is initially small, red, and macular but becomes larger and petechial. It spreads for 2–3 days. In some cases there is splenomegaly, hepatomegaly, jaundice, gangrene, myocarditis, or uremia.

B. Laboratory Findings: Leukocytosis, proteinuria, and hematuria are common. Owing to endothelial damage, there is early activation of platelets, coagulation pathways, and fibrinolysis. Rickettsiae can sometimes be isolated in special laboratories from blood obtained in the first few days of illness. A rise in antibody titer during the second week of illness can be detected by specific complement fixation, immunofluorescence, and microagglutination tests or by the Weil-Felix reaction with *Proteus* OX19 and OX2. Antibody response may be suppressed if antimicrobial drugs are given very early.

Differential Diagnosis

The early signs and symptoms of Rocky Mountain spotted fever are shared with many other infections. The rash may be confused with that of measles, typhoid, or meningococcemia. The suspicion of the latter requires blood cultures and cerebrospinal fluid examination. Infection with *Ehrlichia canis* (ehrlichosis), a leukocytic rickettsiosis resulting from a tick bite, may resemble Rocky Mountain spotted fever.

Prevention

Protective clothing, tick-repellent chemicals, and the removal of ticks at frequent intervals are helpful. Vaccines of inactivated *R rickettsii* grown in eggs or in cell culture have given moderate protection but were not commercially available in the USA or Canada in 1990.

Treatment & Prognosis

In mild, untreated cases, fever subsides at the end of the second week. The response to chloramphenicol or tetracycline (see Chapter 31) is prompt if the drugs are started early.

The mortality rate for Rocky Mountain spotted fever varies strikingly with age. In untreated elderly persons it may be 70%; in children, less than 20%.

Durack DT: Rus in urbe: Spotted fever comes to town. N Engl J Med 1988;318:1388.

Melnick CG et al: Rocky Mountain spotted fever: Clinical, laboratory and epidemiologic features in 262 cases. J Infect Dis 1984;150:480.

2. OTHER SPOTTED FEVERS

Tick-borne rickettsial infections in Africa, Asia, and Australia may resemble Rocky Mountain spotted fever but cover a wide spectrum from very mild to very severe. In many cases, a local lesion develops at the site of the tick bite (eschar), often with painful enlargement of the regional lymph nodes.

RICKETTSIALPOX

Rickettsia akari is a parasite of mice, transmitted by mites (*Allodermanyssus sanguineus*). Upon close contact of mice with humans, infected mites may transmit the disease to humans. Rickettsialpox has an incubation period of 7–12 days. The onset is sudden, with chills, fever, headache, photophobia, and disseminated aches and pains. The primary lesion is a red papule that vesicates and forms a black eschar. Two to 4 days after onset of symptoms, a widespread papular eruption appears that becomes vesicular and forms crusts that are shed in about 10 days. Early lesions may resemble those of chickenpox.

Leukopenia and a rise in antibody titer with rickettsial antigen in complement fixation tests are often present. However, the Weil-Felix test is negative.

Even without treatment, the disease is fairly mild and self-limited. Control requires the elimination of mice from human habitations after insecticide has been applied to suppress the mite vectors.

SCRUB TYPHUS (Tsutsugamushi Disease)

Essentials of Diagnosis

- Exposure to mites in endemic area of Southeast Asia, the western Pacific, and Australia.
- Black eschar at site of bite, with regional and generalized lymphadenopathy.
- Conjunctivitis and a short-lived macular rash.
- Frequent pneumonitis, encephalitis, and cardiac failure.

- Laboratory confirmation with agglutinins to *Proteus* OXK and specific antibodies by immunofluorescence.

General Considerations

Scrub typhus is caused by *Rickettsia tsutsugamushi (R orientalis)*, which is principally a parasite of rodents transmitted by mites. The infectious agent can be transmitted by transovarian transmission. The mites may spend much of their life cycle on vegetation but require a blood meal to complete maturation. At that point, humans coming in contact with infested vegetation are bitten by mite larvae and are infected.

Clinical Findings

A. Symptoms and Signs: After an incubation period of 1–3 weeks, there is a nonspecific prodrome, with malaise, chills, severe headache, and backache. At the site of the mite bite a papule develops that forms a flat black eschar. The regional lymph nodes are enlarged and tender, and there may be generalized adenopathy. Fever rises gradually, and a generalized macular rash appears at the end of the first week of fever. The rash is most marked on the trunk and may be fleeting or may last for a week. The patient appears obtunded and confused. During the second or third week, pneumonitis, myocarditis, and cardiac failure may develop.

B. Laboratory Findings: Blood obtained during the first few days of illness may permit isolation of the rickettsia by mouse inoculation in specialized laboratories. The Weil-Felix test usually shows a rising titer to *Proteus* OXK during the second week of illness. The complement fixation test is often unsatisfactory, but immunofluorescence with specific antigens is diagnostic.

Differential Diagnosis

Leptospirosis, typhoid, dengue, malaria, and other rickettsial infections may have to be considered. When the rash is fleeting and the eschar not evident, laboratory results are the best guide to diagnosis.

Prevention

Repeated application of long-acting miticides can make endemic areas safe. When this is not possible, insect repellents on clothing and skin provide some protection. For short exposure, chemoprophylaxis with chloramphenicol can prevent the disease but permits infection. No effective vaccines are available at present.

Treatment & Prognosis

Without treatment, fever may subside spontaneously after 2 weeks, but the mortality rate may be 10–30%. Early treatment can virtually eliminate deaths.

Chayakul P, Panich V, Silpapojakul K: Scrub typhus pneumonitis: An entity which is frequently missed. Quart J Med 1988;68:595.

TRENCH FEVER

Trench fever is a self-limited, louse-borne relapsing febrile disease caused by *Rochalimaea (Rickettsia) quintana*. This organism grows extracellularly in the louse intestine and is excreted in feces. Humans are infected when infected louse feces enter defects in skin. No animal reservoir except humans has been demonstrated.

This disease has occurred in epidemic forms in louse-infested troops and civilians during wars and in endemic form in Central America. Onset is abrupt, with fever lasting 3–5 days, often followed by relapses. The patient becomes weak and complains of severe pain behind the eyes and in the back and legs. Lymphadenopathy and splenomegaly may appear, as well as a transient maculopapular rash. Subclinical infection is frequent, and a carrier state may occur. The differential diagnosis includes dengue, leptospirosis, malaria, relapsing fever, and typhus fever.

R quintana is the only rickettsia that has been grown on artificial media without living cells. The organism can be cultivated on agar containing 10% fresh blood and has been recovered from blood cultures of patients. The Weil-Felix test is negative, but a specific complement fixation test and a specific enzyme immunoassay are available.

The illness is self-limited, and recovery regularly occurs without treatment.

Q FEVER

Essentials of Diagnosis

- An acute or chronic febrile illness with severe headache, cough, prostration, and abdominal pain.
- Extensive pneumonitis, hepatitis, or encephalopathy; rarely endocarditis.
- Exposure to sheep, goats, cattle, or their products.

General Considerations

Coxiella burnetii is unique among rickettsiae in that it is usually transmitted to humans not by arthropods but by inhalation of infectious aerosols or ingestion of infected milk. It is a parasite of cattle, sheep, and goats, in which it produces mild or subclinical infection. It is excreted by cows and goats principally through the milk and placenta and by sheep through feces, placenta, and milk. Dry feces and milk, dust contaminated with them, and the tissues of these animals contain large numbers of infectious organisms that are spread by the airborne route. Inhalation of contaminated dust and of droplets from infected animal tissues is the main source of human infection. There is an occupational risk for animal handlers, slaughterhouse workers, veterinarians, etc. *Coxiella* is resistant to heat and drying, perhaps because the organism forms endospore-like structures. Thus, it survives in dust, on the fleece of infected animals, or in inadequately pasteurized milk. Spread from one human to another does not seem to occur even in the presence of florid pneumonitis, but fetal infection can occur.

Clinical Findings

A. Symptoms and Signs: After an incubation period of 1–3 weeks, a febrile illness develops with headache, prostration, and muscle pains, occasionally with a nonproductive cough, abdominal pains, or jaundice. Physical signs of pneumonitis are slight. Hepatitis may be severe. Endocarditis occurs rarely but must always be considered in cases of culture-negative endocarditis with a suggestive epidemiologic background. At times, signs of encephalopathy are present. The clinical course may be acute or chronic and relapsing.

B. Laboratory Findings: Laboratory examination often shows leukopenia and a diagnostic rise in specific complement-fixing antibodies to *Coxiella* phase 2. The Weil-Felix test is negative. Liver function tests are often abnormal. In Q fever endocarditis, there is a titer of 1:200 or more by complement fixation or immunofluorescence with phase I antigen of *C burnetii*. Isolation of the organism from blood or sputum is rarely attempted.

C. Imaging: Radiographs of the chest show variable pulmonary infiltration.

Differential Diagnosis

Viral, mycoplasmal, and bacterial pneumonias; viral hepatitis; brucellosis; tuberculosis; psittacosis; and other animal-borne diseases must be considered. The history of exposure to animals or animal dusts or tissues (eg, in slaughterhouses) should lead to appropriate specific serologic tests.

Prevention

Prevention must be based on detection of the infection in livestock, reduction of contact with infected animals or dusts contaminated by them, special care during contact with animal tissues, and effective pasteurization of milk. A vaccine of formalin-inactivated phase 1 *Coxiella* is being developed for persons at high risk of infection and appears to be protective.

Treatment & Prognosis

Treatment with tetracyclines can suppress symptoms and shorten the clinical course but does not always eradicate the infection. Even in untreated patients, the mortality rate is usually low, except with endocarditis.

Sawyer LA, Fishbein DB, McDade JE: Q fever: Current concepts. Rev Infect Dis 1987;9:935.

Infectious Diseases: Bacterial & Chlamydial

26

Henry F. Chambers, MD, Moses Grossman, MD, & Ernest Jawetz, MD, PhD

INFECTIONS CAUSED BY GRAM-POSITIVE BACTERIA

STREPTOCOCCAL INFECTIONS

1. PHARYNGITIS

Essentials of Diagnosis

- Abrupt onset of sore throat, fever, malaise, nausea, and headache.
- Throat red and edematous, with or without exudate; cervical nodes tender.
- Diagnosis confirmed by culture of throat or skin, rapid reagin test.

General Considerations

Beta-hemolytic streptococci, classically group A, are the most common bacterial cause of exudative pharyngitis. *Mycoplasma*, *Chlamydia* (TWAR strain), and viruses have also been isolated from patients with pharyngitis, but their clinical significance remains to be clarified. Transmission is by droplets of infected secretions. If group A streptococci produce erythrogenic toxin, they may cause scarlet fever rashes in susceptible persons.

Clinical Findings

A. Symptoms and Signs: "Strep throat" is characterized by a sudden onset of fever, sore throat, severe pain on swallowing, tender cervical adenopathy, malaise, and nausea. The pharynx, soft palate, and tonsils are red and edematous, and there may be a purulent exudate. The rash of scarlet fever is diffusely erythematous, with superimposed fine red papules, and is most intense in the groin and axillas. It blanches on pressure, may become petechial, and fades in 2–5 days, leaving a fine desquamation. In scarlet fever, the face is flushed, with circumoral pallor; and the tongue is coated, with enlarged red papillae (strawberry tongue).

B. Laboratory Findings: Leukocytosis with an increase in polymorphonuclear neutrophils is a regular early finding. Throat culture and rapid antigen detection tests each have a sensitivity of 70–80%. Antibody levels may remain elevated for months after the infection. Antistreptolysin O is the most commonly elevated antibody.

Complications

The suppurative complications of streptococcal sore throat include sinusitis, otitis media, mastoiditis, peritonsillar abscess, and suppuration of cervical lymph nodes, among others.

Nonsuppurative complications are rheumatic fever (0.05–3%) and glomerulonephritis (0.2–20%). Rheumatic fever may follow recurrent episodes of pharyngitis with any type of group A streptococci and begins 1–4 weeks after the onset of streptococcal sore throat. Glomerulonephritis follows a single infection with a nephritogenic strain of *Streptococcus* group A (eg, types 4, 12, 2, 49, and 60), more commonly on the skin than in the throat, and begins 1–3 weeks after the onset of the infection.

Differential Diagnosis

Streptococcal sore throat resembles (and cannot be reliably distinguished clinically from) pharyngitis caused by adenoviruses, Epstein-Barr virus, and other agents. Pharyngitis accompanied by generalized lymphadenopathy, splenomegaly, atypical lymphocytosis, and a positive serologic test (eg, Monospot) distinguishes mononucleosis from streptococcal pharyngitis. Diphtheria is characterized by a more confluent pseudomembrane; candidiasis shows white patches of exudate and less erythema; and necrotizing ulcerative gingivostomatitis (Vincent's fusospirochetal disease) presents with shallow ulcers in the mouth. The petechial rash of scarlet fever may mimic meningococcemia, sunburn, drug reactions, rubella, echovirus infections, and toxic shock syndrome.

Treatment

A. Specific Measures: Antimicrobial therapy has a minimal effect on resolution of symptoms. Because its main purpose is prevention of complications, therapy may be withheld pending culture or antigen test results. Throat culture and rapid antigen detection tests each have a sensitivity of 70–80%. However, because these tests are relatively insensitive, when clinical suspicion is high (eg, presence of exudative pharyngitis, tender adenopathy, high fever, and absence of cough and rhinorrhea) and the risk of therapy is low (eg, no drug allergy), antimicrobial therapy may be given without laboratory evaluation.

1. Benzathine penicillin G, 1.2 million units intramuscularly as a single dose, is optimal therapy and usually eradicates the streptococci.

2. Penicillin V potassium, 500 mg orally 4 times a day for 10 days, is effective, but this regimen is not easily enforced, since the patient becomes asymptomatic in 2–4 days.

3. Patients hypersensitive to penicillin may be treated with erythromycin, 0.5 g 4 times daily (40 mg/kg/d) for 10 days.

B. General Measures: Acetaminophen and gargling with warm saline solution relieves sore throat. Bed rest is desirable until the patient is afebrile. Diet may be modified to reduce discomfort, and fluids may be forced during fever.

Prevention of Recurrent Rheumatic Fever

Patients who have had rheumatic fever should be treated with a continuous course of antimicrobial prophylaxis for at least 5 years. Benzathine penicillin, 1.2 million units as a single intramuscular injection every 4 weeks, is the regimen of choice. Sulfadiazine, 1 g orally daily, or penicillin G, 500 mg orally daily, is also acceptable, but less reliable, as a prophylactic regimen.

Centor RM, Meier FA, Dalton HP: Throat cultures and rapid tests for diagnosis of group A streptococcal pharyngitis. Ann Intern Med 1986;105:892. (Review of test strategy and treatment recommendations.)

Huovinen P et al: Pharyngitis in adults: The presence and co-existence of viruses and bacterial organisms. Ann Intern Med 1989;110:612. (Viruses, *Chlamydia pneumoniae*, and *Mycoplasma* may cause adult pharyngitis.)

Massell BF, et al: Penicillin and the marked decrease in morbidity and mortality from rheumatic fever in the United States. New Engl J Med 1988;318:280.

2. STREPTOCOCCAL SKIN INFECTIONS

Essentials of Diagnosis

- Fever.
- Erysipelas with tender, edematous, erythematous skin.
- Impetigo.
- Tender cellulitis with rapidly advancing borders.

General Considerations

Unlike staphylococci, aerobic streptococci are not part of normal skin flora. Streptococcal skin infections usually result from colonization of normal skin by contact with other infected individuals or by preceding streptococcal respiratory infection.

Clinical Findings

A. Symptoms and Signs: Impetigo is a focal, vesicular, pustular lesion with a thick, amber-colored crust that has a "stuck-on" appearance.

Erysipelas is a painful superficial cellulitis that frequently involves the face. It is well demarcated from the surrounding normal skin and is likely to affect skin with impaired lymphatic drainage, such as edematous lower extremities or following surgical procedures.

B. Laboratory Findings: Cultures obtained from a wound or pustule are likely to grow group A streptococci. Other cultures of the skin (eg, direct cultures or tissue fluid aspirated from an area of cellulitis or erysipelas) rarely are positive. Blood cultures should be obtained in patients with fever and systemic manifestations of infection. Serologic tests are not useful acutely but may provide evidence of recent streptococcal infection in patients with glomerulonephritis. Antihyaluronidase is the most common elevated antibody.

Treatment

Parenteral antibiotics are indicated for patients with fever, facial erysipelas, bacteremia, or systemic signs of infection. Penicillin, the drug of choice, may be given as procaine penicillin, 600,000 units intramuscularly every 12 hours, or aqueous penicillin, 1 million units intravenously every 4 hours.

Cutaneous infections caused by staphylococci may at times be difficult to differentiate from streptococcal infections. Co-infection with staphylococci also occurs. Therefore, initial therapy for severely ill patients or those who have risk factors for staphylococcal infection (eg, intravenous drug use, wound infection, diabetes) should include an agent—such as nafcillin, 1.5 g intravenously every 6 hours—that also is active against *Staphylococcus aureus*.

In the penicillin-allergic patient without anaphylaxis or other serious reaction to penicillin, cefazolin, 500 mg intravenously or intramuscularly every 8 hours, may be used. In the patient with a serious penicillin allergy, vancomycin, 1000 mg intravenously every 12 hours, should be used.

Patients who do not require parenteral therapy may be treated with penicillin V potassium, 500 mg orally, or erythromycin, 500 mg orally, 4 times daily for 7–10 days.

Hook EW et al: Microbiologic evaluation of cutaneous cellulitis in adults. Arch Intern Med 1986;146:295. (Low yield of cultures in diagnosis.)

3. OTHER GROUP A STREPTOCOCCAL INFECTIONS

Arthritis, pneumonia, empyema, and endocarditis are relatively uncommon infections that may be caused by group A streptococci.

Arthritis generally occurs in association with cellulitis. In addition to intravenous therapy with penicillin G, 2 million units every 4 hours (or cefazolin or vancomycin in doses recommended above for penicillin-allergic patients), frequent percutaneous needle aspiration should be performed to remove accumulated fluid. Open surgical drainage usually is not necessary unless the hip or shoulder is infected, because these are less amenable to percutaneous drainage.

Pneumonia and **empyema** often are characterized by extensive tissue destruction and an aggressive, rapidly progressive clinical course associated with significant morbidity and mortality rates. Besides high-dose penicillin, chest tube drainage is indicated for treatment of empyema.

Group A streptococci can cause **endocarditis.** This complication should be suspected when bacteremia accompanies pneumonia, particularly if there are multiple infiltrates on chest x-ray (suggesting septic pulmonary embolization) or if the patient abuses parenteral drugs. The tricuspid valve is most commonly involved. A patient with suspected endocarditis should be treated with 4 million units of penicillin G every 4 hours for 4 weeks. Vancomycin, 1000 mg every 12 hours, is recommended for persons allergic to penicillin.

Barg NL et al: Group A streptococcal bacteremia in intravenous drug users. Am J Med 1985;78:569. (Forty cases—including 11 of endocarditis—and implications for therapy.)

4. NON-GROUP A STREPTOCOCCAL INFECTIONS

Non-group A streptococci produce a spectrum of disease similar to that resulting from infection with group A streptococci. Some non-group A streptococci are β-hemolytic (eg, groups B, C, and G). These are differentiated from group A streptococci on the basis of biochemical, serologic, or other laboratory tests. The treatment of infections caused by these strains is the same as for group A streptococci.

Group B streptococci are an important cause of sepsis, bacteremia, and meningitis in the neonate. This organism, which is part of the normal vaginal flora, may cause septic abortion, endometritis, or peripartum infections and, less commonly, cellulitis, bacteremia, and endocarditis in adults. Treatment of infections caused by group B streptococci is with either penicillin or vancomycin in doses recommended for group A streptococci. Because of in vitro synergism, some authorities recommend the addition of low-dose gentamicin, 1 mg/kg every 8 hours.

Viridans streptococci, which are nonhemolytic or α-hemolytic (ie, producing a green zone of hemolysis on blood agar), are part of the normal oral flora. Although these strains may produce pyogenic infection virtually at any site, they are most notable as the leading cause of native valve endocarditis (see Chapter 23).

Group D streptococci include *Streptococcus bovis* and enterococci. *S bovis* is a cause of endocarditis in association with bowel cancer or cirrhosis. Endocarditis caused by *S bovis* is treated like viridans streptococci.

Enterococci have been classified into a genus separate from other streptococci. Two species, *S faecalis* and *Enterococcus faecium,* are recognized. Enterococci cause wound infections, urinary tract infections, bacteremia, and endocarditis. Until recently, enterococci were uniformly susceptible to penicillin, vancomycin, and gentamicin. Strains resistant to each of these antibiotics have been reported from a few medical centers in France and the United States. The need for routine susceptibility testing of enterococci remains to be determined. Except for endocarditis, enterococcal infections can still be treated with penicillin, 3 million units every 6 hours; ampicillin (which is slightly more active than penicillin in vitro), 2 g every 6 hours; or vancomycin, 1 g every 12 hours. Because these antibiotics are not bactericidal for enterococci, gentamicin in a dose of 1 mg/kg every 8 hours must be used in combination to cure endocarditis. Combination therapy might also be considered for treatment of more serious enterococcal infections such as osteomyelitis, very serious soft tissue infections, or bacteremia, especially in the immunocompromised host.

Bush LM et al: High level penicillin resistance among isolates of enterococci: Implication for treatment of enterococcal infections. Ann Intern Med 1989;110:515. (Efficacy of vancomycin but not penicillin.)

Opal SM et al: Group B streptococcal sepsis in adults and infants : Contrasts and comparisons. Arch Intern Med 1988;148:641. (Descriptive study and association with underlying disease.)

Venezio ER et al: Group G streptococcal endocarditis and bacteremia. Am J Med 1986;81:29.

PNEUMOCOCCAL INFECTIONS

1. PNEUMOCOCCAL PNEUMONIA

Essentials of Diagnosis

- Productive cough, fever, rigors, dyspnea, pleurisy.
- Consolidating lobar pneumonia on chest x-ray.
- Lancet-shaped gram-positive diplococci on gram-stain of sputum.

General Considerations

The pneumococcus is the most common cause of community-acquired pyogenic bacterial pneumonia. Alcoholism, infection by HIV, sickle cell disease, splenectomy, and hematologic disorders are predisposing factors. The mortality rate remains high in the setting of advanced age, multilobar disease, severe hypoxemia, extrapulmonary complications, and bacteremia.

Clinical Findings

A. Symptoms and Signs: The illness typically evolves over a period of a few days. The patient presents with findings of high fever, productive cough, occasionally hemoptysis, and pleuritic chest pain.

B. Laboratory Findings: Classically, pneumococcal pneumonia is a lobar pneumonia with radiographic signs of consolidation and occasionally effusion. Infiltrates may cause a somewhat patchy appearance within a lobe, as in bronchopneumonia.

Gram's stain of sputum should be examined in all cases. Adequately collected samples (with < 10 epithelial cells and > 25 polymorphonuclear leukocytes per high power field) show gram-positive diplococci 80–90% of the time. Sputum culture alone is less sensitive than Gram's stain. Blood cultures may be positive in up to 25% of cases, with an even higher percentage in HIV-infected patients.

Complications

Parapneumonic (sympathetic) effusion is common and may cause recurrence or persistence of fever 3 or 4 days into therapy. These sterile fluid accumulations will resolve on their own and need no specific therapy. Pleural empyema is an infrequent complication, occurring in 5% or less of cases.

A sympathetic effusion, often asymptomatic, may sometimes collect in the pericardium. Pneumococcal pericarditis is a rare and potentially lethal complication that can cause tamponade.

Pneumococcal endocarditis usually infects the aortic valve and often occurs in association with meningitis and pneumonia. Heart failure and embolic stroke may be present.

Treatment

A. Specific Measures: Although penicillin resistance does occur, the pneumococcal strains usually are sensitive to penicillin. Uncomplicated pneumococcal pneumonia (ie, arterial Po_2 greater than 60 mm Hg, no coexisting medical problems, and single-lobe disease without signs of extrapulmonary infection) may be treated on an outpatient basis with penicillin V potassium, 500 mg orally 4 times a day for 7–10 days. For penicillin-allergic patients, either erythromycin, 500 mg orally 4 times a day, or trimethoprim-sulfamethoxazole, one double-strength tablet

(320 mg trimethoprim and 1600 mg sulfamethoxazole) orally twice a day, may be used.

More seriously ill patients or those with other medical problems should be admitted and treated with procaine penicillin, 600,000 units intramuscularly every 12 hours, or aqueous penicillin G, 1 million units intravenously every 4 hours. For penicillin-allergic patients without anaphylaxis or other serious reactions, cefazolin, 500 mg either intravenously or intramuscularly every 8 hours, is effective. For serious penicillin or cephalosporin allergy, vancomycin, 30 mg/kg/d, up to 2000 mg total, in 2 divided doses, can be used. Trimethoprim-sulfamethoxazole given intravenously with doses of 10 mg/kg/d of the trimethoprim component divided into 3 doses also is effective. Intravenous erythromycin, though effective, is generally less well tolerated because of phlebitis.

B. Treatment of Complications: If empyema is suspected, thoracentesis should be performed to document this complication. Chest tube drainage is usually required in this setting.

Echocardiography should be done if pericardial effusion is suspected. Patients with pericardial effusion who are responding to therapy and have no signs of tamponade may be followed and treated with indomethacin, 50 mg 3 times daily, for pain. In patients with increasing effusion, unsatisfactory clinical response, or evidence of tamponade, pericardiocentesis should be performed to determine if the pericardial space is infected. If the fluid is infected, it must be drained either percutaneously (by tube placement or needle aspiration), by placement of a pericardial window, or by pericardiectomy. Needle aspiration alone tends to be a temporizing measure, and further drainage procedures often are necessary. Pericardiectomy eventually may be necessary to prevent or treat constrictive pericarditis, a common sequela of bacterial pericarditis.

Endocarditis should be treated with 24 million units of penicillin G (or vancomycin for penicillin-allergic patients) for 4 weeks. Mild heart failure may respond to medical therapy alone, such as digoxin and diuretics. Moderate to severe heart failure is an indication for prosthetic valve implantation. Hemodynamic compromise should prompt consultation regarding prosthetic valve implantation. Delaying valve implantation in order to complete a full course of therapy is ill-advised, because heart failure, not recurrence of infection, is responsible for morbidity and deaths.

Pallares R et al: Risk factors and response to antibiotic therapy in adults with bacteremic pneumonia caused by penicillin-resistant pneumococci. N Engl J Med 1987; 317:18. (Therapeutic failure with penicillins against strains having MICs > 2 μg/mL.)

Polsky B et al: Bacterial pneumonia in patients with acquired immunodeficiency syndrome. Ann Intern Med 1986; 104:38.

2. PNEUMOCOCCAL MENINGITIS

Essentials of Diagnosis
- Fever, headache, altered mental status.
- Meningismus.
- Gram-positive diplococci on Gram stain of cerebrospinal fluid.

General Considerations
Streptococcus pneumoniae is the most common cause of meningitis in adults and the second most common cause of meningitis in children over the age of 6 years. Head trauma, cerebrospinal fluid leaks, and sinusitis may precede pneumococcal meningitis.

Clinical Findings
A. Symptoms and Signs: The onset is rapid, with fever, headache, and altered mentation. Pneumonia may be present. Compared to meningitis caused by the meningococcus, pneumococcal meningitis lacks a rash, and focal neurologic deficits and obtundation are more prominent features.

B. Laboratory Findings: The cerebrospinal fluid typically has more than 1000 white blood cells per microliter, over 60% of which are polymorphonuclear leukocytes; the glucose concentration is less than 40 mg/dL, or less than 50% of the simultaneous serum concentration; the protein usually exceeds 150 mg/dL. Not all cases of meningitis will have these typical findings, and alterations in cerebrospinal fluid cell counts and chemistries may be surprisingly minimal, overlapping with those of aseptic meningitis.

Gram's stain of cerebrospinal fluid shows gram-positive cocci in 80–90% of cases, and in untreated cases blood or cerebrospinal fluid cultures are almost always positive. Tests such as counterimmunoelectrophoresis or latex agglutination to detect pneumococcal antigens in cerebrospinal fluid are less sensitive than culture and Gram's stain and usually are not positive if these are negative. Antigen detection tests may be helpful in establishing the diagnosis in the patient who has been partially treated and in whom cultures and stains are negative.

Treatment
Penicillin G, 4 million units intravenously every 4 hours for 14 days, is recommended. In the penicillin-allergic patient, chloramphenicol, 100 mg/kg/d (up to 6 g) in 4 divided doses, is also effective. Third-generation cephalosporins are probably as effective as penicillin. Ceftriaxone, 4 g/d in one or 2 divided doses, is an effective alternative to penicillin or chloramphenicol.

Penicillin-resistant pneumococci (MIC > 0.1 µg/mL) are rare, but their prevalence may be increasing. The oxacillin disk method is recommended to screen blood and cerebrospinal fluid isolates for resistance. The best therapy for penicillin-resistant strains is not known. Ceftriaxone, 2-4 g/d, chloramphenicol, 100 mg/kg/d (provided the strain is susceptible), or vancomycin, 1 g every 12 hours, may be used.

STAPHYLOCOCCUS AUREUS INFECTIONS

1. SKIN & SOFT TISSUE INFECTIONS

Essentials of Diagnosis
- Localized erythema with induration and fluctuance.
- Abscess formation.
- Folliculitis.
- Gram's stain of pus with gram-positive cocci in clusters; cultures usually positive.

General Considerations
Most staphylococci found on cultures of normal skin belong to the Staphylococcus epidermidis group; if Staphylococcus aureus is found, it is usually isolated only transiently and not as normal skin flora. S aureus tends to cause more localized skin infections than streptococci, and abscess formation is common.

Clinical Findings
A. Symptoms and Signs: S aureus skin infections may begin around one or more hair follicles, causing folliculitis. These infections may progress to form boils (or furuncles) or spread to involve a more extensive area of skin and deeper subcutaneous tissue (ie, a carbuncle). Myositis or fasciitis may rarely occur, often in association with a deep wound or other inoculation or injection.

B. Laboratory Findings: Cultures of the wound or abscess material will almost always yield the diagnosis. In patients with fever or other systemic signs of infection, blood cultures should be obtained to document the occurrence of bacteremia, because this connotes more serious disease, with risk of endocarditis, osteomyelitis, or metastatic seeding of other sites. If signs or symptoms point to involvement of other sites (eg, joints, pleural fluid), appropriate cultures of these sites should also be taken.

Treatment
Proper drainage of abscess fluid or other focal infections is the mainstay of therapy. For infections localized to the skin, drainage alone may be all that is needed, whereas antibiotic therapy alone is unlikely to be effective if collections of infected material are undrained.

For uncomplicated skin infections, oral therapy is satisfactory. An oral penicillinase-resistant penicillin or cephalosporin, such as dicloxacillin or cephalexin, 500 mg 4 times a day for 7–10 days, is the drug of choice unless the organism is known not to produce β-lactamase, in which case penicillin should be used.

Erythromycin, 500 mg 4 times a day, may be used in the penicillin-allergic patient.

For more complicated infections with extensive cutaneous or deep tissue involvement or fever, parenteral therapy is indicated initially. A penicillinase-resistant penicillin such as nafcillin or oxacillin at a dose of 1.5 g every 6 hours intravenously is the drug of choice. In allergic patients without a serious reaction, cefazolin, 500 mg intravenously or intramuscularly every 8 hours, can be used. In patients with a serious allergy to β-lactam antibiotics or if the strain is methicillin-resistant, vancomycin, 1000 mg intravenously every 12 hours, is the drug of choice.

Lutomski DM et al: Microbiology of adult cellulitis. J Fam Pract 1988;26:45. (Staphylococci and streptococci, often together.)

2. OSTEOMYELITIS

S aureus is the cause of approximately 60% of all cases of osteomyelitis. Osteomyelitis may be caused by direct inoculation, as may occur in an open fracture or as a result of surgery; by extension from a contiguous focus of infection or open wound; or, more commonly, by hematogenous spread from a primary source elsewhere. Any bone may be involved, but the long bones and vertebrae are the usual sites.

Clinical Findings

A. Symptoms and Signs: The infection may be indolent, with an insidious onset accompanied by vague pain over the site of infection, progressing to local tenderness. Fever may be absent in up to a third of cases. Abscess formation is a late and unusual manifestation. Draining sinus tracts may be present in chronic infections or those occurring in association with foreign body implants.

B. Laboratory Findings: The diagnosis is established by isolation of *S aureus* from the blood or bone of a patient with signs and symptoms of focal bone infection. Blood culture will be positive in approximately 60% of untreated cases of staphylococcal osteomyelitis. Bone biopsy and culture should be performed if blood cultures are not positive.

C. Imaging: Bone scan and gallium scan, each with a sensitivity of approximately 95% and a specificity of 60–70%, are useful in identifying or confirming the site of bone infection. Plain bone films are abnormal early in the course of acute infection in a third of cases but will become abnormal in most cases even with appropriate and effective therapy. Computed tomography is only slightly more sensitive than plain films but can be useful in localizing associated abscesses. MRI is somewhat less sensitive than bone scan but has a specificity of 90%. Myelography or magnetic resonance imaging is indicated when epi-

dural abscess is suspected in association with vertebral osteomyelitis.

Treatment

Prolonged therapy is required to cure staphylococcal osteomyelitis. Durations of 4–6 weeks or longer are recommended. Although oral regimens can be effective, parenteral regimens are advised for the first 2–4 weeks of therapy. Nafcillin or oxacillin, 9–12 g/d in 6 divided doses, is the drug of choice. Cefazolin, 1 g every 8 hours, also is effective. Vancomycin, 1 g every 12 hours, may be used for the penicillin-allergic patient.

Oral regimens are dicloxacillin or cephalexin, 1 g every 6 hours. Trimethoprim-sulfamethoxazole, 320/1600 mg, or ciprofloxacin, 750 mg twice a day, may be effective alternatives.

Because rifampin can penetrate into infected bone and because studies have shown improved results with rifampin combinations in animal models of osteomyelitis, some authorities recommend that rifampin be added to the regimen for treatment of staphylococcal osteomyelitis. The dose is 300 mg twice a day.

Gupta NC, Prezio JA: Radionuclide imaging in osteomyelitis. Semin Nucl Med 1988;28:287. (Sensitivity and specificity.)

Waldvogel FA, Vasey H: Osteomyelitis: The past decade. New Engl J Med 1980;303:360. (Still timely review.)

3. STAPHYLOCOCCAL BACTEREMIA

S aureus readily invades the bloodstream and infects sites distant from the primary focus. The primary site of infection may be relatively minor or even inapparent. Deep infections, such as endocarditis, may present as unexplained bacteremia. Therefore, whenever *S aureus* is recovered from blood culture, the possibility of endocarditis, osteomyelitis, or other metastatic deep infection must be considered. For this reason, parenteral antibiotics are recommended as initial therapy for staphylococcal bacteremia until the sites and severity of infection have been defined, so that the appropriate treatment can be determined.

The appropriate duration of therapy for uncomplicated bacteremia arising from a removable source (eg, intravenous device) or drainable focus (eg, skin abscess) has not been well defined. Although 2 weeks of parenteral therapy is the usual recommendation, shorter courses and oral regimens may be successful. Moreover, approximately 10% or more of patients still relapse, usually with endocarditis, even if treated for 2 weeks.

Because of the tendency of staphylococcal bacteremia to relapse—and based on the impression that longer courses of therapy reduce the relapse rate—a minimum of 10–14 days of nafcillin or oxacillin, 1.5 g intravenously every 4–6 hours, cefazolin, 500–

1000 mg every 8 hours, or vancomycin, 1000 mg every 12 hours, is recommended for uncomplicated staphylococcal bacteremia. Longer courses of either parenteral or oral therapy may be considered for patients (eg, those with diabetes, immunocompromised persons) at risk for late complications from bacteremia.

Ehni WF, Reller B: Short-course therapy for catheter-associated *Staphylococcus aureus* bacteremia. Arch Intern Med 1989;149:533.

4. TOXIC SHOCK SYNDROME

Some strains of staphylococci elaborate toxins that can cause 3 important entities: "scalded skin syndrome" in children, toxic shock syndrome in adults, and enterotoxin food poisoning. Toxic shock syndrome is characterized by abrupt onset of high fever, vomiting, and watery diarrhea. Sore throat, myalgias, and headache are often complaints. Hypotensive shock with renal and cardiac failure is an ominous manifestation in severe cases. A diffuse macular erythematous rash and nonpurulent conjunctivitis are common, and desquamation, especially of palms and soles, is typical as the victim recovers. Reported fatality rates vary and may be as high as 15%. Although toxic shock syndrome has occurred in children and in males, the great majority of cases (90% or more) have been reported in women of childbearing age. Of these, 95% have begun within 5 days of the onset of a menstrual period in women who have used tampons. If a woman recovers from the syndrome, she should stop using tampons. Outbreaks have also developed in surgical patients.

S aureus has been isolated from various sites, including the nasopharynx, vagina, or rectum or from wounds, but blood cultures are negative. Toxic shock syndrome is most often caused by toxic shock syndrome toxin-1 (TSST-1), although not all strains causing toxic shock syndrome produce TSST-1.

Important aspects of treatment include rapid rehydration, antistaphylococcal drugs, management of renal or cardiac insufficiency, and removal of sources of toxin, eg, removal of tampon, drainage of abscess.

Recently, a toxic shock-like syndrome has been reported in association with group A streptococcal infections. This syndrome is characterized by invasive skin or soft tissue infection, shock, myositis, adult respiratory distress syndrome, and renal failure. This syndrome differs from staphylococcal toxic shock syndrome in several respects. Bacteremia, which is uncommon in staphylococcal toxic shock, occurs in half or more of patients. Skin rashes and desquamation may be absent in the streptococcal syndrome. Exotoxin A, an erythrogenic exotoxin that produces scarlet fever, may mediate the systemic toxicity of the streptococcal syndrome.

Bartlett P et al: Toxic shock syndrome associated with surgical wound infections. JAMA 1982;247:1448.

Hirsch ML, Kass EH: An annotated bibliography of toxic shock syndrome. Rev Infect Dis 1986;8(Suppl 1):1. (Synopsis of 173 papers from 1924 to 1985.)

Kass EH, Parsonnet J: On the pathogenesis of toxic shock syndrome. Rev Infect Dis 1987;9(Suppl 5):S482.

Stevens DL et al: Severe group A streptococcal infections associated with toxic shock-like syndrome and scarlet fever toxin A. N Engl J Med 1989;321:1.

CLOSTRIDIAL DISEASES

1. CLOSTRIDIAL MYONECROSIS (Gas Gangrene)

Essentials of Diagnosis

- Sudden onset of pain and edema in an area of wound contamination.
- Brown to blood-tinged watery exudate, with skin discoloration of surrounding area.
- Gas in the tissue by palpation or x-ray.
- Gram-positive rods in culture or smear of exudate.
- Prostration and systemic toxicity.

General Considerations

Gas gangrene or clostridial myonecrosis is produced by entry of one of several clostridia (*Clostridium perfringens, Clostridium ramosum, Clostridium bifermentans, Clostridium histolyticum, Clostridium novyi*, etc) into devitalized tissues. Toxins produced under anaerobic conditions result in shock, hemolysis, and myonecrosis.

Clinical Findings

A. Symptoms and Signs: The onset of gas gangrene is usually sudden, with rapidly increasing pain in the affected area, fall in blood pressure, and tachycardia. Fever is present, but not proportionate to the severity of the inflammation. In the last stages of the disease, severe prostration, stupor, delirium, and coma occur.

The wound becomes swollen, and the surrounding skin is pale. Fluid accumulation beneath produces a foul-smelling brown, blood-tinged serous discharge. As the disease advances, the surrounding tissue changes from pale to dusky and finally becomes deeply discolored, with coalescent, red, fluid-filled vesicles. Gas may be palpable in the tissues. In clostridial sepsis, hemolysis and jaundice are common, often complicated by acute renal failure.

B. Laboratory Findings: Gas gangrene is a clinical diagnosis, and empiric therapy is indicated whenever the clinical picture is present. Radiographic studies may show gas within the soft tissues, but this not sufficient to make the diagnosis because other organisms may produce gas. The smear, which typically shows a remarkable absence of neutrophils, is very suggestive if gram-positive rods are present. Anaerobic culture confirms the diagnosis.

Differential Diagnosis

Other types of infection can cause gas formation in the tissue, eg, *Enterobacter, Escherichia,* and mixed anaerobic infections including *Bacteroides* and peptostreptococci. Clostridia may produce serious puerperal infection with hemolysis.

Treatment

A. Specific Measures: Give penicillin G, 2 million units every 3 hours as a bolus into an intravenous infusion. Although other agents (eg, tetracycline, clindamycin, metronidazole, chloramphenicol, cefoxitin) are active against Clostridium spp in vitro and probably in vivo as well, their clinical efficacy has not been demonstrated.

B. Surgical Measures: Adequate surgical debridement and exposure of infected areas is essential. Radical surgical excision may be necessary.

Cline KA, Turnbull TL: Clostridial myonecrosis. Ann Emerg Med 1985;14:459. (Clinical features and management.)

TETANUS

Essentials of Diagnosis

- Jaw stiffness followed by spasms of jaw muscles (trismus).
- Stiffness of the neck and other muscles, dysphagia, irritability, hyperreflexia.
- Finally, painful convulsions precipitated by minimal stimuli.
- History of wound and possible contamination.

General Considerations

Tetanus is an acute intoxication by the neurotoxin elaborated by *Clostridium tetani.* Spores of this organism are ubiquitous in soil. When introduced into a wound, spores may germinate. The vegetative bacteria elaborate a toxin, tetanospasmin, that blocks the action of inhibitory mediators at spinal synapses and interferes with neuromuscular transmission. As a result, minor stimuli result in uncontrolled spasms, and reflexes are enormously exaggerated. The incubation period is 5 days to 15 weeks, with the average being 8–12 days.

In the United States, most cases occur in unvaccinated individuals. Persons at risk are the elderly, migrant workers, newborns, and intravenous drug users.

Clinical Findings

A. Symptoms and Signs: Occasionally, the first symptom is pain and tingling at the site of inoculation, followed by spasticity of the group of muscles nearby, and this may be all that happens. More frequently, however, the presenting symptoms are stiffness of the jaw, neck stiffness, dysphagia, and irritability. Hyperreflexia develops later, with spasms of the jaw muscles (trismus) or facial muscles and rigidity and spasm of the muscles of the abdomen, neck, and back. Painful tonic convulsions precipitated by minor stimuli are common. The patient is awake and alert during the entire course of the illness. During convulsions, spasm of the glottis and respiratory muscles render the patient unable to breathe, and cyanosis and asphyxia may ensue. The temperature is only slightly elevated, if at all.

B. Laboratory Findings: The diagnosis of tetanus is made clinically.

Differential Diagnosis

Tetanus must be differentiated from various acute central nervous system infections. Trismus may occasionally develop with the use of phenothiazines. Strychnine poisoning should also be considered.

Complications

Airway obstruction and anoxia are common. Urinary retention and constipation may result from spasm of the sphincters. Respiratory arrest and cardiac failure are late, life-threatening events.

Prevention

Tetanus is completely preventable by active immunization, which should be universal. Immunizations for children include tetanus toxoid, usually as DTP (see Table 23–4 for schedule). For primary immunization of adults, tetanus toxoid (usually as combined tetanus toxoid and diphtheria toxoid, since adults should also be immunized against diphtheria) is administered as 2 doses 4–6 weeks apart, with a third dose 6–12 months later. Booster doses are given every 10 years or at the time of major injury if it occurs more than 5 years after a dose.

Passive immunization should be used in nonimmunized individuals and those whose immunization status is uncertain whenever the wound is contaminated or likely to have devitalized tissue. Tetanus immune globulin, 250 units, is given intramuscularly. Active immunization with tetanus toxoid should be started concurrently. Table 26–1 provides a guide to prophylactic management.

Adequate debridement of wounds is an essential preventive measure. In suspect cases, benzathine penicillin G, 1.2 million units intramuscularly, may be a reasonable adjunctive measure.

Treatment

A. Specific Measures: Give tetanus immune globulin, 5000 units intramuscularly.

B. General Measures: Place the patient at bed rest and minimize stimulation. Sedation and paralysis

Table 26–1. Guide to tetanus prophylaxis in wound management (United States, 1985). (Modified from *MMWR* 1985;34: 405.)

History of Absorbed Tetanus Toxoid (Doses)	Clean, Minor Wounds		All Other Wounds[1]	
	Td	**TIG**	**Td**	**TIG**
Unknown or <3	Yes	No	Yes	Yes
≥3	No[2]	No	No[3]	No

Td = tetanus toxoid and diphtheria toxoid, adult form. Use only this preparation (Td-adult) in children older than 6 years.
TIG = tetanus immune globulin.
[1] Such as, but not limited to, wounds contaminated with dirt, feces, soil, saliva, etc; puncture wounds; avulsions; and wounds resulting from missiles, crushing, burns, and frostbite.
[2] Yes, if more than 10 years since last dose.
[3] Yes, if more than 5 years since last dose. (More frequent boosters are not needed and can accentuate side effects.)

often are necessary. Experience from areas of high incidence suggests that most tetanic spasms can be eliminated by treatment with chlorpromazine (50–100 mg 4 times daily) or diazepam combined with a sedative (amobarbital, phenobarbital, or meprobamate). Mild cases of tetanus can be controlled with one or the other rather than both. Only rarely is general curarization required. A course of intravenous penicillin, 20 million units daily, is recommended to eliminate organisms that may be producing toxin at the site of infection.

Tracheostomy may be required for laryngeal spasm. Assisted respiration is required along with curarization.

Prognosis

The mortality rate is higher in very small children and very old people; with shorter incubation periods; with shorter intervals between onset of symptoms and the first convulsion; and with delay in treatment. If trismus develops early, the prognosis is grave. The overall mortality rate is about 40%. Contaminated lesions about the head and face are more dangerous than wounds on other parts of the body.

If the patient survives, recovery is complete.

Centers for Disease Control. General guidelines on immunizations. Ann Intern Med 1989;111:133.
Centers for Disease Control. Tetanus: United States 1987 and 1988. MMWR 1990;39:37. (Epidemiology of tetanus and occurrence in persons over age 50.)

BOTULISM

Essentials of Diagnosis

- Sudden onset of cranial nerve paralysis, diplopia, dry mouth, dysphagia, dysphonia, and muscle weakness progressing to respiratory paralysis.
- History of recent ingestion of home-canned,

smoked, or unusual foods. Demonstration of toxin in serum or food.

General Considerations

Botulism is food poisoning usually caused by ingestion of preformed toxin (usually type A, B, or E) of *Clostridium botulinum,* a strict anaerobic spore-forming bacillus found widespread in soil. Canned, smoked, or vacuum-packed anaerobic foods are involved—particularly home-canned vegetables, smoked meats, and vacuum-packed fish. Infant botulism and wound botulism differ in that organisms present in the gut or wound, respectively, elaborate toxin in vivo. The toxins block the release of acetylcholine from nerve endings. Clinically, early nervous system involvement leads to respiratory paralysis. The mortality rate in untreated cases is high.

Clinical Findings

A. Symptoms and Signs: Twelve to 36 hours after ingestion of the toxin, visual disturbances appear, particularly diplopia and loss of power of accommodation. Other symptoms are dry throat and mouth, dysphagia, and dysphonia. There may be nausea and vomiting, particularly with type E toxin. Muscle weakness is apparent. Ptosis, cranial nerve palsies with impairment of extraocular muscles, fixed dilated pupils, and dry mouth are characteristic. Respiration is impaired, but the sensorium remains clear and the temperature normal. Respiratory paralysis may lead to death unless mechanical assistance is provided.

Infant botulism. Infants in the first few months of life may present with weakness, generalized hypotonicity, and electromyographic findings compatible with botulism. Both botulinus organisms and toxin are found in the stool but not in serum. Honey fed to infants under 1 year of age has been incriminated in this syndrome.

B. Laboratory Findings: Toxin in the patient's serum and in suspected foods may be shown by mouse inoculation and identified with specific antiserum.

Differential Diagnosis

Cranial nerve involvement suggests bulbar poliomyelitis, myasthenia gravis, stroke, infectious neuronitis, secondary syphilis, or tick paralysis. Nausea and vomiting may suggest intestinal obstruction or other types of food poisoning.

Complications

Aspiration pneumonia, infection, and respiratory paralysis are the usual causes of death.

Prevention

Home-canned vegetables must be sterilized to destroy spores. Sterilization standards for commercial canned or vacuum-packed foods must be strictly enforced. Boiling food for 20 minutes can inactivate the toxin, but punctured or swollen cans or jars with defective seals should be discarded. Early and adequate treatment of wounds prevents wound botulism.

Treatment

As soon as the clinical diagnosis of botulism is suspected, the physician should contact the state health authorities for advice and help with procurement of botulinus antitoxin from the Centers for Disease Control and for help if needed with assays for toxin in the patient's serum or stool as well as the suspected food item. During off hours the CDC provides assistance via a recorded message at (404) 639–3753.

Respiratory failure is managed with intubation and mechanical ventilation. Prompt recognition and treatment of pneumonia also is important. Give nothing by mouth while swallowing difficulty persists. Parenteral fluids or alimentation should be given as necessary.

The removal of unabsorbed toxin from the gut may be attempted if it can be done very soon after ingestion of the suspected toxin. Any remnants of suspected foods must be saved for analysis. Persons who might have eaten the suspected food must be located and observed. If the patient survives the attack of botulism, there are no neurologic residua.

Bartlett JC: Infant botulism in adults. N Engl J Med 1986;315:254. (Adult case due to in vivo toxin production.)

ANTHRAX

Anthrax is a disease of sheep, cattle, horses, goats, and swine caused by *Bacillus anthracis*, a gram-positive spore-forming aerobic rod transmitted to humans by entry through broken skin or mucous membranes or, less commonly, by inhalation. Human infection is rare. It is an occupational disease most apt to occur in farmers, veterinarians, and tannery and wool workers.

Clinical Findings

A. Symptoms and Signs:

1. Cutaneous anthrax ("malignant pustule")–An erythematous papule appears on an exposed area of skin and becomes vesicular, with a purple to black center. The area around the lesion is swollen or edematous and surrounded by vesicles. The center of the lesion finally forms a necrotic eschar and sloughs. Regional adenopathy, variable fever, malaise, headache, and nausea and vomiting may be present. After the eschar sloughs, hematogenous spread and sepsis may occur, at times manifested by shock, cyanosis, sweating, and collapse. Hemorrhagic meningitis may also occur.

Anthrax sepsis sometimes develops without a skin lesion.

2. Pulmonary anthrax ("woolsorter's disease")–This follows the inhalation of spores from hides, bristles, or wool. It is characterized by fever, malaise, headache, dyspnea, and cough; congestion of the nose, throat, and larynx; and evidence of pneumonia or mediastinitis.

B. Laboratory Findings: The white count may be elevated or low. Sputum or blood culture may be positive for *B anthracis*. Smears of skin lesions show gram-positive encapsulated rods, and cultures should be attempted. Antibodies may be detected by an indirect hemagglutination test.

Treatment

Give penicillin G, 10 million units intravenously daily; or, in mild, localized cases, tetracycline, 0.5 g orally every 6 hours.

Centers for Disease Control. Human cutaneous anthrax: North Carolina 1987. MMWR 1988;37:413. (Case report, occupational risk, and prevention.)

DIPHTHERIA

Essentials of Diagnosis

- Tenacious gray membrane at portal of entry.
- Sore throat, nasal discharge, hoarseness, malaise, fever.
- Myocarditis, neuritis.
- Culture confirms the diagnosis.

General Considerations

Diphtheria is an acute infection, caused by *Corynebacterium diphtheriae*, that usually attacks the respiratory tract but may involve any mucous membrane or skin wound. The organism is spread chiefly by respiratory secretions from patients with disease or healthy carriers. The incubation period is 2–7 days. Myocarditis and neuritis are important exotoxin-mediated complications. This exotoxin inhibits elongation factor, which is required for protein synthesis.

Diphtheria has almost disappeared as a result of effective vaccination programs. Many cases that now occur are in unvaccinated populations such as the elderly, migrant workers, and immigrants.

Clinical Findings

A. Symptoms and Signs: Nasal, laryngeal, pharyngeal, and cutaneous forms of diphtheria occur. Nasal infection produces few symptoms other than a nasal discharge. Laryngeal infection is characterized by upper airway and bronchial obstruction. In pharyngeal diphtheria, the most common form, a tenacious gray membrane covers the tonsils and pharynx. Mild sore throat, fever, and malaise are followed by toxemia and prostration.

Myocarditis and neuritis are the most common and most serious complications. Myocarditis causes cardiac arrhythmias, heart block, heart failure, and circulatory collapse. Toxic neuritis usually involves the cranial nerves first, producing diplopia and strabismus, slurred speech, and difficulty swallowing. Aspiration of oropharyngeal secretions can cause secondary pneumonia.

B. Laboratory Findings: Because laboratory findings are not distinctive, the diagnosis often is made clinically. The diagnosis can be confirmed by culture of the organism.

Differential Diagnosis

Diphtheria must be differentiated from streptococcal pharyngitis, infectious mononucleosis, adenovirus or herpes simplex infection, Vincent's infection, and candidiasis. A presumptive diagnosis of diphtheria must be made on clinical grounds without waiting for laboratory verification, since emergency treatment is needed.

Prevention

Active immunization with diphtheria toxoid is part of routine childhood immunization (usually as DTP) with appropriate booster injections. The immunization schedule for adults is the same as for tetanus. In order to avoid major reactions, only the "adult type" toxoid (Td) should be used.

Susceptible persons exposed to diphtheria should receive a booster dose of toxoid (start active immunization if not previously immune), erythromycin or penicillin, and daily throat inspections.

Treatment

A. Specific Measures: Antitoxin, which is prepared from horse serum, must be given in all cases when diphtheria is suspected. Conjunctival and skin tests for sensitivity to horse serum should be done and desensitization carried out if necessary.

The dose of antitoxin, given intravenously, for mild early pharyngeal or laryngeal disease is 20–40 thousand units; for moderate nasopharyngeal disease, 40–60 thousand units; for severe, extensive, or late (3 days or more) disease, 80–100 thousand units. Diphtheria equine antitoxin can be obtained from the Centers for Disease Control.

Antibiotics are a useful adjunct to antitoxin. Penicillin or erythromycin, 500 mg orally 4 times daily for 7–10 days, is equally effective.

B. Treatment of Complications: Therapy of myocarditis is supportive and may include maintaining careful fluid balance, supplemental oxygen, digoxin, antiarrhythmic agents, treatment of heart block, and pressor support.

Removal of membrane by direct laryngoscopy or bronchoscopy may be necessary to prevent or alleviate airway obstruction. Nasogastric feeding is indicated for patients unable to swallow. Secondary pneumonia should be treated with appropriate antimicrobials and may require intubation and ventilatory support.

C. Treatment of Carriers: Eradication of organisms from a carrier is difficult. Erythromycin followed by a course of penicillin may be successful. Tonsillectomy is a last resort.

Rappuoli R, Perugini M, Falsen E: Molecular epidemiology of the 1984–1986 outbreak of diphtheria in Sweden. N Engl J Med 1988;318:12. (A virulence factor in addition to toxin is implicated.)

INFECTIONS CAUSED BY GRAM-NEGATIVE BACTERIA

BORDETELLA PERTUSSIS INFECTION (Whooping Cough)

Essentials of Diagnosis

- Paroxysmal cough ending in a high-pitched inspiratory "whoop."
- Two-week prodromal catarrhal stage of malaise, cough, coryza, and anorexia.
- Predominantly in infants under age 2 years.
- Absolute lymphocytosis. Culture confirms diagnosis.

General Considerations

Pertussis is an acute infection of the respiratory tract caused by *Bordetella pertussis* that is transmitted by respiratory droplets. The incubation period is 7–17 days. Infants are most commonly infected; half of all cases occur before age 2 years.

Clinical Findings

A. Symptoms and Signs: Physical findings are minimal or absent. Fever, if present, is low-grade. The symptoms of classic pertussis last about 6 weeks and are divided into 3 consecutive stages.

The catarrhal stage is characterized by its insidious onset, with lacrimation, sneezing, and coryza, anorexia and malaise, and a hacking night cough that tends to become diurnal. The paroxysmal stage follows. Rapid consecutive coughs usually followed by a deep, hurried, high-pitched inspiration (whoop) are typical. Paroxysms may involve 5–15 coughs between breaks and may occur up to 50 times in 24 hours. Stimuli such as fright or anger, crying, sneezing, inhalation of irritants, and overdistention of the stomach may produce the paroxysms. The cough is productive of copious amounts of thick mucus. Vomiting is common during the paroxysms.

The convalescent stage usually begins 4 weeks after onset of the illness with a decrease in the frequency and severity of paroxysms of cough.

B. Laboratory Findings: The white blood cell

count is usually 15–20 thousand/μL (rarely, as high as 50,000/μL), 60–80% of which are lymphocytes. The clinical diagnosis can be confirmed by culture with Bordet-Gengou or other special medium. A specific immunofluorescent stain of the nasopharyngeal swab dried onto a slide may aid in the diagnosis. The organism is recovered in only about half of clinically diagnosed patients.

Differential Diagnosis

B pertussis infection may resemble viral pneumonia, influenza, or acute bronchitis. Respiratory chlamydial infections may produce a syndrome resembling pertussis in infants under 4 months of age. The lymphocytosis may suggest acute leukemia.

Complications

Asphyxia is the most common complication. It may lead to convulsions and cerebral anoxia. Increased intracranial pressure during a paroxysm may produce cerebral hemorrhage. Pneumonia, atelectasis, interstitial and subcutaneous emphysema, and pneumothorax may occur as a result of damaged respiratory mucosa, inspissated mucus, or increased intrathoracic pressure.

Prevention

Active immunization with pertussis vaccine is recommended for all infants, usually combined with diphtheria and tetanus toxoids (DTP). The newborn derives little or no immunity from the mother. Because of the mildness of the disease in older individuals, neither primary nor booster immunization is recommended after age 6 years. Occasionally, neurologic disturbances may occur after DTP injection. Such rare individuals should subsequently receive DT immunization without the pertussis component (see Chapter 23).

Infants and susceptible adults with significant exposure to pertussis should receive prophylaxis with erythromycin (40 mg/kg/d). Those previously immunized should receive a booster dose of vaccine.

Treatment

Erythromycin, 500 mg 4 times a day orally for 10 days, shortens the duration of carriage. It also may diminish the severity of coughing paroxysms.

Bergquist SO et al: Erythromycin in the treatment of pertussis: A study of bacteriologic and clinical effects. Pediatr Infect Dis 1987;6:458.

Centers for Disease Control: Pertussis surveillance: United States, 1986-1988. MMWR 1990;39:57. (Increased incidence, sensitivity and specificity of markers, and insensitivity of culture.)

Griffin MR et al: Risk of seizures and encephalopathy after immunization with the diphtheria-tetanus-pertussis vaccine. JAMA 1990;263:1641. (Safety is documented.)

MENINGOCOCCAL MENINGITIS

Essentials of Diagnosis

- Fever, headache, vomiting, confusion, delirium, convulsions.
- Petechial rash of skin and mucous membranes.
- Neck and back stiffness with positive Kernig and Brudzinski signs.
- Purulent spinal fluid with gram-negative intracellular and extracellular organisms.
- Culture of cerebrospinal fluid, blood, or petechial aspiration confirms the diagnosis.

General Considerations

Meningococcal meningitis is caused by *Neisseria meningitidis* of groups A, B, C, Y, W-135, and others. Up to 40% of persons are nasopharyngeal carriers of meningococci, but relatively few develop disease. Infection is transmitted by droplets. The clinical illness may take the form of meningococcemia (a fulminant form of septicemia without meningitis), both meningococcemia and meningitis, or predominantly meningitis. Chronic recurrent meningococcemia with fever, rash, and arthritis can occur. The development of meningococcal disease is favored by complement deficiencies (especially C7–C9).

Clinical Findings

A. Symptoms and Signs: High fever, chills, and headache; back, abdominal, and extremity pains; and nausea and vomiting are present. In severe cases, rapidly developing confusion, delirium, seizures, and coma and shock occur.

Nuchal and back rigidity are present, with positive Kernig and Brudzinski signs. A petechial rash is found in most cases. Petechiae may vary from pinhead-sized to large ecchymoses or even areas of skin gangrene that may later slough if the patient survives. These petechiae are found in any part of the skin, mucous membranes, or the conjunctiva but never in the nail beds, and they usually fade in 3–4 days.

Shock may develop rapidly and is a bad prognostic sign.

B. Laboratory Findings: Lumbar puncture reveals a cloudy to frankly purulent cerebrospinal fluid, with elevated pressure, increased protein, and decreased glucose content. The fluid usually contains more than 1000 cells/μL, with polymorphonuclear cells predominating and containing gram-negative intracellular diplococci. The absence of organisms in a gram-stained smear of the cerebrospinal fluid sediment does not rule out the diagnosis. The capsular polysaccharide can often be demonstrated in cerebrospinal fluid or urine by latex agglutination. The organism is usually demonstrated by smear or culture of the cerebrospinal fluid, oropharynx, blood, or aspirated petechiae.

Disseminated intravascular coagulation is an important complication of meningococcal infection. Prothrombin time and partial thromboplastin time are prolonged, fibrin dimers are elevated, fibrinogen is low, and the platelet count is low.

Differential Diagnosis

Meningococcal meningitis must be differentiated from other bacterial and viral meningitides. In small infants and in the elderly, the presentation may be vague, without fever or stiff neck.

Rickettsial or echovirus infection and, rarely, other bacterial infections (eg, staphylococcal infections) may also produce a petechial rash.

Complications

Arthritis, cranial nerve damage (especially the eighth nerve, with resulting deafness), and hydrocephalus may occur as complications. Myocarditis, nephritis, and disseminated intravascular coagulation may occur in severe cases.

Prevention

Effective polysaccharide vaccines for groups A, C, Y, and W-135 are available. A and C vaccine has reduced the incidence of infections with these meningococcus groups in military recruits. The vaccines are effective for control of epidemics in civilian populations.

Outbreaks in closed populations are best controlled by eliminating meningococcal carriage. Rifampin is the drug of choice in dosages as follows: 600 mg twice a day for 2 days for adults; 10 mg/kg twice a day for 2 days for children 1 month to 12 years; 5 mg/kg twice a day for 2 days for infants.

Household members exposed to a person with meningococcal meningitis are at increased risk and should be given rifampin prophylaxis for 2 days. Day-care center contacts are treated in the same manner. School and work contacts need not be treated. Hospital contacts should be treated if intensive and intimate exposure has occurred, eg, given mouth-to-mouth resuscitation.

Accidentally discovered carriers without known close contact with meningococcal disease do not require prophylactic antimicrobials.

Treatment

A. Specific Measures: Blood cultures must be obtained and intravenous antimicrobial therapy started immediately, even before lumbar puncture if necessary. If *N meningitidis* is established or strongly suspected as the infectious agent, aqueous penicillin G is the antibiotic of choice (24 million units/24 h) in divided doses every 4 hours. In penicillin-allergic patients or those in whom *Haemophilus influenzae* or gram-negative meningitis is a consideration, ceftriaxone, 4 g intravenously once a day, should be used. Chloramphenicol, 1 g every 6 hours, is an alternative in the severely penicillin- or cephalosporin-allergic patient.

Treatment should be continued in full doses by the intravenous route until the patient is afebrile for 5 days.

In the past, the recommended duration of therapy has been 7–10 days. More recent studies suggest that shorter courses—as few as 4 days if ceftriaxone is used—are also effective.

B. General Measures: Vital signs must be closely monitored. Hypovolemic shock is the most serious complication of meningococcal infections. Volume expansion with isotonic electrolyte solution is the initial approach. Dopamine is added to the infusion if the patient fails to respond. Ventilatory assistance may be required.

Obtundation or deterioration in mental status may result from cerebral edema and increased intracranial pressure. Intravenous mannitol (2 g/kg) may temporarily decrease the intracranial pressure. The role of corticosteroids is controversial.

Heparinization may be useful if there is evidence of disseminated intravascular coagulation and bleeding. An initial dose of 50 units/kg intravenously is given; thereafter, an attempt is made to keep the partial thromboplastin time at 11/2 times control.

Tuncer AM et al: Once daily ceftriaxone for meningococcemia and meningococcal meningitis. Pediatr Infect Dis J 1985;7:711. (Once daily ceftriaxone, 100 mg/kg, for 4 days was as effective as multiple-dose penicillin.)

Viladrich PF et al: Four days of penicillin for meningococcal meningitis. Arch Intern Med 1986;146:2380. (Short course of penicillin shown to be effective.)

INFECTIONS CAUSED BY *HAEMOPHILUS* SPECIES

Haemophilus influenzae type b is primarily a pathogen of children less than 5 years old. Meningitis and epiglottitis, which are almost always caused by type B strains, occur almost exclusively in children. *H influenzae* and other *Haemophilus* species may cause sinusitis, otitis, bronchitis, epiglottis, pneumonitis, cellulitis, arthritis, meningitis, and endocarditis in adults.

In adults, **pneumonia** is one of the more common infections caused by *H influenzae* type b. The presentation is that of a typical bacterial pneumonia, with purulent sputum containing a predominance of gram-negative, pleomorphic rods. Alcoholism, smoking, chronic lung disease, and HIV infection are important risk factors.

Nontypable strains of *H influenzae* and other *Haemophilus* species cause **sinusitis, otitis, and respiratory tract infections.** Alcoholics, smokers, and patients with chronic lung disease are particularly at risk for respiratory infections with these organisms.

Haemophilus species other than *H influenzae* (eg, *H parainfluenzae*, *H aphrophilus*) infrequently cause **endocarditis.**

Although *Haemophilus* species and nontypable strains of *H influenzae* may cause pneumonia, they more frequently colonize the upper respiratory tract. Consequently, in the absence of positive pleural fluid or blood cultures, distinguishing pneumonia from colonization is difficult. Pneumonia from *Haemophilus* species probably is overdiagnosed for this reason.

Beta-lactamase-producing strains are less common in adults than in children. Therefore, for the mildly ill adult patient with sinusitis, otitis, or respiratory tract infection, oral amoxicillin, 500 mg every 8 hours, is adequate. Alternatively, ampicillin, 1–2 g every 6 hours, may be used parenterally.

In the more seriously ill patient (eg, the toxic patient with multilobar pneumonia), use of a second- or third-generation cephalosporin—cefuroxime, 750–1500 mg every 8 hours, or ceftriaxone, 1 g/d—is advisable pending determination of whether the infecting strain is a β-lactamase producer. Trimethoprim-sulfamethoxazole, administered based on a dose of 10 mg/kg/d of trimethoprim, can be used for the penicillin-allergic patient.

Epiglottitis, although rare, does occur in adults. It is characterized by an abrupt onset of high fever, drooling, and inability to handle secretions. Stridor and respiratory distress result from laryngeal obstruction. Early, elective intubation is recommended because airway obstruction may progress unpredictably and rapidly. The diagnosis is best made by direct visualization of the cherry-red, swollen epiglottis at laryngoscopy. Because laryngoscopy may provoke laryngospasm and obstruction, it should be performed in an intensive care unit or similar setting, and only at the time of intubation. Cefuroxime, 1.5 g every 8 hours, or ceftriaxone, 2 g every 24 hours, is the drug of choice. Trimethoprim-sulfamethoxazole (see above for dosage) or chloramphenicol, 4 g/d, may be used in the patient with serious penicillin allergy.

Meningitis—also rare in adults—becomes a consideration in the patient who has meningitis associated with sinusitis or otitis. The presentation is the same as that of other bacterial meningitides. Initial therapy of suspected *H influenzae* meningitis should be with ceftriaxone, 4 g/d in one or 3 divided doses, until the strain is proved not to produce β-lactamase. Cefuroxime probably should not be used because it sterilizes the cerebrospinal fluid culture less rapidly than ceftriaxone. Chloramphenicol, 100 mg/kg/d in 4 divided doses, can be used, but only if the patient has a serious, life-threatening allergy to β-lactam antibiotics.

Schaad WB et al: A comparison of ceftriaxone and cefuroxime for treatment of bacterial meningitis in children. N Engl J Med 1990;322:141. (Ceftriaxone sterilizes the cerebrospinal fluid more rapidly than cefuroxime.)

LEGIONNAIRES' DISEASE

Essentials of Diagnosis

- Patients are generally immunocompromised, smokers, or have chronic lung disease.
- Scant sputum production, pleuritic chest pain, toxic appearance.
- Chest x-ray shows focal patchy infiltrates, which may progress to multiple lobes and consolidation.
- Gram's stain of sputum shows few polymorphonuclear leukocytes, or polymorphonuclear leukocytes and no organisms.
- Relatively common cause of nosocomial infections and outbreaks.

General Considerations

Legionella infection is a common cause of community-acquired pneumonia. In some series, 10% or more of community-acquired pneumonias and nosocomial pneumonias may be caused by *Legionella* spp. Legionnaires' disease is more common in immunocompromised persons, in smokers, and in those with chronic lung disease.

Clinical Findings

A. Symptoms and Signs: Legionnaires' disease is one of the atypical pneumonias, so called because a Gram-stained smear of sputum does not show organisms. However, many features of legionnaires' disease are more like typical pneumonia, with high fevers, a "toxic" appearance of the patient, pleurisy, and even purulent sputum (without organisms). Classically, this pneumonia is caused by *Legionella pneumophila*, though other species can cause disease that is clinically indistinguishable.

B. Laboratory Findings: Legionellosis is best diagnosed by isolation of the organism from culture onto charcoal-yeast extract agar. Culture is about 80% sensitive and permits identification of infections caused by species and serotypes other than *L pneumophila* serotype 1. The organism may also be detected in tissue, pleural fluid, or other infected material by staining techniques. Staining with Dieterle's silver stain is a reliable technique for identifying *Legionella* spp in tissue. Direct fluorescent antibody (DFA) staining, which is less sensitive than culture, may also be useful but is limited to detection of infections caused by *L pneumophila* serotype 1. Urinary antigen detection tests are available. Although sensitive, they lack of specificity because they may be positive in colonized patients or remain positive long after infection. Suspected cases of legionellosis can be confirmed by a 4-fold rise in antibody titer from acute to convalescent serum or by a convalescent serum titer of 1:128 or greater. Like the DFA and antigen tests, only infections due to *L pneumophila* serotype 1 are detected by serology.

Treatment

The drug of choice for treatment of legionellosis is erythromycin, 2–4 g daily for 14–21 days. Rifampin, 300 mg twice a day in combination with erythromycin, may be synergistic and may be considered for those with severe illness and in immunocompromised hosts, who tend to have more aggressive disease.

Tetracyclines and trimethoprim-sulfamethoxazole occasionally have been used to treat legionellosis, and ciprofloxacin is active in vitro. These agents are of unproved efficacy and should be considered for use only if erythromycin is contraindicated or cannot be tolerated.

GRAM-NEGATIVE BACTEREMIA & SEPSIS

There are several hundred thousand episodes of gram-negative sepsis annually, with a mortality rate that is variable depending upon host factors. Patients with rapidly fatal underlying diseases (neutropenic patients or those immunosuppressed by virtue of an underlying disease or medication) have a mortality rate of 40–60%; patients with ultimately fatal underlying diseases (diseases likely to be fatal in 5 years, such as solid tumors, severe liver disease, and aplastic anemia) have a mortality rate of 15–20%; and patients with no underlying disease have a low mortality rate—5% or less. Gram-negative bacteremia can originate in a number of sites, the most common being the genitourinary system, hepatobiliary tract, gastrointestinal tract, and lungs. Less common sources include intravenous lines, infusion fluids, surgical wounds, surgical drains, and decubitus ulcers.

Clinical Findings

A. Symptoms and Signs: Most patients have fevers and chills, often with an abrupt onset. However, the absence of fever does not exclude the diagnosis of sepsis, since 15% of patients are hypothermic (temperature ≤ 36.4 °C [97.6 °F]) at the onset of sepsis, and 5% of patients never develop a temperature above 37.5 °C (99.6 °F). Hyperventilation with respiratory alkalosis and changes in mental status are important manifestations of sepsis because they occur early in the course of the disease, often before the onset of fevers, chills, or hypothermia. They may be the first clues that sepsis is present. Skin lesions occur commonly and can be quite variable. Ecthyma gangrenosum (a lesion with a necrotic center and surrounding erythema) is seen chiefly in *Pseudomonas* sepsis and is most frequently mentioned in association with gram-negative sepsis, but other lesions also occur. Vesicles, bullae, diffuse erythema, and petechiae

have all been described. Although these lesions are nonspecific, when present in the patient with suspected sepsis they should be scraped with culture and Gram stain—the latter may be the easiest and quickest way to document sepsis if the stain is positive. Hypotension and shock occur in 20–50% of patients and when present are poor prognostic signs. In patients with shock, impaired organ perfusion (brain, heart, kidney) may occur, leading to anuria, nitrogen retention, acidosis, circulatory collapse, and ultimately death if left untreated. Thrombocytopenia occurs in 50% of patients, laboratory evidence of coagulation abnormalities in 10%, and frank DIC in 2–3%.

B. Laboratory Findings: Because the clinical manifestations of sepsis are nonspecific, the diagnosis is confirmed by obtaining a positive blood culture. If a single blood culture is obtained before therapy is started, there is an 80% chance that it will be positive; if 3 blood cultures are obtained over a 24-hour period before instituting therapy, there is a 99% chance that at least one will be positive. Unfortunately, the latter approach is not practical in treating a patient with a potentially life-threatening illness—ie, one *must not delay therapy* in order to obtain positive cultures. A single culture should be drawn and therapy started immediately. It is important to realize, however, that when this is done there is a 20% false-negative rate for blood cultures. Several days later, the patient may be improved and cultures may be negative. In that situation, unless there is another good explanation for the patient's course, one must assume that the patient was indeed septic but had a falsely negative culture, and therapy should then be continued for 10–14 days.

Recent data suggest that culturing larger quantities of blood may increase the yield of positive blood cultures. Thus, obtaining a single large volume (30 mL) of blood for culture before starting therapy and inoculating 3 sets of blood culture bottles (5 mL in each of 3 aerobic and 3 anaerobic bottles) may decrease the false-negative rate from 20% to 5–10%.

Treatment

Several factors are important in the management of patients with sepsis.

A. Reversal of Underlying Disease: Since the outcome of sepsis depends upon the severity of the underlying disease (see above), every effort should be made to reverse that process. This usually means decreasing or stopping immunosuppressive medications and in certain circumstances giving white blood cell transfusions to the neutropenic patient.

B. Identifying the Source of Bacteremia: A careful search for the source of bacteremia should be made. By simply finding the source and either removing it (if it is a line or drain) or draining it (if it is an abscess), it is possible to turn what might be a fatal disease into one that is easily treatable.

C. Supportive Measures: The use of fluids and

pressors for maintaining blood pressure is discussed in Chapter 9; management of disseminated intravascular coagulation is discussed in Chapter 10.

D. Antibiotics: Antibiotics should be given as soon as the diagnosis of sepsis is seriously considered, since delays in therapy have been associated with increased mortality rates. In general, bactericidal antibiotics should be used and should be given intravenously to ensure therapeutic serum levels. Penetration of antibiotics into the site of primary infection is critical for successful therapy—ie, if the infection originates in the central nervous system, antibiotics that penetrate the blood-brain barrier should be used—eg, penicillin, ampicillin, chloramphenicol, and third-generation cephalosporins—but not first-generation cephalosporins or aminoglycosides, which penetrate poorly. Since one cannot distinguish gram-positive from gram-negative bacteremia on clinical grounds, initial therapy should include antibiotics active against both types of organisms.

Therapy can be altered once results of cultures are known. The number of antibiotics necessary to treat sepsis is somewhat controversial and depends upon the underlying disease. Most authorities believe that for patients with rapidly fatal underlying diseases, a combination of antibiotics should be given. Preferably, this combination should be synergistic (see Chapter 31); in patients with nonfatal or ultimately fatal underlying disease, single-drug therapy is adequate.

E. Corticosteroids: At present, there is no role for the use of corticosteroids in the therapy of sepsis or septic shock.

F. Opiate Antagonists: Use of naloxone has been reported to be efficacious in reversing shock in some studies. Unfortunately, study design has not been optimum—only small numbers of patients have been studied, and dosage regimens of naloxone have varied. The efficacy of naloxone in this setting is thus unproved.

G. Immunctherapy: Polyclonal antibodies directed at the core glycolipid area of the cell wall of gram-negative organisms have been helpful in some patients. Further studies using monoclonal antibodies are under way, and this form of immunotherapy holds promise for the future.

Bone RC et al: A controlled clinical trial of high-dose-methylprednisolone in the treatment of severe sepsis and septic shock. N Engl J Med 1987;317:653.

Jacobson MA, Young LS: New developments in the treatment of gram-negative bacteremia. West J Med 1986; 144:185.

Root RK, Sande M: *Septic Shock.* Vol. 4 of *Contemporary Issues in Infectious Diseases.* Churchill Livingstone, 1985.

Veterans Administration Systemic Sepsis Cooperative Study Group: Effect of high-dose glucocorticoid therapy on mortality in patients with clinical signs of systemic sepsis. N Engl J Med 1987;317:659.

Ziegler EJ et al: Treatment of gram-negative bacteremia and shock with human antiserum to a mutant of *Escherichia coli.* N Engl J Med 1982;307:1225.

SALMONELLOSIS

Salmonellosis includes infection by any of approximately 1600 serotypes of salmonellae. Three general clinical patterns are recognized: (1) enteric fever, the best example of which is typhoid fever, due to *Salmonella typhi;* (2) acute enterocolitis, caused by *Salmonella typhimurium* and many other types; and (3) the "septicemic" type, characterized by bacteremia and focal lesions, exemplified by infection with *Salmonella choleraesuis.* Each pattern tends to be associated with certain serotypes. All are transmitted by ingestion of the organism in contaminated food or drink.

1. ENTERIC FEVER (Typhoid Fever)

Essentials of Diagnosis

- Gradual onset of malaise, headache, sore throat, cough, and finally "pea soup" diarrhea or constipation.
- Slow (stepladder) rise of fever to maximum and then slow return to normal.
- Rose spots, relative bradycardia, splenomegaly, and abdominal distension and tenderness.
- Leukopenia; blood, stool, and urine culture positive for *Salmonella typhi* (group D)

General Considerations

Enteric fever is a clinical syndrome of constitutional symptoms, headache, and gastrointestinal symptoms that can be caused by any *Salmonella* species. When *S typhi,* which is most common, causes enteric fever, it is called typhoid fever. Infection begins when organisms penetrate the intestinal wall and invade mesenteric lymph nodes and the spleen. Bacteremia occurs, and the infection then localizes principally in the lymphoid tissue of the small intestine (particularly within 60 cm of the ileocecal valve). Peyer's patches become inflamed and may ulcerate, with involvement greatest during the third week of disease. The organism may localize in the lungs, gallbladder, kidneys, or central nervous system. Infection is transmitted by consumption of contaminated food or drink. The sources of most infections are chronic carriers with persistent gallbladder or urinary tract infections. The incubation period is 5–14 days.

Clinical Findings

A. Symptoms and Signs: The onset is usually insidious but in children may be abrupt, with chills and high fever. During the prodromal stage, there is increasing malaise, headache, cough, and sore throat, often with abdominal pain and constipation, while the fever ascends in a stepwise fashion. After about 7–10 days, the fever reaches a plateau and the patient is much more ill, appearing exhausted and often prostrated. There may be marked constipation, "pea soup" diarrhea, or marked abdominal distention. If there are no complications, the patient's condition will gradually improve over 7–10 days. However, relapse may occur for up to 2 weeks after defervescence.

During the early prodrome, physical findings are few. Later, splenomegaly, abdominal distention and tenderness, relative bradycardia, dicrotic pulse, and occasionally meningismus appear. The rash (rose spots) commonly appears during the second week of disease. The individual spot, found principally on the trunk, is a pink papule 2–3 mm in diameter that fades on pressure. It disappears in 3–4 days.

B. Laboratory Findings: Typhoid fever is best diagnosed by isolation of the organism from blood culture, which is positive in the first week of illness in 80% of patients who have not taken antimicrobials. The rate of blood culture positivity declines thereafter, but one-fourth or more of patients still have positive blood cultures in the third week. Culture of bone marrow may be positive when blood cultures are not. Positive stool culture is not reliable because it may be positive in gastroenteritis without typhoid fever.

Serologic studies may occasionally be useful if blood cultures are negative. However, serology is less reliable than culture because some patients may fail to have a rise in antibody titer and others may have a nonspecific anamnestic antibody response after a nontyphoidal infection.

Differential Diagnosis

Enteric fever can be produced by a number of *Salmonella* species (eg, *Salmonella paratyphi*). It must be distinguished not only from other diarrheal illnesses but also from numerous other infections that may have few localizing findings. Examples include tuberculosis, infective endocarditis, brucellosis, and Q fever. Often there is a history of recent travel, and viral hepatitis, malaria, or amebiasis may be in the differential diagnosis.

Complications

Complications occur in about 30% of untreated cases and account for 75% of all deaths. Intestinal hemorrhage, manifested by a sudden drop in temperature and signs of shock followed by dark or fresh blood in the stool, or intestinal perforation, accompanied by abdominal pain and tenderness, is most likely to occur during the third week. Less frequent complications are urinary retention, pneumonia, thrombophlebitis, myocarditis, psychosis, cholecystitis, nephritis, osteomyelitis, and meningitis.

Prevention

Immunization is not always effective but should be provided for household contacts of a typhoid carrier, for travelers to endemic areas, and during epidemic outbreaks. Vaccine is administered in 2 injections subcutaneously, not less than 4 weeks apart.

Adequate waste disposal and protection of food and water supplies from contamination are important public health measures to prevent salmonellosis. Carriers must not be permitted to work as food handlers.

Treatment

A. Specific Measures: Ampicillin, chloramphenicol, and trimethoprim-sulfamethoxazole may be effective. All can be given orally or intravenously depending on the patient's condition. Because resistance to ampicillin and chloramphenicol is common, trimethoprim-sulfamethoxazole, administered as 10 mg/kg/d of trimethoprim, is probably the first choice. Ceftriaxone, 2 g once a day, also is effective. The newer quinolones, such as ciprofloxacin, 750 mg twice a day, are active in vitro and may also be effective, but their use is contraindicated in children and pregnant women.

B. Treatment of Carriers: Chemotherapy often is ineffective in eradicating the carrier state. While treatment of carriage with ampicillin, trimethoprim-sulfamethoxazole, or chloramphenicol may be successful, one recent study suggests that ciprofloxacin, 750 mg twice a day for 4 weeks, is highly effective. Cholecystectomy may also be effective.

Prognosis

The mortality rate of typhoid fever is about 2% in treated cases. Elderly or debilitated persons are likely to do poorly. The course is milder in children.

With complications, the prognosis is poor. Relapses occur in up to 15% of cases. A residual carrier state frequently persists in spite of chemotherapy.

Ferreccio C: Efficacy of ciprofloxacin in the treatment of chronic typhoid carriers. J Infect Dis 1988;157:1235. (Carrier state eliminated in 11 of 12 patients.)

Keusch GT: Antimicrobial therapy for enteric fever and typhoid fever: State of the art. Rev Infect Dis 1988; 10(Suppl 1):S199. (Experience with quinolones.)

Soe GB et al: Treatment of typhoid fever and other systemic salmonelloses with cefotaxime, ceftriaxone, cefoperazone, and other newer cephalosporins. Rev Infect Dis 1987;9:719. (Relapse rates of approximately 5%.)

2. *SALMONELLA* GASTROENTERITIS

By far the most common form of salmonellosis is acute enterocolitis. Numerous *Salmonella* species may cause enterocolitis. The incubation period is 8–48 hours after ingestion of contaminated food or liquid.

Symptoms and signs consist of fever (often with

chills), nausea and vomiting, cramping abdominal pain, and diarrhea, which may be bloody, lasting 3–5 days. Differentiation must be made from viral gastroenteritis, food poisoning, shigellosis, amebic dysentery, acute ulcerative colitis, and acute surgical abdominal conditions. The organisms can be cultured from the stools, but not from blood.

The disease is usually self-limited, but bacteremia with localization in joints or bones may occur, especially in young infants and in patients with sickle cell disease.

Treatment of uncomplicated enterocolitis is symptomatic only. Young, malnourished, or immunocompromised infants, severely ill patients, those with sickle cell disease, and those with suspected bacteremia should be treated with trimethoprim-sulfamethoxazole (one double-strength tablet twice a day), ampicillin (100 mg/kg intravenously or orally), or ciprofloxacin (750 mg twice a day).

3. *SALMONELLA* BACTEREMIA

Rarely, *Salmonella* infection may be manifested by prolonged or recurrent fevers accompanied by bacteremia and local infection in bone, joints, pleura, pericardium, lungs, or other sites. Serotypes other than *S typhi* usually are isolated. This complication tends to occur in immunocompromised persons and is seen in HIV-infected individuals, who frequently have bacteremia without an obvious source. Treatment is the same as for typhoid fever, plus drainage of any abscesses. In HIV-infected patients, relapse is common, and lifelong suppressive therapy may be needed. Ciprofloxacin, 750 mg twice a day, is effective both for therapy and, at lower doses, for suppression.

Jabcoson MA et al: Ciprofloxacin for *Salmonella* bacteremia in the acquired immunodeficiency syndrome (AIDS). Ann Intern Med 1989;110:1027. (Small series demonstrating efficacy.)

SHIGELLOSIS

Essentials of Diagnosis

- Diarrhea, often with blood and mucus.
- Cramps. Fever, malaise, prostration.
- White blood cells in stools; organism isolated on stool culture.

General Considerations

Shigella dysentery is a common disease, often self-limited and mild but occasionally serious, particularly in the first 3 years of life. Poor sanitary conditions promote the spread of *Shigella*. *Shigella sonnei* is the leading cause of this illness in the USA, followed by *Shigella flexneri*. *Shigella dysenteriae* causes the most serious form of the illness. Shigellae are invasive organisms: The infective dose is 10^2–10^3 organisms. Recently, there has been a rise in strains resistant to multiple antibiotics.

Clinical Findings

A. Symptoms and Signs: The illness usually starts abruptly, with diarrhea, lower abdominal cramps, and tenesmus. The diarrheal stool often is mixed with blood and mucus. Systemic symptoms are fever, chills, anorexia and malaise, and headache. The patient becomes progressively weaker and more dehydrated. The abdomen is tender. Sigmoidoscopic examination reveals an inflamed, engorged mucosa with punctate, sometimes large areas of ulceration.

B. Laboratory Findings: The stool shows many leukocytes (even gross pus) and many red blood cells (or gross blood). Stool culture is positive for shigellae in most cases, blood culture in 2–3%.

Differential Diagnosis

Bacillary dysentery must be distinguished from *Salmonella* enterocolitis, enterotoxigenic *E coli*, *Campylobacter enteritis*, *Y enterocolitica*. Amebic dysentery may be similar clinically and is diagnosed by finding amebas in the fresh stool specimen. Ulcerative colitis in the adolescent and adult is an important cause of bloody diarrhea.

Complications

Dehydration, acidosis, and electrolyte imbalance occur in infancy. Temporary disaccharidase deficiency may follow the diarrhea. Arthritis is an uncommon complication.

Treatment

A. Specific Measures: Treatment of dehydration and hypotension is lifesaving in severe cases. The current antimicrobial treatment of choice is trimethoprim-sulfamethoxazole (one double-strength tablet twice a day), or ciprofloxacin (750 mg twice a day; contraindicated in children and pregnant women). Shigellae resistant to ampicillin are common, but if the isolate is susceptible, a dose of 500 mg 4 times a day is also effective. Amoxicillin, which is less effective, should not be used. A single dose of a quinolone (eg, norfloxacin, 400 mg, or ciprofloxacin, 750 mg) may be as effective as a 5-day courses of therapy with other drugs.

B. General Measures: Parenteral hydration and correction of acidosis and electrolyte disturbances are essential in all moderately or severely ill patients.

Antispasmodics (eg, tincture of belladonna) are helpful when cramps are severe. Drugs that inhibit intestinal peristalsis (paregoric, diphenoxylate with atropine) may ameliorate symptoms but prolong fever, diarrhea, and excretion of *Shigella* in feces. Appropriate precautions should be taken both in the hospital and in the home to limit spread of infection.

Gotuzzo E et al: Comparison of single dose treatment with norfloxacin and standard five-day treatment with trimethoprim/sulfamethoxazole for acute shigellosis in adults. Antimicrob Agents Chemother 1989;33:1101. (No advantage of either regimen over the other.)

CHOLERA

Essentials of Diagnosis

- Sudden onset of severe, frequent diarrhea, up to 1 L per hour.
- The liquid stool (and occasionally vomitus) is gray, turbid, and without fecal odor, blood, or pus ("rice water stool").
- Rapid development of marked dehydration, acidosis, hypokalemia, and hypotension.
- History of sojourn in endemic area or contact with infected person.
- Positive stool cultures and agglutination of vibrios with specific sera.

General Considerations

Cholera is an acute diarrheal illness caused by certain serotypes of *Vibrio cholerae*. The disease is toxin-mediated, and fever is unusual. The toxin activates adenylate cyclase in intestinal epithelial cells of the small intestines. This produces hypersecretion of water and chloride ion and a massive diarrhea of up to 15 L per day. Death results from profound hypovolemia, which is most likely to occur in infants and the elderly.

Cholera is rarely seen in the United States. It usually occurs in epidemics under conditions of crowding, war, and famine, and in refugee camps, where sanitation typically is inadequate. Infection is acquired from ingestion of contaminated food or water.

Clinical Findings

A. Symptoms and Signs: Cholera is characterized by a sudden onset of severe, frequent diarrhea (up to 1 L per hour). The liquid stool (and occasionally vomitus) is gray, turbid, and without fecal odor, blood, or pus ("rice water stool"). Marked dehydration, acidosis, hypokalemia, and hypotension develop rapidly.

B. Laboratory Findings: Stool cultures are positive, and agglutination of vibrios with specific sera can be demonstrated.

Prevention

A vaccine is available but confers short-lived, limited protection. The vaccine is required for entry or after travel into some countries. It is administered in 2 doses 1–4 weeks apart. A booster dose every 6 months is recommended for persons remaining in areas where cholera is a hazard.

Vaccination programs are expensive and not particularly effective in managing outbreaks of cholera.

When outbreaks occur, efforts should be directed toward establishing clean water and food sources and proper waste disposal. Often this is not possible given the resources available. Good handwashing to minimize cross-contamination in households and treatment of cases as they occur are inexpensive, practical, and probably effective measures.

Treatment

Treatment is by replacement of fluids. In mild or moderate illness, oral rehydration usually is adequate and has dramatically decreased the mortality rate in developing countries. A simple oral replacement fluid can be made from 1 teaspoon of table salt and 4 heaping teaspoons of sugar added to 1 L of water. Intravenous fluids are indicated for persons in shock or those with other signs of severe hypovolemia and those who cannot take adequate fluids orally. Either lactated Ringer's injection or an intravenous fluid containing 4 g of NaCl, 1 g of KCl, 5.4 g of sodium lactate, and 8 g of glucose per liter is satisfactory.

Antimicrobial therapy will shorten the course of illness. Several antimicrobials are active against V cholerae, including tetracycline, ampicillin, chloramphenicol, trimethoprim-sulfamethoxazole, and fluoroquinolones. Multiple antibiotic resistance does occur, so susceptibility testing, if available, is advisable.

Morris JG Jr, Black RE: Cholera and other vibrioses in the United States. N Engl J Med 1985;312:343.

BRUCELLOSIS

Essentials of Diagnosis

- Insidious onset: easy fatigability, headache, arthralgia, anorexia, sweating, irritability.
- Intermittent fever, especially at night, which may become chronic and undulant.
- Cervical and axillary lymphadenopathy; hepatosplenomegaly.
- Lymphocytosis, positive blood culture, elevated agglutination titer.

General Considerations

The infection is transmitted from animals to humans. *Brucella abortus* (cattle), *Brucella suis*, (hogs), and *Brucella melitensis* (goats) are the main agents. Transmission to humans occurs by contact with infected meat (slaughterhouse workers), placentae of infected animals (farmers, veterinarians), or ingestion of infected unpasteurized milk or cheese. The incubation period varies from a few days to several weeks. The disorder may become chronic and persist for years. In the USA, brucellosis is very rare except in the midwestern states (from B suis) and in visitors or immigrants from countries where brucellosis is endemic (eg, Mexico, Spain, South American countries).

Clinical Findings

A. Symptoms and Signs: The onset may be acute, with fever, chills, and sweats, but typically is insidious. It may be weeks before the patient seeks medical care for weakness, weight loss, low-grade fevers, sweats, and exhaustion upon minimal activity. Symptoms also include headache, abdominal pains with anorexia and constipation, and arthralgia. Epididymitis occurs in 10% of cases. The chronic form may assume an undulant nature, with periods of normal temperature between acute attacks; symptoms may persist for years, either continuously or intermittently.

Physical findings are minimal. Half of cases have peripheral lymph node enlargement and splenomegaly; hepatomegaly is less common.

B. Laboratory Findings: Early in the course of infection, the organism can be recovered from the blood, cerebrospinal fluid, urine, and bone marrow; later, this may be difficult. Because the organism is slow-growing, cultures should be incubated for 21 days before being read as negative. The diagnosis often is made not by culture but by serologic testing. Rising serologic titers or an absolute agglutination titer of greater than 1:100 supports the diagnosis.

Differential Diagnosis

Brucellosis must be differentiated from any other acute febrile disease, especially influenza, tularemia, Q fever, and enteric fever. In its chronic form it resembles Hodgkin's disease, tuberculosis, and malaria.

Complications

The most frequent complications are bone and joint lesions such as spondylitis and suppurative arthritis (usually of a single joint), subacute infective endocarditis, encephalitis, and meningitis. Less common complications are pneumonitis with pleural effusion, hepatitis, and cholecystitis. Abortion in humans is no more common with this disease than with any other acute bacterial disease during pregnancy. Pancytopenia is rare.

Treatment

Single-drug regimens are not recommended because the relapse rate may be as high as 50%. Combination regimens of 2 or 3 drugs are more effective. Either (1) doxycycline plus rifampin or streptomycin (or both) (2) trimethoprim-sulfamethoxazole plus rifampin or streptomycin (or both) are effective in doses as follows for 21 days: (1) doxycycline, 100–200 mg/d in divided doses; trimethoprim 320 mg/d plus sulfamethoxazole 1600 mg/d in divided doses; rifampin, 600–1200 mg/d; and streptomycin, 500 mg intramuscularly twice a day. Longer courses of therapy (eg, several months) may be required to cure relapses or meningitis.

Rahman A et al: The nature of human brucellosis in Kuwait: Study of 379 cases. Rev Infect Dis 1988;10:211. (Superiority of combinations—particularly a triple-drug regimen of tetracycline, streptomycin, and rifampin.)

TULAREMIA

Essentials of Diagnosis

- Fever, headache, nausea, and prostration.
- Papule progressing to ulcer at site of inoculation.
- Enlarged regional lymph nodes.
- History of contact with rabbits, other rodents, and biting arthropods (eg, ticks in summer) in endemic area.
- Serologic tests or culture of ulcer, lymph node aspirate, or blood confirm the diagnosis.

General Considerations

Tularemia is an infection of wild rodents—particularly rabbits and muskrats—with *Francisella (Pasteurella) tularensis*. Humans usually acquire the infection by contact with animal tissues (eg, trapping muskrats, skinning rabbits) or from ticks. Infection in humans often produces a local lesion and widespread organ involvement but may be entirely asymptomatic. The incubation period is 2–10 days.

Clinical Findings

A. Symptoms and Signs: Fever, headache, and nausea begin suddenly, and a local lesion—a papule at the site of inoculation—develops and soon ulcerates. Regional lymph nodes may become enlarged and tender and may suppurate. The local lesion may be on the skin of an extremity (ulceroglandular) or in the eye. Pneumonia may develop from hematogenous spread of the organism or may be primary after inhalation of infected aerosols. Following ingestion of infected meat or water, an enteric form (typhoidal) may be manifested by enteritis, stupor, and delirium. In any type of involvement, the spleen may be enlarged and tender and there may be rashes, generalized aches, and prostration.

B. Laboratory Findings: Culture of blood, an ulcerated lesion, or lymph node aspirate usually is negative unless inoculated special media are used. For this reason and because cultures of *F tularensis* may be hazardous to laboratory personnel, the diagnosis is usually made serologically. A positive agglutination test (> 1:80) develops in the second week after infection and may persist for several years.

Differential Diagnosis

Tularemia must be differentiated from rickettsial and meningococcal infections, cat-scratch disease, infectious mononucleosis, and various pneumonias and fungal diseases. Epidemiologic considerations and rising agglutination titers are the chief differential point.

Complications

Hematogenous spread to any organ may produce severe problems, particularly meningitis, perisplenitis, pericarditis, and pneumonia.

Treatment

Streptomycin, 0.5 g intramuscularly every 6–8 hours, together with tetracycline 0.5 g orally every 6 hours, is administered until 4–5 days after the patient becomes afebrile. Chloramphenicol may be substituted for tetracycline in the same dosage.

Evans ME et al: Tularemia: A 30-year experience with 88 cases. Medicine 1985;64:251. (With photographs.)

Penn RL, Kinasewitz GT: Factors associated with a poor outcome in tularemia. Arch Intern Med 1987;147:265. (Role of underlying illness and importance of early therapy, which should include an aminoglycoside.)

PLAGUE

Essentials of Diagnosis

- Sudden onset of high fever, malaise, muscular pains, and prostration.
- Axillary or inguinal lymphadenitis (bubo).
- Bacteremia, sepsis, and pneumonitis may occur.
- History of exposure to rodents in endemic area.
- Positive smear and culture from bubo and positive blood culture.

General Considerations

Plague is an infection of wild rodents with *Yersinia (Pasteurella) tularensis,* a small gram-negative rod. It is transmitted among rodents and to humans by the bites of fleas or from ingestion of feces of fleas. Persons usually acquire the infection by contact with rodents and fleas from a plague-endemic area. If a plague victim develops pneumonia, the infection can be transmitted by droplets to other persons and an epidemic may be started in this way. The incubation period is 2–10 days.

Following the flea bite, the organisms spread through the lymphatics to the lymph nodes, which become greatly enlarged (bubo). They may then reach the bloodstream to involve all organs. When pneumonia or meningitis develops, the outcome is often fatal.

Clinical Findings

A. Symptoms and Signs: The onset is sudden, with high fever, malaise, tachycardia, intense headache, and generalized muscular aches. The patient appears profoundly ill. Delirium may ensue. If pneumonia develops, tachypnea, productive cough, blood-tinged sputum, and cyanosis also occur. Meningeal signs may develop. A pustule or ulcer at the site of inoculation and signs of lymphangitis may occur. Axillary, inguinal, or cervical lymph nodes become enlarged and tender and may eventually suppurate and drain. With hematogenous spread, the patient may rapidly become toxic and comatose, with purpuric spots (black plague) appearing on the skin.

Primary plague pneumonia results from the inhalation of bacilli in droplets coughed up by another patient with plague pneumonia. This is a fulminant pneumonitis with bloody, frothy sputum and sepsis and is usually fatal unless treatment is started within a few hours of onset.

B. Laboratory Findings: The plague bacillus may be found in smears from aspirates of buboes examined with Gram's stain. Cultures from bubo aspirate or pus and blood are positive but may grow slowly. In convalescing patients, an antibody titer rise may be demonstrated by agglutination tests.

Differential Diagnosis

The lymphadenitis of plague is most commonly mistaken for the lymphadenitis accompanying staphylococcal or streptococcal infections of an extremity, sexually transmitted diseases such as lymphogranuloma venereum or syphilis, and tularemia. The systemic manifestations resemble those of enteric or rickettsial fevers, malaria, or influenza. The pneumonia resembles other bacterial pneumonias.

Prevention

Periodic surveys of rodents and their ectoparasites in endemic areas provide guidelines for the need for extensive rodent and flea control measures. Endemic areas in the United States areas include California, Nevada, Arizona, and particularly New Mexico.

Drug prophylaxis may provide temporary protection for persons exposed to the risk of plague infection, particularly by the respiratory route. Tetracycline hydrochloride, 500 mg orally 1–2 times daily for 5 days, can accomplish this.

Plague vaccines—both live and killed—have been used for many years, but their efficacy is not clearly established. They are given as directed by the manufacturer.

Treatment

Therapy must be started promptly when plague is suspected. Give streptomycin, 1 g intramuscularly, immediately, and then 0.5 g intramuscularly every 6–8 hours. Tetracycline, 2 g daily orally (parenterally if necessary), is given at the same time. Intravenous fluids, pressor drugs, oxygen, and intubation and mechanical ventilation are used as required. Patients with plague pneumonia should be strictly isolated.

Welty TK: Plague. Am Fam Physician. 1986; 33(6):159. (Presentation, diagnosis, therapy, and prevention.)

GONOCOCCAL INFECTIONS

Essentials of Diagnosis

- Purulent urethral discharge, especially in men, with dysuria, yielding positive smear.

- Epididymitis, prostatitis, periurethral inflammation, proctitis in men.
- Cervicitis in women with purulent discharge, or asymptomatic, yielding positive culture. Vaginitis, salpingitis, proctitis in women.
- Disseminated disease with fever, rash, tenosynovitis, and arthritis.
- Gram-negative intracellular diplococci seen in a smear or cultured from any site, particularly the urethra, cervix, pharynx, and rectum.

General Considerations

Gonorrhea is the most prevalent reportable communicable disease in the USA, with an estimated 2.5 million or more infectious cases annually. It is caused by *Neisseria gonorrhoeae*, a gram-negative diplococcus typically found inside polymorphonuclear cells. It is most commonly transmitted during sexual activity and has its greatest incidence in the 15- to 29-year-old age group. The incubation period is usually 2–8 days.

Differential Diagnosis

The chief alternatives to acute gonococcal urethritis or cervicitis are nongonococcal urethritis; cervicitis or vaginitis due to *Chlamydia trachomatis, Gardnerella (Haemophilus) vaginalis, Trichomonas, Candida,* and many other agents associated with sexually transmitted diseases; pelvic inflammatory disease, arthritis, proctitis, and skin lesions. Often, several such agents coexist in a patient. Reiter's disease (urethritis, conjunctivitis, arthritis) may mimic gonorrhea or coexist with it.

Prevention

Prevention is based on education, mechanical or chemical prophylaxis, and early diagnosis and treatment. The condom, if properly used, can reduce the risk of infection. Effective drugs taken in therapeutic doses within 24 hours of exposure can abort an infection, but prophylaxis with penicillin is ineffective and contributes to the selection of penicillinase-producing gonococci.

Ophthalmic infection of the newborn is prevented by the instillation of 0.5% erythromycin ointment, 1% tetracycline ointment, or 1% silver nitrate solution into each conjunctival sac immediately after birth. Ceftriaxone, 125 mg intramuscularly once, is effective against both eye and systemic infections.

Treatment

Therapy typically is administered before antimicrobial susceptibilities are known. The choice of which regimen to use should be based on the prevalence of penicillin-resistant organisms within the community and should be made in consultation with the local health department. When the prevalence is 1% or greater, ceftriaxone is the preferred agent.

A. Uncomplicated Gonorrhea: All sexual partners should be treated. For urethritis or cervicitis, give procaine penicillin G, 4.8 million units intramuscularly once with probenecid, 1 g orally once; amoxicillin, 3 g orally, plus probenecid, 1 g orally, once; or ceftriaxone, 125–250 mg intramuscularly once. Anal gonorrhea in women responds to the same drugs, but in males only ceftriaxone is effective. Pharyngeal gonorrhea responds to ceftriaxone in the same dosage or to trimethoprim-sulfamethoxazole, 9 regular strength tablets orally for 5 days.

Since coexistent chlamydial infection is common, the above courses should be followed by erythromycin or tetracycline, 500 mg 4 times daily orally, for 7 days. The latter is sometimes given concurrently.

B. Penicillin-Resistant Gonorrhea: β-Lactamase-producing gonococci are increasing in frequency. For such infections, give ceftriaxone, 125–250 mg intramuscularly once, or spectinomycin, 2 g intramuscularly once.

C. Follow-Up: Urethral, rectal, or pharyngeal specimens should be obtained from men 1 week after treatment. Cervical, rectal, or pharyngeal specimens should be obtained from women 7–14 days after completion of treatment. Serologic tests for syphilis should also be obtained.

D. Treatment of Other Infections: Salpingitis, prostatitis, bacteremia, arthritis, and other complications in adults should be treated with penicillin G, 10 million units intravenously daily, for 5 days. Ceftriaxone, 2 g intravenously daily for 5 days, also is effective.

Postgonococcal urethritis or cervicitis, usually caused by Chlamydia, is treated with tetracycline or erythromycin, 0.5 g orally 4 times daily, for 7–10 days. Pelvic inflammatory disease requires cefoxitin, 2 g parenterally every 8 hours. Concurrent treatment for chlamydial infection also is indicated. Alternative drug choices exist.

Centers for Disease Control: Antibiotic resistant strains of *N gonorrhoeae:* Policy guidelines for detection, management and control. MMWR 1987;36(Suppl 5S). (Recommendations for therapy of gonococcal urethritis, cervicitis, etc.)

Judson FN. Management of antibiotic-resistant *Neisseria gonorrhoeae.* Ann Intern Med 1989;110:5. (Ceftriaxone, 125 mg, as single-dose therapy.)

1. GONOCOCCAL URETHRITIS & CERVICITIS

In men, there is initially burning on urination and a serous or milky discharge. One to 3 days later, the urethral pain is more pronounced and the discharge becomes yellow, creamy, and profuse, sometimes blood-tinged. Without treatment, the disorder may regress and become chronic or progress to involve the prostate, epididymis, and periurethral glands with acute, painful inflammation. This in turn becomes chronic, with prostatitis and urethral strictures. Rectal infection is common in homosexual men. Unusual sites of primary infection (eg, the pharynx) must always be considered. Systemic involvement is listed below. Asymptomatic infection is common.

In women, dysuria, frequency, and urgency may occur, with a purulent urethral discharge. Vaginitis and cervicitis with inflammation of Bartholin's glands are common. Most often, however, the infection is asymptomatic, with only slightly increased vaginal discharge and moderate cervicitis on examination. Infection may remain as a chronic cervicitis—a main reservoir of gonococci in any community. It may progress to involve the uterus and tubes with acute and chronic salpingitis and with ultimate scarring of tubes and sterility. In pelvic inflammatory disease, anaerobes and chlamydiae often accompany gonococci. Rectal infection is common both as spread of the organism from the genital tract and as a result of infection by anal coitus. Systemic involvement is listed below.

Smears of urethral discharge in men, especially during the first week after onset, usually show typical gram-negative diplococci in polymorphonuclear leukocytes. Smears are less often positive in women. Cultures are essential in all cases where gonorrhea is suspected and gonococci cannot be shown in gram-stained smears. This applies particularly to cervical, rectal, pharyngeal, and joint specimens. Specimens of pus or secretions are streaked on a selective medium such as Thayer-Martin or Transgrow. The latter is suitable for transport if a laboratory is not immediately available. The medium must be 20 °C when inoculated and must be incubated at 37 °C in a 10% CO_2 atmosphere (closed Transgrow bottle; Thayer-Martin in candle jar). Colonies are identified by oxidase test, Gram's stain, or immunofluorescence. No good serologic test is available.

2. DISSEMINATED GONOCOCCAL DISEASE

Systemic complications follow the dissemination of gonococci from the primary site via the bloodstream. Gonococci that produce bacteremia and dissemination are resistant to serum but usually sensitive to penicillin. They belong to certain nutritionally deficient auxotypes. In contrast, strains producing local gonorrhea are susceptible to the bactericidal action of serum but often drug-resistant. Gonococcal bacteremia is associated with intermittent fever, arthralgia, and skin lesions ranging from maculopapular to pustular or hemorrhagic, which tend to be few in number and peripherally located. Rarely, gonococcal endocarditis or meningitis develops. Arthritis and tenosynovitis are common complications, particularly involving the knees, ankles, and wrists. Several joints are commonly involved. Gonococci can be isolated from less than half of patients with gonococcal arthritis. In

the others, some immunologic reaction may be responsible.

Disseminated meningococcemia may cause a similar syndrome.

Rompalo AM et al: The acute arthritis-dermatitis syndrome: The changing importance of *Neisseria gonorrhoeae* and *Neisseria meningitidis*. Arch Intern Med 1987;147:281. (Clinical similarity of meningococcemia to disseminated gonococcal infection, and possible increase in incidence of the former.)

3. GONOCOCCAL CONJUNCTIVITIS

The most common form of eye involvement is direct inoculation of gonococci into the conjunctival sac. In adults, this occurs by autoinoculation of a person with genital infection. The purulent conjunctivitis may rapidly progress to panophthalmitis and loss of the eye unless treated promptly. A single 1-g dose of ceftriaxone is effective.

Haimovici R, Roussel TJ: Treatment of gonococcal conjunctivitis with single dose intramuscular ceftriaxone. Am J Ophthalmol 1989;107:511. (Sterile cultures 6 hours after treatment.)

CHANCROID

Chancroid is a sexually transmitted disease caused by the short gram-negative bacillus *Haemophilus ducreyi*. Nonvenereal inoculation has occurred in medical personnel through contact with chancroid patients. The incubation period is 3–5 days.

The initial lesions at the site of inoculation is a vesicopustule that breaks down to form a painful, soft ulcer with a necrotic base, surrounding erythema, and undermined edges. Multiple lesions—started by autoinoculation—and inguinal adenitis often develop. The adenitis is usually unilateral and consists of tender, matted nodes of moderate size with overlying erythema. These may become fluctuant and rupture spontaneously. With lymph node involvement, fever, chills, and malaise may develop. No external signs may be evident in women, although they can serve as sources of infection for contacts.

Swabs from lesions are best cultured on chocolate agar with 1% Isovitalex and vancomycin, 3 mg/mL, to yield *H ducreyi*. Mixed sexually transmitted disease is very common (including syphilis and herpes), as is infection of the ulcer with fusiforms, spirochetes, and other organisms.

Balanitis and phimosis are frequent complications.

Chancroid must be differentiated from other genital ulcers. The chancre of syphilis, by contrast, is clean and painless, with a hard base.

Treatment is with erythromycin, 0.5 g orally 4 times daily for 7 days; or trimethoprim-sulfamethoxazole, one double-strength tablet twice daily for 7 days. Single-dose regimens are also effective: trimethoprim-sulfamethoxazole, 3 double-strength tablets; ciprofloxacin, 500 mg; or ceftriaxone, 250 mg intramuscularly.

Schmid GP: The treatment of chancroid. JAMA 1986; 255:1757. (Efficacy of single- and multiple-dose regimens.)

Bodhidatta L et al: Evaluation of 500 mg and 1000 mg doses of ciprofloxacin for the treatment of chancroid. Antimicrob Agents Chemother 1988;32:723. (Cure rates of 93–100%.)

GRANULOMA INGUINALE

Granuloma inguinale is a chronic, relapsing granulomatous anogenital infection due to *Calymmatobacterium (Donovania) granulomatis*. The pathognomonic cell, found in tissue scrapings or secretions, is large (25–90 μm) and contains intracytoplasmic cysts filled with bodies (Donovan bodies) that stain deeply with Wright's stain.

The incubation period is 8 days to 12 weeks.

The onset is insidious. The lesions occur on the skin or mucous membranes of the genitalia or perineal area. They are relatively painless infiltrated nodules that soon slough. A shallow, sharply demarcated ulcer forms, with a beefy-red friable base of granulation tissue. The lesion spreads by contiguity. The advancing border has a characteristic rolled edge of granulation tissue. Large ulcerations may advance onto the lower abdomen and thighs. Scar formation and healing may occur along one border while the opposite border advances. The process may become indolent.

The characteristic Donovan bodies are found in scrapings from the ulcer base or on histologic sections. The microorganism may also be cultured on special media.

Superinfection with spirochete-fusiform organisms is common. The ulcer then becomes purulent, painful, foul-smelling, and extremely difficult to treat.

Several therapies are available. Because of the indolent nature of the disease, duration of therapy tends to be relatively long. Erythromycin or tetracycline, 500 mg 4 times a day for 21 days is effective. Ampicillin, 500 mg 4 times a day, also is effective, but up to 12 weeks of therapy may be necessary.

Since other sexually transmitted diseases frequently coexist, cultures for these and a serologic test for syphilis must be performed.

Faro S: Lymphogranuloma venereum, chancroid, granuloma inguinale. Obstet Gynecol Clin North Am 1989; 16:517. (Presentation, diagnosis, and therapy.)

CAT-SCRATCH DISEASE

Essentials of Diagnosis

- A primary infected ulcer or papule-pustule at site of inoculation (30% of cases).
- Regional lymphadenopathy that often suppurates.
- History of scratch by cat at involved area.
- Positive intradermal test.

General Considerations

This is an acute infection that occurs worldwide and is more common in children and young adults in contact with cats and dogs. It may be transmitted by a scratch or other injury, but some proved cases lack such a history. The cause (based on morphologic and immunologic evidence) appears to be a small gram-negative bacterium seen in lesions, especially on the walls of capillaries and inside macrophages.

Clinical Findings

A. Symptoms and Signs: A few days after the scratch, about one-third of patients develop a primary lesion at the site of inoculation. This primary lesion appears as an infected, scabbed ulcer or a papule with a central vesicle or pustule. One to 3 weeks later, symptoms of generalized infection appear (fever, malaise, headache), and the regional lymph nodes become enlarged without evidence of lymphangitis. The nodes may be tender and fixed, with overlying inflammation; or nontender, discrete, and without evidence of surrounding inflammation. Suppuration may occur, with the discharge of sterile pus. While the course is usually benign, some adults have fever and severe systemic symptoms for weeks.

Lymph node enlargement must be differentiated from that of lymphoma, tuberculosis, lymphogranuloma venereum, and acute bacterial infection.

B. Laboratory Findings: The sedimentation rate is elevated, the white blood cell count is usually normal, and the pus from the nodes is sterile. Intradermal skin testing with antigen prepared from the pus is positive (tuberculinlike reaction) in most cases. Lymph node morphology is fairly characteristic; excisional biopsy confirms the diagnosis.

Complications

Encephalitis occurs rarely. Macular or papular rashes and erythema nodosum are occasionally seen. A disseminated form has been described in HIV-infected persons and other immunocompromised individuals.

Treatment

In immunocompetent individuals, antimicrobial therapy is unnecessary since symptoms resolve without treatment in one or 2 weeks. Therapy for disseminated disease is not well defined, but isoniazid, rifampin, or erythromycin may be active (anecdotal evidence).

English CK et al: Cat-scratch disease: Isolation and culture of the bacterial agent. JAMA 1988;259:1347. (Culture and susceptibility testing of an isolate that appeared to be derived from a cell wall-defective variant.)

Koehler JE et al: Cutaneous vascular lesions and disseminated cat-scratch disease in patients with the acquired immunodeficiency syndrome (AIDS) and AIDS-related complex. Ann Intern Med 1988;109:449. (Four cases and response to therapy.)

ANAEROBIC INFECTIONS

A large majority of the bacteria that make up the normal human flora are anaerobes. Prominent members of the normal microbial flora of the mouth (anaerobic spirochetes, *Bacteroides*, fusobacteria), the skin (anaerobic diphtheroids), the large bowel (*Bacteroides*, anaerobic streptococci, clostridia), and the female tract (*Bacteroides*, anaerobic streptococci, fusobacteria) may produce disease when displaced from their normal sites into tissues or closed body spaces.

Certain characteristics are suggestive of anaerobic infections: (1) They tend to involve mixtures of organisms, frequently several anaerobes. (2) They tend to form closed-space infections, either in discrete abscesses (lung, brain, pleura, peritoneum) or by burrowing through tissue layers. (3) Pus from anaerobic infections often has a foul odor. (4) Septic thrombophlebitis and metastatic suppurative lesions are frequent and often require surgical drainage in addition to antimicrobial therapy. (Most of the important anaerobes except *Bacteroides fragilis* are highly sensitive to penicillin G, but the diminished blood supply that favors proliferation of anaerobes because of reduced tissue oxygenation also interferes with the delivery of antimicrobials to the site of anaerobic infection.) (5) Bacteriologic examination may yield negative results or only inconsequential aerobes unless rigorous anaerobic culture conditions are used, employing collection methods and media suitable for fastidious organisms.

The following is a brief listing of important types of infections that are most commonly caused by anaerobic organisms. Treatment of all these infections consists of surgical exploration and judicious excision in conjunction with administration of antimicrobial drugs.

Upper Respiratory Tract

Bacteroides melaninogenicus together with anaerobic spirochetes is commonly involved in periodontal infections. These organisms, fusobacteria, and peptostreptococci are responsible for a substantial percentage of cases of chronic sinusitis and probably of peritonsillar abscess, chronic otitis media, and mastoiditis. Hygiene and drainage are usually more important in treatment than antimicrobials, but penicillin G is the drug of choice, 1–2 million units intravenously every 4 hours if parenteral therapy is required or 0.5 g orally 4 times daily for less severe infections. In the penicillin-allergic patient, clindamycin can be used (600 mg intravenously every 8 hours or 300 mg orally every 6 hours).

Chest Infections

Aspiration of saliva (which contains 10^8 anaerobic organisms per milliliter in addition to aerobes) may lead to pneumonitis, necrotizing pneumonia, lung abscess, and empyema. While polymicrobial infection is the rule, anaerobes—particularly *B melaninogenicus*, fusobacteria, and peptostreptococci—are common etiologic agents. Most of these organisms are susceptible to penicillin G and tend to respond to drug treatment combined with surgical drainage when indicated.

Penicillin-resistant *B fragilis* and *B melaninogenicus* are found in about 20% of anaerobic chest infections, but these still usually respond to penicillin G, 10 million units daily intravenously. Alternative drugs of equal efficacy include clindamycin and chloramphenicol.

Central Nervous System

While anaerobes only rarely produce meningitis, they are a common cause of brain abscess, subdural empyema, or septic central nervous system thrombophlebitis. The organisms reach the central nervous system by direct extension from sinusitis, otitis, or mastoiditis or by hematogenous spread from chronic lung infections. Antimicrobial therapy—eg, 20 million units intravenously, either alone or in combination with chloramphenicol, 50 mg/kg/d in 4 divided doses, or metronidazole, 750 mg intravenously every 8 hours—is an important adjunct to surgical drainage. It appears that some small multiple brain abscesses can be treated with antibiotics alone for 6–8 weeks and may heal without surgical drainage.

Intra-abdominal Infections

In the colon there are up to 10^{11} anaerobes per gram of content—predominantly *B fragilis*, clostridia, and peptostreptococci. These organisms play a central etiologic role in most intra-abdominal abscesses following trauma to the colon, diverticulitis, appendicitis, or perirectal abscess and may also participate in hepatic abscess and cholecystitis, often in association with aerobic coliform bacteria.

The gallbladder wall may be infected with clostridia as well. Infections associated with perforation of the lower bowel are usually polymicrobial. The bacteriology includes anaerobes as well as enteric gram-negative rods and on occasion enterococci. Therapy should be directed at all of these organisms in the seriously ill patient and may require multiple drugs. Antibiotics reliably active against *B fragilis* include metronidazole, chloramphenicol, imipenem, ampicillin-sulbactam (Unasyn) and ticarcillin-clavulanic acid (Timentin). Cefoxitin, cefotetan, and clindamycin are active against 80–90% of strains, but third-generation cephalosporins have poor activity, inhibiting only 50% of isolates.

A number of options are available for the treatment of these mixed infections. One common regimen includes ampicillin (or vancomycin) to treat the enterocci, metronidazole to cover anaerobes, and gentamicin for enteric gram-negative rods. Other examples might include imipenem alone (very expensive), ampicillin-sulbactam alone or in combination with gentamicin, clindamycin with gentamicin, and cefoxitin or cefotetan alone or with gentamicin.

Although the normal flora of the upper intestinal tract is more sparse than that of the colon, anaerobes comprise a large portion of it.

Female Genital Tract & Pelvic Infections

The normal flora of the vagina and cervix includes several species of *Bacteroides,* peptostreptococci, group B streptococci, lactobacilli, coliform bacteria, and, occasionally, spirochetes and clostridia. These organisms commonly cause genital tract infections and may disseminate from there.

While salpingitis is commonly caused by gonococci and chlamydiae, tubo-ovarian and pelvic abscesses are associated with anaerobes in a majority of cases. Postpartum infections may be caused by aerobic streptococci or staphylococci, but in most instances anaerobes are found, and the most severe cases of postpartum or postabortion sepsis are associated with clostridia and *Bacteroides.* These have a high mortality rate, and treatment requires both antimicrobials directed against anaerobes and coliforms (see above) and abscess drainage or early hysterectomy.

Bacteremia & Endocarditis

Anaerobes are responsible for 5–10% of cases of bacteremia seen in general hospitals. Most of these originate from the gastrointestinal tract, the oropharynx, decubitus ulcers, and the female genital tract and—until now—have been associated with a high mortality rate. Endocarditis due to anaerobic and microaerophilic streptococci and *Bacteroides* originates in the same sites. Rigorous anaerobic cultures to identify the causative organism and institute specific and adequate treatment are essential in patients whose "routine" blood cultures have remained negative but who are suspected clinically of having endocarditis. Most cases of streptococcal endocarditis can be effectively treated with 12–20 million units of penicillin G daily, but optimal therapy of other types of anaerobic bacterial endocarditis must rely on laboratory guidance. Anaerobic corynebacteria *(Propionibacterium),* clostridia, and *Bacteroides* occasionally cause endocarditis. *Bacteroides* bacteremia may cause disseminated intravascular coagulation.

Skin & Soft Tissue Infections

Anaerobic infections in the skin and soft tissue usually follow trauma, inadequate blood supply, or surgery and are commonest in areas that are contaminated by oral or fecal flora. There is often rapidly progressive tissue necrosis and a putrid odor.

Bacterial synergistic gangrene is a painful ulcerating lesion that commonly follows laparotomy performed as part of the management of intra-abdominal infections but produces little fever or systemic toxicity. It is usually caused by a mixture of anaerobic streptococci and *Staphylococcus aureus.* It requires wide excision of the discolored skin and (later) skin grafts, but recovery is the rule.

Synergistic necrotizing cellulitis progresses more rapidly, with high fever and often positive blood cultures for peptostreptococci, *Bacteroides,* and aerobic gram-negative bacteria. It occurs with greatest frequency on the perineum and the lower extremities and has a high mortality rate. Excision of necrotic tissue must be combined with antimicrobial drugs to attempt early control.

Necrotizing fasciitis is a mixed anaerobic or aerobic infection that rapidly dissects deep fascial planes and produces severe toxicity with a mortality rate of up to 30%. Anaerobic streptococci and *S aureus* are the commonest etiologic organisms. Extensive surgical incisions through fascial planes are needed.

Nonclostridial crepitant cellulitis is an infection of subcutaneous or deeper tissues with peptostreptococci and coliform bacteria that leads to gas formation in tissue, with minimal toxicity, lack of muscle involvement, and a good prognosis. Improved perfusion, incision and drainage, and antimicrobial drugs are often successful.

Differentiation of these syndromes on clinical grounds is difficult. Because the infections are often polymicrobial and because the patients are usually acutely ill, broad-spectrum antibiotics active against both anaerobes and gram-positive and gram-negative aerobes are instituted (eg, vancomycin plus metronidazole plus gentamicin or tobramycin). Once the bacteriology has been defined by culture, antibiotics specific for isolated organisms can be given. Antibiotics are given for about a week after progressive tissue destruction has been controlled and the margins of the wound remain free of inflammation.

Bartlett JG: Anaerobic bacterial infections of the lung. Chest 987;91:901.

Brook I: Anaerobic bacterial bacteremia: 12-year experience in two military hospitals. J Infect Dis 1989;160:1071.

Styrt B, Gorbach SL: Recent developments in the understanding of the pathogenesis and treatment of anaerobic infections. (Two parts.) N Engl J Med 1989;321:240, 298.

ACTINOMYCOSIS

Actinomyces israelii and other species of *Actinomyces* occur in the normal flora of the mouth and tonsillar crypts. They are anaerobic, gram-positive, branching filamentous bacteria (1 μm in diameter) that may fragment into bacillary forms. When introduced into traumatized tissue and associated with other anaerobic bacteria, these actinomycetes become pathogens.

The most common site of infection is the cervicofacial area (about 60% of cases). Infection typically follows extraction of a tooth or other trauma. Lesions may develop in the gastrointestinal tract or lungs following ingestion or aspiration of the fungus from its endogenous source in the mouth.

Cervicofacial actinomycosis develops slowly. The area becomes markedly indurated, and the overlying skin becomes reddish or cyanotic. The surface is irregular ("lumpy jaw"). Abscesses developing within and eventually draining to the surface persist for long periods. Sulfur granules—masses of filamentous organisms—may be found in the pus. There is usually little pain unless there is marked secondary infection. Trismus indicates that the muscles of mastication are involved. Radiography reveals eventual involvement of the bone, with rarefaction as well as some proliferation of the underlying bone.

Thoracic actinomycosis begins with fever, cough, and sputum production. The patient becomes weak, loses weight, and may have night sweats and dyspnea. Pleuritic pain may be present. Multiple sinuses may extend through the chest wall, to the heart, or into the abdominal cavity. Ribs may be involved. Radiography shows areas of consolidation and the frequent presence of pleural effusion. Occasionally, cervicofacial or thoracic disease may result in central nervous system complications, most commonly brain abscesses or meningitis.

Abdominal actinomycosis usually causes pain in the ileocecal region, spiking fever and chills, intestinal colic, vomiting, and weight loss and may be confused with Crohn's disease. Irregular masses in the ileocecal area or elsewhere in the abdomen may be palpated. Pelvic inflammatory disease caused by actinomycetes is associated with prolonged use of an intrauterine contraceptive device. Sinuses draining to the exterior may develop. Radiography may reveal the mass or enlarged viscera. Vertebrae and pelvic bones may be invaded.

The sedimentation rate may be elevated in patients with progressive disease. Anemia and leukocytosis are usually present. The anaerobic, gram-positive organism may be demonstrated as a granule or as scattered branching gram-positive filaments in the pus. Anaerobic culture is necessary to distinguish *Actino-* *myces* species from *Nocardia* species. Specific identification by culture is necessary to avoid confusion with nocardiosis, because specific therapy differs radically.

Penicillin G is the drug of choice. Ten to 20 million units are given via a parenteral route for 2–4 weeks, followed by oral penicillin V, 500 mg 4 times daily.

Sulfonamides such as sulfamethoxazole may be an alternative regimen at a total daily dosage of 2–4 g. Response to therapy is slow. Therapy should be continued for weeks to months after clinical manifestations have disappeared in order to ensure cure. Surgical procedures such as drainage and resection may be beneficial.

With penicillin and surgery, the prognosis is good. The difficulties of diagnosis, however, may permit extensive destruction of tissue before the diagnosis is identified and therapy is started.

Smego RA Jr. Actinomycosis of the central nervous system. Rev Infect Dis 1987;9:855. (Review of cases, prognosis, and therapy.)

NOCARDIOSIS

Nocardia asteroides and *Nocardia brasiliensis*, aerobic filamentous soil bacteria, cause pulmonary and systemic nocardiosis. Bronchopulmonary abnormalities (eg, alveolar proteinosis) predispose to colonization, but infection is unusual without underlying cellular immunodeficiency.

Pulmonary involvement usually begins with malaise, loss of weight, fever, and night sweats. Cough and production of purulent sputum are the chief complaints. Radiography may show infiltrates accompanied by pleural effusion. The lesions may penetrate to the exterior through the chest wall, invading the ribs.

Dissemination may involve any organ. Abscesses in the brain and subcutaneous nodules are most frequent. Dissemination is seen exclusively in immunocompromised patients, such as those receiving chronic corticosteroid therapy.

N asteroides is usually found as delicate, branching, gram-positive filaments that may be partially acid-fast. Identification is made by culture.

Therapy is initiated with intravenous trimethoprim-sulfamethoxazole and continued with oral trimethoprim-sulfamethoxazole, one double-strength tablet twice a day. In experimental cerebral nocardiosis of the rat, imipenem-cilastatin and amikacin appear more effective than trimethoprim-sulfamethoxazole or minocycline for treatment. Surgical procedures such as drainage and resection may be needed as adjunctive therapy.

Response may be slow, and therapy must be continued for at least 6 months. The prognosis in systemic nocardiosis is poor when diagnosis and therapy are delayed.

Gombert ME et al: Therapy of experimental cerebral nocardiosis with imipenem, amikacin, trimethoprim-sulfamethoxazole, and minocycline. Antimicrob Agents Chemother 1986;30:270. (Imipenem and amikacin have similar efficacy, followed by TMP-SMZ, then minocycline.)

Wilson JP et al. *Nocardia* infections in renal transplant recipients. Medicine 1989;68:38. (Review of the literature.)

INFECTIONS CAUSED BY MYCOBACTERIA

NONTUBERCULOUS ATYPICAL MYCOBACTERIAL DISEASES

About 10% of mycobacterial infections seen in clinical practice are caused not by *Mycobacterium tuberculosis* but by atypical mycobacteria. These organisms have distinctive laboratory characteristics, occur ubiquitously in the environment, are not communicable from person to person, and are often strikingly resistant to antituberculous drugs. Some representative species and clinical presentations are discussed briefly here.

Pulmonary Infections

Pulmonary disease can be produced by a number of different atypical mycobacterial species. *Mycobacterium kansasii* can produce clinical disease resembling tuberculosis, but the illness progresses more slowly. Most such infections occur in patients with preexisting lung disease, though 40% of patients have no known pulmonary disease. Microbiologically, *M kansasii* is similar to *M tuberculosis* and is sensitive to the same drugs that are active against *M tuberculosis*. Therapy with isoniazid, ethambutol, and rifampin for 2 years (or 1 year after sputum conversion) has been highly successful.

The *Mycobacterium avium-intracellulare* (MAI) complex produces asymptomatic colonization or a wide spectrum of diseases, including coin lesions, bronchitis in patients with chronic lung disease, and invasive pulmonary disease that is often cavitary and occurs in patients with underlying lung disease. It is a particularly common cause of pulmonary disease, positive blood cultures, and systemic symptoms in patients with AIDS. These organisms are usually highly drug-resistant and may require as many as 5 drugs for effective therapy. Agents that may be active against the MAI complex of organisms include rif-

ampin, rifabutine (formerly ansamycin, a rifampin analogue), cycloserine, ethionamide, clofazimine, ethambutol, amikacin, and ciprofloxacin. Because of the toxicity of treatment, antimycobacterial therapy is limited to patients with invasive pulmonary disease or AIDS patients with severe systemic symptoms such as disabling fever, fatigue, and weight loss. Generally colonized patients, coin lesions that have been resected, and bronchitis do not require therapy.

Less common causes of pulmonary disease include *Mycobacterium xenopi*, *Mycobacterium szulgai*, and *Mycobacterium gordonae*. These organisms have variable sensitivities, and treatment is based on results of sensitivity tests. *Mycobacterium fortuitum* and *Mycobacterium chelonei* also can cause pneumonia.

Lymphadenitis

Most cases of lymphadenitis (scrofula) in adults are caused by *Mycobacterium tuberculosis* and are a manifestation of disseminated disease. In children, the majority of cases are caused by nontuberculous mycobacterial species, with *Mycobacterium scrofulaceum* being the most common cause. *Mycobacterium kansasii*, *Mycobacterium bovis*, *Mycobacterium chelonei, and Mycobacterium fortuitum* are less common causes. Unlike disease caused by *M tuberculosis*, which requires systemic therapy for 9 months, infection with nontuberculous mycobacteria can be successfully treated by surgical excision without antituberculous therapy.

Skin & Soft Tissues

Skin and soft tissue infections such as abscesses, septic arthritis, and osteomyelitis can result from direct inoculation or hematogenous dissemination or may occur as a complication of surgery.

M chelonei and *M fortuitum* are frequent causes of this type of infection. Most cases occur in the extremities and initially present as nodules. Ulceration with abscess formation often follows. The organisms are resistant to the usual antituberculous drugs but may be sensitive to a variety of antibiotics, including erythromycin, doxycycline, amikacin, cefoxitin, sulfonamides, imipenem, and ciprofloxacin. Therapy includes surgical debridement along with drug therapy. Initially, parenteral drugs are given for several weeks, and this is followed by an oral regimen to which the organism is sensitive. The duration of therapy is variable but usually continues for several months after the soft tissue lesions have healed.

Mycobacterium marinum infection (''swimming pool granuloma'') presents as a nodular skin lesion following exposure to nonchlorinated water. The lesions respond to therapy with doxycycline, minocycline, or trimethoprim-sulfamethoxazole.

Mycobacterium ulcerans infection (Buruli ulcer) is seen mainly in Africa and Australia and produces a large ulcerative lesion. Therapy consists of surgical excision and skin grafting.

Iseman MD et al: Diseases due to *Mycobacterium avium-intracellulare*. Chest 1985;87:1395.

Jacobson MA: Mycobacterial diseases: Tuberculosis and *Mycobacterium avium* complex. Infect Dis Clin North Am 2:465,1988. (Epidemiology, diagnosis, and therapy is discussed for these diseases in AIDS patients.)

Woods GL, Washington JA: Mycobacteria other than *M tuberculosis:* Review of microbiologic and clinical aspects. Rev Infect Dis 1987;9:275.

MYCOBACTERIUM TUBERCULOSIS INFECTIONS

Although *Mycobacterium tuberculosis* most commonly causes pulmonary infection (see Chapter 7), this organism can cause disease virtually anywhere in the body. Extrapulmonary infection, which accounts for approximately 15% of all tuberculosis, is particularly common in HIV-infected individuals. Tuberculosis adenitis, pleural effusion, urinary tract infection, peritonitis, bone and joint infection, and meningitis are the more common extrapulmonary infections. Disseminated disease is present in 5–10% of extrapulmonary cases.

Clinical findings and treatment of tuberculosis are considered in chapters pertaining to the organ system infected. Generally speaking, regimens that are effective for pulmonary tuberculosis also are effective in extrapulmonary disease. Meningitis, with its special problems of drug penetration into the cerebrospinal fluid and its tendency to cause serious neurologic deficit, is discussed below.

Chaisson RE, Slutkin G: Tuberculosis and human immunodeficiency virus infection. J Infect Dis 1989;159:96. (Clinical review.)

TUBERCULOUS MENINGITIS

Essentials of Diagnosis

- Gradual onset of listlessness, irritability, and anorexia.
- Headache, vomiting, coma, convulsions; neck and back rigidity.
- Tuberculosis focus may be evident elsewhere.
- Cerebrospinal fluid shows several hundred lymphocytes, low glucose, and high protein.

General Considerations

Tuberculous meningitis is caused by rupture of a meningeal tuberculoma resulting from earlier hematogenous seeding of a tubercle bacilli from a pulmonary focus, or it may be a consequence of miliary spread. Its greatest incidence is in children aged 1–5 years.

Clinical Findings

A. Symptoms and Signs: The onset is usually gradual, with listlessness, irritability, anorexia, and fever, followed by headache, vomiting, convulsions, and coma. In older patients, headache and behavioral changes are prominent early symptoms. Nuchal rigidity, opisthotonos, and paralysis occur as the meningitis progresses. Cranial nerve palsies may result from inflammation of the basilar meninges. Evidence of active tuberculosis elsewhere or a history of prior tuberculosis is present in up to 75% of patients.

B. Laboratory Findings: The spinal fluid is frequently yellowish, with increased pressure, 100–500 cells/μL (early, polymorphonuclear neutrophils; later, lymphocytes), increased protein, and decreased glucose. Acid-fast stains of cerebrospinal fluid usually are negative, and cultures also may be negative in at least 25% of cases. Chest x-ray often reveals a tuberculosis focus.

Differential Diagnosis

Tuberculous meningitis may be confused with any other type of meningitis, but the gradual onset, the predominantly lymphocytic pleocytosis of the spinal fluid, and evidence of tuberculosis elsewhere often point to the diagnosis.

Fungal and other granulomatous meningitides or rare neoplasms must be considered also.

Complications

Stroke, cranial nerve palsies, seizures, mental impairment, and abnormal behavior may occur. The incidence of these complications increases the later therapy is started.

Prevention

Early identification of tuberculin converters and children with primary tuberculosis—and treatment with isoniazid at that stage—is the key to preventing tuberculous meningitis.

Treatment

Untreated tuberculous meningitis is usually fatal within several weeks after onset. Presumptive diagnosis followed by early, empiric antituberculous therapy is essential for survival and to minimize sequelae. Even if cultures are not positive, a full course of therapy may be warranted if the clinical setting is suggestive of tuberculous meningitis.

Regimens that are effective for pulmonary tuberculosis are effective also for tuberculous meningitis. Rifampin, isoniazid, and pyrazinamide all penetrate into cerebrospinal fluid well. The penetration of ethambutol is more variable, but therapeutic concentrations can be achieved, and the drug has been successfully used for meningitis. Aminoglycosides penetrate less well. An effective 4-drug short-course regimen consists of giving isoniazid, 300 mg/d, and rifampin, 600 mg/d, for 6 months, plus pyrazinamide, 25 mg/kg/d in 2 divided doses, and ethambutol, 15 mg/kg/d, for the first 2 months. The same doses of isoniazid and rifampin may also be given as a 2-drug regimen for 9 months. Other regimens may also be effective, but they are less reliable and generally must be given for longer periods.

Patients should be monitored for drug toxicities, which consist chiefly of hepatitis, rash, and gastrointestinal intolerance. Toxicity from ethambutol is unusual at the 15 mg/kg/d dose in the patient with normal renal function. Pyridoxine, 50 mg daily, will prevent peripheral neuropathy from isoniazid and should be given to patients at risk for this side effect (eg, alcoholics, diabetics, HIV-infected persons).

Some authorities recommend the addition of corticosteroids for patients with focal deficits or altered mental status. Prednisone, 60 mg/d for 1–2 weeks, then discontinued in a tapering regimen over 4 weeks, may be used.

LEPROSY

Essentials of Diagnosis

- Pale, anesthetic macular—or nodular and erythematous—skin lesions.
- Superficial nerve thickening with associated anesthesia.
- History of residence in endemic area in childhood.
- Acid-fast bacilli in skin lesions or nasal scrapings, or characteristic histologic nerve changes.

General Considerations

Leprosy is a chronic infectious disease caused by the acid-fast rod *Mycobacterium leprae*. The mode of transmission probably is respiratory and involves prolonged exposure in childhood. Only rarely have adults become infected. The disease is endemic in tropical and subtropical Asia, Africa, Central and South America and the Pacific regions, and the southern USA.

Clinical Findings

A. Symptoms and Signs: The onset is insidious. The lesions involve the cooler body tissues: skin, superficial nerves, nose, pharynx, larynx, eyes, and testicles. Skin lesions may occur as pale, anesthetic macular lesions 1–10 cm in diameter; discrete erythematous, infiltrated nodules 1–5 cm in diameter; or a diffuse skin infiltration. Neurologic disturbances are manifested by nerve infiltration and thickening, with resultant anesthesia, neuritis, and paresthesia. Trophic ulcers and bone resorption and shortening of digits ensue. In untreated cases, disfigurement due to the skin infiltration and nerve involvement may be extreme.

The disease is divided clinically and by laboratory tests into 2 distinct types: lepromatous and tuberculoid. The lepromatous type occurs in persons with defective cellular immunity. The course is progressive and malignant, with nodular skin lesions; slow, sym-

metric nerve involvement; abundant acid-fast bacilli in the skin lesions; and a negative lepromin skin test. In the tuberculoid type, cellular immunity is intact and the course is benign and nonprogressive, with macular skin lesions, severe asymmetric nerve involvement of sudden onset with few bacilli present in the lesions, and a positive lepromin skin test. Intermediate ("borderline") cases are frequent. Eye involvement (keratitis and iridocyclitis), nasal ulcers, epistaxis, anemia, and lymphadenopathy may occur.

B. Laboratory Findings: Laboratory confirmation of leprosy requires the demonstration of acid-fast bacilli in scrapings from slit skin smears or the nasal septum. Biopsy of skin or of a thickened involved nerve also gives a typical histologic picture.

M leprae has not been grown in culture media, but it multiplies in experimentally injected mouse foot pads and in armadillos.

Differential Diagnosis

The skin lesions of leprosy often resemble those of lupus erythematosus, sarcoidosis, syphilis, erythema nodosum, erythema multiforme, cutaneous tuberculosis, and vitiligo. Nerve involvement may require differentiation from syringomyelia and scleroderma.

Complications

Renal failure from amyloidosis may occur with long-standing disease.

Treatment

Combination therapy is recommended for treatment of all types of leprosy. Single-drug treatment is accompanied by emergence of resistance, and some untreated patients may be infected with dapsone-resistant organisms. For borderline and lepromatous cases, a 3-drug regimen such as dapsone, 50–100 mg/d, clofazimine, 50 mg/d, and rifampin, 10 mg/kg/d (up to 600 mg/d), all given orally, should be used. Ethionamide, 250–375 mg/d, may be substituted for clofazimine. For indeterminate and tuberculoid leprosy, the dapsone-rifampin combination is recommended for at least 6 months, followed by a course of dapsone alone.

Because of the tendency for relapse, treatment must be continued for years—up to 5 years for the tuberculoid type. The large number of organisms that are present and defective immunity in lepromatous leprosy may require lifelong therapy. Isolation of patients under treatment is not necessary.

Two reactional states—erythema nodosum leprosum and reversal reactions—may occur as a consequence of therapy. The reversal reaction, typical of borderline lepromatous leprosy, probably results from enhanced host immunity. Skin lesions and nerves become swollen and tender, but systemic manifestations are not seen. Erythema nodosum leprosum, typical of lepromatous leprosy, is a consequence of immune injury from antigen-antibody complex deposition in skin and other tissues; in addition to skin and nerve manifestations, fever and systemic involvement may be seen. High-dose corticosteroids or thalidomide, 300 mg/d (in the nonpregnant patient only), is effective for erythema nodosum leprosum. Corticosteroids are indicated for treatment of reversal reactions. Therapy for leprosy should not be discontinued during treatment of reactional states.

Freerksen E, Rosenfeld M, Spannuth G: New forms of multidrug therapy for the treatment of leprosy. Chemotherapy 1989;35:133. (Promising new 3-drug regimens.)

INFECTIONS CAUSED BY *CHLAMYDIA*

Chlamydiae are a large group of obligate intracellular parasites closely related to gram-negative bacteria. They are assigned to 3 species—*Chlamydia trachomatis, Chlamydia psittaci,* and *Chlamydia pneumoniae*—on the basis of intracellular inclusions, sulfonamide susceptibility, antigenic composition, and disease production. *C psittaci* causes psittacosis in humans and many animal diseases. *Chlamydia pneumoniae,* TWAR strain, is a newly identified species that caused respiratory tract infections. *C trachomatis* causes many different human infections involving the eye (trachoma, inclusion conjunctivitis), the genital tract (lymphogranuloma venereum, nongonococcal urethritis, cervicitis, salpingitis), or the respiratory tract (pneumonitis). A few specific diseases are described.

CHLAMYDIA TRACHOMATIS INFECTIONS

1. LYMPHOGRANULOMA VENEREUM

Essentials of Diagnosis

- Evanescent primary genital lesion.
- Lymph node enlargement, softening, and suppuration, with draining sinuses.
- Proctitis and rectal stricture in women or homosexual men.
- Positive complement fixation test.

General Considerations

Lymphogranuloma venereum is an acute and chronic sexually transmitted disease caused by *Chlamydia trachomatis* types L1–L3. After the genital lesion disappears, the infection spreads to lymph channels and lymph nodes of the genital and rectal areas. The disease is acquired during intercourse or through contact with contaminated exudate from active le-

sions. The incubation period is 5–21 days. Inapparent infections and latent disease are not uncommon in promiscuous individuals.

Clinical Findings

A. Symptoms and Signs: In men, the initial vesicular or ulcerative lesion (on the external genitalia) is evanescent and often goes unnoticed. Inguinal buboes appear 1–4 weeks after exposure, are often bilateral, and have a tendency to fuse, soften, and break down to form multiple draining sinuses, with extensive scarring. In women, the genital lymph drainage is to the perirectal glands. Early anorectal manifestations are proctitis with tenesmus and bloody purulent discharge; late manifestations are chronic cicatrizing inflammation of the rectal and perirectal tissue. These changes lead to obstipation and rectal stricture and, occasionally, rectovaginal and perianal fistulas. They are also seen in homosexual men.

Systemic invasion may occur, causing fever, arthralgia, arthritis, skin rashes, conjunctivitis, and iritis. Nervous system invasion causes headache and meningeal irritation. Pneumonia can develop in laboratory workers who inhale aerosols of the organisms.

B. Laboratory Findings: The complement fixation test may be positive, but cross-reaction with other chlamydiae occurs. Although a positive reaction may reflect remote infection, high titers usually indicate active disease. Specific immunofluorescence tests for IgM are more specific for acute infection.

Differential Diagnosis

The early lesion of lymphogranuloma venereum must be differentiated from the lesions of syphilis, genital herpes, and chancroid; lymph node involvement must be distinguished from that due to tularemia, tuberculosis, plague, neoplasm, or pyogenic infection; rectal stricture must be differentiated from that due to neoplasm and ulcerative colitis.

Treatment

The antibiotics of choice are the tetracyclines, 0.25–0.5 g orally 4 times daily, or doxycycline, 0.1 g twice daily for 10–20 days. Erythromycin, 500 mg 4 times a day, or trimethoprim-sulfamethoxazole, 160/800 mg twice a day for 14 days, also is effective.

Quinn TC et al: *Chlamydia trachomatis* proctitis. N Engl J Med 1981;305:195.

Walzer PD, Armstrong D: Lymphogranuloma venereum presenting as supraclavicular and inguinal lymphadenopathy. Sex Transm Dis 1977;4:12.

2. CHLAMYDIAL URETHRITIS & CERVICITIS

Some males develop symptomatic or asymptomatic anterior urethritis from which gonococci cannot be isolated by available laboratory tests. This is referred to as nongonococcal urethritis. *Chlamydia trachomatis* immunotypes D-K can be isolated in about 50% of such cases by appropriate techniques. In other cases, a *Mycoplasma, Ureaplasma urealyticum,* can be grown as a possible etiologic agent. In still others, gonococcal urethritis is diagnosed and treated; afterward, gonococci can no longer be found, but postgonococcal urethritis persists. Some of the latter cases can be attributed to chlamydiae or mycoplasmas that were present originally in a mixed infection. Occasionally, epididymitis, prostatitis, or proctitis is caused by chlamydial infection.

The female sexual partners of men with chlamydial nongonococcal urethritis often are infected with the same organisms symptomatically or asymptomatically. Chlamydiae are often recovered from the cervix, and there may be overt cervicitis, salpingitis, or pelvic inflammatory disease. Males or females with genital chlamydial infection may infect the eye through finger contact and develop a follicular conjunctivitis ("inclusion conjunctivitis") that may become chronic and lead to pannus formation.

Diagnosis often is clinical and by exclusion, ie, failure to identify gonococci in a patient with urethritis or cervicitis. The urethral or cervical discharge tends to be less painful, less purulent, and more watery in chlamydial versus gonococcal infection. Absence of gram-negative intracellular diplococci in urethral discharge from a male is very suggestive of chlamydial infection. Culture is reliable but sometimes unavailable. Rapid monoclonal immunofluorescent antibody detection methods are about 75% sensitive.

Therapy often must be given presumptively. Effective treatment regimens are tetracycline or erythromycin, 500 mg 4 times a day, or doxycycline, 100 mg twice daily, for 7–10 days. Trimethoprim-sulfamethoxazole, 160/800 mg twice a day, is acceptable but may be less effective than tetracyclines or erythromycin. Erythromycin is the drug of choice in the pregnant patient.

CHLAMYDIA PSITTACI & PSITTACOSIS (Ornithosis)

Essentials of Diagnosis

- Fever, chills, malaise, prostration; cough, epistaxis; occasionally, rose spots and splenomegaly.
- Atypical pneumonia with slightly delayed appearance of signs of pneumonitis. Isolation of chlamydiae or rising titer of complement-fixing antibodies.
- Contact with infected bird (psittacine, pigeons, many others) 7–15 days previously.

General Considerations

Psittacosis is acquired from contact with birds (par-

rots, parakeets, pigeons, chickens, ducks, and many others).

Clinical Findings

A. Symptoms and Signs: In psittacosis, the onset is usually rapid, with fever, chills, headache, backache, malaise, myalgia, epistaxis, dry cough, and prostration. Signs include those of pneumonitis, alteration of percussion note and breath sounds, and rales. Pulmonary findings may be absent early. Rose spots, splenomegaly, and meningismus are occasionally seen. Delirium, constipation or diarrhea, and abdominal distress may occur. Dyspnea and cyanosis may occur later. Endocarditis, which is culture-negative, may occur.

B. Laboratory Findings: The organism is rarely isolated from cultures. The diagnosis is usually made serologically; antibodies appear during the second week and can be demonstrated by complement fixation or immunofluorescence. Antibody response may be suppressed by early chemotherapy.

C. Imaging: The radiographic findings in typical psittacosis are those of atypical pneumonia, which tends to be interstitial and diffuse in appearance, though consolidation can occur. Psittacosis is indistinguishable from other bacterial or viral pneumonias by radiography.

Differential Diagnosis

This disease can be differentiated from acute viral, mycoplasmal, or rickettsial pneumonias only by the history of contact with potentially infected birds and by laboratory tests. Rose spots and leukopenia suggest typhoid fever. Psittacosis is in the differential diagnosis of culture-negative endocarditis.

Treatment

Treatment consists of giving tetracycline, 0.5 g orally every 6 hours or 0.5 g intravenously every 12 hours, for 14–21 days.

McPhee SJ, Erb B, Harrington W: Psittacosis. West J Med 1987;146:91. (Microbiology, epidemiology, and clinical review.)

CHLAMYDIA PNEUMONIAE, TWAR STRAIN

Chlamydia pneumoniae is a newly recognized species that was initially thought to be related to *C psittaci.* Studies have shown that it is morphologically, serologically, and genetically unique.

C pneumoniae is more difficult to isolate in culture than *C trachomatis* or *C psittaci,* and diagnosis often has been based on serology. Difficulty in culturing the organism has hampered efforts to define precisely the clinical disease caused by it. Nevertheless, TWAR strains clearly can cause upper and lower respiratory tract infections that can be severe. The clinical presentation of pneumonia is that of an atypical pneumonia, resembling that caused by *Mycoplasma pneumoniae*. It has been estimated that up to 10% of pneumonias may be associated with TWAR strains.

Like *C psittaci*, TWAR strains are resistant to sulfonamide drugs. Erythromycin or tetracycline, 500 mg 4 times a day for 10–14 days, appears to be effective therapy.

Grayston JT: *Chlamydia pneumoniae*, strain TWAR. Chest 1989;95:664. (Microbiology, epidemiology, clinical review.)

Grayston JT et al: A new *Chlamydia psittaci* strain, TWAR, isolated in respiratory tract infection. N Engl J Med 1986;315:161. (First study suggesting *Chlamydia* as a respiratory tract pathogen.)

Infectious Diseases: Spirochetal

Richard A. Jacobs, MD, PhD

SYPHILIS

NATURAL HISTORY & PRINCIPLES OF DIAGNOSIS & TREATMENT

Syphilis is a complex infectious disease caused by *Treponema pallidum,* a spirochete capable of infecting almost any organ or tissue in the body and causing protean clinical manifestations (Table 27–1). Transmission occurs most frequently during sexual contact, through minor skin or mucosal lesions; sites of inoculation are usually genital but may be extragenital. The organism is extremely sensitive to heat and drying but can survive for days in fluids; therefore, it can be transmitted in blood from infected persons. Syphilis can be transferred via the placenta from mother to fetus after the tenth week of pregnancy (congenital syphilis).

The immunologic response to infection is complex, but it provides the basis for most clinical diagnoses. The infection induces the synthesis of a number of antibodies, some of which react specifically with pathogenic treponemes and some with components of normal tissues (see below). If the disease is untreated, sufficient defenses develop to produce a relative resistance to reinfection; however, in most cases these immune reactions fail to eradicate existing infection and may contribute to tissue destruction in the late stages. Patients treated early in the disease are fully susceptible to reinfection.

The natural history of acquired syphilis is generally divided into 2 major clinical stages: early (infectious) syphilis and late syphilis. The 2 stages are separated by a symptom-free latent phase during the first part of which (early latency) the infectious stage is liable to recur. Infectious syphilis includes the primary lesions (chancre and regional lymphadenopathy); the secondary lesions (commonly involving skin and mucous membranes, occasionally bone, central nervous system, or liver); relapsing lesions during early latency; and congenital lesions. The hallmark of these lesions is an abundance of spirochetes; tissue reaction is usually minimal. Late syphilis consists of so-called benign (gummatous) lesions involving skin, bones, and viscera; cardiovascular disease (principally aortitis); and a variety of central nervous system and ocular syndromes. These forms of syphilis are not contagious. The lesions contain few demonstrable spirochetes, but tissue reactivity (vasculitis, necrosis) is severe and suggestive of hypersensitivity phenomena.

As a result of intensive public health efforts during and after World War II, there was a reduction in the incidence of infectious syphilis. With the marked increase in all sexually transmitted diseases since the 1970s, there has been a rise in the number of reported cases of syphilis. In the 1980s, the incidence of infectious syphilis was particularly high among homosexual males. There has also been a dramatic increase in congenital syphilis. Reinfection in treated persons is common. No appreciable rise in the incidence of congenital syphilis has been reported yet.

Laboratory Diagnosis

Since the infectious agent of syphilis cannot be cultured in vitro, diagnostic measures must rely mainly on serologic testing, microscopic detection of *T pallidum* in lesions, and other examinations (biopsies, lumbar puncture, x-rays) for evidence of tissue damage.

A. Serologic Tests for Syphilis: (Table 27–2.) There are 2 general categories of serologic tests for syphilis: (1) nontreponemal tests, which use a component of normal tissue (eg, beef heart cardiolipin) as an antigen to measure nonspecific antibodies (reagin) formed in the blood of patients with syphilis; and (2) treponemal tests, which employ live or killed *T pallidum* as antigen to detect antibodies specific for pathogenic treponemes.

1. Nontreponemal antigen tests–Commonly employed nontreponemal antigen tests are of 2 types: flocculation (VDRL, RPR) and complement fixation (Kolmer, Wassermann). The flocculation tests are easy, rapid, and inexpensive to perform and are therefore used primarily for routine (often automated) screening for syphilis. Quantitative expression of the reactivity of the serum, based upon titration of dilutions of serum, may be valuable in establishing the diagnosis and in evaluating the efficacy of treatment.

The VDRL test (the nontreponemal test in widest

Table 27–1. Stages of syphilis and common clinical manifestations.

Primary syphilis
  Genital ulcer: painless ulcer with clean base and firm indurated boarders
  Regional lymphadenopathy
Secondary syphilis
  Skin and mucous membranes
    Rash: diffuse (including palms and soles), macular, papular, pustular, and combinations
    Condylomata lata
    Mucous patches: painless, silvery ulcerations of mucous membrane with surrounding erythema.
  Generalized lymphadenopathy
  Constitutional symptoms
    Fever, usually low-grade
    Malaise
    Anorexia
    Arthralgias and myalgias
  Central nervous system
    Asymptomatic
    Symptomatic
      Headache
      Meningitis
      Cranial neuropathies (II–VIII)
  Ocular
    Iritis
    Iridocyclitis
  Other
    Renal: glomerulonephritis, nephrotic syndrome
    Liver: hepatitis
    Bone and joint: arthritis, periostitis
Late syphilis
  Late benign (gummatous): granulomatous lesion usually involving skin, mucous membranes and bones, but any organ can be involved.
  Cardiovascular
    Aortic insufficiency
    Coronary ostial stenosis
    Aortic aneurysm
  Neurosyphilis
    Asymptomatic
    Meningovascular
      Seizures
      Hemiparesis or hemiplegia
    Tabes dorsalis
      Impaired proprioception and vibratory sensation
      Argyll Robertson pupil
      Shooting pains
      Ataxia
      Romberg's sign
      Urinary and fecal incontinence
      Charcot joint
      Cranial nerve involvement (II–VIII)
    General paresis
      Personality changes
      Hyperactive reflexes
      Argyll Robertson pupil
      Decreased memory
      Slurred speech
      Optic atrophy

Table 27–2. Percentage of patients with positive serologic tests for syphilis.[1]

Test	Stage		
	Primary	Secondary	Tertiary
VDRL[2]	70–75%	99%	75%
FTA-ABS[3]	85–95%	100%	98%

[1] Based on untreated cases.
[2] VDRL = Venereal Disease Research Laboratory test.
[3] FTA-ABS = Fluorescent treponemal antibody test.

factory response to treatment. These serologic tests are not highly specific and must be closely correlated with other clinical and laboratory findings. The tests are positive in patients with non-sexually transmitted treponematoses (see below). More importantly, "false-positive" serologic reactions are frequently encountered in a wide variety of nontreponemal states, including collagen diseases, infectious mononucleosis, malaria, febrile diseases, leprosy, drug addiction, old age, and perhaps pregnancy. False-positive reactions are usually of low titer and transient and may be distinguished from true positives by specific treponemal antibody tests. The rapid plasma reagin (RPR) test is a simple, rapid, and reliable substitute for the traditional VDRL test. RPR titers are often higher than VDRL titers and thus are not comparable. The RPR test is suitable for automated screening.

2. Treponemal antibody tests– The fluorescent treponemal antibody absorption (FTA-ABS) test is the most widely employed treponemal test. It measures antibodies capable of reacting with killed *T pallidum* after absorption of the patient's serum with extracts of nonpathogenic treponemes. The FTA-ABS test is of value principally in determining whether a positive nontreponemal antigen test is "false-positive" or is indicative of syphilis. Because of its great sensitivity, particularly in the late stages of the disease, the FTA-ABS test is also of value when there is clinical evidence of syphilis but the nontreponemal serologic test for syphilis is negative. The test is positive in most patients with primary syphilis and in virtually all with secondary syphilis, and it usually remains positive permanently in spite of successful treatment. False-positive FTA-ABS tests occur rarely in systemic lupus erythematosus and in other disorders associated with abnormal globulins. A treponemal passive hemagglutination (TPHA) test is comparable in specificity and sensitivity to the FTA-ABS test but may become positive somewhat later in infection.

Final decisions about the significance of the results of serologic tests for syphilis must be based upon a total clinical appraisal.

B. Microscopic Examination: In infectious syphilis, *T pallidum* may be shown by darkfield microscopic examination of fresh exudate from lesions or material aspirated from regional lymph nodes. The darkfield examination requires considerable experi-

use) generally becomes positive 4–6 weeks after infection, or 1–3 weeks after the appearance of a primary lesion; it is almost invariably positive in the secondary stage. The VDRL titer is usually high (> 1:32) in secondary syphilis and tends to be lower (< 1:4) or even negative in late forms of syphilis. A falling titer in treated early or latent syphilis suggests a satis-

ence and care in the proper collection of specimens and in the identification of pathogenic spirochetes by observing characteristic features of morphology and motility. Repeated examinations may be necessary. Spirochetes usually are not found in late syphilitic lesions by this technique.

An immunofluorescent staining technique for demonstrating *T pallidum* in dried smears of fluid taken from early syphilitic lesions is available. Slides are fixed and treated with fluorescein-labeled antitreponemal antibody that has been preabsorbed with nonpathogenic treponemes. The slides are then examined for fluorescing spirochetes in an ultraviolet microscope. Because of its simplicity and convenience to physicians (slides can be mailed), this technique has replaced darkfield microscopy in most health departments and medical center laboratories.

C. Spinal Fluid Examination: Cerebrospinal fluid findings in neurosyphilis are variable. In "classic" cases there is an elevation of total protein, lymphocytic pleocytosis, and a positive cerebrospinal fluid reagin test (VDRL). However, cerebrospinal fluid may be completely normal in neurosyphilis, and the VDRL may be negative. In one recent study, 25% of patients with primary or secondary syphilis in whom *T pallidum* was isolated from cerebrospinal fluid had a normal cerebrospinal fluid examination. In later stages of syphilis, normal cerebrospinal fluid analysis in the presence of infection can occur, but it is unusual. Because false-positive reagin tests rarely occur in the cerebrospinal fluid, a positive test confirms the presence of neurosyphilis. Because the cerebrospinal fluid VDRL may be negative in neurosyphilis, *a negative test does not exclude neurosyphilis.*

Cerebrospinal fluid examination is highly recommended in all cases of secondary syphilis or latent syphilis not previously adequately treated. Asymptomatic neurosyphilis (ie, positive cerebrospinal fluid findings without symptoms) requires prolonged penicillin treatment as given for symptomatic neurosyphilis. Adequate treatment is indicated by gradual decrease in cerebrospinal fluid cell count, protein concentration, and VDRL titer. Rarely, serologic tests of cerebrospinal fluid may remain positive for years after adequate treatment of neurosyphilis even though all other parameters have returned to normal. In the presence of high-titer serum FTA-ABS, there may be a positive FTA test on cerebrospinal fluid in the absence of neurosyphilis.

Treatment

A. Specific Measures:

1. Penicillin, as benzathine penicillin G or aqueous procaine penicillin G, is the drug of choice for all forms of syphilis and other spirochetal infections. Effective tissue levels must be maintained for several days or weeks because of the spirochete's long generation time. Penicillin is highly effective in early infections and variably effective in the late stages. The principal contraindication is hypersensitivity to the penicillins. The recommended treatment schedules are included below in the discussion of the various forms of syphilis.

2. Other antibiotic therapy–Oral tetracyclines and erythromycins are effective in the treatment of syphilis for patients who are sensitive to penicillin. Tetracycline, 30–40 g, or erythromycin, 30–40 g, is given over a period of 10–15 days in early syphilis; twice as much is recommended for syphilis of more than 1 year's duration. Experience with these drugs in the treatment of syphilis is limited, and some failures have been reported. Careful follow-up is therefore mandatory.

B. Local Measures (Mucocutaneous Lesions): Local treatment is usually not necessary. No local antiseptics or other chemicals should be applied to a suspected syphilitic lesion until specimens for microscopy have been obtained.

C. Public Health Measures: Patients with infectious syphilis must abstain from sexual activity until rendered noninfectious by antibiotic therapy. All cases of syphilis must be reported to the appropriate public health agency for assistance in identifying, and treating contacts.

D. Epidemiologic Treatment: Patients who have been exposed to infectious syphilis within the preceding 3 months may be infected but seronegative and thus should be treated as for early syphilis. Others at high risk for infection—ie, those with other sexually transmitted diseases—should undergo serologic tests for syphilis. The present recommended therapy for gonorrhea (ceftriaxone and doxycycline) is probably effective against incubating syphilis. If alternative regimens are used to treat gonorrhea, follow-up serologic studies should be performed in 3 months.

Complications of
Specific Therapy

The Jarisch-Herxheimer reaction is ascribed to the sudden massive destruction of spirochetes by drugs and release of toxic products and is manifested by fever and aggravation of the existing clinical picture. It is most likely to occur in early syphilis. Treatment should not be discontinued unless the symptoms become severe or threaten to be fatal or unless syphilitic laryngitis, auditory neuritis, or labyrinthitis is present, where the reaction may cause irreversible damage.

The reaction may be prevented or modified by simultaneous administration of antipyretics. It usually begins within the first 24 hours and subsides spontaneously within the next 24 hours of penicillin treatment.

Follow-Up Care

Patients who receive treatment for early syphilis should be followed clinically and with periodic quantitative VDRL tests for at least 1 year. Patients with all other types of syphilis should be under similar observation for 2 or more years.

Prevention

Avoidance of sexual contact is the only completely reliable method of prophylaxis but is an impractical public health measure for obvious reasons.

A. Mechanical: The standard rubber condom is effective but protects covered parts only. The exposed parts should be washed with soap and water as soon after contact as possible. This applies to both sexes.

B. Antibiotic: If there is known exposure to infectious syphilis, abortive penicillin therapy may be used. Give 2.4 million units of procaine penicillin G intramuscularly. Treatment of gonococcal infection with penicillins, tetracyclines, and ceftriaxone is probably effective against incubating syphilis in most cases. However, other antimicrobial agents (eg, spectinomycin) may be ineffective in aborting preclinical syphilis. In view of the increasing use of antibiotics other than penicillin for gonococcal disease, patients treated for gonorrhea should have a serologic test for syphilis 3–6 months after treatment.

Course & Prognosis
(See Table 27–3.)

The lesions associated with primary and secondary syphilis are self-limiting and resolve with few or no residua. Late syphilis may be highly destructive and permanently disabling and may lead to death. With treatment, the nontreponemal serologic tests usually return to negative in early syphilis. In late latent and late syphilis, serofastness is not uncommon even after adequate treatment. In broad terms, if no treatment is given, about one-third of people infected with syphilis will undergo spontaneous cure, about one-third will remain in the latent phase throughout life, and about one-third will develop serious late lesions.

Brown ST et al: Serological response to syphilis treatment. JAMA 1985;253:1296.
Centers for Disease Control 1989: Sexually transmitted diseases: Treatment guidelines 1989. MMWR 1989;38:S8.
Jackman JD Jr, Radolf JD: Cardiovascular syphilis. Am J Med 1989;87:425.
Lukehart SA et al: Invasion of the central nervous system by *Treponema pallidum:* Implications for diagnosis and treatment. Ann Intern Med 1988;109:855.
Musher DM: How much penicillin cures early syphilis? Ann Intern Med 1988;109:849.

CLINICAL STAGES OF SYPHILIS

1. PRIMARY SYPHILIS

Essentials of Diagnosis

● History of sexual contact (often unreliable).
● Painless ulcer on genitalia, perianal area, rectum, pharynx, tongue, lip, or elsewhere 2–6 weeks after exposure.
● Nontender enlargement of regional lymph nodes.
● Fluid expressed from lesion contains *T pallidum* by immunofluorescence or darkfield microscopy.
● Serologic test for syphilis often positive.

General Considerations

This is the stage of invasion and may pass unrecognized. The typical lesion is the chancre at the site or sites of inoculation, most frequently located on the penis, labia, cervix, or anorectal region. Anorectal lesions are especially common among male homosexuals. The primary lesion occurs occasionally in the oropharynx (lip, tongue, or tonsil) and rarely on the breast or finger. The chancre starts as a small erosion 10–90 days (average, 3–4 weeks) after inoculation that rapidly develops into a painless superficial ulcer with a clean base and firm, indurated margins, associated with enlargement of regional lymph nodes, which are rubbery, discrete, and nontender. Bacterial infection of the chancre may occur and may lead to pain. Healing occurs without treatment, but a scar may form, especially with secondary bacterial infection.

Table 27–3. Natural course of untreated syphilis.

Stage of Disease	Likelihood of Developing Clinical Manifestations (%)	Comment
Latent	24%	90% of relapses occur in first year after infection.
Late Benign (gummatous)	15%	Many patients have more than one late manifestation.
Cardiovascular	10%	Only seen in those who develop syphilis after 15 years of age. Pathologic findings more common, ie, 50–80%.
Neurosyphilis	6.5%	Asymptomatic neurosyphilis has been reported in 8–40%.

Laboratory Findings

The serologic test for syphilis is usually positive 1–2 weeks after the primary lesion is noted; rising titers are especially significant when there is a history of previous infection. Immunofluorescence or dark-field microscopy shows treponemes in at least 95% of chancres. The spinal fluid is normal at this stage.

Differential Diagnosis

The syphilitic chancre may be confused with chancroid, lymphogranuloma venereum, genital herpes, or neoplasm. Any lesion on the genitalia should be considered a possible primary syphilitic lesion.

Treatment

Benzathine penicillin G, 2.4 million units intramuscularly in the gluteal area, is given once. For the penicillin-allergic patient (who is not pregnant), doxycycline, 100 mg orally twice daily for 2 weeks, or tetracycline, 500 mg orally 4 times a day for 2 weeks, can be used. If tetracyclines cannot be given, erythromycin, 500 mg orally 4 times a day for 2 weeks, can be substituted.

2. SECONDARY SYPHILIS

Essentials of Diagnosis

- Generalized maculopapular skin rash.
- Mucous membrane lesions, including patches and ulcers.
- Weeping papules (condylomas) in moist skin areas.
- Generalized nontender lymphadenopathy.
- Fever.
- Meningitis, hepatitis, osteitis, arthritis, iritis.
- Many treponemes in scrapings of mucous membrane or skin lesions by immunofluorescence or darkfield microscopy.
- Serologic tests for syphilis always positive.

General Considerations & Treatment

The secondary stage of syphilis usually appears a few weeks (or up to 6 months) after development of the chancre, when sufficient dissemination of *T pallidum* has occurred to produce systemic signs (fever, lymphadenopathy) or infectious lesions at sites distant from the site of inoculation. The most common manifestations are skin and mucosal lesions. The skin lesions are nonpruritic, macular, papular, pustular, or follicular (or combinations of any of these types), though the maculopapular rash is the most common. The skin lesions usually are generalized; involvement of the palms and soles is especially suspicious. Annular lesions simulating ringworm are observed in blacks. Mucous membrane lesions range from ulcers and papules of the lips, mouth, throat, genitalia, and anus (''mucous patches'') to a diffuse redness of the pharynx. Both skin and mucous membrane lesions are highly infectious at this stage. Specific lesions—**condylomata lata**—are fused, weeping papules on the moist areas of the skin and mucous membranes.

Meningeal (aseptic meningitis or acute basilar meningitis), hepatic, renal, bone, and joint invasion, with resulting cranial nerve palsies, jaundice, nephrotic syndrome, and periostitis may occur. Alopecia (moth-eaten appearance), iritis, and iridocyclitis may also occur. A transient myocarditis may be manifested by temporary electrocardiographic changes.

All serologic tests for syphilis are positive in almost all cases. The cutaneous and mucous membrane lesions often show *T pallidum* on microscopic examination. There is usually a transient cerebrospinal fluid involvement, with pleocytosis and elevated protein, though only 5% of cases have positive serologic cerebrospinal fluid reactions. There may be evidence of hepatitis or nephritis (immune complex type). Circulating immune complexes exist in the blood and are deposited in blood vessel walls.

Skin lesions may be confused with the infectious exanthems, pityriasis rosea, and drug eruptions. Visceral lesions may suggest nephritis or hepatitis due to other causes. The diffusely red throat may mimic other forms of pharyngitis.

Treatment is as for primary syphilis unless central nervous system disease is present, in which case treatment is as for neurosyphilis (see below). Isolation of the patient is important.

Fiumara NJ: Treatment of secondary syphilis: An evaluation of 204 patients. Sex Transm Dis 1977;4:96.

3. RELAPSING SYPHILIS

The essentials of diagnosis are the same as in secondary syphilis.

The lesions of secondary syphilis heal spontaneously, but secondary syphilis may relapse if undiagnosed or inadequately treated. These relapses may include any of the findings noted under secondary syphilis: skin and mucous membrane, neurologic, ocular, bone, or visceral. Unlike the usual asymptomatic neurologic involvement of secondary syphilis, neurologic relapses may be fulminating, leading to death. Relapse is almost always accompanied by a rising titer in quantitative serologic tests; indeed, a rising titer may be the first or only evidence of relapse. About 90% of relapses occur during the first year after infection.

Treatment is as for primary syphilis unless central nervous system disease is present.

4. LATENT (''HIDDEN'') SYPHILIS

Essentials of Diagnosis

- No physical signs.

- History of syphilis with inadequate treatment.
- Positive treponemal serologic tests for syphilis.

General Considerations & Treatment

Latent syphilis is the clinically quiescent phase during the interval after disappearance of secondary lesions and before the appearance of tertiary symptoms. Early latency is defined as the first 4 years after infection, during which time infectious lesions may recur ("relapsing syphilis"); after 4 years, the patient is said to be in the late latent phase. Transmission to the fetus, however, can probably occur in any phase. There are (by definition) no clinical manifestations during the latent phase, and the only significant laboratory findings are positive serologic tests. A diagnosis of latent syphilis is justified only when the cerebrospinal fluid is entirely negative, x-ray and physical examination shows no evidence of cardiovascular involvement, and false-positive tests for syphilis have been ruled out. The latent phase may last from months to a lifetime.

It is important to differentiate latent syphilis from a false-positive serologic test for syphilis, which can be due to the many causes listed above.

Treatment is with benzathine penicillin G, 2.4 million units 3 times at 7-day intervals (total dose, 7.2 million units). In the penicillin-allergic patient, give tetracycline, 0.5 g orally 4 times a day for 30 days. If there is evidence of cerebrospinal fluid involvement, treat as for neurosyphilis. Only a small percentage of serologic tests will be appreciably altered by treatment with penicillin. The treatment of this stage of the disease is intended to prevent the late sequelae.

Ducas J, Robson HG: Cerebrospinal fluid penicillin levels during therapy for latent syphilis. JAMA 1981;246:2583.

5. LATE (TERTIARY) SYPHILIS

Essentials of Diagnosis

- Infiltrative tumors of skin, bones, liver (gummas).
- Aortitis, aneurysms, aortic insufficiency.
- Central nervous system disorders, including meningovascular and degenerative changes, paresthesias, shooting pains, abnormal reflexes, dementia, or psychosis.

General Considerations

This stage may occur at any time after secondary syphilis, even after years of latency, and is seen in about one-third of untreated patients (Table 27–3). Late lesions probably represent, at least in part, a delayed hypersensitivity reaction of the tissue to the organism and are usually divided into 2 types: (1) a localized gummatous reaction, with a relatively rapid onset and generally prompt response to therapy ("be-

nign late syphilis"); and (2) diffuse inflammation of a more insidious onset that characteristically involves the central nervous system and large arteries, is often fatal if untreated, and is at best arrested by treatment. Gummas may involve any area or organ of the body but most often the skin or long bones. Cardiovascular disease is usually manifested by aortic aneurysm, aortic insufficiency, or aortitis. Various forms of diffuse or localized central nervous system involvement may occur.

Late syphilis must be differentiated from neoplasms of the skin, liver, lung, stomach, or brain; other forms of meningitis; and primary neurologic lesions.

Treatment is as for latent syphilis. Reversal of positive serologic tests does not usually occur. A second course of penicillin therapy may be given if necessary. There is no known method for reliable eradication of the treponeme from humans in the late stages of syphilis. Viable spirochetes are occasionally found in the eyes, in cerebrospinal fluid, and elsewhere in patients with "adequately" treated syphilis, but claims for their capacity to cause progressive disease are speculative.

Although almost any tissue and organ may be involved in late syphilis, the following are the most common types of involvement.

Skin

Cutaneous lesions of late syphilis are of 2 varieties: (1) multiple nodular lesions that eventually ulcerate or resolve by forming atrophic, pigmented scars; and (2) solitary gummas that start as painless subcutaneous nodules, then enlarge, attach to the overlying skin, and eventually ulcerate.

Mucous Membranes

Late lesions of the mucous membranes are nodular gummas or leukoplakia, highly destructive to the involved tissue.

Skeletal

Bone lesions are destructive, causing periostitis, osteitis, and arthritis with little or no associated redness or swelling but often marked myalgia and myositis of the neighboring muscles. The pain is especially severe at night.

Eyes

Late ocular lesions are gummatous iritis, chorioretinitis, optic atrophy, and cranial nerve palsies, in addition to the lesions of central nervous system syphilis.

Respiratory System

Respiratory involvement by late syphilis is caused by gummatous infiltrates into the larynx, trachea, and pulmonary parenchyma, producing discrete pulmonary densities. There may be hoarseness, respiratory distress, and wheezing secondary to the gummatous lesion itself or to subsequent stenosis occurring with healing.

Gastrointestinal System

Gummas involving the liver produce the usually benign, asymptomatic hepar lobatum. Occasionally a picture resembling Laennec's cirrhosis is produced by liver involvement. Infiltration into the stomach wall causes "leather bottle" stomach with epigastric distress, inability to eat large meals, regurgitation, belching, and weight loss.

Cardiovascular System

Cardiovascular lesions (10–15% of late syphilitic lesions) are often progressive, disabling, and life-threatening. Central nervous system lesions are often present also. Involvement usually starts as an arteritis in the supracardiac portion of the aorta and progresses to cause one or more of the following: (1) Narrowing of the coronary ostia with resulting decreased coronary circulation, angina, cardiac insufficiency, and acute myocardial infarction. (2) Scarring of the aortic valves, producing aortic insufficiency with its water-hammer pulse, aortic diastolic murmur, frequently aortic systolic murmur, cardiac hypertrophy, and eventually congestive heart failure. (3) Weakness of the wall of the aorta, with saccular aneurysm formation and associated pressure symptoms of dysphagia, hoarseness, brassy cough, back pain (vertebral erosion), and occasionally rupture of the aneurysm. Recurrent respiratory infections are common as a result of pressure on the trachea and bronchi.

Treatment of cardiac problems requires first consideration, after which penicillin G is given as for latent syphilis.

Neurosyphilis

Neurosyphilis (15–20% of late syphilitic lesions; often present with cardiovascular syphilis) is also a progressive, disabling, and life-threatening complication. It develops more commonly in men than in women and in whites than in blacks. There are 4 clinical types.

(1) Asymptomatic neurosyphilis: This form is characterized by spinal fluid abnormalities (positive spinal fluid serology, increased cell count, occasionally increased protein) without symptoms or signs of neurologic involvement.

(2) Meningovascular syphilis: This form is characterized by meningeal involvement or changes in the vascular structures of the brain (or both), producing symptoms of low-grade meningitis (headache, irritability); cranial nerve palsies (basilar meningitis); unequal reflexes; irregular pupils with poor light and accommodation reflexes; and, when large vessels are involved, cerebrovascular accidents. The cerebrospinal fluid shows increased cells (100–1000/μL), elevated protein, and usually a positive serologic test

for syphilis. The symptoms of acute meningitis are rare in late syphilis.

(3) Tabes dorsalis: This form is a chronic progressive degeneration of the parenchyma of the posterior columns of the spinal cord and of the posterior sensory ganglia and nerve roots. The symptoms and signs are impairment of proprioception and vibration sense, Argyll Robertson pupils (which react poorly to light but well to accommodation), and muscular hypotonia and hyporeflexia. Impairment of proprioception results in a wide-based gait and inability to walk in the dark. Paresthesias, analgesia, or sharp recurrent pains in the muscles of the leg ("shooting" or "lightning" pains) may occur. Crises are also common in tabes: gastric crises, consisting of sharp abdominal pains with nausea and vomiting (simulating an acute abdomen); laryngeal crises, with paroxysmal cough and dyspnea; urethral crises, with painful bladder spasms; and rectal and anal crises. Crises may begin suddenly, last for hours to days, and cease abruptly. Neurogenic bladder with overflow incontinence is also seen. Painless trophic ulcers may develop over pressure points on the feet. Joint damage may occur as a result of lack of sensory innervation (Charcot joint). The cerebrospinal fluid may have a normal or increased cell count (3–200/μL), elevated protein, and variable results of serologic tests.

(4) General paresis: This is generalized involvement of the cerebral cortex with insidious onset of symptoms. There is usually a decrease in concentrating power, memory loss, dysarthria, tremor of the fingers and lips, irritability, and mild headaches. Most striking is the change of personality; the patient becomes slovenly, irresponsible, confused, and psychotic. Combinations of the various forms of neurosyphilis (especially tabes and paresis) are not uncommon. The cerebrospinal fluid findings resemble those of tabes dorsalis.

Special considerations in treatment of neurosyphilis. It is most important to prevent neurosyphilis by prompt diagnosis, adequate treatment, and follow-up of early syphilis. Indications for lumbar puncture vary depending upon stage of the disease. In early syphilis (primary and secondary syphilis and early latent syphilis of less than 1 year's duration), cerebrospinal fluid abnormalities occur commonly, but neurosyphilis rarely develops in patients who have received the standard therapy outlined above. Thus, unless clinical signs and symptoms of neurosyphilis are present, a lumbar puncture in early syphilis is not recommended as part of the routine evaluation. In theory, all patients with syphilis of more than 1 year's duration should have a lumbar puncture. This is rarely strictly adhered to, and each case is usually individualized. Cerebrospinal fluid evaluation is strongly suggested in the later stages of syphilis if neurologic signs and symptoms are present; therapy other than with penicillin is to be given; if the patient is HIV-positive; if serum nontreponemal antibody titers are 1:32 or higher; or if there is evidence of active syphilis at other sites (aortitis, iritis, optic atrophy, etc). In the presence of definite cerebrospinal fluid or neurologic abnormalities, treat for neurosyphilis. The pretreatment clinical and laboratory evaluation should include neurologic, ocular, psychiatric, and cerebrospinal fluid examinations.

The regimen of 2.4 million units of benzathine penicillin intramuscularly weekly for 3 consecutive weeks results in low to undetectable cerebrospinal fluid levels of penicillin, and treatment failures have been described when this regimen has been used to treat neurosyphilis. For these reasons, present recommendations for the therapy of neurosyphilis employ higher doses of short-acting penicillin in order to achieve better penetration and higher levels of drug in the cerebrospinal fluid. Recommended regimens include 2–4 million units of aqueous crystalline penicillin G intravenously every 4 hours for 10–14 days. Alternatively, 2–4 million units of procaine penicillin can be given intramuscularly once daily along with 500 mg of probenecid orally 4 times daily, both for 10–14 days. Many experts recommend 2.4 million units of benzathine penicillin intramuscularly once weekly for 3 weeks as additional therapy. Alternative therapy to penicillin has not been established for treatment of neurosyphilis, and patients with a history of penicillin allergy should be skin-tested and desensitized.

All patients should have spinal fluid examinations at 6-month intervals until the cell count is normal. Response may be gauged by clinical improvement and effective and persistent reversal of cerebrospinal fluid changes. A second course of penicillin therapy may be given if the cell count has not decreased at 6 months or is not normal at 2 years. Not infrequently, there is progression of neurologic symptoms and signs despite high and prolonged doses of penicillin. It has been postulated that these treatment failures are related to the unexplained persistence of viable *T pallidum* in central nervous system or ocular lesions in at least some cases.

Rein MF: Treatment of neurosyphilis. JAMA 1981; 246:2613.
Tramont EC: Persistence of *T pallidum* following penicillin G therapy. JAMA 1976;236:2206.

6. SYPHILIS IN HIV-INFECTED PATIENTS

Because syphilis has variable clinical manifestations and an unpredictable course, evaluation of case reports of unusual clinical or laboratory manifestations of syphilis in HIV-infected patients is difficult. Nonetheless, recent reports have suggested that in this situation syphilis may have an accelerated course, serologic response to infection may be blunted, and treatment failures with benzathine penicillin may oc-

cur more commonly. Because of concern about false-negative serologic tests, if the diagnosis of syphilis is suggested on clinical grounds but reagin tests are negative, alternative tests should be performed. These tests include darkfield examination of lesions and direct fluorescent antibody staining for *T pallidum* of lesion exudate or biopsy specimens. Treatment failures with presently recommended regimens of benzathine penicillin have been documented in HIV-infected patients. In one study, 3 of 4 patients treated with 2.4 million units of benzathine penicillin for secondary syphilis failed therapy, and all 3 were HIV-positive. Although no change in the therapy of early syphilis in patients co-infected with HIV is officially recommended, some feel that more aggressive therapy is indicated in this setting. The best treatment regimen—either 3 doses of 2.4 million units of benzathine penicillin at weekly intervals or 2.4 million units of procaine penicillin intramuscularly for 10 consecutive days, plus probenecid, 500 mg 4 times daily—is yet to be determined. Similarly, for symptomatic or asymptomatic neurosyphilis in HIV-infected patients, benzathine penicillin regimens should not be used; either aqueous penicillin intravenously or procaine penicillin intramuscularly for 10 days, as described above, should be given.

Follow-up is important in all patients with syphilis. In patients infected with HIV, nontreponemal quantitative tests should be repeated at 1, 2, and 3 months and thereafter at 3-month intervals until titers have stabilized. If titers have not fallen 2-fold by 3 months in primary syphilis or 6 months in secondary syphilis or if there is a 4-fold or greater increase in titer, the patient should have a spinal fluid examination and be re-treated. In patients with neurosyphilis, cerebrospinal fluid examination is recommended at least every 6 months until serologic parameters have stabilized as described above.

Berry CD et al: Neurologic relapse after benzathine penicillin therapy for secondary syphilis in a patient with HIV infection. N Engl J Med 1987;316:1587.
Johns DR, Tierney M, Felsenstein D: Alteration in the natural history of neurosyphilis by concurrent infection with the human immunodeficiency virus. N Engl J Med 1987;316:1569.
Lukehart SA et al: Invasion of the central nervous system by *Treponema pallidum:* Implications for diagnosis and treatment. Ann Intern Med 1988;109:855.
Recommendations for diagnosing and treating syphilis in HIV-infected patients. MMWR 1988;37:600.

7. SYPHILIS IN PREGNANCY

All pregnant women should have a nontreponemal serologic test for syphilis at the time of the first prenatal visit. Seroreactive patients should be evaluated promptly. Such evaluation includes the history (including prior therapy), a physical examination, a quantitative nontreponemal test, and a confirmatory treponemal test. If the FTA-ABS test is nonreactive and there is no clinical evidence of syphilis, treatment may be withheld. Both the quantitative nontreponemal test and the FTA-ABS test should be repeated in 4 weeks. If the diagnosis of syphilis cannot be excluded with reasonable certainty, the patient should be treated as outlined below.

Patients for whom there is documentation of adequate treatment for syphilis in the past need not be re-treated unless there is clinical or serologic evidence of reinfection (eg, 4-fold rise in titer of a quantitative nontreponemal test).

In women suspected of being at increased risk for syphilis, a second nontreponemal test should be performed during the third trimester.

The preferred treatment is with penicillin in dosage schedules appropriate for the stage of syphilis (see above). Penicillin prevents congenital syphilis in 90% of cases, even when treatment is given late in pregnancy.

Penicillin in the dosage regimens appropriate for the stage of disease is the treatment of choice for syphilis in pregnancy. Tetracycline and doxycycline are contraindicated in pregnancy, and erythromycin is associated with a high risk of failure in the fetus. Women with a history of penicillin allergy should be skin-tested and desensitized if necessary.

The infant should be evaluated immediately, as noted below, and at 6–8 weeks of age.

Centers for Disease Control 1989: Sexually transmitted diseases: Treatment guidelines 1989. MMWR 1989; 38(Suppl 8):1.
Jones JE Jr, Harris RE: Diagnostic evaluation of syphilis during pregnancy. Obstet Gynecol 1979;124:705.
Mescola L et al: Inadequate treatment of syphilis in pregnancy. Am J Obstet Gynecol 1984;150:945.

8. CONGENITAL SYPHILIS

Congenital syphilis is a transplacentally transmitted infection that occurs in infants of untreated or inadequately treated mothers. The physical findings at birth are quite variable: The infant may have many or only minimal signs or even no signs until 6–8 weeks of life (delayed form). The most common findings are on the skin and mucous membranes—serous nasal discharge (snuffles), mucous membrane patches, maculopapular rash, condylomas. These lesions are infectious; *T pallidum* can easily be found microscopically, and the infant must be isolated. Other common findings are hepatosplenomegaly, anemia, or osteochondritis. These early active lesions subsequently heal, and if the disease is left untreated it produces the characteristic stigmas of syphilis—interstitial keratitis, Hutchinson's teeth, saddle nose, saber shins, deafness, and central nervous system involvement.

The serologic evaluation for syphilis in newborn infants is complicated by the transplacental acquisition of maternal antibody (IgG). Evaluation of a newborn suspected of having congenital syphilis includes the history of maternal therapy, a careful physical examination, hematocrit (for possible anemia), a cerebrospinal fluid examination, and x-rays of long bones. It is particularly important to follow the infant every 2–3 weeks over a period of 4 months to watch for developing physical signs; a sustained rise or fall in VDRL titer during this time will reveal the need for treatment. If available, an FTA-ABS test on the purified 19S-IgM fraction of serum should be obtained. If positive, it is confirmatory of congenital syphilis.

Infants should be treated at birth if maternal treatment was inadequate, unknown, or done with drugs other than penicillin or if adequate follow-up of the infant cannot be ensured.

Therapy for congenital syphilis is 100,000–150,000 units/kg of aqueous crystalline penicillin G daily given in 2 or 3 divided doses intravenously, or 50,000 units/kg of procaine penicillin daily given as a single intramuscular injection for 10–14 days.

The quantitative nontreponemal test (VDRL) should be repeated 3, 6, and 12 months after therapy to establish falling titers. If titers fail to fall or increase at 6 months, the child should be re-treated.

Bryan EM, Nicholson E: Congenital syphilis. Clin Pediatr 1981;20:81.
Mescola L et al: Congenital syphilis revisited. Am J Dis Child 1985;139:575.

NON-SEXUALLY TRANSMITTED TREPONEMATOSES

A variety of treponemal diseases other than syphilis occur endemically in many tropical areas of the world. They are distinguished from disease caused by *T pallidum* by their nonsexual transmission, their relatively high incidence in certain geographic areas and among children, and their tendency to produce less severe visceral manifestations. As in syphilis, organisms can be demonstrated in infectious lesions with darkfield microscopy or immunofluorescence but cannot be cultured in artificial media; the serologic tests for syphilis are positive; the diseases have primary, secondary, and sometimes tertiary stages; and penicillin is the drug of choice. There is evidence that infection with these agents may provide partial resistance to syphilis and vice versa. Treatment with penicillin in doses appropriate to primary syphilis (eg, 2.4 million units of benzathine penicillin G intramuscularly) is generally curative in any stage of the non-sexually transmitted treponematoses. In cases of penicillin hypersensitivity, tetracycline is usually the recommended alternative.

YAWS
(Frambesia)

Yaws is a contagious disease largely limited to tropical regions that is caused by *Treponema pertenue*. It is characterized by granulomatous lesions of the skin, mucous membranes, and bone. Yaws is rarely fatal, though if untreated it may lead to chronic disability and disfigurement. Yaws is acquired by direct nonsexual contact, usually in childhood, although it may occur at any age. The "mother yaw," a painless papule that later ulcerates, appears 3–4 weeks after exposure. There is usually associated regional lymphadenopathy. Six to 12 weeks later, similar secondary lesions appear and last for several months or years. Painful ulcerated lesions on the soles are frequent and are called "crab yaws." Late gummatous lesions may occur, with associated tissue destruction involving large areas of skin and subcutaneous tissues. The late effects of yaws, with bone change, shortening of digits, and contractions, may be confused with similar changes occurring in leprosy. Central nervous system, cardiac, or other visceral involvement is rare.

Burke JP et al (editors): International symposium on yaws and other endemic treponematoses. Rev Infect Dis 1985;7:217.

PINTA

Pinta is a non-sexually transmitted spirochetal infection caused by *Treponema carateum*. It occurs endemically in rural areas of Latin America, especially in Mexico, Colombia, and Cuba, and in some areas of the Pacific. A nonulcerative, erythematous primary papule spreads slowly into a papulosquamous plaque showing a variety of color changes (slate, lilac, black). Secondary lesions resemble the primary one and appear within a year after it. These appear successively, new lesions together with older ones; are commonest on the extremities; and later show atrophy and depigmentation. Some cases show pigmentary changes and atrophic patches on the soles and palms, with or without hyperkeratosis, that are indistinguishable from "crab yaws." Very rarely, central nervous system or cardiovascular disease is observed late in the course of infection.

ENDEMIC SYPHILIS

Endemic syphilis is an acute or chronic infection caused by an organism indistinguishable from *T pallidum*. It has been reported in a number of countries, particularly in the eastern Mediterranean area, often with local names: bejel in Syria, Saudi Arabia, and Iraq; and dichuchwa, njovera, and siti in Africa. It also occurs in Southeast Asia. The local forms have distinctive features. Moist ulcerated lesions of the skin or oral or nasopharyngeal mucosa are the most common manifestations. Generalized lymphadenopathy and secondary and tertiary bone and skin lesions are also common. Deep leg pain points to osteoperiostitis. Cardiovascular and central nervous system involvement is rare.

Pace JL, Csonka GW: Endemic non-venereal syphilis (bejel) in Saudi Arabia. Br J Vener Dis 1984;60:293.

MISCELLANEOUS SPIROCHETAL DISEASES

RELAPSING FEVER

Relapsing fever is endemic in many parts of the world. The main reservoir is rodents, which serve as the source of infection for ticks (eg, *Ornithodoros*). The distribution and seasonal incidence of the disease are determined by the ecology of the ticks in different areas. In the USA, infected ticks are found throughout the West, especially in mountainous areas, but clinical cases are uncommon in humans.

The infectious organism is a spirochete, *Borrelia recurrentis*. It may be transmitted transovarially from one generation of ticks to the next. The spirochetes occur in all tissues of the tick, and humans can be infected by tick bites or by rubbing crushed tick tissues or feces into the bite wound. Tick-borne relapsing fever is endemic but is not transmitted from person to person. Different species (or strain) names have been given to *Borrelia* in different parts of the world where the organisms are transmitted by different ticks.

When an infected person harbors lice, the lice become infected with *Borrelia* by sucking blood. A few days later, the lice serve as a source of infection for other persons. Large epidemics may occur in louse-infested populations, and transmission is favored by crowding, malnutrition, and cold climate.

Clinical Findings

A. Symptoms and Signs: There is an abrupt onset of fever, chills, tachycardia, nausea and vomiting, arthralgia, and severe headache. Hepatomegaly and splenomegaly may develop, as well as various types of rashes. Delirium occurs with high fever, and there may be various neurologic and psychic abnormalities. The attack terminates, usually abruptly, after 3–10 days. After an interval of 1–2 weeks, relapse occurs, but often it is somewhat milder. Three to 10 relapses may occur before recovery.

B. Laboratory Findings: During episodes of fever, large spirochetes are seen in blood smears stained with Wright's or Giemsa's stain. The organisms can be cultured in special media but rapidly lose pathogenicity. The spirochetes can multiply in injected rats or mice and can be seen in their blood.

A variety of anti-*Borrelia* antibodies develop during the illness; sometimes the Weil-Felix test and nontreponemal serologic test for syphilis may also be positive. Cerebrospinal fluid abnormalities occur in patients with meningeal involvement. Mild anemia and thrombocytopenia are common, but the white blood cell count tends to be normal.

Differential Diagnosis

The manifestations of relapsing fever may be confused with malaria, leptospirosis, meningococcemia, yellow fever, typhus, or rat-bite fever.

Prevention

Prevention of tick bites (as described for rickettsial diseases) and delousing procedures applicable to large groups can prevent illness. Arthropod vectors should be controlled if possible.

An effective means of chemoprophylaxis has not been developed.

Treatment

A single dose of tetracycline or erythromycin, 0.5 g orally, or a single dose of procaine penicillin G, 600,000 units intramuscularly, probably constitutes adequate treatment. Alternatively, 0.5 g of tetracycline or erythromycin can be given 4 times daily for 5–10 days. Jarisch-Herxheimer reactions may occur and must be managed.

Prognosis

The overall mortality rate is usually about 5%. Fatalities are most common in old, debilitated, or very young patients. With treatment, the initial attack is shortened and relapses are largely prevented.

Butler T et al: *Borrelia recurrentis* infection. J Infect Dis 1978;137:573.
Edell TA et al: Tick-borne relapsing fever in Colorado. JAMA 1979;241:2279.
Malison MD: Relapsing fever. JAMA 1979;241:2819.

RAT-BITE FEVER
(Spirillary Rat-Bite Fever, Sodoku)

Rat-bite fever is an uncommon acute infectious disease caused by *Spirillum minor*. It is transmitted to humans by the bite of a rat. Inhabitants of rat-infested slum dwellings and laboratory workers are at greatest risk.

Clinical Findings

A. Symptoms and Signs: The original rat bite, unless secondarily infected, heals promptly, but 1 to several weeks later the site becomes swollen, indurated, and painful; assumes a dusky purplish hue; and may ulcerate. Regional lymphangitis and lymphadenitis, fever, chills, malaise, myalgia, arthralgia, and headache are present. Splenomegaly may occur. A sparse, dusky-red maculopapular rash appears on the trunk and extremities in many cases, and there may be frank arthritis.

After a few days, both the local and systemic symptoms subside, only to reappear again in a few more days. This relapsing pattern of fever of 24–48 hours alternating with an equal afebrile period may persist for weeks. The other features, however, usually recur only during the first few relapses.

B. Laboratory Findings: Leukocytosis is often present, and the nontreponemal test for syphilis is often falsely positive. The organism may be identified in darkfield examination of the ulcer exudate or aspirated lymph node material; more commonly, it is observed after inoculation of a laboratory animal with the patient's exudate or blood. It has not been cultured in artificial media.

Differential Diagnosis

Rat-bite fever must be distinguished from the rat bite-induced lymphadenitis and rash of streptobacillary fever. Reliable differentiation requires an increasing titer of agglutinins against *Streptobacillus moniliformis* or identification of the causative organism. Rat-bite fever must also be distinguished from tularemia, rickettsial disease, *Pasteurella multocida* infections, and relapsing fever by identification of the causative organism.

Treatment

Treat with procaine penicillin G, 300,000 units intramuscularly every 12 hours; or tetracycline hydrochloride, 0.5 g every 6 hours for 2–3 days. Give supportive and symptomatic measures as indicated.

Prognosis

The reported mortality rate about 10% should be markedly reduced by prompt diagnosis and antimicrobial treatment.

Cole JS et al: Rat-bite fever. Ann Intern Med 1969;71:979.

LEPTOSPIROSIS

Leptospirosis is an acute and often severe infection that frequently affects the liver or other organs and is caused by serovars of *Leptospira interrogans*. The 3 most common serovars of infection are *Leptospira icterohaemorrhagiae* of rats, *Leptospira canicola* of dogs, and *Leptospira pomona* of cattle and swine. Several other varieties can also cause the disease, but *L icterohaemorrhagiae* causes the most severe illness. The disease is worldwide in distribution, and the incidence is higher than usually supposed. The leptospires are often transmitted to humans by the ingestion of food and drink contaminated by the urine of the reservoir animal. The organism may also enter through minor skin lesions and probably via the conjunctiva. Many infections have followed bathing in contaminated water. The disease is an occupational hazard among sewer workers, rice planters, abattoir workers, and farmers. The incubation period is 2–20 days.

Clinical Findings

A. Symptoms and Signs: Anicteric leptospirosis is the more common and milder form of the disease and is often biphasic. The initial or "septicemic" phase begins with abrupt fever to 39–40 °C (102.2–104 °F), chills, abdominal pain, severe headache, and myalgias, especially of the calf muscles. There is marked conjunctival suffusion. Leptospires can be isolated from blood, cerebrospinal fluid, and tissues. Following a 1- to 3-day period of improvement in symptoms and absence of fever, the second or "immune" phase begins. Leptospires are absent from blood and cerebrospinal fluid but are still present in the kidney, and specific antibodies appear. A recurrence of symptoms is seen in the first phase of disease and with the onset of meningitis. Uveitis, rash, and adenopathy may occur. The illness is usually self-limited, lasting 4–30 days, and complete recovery is the rule.

Icteric leptospirosis (Weil's syndrome) (usually caused by *L icterohaemorrhagiae*) is the most severe form of the disease, characterized by impaired renal and hepatic function, abnormal mental status, hypotension, and a 5–10% mortality rate. Signs and symptoms are continuous and not biphasic.

Pretibial fever, a mild form of leptospirosis caused by *Leptospira autumnalis,* occurred during World War II at Fort Bragg, USA. In pretibial fever, there is patchy erythema on the skin of the lower legs or generalized rash occurring with fever.

Leptospirosis with jaundice must be distinguished from hepatitis, yellow fever, and relapsing fever.

B. Laboratory Findings: The leukocyte count may be normal or as high as 50,000/μL, with neutrophils predominating. The urine may contain bile, protein, casts, and red cells. Oliguria is not uncommon, and in severe cases uremia may occur. In cases with meningeal involvement, organisms may be found in the cerebrospinal fluid during the first 10 days of illness. Early in the disease, the organism may be identified by darkfield examination of the patient's blood or by culture on a semisolid medium (eg, Fletcher's EMJH). Cultures take 1–6 weeks to become positive. The organism may also be grown from the urine from the tenth day to the sixth week. Specific agglutination titers develop after 7 days and may persist at high levels for many years; specific serologic tests are of particular value in diagnosis of the milder,

anicteric forms and of aseptic meningitis. A rapid diagnosis can be made by the determination of specific IgM with the DOT-ELISA method. Serum CPK is usually elevated in leptospirosis patients and normal in hepatitis patients.

Complications

Myocarditis, aseptic meningitis, renal failure, and massive hemorrhage are not common but are the usual causes of death. Iridocyclitis may occur.

Treatment

Various antimicrobial drugs, including penicillin and tetracyclines, show antileptospiral activity. Penicillin (eg, 6 million units daily intravenously) is said to be beneficial in severe leptospirosis, especially if started within the first 4 days of illness. Jarisch-Herxheimer reactions may occur. Observe for evidence of renal failure, and treat as necessary. Effective prophylaxis consists of doxycycline, 200 mg orally, given once weekly during the risk of exposure.

Prognosis

Without jaundice, the disease is almost never fatal. With jaundice, the mortality rate is 5% for those under age 30 and 30% for those over age 60.

McLain JB et al: Doxycycline therapy for leptospirosis. Ann Intern Med 1984;100:696.

Pappas MG et al: Rapid serodiagnosis of leptospirosis using IgM-specific DOT-ELISA. Am J Trop Med Hyg 1985; 34:346.

Takafuji ET et al: An efficacy trial of doxycycline chemoprophylaxis against leptospirosis. N Engl J Med 1984; 310:497.

Watt G et al: Placebo-controlled trial of intravenous penicillin for severe and late leptospirosis. Lancet 1988;1:433.

LYME DISEASE
(Lyme Borreliosis)

Essentials of Diagnosis

- Erythema migrans, a flat or slightly raised red lesion that expands with central clearing.
- Headache or stiff neck.
- Arthralgias, arthritis, and myalgias; arthritis is often chronic and recurrent.

General Considerations

This illness, named after the town of Old Lyme, Connecticut, is caused by the spirochete *Borrelia burgdorferi* and is transmitted to humans by ixodid ticks that are part of the *Ixodes ricinus* complex. Lyme disease is being increasingly recognized and has now been reported in most regions of the USA. The vector is *Ixodes dammini* in the Northeast and Midwest, *Ixodes pacificus* on the West Coast of the USA, *Ixodes scapularis* in the southeastern United

States, *Ixodes ricinus* in Europe, and *Ixodes persulcatus* in Asia. The disease also occurs in Australia (vector unknown). Mice and deer make up the major animal reservoir of *B burgdorferi*, but other rodents and birds may also be infected.

Ticks feed once during each of their 3 stages of life. Larval ticks feed in late summer, nymphs in the following spring and early summer, and adults during the fall. The preferred host for the nymphs and larvae is the white-footed mouse. This animal is tolerant of infection—a fact that is critical in maintaining infection, since the mouse can remain spirochetemic and transmit the agent to the larvae the following spring after being infected by the nymphal form in early summer. Adult ticks prefer the white-tailed deer as host. Most infections occur in the summer, when tick exposure is high and adult ticks are active. Any stage of the tick, however, can transmit disease.

Under experimental conditions, ticks must feed for 24 hours or longer to transmit infections. In addition, the percentage of ticks infected varies on a regional basis. In the Northeast and Midwest, 15–50% of *I dammini* ticks are infected with the spirochete; in the Western United States, only 2% of *I pacificus* are infected. There are important epidemiologic features in assessing the likelihood that tick exposure will result in disease. Exposure to *I pacificus* is unlikely to result in disease, since so few ticks are infected, but this is not true of exposure to *I dammini*. Eliciting a history of brushing a tick off the skin (ie, the tick was not feeding) or removing a tick on the same day as exposure (ie, the tick did not feed long enough) decreases the likelihood that infection will develop, since ticks must feed for 24 hours to transmit disease.

Ixodes ticks are smaller than the more common dog ticks *(Dermacentor variabilis)*. Larvae are less than 1 mm in size, and the adult female is 2–3 mm in size, with a red body and black legs. After a blood meal, ticks can reach 2–3 times their unengorged size. Because the tick is so small, the bite is usually painless and goes unnoticed. After feeding, the tick drops off in 2–4 days. If a tick is found, it should be removed immediately. The best way to accomplish this is to grab the mouth part—not the body—where it enters the skin with a fine-tipped tweezers and pull firmly and repeatedly until the tick releases its hold. Saving the tick in a bottle of alcohol for future identification may be useful, especially if symptoms develop.

Congenital infection has been documented, but the exact frequency and manifestations have not been clearly defined. Similarly, because the organism can be latent, it is not known if women infected prior to becoming pregnant can activate the disease and transmit infection to the fetus. In one retrospective study, 5 of 19 pregnancies complicated by Lyme disease resulted in an adverse outcome, but all of the outcomes were different and could not be conclusively linked to infection.

Clinical Findings

The typical clinical description of Lyme disease divides the illness into 3 stages: stage 1, flulike symptoms and a typical skin rash (erythema migrans); stage 2, weeks to months later, Bell's palsy or meningitis; and stage 3, months to years later, arthritis. The problem with this simplified scheme is that there is a great deal of overlap, and the skin, central nervous system, and musculoskeletal system can be involved early or late. A more accurate classification divides disease into early and late manifestations and specifies whether disease is localized or disseminated.

A. Symptoms and Signs:

1. Stage 1, early localized infection–Stage 1 infection is characterized by erythema migrans. About 1 week after the tick bite (range, 3–30 days), a flat or slightly raised red lesion appears at the site, which is commonly in areas of tight clothing such as the groin, thigh, or axilla. This lesion expands over several days, with central clearing. About 20% of patients either do not have typical skin lesions or the lesions go unnoticed. A flulike illness with fever, chills, and myalgia occurs in about half of patients. Even without treatment, the signs and symptoms of erythema migrans resolve in 3–4 weeks.

2. Stage 2, early disseminated infection–In stage 2, the spirochete may spread in the patient's blood or lymph to cause a wide variety of signs and symptoms. This usually occurs within days to weeks after inoculation of the organism. The most common manifestations involve the skin, central nervous system, and musculoskeletal system. In about half of patients, secondary lesions develop that are not associated with a tick bite. These lesions are similar in appearance to the primary lesion but are usually smaller. Headache and stiff neck can occur, as well as migratory pains in joints, muscles, and tendons. Fatigue and malaise are common. Generally, the neurologic and musculoskeletal symptoms are intermittent and last only hours, whereas fatigue is persistent. After hematogenous spread, the organism sequesters itself in certain areas and produces focal symptoms. Some patients experience cardiac (4–10% of patients) or neurologic (10–20% of patients) manifestations. Involvement of the heart includes myocarditis, with arrhythmias and heart block. Neurologic disease is most commonly manifested as aseptic meningitis, Bell's palsy, or encephalitis. Peripheral neuropathy (sensory or motor), transverse myelitis, and mononeuritis multiplex have also been described. Rarely, panophthalmitis can occur.

3. Stage 3, late persistent infection–Stage 3 infection occurs months to years after the initial infection and again primarily manifests itself as musculoskeletal, neurologic, and skin disease. Up to 60% of patients develop musculoskeletal complaints. Clinical manifestations are quite variable and include (1) joint and periarticular pain without objective findings; (2) frank arthritis, mainly of large joints, that is chronic or recurrent over years (recurrences become less severe, less frequent, and shorter with time); and (3) chronic synovitis, which may result in permanent disability. Both the central and peripheral nervous system may be involved. Encephalomyelitis—with cognitive dysfunction, spastic paraparesis, ataxia, and bladder dysfunction—has been described but is rare. More commonly, a peripheral neuropathy with radicular pain or distal paresthesias may occur. The cutaneous manifestation of late infection, which can occur up to 10 years after infection, is acrodermatitis chronicum atrophicans. It has been described mainly in Europe and only rarely in the United States. There is usually bluish-red discoloration of a distal extremity with associated swelling. These lesions become atrophic and sclerotic with time and eventually resemble localized scleroderma.

B. Laboratory Findings: The diagnosis of Lyme disease is usually confirmed by detection of specific antibodies to *B burgdorferi* in serum, either by indirect immunofluorescence assay (IFA) or enzyme-linked immunosorbent assay (ELISA); the latter is now preferred, because it is more sensitive and specific. IgM antibody appears first and peaks 3–6 weeks after onset of symptoms. IgG occurs later and requires a 4-fold rise or fall in titer to confirm the diagnosis. In early disease, up to 50% of patients may be antibody-negative. In later stages, most patients are antibody-positive, but up to 5% may be seronegative. Newer tests (antibody-capture ELISA) appear to be more sensitive in stage 1 disease (90% positivity rate), but clinical experience is limited. Antibiotic therapy of early disease may abort seroconversion.

Caution should be exercised in basing the diagnosis of Lyme disease on serologic testing. In addition to the lack of sensitivity of the available tests as noted above, interlaboratory variation in test results is a major problem. In one study, aliquots of serum were sent to different laboratories, and there was a marked difference in reported test results, with known positive serum being identified in less than half of cases. When a second specimen of the same serum was sent 2 weeks later, 8 of 18 laboratories reported a 4-fold difference in titers. These data demonstrate the difficulty in making the diagnosis of Lyme disease by serologic testing and emphasize the need for national standards.

B burgdorferi has rarely been cultured from blood, cerebrospinal fluid, or erythema chronicum migrans lesions. Special silver staining of chronically inflamed synovial tissue demonstrates spirochetes in one-third of patients.

Treatment

Antibiotic sensitivity of *B burgdorferi* has been established in vitro. Tetracycline is effective against the spirochete, but penicillin is only moderately so. Erythromycin is effective in vitro but has been disappointing in clinical trials. Ampicillin, ceftriaxone, and imipenem are also effective in vitro, but aminoglycosides, ciprofloxacin, and rifampin are not.

Present recommendations for therapy are outlined in Table 27–4. For early disease, tetracycline, 250 mg 4 times daily, or doxycycline, 100 mg twice daily for 10–30 days, is the treatment of choice. Amoxicillin

Table 27–4. Treatment of Lyme disease.

Manifestation	Drug and Dosage	Pediatric Dosage
Erythema migrans	Doxycycline, 100 mg BID for 10–30 days; or tetracycline, 250–500 mg QID for 10–30 days; or amoxicillin, 250–500 mg TID for 10–30 days; or erythromycin, 250 mg QID for 10–30 days.	Amoxicillin, 20–40 mg/kg/d for 10–30 days; or erythromycin, 30 mg/kg/d for 10–30 days
Neurologic disease Bell's palsy	Doxycycline, tetracycline, or amoxicillin as above for 1 month	Amoxicillin, 20–40 mg/kg/d for 1 month
Other central nervous system disease	Ceftriaxone, 2 g IV once daily for 14 days; or penicillin G, 20 million units/d IV in 6 divided doses for 14 days	Ceftriaxone, 50–80 mg/kg/d for 14 days; penicillin, 250–400 units/kg/d IV in divided doses for 14 days
Cardiac disease First-degree block (PR < 0.3 s)	Doxycyline, tetracycline, or amoxicillin as above for 10–30 days	Amoxicillin as above for 10–30 days
High-degree atrioventricular block	Ceftriaxone or penicillin G as above for 14 days	Penicillin G or ceftriaxone as above for 14 days
Arthritis Oral dosage	Doxycycline, tetracycline, or amoxicillin as above for 1 month	Amoxicillin as above for 1 month
Parenteral dosage	Ceftriaxone or penicillin G as above for 14 days	Penicillin G as above for 14 days
Acrodermatitis	Doxycyline, tetracycline, or amoxicillin orally as above for 30 days	Tetracycline as above for 1 month

is suggested for children and those who cannot take tetracycline. Erythromycin is less effective. For disseminated stage 2 disease, oral medication—doxycycline or amoxicillin—can be used for Bell's palsy. If other central nervous system manifestations are present (meningitis), ceftriaxone is given intravenously. Intravenous penicillin is also effective for central nervous system disease, but ceftriaxone penetrates into the cerebrospinal fluid better and can be given once daily. Mild cardiac disease (PR < 0.3 s) can be treated with oral agents, but high-degree atrioventricular block should be treated with either intravenous ceftriaxone or penicillin. Therapy of arthritis is difficult because some patients fail to respond to any therapy and others who do respond do so slowly. Initial studies suggested that intravenous penicillin was superior to benzathine penicillin. In one small study, ceftriaxone appeared to be superior to intravenous penicillin. In a recent study, however, oral agents (doxycycline or amoxicillin) were just as effective as intravenous regimens (penicillin or ceftriaxone). A reasonable approach to the patient with Lyme arthritis is to start with oral therapy and if this fails to switch to an intravenous agent.

Unresolved issues with respect to therapy include the role of prophylaxis following tick bites and the role of therapy in pregnancy. In one study comparing penicillin V to placebo, there was no beneficial effect of antibiotic therapy in preventing Lyme disease following exposure. The number of patients studied was small, and the number who developed Lyme disease was less than expected. Data for treatment in pregnancy are limited. Because of the failure of oral agents to prevent fetal infection in one case, some have recommended intravenous penicillin in this setting.

Berardi VP, Weeks KE, Steere AC: Serodiagnosis of early Lyme disease: Analysis of IgM and IgG antibody responses by using an antibody-capture enzyme immunoassay. J Infect Dis 1988;158:754.

Malawista SE, Steere AC: Lyme disease: Infectious in origin, rheumatic in expression. Adv Intern Med 1986; 31:147.

Luft BJ, Dattwyler RJ: Borreliosis. Page 56 in: *Current Clinical Topics in Infectious Diseases*, vol 10. Remington JS, Swartz MN (editors). Blackwell Scientific Publications, 1989.

Luger SW, Krauss E: Serologic tests for Lyme disease: Interlaboratory variability. Arch Intern Med 1990; 150:761.

Lyme disease. Rev Infect Dis 1989;11(Suppl 6). [Entire issue.]

McAlister HF et al: Lyme carditis: An important cause of reversible heart block. Ann Intern Med 1989;110:339.

Steere AC: Lyme disease. N Engl J Med 1989;321:586.

Treatment of Lyme disease. Med Lett Drugs Ther 1989;31:57.

Infectious Diseases: Protozoal

28

Robert S. Goldsmith, MD, MPH, DTM&H

AFRICAN TRYPANOSOMIASIS (Sleeping Sickness)

African trypanosomiasis is caused by *Trypanosoma brucei rhodesiense* and *Trypanosoma brucei gambiense*, both hemoflagellates. The organisms are transmitted by bites of tsetse flies (*Glossina* species), which inhabit shaded areas along streams and rivers. Human disease occurs locally throughout tropical Africa from south of the Sahara to about 20° south latitude. *T b gambiense* infections are in the moist sub-Saharan savannah and riverine forests of west and central Africa up to the eastern Rift Valley. *T b rhodesiense* occurs to the east of the Rift Valley in the savannah of east and southeast Africa and along the shores of Lake Victoria. The annual incidence of cases is estimated to be 10,000–20,000.

T b rhodesiense infection is primarily a zoonosis of game animals; humans are infected sporadically. Humans are the principal mammalian host for *T b gambiense*, but recent information suggests an animal reservoir as well.

Clinical Findings

A. Symptoms and Signs: *T b rhodesiense* infections go through the following 3 stages, are much more virulent, and untreated patients die within weeks to a year. In *T b gambiense* infections, however, chancres do not appear and the hemolymphatic stage is usually absent or goes unnoticed; when symptoms do become manifest after weeks to years, they are initially so mild that they are often ignored by the patient.

1. The trypanosomal chancre–This is a local pruritic, painful inflammatory reaction (3–10 cm) with regional lymphadenopathy that appears about 48 hours after the tsetse fly bite and lasts 2–4 weeks.

2. The hemolymphatic stage–This stage usually begins 3–10 days later with invasion of the bloodstream and reticuloendothelial system. High fever, severe headache, joint pains, and malaise recur at irregular intervals corresponding to waves of parasitemia. Between febrile episodes there are symptom-free periods that last up to 2 weeks. Transient rashes may appear, often pruritic and papular or circinate. There may be tachycardia, myalgias and arthralgias, mild enlargement of the liver and spleen, and edema (peripheral, pleural, ascites, etc). Enlarged, rubbery, and painless lymph nodes occur in 75% of patients.

In *T b gambiense*, only the posterior cervical group (Winterbottom's sign) may be enlarged. With progression of the disease, there is increasing weight loss and debilitation. Signs of myocardial involvement may appear early in Rhodesian infection, and the patient may succumb to myocarditis before signs of central nervous system invasion appear.

3. The meningoencephalitic stage–This stage appears within a few weeks or months of onset of Rhodesian infection but in Gambian sleeping sickness develops more insidiously, starting 6 months to several years after onset. Insomnia, anorexia, personality changes, apathy, and headaches are among the early findings. A variety of motor or tonus disorders may develop, including tremors and disturbances of speech, gait, and reflexes; somnolence appears late. The patient becomes severely emaciated and, finally, comatose. Death often results from secondary infection.

B. Laboratory Findings: Definitive diagnosis is by finding the organism in the bite lesion (rare), blood, lymph node aspirate, or cerebrospinal fluid. Because the number of trypanosomes in the blood fluctuates in waves and because the organisms are undetectable about 3 out of 5 days, specimens should be examined daily for 15 days (1) for motile organisms in wet films, (2) after Giemsa staining of thick and thin films, and (3) after concentration by centrifugation of heparinized blood (trypanosomes are concentrated in the buffy coat). Other diagnostic techniques employing blood samples include Millipore filtration, DEAE-cellulose anion exchange, and inoculation of culture medium. The most sensitive approach has been intraperitoneal inoculation of blood into laboratory rodents. A recently reported xenodiagnostic method in which *Glossina* fed on patient blood through a membrane was more sensitive than use of inoculated rats. Lymph nodes selected for aspiration should still be soft (ie, not fibrosed). The cerebrospinal fluid contains increased numbers of cells (lymphocytes) and an increased protein concentration. Wet films and stained smears of centrifuged cerebrospinal fluid (double centrifugation is at least twice as sensitive as single centrifugation—850 *g* for 10 minutes followed by 15,000 *g* for 1 minute—) may show trypanosomes in advanced cases; the fluid should be inoculated also into an experimental animal and culture medium. Serologic tests become positive about 12 days after onset of infection. Titers of circulating antibody fluctuate and, after high parasitemia, brief periods of excess antigen may depress antibody titers below detectable levels. In addition, in the late meningoencephalitic phase, both serologic titers and parasitemia may fall below demonstrable levels. ELISA and immunofluorescent tests of CSF may prove useful in late disease.

Other findings include anemia, increased sedimentation rate, thrombocytopenia, reduced total serum protein, increased serum globulin, and an elevated IgM level. The latter begins to rise shortly after infection and may reach 10–20 times normal. However, normal or low levels of IgM in acute disease do not rule out the infection. In central nervous system involvement, an elevated IgM in the cerebrospinal fluid is pathognomonic for the meningoencephalitic stage of trypanosomiasis, except that false-negative results have been reported.

Differential Diagnosis

Trypanosomiasis may be mistaken for a variety of other diseases, including malaria, influenza, pneumonia, infectious mononucleosis, leukemia, Hodgkin's disease, the arbovirus encephalitides, cerebral tumor, and various psychoses. Serologic tests for syphilis may be falsely positive in trypanosomiasis.

Prevention

Individual prevention in endemic areas should include wearing long sleeves and trousers, avoiding dark-colored clothing, and using mosquito nets while sleeping. Repellents have no effect. Pentamidine is used in chemoprophylaxis only against the Gambian type. In *T b rhodesiense* infection, pentamidine may suppress early symptoms, resulting in recognition of the disease too late in its course for effective treatment. Excretion of pentamidine is slow; therefore, one intramuscular injection (4 mg/kg, maximum 300 mg) protects for 3–6 months. The drug is potentially toxic and should only be used for persons at high risk (ie, those with constant, heavy exposure to tsetse flies in areas with known transmission of Gambian disease). Performing serologic tests every 6 months during exposure and for 3 years afterward is the safest method for detecting the disease at an early stage.

Treatment

A. Specific Measures: Suramin (drug of choice) and pentamidine (alternative drug) are used in the hemolymphatic stage of infection; however, because these drugs do not pass the blood-brain barrier, they are not used when the central nervous system is involved—melarsoprol instead is the drug of choice for the latter infections. Since each of the drugs frequently causes severe adverse reactions, they should be administered by experienced persons. For details of dosages and drug administration, see the references. In the USA, suramin and melarsoprol are available only from the CDC Drug Service, Centers for

Disease Control, Atlanta, GA 30333. Telephone: (404) 639–3670; (404) 639–2888 evenings, weekends, and holidays. α-Difluoromethylornithine, an inhibitor of ornithine decarboxylase, is being tested clinically and appears promising for the clearing of both peripheral and central nervous system parasites.

B. General Measures: Good nursing care, treatment of anemia and concurrent infections, and correction of malnutrition are essential in the management of advanced trypanosomiasis. Following treatment, patients should be monitored for signs of central nervous system involvement at 3- and then 6-month intervals for 3 years.

Prognosis

Most patients recover following treatment with pentamidine or suramin for hemolymphatic disease. Generally, with early treatment of central nervous system disease, most patients treated with melarsoprol will recover, though relapses occur in about 2%; if therapy is started late, irreversible brain damage or death is common. If African trypanosomiasis is untreated, most persons will die.

Bales JD Jr et al: Treatment of arsenical refractory Rhodesian sleeping sickness in Kenya. Ann Trop Med Parasitol 1989; 83(Suppl 1):111.

de Raadt P: African trypanosomiasis. In: *Tropical Medicine and Parasitology*. Goldsmith R, Heyneman D (editors). Appleton & Lange, 1989.

Dukes P et al: A new method of isolating *Trypanosoma brucei gambiense* from sleeping sickness patients. Trans R Soc Trop Med Hyg 1989;83:636.

Pepin J et al: An open clinical trial of nifurtimox for arseno-resistant *Trypanosoma brucei gambiense* sleeping sickness in central Zaire. Trans R Soc Trop Med Hyg 1989;83:514.

Petru AM et al: African sleeping sickness in the United States: Successful treatment with eflornithine. Am J Dis Child 1988;142:224.

AMERICAN TRYPANOSOMIASIS (Chagas' Disease)

Chagas' disease is caused by *Trypanosoma cruzi*, a protozoan parasite of humans and wild and domestic animals. *T cruzi* occurs only in the Americas; it is found in wild animals from southern South America to northern Mexico, Texas, and the southwestern USA. Though human infection is less widespread, an estimated 12 million people are infected, mostly in rural areas. In many countries of Latin America, particularly South America, Chagas' disease is the most important cause of heart disease. The infection is rare in the southern and southwestern USA.

T cruzi is transmitted by many species of triatomine bugs that become infected by ingesting blood with circulating trypanosomes from infected animals or humans. Multiplication occurs in the digestive tract of the bug; infective forms are eliminated in feces.

Infection in humans is through "contamination" with bug feces; the parasite penetrates the skin (generally through the bite wound) or the conjunctiva. Transmission can also occur by blood transfusion or in utero.

The trypanosomes first multiply close to the point of entry. They then enter the bloodstream as trypanosomes and later invade the heart and other tissues, where they assume a leishmanial form. Multiplication causes cellular destruction, inflammation, and fibrosis. Infection continues for many years, probably for life.

Clinical Findings

A. Symptoms and Signs: Most infected persons are asymptomatic. The **acute stage,** seen principally in children, lasts 2–4 months and leads to death in up to 10% of cases. The earliest findings are at the site of inoculation either in the eye—Romăna's sign (unilateral bipalpebral edema, conjunctivitis, local lymphadenopathy)—or in the skin—a chagoma (furunclelike lesion with local lymphadenopathy). Subsequent findings include fever, malaise, headache, hepatomegaly, mild splenomegaly, and generalized lymphadenopathy. Acute myocarditis may lead to biventricular failure, but arrhythmias are rare. Meningoencephalitis is limited to young children and is often fatal.

A **latent period** may last from 10 to 30 years in which the patient is asymptomatic but in which serologic tests and sometimes parasitologic examination confirm the presence of the infection.

The **chronic stage** is usually manifested by cardiac disease in the third and fourth decades of life, characterized by arrhythmias, congestive heart failure (mainly right-sided), and thromboembolic phenomena arising from a ventricle. Sudden cardiac arrest in young persons may occur and is attributed to ventricular fibrillation. Megacolon and megaesophagus, caused by damage to nerve plexuses in the bowel or esophageal wall, occur in some areas of Chile, Argentina, and Brazil; symptoms include dysphagia, regurgitation, and constipation.

B. Laboratory Findings: Appropriate selection of tests allows a definitive parasitologic diagnosis in most acute cases and in up to 40% of chronic ones. In the acute stage, trypanosomes should be looked for by examination of anticoagulated fresh blood for motile organisms and by examination of the following stained preparations: thick blood films, buffy coat after centrifugation of 5–10 mL of heparinized blood, and the sediment after centrifuging the supernatant of clotted blood. In the chronic stage, the parasite can only be detected by culture or xenodiagnosis. The latter consists of permitting uninfected laboratory-reared bugs of the local major vector to feed on the patients and then examining their intestinal contents for trypanosomes. In both acute and chronic infection, blood should also be cultured using Nicolle-Novy-MacNeal medium and inoculated into labora-

tory mice or rats 3–10 days old. *Trypanosoma rangeli,* a nonpathogenic blood trypanosome also found in humans in Central America and northern South America, must not be mistaken for *T cruzi.* Several serologic tests are available and are of presumptive value when positive; when possible, more than one test should be used. Antibodies of the IgM class are usually elevated in the acute stage but normal in the chronic stage. The most important electrocardiographic abnormalities are complete right bundle branch block, conduction defects, and arrhythmias. In certain regions of South America, radiologic examination may show cardiac enlargement with characteristic apical aneurysms, megaesophagus, or megacolon.

Treatment

Treatment of Chagas' diseases is unsatisfactory. Cures are usually possible only in the acute phase. In the chronic phase, although parasitemia and xenodiagnosis become negative, treatment does not alter the serologic reaction, cardiac function, or progression of the disease. Benznidazole (not available in the USA) is preferred over nifurtimox in treatment; both drugs have shown clastogenic effects during treatment.

Nifurtimox is given orally in a dosage of 8–16 mg/kg/d in 3 divided doses for 50–120 days. It generally produces anorexia, weight loss, tremors, and peripheral neuritis. Hallucinations and convulsions are rare. In the USA, nifurtimox is available only from the Parasitic Disease Drug Service, Centers for Disease Control, Atlanta 30333 (call (404) 488–4240).

Ketoconazole has promoted parasitologic cure of mice and should be tried in humans. In advanced cardiac failure, diuretics are usually very effective, but digoxin is not well tolerated. Arrhythmias require selected use of intravenous lidocaine, quinidine, procainamide, or amiodarone.

Prognosis

Acute infections in infants and young children are often fatal, particularly when the central nervous system is involved. Adults with chronic cardiac infections also may ultimately succumb to the disease.

Kirchhoff LV: Is *Trypanosoma cruzi* a new threat to our blood supply? Ann Intern Med 1989;111:773.

Marr JJ, Docampo R: Chemotherapy for Chagas' disease: A perspective of current therapy and considerations for future research. Rev Infect Dis 1986;8:884.

McCabe RE, Remington JS, Araujo FG: Ketoconazole promotes parasitological cure of mice infected with *Trypanosoma cruzi.* Trans R Soc Trop Med Hyg 1987;81:613.

Palacios-Pru E et al: Ultrastructural characteristics of different stages of human chagasic myocarditis. Am J Trop Med Hyg 1989;41:29.

Prata A: American trypanosomiasis (Chagas' disease). In: *Tropical Medicine and Parasitology.* Goldsmith R, Heyneman D (editors). Appleton & Lange, 1989.

AMEBIASIS

Essentials of Diagnosis

● Mild to moderate amebic colitis: recurrent diarrhea and abdominal cramps, sometimes alternating with constipation. Mucus may be present but no blood.

● Severe amebic colitis: semiformed to liquid stools streaked with blood and mucus; fever; colic; prostration. In fulminant cases, ileus, perforation, peritonitis, hemorrhage.

● Hepatic amebiasis: hepatic enlargement, pain, and tenderness; fever. Laboratory findings: amebas in stools or in abscess aspirate. Serologic tests positive with severe colitis or hepatic abscess. Imaging methods show size and location of abscess.

General Considerations

Amebiasis is caused by the protozoan parasite *Entamoeba histolytica*. The organisms either live as commensals in the lumen of the large intestine without causing disease (the asymptomatic chronic carrier) or invade the colon wall causing acute dysentery or chronic diarrhea of variable severity. The organisms may also be carried by the blood to the liver, where they may produce hepatic abscesses. Rarely, they are carried to the lungs, brain, or other organs or invade the perianal skin.

The infection is present worldwide but is most prevalent and severe in tropical areas, where rates may exceed 40% under conditions of crowding, poor sanitation, and poor nutrition. It is estimated that invasive amebiasis causes between 40,000 and 100,000 deaths annually worldwide. In temperate areas, however, amebiasis tends to be asymptomatic or a mild, chronic infection that often remains undiagnosed. In the USA, seropositive rates up to 2–5% have been reported in some populations.

E histolytica exists as 2 forms in the lumen and mucosal crypts of the large bowel: cysts (10–14 μm) and motile trophozoites (12–50 μm). In the absence of diarrhea, trophozoites encyst in the large bowel. Trophozoites passed into the environment die rapidly, but cysts remain viable in soil and water for several weeks to months at appropriate temperature and humidity.

Humans are the only established host and are universally susceptible. Only cysts are infectious, since after ingestion they survive gastric acidity whereas trophozoites are destroyed.

Transmission generally occurs through ingestion of cysts from fecally contaminated food or water. Flies and other arthropods also serve as mechanical vectors; to an undetermined degree, transmission results from contamination of food by the hands of food handlers. Where human excrement is used as fertilizer, it is often a source of food contamination. Person-to-person contact is also important in transmission; therefore, all household members as well as an infected person's sexual partner should have their stools examined. Sexual transmission of *E histolytica* and other intestinal protozoa has reached epidemic proportions among male homosexuals in some temperate urban areas, but these infections are predominantly nonpathogenic. In closed institutions such as mental hospitals, prevalence rates as high as 50% have been reported. Amebiasis is rarely epidemic, but urban outbreaks have occurred because of common-source water contamination.

It is undetermined whether strains differ with regard to invasiveness or whether all strains under the right conditions can become invasive. The circumstances under which commensals become invasive are little understood. Malnutrition and alcoholism probably predispose to enhanced virulence. Corticosteroids and other immunosuppressive drugs often convert a commensal infection to an invasive one. Women in late pregnancy and the puerperium are especially susceptible. Isoenzyme analysis of isolates has shown 22 zymodemes from different parts of the world, of which 9 have been associated with tissue invasiveness. Tissue invasion elicits both humoral (IgM and IgG) antibodies and a cellular immune response, but humoral antibody titers do not correlate with protective immunity.

The characteristic intestinal lesion is the amebic ulcer, which can occur anywhere in the large bowel (including the appendix) and sometimes in the terminal ileum but predominates in the cecum, descending colon, and the rectosigmoid colon—areas of greatest fecal stasis. Trophozoites invade the colonic mucosa by means of their ameboid movement and proteolytic secretions and induce necrosis to form the characteristic flask-shaped ulcers. Ulcers are usually limited to the muscularis, but if penetration to the serous layer occurs, bowel perforation, local abscess, or generalized peritonitis may result. In fulminating cases, ulceration may be extensive, and the bowel becomes thin and friable. Hepatic abscesses range from a few millimeters to 15 cm or larger, usually are single but may be multiple, occur more often in the right lobe (particularly the upper portion), and are more common in men.

Clinical Findings

A. Symptoms and Signs: Amebiasis can be classified into intestinal and extraintestinal disease and further subdivided into the clinical syndromes described below. Some patients have an acute onset of severe diarrhea as early as 8 days (commonly 2–4 weeks) after infection. Others may have an asymptomatic or mild intestinal infection for months to several years before either intestinal symptoms or liver abscess appears. Transition may occur from one type of intestinal infection to another, and each may give rise to hepatic abscess, or the intestinal infection may clear spontaneously.

1. Intestinal amebiasis–

a. Asymptomatic infection–In most infected

persons, the organism lives as a commensal, and the patient is without symptoms.

b. Mild to moderate colitis (nondysenteric colitis)–A few stools a day are passed that are semiformed and have a strong fetid odor; mucus may be present but no blood. There may be abdominal cramps, flatulence, chronic fatigue, and weight loss. Periods of remission and recurrence may last days to weeks or longer; during remissions, the patient may have constipation. Abdominal examination may show hyperperistalsis and tenderness and fullness due to gaseous distention of the colon. In some patients with chronic infection, the colon is thick and palpable, particularly over the cecum and descending colon.

c. Severe colitis (dysenteric colitis)–As the severity of intestinal infection increases, the number of stools increases, they change from semiformed to liquid with an unpleasant odor, and streaks of blood and mucus begin to appear. With larger numbers of stools, 10–20 or more, little fecal material is present, but blood (fresh or dark), mucus, and bits of necrotic tissue become increasingly evident. With increasing severity, the patient may become prostrate and show signs of toxicity, with fever up to 40.5°C, and have colic, tenesmus, vomiting, generalized abdominal tenderness, and nonspecific hepatic enlargement and tenderness. Rare complications include appendicitis, bowel perforation (followed by peritonitis, pericolonic abscess, retroperitoneal fecal cellulitis, fistula to the abdominal surface), and fulminating colitis (with paralytic ileus, hypotension, massive mucosal sloughing, and hemorrhage). Death may follow.

d. Localized ulcerative lesions of the colon– Bowel ulcerations limited to the rectal area may result in passage of formed stools with bloody exudate. Ulcerations limited to the cecum may induce mild diarrhea and simulate acute appendicitis. Amebic appendicitis, in which the appendix is extensively involved but not the remainder of the large bowel, is rare.

e. Localized granulomatous lesions of the colon (ameboma)–This occurs as a result of excessive production of granulation tissue in response to amebic infection, either in the course of dysentery or slowly in chronic intestinal infection. These masses may present as an irregular tumor (single or multiple) that projects into the bowel or as an annular constricting mass up to several centimeters in length. Clinical findings (pain, obstructive symptoms, and hemorrhage) and x-ray findings may simulate bowel carcinoma or lymphogranuloma venereum. At endoscopy, the mass is deep red and bleeds easily, and biopsy specimens show granulation tissue and *E histolytica*. Antiamebic drugs are usually adequate in treatment; surgical removal of the lesion without prior or immediate postoperative drug therapy is likely to result in death of the patient.

2. Extraintestinal amebiasis–

a. Hepatic amebiasis–Amebic liver abscess, although a relatively infrequent consequence of intestinal amebiasis, is not uncommon given the large number of intestinal infections. A large proportion of patients with liver abscess do not have concurrent intestinal symptoms, nor can they recall having had chronic intestinal symptoms. The onset of symptoms can be sudden or gradual, ranging from a few days to many months. Cardinal manifestations are fever (often high), pain (continuous, stabbing, or pleuritic, and sometimes severe), and an enlarged and tender liver. Patients may also experience malaise or prostration, sweating, chills, anorexia, and weight loss. The liver enlargement may present subcostally, in the epigastrium, as a localized bulging of the rib cage, or, as a result of enlargement against the dome of the diaphragm, it may produce coughing and findings at the right lung base (dullness to percussion, rales, and diminished breath sounds). Intercostal tenderness is common. Localizing signs on the skin may be an area of edema or a point of maximum tenderness. Without prompt treatment, the hepatic abscess may rupture into the pleural, peritoneal, or pericardial space or other contiguous organs, and death may follow.

b. Nonspecific hepatic enlargement–A low-grade, nonspecific enlargement of the liver—in which amebic liver infection is not present—may accompany invasive amebic bowel disease. It disappears with eradication of the amebic bowel infection but without use of specific drugs required to eradicate an amebic liver infection.

3. Other extraintestinal infections–Skin infections may develop in the perianal area. Metastatic infection may rarely occur throughout the body, particularly the lungs, brain, perianal skin, and genitalia.

B. Laboratory Findings:

1. Intestinal amebiasis–Three specimens obtained under optimal conditions and examined by skilled personnel will generally detect only 80% of amebic infections. Three additional tests will raise the diagnosis rate to about 90%. Trophozoites predominate in liquid stools, cysts in formed stools.

A standard procedure is to collect 3 specimens at 2-day intervals or longer, with one of the 3 obtained after a laxative such as (1) sodium sulfate or phosphate (Fleet's Phospho-Soda), 30–60 g in a glass of water; or (2) bisacodyl (Dulcolax, 5–15 mL). Oil laxatives such as mineral oil should not be used. Specimens should be collected in a clean container without having come in contact with urine or toilet bowl water. Because trophozoites rapidly autolyze, specimens should be examined within about 30 minutes or should immediately be mixed with a preservative.

If the patient has received specific therapy, antibiotics, antimalarials, antidiarrheal preparations containing bismuth or kaolin, magnesium hydroxide, barium, or mineral oil, specimen collection should be delayed 10–14 days.

On sigmoidoscopic examination, no findings are

typical in mild intestinal disease; in severe disease, ulcers may be found that are 1 mm to 2 cm across, with intact intervening mucosa. If present, exudate should be collected with a glass pipette (not with cotton) or by scraping with a metal curet and examined immediately. The colon should not be cleansed before sigmoidoscopy, since this washes exudate from ulcers and destroys trophozoites. In some centers, rectal biopsy has enhanced diagnosis; the specimens are best examined by immunofluorescence methods. Where possible, in vitro culture of amebas can be attempted.

Finding trophozoites that contain ingested red blood cells is diagnostic for invasive *E histolytica*, but they may be confused with the occasional macrophage that also contains red blood cells. *E histolytica* cysts and trophozoites must be differentiated from the other pathogenic and nonpathogenic intestinal protozoa.

In dysentery, the white blood cell count can reach 20,000 or higher, but it is not elevated in mild colitis. A low-grade eosinophilia is occasionally present.

Serologic testing for amebiasis is specific and usually positive if there has been substantial tissue invasion (as occurs in severe intestinal infection); in mild or asymptomatic intestinal infection, few patients are positive. The indirect hemagglutination test is sensitive and apparently produces no false-positive reactions. Positive titers persist for several years after successful treatment. The agar gel methods, though less sensitive, are rapidly conducted laboratory tests that measure current invasion; the tests become negative within about 3–6 months after eradication of infection. ELISA, DNA probes, and other methods continue to be evaluated for detection of the organism or its antigen in stool or liver abscess aspirate.

2. Hepatic abscess–The size and location of abscess can be determined by ultrasonography (usually round or oval lesions, abrupt transition from normal liver to the lesion, hypoechoic center with diffuse echoes throughout the abscess), CT (well-defined, round, low-density lesions with an internal, unhomogeneous structure), and radioisotope scanning. After intravenous injection of contrast material, CT may show a hyperdense halo around the periphery of the abscess. Elevation of the right dome of the diaphragm, with diminished motility, is well demonstrated by chest x-ray, fluoroscopy, and ultrasound. Serologic tests are usually positive, but stools often no longer contain the parasite. The white count ranges from 15,000 to 25,000/μL. Eosinophilia is not present. Liver function test abnormalities, when present, are usually low-grade. In many patients, aspiration is indicated for diagnosis and, if the abscess is large, for therapy as well to prevent rupture. The risks are hemorrhage and bacterial infection; therefore, aspiration should be done under strict aseptic conditions. Divide the aspirate into serial 30- to 50-mL aliquots, but examine only the last sample, as organisms are found only at the edge of the abscess.

Differential Diagnosis

Amebiasis should be considered in most cases of acute or chronic diarrhea (including cases associated with only mild changes in bowel habits in patients who have an exposure history), liver abscess, and annular lesions of the colon. The infection is more likely to occur in persons residing in or travelers returning from endemic areas, in individuals intimately associated with known cases, and in homosexual men. All patients with presumed inflammatory bowel disease should be tested by stool examination and serology because of the risk of overwhelming amebic disease if corticosteroid therapy were to be given.

Treatment

The choice of drug depends on the type of clinical presentation and the site of drug action. Treatment may require the concurrent or sequential use of several drugs. Table 28–1 outlines a preferred and an alternative method of treatment for each clinical type of amebiasis.

The **tissue amebicides** dehydroemetine and emetine act on organisms in the bowel wall and in other tissues but not on amebas in the bowel lumen. Chloroquine is active principally against amebas in the liver. The **luminal amebicides** diloxanide furoate, iodoquinol, and paromomycin act on organisms in the bowel lumen but are ineffective against amebas in the bowel wall or other tissues. Oral tetracycline inhibits the bacterial associates of *E histolytica* and thus has an indirect effect on amebas in the bowel lumen and bowel wall but not in other tissues. Given parenterally, antibiotics have little antiamebic activity at any site. Metronidazole is unique in that it is effective both in the bowel lumen and in the bowel wall and other tissues. However, metronidazole when used alone for bowel infections is not sufficient as a luminal amebicide, for it fails to cure up to 50% of infections. Metronidazole also reaches the central nervous system.

A. Asymptomatic Intestinal Infection: Cure rates with a single course of diloxanide furoate or iodoquinol are 80–85%. Usually in asymptomatic infection, a tissue amebicidal drug is not given to prevent liver infection. Other alternatives for treatment or re-treatment are paromomycin or metronidazole plus iodoquinol or diloxanide furoate.

B. Mild to Moderate Intestinal Infection: When iodoquinol is used, concomitant use of tetracycline probably increases intestinal cure rates. It is less well established that adding a tetracycline to diloxanide furoate therapy increases effectiveness. Chloroquine is used to destroy trophozoites carried to the liver or to eradicate an undetected early-stage amebic liver abscess; the minimum dose needed to accomplish this is not known. In endemic areas where intestinal infection and reinfection are common yet hepatic abscess is rare (eg, in urban communities where intesti-

Table 28-1. Treatment of amebiasis.

	Drug(s) of Choice	Alternative Drug(s)
Asymptomatic intestinal infection	Diloxanide furoate[1,2]	Iodoquinol (diiodohydroxyquin)[3]
Mild to moderate intestinal infection (non-dysenteric colitis)	(1) Metronidazole[4] **plus** (2) Diloxanide furoate[1,2] or iodoquinol[3]	(1) Diloxanide furoate[1,2] or iodoquinol[3] **plus** (2) A tetracycline[5] **followed by** (3) Chloroquine[6] **or** (1) Paromomycin[7] **followed by** (2) Chloroquine[6]
Severe intestinal infection (dysentery)	(1) Metronidazole[8] **plus** (2) Diloxanide furoate[1,2] or iodoquinol[3] **If parenteral therapy is needed initially** (1) Intravenous metronidazole[9] until oral therapy can be started (2) Then give oral metronidazole[8] plus diloxanide furoate[1,2] or iodoquinol[3]	(1) A tetracycline[5] **plus** (2) Diloxanide furoate[1,2] or iodoquinol[3] **followed by** (3) Chloroquine[10] **or** (1) Dehydroemetine[1,11] or emetine[11] **followed by** (2) A tetracycline[5] plus diloxanide furoate[1,2] or iodoquinol[3] **followed by** (3) Chloroquine[10]
Hepatic abscess	(1) Metronidazole[8,9] **plus** (2) Diloxanide furoate[1,2] or iodoquinol[3] **followed by** (3) Chloroquine[10]	(1) Dehydroemetine[1,12] or emetine[12] **plus** (2) Chloroquine[13] **plus** (3) Diloxanide furoate[1,2] or iodoquinol[3]
Ameboma or extraintestinal infection	As for hepatic abscess, but not including chloroquine	As for hepatic abscess, but not including chloroquine

[1] Available in the USA only from the CDC Drug Service, Centers for Disease Control, Atlanta 30333. Telephone requests may be made by calling the central number (404) 639-3670 days; (404) 639-2888 nights, weekends, and holidays (emergencies only).

[2] Diloxanide furoate, 500 mg 3 times daily with meals for 10 days (for children, 20 mg/kg in 3 divided doses daily for 10 days).

[3] Iodoquinol (diiodohydroxyquin), 650 mg 3 times daily for 21 days (for children, 30-40 mg/kg [maximum 2 g] in 3 divided doses daily for 21 days).

[4] Metronidazole, 750 mg 3 times daily for 10 days (for children, 35 mg/kg in 3 divided doses daily for 10 days).

[5] A tetracycline—eg, oxytetracycline, 250 mg 4 times daily for 10 days; in severe dysentery, give 500 mg 4 times daily for the first 5 days, then 250 mg 4 times daily for 5 days. Tetracycline should not be used during pregnancy or in children under 8 years of age; in older children, give 20 mg/kg in 4 divided doses daily for 10 days).

[6] Chloroquine, 500 mg (salt) daily for 7 days (for children, 16 mg/kg [salt] daily for 7 days).

[7] Paromomycin, 25-30 mg/kg (base) (maximum 3 g) in 3 divided doses after meals daily for 5-10 days (for children, the same dosage). Use only for mild disease.

[8] Metronidazole, 750 mg 3 times daily for 5-10 days (for children, 35-50 mg/kg in 3 divided doses daily for 10 days).

[9] An intravenous metronidazole is available; change to oral medication as soon as possible. See manufacturer's recommendation for dosage.

[10] Chloroquine, 500 mg (salt) daily for 14 days (for children, 16 mg/kg [salt] daily for 14 days).

[11] Dehydroemetine or emetine, 1 mg/kg subcut (preferred) or IM daily for the least number of days necessary to control severe symptoms (usually 3-5 days) (maximum daily dose for dehydroemetine is 90 mg; for emetine, 65 mg). For children, the daily dose is divided into 2 parts. Because of potential cardiac drug toxicity, patients should remain sedentary during treatment.

[12] Dehydroemetine or emetine, 1 mg/kg subcut (preferred) or IM daily for 8-10 days (maximum daily dose for dehydroemetine is 90 mg; for emetine, 65 mg). For children, the daily dose is divided into 2 parts. Because of potential cardiac drug toxicity, patients should remain sedentary during treatment.

[13] Chloroquine, 500 mg (salt) twice daily for 2 days orally or IM and then 500 mg orally daily for 21 days (for children, 16 mg/kg [salt] daily for 21 days).

nal amebiasis is sexually transmitted among male homosexuals but hepatic amebiasis is uncommon), it is probably unnecessary to use chloroquine in the treatment of mild intestinal disease.

C. Severe Intestinal Infection: Fluid and electrolyte therapy and opiates to control bowel motility are necessary adjuncts in severe amebic dysentery.

D. Hepatic Abscess: Hospitalization and bed rest are necessary. When metronidazole is given for 10 days, early or late treatment failure occurs rarely. If a satisfactory clinical response has not occurred within 2-3 days, especially if the abscess has been adequately drained, therapy should be changed to the alternative mode of treatment: dehydroemetine (or emetine) plus chloroquine. When the clinical response to metronidazole is adequate, it is suggested that a 2-week course of chloroquine follow to prevent late failures. The need for adding this course of chloroquine remains to be evaluated. Either mode of treatment also requires a luminal amebicide (diloxanide furoate or iodoquinol), whether or not the organism is found in the stool. Antibiotics are added only when there is concomitant bacterial liver abscess, which is rare. Metronidazole is highly effective against anaerobic bacteria, a major cause of bacterial liver abscesses.

Since a comparative trial of metronidazole with and without aspiration has not been reported, the indications for therapeutic aspiration are still controversial. Aspiration is clearly indicated when the diagnosis is in doubt, if rupture of a large abscess is impending, or if there is a lack of response to therapy.

E. Adverse Drug Reactions: Metronidazole often induces transient nausea or vomiting; if alcohol is taken during or shortly after treatment, a disulfiram-like reaction may occur. Metronidazole may be carcinogenic; however, some authorities consider the drug to be essentially free of cancer risk. Dehydroemetine and emetine cause nausea, vomiting, and pain at the injection site. They are general protoplasmic poisons having adverse effects on many tissues (particularly the heart) and a narrow range between therapeutic and toxic effects; dehydroemetine may be the safer of the 2 drugs. The tetracyclines should not be used for children under age 8 years or for pregnant women; use erythromycin stearate instead, even though it is less effective. Iodoquinol may cause mild, transient diarrhea; neurotoxicity has not been reported at standard doses. Flatulence is common with diloxanide furoate.

Follow-Up Care

In follow-up, examine at least 3 stools at 2- to 3-day intervals, starting 2–4 weeks after the end of treatment. For some patients, sigmoidoscopy and reexamination of stools within 3 months may be indicated.

Postdysenteric colitis is an uncommon sequela of severe amebic colitis. Following adequate treatment, diarrhea continues and the mucosa may be reddened and edematous, but no ulcers or organisms are found. Most such cases are self-limited, with permanent remission in weeks to months. Uncommonly, the diarrhea may be profound and unremitting and in some instances probably represents ulcerative colitis triggered by the amebic infection.

Prevention & Control

Efforts at prevention depend upon safe water supplies, sanitary disposal of human feces, adequate cooking of foods to destroy cysts, protection of foods from fly contamination, washing hands after defecation and before preparing or eating foods, and, in endemic areas, avoidance of foods that cannot be cooked or peeled. Water supplies can be boiled (briefly) or treated with iodine (0.5 mL tincture of iodine per liter for 20 minutes, or longer if the water is cold). Disinfection dips for fruits and vegetables are not advised, and no drug is safe or effective in prophylaxis.

Prognosis

The mortality rate from untreated amebic dysentery, hepatic abscess, or ameboma may be high. With modern chemotherapy instituted early in the course of the disease, the prognosis is good.

Greenstein AJ, Sachar DB: Pyogenic and amebic abscesses of the liver. Semin Liver Dis 1988;8:210.

Guerrant RL: Amebiasis: Introduction, current status, and research questions. Rev Infect Dis 1986;8:218. (Review.)

Ravdin JI (editor): *Amebiasis: Human Infection by Entamoeba histolytica.* Churchill Livingstone, 1988.

Rustgi AK, Richter JM: Pyogenic and amebic liver abscess. Med Clin North Am 1989;73:847.

Salata RA, Radvin J: Review of the human immune mechanism directed against *Entamoeba histolytica.* Rev Infect Dis 1986;8:261. (Includes review of serologic methods.)

PATHOGENIC FREE-LIVING AMEBAS

Primary Amebic Meningoencephalitis

Primary amebic meningoencephalitis is a fulminating, purulent meningoencephalitis that resembles bacterial meningitis and is rapidly fatal. More than 130 cases have been recognized, mostly in children and young adults. The responsible organisms are free-living ameboflagellates of the genus *Naegleria*, most cases due to *Naegleria fowleri*.

N fowleri is a thermophilic organism found in fresh and polluted warm lake water, domestic water supplies, swimming pools, thermal water, and sewers. Most patients give a history of exposure to fresh water; dust is also a possible source of infection. Nasal and throat swabs have shown that there is a human carrier state, and serologic surveys suggest that inapparent infections occur.

The organism apparently invades the central nervous system through the cribriform plate. The incubation period varies from 1 to 14 days. Early symptoms include headache, fever, and lethargy, often associated with rhinitis and pharyngitis. Vomiting, disorientation, and other signs of meningoencephalitis develop within 1 or 2 days, followed by coma and then death on the fifth or sixth day. At autopsy, some victims have a nonspecific myocarditis.

Lumbar or ventricular fluid contains several hundred to 25,000 leukocytes/μL (50–100% neutrophils) and erythrocytes (up to several thousand/μL). Protein is usually moderately elevated and glucose moderately reduced. If conventional examinations for bacteria and fungi are negative, the fluid must then be examined for free-living amebas to make the specific diagnosis. A wet mount examined by an ordinary optical microscope with the aperture restricted or condenser down will enhance contrast and refractility; a warm stage is not needed. The fluid should not be centrifuged or refrigerated, as this tends to immobilize the amebas. Their brisk motility distinguishes them from leukocytes of various types, which they closely resemble. Culture and mouse inoculation studies should be performed. Serologic testing for antibody and circulating antigen is experimental.

Precise species identification is based on morphology, demonstration of flagellate transformation (*Naegleria* only), and various immunologic studies.

Only 2 well-documented survivors have been reported. One was treated with intravenous and intrathecal amphotericin B and the other with a combination of amphotericin B, miconazole, and rifampin. Experimental studies have shown a marked synergistic effect between amphotericin B and either tetracycline or rifampin.

Acanthamoeba Infections

Free-living amebas of the genus *Acanthamoeba* are found in soil and in fresh, brackish, and thermal water as trophozoites (15–45 μm) or cysts (10–25 μm). Several species have been recognized only recently as human pathogens that cause a number of poorly defined syndromes: (1) a subacute and chronic focal granulomatous necrotizing meningoencephalitis that invariably has led to death in weeks to months, (2) skin lesions that resemble deep fungal infections, (3) granulomatous dissemination to many tissues, and (4) uveitis or chronic keratitis that may lead to blindness. Portals of entry may include the skin, eyes, or respiratory tract. A commensal nasal carrier state is established. Immunocompromised patients may have increased susceptibility.

In the encephalitis syndrome, cerebrospinal fluid lymphocytosis has been described. Antemortem diagnosis has been made via biopsy specimens. The presence of cysts or mitotic division in tissue section may be pathognomonic of *Acanthamoeba* infection. Serology may be helpful.

More than 200 cases of *Acanthamoeba* keratitis have been identified in the USA since 1981, most associated with wearing contact lenses, penetrating corneal trauma, or exposure to contaminated water. The clinical features suggestive of *Acanthamoeba* keratitis are (1) severe ocular pain, (2) partial or 360-degree paracentral stromal ring infiltrate on ophthalmologic examination, (3) recurrent corneal epithelial breakdown, and (4) a corneal lesion refractory to the usual medications. Typically, the keratitis progresses slowly over months. The diagnosis can be confirmed by vigorously scraping the cornea with a swab or platinum-tipped scapula; the material is microscopically examined after staining with Giemsa's or trichrome stain or by immunofluorescent techniques and

is also placed in culture on nonnutrient agar seeded with Escherichia coli.

There is no effective treatment for the meningoencephalitis. In vitro studies show that some strains are sensitive to ketoconazole, miconazole, sulfonamides, clotrimazole, pentamidine, paromomycin, flucytosine, and other drugs but not to amphotericin B.

Although there is no specific treatment for *Acanthamoeba* keratitis, a number of antimicrobials have been effective. One approach is with systemic ketoconazole and topical propamide isethionate, miconazole, clotrimazole, and neomycin-polymyxin. If medical treatment fails, penetrating keratoplasty may be necessary to excise diseased tissue. Prevention requires use of disinfectant solutions to clean contact lenses; a recent report, however, showed that they were inadequate in destroying *Acanthamoeba* cysts when used for less than 6 hours.

Bia FJ, Barry M: Parasitic infections of the central nervous system. Neurol Clin 1986;4:171.

Brandt FH, Ware DA, Visvesvara GS: Viability of *Acanthamoeba* cysts in ophthalmic solutions. Appl Environ Microbiol 1989;55:1144.

Ferrante A: Amphotericin B doses for primary amoebic meningoencephalitis. Lancet 1986;2:35.

Moore MB: *Acanthamoeba* keratitis. (Editorial.) Arch Ophthalmol 1988;106:1181.

Tripathi RC, Monninger RHG, Tripathi BJ: Contact lens-associated *Acanthamoeba* keratitis: A report from the USA. Fortschr Ophthalmol 1989;86:67.

BABESIOSIS
(Piroplasmosis)

Babesia are tick-borne protozoal parasites of wild and domestic animals worldwide. Babesiosis in humans is a rare intraerythrocytic infection caused by 2 *Babesia* species. The infection has been recognized only in Europe *(Babesia divergens)* and North America *(Babesia microti),* with most infections reported from the northeastern coastal region of the USA. Known endemic areas are Nantucket, Martha's Vineyard, Shelter Island, and parts of Long Island. Natural hosts for *B microti* include the white-footed mouse and the meadow vole. Serosurveys show frequent subclinical *B microti* infections. Humans are infected as a result of *Ixodes* tick bites, but transmission from blood transfusion has also been reported. Without passing through an exoerythrocytic stage, the parasite enters the red blood cell and multiplies, resulting in cell rupture followed by infection of other cells. Splenectomized, elderly, or immunosuppressed persons are the most likely to have severe manifestations.

The incubation period is 1–4 weeks, but patients usually do not recall the tick bite. *B microti* infection lasts a few weeks to a month; the illness is characterized by irregular fever, chills, headache, diaphoresis, myalgia, and fatigue but is without malarialike periodicity of symptoms. Most patients have a moderate hemolytic anemia, and some have hepatosplenomegaly. Although parasitemia may continue for months, with or without symptoms, the disease is self-limited and most patients recover without sequelae.

Only a few *B divergens* infections have been reported, all in splenectomized patients. These infections progress rapidly with high fever, severe hemolytic anemia, jaundice, hemoglobinuria, and renal failure; death usually follows.

Diagnosis is by identification of the intraerythrocytic parasite on Giemsa-stained thick or thin blood smears; no gametocytes and no intracellular pigment are seen. Repeated smears may be necessary. The organism must be differentiated from malarial parasites, particularly *Plasmodium falciparum*. Isolation of the parasite can be attempted by inoculating patient blood into hamsters or gerbils. Serologic tests are available; serologic cross-reactions occur between *Babesia* and malaria parasites, but antibody titers are generally highest to the infecting organism.

No drug treatment is satisfactory. The only patients who have recovered from *B divergens* infections have been managed with blood transfusions and renal dialysis. As *B microti* infections in patients with intact spleen are usually self-limiting, most infections can be treated symptomatically. In splenectomized patients, however, limited experience suggests that quinine (650 mg 3 times a day for 7 days) plus clindamycin (1.2 g twice daily parenterally or 600 mg 3 times a day orally for 7 days) may be useful; exchange transfusion has also been successful in several patients.

Centers for Disease Control: Babesiosis—Connecticut. JAMA 1989;262:2067.
Raoult D et al: Babesiosis, pentamidine, and cotrimoxazole. (Letter.) Ann Intern Med 1987;107:944. (Successful treatment of *B divergens* in a nonsplenectomized patient.)
Ruebush TK II: Babesiosis. In: *Tropical Medicine and Parasitology.* Goldsmith R, Heyneman D (editors). Appleton & Lange, 1989.
Smith RP et al: Transfusion-acquired babesiosis and failure of antibiotic treatment. JAMA 1986;256:2276.

BALANTIDIASIS

Balantidium coli is a large ciliated intestinal protozoon found worldwide, but particularly in the tropics. Infection results from ingestion of cysts passed in stools of humans or swine, the reservoir hosts. In the new host, the cyst wall dissolves and the trophozoite may invade the mucosa and submucosa of the terminal ileum and large bowel, causing abscesses and irregularly rounded ulcerations. Many infections are asymptomatic and probably need not be treated. Chronic recurrent diarrhea, alternating with constipation, is most common, but severe dysentery with bloody mucoid stools, tenesmus, and colic may occur

intermittently. Diagnosis is made by finding trophozoites in liquid stools and cysts in formed stools. The treatment of choice is tetracycline hydrochloride, 500 mg 4 times daily for 10 days. The alternative drug is iodoquinol (diiodohydroxyquin), 650 mg 3 times daily for 21 days. Occasional success has also been reported with metronidazole (750 mg 3 times daily for 5 days) or paromomycin (25–30 mg/kg [base] in 3 divided doses for 5–10 days).

In properly treated mild to moderate symptomatic cases, the prognosis is good, but in spite of treatment, fatalities have occurred in severe infections as a result of intestinal perforation or hemorrhage.

Knight R: Giardiasis, isosporiasis and balantidiasis. Clin Gastroenterol 1978;7:31.
Ladas SD et al: Invasive balantidiasis presented as chronic colitis and lung involvement. Dig Dis Sci 1989;34:1621.

COCCIDIOSIS: ISOSPORIASIS, CRYPTOSPORIDIOSIS, SARCOCYSTOSIS

Coccidiosis is an intestinal infection usually accompanied by diarrhea and abdominal discomfort and caused by coccidia of 3 genera: *Isospora, Cryptosporidium,* and *Sarcocystis.* These infections occur worldwide but except for *Cryptosporidium* are recognized only sporadically.

General Considerations

A. Isosporiasis: Isosporiasis, caused by *Isospora belli,* is considered host-specific for humans, with transmission directly from person to person. Infection is by the fecal-oral route following ingestion of oocysts. Sporozoites excyst and invade jejunal and duodenal epithelial cells, in which they undergo both a sexual and an asexual cycle, resulting in the liberation of unsporulated oocysts, 20–30 × 10–20 μm, into the feces.

The incubation period is 7–11 days. Some patients remain asymptomatic. Most symptomatic infections follow a benign, self-limited course lasting a few weeks or months. The principal findings are diarrhea, abdominal pain, flatulence, low-grade fever, vomiting, malaise, and anorexia. Infrequently, the disease is protracted or recurrent; when severe, there may be intense diarrhea, steatorrhea, malabsorption, and weight loss. Several deaths have been reported. Isosporiasis, sometimes severe, is seen in AIDS.

The diagnosis is made by finding the parasite in feces or duodenal aspirates or by duodenal biopsy. Diagnosis by stool examination is often difficult, for the organisms may be scanty even in the presence of significant symptoms. The laboratory should be notified of the need to search for the organisms, so that special concentration techniques will be used. Because of their buoyancy, oocysts must be looked for just beneath the coverslip of the preparation. Although the peroral duodenal string test or duodenal aspiration may also assist in diagnosis, frequently diagnosis can be made only after duodenal biopsy and search of multiple serial sections. Up to 50% of patients with isosporiasis have eosinophilia.

B. Cryptosporidiosis: *Cryptosporidium,* which causes diarrhea in many animal species, has only recently been recognized worldwide as a cause of sporadic mild diarrhea in all ages, acute childhood diarrhea (particularly in developing countries), traveler's diarrhea, and severe diarrhea in immunocompromised persons, particularly those with AIDS. Outbreaks in day care centers, clustering in families, and water-borne outbreaks have been reported. Stool surveys and duodenal aspiration in immunocompetent persons show an asymptomatic carrier state. Although it remains unsettled whether more than one species exists, currently, *C parvum* is considered the agent responsible for infection in humans.

Fecal-oral transmission is from animals to humans, and human-to-human transmission is presumed to occur. Oocysts (about 4 μm in diameter) passed in stool are fully sporulated and infectious; infection occurs as a result of their ingestion. The incubation period appears to be 2–10 days.

In humans, as well as animals, the full life cycle of *Cryptosporidium* occurs within a single host—asexual and sexual proliferation and parasite amplification. The organisms attach to the microvillous borders of enterocytes of the small bowel and also are found free in mucosal crypts. The host cell membrane deteriorates, leaving the parasitic membrane in direct contact with epithelial cell cytoplasm. The organisms are not, however, invasive into the tissues. Voluminous secretory diarrhea results, but the mechanism has not been elucidated. In AIDS, the organism has also been found in extraintestinal sites.

In immunocompetent persons, infection varies from no symptoms to mild enteritis to marked watery diarrhea (up to 10 stools daily) without mucus or gross or microscopic blood. Accompanying findings may include low-grade fever, malaise, nausea, vomiting, abdominal cramps, and, sometimes, anorexia and weight loss. The infection is generally self-limited and lasts a few days to about 2 weeks. Occasionally described are a malabsorption state or marked dehydration and failure to thrive in children.

In immunologically deficient patients—especially those with AIDS—the illness is characterized by chronic, profuse, choleralike watery diarrhea and by fever, severe malabsorption, marked weight loss, and lymphadenopathy. The diarrhea may recur or persist for months and contribute to death. In AIDS, infection may involve any part of the gastrointestinal tract, and multisystem involvement has been described.

Diagnosis is by detection of oocysts in stool by a variety of flotation or concentration methods or by mucosal biopsy, followed by special staining methods that use modifications of the acid-fast stain (routine fecal staining methods do not detect the organism). Three stools should be examined over 5 days, and the laboratory should be notified that *Cryptosporidium* and *Isospora* are being sought. A fluorescein-labeled IgG monoclonal antibody test has recently become available to detect the oocysts. Serologic tests are available but are not useful in diagnosing acute disease. Radiologic changes have been reported in the stomach, intestines, and bile ducts in severe disease. In AIDS patients, the organism should also be looked for in sputum and specimens obtained from lung tissue.

C. Sarcocystosis: *Sarcocystis* is a 2-host coccidian. Human disease occurs as 2 syndromes, both rare: (1) an enteric infection in which humans are the definitive host and (2) a muscle infection in which humans are an intermediate host. In the enteric form, sporocysts passed in human feces are not infective for humans but must be ingested by cattle or pigs. Humans become infected by eating poorly cooked beef or pork containing oocysts of *Sarcocystis bovihominis* or *Sarcocystis suihominis,* respectively. (Formerly, the causative agent was known as *Isospora hominis.*) Organisms enter intestinal epithelial cells and are transformed into oocysts that release sporocysts into the feces. Clinically, the intestinal infection is often asymptomatic or causes mild, protracted diarrhea. Diagnosis is by stool examination using a fecal flotation method.

The muscle form of sarcocystosis results when humans ingest sporocysts in feces from an infected carnivore that has eaten prey which harbored sarcocysts. The sporocysts liberate sporozoites that invade the intestinal wall and are disseminated to skeletal muscle. This results in subcutaneous and muscular inflammation lasting several days to 2 weeks and the finding of swellings at these sites, sometimes associated with eosinophilia. Sarcocysts are often asymptomatic, however, such as those found incidentally at autopsy in cardiac muscle.

Treatment

In **isosporiasis,** instances of effective treatment have been described using (1) sulfadiazine, 4 g, and pyrimethamine, 35–75 mg, in 4 divided doses daily for 3 weeks; or (2) trimethoprim (160 mg) and sulfamethoxazole (800 mg) 4 times daily for 10 days and then twice daily for 3 weeks. In AIDS patients, recurrence has been prevented by weekly prophylactic use of an alternative drug (see Pape reference, below). Efficacy in primary infection has also been reported for furazolidone (400 mg/d for 10 days), metronidazole, and quinacrine.

Cryptosporidiosis in immunologically competent individuals is a self-limiting disease. In **sarcocystosis** and in cryptosporidiosis in immunologically incompetent persons, no treatment has been successful, although in the latter infection spiramycin (1 g 3 times daily), zidovudine (AZT), and eflornithine have sometimes been reported to be of value. Supportive treatment includes fluid and electrolyte replacement and, in chronic cases, parenteral nutrition.

Crawford FG, Vermund SH: Human cryptosporidiosis. Crit Rev Microbiol 1988;16:113.

Greenberg RE et al: Resolution of intestinal cryptosporidiosis after treatment of AIDS with AZT. Gastroenterology 1989;97:1327.

Pape JW, Verdier R-I, Johnson WD Jr: Treatment and prophylaxis of *Isospora belli* infection in patients with the acquired immunodeficiency syndrome. N Engl J Med 1989;320:1044.

Rolston KVI, Fainstein V, Bodey GP: Intestinal cryptosporidiosis treated with eflornithine: A prospective study among patients with AIDS. J Acquir Immune Defic Syndr 1989;2:426.

S'aez-Llorens X et al: Spiramycin vs. placebo for treatment of acute diarrhea caused by *Cryptosporidium*. Pediatr Infect Dis 1989;8:136.

Soave R, Johnson WD: *Cryptosporidium* and *Isospora belli* infections. J Infect Dis 1988;157:225.

Tzipori S: Cryptosporidiosis in perspective. Adv Parasitol 1988;27:63.

Wittenberg DF, Miller NM, van den Ende J: Spiramycin is not effective in treating *Cryptosporidium* diarrhea in infants: Results of a double-blind randomized trial. J Infect Dis 1989;159:131.

GIARDIASIS

Essentials of Diagnosis

- Most infections are asymptomatic.
- In some cases, acute or chronic diarrhea, mild to severe, with bulky, greasy, frothy, malodorous stools, free of blood and pus.
- Upper abdominal discomfort, cramps, distention, excessive flatus, and lassitude.
- Cysts and occasionally trophozoites in stools.
- Trophozoites in duodenal fluid.

General Considerations

Giardiasis is a protozoal infection of the upper small intestine caused by the flagellate *Giardia lamblia*. The parasite occurs worldwide and is nearly universal in children in developing countries. In the USA and Europe, the infection is considered the most common intestinal protozoal pathogen. Persons of all ages are affected, but occurrence is particularly high among children.

The organism occurs in feces as a symmetric, heart-shaped flagellated trophozoite measuring $10-25 \times 6-12$ μm and as a cyst measuring $8-13 \times 6-11$ μm. Only the cyst form is infectious by the oral route; trophozoites are destroyed by gastric acidity. Humans are the reservoir for *Giardia*, but dogs and beavers have been implicated as a zoonotic source of infection.

Most infections are sporadic, resulting from cysts transmitted as a result of fecal contamination of water or food, by person-to-person contact, or by anal-oral sexual contact. Multiple infections are common in households, and outbreaks occur in nursery schools and mental institutions and as a result of contamination of water supplies. Giardiasis is a well-recognized problem in special groups including travelers, campers, male homosexuals, and persons with impaired immune states.

After the cysts are ingested, trophozoites emerge in the duodenum and jejunum. They can cause epithelial damage, atrophy of villi, hypertrophic crypts, and extensive cellular infiltration of the lamina propria by lymphocytes, plasma cells, and neutrophils. It is likely that hypogammaglobulinemia, low secretory IgA levels in the gut, achlorhydria, and malnutrition favor the development of infection.

Clinical Findings

A. Symptoms and Signs: A large proportion of infected persons remain asymptomatic cyst carriers, and their infection clears spontaneously. The clinical forms of giardiasis are (1) acute diarrhea, (2) chronic diarrhea, and (3) malabsorption syndrome. The incubation period is usually 1–3 weeks but may be longer. The illness may begin gradually or suddenly. The acute phase may last days or weeks, but it is usually self-limited, although cyst excretion may continue. In a few patients, the disorder may become chronic and last for years, but it does not appear to last indefinitely.

In both the acute and chronic forms, diarrhea ranges from mild to severe; most often it is mild. There may be no complaints other than of one bulky, loose bowel movement a day, often after breakfast. With larger numbers of movements, the stools become increasingly watery and may contain mucus but are usually free of blood and pus; they are copious, frothy, malodorous, and greasy, tending to float in the toilet bowl. The diarrhea may be daily or recurrent; if recurrent, stools may be normal to mushy during intervening days, or the patient may be constipated. Weight loss and weakness may occur. Less common are anorexia, nausea and vomiting, midepigastric discomfort and cramps (often after meals), belching, flatulence, borborygmus, and abdominal distention. Low-grade fever is infrequent, and headache, urticaria, and myalgia are rare.

A malabsorption syndrome occasionally develops in the acute or chronic stage that may result in marked weight loss and debility. Findings may include fat- and protein-losing enteropathy and vitamin B_{12}, D-xylose, and lactase deficiency. The latter may persist for a long time in persons apparently cured after specific treatment.

B. Laboratory Tests: Diagnosis is by identifying cysts or trophozoites in feces or duodenal fluid. Detection can be difficult, because the number of cysts passed varies considerably from day to day, and at the onset of infection, patients may have symptoms for about a week before organisms can be detected.

If clinically warranted, diagnostic accuracy can be increased by proceeding as follows: (1) routine stool examinations → (2) examination of upper intestinal fluid by the duodenal string test (Entero-Test) or by duodenal aspiration → (3) duodenal biopsy examined after permanent staining. Duodenal biopsy is rarely done, however; most workers prefer instead an empiric course of treatment after presumptive diagnosis. Three stool specimens should be examined at intervals of 2 days or longer. Unless they can be submitted within an hour, specimens should be preserved immediately in a fixative. Purges do not increase the likelihood of finding the organism. Use of barium, antibiotics, antacids, kaolin products, or oily laxatives may temporarily reduce the number of parasites or interfere with detection, requiring a delay in further examination for about 10 days. Duodenal aspirate should be concentrated by centrifugation at 500 rpm for 5 minutes and be examined by wet mount and after permanent staining. Biopsy specimens should first be pressed onto a slide to obtain a mucosal imprint for staining and then be sectioned for histologic examination.

Serologic tests for circulating antibody and coproantigen are being developed. Radiologic examination of the small bowel is usually normal in asymptomatic and mildly ill persons but may show nonspecific findings of altered motility, thickened mucosal folds, and barium column segmentation in patients with marked symptoms.

Treatment

A. Specific Measures: Symptomatic patients should be treated; asymptomatic patients should also be treated, since they can transmit the infection to others and may occasionally become symptomatic themselves. In selected instances of asymptomatic infection, it may be best to wait a few weeks before starting treatment to see if the infection will clear spontaneously.

Treatment can be carried out effectively with tinidazole, metronidazole, quinacrine, or furazolidone. Occasional treatment failures require re-treatment with an alternative drug. Tinidazole, where available, is the drug of choice, based on reports that it is effective as a single dose.

In follow-up, it is best to wait about 2 weeks before rechecking 2 or more stools at weekly intervals.

All of these drugs occasionally have unpleasant side effects. The potential carcinogenicity of furazolidone, metronidazole, and tinidazole appears to be negligible based on 2 decades of use.

1. Metronidazole (Flagyl)–Adults receive 250 mg 3 times daily for 5–10 days; children receive 5 mg/kg 3 times daily for 5 days. Cure rates are generally between 85 and 95%. Metronidazole may cause gastrointestinal symptoms, headache, and a metallic taste. Patients must be warned that alcohol may cause a disulfiramlike reaction. Liquid suspensions for pediatric use are available only outside the USA.

2. Quinacrine (mepacrine, Atabrine)–For adults and children over 8 years of age, give 100 mg 3 times daily after meals for 5–7 days; for younger children, give 2 mg/kg 3 times daily (maximum 300 mg/d) for 5–7 days. The drug has a bitter taste, and young children tend to tolerate it poorly. Cure rates are 80–95%. Gastrointestinal symptoms, headache, and dizziness are common; harmless yellowing of the skin is infrequent. Toxic psychosis and exfoliative dermatitis, which are rare, may be severe and longlasting. Quinacrine is contraindicated in psoriasis or in persons with a history of psychosis.

3. Furazolidone (Furoxone)–This is the most convenient pediatric drug, dispensed as a suspension. Adults receive 100 mg (children, 1.25 mg/kg) 4 times daily for 10 days. Cure rates range from 72 to 90%. Gastrointestinal symptoms, fever, headache, rash, and a disulfiramlike reaction with alcohol occur. Furazolidone can cause mild hemolysis in glucose-6-phosphate dehydrogenase-deficient persons and rarely causes hypersensitivity reactions.

4. Tinidazole (Fasigyn) (not available in the USA), 2 g given once, has had reported cure rates of 90–100%. Adverse reactions consist of mild gastrointestinal side effects in about 10% of patients; headache and vertigo are less common.

B. Prevention: There is no effective chemoprophylaxis for giardiasis. Prevention is as for amebiasis (above).

Prognosis

With treatment and successful eradication of the infection, there are no sequelae. Without treatment, severe malabsorption may rarely contribute to death from other causes.

Dupont HL, Sullivan PS: Giardiasis: The clinical spectrum, diagnosis and therapy. Pediatr Infect Dis 1986;5:131.

Erlandsen SL, Meyer EA (editors): *Giardia* and Giardiasis. Plenum Press, 1984.

Goka AKJ et al: The relative merits of faecal and duodenal juice microscopy in the diagnosis of giardiasis. Trans R Soc Trop Med Hyg 1990;84:66.

Pickering LK, Engelkirk PG: *Giardia lamblia*. Pediatr Clin North Am 1988;35:565.

Rosoff JD et al: Stool diagnosis of giardiasis using a commercially available enzyme immunoassay to detect *Giardia*-specific antigen 65 (GSA 65). J Clin Microbiol 1989; 27:1997.

LEISHMANIASIS

Leishmaniasis is infection by species of the genus *Leishmania*. The disease is a zoonosis transmitted by bites of sandflies (*Phlebotomus* species) from wild or domestic animal reservoirs to humans—except in the case of Indian kala-azar, which is transmitted from human to human. Leishmaniae have 2 distinct forms in their life cycle: (1) In mammalian hosts, the parasite is found in its amastigote form (2–3 mm in length) within mononuclear phagocytes. (2) In the sandfly vector, the parasite converts to and is then transmitted as a flagellated extracellular promastigote.

Over 1 million cases of leishmaniasis are estimated to occur in the tropical and temperate zones each year. The clinical manifestations may be classified as (1) visceral, (2) cutaneous, and (3) mucocutaneous. Severity of infection ranges from subclinical or minimally pathogenic (self-healing or easily treated) to severely incapacitating, metastasizing, mutilating, and fatal. Evidence is accumulating that in HIV-infected persons, visceral leishmaniasis is an opportunistic infection.

Laboratory Tests

Laboratory methods for diagnosis of leishmaniasis vary by species of infecting organism. Definitive diagnosis is achieved by finding the parasite—either the amastigote in stained smears or biopsies, or the motile promastigote in culture. Serologic and skin tests provide only indirect evidence of infection.

A. Culture: To inoculate culture medium (NNN, Schneider's insect medium, and others), tissue from a biopsy specimen is preferable, but fluid aspirated from under the margin of a lesion can also be used.

B. Staining of Smears and Biopsy Sections: To demonstrate organisms, stained smears of scrapings (preparation is by cleaning and disinfecting, puncturing, and then scraping the lesion) and touch preparations from a fresh biopsy are superior to stained biopsy sections.

C. Serologic and Skin Tests: See below under individual forms of the disease.

Treatment

Treatment remains inadequate because of drug toxicity, long courses required, and frequent need for hospitalization. The drug of choice is sodium antimony gluconate (sodium stibogluconate). Alternative drugs for some forms of infection are amphotericin B and pentamidine.

A. Sodium Antimony Gluconate (Sodium Stibogluconate): Treatment is started with a 200-mg test dose, followed by 20 mg Sb^5/kg/d (maximum, 850 mg/d) in 2 or 3 divided doses as a 5% solution intramuscularly (preferred) or intravenously for 4 weeks. Hospitalization may be necessary. Relapses should be treated at the same dosage level for at least twice the previous duration. This dosage is based on the 1984 recommendations by WHO that indicate (1) there is no pharmacologic basis for a rest period between courses and (2) antimony is less toxic when divided into 2 or 3 equally spaced doses (ie, at 8- or 12-hour intervals). Only fresh solutions of antimony should be used; the ampules must be stored away from heat. Intravenous injections must be given

slowly over 5 minutes through a 22- or 23-gauge needle. On an equal-weight basis, children require more antimony than adults and tolerate it better. In the USA, the drug is available only from the CDC Drug Service, Centers for Disease Control, Atlanta 30333 ([404]) 639–3670).

B. Pentamidine Isethionate: Pentamidine isethionate, 2–4 mg/kg intramuscularly (preferable) or intravenously, is given daily or on alternate days (up to 15 injections). For adverse reactions, see Pneumocystosis (below).

C. Amphotericin B: Amphotericin B is dissolved in 500 mL of 5% dextrose and injected slowly intravenously over 6 hours on alternate days. The initial dose of 0.25 mg/kg/d is gradually increased to 1 mg/kg/d ($0.25 \rightarrow 0.5 \rightarrow 1$) until a total of about 30 mg/kg is given. Patients must be closely monitored in hospital, because side effects may be severe.

Berman JD: Chemotherapy for leishmaniasis: Biochemical mechanisms, clinical efficacy, and future strategies. Rev Infect Dis 1988;10:560.

Goldsmith R, Heyneman D (editors): Leishmaniases. In: *Tropical Medicine and Parasitology*. Appleton & Lange, 1989.

Grimaldi G Jr, Tesh RB, McMahon-Pratt D: A review of the geographic distribution and epidemiology of leishmaniasis in the New World. Am J Trop Med Hyg 1989;41:687.

Montalban C et al: Visceral leishmaniasis (kala-azar) as an opportunistic infection in patients infected with the human immunodeficiency virus in Spain. Rev Infect Dis 1989;11:655.

Peters W, Killick-Kendrick R (editors): *The Leishmaniases*. Vol I: *Biology and Epidemiology*. Vol II: *Clinical Aspects and Control*. Academic Press, 1987.

World Health Organization: *Report of a WHO Expert Committee: The Leishmaniases*. WHO Tech Rep Ser No. 701, 1984.

1. VISCERAL LEISHMANIASIS (Kala-Azar)

Visceral leishmaniasis is caused mainly by the *Leishmania donovani* complex: (1) *L d donovani* (eastern India, Bangladesh, Sudan, Ethiopia, Kenya, scattered foci in central Africa, Soviet Central Asia, and China), (2) *L d infantum* (Mediterranean littoral, Middle East, Iran, Afghanistan, Pakistan), and (3) *L d chagasi* (South America, chiefly Brazil). In each locale, the disease has its own peculiar clinical and epidemiologic features; India, China, and east Africa have had epidemics. Although humans are the major reservoir, animal reservoirs such as the dog, other canids, and rodents are important. The incubation period is usually 4–6 months (range, 10 days to 24 months). Both *L tropica* in Africa and *L mexicana amazonensis* in Brazil have been shown to cause visceral leishmaniasis in a few patients.

A local nonulcerating nodule at the site of the bite

may precede systemic manifestations but usually is inapparent. The onset may be acute or insidious. Fever often peaks twice daily, with chills and sweats, weakness, weight loss, cough, or diarrhea. The spleen progressively becomes huge, hard, and nontender. The liver is somewhat enlarged, and generalized lymphadenopathy is common. Hyperpigmentation of skin, especially on the hands, feet, abdomen, and forehead, is marked in light-skinned patients. In blacks, there may be warty eruptions or skin ulcers. Petechiae, bleeding from the nose and gums, jaundice, and ascites may occur. In some regions, oral and nasopharyngeal or cutaneous manifestations occur without visceral involvement. Wasting is progressive; death, often due to intercurrent infection, occurs within months to 1–2 years.

Post-kala-azar dermal leishmaniasis may appear 1–2 years after apparent cure (up to 10 years in India and China). It may simulate leprosy, as multiple hypopigmented macules or nodules develop on preexisting lesions. Erythematous patches may appear on the face. Leishmaniae are present in the skin. The condition is often unresponsive to antimony therapy.

Diagnosis is by demonstrating the organism in buffy coat preparations of blood; on stained smears of aspirates of sternal marrow or iliac crest, liver, lymph nodes, or spleen; and by culture. The immunofluorescent antibody test (positive titer, 1:128) has few false-positive reactions. The leishmanin skin test is always negative during active disease and becomes positive months to years after recovery. Other characteristic findings are progressive leukopenia (seldom over 3000/μL after the first 1–2 months), with lymphocytosis and monocytosis, normochromic anemia, and thrombocytopenia. There is a marked increase in total protein up to or greater than 10 g/dL owing to an elevated IgG fraction; serum albumin is 3 g/dL or less. Liver function tests show hepatocellular damage. Proteinuria may be present.

The differential diagnosis includes leukemia, lymphoma, tuberculosis, brucellosis, malaria, typhoid, schistosomiasis, African trypanosomiasis, infective endocarditis, cirrhosis, and other entities.

Sodium antimony gluconate is the drug of choice. Most patients respond readily, but prolonged treatment may be required, especially in the Sudan, Kenya, and India. Failure after repeated courses should lead to use of pentamidine or amphotericin B.

Without treatment, the case-fatality rate can reach 90%. Early diagnosis and treatment reduces the mortality rate to 2–5%.

Badaro R et al: Treatment of visceral leishmaniasis with pentavalent antimony and interferon gamma. N Engl J Med 1990;322:16.
Mebrahtu Y et al: Visceral leishmaniasis unresponsive to pentostam caused by Leishmania tropica in Kenya. Am J Trop Med Hyg 1989;41:289.
Rees PH et al: The treatment of kala-azar: A review with comments drawn from experience in Kenya. Trop Geogr Med 1985;37:37.
Thakur CP et al: Rationalisation of regimens of treatment of kala-azar with sodium stibogluconate in India: A randomised study. Br Med J 1988;296:1557.

2. CUTANEOUS LEISHMANIASIS

Agents of Old World cutaneous leishmaniasis are (1) L tropica (Middle East, India, USSR [Turkmenistan], Afghanistan, Armenia, Greece), (2) L major (Middle East, Arabian peninsula, USSR [Turkmenistan], Afghanistan, Africa [north, east, sub-Sahara, Senegal, Sudan, Kenya]), and (3) L aethiopica (Ethiopian highlands, Kenya).

Agents of New World cutaneous leishmaniasis are L mexicana mexicana (Mexico [Yucatan], Belize, Guatemala), (2) L m amazonensis (Brazil [Amazon basin], Venezuela), (3) other members of the L m mexicana complex (South America), and (4) the L braziliensis complex (Central and South America). The L d donovani complex sometimes causes cutaneous lesions without visceral manifestations.

Lesions can be single or multiple. Cutaneous swellings appear 2 to several months after sandfly bites, may ulcerate and discharge pus, or may remain dry. The lesions are painless unless secondarily infected. Systemic symptoms are rare, but a low-grade fever of short duration may be present at the onset. Healing may occur spontaneously in months to 1–3 years, the rate varying by species. Contraction of scars can cause deformities and disfigurement, especially if lesions are on the face.

In the Old World, L major infections occur in dry or desert rural areas and are characterized by a wet, rapidly ulcerating sore; L tropica infection is urban and chronic and produces a dry sore that ulcerates slowly or not at all. Most New World cutaneous lesions are ulcers, but vegetative, verrucous, or nodular lesions may occur also. L m mexicana ("chiclero's ulcer") produces destructive lesions on the ear cartilage. Up to 80% of L b braziliensis cutaneous lesions progress to espundia (see below); some L braziliensis complex strains also show a chain of palpable local lymph nodes. In addition to cutaneous lesions, L aethiopica and L m amazonensis may also cause diffuse cutaneous leishmaniasis, a chronic, disseminated form that resembles leprosy; it is associated with anergy and skin tests are negative, but amastigotes are abundant. Leishmaniasis recidivans is a relapsing form in which slow spread of ulcers and scarring can be extensive. It is caused by L tropica and is associated with hypersensitivity; the skin test is strongly positive, and amastigotes are scarce.

Leishmania species cannot be detected in purulent discharge but may be seen in stained scrapings from the cleaned edge of the ulcer or in material aspirated after the injection of saline under the margin of the ulcer. Under sterile conditions, aspirate may be inoculated into culture or hamsters. The skin test is positive early. Serologic tests are often unreliable.

Cutaneous leishmaniasis in the Old World is normally self-healing and confers protection. Lesions should be kept clean and antibiotics used if secondary infection of lesions occurs. Travelers not returning to endemic areas or persons whose lesions are large or numerous should be treated either with physical measures (cryotherapy, heat treatment, electrocoagulation, surgical removal) or with chemotherapy: (1) intralesional (sodium antimony gluconate, emetine) or (2) parenteral (sodium antimony gluconate is preferred; pentamidine or amphotericin B is used for failures). See references for details on treatment.

In New World *L mexicana* infections from Mexico and Central America, solitary nodules or ulcers in inconspicuous sites generally will heal spontaneously, but metronidazole, 750 mg 3 times daily for 10 days, can be tried. Lesions on the ear, face, or hands should be treated with sodium antimony gluconate but usually require only a 12- to 14-day course. Cutaneous lesions acquired in regions of mucocutaneous leishmaniasis may be due to *L braziliensis* and should be treated with a full course of sodium antimony gluconate. See references for information on treatment of lesions acquired in other areas and for treatment of diffuse cutaneous and recidivans leishmaniasis.

Ballou WR et al: Safety and efficacy of high-dose sodium stibogluconate therapy of American cutaneous leishmaniasis. Lancet 1987;2:13.

El-On J et al: Topical treatment of cutaneous leishmaniasis. J Invest Dermatol 1986;87:284.

Kubba R, Al-Gindan Y: Leishmaniasis. Dermatol Clin 1989;7:331.

Viallet J, MacLean JD, Robson H: Response to ketoconazole in two cases of long-standing cutaneous leishmaniasis. Am J Trop Med Hyg 1986;35:491.

3. MUCOCUTANEOUS LEISHMANIASIS (Espundia)

Leishmania b braziliensis causes severe naso-oral lesions in lowland forest areas of South America and Central America north to Belize. The initial lesion, single or multiple, is on exposed skin; at first it is papular (can be pruriginous or painful), then nodular, and later may ulcerate or become wartlike or papillomatous. Local healing follows, with scarring within several months to a year. Subsequent naso-oral involvement occurs in a small proportion of patients either by direct extension or, more often, metastatically to the mucosa. It may appear concurrently with the initial lesion, shortly after healing, or after many years. The mucosa of the anterior part of the nasal septum is generally the first area to be involved. Extensive destruction of the soft tissues and cartilage of the nose, oral cavity, and lips may follow and may

extend to the larynx and pharynx. Gross and hideous destruction and marked suffering can result. Severe bacterial infection is common. Regional lymphangitis, lymphadenitis, fever, weight loss, keratitis, and anemia may be present.

Diagnosis is by finding amastigotes in scrapings, biopsy specimens, or aspirated tissue fluid; the organism grows with difficulty in culture or after inoculation of hamsters. The leishmanin skin test is useful if it produces a fully developed papule in 2–3 days that disappears after a week. Antibodies are detectable in most cases and disappear with cure. The main considerations in the differential diagnosis are paracoccidioidomycosis, lethal midline granuloma, lymphoma, and nasopharyngeal carcinoma, which are distinguishable by biopsy.

In treatment, at least one full course of sodium antimony gluconate is given. Corticosteroids may be needed to control local inflammation due to release of antigens. If antimony treatment fails, amphotericin B is used. Antibiotics are usually needed to treat associated bacterial or fungal infection.

Marsden PD: Mucosal leishmaniasis ("espundia" Escomel, 1911). Trans R Soc Trop Med Hyg 1986;80:859.

MALARIA

Essentials of Diagnosis

- History of exposure in a malaria-endemic area.
- Periodic attacks of sequential chills, fever, and sweating.
- Headache, myalgia, splenomegaly; anemia, leukopenia.
- Characteristic parasites in erythrocytes, identified in thick or thin blood films.
- Complications of falciparum malaria: Cerebral findings (mental disturbances, neurologic signs, convulsions), hemolytic anemia, hyperpyrexia, dysenteric or choleralike stools, dark urine, anuria.

General Considerations

Four species of the genus *Plasmodium* are responsible for human malaria: *Plasmodium vivax, Plasmodium malariae, Plasmodium ovale,* and *Plasmodium falciparum.* Although the disease has been eradicated from most temperate zone countries, it continues to be endemic in many parts of the tropics and subtropics, and imported cases occur in the USA and other countries free of transmission. Malaria is present in parts of Mexico, Haiti, Central and South America, Africa, the Middle East, the Indian subcontinent, southeast Asia, China, and Oceania. *P vivax* and *P falciparum* are responsible for most infections and are found throughout the malaria belt. *P malariae* is widely distributed but is less common. *P ovale* is rare, but in West Africa it seems to replace *P vivax.*

Malaria is transmitted from human to human by

the bite of infected female *Anopheles* mosquitoes. Congenital transmission and transmission by blood transfusion also occur. There are no animal reservoirs for human malaria.

The mosquito becomes infected by taking blood containing the sexual forms of the parasite (micro- and macrogametocytes). After a developmental phase in the mosquito, sporozoites develop that are inoculated into humans when the mosquito next feeds. The first stage of development in humans, the exoerythrocytic stage, takes place in the liver. Subsequently, parasites escape from the liver into the bloodstream, invade red blood cells, multiply, and 48 hours later (or 72 with *P malariae*) cause the red cells to rupture, releasing a new crop of parasites (merozoites). Within the bloodstream, this cycle of invasion, multiplication, and red cell rupture may be repeated many times. Symptoms do not appear until several of these erythrocytic cycles have been completed.

The incubation period for *P falciparum* is approximately 12 days (range, 9–25 days); for *P vivax* and *P ovale*, 14 days (range, 8–27 days [initial attacks for some temperate strains may not occur for up to 8 months]); and for *P malariae*, 30 days (range, 16 days to 8 weeks). If untreated, *P falciparum* infections usually terminate spontaneously in 6–8 months but can persist for up to 1½ years; *P vivax* and *P ovale* infections can persist without treatment for as long as 5 years; and *P malariae* infections have lasted for as long as 50 years.

P falciparum and *P malariae* have only one cycle of liver cell invasion and multiplication. Liver infection ceases spontaneously in less than 4 weeks; thereafter, multiplication is confined to the red cells. Thus, treatment that eliminates these species from the red cells will cure the infection. *P vivax* (and presumably *P ovale*) have, however, a dormant hepatic stage (the hypnozoite) that is responsible for subsequent relapses. Cure of *P vivax* and *P ovale* infections, therefore, requires treatment to eradicate parasites both from the red cells and from the liver.

Clinical Findings

A. Symptoms and Signs: Typical malarial attacks show sequential shaking chills (the cold stage); fever (the hot stage) to 41 °C (105.8 °F) or higher; and marked diaphoresis (the sweating stage). A full attack lasts 4–8 hours. Attacks may be accompanied by fatigue, headache, dizziness, gastrointestinal symptoms (anorexia, nausea, slight diarrhea, vomiting, abdominal cramps), myalgia, arthralgia, backache, and dry cough.

Either from the onset of symptoms or with progression of the disease, the attacks may show an every-other-day (tertian) periodicity in vivax, ovale, or falciparum malaria or an every-third-day (quartan) periodicity in malariae malaria. Regular periodicity reflects synchronous parasite maturation, red cell rup-

ture, and release of merozoites. Splenomegaly usually appears when acute symptoms have continued for 4 or more days; the liver is frequently mildly enlarged. The patient may be tired between attacks but otherwise feels well. After this primary episode, there is often a latent period followed by a recurrence.

P falciparum infection is more serious than the others because of the high frequency of severe or fatal complications, which sometimes occur within 24 hours. Complications can be anticipated if parasitemia exceeds 100,000/μL of red blood cells or if many cells (> 10%) contain more than one parasite. Complications, variously combined, include the following: (1) cerebral malaria with edema (headache, mental disturbances, neurologic signs, convulsions, delirium, coma); (2) hyperpyrexia; (3) hemolytic anemia; (4) acute pulmonary edema, with profound difficulties with oxygenation; (5) acute tubular necrosis and renal failure, with production of dark urine (blackwater fever); (6) acute hepatopathy, with centrilobular necrosis and marked jaundice; (7) major problems with water and electrolyte imbalance, including hypovolemia; (8) hypoglycemia (can occur even when patient is receiving a 5% glucose infusion); (9) an acute adrenal insufficiency-like state (low blood pressure, thin and rapid pulse, pale and clammy skin, hemoconcentration, shock); (10) cardiac dysrhythmias; and (11) gastrointestinal syndromes (choleralike, bacillary dysentery-like, hemorrhage). A form of nephrosis may occur in *P malariae* infection. Tropical splenomegaly is an immunologic disorder related to chronic malaria.

B. Laboratory Findings: The thick and thin blood film, stained with Giemsa's stain, is the mainstay of diagnosis. The thin film is used primarily for species differentiation after the presence of an infection is detected on a thick film. Because the level of parasitemia varies from hour to hour—especially for *P falciparum* infections, in which parasites may not be found—blood should be examined at 6- to 8-hour intervals for 2–3 days, during and between febrile spikes. In all but *P falciparum* infections, the number of red cells infected seldom exceeds 2% of the total cells. A severe parasitemia in falciparum malaria is 10%, but levels may reach 20–30% or more. During paroxysms, there may be transient leukocytosis; leukopenia develops subsequently, with a relative increase in large mononuclear cells. Hepatic function tests often become abnormal, but the tests revert to normal with treatment or spontaneous recovery. Hemolytic jaundice and thrombocytopenia may develop in severe infections.

Serologic tests are not used in the diagnosis of acute malaria but may be of value occasionally in investigation of recurrent febrile illness and in recognition of infection in persons returning from a malarious area. A titer of 1:64 in the indirect immunofluorescence test indicates that the patient has acquired malaria at some time in the past.

Table 28–2. Prevention of malaria in travelers.[1]

To prevent attacks of all forms of malaria and to eradicate *Plasmodium falciparum* and *P malariae* infections[2]

A. In areas free of falciparum malaria resistant to chloroquine (ie, Central America, the Caribbean, and the Middle East):
- Chloroquine phosphate,[3] 500 mg (salt) once weekly starting 1 week before entering the endemic area, while there, and for 4 weeks after leaving.

B. In areas where falciparum malaria is resistant to chloroquine (ie, all other malarious areas of the world):
- Preferred method: Mefloquine,[4] 250 mg (salt) once weekly starting 1 week before entering the endemic area, while there, and for 4 weeks after leaving.
- First alternative: Chloroquine and Fansidar.[5] Give chloroquine at the above schedule. Give 3 tablets of Fansidar as a single dose once only in self-treatment of febrile illness if medical care is not immediately available.
- Second Alternative: Chloroquine plus doxycycline.[6] Give chloroquine at the above schedule. Give 100 mg of doxycycline daily during exposure and for 4 weeks afterward.

To eradicate *Plasmodium vivax* and *P ovale* infections[2]
- Primaquine phosphate,[7] 26.3 mg (salt) daily for 14 days.

---

[1] A single dose of all drugs used in prophylaxis (except for Fansidar) should be tested while the patient is still at home to detect possible idiosyncratic reactions. See text for additional comments on indications and adverse reactions of the drugs. For additinal information and advice on prophylaxis, see references or call the Centers for Disease Control, Atlanta; (404) 332-4555 for recorded announcements; (404) 488-4046 for answers to questions.

[2] The blood schizonticides (chloroquine, mefloquine, doxycycline), when taken for 4 weeks after leaving an endemic area, are curative for sensitive *P falciparum* and *P malariae* infections, but primaquine is needed to eradicate the persistent liver stages of *P vivax* and *P ovale*.

[3] Chloroquine phosphate: 500 mg (salt) = 300 mg (base). Can be used in pregnancy and by young children. Weekly pediatric dose is 8.3 mg/kg (salt) = 5 mg/kg (base), up to maximum adult dose of 500 mg (salt).

[4] Mefloquine hydrochloride: 250 mg (salt) tablet = 228 mg (base). Take with one-half glass of water after eating. Not recommended in pregnancy, for children under 15 kg, or under certain other conditions (see text). Pediatric dose: 15–19 kg, one-fourth tablet; 20–30 kg, one-half tablet; 31–45 kg, three-fourths tablet; > 45 kg, 1 tablet.

[5] Fansidar: One Fansidar tablet = pyrimethamine (25 mg), sulfadoxine (500 mg). Contraindicted in pregnancy at term, in patients with known sulfonamide or pyrimethamine intolerance, and in infants less than 2 months of age. Pediatric dose: 5–10 kg, one-half tablet; 11–20 kg, 1 tablet; 21–30 kg, 1½ tablets; 31–45 kg, 2 tablets; > 45 kg, 3 tablets.

[6] Doxycycline: Contraindicated in pregnancy and for children under 8 years of age. Side effects include photosensitivity (use sunscreens that contain phenoxybenzone or anthranilates that absorb ultraviolet A radiation, and avoid as much direct sun exposure as possible), gastrointestinal symptoms (the drug should be taken with a meal), and candidal vaginitis. Pediatric dose: > 8 years, 2 mg/kg/d up to adult dose of 100 mg.

[7] Primaquine phosphate: 26.3 mg (salt) = 15 mg (base). Start primaquine only after returning home—during the last 2 week of chemoprophylaxis. See text regarding the following: (a) The drug should be used only for persons who have a high probability of exposure to *P vivax* or *P ovale* infection. (b) Before use, patients should be screened for G6PD deficiency. Primaquine is contraindicated in pregnancy. An alternative regimen for adults who have been taking chloroquine in prophylaxis is combined chloroquine phosphate 500 mg (salt) and primaquine phosphate 78.9 mg (salt) weekly for 8 weeks. Pediatric dosage: 0.5 mg (salt)/kg = 0.3 (base)/kg once daily for 14 days.

Differential Diagnosis

Uncomplicated malaria must be distinguished from a variety of other causes of fever, splenomegaly, anemia, or hepatomegaly. Often considered are influenza, urinary tract infections, typhoid fever, infectious hepatitis, dengue, kala-azar, amebic liver abscess, leptospirosis, and relapsing fever. Malaria complications can mimic many diseases.

Drugs Used in Treatment & Chemoprophylaxis (Tables 28–2 and 28–3)

Consultation with a center working on malaria is important for obtaining up-to-date information on malaria prophylaxis and treatment. Sources of information and advice in the USA include state health departments and the Malarial Branch, Centers for Disease Control, in Atlanta, Georgia: For recorded information on prophylaxis, (404) 332–4555; for questions about management of acute attacks or on prophylaxis, (404) 488–4046 (emergencies, (404) 639–2888).

A. Drug Classification: By chemical groups, some of the major antimalarial drugs are as follows:

4-aminoquinolines—chloroquine, hydroxychloroquine, amodiaquine;* diaminopyrimidines—pyrimethamine, trimethoprim; biguanides—proguanil* (chlorguanide); 8-aminoquinolines—primaquine; *Cinchona* alkaloids—quinine; sulfonamides—sulfadoxine, sulfalene, sulfamethoxazole; sulfones—dapsone; 4-quinoline-carbinolamines—mefloquine; and antibiotics—tetracycline, doxycycline. Pyrimethamine and proguanil are known as antifolates, since they inhibit dihydrofolate reductase of plasmodia. Drug combinations that have come into use for treatment of *P falciparum* malaria resistant to chloroquine include Fansidar (pyrimethamine plus sulfadoxine) and Maloprim* (pyrimethamine plus dapsone).

The effectiveness of antimalarial drugs differs with different species of the parasite and with different stages of the life cycle. Drugs that act in the liver to eliminate developing exoerythrocytic schizonts or latent hypnozoites are called **tissue schizonticides** (eg, primaquine). Those that act on blood schizonts are **blood schizonticides** or **suppressive agents** (eg,

---

* Not available in the USA but available in some other countries.

Table 28–3. Treatment of malaria in nonimmune adult populations.

Treatment[1] of all species (except chloroquine-resistant *P falciparum*

- **Oral treatment of *P falciparum*[2] or *P malariae:*** Chloroquine phosphate, 1 g (salt)[3,4] as initial dose, then 0.5 g at 6, 24, and 48 hours.
- **Oral treatment of *P vivax* or *P ovale:*** Chloroquine[3,4] as above, followed by 0.5 g on days 7 and 14, plus primaquine phosphate, 26.3 mg (salt)[5] daily for 14 days starting about the fourth day.
- **Parenteral treatment of severe attacks:** Quinine dihydrochloride[7] or quinidine gluconate.[8] Start oral chloroquine therapy as soon as possible; when the patient is well, give primaquine[4,5] if the infection is due to *P vivax* or *P ovale.*

or

Chloroquine hydrochloride, 250 mg (salt)[10] IM, and repeat every 6 hours. Start oral chloroquine therapy as soon as possible; when the patient is well, give primaquine[4,5] if the infection is due to *P vivax* or *P ovale.*

Treatment[1] of *P falciparum* strains resistant to chloroquine
A. Oral treatment:

- Quinine sulfate, 650 mg 3 times daily for 3–7 days,[6] plus one of the following: Pyrimethamine 75 mg and sulfadoxine 1500 mg (= 3 tabs Fansidar) once

or

Tetracycline[9], 250–500 mg 4 times daily for 7 days,

or

Doxycycline,[9] 100 mg twice daily for 7 days,

or

Clindamycin, 900 mg 3 times daily for 3 days,

or

Pyrimethamine, 25 mg twice daily for 3 days, and sulfadiazine, 500 mg 4 times daily for 5 days
- Mefloquine,[11] 1250 mg once

B. Parenteral treatment of severe attacks:

- Quinine dihydrochloride[7] or quinidine gluconate.[8] Start oral therapy with quinine plus a second drug (as above) as soon as possible.

---

[1] See text for cautions and contraindications pertaining to each drug.

[2] In falciparum malaria, if the patient has not shown a response to conventional oral doses of chloroquine (within 48–72 hours for mild infections, 24 hours for severe infections), parasitic resistance to chloroquine should be considered; chloroquine should be stopped and quinine started.

[3] 500 mg chloroquine phosphate = 300 mg base.

[4] Chloroquine alone is curative for *P malariae* and sensitive strains of *P falciparum,* but primaquine is needed to eradicate the persistent liver stages of *P vivax* and *P ovale.* Start primaquine after the patient has recovered from the acute illness; continue cloroquine weekly during primaquine therapy. Patients should be screened for G6PD deficiency before use of primaquine. An alternative method for primaquine therapy is combined primaquine 78.9 mg (salt) and chloroquine 0.5 g (salt) weekly for 8 weeks.

[5] 26.3 mg of primaquine phosphate = 15 mg primaquine base.

[6] Although quinine sulfate is usually given orally for 3 days, it should be continued for 7 days for infections from Thailand, where diminished sensitivity to quinine has been noted.

[7] Quinine dihydrochloride for intravenous use is available in the USA from the Centers for Disease Control, Atlanta 30333. Telephone (404) 488-4046 during the day; (404) 639-2888 nights, weekends, and holidays (emergencies only). Give 10 mg/kg in 500 mL of normal saline or 5% glucose solution IV slowly over 4 hours; repeat every 8 hours until oral therapy is possible (maximum, 1800 mg/d). Blood pressure and ECG should be monitored constantly to detect arrhythmia or hypotension. For infections from Southeast Asia, if it is known with certainty that the patient has not already taken the medication, a higher initial loading dose of quinine is given (20 mg/kg). Caution is required in treating patients with quinine who previously have been taking mefloquine as prophylaxis.

[8] In an emergency, when parenteral quinine is unavailable, quinidine gluconate can be used. A 10 mg/kg (maximum, 600 mg) loading dose is diluted in 300 mL normal saline and administered over 1 hour followed by continuous administration of 0.02 mg/kg/min (maximum, 10 mg/kg every 8 hours) until oral quinine therapy is possible. Blood pressure and ECG should be monitored constantly; widening of the QRS interval or lengthening of the QT (QT uncorrected > 0.6 ms) requires discontinuation.

[9] Contraindicated in children under the age of 8 years and in pregnant women.

[10] 250 mg of chloroquine hydrochloride (salt) = 200 mg (base); parenteral use of the drug is contraindicated in young children.

[11] Serious side effects can occur rarely. See text for cautions and contraindications. Mefloquine must not be given with quinine.

---

chloroquine, amodiaquine, proguanil, pyrimethamine, mefloquine, quinine). **Gametocides** are drugs that prevent infection of mosquitoes by destroying gametocytes in the blood (eg, primaquine for *P falciparum* and chloroquine for *P vivax, P malariae,* and *P ovale*). **Sporonticidal** agents are drugs that render gametocytes noninfective in the mosquito but do not destroy the gametocytes (eg, pyrimethamine, proguanil).

None of the drugs prevent infection (ie, are true causal prophylactic drugs), except for the **antifolates** (pyrimethamine and proguanil), which prevent matu-

ration of the early *P falciparum* hepatic schizonts. Blood schizonticides, however, which destroy circulating plasmodia, prevent attacks and when used for sufficient time (4 weeks) are curative for *P falciparum* and *P malariae* malaria. Primaquine, which destroys the persisting liver hypnozoites of *P vivax* and *P ovale,* prevents relapses from these parasites and thus effects radical cure.

B. Parasite Resistance to Drugs:
1. *P falciparum* resistance—
a. Chloroquine-resistant strains of *P falciparum* have been confirmed or are probably present in

all malarious areas except in the Caribbean, Central America west of the Panama Canal, and the Middle East, including Egypt. Sometimes these strains are only partially resistant to the drug, as manifested by temporary subsidence of symptoms and transient decrease in asexual parasitemia, followed by return of both after several days to weeks.

b. Resistance to pyrimethamine-sulfadoxine (Fansidar) is present in parts of the Amazon basin of South America, sub-Saharan Africa, and Southeast Asia (widespread in Thailand, Burma, and Cambodia).

c. Resistance to pyrimethamine or proguanil when used alone is common in most endemic areas, but the degree and distribution are not accurately known.

d. Rarely, strains in southeast Asia have shown decreased sensitivity to quinine or mefloquine.

2. *P vivax* resistance–
a. Resistance of *P vivax* blood schizonts to antifolate drugs, including the pyrimethamine-containing drugs Fansidar and Maloprim, has been reported in many areas of the world, particularly southeast Asia.

b. Partial resistance of some strains of *P vivax* hepatic schizonts to primaquine in areas of the southwest Pacific and Thailand may require for cure a larger dose (30 mg of base for 14 days).

c. Two recent reports suggest for the first time possible *P vivax* blood schizonts resistant to chloroquine.

3. *P ovale* and *P malariae*–These forms have not shown resistance.

C. Indications, Limitations, and Adverse Side Effects of Selected Drugs:
1. Chloroquine phosphate–Chloroquine (Aralen) is used in chemoprophylaxis to prevent attacks (to suppress symptoms) of all forms of malaria except for disease due to resistant strains of *P falciparum*. However, in *P vivax* and *P ovale* infections, which have a persistent liver phase, delayed initial attacks or relapses may occur after chloroquine is stopped. Use of primaquine eradicates the liver phase.

Chloroquine is also the drug of choice for treating acute attacks of malaria, but cure occurs only with *P falciparum* and *P malariae*. Cure for *P vivax* and *P ovale* requires primaquine.

Although capable of causing ocular damage when used in large doses for prolonged periods for collagen disease, chloroquine is usually well tolerated when used for malaria prophylaxis or treatment. Gastrointestinal symptoms, mild headache, pruritus (especially in blacks), dizziness, blurred vision, anorexia, malaise, and urticaria may occur; taking the drug after meals or in divided twice-weekly doses may reduce side effects. For some persons, the related compound hydroxychloroquine sulfate (Plaquenil) may be better tolerated at a dosage of 400 mg of the salt weekly and for 4 weeks after leaving the endemic area. Chloroquine hydrochloride is available

for intramuscular administration, but oral treatment should be started as soon as possible. The drug should not be used in young children, in whom it may cause hypotension or sudden death.

Rare reactions from oral chloroquine include impaired hearing, psychosis, convulsions, blood dyscrasias, skin reactions, and hypotension. A total cumulative dosage of 100 g (base) theoretically may be critical in the development of ocular, ototoxic, and myopathic effects. A WHO paper, however, presented the view that weekly administration of 0.5 g (of salt) of chloroquine could be continued for 6 years. Baseline and periodic follow-up ophthalmologic examinations should be done if chemotherapy is to be continued for years. Chloroquine is safe to use in pregnancy and for young children. It is contraindicated in patients with psoriasis.

Certain antacids and antidiarrheal agents (kaolin, calcium carbonate, and magnesium trisilicate) have been shown to interfere with absorption of chloroquine and should not be taken within about 4 hours of taking the drug.

2. Mefloquine hydrochloride–Mefloquine, a quinoline methanol derivative, recently was approved for use in the USA. It is effective against the blood schizonts of all forms of malaria, including most but not all chloroquine-resistant or multidrug-resistant strains of *P falciparum*. The drug has little effect on the liver forms of the parasites or on gametocytes.

Information about side effects with prophylactic doses is still limited, and new findings may emerge. Most reports are of mild and transient gastrointestinal symptoms and dizziness. However, central nervous system toxicity (vertigo, restlessness, light-headedness, disorientation, psychosis, and seizures) has been reported only rarely with prophylactic doses. At the higher doses used in treatment, one estimate is that central nervous system toxicity may occur in about 1% of patients. The terminal half-life of mefloquine varies from 1 week to more than 4 weeks, and side effects have persisted in patients for up to 2 weeks.

Mefloquine is contraindicated in children under 15 kg; in pregnant women; in persons with a history of epilepsy or psychiatric disorder; in travelers using beta-blockers, calcium-channel blockers, or other drugs that may prolong or otherwise alter cardiac conduction; and in travelers involved in tasks requiring fine coordination and spatial discrimination (eg, airline pilots). Women should take contraceptive precautions while taking mefloquine and for 2 months after the last dose. The pediatric dose has not been approved by FDA. Extreme caution is required if quinine is used to treat malaria in persons who have been taking mefloquine prophylaxis.

3. Primaquine phosphate–Primaquine is used (1) to prevent relapse of disease by eliminating persistent liver forms of *P vivax* or *P ovale* ("radical cure") in patients who have had an acute attack and (2) for prophylactic use for individuals returning from an endemic area who have probably been exposed to malaria. In persons with a low probability of exposure, it is preferable to avoid possible primaquine toxicity by not giving the drug but instead advising patients to be evaluated in the event of malarialike symptoms, which usually occur in the first 2 years after infection but can occur up to 4 years after infection.

Primaquine is generally well tolerated. Occasional side effects of the drug are gastrointestinal disturbances, headache, dizziness, or neutropenia. Primaquine should not be used in pregnancy.

All patients should be tested for glucose-6-phosphate dehydrogenase (G6PD) deficiency before therapy is begun and followed carefully during treatment; this is because primaquine may cause mild, self-limited hemolysis or marked hemolysis or methemoglobinemia. G6PD deficiency is most common among blacks or persons of Mediterranean or Asian ancestry. Stop the drug if reddening or darkening of the urine occurs. For individuals deficient in G6PD, it is usually safe to give primaquine phosphate, 78.9 mg (45 mg base) weekly, and chloroquine phosphate, 0.5 g (0.3 g base) weekly, for 8 weeks. However, for persons suspected of having the Mediterranean or Canton forms of G6PD deficiency, it may be preferable not to give primaquine but to treat attacks of malaria with chloroquine as they occur.

Primaquine is also used occasionally to eliminate gametocytes of *P falciparum* from patients and thus prevent their transmission to mosquitoes.

4. Quinine—Oral quinine sulfate is used to treat malaria due to chloroquine-resistant strains of *P falciparum*. Although quinine alone will control an acute attack, in many infections—particularly with strains from southeast Asia—it fails to prevent recurrence. Addition of one of several drugs (Table 28–3) lowers the rate of recurrence.

Parenteral quinine (dihydrochloride) is used in the treatment of severe attacks of malaria due to *P falciparum* strains sensitive or resistant to chloroquine. The drug is given only intravenously at a slow rate (Table 28–3). It should be used with extreme caution and only for patients who cannot take the medication orally; appropriate oral therapy should be started as soon as possible.

Quinine toxicity (cinchonism) includes nausea, vomiting, diarrhea, abdominal pain, tinnitus, decreased auditory acuity, blurred vision, and, less often, hypotension or hives or other allergic reactions. Severe toxicity, including agranulocytosis, thrombocytopenia, hypoprothrombinemia, or massive acute hemolysis and renal failure (blackwater fever), is very rare. Desired plasma quinine levels are about 5–10 mg/mL. Plasma quinine determinations and reduction in dosage to avoid serious toxicity are crucial in patients with renal insufficiency. When given intravenously, quinine can cause hypotension or hypoglycemia, both of which can be severe.

5. Pyrimethamine-sulfadoxine (Fansidar)— Fansidar is supplied as tablets that contain pyrimethamine (25 mg) and sulfadoxine (500 mg). The drug is used in presumptive self-treatment of malaria—ie, in the event of malarialike symptoms that cannot be immediately diagnosed and managed by a local physician, the patient decides when to self-treat with a single dose (3 tablets for adults). *It is imperative, however, that medical follow-up be sought promptly.* Fansidar is no longer used for continuing prophylaxis because of its potential for severe toxicity (eg, Stevens-Johnson syndrome, toxic epidermal necrolysis, death).

Fansidar in single-dose treatment is contraindicated for individuals with known sulfonamide sensitivity and in infants under 2 months of age. It should be used with caution in the presence of impaired renal or hepatic function, in patients with G6PD deficiency (hemolysis occurs in some), and in those with severe allergic disorders or bronchial asthma.

Chemoprophylaxis (See Table 28–2 for methods and dosages.)

Adults and children at whatever age, including breast-fed infants, require prophylaxis, but no method is 100% effective. Travelers to malarious areas must be warned that malaria is a possible diagnosis if they develop fever and other symptoms even when taking prophylaxis regularly. Symptoms can occur as early as 8 days after initial exposure. Travelers should also be reminded of the need to use other protective measures when mosquitoes are biting (chiefly between dusk and dawn)—eg, wear clothing that covers most of the body, apply insect repellents (N,N-diethyl-m-toluamide (deet)) and reapply it at frequent intervals (1–2 hours); use mosquito nets and screens; and spray living and sleeping quarters with a pyrethrum-containing flying-insect spray to kill mosquitoes.

Toxic encephalopathy has recently been recognized in some persons exposed to deet. This can be minimized by the following precautions: Apply repellent sparingly and only to exposed skin or clothing; avoid application of products with high concentrations (up to 95%) to the skin (particularly that of children); do not inhale; and do not get into eyes, mouth, on wounds, or on irritated skin. Wash the skin after coming indoors.

A. Chemoprophylaxis in Regions Where *P falciparum* Is Sensitive to 4-Aminoquinolines:

1. Drug of choice—Chloroquine prevents attacks for all forms of malaria and is curative for *P falciparum* and *P malariae* when taken for 4 weeks after leaving the endemic area. Primaquine is needed to provide cure of *P vivax* and *P ovale* (ie, to eliminate the continuing liver stages of these parasites). Pregnant women should take chloroquine throughout their pregnancy and only start primaquine after parturition.

2. Alternative drugs—For persons who cannot

take chloroquine, hydroxychloroquine sulfate can be tried (see above under chloroquine). Other alternatives are mefloquine and doxycycline.

3. Proguanil* (Chlorguanide,* Paludrine*)– The status of proguanil in chemoprophylaxis is uncertain, as drug-resistant strains of *P vivax* and *P falciparum* usually appear wherever the drug is extensively used; nevertheless, some evidence suggests that proguanil remains effective against pre-erythrocytic stages when effectiveness is lost against blood forms. The prophylactic dose of proguanil is 100 mg (200 mg for a limited period in highly endemic areas) daily and for 4 weeks after departure from the endemic area; when necessary, primaquine is used to eradicate *P vivax* and *P ovale*. Rarely reported side effects are nausea, vomiting, and mouth ulcers.

In sub-Saharan Africa, chloroquine (0.5 g weekly) and proguanil (200 mg daily) while exposed and for 4 weeks afterward are recommended by many workers. Primaquine may be indicated on returning home (see Primaquine, above).

4. Pyrimethamine (Daraprim)– Pyrimethamine alone is no longer used in prophylaxis because of the widespread resistance of *P falciparum* and *P vivax*.

5. Amodiaquine* (Basoquin, Camoquin,* Flavoquine)– Amodiaquine, a 4-aminoquinoline similar in structure to chloroquine, has been shown to cause agranulocytosis and toxic hepatitis and is no longer recommended for prophylaxis.

6. Prophylaxis for children and pregnant women– Children of all ages and pregnant women should be protected; malaria infection during pregnancy may be particularly severe. Drugs contraindicated in pregnancy are doxycycline, mefloquine, and primaquine. Doxycycline is also contraindicated in children under 8 years of age, mefloquine in those under 15 kg, and Fansidar in children under 2 months. Therefore, in children and pregnant women, prescribe weekly chloroquine or hydroxychloroquine with Fansidar to be carried and taken in self-treatment as described above.

7. Chemoprophylaxis for indigenes in endemic areas– Chemoprophylaxis is recommended for semi-immune pregnant women, but *mass* prophylaxis of children under 5 years is not recommended.

B. Chemoprophylaxis in Regions Where *P falciparum* Is Resistant to Chloroquine: Prophylaxis is taken weekly while in the endemic area and for 4 weeks afterward. On returning home, primaquine is given to eradicate persistent liver stages of *P vivax* or *P ovale* if there has been significant exposure to these parasites. For additional details on the following drugs and on primaquine, see Table 28–2 and under the individual drugs (above).

1. Drug of choice– Mefloquine is the drug of

choice. It recently became available in the USA. Note its contraindications.

2. First Alternative– Chloroquine phosphate plus Fansidar. Chloroquine is taken weekly. A single dose of Fansidar (3 tablets) is carried and is only taken as self-treatment for a febrile illness when medical care is not immediately available (see above under Fansidar for appropriate usage). Because of the high level of Fansidar resistance as well as chloroquine resistance in Thailand, Burma, and Cambodia, these 2 drugs cannot be used in those areas.

3. Second alternative– Chloroquine plus doxycycline. Chloroquine is taken weekly, and doxycycline is taken daily. Doxycycline is effective against *P falciparum* strains resistant to chloroquine, but doxycycline's side effects can be a problem for some persons (see Table 28–2). Some workers (Med Lett Drugs Ther 1990;31:13) prescribe doxycycline without addition of chloroquine. FDA considers use of doxycycline investigational.

4. Sub-Saharan Africa– Chloroquine phosphate is taken weekly and proguanil daily (200 mg).

Treatment of Acute Attacks
(See Table 28–2 for dosages.)

A. Treatment of All Forms of Malaria Except *P falciparum* Strains Resistant to Chloroquine and Other Drugs:

1. Elimination of asexual erythrocytic parasites– Infection by all 4 species of malaria is treated with oral chloroquine.

In monitoring the therapeutic response, it is essential also to determine the density of parasites on the blood smear (as a measure of the severity of infection) and to recheck the patient at regular intervals. If symptoms caused by *P falciparum* do not begin to respond to chloroquine within about 48 hours or if there is increasing asexual parasitemia after 1–2 days (in the presence of adequate drug ingestion and retention), parasite resistance to the drug must be assumed and treatment changed to quinine and another drug (Table 28–3).

If patients cannot effectively absorb the drug because of vomiting or severe diarrhea—or if they are comatose or have a high parasite count (100,000/μL, or parasites in 1–2% of red cells)—give quinine or quinidine gluconate intravenously (Table 28–3) and start oral treatment with chloroquine as soon as possible. Chloroquine hydrochloride intramuscularly (contraindicated in young children) is a more toxic alternative parenteral drug.

2. Eradication of *P vivax* or *P ovale* infections– This is accomplished with a standard course of primaquine.

3. Elimination of persistent gametocytemia– Gametocytes of *P vivax*, *P ovale*, and *P malariae* are eliminated by chloroquine. Gametocytes of *P falciparum* are eliminated by a single dose of 26.3 mg of primaquine salt.

---

* Not available in the USA but available in some other countires.

4. Treatment of semi-immunes–Treatment of attacks in semi-immune patients generally requires shorter courses.

B. Treatment of Falciparum Malaria Acquired in Areas Where *P falciparum* Is Resistant to Chloroquine: Start treatment with oral quinine and a second drug (Table 28–3). Quinine is a rapidly acting blood schizonticide, whereas the other drugs are slower-acting. Fansidar should not be used in areas of Southeast Asia where resistance to the drug commonly occurs. If the patient is severely ill, begin with parenteral quinine or quinidine gluconate and start oral quinine as soon as possible. For other details on quinine administration, see above.

Special Measures for Treatment of Severe *P falciparum* Malaria

For details on the management of severe and complicated falciparum malaria, see the WHO review article (1986) cited below. Corticosteroids were recently shown to be deleterious in cerebral malaria and should no longer be used. Heparin therapy is also no longer recommended, since its use may be hazardous and since its indication—ie, disseminated intravascular coagulation—is rare in severe malaria. If there is proof of disseminated intravascular coagulation, however, heparin therapy may be considered. Rehydration of the patient should be carried out with caution, particularly in the first 24 hours, since overhydration may precipitate pulmonary edema. In general, 2–3 L of fluid is required the first day, followed by 10–20 mL/kg/d; intake and output should be carefully recorded. Dialysis may be necessary for renal failure. Blood glucose levels should be monitored during the acute and early convalescent period, since hypoglycemia (unrelated to starvation) may be severe and life-threatening, especially during quinine therapy. Anticonvulsants (diazepam) may be needed; hyperpyrexia should be controlled symptomatically. Severe anemia is an indication for transfusion of packed red blood cells. Recent reports suggest that the survival of patients with parasitemias greater than $10^6/\mu L$ may be increased by exchange transfusion.

Follow-Up for *P falciparum* Malaria

Blood films should be checked daily until parasitemia clears; check weekly thereafter for 4 weeks to observe for recrudescence of infection.

Prognosis

The uncomplicated and untreated primary attack of *P vivax, P ovale,* or *P falciparum* malaria usually lasts 2–4 weeks; that of *P malariae* about twice as long. Each type of infection may subsequently relapse (once or many times) before the infection terminates spontaneously. With modern antimalarial drugs, the prognosis is good for most malaria infections, but in *P falciparum* infections, when severe complications

such as cerebral malaria and blackwater fever develop, the prognosis is poor even with treatment.

Bradley DJ, Phillips-Howard PA: Prophylaxis against malaria for travellers from the United Kingdom. Br Med J 1989;299:1087.

Bruce-Chwatt LJ et al (editors): *Chemotherapy of Malaria,* 2nd ed. World Health Organization Monograph Series No. 27, 1986.

Centers for Disease Control: Recommendations for the prevention of malaria among travelers. MMWR 1990;39:1.

Gilles HM: Malaria—An overview. J Infect 1989;18:11.

Haworth J: Malaria in man: Its epidemiology, clinical aspects and control. Trop Dis Bull 1989;86:R1.

Herwaldt BL et al: Antimalarial agents: Specific chemoprophylaxis regimens. Antimicrob Agents Chemother 1988;32:953.

Krogstad D et al: Antimalarial agents: Specific treatment regimens. Antimicrob Agents Chemother 1988;32:957.

Mefloquine for malaria. Med Lett Drugs Ther 1990;31:13.

Patches LC, Campbell CC, Williams SB: Neurologic reactions after therapeutic dose of mefloquine. N Engl J Med 1989;321;1415.

WHO Malaria Action Programme: Severe and complicated malaria. Trans Roy Soc Trop Med Hyg 1986;80 (Suppl):1.

PNEUMOCYSTOSIS
(*Pneumocystis carinii* Pneumonia)

Essentials of Diagnosis

- Fever, dyspnea, nonproductive cough, cyanosis.
- Bilateral diffuse alveolar disease, usually without hilar adenopathy by chest x-ray.
- Absence of rales and other pulmonary physical findings.
- Reduced partial pressure of oxygen.
- *Pneumocystis carinii* in lung tissue or fluid.

General Considerations

Serologic surveys indicate that *P carinii* infection occurs as an asymptomatic process in most of the population by a young age. Overt infection, pneumocystosis, is an acute interstitial plasma cell pneumonia. The disease occurs worldwide; although rare in the general population, it occurs in larger numbers among 2 groups: (1) as epidemics of primary infections among prematures or among debilitated or marasmic infants on hospital wards or in nursing homes, and (2) as sporadic cases among older children and adults who have an abnormal or altered immune status. Infection in the latter group is assumed to be due to reactivation of latent infection in the presence of immunosuppression. Cases occur generally in patients with cancer or severe malnutrition and debility, in patients treated with immunosuppressive or cytotoxic drugs or irradiation for the management of organ transplants and cancer, patients receiving adrenocorticosteroid therapy, and patients with acquired immunodeficiency syndrome (AIDS) (see Chapter 24). In the USA, *Pneumocystis* pneumonia occurs in about 80% of AIDS patients and is a major cause of death.

The organism, often considered to be a protozoan with intra- and extracellular stages, has 3 forms: cysts, sporozoites, and trophozoites. The thick-walled cyst is 4–6 μm in diameter and contains 8 sporozoites; when released from the cyst, these sporozoites become pleomorphic trophozoites, which are 2–5 μm in diameter. Recent genetic analysis indicates that the organism may be a fungus. Although the mode of transmission in primary infection is unknown, some evidence suggests airborne transmission. Following asymptomatic primary infection, latent and presumably inactive organisms are sparsely distributed in the alveoli. With symptomatic pulmonary disease in AIDS patients, dissemination can occur.

Clinical Findings

A. Symptoms and Signs: With rare exceptions, findings are limited to the pulmonary parenchyma. In the sporadic form of the disease associated with deficient cell-mediated immunity, the onset is abrupt, with high fever, tachypnea, shortness of breath, mild nonproductive cough, intercostal retractions, and cyanosis. Pulmonary physical findings may be slight (including no rales) and disproportionate to the degree of illness and to the radiologic findings. Without treatment, the course is usually one of rapid deterioration and death. In adult disease, patients may present with spontaneous pneumothorax. In the infantile form of the disease, the patient is generally free of fever and may show eosinophilia.

B. Laboratory Findings: In screening, chest radiographs most often show diffuse "interstitial" infiltration. However, there may be heterogeneous distribution of infiltrate, diffuse or focal consolidation, cystic changes, nodules, or cavitation within nodules; 5–10% of patients with *P carinii* pneumonia have normal chest films. Typically there is reduction in vital and total lung capacity. The blood gases usually show severe hypoxemia with minimal (or no) CO_2 retention, resulting in uncompensated respiratory alkalosis. The single-breath diffusing capacity for carbon monoxide shows impaired diffusion and is a particularly sensitive and useful test. Gallium lung scanning (sensitivity > 95%, specificity 20%) shows diffuse uptake; the test should be reserved for those with normal chest films and normal pulmonary function. Isolated elevation of serum LDH may occur. Lymphopenia is common. Serologic tests, including tests to detect antigenemia, are not helpful in diagnosis.

Specific diagnosis depends on morphologic demonstration of the organisms in clinical specimens using specific stains. Although patients rarely spontaneously produce sufficient sputum for examination, adequate specimens can usually be obtained with induced sputum by having patients inhale an aerosol of hypertonic saline produced by an ultrasonic nebulizer. Additional techniques for obtaining specimens include bronchoalveolar lavage (sensitivity 90–97%) and transbronchial lung biopsy (94–97%). Open lung biopsy and needle lung biopsy are less frequently done.

Treatment

Trimethoprim-sulfamethoxazole (TMP-SMZ) and pentamidine isethionate are equally effective, and both can have severe adverse reactions. In non-AIDS patients, the former drug is preferred because of its lower incidence of side effects. In AIDS patients, however, side effects are equivalent, and the choice of agent therefore depends on other factors (eg, TMP-SMZ is used in preexisting renal disease; pentamidine, if fluid must be restricted or if there is a history of sulfonamide drug sensitivity). Therapy should be continued with the selected drug for at least 5–10 days before one considers changing agents. Arterial blood gases and chest films should be monitored.

The dosage of trimethoprim-sulfamethoxazole is TMP 20 mg/kg and SMZ 100 mg/kg given orally or intravenously daily in 4 divided doses for 14–21 days. When possible, blood levels should be monitored; optimum peak therapeutic blood levels are 3–5 μg/mL of TMP and 100–150 μg/mL of SMZ. If necessary, an intravenous preparation can be used (follow the manufacturer's directions). Sulfonamide precautions must be observed. Patients with AIDS have a high frequency of hypersensitivity reactions—fever, rashes (sometimes severe), malaise, neutropenia, hepatitis, nephritis, thrombocytopenia, and hyperbilirubinemia.

Pentamidine causes side effects in nearly 50% of patients. Pain at the injection site is common; infrequently, a sterile abscess can develop. Occasional reactions include rash, abnormal liver function tests, serum folate depression, and hypocalcemia. Hypoglycemia (often clinically inapparent), hyperglycemia, and delayed azotemia may occur. Rarely, a variety of other severe adverse reactions may occur, including neutropenia, thrombocytopenia, ventricular arrhythmias, and fatal pancreatitis. Inadvertent rapid intravenous infusion may cause precipitous hypotension. Pentamidine isethionate is administered intravenously (preferred) or intramuscularly as a single dose of 4 mg (salt)/kg/d for 14–21 days. To avoid injection site abscesses, most workers administer the drug only intravenously by diluting it in 100 mL of fluid and giving it slowly over 1 hour.

Clinical trials of aerosolized pentamidine continue in treatment and prophylaxis. When aerosolized, pentamidine is minimally absorbed and, for the most part, systemic toxicity is avoided; infrequent side effects are cough, bronchospasm, and bronchial bleeding. Pretreatment with bronchodilators may be useful. Failures with inhaled pentamidine tend to be in the upper lobes. When used in treatment, the aerosol should not be used alone but in conjunction with oral or parenteral medication.

α-Difluoromethylornithine, trimetrexate with or without sulfadiazine, clindamycin with primaquine, and dapsone with trimethoprim are investigational therapies. Corticosteroids in conjunction with antimicrobials are being evaluated in severe disease.

Because of the hypoxia usually associated with this disease, oxygen therapy may be indicated to maintain the Po_2 at 70 mm Hg or higher. The fraction of inspired oxygen (Fio_2) should be kept below 50% if possible to avoid oxygen toxicity.

Prophylaxis

The recommendation from the Centers for Disease Control is that prophylaxis be provided for all HIV-infected adults who have had an episode of pneumocystosis. Prophylaxis should also be initiated for those who have never had an episode if their T-helper lymphocytes are less than $200/\mu L$ or less than 20% of total lymphocytes. The treatment IND approved for use in the USA for aerosol pentamidine is a 300-mg dose every 4 weeks, with delivery recommended via the Respirgard II jet nebulizer. The dose is diluted in 6 mL of sterile water and delivered at 6 L/min from a 50-psi compressed air source until the reservoir is dry. Further information is available from (800) 727–7003. Although less extensively studied, prophylaxis is also possible with oral TMP (160 mg) and SMZ (800 mg) twice daily plus 5 mg of leucovorin once daily.

Chemoprophylaxis for high-risk non-AIDS immunocompromised patients consists of oral TMP (5 mg/kg) and SMZ (25 mg/kg) in 2 divided doses daily. Persons with G6PD deficiency should not receive such prophylaxis.

Prognosis

In the absence of early and adequate treatment, the fatality rate for the endemic infantile form of pneumocystosis is 20–50%; for the sporadic form in immunodeficient persons, the fatality rate is nearly 100%. Early treatment reduces the mortality rate to about 3% in the former and 25% in the latter forms of infection. Without prophylaxis, recurrences are common.

Centers for Disease Control: Guidelines for prophylaxis against *Pneumocystis carinii* pneumonia for persons infected with human immunodeficiency virus. MMWR 1989;38:1.

Gazzard BG: *Pneumocystis carinii* pneumonia and its treatment in patients with AIDS. J Antimicrob Chemother 1989;23(Suppl A):67.

Luce JM, Hopewell PC: Aerosolized pentamidine for *Pneumocystis carinii* pneumonia. Chest 1989;96:713-714.

Masur H, Kovacs JA: Treatment and prophylaxis of *Pneumocystis carinii* pneumonia. Infect Dis Clin North Am 1988;2:419

McCabe RE: Diagnosis of pulmonary infections in immuno-

compromised patients. Med Clin North Am 1988; 72:1067.

Rankan JA, Collman R, Daniele RP: Acquired immune deficiency syndrome and the lung. Chest 1988:94:155.

Toma E et al: Clindamycin with primaquine for *Pneumocystis carinii* pneumonia. Lancet 1989;1:1046.

Trimetrexate for *Pneumocystis carinii* pneumonia. Med Lett Drugs Ther 1989;31:5.

TOXOPLASMOSIS

Essentials of Diagnosis

Acute primary infection:
- Fever, malaise, headache, lymphadenopathy (especially cervical), myalgia, arthralgia, stiff neck, sore throat; occasionally, rash, hepatosplenomegaly, retinochoroiditis, confusion; in various combinations.
- Positive serologic tests with high and rising IgG and IgM.
- Isolation of *Toxoplasma gondii* from blood or body fluids; tachyzoites in histologic sections of tissue or cytologic preparations of body fluids.

Acute primary or recrudescent infection in immunocompromised patients:
- Retinochoroiditis, encephalitis, pneumonitis, myocarditis; sometimes other findings as above.
- Positive IgG titers moderately high; IgM antibody usually absent.
- Laboratory findings as above.

General Considerations

T gondii, an obligate intracellular protozoan, is found worldwide in humans and in many species of animals and birds. The parasite is a coccidian of cats, the definitive host, and exists in 3 forms: The trophozoite (tachyzoite) is the rapidly proliferating form seen in the tissues and body fluids in the acute stage. The trophozoites can enter and multiply in most mammalian nucleated cells. The cyst (bradyzoite), containing viable trophozoites, is the latent form that can persist indefinitely in the host in the chronic stage and is found particularly in muscle and nerve tissue. The oocyst is the form passed only in the feces of the cat family. In the intestinal epithelium of cats, a sexual cycle occurs, with subsequent release of oocysts. Human infection results from (1) ingestion of oocysts (from soil by soil-eating children or by careless handling of cat litter), (2) ingestion of cysts in raw or undercooked meat, (3) transplacental transmission, or, rarely, (4) direct inoculation of trophozoites, as in blood transfusion.

Clinical Findings

A. Symptoms and Signs: Over 80% of primary infections are asymptomatic. The incubation period for symptomatic persons is 1–2 weeks.

The clinical manifestations of toxoplasmosis may be grouped into 4 syndromes:

1. Primary infection in the normal host–Most infections are acute, mild, febrile multisystem illnesses that resemble infectious mononucleosis. Lymphadenopathy, particularly of the head and neck, is the most common finding. Other features in various combinations are malaise, myalgia, arthralgia, headache, sore throat, and maculopapular or urticarial rash. Hepatomegaly may occur. Rarely, severe cases are complicated by pneumonitis, meningoencephalitis, hepatitis, myocarditis, and retinochoroiditis. Symptoms may fluctuate, but most patients recover spontaneously over 1–2 months. Generally, on recovery, both asymptomatic and symptomatic infections persist as chronic infections.

2. Congenital infection–Congenital transmission occurs only as a result of infection (generally asymptomatic) in a nonimmune woman during pregnancy. Infection has been detected in up to 1% of women during pregnancy; 15–60% of such infections, varying by trimester, are transmitted to the fetus, but only a small percentage result in abortions or stillbirths or in active disease in premature or full-term, liveborn infants. Though fetal infection may occur in any trimester, it is more severe early in pregnancy.

Signs of congenital toxoplasmosis may be present at birth or may develop during the first months of life: central nervous system disorders (microcephaly, internal hydrocephalus, seizures, retinochoroiditis, cerebral calcifications), hepatosplenomegaly, pneumonitis, rash, fever, jaundice, anemia, and thrombocytopenia. Psychomotor and learning disorders, hearing loss, mental retardation, and retinochoroiditis may not be apparent for years.

3. Retinochoroiditis–This develops gradually weeks to years after congenital infection (the preponderant form, which is generally bilateral) or rarely after an acquired infection in a young child (generally unilateral). Primary infections in older children and adults rarely progress to retinochoroiditis. The inflammatory process persists for weeks to months as focally necrotic retinal lesions with blurred margins. Visual defects include blurring, central defects, and scotomas. Rarely, progression may result in glaucoma and blindness. With healing, white or dark-pigmented scars may result.

4. Primary infection or reactivated disease in the immunologically compromised host–This may present as disseminated disease or in specific organs (eg, myocarditis, pneumonitis), particularly in patients given immunosuppressive drugs or patients with lymphoreticular, hematologic, or other cancers or with AIDS. In AIDS, central nervous system involvement (diffuse or focal encephalitis or mass lesions and accompanying meningoencephalitis) occurs in up to 30% of seropositive patients. Other AIDS patients may present with infections in other organs or with disseminated disease.

B. Laboratory Findings: Diagnosis depends principally on serologic tests, which are sensitive and reliable. However, toxoplasmosis can be diagnosed occasionally by histologic examination of tissue or isolation of the parasite in mice or tissue culture. Cysts or trophozoites may be directly identified by staining blood (buffy coat from centrifuged heparinized blood), bone marrow aspirates, cerebrospinal fluid sediment, sputum, and other tissue or body fluids or placental tissue. The demonstration of cysts does not establish a causal relationship to clinical illness, since cysts may be found in both acute and chronic infections. However, only finding tachyzoites in blood or body fluids confirms active infection. In the placenta, fetus, or newborn, the presence of cysts indicates congenital infection. Leukocyte counts are normal or reduced, often with lymphocytosis or monocytosis with rare atypical cells, but there is no heterophil antibody. Chest radiographs may show interstitial pneumonia.

Serologic tests—the Sabin-Feldman dye test and the indirect hemagglutination, indirect immunofluorescence (IFA), ELISA, and other tests—can be done on blood, cerebrospinal fluid, aqueous humor, and other body fluids. The dye test, which is extremely sensitive and specific, is the standard, but it is rarely used because of laboratory safety factors. The ELISA and IFA tests permit separation of IgM and IgG antibody. In the IFA test for IgM, antibody appears 1–2 weeks after start of infection, reaches a peak at 6–8 weeks, and then gradually declines; low titers persist for life in most patients; but in some, high titers persist. False-positive and false-negative tests can occur with the IFA test; the former can be avoided by use of IgM capture tests.

The following are selected serologic findings in specific toxoplasmosis syndromes:

1. Acute infection in immunocompetent persons–The diagnosis is established by seroconversion from negative to positive, by a 4-fold rise in serologic titers by any test, or by a single high titer (1:160) of IgM antibody. A presumptive diagnosis is based on a single IgM titer of over 1:64 and a very high IgG titer (> 1:1000). A negative dye or comparable test for IgG virtually excludes the diagnosis of acute toxoplasmosis.

2. Recrudescent infection in immunosuppressed patients–Although definitive diagnosis is only by finding *Toxoplasma* organisms in cerebrospinal fluid (Wright-Giemsa stain) or by brain biopsy, to avoid the latter, empiric antibiotic treatment is generally started after presumptive evidence is obtained by CT scan or MRI. Antibody titers cannot be depended on, since most patients have IgG titers that reflect past infection, significant rises are infrequent, and IgM antibody is rare. Absence of IgG is strong evidence against the diagnosis of central nervous system toxoplasmosis. Rarely, *Toxoplasma* antigen or a rise in serologic titers has been shown in cerebrospinal fluid.

3. Toxoplasmic retinochoroiditis–This is usually associated with stable, usually low IgG titers and no IgM antibody. If IgG antibody in aqueous humor is higher than in the serum, the diagnosis is supported.

4. Congenital toxoplasmosis–An IgG titer in excess of 1:1000 or rising titers are presumptively diagnostic, but low titers are sometimes found. Confirmation is by a test for IgM and finally the isolation of *Toxoplasma*. IgG but not IgM is transferred across the intact placenta; if a leak occurs in the placenta, the IgM transferred has a half-life of 3–5 days.

Where available, the following new methods may be useful in diagnosis: Testing for antigenemia has been used to demonstrate acute infection, and lymphocyte transformation to *Toxoplasma* antigens has provided a specific and sensitive indicator of prior infection.

Differential Diagnosis

In acute febrile disease, consider cytomegalovirus infection, infectious mononucleosis, and other causes of pneumonitis, myocarditis, myositis, hepatitis, and splenomegaly. With lymphadenopathy, consider sarcoidosis, tuberculosis, tularemia, lymphoma, Hodgkin's disease, and metastatic carcinoma. With encephalitis in the immunosuppressed host, consider herpes simplex, cytomegalovirus infection, other viral encephalitides, multifocal leukoencephalopathy, fungal encephalitis, hemorrhage, psychosis, and neoplasms.

Treatment

Asymptomatic infections in normal hosts are not treated except in children under 5 years of age, who are treated to avoid possible occurrence of retinochoroiditis.

Symptomatic patients should be treated until manifestations of the illness have subsided and there is serologic evidence that immunity has been acquired.

Although most episodes of **retinochoroiditis** are self-limited, treatment is generally given because the clinical course cannot be predicted with certainty. Corticosteroids are commonly prescribed for their anti-inflammatory action.

Immunocompromised patients with active infection (primary or recrudescent) must be treated. Therapy should continue for 4–6 weeks after cessation of symptoms—which may require up to a 6-month course, to be followed by drug prophylaxis as long as immunosuppression persists. In **AIDS** patients, treatment should be continued indefinitely. Chronic asymptomatic infection in these patients usually need not be treated, but prophylaxis may be started after a significant increase in antibody titer is noted.

Treatment is also indicated in **congenitally infected infants** with or without symptoms.

Treatment of women who become infected during **pregnancy** is controversial because of possible toxic effects on the fetus. Because early treatment reduces (but does not eliminate) the incidence of fetal infection, most workers feel that treatment is justified.

For details on management of congenital infections and those occurring during pregnancy, see specialized texts.

The treatment of choice is pyrimethamine, 75 mg/d for 3 days, then 25 mg daily, plus either trisulfapyrimidines (2–6 g/d in 4 divided doses) or sulfadiazine (100 mg/kg/d (maximum 6 g/d) in 4 divided doses); continue this treatment for 3–4 weeks. Folinic acid (calcium leucovorin), 10 mg/d in divided doses, is given to avoid the hematologic effects of pyrimethamine-induced folate deficiency. Platelet and white blood cell counts should be performed at least twice weekly. Screen patients for a history of sulfonamide sensitivity; if a reaction occurs with treatment, see references on how to proceed with treatment.

Spiramycin is in use in Europe at a dosage of 2–4 g in 4 divided doses. Although safe and effective in pregnancy, the drug does not reach the fetus. It is not effective in encephalitis. Trimethoprim-sulfamethoxazole is being used but with unreliable results. Clindamycin (300 mg 4 times daily) may be a useful alternative therapy; because it concentrates in the choroid, it is used in the treatment of ocular disease. Corticosteroids may also be required in the management of ocular disease.

See the Israelski reference below for dosages and approach to therapy of AIDS patients, in whom sulfonamide sensitivity is common. Primary therapy is continued for at least 6 weeks with higher doses of pyrimethamine and folinic acid; daily chronic suppressive therapy is given thereafter.

Prevention

Freezing of meat to $-20\,°C$ for 2 days or heating to $60\,°C$ kills cysts in tissues. Under appropriate environmental conditions, oocysts passed in cat feces can remain infective for a year or more. Thus, children's play areas, including sandboxes, should be protected from cat and dog feces; hand washing is indicated after contact with soil potentially contaminated by animal feces. Indoor cats should be fed only dry, canned, or cooked meat. Litter boxes should be changed daily, as freshly deposited oocysts are not infective for 48 hours.

Pregnant women should have their serum examined for *Toxoplasma* antibody. If the IgM test is negative but an IgG titer is present and less than 1:1000, no further evaluation is necessary. Those with negative titers should take measures to prevent infection—preferably by having no further contact with cats and by thoroughly cooking meat. Hands should be washed after handling raw meat and before eating or touching the face.

Prognosis

The outlook for acute toxoplasmosis in adults is excellent as long as the patient is immunocompetent. Acute infection in young children, however, may be followed by an attack (or by repeated attacks) of retinochoroiditis; treatment appears to reduce the frequency of attacks. Treatment of immunosuppressed patients usually results in improvement if begun early, but recrudescence is common. Chronic asymptomatic infection, as indicated by a persistent antibody titer, is usually benign.

Carrazana EJ, Rossitch E Jr, Samuels MA: Cerebral toxoplasmosis in the acquired immune deficiency syndrome. Clin Neurol Neurosurg 1989;91:291.

Daffos F et al: Prenatal management of 746 pregnancies at risk for congenital toxoplasmosis. N Engl J Med 1988;318:271.

Derouin F et al: Laboratory diagnosis of pulmonary toxoplasmosis in patients with acquired immunodeficiency syndrome. J Clin Microbiol 1989;27:1661.

Editorial: Toxoplasmosis in immunocompromised patients. Eur J Clin Microbiol 1987;6:1.

Frankel J: Toxoplasmosis. In: Tropical Medicine and Parasitology. Goldsmith R, Heyneman D (editors). Appleton & Lange, 1989.

Israelski DM, Remington JS: Toxoplasmic encephalitis in patients with AIDS. Infect Dis Clin North Am 1988; 2:429.

Jackson MH, Hutchison WM: The prevalence and source of Toxoplasma infection in the environment. Adv Parasitol 1989;28:55.

McCabe RE et al: Clinical spectrum in 107 cases of toxoplasmic lymphadenopathy. Rev Infect Dis 1987;9:754.

Steahly LP: Laser treatment of toxoplasmosis. Ann Ophthalmol 1989;21:36.

REFERENCES

Adams ARD, Maegraith BG: Clinical Tropical Diseases, 8th ed. Blackwell, 1984.

Beaver PC, Jung RC, Cupp EW: Clinical Parasitology, 9th ed. Lea & Febiger, 1984.

Benenson AS (editor): Control of Communicable Diseases in Man, 15th ed. Lucas, 1990.

Bia FJ, Barry M: Parasitic infections of the central nervous system. Neurol Clin 1986;4:171.

Binford CH, Connor DH (editors): Pathology of Tropical and Extraordinary Diseases. Vols 1 and 2. Armed Forces Institute of Pathology, 1976.

Brown HW, Neva FA: Basic Clinical Parasitology, 5th ed. Appleton-Century-Crofts, 1983.

Campbell WC, Rew RS (editors): Chemotherapy of Parasitic Disease. Plenum, 1986.

Cook GC: Tropical Gastroenterology. Oxford Medical Publications, 1980.

Drugs for Parasitic Infections. Med Lett Drugs Ther 1990;32:23.

Goldsmith RS: Clinical pharmacology of the anthelmintic drugs. Chap 55 in: Basic & Clinical Pharmacology, 4th ed. Katzung BG (editor). Appleton & Lange, 1989.

Goldsmith RS, Heyneman D (editors): Tropical Medicine and Parasitology. Appleton & Lange, 1989.

Leech JH, Sande MA, Root RK (editors): Contemporary Issues in Infectious Diseases: Parasitic Infections. Churchill Livingstone, 1988.

Mandell WF, Neu HC: Parasitic infections: Therapeutic considerations. Med Clin North Am 1988;72:669.

Manson-Bahr PEC, Apted FIC: Manson's Tropical Diseases, 19th ed. Bailliegre Tindall, 1988.

Markell EK, Voge M, John DT (editors): Medical Parasitology, 6th ed. Saunders, 1986.

Sharma S: Drugs for parasitic diseases. Drugs for Today 1989;25:249.

Strickland GT: Hunter's Tropical Medicine, 6th ed. Saunders, 1984.

White NJ: Antiparasitic drugs in children. Clin Pharmacokinet 1989;17:138.

Warren KS, Mahmoud AAF: Tropical and Geographic Medicine, 2nd ed. McGraw-Hill, 1990.

WHO: Prevention and control of intestinal parasitic infections. Report of a WHO expert committee. WHO Tech Rep Ser 1987;749:1.

Infectious Diseases: Helminthic 29

Robert S. Goldsmith, MD, MPH, DTM&H

TREMATODE (FLUKE) INFECTIONS

SCHISTOSOMIASIS (Bilharziasis)

Essentials of Diagnosis

- Acute phase: Abrupt onset (2–6 weeks postexposure) of abdominal pain, weight loss, headache, malaise, chills, fever, myalgia, diarrhea (sometimes bloody), dry cough, hepatomegaly, and eosinophilia.
- Chronic phase: Either (1) diarrhea, abdominal pain, blood in stool, hepatomegaly or hepatosplenomegaly, and bleeding from esophageal varices (*Schistosoma mansoni* or *Schistosoma japonicum* infection); or (2) terminal hematuria, urinary frequency, and urethral and bladder pain (*Schistosoma haematobium* infection).
- Depending on species, characteristic eggs in feces, urine, or scrapings or biopsy of rectal or bladder mucosa.

General Considerations

Schistosomiasis, which infects more than 200 million persons worldwide, is caused mainly by 3 blood flukes (trematodes). *S mansoni*, which causes intestinal schistosomiasis, is widespread in Africa and occurs in the Arabian peninsula, northeastern South America, and the Caribbean (including Puerto Rico but not Cuba). Vesical (urinary) schistosomiasis, caused by *S haematobium*, is found throughout the Middle East and Africa. Asiatic intestinal schistosomiasis, due to *S japonicum,* is important in China and the Philippines, and a small focus is present in Sulawesi, Indonesia, but transmission in Japan has been interrupted. A number of schistosome species of animals sometimes infect humans, including *Schistosoma intercalatum* in central Africa and *Schistosoma mekongi* in the Mekong delta in Thailand, Cambodia, and Laos.

Mammals are important reservoirs for *S japonicum.* Humans are the main reservoir for *S mansoni* and *S haematobium;* the few animal species infected with *S mansoni* are not epidemiologically important.

In the life cycle involving humans, the adult worms live in terminal venules of the bowel (*S mansoni, S japonicum*) or bladder (*S haematobium*). When eggs passed in feces or urine reach fresh water, a larval form is released that subsequently infects snails, the intermediate host. After development, infective larvae (cercariae) leave the snails, enter water, and infect exposed persons through the skin or mucous membranes. After penetration, the cercariae become schistosomula larvae that reach the portal circulation in the liver, where they rapidly mature. After a few weeks, adult worms pair, mate, and migrate mainly to terminal venules of specific veins, where females deposit their eggs. By means of their lytic secretions, some eggs reach the lumen of the bowel or bladder and are passed with feces or urine. Others are retained in the bowel or bladder wall, while still others are carried in the circulation to the liver, lung, and (less often) to other tissues. Except for the allergic response in the acute syndrome (see below), disease is primarily due to delayed hypersensitivity. Antigens released by the eggs stimulate a local granulomatous response, followed by a strong fibrotic reaction. Live worms produce no lesions and rarely cause symptoms. The type or degree of tissue damage and symptoms varies with the intensity of infection (worm burden), the degree of host activity, the site of egg deposition, and the duration of infection.

S mansoni adults migrate to the inferior mesenteric veins of the large bowel and *S japonicum* to the superior and inferior mesenteric veins in the large and small bowel. Ulcers and polyps (common only in Egypt) result from granuloma formation and fibrosis in the bowel wall. Egg accumulation in the liver can result in periportal fibrosis and portal hypertension of the presinusoidal type, but liver function typically remains intact even in advanced disease. Massive embolization of eggs to the lungs may result in endarteritis, pulmonary hypertension, and cor pulmonale. Because greater numbers of eggs are produced by *S japonicum,* the resulting disease is often more severe.

Adult *S haematobium* mature in the venous plexus of the bladder, rectum, prostate, and uterus. Ulcers and polyps result from granuloma formation and fibrosis in the bladder wall, and eggshell remnants may calcify. Stricture or distortion of the ureteral orifices of terminal ureters may result in hydroureter, hydronephrosis, and ascending infection. Lesions in the pelvic organs rarely cause extensive fibrosis and infection. Eggs are carried to the liver or lungs, but severe pathology is uncommon.

In size, adult *S mansoni* are 6–13 × 1 mm. The prepatent period—from cercarial penetration until appearance of eggs in feces—is about 50 days. The life span of the worms ranges from 5 to 30 years or more.

Clinical Findings

A. Symptoms and Signs: The great majority of infected persons have light infections and are asymptomatic.

1. Cercarial dermatitis–Following cercarial penetration, clinical findings progress from an itchy erythematous or petechial rash to macules and papules that last up to 5 days. This syndrome is uncommon with human schistosome infections. Instead, most recognized cases occur worldwide in fresh or marine water and are due to skin invasion by bird or nonhuman cercariae, schistosomes that do not mature in humans.

2. Acute schistosomiasis (Katayama fever)– This syndrome, primarily an allergic response to the developing schistosomes, may occur with the 3 schistosomes (rare with *S haematobium*) and usually is not seen in indigenes. The incubation period ranges from 2 to 7 weeks and the severity of illness from mild to (rarely) life-threatening. In addition to fever, malaise, urticaria, diarrhea (sometimes bloody), myalgia, dry cough, and marked eosinophilia, the liver and spleen may be temporarily enlarged. The patient again becomes asymptomatic in 2–8 weeks. It is not established that drug treatment is safe during the acute stage because release of antigens from dying immature worms may severely exacerbate symptoms.

3. Chronic (hepatosplenic) schistosomiasis– This stage begins 6 months to several years after infection. Early in *S mansoni* and *S japonicum* infections, findings include diarrhea, abdominal pain, blood in stool, and hepatomegaly. With subsequent slow progression over 5–15 years or longer, the following may appear: anorexia, weight loss, weakness, polypoid intestinal tumors, and features of portal hypertension, in which the liver gradually contracts and the spleen enlarges. Chronic salmonellosis or the nephrotic syndrome may also occur.

Early symptoms of urinary tract disease are frequency and dysuria, followed by terminal hematuria and proteinuria. Frank hematuria may be recurrent; obstruction of the ureteral orifices may lead to hydronephrosis. Sequelae may include bladder polyp formation, cystitis, chronic *Salmonella* infection, pyelitis, pyelonephritis, urolithiasis, nephrotic syndrome, renal failure, and death. Severe liver, lung, genital, or neurologic disease is rare. Many cases of bladder cancer have been associated with vesicular schistosomiasis.

4. Complications–

a. Portal hypertension may result in splenomegaly, pancytopenia, esophageal varices, and variceal bleeding. Abnormal liver function, jaundice, ascites, and hepatic coma are end-stage findings.

b. Cor pulmonale is manifested by right-sided heart failure and clubbing.

c. Colonic polyposis is manifested by bloody diarrhea, anemia, hypoalbuminemia, and clubbing.

d. Other large bowel complications include stricture, granulomatous masses, and *Salmonella* infection.

e. Ectopic eggs and worms may cause manifestations related to the spinal cord or brain (transverse myelitis, epilepsy, optic neuritis).

B. Laboratory Findings:

1. Eggs–Definitive diagnosis is made by finding characteristic eggs in excreta or by mucosal or liver biopsy. In *S haematobium* infection, eggs may be found in the urine or, less frequently, in the stools. Eggs are sought in urine specimens collected between 9:00 AM and 2:00 PM or in 24-hour collections. They are processed either by examination of the sediment or preferably by membrane filtration. Occasionally, eggs are sought by vesical mucosa biopsy. In *S mansoni* and *S japonicum* infections, eggs may be found in stool specimens by direct examination, but some form of concentration is usually necessary; repeated examinations are often needed to find eggs in light infections. If results are negative—in selected cases only (because of the risk of biopsy)—proceed to rectal mucosal biopsy of suspicious lesions or take biopsy specimens at 2–3 sites of normal mucosa. Biopsy specimens should be examined as crush preparations between 2 glass slides. Rarely, liver biopsy may be necessary to make the diagnosis.

2. Serologic tests–Screening for infection is possible by skin or serologic testing, but neither is sufficiently sensitive or specific to be used as the sole criterion for diagnosis.

3. Other tests–Eosinophilia, common during the acute stage, usually is absent or low-grade in the chronic stage. With hepatosplenic schistosomiasis, the wedged hepatic vein pressure is normal (consistent with presinusoidal portal hypertension), and ultrasound examination of the liver shows the pathognomonic pattern of Symmers' fibrosis.

In schistosomiasis due to *S haematobium*, microscopic hematuria may be present. In advanced disease, cystoscopy may show "sandy patches," ulcers, and areas of squamous metaplasia; and lower abdominal x-rays may show calcification of the bladder wall or ureters.

Differential Diagnosis

Early intestinal schistosomiasis may be mistaken for amebiasis, bacillary dysentery, or other causes of diarrhea and dysentery. Later, the various causes of portal hypertension or of bowel polyps must be considered. In endemic areas, vesical schistosomiasis must be differentiated from other causes of hematuria, dysuria, prostatic disease, genitourinary tract cancer, and bacterial infections of the urinary tract.

Treatment

A. Medical Treatment: (Table 29–1.) Treatment should be given only if live ova are identified. The safety and effectiveness of current drugs make it possible to treat all infections orally and without concern for serious side effects. Praziquantel can be used to treat all species; alternative drugs are oxamniquine for *S mansoni* and metrifonate for *S haematobium*.

After treatment, periodic laboratory follow-up for continued passage of eggs is essential, starting at 3 months and continuing at intervals for 1 year. If eggs are found, their viability should be determined, since dead eggs are passed for some months.

1. Praziquantel–Cure rates at 6 months for *S haematobium*, *S mansoni*, and *S japonicum* infections are 87%, 80%, and 84%, respectively, with marked reduction in ovum counts in those not cured.

The manufacturer's recommended dosage for treatment of all forms of schistosomiasis is 20 mg/kg 3 times daily for 1 day. Lower dosages have been reported to be highly effective in some parts of the world for *S haematobium* (40 mg/kg once) or *S mansoni* (20 mg/kg twice in 1 day). Tablets are taken with water after a meal and should not be chewed. The interval between doses should be no less than 4 and no more than 6 hours.

Mild and transient side effects persisting for hours to 1 day are common and include malaise, headache, dizziness, and anorexia. Less frequent are fatigue, drowsiness, nausea, vomiting, generalized abdominal pain, loose stools, pruritus, urticaria, arthralgia and myalgia, and low-grade fever. The drug is well tolerated by patients in the hepatosplenic stage of advanced schistosomiasis. It should not be used in pregnancy, and because of drug-induced dizziness, patients should not drive and should be cautioned if their work requires physical coordination or alertness. In areas where cysticercosis may coexist with a schistosomal infection being treated with praziquantel, treatment is best conducted in a hospital.

2. Metrifonate–Metrifonate is a highly effective alternative drug for the treatment of *S haematobium* infections only. The dosage is 7.5–10 mg/kg (maximum 600 mg) once and then repeated twice at 2-week intervals. Cure rates range from 44% to 93%. Those not cured show marked reduction in ovum counts. Side effects range from none to mild and transient findings, including gastrointestinal symptoms, headache, bronchospasm, weakness, and vertigo. Metrifonate is not available in the USA.

3. Oxamniquine is a highly effective alternative drug for *S mansoni* infections only and is safe in

advanced (hepatosplenic) disease. The dosage for strains of *S mansoni* in the western hemisphere is 12–15 mg/kg given once; for children under 30 kg, 20 mg/kg is given in 2 divided doses in 1 day, with an interval of 2–8 hours between doses. Cure rates are 70–95% with a marked reduction in egg excretion in those not cured. For most African strains, the total dosage for adults and children varies by region from 40 to 60 mg/kg in divided doses over 2–3 days. Dizziness persisting for about 6 hours is a common side effect. Less frequent are drowsiness, nausea and vomiting, diarrhea, abdominal pain, and headache. An orange or red discoloration of the urine may occur. Rarely reported is central nervous system stimulation with behavioral changes, hallucinations, or seizures; patients should be observed for 2 hours after ingestion of the drug for appearance of these findings. Since the drug makes some patients dizzy or drowsy, it should be used with caution in patients whose work or activity requires mental alertness. The drug has shown mutagenic and embryocidal effects and is contraindicated in pregnancy.

B. Surgical Measures: In selected instances, corrective surgery may be indicated for removal of polyps. For bleeding esophageal varices, sclerotherapy is the treatment of choice. As a last resort in patients who have repeated bleeding, splenorenal anastomosis is done rather than portacaval shunts, which are associated with a high level of chronic portal systemic encephalopathy. Distal splenorenal shunt and esophagogastric devascularization with splenectomy may be a more successful procedure. Severe pancytopenia is an indication for splenectomy. Filtering of *S mansoni* adults from the portal system should be considered whenever splenectomy is contemplated. Surgery may be required for obstructive uropathy.

Prognosis

With treatment, as long as reinfection does not occur, the prognosis is excellent in early and light infections. There may be shrinkage or elimination of bladder and bowel ulcerations, granulomas, and polyps. In advanced disease with extensive involvement of the intestines, liver, bladder, or other organs, the outlook is poor even with treatment.

Andrade ZA: Pathology of human schistosomiasis. Mem Inst Oswaldo Cruz 1987;82(Suppl 4):17.

Archer S: The chemotherapy of schistosomiasis. Annu Rev Pharmacol Toxicol 1985;25:485.

Chen MG, Mott KE: Progress in assessment of morbidity due to *Schistosoma haematobium* infection. Trop Dis Bull 1989;86:R2.

De Cock KM: Progress Report: Hepatosplenic schistosomiasis: A clinical review. Gut 1986;27:734.

Harries AD, Cook GC: Acute schistosomiasis (Katayama fever): Clinical deterioration after chemotherapy. J Infect 1987;14;159.

Hatz C et al: Ultrasound scanning for detecting morbidity

Table 29–1. Drugs for the treatment of helminthic infections.

Infecting Organism	Drug of Choice	Alternative Drugs
Roundworms (nematodes)		
Ascaris lumbricoides (roundworm)	Pyrantel pamoate	Piperazine, mebendazole, levamisole,[1] or albendazole[1]
Trichuris trichiura (whipworm)	Mebendazole	Oxantel-pyrantel pamoate[1] or albendazole[1]
Necator americanus (hookworm) *Ancylostoma duodenale* (hookworm)	Pyrantel pamoate[2] or mebendazole	Albendazole,[1] tetrachloroethylene,[1] or levamisole[1]
Combined infection with *Ascaris, Trichuris,* and hookworm	Mebendazole or albendazole[1]	Oxantel-pyrantel pamoate[1]
Combined infection with *Ascaris* and hookworm	Mebendazole or pyrantel pamoate	Albendazole[1]
Strongyloides stercoralis (threadworm)	Thiabendazole	Albendazole, [1,3,4] mebendazole,[2,4] or ivermectin[1,3,4,6]
Enterobius vermicularis (pinworm)	Mebendazole or pyrantel pamoate	Albendazole[1]
Trichinella spiralis (trichinosis)	Thiabendazole[4] or mebendazole;[2,4] add corticosteroids for severe infection	Albendazole;[1,3,4] add corticosteroids for severe infection
Trichostrongylus species	Pyrantel pamoate[2] or mebendazole[2]	Levamisole[1]
Cutaneous larva migrans (creeping eruption)	Thiabendazole	Albendazole[1,3,4]
Visceral larva migrans	Thiabendazole[2,4] or albendazole[1,2,4]	Mebendazole[2,4] or ivermectin[1,3,4,6]
Angiostrongylus cantonensis	Levamisole[1,4]	Albendazole[1,2,4]
Wuchereria bancrofti (filariasis), *Brugia malayi* (filariasis), tropical eosinophilia, and *Loa loa* (loiasis)	Diethylcarbamazine[5]	Ivermectin[1,3,4,6]
Onchocerca volvulus (onchocerciasis)	Ivermectin[3,6]	Diethylcarbamazine[5] plus suramin[7]
Dracunculus medinensis (guinea worm)	Metronidazole[2]	Thiabendazole[2] or mebendazole[2]
Capillaria philippinensis (intestinal capillariasis)	Albendazole[1]	Thiabendazole[2] or mebendazole[2]
Flukes (trematodes)		
Schistosoma haematobium (bilharziasis)	Praziquantel	Metrifonate[1]
Schistosoma mansoni	Praziquantel	Oxamniquine
Schistosoma japonicum	Praziquantel	None
Clonorchis sinensis (liver fluke) *Opisthorchis* species	Praziquantel[2]	Mebendazole[2,4] or albendazole[1,3,4]
Paragonimus westermani (lung fluke)	Praziquantel[2]	Bithionol[7]
Fasciola hepatica (sheep liver fluke)	Bithionol[7]	Praziquantel;[2,4] emetine or dehydroemetine[7]
Fasciolopsis buski (large intestinal fluke)	Praziquantel[2] or niclosamide[2]	Dichlorophen,[1,4] tetrachloroethylene,[1] or bephenium[1]
Heterophyes heterophyes and *Metagonimus yokogawai* (small intestinal flukes)	Praziquantel[2] or niclosamide[2]	Bephenium[1] or tetrachloroethylene[1]
Tapeworms (cestodes)		
Taenia saginata (beef tapeworm)	Niclosamide or praziquantel[2]	Dichlorophen,[1] paromomycin,[2] or mebendazole[2,4]
Diphyllobothrium latum (fish tapeworm)	Niclosamide or praziquantel[2]	Dichlorophen[1] or paromomycin[2]
Taenia solium (pork tapeworm)	Niclosamide	Praziquantel[2]
Cysticercosis (pork tapeworm larval stage)	Praziquantel[2,3]	Albendazole[1,3,4] or metrifonate[1,3,4]
Hymenolepis nana (dwarf tapeworm)	Praziquantel[2]	Niclosamide or paromomycin[2]
Hymenolepis diminuta (rat tapeworm) *Dipylidium caninum* (dog tapeworm)	Niclosamide	Praziquantel[2,4]
Echinococcus granulosus (hydatid disease) *Echinococcus multilocularis*	Albendazole[1,3,4]	Mebendazole[2,3,4]

[1] Not available in the USA; available in some other countries.
[2] Available in the USA but not labeled for this indication.
[3] Undergoing clinical investigation.
[4] Effectiveness not established or not at a high level.
[5] Available in the USA from Lederle Laboratories, (914) 735–5000.
[6] Available from Merck Sharpe & Dohme, (215) 661–7300.
[7] Available in the USA only from the Parasitic Disease Drug Service, Parasitic Diseases Branch, Centers for Disease Control, Atlanta 30333. Telephone (404) 488–4240 during the day, (404) 639–2888 nights, weekends, and holidays (emergencies only).

due to *Schistosoma haematobium* and its resolution following treatment with different doses of praziquantel. Trans R Soc Trop Med Hyg 1990;84:84.

Masry NA, Bassily S, Farid Z: A comparison of the efficacy and side effects of various regimens of praziquantel for the treatment of schistosomiasis. Trans R Soc Trop Med Hyg 1988;82:719.

FASCIOLOPSIASIS

The large intestinal fluke, *Fasciolopsis buski,* is a common parasite of humans and pigs in central and south China, Taiwan, Southeast Asia, Indonesia, eastern India, and Bangladesh. When eggs shed in stools reach water, they hatch to produce free-swimming larvae that penetrate and develop in the flesh of snails. Cercariae subsequently escape from the snails and encyst on various water plants. Humans are infected by eating these plants uncooked (usually water chestnuts, bamboo shoots, or caltrops). Adult flukes (length 2–7.5 cm) mature in about 3 months and live in the small intestine attached to the mucosa or buried in mucous secretions.

After an incubation period of several months, manifestations of gastrointestinal irritation appear in all but light infections. Symptoms in severe infections include nausea, anorexia, upper abdominal pain, and diarrhea, sometimes alternating with constipation. Ascites and edema of the face and lower extremities may occur later. Intestinal stasis, ileus, and partial obstruction have been described.

Diagnosis depends on finding characteristic eggs (that must be distinguished from *Fasciola* and various echinostome eggs) or, occasionally, flukes in the stools. Leukocytosis with moderate eosinophilia is common. No serologic test is available. Because the adult worms live for only 6 months, absence from the endemic area for a longer period makes the diagnosis unlikely.

The drug of first choice is praziquantel as a single 25 mg/kg dose. Alternative drugs are tetrachloroethylene, administered as for hookworm disease, and niclosamide, administered as for taeniasis but given every other day for 3 doses.

In rare cases—particularly in children—heavy infections with severe toxemia have resulted in death from cachexia or intercurrent infection. With these exceptions, the prognosis is excellent with proper treatment.

Idris M et al: The treatment of fasciolopsiasis with niclosamide and dichlorophen. J Trop Med Hyg 1980;83:71.

Taraschewski H et al: Effects of praziquantel on human intestinal flukes (*Fasciolopsis buski* and *Heterophyes heterophyes*). Zbl Bakt Hyg A 1986;262:542.

FASCIOLIASIS

Infection by *Fasciola hepatica*, the sheep liver fluke, results from ingestion of encysted metacercariae on watercress or other aquatic vegetables or in water. A wide range of herbivorous mammals are reservoir hosts. The disease in humans probably occurs worldwide but is most prevalent in sheep-raising countries, particularly where raw salads are eaten. The infection has been reported from Europe, mainland USA, Hawaii, the West Indies, the Middle East, China, Siberia, and North, East and South Africa. Eggs of the worm, passed in host feces, release a miracidium that infects snails; the snails subsequently release cercariae that in turn encyst on vegetation to complete the life cycle. The leaf-shaped adult flukes measure 3 cm × 1.5 cm.

In infection in humans, metacercariae excyst from eggs, penetrate and migrate through the liver, and mature in the bile ducts, where they cause inflammatory and obstructive changes. Although the infection is usually mild, 3 clinical syndromes can develop: acute, chronic latent, and chronic obstructive. The acute illness, associated with migration of immature larvae through the liver, shows an enlarged and tender liver, high fever, leukocytosis, and marked eosinophilia (to 90%). Pain may be present in the epigastrium or right upper quadrant, and the patient may experience headache, anorexia, and vomiting. In severe illnesses, the patient may be prostrated, wasted, and jaundiced. Anemia and a variety of allergic symptoms, including myalgia and urticaria, may be present. Hypergammaglobulinemia is common; other liver function tests may be abnormal. Early diagnosis is difficult in the acute phase, because eggs are not found in the feces for 3–4 months.

In the chronic latent phase, many persons are free of symptoms. Others have variable degrees of hepatomegaly and other acute-phase findings. The chronic obstructive phase takes place if the extrahepatic bile ducts are occluded, producing a clinical picture similar to that of choledocholithiasis. Occasionally, adult flukes migrate and produce lesions and symptoms in ectopic sites.

Diagnosis is by detecting characteristic eggs in the feces; repeated examinations may be necessary. Sometimes the diagnosis can only be made by finding eggs in biliary drainage and, in rare instances, only after liver biopsy or at surgical exploration. Spurious (transient) infections can occur as a result of ingestion of egg-containing cow or sheep liver. Serologic tests are often useful in diagnosis, particularly in the acute phase. Cross-reactions occur with other helminths.

Bithionol, given as for paragonimiasis, is the drug of choice but is only moderately effective. Side effects occur in up to 40% of patients. Reports on the effectiveness of praziquantel have been variable. Although the drug has been generally ineffective when used for 1–2 days, it should be tried on an investigational basis at a dose of 25 mg/kg 3 times daily for 7 days, with a 4- to 6-hour interval between doses. If bithionol or praziquantel are not effective, give dehydroemetine or emetine hydrochloride in dosages used for amebic liver abscess (see Table 28–1); both drugs are potentially toxic, but dehydroemetine may be less so. Triclabendazole, a veterinary fasciolicide, has recently been reported to be useful in several studies, but its safety and effectiveness need to be determined. For any of the drugs, the destruction of parasites followed by release of antigen in sensitized patients may evoke clinical symptoms.

Bithionol and dehydroemetine are available in the USA only from the Parasitic Disease Drug Service, Centers for Disease Control, Atlanta 30333.

In endemic areas, aquatic plants should not be eaten raw; washing does not destroy the metacercariae, but cooking will. Drinking water must be boiled or purified.

Bassily S et al: Sonography in diagnosis of fascioliasis. (Letter.) Lancet 1989;1:1270.

Farag H et al: Bithionol (Bitin) treatment in established fascioliasis in Egyptians. J Trop Med Hyg 1988;91:240.

Farid Z, Kamal M, Woody J: Treatment of acute toxaemic fascioliasis. Trans R Soc Trop Med Hyg 1988;82:299.

Farid Z, Kamal M, Mansour N: Praziquantel and *Fasciola hepatica* infection. Trans R Soc Trop Med Hyg 1989; 83:813.

Loutan L et al: Single treatment of invasive fascioliasis with triclabendazole. (Letter.) Lancet 1989;2:383.

CLONORCHIASIS & OPISTHORCHIASIS

Infection by *Clonorchis sinensis,* the Chinese liver fluke, is endemic in areas of Japan, Korea, China, Taiwan, and southeast Asia. Opisthorchiasis is caused by worms of the genus *Opisthorchis,* generally either *O felineus* (central, eastern, and southern Europe, east Asia, southeast Asia, India) or *O viverrini* (Thailand, Laos, Vietnam). Clinically and epidemiologically, opisthorchiasis and clonorchiasis are identical.

Certain snails are infected when they ingest eggs shed into water in human or animal feces. Larval forms escape from the snails, penetrate the flesh of various freshwater fish, and encyst. Fish-eating mammals, including dogs and cats, are of great importance in maintaining the natural cycle. Human infection results from eating such fish, either raw or undercooked. Pickling, smoking, or drying may not suffice to kill the metacercariae. In humans, the ingested parasites excyst in the duodenum and ascend the bile ducts into the medium and small bile capillaries, where they mature and remain throughout their lives, shedding eggs in the bile. In the chronic stage of infection, there is progressive bile duct thickening, periductal fibrosis, dilatation, biliary stasis, and secondary infection. Little fibrosis occurs in the portal tracts.

Most patients harbor few parasites and are asymptomatic. Among symptomatic patients, an acute and chronic syndrome occurs. Acute symptoms follow entry of immature worms into the biliary ducts and may persist for several months. Findings include malaise, low-grade fever, marked leukocytosis and eosinophilia, an enlarged, tender liver, and pain in the hepatic area or epigastrium. The acute syndrome is difficult to diagnose, since ova may not appear in the feces until 3–4 weeks after onset of symptoms.

In chronic infections, findings include weakness, anorexia, epigastric pain, diarrhea, prolonged low-grade fever, progressive hepatomegaly, and intermittent episodes of right upper quadrant pain and localized hepatic area tenderness.

Complications include intrahepatic bile duct calculi that may lead to recurrent pyogenic cholangitis, biliary abscess, or endophlebitis of the portal-venous branches. Although focal initially, this may gradually result in destruction of the liver parenchyma, fibrosis, and, in a few patients, cirrhoses with ascites, anasarca, and jaundice. Flukes may also enter the gallbladder or the pancreatic duct, causing acute pancreatitis. Cholangiocarcinoma has been linked with prolonged *Clonorchis* infection.

Diagnosis is by finding characteristic eggs in stools or duodenal aspirate. During the chronic stage, leukocytosis varies according to intensity of infection; eosinophilia may be present. In advanced disease, (1) liver function tests will indicate parenchymal damage; (2) CT and sonography may show diffuse dilatation of small intrahepatic bile ducts with no or minimal dilatation of the large intra- and extrahepatic ducts; and (3) transhepatic cholangiograms may show alternating stricture and dilatation of the biliary tree. Serologic tests are sometimes available.

The drug of choice is praziquantel. With a dosage of 25 mg/kg 3 times daily for 2 days (with a 4- to 6-hour interval between doses), cure rates over 95% can be anticipated for *Clonorchis* infections. One day of treatment may be sufficient for *Opisthorchis* infections. (For side effects, see Schistosomiasis, above.) Albendazole, undergoing early clinical trials, may prove to be a useful alternative drug; a dosage of 400 mg twice daily for 3–7 days can be tried.

The disease is rarely fatal, but patients with advanced infections and impaired liver function may succumb more readily to other diseases. The prognosis is good for light to moderate infections.

Lim JH et al: Clonorchiasis: Sonographic findings in 59 proven cases. AJR 1989;152:761.

Riganti M et al: Human pathology of *Opisthorchis viverrini* infection: A comparison of adults and children. Southeast Asian J Trop Med Public Health 1989;20:95.

Rim HJ: The current pathobiology and chemotherapy of clonorchiasis. Korean J Parasitol 1986;24(Suppl):1.

Yangco BG et al: Clinical study evaluating efficacy of praziquantel in clonorchiasis. Antimicrob Agents Chemother 1987;31:135.

PARAGONIMIASIS

Paragonimus westermani, the lung fluke, commonly infects humans throughout the Far East; foci are also present in West Africa, southeast Asia, South Asia, the Pacific Islands, Indonesia, and New Guinea. Many carnivores and omnivores in addition to humans serve as reservoir host for the adult fluke (8–16 × 4–8 × 3–5 mm). A number of other *Paragonimus* species can also infect humans in China, Japan, and Central and South America.

Eggs reaching water, either in sputum or feces, hatch in 3–6 weeks. Released miracidia penetrate and develop in snails. Emergent cercariae encyst in the tissues of crabs and crayfish. When these crustaceans are eaten raw or pickled, when crabs are crushed and food, vessels, or fingers are contaminated by metacercariae that are later ingested, or when drinking water is contaminated by metacercariae, immature flukes excyst in the small intestine and penetrate the peritoneal cavity. Most migrate through the diaphragm and enter the peripheral lung parenchyma; some may lodge in the peritoneum, the intestinal wall, the liver, the skin, or other tissues but most often they lodge in the brain. In the lungs, the parasite becomes encapsulated by granulomatous fibrous tissue, reaching up to 2 cm in diameter. The lesion, which usually opens into a bronchiole, may subsequently rupture, resulting in expectoration of eggs, blood, and inflammatory cells. Eggs from lung cysts may also enter the general circulation and be carried throughout the body, where they produce granulomas in the tissues.

The incubation period ranges from 1 month to 2 years. The majority of light and moderate infections are asymptomatic. In symptomatic patients, there is low-grade fever and dry cough, initially; subsequently, a rusty, blood-flecked viscous sputum may be produced, or hemoptysis may occur. Pleuritic chest pain is common. The condition is chronic and slowly progressive. Dyspnea, signs of bronchitis and bronchiectasis, weakness, malaise, and weight loss may be seen in heavy infections. Parasites in the peritoneal cavity or intestinal wall may cause abdominal pain, diarrhea, or dysentery. Those in the central nervous system, depending on their location, may provoke seizures, palsies, or meningoencephalitis. Migratory subcutaneous nodules (a few millimeters to 10 cm in diameter) occur with about 10% of *P westermani* infections and up to 60% of *Paragonimus skrjabini* infections.

Diagnosis is by finding characteristic eggs in sputum, feces, or pleural fluid or adult flukes in subcutaneous nodules or other surgical specimens. Serologic tests are available. Eosinophilia and low-grade leukocytosis are common. Chest x-rays may show a patchy infiltrate, nodular shadows, calcified spots, or pleural thickening or effusion. Cerebral paragonimiasis can result in intracranial calcifications.

Praziquantel is the drug of choice (25 mg/kg after meals 3 times daily for 3 days, with a 4- to 6-hour interval between doses). (For side effects, see above under Schistosomiasis.) Bithionol is the alternative drug (30–50 mg/kg, given on alternate days for 10–15 doses [20–30 days]; the daily dose should be divided into a morning and evening dose). Side effects are frequent but generally mild and transient. Gastrointestinal symptoms, particularly diarrhea, occur in most patients. Liver function should be tested serially. Bithionol is available in the USA only from the Parasitic Disease Drug Service, Centers for Disease Control, Atlanta 30333. Antibiotics may be necessary to control secondary pulmonary infection. Cure rates of over 90% can be anticipated for both praziquantel and bithionol.

In the acute stage of cerebral paragonimiasis, particularly meningitis, bithionol or praziquantel may be effective. In the chronic stage, when the drug by itself is unlikely to be effective (though it should be tried), surgical removal of parasites is indicated when possible.

Johnson RJ et al: Paragonimiasis: Diagnosis and the use of praziquantel in treatment. Rev Infect Dis 1985;7:200.

Singh TS, Mutum SS, Razaque MA: Pulmonary paragonimiasis: Clinical features, diagnosis and treatment of 39 cases in Manipur. Trans R Soc Trop Med Hyg 1986;80:967.

Udonsi JK: Clinical field trials of praziquantel in pulmonary paragonimiasis due to *Paragonimus uterobilateralis* in endemic populations of the Igwun Basin, Nigeria. Trop Med Parasitol 1989;40:65.

CESTODE INFECTIONS

TAPEWORM INFECTIONS
(See also Cysticercosis
and Echinococcosis, below.)

Classification

Six tapeworms infect humans frequently. The large tapeworms are *Taenia saginata* (the beef tapeworm, up to 25 m in length), *Taenia solium* (the pork tapeworm, 7 m), and *Diphyllobothrium latum* (the fish tapeworm, 10 m). The small tapeworms are *Hymenolepis nana* (the dwarf tapeworm, 25–40 mm), *Hymenolepis diminuta* (the rodent tapeworm, 20–60 cm), and *Dipylidium caninum* (the dog tapeworm, 10–70 cm). Four of the tapeworms occur worldwide; the pork and fish tapeworms have more limited distribution. Humans are the only definitive host of *T saginata, T solium,* and *H nana.*

An adult tapeworm consists of a head (scolex), a neck, and a chain of individual segments (proglottids).

The scolex is the attachment organ and generally lodges in the upper part of the small intestine.

Multiple infections are the rule for small tapeworms and may occur for *D latum;* however, it is rare for a person to harbor more than one or 2 of the taeniae.

A. Beef Tapeworm: The infection is highly endemic in parts of the Far East, central and eastern Africa, and southern USSR, but occurs in most countries with cattle husbandry. Gravid segments of *T saginata* detach themselves from the chain and are passed in feces to soil. When proglottids or eggs are ingested by grazing cattle, the eggs hatch to release embryos that encyst in muscle as cysticerci. Humans are infected by eating undercooked beef containing viable cysticerci. In the human intestines, the cysticercus develops into an adult worm.

B. Pork Tapeworm: This tapeworm is particularly prevalent in Mexico, Latin America, the Iberian Peninsula, the Slavic countries, Africa, southeast Asia, India, and China. In the USA and Canada, the infection is rare, usually occurring in imported cases. The worm is no longer found in northwestern Europe. The life cycle of *T solium* is similar to that of *T saginata* except that the pig is the host of the larval stage. Humans become infected when they eat undercooked pork. Humans are also the intermediate host when they become infected with the larval stage (see Cysticercosis, below) by accidentally ingesting eggs in human feces. Transmission of eggs may occur as a result of autoinfection (hand to mouth), direct person-to-person transfer, or ingestion of food or drink contaminated by eggs.

C. Fish Tapeworm: *D latum* is found in temperate and subarctic lake regions in many areas of the world, including Europe, the USA, Alaska and Canada, Japan, the Middle East, central and southern Africa, and southern South America. Eggs passed in human feces that reach water are taken up first by crustaceans that in turn are eaten by fish, both of which are intermediate hosts. Human infection results from eating raw or inadequately cooked brackish or freshwater fish, including salmon.

D. Dwarf Tapeworm: The *H nana* life cycle is unusual in that both larval and adult stages are found in the human intestine and there is no intermediate host. Eggs passed in the feces are immediately infective. Egg transmission is in most cases directly from person to person and only infrequently by fomites, water, or food. Internal autoinfection occurs when larvae hatch within the intestine, invade the mucosa, develop for a time, and then return to the lumen to mature.

E. Rodent Tapeworm: *H diminuta* is a common parasite of rodents. Many arthropods (eg, rat fleas, beetles, and cockroaches) serve as intermediate hosts. Humans are infected by accidentally swallowing the infected arthropods, usually in cereals or stored products.

F. Dog Tapeworm: *D caninum* infection generally occurs in young children in close association with infected dogs or cats. Transmission results from swallowing the infected intermediate hosts, ie, fleas or lice.

Clinical Findings

A. Signs and Symptoms:

1. Large tapeworms–Large tapeworm infections are generally asymptomatic. Occasionally, vague gastrointestinal symptoms (eg, nausea, diarrhea, abdominal pain) and systemic symptoms (eg, fatigue, hunger, dizziness) have been attributed to the infections. Vomiting of proglottid segments or obstruction of the bile duct, pancreatic duct, or appendix is rare.

Some persons (mostly Scandinavian residents) who harbor the fish tapeworm develop a hyperchromic macrocytic megaloblastic anemia accompanied by thrombocytopenia and mild leukopenia. Gastric acidity is normal. The anemia is a result of the worm's competing with the host for vitamin B_{12}. Clinical findings include glossitis, dyspnea, tachycardia, and neurologic findings (weakness, numbness, paresthesias, disturbances of motility and coordination, and impairment of vibration and position senses).

2. Small tapeworms–Light infections are generally asymptomatic. Heavy infections, particularly with *H nana,* may cause diarrhea, abdominal pain, anorexia, vomiting, weight loss, and irritability, particularly in young children.

B. Laboratory Findings:
Infection by a beef or pork tapeworm is often discovered by the patient finding segments in stool, clothing, or bedding. To determine the species, proglottid segments are either flattened between glass slides and examined microscopically for anatomic detail or differentiated by enzyme electrophoresis of glucose phosphate isomerase. Eggs are only infrequently present in stools, but the perianal cellophane tape test, as used to diagnose pinworm, is sometimes useful in detecting *T saginata* eggs. However, *Taenia* eggs look alike and do not permit species differentiation.

Fish tapeworm is diagnosed by finding characteristic operculated eggs in stool; repeat examinations may be necessary. Proglottids are passed occasionally, and their internal morphology is also diagnostic. The presence of hydrochloric acid in the stomach differentiates the anemia from pernicious anemia; in both conditions, the Schilling test is abnormal.

H nana and *H diminuta* infections are diagnosed by finding characteristic eggs in feces; proglottids are usually not seen. *D caninum* infection is diagnosed by detection of proglottids (the size of melon seeds) in feces or after their active migration through the anus.

Serologic tests are not available for tapeworm infections.

Treatment

A. Specific Measures:

1. *T saginata* and *D latum*–The drug of choice is a single dose of niclosamide. Cure rates over 95% can be anticipated with the following dosages: adults, 4 tablets (2 g); children weighing more than 34 kg, 3 tablets; children 11–34 kg, 2 tablets. The drug is given in the morning before the patient has eaten. The tablets *must be chewed thoroughly* and swallowed with water. Eating may be resumed in 2 hours. Niclosamide usually produces no side effects.

Praziquantel in a single dose of 10 mg/kg is the alternative drug. At this low dose, side effects (see under Schistosomiasis, above) are minimal.

Pre- and posttreatment purges are not used for either drug. The anemia and neurologic manifestations of *D latum* respond to vitamin B_{12} as used in treatment of pernicious anemia.

2. *T solium*–The choice of drugs and methods of treatment are as above. For both drugs, it may be useful to give a moderate purgative 2–3 hours after treatment to rapidly eliminate segments from the bowel. The patient must be instructed about the need for careful washing of the hands and perianal area and for safe disposal of feces for 4 days following therapy.

3. *H nana*–Praziquantel, the drug of choice, produces 95% cure rates with a single 25 mg/kg dose. Niclosamide, the alternative drug, produces cure rates of 75% when given at the above dosage for 5–7 days; some workers repeat the course 5 days later.

4. *H diminuta* and *D caninum*–Treatment is with niclosamide or praziquantel in dosages as for *H nana*. Cure rates are not established.

B. Follow-Up Care: In treatment of large tapeworm infections, a disintegrating worm is usually passed within 24–48 hours of treatment. Since efforts are not generally made to recover and identify the scolex, cure can be presumed only if regenerated segments have not reappeared 3–5 months later. If it is preferred that parasitic cure be established immediately, the head (scolex) must be found in posttreatment stools. A laxative is given 2 hours after treatment, and stools must be collected in a preservative for 24 hours. To facilitate examination, toilet paper must be disposed of separately.

Prognosis

Because the prognosis is often poor in cerebral cysticercosis, *T solium* infections must be immediately eradicated.

Chunge CN: Praziquantel for the treatment of tapeworms in Kenya. East Afr Med J 1987;64:672.

Fan PC et al: Studies on taeniasis in Taiwan. V. Field trial on evaluation of therapeutic efficacy of mebendazole and praziquantel against taeniasis. Southeast Asian J Trop Med Public Health 1986;17:82

CYSTICERCOSIS

Essentials of Diagnosis

- History of exposure in an endemic region; concomitant or past intestinal infection by *Taenia solium*.
- Seizures, signs of intracranial hypertension, signs of a focal space-occupying central nervous system lesion.
- Subcutaneous or muscular nodules (5–10 mm); calcified lesions on x-rays of soft tissues.
- Calcified or uncalcified cysts by CT scan; positive serologic tests.

General Considerations

Human cysticercosis is infection by the larval (cysticercus) stage of the tapeworm *T solium* (see above), which forms cysts in the tissues. Locations of cysts in order of frequency are the central nervous system, the subcutaneous tissues and striated muscle, the globe of the eye, and, rarely, other tissues. Cysts reach 5–10 mm in soft tissues but may be larger in the central nervous system. Cysticerci complete their development within 3–4 months after larval entry and can live for many years. The parasite causes little or no inflammatory reaction until it dies, at which time the cyst capsule becomes distended with fluid and increases in size; subsequently, it is replaced by fibrous tissue or undergoes calcification. Both living and calcified cysts may be present in the same organ.

Clinical Findings

A. Signs and Symptoms: Up to 50% of central nervous system cysticerci are asymptomatic; cysticerci in other locations are usually asymptomatic as well, even in the presence of heavy infection.

1. Neurocysticercosis–One or more of the following syndromes (in order of frequency) may be present: (a) Epilepsy. (b) Intracranial hypertension (intense headache, nausea, vomiting, papilledema, diplopia, progressive loss of visual acuity leading to blindness). (c) Mental disturbances. (d) Meningeal syndrome: The basilar membranes, principally the arachnoid, are affected. Extensive adhesive arachnoiditis may be manifested by intracranial hypertension, obstructive hydrocephalus, arterial thrombosis, and cranial nerve involvement, most often the optic nerve. (e) Ventricular cysts: Cysts may float freely within the ventricles or cerebral aqueduct or may be attached to the ventricular wall. They are usually asymptomatic but can cause increased intracranial pressure as a result of intermittent or total blockage. (f) Racemose cysts: These are rare aberrant forms that are multiple-branched, nonencysted, lack a scolex, and may reach over 10 cm in diameter. They generally are found in the ventricular and subarachnoid spaces, where they cause marked adhesive arachnoiditis and often obstructive hydrocephalus. (g)

Spinal cord cysts: These can be extraspinal or in-traspinal and cause arachnoiditis or pressure symptoms.

2. Ophthalmocysticercosis—Usually there is a single cyst. Presenting symptoms include periorbital pain, scotomas, and progressive deterioration of visual acuity. Findings include disk hemorrhage and edema, retinal detachment, iridocyclitis, and chorioretinitis.

3. Subcutaneous and muscular cysticerco-sis—These cysts present as fixed nodules that tend to appear at different times. Some nodules will collapse and disappear and then may reappear after a period of time.

B. Laboratory Tests: Definitive diagnosis of neurocysticercosis is by finding the parasite on histologic section of specimens removed by excisional biopsy of skin or subcutaneous tissues (not of brain tissue). Patients should be thoroughly examined by palpation for pea-sized nodules. Presumptive diagnosis is by the following tests.

1. Imaging—Plain radiographs of soft tissues may detect oval or linear calcified lesions (4–10 × 2–5 mm). The lesions are usually multiple, sometimes in the hundreds, and the long axes of the cysts are nearly always in the plane of the surrounding muscle fibers.

Plain skull films may demonstrate intracranial hypertension as well as one or more cerebral calcifications (generally 5–10 mm; sometimes 1–2 mm when only the scolex is calcified). Computed tomography is the most useful procedure, as it detects both uncalcified and calcified cysts, edema, intracranial hypertension, and enhancement signs when contrast medium is used. Often a combination of different CT images is found, owing to different stages of development among cysticerci. MRI is useful. Spinal cysticercosis is evaluated by myelography or MRI.

2. Immunologic tests—Immunologic tests are useful adjuncts in diagnosis. Differentiation of cysticercosis from echinococcosis is possible by the immunoelectrophoresis and agar gel double diffusion tests but not by the indirect hemagglutination test. Sometimes a patient may have a positive blood test but a negative test on cerebrospinal fluid; even a negative test with both fluids does not rule out cysticercosis. Patients presenting with only calcified lesions are generally serologically negative.

3. Other tests—The cerebrospinal fluid in neuro-cysticercosis typically shows increased protein, decreased glucose, and a cellular reaction consisting mainly of lymphocytes and eosinophils; eosinophilia over 20% is diagnostically important. Though the patient usually no longer harbors a tapeworm at the time cysticercosis is diagnosed, stools should be examined over several days by the patient for the passage of proglottids and by the laboratory for proglottids and eggs.

Treatment

When living parasites are present in the central nervous system, medical treatment with praziquantel (which crosses the blood-brain barrier) is usually preferred to surgical removal of the lesion. However, praziquantel has no effect on calcified parasites, whether or not the patient is symptomatic.

A. Specific Measures:

1. Praziquantel—The dosage for praziquantel is 50 mg/kg/d for 14 days or 75 mg/kg/d for 10 days; the daily dose is divided into 3 parts. To avoid or diminish the inflammatory reaction that follows death of parasites in brain tissue, a steroid such as prednisone, 30 mg/d in 2–3 divided doses, starting 1–2 days before praziquantel and continuing for 3–4 days afterward, should be given. Others advocate use of steroids only for selected patients, based on the initial response to praziquantel. Use of anticonvulsant drugs must be continued during praziquantel treatment and probably for a considerable time afterward.

Side effects, which occur in about one-third of patients treated with combined praziquantel and steroids—and in about 90% given praziquantel without steroids—include increased intracranial pressure, headache, vomiting, mental changes, and convulsions. The side effects are usually mild and generally subside within 48–72 hours. In some cases, however, severity may require the following additional measures: (1) steroids in higher doses, (2) mannitol, (3) anticonvulsants if not used concomitantly, and (4) diuretics.

Fifty percent of praziquantel-treated patients are clinically cured (clearing of symptoms and disappearance of lesions by cerebral tomograms). Of the remainder, many have amelioration of symptoms, including intracranial hypertension and seizures. In ventricular and spinal cysticercosis, however, little or no response is achieved. When hydrocephalus is present, surgical shunt is required, even where the parasites have been destroyed.

At 3 months, the patient should be assessed clinically and by cerebral tomograms to determine whether a second treatment is necessary.

2. Other drugs—Albendazole (15 mg/kg/d for 30 days) may be as effective, but few studies are available as yet. Shorter courses are being tried. The importance of corticosteroids in concurrent treatment has not been evaluated.

3. Surgery—Surgery has successfully removed orbital, cisternal, and ventricular cysts and, if accessible, cerebral, meningeal, or spinal cord cysts. Ocular cysticercosis is treated by surgical removal of cysts. Praziquantel is contraindicated for a cyst attached to the retina, as destruction of the larva may damage the retina irreversibly.

B. General Measures: Symptomatic treatment of neurocysticercosis is based on the use of steroids for cerebral edema and anticonvulsants for seizures.

Prognosis

The fatality rate for untreated neurocysticercosis is about 50%; survival time from onset of symptoms ranges from days to many years. Drug treatment has reduced the mortality rate to 6–16%. Surgical procedures to relieve intracranial hypertension along with use of steroids to reduce edema improve the prognosis for those not effectively treated by praziquantel.

Alarcon F et al: Neurocysticercosis: Short course of treatment with albendazole. Arch Neurol 1989;46:1231.
Cook GC: Neurocysticercosis: Parasitology, clinical presentation, diagnosis, and recent advances in management. Q J Med 1988;68:575.
Del Brutto OH, Sotelo J: Neurocysticercosis: An update. Rev Infect Dis 1988;10:1075-1087.
Moodley M, Moosa A: Treatment of neurocysticercosis: Is praziquantel the new hope? Lancet 1989;1:262.
Tsang VCW, Brand JA, Boyer AE: An enzyme-linked immunoelectrotransfer blot assay and glycoprotein antigens for diagnosing human cysticercosis (Taenia solium). J Infect Dis 1989;159:50. (New, specific diagnostic test.)
Vazquez ML, Jung H, Sotelo J: Plasma levels of praziquantel decrease when dexamethasone is given simultaneously. Neurology 1987;37:1561. (Possible decreased efficacy if steroids are given.)

ECHINOCOCCOSIS/HYDATIDOSIS
(Hydatid Disease)

Human echinococcosis results from parasitism by the larval stage of 2 *Echinococcus* species: *Echinococcus granulosus* (cystic hydatid disease) and *Echinococcus multilocularis* (alveolar hydatid disease). Very rarely, *Echinococcus vogeli* (polycystic hydatid disease) has been reported from northern South America and Panama. Echinococcosis is a zoonosis in which humans are an intermediate host of the larval stage of the parasite. The definitive host is a carnivore (all of which, except for the lion, are Canidae) that harbors the adult tapeworm in the small intestine; the carnivore becomes infected by ingesting the larval form in tissue of the intermediate host. The intermediate hosts, chiefly herbivorous mammals but including humans, become infected by ingesting tapeworm eggs passed in carnivore feces. The larval stage is referred to as a hydatid cyst.

1. CYSTIC HYDATID DISEASE
(Unilocular Hydatid Disease)

Essentials of Diagnosis

- Avascular cystic tumor of liver, lung, or, infrequently, bone, brain, or other organs as detected by imaging procedures.
- Positive serologic tests.
- History of exposure to dogs associated with livestock in a hydatid-endemic region.

General Considerations

Human infection with *E granulosus* occurs principally where dogs are used to herd grazing animals, particularly sheep. The disease is common throughout southern South America, the Mediterranean littoral and the Middle East, central Asia, and East Africa. Foci of endemicity are in eastern Europe, Russia, Australasia, India, and the United Kingdom. In North America, endemic foci have been reported from the western USA, the lower Mississippi valley, Alaska, and northwestern Canada.

There are at least 2 geographic strains of the parasite. The pastoral strain—which is more pathogenic to humans—has a transmission cycle in which dogs are the definitive host, and sheep (usually) but also cattle, hogs, and other domestic livestock are intermediate hosts. The sylvatic, or northern, strain is maintained in wolves and wild ungulates (moose and reindeer) in northern Alaska, Canada, Scandinavia, and Eurasia.

Human infection occurs when eggs passed in dog feces are accidentally swallowed. Embryos liberated from the eggs penetrate the intestinal mucosa, enter the portal bloodstream, and are carried to the liver where they are trapped and become hydatid cysts (65% of all cysts). Some larvae reach the lung (25%) and develop into pulmonary hydatids. Infrequently, cysts form in the brain, bones, skeletal muscles, kidneys, spleen, or other tissues. Cysts of the sylvatic strain tend to localize in the lungs.

The cyst wall has 3 layers: an inner germinal layer that gives rise within the cyst to germinal elements, a supporting intermediate layer, and an outer layer produced by the host. In the liver, cysts may increase in size 1–5 cm in diameter per year and become enormous, but symptoms generally do not develop until they reach about 10 cm. Some cysts die spontaneously. Part or all of the inner layer of some hepatic or splenic cysts may calcify, which does not necessarily mean cyst death.

Clinical Findings
A. Symptoms and Signs: A liver cyst may remain silent for 10–20 or more years until it becomes large enough to be palpable, to be visible as an abdominal swelling, to produce pressure effects, or to produce symptoms due to leakage or rupture. There may be right upper quadrant pain, nausea, and vomiting. The effects of pressure may result in cholangitis and secondary infection, which may lead to obstructive jaundice, cirrhosis, and portal hypertension. If a cyst ruptures suddenly, anaphylaxis and death may occur. If fluid and hydatid particles escape slowly, allergic manifestations may result, including a rise in the eosinophil count. Rupture can occur into the pleural, pericardial, or peritoneal space or into the duodenum, colon, or renal pelvis. Dissemination of germinal elements may be followed by the development of multiple secondary cysts. A characteristic clinical syn-

drome may follow intrabiliary extrusion of cyst contents—jaundice, biliary colic, and urticaria.

Pulmonary cysts cause no symptoms until they leak; become large enough to obstruct a bronchus, causing segmental collapse; or erode a bronchus and rupture. Brain cysts produce symptoms earlier and may cause seizures or symptoms of increased intracranial pressure. Cysts in the bone marrow or spongiosa do not have a host layer, are irregular in shape, erode osseous tissue, and may present as pain or as spontaneous fracture. The bones most often affected are the vertebrae; many of these cases develop epidural extension with compression of the spinal cord and paraplegia. Because 20% of patients have multiple cysts, each patient should be screened for cysts in the liver, spleen, kidneys, lungs, brain, bones, skin, tongue, vitreous, and other tissues.

B. Imaging: Sonography and CT scan are most commonly used to detect a cystic mass in the liver. Nearly pathognomonic is the presence within a hydatid cyst of daughter cysts; they must be distinguished, however, from blood clots within the cavity of simple cysts. The mass can also be defined by scintillation scan or by angiography (which would rarely be used), which may show the "halo" sign. Spotty calcified densities or a calcified cyst wall may be seen in the liver or spleen. Chest films may show a pulmonary lesion, but calcification of the wall does not occur. An intravenous urogram or full body bone scan may detect other cysts at other sites.

C. Laboratory Findings: Several serologic tests (indirect hemagglutination, indirect immunofluorescence, ELISA) are useful for screening for serum antibody. False-negative reactions may occur in 5–10% of liver cysts and up to 50% of lung cysts. In addition, false-positive cross-reactions may occur with other helminthic infections, liver cirrhosis, and cancer. Persons positive in the screening test should be tested by one of several methods to detect arc 5; its presence is considered diagnostic except for cross-reactions with *T solium* infections. A new test by immunoblot assay was reported to be 100% specific and 91% sensitive. Persons from whom cysts have been completely removed and carriers of dead cysts may become seronegative. The Casoni intracutaneous skin test has been abandoned because of poor specificity.

Eosinophilia is uncommon except after cyst rupture. Liver function tests are usually normal. Diagnostic aspiration of suspected hydatid cysts should never be undertaken because of the danger of leakage with secondary spread or anaphylaxis. Confirmation of the diagnosis is possible only by examination of cyst contents after surgical removal.

Differential Diagnosis

Noninfected hydatid cysts of the liver need to be differentiated from simple (epithelial cysts); infected cysts, from bacterial and amebic abscesses. Hydatid cysts in any site may be mistaken for a variety of malignant and nonmalignant tumors and cysts. In the lung, a cyst may be confused with an advanced tubercular lesion. Allergic symptoms arising from cyst leakage may resemble those associated with many other diseases.

Treatment & Prevention

A. Surgical Treatment: The current definitive treatment is surgical removal of cysts if their location and the patient's general condition permit. All lung cysts should be removed but not all liver cysts. Whether newly available chemotherapy should alter this position will depend upon the results of long-term follow-up of patients treated only with a drug. Decision-making must take into account that surgical mortality rates range from 1% to 4%, and recurrences after surgery are about 10%. Operative treatment of liver cysts involves 2 major problems: (1) selection of a method to sterilize and remove cyst contents without spillage, and (2) management of the remaining cavity. Germicidal solutions include cetrimide (5%), hypertonic saline (20%), silver nitrate (0.5%), and sodium hypochlorite (3.75%). If spillage occurs during surgery, albendazole, mebendazole, or praziquantel (which kills protoscoleces) may be useful. For the treatment of bone cysts, curettage, lavage, and instillation of chemical sterilization substances are indicated.

B. Drug Treatment:

1. Albendazole–Albendazole is much more readily absorbed than mebendazole; this permits a substantially lower dosage of albendazole to be used, yet its active metabolite, the sulfoxide, reaches effective concentrations in cyst wall and fluid. A current regimen is 4 tablets (800 mg) daily for three 28-day courses, with 2-week rest periods between courses. Among 253 patients treated in multiple studies, the outcomes for liver and lung cysts were, respectively, as follows: cured (33%, 40%), improved (44%, 37%), no change (21%, 22%), and worse (2%, 1%). However, most patients were not followed long enough to permit evaluation for recurrences (4 occurred among the 29 persons followed over 2 years). Bone cysts may prove more refractory to treatment. In the 3-month courses, drug side effects include fever, headache, nausea, vomiting, alopecia, cyst leakage (with an anaphylactic reaction in one patient), and reversible leukopenia and transaminase elevations (17%).

2. Mebendazole–When mebendazole was used at high doses for several months, marked regression and apparent death of cysts occurred in some patients. In others, cysts were either stable or continued to grow and if removed were viable. The dosage is 50 mg/kg/d in 3 divided doses for 3 months, with many patients requiring repeated courses. When possible, mebendazole levels should be monitored; serum levels in excess of 100 mg/L 1–2 hours after an oral dose may be necessary for parasite killing. In unresponsive cases, it is possible that plasma levels of mebendazole are insufficient; some researchers, therefore, give up to 200 mg/kg/d. Occasional side effects with treatment include pruritus, rash, alopecia, reversible leukopenia, gastric irritation, musculoskeletal pain, fever, and acute pain in the cyst area; 6 cases of glomerulonephritis and 3 of agranulocytosis (with one death) have been reported.

Under evaluation are pre- and postsurgical use of albendazole to reduce risk of recurrence due to operative spillage.

C. Prevention: In endemic areas, prevention is by prophylactic treatment of pet dogs with 5 mg/kg of praziquantel at monthly intervals to remove adult tapeworms and by health education to prevent feeding of offal to dogs.

Prognosis

Most liver and lung cysts often can be removed surgically without great difficulty, but in patients with cysts in less accessible sites the prognosis is less favorable. The prognosis is always grave when there has been spillage and the development of secondary cysts. About 15% of untreated patients eventually die because of the disease or its complications.

2. ALVEOLAR HYDATID DISEASE (Multilocular Hydatid Disease)

Alveolar hydatid disease results from infection by the larval form of *Echinococcus multilocularis*. The life cycle involves foxes as definitive host and microtine rodents as intermediate host. Domestic dogs and cats can also become infected with the adult tapeworm when they eat infected wild rodents. Human infection is by accidental ingestion of tapeworm eggs passed in fox or dog feces. The disease in humans has been reported in parts of central Europe, much of Siberia, northwestern Canada, and western Alaska. A single case has been reported in Minnesota. The primary localization of alveolar cysts is in the liver, where they may extend locally or metastasize to other tissues. The larval mass has poorly defined borders and behaves like a neoplasm; it infiltrates and proliferates indefinitely by exogenous budding of the germinative membrane, producing an alveoluslike pattern of microvesicles. X-rays show hepatomegaly and characteristic scattered areas of radiolucency often outlined by 2- to 4-mm calcific rings. Serologic tests are the same as for cystic hydatid disease and cannot distinguish between the species. Treatment is by surgical removal of the entire larval mass, when possible. Ninety percent of patients with nonresectable masses die within 10 years. Long-term mebendazole therapy (40 mg/kg/d) inhibits growth of the parasite and has extended patient survival, but larval tissue is not completely destroyed.

Choudhuri G et al: Poor responses to long-term albendazole therapy of hydatid liver cysts. Scand J Infect Dis 1989;21:323.

Horton RJ: Chemotherapy of *Echinococcus* infection in man with albendazole. Trans R Soc Trop Med Hyg 1989; 83:97.

Maddison SE et al: A specific diagnostic antigen of *Echinococcus granulosus* with an apparent molecular weight of 8 KDA. Am J Trop Med Hyg 1989;40:377.

Taylor DH, Morris DL: The current management of hydatid disease. Br J Clin Pract 1988;42:401.

NEMATODE (ROUNDWORM) INFECTIONS

ANISAKIASIS

Anisakiasis is larval invasion of the stomach or intestinal wall by anisakid nematodes. In the acute form, the infection may mimic surgical abdomen; in the chronic form, mild symptoms may persist for weeks to years.

Definitive hosts are marine mammals. Eggs discharged with feces are ingested by crustaceans, in which larvae develop that are infective for squids, mackerel, herring, cod, rockfish (red snapper), salmon, tuna, and other marine fish. In the fish, the larvae pass to the peritoneum and musculature and are able to transfer from fish to fish along the food chain. Eventually, the larvae within the fish intermediate host are ingested by a marine mammal and mature to the adult stage (20–30 × 0.4–0.6 mm).

Humans are infected when they ingest larvae in marine fish or in squid eaten raw, undercooked, salted, or lightly pickled. Although the larvae sometimes develop to the adult stages, gravid females are not found in humans. The infection occurs worldwide, but most cases have been reported in Japan and the Netherlands, with a few in the United States, Scandinavia, Chile, and other fish-eating countries. Regional foods eaten raw such as sashimi in Japan, pickled herring in the Netherlands, and seviche in Latin America are common vehicles of infection.

Clinical Findings

A. Symptoms and Signs: Most ingested larvae probably fail to cause infection and are passed in feces or, rarely, migrate up the esophagus or are coughed up and expectorated. Larvae liberated in the stomach attach to and partially penetrate either the gastric or the intestinal mucosa, which may ulcerate locally. Many acute cases are not diagnosed and go on to a chronic course. Rarely, worms penetrate the gut wall, enter the peritoneal cavity, and migrate.

1. Acute gastric anisakiasis–Within 4 hours,

the patient experiences nausea, vomiting, and epigastric pain that progressively becomes more severe. Hematemesis is rare.

2. Acute intestinal anisakiasis–Within 1–7 days, colicky pain appears in the lower abdomen, often localized at the ileocecal region, accompanied by diarrhea, nausea, vomiting, and mild fever.

3. Chronic disease–For weeks to several years, symptoms may continue that mimic gastric ulcer, gastritis, gastric tumor, bowel tumor or bowel inflammation. An eosinophilic abscess and granuloma then form, and the parasite dies.

B. Laboratory Findings: Stools may show occult blood. Mild leukocytosis and eosinophilia may be present. In chronic cases, ELISA and RAST serologic tests, if available, may be useful.

C. Imaging and Endoscopy: In acute infection, the larvae sometimes can be seen and removed endoscopically from the stomach. X-rays of the stomach may show a localized edematous, ulcerated area with a thickened wall, decreased peristalsis, and rigidity. Double contrast technique may show the threadlike larvae. Small bowel x-rays may show thickened mucosa and segments of stenosis with proximal dilatation. In the chronic stage, x-rays and endoscopy of the stomach—but not of the bowel—may be helpful.

In chronic infection, the diagnosis is often made only at laparotomy with surgical removal of the parasite.

Prevention & Treatment

Prevention is by avoidance of ingestion of raw or incompletely cooked marine fish or squid, especially salmon, rockfish, herring, and mackerel. Larvae within fish may with difficulty be seen as colorless, tightly coiled or spiraled worms in 3-mm whorls or as reddish or pigmented larvae lying open in muscles or viscera. The larvae are killed by temperatures about 60 °C or by freezing at −20 °C for 24 hours. Smoking procedures that do not bring the temperature to 60 °C and salt-curing are not reliable. The preferred public health measure is freezing before marketing, as is done with herring in Holland and on most tuna boats.

Except where larvae can be removed by fiberoptic gastroscopy, treatment of acute and chronic lesions is limited to symptomatic measures or surgical excision of the worm in severe cases. There is no drug treatment.

Kliks MM: Update on anisakiasis in the U.S. JAMA 1986;255:2605.

McKerrow JM, Sakanari J, Deardorff TL: Anisakiasis: Revenge of the sushi parasite. (Letter.) N Engl J Med 1988;319:1228.

Oshima T: Anisakiasis: Is the sushi bar guilty? Parasitology Today 1987;3:44.

Sugimachi K et al: Acute gastric anisakiasis. Analysis of 178 cases. JAMA 1985;253:1012.

Schantz PM: The dangers of eating raw fish. N Engl J Med 1989;320:1143.

Wittner M et al: Eustromgylidiasis: A parasitic infection acquired by eating sushi. N Engl J Med 1989;320:1124.

ANGIOSTRONGYLIASIS

1. ANGIOSTRONGYLIASIS CANTONENSIS (Eosinophilic Meningoencephalitis)

A nematode of rats, *Angiostrongylus cantonensis*, is the causative agent of a form of eosinophilic meningoencephalitis. It has been reported from Hawaii and other Pacific islands, south and southeast Asia, Japan, Australia, Egypt, Madagascar, Cuba, and Puerto Rico.

Human infection results from the ingestion of infected larvae contained in raw food—either infected mollusks (the intermediate host) or transport hosts (crabs, shrimp, fish) that have ingested mollusks. Drinking water and fresh vegetables can also become contaminated with infective larvae, as can fingers during the collection and preparation of snails for cooking.

The incubation period is about 2 weeks. The larvae (0.5 × 0.025 mm) usually invade the central nervous system, producing findings of meningoencephalitis, including headache, fever, neck stiffness, nausea and vomiting, and multiple neurologic findings, particularly asymmetric transient paresthesias and cranial and other nerve palsies. A characteristic feature is spinal fluid pleocytosis, consisting largely of eosinophils. Occasionally, the parasite can be recovered from spinal fluid. Peripheral eosinophilia with a low-grade leukocytosis are common. Serologic and skin tests are not specific. Ocular infection has been reported from Thailand.

No specific treatment is available; however, levamisole or albendazole can be tried. Corticosteroids have not influenced the course of the disease. The illness usually persists for weeks to months, the parasite dies, and the patient then recovers spontaneously, usually without sequelae. However, fatalities have been recorded.

2. ANGIOSTRONGYLIASIS COSTARICENSIS

Angiostrongylus costaricensis has been identified in humans in Mexico, Central America, Venezuela, Brazil, and the USA (Texas). The known geographic range of the parasite in rats (the definitive host) extends from northern South America to Texas. The intermediate host is a slug that contaminates human food with infective larvae. In humans, adult worms mature in the mesenteric vessels, where they cause arteritis, thrombosis, and ischemic necrosis. Eggs lodging in capillaries give rise to eosinophilic granulomas, most commonly in the appendix but also in the terminal ileum, the cecum, the first part of the ascending colon, and the regional lymph nodes. Findings include fever, right lower quadrant abdominal pain and a mass, leukocytosis, and eosinophilia. Bowel complications consist of incomplete or complete obstruction and infarction. No serologic test is available. The disease usually simulates acute appendicitis, which can in fact be caused by the parasite. Intra-abdominal mass can mimic tumor. There is no specific treatment. Operative treatment is frequently necessary.

Campbell BG, Little MD: The finding of *Angiostrongylus cantonensis* in rats in New Orleans. Am J Trop Med Hyg 1988;38:568. (The first report of the parasite from North America.)

Ishii AI et al: In vivo efficacy of levamisole against larval stages of *Angiostrongylus cantonensis* and *A costaricensis*. Southeast Asian J Trop Med Public Health 1989;20:109.

Koo J, Pien F, Kliks MM: *Angiostrongylus (Parastrongylus)* eosinophilic meningitis. Rev Infect Dis 1988; 10: 1155.

Silvera CT et al: Angiostrongyliasis: A rare cause of gastrointestinal hemorrhage. Am J Gastroenterol 1989; 84:329.

ASCARIASIS

Essentials of Diagnosis

- Pulmonary phase: Transient cough, dyspnea, wheezing; allergic findings (eosinophilia, urticaria, asthma); transient pulmonary infiltrates.
- Intestinal phase: Vague upper abdominal discomfort; occasional vomiting, abdominal distention.
- Eggs in stools; worms passed per rectum, nose, or mouth.

General Considerations

Ascaris lumbricoides is the most common of the intestinal helminths. It is cosmopolitan in distribution and is found in high prevalence wherever there are low standards of hygiene and sanitation or where human feces are used as fertilizer. The infection is specific for humans and occurs in all age groups. Heavy worm burdens, however, are usually seen only in children; there is evidence of resistance to superinfection in adults.

Adult worms live in the upper small intestine. After fertilization, the female produces enormous numbers of eggs that pass in feces. Direct transmission between humans does not occur, as the eggs must remain on the soil for 2–3 weeks before they become infective. Thereafter, they can survive for years. Infection occurs through ingestion of mature eggs in fecally contaminated food and drink. The eggs hatch in the small intestine, releasing motile larvae that penetrate the wall of the small intestine and reach the right heart via the mesenteric venules and lymphatics. From the heart they move to the lung, burrow through the alveolar walls, and migrate up the bronchial tree into the pharynx, down the esophagus, and back to the small intestine. Egg production begins 60–75 days after ingestion of infective eggs. Adult worms (20–40 cm × 3–6 mm) live for 1 year or more.

Clinical Findings

A. Symptoms and Signs: Migrating larvae in the lung cause capillary and alveolar damage, which may result in low-grade fever, cough, blood-tinged sputum, wheezing, rales, dyspnea, substernal pain, areas of local pulmonary consolidation, and allergic findings (eosinophilia, urticaria, asthma, angioneurotic edema). Rarely, larvae lodge ectopically in the brain, kidney, eye, spinal cord, etc, and may cause unusual symptoms.

Small numbers of adult worms in the intestine usually produce no symptoms. With heavy infection, vague abdominal discomfort (preprandial or postprandial) and colic may occur, particularly in children. Adult worms may also migrate with heavy infections; they may be coughed up, vomited, or passed out through the nose. They may also force themselves into the common bile duct, pancreatic duct, appendix, diverticula, and other sites, which may lead to cholangitis, cholecystitis, pyogenic liver abscess, or pancreatitis. With very heavy infestations, masses of worms may cause intestinal obstruction, volvulus, or intussusception. During typhoid fever, worms may penetrate the weakened bowel wall.

Because anesthesia stimulates the worms to become hypermotile, they should be removed in advance for patients undergoing elective surgery.

B. Imaging: During the pulmonary phase, chest radiographs may show scattered, patchy, ill-defined asymmetric infiltrations (Löffler's pneumonia). Intestinal infection is sometimes established by chance, when radiologic examination of the abdomen (with or without barium) shows the presence of worms.

C. Laboratory Findings: Diagnosis usually depends upon finding the characteristic eggs in feces. Occasionally, an adult worm spontaneously passed per rectum or orally reveals an unsuspected infection.

Serologic tests are not useful, because of low specificity. There are no hematologic alterations during the intestinal phase.

During the pulmonary phase, eosinophils may reach 30–50% and remain high for about a month; larvae are occasionally found in sputum.

Differential Diagnosis

Pulmonary ascariasis with eosinophilia must be differentiated from nonparasitic causes (asthma, Löffler's syndrome, eosinophilic pneumonia, systemic lupus erythematosus, Hodgkin's disease) and parasitic causes (tropical pulmonary eosinophilia, toxocariasis, strongyloidiasis, hookworm disease, paragonimiasis). *Ascaris*-induced pancreatitis, appendicitis, diverticulitis, etc, must be differentiated from other causes of inflammation of these tissues. Postprandial dyspepsia may simulate duodenal ulcer, hiatal hernia, gallbladder disease, or pancreatic disease.

Treatment

Pyrantel pamoate is the treatment of choice. None of the drugs listed below require pre- or posttreatment purges. Stools should be rechecked at 2 weeks and patients re-treated until all ascarids are removed. Ascariasis, hookworm, and trichuriasis infections, which often occur together, may be treated simultaneously by mebendazole, albendazole, or oxantel-pyrantel pamoate. Ascariasis and hookworm combined may be treated with mebendazole, pyrantel, or albendazole. In the treatment of biliary ascariasis, endoscopic removal of the worm under ultrasonographic guidance is often successful.

A. Pyrantel Pamoate: Pyrantel pamoate as a single oral dose of 10 mg base/kg (maximum, 1 g) results in 85–100% cure rates. It may be given before or after meals. Infrequent side effects include vomiting, diarrhea, headache, dizziness, drowsiness, and rash.

B. Piperazine: The dosage for piperazine (as the hexahydrate) is 75 mg/kg body weight (maximum, 3.5 g) for 2 days in succession, giving the drug orally before or after breakfast. For heavy infestations, treatment should be continued for 4 days in succession or the 2-day course should be repeated after 1 week.

Gastrointestinal symptoms and headache occur occasionally; central nervous system symptoms (temporary ataxia and exacerbation of seizures) are rare. Allergic symptoms have been attributed to piperazine. The drug should not be used for patients with hepatic or renal insufficiency or with a history of seizures or chronic neurologic disease. Piperazine may be used in the last trimester of pregnancy.

C. Mebendazole: Mebendazole is highly effective when given in a dosage of 100 mg twice daily before or after meals for 3 days. Gastrointestinal side effects are infrequent, but worms may appear occasionally at the nose or mouth of children under age 5. The drug is contraindicated in pregnancy, and experience is limited in children under age 2 years.

D. Other Drugs: Albendazole, when given as a single 400-mg dose, resulted in high cure rates (over 95%) among persons with light infections; in heavy infection, the rates were 85–90%. Thus, heavy infections will require a longer course, perhaps 2–3 days.

Levamisole is highly effective as a single oral dose of 150 mg (children, 3 mg/kg). Occasional mild and transient side effects are nausea, vomiting, abdominal pain, headache, and dizziness.

Albendazole, levamisole, and oxantel-pyrantel pamoate are not available in the USA.

Prognosis

The complications caused by wandering adult worms, plus the possibility of intestinal obstruction, require that all *Ascaris* infections be treated and completely eradicated.

Khuroo MS et al: Sonographic appearances in biliary ascariasis. Gastroenterology 1987;93:267.

Latham MC: Ascariasis. Lancet 1989;1:1270.

Leung JW, Chung SC: Endoscopic management of biliary ascariasis. Gastrointest Endosc 1988:34:318.

Wiersma R, Hadley GP: Small bowel volvulus complicating intestinal ascariasis in children. Br J Surg 1988;75:86.

CUTANEOUS LARVA MIGRANS (Creeping Eruption)

Creeping eruption, prevalent throughout the tropics and subtropics, is caused by larvae of the dog and cat hookworms, *Ancylostoma braziliense* and *Ancylostoma caninum*. A number of other animal hookworms have rarely been implicated. Human infection is common in southeastern USA, particularly where people come in contact with moist sandy soil (beaches, children's sand piles) contaminated by dog or cat feces.

At the site of larval entry, particularly on the hands or feet, up to several hundred minute, intensely pruritic erythematous papules appear. Two to 3 days later, serpiginous eruptions appear as the larvae migrate at a rate of several millimeters a day; the parasite lies slightly ahead of the advancing border. The process continues for weeks to a year, and the lesions may remain severely pruritic, vesiculate, and become encrusted and secondarily infected. Without treatment, the larvae eventually die and are absorbed.

The diagnosis is based on the characteristic appearance of the lesions and the frequent presence of eosinophilia. Biopsy is usually not indicated.

Simple transient cases may not require treatment. In severe cases, the larvae must be killed to provide relief. Thiabendazole, given as for strongyloidiasis, is very effective and the drug of choice. Progression of the lesions and itching are usually stopped within 48 hours, but if active lesions are still present at that time, repeat treatment. Thiabendazole cream (15% in a hygroscopic base) applied topically daily for 5 days may also be effective. As an alternative drug for patients who cannot tolerate thiabendazole, albendazole at a dosage of 400 mg daily for 3–7 days should be tried. Antihistamines are helpful in controlling pruritus, and antibiotic ointments may be necessary to treat secondary infections.

Leicht SS, Youngberg GA: Cutaneous larva migrans. Am Fam Physician (June) 1987;35:163.

Torres RJR et al: Treatment of cutaneous larva migrans with albendazole: Preliminary report. Rev Inst Med Trop (São Paulo) 1989;31:56.

Williams HC, Monk B: Creeping eruption stopped in its tracks by albendazole. Clin Exp Dermatol 1989;14:355.

DRACUNCULIASIS
(Guinea Worm Infection,
Dracunculosis, Dracontiasis)

Dracunculus medinensis infection is found only in humans. It occurs in the Indian subcontinent; west and central Africa (Cameroon to Mauritania, Uganda, southern Sudan); and Saudi Arabia, Iran, and Yemen. All ages are affected, and the prevalence may reach 60% in some areas.

Infection is by swallowing water containing the infected intermediate host, the crustacean *Cyclops* (water fleas). Larvae escape from the crustacean and mature in subcutaneous connective tissue. After mating, the male worm dies and the gravid female (1 m or more) moves to the surface of the body, where its head reaches the dermis and provokes a blister that ruptures on contact with water. Intermittently over 2–3 weeks, the uterus discharges great numbers of larvae, whenever the ulcer comes in contact with water. The larvae are eaten by the water fleas. Most adult worms are gradually extruded; some worms retract and reemerge; and others die in the tissues, disintegrate, and may provoke a severe inflammatory reaction. Infection does not induce protective immunity.

Clinical Findings

A. Symptoms and Signs: The incubation period is 9–14 months. Infection may be single or multiple. Several hours before the head appears at the skin surface, local erythema, burning, pruritus, and tenderness often develop at the site of emergence. There may also be a 24-hour systemic allergic reaction (generalized urticaria and pruritus, fever, nausea, vomiting, and dyspnea). After rupture, the tissues surrounding the ulceration frequently become indurated, reddened, and tender. Because most lesions appear on the leg or foot, patients often must give up walking and working. Uninfected ulcers heal in 4–6 weeks.

B. Laboratory Findings: When an emerging adult worm is not visible in the ulcer or under the skin, the diagnosis may be made by detection of larvae in smears from discharging sinuses. Immersion of an ulcer in cold water stimulates larval expulsion. Eosinophilia is usually present. Skin and serologic tests are not useful. Calcified worms can be recognized on radiographs.

Complications

Secondary infections, including tetanus, are common. Deep "cold" abscesses may result at the sites of dying worms; ankle and knee joint infections with resultant deformity are common complications. If the worm is broken during removal, sepsis almost always results, leading to cellulitis, abscess formation, or septicemia. The worm rarely reaches ectopic sites.

Treatment

All persons in an endemic area should be actively immunized against tetanus.

A. General Measures: The patient should be at bed rest with the affected part elevated. Cleanse the lesion, control secondary infection with antibiotics, and change dressings daily.

B. Manual Extraction: Traditional extraction of emerging worms by gradually rolling them out a few centimeters each day on a small stick is still useful, especially when done along with chemotherapy.

C. Chemotherapy: Two drugs—metronidazole and thiabendazole—are effective (failure rate, 25%) both in alleviating symptoms (due to their anti-inflammatory action) and in reducing the duration of infection (by expediting spontaneous extrusion of worms or facilitating their manual extraction). The drugs do not kill the adult or larvae.

1. Metronidazole, 250 mg 3 times daily for 10 days, may cause mild gastrointestinal symptoms, headache, fatigue, and a bitter taste. The drug produces disulfiramlike reactions when alcohol is ingested.

2. Thiabendazole, 25 mg/kg twice daily for 2–3 days after meals, frequently causes side effects, sometimes severe (see under Strongyloidiasis, above).

D. Surgical Removal: Preemergent female worms can be surgically removed intact under local anesthesia if not firmly embedded in deep fascia or around tendons. Abscesses should be incised.

The disease can be prevented by use of only noncontaminated drinking water, either by community action to ensure safe potable water or by individual action in households—boiling, filtering through a cloth, or treating water with temephos. Because only humans are infected by the parasite and transmission can be relatively easily interrupted, the potential exists for eradication of the disease. Such a program is currently in progress.

Hopkins DR: Dracunculiasis eradication: The tide has turned. Lancet 1988;2:148.

Kake OO, Elemile T, Enahoro F: Controlled comparative trial of thiabendazole and metronidazole in the treatment of dracontiasis. Ann Trop Med Parasitol 1983; 77:151.

Sullivan JJ, Long EG: Synthetic-fibre filters for preventing dracunculiasis: 100 versus 200 micrometres pore size. Trans R Soc Trop Med Hyg 1988;82:465.

ENTEROBIASIS
(Pinworm Infection)

Essentials of Diagnosis

- Nocturnal perianal and vulval pruritus, insomnia, irritability, restlessness.
- Vague gastrointestinal symptoms.

● Eggs demonstrable by cellulose tape test; worms visible on perianal skin or in stool.

General Considerations

Enterobius vermicularis (8–13 mm) is common worldwide. Humans are the only host. Young children are affected more often than adults, and multiple infections occur frequently in households with young children.

The adult worms inhabit the cecum and adjacent bowel areas, lying loosely attached to the mucosa. Gravid females migrate through the anus to the perianal skin and deposit eggs in large numbers. The eggs become infective in a few hours and may then infect others or be autoinfective, if transferred to the mouth by contaminated food, drink, fomites, or hands. After being swallowed, the eggs hatch in the duodenum, and the larvae migrate down to the cecum. Retroinfection occasionally occurs when the eggs hatch on the perianal skin and the larvae migrate through the anus into the large intestine. The development of a mature ovipositing female from an ingested egg requires about 3–4 weeks. Eggs remain viable for 2–3 weeks outside the host. The life span of the worm is 30–45 days.

Clinical Findings

A. Symptoms and Signs: Many patients are asymptomatic. The most common and important symptom is perianal pruritus (particularly at night), due to the presence of the female worms or deposited eggs. Insomnia, restlessness, enuresis, and irritability are common symptoms, particularly in children. Many mild gastrointestinal symptoms have also been attributed to enterobiasis, but the association is difficult to prove. At night, worms may occasionally be seen near the anus. Perianal scratching may result in excoriation and impetigo. Adults sometimes report a "crawling" sensation in the anal area. Rarely, worm migration results in ectopic inflammation or granulomatous reaction (including appendicitis) or, in young girls, vulvovaginitis, urethritis, endometritis, salpingitis, and pelvic granuloma. Recurrent urinary tract infections have also been associated with the infection.

B. Laboratory Findings: Diagnosis is by finding eggs on the perianal skin (eggs are seldom found on stool examination). The most reliable method is by applying a short strip of sealing cellulose pressure-sensitive tape (eg, Scotch Tape) to the perianal skin and then spreading the tape on a slide for low-power microscopic study. Three such preparations made on consecutive mornings before bathing or defecation will establish the diagnosis in about 90% of cases. Before the diagnosis can be ruled out, 5–7 such examinations are necessary. Nocturnal examination of the perianal area or gross examination of stools may reveal adult worms, which should be placed in preservative or saline for laboratory examination. The

worms can sometimes be seen on anoscopy. Eosinophilia is rare.

Differential Diagnosis

Pinworm pruritus must be distinguished from similar pruritus due to mycotic infections, allergies, hemorrhoids, proctitis, fissures, strongyloidiasis, and other conditions.

Treatment

A. General Measures: Symptomatic patients should be treated, and in some situations all members of the patient's household should be treated concurrently, since for each overt case there are usually several inapparent cases. However, treatment of all nonsymptomatic cases is not necessary. Careful washing of hands with soap and water after defecation and again before meals is important. Fingernails should be kept trimmed close and clean and scratching of the perianal area avoided. Ordinary washing of bedding will usually kill pinworm eggs. Recurrence is frequent in children because of continued exposure outside the home.

B. Specific Measures: Treatment with the following drugs should be repeated at 2 and 4 weeks.

1. Pyrantel pamoate is a highly effective oral drug (with cure rates of over 95%) and a drug of choice. It is administered as a 10-mg (base)/kg (maximum, 1 g) dose. It may be given before or after meals. Infrequent side effects include vomiting, diarrhea, headache, dizziness, drowsiness, and rash.

2. Mebendazole is highly effective and also a drug of choice. It is administered as a 100-mg oral dose, irrespective of body weight. It may be given with or without food and should be chewed for best effect. Gastrointestinal side effects are infrequent. The drug should not be used in pregnancy.

3. Other drugs—Albendazole (not available in the USA) achieves 100% cure rates when given as a 400-mg dose. Piperazine is not recommended, because treatment requires 1 week. Thiabendazole is not recommended, because it causes frequent side effects which are in rare instances severe and life-threatening.

Prognosis

Although annoying, the infection is benign. Cure is readily attainable with one of several effective drugs, but reinfection is common.

Budd JS, Armstrong C: Role of *Enterobius vermicularis* in the aetiology of appendicitis. Br J Surg 1987;74:748.

Jones JE: Pinworms. Am Fam Physician (Sept) 1988; 38:159.

Knuth KR et al: Pinworm infestation of the genital tract. Am Fam Physician (Nov) 1988;38:127.

FILARIASIS

Filariasis is caused by 3 filiarial nematodes: *Wuchereria bancrofti, Brugia malayi,* or *Brugia timori. W bancrofti* is widely distributed in the tropics and subtropics of both hemispheres and on Pacific islands and is transmitted by *Culex, Aedes,* and *Anopheles* mosquitoes. *B malayi* is transmitted by *Mansonia* and *Anopheles* mosquitoes of south India, Sri Lanka, southeast Asia, south China, the northern coastal areas of China, and South Korea. *B timori* is found on the southeast islands of Indonesia.

No animal reservoir hosts are known for *W bancrofti* or *B timori*; cats, monkeys, and other animals may harbor *B malayi*. Mosquitoes become infected by ingesting microfilariae with a blood meal; at subsequent feedings, they can infect new susceptible hosts. Over months, adult worms (females, 8–9 cm × 0.2–0.3 mm) mature and live in or near superficial and deep lymphatics and lymph nodes and produce large numbers of viviparous circulating microfilariae, which may be seen in the blood starting 6–12 months after infection.

Pathologic changes in lymph vessels are due to host immunologic reactions to developing and mature worms. Living microfilariae generally cause no lesions, with the exception of tropical pulmonary eosinophilia. Rapid death of microfilariae, however, does produce findings (see below), and an abscess may form at the site of a dying adult worm.

Dirofilariasis, infection by *Dirofilaria immitis,* the dog heartworm, has been reported in the USA, Japan, and Australia. Nodules have been found in the skin or as solitary 1–2 cm "coin" lesions in the periphery of the lungs. The serologic test for filariasis is positive. Several other species of filarial worms infect humans—*Mansonella perstans, Mansonella streptocerca,* and *Mansonella ozzardi*—but usually without causing important findings.

Tropical pulmonary eosinophilia is probably due to sequestered microfilariae of *W bancrofti* or *B malayi* in the lungs. The condition is characterized by miliary lesions on chest films, episodic asthmatic coughing or wheezing, eosinophilia, high IgE levels, positive serologic tests, and a response to diethylcarbamazine treatment.

Clinical Findings

A. Symptoms and Signs: Many infections remain asymptomatic. In early cases, episodes of fever, with or without inflammation of lymphatics and nodes, occur at irregular intervals and last for several days. With progression, funiculitis, epididymitis, and orchitis as well as involvement of pelvic, abdominal, or retroperitoneal lymphatics may also occur intermittently. Lymph node enlargement may persist.

Later in the disease, obstructive phenomena occur as a result of interference with normal lymphatic flow and include hydrocele, scrotal lymphedema, lymphatic varices, and elephantiasis, particularly of the extremities, genitals, and breasts. Chyluria may result from rupture of distended lymphatics into the urinary tract.

B. Laboratory Findings: Diagnosis is by finding microfilariae in the blood. They are rare in the first 2–3 years, abundant as the disease progresses, and again rare in the obstructive stage. Microfiliariae of *W bancrofti* are found in the blood chiefly at night (nocturnal periodicity 10 PM to 2 AM), except for a nonperiodic variety in the South Pacific. *B malayi* microfilariae are usually nocturnally periodic but in southeast Asia may be present at all times, with a slight nocturnal rise. Anticoagulated blood specimens are collected at times related to the periodicity of the local strain. Specimens may be stored at ambient temperatures until examined in the morning by wet film for motile larvae and by Giemsa-stained thin smears for specific morphology. If these are negative, the blood specimens should be concentrated by the Knott concentration or membrane filtration technique. If all are negative, oral administration of 12 mg/kg of diethylcarbamazine often produces positive blood specimens when examined in 1 hour. This test must be done with extreme caution in areas where onchocerciasis or loiasis may be present.

Serologic tests may be helpful in diagnostic screening, but false-positive and false-negative reactions occur. An indirect hemagglutination titer of 1:128 and a bentonite flocculation titer of 1:5 in combination are considered minimum significant titers. Lymphangiography is helpful in differential diagnosis.

Treatment, Prevention, Prognosis

See references for detailed information on treatment and drug side effects.

Diethylcarbamazine, given during a quiescent period between attacks, rapidly kills blood microfilariae but only slowly kills or injures adult worms. Cure may require multiple 3- to 4-week courses (2 mg/kg 3 times a day after meals, starting with small doses, and gradually increasing over 3–4 days). In the USA, the drug is only available from the manufacturer, Lederle Laboratories, (914) 735–5000. General measures include bed rest during acute inflammatory episodes, antibiotics for secondary infection, and use of elastic stockings and pressure bandages for leg edema and suspensory bandaging for orchitis and epididymitis. Surgery is sometimes useful for hydroceles and for removal of elephantoid tissue at some sites. Small hydroceles may benefit from a locally injected sclerosing agent.

Ivermectin shows promise in drug treatment of filariasis, resulting in death of microfilariae but apparently not of adult worms. In prophylaxis, 50 mg of diethylcarbamazine monthly may be useful.

The prognosis is good with treatment of early and mild cases but not in advanced infection.

Connor DH, Palmieri JR, Gibson DW: Pathogenesis of lymphatic filariasis in man. Z Parasitenkd 1986;72:13.

Enright T, Chua S, Lim DT: Pulmonary eosinophilic syndromes. Ann Allergy 1989;62:277.

Kumaraswami V et al: Ivermectin for the treatment of *Wuchereria bancrofti* filariasis. JAMA 1988;259;3150.

Markell EK: Filariasis: Bancroftian, Malayan, and Timoran. In: *Tropical Medicine and Parasitology.* Goldsmith R, Heyneman D (editors). Appleton & Lange, 1989.

Orihel TC, Isbey EK: *Dirofilaria striata* infection in a North Carolina child. Am J Trop Med Hyg 1990;42:124.

Ottesen EA: Filariasis now. Am J Trop Med Hyg 1989;41:9.

WHO Expert Committee on Filariasis: *Lymphatic Filariasis, Fourth Report.* Technical Report Series No. 702. World Health Organization, 1984.

GNATHOSTOMIASIS

Gnathostomiasis is infection by the larval stage of *Gnathostoma spinigerum.* Most common in Thailand and Japan, it is also reported from southeast Asia, China, India, Mexico, and Israel. Humans are infected by ingestion of larvae in raw, marinated, or inadequately cooked freshwater fish, chicken or other fowl, frogs, or rarely pork.

Within 24–48 hours, larval migration through the intestinal wall can cause acute epigastric pain, vomiting, urticaria, and eosinophilia. The worm then migrates to subcutaneous and other tissues but is unable to mature. Most common is a pruritic subcutaneous swelling up to 25 cm across, occasionally accompanied by stabbing pain. The swelling may remain in one area for days or weeks, or move continuously. Occasionally the worm becomes visible under the skin.

Internal organs and the eye may also be invaded. Spontaneous pneumothorax, leukorrhea, hematemesis, hematuria, hemoptysis, paroxysmal coughing, and edema of the pharynx with dyspnea have been reported as complications. Invasion of the brain can result in encephalitis, paralysis, subarachnoid hemorrhage, cerebrospinal fluid eosinophilia, and other findings. Spinal cord invasion can result in myelitis and severe nerve root pain.

Marked eosinophilia is common. Serodiagnosis by immunoblot assay or ELISA is promising. Skin and serologic tests are unsatisfactory.

Treatment and definitive diagnosis are by surgical removal of the worm when it appears close to the skin surface or in the eye. Although chemotherapy has not proved successful, diethylcarbamazine (as for filariasis), thiabendazole, or albendazole should be tried. Courses of prednisolone have provided temporary relief of symptoms.

Akao N et al: Immunoblot analysis of human gnathostomiasis. Ann Trop Med Parasitol 1989;83:635.

Martinez-Cruz JM et al: [Gnathostomiasis in Mexico.] Salud Publica de Mexico 1989;31:541.

HOOKWORM DISEASE

Essentials of Diagnosis

Early findings (not commonly recognized):
- Dermatitis: pruritic, erythematous, papulovesicular eruption at site of larval invasion.
- Pulmonary migration of larvae: transient episodes of coughing, asthma, fever, blood-tinged sputum, marked eosinophilia.

Later findings:
- Intestinal symptoms: anorexia, diarrhea, abdominal discomfort.
- Anemia (hypochromic microcytic): fatigue, apathy, pallor, deformed nails, dyspnea on exertion, palpitations, syncope, peripheral edema, heart failure.
- Characteristic eggs and occult blood in the stool.

General Considerations

Hookworm disease, widespread in the moist tropics and subtropics, is caused by *Ancylostoma duodenale* and *Necator americanus.* Probably a quarter of the world's population is infected, and in many areas hookworms are a major cause of general debility, retardation of growth of children, and increased susceptibility to infections. Deaths of many children occur from infections that could normally be tolerated, such as malaria, measles, and those that cause diarrhea.

In the Western Hemisphere and tropical Africa, *Necator* was the prevailing species, and in the Far East, India, China, and the Mediterranean area, *Ancylostoma* was prevalent, but both species have now become widely distributed. Infection is rare in regions with less than 40 inches of rainfall annually. Humans are the only host for both species.

The adult worms are approximately 1 cm long. Eggs produced by female worms are passed in the stool and must fall on warm, moist soil if hatching followed by larval development is to take place. Larvae remain infective for hours to about a week, depending on environmental conditions. Following skin penetration, the larvae migrate in the bloodstream to the pulmonary capillaries, break into alveoli, and then are carried by ciliary action upward to the bronchi, trachea, and mouth. After being swallowed, they reach and attach to the mucosa of the upper small bowel, where they develop into adult worms. *Ancylostoma* infection can probably also be acquired by ingestion of the larvae in food or water. Adult *Ancylostoma* survive about a year; *Necator,* about 3–5 years.

Clinical Findings

A. Symptoms and Signs: Ground itch, the first manifestation of infection, is a pruritic erythematous dermatitis, either maculopapular or vesicular, that follows skin penetration of the infective larvae. Severity is a function of the number of invading larvae and the sensitivity of the host. Scratching may result in secondary infection. *Strongyloides* infection and creeping eruption caused by nonhuman hookworm species must be considered in the differential diagnosis at this stage.

The pulmonary phase, in which there is larval migration through the lungs, is sometimes characterized by dry cough, asthmatic wheezing, blood-tinged sputum, and low-grade fever.

Two or more weeks after skin invasion, maturing and adult worms attach to the mucosal villi of the duodenum and upper jejunum. In heavy infections, worms may reach the ileum. A large proportion of patients who have light infections and adequate iron intake remain asymptomatic. In heavy infections, however, there may be anorexia, diarrhea, vague abdominal pain, and ulcerlike epigastric symptoms. Severe illness results from blood loss caused by worms sucking blood at their attachment sites. Depending on the host's dietary intake of iron, severe anemia may result if 30 or more *Ancylostoma* or 100 or more *Necator* worms are present. Marked protein loss may also occur, resulting in hypoalbuminemia and edema. There are conflicting reports of malabsorption in some severe cases. Severe anemia may result in pallor, thinning of the hair, deformed nails, pica, cardiac decompensation, edema, ascites, and other clinical manifestations. Young children are especially likely to be seriously affected; a protuberant abdomen is common, and kwashiorkor may be precipitated. Stunted growth and possibly some degree of mental retardation may occur.

Reduction in worm loads after the first decade of life suggests that a moderate degree of immunity develops.

B. Laboratory Findings: Diagnosis depends upon demonstration of characteristic eggs in the feces. The stool usually contains occult blood. The hypochromic microcytic anemia can be severe, with hemoglobin levels as low as 2 g/dL and a low serum iron and a high iron-binding capacity. Worm burdens can be estimated by quantitative egg counts: light infections, up to 2000 ova per gram of feces; moderate, 2000–5000; heavy, over 5000. Eosinophilia (as high as 30–60% of a total white blood count reaching 17,000/μL) is usually present in the pulmonary migratory phase of infection but is not marked in the chronic stage.

Treatment

A. General Measures: The availability of safe anthelmintics makes it reasonable to treat all patients initially, irrespective of the intensity of infection. Re-treatment is often necessary at 2-week intervals until the worm burden is reduced to a low level as estimated by semiquantitative egg counts. Eradication of infection is not essential, since light infections do not injure the well-nourished patient and iron loss is replaced if the patient is receiving adequate dietary iron.

If anemia is present, provide iron medication and a diet high in protein and vitamins: continue for at least 3 months after the anemia has been corrected in order to replace iron stores. Blood transfusion may be necessary if anemia is severe.

B. Specific Measures: If ascariasis and hookworm infections are both present, give either mebendazole or pyrantel for the combined infection.

1. Pyrantel pamoate is a drug of choice. In *A duodenale* infections, when given as a single dose, 10 mg (base)/kg (maximum 1 g), it produces cures in 76–98% of cases and a marked reduction in the worm burden in the remainder. However, for *N americanus* infections, a single dose may give a satisfactory cure rate in light infection, but for moderate or heavy infection a 3-day course is necessary. If the species is unknown, treat as for necatoriasis. Side effects are infrequent, mild, and transient, including gastrointestinal symptoms, drowsiness, and headache. The drug is given before or after meals, without purges.

2. Mebendazole is also a drug of choice for treatment of *Necator* and *Ancylostoma* infections. When given at a dosage of 100 mg twice daily for 3 days, reported cure rates for both species range from 35 to 95%. The drug is given before or after meals, without purges. Therapy is remarkably free of side effects; gastrointestinal symptoms occur infrequently. The drug should not be used in pregnancy, and experience with the drug in children under 2 years is limited.

3. Albendazole, given orally once only at a dosage of 400 mg, resulted in the cure of 86–95% of patients with *Ancylostoma* infection and markedly reduced the worm burden in those not cured. Because cure rates for single-dose treatments of *Necator* infection were 33–90%, treatment should be continued for 2–3 days, especially in heavy infections.

4. Other drugs–Tetrachloroethylene and bephenium hydroxynaphthoate are moderately effective against both hookworm species but are more difficult to use and have more frequent side effects. Neither drug is marketed in the USA.

Prognosis

If the disease is recognized before serious secondary complications appear, the prognosis is favorable. With iron therapy, improved nutrition, and administration of an anthelmintic, complete recovery is the rule.

Behnke JM: Do hookworms elicit protective immunity in man? Parasitol Today 1987;3:200.

Crompton DWT: Hookworm disease: Current status and new directions. Parasitol Today 1989;5:1.

Gilman RH: Hookworm disease: Host-pathogen biology. Rev Infect Dis 1982;4:824.

Rossignol JF, Maisonneuve H: Albendazole: Placebo-controlled study in 870 patients with intestinal helminthiasis. Trans R Soc Med Hyg 1983;77:707.

LOIASIS

Loiasis is a chronic filarial disease caused by infection with *Loa loa*. The infection occurs in humans and monkeys in rain and swamp forest areas of West Africa from Nigeria to Angola and throughout the Congo river watershed of central Africa eastward to southwest Sudan and western Uganda. The vector and intermediate hosts are female *Chrysops* spp, day-biting flies (about 10 AM to 4 PM) that become infected when they ingest a blood meal that contains microfilariae. When the fly feeds again, it can infect a new host.

Clinical Findings

A. Symptoms and Signs: Though often asymptomatic, the infection can be manifested by Calabar swellings or temporary appearance of worms beneath the skin or conjunctiva. Symptoms are a hypersensitivity response to the adult worms (females, 4–7 cm × 0.5 mm), which live for years. Calabar swellings are subcutaneous edematous reactions, 3–10 cm in diameter, nonpitting and nonerythematous but at times somewhat painful. The swellings may migrate a few centimeters for 2–3 days or stay in place before they subside; at irregular intervals, they recur at the same or different sites, but only one appears at a time. When near joints, they may be temporarily disabling. Systemic symptoms include urticaria, erythema, pruritus, low-grade fever, and edema of an extremity. Migration across the eye may be asymptomatic or may produce pain, intense conjunctivitis, and eyelid edema. Dying adult worms may elicit small nodules or local sterile abscesses.

Microfilariae in the blood do not induce symptoms. Rarely, however, they enter the central nervous system and may cause encephalitis, myelitis, or jacksonian seizures; the larvae can also induce lesions in the retina, heart, and other tissues.

Natives generally have a mild form of the infection, often showing only microfilaremia and being otherwise asymptomatic; by contrast, the disease among visitors is more often characterized by hyperreactive allergic symptoms (frequent and debilitating Calabar swellings, high peripheral eosinophilia, hypergammaglobulinemia, increased serum IgE), sometimes with no detectable microfilaremia.

B. Laboratory Findings: Specific diagnosis is by finding characteristic microfilariae in daytime blood specimens by concentration methods; in order of increasing sensitivity, they are (1) thick films, (2) Knott's concentration, and (3) Nuclepore filtration. Finding microfilariae, however, is unreliable. Presumptive diagnosis that permits treatment is based on Calabar swellings, a history of residence in an endemic area, and marked eosinophilia (40% or greater). Serologic tests may be helpful, but cross-reactions occur with other filarial diseases.

Treatment & Prognosis

See references for details on diethylcarbamazine treatment, since side effects may be severe and rarely life-threatening. Reactions are more likely with pretreatment microfilariae counts greater than 25/μL. Surgical removal of adult worms from the eye or skin is not recommended.

Diethylcarbamazine appears to be useful in prophylaxis for persons whose risk of exposure in an endemic area is high. It is not indicated, however, for the casual traveler or for persons who might previously have acquired any of the filarial infections. At the recommended dose of 300 mg weekly, it is safe and without significant side effects.

Most infections run a benign course, but some are accompanied by severe and temporarily disabling symptoms. The prognosis is excellent with treatment. Fatal encephalitis has rarely occurred from the infection or following diethylcarbamazine treatment.

Jaccard A, Lortholary O, Visser H: Diethylcarbamazine and human loiasis. (Letter.) N Engl J Med 1989;320:320.

Loa loa—a pathogenic parasite. (Editorial.) Lancet 1986; 2:554.

Markell EK: Loiasis. In: *Tropical Medicine and Parasitology*. Goldsmith R, Heyneman D (editors). Appleton & Lange, 1989.

Nutman TB et al: Immunologic correlates of the hyperresponsive syndrome of loiasis. J Infect Dis 1988;157:544. (Entree to the literature on the clinical differences between the disease in natives and visitors.)

ONCHOCERCIASIS

Onchocerciasis is a chronic filarial disease caused by *Onchocerca volvulus*. Primary findings are subcutaneous nodules that contain adult worms and skin and eye changes that result from dead or dying microfilariae. Heavy infection leads to chronic pruritus, disfiguring skin lesions, visual impairment, and debility. An estimated 20–50 million persons are infected, of whom 0.5 million are blinded by the condition. The infection occurs in many parts of tropical Africa and in localized areas of the southwestern Arabian peninsula, southern Mexico, Guatemala, Venezuela, Colombia, and northwestern Brazil.

Humans are the only important host. The vector and intermediate host are *Simulium* flies, day biters, which become infected by ingesting microfilariae with a blood meal; at subsequent feedings, they can infect new susceptible hosts.

Clinical Findings

A. Symptoms and Signs: Adult worms, which live for years, typically are in fibrous subcutaneous nodules that are painless, freely movable, and 0.5–1 cm in diameter. Within 10–20 months after infection (range, 7–24 months), female worms begin to release motile microfilariae into the skin, subcutaneous tissues, lymphatics, and eyes; microfilariae are occasionally seen in the urine but rarely in blood or cerebrospinal fluid. Skin manifestations are localized or cover large areas. Pruritus may be severe, leading to scratching, skin excoriation, and lichenification; other findings include pigmentary changes, papules, scaling, atrophy, pendulous skin, and acute inflammation. There may be marked enlargement of femoral and inguinal nodes and generalized lymph node enlargement. Microfilariae in the eye may lead to visual impairment and blindness; findings include itching, photophobia, corneal opacities (punctate keratitis), sclerosing keratitis, anterior uveitis (with secondary glaucoma), cataract, chorioretinitis, and optic neuritis.

B. Laboratory Findings: Diagnosis is by demonstrating microfilariae in skin snips or shavings, in the cornea or anterior chamber by slit lamp examination, or after aspiration of nodules. When microfilariae are absent, a small challenge dose of diethylcarbamazine may facilitate the diagnosis (see references for method). Adult worms may be recovered in excised nodules. Skin and serologic tests are usually positive, but cross-reactions occur with other forms of filariasis. Eosinophilia (15–50%) is common.

Treatment & Prognosis

For details on drug usage and side effects, see references. Nodules on or near the head should be removed surgically. The preferred drug in treatment is a single dose of ivermectin, which is given by weight; this results in a dose between 120 and 230 μg/kg. Skin and eye microfilaria counts drop rapidly—without inducing the severe adverse reactions of diethylcarbamazine (except in about 1% of persons)—and remain low for 6–12 months. As the drug does not, however, kill the adult worms, treatment needs to be repeated at intervals to be determined, probably yearly. Ivermectin is not marketed but is available on a compassionate use basis from the manufacturer (Merck Sharp & Dohme). Alternative treatment is by combined use of diethylcarbamazine and suramin; however, these drugs frequently induce severe adverse reactions.

With treatment, some skin and ocular lesions improve, and ocular progression is prevented. The prognosis is unfavorable only for those patients who are seen for the first time with already far-advanced ocular onchocerciasis.

Awadzi K: Onchocerciasis. In: *Tropical Medicine and Parasitology.* Goldsmith R, Heyneman D (editors). Appleton & Lange, 1989.
Dadzie KY et al: Changes in ocular onchocerciasis four and twelve months after community-based treatment with ivermectin in a holoendemic onchocerciasis focus. Trans R Soc Trop Med Hyg 1990;84:103.
O'Day J, Mackenzie CD: Ocular onchocerciasis: Diagnosis and current clinical approaches. Trop Doct 1985;15:87.
Taylor HR, Greene BM: The status of ivermectin in the treatment of human onchocerciasis. Am J Trop Med Hyg 1989;40:460.
Taylor HR et al: Ivermectin treatment of patients with severe ocular onchocerciasis. Am J Trop Med Hyg 1989;40:494.

STRONGYLOIDIASIS

Essentials of Diagnosis

- Pruritic dermatitis at sites of larval penetration. Diarrhea, epigastric pain, nausea, malaise, weight loss.
- Cough, rales, transient pulmonary infiltrates. Eosinophilia; characteristic larvae in stool specimens, duodenal aspirate, or sputum.
- Hyperinfection syndrome: Severe diarrhea, malabsorption, bronchopneumonia, pulmonary infiltrates, ileus, cachexia.

General Considerations

Strongyloidiasis is an infection caused by *Strongyloides stercoralis* (2–2.5 mm × 30–50 mm). The major symptoms result from adult parasitism, principally in the duodenum and jejunum, or from larval migration through pulmonary and cutaneous tissues.

The parasite is an infection of humans, but dogs, cats, and primates have been found naturally infected with strains indistinguishable from those of humans. The disease is endemic in tropical and subtropical regions; although the prevalence is generally low, in some areas disease rates exceed 25%. In temperate areas, including the USA, the disease occurs sporadically. Multiple infections in households are common, and prevalence in institutions, particularly mental institutions, may be high. Hospital staff should be protected from contact with feces and sputum from infected patients.

The parasite is uniquely capable of maintaining its life cycle both within the human host and in soil. Infection occurs when filariform larvae in soil penetrate the skin, enter the bloodstream, and are carried to the lungs, where they escape from capillaries into alveoli and ascend the bronchial tree to the glottis. The larvae are then swallowed and carried to the duodenum and upper jejunum, where maturation to the adult stage takes place. The parasitic female, generally held to be parthenogenetic, matures and lives embedded in the mucosa, where its eggs are laid and hatch. Rhabditiform larvae, which are noninfective, emerge, and most migrate into the intestinal lumen to leave the host via the feces. The life span of the adult worm may be as long as 5 years.

In the soil, the rhabditiform larvae metamorphose into the infective (filariform) larvae. However, the parasite also has a free-living cycle in soil, in which some rhabditiform larvae develop into adults that produce eggs from which rhabditiform larvae emerge to continue the life cycle.

Autoinfection, which probably occurs at a low rate

in most infections, is an important factor in determining worm burden and is responsible for persistence of asymptomatic or symptomatic strongyloidiasis in individuals for many years after they leave an endemic area. Internal autoinfection takes place in the lower bowel when some rhabditiform larvae, instead of passing with the feces, develop into filariform larvae that penetrate the intestinal mucosa, enter the intestinal lymphatic and portal circulation, are carried to the lungs, and return to the small bowel to complete the cycle. This process is accelerated by constipation and other conditions that reduce bowel motility. In addition, an external autoinfection cycle can occur as a result of fecal contamination of the perianal area.

In the hyperinfection syndrome, autoinfection is greatly increased, resulting in a marked increase in the intestinal worm burden and in massive dissemination of filariform larvae to the lungs and most other tissues, where they can cause local inflammatory reactions and granuloma formation. Occasionally, in the lungs and elsewhere, larvae metamorphose into adults. Hyperinfection is generally initiated under conditions of depressed host cellular immunity, especially in debilitated, malnourished persons and in patients receiving immunosuppressive therapy, particularly corticosteroids. It is rare, however, in AIDS. The syndrome can also occur in individuals who show no obvious predisposing cause. Penetration of the bowel wall by filariform larvae can result in polymicrobial gram-negative septicemia.

Clinical Findings

A. Signs and Symptoms: The time from penetration of the skin by filariform larvae until rhabditiform larvae appear in the feces is 3–4 weeks. The severity of infection ranges from asymptomatic to fatal. Although an acute syndrome can sometimes be recognized in which cutaneous symptoms are followed by pulmonary and then intestinal symptoms, most patients have chronic symptoms that continue for years or sometimes for life. Symptoms may be continuous, or exacerbations may recur at irregular intervals.

1. Cutaneous manifestations–In acute infection, filariform larvae usually invade the skin of the feet. The reaction in unsensitized patients may be minimal, with only a macule or papule, but in sensitized patients there may be focal edema, inflammation, petechiae, serpiginous or urticarial tracts, and intense itching. In chronic infections, stationary urticaria or larva currens, characterized by transient eruptions that migrate in serpiginous tracts, may occur.

2. Intestinal manifestations–Symptoms range from mild to severe, the most common being diarrhea, abdominal pain, and flatulence. Anorexia, nausea, vomiting, and epigastric tenderness may be present. The diarrhea may alternate with constipation, and in severe cases the feces contain mucus and blood. The pain is often epigastric in location and may mimic the burning, dull cramp, or ache of duodenal ulcer. Malabsorption or a protein-losing enteropathy can result from a large intestinal worm burden.

3. Pulmonary manifestations–With migration of larvae through the lungs, bronchi, and trachea, there may be a dry cough and throat irritation without further difficulty or a low-grade fever, bronchitis, dyspnea, wheezing, asthma, and hemoptysis. As the disease becomes more marked, bronchopneumonia and pleural effusion can occur, accompanied by progressive dyspnea; the cough may become productive of an odorless, mucopurulent sputum; miliary abscesses can develop.

4. Other findings–Severe infection may present with fever, malaise, and weakness leading to prostration and emaciation.

5. Hyperinfection syndrome–Massive increase in the intestinal worm burden with intense dissemination of larvae to the lungs and other tissues can result in the following complications: severe diarrhea with generalized abdominal pain and distention, malabsorption, bronchopneumonia, pleural effusion, pericarditis and myocarditis, hepatic granulomas, cholecystitis, ulcerating lesions at all levels of the gastrointestinal tract, paralytic ileus, perforation and peritonitis, gram-negative septicemia, meningitis, cachexia, shock, and death.

B. Laboratory Findings:

1. Detection of eggs and larvae–Eggs are seldom found in feces. Diagnosis is by finding the larval stages in feces or duodenal fluid. Rhabditiform larvae may be found in recently passed stool specimens; filariform larvae will be present in specimens held in the laboratory for some hours. Three specimens, preserved or unpreserved, should be collected at 2-day intervals or longer, since the number of larvae in feces may vary considerably from day to day. Each specimen should be examined by direct microscopy, and one or more should be processed by the Baermann concentration method to increase sensitivity of testing. Stool specimens used in the Baermann procedure must be unpreserved; they can be received in the laboratory up to 48 hours after passage if held at refrigerated but nonfreezing temperatures. Unpreserved stool specimens can also be put into culture for 7–10 days to increase the number of larvae.

Although larvae cannot be found in the stools of 25% or more of infected patients, the diagnosis can often be made by examination of duodenal mucus for rhabditiform larvae or ova. Mucus is obtained by means of the duodenal string test or by duodenal intubation and aspiration. Duodenal biopsy is seldom indicated but will confirm the diagnosis in most patients. Occasionally, filariform or rhabditiform larvae can be detected in sputum during the pulmonary phase.

2. Serologic and hematologic findings–In chronic low-grade intestinal strongyloidiasis, the white blood cell count is often normal, with a slightly elevated percentage of eosinophils. However, with increasing larval migration, eosinophilia may reach 50% and leukocytosis 20,000/μL. Mild anemia may be present. Serum IgE immunoglobulins may be elevated. New ELISA and immunofluorescent serologic tests are promising.

3. Imaging–Small bowel x-rays early in the disease may show inflammation and irritability, with prominent mucosal folds; there may be bowel dilatation, delayed emptying, and ulcerative duodenitis. Later in the disease, the findings can resemble those in nontropical and tropical sprue, or there may be narrowing, rigidity, and diminished peristalsis. During pulmonary migration of larvae, fine nodularity or irregular patches of pneumonitis may be seen.

4. Hyperinfection–In the hyperinfection syndrome, there may also be findings of hypoproteinemia, malabsorption, and abnormal liver function. Ova and rhabditiform and filariform larvae may be present in sputum, and filariform larvae in the urine; eosinopenia, when present, is thought to be an unfavorable prognostic sign.

Differential Diagnosis

Because of varied signs and symptoms, the diagnosis of strongyloidiasis is often difficult, especially in nonendemic areas. The disease should always be considered in patients with unexplained eosinophilia. Eosinophilia plus one or more of the following factors should further enhance consideration of the diagnosis: endemic area exposure, duodenal ulcer-like pain, persistent or recurrent diarrhea, recurrent coughing or wheezing, and transient pulmonary infiltrates. The duodenitis and jejunitis of strongyloidiasis can mimic giardiasis, cholecystitis, and pancreatitis. Transient pulmonary infiltrates must be differentiated from tropical pulmonary eosinophilia and Löffler's syndrome. The diagnosis should be considered among the many causes of malabsorption in the tropics.

Treatment

Since *Strongyloides* can multiply in humans, treatment should continue until the parasite is eradicated. Patients receiving immunosuppressive therapy should be examined for the presence of the infection before and probably at intervals during treatment. In concurrent infection with *Strongyloides* and *Ascaris* or hookworm (which is common), eradicate *Ascaris* and hookworms first and *Strongyloides* subsequently.

A. Thiabendazole: Thiabendazole is the drug of choice. An oral dose of 25 mg/kg (maximum, 1.5 g) is given after meals twice daily for 2–3 days. A 5- to 7-day course of treatment is needed for disseminated infections. Tablet and liquid formulations are available; tablets should be chewed. Side effects, including headache, weakness, vomiting, vertigo, and decreased mental alertness, occur in as many as 30% of patients and may be severe. These symptoms are lessened if the drug is taken after meals. Other potentially serious side effects occur rarely. Erythema multiforme and the Stevens-Johnson syndrome have been associated with thiabendazole therapy; several fatalities have occurred.

B. Alternative Drugs: Albendazole is undergoing clinical trials. At a dosage of 400 mg twice daily for 3 days and repeated in 1 week, cure rates in several studies reached about 80%. At this dosage, the drug is nearly free of side effects. If thiabendazole cannot be tolerated, mebendazole (500 mg 3 times daily for 14 days), cambendazole, ivermectin, or levamisole can be tried, but their efficacy is based on limited trials.

Prognosis

The prognosis is favorable except in the hyperinfection syndrome. Infections associated with emaciation, advanced liver disease, cancer, immunologic disorders, or the use of immunosuppressive drugs may be difficult to treat. In selected instances, a 2-day course of treatment with thiabendazole once monthly can be tried to control infections that cannot be eradicated.

Chanthavanich P et al: Repeated doses of albendazole against strongyloidiasis in Thai children. Southeast Asian J Trop Med Public Health 1989;20:221.

Cook GC: *Strongyloides stercoralis* hyperinfection syndrome: How often is it missed? Q J Med 1987;64:624.

Grove DI (editor): Strongyloidiasis: A major roundworm infection in man. Taylor & Francis, 1989.

Naquira C et al: Ivermectin for human strongyloidiasis and other intestinal helminths. Am J Trop Med Hyg 1989;40:304.

Neva FA: Biology and immunology of human strongyloidiasis. J Infect Dis 1986;153:397.

TRICHINOSIS
(Trichinelliosis, Trichinellosis)

Essentials of Diagnosis

- History of ingestion of raw or inadequately cooked pork, boar, or bear.
- First week: diarrhea, cramps, malaise.
- Second week to 1–2 months: muscle pain and tenderness, fever, periorbital and facial edema, conjunctivitis.
- Eosinophilia and elevated serum enzymes. Positive serologic tests. Larvae in muscle biopsy.

General Considerations

Trichinosis is caused by *Trichinella spiralis*. Adult worms (2–3.6 mm × 75–90 μm) live in the intestines of humans, pigs, bears, rats, and most carnivores, including marine animals; fowl are resistant to infection. Viviparous larvae enter striated muscle, encyst, and live for years. In the natural life cycle, these larvae develop into a new generation of adults when parasitized muscle is ingested by a new host. Pigs generally become infected by feeding on uncooked food scraps or, less often, by eating infected rats.

Human infections occur sporadically or in outbreaks. Infection is usually acquired by eating encysted larvae in raw or uncooked pork or pork products. Ground beef has also been a source of infection when adulterated with pork or inadvertently contaminated in a common meat grinder. In some cases, the source of infection is the flesh of wild animals, particularly bear, walrus, or bush pigs.

Gastric juices liberate the encysted larvae. They rapidly mature and mate, and the adult female then burrows into the mucosa of the small intestine. Within 4–5 days, the female begins to discharge larvae that are disseminated via the lymphatics and bloodstream to most body tissues. Larvae that reach striated muscle encyst and remain viable for months to years; those that reach other tissues are rapidly destroyed.

Trichinosis is present wherever pork is eaten but is a greater problem in many temperate areas than in the tropics. In the USA, there has been a marked reduction in the prevalence of trichinosis both in humans and in pigs. Less than 100 human cases are reported per year, but many mild or asymptomatic infections are undetected or misdiagnosed.

Clinical Findings

A. Symptoms and Signs: The incubation period is generally from 2 to 7 days (range, 12 hours to 28 days). Severity depends upon the intensity of infection, the tissues invaded, the immune status of the host, the age of the host (children have less severe infections), and perhaps the strain of the parasite. Infection ranges from (1) asymptomatic to (2) a mild febrile illness with one or more mild, short-lasting symptoms to (3) a severe progressive illness with multiple system involvement that in rare cases is fatal.

1. Intestinal stage–When present, intestinal symptoms persist for 1–7 days: diarrhea, abdominal cramps, and malaise are the major findings; nausea and vomiting occur less frequently; and constipation is uncommon. Fever and leukocytosis are rare during the first week.

2. Muscle invasion stage–This begins at the end of the first week and lasts about 6 weeks, corresponding with the death of the adult worms. Parasitized muscles show an intense inflammatory reaction. Clinical findings include fever (low-grade to marked); muscle pain (especially upon movement) and muscle tenderness, edema, and spasm; periorbital and facial edema; sweating; photophobia and conjunctivitis; weakness or prostration; pain on swallowing; dyspnea, coughing, and hoarseness; subconjunctival, retinal, and nail splinter hemorrhages; and rashes and formication. The most frequently parasitized muscles and sites of findings are the masseters, the tongue, the diaphragm, the intercostal muscles, and the extraocular, laryngeal, paravertebral, nuchal, deltoid, pectoral, gluteus, biceps, and gastrocnemius muscles. Inflammatory reactions around larvae that reach tissues other than muscle may result in a broad range of findings, including the development of meningitis, encephalitis, myocarditis, bronchopneumonia, nephritis, and peripheral and cranial nerve disorders.

3. Convalescent stage–This generally begins in the second month but in severe infections may not begin before 3 months or longer. Vague muscle pains and malaise may persist for several more months. Permanent muscular atrophy has been reported.

B. Laboratory Findings: The diagnosis is supported by findings of eosinophilia, elevated serum muscle enzymes (CPK, AST), and positive serologic tests; confirmation is by detection of larvae in muscle biopsy specimens.

Leukocytosis and eosinophilia appear during the second week after ingestion of infected meat. The proportion of eosinophils rises to a maximum of 20–90% in the third or fourth week and then slowly declines to normal over the next few months.

Serologic tests can detect most clinically manifest cases but are not sufficiently sensitive to detect low-level infections (ie, a few larvae per gram of ingested muscle). More than one test should be used and then repeated to observe for seroconversion or for a rising titer. The bentonite flocculation (BF) test (positive titer, ≥ 1:5) is highly sensitive and is considered nearly 100% specific. It becomes positive in the third or fourth week, and reaches a maximum titer at about 2 months, and generally reverts to negative in 2–3 years. The immunofluorescence test (positive titer > 16) is also highly sensitive, though less specific than the BF test; it may become positive in the second week. The ELISA test is also showing high sensitivity and specificity. The intradermal test is no longer recommended, as it may remain positive for years and batches of antigen vary in potency.

Adult worms may be looked for in feces, though they are seldom found. In the second week, there are occasional larvae in blood, duodenal washings, and, rarely, in centrifuged spinal fluid. In the third to fourth weeks, biopsy of skeletal muscle may be definitive (particularly gastrocnemius and pectoralis), preferably at a site of swelling or tenderness. Portions of the specimen should be examined microscopically by compression between glass slides, by digestion, and by preparation of multiple histologic sections. If the biopsy is done too early, larvae may not be detectable. Myositis even in the absence of larvae is a significant finding.

Nonspecific laboratory findings include elevation of serum enzymes (creatinine phosphokinase, lactate dehydrogenase, serum aspartate aminotransferase [AST or SGOT], and serum aldolase). Absence of an elevated sedimentation rate is a useful diagnostic clue. There may be a marked hypergammaglobulinemia with reversal of the albumin-globulin ratio.

C. Imaging: Chest films during the acute phase may show disseminated or localized infiltrates. Late calcification of muscle cysts cannot be detected radiologically.

Complications

The more important complications are allergic granulomatous reactions in the lungs, encephalitis, and cardiac failure.

Differential Diagnosis

Because of its protean manifestations, trichinosis may resemble many other diseases. Eosinophilia, muscle pain and tenderness, and fever should lead the physician to consider collagen vascular disorders.

Prevention

The frequency and intensity of infection in the USA and other countries have been significantly reduced by public health measures to prevent feeding of uncooked garbage to hogs and by animal inspection (not in the USA). The chief safeguard against trichinosis is adequate cooking of pork at the newly recommended temperature of 77 °C. Alternatively, larvae can be made nonviable by freezing meat at −15 °C (5 °F) for 20 days. Recent reports indicate that *T spiralis* in Arctic sylvatic animals is resistant to freezing.

Treatment

Treatment is principally supportive, since in most cases recovery is spontaneous without sequelae. If the patient is still in the intestinal phase, thiabendazole is indicated at an oral dosage of 25 mg/kg (maximum 1.5 g) twice daily after meals for 3–5 days. Side effects may occur (see Strongyloidiasis, above). Unless the patient is severely ill, corticosteroids are contraindicated in the intestinal phase.

In the muscle invasion stage, severe infections require hospitalization and high doses of corticosteroids for 24–48 hours, followed by lower doses for several days or weeks to control symptoms. Thiabendazole has been tried in the muscle stage with equivocal relief of muscle pain or tenderness or lysis of fever. Further trials are recommended.

Initial reports suggest some success for mebendazole against adult worms in the intestinal tract, migrating larvae, and larvae in muscle using the following schedule: 200–400 mg 3 times daily for 3 days, followed by 400–500 mg 3 times daily for 10 days. Albendazole (400 mg twice daily for 15 days) is also undergoing clinical tests.

Prognosis

Death is rare—sometimes within 2–3 weeks in overwhelming infections, more often in 4–8 weeks from a major complication such as cardiac failure or pneumonia.

Bailey TM, Schantz PM: Trends in the incidence and transmission patterns of trichinosis in humans in the United States: Comparisons of the periods 1975–1981 and 1982–1986. Rev Infect Dis 1990;12:5.

Campbell WC (editor): *Trichinella and Trichinosis*. Plenum Press, 1983.

Fröscher W et al: Chronic trichinosis: Clinical, bioptic, serological, and electromyographic observations. Eur Neurol 1988;28:221.

Levin ML: Treatment of trichinosis with mebendazole. Am J Trop Med Hyg 1983;32:980.

TRICHURIASIS
(Trichocephaliasis, Whipworm)

Essentials of Diagnosis

- Most infections are silent; heavy infections may cause chronic diarrhea, lower abdominal cramps, flatulence, hematochezia, tenesmus, and rectal prolapse.
- Characteristic barrel-shaped eggs and (less commonly) adult worms are found in the stool.

General Considerations

Trichuris trichiura is a common intestinal parasite of humans throughout the world, particularly in the subtropics and tropics. Persons of all ages are affected, but infection is heaviest and most frequent in children. The slender worms, 30–50 mm in length, attach by means of their anterior whiplike end to the mucosa of the large intestine, particularly to the cecum. Eggs are passed in the feces but require 2–4 weeks for larval development after reaching the soil before becoming infective; thus, person-to-person transmission is not possible. Infections are acquired by ingestion of the infective egg. The larvae hatch in the small intestine and mature in the large bowel but do not migrate through the tissues.

Clinical Findings

A. Symptoms and Signs: Light (fewer than 10,000 eggs per gram of feces) to moderate infections rarely cause symptoms. Heavy infections (30,000 or more eggs per gram of feces) may be accompanied by abdominal cramps, tenesmus, diarrhea, distention, flatulence, nausea, vomiting, and weight loss. Rectal prolapse and hematochezia or chronic occult blood loss may also occur, most often in malnourished young children. Sometimes, adult worms are seen in stools. Invasion of the appendix, with resulting appendicitis, is rare.

B. Laboratory Findings: Diagnosis is by identification of characteristic eggs and, sometimes, adult worms in stools. Eosinophilia (5–20%) is common with all but light infections. Severe hypochromic microcytic anemia may be present with heavy infections.

Treatment

A. Mebendazole: Patients with asymptomatic light infections do not require treatment. For those with heavier or symptomatic infections, give mebendazole, 100 mg twice daily before or after meals for 3 days. It may be therapeutically advantageous for the tablets to be chewed before swallowing. Cure rates of 60–80% and higher are reported after one course of treatment, with marked reduction in ova counts in the remaining patients. For severe trichuriasis, a longer course of treatment (up to 6 days) or a repeat course will often be necessary. Gastrointestinal side effects from the drug are rare. The drug is contraindicated in pregnancy, and experience with it is limited in children under age 2.

B. Albendazole: Albendazole, given orally at a single dose of 400 mg, has resulted in cure rates of 33–90%, with marked reduction in egg counts in those not cured. An appropriate dosage to achieve higher cure rates in moderate to heavy infections remains to be determined, but daily treatment for 2–3 days can be tried. Albendazole is not available in the USA.

C. Oxantel Pamoate: Oxantel pamoate is an analogue of pyrantel pamoate and acts only on *T trichiura*. Cure rates of 57–100% have been reported in various trials. One treatment schedule is 15 mg/kg (base) daily for 2 days for patients with mild to moderate intensity of infection. For patients with severe infection, give 10 mg/kg (base) daily for 5 days. Oxantel is not available in the USA.

D. Thiabendazole: Thiabendazole should *not* be used, because it is not effective and is potentially toxic.

Bundy DA, Cooper ES: *Trichuris* and trichuriasis in humans. Adv Parasitol 1989;28:107.
Davis M, Matteson R, Williams WC: Radiographic and endoscopic findings in human whipworm infection (*Trichuris trichiura*). J Clin Gastroenterol 1986;8:700.
Sebastian VJ, Bhattacharya S, Ray S: Mebendazole retention enema for severe *Trichuris trichiura* (whipworm) infection: A case report. J Trop Med Hyg 1989;92:39.

VISCERAL LARVA MIGRANS (Toxocariasis)

Most cases of visceral larva migrans are due to *Toxocara canis*, an ascarid of dogs and other canids, but in a few cases *Toxocara cati* in domestic cats has been implicated and rarely *Belascaris procyonis* of raccoons. The adult worms live in the intestinal tracts of their respective hosts and release large numbers of eggs in the stool.

The reservoir mechanism for *T canis* is latent infections in female dogs which are reactivated during pregnancy. Transmission from mother to puppies is via the placenta and milk. Most eggs passed to the environment are from puppies (2 weeks to 6 months) and lactating bitches (up to 6 months after parturition). The life cycle of *T cati* is similar, but transplacental transmission does not occur.

Human infections are sporadic and probably occur worldwide. Infection is generally in dirt-eating young children who ingest *T canis* eggs from soil or sand contaminated with dog feces, most often from puppies. Direct contact with infected animals does not produce infection, as the eggs require a 3- to 4-week extrinsic incubation period to become infective; thereafter, eggs in soil remain infective for months to years. In humans, hatched larvae are unable to mature and continue to migrate through the tissues for up to 6 months. Eventually they lodge in various organs, particularly the lungs and liver, less often the brain, eyes, and other tissues, where they produce eosinophilic granulomas up to 1 cm in diameter.

Clinical Findings

A. Acute Infection: Fever, cough, wheezing, hepatomegaly, and sometimes splenomegaly and lymphadenopathy are present. A variety of other findings may occur when other organs are invaded. The acute phase may last 2–3 weeks, but resolution of all physical and laboratory findings may take up to 18 months.

Leukocytosis is marked (may exceed 100,000/μL), with 30–80% due to eosinophils. Hyperglobulinemia occurs when the liver is extensively invaded and is a useful clue in diagnosis. An ELISA test is the most specific (92%) and sensitive (78%) serologic test and permits a presumptive diagnosis. Nonspecific isohemagglutinin titers (anti-A and anti-B) are usually greater than 1:1024. Chest radiographs may show infiltrates. With central nervous system involvement, the cerebrospinal fluid may show eosinophils. No parasitic forms can be found by stool examination.

Specific diagnosis can only be made by liver biopsy or by direct biopsy of a granuloma at laparoscopy, but the procedures are seldom justified.

B. Ocular Toxocariasis: Most cases occur in children, most commonly aged 5–10 years, who present with visual loss. The principal pathologic entity is eosinophilic granuloma of the retina that resembles retinoblastoma. Until the recent development of the ELISA test, this resulted in the enucleation of many eyes. The most common clinical findings are a diffuse, painless endophthalmitis; posterior pole granuloma; and a peripheral inflammatory mass. Uncommonly seen are an iris nodule, optic nerve granuloma, uniocular pars planitis, and a migrating retinal nematode. Ocular toxocariasis is generally not associated with peripheral eosinophilia, hypergammaglobulinemia, or isohemagglutinin elevation. Serum ELISA tests may be positive, but a negative test does not rule out the diagnosis. If doubt exists about whether a patient with a positive serum ELISA test has retinoblastoma, examination of the vitreous humor for ELISA antibody and eosinophils can be helpful. High-resolution CT scanning of the orbit should be done.

Prevention, Treatment, & Prognosis

Disease in humans is best prevented by periodic treatment of puppies, kittens, and nursing dog and cat mothers, starting at 2 weeks postpartum, repeating at weekly intervals for 3 weeks and then every 6 months. Children should be supervised to prevent dirt-eating; their hands should be washed after playing in soil and sand; and play areas should be protected from animal feces.

A. Acute Infection: There is no specific treatment, but thiabendazole, mebendazole, albendazole, or ivermectin should be tried. Corticosteroids, antibiotics, antihistamines, and analgesics may be needed to provide symptomatic relief. Symptoms may persist for months but generally clear within 1–2 years, and the ultimate prognosis is usually good.

B. Ocular Toxocariasis: Treatment includes corticosteroids (subconjunctival applications may be preferable to oral usage), vitrectomy for vitreous traction, laser photocoagulation, and an anthelmintic drug. Partial or total permanent visual impairment is rare.

Dinning WJ et al: Toxocariasis: A practical approach to management of ocular disease. Eye 1988;2:580.

Gillespie SH: Human toxocariasis. J Appl Bacteriol 1987;63:473.

Schantz PM: *Toxocara* larva migrans now. Am J Trop Med Hyg 1989;41:21

Sturchler D et al: Thiabendazole vs. albendazole in treatment against toxocariasis: A clinical trial. Ann Trop Med Parasitol 1989;83:473.

Taylor MR et al: The expanded spectrum of toxocaral disease. Lancet 1988;1:692-695.

REFERENCES
(See also Chapter 28 references.)

Cook GC: The clinical significance of gastrointestinal helminths: A review. Trans R Soc Trop Med Hyg 1986; 80:675.

Edwards G, Breckenridge AM: Clinical pharmacokinetics of anthelmintic drugs. Clin Pharmacokinet 1988;15:67.

Goldsmith R, Heyneman D (editors): *Tropical Medicine and Parasitology*. Appleton & Lange, 1989.

Hillyer GV, Hopla CE (editors): *Trematode Zoonoses.* Vol 3 of: *Parasitic Zoonoses.* Section C of: *CRC Handbook Series in Zoonoses.* Steele JH (editor). CRC Press, 1982.

King CH, Mahmoud AAF: Drugs five year later: Praziquantel. Ann Intern Med 1989;110:290.

Mahmoud AAF: Praziquantel for the treatment of helminthic infections. Adv Intern Med 1987;32:193.

Reeder MM, Palmer PE (editors): *The Radiology of Tropical Disease With Epidemiological, Pathological, and Clinical Correlation*. Williams & Wilkins, 1980.

Schantz PM: Improvements in the serodiagnosis of helminthic zoonoses. Vet Parasitol 1987;25:95.

Sharma S: Treatment of helminth diseases: Challenges and achievements. Prog Drug Res 1987;31:9.

Stephenson LS et al: Treatment with a single dose of albendazole improves growth of Kenyan schoolchildren with hookworm, *Trichuris trichiura*, and *Ascaris lumbricoides* infections. Am J Trop Med Hyg 1989;41:78.

30

Infectious Diseases: Mycotic*

Harry Hollander, MD, & Carlyn Halde, MD

Fungal infections have assumed an increasingly important role as use of broad-spectrum antimicrobial agents has increased and the number of immunodeficient patients has risen. Some pathogens (eg, *Cryptococcus, Candida, Fusarium*) virtually never cause serious disease in normal hosts. Other endemic fungi (eg, *Histoplasma, Coccidioides, Paracoccidioides*) commonly cause disease in normal hosts but tend to be more aggressive in immunocompromised ones.

The major fungal diseases are discussed in this chapter.

CANDIDIASIS

Essentials of Diagnosis

- Common normal flora but opportunistic pathogen.
- Gastrointestinal mucosal disease, particularly esophagitis, most common.
- Transient fungemia usually clears.
- Disseminated visceral disease in severely immunocompromised patient.

General Considerations

Candida albicans can be cultured from the mouth, vagina, and feces of most people. Cutaneous and oral lesions are discussed in Chapters 4 and 11, respectively. The risk factors for invasive candidiasis include cellular immunodeficiency, prolonged neutropenia, diabetes mellitus, broad-spectrum antibiotic therapy, the presence of intravascular catheters (especially when providing total parenteral nutrition), and intravenous drug use. When no other underlying cause is found, persistent oral candidiasis should arouse a suspicion of HIV infection; over the course of their disease, AIDS patients will almost without exception have candidiasis as a complication.

Clinical Findings & Treatment

Esophageal involvement is the most frequent type of invasive mucosal disease. Individuals present with substernal odynophagia, gastroesophageal reflux, or nausea without substernal pain. Examination reveals oral candidiasis only 50% of the time. Diagnosis is best confirmed by endoscopy with biopsy and culture, since radiographically the condition may be difficult

to distinguish from esophagitis caused by infection with cytomegalovirus or herpes simplex virus. Therapy depends upon the severity of disease. If patients are able to swallow and take adequate amounts of fluid orally, ketoconazole, 200–400 mg/d, will usually suffice. In the individual who is more ill, a 10- to 14-day course of amphotericin B at a dose of 0.3 mg/kg/d usually results in resolution.

Candidal funguria usually resolves with discontinuance of antibiotics or removal of bladder catheters; rarely, since renal clearance of ketoconazole is low, bladder irrigation with 5 mg/d of amphotericin may be necessary. Fluconazole achieves excellent urinary levels and will probably provide an excellent alternative.

Candidal fungemia may represent a benign, self-limited process or may be a sign of serious disseminated disease. If fungemia resolves with removal of intravascular catheters, there are often no further complications, though some would recommend a short course of intravenous amphotericin B to a total dose of 200–500 mg. If fungemia is documented repeatedly or if *Candida* is isolated from other sites, the patient is considered to have disseminated disease even if no other clinical stigmas are present. Important clinical findings in disseminated candidiasis are fluffy white retinal infiltrates that extend into the vitreous and raised, erythematous skin lesions that may be painful. However, these are insensitive findings seen in less than 50% of cases. Other organ system involvement in disseminated disease may include the brain, meninges, and myocardium. Amphotericin B to a total dose of 1 g is the agent of choice. Flucytosine, 150 mg/kg/d orally in 4 divided doses, is added if central nervous system involvement occurs. Culture of skin lesions has a good diagnostic yield if fungemia is not documented, as is the case about 50% of the time. Unfortunately, serologic tests for *Candida* have not proved helpful in differentiating transient fungemia from disseminated disease.

Candidal endocarditis rarely is a complication of transient fungemia. It usually results from direct inoculation at the time of open heart surgery or repeated inoculation with intravenous drug use. Splenomegaly and petechiae are common, and there is a predilection for large-vessel embolization. Nonalbicans species such as *Candida parapsilosis* and *Candida tropicalis* may be important etiologic agents. As in other forms

---

* Superficial mycoses are discussed in Chapter 4.

of fungal endocarditis, blood cultures have a low sensitivity of approximately 20%. The diagnosis is established definitively by culturing *Candida* from emboli or from large vegetations at the time of valve replacement. Valve destruction (usually aortic or mitral) is common, and surgical therapy is necessary in addition to a prolonged course of amphotericin therapy, usually to a total dose of 1–1.5 g intravenously.

A newly recognized form of disseminated disease is hepatosplenic candidiasis. This results from aggressive chemotherapy and prolonged neutropenia in patients with underlying hematologic cancers. Patients typically present with fever and variable abdominal pain weeks after chemotherapy, when neutrophil counts have recovered. Blood cultures are generally negative. Liver function tests reveal an alkaline phosphatase elevation that may be marked. CT scanning of the abdomen shows hepatosplenomegaly, most often with multiple low-density defects in the liver. Diagnosis is established by liver biopsy and culture. Amphotericin B is given to a total dose of 1 g intravenously.

In all forms of invasive candidiasis, an important element of therapy is reversal of the underlying predisposing factor when possible.

Bross J et al: Risk factors for nosocomial candidemia: A case-control study in adults without leukemia. Am J Med 1989;87:614. (Role of antibiotics and central venous catheters.)

Thaler M et al: Hepatic candidiasis in cancer patients: The evolving picture of the syndrome. Ann Intern Med 1988;108:88.

HISTOPLASMOSIS

Essentials of Diagnosis

- Epidemiologically linked to bird feather and bat exposure.
- Asymptomatic to severe respiratory symptoms with malaise, fever, cough, and chest pain.
- Ulceration of naso- and oropharynx.
- Hepatomegaly, splenomegaly, and lymphadenopathy.
- Positive skin test; positive serologic findings; small budding fungus cells found within reticuloendothelial cells; culture confirms diagnosis.

General Considerations

Histoplasmosis is caused by *Histoplasma capsulatum,* a mold that has been isolated from soil in endemic areas (central and eastern USA, eastern Canada, Mexico, Central America, South America, Africa, and southeast Asia). Infection presumably takes place by inhalation of spores. These convert into small budding cells that are engulfed by phagocytic cells in the lungs. The organism proliferates and may be carried hematogenously to other organs.

Clinical Findings

A. Symptoms and Signs: Most cases of histoplasmosis are asymptomatic or mild and so are unrecognized. Past infection is recognized by the development of a positive histoplasmin skin test and occasionally by pulmonary and splenic calcification. Symptomatic infections may present with mild influenza-like illness, often lasting 1–4 days. Signs and symptoms of pulmonary involvement are usually absent even in patients who subsequently show areas of calcification on chest x-ray. Moderately severe infections are frequently diagnosed as atypical pneumonia. These patients have fever, cough, and mild chest pain lasting 5–15 days. Physical examination is usually negative. Radiographic findings are variable and nonspecific.

Severe infections occur in several forms: (1) Acute histoplasmosis frequently occurs in epidemics. It is a severe disease manifested by marked prostration, fever, and relatively few pulmonary complaints even when x-rays show pneumonia. The illness may last from 1 week to 6 months but is almost never fatal. (2) Acute progressive histoplasmosis is usually fatal within 6 weeks or less. Symptoms usually consist of fever, dyspnea, cough, loss of weight, and prostration. Diarrhea is usually present in children. Ulcers of the mucous membranes of the oropharynx may be present. The liver and spleen are nearly always enlarged, and all the organs of the body are involved. (3) Chronic progressive histoplasmosis is usually seen in older patients with chronic obstructive lung disease and in immunocompromised patients. The lungs show chronic progressive changes, often with cavities. Clinically, chronic histoplasmosis appears to be primarily confined to the lungs, though any organ may be involved in the terminal stage. (4) In contrast, disseminated disease in the profoundly immunocompromised host usually represents reactivation of prior infectious foci. This form is commonly seen in patients with underlying HIV infection and is characterized by fever and multiple organ system failure. Chest x-rays may show a miliary pattern.

B. Laboratory Findings: In the moderately to severely ill patient, the sedimentation rate is elevated. Leukopenia may be present, with normal differential count or neutropenia. Most patients with progressive disease show anemia of chronic disease. In pulmonary disease, sputum culture is rarely positive; in contrast, blood or bone marrow cultures from immunocompromised patients with acute disseminated disease are positive over 50% of the time. A new antigen assay has a sensitivity of greater than 90% for disseminated disease in AIDS patients. The sensitivity of screening immunodiffusion or complement fixation serologic tests is better than 95% in pulmonary disease but only 70% in disseminated histoplasmosis in immunocompromised patients. Since skin test reactivity may persist for years following infection, it is generally not useful for establishing the diagnosis. Skin testing may also interfere with subsequent serologic diagnosis.

Treatment

Self-limited pulmonary disease requires no specific therapy. Resection is rarely necessary. Amphotericin B (see Chapter 31) in a low total dose (150–500 mg) has given excellent results in severe acute pulmonary disease. For disseminated disease, a total of 2–3 g of amphotericin B is given. Relapses are not uncommon, especially in the setting of underlying HIV infection. For immunocompromised patients, maintenance ketoconazole is given after initial intravenous amphotericin B therapy. Itraconazole is also proving to be useful in both acute and maintenance therapy. Ketoconazole, 400–600 mg orally daily for several months, is an alternative for progressive pulmonary disease.

Graybill JR: Histoplasmosis in AIDS. J Infect Dis 1988;158:841. (Unique features in this population.)

Wheat LJ: Systemic fungal infections: Diagnosis and treatment: 1. Histoplasmosis. Infect Dis Clin North Am 1988;2:841.

Wheat LJ et al: *Histoplasma capsulatum* polysaccharide antigen detection in diagnosis and management of disseminated histoplasmosis in patients with acquired immunodeficiency syndrome. Am J Med 1989; 87:396.

COCCIDIOIDOMYCOSIS

Essentials of Diagnosis

- Influenzalike illness with malaise, fever, backache, headache, and cough.
- Arthralgia and periarticular swelling of knees and ankles. Erythema nodosum or erythema multiforme. Dissemination may result in meningitis or granulomatous lesions in any organ.
- X-ray findings vary widely from pneumonitis to cavitation.
- Serologic tests useful; sporangia containing endospores demonstrable in sputum or tissues.

General Considerations

Coccidioidomycosis should be considered in the diagnosis of any obscure illness in a patient who has lived in or visited an endemic area.

Infection results from the inhalation of arthroconidia of *Coccidioides immitis,* a mold that grows in soil in certain arid regions of the southwestern USA, in Mexico, and in Central and South America.

About 60% of infections are subclinical and unrecognized other than by the subsequent development of a positive coccidioidin skin test. In the remaining cases, symptoms may be of severity warranting medical attention. Fewer than 1% of immunocompetent hosts show dissemination, but among these patients the mortality rate is high.

Clinical Findings

A. Symptoms and Signs: Symptoms of primary coccidioidomycosis occur in about 40% of infections. These vary from mild to severe and prostrating and may be very nonspecific. The onset (after an incubation period of 10–30 days) is usually that of a respiratory tract illness with fever and occasionally chills. Pleuritic pain is common. Nasopharyngitis may be followed by bronchitis accompanied by a dry or slightly productive cough. Weakness and anorexia may become marked, leading to prostration. A morbilliform rash may appear 1–2 days after the onset of symptoms.

Arthralgia accompanied by periarticular swellings, often of the knees and ankles, is common. Erythema nodosum may appear 2–20 days after onset of symptoms. Erythema multiforme may also occur rarely. Persistent pulmonary lesions, varying from cavities and abscesses to parenchymal nodular densities or bronchiectasis, occur in about 5% of diagnosed cases.

About 0.1% of white and 1% of nonwhite patients are unable to localize or control infection caused by *C immitis.* Symptoms in progressive coccidioidomycosis depend upon the site of dissemination. Any organ may be involved. Pulmonary findings usually become more pronounced, with mediastinal and hilar lymph node enlargement, cough, and increased sputum production. Pulmonary abscesses may rupture into the pleural space, producing an empyema. Extension to bones and skin may take place, and pericardial and myocardial extension is not unusual. Dissemination may be associated with fungemia, characterized clinically by a diffuse miliary pattern on chest x-ray and by early death. The course may be particularly rapid in immunosuppressed patients.

Bone lesions most often occur at bony prominences. Meningitis occurs in 30–50% of cases of dissemination. Subcutaneous abscesses and verrucous skin lesions are especially common in fulminating cases. Lymphadenitis may occur and may progress to suppuration. Mediastinal and retroperitoneal abscesses are not uncommon.

B. Laboratory Findings: In primary coccidioidomycosis, there may be moderate leukocytosis and eosinophilia and an elevated sedimentation rate. A persisting elevated or increasing sedimentation rate is a sign of progressive disease. The coccidioidin skin test becomes positive early after infection and may remain positive for years. Serologic testing is useful for both diagnosis and prognosis. The immunodiffusion test (CIE) is useful for screening, but the complement fixation test is needed for confirmation and quantitation. A persistent rising complement fixation tier ($\geq$ 1:8) is suspicious for disseminated disease. Demonstrable antibodies in spinal fluid are pathognomonic for coccidioidal meningitis. Spinal fluid findings include increased cell count with lymphocytosis and reduced glucose. Sporangia filled with endospores may be found in clinical specimens. These should be cultured only by trained technicians using strict safety precautions because of the danger of laboratory infection. Blood cultures in appropriate media are positive in about 30% of cases of acutely disseminated disease. Spinal fluid culture is positive in approximately 30% of meningitis cases.

C. Imaging: Radiographic findings vary, but patchy, nodular pulmonary infiltrates and thin-walled cavities are most common. Hilar lymphadenopathy may be visible. There may be pleural effusions and lesions in bone.

Complications

Pulmonary infiltrates persisting for 6 or more weeks should be suspected of possible progression, especially with increase in area, enlargement of mediastinal and hilar nodes, cavity enlargement, and hemoptysis. Progressive disease is more likely to appear in blacks, Filipinos, and Mexicans. Immunodeficient patients, including those with HIV infection, and pregnant women of any race are also more vulnerable to dissemination.

Treatment

General symptomatic therapy is given as needed for disease limited to the chest with no evidence of progression. For progressive pulmonary or extrapulmonary disease, amphotericin B intravenously has proved effective in some patients (see Chapter 31). Therapy should be continued to a total dose of 2.5–3 g. For meningitis, systemic maintenance amphotericin B may be required for the lifetime of the individual as guided by symptoms and spinal fluid complement fixation titers. Intrathecal amphotericin B, 1–5 mg monthly, may be needed if systemic therapy fails. Oral ketoconazole, 200–800 mg daily 1–2 hours before breakfast, is an alternative for disease limited to the chest; however, therapy must be continued for 6 months or longer in order to prevent relapse. Itraconazole also has potent activity against this organism; preliminary results are promising for nonmeningeal disease.

Thoracic surgery is occasionally indicated for giant, infected, or ruptured cavities. Surgical drainage is also useful for subcutaneous abscesses. Amphotericin B is advisable following extensive surgical manipulation of infected tissue.

Prognosis

The prognosis in the case of limited disease is good, but persistent pulmonary cavities may cause complications. Nodules, cavities, and fibrotic residuals may rarely progress after long periods of stability or regression. Disseminated and meningeal forms still have significant mortality rates.

Ampel NM, Wieden MA, Galgiani JN: Coccidioidomycosis: Clinical update. Rev Infect Dis 1989;11:897.

Bronneman DA et al: Coccidioidomycosis in the acquired immunodeficiency syndrome. Ann Intern Med 1987; 106:372.

Gaglia JN et al: Ketoconazole therapy of progressive coccidioidomycosis: Comparison of 400 mg and 800 mg doses and observations at higher doses. Am J Med 1988;84:603.

CRYPTOCOCCOSIS

Essentials of Diagnosis

- Most common cause of fungal meningitis.
- Predisposing factors: lymphoid cancer, corticosteroids, HIV infection.
- Culture, demonstration of capsular antigen diagnostic.

General Considerations

Cryptococcosis is caused by *Cryptococcus neoformans,* an encapsulated budding yeast that has been found worldwide in soil and on dried pigeon dung.

Infections are acquired by inhalation. In the lung, the infection may remain localized, heal, or disseminate. Immunocompetent hosts rarely develop clinically apparent cryptococcal pneumonia. Progressive lung disease and dissemination most often occur in the setting of cellular immunodeficiency, including underlying hematologic cancer, long-term corticosteroid therapy, or HIV infection.

Clinical Findings

A. Symptoms and Signs: Disseminated disease may involve any organ, but central nervous system disease usually predominates. Headache is usually the first symptom of meningitis. Confusion and cranial nerve abnormalities may be seen as the disease progresses. Nuchal rigidity and meningeal signs are seen about 50% of the time but are uncommon in HIV-infected patients with this complication. Intracerebral mass lesions (cryptococcomas) are rarely seen. Obstructive hydrocephalus may complicate the course.

B. Laboratory Findings: Mild anemia, leukocytosis, and increased sedimentation rate are found. Spinal fluid findings include increased pressure, variable pleocytosis, budding encapsulated fungus cells, increased protein, and decreased glucose. Cryptococcal antigen in cerebrospinal fluid and culture establish the diagnosis 90% of the time. As many as 50% of AIDS patients may have no pleocytosis. These patients have a high incidence of extrameningeal disease, so that fungal blood culture and serum cryptococcal antigen tests are diagnostically helpful.

Treatment

A combination of amphotericin B (0.3 mg/kg/d administered as for coccidioidomycosis) and flucytosine, 150 mg/kg/d orally or intravenously divided into 4 equal doses and given every 6 hours, is as effective as higher doses of amphotericin B alone and may cause less toxicity. However, flucytosine may not be tolerated, particularly in AIDS patients, because of diarrhea and leukopenia. Intrathecal amphotericin B may be necessary if sterilization of fluid has not occurred after several weeks of therapy and clinical deterioration has taken place. Ventricular shunting may be important if hydrocephalus is a complication. In non-HIV-related cryptococcal meningitis, amphotericin B therapy is usually continued to a total dose of 1.5–2 g. Therapy is generally continued if cerebrospinal fluid cultures remain positive or cerebrospinal fluid antigen titers remain greater than 1:8. In AIDS patients, it may be very difficult to achieve such a low cerebrospinal fluid titer. Thus, the end points for amphotericin B therapy are clinical response and culture negativity of the cerebrospinal fluid.

After treatment of a bout of AIDS-related cryptococcal meningitis, it is extremely important to begin some form of maintenance antifungal therapy. Without this, the rate of relapse is greater than 50%. Maintenance schedules can utilize either amphotericin B, 1 mg/kg/wk in one dose or 2 divided doses, or fluconazole, 200 mg orally daily. The availability of fluconazole also promises to revolutionize the therapy of acute bouts of cryptococcal meningitis. In the AIDS population, at a daily dose of 200–400 mg, this agent has a response rate approximately equivalent to that of amphotericin B used alone.

Prognosis

Factors that indicate a poor prognosis include lymphoid cancer, lack of spinal fluid pleocytosis, high initial antigen titer in either serum or cerebrospinal fluid, and the presence of extraneural disease. These factors may not be predictive in AIDS-related cryptococcal meningitis.

Byrne WR, Wajszccuk CP: Cryptococcal meningitis in the acquired immunodeficiency syndrome (AIDS): Successful treatment with fluconazole after failure of amphotericin B. Ann Intern Med 1988;108:384.

Chuck SL, Sande MA: Infections with *Cryptococcus neoformans* in the acquired immune deficiency syndrome. N Engl J Med 1989;321:794.

Dismukes WE et al: Treatment of cryptococcal meningitis with combination amphotericin B and flucytosine for four as compared with six weeks. N Engl J Med 1987;317:334.

ASPERGILLOSIS

Aspergillus fumigatus is the usual cause of aspergillosis, though many species may cause a wide spectrum of disease. Burn eschar and detritus in the external ear canal are often colonized by these fungi. Clinical illness results either from an aberrant immunologic response or tissue invasion.

Allergic bronchopulmonary aspergillosis leads to severe asthma and transient pulmonary infiltrates. This diagnosis should be considered when asthma and fleeting infiltrates are accompanied by eosinophilia, high levels of IgE, and *Aspergillus* precipitins in the blood. The disease characteristically has a waxing and waning course with gradual improvement over time. For acute exacerbations, oral prednisone is begun at a dose of 1 mg/kg/d and then tapered slowly over several months. Antifungal agents do not have a role in the management of allergic aspergillosis.

Important invasive manifestations may be seen in immunocompetent adults. These include chronic sinusitis and colonization of preexisting pulmonary cavities. Sinus disease may require long courses of antibiotics as well as surgical debridement. Aspergillomas of the lung may be found by incidental radiographic studies but may also present with significant hemoptysis. Intracavitary instillation of amphotericin B and bronchoscopic removal have been tried, but the most effective therapy for symptomatic aspergilloma remains surgical resection.

Life-threatening invasive disease most commonly occurs in profoundly immunodeficient patients, particularly those with prolonged severe neutropenia. AIDS patients do not have an increased incidence of invasive aspergillosis. Pulmonary disease is most common, with patchy infiltration leading to a severe necrotizing pneumonia. There is often distal infarction as the organism grows into blood vessels. Late in the course, there may be hematogenous dissemination to the central nervous system, skin, and other organs. Early diagnosis and reversal of any correctable immunosuppression are essential. Blood cultures have very low yield. In contrast to allergic aspergillosis, serologic tests and antigen detection have low sensitivities for invasive disease. Isolation of *Aspergillus* from pulmonary secretions does not necessarily imply invasive disease. Therefore, the mainstay of diagnosis is demonstration of *Aspergillus* in tissue. Histologically, one sees branched septate hyphae. Biopsy specimens will not invariably grow the organism.

When severe invasive aspergillosis is considered clinically or microbiologically, rapid institution of high doses of amphotericin B may be life-saving (see Chapter 31). After a test dose, the total daily dose is increased to 0.8–1 mg/kg/d intravenously as tolerated for the first several weeks of therapy. Thereafter, more traditional doses of 0.6 mg/kg/d are continued until a total dose of at least 2 g has been reached. The addition of flucytosine is of unclear benefit. Itraconazole has activity against *Aspergillus,* and initial clinical experience is favorable. Until more data accumulate, amphotericin B should remain the first-line drug for invasive disease. The mortality rate of pulmonary or disseminated disease in the immunocompromised patient still approaches 50%.

Denning DW et al: Treatment of invasive aspergillosis with itraconazole. Am J Med 1989;86:791. (Excellent responses in 12 of 20 patients.)

Slavin RG, Gottlieb CC, Avioli LV: Grand rounds: Allergic bronchopulmonary aspergillosis. Arch Intern Med 1986;146:1799.

MUCORMYCOSIS

The term "mucormycosis" (zygomycosis, phycomycosis) is applied to opportunistic infections caused by members of the genera *Rhizopus, Mucor, Absidia,* and *Cunninghamella*. Predisposing conditions include diabetic acidosis and treatment with steroids or cytotoxic drugs. These organisms appear in tissues as broad, branching nonseptate hyphae. Biopsy is almost always required for diagnosis. Invasive disease of the sinuses, orbits, and the lungs may be noted. Widely disseminated disease has been more commonly seen recently in patients who have received aggressive chemotherapy. The diagnosis should be considered in acidotic diabetic patients with black necrotic lesions of the nose or sinuses or with new cranial nerve abnormalities. High-dosage amphotericin B therapy initiated early, control of diabetes or other underlying conditions, and extensive surgical removal of necrotic, nonperfused tissue are essential. The prognosis is poor, with a 30–50% mortality rate for localized disease and higher rates in disseminated cases.

Ingram CW et al: Disseminated zygomycosis: Report of four cases and review. Rev Infect Dis 1989;2:741. (Must be considered in immunocompromised patients. Prognosis very poor.)
Parfrey NA: Improved diagnosis and prognosis of mucormycosis: A clinicopathologic study of 33 cases. Medicine 1986;65:113.

BLASTOMYCOSIS

Blastomyces dermatitidis causes this chronic systemic fungus infection. The disease occurs more often in men and in a geographically delimited area of the central and eastern USA and Canada. A few cases have been found in Mexico and Africa.

Pulmonary infection may be asymptomatic. When dissemination takes place, lesions are most frequently seen on the skin, in bones, and in the urogenital system.

Cough, moderate fever, dyspnea, and chest pain are evident in symptomatic patients. These may resolve or progress, with bloody and purulent sputum production, pleurisy, fever, chills, loss of weight, and prostration. Radiologic studies usually reveal infiltrates and enlarged mediastinal nodes. Raised, verrucous cutaneous lesions that have an abrupt downward sloping border are usually present in disseminated blastomycosis. The border extends slowly, leaving a central atrophic scar. These lesions persist untreated for long periods, mimicking skin cancer.

Bones—often the ribs and vertebrae—are frequently involved. Lesions appear to be both destructive and proliferative on radiography. Epididymitis, prostatitis, and other involvement of the male urogenital system may occur. Central nervous system involvement is uncommon.

Laboratory findings usually include leukocytosis, anemia, and elevated sedimentation rate. The organism is found in clinical specimens as a thick-walled cell 5–20 mm in diameter that may have a single bud. It grows readily on culture. Serologic tests are not well standardized.

Amphotericin B (see Chapter 31) in a total dose of 1.5–2 g intravenously is the best drug for treatment of severe or progressive disease. Ketoconazole at a daily dose of 200–600 mg is an effective alternative in immunocompetent patients with nonmeningeal disease. Large abscesses or bronchopleural fistulas rarely require drainage.

Careful follow-up for early evidence of relapse should be made for several years so that therapy may be resumed or another drug instituted. Patients with limited cutaneous lesions have the best prognosis.

Bradshur RW: Systemic fungal infections: Diagnosis and treatment: 1. Blastomycosis. Rev Infect Dis 1989;2:741.
National Institute of Allergy and Infectious Diseases Mycoses Study Group: Treatment of blastomycosis and histoplasmosis with ketoconazole: Results of a prospective randomized clinical trial. Ann Intern Med 1985;103:861.

PARACOCCIDIOIDOMYCOSIS
(South American Blastomycosis)

Paracoccidioides brasiliensis infections have been found only in patients who have resided in South or Central America or Mexico. Long asymptomatic periods enable patients to travel far from the endemic areas. Ulceration of the naso- and oropharynx is usually the first symptom. Papules ulcerate and enlarge both peripherally and deeper into the subcutaneous tissue. Differential diagnosis includes mucocutaneous leishmaniasis and syphilis. Extensive coalescent ulcerations may eventually result in destruction of the epiglottis, vocal cords, and uvula. Extension to the lips and face may occur. Eating and drinking are extremely painful. Skin lesions may occur, usually on the face. Variable in appearance, they may have a necrotic central crater with a hard hyperkeratotic border. Lymph node enlargement may follow mucocutaneous lesions, eventually ulcerating and forming draining sinuses. Lymph node enlargement may be the presenting symptom, with subsequent suppuration and rupture through the skin. In some patients, hepatosplenomegaly is noted. Cough, sometimes with sputum, indicates pulmonary involvement, but the signs and symptoms are often mild, even though radiographic findings indicate severe parenchymatous changes in the lungs. The extensive ulceration of the upper gastrointestinal tract may prevent sufficient intake and result in cachexia.

Laboratory findings are nonspecific. Serology by immunodiffusion is positive in 98% of cases. Complement fixation titers correlate with progressive disease and fall with effective therapy. The fungus is found in clinical specimens as a spherical cell that may have many buds arising from it. If direct examination does not reveal the organism, biopsy with Gomori staining may be helpful.

Oral ketoconazole, 200–400 mg daily 1–2 hours before breakfast, generally results in a clinical response within 1 month and effective control after 6 months. The rare relapse responds to resumed ketoconazole therapy. Itraconazole, 100 mg orally daily, also is effective.

Restrepo A et al: Itraconazole in the treatment of paracoccidioidomycosis: A preliminary report. In: First International Symposium on Itraconazole. Rev Infect Dis 1987;9(Suppl 1):S51.
Restrepo A et al: Treatment of paracoccidioidomycosis with ketoconazole: A three-year experience. (In: Symposium on ketoconazole therapy.) Am J Med 1983;74(Suppl 1B):48.

SPOROTRICHOSIS

Sporotrichosis is a chronic fungal infection caused by *Sporothrix schenckii*. It is worldwide in distribution; most patients have had contact with soil, plants, or decaying wood. Infection takes place when the organism is inoculated into the skin—usually on the hand, arm, or foot.

The most common form of sporotrichosis begins with a hard, nontender subcutaneous nodule. This later becomes adherent to the overlying skin and ulcerates. Within a few days to weeks, similar nodules usually develop along the lymphatics draining this area, and these may ulcerate. The lymphatic vessels become indurated and are easily palpable. Blood-borne dissemination is rare, and the general health of the patient is not affected.

Disseminated sporotrichosis is rare in the immunocompetent host but may present with lung, bone, joint, and central nervous system involvement in immunocompromised patients.

Cultures are needed to establish diagnosis. Serologic tests may be useful for diagnosis of disseminated disease.

Potassium iodide taken orally in increasing dosage is the treatment of choice for cutaneous disease. Give as the saturated solution, 5 drops 3 times a day after meals, increasing by 1 drop per dose until 40 drops 3 times a day are being given. Continue until signs of the active disease have disappeared. The dosage is then decreased by 1 drop per dose until 5 drops are being given, and then is discontinued. Care must be taken to reduce the dosage if signs of iodism appear or thyroid disease is present. Amphotericin B intravenously, 1.5–2 g (see Chapter 31), has been effective in systemic infection. It appears that itraconazole will supplant iodide as the therapy of choice for cutaneous disease. Surgery is usually contraindicated except for simple aspiration of secondary nodules.

The prognosis is good for all forms of sporotrichosis except the disseminated type.

Gullberg RM et al: Sporotrichosis: Recurrent cutaneous, articular, and central nervous system infection in a renal transplant recipient. Rev Infect Dis 1987;9:369.
Scott EN et al: Serologic studies in the diagnosis and management of meningitis due to *Sporothrix schenckii*. N Engl J Med 1987;317:935.

CHROMOMYCOSIS

Chromomycosis is a chronic, principally tropical cutaneous infection caused by several species of closely related black molds (*Fonsecaea* sp and *Phialophora* sp).

Lesions are slowly progressive and occur most frequently on a lower extremity. The lesion begins as a papule or ulcer. Over months to years, papules enlarge to become vegetating, papillomatous, verrucous elevated nodules. Satellite lesions may appear along the lymphatics. There may be secondary bacterial infection. Elephantiasis may result.

The fungus is seen as brown, thick-walled, spherical, sometimes septate cells in pus. The type of reproduction found in culture determines the species.

Surgical excision is the treatment of choice for early lesions. Medical therapy is generally disappointing, but flucytosine, 150 mg/kg/d, alone or in combination with ketoconazole, 200–400 mg orally, has been successful in some cases. Itraconazole, 100–400 mg/d orally, has also resulted in some clinical responses.

Borelli D: A clinical trial of itraconazole in the treatment of deep mycoses and leishmaniasis. In: First International Symposium on Itraconazole. Rev Infect Dis 1987; 9(Suppl 1):S57.
McGinnis MR: Chromoblastomycosis and phaeohyphomycosis: New concepts, diagnosis, and mycology. J Am Acad Dermatol 1983;8:1.

MYCETOMA
(Maduromycosis & Actinomycetoma)

Maduromycosis is the term used to describe mycetoma caused by the true fungi. Actinomycotic mycetoma is caused by *Nocardia* and *Actinomadura* spp. The disease begins as a papule, nodule, or abscess that over months to years progresses slowly to form multiple abscesses and sinus tracts ramifying deep into the tissue. Secondary bacterial infection may result in large open ulcers. Radiographs may show destructive changes in the underlying bone. The agents occur as white, yellow, red, or black granules in tissue or pus. Microscopic examination assists in the diagnosis.

The prognosis is good for patients with actinomycetoma, since they usually respond well to sulfonamides and sulfones, especially if treated early. Give trimethoprim-sulfamethoxazole, 160/800 mg orally twice a day. Dapsone, 100 mg twice daily after meals, has also been reported to be effective. Streptomycin, 14 mg/kg/d intramuscularly, may be useful during the first month of therapy. All other medications must be taken for months and continued for several months after clinical cure to prevent relapse. Debridement assists healing.

The prognosis for maduromycosis is poor. Early trials indicate that itraconazole may be useful. Surgical excision of early lesions may prevent spread. Amputation is necessary in far-advanced cases.

Borelli D: A clinical trial of itraconazole in the treatment of deep mycoses and leishmaniasis. In: First International Symposium on Itraconazole. Rev Infect Dis 1987; 9(Suppl 1):S57.

MYCOTIC KERATITIS

Candida albicans, Fusarium, and *Aspergillus* are most often responsible for mycotic keratitis. Trauma to the cornea followed by corticosteroid and antibiotic therapy is often a predisposing factor. Prompt withdrawal of corticosteroids, removal of the infected necrotic tissue, and application of natamycin or ketoconazole are useful in management. Amphotericin B and flucytosine are used for fungal endophthalmitis.

OTHER OPPORTUNISTIC MOLD INFECTIONS

Fungi previously considered to be harmless colonizers are emerging as significant pathogens in immunocompromised patients. Infection in cancer patients, particularly those with hematologic cancer, is most common. Infection may be localized in the skin, lungs, or sinuses, or widespread disease may appear with lesions in multiple organs. Colonization of tuberculosis cavities may cause minimal symptoms or may precede dissemination with meningitis or brain abscesses. Endocarditis occurs more commonly in intravenous drug abusers. Sinus infection may cause bony erosion. Infection in subcutaneous tissues following traumatic implantation may develop as a well-circumscribed cyst or as an ulcer.

Nonpigmented septate hyphae are seen in tissue and are indistinguishable from those of *Aspergillus* when infections are due to *Pseudallescheria boydii* or species of *Fusarium, Paecilomyces, Penicillium,* or other hyaline molds. Spores or mycetoma-like granules are rarely present in tissue.

Infection by any of a number of black molds is designated as phaeohyphomycosis. These black molds are common in the environment, especially on decaying vegetation, and do not cause infection in the normal host, although some black molds, as well as

Table 30–1. Agents for systemic mycoses.

Drug	Dosing	Renal Clearance?	CSF Penetration?	Toxicities	Spectrum of Activity
Amphotericin B	0.3–1 mg/kg/d IV	No	Poor	Rigors, fever, azotemia, hypokalemia, renal tubular acidosis, anemia	All major pathogens except *Pseudallescheria,* some nonalbicans *Candida*
Flucytosine (5-FC)	150 mg/kg/d orally in 4 divided doses	Yes	Yes	Leukopenia, rash, diarrhea, hepatitis	Cryptococcosis,[1] candidiasis,[1] chromomycosis
Ketoconazole	200–800 mg/d orally in 1 or 2 doses	No	Yes	Anorexia, nausea, suppression of testosterone and cortisol, rash, hepatitis	Nonmeningeal histoplasmosis and coccidioidomycosis, blastomycosis, paracoccidioidomycosis, mucosal candidiasis (except urinary)
Fluconazole	200–400 mg/d as single dose IV or orally	Yes	Yes	Nausea	Mucosal candidiasis (including urinary), cryptococcosis
Itraconazole[2]	100–400 mg/d orally as single dose	No	Yes	Nausea	Same as ketoconazole plus sporotrichosis, aspergillosis, chromomycosis

[1] In combination with amphotericin B.
[2] Not licensed in USA.

some hyaline molds, are allergens. In tissues of patients with phaeohyphomycosis, the mold is seen as black or faintly brown hyphae, yeast cells, or both. Culture on appropriate medium is needed to identify the agent. Some isolates are sensitive to antifungal antibiotics.

Adam RD et al: Phaeohyphomycosis caused by the fungal genera *Bipolaris* and *Exserohilum:* A report of 9 cases and review of the literature. Medicine 1986;65:203.

Anaissie E et al: The emerging role of *Fusarium* infections in patients with cancer. Medicine 1988;67:77.

Anaissie E et al: New spectrum of fungal infections in patients with cancer. Rev Infect Dis 1989;11:369.

Travis LB, Roberts GD, Wilson WR: Clinical significance of *Pseudallescheria boydii:* A review of 10 years experience. Mayo Clin Proc 1985;60:531.

ANTIFUNGAL THERAPY

With recent advances in drug development, the field of antifungal chemotherapy is changing rapidly. In addition to the newer imidazoles, novel classes of agents are beginning to undergo clinical trials. Table 30–1 summarizes the major properties of currently available antifungal agents and the other imidazole (itraconazole) that is likely to be licensed within the next several years.

REFERENCES

Bodey GP: Topical and systemic antifungal agents. Med Clin North Am 1988;72:637.

Dismukes WE: Azole antifungal drugs: Old and new. Ann Intern Med 1988;109:177.

Anti-infective Chemotherapeutic & Antibiotic Agents

31

Richard A. Jacobs, MD, PhD, & Ernest Jawetz, MD, PhD

Some Rules for Antimicrobial Therapy

Antimicrobial drugs are used on a very large scale, and their proper use gives striking therapeutic results. On the other hand, they can create serious untoward reactions and should therefore be administered only upon proper indication.

Drugs of first choice and alternative drugs are presented in Table 31–1.

The following steps are required in each patient considered for antibiotic therapy.

A. Etiologic Diagnosis: Formulate an etiologic diagnosis based on clinical observations. Microbial infections are best treated early. The physician must decide on clinical grounds (1) whether the patient has a microbial infection that can be favorably influenced by antimicrobial drugs and (2) the kind of pathogen most probably causing such infection ("best guess").

B. "Best Guess": (Tables 31–2 and 31–3.) Select a specific antimicrobial drug on the basis of past experience for empiric therapy. Based on a "best guess," the physician should choose a drug or combination of drugs that is likely to be effective against the suspected pathogens.

C. Laboratory Control: Before beginning antimicrobial drug treatment, obtain specimens for laboratory examination to determine the causative infectious organism and, if desirable, its susceptibility to antimicrobial drugs.

D. Clinical Response: Based on the clinical response of the patient, evaluate the laboratory reports and consider the desirability of changing the antimicrobial drug regimen. Laboratory results should not overrule clinical judgment. Isolation of an organism that confirms the initial clinical impression is useful. Conversely, laboratory results may contradict the initial clinical impression and compel its reconsideration. If the specimen was obtained from a site that is normally devoid of bacterial flora and not exposed to the external environment (eg, blood, cerebrospinal fluid, pleural fluid, joint fluid), the recovery of a microorganism is a significant finding even if the organism recovered is different from the clinically suspected etiologic agent, and this may force a change in treatment. On the other hand, isolation of unex-

pected microorganisms from the respiratory tract, gut, or surface lesions (sites that have a complex flora) must be critically evaluated before drugs are abandoned that were judiciously selected on the basis of an initial "best guess" for empiric treatment.

E. Drug Susceptibility Tests: Some microorganisms are fairly uniformly susceptible to certain drugs; if such organisms are isolated from the patient, they need not be tested for drug susceptibility. For example, group A hemolytic streptococci and most pneumococci and clostridia respond predictably to penicillin. On the other hand, some organisms (eg, enteric gram-negative rods) are so variable in response as to warrant drug susceptibility testing when they are isolated from a significant specimen.

Antimicrobial drug susceptibility tests may be done on solid media as "disk tests," in broth in tubes, or in wells of microdilution plates. The latter method yields results expressed as MIC (minimal inhibitory concentration), and the technique can be modified to give MBC (minimal bactericidal concentration) results. In some infections, the MIC or MBC permits a better estimate of the amount of drug required for therapeutic effect in vivo.

Disk tests usually indicate whether an isolate is susceptible or resistant to serum concentrations of drug achieved in vivo with conventional dosage regimens, thus providing valuable guidance in selecting therapy. When there appear to be marked discrepancies between test results and clinical response of the patient, the following possibilities must be considered:

1. Selection of an inappropriate drug, dosage, or route of administration.

2. Failure to drain a collection of pus or to remove a foreign body.

3. Failure of a poorly diffusing drug to reach the site of infection (eg, central nervous system) or to reach intracellular phagocytosed bacteria.

4. Superinfection in the course of prolonged chemotherapy. After suppression of the original infection or of normal flora, a second type of microorganism may establish itself against which the originally selected drug is ineffective.

5. Emergence of drug-resistant or tolerant organisms.

6. Participation of 2 or more microorganisms

Table 31–1. Drugs of choice for suspected or proved microbial pathogens, 1990–1991.
(± = alone or combined with)

Suspected or Proved Etiologic Agent	Drug(s) of First Choice	Alternative Drug(s)
Gram-negative cocci		
Moraxella (*Branhamella*) *catarrhalis*	Amoxicillin-clavulanic acid or TMP-SMZ[1]	Newer cephalosporins,[2] erythromycin,[3] tetracycline[4]
Gonococcus	Ceftriaxone	Penicillin,[5] ampicillin, or amoxicillin + probenecid
Meningococcus	Penicillin[5]	Newer cephalosporins,[2] ampicillin, chloramphenicol
Gram-positive cocci		
Pneumococcus (*Streptococcus pneumoniae*)	Penicillin[5]	Erythromycin,[3] cephalosporin,[6] vancomycin
Streptococcus, hemolytic, groups A, B, C, G	Penicillin[5]	Erythromycin,[3] cephalosporin,[6] vancomycin
Streptococcus viridans	Penicillin[5] ± aminoglycosides[7]	Cephalosporin,[6] vancomycin
Staphylococcus, methicillin-resistant	Vancomycin ± gentamicin or rifampin (or both)	TMP-SMZ, ciprofloxacin
Staphylococcus, non-penicillinase-producing	Penicillin	Cephalosporin, vancomycin
Staphylococcus, penicillinase-producing	Penicillin-resistant penicillin[8]	Vancomycin, cephalosporin[6]
Streptococcus faecalis (enterococcus)	Ampicillin + gentamicin	Vancomycin + gentamicin
Gram-negative rods		
Acinetobacter	Aminoglycoside[7] ± imipenem	Minocycline, TMP-SMZ[1]
Bacteroides, oropharyngeal strains	Penicillin,[5] clindamycin	Metronidazole, cephalosporin[2,6]
Bacteroides, gastrointestinal strains	Metronidazole	Cefoxitin, chloramphenicol, clindamycin
Brucella	Tetracycline[4] ± streptomycin	TMP-SMZ[1]
Campylobacter	Erythromycin[3]	Tetracycline,[4] ciprofloxacin
Enterobacter	TMP-SMZ,[1] aminoglycoside[7]	Imipenem, newer cephalosporin[2]
Escherichia coli (sepsis)	Aminoglycoside,[7] newer cephalosporin[2]	Ampicillin, TMP-SMZ[1]
Escherichia coli (first urinary infection)	Sulfonamide,[9] TMP-SMZ[1]	Ampicillin, cephalosporin[6]
Haemophilus (meningitis, respiratory infections)	Newer cephalosporins[2]	Ampicillin and chloramphenicol
Klebsiella	Newer cephalosporins[2]	TMP-SMZ,[1] aminoglycoside[7]
Legionella sp (pneumonia)	Erythromycin[3] ± rifampin	TMP-SMZ[1]
Pasteurella (*Yersinia*) (plague, tularemia)	Streptomycin, tetracycline[4]	Chloramphenicol
Proteus mirabilis	Ampicillin	Newer cephalosporins,[2] aminoglycoside[7]
Proteus vulgaris and other species	Newer cephalosporins[2]	Aminoglycoside[7]
Pseudomonas aeruginosa	Aminoglycoside[7] + antipseudomonal penicillin[10]	Ceftazidime or cefoperazone ± aminoglycoside; imipenem ± aminoglycoside; aztreonam
Pseudomonas pseudomallei (melioidosis)	Ceftazidime	Chloramphenicol, tetracycline,[4] TMP-SMZ[1]
Pseudomonas mallei (glanders)	Streptomycin + tetracycline[4]	Chloramphenicol + streptomycin
Salmonella	Ceftriaxone	TMP-SMZ,[1] ciprofloxacin, ampicillin, chlorampenicol
Serratia, *Providenica*	Newer cephalosporins,[2] aminoglycoside[7]	TMP-SMZ[1]
Shigella	TMP-SMZ[1]	Ampicillin, tetracycline,[4] ciprofloxacin, chloramphenicol
Vibrio (cholera, sepsis)	Tetracycline[4]	TMP-SMZ[1]
Gram-positive rods		
Actinomyces	Penicillin[5]	Tetracycline[4]
Bacillus (eg, anthrax)	Penicillin[5]	Erythromycin[3]
Clostridium (eg, gas gangrene, tetanus)	Penicillin[5]	Metronidazole, chloramphenicol, clindamycin
Corynebacterium diphtheriae	Erythromycin[3]	Penicillin[5]
Corynebacterium, JK strain	Vancomycin	Ciprofloxacin
Listeria	Ampicillin ± aminoglycoside[7]	TMP-SMZ[1]
Acid-fast rods		
Mycobacterium tuberculosis	INH + rifampin + pyrazinamide	Other antituberculous drugs
Mycobacterium leprae	Dapsone + rifampin, clofazimine	Ethionamide
Mycobacterium kansasii	INH + rifampin + ethambutol	Other antituberculous drugs
Mycobacterium avium-intracellulare	Ethambutol + rifampin + clofazimine + ciprofloxacin + amikacin	Other antituberculous drugs

Table 31–1 (cont'd). Drugs of choice for suspected or proved microbial pathogens, 1990–1991.
($\pm$ = alone or combined with)

Suspected or Proved Etiologic Agent	Drug(s) of First Choice	Alternative Drug(s)
Mycobacterium fortuitum-chelonei	Amikacin + doxycycline	Cefoxitin, erythromycin, sulfonamide
Nocardia	Sulfonamide,[9] TMP-SMZ[1]	Minocycline
Spirochetes		
Borrelia (Lyme disease, relapsing fever)	Tetracycline,[4] ceftriaxone	Penicillin,[5] erythromycin[3]
Leptospira	Penicillin[5]	Tetracycline[4]
Treponema (syphilis, yaws, etc)	Penicillin[5]	Erythromycin,[3] tetracycline[4]
Mycoplasmas	Erythromycin[3] or tetracycline[4]	
Chlamydiae (*C trachomatis, C psittaci, C pneumoniae*)	Tetracycline[4]	Erythromycin[3]
Rickettsiae	Tetracycline[4]	Chloramphenicol

[1] TMP-SMZ is a mixture of 1 part trimethoprim and 5 parts sulfamethoxazole.
[2] Newer cephalosporins (1990) include cefotaxmine, cefuroxime, ceftriaxone, ceftazidime, ceftizoxime, and others.
[3] Erythromycin estolate is best absorbed orally but carries the highest risk of hepatitis; erythromycin stearate and erythromycin ethylsuccinate are also available.
[4] All tetracyclines have similar activity against microorganisms. Dosage is determined by rates of absorption and excretion of various preparations.
[5] Penicillin G is preferred for parenteral injection; penicillin V for oral administration—to be used only in treating infections due to highly sensitive organisms.
[6] Older cephalosporins are cephalothin, cefazolin, cephapirin, and cefoxitin for parenteral injection; cephalexin and cephradine can be given orally.
[7] Aminoglycosides—gentamicin, tobramycin, amikacin, netilmicin—should be chosen on the basis of local patterns of susceptibility.
[8] Parenteral nafcillin or oxacillin; oral dicloxacillin, cloxacillin, or oxacillin.
[9] Oral sulfisoxazole and trisulfapyrimidines are highly soluble in urine; parenteral sodium sulfadiazine can be injected intravenously in treating severely ill patients.
[10] Antipseudomonal penicillins: ticarcillin, carbenicillin, mezlocillin, azlocillin, pipericillin.
[11] First choice for previously untreated urinary tract infection is a highly soluble sulfonamide (see Note 9). TMP-SMZ (see Note 1) is acceptable.

in the infectious process, of which only one was originally detected and used for drug selection.

F. Adequate Dosage: Adequacy of therapy is usually assessed by a favorable clinical response. In most infections, either a bacteriostatic or a bactericidal agent can be used. In some infections (eg, infective endocarditis), it is mandatory to kill the infecting organism to achieve a cure, and proper choice of drug and dose can be judged by "serum assay." Two days after initiation of a drug regimen, serum is obtained from the patient 1–2 hours after a drug dose. Dilutions of this serum are inoculated with the organism originally isolated from the patient, and antibacterial activity is estimated. If an adequate dose of a proper drug is being given, the serum will be bactericidal in a dilution of 1:4 or more. When potentially toxic drugs (eg, aminoglycosides, vancomycin) are used, the serum levels of the drug should be measured to avoid toxicity and ensure appropriate dosage. In patients with altered clearance of drugs, the dose or frequency of administration must be adjusted. This can sometimes be done by reference to dosage nomograms or formulas, but it is best to measure levels directly and adjust therapy accordingly.

In renal failure, dosage must be adjusted as shown in Table 31–4.

G. Duration of Antimicrobial Therapy: Generally, effective antimicrobial treatment results in reversal of the clinical and laboratory parameters of active infection and marked clinical improvement. However, varying periods of treatment may be required for cure. This is influenced by such factors as (1) the type of infecting organism (bacterial infections can be cured more rapidly than fungal or mycobacterial ones), (2) the location of the process (eg, endocarditis and osteomyelitis require prolonged therapy), and (3) the immunocompetence of the patient.

The following examples are illustrative: Streptococcal pharyngitis requires 10 days of effective penicillin levels to eradicate the organism. Acute uncomplicated gonococcal urethritis can be cured in males in 24 hours. Endocarditis due to viridans streptococci is curable in 2–4 weeks; that caused by staphylococci requires 4–6 weeks of treatment. Acute uncomplicated cystitis in women often responds to a single dose of drug.

To minimize untoward reactions from drugs and the risk of superinfection, treatment should be continued only as long as needed to eradicate the infection.

H. Adverse Reactions: All antimicrobials can cause adverse effects. Most commonly these are (1) hypersensitivity reactions (eg, fever, rashes, anaphylaxis), (2) direct toxicity (eg, diarrhea, vomiting, impairment of renal or hepatic function, neurotoxicity), or (3) superinfection by drug-resistant microorganisms. Physicians prescribing antimicrobials must be familiar with the adverse effects associated with specific drugs.

Table 31-2. Initial antimicrobial therapy for acutely ill adults pending identification of causative organism.

Suspected Clinical Diagnosis	Likely Etiologic Agents	Drugs of Choice	Alternative Drugs
(a) Meningitis, bacterial	Pneumococcus, meningococcus	Penicillin G, 4 million units IV every 4 hours	Chloramphenicol, 0.5 g IV every 6 hours, or cefuroxime, 1.5 g IV every 6 hours, or cefotaxine,[2] 3 g IV every 6 hours
(b) Meningitis, postoperative or posttraumatic	*Staphylococcus aureus*, pneumococcus, gram-negative bacteria	Penicillin G as in (a) + nafcillin, 1.5 g IV every 4 hours, + gentamicin,[1] 1.7 mg/kg IV every 8 hours, + gentamicin,[1] 8 mg intrathecally once daily	Vancomycin, 10 mg/kg every 8 hours, + cefotaxime,[2] 3 g IV every 6 hours
(c) Brain abscess	Mixed anaerobes, pneumococci, streptococci	Penicillin G as in (a) + chloramphenicol as in (a) or metronidazole, 500 mg IV 3 times daily, + cefotaxine as in (a)	Metronidazole, 500 mg IV 3 times daily, + penicillin G as in (a)
(d) Pneumonia, acute, community-acquired, severe	Pneumococci, *Mycoplasma pneumoniae*	Erythromycin, 0.5 g orally or IV 4 times daily	Penicillin G, 1 million units IV every 4 hours
(e) Pneumonia, postoperative	*S aureus*, *Klebsiella*, mixed anaerobes	Nafcillin as in (b) + gentamicin[1] as in (b) + penicillin G as in (d)	Cefotaxime,[2] 2 g IV every 8–12 hours
(f) Pneumonia in chronic lung disease, aspiration	Pneumococci, *Haemophilus influenzae*, *S aureus*, mixed anaerobes	Ampicillin, 1 g IV every 6 hours, + nafcillin as in (b)	Cefuroxime,[2] 1.5 g IV every 8 hours
(g) Endocarditis, acute (including prosthetic or IV drug user)	*S aureus*, *Streptococcus faecalis*, gram-negative aerobic bacteria	Penicillin G as in (a) + nafcillin as in (b) + gentamicin[1] as in (b)	Gentamicin[1] as in (b) + vancomycin as in (b)
(h) Septic thrombophlebitis (eg, IV tubing, IV shunts)	*S aureus*, gram-negative aerobic bacteria	Nafcillin as in (b) + gentamicin[1] as in (b)	Vancomycin, 20–30 mg/kg/d in 2 or 3 divided doses, + gentamicin[1] as in (b)
(i) Osteomyelitis	*S aureus*	Nafcillin as in (b)	Vancomycin as in (b)
(j) Septic arthritis	*S aureus*, *Neisseria gonorrhoeae*	Ceftriaxone, 1 g IV daily	Nafcillin as in (b) + penicillin G as in (a)
(k) Urinary tract infection, first episode, community-acquired	*Escherichia coli*	Sulfisoxazole, 1 g orally 4 times daily for 1–3 days	Ampicillin, 0.5 g orally 4 times daily for 1–3 days
(l) Pyelonephritis with flank pain and fever (recurrent UTI)	*E coli*, *Klebsiella*, *Enterobacter*, *Pseudomonas*	Gentamicin[1] as in (b)	Cefotaxime as in (e)
(m) Suspected sepsis in neutropenic patient receiving cancer chemotherapy	*S aureus*, *Pseudomonas*, *Klebsiella*, *E coli*	Ticarcillin, 18 g IV daily, + tobramycin,[1] 1.7 mg/kg every 8 hours	Ceftazidime, 2 g IV every 8 hours, + vancomycin as in (b) + tobramycin
(n) Intra-abdominal sepsis (eg, postoperative, peritonitis, cholecystitis)	Gram-negative aerobic bacteria, *Bacteroides*, anaerobic bacteria, streptococci, clostridia	Ampicillin as in (f) + gentamicin[1] as in (b) + metronidazole as in (c)	Clindamycin, 600 mg IV every 8 hours, + gentamicin[1] as in (b)

[1] Depending on local drug susceptibility pattern, use tobramycin, 5–7 mg/kg/d, or amikacin, 15 mg/kg/d, in place of gentamicin.
[2] Cefotaxime, cefuroxime, ceftriaxone, ceftazidime, ceftizoxime, cefoperazone, or others, depending on local susceptibility patterns (see text).

When an adverse reaction develops, the physician must assess its severity and prognosis in the context of the infection being treated. If the infection is life-threatening and treatment cannot be stopped, the reactions may be managed symptomatically (especially if mild) or another drug may be chosen that does not cross-react with the offending one (Table 31–1). If the infection is less severe, it may be possible to stop all antimicrobials and follow the patient carefully.

I. Oral Antibiotics: Food does not significantly influence the bioavailability of most oral antibiotics. Exceptions include tetracycline and the quinolones, which are chelated by heavy metals and thus should be given between meals.

J. Intravenous Antibiotics: When an antibiotic must be administered intravenously (eg, for life-threatening infection or to sustain very high blood levels), the following cautions should be observed:

Table 31–3. Examples of empirical choices of antimicrobials for adult outpatient infections.

Suspected Clinical Diagnosis	Likely Etiologic Agents	Drug of Choice	Alternative Drugs
Erysipelas, impetigo, cellulitis, ascending lymphangitis	Group A streptococcus	Phenoxymethyl penicillin, 0.5 g orally 4 times daily	Erythromycin, 0.5 g orally 4 times daily, or cephalexin, 0.5 g orally 4 times daily for 7–10 days.
Furuncle with surrounding cellulitis	Staphylococcus aureus	Dicloxacillin, 0.5 g orally 4 times daily for 7–10 days	Cephalexin, 0.5 g orally 4 times daily for 7–10 days.
Pharyngitis	Group A streptococcus	Phenoxymethyl penicillin, 0.5 g orally 4 times daily for 10 days.	Erythromycin, 0.5 g orally 4 times daily for 10 days.
Otitis media	Streptococcus pneumoniae, Haemophilus influenzae, Branhamella catarrhalis	Ampicillin, 0.5 g orally 4 times daily; amoxicillin, 0.5 g orally 3 times daily; or TMP-SMZ,[1] 1 double-strength tablet twice daily for 10 days.	Augmentin,[2] 0.5 g orally 3 times daily; cefuroxime, 0.5 orally twice daily; cefixime, 0.2–0.4 g daily for 10 days
Acute sinusitis	S pneumoniae, H influenzae, B catarrhalis	Ampicillin, 0.5 g orally 4 times daily; amoxicillin, 0.5 g orally 3 times daily; or TMP-SMZ,[1] double-strength tablets twice daily for 10 days.	Augmentin,[2] 0.5 g orally 3 times daily; cefuroxime, 0.5 g orally twice daily; cefixime, 0.2–0.4 g daily for 10 days
Acute bronchitis	S pneumoniae, H influenzae	Tetracycline, 0.5 g orally 4 times daily; erythromycin, 0.5 g orally 4 times daily; ampicillin, 0.5 g orally 4 times daily.	TMP-SMZ,[1] 1 double-strength tablet twice daily for 10 days.
Aspiration pneumonia	Mixed oropharyngeal flora, including anaerobes	Phenoxymethyl penicillin, 0.5 g orally 4 times daily for 10–14 days.	Clindamycin, 0.35 g orally 4 times daily for 10–14 days.
Pneumonia	S pneumoniae, Mycoplasma pneumoniae, Legionella pneumophila	Erythromycin, 0.5 g orally 4 times daily for 10–14 days.	Phenoxymethyl penicillin, 0.5 g orally 4 times daily for 10 days.
Cystitis	Escherichia coli, Klebsiella pneumoniae, Proteus spp, Staphylococcus saprophyticus	Amoxacillin, 3 g as a single dose; TMP-SMZ,[1] double-strength, 2 tablets as a single dose; sulfasoxazole, 1 g orally 4 times daily for 1–3 days.	Ampicillin, 0.5 g orally 4 times daily for 1–3 days; TMP-SMZ,[1] 1 double-strength tablet twice daily for 1–3 days.
Pyelonephritis	E coli, K pneumoniae, Proteus spp, S saprophyticus	TMP-SMZ,[1] 1 double-strength tablet twice daily for 10 days.	Ampicillin, 0.5 g orally 4 times daily for 10 days.
Gastroenteritis	Salmonella, Shigella, Campylobacter, Entamoeba histolytica	See Note 3.	
Urethritis	Neisseria gonorrhoeae, Chlamydia trachomatis	Ceftriaxone, 125–250 mg IM once for N gonorrhoeae; tetracycline, 0.5 g orally 4 times daily for 7 days; or doxycycline, 100 mg twice daily for 7 days for C trachomatis.	Amoxicillin, 3 g orally with 1 g of probenecid orally as a single dose for N gonorrhoeae; erythromycin, 0.5 g orally 4 times daily for 7 days for C trachomatis.
Pelvic inflammatory disease	N gonorrhoeae, C trachomatis, anaerobes, gram-negative rods	Ceftriaxone, 125–250 mg IM once, followed by doxycycline, 100 mg orally twice daily for 10–14 days.	Cefoxitin, 2 g IM, with probenecid, 1 g orally, followed by doxycycline, 100 mg orally twice daily for 10–14 days.
Syphilis	Treponema pallidum		
Early syphilis (primary, secondary, or latent of less than 1 year's duration)		Benzathine penicillin G, 2–4 million units IM once.	Tetracycline, 0.5 g orally 4 times daily; or erythromycin, 0.5 g orally 4 times daily for 15 days.
Latent of more than 1 year's duration or cardiovascular syphilis		Benzathine penicillin G, 2.4 million units IM per week for 3 weeks.	Tetracycline, 0.5 g orally 4 times daily; or erythromycin, 0.5 g orally 4 times daily for 30 days.
Neurosyphilis		Aqueous penicillin G, 12–24 million units/d IV for 10 days; or procaine penicillin G, 2–4 million units/d IM, plus probenecid, 500 mg orally 4 times daily, both for 10 days.	Tetracycline, 0.5 g orally 4 times daily; or erythromycin, 0.5 g orally 4 times daily for 30 days.

[1] TMP-SMZ is a fixed combination of 1 part trimethoprim and 5 parts sulfamethoxazole. Single-strength tablets (ss): 80 mg TMP, 400 mg SMZ; double-strength tablets (ds): 160 mg TMP, 800 mg SMZ.
[2] Augmentin is a combination of amoxicillin, 250 mg or 500 mg, plus 125 mg of clavulanic acid.
[3] The diagnosis should be confirmed by culture before therapy. Salmonella gastroenteritis does not require therapy. For Shigella, give TMP-SMZ double-strength tablets twice daily for 5 days; or ampicillin, 0.5 g orally 4 times daily for 5 days; or ciprofloxacin, 0.5 orally twice daily for 5 days. For Campylobacter, give erythromycin, 0.5 g orally 4 times daily for 5 days; or ciprofloxacin, 0.5 g orally 4 times daily for 5 days. For E histolytica, give metronidazole, 750 mg orally 3 times daily for 5–10 days, followed by diiodohydroxyquin, 600 mg 3 times daily for 3 weeks.

Table 31–4. Use of antibiotics in patients with renal failure[1] and hepatic failure.

| | Principal Mode of Excretion or Detoxification | Approximate Half-Life in Serum | | Proposed Dosage Regimen in Renal Failure[2] | | | Removal of Drug by Hemodialysis | Dose after Hemodialysis | Dosage in Hepatic Failure |
		Normal	Renal Failure[2]	Initial Dose[3]	Maintenance Dose			
Penicillin G	Tubular secretion	0.5 hours	7–10 hours	1–2 million units	1 million units every 8 hours	Yes	500,000 units	No change
Ampicillin	Tubular secretion	0.5–1 hours	8–12 hours	1 g	1 g every 8–12 hours	Yes	1 g	No change
Carbenicillin	Tubular secretion	1 hour	16 hours	4 g	2 g every 12 hours	Yes	2 g	No change
Ticarcillin	Tubular secretion	1.1 hour	15–20 hours	3 g	2 g every 6–8 hours	Yes	1 g	No change
Azlocillin, mezlocillin, piperacillin	Renal, 50–70%; biliary, 20–30%	1 hour	3–6 hours	3 g	2 g every 6–8 hours	Yes	1 g	1–2 g every 8 hours
Nafcillin	Liver, 80%; kidney, 20%	0.75 hours	1.5 hours	1.5 g	1.5 g every 5 horus	No	None	1–1.5 g every 12 hours
Vancomycin	Glomerular filtration	6 hours	6–10 days	1 g	1 g every 6–10 days based on serum levels[4]	No	None	No change
Chloramphenicol	Mainly liver	3 hours	4 hours	0.5 g	0.5 g every 6 hours	Yes	0.5 g	0.25–0.5 g every 12 hours
Erythromycin	Mainly liver	1.5 hours	1.5 hours	0.5–1 g	0.5–1 g every 6 hours	No	None	0.25–0.5 g every 6 hours
Clindamycin	Liver	2–4 hours	2–4 hours	0.6 g IV	0.6 g every 8 hours	No	None	0.3–0.6 g every 8 hours
Trimethoprim-sulfamethoxazole	Some liver	TMP 10–12 hours; SMZ, 8–10 hours	TMP 24–48 hours; SMZ 18–24 hours	320 mg TMP + 1600 mg SMZ	80 mg TMP + 400 mg SMZ every 12 hours	Yes	80 mg TMP + 400 mg SMZ	No change
Metronidazole	Liver	6–10 hours	6–10 hours	0.5 g IV	0.5 g every 8 hours	Yes	0.25 g	0.25 g every 12 hours
Aztreonam	Renal	1.7 hours	6 hours	1–2 g	0.5–1 g every 6–8 hours	Yes	0.5–1 g	No change
Acyclovir	Renal	2.5–3.5 hours	20 hours	2.5 mg/kg	2.5 mg/kg every 24 hours	Yes	2.5 mg/kg	No change
Imipenem	Glomerular filtration	1 hour	3 hours	0.5 g	0.25–0.5 g every 12 hours	Yes	0.25–0.5 g	No change

[1] For cephalosporins, see text and Table 31–7; for aminoglycosides, see Table 31–8.
[2] Considered here to be marked by creatinine clearance of 10 mL/min or less.
[3] For a 70-kg adult with a serious systemic infection.
[4] When serum levels reach 5–10 μg/mL, another dose should be given.

(1) Give in neutral solution (pH 7.0–7.2) of sodium chloride (0.9%) or dextrose (5%) in water.

(2) Give alone without admixture of any other substance in order to avoid chemical and physical incompatibilities (which are frequent). Help from the clinical pharmacist will avoid physiologic incompatibilities, a few of which are mentioned in the discussions of individual drugs.

(3) Administer by intermittent (every 2–6 hours) addition to the intravenous infusion ("bolus injection") to avoid inactivation (by temperature, changing pH, etc) and prolonged vein irritation from high drug concentration, which favors thrombophlebitis.

(4) Peripheral infusion sites must be changed every 48–72 hours to reduce the chance of superinfection.

K. Cost of Antibiotics: Because of the widespread use of antibiotics, the cost of these agents can be substantial both to institutions and to individuals. Cost should not be the only determinant in choosing antibiotics, but if several drugs with equal efficacy and toxicity are available, one should choose the least expensive. Table 31–5 lists the cost of commonly used antibiotics.

Bennett WM et al: Drug prescribing in renal failure: Dosing guidelines for adults. Am J Kidney Dis 1983;3:155.

Calderwood SB, Moellering RC: Common adverse effects of antibacterial agents on major organ systems. Surg Clin North Am 1980;60:65.

Mills J, Barriere SL, Jawetz E: Clinical use of antimicrobials. Chapter 52 in: *Basic & Clinical Pharmacology*, 4th ed. Katzung BG (editor). Appleton & Lange, 1989.

Neu HC (guest editor): Impact of the patient at risk on current and future antimicrobial therapy. Am J Med 1984;76(No. 5A).

PENICILLINS

The penicillins are a large group of antimicrobial substances, all of which share a common chemical nucleus (6-aminopenicillanic acid) that contains a β-lactam ring essential to their biologic activity. All β-lactam antibiotics inhibit formation of microbial cell walls.

Penicillins fall into 4 major categories, discussed below.

Antimicrobial Action & Resistance

The initial step in penicillin action is the binding of the drug to receptors—penicillin-binding proteins—some of which are transpeptidation enzymes. The penicillin-binding proteins of different organisms differ in number and in affinity for a given drug. After penicillins have attached to receptors, peptidoglycan synthesis is inhibited because the activity of transpeptidation enzymes is blocked. The final bactericidal action is the removal of an inhibitor of the autolytic enzymes in the cell wall, which activates the enzymes and results in cell lysis. Organisms that are defective in autolysin function are inhibited but not killed by β-lactam antibiotics ("tolerance"). Organisms that produce β-lactamases (penicillinases) are resistant to some penicillins because the β-lactam ring is broken and the drug inactivated. Only organisms that are actively synthesizing peptidoglycan (in the process of multiplication) are susceptible to β-lactam antibiotics. Nonmultiplying organisms or those lacking cell walls (L forms) are not susceptible but may act as "persisters."

Microbial resistance to penicillins is caused by 4 factors:

1. Production of β-lactamases, eg, by staphylococci, gonococci, *Haemophilus* species, coliform organisms.

2. Lack of penicillin receptors (eg, resistant pneumococci) or impermeability of cell envelope, so that penicillins cannot reach receptors (eg, metabolically inactive bacteria).

3. Failure of activation of autolytic enzymes in the cell wall; "tolerance," eg, in staphylococci, group B streptococci.

4. The presence of cell wall-deficient (L) forms or mycoplasmas, which do not synthesize peptidoglycans.

1. NATURAL PENICILLINS

The natural penicillins include forms of penicillin G for parenteral administration (aqueous crystalline, procaine, and benzathine penicillin G) or for oral administration (penicillin G and phenoxymethyl penicillin [penicillin V]). They are most active against gram-positive organisms, less active against gram-negatives, and susceptible to hydrolysis by β-lactamases. They are used for infections caused by pneumococci, streptococci, meningococci, non-β-lactamase-producing staphylococci and gonococci, *Treponema pallidum* and other spirochetes, *Bacillus anthracis* and other gram-positive rods, clostridia, *Actinomyces,* and most anaerobes except β-lactamase-producing strains, eg, *Bacteroides fragilis* (Table 31–1).

Pharmacokinetics & Administration

While aqueous crystalline penicillin G can be given intramuscularly or intravenously, the intravenous route, by intermittent bolus injection or continuous infusion, is often preferred to avoid local pain. After parenteral administration, penicillin is widely distributed in tissues. An intravenous dose of 1 million units of penicillin G produces a peak serum level of 10 μg/mL. (One million units of penicillin G equals 0.6 g.) Levels equal to those in serum occur in many tissues, but lower levels prevail in the eye, prostate,

Table 31–5. Costs of antibiotics. (Based on costs at the University of California, San Francisco, 1990.)

	Unit Cost	Dose per Day[1]	Daily Cost of Therapy[2]
Intravenous			
Penicillin (1 million units)	$ 0.46	12 million units	$18.16 (q4h); $14.64 (q6h)
Ampicillin (2 g)	$ 0.93	100 mg/kg	$16.34 (q4h); $12.66 (q6h)
Nafcillin (2 g)	$ 2.22	100 mg/kg	$21.52 (q4h); $17.82 (q6h)
Vancomycin (0.5 g)	$ 6.50	25 mg/kg	$29.81 (q8h); $27.96 (q12h)
Clindamycin (0.6 g)	$ 6.89	2400 mg	$34.54 (q8h); $32.80 (q12h)
Metronidazole (0.5 g)	$ 1.48	30 mg/kg	$13.00 (q8h); $11.16 (q12h)
Ticarcillin (3 g)	$ 6.20	250 mg/kg	$49.84 (q4h); $46.14 (q6h)
Mezlocillin (3 g)	$ 7.80	250 mg/kg	$45.58 (q4h); $40.14 (q6h)
Pipericillin (3 g)	$ 7.20	250 mg/kg	$42.53 (q4h); $37.94 (q6h)
Cefazolin (1 g)	$ 1.70	50 mg/kg	$12.43 (q8h)
Cefuroxime (1.5 g)	$10.57	50 mg/kg	$28.23 (q8h) $26.38 (q12h)
Ciprofloxacin (0.5 g) (0.75 g)	$ 1.86 $ 3.54	Note[3] Note[3]	$ 3.72 $ 7.08
Cefoxitin (1 g)	$ 6.87	50 mg/kg	$36.42 (q6h); $27.70 (q8h)
Ceftizoxime (1 g)	$ 7.91	50–75 mg/kg	$37.33 (q8h); $35.58 (q12h)
Ceftazidime (1 g)	$11.17	50–75 mg/kg	$51.77 (q8h)
Aztreonam (1 g)	$ 9.56	50–75 mg/kg	$47.18 (q6h); $45.33 (q8h)
Imipenem (0.5 g)	$15.07	50 mg/kg	$129.50 (q6h); $127.65 (q8h)
Trimethoprim-sulfamethoxazole (0.32 g TMP in 20 mL)	$ 5.24	7.5–10 mg/kg TMP	$17.57 (q8h); $15.71 (q12h)
Gentamicin (80 mg)	$ 0.18	4.5 mg/kg	$ 8.17 (q8h)
Tobramycin (80 mg)	$ 5.21	4.5 mg/kg	$26.62 (q8h)
Amikacin (0.5 g)	$28.38	15 mg/kg	$63.85 (q8h)
Oral			
Phenoxymethyl penicillin (0.5 g)	$ 0.14	30 mg/kg	$ 0.56
Ampicillin (0.5 g)	$ 0.15	30 mg/kg	$ 0.60
Amoxicillin (0.5 g)	$ 0.25	30 mg/kg	$ 1.00
Augmentin (0.5 g amoxicillin plus 0.125 g clavulanic acid)	$ 1.45	30 mg/kg	$ 5.80

Table 31–5 (cont'd). Costs of antibiotics. (Based on costs at the University of California, San Francisco, 1989.)

	Unit Cost	Dose per Day[1]	Daily Cost of Therapy[2]
Trimethoprim-sulfamethoxazole (80 mg TMP and 400 mg SMZ)	$ 0.16	5 mg/kg TMP	$ 0.64
Cephalexin (0.5 g)	$ 1.10	30 mg/kg	$ 4.40
Cefaclor (0.5 g)	$ 2.35	30 mg/kg	$ 7.05
Cefixime (0.4 g)	$ 4.14	400 mg	$ 4.14
Cefuroxime axetil (0.5 g)	$ 3.71	15 mg/kg	$ 7.42
Tetracycline (0.5 g)	$ 0.06	30 mg/kg	$ 0.24
Ciprofloxacin[3] (0.5 g)	$ 1.86	See footnote 3	$ 3.72
(0.75 g)	$ 3.54	See footnote 3	$ 7.08
Doxycycline (0.1 g)	$ 1.34	3 mg/kg	$ 2.68

[1] Dose based on a 70-kg individual with normal renal function.
[2] Daily cost for intravenous antibiotics includes acquisition cost, preparation costs, and administration costs (including the cost of tubing, bags, and controllers).
[3] The dosage of ciprofloxacin is either 0.5 mg twice daily (total 1 g) or 0.75 mg twice daily (total 1.5 g).

and central nervous system. However, with acute inflammation of the meninges (eg, in bacterial meningitis), penicillin G levels in the cerebrospinal fluid exceed 0.2 μg/mL with a daily parenteral dose of 20 million units. This level is more than is required to kill sensitive pneumococci and meningococci. Consequently, systemically administered penicillin G is adequate to treat meningitis caused by these organisms.

Special dosage forms of penicillin permit delayed absorption to yield low blood and tissue levels for long periods, eg, benzathine penicillin G. After a single intramuscular injection of 1.2 million units (0.9 g), serum levels in excess of 0.02 μg/mL are maintained for 10 days and levels in excess of 0.004 μg/mL for 3 weeks. The latter is sufficient to protect against β-hemolytic streptococcal infection; the former, to treat an established infection with these organisms. Procaine penicillin also has delayed absorption. After intramuscular injection of 1–2 million units (1–2 g), serum levels of 0.1 μg/mL persist for 18–24 hours.

Phenoxymethyl penicillin (penicillin V) is the oral penicillin of choice. It is more acid-stable than oral penicillin G and gives higher serum levels. A 250-mg dose results in serum levels of 2–3 μg/mL.

Most of the absorbed penicillin is rapidly excreted by the kidneys into the urine; small amounts are excreted by other routes. About 10% of renal excretion is by glomerular filtration and 90% by tubular secretion. Tubular secretion can be partially blocked by probenecid (Benemid), 0.5 g (10 mg/kg) every 6 hours orally, to achieve higher systemic levels. Renal clearance is less efficient in the newborn. Individuals with impaired renal function likewise tend to maintain higher penicillin levels longer, and the dose should be reduced in moderate to severe renal failure. One commonly used formula for calculating the maximum daily dose of penicillin in millions of units in patients with a creatinine clearance of less than 40 mL/min is as follows (see also Table 31–4):

$$\text{Dosage} = 3.2 + \frac{\text{Creatinine clearance}}{7}$$

Renal excretion of penicillin results in very high levels in the urine. Thus, systemic daily doses of 10 million units (6 g) of penicillin may yield urine levels of 500–3000 μg/mL; this is enough to suppress not only gram-positive but also many gram-negative bacteria in the urine (provided they produce little β-lactamase).

Penicillin is also excreted into sputum and milk to levels of 3–15% of those present in the serum. This is the case in both humans and cattle. The presence of penicillin in the milk of cows treated for mastitis presents a problem for those who drink milk and are allergic to penicillin.

Clinical Uses

Most infections caused by organisms sensitive to penicillin will respond to aqueous penicillin G in daily doses of 0.6–5 million units (0.36–3 g) administered intramuscularly or intravenously every 4–6 hours. For severe or life-threatening infections (meningitis, endocarditis), much larger doses (10–24 million units) should be given by intermittent intravenous infusion every 2–4 hours.

Penicillin V is indicated only in minor infections such as mild respiratory infections, pharyngitis, and skin and soft tissue infections. The usual dose is 1–2 g/d.

A single injection of 1.2 million units of benzathine penicillin intramuscularly is satisfactory for treatment of β-hemolytic streptococcal pharyngitis. An injection of 1.2–2.4 million units every 3–4 weeks provides satisfactory prophylaxis for rheumatics against reinfection with group A streptococci. Syphilis can be treated with benzathine penicillin, 2.4 million units intramuscularly weekly for 1–3 weeks, depending on the stage of the disease (see Table 31–3).

Procaine penicillin is used primarily for treatment of uncomplicated pneumococcal pneumonia in a dose of 600,000 units twice a day and for treatment of uncomplicated penicillin-sensitive gonorrhea in a single intramuscular dose of 4.8 million units with 1 g of probenecid orally.

Penicillins should not be given intrathecally because they are neurotoxic and can cause seizures. Penicillins are highly sensitizing and should not be applied to the skin.

2. EXTENDED-SPECTRUM PENICILLINS

The extended-spectrum group of penicillins includes the aminopenicillins ampicillin and amoxicillin; the carboxypenicillins carbenicillin and ticarcillin; and the ureidopenicillins piperacillin, azlocillin, and mezlocillin. These drugs are all susceptible to destruction by staphylococcal (and other) β-lactamases. They tend to be active against many gram-negative rods but less active against gram-positive bacteria than the natural penicillins.

Antimicrobial Activity

Ampicillin and amoxicillin are active against most strains of *E coli*, *Proteus mirabilis*, *Salmonella*, *Listeria*, and non-β-lactamase-producing strains of *Haemophilus influenzae* but inactive against most strains of *Klebsiella*, *Pseudomonas*, *Serratia*, *Enterobacter*, and indole-positive *Proteus*. While these drugs are less active than penicillin in vitro against pneumococci

and streptococci, they are clinically effective in treating infections caused by these organisms. They are more active than penicillin G against enterococci.

Carbenicillin extends the activity of ampicillin to include many strains of *Pseudomonas*, *Enterobacter*, *Serratia*, and indole-positive *Proteus*, but it has poor activity against most strains of *Klebsiella*. Ticarcillin is similar to carbenicillin but is 2–4 times more active against *Pseudomonas*. Neither drug is effective against enterococci.

The ureidopenicillins are similar to carbenicillin and ticarcillin but exhibit slight differences in activity against gram-negative organisms. Piperacillin is more active than ticarcillin against *P aeruginosa* and *Klebsiella*, but otherwise its spectrum of activity is similar to that of ticarcillin. Mezlocillin is similar in activity to piperacillin but slightly less active against *P aeruginosa*. Azlocillin is as active as piperacillin against *P aeruginosa* but less active than the other ureidopenicillins against most other gram-negative organisms.

The extended-spectrum penicillins are active against most anaerobes. Ampicillin and amoxicillin are not active against β-lactamase-producing strains of *Bacteroides fragilis*—in contrast to the other drugs in this class at high concentrations.

Pharmacokinetics & Administration

Ampicillin can be given orally or parenterally. The usual oral dose is 1–2 g/d (15–50 mg/kg/d), resulting in serum levels of 4–6 μg/mL. Intravenous doses range from 20 to 200 mg/kg/d (the higher doses required in meningitis), resulting in serum levels of up to 40 μg/mL. Amoxicillin is given orally only, in doses of 25–100 mg/kg/d, usually as 250- or 500-mg tablets 3 times daily, and is absorbed better than ampicillin, resulting in serum levels twice as high as those achieved with ampicillin. Bacampicillin, an esterified form of ampicillin that is hydrolyzed to release ampicillin, is well absorbed and can be given twice daily in a dose of 400–800 mg.

Carbenicillin is given intravenously (400–500 mg/kg/d) in doses of 5 g every 4 hours. The other carboxy- and ureidopenicillins are given intravenously (200–300 mg/kg/d) in doses of 3–4 g every 4–6 hours, resulting in serum levels of 250–300 μg/mL. Oral indanyl sodium carbenicillin is suitable only for treatment of urinary tract infections in a dose of 1–2 tablets (382 mg per tablet) every 6 hours.

Dosage adjustments in renal failure are required for the extended-spectrum penicillins and are summarized in Table 31–4.

Clinical Uses

Ampicillin is given orally for minor infections, such as bronchitis, sinusitis, otitis, or urinary tract infections. It is given intravenously for pneumonia, meningitis, bacteremia, or endocarditis. In meningitis in the neonate or elderly, ampicillin is given concurrently with a second- or third-generation cephalosporin to cover *Listeria*. For *Haemophilus influenzae* infections, ampicillin is given concurrently with chloramphenicol or a third-generation cephalosporin until β-lactamase production can be excluded by laboratory test. Typhoid or paratyphoid fever, caused by susceptible *Salmonella* species is treated with ampicillin, 6–12 g/d intravenously. *Shigella* dysentery can be treated with oral ampicillin. Uncomplicated gonorrhea due to non-β-lactamase-producing strains of *Neisseria gonorrhoeae* responds to a single oral dose of 3.5 g of ampicillin with 1 g of probenecid.

Amoxicillin is frequently used for urinary tract infections, sinusitis, otitis, bronchitis, and uncomplicated gonorrhea (a single dose of 3 g with probenecid). Because of its better absorption from the intestinal tract, less drug remains in the intestine, and amoxicillin is thus less effective than ampicillin for shigellosis. Carbenicillin is rarely used because of its large sodium load and the coagulation abnormalities that have been associated with its use. Although ticarcillin, mezlocillin, azlocillin, and piperacillin have been used as single drugs, they are commonly used in combination with an aminoglycoside to treat serious infections and as empiric therapy in the febrile neutropenic patient.

3. PENICILLINS COMBINED WITH BETA-LACTAMASE INHIBITORS

The addition of β-lactamase inhibitors (clavulanic acid, sulbactam) can prevent inactivation of the parent penicillin by bacterial β-lactamases. Augmentin (amoxicillin, 250 mg or 500 mg, plus 125 mg of clavulanic acid), Timentin (ticarcillin, 3 g, plus 100 mg of clavulanic acid), and Unasyn (ampicillin, 1 g, plus 500 mg of sulbactam) are available. Augmentin is given orally and the others intravenously. In general, the β-lactamase inhibitors effectively inactivate β-lactamases produced by anaerobes, *Staphylococcus aureus, Haemophilus influenzae, Branhamella catarrhalis,* and *Neisseria gonorrhoeae* but are variably and unpredictably effective against β-lactamases produced by aerobic enteric gram-negative rods and pseudomonads.

Augmentin, because of its high cost, is used to treat refractory cases of sinusitis and otitis that have not responded to less costly agents and may be useful in animal and human bites. The roles of Timentin and Unasyn are not well defined at present. One possible application of these agents would be to use them alone or in combination with an aminoglycoside to treat polymicrobial infections such as peritonitis from a ruptured viscus, osteomyelitis in a diabetic patient, or traumatic osteomyelitis.

The dosage regimens of these drugs are the same as those of the parent drugs.

4. PENICILLINASE-RESISTANT PENICILLINS

Methicillin, oxacillin, cloxacillin, dicloxacillin, nafcillin, and others are relatively resistant to destruction by β-lactamases produced by staphylococci and are limited to the treatment of infections with such organisms. They are less active than natural penicillins against gram-positives and inactive against gram-negatives.

Oxacillin, cloxacillin, dicloxacillin, and nafcillin are given orally in doses of 0.25–0.5 g every 4–6 hours in mild or localized staphylococcal infections (50–100 mg/kg/d for children).

For serious systemic staphylococcal infections, nafcillin, 6–12 g/d, is given intravenously in 4–6 divided doses (50–100 mg/kg/d for children). Eighty percent of administered nafcillin is excreted into the biliary tract and only 20% by tubular secretion. Thus, the action and dose of nafcillin are little affected by renal failure.

5. ADVERSE EFFECTS OF PENICILLINS

The penicillins undoubtedly possess less direct toxicity than other antibiotics. Most of the serious side effects are due to hypersensitivity.

Allergy

All penicillins are cross-sensitizing and cross-reacting. Any preparation containing penicillin may induce sensitization, including foods or cosmetics. In general, sensitization occurs in proportion to the duration and total dose of penicillin received in the past. The responsible antigenic determinants appear to be degradation products of penicillins, particularly penicilloic acid and products of alkaline hydrolysis (minor antigenic determinants) bound to host protein. Skin tests with penicilloyl-polylysine, with minor antigenic determinants, and with undegraded penicillin can identify most hypersensitive individuals. Among positive reactors to skin tests, the incidence of subsequent immediate severe penicillin reactions is high. Although many persons develop IgG antibodies to antigenic determinants of penicillin, the presence of such antibodies is not correlated with allergic reactivity (except for rare instances of hemolytic anemia), and serologic tests have little predictive value. A history of a penicillin reaction in the past is not reliable. Only one-fourth of patients with a history of penicillin allergy have an adverse reaction when challenged with the drug. The decision to administer penicillin or related drugs (other β-lactams) to patients with an allergic history depends upon the severity of the reported reaction, the severity of the infection being treated, and the availability of alternative drugs. For patients with a history of severe reaction (anaphylaxis), alternative drugs should be used. In the rare situations when there is a strong indication for using penicillin (eg, syphilis in pregnancy) despite a history of severe reaction, desensitization can be attempted. If the history is unclear or the reaction mild (rash), the patient may be rechallenged with penicillin or may be given another β-lactam antibiotic.

Allergic reactions may occur as typical anaphylactic shock, typical serum sickness type reactions (urticaria, fever, joint swelling, angioneurotic edema, intense pruritus, and respiratory embarrassment occurring 7–12 days after exposure), and a variety of skin rashes, oral lesions, fever, interstitial nephritis, eosinophilia, hemolytic anemia, other hematologic disturbances, and vasculitis. The incidence of hypersensitivity to penicillin is estimated to be 1–5% among adults in the USA but is negligible in small children. Acute anaphylactic life-threatening reactions are fortunately very rare (0.05%). Ampicillin produces maculopapular skin rashes more frequently than other penicillins, but some ampicillin rashes are not allergic in origin. Methicillin and other penicillins can induce nephritis with primary tubular lesions associated with anti-basement membrane antibodies. Nafcillin is less nephrotoxic than methicillin.

Individuals known to be hypersensitive to penicillin can at times tolerate the drug during corticosteroid administration.

Toxicity

Since the action of penicillin is directed against a unique bacterial structure, the cell wall, it is virtually without effect on animal cells. The toxic effects of penicillin G are due to the direct irritation caused by intramuscular or intravenous injection of exceedingly high concentrations (eg, 1 g/mL). Such concentrations may cause local pain, induration, thrombophlebitis, or degeneration of an accidentally injected nerve. All penicillins are irritating to the central nervous system. There is no indication for intrathecal administration at present. In rare cases, a patient with renal insufficiency receiving large doses may exhibit signs of cerebrocortical irritation as a result of passage of unusually large amounts of penicillin into the central nervous system. With doses of this magnitude, direct cation toxicity (Na^+, K^+) can also occur. Potassium penicillin G contains 1.7 meq of K^+ per million units (2.8 meq/g), and potassium may accumulate in renal failure. Carbenicillin contains 4.7 meq of Na^+ per gram—a risk in heart failure.

Large doses of penicillins given orally may lead to gastrointestinal upset, particularly nausea and diarrhea. This is most pronounced with the broad-spectrum penicillins—ampicillin or amoxicillin—and may be due to overgrowth of staphylococci, *Pseudomonas*, clostridia, or yeasts or to toxin production by *C difficile*. Superinfections in other organ systems may occur with penicillins as with any other antibiotic. Methicillin, nafcillin, and carbenicillin can cause granulocy-

topenia. Carbenicillin and ticarcillin can produce hypokalemic alkalosis and elevation of serum transaminases and can damage platelets or induce hemostatic defects leading to bleeding tendency.

Donowitz GR, Mandell GL: Beta-lactam antibiotics. (2 parts.) N Engl J Med 1988;318:419, 490.

Eliopoulos GM, Moellering RC: Azlocillin, mezlocillin, and piperacillin: New broad-spectrum penicillins. Ann Intern Med 1982;97:755.

Parker CW: Drug allergy. (3 parts.) N Engl J Med 1975;292:511, 732, 957.

Wendel GD et al: Penicillin allergy and desensitization in serious infections during pregnancy. N Engl J Med 1985;312:1229.

Wright AJ, Wilkowske CJ: The penicillins. Mayo Clin Proc 1987;62:806.

CEPHALOSPORINS (Tables 31–6 and 31–7)

The cephalosporins are structurally related to the penicillins. They consist of a β-lactam ring attached to a dihydrothiazoline ring. Substitutions of chemical groups at various positions on the basic structure have resulted in a proliferation of drugs with varying pharmacologic properties and antimicrobial activities.

The mechanism of action of cephalosporins is analogous to that of the penicillins: (1) binding to specific penicillin-binding proteins that serve as drug receptors on bacteria, (2) inhibition of cell wall synthesis, and (3) activation of autolytic enzymes in the cell wall that result in bacterial death. Resistance to cephalosporins may be due to poor permeability of the drug into bacteria, lack of penicillin-binding proteins, or degradation by β-lactamases.

Cephalosporins have been divided into 3 major groups or "generations" (Table 31–6) based mainly on their antibacterial activity: First-generation cephalosporins have good activity against aerobic gram-positive organisms and many community-acquired gram-negative organisms; second-generation drugs have a slightly extended spectrum against gram-negative bacteria, and some are active against anaerobes;

Table 31–6. Major groups of cephalosporins.

First Generation	Second Generation	Third Generation
Cephalothin	Cefamandole	Cefotaxime
Cephapirin	Cefuroxime	Ceftizoxime
Cefazolin	Cefonicid	Ceftriaxone
Cefalexin[1]	Ceforanide	Ceftazidime
Cephradine[1]	Cefaclor[1]	Cefoperazone
Cefadroxil[1]	Cefoxitin	Moxalactam
	Cefotetan	Cefixime[1]
	Cefuroxime axetil[1]	
	Cefmetazole	

[1] Oral agents.

Table 31–7. Pharmacology of the cephalosporins.

Drug	Peak Serum Level (μg/mL) After 1 g IV	Serum Half-Life (min)	Total Daily Dose (mg/kg)	Dosage Interval (hours)	Dosage Adjustments in Renal Failure		
					Moderate (Cl$_{cr}$ 10–50 mL/min)	Severe (Cl$_{cr}$ < 10 mL/min)	Post-hemodialysis Dose
Cephalothin, cephapirin	40–60	40	50–200	4–6	1–2 g every 6–12 hours	1 g every 12 hours	1 g
Cefazolin	90–120	90	25–100	8	0.5–1 g every 12 hours	0.5 g daily	0.5 g
Cephalexin, cephradine[1]	15–20	50–60	15–30	6	0.25–0.5 g every 8–12 hours	0.25–0.5 g daily	0.5 g
Cefadroxil[1]	15	75	15–30	12–24	1 g daily	0.5 g daily	0.5 g
Cefamandole	60–80	45	75–200	6–8	1 g every 12 hours	1–2 g daily	0.5 g
Cefuroxime	80–100	80	50	6–12	1 g every 12 hours	1–2 g daily	0.5 g
Cefuroxime axetil[1]	6–8	75	5–15	12	0.5 g every 24 hours	0.25 g daily	0.25 g
Cefonicid	200–250	240	15–30	24	0.5 g daily	1 g every 72 hours	0.25 g
Ceforanide	125	180	15–30	12	1 g daily	1 g every 48 hours	0.25 g
Cefaclor[1]	15–20	50	20–40 children, 10–15 adults	6–8	0.5 g every 8–12 hours	0.25–0.5 g every 12–24 hours	0.25–0.5 g
Cefixime[1]	3–5	180–240	8 (with maximum of 0.4 g/d total)	12–24	0.4 g daily	0.1 g daily	None
Cefotetan	60–80	150	50–100	8–12	1 g every 8–12 hours	0.5–1 g daily	0.5 g
Cefotaxime	40–60	60	50–75	6–8	1–2 g every 6–8 hours	1–2 g every 12 hours	1–2 g
Cefoxitin	60–80	60	50–100	6–8	1 g every 12 hours	1–2 g daily	0.5 g
Cefmetazole	70–100	60–80	50–100	6–8	1–2 g every 12–24 hours	1–2 g every 24–48 hours	1 g
Ceftizoxime	80–100	100	5–75	8–12	0.5–1 g every 8–12 hours	0.25–0.5 g every 12–24 hours	0.5 g
Ceftriaxone	150	480	30–50	12–24	1–2 g daily	1–2 g daily	None
Ceftazidime	100–120	120	50–75	8–12	1 g every 8–12 hours	0.5–1 g daily	0.5 g
Cefoperazone	150	120	30–200	8–12	1–2 g every 12 hours	1–2 g every 12 hours	None
Moxalactam	60–100	120	50–200	6–12	0.5–1 g every 12 hours	0.25–0.5 g every 12 hours	0.5 g

[1] Oral agents. Serum levels based on 0.5 g oral dose.

and third-generation cephalosporins have less activity against gram-positives but are extremely active against most gram-negative bacteria. Not all cephalosporins fit neatly into this grouping, and there are exceptions to the general characterization of the drugs in the individual classes; however, the generational classification of cephalosporins is useful for discussion purposes.

Both parenteral and oral cephalosporins—especially second- and third-generation agents—are quite costly (Table 31–5). Because of their broad spectrum of activity and low toxicity, these drugs are used to treat many infections. As discussed below, cephalosporins are rarely the drug of first choice (see Tables 31–2 and 31–3), but they are useful in certain specific

clinical settings. Because of their cost, their broad spectrum of activity, and concerns about selecting for resistant organisms, the use of cephalosporins should be limited to those situations in which clear-cut superiority over less expensive drugs with more narrow spectrums of activity has been demonstrated.

1. FIRST-GENERATION CEPHALOSPORINS

Antimicrobial Activity

These drugs are very active against gram-positive cocci, including pneumococci, viridans streptococci, group A hemolytic streptococci, and *S aureus*. Like all cephalosporins, they are inactive against enterococci and methicillin-resistant staphylococci. Among gram-negative bacteria, *E coli, K pneumoniae,* and *P mirabilis* are usually sensitive except for some hospital-acquired strains. There is very little activity against such gram-negatives as *P aeruginosa,* indole-positive *Proteus* sp, *Enterobacter* spp, *Serratia marcescens, Citrobacter* spp, and *Acinetobacter* spp. Anaerobic cocci are usually sensitive, but *Bacteroides fragilis* is not.

Pharmacokinetics & Administration

A. Oral: Cephalexin, cephradine, and cefadroxil are variably absorbed from the gut. Urine levels of these drugs are several hundred times higher than serum levels, but concentrations in other tissues are variable and usually lower than in the serum. Cefadroxil, because of its longer half-life, can be given twice daily. Dosage adjustment is required in renal insufficiency.

B. Intravenous: Cefazolin is preferred over cephalothin and cephapirin because it has a longer half-life, requires less frequent dosing, and achieves higher serum levels. In renal insufficiency, all of these agents require dosage adjustments.

C. Intramuscular: Both cephapirin and cefazolin can be given intramuscularly, but pain on injection is less with cefazolin.

Clinical Uses

Although the first-generation cephalosporins have a broad spectrum of activity and are relatively nontoxic, they are rarely the drugs of choice. Oral drugs are indicated for treatment of urogenital infections in patients who are allergic to sulfonamides or penicillins, and they can be used for minor staphylococcal infections in penicillin-allergic patients. Oral cephalosporins may also be preferred for minor polymicrobial infections (eg, cellulitis, soft tissue abscess). Oral cephalosporins should not be relied on in serious systemic infections.

Intravenous first-generation cephalosporins penetrate most tissues well and are the drugs of choice for surgical prophylaxis, particularly surgery undertaken for placement of a prosthesis. More expensive second- and third-generation cephalosporins offer no advantage over the first-generation drugs for surgical prophylaxis and should not be used for that purpose.

Other major uses of intravenous first-generation cephalosporins include infections for which they are the least toxic drugs (eg, *Klebsiella* infections) and infections in persons with a history of *mild* penicillin allergy (not anaphylaxis).

First-generation cephalosporins do not penetrate the cerebrospinal fluid and cannot be used to treat meningitis.

2. SECOND-GENERATION CEPHALOSPORINS

Second-generation cephalosporins are a heterogeneous group with marked individual differences in activity, pharmacokinetics, and toxicity. In general, all are active against organisms also covered by first-generation drugs, but they have an extended gram-negative coverage. *Enterobacter* spp, indole-positive *Proteus,* and *Klebsiella* spp (including cephalothin-resistant strains) are usually sensitive. Cefamandole, cefuroxime, cefonicid, ceforanide, cefuroxime axetil, and cefaclor are active against *H influenzae,* including β-lactamase-producing strains but have little activity against *Serratia* and *B fragilis*. In contrast, cefoxitin and cefotetan are active against *B fragilis* and some strains of *Serratia* but have poor activity against *Enterobacter* and *H influenzae*. Cefmetazole is similar in activity to cefoxitin and cefotetan but has more activity against *H influenzae*. Against gram-positive organisms, these drugs are less active than the first-generation cephalosporins. Like the latter, second-generation drugs have no activity against *P aeruginosa* or enterococci.

Pharmacokinetics & Administration

A. Oral: Only cefaclor and cefuroxime axetil can be given orally. Cefaclor is available as capsules (0.25 or 0.5 g) and in suspension (0.125 or 0.25 g/5 mL). Cefuroxime axetil releases cefuroxime after absorption. Its longer half-life permits twice-daily dosing. It is available only in tablet form, and absorption is enhanced when it is taken with food (as is not the case with many other oral antibiotics).

B. Intravenous and Intramuscular: Because of differences in drug half-life and protein binding, peak serum levels achieved and dosing intervals vary greatly for this group of drugs (Table 31–7). Drugs with shorter half-lives (cefoxitin, cefamandole) require higher doses and more frequent dosing than drugs with longer half-lives (cefuroxime, cefonicid, ceforanide, cefotetan). Dosage adjustments are required with renal impairment.

Clinical Uses

Because of their activity against β-lactamase-producing *H influenzae* and *B catarrhalis,* cefaclor and cefuroxime axetil can be used to treat sinusitis and otitis media in patients who are allergic to ampicillin or amoxicillin or have not responded to treatment with those drugs. Cefuroxime is the only second-generation cephalosporin that crosses the blood-brain barrier in sufficient amounts to be useful for treatment of meningitis. It is often used to treat serious *H influenzae* infections, including meningitis. For meningitis in neonates, it should be combined with ampicillin to cover possible *Listeria monocytogenes* infections and should be given every 6 hours.

Because of their activity against *B fragilis,* cefoxitin, cefmetazole, and cefotetan can be used to treat mixed anaerobic infections, eg, peritonitis and diverticulitis. Cefonicid and ceforanide have been promoted for use in surgical prophylaxis, but there is no evidence that they are more effective than first-generation cephalosporins, and they tend to be more expensive. Cefamandole, like cefuroxime, may be useful for the treatment of community-acquired pneumonia, but it has few other uses.

3. THIRD-GENERATION CEPHALOSPORINS

Antimicrobial Activity

These drugs are active against staphylococci (not methicillin-resistant strains) but less so than first-generation cephalosporins. They have no activity against enterococci but do inhibit nonenterococcal streptococci. A major advantage of these cephalosporins is their expanded gram-negative coverage. In addition to organisms inhibited by other cephalosporins, they are consistently active against *Enterobacter* spp, *Citrobacter freundii, Serratia marcescens, Providencia* spp, *Haemophilus* spp, and *Neisseria* spp, including β-lactamase-producing strains. Two drugs—ceftazidime and cefoperazone—have good activity against *P aeruginosa,* whereas the others inhibit only 40–60% of strains. *Listeria* spp, *Acinetobacter* spp, and non-aeruginosa strains of *Pseudomonas* are variably sensitive to third-generation cephalosporins. Activity against *B fragilis* is variable, and these agents should not be relied upon to treat serious infections by this organism.

Cefixime, the only oral agent in this group, is more active than cefuroxime axetil but is not as active as parenteral third-generation cephalosporins against gram-negative organisms such as *Pseudomonas, Enterobacter* spp, *Morganella,* and *Serratia marcescens.* It has very poor activity against *S aureus* and *S epidermidis* and, like other members of this class, is inactive against enterococci and *L monocytogenes.*

Pharmacokinetics & Administration

These agents penetrate well into body fluids and tissues and—except for cefoperazone—reach levels in the cerebrospinal fluid that exceed those needed to inhibit most pathogens, including gram-negative rods. The half-lives of these drugs are variable, which accounts for the differences in dosing intervals (Table 31–7). Cefoperazone and ceftriaxone are eliminated primarily by biliary excretion, and no dosage adjustment is required in renal insufficiency. The other drugs are eliminated by the kidney and thus require dosage adjustments in renal insufficiency.

Clinical Uses

Because of their penetration into the cerebrospinal fluid, third-generation cephalosporins—except cefoperazone—can be used to treat meningitis. Meningitis due to pneumococci, meningococci, *H influenzae,* and susceptible enteric gram-negative rods has been successfully treated. In neonatal meningitis, third-generation cephalosporins should be combined with ampicillin until *L monocytogenes* has been excluded as the etiologic agent. Because of the high minimum inhibitory concentration of third-generation cephalosporins against *Pseudomonas,* these drugs are not recommended in meningitis caused by this organism. The dosage for meningitis should be near the top of the recommended range, because cerebrospinal fluid levels of these drugs are only 10–20% of serum levels.

Apart from meningitis, other potential indications include (1) infections in which cephalosporins are the least toxic agent available; (2) sepsis of unknown cause in the immunocompetent patient; and (3) fever in the immunocompromised neutropenic patient, in which case the drug should be given in combination with an aminoglycoside.

Cefixime, because of its long half-life, can be given once daily. For improved compliance, this may be advantageous in treating sinusitis and otitis in children.

Because of the high cost of third-generation cephalosporins, their use should be limited. When they are used empirically, therapy can be changed to the most efficacious, least toxic, and least expensive drug once the etiologic agent has been identified.

Barriere SL, Flaherty JF: Third-generation cephalosporins: A critical evaluation. Clin Pharmacol 1984;3:351.

Donowitz GR, Mandell GL: Beta-lactam antibiotics. (2 parts.) N Engl J Med 1988;318:419, 490.

Mandell GL, Douglas G, Bennett JE: Cephalosporins. Chapter 18, pp 180–187, in: *Principles and Practice of Infectious Diseases,* 3rd ed. Wiley, 1985.

Neu HC: New antibiotics: Areas of appropriate use. J Infect Dis 1987;155:403.

ADVERSE EFFECTS OF CEPHALOSPORINS

Allergy

Cephalosporins are sensitizing, and a variety of hypersensitivity reactions occur, including anaphylaxis, fever, skin rashes, nephritis, granulocytopenia, and hemolytic anemia. The frequency of cross-allergy between cephalosporins and penicillins is not known but is estimated to be about 6–10%. Persons with a history of anaphylaxis to penicillins should not receive cephalosporins.

Toxicity

Local pain can occur after intramuscular injection, or thrombophlebitis after intravenous injection. Hypoprothrombinemia is a frequent adverse effect (40–68%) of cephalosporins that have a methylthio-tetrazole group (eg, cefamandole, moxalactam, cefmetazole, cefoperazone, cefotetan). Prophylactic administration of vitamin K, 10 mg twice weekly, can prevent this complication. Moxalactam interferes with platelet function and has been associated with severe bleeding. Drugs containing the methylthiotetrazole ring can also cause severe disulfiramlike reactions, and use of alcohol or medications containing alcohol (eg, theophylline) must be avoided.

Superinfection

Many newer cephalosporins have little activity against gram-positive organisms, particularly staphylococci and enterococci. Superinfection with these organisms—as well as with fungi—may occur.

NEW BETA-LACTAM DRUGS

Monobactams

These are drugs with a monocyclic β-lactam ring that are resistant to β-lactamases and active against gram-negative organisms (including *Pseudomonas*) but have no activity against gram-positive organisms or anaerobes. Aztreonam resembles aminoglycosides in activity. The usual dose is 1–2 g intravenously every 6–8 hours, providing peak serum levels of 100 μg/mL. Clinical uses of aztreonam are limited because of the availability of third-generation cephalosporins with a broader spectrum of activity and minimal toxicity. Despite the structural similarity of aztreonam to other β-lactam drugs, it does not appear to cross-react with them. Thus, it can be used in patients with penicillin allergy.

Carbapenems

This new class of drugs is structurally related to β-lactam antibiotics. Imipenem, the first drug of this type, has a wide spectrum with good activity against many gram-negative rods (including *P aeruginosa*) and gram-positive organisms and anaerobes, with the exception of *Pseudomonas cepacia, Pseudomonas maltophilia, S faecium,* and most methicillin-resistant *S aureus* and *S epidermidis.* It is resistant to β-lactamases but is inactivated by dipeptidases in renal tubules. Consequently, it must be combined with cilastatin, a dipeptidase inhibitor, for clinical use.

The half-life of imipenem is 1 hour. Penetration into body tissues and fluids, including the cerebrospinal fluid, is good. The usual dose is 0.5–1 g intravenously every 6 hours. Dosage adjustment is required in renal insufficiency. For patients with creatinine clearances of 10–30 mL/min, one-half the usual dose is given; for those with clearances of 10 mL/min, 0.5 g is given every 12 hours. An additional dose is given after hemodialysis.

The role of imipenem in therapy has not been defined. Because of its high cost and broad spectrum of activity, it should not be routinely used as first-line therapy unless the organism causing infection is multidrug-resistant and is known to be sensitive to imipenem. *Pseudomonas* may rapidly develop resistance to imipenem. The use of imipenem alone or in combination with an aminoglycoside in febrile neutropenic patients is under investigation.

The most common adverse effects of imipenem are nausea, vomiting, diarrhea, reactions at the infusion site, and skin rashes. Seizures can occur, especially in patients with impaired renal function. Patients allergic to penicillins may be allergic to imipenem as well.

Barriere SL, Flaherty JF: Third-generation cephalosporins: A critical evaluation. Clin Pharm 1984;3:351.

Mandell GL, Douglas G, Bennett JE: Chapter 18, p 180, in: *Principles and Practice of Infectious Diseases,* 3rd ed. Wiley, 1985.

Neu HC: New antibiotics: Areas of appropriate use. J Infect Dis 1987;155:403.

Neu HC (editor): Advances in cephalosporin therapy: Beyond the third generation. Am J Med 1985;79(Suppl 2A):1.

Remington JS (editor): Carbapenems: A new class of antibiotics. Am J Med 1985;78(Suppl 6A):1.

ERYTHROMYCIN GROUP (Macrolides)

The erythromycins are a group of closely related compounds characterized by a macrocyclic lactone ring to which various sugars are attached.

Antimicrobial Activity

Erythromycins inhibit protein synthesis by binding to the 50S subunit of bacterial ribosomes. They are bacteriostatic or bactericidal for gram-positive organisms, including pneumococci, streptococci, and corynebacteria in a concentration of 0.02–2 μg/mL. Chlamydiae, mycoplasmas, *Legionella,* and *Campylobacter* are also susceptible. There is complete cross-resistance among all members of the group. Activity is enhanced at alkaline pH.

Pharmacokinetics & Administration

Preparations for oral use include erythromycin base, erythromycin stearate, estolate, and ethyl succinate. The base is most acid-stable and the estolate is the best-absorbed of the oral forms. Clinically, however, none of the oral preparations have any advantage over others. The usual adult oral dose is 250–500 mg 4 times daily (for children, 40 mg/kg/d), resulting in serum levels of 1–2 μg/mL. Erythromycins are excreted largely in the bile; only 5% is excreted in the urine, and no adjustment is therefore required in renal failure.

Erythromycin lactobionate and gluceptate are available for intravenous use. The usual dose is 250–500 mg every 6 hours, but larger doses (1 g every 6 hours) are used initially in the treatment of legionnaires' disease.

Clinical Uses

Erythromycins are drugs of choice for infections caused by *Legionella, Mycoplasma, Corynebacterium* (including diphtheria and bacteremia), and *Chlamydia* (including ocular, respiratory, and genital infections). They are effective in streptococcal and pneumococcal disease and for endocarditis prophylaxis in dental procedures in penicillin-allergic patients. They can also be used in combination with sulfisoxazole for acute otitis media; with neomycin in prophylaxis for bowel surgery; and for therapy of syphilis in penicillin-allergic patients. When administered early, erythromycin may shorten the course of *Campylobacter* enteritis. Spiramycin may be useful in treating acute toxoplasmosis in pregnant women in the first trimester and congenital toxoplasmosis.

Adverse Effects

Nausea, vomiting, and diarrhea may occur after oral intake. Erythromycins—particularly the estolate—can produce acute cholestatic hepatitis (fever, jaundice, impaired liver function), probably as a hypersensitivity reaction. Most patients recover, but hepatitis recurs if the drug is readministered. Erythromycins can increase the effects of oral anticoagulants and of digoxin.

Wilson WR, Cockerill FR III: Tetracyclines, chloramphenicol, erythromycin, and clindamycin. Mayo Clin Proc 1987;62:906.

TETRACYCLINE GROUP

The tetracyclines are a large group of drugs with common basic chemical structures, antimicrobial activity, and pharmacologic properties. Microorganisms resistant to this group show extensive cross-resistance to all tetracyclines.

Antimicrobial Activity

Tetracyclines are inhibitors of protein synthesis and are bacteriostatic for many gram-positive and gram-negative bacteria. They are strongly inhibitory for the growth of mycoplasmas, rickettsiae, chlamydiae, spirochetes, and some protozoa (eg, amebas). Equal concentrations of all tetracyclines in blood or tissue have approximately equal antimicrobial activity. However, there are great differences in the susceptibility of different strains of a given species of microorganism, and laboratory tests are therefore important. Because of the emergence of resistant strains, tetracyclines have lost some of their former usefulness. *Proteus* and *Pseudomonas* are regularly resistant; among coliform bacteria, *Bacteroides,* pneumococci, staphylococci, streptococci, shigellae, and vibrios, strains resistant to tetracyclines are increasingly common.

Pharmacokinetics & Administration

Tetracyclines are absorbed irregularly from the gut. Absorption is impaired by dairy products, aluminum hydroxide gels (antacids), and chelation with divalent cations, eg, Ca^{2+} or Fe^{2+}. Absorption is least with chlortetracycline (30%); intermediate with tetracycline, oxytetracycline, and demeclocycline (60–80%); and highest with doxycycline and minocycline (95% or more). An oral dose of 250 mg of tetracycline hydrochloride gives serum levels of 2–3 μg/mL, and 100 mg of doxycycline gives serum levels of 1–2 μg/mL. Tetracyclines are widely distributed in tissues, but levels in the central nervous system, cerebrospinal fluid, and joint fluid are only 5–15% of serum levels.

The usual dose of tetracyclines is 250–500 mg 4 times daily. Doxycycline and minocycline are given as 100 mg twice daily and demeclocycline and methacycline as 150 mg 4 times daily or 300 mg twice daily.

Tetracyclines are metabolized in the liver and concentrated in bile. Excretion is mainly through bile and urine. All tetracyclines—except doxycycline—accumulate in renal insufficiency and are antianabolic in high doses. Doxycycline requires no dosage adjustment in renal failure; the other tetracyclines should be avoided or given in reduced dosage.

For patients unable to take oral medication, some tetracyclines are formulated for parenteral administration in doses similar to the oral ones. A 1% topical tetracycline ointment is available for conjunctival infections.

Clinical Uses

Tetracyclines are the drugs of choice for chlamydial, rickettsial, and *Vibrio* infections and some spirochetal infections. Sexually transmitted diseases in which chlamydiae often play a role—endocervicitis, urethritis, proctitis, and epididymitis—should be treated with a tetracycline for 10–14 days. Pelvic inflammatory disease is often treated with doxycycline plus cefoxitin. Other chlamydial infections (psittacosis, lymphogranuloma venereum, trachoma) and sexually transmitted disease (granuloma inguinale) also respond to tetracyclines. Other uses include treatment of acne, urinary tract infections, exacerbations of bronchitis, Lyme disease and relapsing fever, brucellosis and tularemia (often in combination with streptomycin), cholera, mycoplasmal pneumonia, and infections caused by *Mycobacterium marinum* and *Pasteurella multocida* (often after an animal bite). Tetracycline has also been used in combination with other drugs for amebiasis and falciparum malaria.

Minocycline achieves a high concentration in the saliva and can be used for eradication of meningococci in carriers who cannot tolerate rifampin. Tetracycline ointment is effective prophylaxis against gonococcal and chlamydial ophthalmia neonatorum in newborns.

Adverse Effects

A. Allergy: Hypersensitivity reactions with fever or skin rashes are uncommon.

B. Gastrointestinal Side Effects: Gastrointestinal side effects, especially diarrhea, nausea, and anorexia, are common. These can be diminished by reducing the dose or by administering tetracyclines with food or carboxymethylcellulose, but sometimes they force discontinuance of the drug. After a few days of oral use, the gut flora is modified so that drug-resistant bacteria and yeasts become prominent. This may cause functional gut disturbances, anal pruritus, and even enterocolitis with shock and death.

C. Bones and Teeth: Tetracyclines are bound to calcium deposited in growing bones and teeth, causing fluorescence, discoloration, enamel dysplasia, deformity, or growth inhibition. Therefore, tetracyclines should not be given to pregnant women or children under 6 years of age.

D. Liver Damage: Tetracyclines can impair hepatic function or even cause liver necrosis, particularly during pregnancy, in the presence of preexisting liver damage, or with doses of more than 3 g intravenously.

E. Kidney Damage: Outdated tetracycline preparations have been implicated in renal tubular acidosis and other forms of renal damage. Tetracyclines may increase blood urea nitrogen when diuretics are administered.

F. Other: Vaginal candidiasis is a common complication of tetracycline therapy. Tetracyclines—principally demeclocycline—may induce photosensitization, especially in fair-skinned individuals. Intravenous injection may cause thrombophlebitis, and intramuscular injection may induce local inflammation with pain. Minocycline induces vestibular reactions (dizziness, vertigo, nausea, vomiting), with a frequency of 35–70% after doses of 200 mg daily. Demeclocycline inhibits antidiuretic hormone.

Wilson WR, Cockerill FR III: Tetracyclines, chloramphenicol, erythromycin, and clindamycin. Mayo Clin Proc 1987;62:906.

CHLORAMPHENICOL

Antimicrobial Activity

Chloramphenicol is active against many gram-positive and gram-negative bacteria and rickettsiae. It binds to the 50S subunit of ribosomes and inhibits protein synthesis. It is bacteriostatic for most organisms but bactericidal for *Streptococcus pneumoniae*, *Haemophilus influenzae*, and *Neisseria meningitidis*.

This bactericidal activity accounts for the efficacy of chloramphenicol in the treatment of meningitis caused by these organisms.

Pharmacokinetics & Administration

For most systemic infections, chloramphenicol, 30 mg/kg/d, is given intravenously, but meningitis in adults may require 50 mg/kg/d in 4 divided doses. The dose for meningitis in children is up to 100 mg/kg/d, but in neonates not more than 25 mg/kg/d should be given. With a 500-mg intravenous dose, serum levels reach 5–10 μg/mL. Since the intravenous preparation chloramphenicol sodium succinate must be hydrolyzed to active drug by the liver, it yields somewhat lower levels than the oral form. A 500-mg oral dose gives serum levels of 10 μg/mL.

Chloramphenicol is widely distributed in tissues, including the eye and central nervous system. Cerebrospinal fluid levels are 70–80% of serum levels, and the levels in brain tissue may even exceed those in serum.

Chloramphenicol is metabolized in the liver, and less than 10% is excreted unchanged in the urine. Thus, no dosage adjustment is needed in renal insufficiency. Patients with liver disease may accumulate the drug, and levels should be monitored.

Clinical Uses

Because of potential toxicity and the availability of other effective drugs (eg, cephalosporins), chloramphenicol is a possible choice only in the following circumstances: (1) Symptomatic *Salmonella* infections, eg, typhoid fever. Many strains of *Salmonella* are resistant to chloramphenicol, and trimethoprim-sulfamethoxazole is often used. (2) Serious infections with *Haemophilus influenzae,* eg, meningitis, epiglottitis, pneumonia. However, cefuroxime, cefotaxime, or ceftriaxone may be considered drugs of choice. (3) Meningococcal or pneumococcal infections of the central nervous system in patients hypersensitive to β-lactam drugs. (4) Anaerobic or mixed infections in the central nervous system, eg, brain abscess. (5) Topical chloramphenicol is occasionally used in ophthalmic infections. Rarely, chloramphenicol is used as an alternative to tetracyclines in rickettsial infections.

Adverse Effects

Nausea, vomiting, and diarrhea occur infrequently. The most serious adverse effects pertain to the hematopoietic system. Adults taking chloramphenicol in excess of 50 mg/kg/d regularly exhibit disturbances in red cell maturation within 1–2 weeks. There is anemia, rise in serum iron concentration, reticulocytopenia, and the appearance of vacuolated nucleated red cells in the bone marrow. These changes regress when the drug is stopped and are not related to the rare aplastic anemia.

Serious aplastic anemia is a rare consequence of chloramphenicol administration and represents a specific, probably genetically determined individual defect. It is seen more frequently with prolonged or repeated use. It tends to be irreversible. It has been estimated that fatal aplastic anemia occurs in one of 25–40 thousand courses of chloramphenicol treatment. Hypoplastic anemia may be followed by the development of leukemia.

Chloramphenicol inhibits the metabolism of certain drugs. Thus, it may prolong the action and raise the blood concentration of tolbutamide, phenytoin, chlorpropamide, and warfarin sodium (Coumadin).

Chloramphenicol is specifically toxic for newborns, particularly premature infants. Because they lack the mechanism for detoxification of the drug in the liver, the drug may accumulate, producing the highly fatal "gray syndrome," with vomiting, flaccidity, hypothermia, and collapse. In full-term infants, the dose should be limited to less than 50 mg/kg/d; in prematures, the dose should be less than 30 mg/kg/d if the drug is employed at all.

AMINOGLYCOSIDES

Aminoglycosides are a group of bactericidal drugs sharing chemical, antimicrobial, pharmacologic, and toxic characteristics. At present, the group includes streptomycin, neomycin, kanamycin, amikacin, gentamicin, tobramycin, sisomicin, netilmicin, and others. All these agents inhibit protein synthesis in bacteria by attaching to and inhibiting the function of the 30S subunit of the bacterial ribosome. Resistance is based on (1) a deficiency of the ribosomal receptor (chromosomal mutant); (2) the enzymatic destruction of the drug (plasmid-mediated transmissible resistance of clinical importance) by acetylation, phosphorylation, or adenylylation; or (3) a lack of permeability to the drug molecule or failure of active transport across cell membranes. (This can be chromosomal, eg, streptococci are relatively impermeable to aminoglycosides; or plasmid-mediated, eg, in gram-negative enteric bacteria.) Anaerobic bacteria are resistant to aminoglycosides because transport across the cell membrane is an oxygen-dependent energy-requiring process.

All aminoglycosides are more active at alkaline than at acid pH. All are potentially ototoxic and nephrotoxic, though to different degrees. All can accumulate in renal insufficiency; therefore, dosage adjustments must be made in patients with renal dysfunction (see Table 31–8).

Aminoglycosides are used most widely against gram-negative enteric bacteria or when there is a suspicion of sepsis. Although aminoglycosides demonstrate in vitro activity against many gram-positive bacteria, they should never be used alone to treat infections caused by these organisms—both because

there is no clinical experience with the treatment of such infections and because less toxic alternatives are available. In the treatment of bacteremia or endocarditis caused by fecal streptococci or by some gram-negative bacteria, the aminoglycoside is given together with a β-lactam drug to enhance permeability and facilitate the entry of the aminoglycoside. Aminoglycosides are selected according to recent susceptibility patterns in a given area or hospital until susceptibility tests become available on a specific isolate.

General Properties of Aminoglycosides

Because of the similarities of the aminoglycosides, a summary of properties is presented briefly.

A. Physical Properties: Aminoglycosides are water-soluble and stable in solution. If they are mixed in solution with β-lactam antibiotics, they may form complexes and lose some activity.

B. Absorption, Distribution, Metabolism, and Excretion: Aminoglycosides are well absorbed after intramuscular or intravenous injection, but they are not absorbed from the gut. They are distributed widely in tissues and penetrate into pleural, peritoneal, or joint fluid in the presence of inflammation. They diffuse poorly into the eye, prostate, bile, central nervous system, or spinal fluid after parenteral injection.

There is no significant metabolic breakdown of aminoglycosides. The serum half-life is 2–3 hours. Excretion is almost entirely by glomerular filtration. Urine levels usually are 10–50 times higher. Aminoglycosides are removed fairly effectively by hemodialysis but irregularly by peritoneal dialysis.

C. Dose and Effect of Impaired Renal Function: In persons with normal renal function, the dose of kanamycin or amikacin is 15 mg/kg/d; that for gentamicin or tobramycin is 4.5–6 mg/kg/d, usually injected in 3 equal amounts every 8 hours.

In persons with impaired renal function, excretion is diminished and there is the danger of drug accumulation with increased side effects. Therefore, if the interval is kept constant, the dose has to be reduced, or the interval must be increased if the dose is kept constant. Nomograms have been constructed relating creatinine clearance to adjustments of treatment regimens. One widely used nomogram is shown in Table 31–8. Because aminoglycoside levels vary considerably in different patients with similar creatinine values, serum drug levels should be monitored to avoid severe toxicity, especially when renal function is rapidly changing.

D. Adverse Effects: All aminoglycosides can cause varying degrees of ototoxicity and nephrotoxicity. Ototoxicity, though rare, is worrisome because it is often irreversible and is cumulative with repeated use of the drug. Ototoxicity can present either as hearing loss (cochlear damage) that is noted first with high-frequency tones, or as vestibular damage, manifested by vertigo, ataxia, and loss of balance. Of

Table 31–8. Dosing of aminoglycosides.[1]

1. Select loading dose in mg/kg (ideal weight) to provide peak serum levels in range listed below for desired aminoglycoside.

Aminoglycoside	Usual Loading Doses	Expected Peak Serum Levels
Tobramycin ⎤ Gentamicin ⎦	1.5–2 mg/kg	4–10 µg/mL
Amikacin ⎤ Kanamycin ⎦	5–7.5 mg/kg	15–30 µg/mL

2. Select maintenance dose (as percentage of chosen loading dose) to continue peak serum levels indicated above according to desired dosing interval and the patient's corrected creatinine clearance.[2]

		Percentage of Loading Dose Required for Dosage Interval Selected		
C(c)cr (mL/min)	Half-Life[3] (hours)	8 hours	12 hours	24 hours
90	3.1	84%	. . .	. . .
80	3.4	80	91%	. . .
70	3.9	76	88	. . .
60	4.5	71	84	. . .
50	5.3	65	79	. . .
40	6.5	57	72	92%
30	8.4	48	63	86
25	9.9	43	57	81
20	11.9	37	50	75
17	13.6	33	46	70
15	15.1	31	42	67
12	17.9	27	37	61
10[4]	20.4	24	34	56
7	25.9	19	28	47
5	31.5	16	23	41
2	46.8	11	16	30
0	69.3	8	11	21

[1] Reproduced, with permission, from Sarubbi FA, Hull JH: Amikacin serum concentrations: Prediction of levels and dosage guidelines. *Ann Intern Med* 1978;**89(Part 1)**:612.
[2] Calculate corrected creatinine clearance [C(c)cr] as follows:

$$C(c)cr \text{ male} = 140 - \text{Age} \div \text{Serum creatinine}$$
$$C(c)cr \text{ female} = 0.85 \times C(c)cr \text{ male}$$

[3] Alternatively, one-half of the chosen loading dose may be given at an interval approximately equal to the estimated half-life.
[4] Dosing for patients with C(c)cr ≤ 10 mL/min should be assisted by measured serum levels.

the commonly used aminoglycosides, amikacin appears to be more ototoxic than gentamicin, tobramycin, or netilmicin. Nephrotoxicity, which occurs more frequently than ototoxicity, is evident with rising serum creatinine levels or reduced creatinine clearance. Nephrotoxicity is usually reversible and occurs with similar frequency with gentamicin, tobramycin, amikacin, and netilmycin.

In very high doses, aminoglycosides can be neurotoxic, producing a curarelike effect with neuromuscular blockade that results in respiratory paralysis. Calcium gluconate or neostigmine can serve as an antidote to this reaction. Rarely, aminoglycosides cause hypersensitivity and local reactions.

Moellering RC, Siegenthaler WE (editors): Aminoglycoside therapy. The new decade: A worldwide perspective. Am J Med 1986;80(Suppl 6B):1.

1. STREPTOMYCIN

Streptomycin is bactericidal for both gram-positive and gram-negative bacteria. However, resistance emerges so rapidly and has become so widespread that only a few specific indications for this drug remain. These are (1) plague and tularemia; (2) endocarditis caused by *S faecalis* or *Streptococcus viridans* (use in conjunction with a penicillin); (3) serious active tuberculosis (use with other antituberculosis drugs); and (4) acute brucellosis (use with tetracycline). The usual adult dose is 15 mg/kg/d (about 1 g/d) injected in one or 2 divided doses intramuscularly. The dose for children is 20–40 mg/kg/d.

Streptomycin exhibits all the adverse effects typically associated with the aminoglycosides. It should not be given concurrently with other aminoglycosides, because excessive ototoxicity may occur.

2. NEOMYCIN & KANAMYCIN

These aminoglycosides are closely related, with similar activity and complete cross-resistance. The related drug paromomycin is used in amebiasis. Systemic use has been abandoned because of oto- and nephrotoxicity.

Ointments containing 1–5 mg/g neomycin, often combined with bacitracin and polymyxin, can be applied to infected superficial skin lesions. The drug mixture covers most staphylococci and gram-negative bacteria likely to be present, but the efficacy of such topical treatment is in doubt. Solutions of neomycin, 2.5–5 mg/mL, have been used for irrigation of infected joints or wounds. The total amount of drug must be kept below 15 mg/kg/d, because absorption can lead to systemic toxicity.

In preparation for elective bowel surgery, 1 g of neomycin is given orally every 6–8 hours for 1–2 days (often combined with erythromycin, 1 g) to reduce aerobic bowel flora. Action on gram-negative anaerobes is negligible. In hepatic coma, the coliform bacteria can be suppressed for prolonged periods by oral neomycin or kanamycin, 1 g every 6–8 hours, during reduced protein intake. This results in diminished ammonia production and intoxication.

Kanamycin is somewhat less toxic than neomycin. It is used for the same indications and in the same doses as neomycin for topical application and oral intake.

In addition to oto- and nephrotoxicity, which can result from systemic absorption, neomycin or kanamycin can give rise to allergic reactions when applied topically to skin or eye. Respiratory arrest has followed the instillation of 3–5 g of kanamycin into the peritoneal cavity after colonic surgery; this can be overcome by neostigmine.

3. AMIKACIN

Amikacin is a semisynthetic derivative of kanamycin. It is relatively resistant to several of the enzymes that inactivate gentamicin and tobramycin, and bacterial resistance is increasing only slowly. Many gram-negative enteric bacteria—including many strains of *Proteus, Pseudomonas, Enterobacter,* and *Serratia*—are inhibited by 1–20 μg/mL of amikacin in vitro. After injection of 500 mg of amikacin intramuscularly every 12 hours (15 mg/kg/d), peak levels in serum are 10–30 μg/mL. Some infections caused by gram-negative bacteria resistant to gentamicin respond to amikacin. Central nervous system infections require intrathecal or intraventricular injection of 5–10 mg daily.

Like all aminoglycosides, amikacin is nephrotoxic and ototoxic (particularly for the auditory portion of the eighth nerve). Its levels should be monitored in patients with renal failure.

Meyer RD: Drugs five years later: Amikacin. Ann Intern Med 1981;95:328.

Sarubbi FA, Hull JH: Amikacin serum concentrations: Prediction of levels and dosage guidelines. Ann Intern Med 1978;89:612.

4. GENTAMICIN

With doses of 4.5–6 mg/kg/d of this aminoglycoside, serum levels reach 3–8 μg/mL—sufficient for bactericidal effect against many strains of staphylococci, coliforms, and other gram-negative organisms. Enterococci are resistant unless a penicillin is also given. Gentamicin may be synergistic with penicillins active against *Pseudomonas, Proteus, Enterobacter, Klebsiella,* and other gram-negatives. Sisomicin resembles the C1a component of gentamicin.

Indications, Dosages, & Routes of Administration

Gentamicin is used in severe infections caused by gram-negative bacteria. Included are sepsis, infected burns, pneumonia, and other serious infections. The dosage is 4.5–6 mg/kg/d intramuscularly (or intravenously) in 3 equal doses. In endocarditis due to viridans streptococci or *S faecalis,* gentamicin in lower doses (3 mg/kg/d in 3 divided doses) is combined with penicillin or ampicillin. In renal insufficiency, the dose should be adjusted according to Table 31–8. About 2–3% of patients develop vestibular dysfunction and loss of hearing when peak serum levels exceed 10 μg/mL. For infected burns or skin lesions, creams containing 0.1% gentamicin are used. Such topical use should be restricted to avoid favoring the development of resistant bacteria in hospitals. In meningitis due to gram-negative bacteria, 1–10 mg of gentamicin has been injected daily intrathecally or intraventricularly in adults. However, in neonatal gram-negative bacillary meningitis the benefit of either of these routes is in doubt, and intraventricular gentamicin is toxic.

Edson RS, Terrell CL: The aminoglycosides: Streptomycin, kanamycin, gentamicin, tobramycin, amikacin, netilmicin, and sisomicin. Mayo Clin Proc 1987;62:916.

5. TOBRAMYCIN

Tobramycin closely resembles gentamicin in antibacterial activity and pharmacologic properties and exhibits partial cross-resistance. Tobramycin may be effective against some gentamicin-resistant gram-negative bacteria. A daily dose of 4.5–6 mg/kg is given in 3 equal amounts intramuscularly or intravenously at intervals of 8 hours. In renal insufficiency, dosage adjustment is necessary (Table 31–8). Tobramycin and gentamicin are potentially ototoxic and nephrotoxic. The frequency of these adverse effects is similar for both drugs.

Netilmicin shares many characteristics with gentamicin and tobramycin and can be given in a dose of 5–7 mg/kg/d. It may be less ototoxic and less nephrotoxic than the other aminoglycosides.

Smith CR et al: Double blind comparison of the nephrotoxicity and auditory toxicity of gentamicin and tobramycin. N Engl J Med 1980;302:1106.

6. SPECTINOMYCIN

Spectinomycin is an aminocyclitol antibiotic (related to aminoglycosides) for intramuscular administration. Its sole application is in the treatment of gonococci producing β-lactamase or of persons with gonorrhea who are hypersensitive to penicillin. One injection of 2 g (40 mg/kg) is given. About 5–10% of gonococci are probably resistant. There is usually pain at the injection site, and there may be nausea and fever.

Rettig PJ et al: Spectinomycin therapy for gonorrhea in prepubertal children. Am J Dis Child 1980;134:359.

POLYMYXINS

The polymyxins are basic polypeptides that are bactericidal for most gram-negative aerobic rods, including *Pseudomonas*. Because of their poor distribution to tissues and substantial toxicity—and in view of the availability of better drugs—they are now rarely considered for systemic administration but are used topically.

Solutions of polymyxin B sulfate, 1 mg/mL, can be applied to infected surfaces; injected into joint spaces, the pleural cavity, or subconjunctivally; or inhaled as aerosols. Ointments containing 0.5 mg/g of polymyxin B sulfate in a mixture with neomycin or bacitracin (or both) are often applied to superficial infected skin lesions. Polymyxins are inactivated by purulent exudates. They rarely cause local sensitization.

Davis SD: Polymyxins, colistin, vancomycin and bacitracin. In: *Antimicrobial Therapy*, 3rd ed. Kagan BM (editor). Saunders, 1980.

ANTITUBERCULOSIS DRUGS

Singular problems exist in the treatment of tuberculosis and other mycobacterial infections, which tend to be exceedingly chronic but may give rise to hyperacute lethal complications. The organisms are frequently intracellular, have long periods of metabolic inactivity, and tend to develop resistance to any one drug. Therefore, combined drug therapy is employed to delay the emergence of this resistance. "First-line" drugs, often employed together in tuberculous meningitis, miliary dissemination, or severe pulmonary disease, are isoniazid, ethambutol, rifampin, and pyrazinamide. A series of "second-line" drugs will be mentioned only briefly. Most patients become noninfectious within 2–4 weeks after effective drug therapy is instituted. In active pulmonary tuberculosis without complications, treatment schedules including isoniazid and rifampin for 6–9 months are satisfactory.

1. ISONIAZID

Isoniazid is the hydrazide of isonicotinic acid (INH), the most active antituberculosis drug. Isoniazid in a concentration of 0.2 µg/mL or less inhibits and kills most tubercle bacilli. However, some "atypical" mycobacteria are resistant. In susceptible large populations of *Mycobacterium tuberculosis*, isoniazid-resistant mutants occur. Their emergence is delayed in the presence of a second drug. There is no cross-resistance between isoniazid and other antituberculosis drugs.

Isoniazid is well absorbed from the gut and diffuses readily into all tissues, including the central nervous system. The inactivation of isoniazid—particularly its acetylation—is under genetic control. However, the speed of isoniazid acetylation has little influence over the selection of drug regimens. Isoniazid and its conjugates are excreted mainly in the urine.

Indications, Dosages, & Routes of Administration

Isoniazid is the most widely used drug in tuberculosis. It should not be given as the sole drug in active tuberculosis. This favors emergence of resistance (up to 30% in some countries). In active, clinically manifest disease, it is given in conjunction with one or more drugs. The usual oral adult dose is 300 mg/d. For children, it is 10–20 mg/kg/d, not to exceed 300 mg/d. In noncompliant patients, it can be given twice weekly in a dose of 15 mg/kg/dose (maximum, 900 mg/dose). In anephric patients, the dose is reduced to 200 mg/d.

Individuals who convert from a negative to a positive tuberculin test but who have no evidence of active disease may be given 10 mg/kg/d (maximum: 300 mg/d) for 6–12 months as prophylaxis against the 5–15% risk of meningitis or miliary dissemination. For this "prophylaxis," isoniazid is given as the sole drug. Other indications for prophylaxis are discussed in Chapter 7.

Toxic reactions to isoniazid include insomnia, restlessness, fever, myalgia, hyperreflexia, and even convulsions and psychotic episodes. Some of these are attributable to a relative pyridoxine deficiency and peripheral neuritis and can be prevented by the administration of pyridoxine, 100 mg/d. Isoniazid can induce hepatitis. Progressive liver damage occurs rarely in patients under age 20; in 1.5% of persons between 30 and 50 years of age; and in 2.5% of older individuals. The risk of hepatitis is greater in alcoholics. Mild elevations (2–3 times normal) of transaminases are common, occurring in 10–20% of patients taking isoniazid. Most physicians do not discontinue the drug unless there is more definite hepatic impairment, with transaminases 3–5 times normal values. Isoniazid can reduce the metabolism of phenytoin, increasing its blood level and toxicity.

2. ETHAMBUTOL

Ethambutol is a synthetic, water-soluble, heat-stable compound, dispensed as the hydrochloride.

Many strains of *M tuberculosis* and of "atypical" mycobacteria are inhibited in vitro by ethambutol, 1–5 μg/mL. The mechanism of action is not known.

Ethambutol is well absorbed from the gut. About 20% of the drug is excreted in feces and 50% in the urine, in unchanged form. Excretion is delayed and dosage adjustment is required in renal insufficiency; with creatinine clearance of 10–30 mL/min, one-half the usual dose is given, and with clearance of less than 10 mL/min, 35% of the usual dose. In meningitis, ethambutol appears in the cerebrospinal fluid.

Resistance to ethambutol emerges fairly rapidly among mycobacteria when the drug is used alone. Therefore, ethambutol, 15 mg/kg, is usually given as a single daily dose in combination with other antituberculosis drugs.

Hypersensitivity to ethambutol occurs infrequently. It may cause a rise in the serum uric acid. The commonest side effects are visual disturbances: reduction in visual acuity, optic neuritis, and perhaps retinal damage occur in some patients receiving ethambutol, 25 mg/kg/d for several months. Most changes are reversible, but periodic visual acuity testing is mandatory when doses above 15 mg/kg/d are used. At lower doses, side effects are rare.

3. RIFAMPIN

Rifampin is a semisynthetic derivative of rifamycin. Rifampin, 1 μg/mL or less, inhibits many gram-positive cocci, meningococci, and mycobacteria in vitro. Gram-negative organisms are often more resistant. Highly resistant mutants occur frequently in susceptible microbial populations (one in 10^6–10^8 bacteria).

Rifampin binds strongly to DNA-dependent bacterial RNA polymerase and thus inhibits RNA synthesis in bacteria. Rifampin penetrates well into phagocytic cells and can kill intracellular organisms. Rifampin sometimes enhances the activity of amphotericin B against various fungi in vitro.

Rifampin given orally is well absorbed and widely distributed in tissues, including the central nervous system. Levels in cerebrospinal fluid are 50% of those in serum. It is excreted mainly through the liver and to a lesser extent in the urine. With oral doses of 600 mg, serum levels exceed 5 μg/mL for 4–6 hours, and urine levels may be 3–20 times higher. No adjustment is needed in renal insufficiency.

In the treatment of tuberculosis, a single oral dose of 600 mg (10–20 mg/kg) is given daily or, in noncompliant patients, 600 mg twice weekly. In order to delay the rapid emergence of resistant microorganisms, combined treatment with other antituberculosis drugs is required. Rifampin is effective for treatment of leprosy (see below). Rifampin, 600 mg twice daily for 2 days, can terminate the meningococcal carrier state, but rifampin-resistant strains emerge in 10% of subjects. Close contacts of children with manifest *H influenzae* infection (eg, in family or day care center) can receive rifampin, 20 mg/kg/d for 4 days, as prophylaxis. Rifampin combined with trimethoprim-sulfamethoxazole can eradicate staphylococcal carriage in the nasopharynx. Combination of rifampin with either penicillin or clindamycin is effective in eradication of group A β-hemolytic streptococci from the pharynx of chronic carriers. Synergistic action of rifampin with nafcillin against staphylococci in vitro is of uncertain clinical significance. With the exception of prophylaxis, rifampin should never be used alone.

Rifampin imparts an orange color to urine, sweat, and contact lenses. Occasional adverse effects include rashes, thrombocytopenia, impaired liver function, light chain proteinuria, and some impairment of immune response. In intermittent administration, rifampin must be given at least twice weekly to avoid a "flu syndrome," anemia, and other adverse affects. Rifampin increases the metabolism of oral anticoagulants and contraceptives and lowers serum levels of methadone, ketoconazole, and chloramphenicol.

4. STREPTOMYCIN

The general pharmacologic features and toxicity of streptomycin are described above. Streptomycin, 1–10 μg/mL, is inhibitory and bactericidal for most tubercle bacilli, whereas most "atypical" mycobacteria are resistant. All large populations of tubercle bacilli contain some streptomycin-resistant mutants. Therefore, streptomycin is employed only in combination with another antituberculosis drug.

Streptomycin penetrates poorly into cells and exerts its action mainly on extracellular tubercle bacilli. Since at any moment 90% of tubercle bacilli are intracellular and thus unaffected by streptomycin, treatment for many months is required.

For combination therapy in tuberculous meningitis, miliary dissemination, and severe organ tuberculosis, streptomycin is given intramuscularly, 0.5–1 g daily (30 mg/kg/d for children) for weeks or months. This is followed by streptomycin, 1 g intramuscularly 2–3 times a week for months.

Prolonged streptomycin treatment may impair vestibular function and result in inability to maintain equilibrium. Later, some compensation usually occurs, so that patients can function fairly well.

5. PYRAZINAMIDE

Pyrazinamide is bactericidal for most *Mycobacterium tuberculosis* strains and also for "atypical" mycobacteria. It is well absorbed after oral administration and is widely distributed in tissues. It penetrates well into the cerebrospinal fluid and achieves levels equal to those in serum. The usual oral dose is 20–30 mg/kg (1.5–2 g) given once daily. In noncompliant patients, 50–70 mg/kg can be given twice weekly. Pyrazinamide is being used with increased frequency in the therapy of tuberculosis because of its demonstrated efficacy in short-course therapy regimens (see below).

The major adverse effect is hepatotoxicity, seen in 1–5% of patients. Nausea, vomiting, drug fever, and hyperuricemia can occur.

6. SHORT-COURSE THERAPY

For uncomplicated pulmonary tuberculosis (and perhaps extrapulmonary disease), treatment for only 6–9 months can be satisfactory *provided that* both isoniazid and rifampin are administered (see Chapter 7). In adults, isoniazid, 300 mg, and rifampin, 600 mg, are given daily for 9 months. Alternatively, isoniazid, rifampin, and pyrazinamide (30 mg/kg/d) can be given for 2 months followed by 4 additional months of isoniazid and rifampin. Ethambutol (15 mg/kg/d) should be included in the regimen if the patient resides in or has come from an area with a high level of drug resistance. In noncompliant patients, twice-weekly administration of drug has been shown to be effective. One such regimen is the use of isoniazid 300 mg and rifampin 600 mg daily for 2 months, followed by twice-weekly administration of isoniazid (15 mg/kg or a maximum dose of 900 mg) and rifampin (10 mg/kg or a maximum of 600 mg), to complete a total of 9 months of therapy.

7. ALTERNATIVE DRUGS IN TUBERCULOSIS TREATMENT

The drugs listed alphabetically below are usually considered only in cases of drug resistance (clinical or laboratory) to "first-line" drugs and when expert guidance is available to deal with toxic side effects.

Aminosalicylic acid (PAS), closely related to *p*-aminobenzoic acid, inhibits most tubercle bacilli in concentrations of 1–5 μg/mL but has no effect on other bacteria.

Aminosalicylic acid is readily absorbed from the gut. Doses of 8–12 g/d orally give blood levels of 10 μg/mL. The drug is widely distributed in tissues (except the central nervous system) and rapidly excreted into the urine.

Common side effects include anorexia, nausea, diarrhea, and epigastric pain. Sodium aminosalicylate may be given parenterally. Hypersensitivity reactions include fever, skin rashes, granulocytopenia, lymphadenopathy, and arthralgias.

Ansamycin—a derivative of rifampin—is more active than the latter against *M tuberculosis, M avium-intracellulare,* and *M fortuitum.* The dose is 0.15–0.5 g/d orally. It is under investigation for mycobacterial infections.

Clofazimine is a phenazine dye used in the treatment of leprosy and is active in vitro against *M avium-intracellulare.* It is given orally as a single daily dose of 100–300 mg for investigational treatment of mycobacterial disease. Adverse effects include nausea, vomiting, abdominal pain, and skin discoloration from red-brown to black.

Cycloserine, 0.5–1 g/d orally, has been used in re-treatment regimens and for primary therapy of highly resistant *M tuberculosis.* It can induce a variety of central nervous system dysfunctions and psychotic reactions. These may be controlled by phenytoin, 100 mg/d orally. In smaller doses (15–20 mg/kg/d), cycloserine has been used in urinary tract infections.

Ethionamide, 0.5–1 g/d orally, has been used in combination therapy but produces marked gastric irritation.

American Thoracic Society: Treatment of tuberculosis and tuberculous infection in adults and children. Am Rev Respir Dis 1986;134:355.

Cohn DL et al: A 62-dose, 6-month therapy for pulmonary and extrapulmonary tuberculosis: Twice weekly, directly observed, and cost-effective regimen. Ann Intern Med 1990;112;407.

Combs DL, O'Brien RJ, Geiter LJ: USPHS tuberculosis short-course chemotherapy trial 21: Effectiveness, toxicity and acceptability—the report of final results. Ann Intern Med 1990;112:397.

Dutt AK, Moers D, Stead WW: Short-course chemotherapy for extrapulmonary tuberculosis. Ann Int Med 1986;104:7.

SULFONAMIDES & ANTIFOLATE DRUGS

Since the demonstration in 1935 of the striking antibacterial activity of sulfanilamide, the molecule has been drastically altered in many ways. More than 150 different sulfonamides have been marketed at one time or another, the modifications being designed principally to achieve greater antibacterial activity, a wider antibacterial spectrum, greater solubility, or more prolonged action. Because of their low cost and their relative efficacy in some common bacterial infections, sulfonamides are still used widely.

Antimicrobial Activity

Sulfonamides are structural analogues of *p*-aminobenzoic acid (PABA) and compete with PABA to block its conversion to dihydrofolic acid. Organisms that require exogenous PABA in the synthesis of folates and pyrimidines are inhibited. Animal cells and some resistant microorganisms can utilize exogenous folate and thus are not affected by sulfonamides.

Trimethoprim, a substituted pyrimidine, inhibits the conversion of dihydrofolic to tetrahydrofolic acid by blocking the enzyme dihydrofolate reductase. It inhibits this enzyme of bacteria 50,000 times more efficiently than the same enzyme of mammalian cells.

Sulfonamides inhibit many gram-positive (including *Nocardia*) and gram-negative organisms. Emerging resistance, particularly among streptococci, gonococci, meningococci, and enteric gram-negative organisms, has limited their use somewhat. Sulfonamides are also active against chlamydiae and such parasites as *Toxoplasma* and *Plasmodium*.

The combination of trimethoprim (TMP) (1 part) plus sulfamethoxazole (SMZ) (5 parts) is bactericidal for such gram-negative rods as *E coli, Klebsiella, Enterobacter, Salmonella,* and *Shigella.* It is also active against many strains of *Serratia, Providencia, Pseudomonas maltophilia, Pseudomonas cepacia, Pseudomonas pseudomallei,* and *Pseudomonas mallei* but not against *Pseudomonas aeruginosa.* It is inactive against anaerobes, enterococci, and group A streptococci but inhibits *S aureus* and *S epidermidis, Branchamella catarrhalis, Haemophilus influenzae, Haemophilus ducreyi,* and some atypical mycobacteria, eg, *M marinum.*

Pharmacokinetics & Administration

Sulfisoxazole is widely used because of its low cost and high solubility. Like other soluble sulfonamides (sulfadiazine, sulfamethoxazole), it is well absorbed from the gut and widely distributed in tissues. For mild infections (eg, urinary tract infections), the usual dose is 0.5–1 g 4 times daily (30–60 mg/kg/ d), while for systemic infections, 100 mg/kg/d is appropriate. A 1-g oral dose of sulfisoxazole yields serum levels of 50–100 μg/mL.

One-half the dose of sulfisoxazole is excreted unchanged in the urine. In mild renal insufficiency, no dosage adjustment is needed; in severe renal failure (creatinine clearance < 5 mL/min), one-third to one-half the usual dose is given.

Insoluble sulfonamides, eg, phthalylsulfathiazole and salicylazosulfapyridine (sulfasalazine), are little absorbed from the gut and are largely excreted in the feces. Phthalylsulfathiazole has been used in the past for preparation of the bowel for surgery (8–15 g/d for 5–7 days). Sulfasalazine is used for ulcerative colitis (6 g/d in 4 doses); it is broken down to sulfapyridine and salicylate in the bowel, and the latter is anti-inflammatory.

For patients who are unable to take oral drugs, some intravenous sulfonamide preparations are available. Most widely used is trimethoprim-sulfamethoxazole. Each vial contains 80 mg TMP + 400 mg SMZ in a volume of 5 mL, which must be diluted in 125 mL of 5% dextrose in water. For many bacterial infections, the dose is 10 mg TMP + 50 mg SMZ/ kg/d in 2–4 doses; for *Pneumocystis carinii* infections, 20 mg TMP + 100 mg SMZ/kg/d is given in 4 doses. This dose is suitable for patients with creatinine clearances above 50 mL/min. Half to three-fourths of that dose is given for patients with creatinine clearances of 10–50 mL/min and one-quarter of the dose for clearances under 5 mL/min.

The topical application of sulfonamides to skin, wounds, or mucous membranes is undesirable because of the high risk of allergic sensitization or reaction. Exceptions are the application of sodium sulfacetamide solution (30%) or ointment (10%) to the conjunctiva and mafenide acetate cream (Sulfamylon) or silver sulfadiazine (Silvadene) to burn wounds.

Clinical Uses

Present indications for sulfonamides include the following:

A. Urinary Tract Infections: Coliform bacteria, the commonest cause of urinary tract infections, often remain susceptible to sulfonamides. "Single-dose" therapy with TMP-SMZ (2 tablets of 80 mg TMP + 400 mg SMZ) is effective in many patients with symptoms of less than a week's duration. Alternatively, 2 such tablets can be given twice daily, or 500 mg sulfisoxazole 4 times daily for 7–10 days. Shorter courses of therapy (ie, 3 days) for simple, uncomplicated urinary tract infections may be as effective as longer courses and are presently under investigation. Since TMP is concentrated in the prostate, TMP-SMZ, 2 tablets twice daily for 10–14 days, is effective in acute prostatitis.

B. Parasitic Infections: TMP-SMZ is effective for prophylaxis and treatment of *P carinii* pneumonia and *Isospora belli* infection. For therapy of *P carinii* pneumonia, 20 mg/kg/d of trimethoprim in 4 divided doses is administered intravenously or orally—depending upon the severity of disease—for 3 weeks. The dose for prophylaxis is 160 mg TMP + 800 mg SMZ twice daily. *I belli* infection in AIDS has been successfully treated with 160 mg TMP + 800 mg SMZ orally 4 times daily for 10 days followed by twice-daily administration for 3 weeks. Treatment with 160 mg TMP + 800 mg SMZ 3 times a week or 500 mg sulfadoxine with 25 mg pyrimethamine once a week has prevented recurrences. Sulfadoxine with pyrimethamine is also used to treat toxoplasmosis and chloroquine-resistant falciparum malaria.

C. Bacterial Infections: Sulfonamides are the drugs of choice for *Nocardia* infections. TMP-SMZ has a wide spectrum in therapy. It penetrates into the cerebrospinal fluid and has been used to treat meningitis caused by gram-negative rods, though third-generation cephalosporins are now preferred. TMP-SMZ is a frequent choice for management of acute sinusitis, otitis media, acute bronchitis, and shigellosis. The usual dose for adults is 160 mg TMP + 800 mg SMZ twice daily for 10 days; for children, it is 5 mg/kg TMP + 25 mg/kg SMZ twice daily. Other uses of TMP-SMZ include treatment of melioidosis *(Pseudomonas pseudomallei)* and infections by *Pseudomonas maltophilia* or *Pseudomonas cepacia;* of chancroid *(Haemophilus ducreyi);* in combination with rifampin for eradication of nasopharyngeal carriage of *S aureus;* for prophylaxis of meningococcal disease when susceptible *Neisseria meningitidis* strains prevail; and for therapy of legionellosis in patients who cannot tolerate or fail to respond to erythromycin.

D. Chlamydial Infections: Sulfonamides effectively suppress trachoma, urethritis, inclusion conjunctivitis, and other manifestations, but erythromycin or tetracyclines are preferred.

E. Leprosy: Certain sulfones are widely used (see below).

Adverse Effects

Sulfonamides produce a wide variety of side effects—due partly to hypersensitivity, partly to direct toxicity—that must be considered whenever unexplained symptoms or signs occur in a patient who may have received these drugs. Except in the mildest reactions, fluids should be forced, and—if symptoms and signs progressively increase—the drugs should be discontinued. Precautions to prevent complications (below) are important.

A. Systemic Side Effects: Fever, skin rashes, urticaria; nausea, vomiting, or diarrhea; stomatitis, conjunctivitis, arthritis, exfoliative dermatitis; bone marrow depression, thrombocytopenia, hemolytic (in G6PD deficiency) or aplastic anemia, granulocytopenia, leukemoid reactions; hepatitis, polyarteritis nodosa, vasculitis, Stevens-Johnson syndrome; psychosis; and many others.

Trimethoprim can evoke similar side effects. It may precipitate folate deficiency.

Application of mafenide to burns may cause severe pain.

B. Urinary Tract Disturbances: Sulfonamides may precipitate in urine, especially at neutral or acid pH, producing hematuria, crystalluria, or even obstruction. They have also been implicated in various types of nephritis and nephrosis. Sulfonamides and methenamine salts should not be given together.

Precautions in the Use of Sulfonamides

(1) There is cross-allergenicity among all sulfonamides. Obtain a history of past administration or reaction. Observe for possible allergic responses.

(2) Keep the urine volume above 1500 mL/d by forcing fluids.

(3) Check hemoglobin, white blood cell count, and differential count once weekly to detect possible disturbances early in high-risk patients.

Cockerill FR III, Edson RS: Trimethoprim-sulfamethoxazole. Mayo Clin Proc 1987;62:921.

SULFONES USED IN THE TREATMENT OF LEPROSY

A number of drugs closely related to the sulfonamides (eg, dapsone; diaminodiphenylsulfone, DDS) have been used effectively in the long-term treatment of leprosy. Dapsone may also be effective for *P carinii* pneumonia in AIDS when combined with trimethoprim. The clinical manifestations of both lepromatous and tuberculoid leprosy can often be suppressed by treatment extending over several years. It appears that 5–30% of *Mycobacterium leprae* organisms were resistant to dapsone in 1990. Consequently, initial combined treatment with rifampin is advocated.

Absorption, Metabolism, & Excretion

All sulfones are well absorbed from the intestinal tract, are distributed widely in all tissues, and tend to be retained in skin, muscle, liver, and kidney. Skin involved by leprosy contains 10 times more drug than normal skin. Sulfones are excreted into the bile and reabsorbed by the intestine. Consequently, blood levels are prolonged. Excretion into the urine is variable, and the drug occurs in urine mostly as a glucuronic acid conjugate. Some persons acetylate sulfones slowly and others rapidly; this requires dosage adjustment.

Dosages & Routes of Administration

See Leprosy, Chapter 26, for recommendations.

Adverse Effects

The sulfones may cause any of the side effects listed above for sulfonamides. Anorexia, nausea, and vomiting are common. Hemolysis, methemoglobinemia, or agranulocytosis may occur. If sulfones are not tolerated, clofazimine can be substituted.

Yawalkar SJ et al: Once-monthly rifampin plus daily dapsone in initial treatment of lepromatous leprosy. Lancet 1982;1:1199.

SPECIALIZED DRUGS AGAINST BACTERIA

1. BACITRACIN

This polypeptide is selectively active against gram-positive bacteria. Because of severe nephrotoxicity upon systemic administration, its use has been limited to topical application on surface lesions, usually in combination with polymyxin or neomycin. Occasionally it is given orally for pseudomembranous colitis caused by toxin-producing *Clostridium difficile* (see below).

2. LINCOMYCIN & CLINDAMYCIN

These drugs resemble erythromycin (although different in structure) and are active against gram-positive organisms (except enterococci). Lincomycin, 0.5 g orally every 6 hours (30–60 mg/kg/d for children), or clindamycin, 0.15–0.3 g orally every 6 hours (10–40 mg/kg/d for children) yields serum concentrations of 2–5 μg/mL. The drugs are widely distributed in tissues. Excretion is through the bile and urine. The drugs are alternatives to erythromycin as substitutes for penicillin. Clindamycin is active against most anaerobes, including *Bacteroides* sp. It is frequently used to treat infections in which anaerobes are significant pathogens (eg, aspiration pneumonia in penicillin-allergic patients; pelvic and abdominal infections), sometimes in combination with an aminoglycoside. Seriously ill patients are given clindamycin, 600 mg (20–30 mg/kg/d) intravenously during a 1-hour period every 8 hours. Success has also been reported in staphylococcal osteomyelitis. In the sulfonamide-allergic patient, high-dose clindamycin therapy (600–1200 mg intravenously every 6 hours or 600 mg orally every 6 hours) in conjunction with pyrimethamine has been used to treat toxoplasmosis of the central nervous system. These drugs are ineffective in meningitis.

Common side effects are diarrhea, nausea, and skin rashes. Impaired liver function and neutropenia have been noted. If 3–4 g is given rapidly intravenously, cardiorespiratory arrest may occur. Bloody diarrhea with pseudomembranous colitis has been associated with the administration of clindamycin and other antibiotics. This antibiotic-associated colitis is due to a necrotizing toxin produced by *C difficile*. The organism is resistant to the antimicrobial, is selected out by its presence, and is favored in its growth and toxin production. *C difficile* is usually susceptible to—and can be treated with—vancomycin (see below), bacitracin, or metronidazole given orally.

Wilson WR, Cockerill FR III: Tetracyclines, chloramphenicol, erythromycin, and clindamycin. Mayo Clin Proc 1987;62:906.

3. METRONIDAZOLE

Metronidazole is an antiprotozoal drug (see Chapter 28) that also has striking antibacterial effects against most anaerobes, including *Bacteroides* sp. It is well absorbed after oral administration, is widely distributed in tissues, and yields serum levels of 4–6 μg/mL after a 250-mg dose. It penetrates well into the cerebrospinal fluid, yielding levels similar to those in serum. The drug is metabolized in the liver, and dosage reduction is required in severe hepatic insufficiency. Metronidazole can be given intravenously.

Metronidazole is employed in amebiasis (see Table 28–1) and in the following circumstances:

(1) *Trichomonas* vaginitis responds to either a single dose (2 g) or to 250 mg orally 3 times daily for 7–10 days. Bacterial vaginosis responds to a single 2-g dose or to 500 mg 3 times daily for 7–10 days.

(2) In anaerobic or mixed infections, metronidazole can be given orally or intravenously, 500 mg 3 times daily (30 mg/kg/d).

(3) As an alternative to oral vancomycin for antibiotic-associated colitis due to *C difficile*, give 500 mg 3 times daily orally. If oral medication is impractical, it is given intravenously. Metronidazole is less expensive than clindamycin or vancomycin.

(4) Preparation of the colon before bowel surgery.

(5) Therapy of brain abscess, often in combination with penicillin or a third-generation cephalosporin.

Adverse effects include stomatitis, nausea, and diarrhea. Ingestion of alcohol while taking metronidazole can result in flushing, hypotension, nausea, and vomiting. With prolonged use at high doses, reversible peripheral neuropathy can develop. Metronidazole has been shown to be carcinogenic in animals and mutagenic for certain bacteria. To date, human studies have not confirmed an increased incidence of cancer after treatment.

Rosenblatt JE, Edson RS: Metronidazole. Mayo Clin Proc 1987;62:1013.

4. VANCOMYCIN

This drug is bactericidal for most gram-positive organisms, particularly staphylococci and enterococci, in concentrations of 0.5–10 μg/mL. Resistant mutants are very rare, and there is no cross-resistance with other antimicrobial drugs. Vancomycin is not absorbed from the gut. It is given orally only for the treatment of antibiotic-associated enterocolitis. For systemic effect the drug must be administered intravenously (20–30 mg/kg/d in 2–3 divided doses). An intravenous injection of 10 mg/kg over a period of 20 minutes yields blood levels of 20–30 μg/mL. Vancomycin is excreted mainly via the kidneys but may accumulate also in liver failure. In renal insufficiency, the half-life may be up to 8 days. Thus, only one dose of 0.5–1 g may be given every 4–8 days to a uremic individual undergoing hemodialysis.

Indications for parenteral vancomycin include the following: (1) Severe staphylococcal infections in penicillin-allergic patients; it is the drug of choice for methicillin-resistant *S aureus* and *S epidermidis* infections. (2) Severe enterococcal infections, often in combination with an aminoglycoside. (3) Other gram-positive infections in penicillin-allergic patients, eg, viridans streptococcal endocarditis. (4) Surgical prophylaxis in penicillin-allergic patients.

In antibiotic-associated enterocolitis, vancomycin, 0.125–0.5 g, is given orally 2–4 times daily.

Vancomycin is irritating to tissues; chills, fever, and thrombophlebitis sometimes follow intravenous injection. The drug is somewhat ototoxic and perhaps nephrotoxic. Rapid infusion may induce diffuse hyperemia ("red man syndrome") and can be avoided by extending infusions over 1 hour or by pretreating with a histamine antagonist such as hydroxyzine.

Hermans PE, Wilhelm MP: Vancomycin. Mayo Clin Proc 1987;62:901.

Sahai J et al: Influence of antihistamine pretreatment on vancomycin-induced red-man syndrome. J Inf Dis 1989;160:876.

Wise RI: The Vancomycin Symposium: Summary and comments. Rev Infect Dis 1981;3(Suppl):S293.

QUINOLONES

The quinolones are synthetic analogues of nalidixic acid. They are active against many gram-positive and gram-negative bacteria. The mode of action of all quinolones involves inhibition of bacterial DNA synthesis by blocking the enzyme DNA gyrase.

The earlier quinolones (nalidixic acid, oxolinic acid, cinoxacin) did not achieve systemic antibacterial levels after oral intake and thus were useful only as urinary antiseptics. The newer fluorinated derivatives (norfloxacin, ciprofloxacin, enoxacin, pefloxacin, and others) have greater antibacterial activity, achieve clinically useful levels in blood and tissues, and have low toxicity.

Antimicrobial Activity

The fluoroquinolones are active against many aerobic bacteria but have little activity against clinically important anaerobes. A majority of gram-negative bacteria are susceptible, including *Pseudomonas aeruginosa, Salmonella, Shigella, Campylobacter, Yersinia, Vibrio, Haemophilus, Brucella,* and *Legionella. Pseudomonas cepacia* and *P maltophilia* tend to be resistant. Most *S aureus* and *S epidermidis,* including methicillin-resistant stains, are sensitive to ciprofloxacin. Streptococci, including *Streptococcus faecalis* (enterococcus), *Streptococcus pneumoniae,* and groups A, B, and D are only moderately sensitive to ciprofloxacin. In vitro, mycobacteria, mycoplasmas, and chlamydiae are sensitive to quinolones, though there is little clinical experience in treating infections caused by these agents with the drug.

Pharmacokinetics & Administration

After oral administration, norfloxacin, ciprofloxacin, enoxacin, pefloxacin, and others are well absorbed and widely distributed in body fluids and tissues, though to different levels. The serum half-life ranges from 3 to 8 hours for different drugs. After ingestion of 400–600 mg, peak serum levels are 1–3 μg/mL for ciprofloxacin and norfloxacin, 4 μg/mL for enoxacin, and 10 μg/mL for ofloxacin. The fluoroquinolones are excreted mainly through the kidney by tubular secretion (which can be blocked by probenecid) and by glomerular filtration. Up to 20% of the dose is metabolized by the liver. In renal insufficiency, half-lives are prolonged, but only slight dosage adjustment is needed.

Clinical Uses

Because of their high cost, broad spectrum of activity, and tendency for some organisms (eg, *P aeruginosa*) to develop resistance, these agents should not be routinely used as first-line therapy when less expensive and less toxic agents are available. Despite their extensive in vitro activity, the exact role of quinolones in therapy has not been clearly defined. Urinary tract infections caused by multidrug-resistant gram-negative organisms that are sensitive to quinolones can be treated with norfloxacin, 400 mg twice daily, or ciprofloxacin, 500 mg twice daily. Ciprofloxacin has been successfully used to treat complicated skin and soft tissues infections, osteomyelitis caused by gram-negative organisms, and malignant otitis externa. Because quinolones are the only available oral agents active against *Campylobacter* and the other major bacterial pathogens associated with diarrhea (*Salmonella, Shigella,* toxigenic *E coli*), both ciprofloxacin and norfloxacin show promise for the therapy of traveler's diarrhea as well as domestically acquired acute diarrhea. Ciprofloxacin has been used to eradicate meningococci from the nasopharynx of carriers. Anecdotal reports have suggested that norfloxacin may be useful for treating falciparum malaria, and both norfloxacin and ciprofloxacin may be effective for prophylaxis in the neutropenic patient. Although some clinical studies have suggested that ciprofloxacin is efficacious in the therapy of lower respiratory tract infections, caution should be exercised since the drug has only marginal activity against *Streptococcus pneumoniae* and failures in treating pneumococcal pneumonia have been reported. Further controlled studies comparing ciprofloxacin to other available agents are needed to define its role.

Adverse Effects

The most prominent adverse effects of the quinolones are nausea, vomiting, and diarrhea. Occasionally, headache, dizziness, insomnia, impaired liver function, and skin rashes have been observed as well as more serious reactions such as anaphylaxis. Superinfections with enterococci and yeasts can develop. Because several fluoroquinolones cause joint damage in young animals, they are not recommended for children or pregnant women. While fluoroquinolones appear to be well tolerated in general, their role—as compared with other drugs—needs to be established.

Genty LO et al: Oral ciprofloxacin vs parenteral cefotaxime in the treatment of different skin and skin structure infections: A multicenter trial. Arch Int Med 1989;149:2579.

Goodman LJ et al: Empiric antimicrobial therapy pf domestically acquired acute diarrhea in urban adults. Arch Int Med 1990;150:541

Lang R et al: Successful treatment of malignant external otitis with oral ciprofloxacin: Report of experience with 23 patients. J Infect Dis 1990;161:537.

Neu HC: New antibiotics: Areas of appropriate use. J Infect Dis 1987;155:403.

Walker RC, Wright AJ: The quinolones. Mayo Clin Proc 1987;62:1007.

URINARY ANTISEPTICS

These drugs exert antimicrobial activity in the urine but have little or no systemic antibacterial effect. Their usefulness is limited to urinary tract infections.

1. NITROFURANTOIN

Nitrofurantoin is bacteriostatic and bactericidal for both gram-positive (including enterococci and staphylococci) and many gram-negative bacteria (not *Serratia marcescens* or *P aeruginosa*) in concentrations of 10–500 μg/mL. Microbial resistance does not emerge rapidly. The activity of nitrofurantoin is greatly enhanced at pH 6.5 or less.

Nitrofurantoin is rapidly absorbed from the gut, but levels in serum and tissues are negligible. Thus, there is no systemic antibacterial effect. Use of the drug is limited to lower urinary tract infections. It is rapidly excreted in urine, where concentrations may be 200–400 μg/mL. In renal failure, there is virtually no excretion into the urine and no therapeutic effect.

The average daily dose in urinary tract infections is 100 mg orally 4 times daily (for children, 5–10 mg/kg/d), taken with food. A single daily dose of 50–100 mg can prevent recurrent urinary tract infections in women.

Oral nitrofurantoin often causes nausea and vomiting. Hemolytic anemia occurs in G6PD deficiency. Hypersensitivity may produce skin rashes and pulmonary infiltration.

2. NALIDIXIC ACID & OXOLINIC ACID

Nalidixic acid is a synthetic urinary antiseptic that inhibits many gram-negative bacteria in concentrations of 1–50 μg/mL but has no effect on *Pseudomonas* or gram-positive organisms. In susceptible bacterial populations, resistant mutants emerge fairly rapidly.

Nalidixic acid is readily absorbed from the gut. In the blood, virtually all drug is firmly bound to protein. Thus, there is no systemic antibacterial action. About 20% of the absorbed drug is excreted in the urine in active form to give urine levels of 20–200 μg/mL, which may produce false-positive tests for glucose.

The dose in urinary tract infections is 1 g orally 4 times daily (for children, 30–60 mg/kg/d). Adverse reactions include nausea, vomiting, rash, drowsiness, visual hallucinations, excitement, and, rarely, increased intracranial pressure with convulsions.

Cinoxacin, a drug related to nalidixic acid, can be effective in urinary tract infections in oral doses of 250 mg 4 times daily or 500 mg twice daily. Because it is more expensive than nalidixic acid and has similar activity, its use is limited.

Brumfitt W, Hamilton-Miller JMT: Sulfonamides, nalidixic acid, oxolinic acid, methenamine and nitrofurans. In: *Antimicrobial Therapy,* 3rd ed. Kagan BM (editor). Saunders, 1980.

3. METHENAMINE MANDELATE & METHENAMINE HIPPURATE

These are salts of methenamine and mandelic acid or hippuric acid. The action of the drug depends on the liberation of formaldehyde from methenamine in the presence of acid. Almost all bacteria are inhibited by formaldehyde, which reaches levels of 200–800 μg/mL after an oral dose of 1 g. Little drug is excreted into the urine in renal insufficiency. Ammonia-producing organisms (eg, *Proteus*) produce an alkaline urine and may be resistant to these drugs. Sulfonamides and methenamine must not be given simultaneously. The usual dose is 2–6 g orally daily.

4. ACIDIFYING AGENTS

Urine with a pH below 5.5 tends to be antibacterial. Many substances can acidify urine and thus produce antibacterial activity. Ammonium chloride, ascorbic acid, methionine, and mandelic acid are sometimes used. The dose must be established for each patient by testing the urine for acid pH with test paper at frequent intervals.

SYSTEMICALLY ACTIVE DRUGS IN URINARY TRACT INFECTIONS

Many antimicrobial drugs are excreted in the urine in very high concentration. For this reason, low and relatively nontoxic amounts of many different antimicrobials can produce effective urine levels. Many penicillins, cephalosporins, aminoglycosides, quinolones, and trimethoprim-sulfamethoxazole can reach very high urine levels and can thus be effective in urinary tract infections.

Jawetz E: Disinfectants and antiseptics. Chapter 51 in: *Basic & Clinical Pharmacology*, 4th ed. Katzung BG (editor). Appleton & Lange, 1989.

ANTIFUNGAL DRUGS

Most antibacterial substances have no effect on pathogenic fungi. Only a few drugs are known to be therapeutically useful in mycotic infections (see Table 30–1).

1. AMPHOTERICIN B

Amphotericin B, 0.1–0.8 µg/mL, inhibits in vitro several organisms producing systemic mycotic disease in humans, including *Histoplasma, Cryptococcus, Coccidioides, Candida, Blastomyces, Sporothrix,* and others. This drug can be used for treatment of these systemic fungal infections. Intrathecal administration is necessary for the treatment of *Coccidioides* meningitis and may be required in meningitis caused by other fungi if systemic therapy fails (eg, *Cryptococcus, Candida*).

There is no absolute consensus on how amphotericin B should be administered or on the proper dosage and duration of therapy. A 1-mg test dose is given intravenously in 200 mL of 5% dextrose in water over 2–4 hours. If no adverse effects occur and the patient is not critically ill, 5 mg is given in 500 mL of 5% dextrose in water over 4–6 hours. Thereafter, the dose is increased by 5–10 mg daily until a final dosage of 0.4–0.75 mg/kg/d is reached. In critically ill patients, the dose is boosted more rapidly, eg, a test dose of 1 mg followed by 0.25 mg/kg; on day 2, 0.5 mg/kg; and on day 3, 0.75 mg/kg. The final dose is usually continued daily (or in double doses on alternate days) for many weeks.

In fungal meningitis, amphotericin B, 0.5 mg, is injected intrathecally 3 times weekly; continuous treatment (many weeks) with an Ommaya reservoir is sometimes employed. Relapses of fungal meningitis occur commonly and can be seen years after completion of therapy. Combined treatment with flucytosine is beneficial in systemic candidiasis and cryptococcal meningitis. Amphotericin B can also be effective in *Naegleria* meningoencephalitis.

Amphotericin B is little removed by hemodialysis and is nephrotoxic.

In patients with Foley catheters in place who have candiduria, amphotericin B bladder irrigations have been used to decrease colony counts. Twenty-five to 50 milligrams of drug is added to 500–1000 mL of sterile water. This solution is used for continuous (30–50 mL/h) or intermittent irrigation (200 mL 4 or 5 times daily with clamping of the catheter for 1/2 to 1 hour).

In impaired renal function, the dose of amphotericin B need not be reduced initially. However, if the serum creatinine reaches 2.5–3 mg/dL, the dose is temporarily lowered (or even stopped for a few days) until renal function recovers. Amphotericin B is then resumed at about one-half the previous dose and increased in 5-mg daily increments as tolerated.

The intravenous administration of amphotericin B usually produces chills, fever, vomiting, and headache. Tolerance may be enhanced by temporary lowering of the dose or by administration of aspirin, diphenhydramine, phenothiazines, meperidine, and corticosteroids. Therapeutically active amounts of amphotericin B commonly impair kidney and liver function and produce anemia (impaired iron utilization by bone marrow). Electrolyte disturbances (hypokalemia, distal renal tubular acidosis), shock, and a variety of neurologic symptoms also occur.

Liposomal amphotericin B, a water-soluble preparation, permits the administration of larger doses with fewer adverse effects. Preliminary results suggest that it may be beneficial for systemic fungal infections in the neutropenic patient, but further studies are needed.

Galles HA, Drew RH, Pickard WW: Amphotericin B: 30 years of clinical experiences. Rev Inf Dis 1990;12:308.
Terrell CL, Hermans PE: Antifungal agents used for deep-seated mycotic infections. Mayo Clin Proc 1987;62:1116.
Lopez-Bernstein G et al: Treatment of systemic fungal infections with liposomal amphotericin B. Arch Intern Med 1989;149:2533.

2. GRISEOFULVIN

Griseofulvin is an antibiotic that can inhibit the growth of some dermatophytes but has no effect on bacteria or on the fungi that cause deep mycoses. Absorption of griseofulvin microsize, 1 g/d, gives blood levels of 0.5–1.5 µg/mL. The absorbed drug has an affinity for skin and is deposited there, bound to keratin. Thus, it makes keratin resistant to fungal growth, and the new growth of hair or nails is free of infection. As keratinized structures are shed, they are replaced by uninfected ones. The bulk of ingested griseofulvin is excreted in the feces. Topical application of griseofulvin has little effect.

Give oral doses of 0.5–1 g/d (for children, 15 mg/kg/d) for 3–5 weeks if only the skin is involved and for 3–6 months or longer if the hair and nails are involved. Griseofulvin is most successful in severe dermatophytosis, particularly if caused by *Trichophyton rubrum,* though some strains are resistant.

An ultramicrosize particle formulation (Gris-PEG) is better absorbed The dose is 0.33–0.66 g orally daily for adults or 7.25 mg/kg/d for children.

Griseofulvin is relatively nontoxic and has a long history of clinical safety. Headache, nausea, vomiting, diarrhea, photosensitivity, and leukopenia have all been reported but are reversible and often will resolve without interruption of therapy. Routine monitoring for adverse effects is not required.

Major indications for use of this drug include tinea capitis, widespread tinea corporis, and tinea unguium (onychomycosis), though success rates in the latter are only 25–30%.

3. NYSTATIN

Nystatin inhibits *Candida* sp upon direct contact. The drug is not absorbed from mucous membranes or gut. Nystatin in ointments, suspensions, etc, can be applied to buccal or vaginal mucous membranes to suppress a local *Candida* infection. After oral intake of nystatin, *Candida* in the gut is suppressed and the drug is excreted in feces. The only indication for the use of nystatin orally is for control of oral candidiasis, especially in immunosuppressed patients.

4. FLUCYTOSINE

Flucytosine inhibits some strains of *Candida, Cryptococcus, Aspergillus, Torulopsis,* and other fungi. Dosages of 3–8 g daily (150 mg/kg/d) orally produce good levels in serum and cerebrospinal fluid. Clinical remissions of meningitis or sepsis due to yeasts have occurred. However, resistant organisms are selected out rapidly, and flucytosine is therefore not employed as a single drug except in urinary tract infections.

In renal insufficiency, flucytosine may accumulate to toxic levels. It is effectively removed by hemodialysis. Toxic effects include bone marrow depression, abnormal liver function, loss of hair, and others. The side effects may be caused by conversion of flucytosine to fluorouracil in the body. Combined use of flucytosine and amphotericin B in systemic candidiasis and cryptococcal meningitis has been shown to be of value.

Bennett JE et al: A comparison of amphotericin alone and combined with flucytosine in the treatment of cryptococcal meningitis. N Engl J Med 1979;301:126.

5. NATAMYCIN

Natamycin is a polyene antifungal drug effective against many different fungi in vitro. When it is combined with appropriate surgical measures, topical application of 5% ophthalmic suspension may be beneficial in the treatment of keratitis caused by *Fusarium, Cephalosporium,* or other fungi. The drug may also be effective in the treatment of oral or vaginal candidiasis. The toxicity after topical application appears to be low.

6. ANTIFUNGAL IMIDAZOLES

These antifungal drugs increase membrane permeability and inhibit lipid and enzyme synthesis.

Clotrimazole, taken orally in 10-mg troches 5 times daily, can suppress oral candidiasis. It is too toxic for systemic use.

Miconazole is active in vitro against *Coccidioides, Candida, Histoplasma, Cryptococcus, Paracoccidioides, Pseudallescheria,* and other fungi. However, it has substantial toxicity and little clinical activity and is rarely used intravenously. It is a drug of choice only for *P boydii* infections in a dose of 30 mg/kg/d in 3 doses. Its major use is as a 2% cream for dermatophytosis and vaginal candidiasis.

Ketoconazole inhibits synthesis of sterols in fungal cell membranes, among other effects. It can be given orally as a single dose, 200–600 mg daily, preferably with food. It is well absorbed and reaches serum levels of 2–4 μg/mL, and it is metabolized in vivo. The dose remains the same in renal or hepatic failure. Absorption is impaired by antacid, cimetidine, or rifampin administration.

Ketoconazole dramatically improves chronic mucocutaneous candidiasis, vaginal candidiasis, paracoccidioidomycosis, and blastomycosis. It also has therapeutic benefits in noncavitary pulmonary histoplasmosis but not in meningitis due to these fungi. In disease of moderate severity, this oral antifungal drug has given encouraging results. However, this drug has been disappointing in the treatment of deep-seated candidal and coccidioidal infections (other than cutaneous lesions) and cryptococcal meningitis, where amphotericin B remains the drug of choice.

Adverse effects include nausea, vomiting, skin rashes, and occasional elevations in transaminase levels. Ketoconazole blocks the synthesis of adrenal steroids and testosterone and can cause gynecomastia and impotence.

Fluconazole, a *bis*-triazole with activity similar to that of miconazole, is water-soluble, which means it can be given both orally and intravenously. It penetrates well into the cerebrospinal fluid and eye and reaches therapeutically significant levels in the urine, making it an attractive agent for the therapy of fungal urinary tract infections due to susceptible organisms. The drug has been shown to be effective in therapy of infections with *Candida, Aspergillus, Cryptococcus, Blastomyces,* and other fungi in animal models, but experience in treating human disease is limited. Fluconazole (100 mg/d) appears to be as efficacious as ketoconazole (400 mg/d) in the therapy of oropharyngeal candidiasis in immunosuppressed patients. Fluconazole (200 mg/d) appears to be effective also in chronic suppressive therapy of cryptococcal meningitis in patients with AIDS. Its use as initial therapy for cryptococcal meningitis and other invasive fungal infections has not been adequately studied and cannot be recommended at present. Its role in prophylaxis in the neutropenic patient is under investigation.

Although pharmacologic properties of the drug and early reports indicating fewer drug interactions than ketoconazole (ie, it may have less of an effect in cyclosporine levels) make fluconazole an attractive agent, it should be emphasized that controlled trials comparing it to existing agents have not been reported, and compared to ketoconazole it is expensive . (One 200-mg tablet of ketoconazole costs $1.37, versus $9.00 for one 100-mg tablet of fluconazole.)

Itraconazole is another oral imidazole with antifungal and pharmacologic properties similar to those of fluconazole. Data on its efficacy in human disease are limited, and the drug requires further study.

Dismukes WE et al: Treatment of systemic mycoses with ketoconazole. Ann Intern Med 1983;98:13.

Fluconazole: A novel advance in therapy for systemic fungal infections. Rev Inf Dis 1990;12(Suppl 3). [Entire issue.]

Hay RJ, Dupont B, Graybill JR (editors): First international symposium on itraconazole. Rev Infect Dis 1987;9(Suppl 1). [Entire issue.]

NIH Mycoses Study Group: Treatment of blastomycosis and histoplasmosis with ketoconazole. Ann Intern Med 1985;103:861.

Restrepo A, Stevens DA, Utz JP (editors): Symposium on ketoconazole. Rev Infect Dis 1980;2:519.

Sugar AM, Sanders C: Oral fluconazole as suppressive therapy of disseminated cryptococcosis in patients with acquired immunodeficiency syndrome. Am J Med 1988; 85:481

ANTIVIRAL CHEMOTHERAPY

Several compounds can influence viral replication and the development of viral disease.

Amantadine is active against influenza A (but not influenza B) and has efficacy both in prophylaxis and therapy of this infection. Amantadine prophylaxis is suggested for the influenza season (6–8 weeks) in patients at increased risk of developing complications of influenza (those with chronic pulmonary and cardiac diseases, persons over 65 years of age, persons with chronic metabolic diseases such as diabetes mellitus and chronic renal failure); in medical personnel who cannot receive vaccine but are capable of transmitting influenza to high-risk patients; if vaccine is not available; and if vaccine strains differ from the strain causing an epidemic. Short-term prophylaxis (2 weeks) is indicated if an outbreak occurs before vaccination has been given. In this setting, amantadine will protect against disease while antibody production is induced and will not interfere with antibody production. Because of its modest therapeutic benefit, high-risk patients and others with influenza A may benefit from treatment with amantadine if it is instituted within 48 hours of the onset of symptoms and continued for 1 week. The usual adult dose is 200 mg orally per day (in persons over 65 years of age, 100 mg). The most marked untoward effects are insomnia, nightmares, and ataxia, especially in the elderly. Amantadine may accumulate and be more toxic in patients with renal insufficiency, and the dosage should be reduced.

Rimantadine is equally effective and perhaps less toxic.

Idoxuridine, 0.1% solution or 0.5% ointment, can be applied topically every 2 hours to the lesions of acute dendritic herpetic keratitis to enhance healing. It is also used, with corticosteroids, for stromal disciform lesions of the cornea to reduce the chance of acute epithelial herpes. Because of its toxicity for the cornea, it must not be used for more than 2–3 weeks.

Trifluridine ointment (1%) is more effective than idoxuridine in herpetic keratitis but also more expensive.

Vidarabine (adenine arabinoside), 3% administered topically, is very effective in herpetic keratitis. Vidarabine, 15 mg/kg/d intravenously, provides systemic treatment for some herpesvirus infections. It is effective in the therapy of herpes zoster infections in immunocompromised patients, for herpes encephalitis, and for neonatal herpes infections. Its use is limited, however, since acyclovir has equal or greater efficacy in these infections. The incidence of cytomegalovirus pneumonia in recipients of bone marrow transplants or kidney transplants has not been reduced by prophylactic vidarabine. Topical vidarabine likewise has no effect on herpetic lesions of skin or mucous membranes.

The untoward effects of vidarabine include rashes, gastrointestinal disturbances, and neurologic abnormalities, including tremors, ataxia, abnormal electroencephalogram, paresthesias, and encephalopathy. All of these are enhanced in renal failure.

Methisazone, 2–4 g orally given within 2 days after exposure to smallpox, protects against clinical disease. The drug is also effective against complications of vaccinia, which continue to occur in military personnel in the USA. The most serious adverse effect is profuse vomiting.

Acyclovir is the least toxic antiviral drug, with therapeutic effects in infections due to herpes simplex and in herpes zoster-varicella infections. In herpes-infected cells, it is selectively active against viral DNA polymerase and thus inhibits virus proliferation. Given intravenously (15 mg/kg/d or 250–500 mg/m^2 every 8 hours), it can prevent and promote healing of mucocutaneous herpes simplex in immunocompromised patients. It can reduce pain, accelerate healing, and prevent dissemination of herpes zoster and varicella in immunocompromised patients. The usual dose for varicella-zoster infections is 30 mg/kg/d in 3 equal doses intravenously. The drug has no effect on establishment of latency, frequency of recurrence, or incidence of postherpetic neuralgia. Acyclovir (30 mg/kg/d in 3 equal doses intravenously) is the drug of choice for herpes encephalitis. Intravenous or oral acyclovir is effective prophylaxis against recurrent mucocutaneous and visceral herpes infections in transplant patients. Intravenous acyclovir may also help in reducing cytomegalovirus infections in seropositive bone marrow and renal transplant patients.

Oral acyclovir, 200 mg 5 times daily, has therapeutic effects similar to those achieved with intravenous acyclovir, particularly in primary genital herpes simplex infections. When taken prophylactically (200 mg 3 times daily or 400 mg twice daily) for 4–6 months, oral acyclovir can reduce the frequency and severity of recurrent lesions during this period. Other possible uses of oral acyclovir include (1) prophylaxis of recurrent herpes simplex infections in renal transplant patients, (2) therapy of herpetic keratitis, (3) prevention and treatment of herpetic whitlow, (4) possibly acceleration of healing of herpes zoster in immunocompetent patients (600–800 mg 5 times daily for 10 days), and (5) therapy of herpes proctitis (400 mg 5 times daily for 10 days).

Topical 5% acyclovir ointment can shorten the period of pain and viral shedding in herpes simplex mucocutaneous oral lesions in immunosuppressed patients but not in patients with normal immunity. Topical acyclovir has largely been replaced by the oral form of the drug.

Serum levels of 2.5 μg/mL are achieved after a 200-mg oral dose, and levels of 35–50 mg/mL are seen after an intravenous infusion of 5 mg/kg. Dosage reduction in renal insufficiency is required. For most infections except encephalitis, the usual dose is 5 mg/kg every 8 hours. For patients with creatinine clearances of 25–50 mL/min, give 5 mg/kg every 12 hours; for clearances of 10–24 mL/min, give 5 mg/kg every 24 hours; and for clearances of 0–10 mL/min, give 2.5 mg/kg every 24 hours. Since hemodialysis reduces serum levels significantly, the daily dose should be given after hemodialysis.

Acyclovir is relatively nontoxic. Precipitation of drug in renal tubules has been described and can best be avoided by maintaining adequate hydration and urine flow. Central nervous system toxicity manifested by confusion, agitation, tremors, and hallucinations has been described.

Foscarnet, an investigational antiviral agent that inhibits DNA polymerase, may be effective in the therapy of herpes simplex infections caused by acyclovir-resistant strains. Studies are presently under way. It may also be useful for ganciclovir-resistant CMV infections.

Ribavirin aerosols sprayed into the respiratory tract early in influenza A and B infection of young adults or respiratory syncytial virus infections of small children resulted in a reduction of symptoms and more rapid recovery. Intravenous ribavirin can significantly lower the fatality rate of Lassa fever.

Zidovudine (Retrovir; formerly azidothymidine [AZT]) is a synthetic thymidine analogue that can be incorporated into DNA by the DNA polymerase (reverse transcriptase) of retroviruses. This terminates chain synthesis of viral DNA. HIV reverse transcriptase is about 100 times more susceptible to inhibition by zidovudine than the DNA polymerase of mammalian cells.

Zidovudine is well absorbed from the gut; peak serum concentrations after 5 mg/kg by mouth are similar to those reached after 2.5 mg/kg intravenously in 1 hour. The drug is metabolized by the liver and excreted in the urine with a half-life of 1 hour. Zidovudine appears to penetrate fairly well into the cerebrospinal fluid.

Zidovudine appears to inhibit retrovirus synthesis and temporarily decrease the morbidity and mortality rates in patients with AIDS or ARC. It has also been shown to slow progression to ARC and AIDS when given in a dose of 1200 mg/d (200 mg every 4 hours) to asymptomatic HIV-positive individuals with fewer than 500 CD4-positive lymphocytes per microliter. Patients with AIDS have a temporary increase in T4 lymphocytes and a reduction in opportunistic infections. In patients with ARC, the increase in T4 lymphocytes persists longer.

The main adverse effects are anemia, granulocytopenia, thrombocytopenia due to bone marrow suppression, and the need for frequent transfusions. There may also be headaches, restlessness, agitation, insomnia, and myopathy. Drugs that interfere with glucuronide conjugation in the liver (eg, acetaminophen, trimethoprim-sulfamethoxazole) will probably increase zidovudine toxicity.

See Chapter 24 for the use of zidovudine in the management of HIV-positive patients.

Dideoxyinosine (ddI), a drug related to zidovudine, is presently under investigation for treatment of AIDS and ARC. After conversion to 5′-triphosphates by cellular enzymes, ddI interferes with reverse transcriptase-mediated production of proviral DNA. Preliminary data suggest that ddI increases CD4 cells and decreases viremia. Major toxicity includes pancreatitis and peripheral neuropathy.

Drugs for cytomegalovirus (CMV) infections. While CMV has long been known as a cause of intrauterine infection and resulting defects, the increasing number of immunocompromised patients—especially those who receive organ transplants or antineoplastic drugs or suffer from AIDS—has drawn attention to the importance of CMV diseases, including retinitis and pneumonia with a high mortality rate.

Ganciclovir (formerly DHPG) is an analogue of acyclovir that has broad antiviral activity, including activity against CMV. Most information about its potential usefulness for the therapy of CMV infections comes from uncontrolled open trials. The drug appears to be efficacious in the therapy of CMV retinitis in AIDS patients and may be useful for therapy of CMV gastroenteritis in these patients. Once therapy is stopped, the relapse rate is high, and long-term maintenance suppressive therapy is required. Therapy of CMV pneumonitis with this agent has been disappointing. Uncontrolled studies of small numbers of patients have suggested that the addition of intravenous immunoglobulin to ganciclovir may improve therapy of CMV pneumonitis. In one of the few prospective, controlled, randomized studies, ganciclovir was found to be no better than placebo for therapy of CMV gastroenteritis (esophagitis, gastritis, duodenitis) in bone marrow transplant patients. CMV viremia and hepatitis are often self-limited diseases, and the role of ganciclovir in treating these syndromes awaits clarification. In addition, ganciclovir has not been studied as a prophylactic agent to prevent CMV infection in high-risk patients, though high-dose intravenous and oral acyclovir has been shown to be effective for this purpose in bone marrow and renal transplant patients.

The initial dose of ganciclovir is usually 2.5 mg/kg every 8 hours or 5 mg/kg every 12 hours, resulting in peak serum levels of 18–24 μg/mL and cerebrospinal fluid levels of 2–2.7 μg/mL. The drug is cleared by the kidneys, and dosage adjustments are required for creatinine clearances less than 50 mL/min. For clearances of 30–50 mL/min, 2.5 mg/kg every 12 hours should be given; for clearances of 10–29 mL/min, 2.5 mg/kg once daily should be given; and for a clearance of less than 10 mL/min, a single daily dose of 1.25 mg/kg is given. Usual maintenance therapy in a patient with normal renal function is 5 mg/kg/d for 5 days a week.

The major adverse effect is neutropenia, which is reversible but requires dosage reduction. Thrombocytopenia, disorientation, nausea, rash, and phlebitis occur less commonly.

Human interferons have been prepared from stimulated lymphocytes or other cells and, more recently, by recombinant DNA technology. When given intravenously, 10^6–10^9 units daily prevented dissemination of early herpes zoster in immunocompromised patients, prevented or delayed reactivation of herpes simplex after trigeminal root section, and suppressed viremia with hepatitis B virus. Interferons may have an adjunctive role in managing certain neoplasms or virus infections. Such preparations exhibit moderate antineoplastic and antiviral effects and, in high doses, significant toxicity. Possible practical use of this material is not yet evident.

Balfour HH et al: Acyclovir halts progression of herpes zoster in immunocompromised patients. N Engl J Med 1983;308:1448.

Collaborative DHPG Treatment Study Group: Treatment of serious cytomegalovirus with DHPG in patients with AIDS and other immunodeficiencies. N Engl J Med 1986;314:801.

Dorsky DI, Crumpacker CS: Drugs five years later: Acyclovir. Ann Intern Med 1987;107:859.

Douglas RG Jr Prophylaxis and treatment of influenza. N Engl J Med 1990;332:443.

Erlich KS et al: Foscarnet therapy for severe acyclovir-resistant herpes simplex virus type 2 infections in patients with the acquired immunodeficiency syndrome (AIDS): An uncontrolled trial. Ann Intern Med 1989;110:710.

Fischl MA et al: The safety and efficacy of zidovudine (AZT) in the treatment of subject with mildly symptomatic human immunodeficiency virus type 1 (HIV) infection: A double blind, placebo-controlled trial. Ann Intern Med 1990;112:727.

Hirsch MS, Schooley RT: Treatment of herpesvirus infections. (2 parts.) N Engl J Med 1983;309:963, 1034.

Jacobson MA, Mills J: Serious cytomegalovirus disease in the acquired immunodeficiency syndrome (AIDS): Clinical findings, diagnosis, and treatment. Ann Intern Med 1988;108:585.

Laskin OL et al: Use of ganciclovir to treat serious cytomegalovirus infections in patients with AIDS. J Infect Dis 1987;155:323.

Mertz GJ et al: Long-term acyclovir suppression of frequently recurring genital herpes simplex virus infection: A multicenter double-blind trial. JAMA 1988;260:201.

Meyers JD et al: Acyclovir for prevention of cytomegalovirus infection and disease after allogeneic marrow transplantation. N Engl J Med 1988;318:70.

Reed EC et al: Ganciclovir for the treatment of cytomegalovirus gastroenteritis in bone marrow transplant patients: A randomized, placebo-controlled trial. Ann Intern Med 1990;112:505.

Straus SE et al: Acyclovir suppression of frequently recurring genital herpes: Efficacy and diminishing need during successive years of treatment. JAMA 1988;260:2227.

Volberding PA et al: Zidovudine in asymptomatic human immunodeficiency virus infection: A controlled trial in persons with fewer than 500 CD4 positive cells per cubic millimeter. N Engl J Med 1990;322:941.

Whitley RJ et al: Vidarabine versus acyclovir therapy in herpes simplex encephalitis. N Engl J Med 1986;314:144.

Yarchoan R et al: Clinical pharmacology of 3'-azido-2',3' dideoxy-thymidine (zidovudine) and related dideoxynucleosides. N Engl J Med 1989;321:726.

ANTIMICROBIAL DRUGS USED IN COMBINATION

Indications

Possible reasons for employing 2 or more antimicrobials simultaneously instead of a single drug are as follows:

(1) Prompt treatment in desperately ill patients suspected of having a serious microbial infection. A good guess about the most probable 2 or 3 pathogens is made, and drugs are aimed at those organisms. Before such treatment is started, adequate specimens must be obtained for identifying the etiologic agent in the laboratory. Suspected gram-negative or staphylococcal sepsis and bacterial meningitis in children are the foremost indications in this category at present.

(2) To delay the emergence of microbial mutants resistant to one drug in chronic infections by the use of a second or third non-cross-reacting drug. The most prominent examples are active tuberculosis of one or more organs, with large microbial populations.

(3) Mixed infections, particularly those following massive trauma or those involving vascular structures. Each drug is aimed at an important pathogenic microorganism.

(4) To achieve bactericidal synergism (see below). In a few infections, eg, enterococcal endocarditis, a combination of drugs is more likely to eradicate the infection than either drug used alone. Unfortunately, such synergism is unpredictable. A given drug pair may be synergistic for only one microbial strain. Occasionally, simultaneous use of 2 drugs permits significant reduction in dose and thus avoids toxicity but still provides satisfactory antimicrobial action.

Disadvantages

The following disadvantages of using antimicrobial drugs in combinations must always be considered:

(1) The doctor may feel that since several drugs are already being given, everything possible has been done for the patient. This attitude leads to relaxation of the effort to establish a specific diagnosis. It may also give a false sense of security.

(2) The more drugs are administered, the greater the chance for drug reactions to occur or for the patient to become sensitized to drugs.

(3) The cost is unnecessarily high.

(4) Antimicrobial combinations often accomplish no more than an effective single drug.

(5) On very rare occasions, one drug may antagonize a second drug given simultaneously. Antagonism resulting in higher morbidity and mortality rates has been observed mainly in bacterial meningitis when a bacteriostatic drug (eg, tetracycline or chloramphenicol) was given prior to or with a bactericidal drug (eg, a penicillin or aminoglycoside). However, antagonism is usually limited by time-dose relationships and is overcome by an excess dose of one of the drugs in the pair and is therefore a very infrequent problem in clinical therapy.

Synergism

Antimicrobial synergism can occur in several types of situations. Synergistic drug combinations must be selected by complex laboratory procedures.

(1) Sequential block of a microbial metabolic pathway by 2 drugs. Sulfonamides inhibit the use of extracellular p-aminobenzoic acid by some microbes for the synthesis of folic acid. Trimethoprim or pyrimethamine inhibits the next metabolic step, the reduction of dihydrofolic to tetrahydrofolic acid. The simultaneous use of a sulfonamide plus trimethoprim is effective in some bacterial infections (eg, urinary tract, enteric) and in some parasitic infections (*Pneumocystis* infection). Pyrimethamine plus a sulfonamide is used in toxoplasmosis and malaria.

(2) One drug may greatly enhance the uptake of a second drug and thereby greatly increase the overall bactericidal effect. Penicillins enhance the uptake of aminoglycosides by enterococci. Thus, a penicillin plus an aminoglycoside may be essential for the eradication of *S faecalis* or *Streptococcus* group B infections, particularly in sepsis or endocarditis. Similarly, ticarcillin plus gentamicin may be synergistic against some strains of *Pseudomonas*. Cell wall inhibitors (penicillins and cephalosporins) may also enhance the entry of aminoglycosides into other gram-negative bacteria and thus produce synergistic effects.

(3) One drug may affect the cell membrane and facilitate the entry of the second drug. The combined effect may then be greater than the sum of its parts. Polymyxins have been synergistic with trimethoprim-sulfamethoxazole or rifampin against *Serratia*, and amphotericin B has been synergistic with flucytosine against *Candida* and *Cryptococcus*.

(4) One drug prevents the inactivation of a second drug by microbial enzymes. Thus, inhibitors of β-lactamase (eg, clavulanic acid) can protect amoxicillin or ticarcillin from inactivation by β-lactamase-producing *H influenzae* and other organisms.

Jawetz E: The doctor's dilemma. In: *Current Clinical Topics in Infectious Diseases.* Remington JS, Swartz MN (editors). McGraw-Hill, 1981.

ANTIMICROBIAL CHEMOPROPHYLAXIS

Anti-infective chemoprophylaxis implies the administration of antimicrobial drugs to prevent infection. In a broader sense, it also includes the use of antimicrobial drugs soon after the acquisition of pathogenic microorganisms (eg, after compound fracture) but before the development of signs of infection.

Useful chemoprophylaxis is limited to the action of a specific drug on a specific organism. An effort to prevent all types of microorganisms in the environment from establishing themselves only selects the most drug-resistant organisms as the cause of a resulting infection. In all proposed uses of prophylactic antimicrobials, the risk of the patient's acquiring an infection must be weighed against the toxicity, cost, inconvenience, and enhanced risk of superinfection resulting from the "prophylactic" drug.

Prophylaxis in Persons of Normal Susceptibility Exposed to a Specific Pathogen

In this category, a specific drug is administered to prevent one specific infection. Outstanding examples are the injection of benzathine penicillin G, 1.2 million units intramuscularly once every 3–4 weeks, to prevent reinfection with group A hemolytic streptococci in patients who have had rheumatic fever; prevention of meningitis by eradicating the meningococcal carrier state with rifampin, 600 mg orally twice daily for 2 days, or minocycline, 100 mg every 12 hours for 5 days; prevention of *H influenzae* disease in contacts of patients with rifampin, 20 mg/kg/d for 4 days; prevention of syphilis by the injection of benzathine penicillin G, 2.4 million units intramuscularly, within 24 hours of exposure; and prevention of plague pneumonia in contacts of plague victims with tetracycline, 0.5 g twice daily for 5 days.

Early treatment of an asymptomatic infection is sometimes called "prophylaxis." Thus, administration of isoniazid, 6–10 mg/kg/d (maximum, 300 mg daily) orally for 6–12 months, to an asymptomatic person who converts from a negative to a positive tuberculin skin test may prevent later clinical active tuberculosis.

Prophylaxis in Persons of Increased Susceptibility

Certain anatomic or functional abnormalities predispose to serious infections. It may be feasible to prevent or abort such infections by giving a specific drug for short periods. Some important examples are listed below:

A. Heart Disease: Persons with abnormalities of heart valves or with prosthetic valves are unusually susceptible to implantation of microorganisms circulating in the bloodstream. Thus, bacterial endocarditis can sometimes be prevented if the proper drug can be used during periods of bacteremia. Large numbers of viridans streptococci are introduced into the circulation during dental procedures and operations on the mouth or throat. At such times, the increased risk warrants the use of a prophylactic antimicrobial drug aimed at viridans streptococci, eg, penicillin V, 2 g orally 1 hour before and 1 g orally 6 hours after the procedure (Shulman et al, 1984). It may be that an aminoglycoside should be given together with penicillin for optimal bactericidal effect in high-risk patients such as those with prosthetic valves. In persons hypersensitive to penicillin or those receiving daily doses

of penicillin for prolonged periods (for rheumatic fever prophylaxis), erythromycin should be given in a dosage of 1 g orally 1 hour before and 0.5 g orally 6 hours after the procedure.

Enterococci cause 5–15% of cases of bacterial endocarditis. They reach the bloodstream from the urinary or gastrointestinal tract or from the female genital tract. During surgical procedures in these areas, persons with heart valve abnormalities can be given prophylaxis directed against enterococci, eg, ampicillin, 2 g intramuscularly or intravenously, plus gentamicin, 1.5 mg/kg intramuscularly, 1 hour prior to the procedure. An optimal follow-up dose may be given 8 hours after the initial dose.

During and after cardiac catheterization, blood cultures may be positive in 10–20% of patients. Many of these persons also have fever, but very few acquire endocarditis. Prophylactic antimicrobials do not appear to influence these events.

B. Respiratory Tract Disease: Persons with functional and anatomic abnormalities of the respiratory tract—eg, emphysema or bronchiectasis—are subject to attacks of "recurrent chronic bronchitis." This is a recurrent bacterial infection, often precipitated by acute viral infections and resulting in respiratory decompensation. The most common organisms are pneumococci and *H influenzae*. Chemoprophylaxis consists of giving tetracycline or ampicillin, 1 g daily orally, during the "respiratory disease season." This is successful only in patients who are not hospitalized; otherwise, superinfection with *Pseudomonas, Proteus,* or yeasts is common. Similar prophylaxis of bacterial infection has been applied to children with cystic fibrosis who are not hospitalized. In spite of this, such children contract complicating infections caused by *Pseudomonas* and staphylococci. The efficacy of aerosolized aminoglycosides in preventing recurrences of infection in cystic fibrosis has not been conclusively demonstrated. Trimethoprim-sulfamethoxazole is effective as a prophylactic against *Pneumocystis* pneumonia in immunocompromised persons.

C. Recurrent Urinary Tract Infection: In certain women who are subject to frequently recurring urinary tract infections, oral intake of nitrofurantoin, 100 mg, or trimethoprim (40 mg)-sulfamethoxazole (200 mg), daily or 3 times weekly; trimethoprim, 100 mg daily; and others may markedly reduce the frequency of symptomatic recurrences.

Some women frequently develop symptoms of cystitis after sexual intercourse. The ingestion of a single dose of antimicrobial drug (100 mg nitrofurantoin, 250 mg cephalexin, etc) can prevent this postcoital cystitis by early inhibition of growth of bacteria moved into the proximal urethra or bladder from the introitus during intercourse.

D. Opportunistic Infections in Severe Granulocytopenia: Patients with leukemia or neoplasm develop profound leukopenia while being given antineoplastic chemotherapy. When the neutrophil count falls below $500/\mu L$, they become unusually susceptible to opportunistic infections, most often gram-negative sepsis. In some cancer centers, such individuals are given a drug combination (antipseudomonal penicillin, aminoglycoside, cephalosporin) directed at the most prevalent opportunists at the earliest sign (eg, fever) of infection. This is continued until the granulocyte count rises again. Retrospective studies suggest that there is some benefit to this procedure.

In other centers, such patients are given drugs to suppress the bowel flora such as oral insoluble antimicrobials (neomycin + polymyxin + nystatin, trimethoprim-sulfamethoxazole, norfloxacin, or ciprofloxacin) during the period of granulopenia to reduce the incidence of gram-negative sepsis. Some benefit has been reported from this approach.

Prophylaxis in Surgery

A major portion of all antimicrobial drugs used in hospitals is employed on surgical services with the stated intent of "prophylaxis." The administration of antimicrobials before and after surgical procedures is sometimes viewed as "banning the microbial world" both from the site of the operation and from other organ systems that suffer postoperative complications. Regrettably, the provable benefit of antimicrobial prophylaxis in surgery is much more limited.

Several general features of "surgical prophylaxis" merit consideration.

(1) In clean elective surgical procedures (ie, procedures during which no tissue bearing normal flora is traversed, other than the prepared skin), the disadvantages of "routine" antibiotic prophylaxis (allergy, toxicity, superinfection) generally outweigh the possible benefits.

(2) Prophylactic administration of antibiotics should generally be considered only if the expected rate of infectious complications approaches or exceeds 5%. An exception to this rule is the elective insertion of prostheses (cardiovascular, orthopedic), where a possible infection would have a catastrophic effect.

(3) If prophylactic antimicrobials are to be effective, a sufficient concentration of drug must be present at the operative site to inhibit or kill bacteria that might settle there. Thus, it is essential that drug administration begin 1–3 hours before operation.

(4) Prolonged administration of antimicrobial drugs tends to alter the normal flora of organ systems, suppressing the susceptible microorganisms and favoring the implantation of drug-resistant ones. Thus, antimicrobial prophylaxis should last only 24 hours after the procedure to prevent superinfection.

(5) Systemic antimicrobial levels usually do not prevent wound infection, pneumonia, or urinary tract infection if physiologic abnormalities or foreign bodies are present.

In major surgical procedures, the administration of a "broad-spectrum" bactericidal drug from just before until 1 day after the procedure has been found effective. First-generation cephalosporins have been most extensively studied and are usually employed for prophylaxis. They are as effective as second- and third-generation cephalosporins for prophylaxis and are much less expensive (see Table 31–5). Thus, cefazolin, 1 g intramuscularly or intravenously given 2 hours before gastrointestinal, pelvic, or orthopedic procedures and again at 2, 10, and 18 hours after the end of the operation, reduces the risk of deep infections at the operative site. Similarly, in cardiovascular surgery, antimicrobials directed at the commonest organisms producing infection are begun just prior to the procedure and continued for 24 hours thereafter. While this prevents drug-susceptible organisms from producing endocarditis, pericarditis, or similar complications, it may favor the implantation of drug-resistant bacteria or fungi.

Other forms of surgical prophylaxis attempt to reduce normal flora or existing bacterial contamination at the site. Thus, the colon is routinely prepared not only by mechanical cleansing through cathartics and enemas but also by the oral administration of insoluble drugs (eg, neomycin, 1 g, plus erythromycin base, 1 g, every 6 hours) for 1 day before operation. In the case of a perforated viscus resulting in peritoneal contamination, there is little doubt that immediate treatment with an aminoglycoside, a penicillin, or clindamycin reduces the impact of seeded infection. Similarly, grossly infected compound fractures or war wounds benefit from a penicillin or cephalosporin plus an aminoglycoside. In all these instances, the antimicrobials tend to reduce the likelihood of rapid and early invasion of the bloodstream and tend to help localize the infectious process—though they generally are incapable of preventing it altogether. The surgeon must be watchful for the selection of the most resistant members of the flora, which tend to manifest themselves 2 or 3 days after the beginning of such "prophylaxis"—which is really an attempt at very early treatment.

In all situations where antimicrobials are administered with the hope that they may have a "prophylactic" effect, the risk from these same drugs (allergy, toxicity, selection of superinfecting microorganisms) must be evaluated daily, and the course of prophylaxis must be kept as brief as possible.

Topical antimicrobials (intravenous tube site catheter, closed urinary drainage, within a surgical wound, acrylic bone cement, etc) may have limited usefulness but must always be viewed with suspicion.

Conte JE Jr, Jacob LS, Pole HC Jr: *Antibiotic Prophylaxis in Surgery.* Lippincott, 1984.

Hughes WT et al: Successful chemoprophylaxis for *Pneumocystis carinii* pneumonitis. N Engl J Med 1977;297:1419.

Jackson GG: Considerations of antibiotic prophylaxis in nonsurgical high risk patients. Am J Med 1981;70:467.

Joshi JH et al: Can antibacterial therapy be discontinued

in persistently febrile granulocytopenic cancer patients? Am J Med 1984;76:450.

Kaiser AB: Antimicrobial prophylaxis in surgery. N Engl J Med 1986;315:1129.

Shulman ST et al: Prevention of bacterial endocarditis. (Committee on Rheumatic Fever and Infective Endocarditis of the Council on Cardiovascular Disease.) Circulation 1984;70:1123A.

REFERENCES

Brown AE, Armstrong D (editors): Symposium on infectious complications of neoplastic disease. (2 parts.) Am J Med 1984;76:413, 631.

Committee on Infectious Diseases: *Report*, 20th ed. American Academy of Pediatrics, 1986.

Jawetz E et al: *Review of Medical Microbiology*, 18th ed. Appleton & Lange, 1989.

Katzung BG (editor): *Basic & Clinical Pharmacology*, 4th ed. Appleton & Lange, 1989.

Man and Drugs in the Third World: The doctor's viewpoint. (Workshop.) Dan Med Bull 1984;31(Suppl 1). [Entire issue.]

Neu HC: Changing patterns of hospital infections—implications for therapy: Changing mechanisms of bacterial resistance. Am J Med 1984;77(1B):11.

Snavely SR, Hodges GR: The neurotoxicity of antibacterial agents. Ann Intern Med 1984;101:92.

Disorders Due to Physical Agents

32

Joseph LaDou, MD, & Richard Cohen, MD, MPH

DISORDERS DUE TO COLD

Cold tolerance varies considerably among individuals. Factors that increase the likelihood of injury from exposure to cold include poor general physical conditioning, nonacclimatization, advanced age, systemic illness, poor tissue oxygenation, and the use of alcohol or other sedative drugs. High wind velocity ("windchill factor") increases the severity of cold injury at low temperatures.

Cold Urticaria

Some persons have a familial or acquired hypersensitivity to cold and may develop urticaria upon even limited exposure to a cold wind. The urticaria usually occurs only on exposed areas, but in markedly sensitive individuals the response can be generalized. Immersion in cold water may result in severe systemic symptoms, including shock. Recognition of the disorder is important because it has been responsible for deaths from swimming in cold water. Familial cold urticaria, manifested as a burning sensation of the skin occurring about 30 minutes after exposure to cold, does not seem to be a true urticarial disorder. In some patients with acquired cold urticaria, the disorder may be associated with the administration of drugs such as griseofulvin or with infections such as infectious mononucleosis. Cold urticaria may occur secondarily to cryoglobulinemia. Cold urticaria may be associated with cold hemoglobinuria as a complication of syphilis. In most cases of acquired cold urticaria, the cause is not known. For diagnosis, an ice cube is usually applied to the skin of the forearm for 4–5 minutes, then removed, and the area is observed for 10 minutes. As the skin rewarms, an urticarial wheal appears at the site and may be accompanied by itching. Histamine and other mediators released in the cold urticaria response are similar to those found in allergic reactions. Cyproheptadine in divided doses of 16–32 mg/d is the drug of choice for cold urticaria.

Raynaud's Phenomenon

See Chapter 9.

SYSTEMIC HYPOTHERMIA

Systemic hypothermia may result from exposure (atmospheric or immersion) to prolonged or extreme cold. The condition may arise in otherwise healthy individuals in the course of occupational or recreational exposure or in victims of accidents.

Systemic hypothermia may follow exposure even to comparatively ordinary temperatures when there is altered homeostasis due to debility or disease. In colder climates, elderly and inactive individuals living in inadequately heated housing are particularly susceptible. Acute alcoholism is commonly a predisposing cause. Patients with cardiovascular or cerebrovascular disease, mental retardation, malnutrition, myxedema, and hypopituitarism are more vulnerable to accidental hypothermia. The use of sedative and tranquilizing drugs may be a contributing factor. Prolonged postoperative hypothermia with increased mortality rates after surgery has been reported, especially in elderly patients. Administration of large amounts of refrigerated stored blood (without rewarming) can cause systemic hypothermia.

Pathogenesis

Systemic hypothermia is a reduction of core (rectal) body temperature below 35 °C. It causes reduced physiologic function—with decreased oxygen consumption and slowed myocardial repolarization, peripheral nerve conduction, gastrointestinal motility, and respirations—as well as hemoconcentration and pancreatitis. The body defends itself against cold exposure by superficial blood vessel constriction and increased metabolic heat production.

Clinical Findings

Early manifestations of hypothermia are not specific. There may be weakness, drowsiness, lethargy, irritability, confusion, and impaired coordination. A lowered body temperature may be the sole finding.

The internal (core) body temperature in accidental hypothermia may range from 25 to 35 °C (77–95 °F). Oral temperatures are useless, so an esophageal or rectal probe that reads as low as 25 °C is required. At core temperatures below 35 °C, the patient may become delirious, drowsy, or comatose and may stop breathing. Indeed, the pulse and blood pressure may be unobtainable, leading clinicians to believe the patient is dead. Metabolic acidosis, pneumonia, pancreatitis, ventricular fibrillation, hypoglycemia or hyperglycemia, coagulopathy, and renal failure may occur. Abnormalities in cardiac rhythm are directly related to the lowering of core temperature. Progression of electrocardiographic abnormalities can also occur, including the pathognomonic "J" wave of Osborn—a second upward wave immediately following the S wave, which has been well described in lead II. Death in systemic hypothermia usually results from cardiac arrest or ventricular fibrillation.

Treatment

Patients with mild hypothermia (rectal temperature > 33 °C) who have been otherwise physically healthy usually respond well to a warm bed or to rapid rewarming with a warm bath or warm packs and blankets. A conservative approach is also usually employed in treating elderly or debilitated patients, using an electric blanket kept at 37 °C (98.6 °F).

Patients with moderate or severe hypothermia (core temperatures of < 32 °C [89.6 °F]) do not have the thermoregulatory shivering mechanism and so require active rewarming with individualized supportive care. Adequate cardiovascular support, acid-base balance, arterial oxygenation, and adequate intravascular volume should be established prior to rewarming to minimize the risk of organ infarction. The methods and rate of active rewarming are controversial. Successful treatment usually includes a combination of active external and internal methods. Aggressive rewarming should be attempted only by those experienced in the methods. *Once begun, CPR should continue until the patient has been rewarmed to at least 32 °C (89.6 °F).* The need for oxygen therapy, endotracheal intubation, controlled ventilation, warmed intravenous fluids, and treatment of metabolic acidosis should be dictated by careful clinical and laboratory monitoring during the rapid rewarming process. Essential laboratory tests include serum amylase, electrolytes, pH, hemoglobin, glucose, blood gases, and urine volume. Cardiac rhythm should be monitored, and cardiac, central vascular, or chest trauma or stimulation (catheter, cannulas, etc) should be avoided unless essential because of the risk of inducing ventricular fibrillation. The patient should be evaluated for trauma and peripheral cold injury (eg, frostbite). Steroids and antibiotics are not routinely given and should be used only if indicated. Core temperature (esophageal preferred over rectal) should be monitored frequently during and after initial rewarm-

ing because of reports of delayed (repeated) hypothermia.

Active external rewarming methods. Although relatively simple and generally available, active external warming methods may cause marked peripheral dilation that predisposes to ventricular fibrillation and hypovolemic shock. Either heated blankets or warm baths may be used for active external rewarming. Rewarming by a warm bath is best carried out in a tub of stirred water at 40–42 °C (104–107.6 °F), with a rate of rewarming of about 1–2 °C/h. It is easier, however, to monitor the patient and to carry out diagnostic and therapeutic procedures when heated blankets are used for active rewarming.

Active internal (core) rewarming methods. Internal rewarming is recommended for patients with severe hypothermia. Repeated peritoneal dialysis may be employed with 2 L of warm (43 °C) potassium-free dialysate solution exchanged at intervals of 10–12 minutes until the core temperature is raised to about 35 °C. The administration of heated, humidified air through a face mask or endotracheal tube may be useful, either alone or as an adjunct to other rewarming techniques. Warm colonic and gastrointestinal irrigations and warmed intravenous fluids are of less value. Extracorporeal blood rewarming methods (eg, femorofemoral bypass) have been effectively employed in some medical centers to provide rapid cardiac rewarming with less likelihood of arrhythmias.

Prognosis

With proper early care, more than 75% of otherwise healthy patients may survive moderate or severe systemic hypothermia. The risk of aspiration pneumonia is great in comatose patients. The prognosis is grave if there are underlying predisposing causes or treatment is delayed.

HYPOTHERMIA OF THE EXTREMITIES

Exposure of the extremities to cold produces immediate localized vasoconstriction followed by generalized vasoconstriction. When the skin temperature falls to 25 °C (77 °F), tissue metabolism is slowed, but the demand for oxygen is greater than the slowed circulation can supply, and the area becomes cyanotic. At 15 °C (59 °F), tissue metabolism is markedly decreased and the dissociation of oxyhemoglobin is reduced; this gives a deceptive pink, well-oxygenated appearance to the skin. Tissue damage occurs at this temperature. Tissue death may be caused by ischemia and thromboses in the smaller vessels or by actual freezing. Freezing (frostbite) does not occur until the skin temperature drops to −10 to −4 °C (14–24.8 °F) or even lower, depending on such factors as wind, mobility, venous stasis, malnutrition, and occlusive arterial disease. Neuropathic sequelae such as pain, numbness, tingling, hyperhidrosis, cold sensitivity of the extremities, and nerve conduction abnormalities may persist for many years after the cold injury.

Prevention

"Keep warm, keep moving, and keep dry." Individuals should wear warm, dry clothing, preferably several layers, with a windproof outer garment. Wet clothing, socks, and shoes should be replaced with dry ones. Extra socks, mittens, and insoles should always be carried in a pack when a person is in cold or icy areas. Cramped positions, constricting clothing, and prolonged dependency of the feet are to be avoided. Arms, legs, fingers, and toes should be exercised to maintain circulation. Wet and muddy ground and exposure to wind should be avoided. Tobacco and alcohol should be avoided when the danger of frostbite is present.

CHILBLAIN
(Pernio)

Chilblains are red, itching skin lesions, usually on the extremities, caused by exposure to cold without actual freezing of the tissues. They may be associated with edema or blistering and are aggravated by warmth. With continued exposure, ulcerative or hemorrhagic lesions may appear and progress to scarring, fibrosis, and atrophy.

Treatment consists of elevating the affected part slightly and allowing it to warm gradually at room temperature. Do not rub or massage injured tissues or apply ice or heat. Protect the area from trauma and secondary infection.

FROSTBITE

Frostbite is injury of the tissues due to freezing. In mild cases, only the skin and subcutaneous tissues are involved; the symptoms are numbness, prickling, and itching. With increasing severity, deep frostbite involves deeper structures, and there may be paresthesia and stiffness. Thawing causes tenderness and burning pain. The skin is white or yellow, loses its elasticity, and becomes immobile. Edema, blisters, necrosis, and gangrene may appear. Scintigraphy has been used to assess the degree of involvement in severe frostbite and to distinguish viable from nonviable tissue.

Treatment

A. Immediate Treatment: Treat the patient for associated systemic hypothermia.

1. Rewarming–Superficial frostbite (frostnip) of extremities in the field can be treated by firm steady

pressure with the warm hand (without rubbing), by placing fingers in the armpits, and, in the case of the toes or heels, by removing footwear, drying feet, rewarming, and covering with adequate dry socks or other protective footwear.

Rapid thawing at temperatures slightly above body heat may significantly decrease tissue necrosis. If there is any possibility of refreezing, the frostbitten part should not be thawed, even if this might mean prolonged walking on frozen feet. Refreezing results in increased tissue necrosis. It has been suggested that rewarming is best accomplished by immersing the frozen portion of the body for several minutes in water heated to 40–42 °C (104–107.6 °F) *(not warmer)*. Water in this temperature range feels warm but not hot to the normal hand. Dry heat (eg, stove or open fire) is more difficult to regulate and is not recommended. After thawing has occurred and the part has returned to normal temperature (usually in about 30 minutes), discontinue external heat. Victims and rescue workers should be cautioned not to attempt rewarming by exercise or thawing of frozen tissues by rubbing with snow or ice water.

2. Protection of the part–Pressure or friction is avoided and physical therapy contraindicated in the early stage. The patient is kept at bed rest with the affected parts elevated and uncovered at room temperature. Casts, dressings, or bandages are not applied. A combination of ibuprofen and aloe vera has been used to prevent dermal ischemia.

3. Anti-infective measures–It is very important to prevent infection after the rewarming process. Protect skin blebs from physical contact. Local infections may be treated with mild soaks of soapy water or povidone-iodine. Whirlpool therapy at temperatures slightly below body temperature twice daily for 15–20 minutes for a period of 3 or more weeks helps cleanse the skin and debrides superficial sloughing tissue. Antibiotics may be required for deep infections.

B. Follow-Up Care: Gentle, progressive physical therapy to promote circulation is important as healing progresses. Buerger's exercises should be instituted as soon as tolerated.

C. Surgery: Early regional sympathectomy (within 36–72 hours) has been reported to protect against the sequelae of frostbite, but the value of this measure is controversial. In general, other surgical intervention is to be avoided. *Amputation should not be considered until it is definitely established that the tissues are dead.* Tissue necrosis (even with black eschar formation) may be quite superficial, and *the underlying skin may sometimes heal spontaneously even after a period of months.*

Prognosis

Recovery from frostbite is most often complete, but there may be increased susceptibility to discomfort in the involved extremity upon reexposure to cold.

IMMERSION SYNDROME
(Immersion Foot or Trench Foot)

Immersion foot (or hand) is caused by prolonged immersion in cool or cold water or mud. The affected parts are first cold and anesthetic. They become hot with intense burning and shooting pains during the hyperemic period and pale or cyanotic with diminished pulsations during the vasospastic period; blistering, swelling, redness, heat, ecchymoses, hemorrhage, or gangrene and secondary complications such as lymphangitis, cellulitis, and thrombophlebitis follow later.

Treatment is best instituted during the stage of reactive hyperemia. Immediate treatment consists of protecting the extremities from trauma and secondary infection and gradual rewarming by exposure to cool air (not ice or heat) without massaging or moistening the skin or immersing it in water. Bed rest is required until all ulcers have healed. Affected parts are elevated to aid in removal of edema fluid, and pressure sites (eg, heels) are protected with pillows. Later treatment is as for Buerger's disease (see Chapter 9).

Edlich RF et al: Cold injuries: Compr Ther 1989;15:13.
Fritz RL, Perrin DH: Cold exposure injuries: Prevention and treatment. Clin Sports Med 1989;8:111.
Lønning PE, Skulberg A, Abyholm F: Accidental hypothermia: Review of the literature. Acta Anaesthesiol Scand 1986;30:601.

DISORDERS DUE TO HEAT

Four medical disorders comprise a spectrum of illness that can result from excessive exposure to hot environments (in order of increasing severity): heat syncope, heat cramps, heat exhaustion, and heat stroke. A stable internal temperature requires a balance between heat production and heat loss, which the hypothalamus regulates by initiating changes in muscle tone, vascular tone, and sweat gland function.

Etiology

Sweat production and evaporation is a major mechanism of heat removal. Conduction (convection)—the direct transfer of heat from the skin to the surrounding air—also occurs, but with diminished efficiency as the ambient temperature rises. The passive transfer of heat from a warmer to a cooler object by radiation accounts for 65% of body heat loss under normal conditions. Radiant heat loss decreases as the temperature of the surrounding environment increases up to 37.2 °C (99 °F), the point at which heat transfer reverses direction. At normal temperatures, evaporation accounts for approximately 20% of the body's heat

loss, but at high temperatures it becomes the major mechanism for dissipation of heat. This mechanism is also limited as humidity increases.

Health conditions that inhibit sweat production or evaporation and increase susceptibility to heat disorders include obesity, generalized skin diseases (miliaria), diminished cutaneous blood flow, dehydration, malnutrition, hypotension, and reduced cardiac output. Medications that impair the sweating mechanism are the anticholinergics, antihistamines, phenothiazines, tricyclic antidepressants, monoamine oxidase inhibitors, and diuretics; reduced cutaneous blood flow results from use of vasoconstrictors and β-adrenergic blocking agents; and dehydration results from use of alcohol. Illicit drugs—eg, phencyclidine, LSD, amphetamines, and cocaine—can cause increased muscle activity and thus generate increased body heat. Drug withdrawal syndrome may have the same effect, as may prolonged seizures.

Prevention

Medical evaluation and monitoring should be used to identify individuals at increased risk of heat disorders. The exposed public should be made aware of the early signs and symptoms of heat disorders. It is not recommended to make salt tablets available for use without medical supervision; close monitoring of fluid and electrolyte intake may be necessary in situations necessitating activity in hot environments. Athletic events should be organized and managed with attention to thermoregulation: the WBGT (wet bulb global temperature) Index should be monitored, water consumption should be encouraged, and medical support should be immediately accessible. Workers should not begin work in hot temperatures without proper acclimatization and should be encouraged to take water frequently.

Protective air-cooled suits have been used successfully in the nuclear power industry for prolonged work in environments up to 60 °C.

Acclimatization is achieved by scheduled regulated exposure to hot environments and by gradually increasing the duration of exposure and the work load, until the body adjusts by starting to produce sweat of lower salt content in greater amounts at lower ambient temperatures. Acclimatization is accompanied by increased plasma volume, cardiac output, and cardiac stroke volume and a slower heart rate.

SPECIFIC SYNDROMES
DUE TO HEAT EXPOSURE

1. HEAT SYNCOPE

Sudden unconsciousness can result from cutaneous vasodilatation with consequent systemic and cerebral hypotension. Systolic blood pressure is usually less than 100 mm Hg, and there is typically a history of vigorous physical activity for 2 hours or more just preceding the episode. The skin is typically cool and moist, and the pulse is weak.

Treatment consists of rest and recumbency in a cool place, with fluids by mouth (or intravenously if necessary).

2. HEAT CRAMPS

Fluid and electrolyte depletion can result in slow, painful skeletal muscle contractions ("cramps") and even severe muscle spasms lasting 1–3 minutes, usually of the muscles most heavily used. Cramping results from salt depletion as sweat losses are replaced with water alone. The skin is moist and cool, and the muscles are tender. There may be muscle twitching. The victim is alert, with stable vital signs, but may be agitated and complaining of pain. The body temperature may be normal or slightly increased. Involved muscle groups are hard and lumpy. There is almost always a history of vigorous activity just preceding the onset of symptoms. Laboratory evaluation may show low serum sodium and hemoconcentration.

The patient should be moved to a cool environment and given oral saline solution (4 tsp of salt per gallon of water) to replace both salt and water. *Because of their slower absorption, salt tablets are not recommended.* The victim may have to rest for 1–3 days with continued dietary salt supplementation before returning to work or resuming heavy activity in the heat.

3. HEAT EXHAUSTION

Heat exhaustion results from prolonged heavy activity with inadequate salt intake in a hot environment and is characterized by dehydration, sodium depletion, or isotonic fluid loss with accompanying cardiovascular changes.

The diagnosis is based on prolonged symptoms and a rectal temperature over 37.8 °C (100 °F), increased pulse rate—usually more than half again the patient's normal rate—and moist skin. Symptoms associated with heat syncope and heat cramps may also be present. The patient may be quite thirsty and weak, with central nervous system symptoms such as headache, fatigue, and, in cases due chiefly to water depletion, anxiety paresthesias, impaired judgment, hysteria, and in some cases psychosis. Hyperventilation secondary to heat exhaustion can lead to respiratory alkalosis. Heat exhaustion may progress to heat stroke if sweating ceases.

Treatment consists of placing the patient in a shaded, cool environment and providing adequate hydration and salt replenishment—orally, if possible. Physiologic saline or isotonic glucose solution can be administered intravenously in severe cases or when oral administration is not appropriate. Intravenous hypertonic saline may be necessary if sodium depletion is severe. At least 24 hours of rest is recommended.

4. HEAT STROKE

Heat stroke is a life-threatening medical emergency resulting from failure of the thermoregulatory mechanism and is manifested by cerebral dysfunction with impaired consciousness, high fever, and absence of sweating. Heat stroke is imminent when the core (rectal) temperature approaches 41 °C (106 °F). Persons at greatest risk are the elderly or chronically infirm or those receiving medications (eg, anticholinergics, antihistamines, phenothiazines) that interfere with heat-dissipating mechanisms. Morbidity or even death can result from cerebral, cardiovascular, hepatic, or renal damage.

Clinical Findings

A. Symptoms and Signs: Failure of the heat dissipation mechanism for any reason results in dizziness, weakness, emotional lability, nausea and vomiting, confusion, delirium, blurred vision, convulsions, collapse, and unconsciousness. The skin is hot and initially covered with perspiration. Later it dries. The pulse is strong initially. Blood pressure may be slightly elevated at first, but hypotension develops later. The core temperature is usually over 41 °C. As with heat exhaustion, hyperventilation can occur, leading to respiratory alkalosis and compensatory metabolic acidosis.

B. Laboratory Findings: Laboratory evaluation reveals dehydration, leukocytosis, elevated BUN, hemoconcentration, and decreased serum potassium, calcium, and phosphorus; urine is concentrated, with elevated protein, tubular casts, and myoglobinuria. Thrombocytopenia, increased bleeding and clotting times, fibrinolysis, and consumption coagulopathy may also be present. Rhabdomyolysis and myocardial, hepatic, or renal damage may be identified by appropriate tests.

Treatment

Treatment is aimed at reducing the core temperature rapidly (within 1 hour) and controlling the secondary effects. Evaporative cooling is rapid and effective and is easily performed in most emergency settings. The patient's clothing should be removed and the entire body sprayed with water (15 °C) while cooled or ambient air is passed across the patient's body with large fans or other means at high velocity (100 ft/min). The patient should be in the lateral recumbent position or supported in a hands-and-knees position to expose as much skin surface as possible to the air. Other alternatives include use of cold wet sheets accompanied by fanning or isopropyl alcohol instead of water.

Immersion in an ice-water bath has often been recommended but is no longer preferred because of its greater potential for complications of hypotension and shivering. Other treatment alternatives include ice packs and iced gastric lavage, although these are much less effective than evaporative cooling.

Treatment should be continued until the rectal temperature drops to 39 °C. The temperature remains stable in most cases, but it should continue to be monitored for 24 hours. Chlorpromazine (25–50 mg intravenously) can be used to control shivering and other muscular activity associated with increased heat load. Aspirin should not be given because of its antiplatelet effect; additionally, it has no effect on the hyperthermia.

Hypovolemic and cardiogenic shock must be carefully distinguished, as either or both may occur. Central venous or pulmonary artery wedge pressure should be monitored. Five percent dextrose in saline (500–1000 mL) may be given without overloading the circulation if hypovolemic shock is present.

The patient should also be observed for renal failure due to rhabdomyolysis, hypokalemia, cardiac arrhythmias, disseminated intravascular coagulation, and hepatic failure. Corticosteroids have not been shown to be of value.

Fluid output should be monitored through the use of an indwelling urinary catheter.

Because sensitivity to high environmental temperature continues in some patients for prolonged periods following an episode of heat stroke, immediate reexposure should be avoided.

American College of Sports Medicine: Position stand on the prevention of injuries during distance running. Med Sci Sports Exerc 1987;19:529.
Knochel JP: Heat stroke and related heat stress disorders. DM (May) 1989;35:303.

BURNS

Over 2 million injuries, 70,000 hospitalizations, and 9000 deaths occur from burns each year in the USA. Burns are the leading cause of accidental death in children and are largely preventable.

Scalds are a common form of thermal injury to children and the elderly that can be partially prevented by regulating water temperatures. Enforcement of the Flammable Fabric Act in the USA has reduced the incidence of flame injury to children. However, loose-fitting clothing of the elderly is a hazard near an open flame. Carelessness with burning cigarettes is a common cause of dwelling fires. Smoke alarms

and other fire safety measures have helped to save lives and prevent injury, but further safety legislation and public education are needed.

CLASSIFICATION

Burns are classified by extent, depth, patient age, and associated illness or injury.

Extent

The "rule of nines" (Fig 32–1) is useful for rapidly assessing the extent of a burn. More detailed charts based on age are available when the patient reaches the burn unit. Therefore, it is important to view the entire patient after cleaning soot to make an accurate assessment, both initially and on subsequent examinations. Only second- and third-degree burns are included in calculating the total burn surface area (TBSA), since first-degree burns usually do not represent significant injury in terms of prognosis or fluid and electrolyte management.

Depth

Judgment of depth of injury is difficult. The **first-degree burn** may be red or gray but will demonstrate excellent capillary refill. First-degree burns are not blistered initially. If the wound is blistered, this represents a partial-thickness injury to the dermis, or a **second-degree burn**. However, a deep second-degree burn may have lost its blister and may actually appear

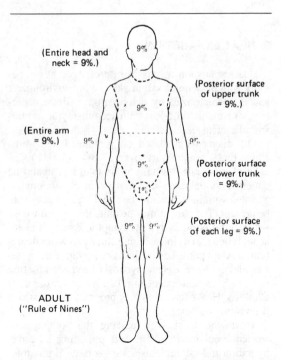

Figure 32–1. Estimation of body surface area in burns.

hyperemic from fixed hemoglobin in the tissue. This redness will not have good refill and will not be as exquisitely sensitive as the hyperemia of the first-degree burn. The line between the partial- and full-thickness injury, or **third-degree burn,** may be indefinite. The initial vasoconstriction of a second-degree burn may make it appear more severe at first. Concerning healing properties of any second- or third-degree burn, the critical factors are blood supply and appendage population. In areas rich in vascularity, hair follicles, and sweat glands, the prospects for reepithelialization are good. Otherwise, even when the dermis is healthy, epithelialization may be slow and more scarring will result.

Age of the Patient

As much as extent and depth of the burn, age of the victim plays a critical part. Even a relatively small burn in an elderly patient or infant may be fatal, as demonstrated in Figs 32–2 and 32–3.

Associated Injuries
& Illnesses

An injury commonly associated with burns is smoke inhalation. The products of combustion, not heat, are responsible for lower airway injury. Burning plastic products produce both hydrochloric acid and hydrocyanic acid. Electrical injury that causes burns may also produce cardiac arrhythmias that require immediate attention. Premorbid physical and psychosocial disorders that complicate recovery from burn injury include cardiac or pulmonary disease, diabetes, alcoholism, drug abuse, and psychiatric illness.

Special Burn Care Units
& Facilities

The American Burn Association and the American College of Surgeons have recommended that major burns be treated in specialized burn care facilities. They also advocate that even moderately severe burns be treated in a specialized facility or hospital where personnel have expertise in burn care. The American Burn Association has classified burn injuries as follows:

A. Major Burn Injuries:

1. Partial-thickness burns over more than 25% of body surface area in adults or 20% in children.

2. Full-thickness burns over more than 10% of surface area in any age group.

3. Deep burns involving the hands, face, eyes, ears, feet, or perineum.

4. Burns complicated by inhalation injury.

5. Electrical and chemical burns.

6. Burns complicated by fractures and other major trauma.

7. Burns in poor-risk patients (extremes of age or intercurrent disease).

B. Moderate Uncomplicated Burn Injuries:

1. Partial-thickness burns over 15–25% of body surface area in adults or 10–20% of body surface area in children.

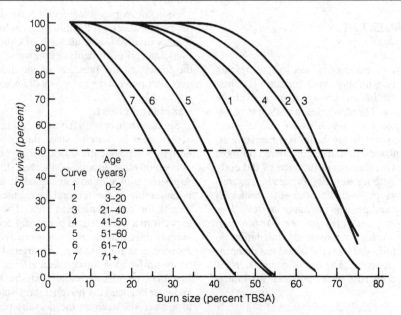

Figure 32–2. Patient survival and burn size according to patient age. (Reproduced, with permission, from Merrell SW et al: Increased survival after major thermal injury. Am J Surg 1987;154:623.)

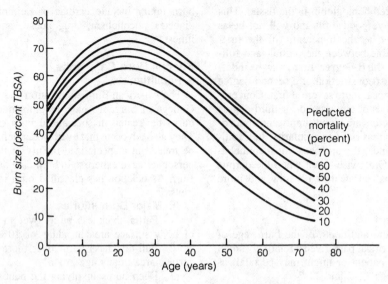

Figure 32–3. Burn size and patient age as predictors of mortality. (Reproduced, with permission, from Merrell SW et al: Increased survival after major thermal injury. AM J Surg 1987;154:623.)

2. Full-thickness burns over 2–10% of body surface area.

3. Burns not involving the specific conditions listed above.

C. Minor Burn Injuries:

1. Partial-thickness burns over less than 15% of body surface area in adults or 10% in children.

2. Full-thickness burns over less than 2% of body surface area.

INITIAL MANAGEMENT

Airway

The physician or emergency medical technician should proceed as with any other trauma. The first priority is to establish an airway, then to evaluate the cervical spine and head injuries, and then to stabilize fractures. *The burn wound itself has a lower priority.* At some point during the initial management, endotracheal intubation should be considered for most major burn cases, regardless of the area of the body involved, for as fluid resuscitation proceeds, generalized edema develops, including the soft tissues of the upper airway and perhaps the lungs as well. *Tracheostomy is rarely indicated for the burn victim,* unless dictated by other circumstances. Inhalation injuries should be followed by serial blood gas determination and bronchoscopy. The use of corticosteroids is contraindicated because of the potential for immunosuppression.

Cooling the Wound

Cooling the victim for up to 20 minutes following the burn has been shown to reduce the depth of injury. Avoid prolonged application of cold water or ice packs to large surfaces, however, since they can cause systemic hypothermia and arrhythmias. Saline soaks at room temperature or cooler should be used. At the scene of an injury, a hose can be used for this purpose. Fire extinguishers and ice are not recommended, as further tissue injury may result.

History

As soon as possible, obtain a detailed history of the circumstances of the injury, including locale, substances involved, and duration of exposure; medications, mental disturbances, confusion resulting from the injury, or the presence of an endotracheal tube may later prevent the recording of an accurate history.

Vascular Access

Simultaneously with the above procedures, venous access must be sought, since the victim of a major burn is in hypovolemic shock. Ideally, a percutaneous intravenous line through nonburned skin is preferred. A peripheral line in an antecubital or subclavian vein is preferable to the femoral vein unless the femoral area is the only nonburned area. The last choice is to perform a well-secured peripheral cutdown. A burn eschar, since it has been flame-sterilized, is an acceptable location for cutdown. An arterial line may also be useful for monitoring mean arterial pressure. The line may be placed initially in the femoral artery and later changed (as peripheral resistance decreases) to a safer site such as the dorsalis pedis, temporal, or radial arteries. Swan-Ganz catheters should be used in patients with preexisting cardiopulmonary disease and in severe burn cases to determine cardiac output and peripheral resistance. Once these parameters have been established, the catheter is usually removed.

FLUID RESUSCITATION

Crystalloids

Generalized capillary leak results from burn injury over more than 25% of the total body surface area. This often necessitates replacement of a large volume of fluid. An intravenous line is recommended in the management of deep partial-thickness and full-thickness burns that cover more than 20% of total body surface area in the adult and 10% in the child.

There are many guidelines for fluid resuscitation, eg, those of Evans, Brooke, Monafo (hypertonic saline), and Parkland (Baxter). In the first 24 hours, all of these fluids deliver approximately 0.5–0.6 meq of sodium per kilogram of body weight per percent of body surface area burned. The total amount of fluid in all but the hypertonic saline formula is roughly the same but differs in distribution. The Parkland formula is currently the most widely used in the USA. It relies upon the use of lactated Ringer's injection, which is available in every emergency room. For adults and children, the fluid requirement in the first 24 hours is estimated as 3–5 mL/kg body weight per percent of body surface area burned (Fig 32–4). The smaller amounts would be used in the elderly or those with less severe burns; the larger amounts would be used in children (who have a larger relative surface-to-volume ratio) and for treatment of deep electrical burns. Four mL/kg body weight per percent of body surface area burned is begun, and this amount is varied according to the patient's response. *Remember that a formula is only a guideline.*

Half the calculated fluid is given in the first 8-hour period. The remaining fluid, divided into 2 equal

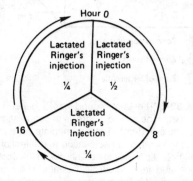

Figure 32–4. Half of the calculated crystalloid formula (lactated Ringer's injection [4mL/kg wt/% TBSA]) is given in the first 8 hours, beginning at the time of the injury. The remainder is given evenly over the ensuing 16 hours.

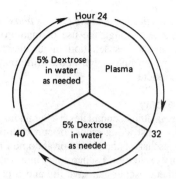

Figure 32–5. The colloid formula (aged plasma or 5% normal serum albumin) [0.3–0.5 mL/kg wt/% TBSA] is given as calculated between hours 24 and 32. In the remaining 16-hour period, 5% dextrose in water is given as needed to maintain a urine output of no less than 30 mL/h.

parts, is delivered over the next 16 hours. An extremely large volume of fluid may be required. For example, an injury over 40% of the total body surface area in a 70-kg victim may require 13 L *in the first 24 hours*. The first 8-hour period is calculated from the hour of injury.

Colloids

After 24 hours, capillary leaks have sealed in the majority of cases, and plasma volume may be restored with colloids (plasma or albumin). The Parkland formula calls for 0.3–0.5 mL/kg body weight per percent of body surface area burned to be given over the first 8-hour period of the second 24 hours. Fluids given in the following 16 hours consist of dextrose in water in quantities sufficient to maintain adequate urine output (Fig 32–5). It is hoped that during the second 24-hour period the vascular system will hold colloids and draw off edema fluid, resulting in diuresis.

Adequacy of Resuscitation

Mental alertness, urinary output, and the vital signs reflect the adequacy of fluid resuscitation. Mental alertness is important because it is the best indicator of adequate cerebral perfusion. Overmedication may cloud the sensorium during the resuscitation phase. Analgesics in the form of small doses of intravenous morphine should be used judiciously so as not to interfere with diagnosis. Renal perfusion is judged by urinary output. Adequate urinary output is 30–50 mL/h in adults and 1 mL/kg body weight/h in children. A smaller output represents inadequate renal perfusion. However, a larger output is unnecessary, and overloading results in edema in every organ.

Monitoring Fluid Resuscitation

A Foley catheter is essential for monitoring urinary

output. *Diuretics have no part in this phase of patient management,* although the use of mannitol may be indicated in the resuscitation of an electrical burn victim in whom myoglobin in the urine may precipitate in the kidneys.

Escharotomy

As edema fluid accumulates, ischemia may develop under any constricting eschar of an extremity. Similarly, an eschar of the thorax or abdomen may limit respiratory excursion. Escharotomy incisions through the anesthetic eschar can save life and limb.

THE BURN WOUND

Treatment of the burn wound is based on several principles: (1) Prevention or delay of infection. (2) Protection from desiccation and further injury of those burned areas that will spontaneously reepithelialize in 7–10 days. (3) Excision and grafting of burned areas that cannot spontaneously reepithelialize during this period.

Systemic Prophylactic Antibiotics

Regardless of the severity of the burn, prophylactic systemic antibiotics are usually not recommended. Their effectiveness is unproved, and they have the disadvantage of favoring the growth of resistant organisms.

Topical Antibiotics

Topical antibiotics delay or prevent infection. An ideal agent would readily penetrate the burn wound eschar, be effective against both gram-negative and gram-positive microorganisms as well as *Candida,* be painless and inexpensive, and have no deleterious side effects. Such an ideal agent does not currently exist. Silver sulfadiazine (Silvadene) is currently the most popular topical agent. It is painless, easy to apply, effective against most *Pseudomonas,* and a fairly good penetrator of eschar, but some microorganisms are resistant to it, and it may cause leukopenia or fever and delay epithelialization.

Mafenide (Sulfamylon) penetrates eschars better than silver sulfadiazine and is more effective against *Pseudomonas.* Mafenide inhibits carbonic anhydrase when used as a 10% solution and results in metabolic acidosis. It also delays epithelialization and may be painful. When it is diluted to a 5% solution, pain and metabolic side effects are lessened. It is useful primarily for deep burns, eg, electrical burns and burns of the ear or nose where cartilage is close to the surface, and when silver sulfadiazine is ineffective. It is best to limit the use of mafenide to no more than 10% of the total body surface area at any given time because of its metabolic effect.

Povidone-iodine is especially useful against *Candida* and both gram-positive and gram-negative microorganisms. However, it penetrates eschar poorly, is very desiccating to the wound surface, and is painful. Also, significantly high blood iodine levels have been demonstrated in patients receiving this agent.

Gentamicin and silver nitrate are no longer recommended as topical agents.

Wound Closure

The goal of therapy after fluid resuscitation is closure of the wound. Nature's own blister is the best cover to protect wounds that spontaneously epithelialize in 7–10 days (ie, superficial second-degree burns). The serum in the blister nurses the surface of the **zone of stasis** until epithelialization takes place (Fig 32–6). Where the blister has been disrupted, human amnion, porcine heterografts (preferably fresh, or frozen and meshed), or collagen composite dressings (Biobrane) can substitute. Cadaver homografts can also serve this purpose if available.

Wounds that will not heal spontaneously in 7–10 days (ie, deep second-degree or third-degree burns) are best treated by excision and autograft; otherwise, granulation and infection may develop. Granulation is nature's signal that attempts to close the wound have failed. A "skin equivalent"—a patient's own skin cells grown in culture into multilayered sheets of epithelium—is currently being tested in some burn centers.

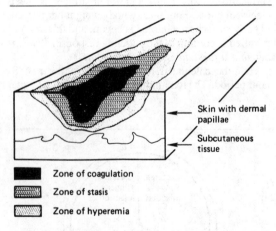

Zone of coagulation

Zone of stasis

Zone of hyperemia

Figure 32–6 The burn wound has 3 general zones of tissue death. The zone of necrosis or coagulation involves irreversible skin death. The intermediate zone of capillary stasis is vulnerable to desiccation and infection that can convert potentially salvageable tissue to full-thickness destruction and irreversible skin death. There is minimal cell involvement in the outermost hyperemic zone. (Modified from Zawacki BE: Reversal of capillary stasis and prevention of necrosis in burns. Ann Surg 1974;180:98. Redrawn, with permission, from Artz CP, Moncrief JA, Pruitt BA: *A Team Approach.* Saunders, 1979.)

PATIENT SUPPORT

During the wound closure phase, the patient must be supported in many ways. Most important is adequate nutrition. Enteral feedings may begin once the ileus of the resuscitation period is relieved, which usually coincides with the subsidence of edema. The large nasogastric sump tube used to decompress stomach contents during resuscitation may now be replaced with a smaller, preferably soft Silastic tube. This will aid in delivering large quantities (4000–6000 kcal/d) that may be required during the wound closure period. The metabolic demands are immense. A useful guide is to provide 25 kcal/kg body weight plus 40 kcal per percent of burn surface area. Fat emulsions (Intralipid) given intravenously are useful during the resuscitation period to span the period of ileus.

Many enteral formulas are available. Eggs are a readily available source of protein and calories and are well tolerated by the patient. In many cases, more than 30 eggs per day are desirable. Early enteral feedings reduce the need for antacids and lessen the likelihood of development of Curling's ulcer, a life-threatening complication of burn injury. Gastric pH and hourly antacid delivery should be monitored during the resuscitation phase. H_2 blockers may be used to reduce acid production; however, undesirable side effects such as leukopenia and confusion in the elderly may result.

Pain plays a major role during the wound closure phase. The patient is more aware of pain during dressing changes and postsurgical periods. Hydrotherapy aids in dressing removal and joint range of motion, but it can be a source of wound contamination. Analgesics are essential, but overuse or underuse may be harmful.

The Burn Team

The burn team consists of a group of highly skilled professionals—nurses, dietitians, physical therapists, occupational therapists, and counselors—who work closely with the physician in providing comprehensive services for the victim from the period of intensive care through recovery and rehabilitation. Careful attention is given to the complex problems encountered during the intensive care and recovery periods, including fluid and electrolyte abnormalities, infection, physical discomfort, malnutrition, immobility, and psychologic suffering.

The residual physical and emotional problems in burn patients, eg, body disfigurement, impaired mobility, persistent itching, decreased ability to perspire, decreased skin sensitivity, and impairment of sexual enjoyment, require long-term committed care.

Boswick JA: Comprehensive rehabilitation after burn injury. Surg Clin North Am 1987;67:159.
Demling RH: Fluid replacement in burned patients. Surg Clin North Am 1987;67:15.
Goodwin CW: Major burns. Chap 9, pp 163–175, in: *Principles of Trauma Care,* 3rd ed. Shires GT (editor). McGraw-Hill, 1985.
Heimbach DM: Early burn excision and grafting. Surg Clin North Am 1987;67:93.
Herndon DN et al: Pulmonary injury in burned patients. Surg Clin North Am 1987;67:3
Jones J, McMullen MJ, Dougherty J: Toxic smoke inhalation: Cyanide poisoning in fire victims. Am J Emerg Med 1987;5:317.
Kagan RJ et al: Serious wound infections in burned patients. Surgery 1985;98:640.
Rubin WD, Mani MM, Hiebert JM: Fluid resuscitation of the thermally injured patient: Current concepts with definition of clinical subsets and their specialized treatment. Clin Plast Surg 1986;13:9.
Warden GD: Outtreatment care of thermal burns. Surg Clin North Am 1987;67:147.

ELECTRIC SHOCK

The possibility of life-threatening electrical injury exists wherever there is electric power or lighting. The amount and type of current, the duration and area of exposure, and the pathway of the current through the body determine the degree of damage. If the current passes through the heart or brain stem, death may occur immediately owing to ventricular fibrillation or apnea. Current passing through skeletal muscle can cause contractions severe enough to result in bone fracture. Delayed electrical injuries include damage to the spinal cord, bone, and cataracts.

Direct current is much less dangerous than alternating current. Alternating current of high voltage with a very high number of cycles per second (hertz, Hz) may be less dangerous than a low voltage with fewer cycles per second. With alternating currents of 25–300 Hz, low voltages (< 220 Hz) tend to produce ventricular fibrillation; high voltages (> 1000 Hz), respiratory failure; intermediate voltages (220–1000 Hz), both. Domestic house current (AC) of 100 volts with low cycles (about 60 Hz) is, accordingly, dangerous to the heart, since it may cause ventricular fibrillation.

Lightning injuries differ from high-voltage electric shock injuries in that lightning usually involves higher voltage, briefer duration of contact, asystole rather than ventricular fibrillation, a shock wave characteristic, and multisystem pathologic involvement.

Electrical burns are of 3 distinct types: flash (arcing) burns, flame (clothing) burns, and the direct heating effect of tissues by the electric current. The latter lesions are usually sharply demarcated, round or oval, painless yellow-brown areas (Joule burn) with inflammatory reaction. There is usually a second burn mark where the current exits the body. The superficial appearance of many discrete burns is deceptive; operation frequently discloses more extensive destruction than anticipated. Little happens for several weeks; sloughing then occurs slowly over a fairly wide area.

Electric shock may produce loss of consciousness. With recovery there may be muscular pain, fatigue, headache, and nervous irritability. The physical signs vary according to the action of the current. Ventricular fibrillation or respiratory failure (or both) can occur; the patient may be unconscious, pulseless, hypotensive, cold and cyanotic, and without respirations.

Electric shock may be a hazard in equipment that is usually considered to be harmless (eg, home appliances and medical equipment). Proper installation, utilization, and maintenance of equipment by qualified personnel should minimize this hazard. Battery-operated devices provide the maximum protection from accidental electric shock. Electrochemical cutaneous burns have been reported with direct current voltages as low as 3 volts.

Treatment

A. Emergency Measures: The victim may be freed from the current in many ways, but the rescuer must be protected. Turn off the power, sever the wire with a dry wooden-handled axe, make a proper ground to divert the current, or drag the victim carefully away by means of dry clothing or a leather belt.

CPR is instituted if breathing and pulses are absent and continued according to the usual AHA protocol.

Lightning injury. Victims of lightning injury, in whom coma may last for a few minutes to several days, should receive prompt and sustained artificial resuscitation. This should be continued as long as there is no clinical evidence of brain death.

B. Hospital Measures: The patient is hospitalized when revived and observed for shock, arrhythmia, sudden cardiac dilatation, hemorrhage, or myoglobinuria. Electroshock injury cases should also be evaluated for blunt trauma, dehydration, acid-base disturbances, and neurologic damage.

The unpredictable damage to deep tissues in electrical burns makes it difficult to assess the fluid requirements for patients who are in shock.

Prognosis

Complications may occur in almost any part of the body but most commonly include sepsis, limb amputation, or neurologic, cardiac, or psychiatric dysfunction.

Cooper MA: Electrical and lightning injuries. Emerg Med Clin North Am 1984;2:489.

Hammond JS, Ward CG: High voltage electrical injuries: Management and outcome of 60 cases. South Med J 1988;81:1351.

IONIZING RADIATION REACTIONS

The effects of ionizing radiation on the body have been observed in clinical use of x-rays and radioactive agents, after occupational or accidental exposure, and following the use of atomic weaponry. The extent of damage due to radiation exposure depends on the quantity of radiation delivered to the body, the dose rate, the organs exposed, the type of radiation (x-rays, neutrons, gamma rays, alpha or beta particles), the duration of exposure, and the energy transfer from the radioactive wave or particle to the exposed tissue. The Chernobyl experience suggests that the best biologic indicators of dose are the duration of the asymptomatic latent period (particularly for nausea or emesis), the severity of early symptoms, the rate of decline of the lymphocyte count, and the number and distribution of dicentric chromosomes in peripheral lymphocytes.

The National Committee on Radiation Protection has set the maximum permissible radiation exposure for occupationally exposed workers over age 18 at 0.1 rem* per week for the whole body (but not to exceed 5 rem per year) and 1.5 rem per week for the hands. (For purposes of comparison, routine chest x-rays deliver from 0.1–0.2 rem.)

Death after acute lethal radiation exposure is usually due to hematopoietic failure, gastrointestinal mucosal damage, central nervous system damage, widespread vascular injury, or secondary infection. The acute radiation syndrome may be dominated by central nervous system, gastrointestinal, or hematologic manifestations depending on dose and survival. Four hundred to 600 cGy of x-ray or gamma radiation applied to the entire body at one time may be fatal within 60 days; death is usually due to hemorrhage, anemia, and infection secondary to hematopoietic injury. Levels of 1000–3000 cGy to the entire body destroy gastrointestinal mucosa; this leads to toxemia and death within 2 weeks. Total body doses above 3000 cGy cause widespread vascular damage, cerebral anoxia, hypotensive shock, and death within 48 hours.

---

* In radiation terminology, a rad is the unit of absorbed dose and a rem is the unit of any radiation dose to body tissue in terms of its estimated biologic effect. Roentgen (R) refers to the amount of radiation dose delivered to the body. For x-ray or gamma ray radiation, rems, rads, and roentgens are virtually the same. For particulate radiation from radioactive materials, these terms may differ greatly (eg, for neutrons, 1 rad equals 10 rems). In the Système International (SI) nomenclature, the rad has been replaced by the gray (Gy), and 1 rad equals 0.01 Gy = 1 cGy. The SI replacement for the rem is the Sievert (Sv), and 1 rem equals 0.01 Sv.

ACUTE (IMMEDIATE) IONIZING RADIATION EFFECTS ON NORMAL TISSUES

Clinical Findings

A. Injury to Skin and Mucous Membranes: Irradiation may cause erythema, epilation, destruction of fingernails, or epidermolysis.

B. Injury to Deep Structures:

1. Hematopoietic tissues–Injury to the bone marrow may cause diminished production of blood elements. Lymphocytes are most sensitive, polymorphonuclear leukocytes next most sensitive, and erythrocytes least sensitive. Damage to the blood-forming organs may vary from transient depression of one or more blood elements to complete destruction.

2. Cardiovascular system–Pericarditis with effusion or constrictive carditis may occur after a period of months or even years. Myocarditis is less common. Smaller vessels (the capillaries and arterioles) are more readily damaged than larger blood vessels.

3. Gonads–In males, small single doses of radiation (200–300 R) cause temporary aspermatogenesis, and larger doses (600–800 R) may cause permanent sterility. In females, single doses of 200 R may cause temporary cessation of menses, and 500–800 R may cause permanent castration. Moderate to heavy irradiation of the embryo in utero results in injury to the fetus or in embryonic death and abortion.

4. Respiratory tract–High or repeated moderate doses of radiation may cause pneumonitis, often delayed for weeks or months.

5. Salivary glands–The salivary glands may be depressed by radiation, but relatively large doses may be required.

6. Mouth, pharynx, esophagus, and stomach–Mucositis with edema and painful swallowing of food may occur within hours or days after onset of irradiation. Gastric secretion may be temporarily (occasionally permanently) inhibited by moderately high doses of radiation.

7. Intestines–Inflammation and ulceration may follow moderately large doses of radiation.

8. Endocrine glands and viscera–Hepatitis and nephritis may be delayed effects of therapeutic radiation. The normal thyroid, pituitary, pancreas, adrenals, and bladder are relatively resistant to low or moderate doses of radiation; parathyroid glands are especially resistant.

9. Brain and spinal cord–The brain and spinal cord may be damaged by high doses of radiation because of impaired blood supply.

10. Peripheral and autonomic nerves–These nerves are highly resistant to radiation.

C. Systemic Reaction (Radiation Sickness): The basic mechanisms of radiation sickness are not known. Anorexia, nausea, vomiting, weakness, exhaustion, lassitude, and in some cases prostration may occur, singly or in combination. Dehydration, anemia, and infection may follow. Radiation sickness associated with x-ray therapy is most likely to occur when the therapy is given in large dosage to large areas over the abdomen, less often when given over the thorax, and rarely when therapy is given over the extremities. With protracted therapy, this complication is rarely significant. The patient's psychologic reaction to the illness or its treatment plays an important role in aggravating or minimizing such effect.

Prevention

Persons handling radiation sources can minimize exposure to radiation by recognizing the importance of time, distance, and shielding. Areas housing x-ray and nuclear materials must be properly shielded. X-ray equipment should be periodically checked for reliability of output, and proper filters should be employed. When feasible, it is advisable to shield the gonads, especially of young persons. Fluoroscopic examination should be performed as rapidly as possible, using an optimal combination of beam characteristics and filtration; the tube-to-table distance should be at least 45 cm, and the beam size should be kept to a minimum required by the examination. Special protective clothing may be necessary to protect against contamination with radioisotopes. In the event of accidental contamination, all clothing should be removed and the body vigorously bathed with soap and water. This should be followed by careful instrument (Geiger counter) check to localize the ionizing radiation.

Emergency Treatment for Radiation Accident Victims

The proliferation of radiation equipment and nuclear energy plants and the increased transportation of radioactive materials necessitate hospital plans for managing patients who are accidentally exposed to ionizing radiation or contaminated with radioisotopes. The plans should provide for effective emergency care and disposition of victims and materials with the least possible risk of spreading radioactive contamination to personnel and facilities.

Treatment

The success of treatment of local radiation effects depends upon the extent, degree, and location of tissue injury. Particulate or radioisotope exposures should be decontaminated in designated confined areas. For many radioisotopes, chelation, blocking, or dilution therapy is indicated (see NCRP No. 65 reference, below). Treatment of systemic reactions is symptomatic and supportive. No truly effective antinauseant drug is available for the distressing nausea that frequently occurs. Chlorpromazine, 25–50 mg given deeply intramuscularly every 4–6 hours as necessary or 10–50 mg orally every 4–6 hours as necessary, may be of value. Dimenhydrinate, 100 mg, or perphenazine, 4–8 mg, 1 hour before and 1 and 4 hours after radiation therapy has been recommended. Simple, palatable foods and emotional support may help.

When radiation dosage levels are sufficient to cause damage to gastrointestinal mucosa, bone marrow, and other important tissues, good medical and nursing care may be lifesaving. Blood and platelet transfusions, bone marrow transplants, antibiotics, fluid and electrolyte maintenance, and other supportive measures may be useful. Recombinant granulocyte-macrophage colony-stimulating factor has been effective in increasing numbers of granulocytes and preventing infection.

CHRONIC (DELAYED) EFFECTS OF EXCESSIVE DOSES OF IONIZING RADIATION

The chronic and delayed effects of radiation may be difficult to evaluate, because they take many years to become apparent. Furthermore, it is difficult to differentiate effects presumed to be due to radiation from abnormal conditions known to occur spontaneously in the population at large.

Skin scarring, atrophy and telangiectasis, obliterative endarteritis, pericarditis, hypothyroidism, pulmonary fibrosis, hepatitis, intestinal stenosis, and nephritis are known to occur following high-dose exposure. The incidence of neoplastic disease, including leukemia, is increased in persons exposed to excessive radiation. The latency period between radiation therapy and the development of cancer may be 30 years or longer. Much of our knowledge of radiation-induced cancer in humans has been derived from follow-up studies of the survivors of the 1945 bombings in Japan during World War II. There is an increased incidence of thyroid cancer in patients who have received radiation therapy to the thymus. Prenatal irradiation may increase the risk of childhood cancer.

Microcephaly and other congenital abnormalities may occur in children exposed in utero, especially if the fetus was exposed during early pregnancy. Carcinogenesis from low-dose ($<$ 10 rem) exposure to adults has not been demonstrated. However, because of age-related differences in sensitivity to radiation, carcinogenesis following childhood exposures has been observed.

Abrams HL, Von Kaenel WE: Medical problems of survivors of nuclear war: Infection and the spread of communicable disease. N Engl J Med 1981;305:1226.

American Medical Association: *A Guide to the Hospital Management of Injuries Arising From Exposure to or Involving Ionizing Radiation.* American Medical Association, 1985.

Brook I: Use of antibiotics in the management of postirradiation wound infection and sepsis. Radiat Res 1988;115:1.

Champlin RE, Kustenburg WE, Gale RP: Radiation accidents and nuclear energy: Medical consequences and therapy. Ann Intern Med 1988;109:730.

Milroy WC: Management of irradiated and contaminated casualty victims. Emerg Med Clin North Am 1984;2:667.

National Council on Radiation Protection and Measurement (NCRP): *Management of Persons Accidentally Contaminated With Radionuclides.* Report No. 65. NCRP, 1985.

Ritenour ER: Health effects of low level radiation: Carcinogenesis, teratogenesis, and mutagenesis. Semin Nucl Med 1986;16:106.

DROWNING

Drowning is the fourth leading cause of accidental death in the USA. The number of deaths due to drowning could undoubtedly be significantly reduced if adequate preventive and first aid instruction programs were instituted.

The asphyxia of drowning is usually due to aspiration of fluid, but it may result from airway obstruction caused by laryngeal spasm while the victim is gasping under water. About 10% of victims develop laryngospasms after the first gulp and never aspirate water ("dry drowning"). The rapid sequence of events after submersion—hypoxemia, laryngospasm, fluid aspiration, ineffective circulation, brain injury, and brain death—may take place within 5–10 minutes. This sequence may be delayed for longer periods if the victim, especially a child, has been submerged in very cold water or if the victim has ingested significant amounts of barbiturates. Immersion in cold water can also cause a rapid fall in the victim's core temperature, so that systemic hypothermia and death may occur before actual drowning.

Past emphasis on differences in the pathophysiology of drowning in fresh water (hypotonic) and seawater (hypertonic), based upon observations in animal models, is of limited clinical significance in humans, since the amount of fluid aspirated is usually small. The primary effect in both cases is perfusion of poorly ventilated alveoli. The clinical presentation in both types of drowning is similar, and *cardiopulmonary resuscitation is the immediate requirement of rescue.*

A number of circumstances or primary events may precede near drowning and must be taken into consideration in management: (1) use of alcohol or other drugs (a contributing factor in an estimated 25% of adult drownings), (2) extreme fatigue, (3) intentional hyperventilation, (4) sudden acute illness (eg, epilepsy, myocardial infarction), (5) head or spinal cord injury sustained in diving, (6) venomous stings by aquatic animals, and (7) decompression sickness in deep water diving.

When first seen, the near-drowning victim may present with a wide range of clinical manifestations. Spontaneous return of consciousness often occurs in otherwise healthy individuals when submersion is very brief. Many other patients respond promptly to immediate ventilation. Other patients, with more severe degrees of near drowning, may have frank pulmonary failure, pulmonary edema, shock, anoxic encephalopathy, cerebral edema, and cardiac arrest. A few patients may be deceptively asymptomatic during the recovery period, only to deteriorate or die as a result of acute respiratory failure within the following 12–24 hours.

Clinical Findings

A. Symptoms and Signs: The patient may be unconscious, semiconscious, or awake but apprehensive, restless, and complaining of headaches or chest pain. Vomiting is common. Examination may reveal cyanosis, trismus, apnea, tachypnea, and wheezing. A pink froth from the mouth and nose indicates pulmonary edema. Cardiovascular manifestations may include tachycardia, arrhythmias, hypotension, cardiac arrest, and circulatory shock. Hypothermia may be present.

B. Laboratory Findings: Urinalysis shows proteinuria, hemoglobinuria, and acetonuria. There is usually a leukocytosis. The Pao_2 is usually decreased and the $Paco_2$ increased or decreased. The blood pH is decreased as a result of metabolic acidosis. Chest x-rays may show pneumonitis or pulmonary edema.

Treatment

A. First Aid: Immediate measures to combat hypoxemia at the scene of the incident—with sustained effective ventilation, oxygenation, and circulatory support—are critical to survival with complete recovery.

1. Standard CPR is initiated if pulse and respirations are absent.

2. Do not waste time attempting to drain water from the victim's lungs, since this measure is most often of no value. The Heimlich maneuver (subdiaphragmatic pressure) may clear the airway in a few persons, especially those who have gagged or vomited while aspirating water. The cervical spine should be immobilized if neck injury is possible.

3. Do not discontinue basic life support for seemingly "hopeless" patients. Complete recovery has been reported after prolonged resuscitation efforts even when victims have had wide, fixed pupils, especially when the patient is hypothermic.

B. Hospital Care: Careful observation of the patient; continuous monitoring of cardiorespiratory function; serial determination of arterial blood gases, pH, and electrolytes; and measurement of urinary output are required. Pulmonary edema may not appear for 24 hours.

1. Ensure optimal ventilation and oxygenation–The danger of hypoxemia exists even in the alert, conscious patient who appears to be breathing normally. Oxygen should be immediately administered at the highest available concentration. Endotra-

cheal intubation and mechanical ventilation are necessary for patients unable to maintain an open airway or normal blood gases and pH. If the victim does not have spontaneous respirations, intubation is required. Oxygen saturation should be maintained at 90% or higher. Positive end-expiratory pressure (PEEP) should be considered when the patient is unable to achieve a Pao_2 greater than 55 mm Hg when receiving less than 50% oxygen. Serial physical examinations and chest x-rays should be carried out to detect possible pneumonitis, atelectasis, and pulmonary edema. Bronchospasm due to aspirated material may require use of bronchodilators. Antibiotics should be given only when there is clinical evidence of infection—not prophylactically.

2. Cardiovascular support–Central venous pressure (or, preferably, pulmonary artery wedge pressure) may be monitored as a guide to determining whether vascular fluid replacement and cardiac drug therapy are needed. If low cardiac output persists after adequate intravascular volume is achieved, pressors should be given. Otherwise, standard therapy for pulmonary edema, cardiogenic or not, is administered.

3. Correction of blood pH and electrolyte abnormalities–Metabolic acidosis is almost invariably present in near-drowning victims. Many authorities feel that patients who have been pulseless should routinely be given intravenous sodium bicarbonate (1 meq/kg) upon admission. All subsequent bicarbonate administration should be based upon arterial blood gas and pH findings. Alkalosis is dangerous and should be avoided.

4. Cerebral injury–Some near-drowning patients may progress to irreversible central nervous system damage despite apparently adequate treatment of hypoxia and shock. Several types of measures to prevent cerebral injury have been employed with varying degrees of success—hypothermia, barbiturates, corticosteroids, osmolar agents (eg, mannitol), and readjustment of ventilatory assistance.

5. Hypothermia–Core temperature should be measured and managed as appropriate (see Systemic Hypothermia, above).

Course & Prognosis

Victims of near drowning who have had prolonged hypoxemia should remain under close hospital observation for 2–3 days after all supportive measures have been withdrawn and clinical and laboratory findings have been stable. Residual complications of near drowning may include intellectual impairment, convulsive disorders, and pulmonary or cardiac disease.

Brooks JG: Near drowning. Pediatrics Rev 1988;10:6.
Pruessner HT et al: Management of the near-drowning victim. Am Fam Physician (May) 1988;37:251.
Shaw KN, Briede CA: Submersion injuries: Drowning and near-drowning. Emerg Clin North Am 1989;7:355.

OTHER DISORDERS DUE TO PHYSICAL AGENTS

DECOMPRESSION SICKNESS
(Caisson Disease, Bends)

Decompression sickness has long been known as an occupational hazard for fliers and for professional divers who are involved in deep-water exploration, rescue, salvage, or construction; and professional divers and their surface supporting teams are familiar with the prevention, recognition, and treatment of this disease. In recent years, the sport of scuba diving has become very popular, and a large number of untrained individuals are exposed to the hazards of decompression sickness.

At low depths the greatly increased pressure (eg, at 30 meters [100 ft] the pressure is 4 times greater than at the surface) compresses the respiratory gases into the blood and other tissues. During ascent from depths greater than 9 meters, gases dissolved in the blood and other tissues escape as the external pressure decreases. The appearance of symptoms depends on the depth and duration of submersion; the degree of physical exertion; the age, weight, and physical condition of the diver; and the rate of ascent. The size and number of gas bubbles (notably nitrogen) escaping from the tissues depends on the difference between the atmospheric pressure and the partial pressure of the gas dissolved in the tissues. The release of gas bubbles and (particularly) the location of their release determine the symptoms.

Decompression sickness also occurs among fliers during rapid ascent from sea level to high altitudes when there is no adequate pressurizing protection. Deep-sea and scuba divers may be vulnerable to air embolism if airplane travel is attempted too soon (within a few hours) after diving.

Predisposing factors include exercise, injury, obesity, dehydration, alcoholic excess, hypoxia, some medications (eg, narcotics, antihistamines), and cold. Reported sequelae include hemiparesis, neurologic dysfunction, and bone damage.

The onset of symptoms occurs within 30 minutes in half of cases and almost invariably within 6 hours. Symptoms, which are highly variable, include pain (largely in the joints), headache, confusion, pruritic rash, visual disturbances, weakness or paralysis, dizziness or vertigo, dyspnea, paresthesias, aphasia, and coma.

Early recognition and prompt treatment are extremely important. Continuous administration of oxygen is indicated as a first aid measure, whether or not cyanosis is present. Aspirin may be given for pain, but narcotics should be used very cautiously,

since they may obscure the patient's response to recompression. Rapid transportation to a treatment facility for recompression, hyperbaric oxygen, hydration treatment of plasma deficits, and supportive measures is necessary not only to relieve symptoms but also to prevent permanent impairment. It has been recommended, however, that decompression symptoms be treated whenever they are seen—even up to 2 weeks postinjury—since it is still possible to completely alleviate symptoms. The physician should be familiar with the nearest compression center. The local public health department or nearest naval facility should be able to provide such information. The National Divers Alert Network (DAN) ([919] 684–8111) provides assistance in the management of underwater diving accidents.

Gorman DF: Decompression sickness and arterial gas embolism in sports scuba divers. Sports Med 1989;8:32.

Hickey DD: Outline of medical standards for divers. Undersea Biomed Res 1984;11:407.

Kizer KW: Diving medicine. Emerg Med Clin North Am 1984;2:513.

Parell GJ et al: Management of inner ear barotrauma caused by scuba diving. Otolaryngol Head Neck Surg 1985; 93:393.

Wirjosemito SA et al: Type II altitude decompression sickness (DCS): US Air Force experience with 133 cases. Aviat Space Environ Med 1989;60:256.

MOUNTAIN SICKNESS

Lack of sufficient time for acclimatization, increased physical activity, and varying degrees of health may be responsible for the acute and chronic disturbances that result from hypoxia at altitudes greater than 2000 meters. Marked individual differences in tolerance to hypoxia exist. Patients with sickle cell disease are at high risk of painful crises from altitude-induced hypoxemia; if they have had no previous mountain exposure, they should be advised to avoid mountains.

Acute Mountain Sickness

Initial manifestations include dizziness, headache, lassitude, drowsiness, chilliness, nausea and vomiting, facial pallor, dyspnea, and cyanosis. Later, there is facial flushing, irritability, difficulty in concentrating, vertigo, tinnitus, visual (retinal hemorrhages may occur) and auditory disturbances, anorexia, insomnia, increased dyspnea and weakness on exertion, increased headaches (due to cerebral edema), palpitations, tachycardia, Cheyne-Stokes breathing, and weight loss. More severe manifestations include pulmonary edema and encephalopathy. Voluntary, periodic hyperventilation may relieve symptoms. In most individuals, symptoms clear within 24–48 hours, but in some instances, if the symptoms are sufficiently persistent or severe, the patient must be returned to lower altitudes. Administration of oxygen will often relieve acute symptoms. Acetazolamide or dexamethasone is recommended therapy at the same dosage schedules as used in prophylaxis. Judicious use of sedatives may be of value for some adults with irritability and insomnia. Preventive measures include adequate rest and sleep the day before travel, reduced food intake, and avoidance of alcohol, tobacco, and unnecessary physical activity during travel. Acetazolamide (Diamox), 250 mg every 8 hours one day before, during, and several days after ascent, may prevent symptoms of acute mountain sickness or alleviate its severity. Dexamethasone, 2–4 mg every 5 hours beginning on the day of ascent, continuing for 3 days at the higher altitude, and then tapering over 5 days, is an alternative, particularly for extreme situations.

Acute High-Altitude Pulmonary Edema

This serious complication usually occurs at levels above 3000 meters. Early symptoms of pulmonary edema may appear within 6–36 hours after arrival at a high-altitude area—dry, incessant cough, dyspnea at rest, and substernal oppression. Later, wheezing, orthopnea, and hemoptysis may occur. Recognition of the early symptoms may enable the patient to climb down (or be assisted) to lower altitudes before incapacitating pulmonary edema develops. An early descent of even 500 or 1000 meters may result in improvement of symptoms. Physical findings include tachycardia, mild fever, tachypnea, cyanosis, prolonged respiration, and rales and rhonchi. The patient may become confused or even comatose, and the entire clinical picture may resemble severe pneumonia. Microthrombi are often found in the pulmonary capillaries. The white count is often slightly elevated, but the blood sedimentation rate is usually normal. Chest x-ray findings vary from irregular patchy infiltration in one lung to nodular densities bilaterally or with transient prominence of the central pulmonary arteries. Transient, nonspecific electrocardiographic changes, occasionally showing right ventricular strain, may occur. Pulmonary arterial blood pressure is elevated, whereas pulmonary wedge pressure is normal. Treatment, which must often be given under field conditions, consists of rest in the semi-Fowler position and administration of 100% oxygen by mask at a rate of 6–8 L/min for 15–30 minutes. *Immediate descent is essential.* To conserve oxygen, lower flow rates may be used for the next 24–48 hours until the victim recovers or can be evacuated to a lower altitude. Treatment for adult respiratory distress syndrome (see Chapter 7) may be required for some patients who have a prolonged course of pulmonary edema. Acetazolamide should be administered if acute mountain sickness is suspected. If bacterial pneumonia exists, appropriate antibiotic therapy should be given.

Preventive measures include education of prospective mountaineers regarding the possibility of serious pulmonary edema, optimal physical conditioning before travel, gradual ascent to permit acclimatization, and a period of rest and inactivity for 1–2 days after arrival at high altitudes. Acetazolamide (Diamox) is recommended for prophylaxis. Prompt medical attention with rest and high-flow oxygen if respiratory symptoms develop may prevent progression to frank pulmonary edema. Persons with a history of high-altitude pulmonary edema should be hospitalized for further observation if possible. Pulmonary embolism and high-altitude bronchitis can also occur. Mountaineering parties at levels of 3000 meters or higher should carry a supply of oxygen and equipment sufficient for several days. Persons with symptomatic cardiac or pulmonary disease should avoid high altitudes.

Acute High-Altitude Encephalopathy

High-altitude encephalopathy appears to be an extension of the central nervous symptoms of acute mountain sickness (see above). It usually occurs at elevations above 2500 meters (8250 ft) and is more common in unacclimated individuals. Clinical findings are due largely to hypoxemia and cerebral edema. Severe headaches, confusion, truncal ataxia, staggering gait, focal deficits, nausea and vomiting, and seizures may progress to obtundation and coma. Papilledema and retinal hemorrhages may be observed in about 50% of patients.

Early recognition of the encephalopathic symptoms is essential. Oxygen should be administered by mask. Dexamethasone may be helpful if descent is impossible. If descent is accomplished as quickly as possible, recovery is usually rapid and complete.

Subacute Mountain Sickness

This occurs most frequently in unacclimatized individuals and at altitudes above 4500 meters. Symptoms, which are probably due to central nervous system anoxia without associated alveolar hyperventilation, are similar to but more persistent and severe than those of acute mountain sickness. There are additional problems of dehydration, skin dryness, and pruritus. The hematocrit may be elevated, and there may be electrocardiographic and chest x-ray evidence of right ventricular hypertrophy. Treatment consists of rest, oxygen administration, and return to lower altitudes.

Chronic Mountain Sickness (Monge's Disease)

This uncommon condition of chronic alveolar hypoventilation, which is encountered in residents of high-altitude communities who have lost their acclimatization to such an environment, is difficult to differentiate clinically from chronic pulmonary disease. The disorder is characterized by somnolence, mental depression, hypoxemia, cyanosis, clubbing of fingers, polycythemia (hematocrit often > 75%), signs of right ventricular failure, electrocardiographic evidence of right axis deviation and right atrial and ventricular hypertrophy, and x-ray evidence of right heart enlargement and central pulmonary vessel prominence. There is no x-ray evidence of structural pulmonary disease. Pulmonary function tests usually disclose alveolar hypoventilation and elevated CO_2 tension but fail to reveal defective oxygen transport. There is a diminished respiratory response to CO_2. Almost complete disappearance of all abnormalities eventually occurs when the patient returns to sea level.

Houston CS: Altitude illness. Emerg Med Clin North Am 1984;2:503.
Jacobson ND: Acute high-altitude illness. Am Fam Physician (Sept) 1988;38:135.
Johnson TS, Rock PB: Current concepts: Acute mountain sickness. N Engl J Med 1988;319:841.
Rabold M: High altitude pulmonary edema: A collective review. Am J Emerg Med 1989;7:426.

MEDICAL EFFECTS OF AIR TRAVEL & SELECTION OF PATIENTS FOR AIR TRAVEL

The decision about whether or not it is advisable for a patient to travel by air depends not only upon the nature and severity of the illness but also upon such factors as the duration of flight, the altitude to be flown, pressurization, the availability of supplementary oxygen and other medical supplies, the presence of attending physicians and trained nursing attendants, and other special considerations. Air carriers in the USA cannot legally allow the use of personal (passenger-supplied) oxygen containers, but most major airlines will supply oxygen upon advance written request from the passenger's physician. Airline policies, charges, and other details must be checked with each carrier. Medical hazards or complications of modern air travel are remarkably uncommon; unless there is some specific contraindication (Table 32–1), air transportation may actually be the best means of moving patients. The most common in-flight emergencies are cardiovascular, syncopal, neuropsychiatric, and abdominal. The Air Transport Association of America defines an incapacitated passenger as "one who is suffering from a physical or mental disability and who, because of such disability or the effect of the flight on the disability, is incapable of self-care; would endanger the health or safety of such person or other passengers or airline employees; or would cause discomfort or annoyance of other passengers."

All commercial airlines retain medical consultants to assist their personnel in making decisions regarding

Table 32–1. Contraindications to commercial air travel.[1]

Cardiovascular
Within 4 weeks after myocardial infarction[2]
Within 2 weeks after cerebrovascular accident
Severe hypertension
Decompensated cardiovascular disease or restricted cardiac reserve[3]
Bronchopulmonary
Pneumothorax
Congenital pulmonary cysts
Vital capacity less than 50%
Eye, ear, nose, and throat
Recent eye surgery
Acute sinusitis or otitis media
Surgical mandibular fixation (permanent wiring of jaw)
Gastrointestinal tract
Less than 10–14 days after abdominal surgery
Acute diverticulitis or ulcerative colitis
Acute esophageal varices
Acute gastroenteritis
Neuropsychiatric
Epilepsy (unless well controlled medically and cabin altitude does not exceed 2500 m [8000 ft])
Previous violent or unpredictable behavior
Recent skull fracture
Brain tumor
Hematologic
Anemia (hemoglobin < 8.5 g/dL or red blood cell count of < 3 million/μL in an adult)
Sickle cell disease (except below 6800-m [22,500-foot] altitude)
Blood dyscrasias with active bleeding (hemophilia, leukemia)
Pregnancy
Beyond 240 days or with threatened miscarriage
Miscellaneous
Need for intravenous fluids or special medical apparatus[2]

---

[1] Slightly modified and reproduced, with permission, from *Mod Med* (June) 1982;**50**:196. Based on recommendations of the American Medical Association in *JAMA* 1982;**247**:1009.
[2] Consultation with an airline flight surgeon is suggested.
[3] In some cases, low-altitude flights can be made without supplemental oxygen in accordance with recommendations of the American College of Chest Physicians.

the transportation of passengers with noticeable symptoms of sickness or injury. Physicians may contact these medical consultants by calling or writing the medical departments of major airlines.

Cardiovascular Disease

A. Cardiac Decompensation: Patients in congestive failure should not fly until they are compensated by appropriate treatment, or unless they are in a pressurized plane with 100% oxygen therapy available during the entire flight.

B. Compensated Valvular or Other Heart Disease: Patients should not fly above 2400–2800 m unless the aircraft is pressurized and oxygen is administered at altitudes of 2400 m or higher.

C. Acute Myocardial Infarction, Convalescent and Asymptomatic: At least 4 weeks of convalescence are recommended even for asymptomatic patients if flying is contemplated. Ambulatory, stabilized, and compensated patients tolerate air travel well. Oxygen should be available.

D. Angina Pectoris: Air travel is inadvisable for patients with severe angina. In mild to moderate cases of angina, air travel may be permitted, especially in pressurized planes. Oxygen should be available.

Respiratory Disease

A. Nasopharyngeal Disorders: Nasal allergies and infections predispose to development of aerotitis. Chewing gum, nasal decongestants, appropriate anti-infective treatment, and avoiding sleep on descent may prevent barotitis.

B. Asthma: Patients with mild asthma can travel without difficulty. Patients with status asthmaticus should not be permitted to fly.

C. Congenital Pulmonary Cysts: Patients should not travel unless cleared by a physician.

D. Tuberculosis: Patients with active, communicable tuberculosis or pneumothorax should not be permitted to travel by air.

E. Other Pulmonary Disorders: Patients may be flown safely unless vital capacity is less than 50% of predicted.

Anemia

If hemoglobin is less than 8–9 g/dL, oxygen should be available. Patients with severe anemia should not travel by air until hemoglobin has been raised to a reasonable level. Patients with sickle cell anemia appear to be particularly vulnerable.

Diabetes Mellitus

Diabetics who do not need insulin or who can administer their own insulin during flight may fly safely. "Brittle" diabetics who are subject to frequent episodes of hypoglycemia should be in optimal control before flying and should carry sugar or candy in case hypoglycemic reactions occur.

Patients With Surgical Problems

Patients convalescing from thoracic or abdominal surgery should not fly until 10 days after surgery, and then only if the wound is healed and there is no drainage.

Colostomy patients may be permitted to travel by air providing they are nonodorous and colostomy bags are emptied before flight.

Patients with large hernias unsupported by a truss or binder should not be permitted to fly in nonpressur-

ized aircraft because of an increased danger of strangulation of the herniated bowel.

Postsurgical or posttraumatic eye cases require pressurized cabins and oxygen therapy to avoid retinal damage due to hypoxia.

Long flights increase the risk of deep vein thrombosis and resulting embolic disease. Prevention includes avoidance of smoking and alcohol, low-dose aspirin, and leg exercises and walking during the flight.

Psychiatric Disorders

Severely psychotic, agitated, or disturbed patients should not be permitted to fly on scheduled airlines even when accompanied by a medical attendant.

Extremely nervous or apprehensive patients may travel by air if they receive adequate sedatives or tranquilizers before and during flight.

Motion Sickness

Patients subject to motion sickness should receive sedatives or antihistamines (eg, dimenhydrinate or meclizine), 50 mg 4 times daily, before and during the flight, or one transdermal scopolamine disk applied behind one ear at least 4 hours before the antiemetic effect is desired. Small meals of easily digested food before and during the flight may reduce the tendency to nausea and vomiting.

Pregnancy

Pregnant women may be permitted to fly during the first 8 months of pregnancy unless there is a history of habitual abortion or premature birth. During the ninth month of pregnancy, air travel is not recommended; if travel is essential, a physician's authorization is required. Infants less than 1 week old should not be flown at high altitudes or for long distances.

AMA Commission on Emergency Medical Services: Medical aspects of transportation aboard commercial aircraft. JAMA 1982;247:1007.

AMA Commission on Emergency Medical Services and Department of Transportation: *Air Ambulance Guidelines,* 2nd ed. DOT HS 806 703. NTS-42, 1986.

Cottrell JJ et al: In-flight medical emergencies: One year experience with the enhanced medical kit. JAMA 1989; 262:1653.

Gong H Jr: Advising patients with pulmonary diseases on air travel. Ann Intern Med 1989;111:349.

Rodenberg H: Prevention of medical emergencies during air travel. Am Fam Physician (Feb) 1988;37:263.

Poisoning

Kent R. Olson, MD

INITIAL EVALUATION OF THE PATIENT WITH POISONING OR DRUG OVERDOSE

Patients with drug overdoses or poisoning may initially present with no symptoms or with varying degrees of overt intoxication. The asymptomatic patient may have been exposed to or may have ingested a lethal dose of a poison but not yet have any manifestations of toxicity. It is always important to (1) quickly assess the potential danger, (2) perform gut decontamination to prevent absorption, and (3) observe the patient for an appropriate interval.

Assess the Danger

If the toxin is known, the danger can be assessed by consulting a text or computerized information resource (eg, POISINDEX) or by calling a regional poison control center (Table 33–1). Assessment will usually take into account the dose ingested (in milligrams per kilogram of body weight), the time interval since ingestion, the presence of any clinical signs, and serum drug or toxin levels. Be aware that the history given by the patient or family may be unreliable.

Gut Decontamination

The choice of gut decontamination procedure depends on the toxin and the circumstances. (See below for more discussion of methods.)

Observation of the Patient

Asymptomatic or mildly symptomatic patients should generally be observed for at least 4–6 hours. After that time, the patient may be discharged if no symptoms have developed and adequate gastric decontamination has been assured (as shown by passage of a charcoal-laden stool). Before discharge, psychiatric evaluation must be performed to assess suicidal risk. Intentional ingestions in adolescent girls should raise the possibility of unwanted pregnancy or sexual abuse in the home.

THE SYMPTOMATIC PATIENT

In symptomatic patients, treatment of life-threatening complications takes precedence over gut decontamination or in-depth diagnostic evaluation. Patients with mild symptoms may deteriorate rapidly, which is why all potentially significant exposures should be observed in an acute care facility. The following complications may occur, depending on the type of poisoning.

COMA

Assessment & Complications

Coma is commonly due to ingestion of large doses of antihistamines and anticholinergics, barbiturates, benzodiazepines, ethanol, opioids, phenothiazines, and tricyclic antidepressants. The most common cause of death in comatose patients is respiratory failure (hypoventilation or apnea), which may occur abruptly. Pulmonary aspiration of gastric contents may also occur, especially in victims who are comatose or convulsing. Hypoxia and hypoventilation may aggravate or even cause other common complications such as arrhythmias, hypotension, and seizures. Thus, protection of the airway and assisted ventilation are the most important treatment measures for any poisoned patient.

Treatment

A. Emergency Management: The initial emergency management of coma can be remembered by the mnemonic *ABCD*, for *A*irway, *B*reathing, *C*irculation, and *D*extrose, thiamine, and maloxone (Table 33–2).

1. Airway–Establish a patent airway by positioning, suction, or insertion of an artificial nasal or oropharyngeal airway. If the patient is deeply comatose or if there is no gag or cough reflex, perform endotracheal intubation. These airway interventions may not be necessary if the patient is intoxicated by an opioid and responds rapidly to intravenous naloxone (see below).

2. Breathing–Clinically assess the quality and depth of respiration, and provide assistance if neces-

Table 33–1. AAPCC-certified regional poison control centers.[1]

The American Association of Regional Poison Control Centers has certified 36 regional poison centers as meeting their minimum operating criteria. Regional poison control centers operate 24 hours a day, utilizing specially trained and dedicated staff with access to a variety of texts, files, and computerized poison information resources. They can also provide immediate telephone consultation with a physician specializing in medical toxicology.

State	Poison Center	Phone Number
Alabama	Alabama Poison Center, Tuscaloosa	(800) 462–0800 (205) 345–0600
	Children's Hospital of Alabama , Birmingham	(800) 292–6678 (205) 933–4050
Arizona	Arizona Poison and Drug Information Center, Tucson	(800) 362–0101 (602) 626–6016
	Samaritan Regional Poison Center, Phoenix	(602) 253–3334
California	Fresno Regional Poison Control Center, Fresno	(800) 346–5922 (209) 445–1222
	Los Angeles County Medical Association Regional Poison Control Center, Los Angeles	(800) 825–2722 (213) 664–1212
	San Diego Regional Poison Center, UC San Diego	(800) 876–4766 (619) 543–6000
	San Francisco Bay Area Regional Poison Center, San Francisco	(800) 523–2222 (415) 476–6600
	UC Davis Medical Center, Regional Poison Center, Sacramento	(800) 342–9293 (916) 453–3692
Colorado	Rocky Mountain Poison and Drug Center, Denver CO	(800) 332–3073 (303) 629–1123
Florida	Florida Poison Information Center, Tampa	(800) 282–3171 (813) 253–4444
Georgia	Georgia Poison Control Center, Atlanta	(800) 282–5846 (404) 589–4400
Kentucky	Kentucky Regional Poison Center, Louisville	(800) 722–5725 (502) 589–8222
Maryland	Maryland Poison Center, Baltimore	(800) 492–2414 (301) 528–7701
Massachusetts	Massachusetts Poison Control System, Boston	(800) 682–9211 (617) 232–2120
Michigan	Blodgett Regional Poison Center, Grand Rapids	(800) 632–2727 (616) 774–7851
	Poison Control Center, Children's Hospital, Detroit	(800) 462–6642 (313) 745–5711
Minnesota	Hennepin Regional Poison Center, Minneapolis	(612) 347–3141
	Minnesota Regional Poison Center, St Paul	(800) 222–1222 (612) 221–2113
Missouri	Cardinal Glennon Children's Hospital Regional Poison Center, St Louis	(800) 392–9111 (314) 772–5200
Montana	Rocky Mountain Poison and Drug Center, Denver CO	(800) 525–5042
Nebraska	Mid-Plains Poison Center, Omaha NE	(800) 642–9999 (402) 390–5400
New Jersey	New Jersey Poison Information and Education System, Newark	(800) 962–1253 (201) 923–0764

Table 33–1 (cont'd). AAPCC-certified regional poison control centers.[1]

State	Poison Center	Phone Number
New Mexico	New Mexico Poison and Drug Information Center, Albuquerque	(800) 432–6866 (505) 843–2551
New York	Long Island Regional Poison Control Center, East Meadow	(516) 542–2323
	New York City Poison Control Center, New York City	(212) 340–4494 (212) 764–7667
Ohio	Central Ohio Poison Center, Columbus	(800) 682–7625 (614) 228–1323
	Regional Poison Control System and Drug and Poison Information Center, Cincinnati	(800) 872–5111 (513) 558–5111
Oregon	Oregon Poison Center, Portland	(800) 452–7165 (503) 279–8968
Pennsylvania	Delaware Valley Regional Poison Center, Philadelphia	(215) 386–2100
	Pittsburgh Poison Center, Pittsburgh	(412) 681–6669
Rhode Island	Rhode Island Poison Center, RI Hospital, Providence	(401) 277–5727
Texas	North Texas Poison Center, Dallas	(800) 441–0040 (214) 590–5000
	Texas State Poison Center, Galveston Houston Austin	(800) 392–8548 (409) 765–9728 (713) 654–1701 (512) 478–4490
Utah	Intermountain Regional Poison Center, Salt Lake City	(800) 456–7707 (801) 581–2151
Washington DC	National Capitol Poison Center, Washington DC	(202) 625–3333
West Virginia	West Virginia Poison Center, Charleston	(800) 642–3625 (304) 348–4211
Wyoming	Rocky Mountain Poison and Drug Center, Denver CO	(800) 442–2702

[1] AAPCC, Regional Certification Committee, 1990.

sary with a bag-valve-mask device or mechanical ventilator. Provide supplemental oxygen. The arterial blood CO_2 tension is useful in determining the adequacy of ventilation. The arterial blood Po_2 determination may reveal hypoxemia, which may be caused by respiratory arrest, bronchospasm, pulmonary aspiration, or noncardiogenic pulmonary edema.

3. Circulation–Measure the pulse and blood pressure, and estimate tissue perfusion (eg, by measurement of urinary output, skin signs, blood pH). Insert

Table 33–2. Initial management of coma.

A	Airway control
B	Breathing
C	Circulation
D	Dextrose 50%, 50–100 mL IV; thiamine, 100 mg IM or IV; and naloxone, 0.4–2 mg IV

an intravenous line, and draw blood for blood count, glucose, electrolytes, and possible toxicologic testing.

4. Dextrose and thiamine–Unless promptly treated, severe hypoglycemia can cause irreversible brain damage. Therefore, in all comatose or convulsing patients, give 50% dextrose, 50–100 mL by intravenous bolus, unless a rapid bedside blood sugar test is available and rules out hypoglycemia. In alcoholic or very malnourished patients who may have marginal thiamine stores, give thiamine, 100 mg intramuscularly or slowly intravenously.

B. Narcotic Antagonists: Naloxone, 0.4–2 mg intravenously, may reverse opioid-induced respiratory depression and coma. If opioid overdose is strongly suspected, give additional doses of naloxone (up to 5–10 mg may be required to reverse potent opioids). *Caution:* Naloxone has a much shorter duration of action (2–3 hours) than most common opioids; repeated doses may be required, and continuous observation for several hours is mandatory.

HYPOTHERMIA

Assessment & Complications

Hypothermia commonly accompanies coma due to opioids, ethanol, hypoglycemic agents, phenothiazines, barbiturates, and other sedative-hypnotics and depressants.

Hypothermic patients may have a barely perceptible pulse and blood pressure and often appear to be dead. Hypothermia may cause or aggravate hypotension, and the hypotension will not reverse until the temperature is normalized.

Treatment

Hypothermia treatment is discussed in Chapter 32. Gradual rewarming is preferred unless the patient is in cardiac arrest.

HYPOTENSION

Assessment & Complications

Hypotension may be due to poisoning with antihypertensive drugs, beta-blockers, calcium channel blocking agents, iron, theophylline, opioids, phenothiazines, barbiturates, and tricyclic antidepressants.

Hypotension in the poisoned or drug-overdosed patient may be caused by venous or arteriolar vasodilatation, depressed cardiac contractility, or a combination of these effects. The only certain way to determine the cause of hypotension in any individual patient is to insert a pulmonary artery catheter and measure the left ventricular filling pressure and then calculate the cardiac output and peripheral vascular resistance. Alternatively, a central venous pressure monitor may indicate a need for further fluid therapy.

Treatment

If cardiac catheterization and CVP monitoring are not practical, keep in mind that most patients respond to empiric treatment (200-mL intravenous boluses of normal saline or other isotonic crystalloid up to total of 1–2 L). If fluid therapy is not successful, give dopamine, 5–15 μg/kg/min by intravenous infusion.

Hypotension caused by certain toxins may respond to specific treatment. For hypotension caused by overdoses of tricyclic antidepressants or related drugs, administer sodium bicarbonate, 1–2 meq/kg by intravenous bolus injection. For beta-blocker overdose, administer glucagon, 0.1 mg/kg by intravenous bolus injection. For calcium antagonist overdose, administer calcium chloride, 15–20 mg/kg intravenously.

HYPERTENSION

Assessment & Complications

Hypertension may be due to poisoning with am-

phetamines, anticholinergics, cocaine, phencyclidine (PCP), phenylpropanolamine, or monoamine oxidase inhibitors (interactions).

Severe hypertension (diastolic blood pressure > 105–110 mm Hg) can result in acute intracranial hemorrhage, myocardial infarction, or aortic dissection. Patients often present with headache, chest pain, or encephalopathy.

Treatment

Treat hypertension if the patient is symptomatic or if the diastolic pressure is greater than 105–110 mm Hg—especially if there is no prior history of hypertension.

Administer phentolamine, 2–5 mg intravenously; nifedipine, 10–20 mg orally; or nitroprusside sodium, 0.5–5 μg/kg/min intravenously. If excessive tachycardia is present, add propranolol, 1–3 mg intravenously, or esmolol 25–50 μg/kg/min intravenously. *Caution:* Do not give beta-blockers alone, since doing so may paradoxically worsen hypertension.

ARRHYTHMIAS

Assessment & Complications

Arrhythmias may occur with a variety of drugs or toxins (Table 33–3). They may also occur as a result of hypoxia, metabolic acidosis, or electrolyte imbalance (eg, hyper- or hypokalemia, hypocalcemia).

Treatment

Arrhythmias are often caused by hypoxia or electrolyte imbalance, and these conditions should be sought and treated. If ventricular arrhythmias persist, administer lidocaine or phenytoin. *Caution:* avoid type IA agents (quinidine, procainamide, disopyramide), which may aggravate arrhythmias caused by tri-

Table 33–3. Common toxins or drugs causing arrhythmias.

Arrhythmia	Common Causes
Sinus bradycardia	Beta blockers, verapamil, organophosphates, digitalis glycosides, opioids, clonidine, sedative-hypnotics.
Atrioventricular block	Beta-blockers, digitalis glycosides, calcium antagonists, tricyclic antidepressants, lithium.
Sinus tachycardia	Theophylline, caffeine, cocaine, amphetamines, phencyclidine, metaproterenol and beta-agonists, iron, anticholinergics, tricyclic antidepressants, antihistamines.
Wide QRS complex	Tricyclic antidepressants, quinidine and type IA antiarrhythmics, type IC antiarrhythmics, phenothiazines, hyperkalemia.

cyclic antidepressants, calcium antagonists, or beta-blockers.

For tachyarrhythmias induced by sympathomimetic agents, use propranolol or esmolol (see doses given above in hypertension section). Wide QRS complex tachycardia in the setting of tricyclic antidepressant overdose (or quinidine and other class IA drugs) should be treated with sodium bicarbonate, 50–100 meq intravenously by bolus injection.

CONVULSIONS

Assessment & Complications

Convulsions may be due to poisoning with amphetamines, antihistamines, camphor, cocaine, isoniazid, lindane, phencyclidine (PCP), phenothiazines, strychnine (rigidity), theophylline, tricyclic antidepressants, or withdrawal from alcohol or sedative-hypnotics.

Convulsions may also be caused by hypoxia, hypoglycemia, hyponatremia, head trauma, central nervous system infection, and idiopathic epilepsy.

Prolonged or repeated convulsions may lead to hypoxia, metabolic acidosis, hyperthermia, and rhabdomyolysis.

Treatment

Administer diazepam, 5–10 mg intravenously, or—if intravenous access is not immediately available—midazolam, 5–10 mg intramuscularly. If convulsions continue, administer phenobarbital, 15–20 mg/kg intravenously over no less than 30 minutes; or phenytoin, 15 mg/kg intravenously over no less than 30 minutes. Both drugs may be used if necessary. Maintenance doses may be required if drug toxicity is expected to last more than 18–24 hours.

Convulsions due to a few drugs and toxins may require antidotes or other specific therapies (as listed in Table 33–4).

Table 33–4. Convulsions requiring special consideration.

Toxin or Drug	Comments
Isoniazid (INH)	Administer pyridoxine, 5–10 g IV.
Lithium	May indicate need for hemodialysis.
Organophosphates	Administer pralidoxime (2-PAM) and atropine.
Strychnine	"Convulsions" are actually spinally mediated muscle spasms and usually require neuromuscular paralysis.
Theophylline	Convulsions indicate need for charcoal hemoperfusion.
Tricyclic antidepressants	Hyperthermia and cardiotoxicity are common complications of repeated convulsions; paralyze early with neuromuscular blockers.

HYPERTHERMIA

Assessment & Complications

Hyperthermia may be due to poisoning with amphetamines, atropine and other anticholinergic drugs, cocaine, dinitrophenol and pentachlorophenol, haloperidol and other neuroleptics, monoamine oxidase inhibitors, phencyclidine (PCP), salicylates, strychnine, and tricyclic antidepressants.

Hyperthermia is a rapidly life-threatening complication. Severe hyperthermia (temperature > 40–41 °C [104–105.8 °F]) may rapidly cause brain damage and multiorgan failure, including rhabdomyolysis, renal failure, and coagulopathy.

Treatment

Treat hyperthermia aggressively by removing all clothing, spraying with tepid water, and fanning the patient. If this is not rapidly effective, as shown by a normal rectal temperature within 30–60 minutes or if there is significant muscle rigidity or hyperactivity, induce neuromuscular paralysis with pancuronium, 0.1 mg/kg intravenously. Once paralyzed, the patient must be intubated and mechanically ventilated. Absence of visible muscular convulsive movements may give the false impression that brain seizure activity has ceased; however, this must be confirmed by electroencephalography.

OTHER TREATMENT

ANTIDOTES

Give "specific" antidotes when there is reasonable certainty of a specific diagnosis (Table 33–5). To effectively negate the physiologic effects of the toxic agent, the antidote must be given promptly. Keep in mind, however, that antidotes frequently have serious side effects of their own. The indications and dosages for specific antidotes are discussed in the respective sections for specific toxins. See also Table 33–6.

DECONTAMINATION OF THE SKIN

Corrosive agents rapidly injure the skin and eyes and must be removed immediately. In addition, many toxins are readily absorbed through the skin, and systemic absorption can only be prevented by rapid action.

Wash the affected areas with copious quantities of lukewarm water or saline. Wash carefully behind the ears, under the nails, and in skin folds. For oily

Table 33–5. Some toxic agents for which there are "specific" antidotes.

Toxic Agent	Specific Antidote
Acetaminophen	Acetylcysteine
Anticholinergics (eg, atropine)	Physostigmine
Anticholinesterases (eg, organo-phosphate pesticides)	Atropine and pralidoxime (2-PAM)
Carbon monoxide	Oxygen
Cyanide	Sodium nitrite, sodium thiosulfate
Digitalis glycosides	Digoxin-specific Fab antibodies
Heavy metals (eg, lead, mercury, iron) and arsenic	Specific chelating agents
Isoniazid	Pyridoxine (vitamin B_6)
Methanol, ethylene glycol	Ethanol (ethyl alcohol)
Opioids	Naloxone (Narcan)
Snake venom	Specific venom antisera

substances (eg, pesticides), wash the skin with plain soap and shampoo the hair.

DECONTAMINATION OF THE EYES

Act quickly to prevent serious damage. Flush the eyes with copious amounts of lukewarm water or saline. (If available, instill local anesthetic drops in the eye before beginning irrigation.) Place the victim supine under a tap or stream of water, and direct the stream so that it will flow across both eyes after running off the nasal bridge. Lift the tarsal conjunctiva to look for undissolved particles and to facilitate irrigation. Continue irrigation for 10 minutes by the clock

Table 33–6. Examples of ineffective or dangerous "antidotes."[1]

"Antidote"	Application	Problems
Amphetamines, caffeine, or doxapram	Nonspecific arousal, eg, sedative overdose	Cardiac arrhythmias, seizures
Mineral oil	Petroleum distillate ingestion	Lipoid pneumonia
Physostigmine	Nonspecific arousal, eg, diazepam overdose, tricyclic antidepressants	Bradycardia, asystole, seizures
"Universal antidote" (burnt toast, tea)	Adsorbent in gut	Ineffective; aspiration; wastes time
Vinegar, other weak acids	Neutralization of alkali burns	Ineffective; may worsen injury

[1] Reproduced, with permission, from Olson KR, Becker CE: Chapter 29 in: *Current Emergency Diagnosis & Treatment*, 3rd ed. Ho MT, Saunders CE (editors). Appleton & Lange, 1990.

or until each eye has been irrigated with at least 1 L of solution. If the toxin is an acid or a base, check the pH of the tears after irrigation, and continue irrigation if the pH is abnormal.

After irrigation is complete, perform fluorescein examination of the eye, using Wood's lamp to identify areas of corneal injury. Patients with serious conjunctival or corneal injury should be immediately referred to an ophthalmologist.

GASTROINTESTINAL DECONTAMINATION

Removal of ingested poisons is an essential part of emergency treatment. However, if more than 60 minutes has passed, induced emesis and gastric lavage are relatively ineffective. Exceptions are ingestion of anticholinergic compounds and salicylates, which often delay gastric emptying, and ingestion of sustained-release or enteric-coated tablets, which may remain intact for several hours.

Gastric emptying is not generally used for ingestion of corrosive agents or petroleum distillates, because further esophageal injury or pulmonary aspiration may result. However, in certain cases, removal of the toxin may be more important than concern over possible complications. Consult a medical toxicologist or regional poison control center (Table 33–1) for advice.

Emesis
Emesis using syrup of ipecac is a convenient and fairly effective way to evacuate gastric contents if given shortly after ingestion. However, it may delay or prevent use of oral activated charcoal.

A. Indications: For removal of poison in conscious, cooperative patients and for promptness, since ipecac can be given in the home in the first few minutes after poisoning.

B. Contraindications: Induced emesis is contraindicated for drowsy, unconscious, or convulsing patients and for patients who have ingested kerosene or other hydrocarbons (danger of aspiration of stomach contents), corrosive poisons, or rapidly acting convulsants (eg, cyclic antidepressants, strychnine, nicotine, camphor).

C. Technique: Give syrup of ipecac, 30 mL (15 mL in children), followed by an 8-oz glass of water. Repeat in 20 minutes if necessary.

Gastric Lavage
A. Indications: Gastric lavage is indicated for removal of ingested poisons when emesis is refused, contraindicated, or unsuccessful; for collection and examination of gastric contents for identification of poison; and for convenient administration of antidotes.

B. Contraindications: Do *not* use lavage for stuporous or comatose patients with absent gag reflexes unless they are endotracheally intubated beforehand.

Some authorities advise against lavage when caustic material has been ingested; others regard it as essential to remove such material from the stomach.

C. Technique: The danger of aspiration pneumonia is reduced by first protecting the airway with endotracheal intubation. Gently insert a lubricated, soft but noncollapsible stomach tube (at least 37–40F) through the mouth or nose into the stomach. Aspirate and save the contents, and then lavage repeatedly with 50–100 mL of fluid until the return fluid is clear. Always remove excess lavage fluid. Use lukewarm tap water or saline. For iron ingestion, use 1–2% bicarbonate solution.

Activated Charcoal

Activated charcoal effectively adsorbs almost all drugs and poisons. Poorly absorbed substances are medicinal iron, lithium, potassium, sodium, cyanide, mineral acids, and alcohols.

A. Indications: Activated charcoal should be used for prompt adsorption of drugs or toxins in the stomach and intestine. Given alone, it may be as effective as or more effective than ipecac-induced emesis.

B. Contraindications: Activated charcoal should not be used for stuporous, comatose, or convulsing patients unless it can be given by gastric tube and the airway is first protected by cuffed endotracheal tube. This substance is contraindicated also for patients with ileus or intestinal obstruction or those who have ingested corrosives for whom endoscopy is planned.

C. Technique: Administer 60–100 g orally or via gastric tube, mixed in aqueous slurry. Repeated doses may be given to ensure gastrointestinal adsorption or to enhance elimination of some drugs (see below).

Catharsis

A. Indications: Catharsis is indicated for removal of unabsorbed poisons, especially those that have passed into the intestine.

B. Contraindications and Cautions: Do not use mineral oil or other oil-based cathartics. Avoid sodium-based cathartics in patients with hypertension, renal failure, and congestive heart failure and magnesium-based cathartics in those with renal failure.

C. Technique: Sodium sulfate 10%, 1–2 mL/kg; magnesium sulfate 10%, 2–3 mL/kg; or sorbitol 70%, 1–2 mL/kg. Combine with activated charcoal, 60–90 g. Alternatives are magnesium citrate or magnesium sulfate.

Whole Bowel Irrigations

Whole bowel irrigation utilizes large volumes of balanced polyethylene glycol-electrolyte solution to push tablets through the intestinal tract. There is no net gain or loss of systemic fluids or electrolytes.

A. Indications: Whole bowel irrigation is particu-

larly effective for massive iron ingestion in which intact tablets persist on abdominal x-ray despite emesis and lavage. It has also been reported to be useful for ingestions of sustained-release and enteric-coated tablets.

B. Contraindications: Same as for cathartics.

C. Technique: Administer the balanced polyethylene glycol-electrolyte solution (CoLyte, Go-LYTELY) into the stomach via gastric tube at a rate of 1–2 L/h until the rectal effluent is clear. Several hours of irrigation may be required.

Increased Drug Removal

A. Forced Diuresis: Forced diuresis is hazardous; the risk of complications (pulmonary edema, electrolyte imbalance) usually outweighs its benefits. Acidic drugs (eg, salicylates, phenobarbital) are more rapidly excreted with an alkaline urine. Acidification (sometimes promoted for amphetamines, PCP) is *not* very effective and is contraindicated in the presence of rhabdomyolysis or myoglobinuria.

B. Dialysis (Hemodialysis or Hemoperfusion): The indications for dialysis are as follows: (1) Known or suspected potentially lethal amounts of a dialyzable drug (Table 33–7). (2) Poisoning with deep coma, apnea, severe hypotension, fluid and electrolyte or acid-base disturbance, or extreme body temperature changes which cannot be corrected by conventional measures. (3) Poisoning in patients with severe renal, cardiac, pulmonary, or hepatic disease

Table 33–7. Recommended use of hemodialysis (HD) and hemoperfusion (HP) in poisoning.

Toxin	Procedure	Indications[1]
Carbamaze-pine	HP	Seizures, severe cardiotoxicity.
Digitoxin	HP	Severe toxicity, Fab not available.
Ethylene gly-col	HD	Acidosis, serum level > 100 mg/dL.
Lithium	HD	Severe symptoms, serum level > 2 meq/L (chronic) or > 4 meq/L (acute).
Methanol	HD	Acidosis, serum level > 50 mg/dL.
Paraquat	HP	Ingestion of known lethal dose.
Phenobarbital	HP	Intractable hypotension, acidosis despite maximal supportive care.
Salicylate	HD	Severe acidosis, CNS symptoms, level > 100 mg/dL (acute) or > 60 mg/dL (chronic).
Theophylline	HP	Seizures, serum level > 90–100 mg/L (acute) or > 40–60 mg/L (chronic).

[1] Contact a regional poison center or a clinical toxicologist before undertaking these procedures. See text for further discussion of indications.

who will not be able to eliminate the toxin by usual mechanisms.

Many of the substances that cannot be removed effectively by aqueous dialysis can be removed by hemoperfusion through specially designed coated charcoal columns. Indications are the same as for dialysis. Peritoneal dialysis may occasionally be employed for acute poisonings when hemodialysis is not available, but it is very inefficient. Dialysis should usually augment rather than replace well-established emergency and supportive measures.

C. Repeat-Dose Charcoal: Repeated doses of activated charcoal, 20–30 g every 3–4 hours, may hasten elimination of some drugs (eg, digitoxin, theophylline, phenobarbital) by adsorbing drug excreted into the gut lumen ("gut dialysis"). However, if sorbitol or other cathartic is used with each dose, large stool volumes may result in dehydration or hypernatremia.

DIAGNOSIS OF POISONING

The identity of the ingested substance is usually known, but occasionally a comatose patient is found with an unlabeled container or refuses or otherwise fails to give a coherent history. By performing a directed physical examination and ordering common clinical laboratory tests, the clinician can often make a tentative diagnosis that may allow empiric interventions or may suggest specific toxicologic tests.

PHYSICAL EXAMINATION

Important diagnostic variables in the physical examination include blood pressure, pulse rate, temperature, pupil size, sweating, and the presence or absence of peristaltic activity. Poisonings with many drugs fit into one of 4 common syndromes.

Sympathomimetic Syndrome

The blood pressure and pulse rate are elevated, though with severe hypertension reflex bradycardia may occur. The temperature is often elevated, pupils are dilated, and the skin is sweaty, though mucous membranes are dry. Patients are usually agitated, anxious, or even psychotic.

Examples: Amphetamines, cocaine, ephedrine and pseudoephedrine, phencyclidine (pupils normal or small), phenylpropanolamine (bradycardia common).

Sympatholytic Syndrome

The blood pressure and pulse rate are decreased and body temperature is low. The pupils are small or even pinpoint. Peristalsis is usually decreased. Patients are usually obtunded or comatose.

Examples: Barbiturates, benzodiazepines and other sedative hypnotics, clonidine and related antihypertensives, ethanol, opioids.

Cholinergic Syndrome

Stimulation of muscarinic receptors causes bradycardia, miosis, sweating, and hyperperistalsis as well as bronchorrhea, wheezing, excessive salivation, and urinary incontinence. Nicotinic receptor stimulation may produce initial hypertension and tachycardia as well as fasciculations and muscle weakness. Patients are usually agitated and anxious.

Examples: Carbamates, nicotine, organophosphates, physostigmine.

Anticholinergic Syndrome

Tachycardia with mild hypertension is common, and the body temperature is often elevated. Pupils are widely dilated. The skin is flushed, hot and dry. Peristalsis is decreased, and urinary retention is common. Patients may have myoclonic jerking or choreoathetoid movements. Agitated delirium is frequently seen, and severe hyperthermia may occur.

Examples: Atropine, scopolamine, other anticholinergics, amantadine, antihistamines, phenothiazines (hypotension, small pupils), tricyclic antidepressants.

CLINICAL LABORATORY TESTS IN MANAGEMENT OF POISONING

The following clinical laboratory tests are recommended for routine screening of the overdosed patient: serum osmolality and osmolar gap, serum electrolytes, serum glucose, serum creatinine, serum urea nitrogen, urinalysis (crystals, hemoglobinuria or myoglobinuria), and electrocardiography. In addition, it is recommended that serum acetaminophen and ethanol levels be determined in all patients with drug overdoses.

OSMOLAR GAP

The osmolar gap is defined and calculation of the gap is described in Table 33–8. It is increased in the presence of large quantities of low-molecular-weight substances, most commonly ethanol. Common poisons associated with increased osmolar gap are acetone, ethanol, ethylene glycol, isopropyl alcohol, methanol, and propylene glycol. The presence of a combined osmolar and elevated anion gap suggests poisoning by methanol or ethylene glycol.

Table 33–8. Use of the osmolar gap in toxicology.[1]

The osmolar gap (Δosm) is determined by subtracting the calculated serum osmolality from the measured serum osmolality.

Calculated osmolality (osm) = 2(Na [meq/L]) +

$$\frac{\text{Glucose (mg/dL)}}{18} + \frac{\text{BUN (mg/dL)}}{2.8}$$

Δosm = Measured osmolality – Calculated osmolality

Serum osmolality may be increased by contributions of circulating alcohols and other low-molecular-weight substances. Since these substances are not included in the calculated osmolality, there will be a gap proportionate to their serum concentration and inversely proportional to their molecular weight:

$$\text{Serum concentration (mg/dL)} \approx \Delta\text{osm} \times \frac{\text{Molecular weight}}{10}$$

For ethanol (the commonest cause of Δosm), a gap of 30 mosm/L indicates an ethanol level of

$$30 \times 45/10 = 138 \approx 140 \text{ mg/dL}$$

	Molecular Weight	Lethal Concentration (mg/dL)	Corresponding Δosm (mosm/L)
Ethanol	46	350	75
Methanol	32	80	25
Ethylene glycol	62	200	35
Isopropanol	60	350	60

[1] Modified from Olson KR, Becker CE: Chapter 29 in: *Current Emergency Diagnosis & Treatment*, 3rd ed. Ho MT, Saunders CE (editors). Appleton & Lange, 1990.
Note: Most laboratories use the freezing point method for calculating osmolality. If the vaporization point method is used, alcohols are driven off and their contribution to osmolality is lost.

ANION GAP

The anion gap is the difference between serum sodium concentration and chloride plus bicarbonate. Common causes of elevated anion gap include some types of metabolic acidosis (see Table 16–3) and poisoning by carbon monoxide, cyanide, ethylene glycol, medicinal iron, isoniazid, methanol, phenformin, and salicylates.

Metabolic acidosis associated with an elevated anion gap is usually due to accumulation of lactic acid or other organic acids. Calculation of the anion gap (normal: 8–12 meq/L) is by the following equation:

$$\text{Anion gap} = Na^+ - (Cl^- + HCO_3^-)$$

One should also check the osmolar gap; combined elevated anion and osmolar gap suggests poisoning by methanol or ethylene glycol.

TOXICOLOGY LABORATORY EXAMINATION

The routine toxicology screen (Table 33–9) is of little value in the initial care of the poisoned patient—on the contrary, it is time-consuming, expensive, and frequently erroneous. Specific quantitative levels of certain drugs may be extremely helpful (Table 33–10), however, especially if specific antidotes or interventions (eg, dialysis, antidotes) would be indicated based upon the results.

If a toxicology screen is required, urine is the best specimen for broad qualitative screening. Blood samples may be saved for possible quantitative testing, but blood is not appropriate for screening purposes since it is relatively insensitive for many common drugs, including psychotropic agents, opioids, and stimulants.

ABDOMINAL X-RAYS

A plain film of the abdomen may reveal radiopaque iron tablets, drug-filled condoms, or other toxic material. Recent studies suggest that few tablets are predictably visible (eg, ferrous sulfate, sodium chloride, calcium carbonate, and potassium chloride). Thus, the x-ray is useful only if positive.

Bryson P: *Critical Review in Toxicology.* Aspens Systems, 1989.

Ellenhorn M, Barceloux D: *Medical Toxicology: Diagnosis and Treatment of Human Poisoning.* Elsevier, 1988.

Goldfrank LR et al (editors): *Goldfrank's Toxicologic Emergencies.* Appleton-Century-Crofts, 1985.

Haddad LM, Winchester JF: *Clinical Management of Poisoning and Drug Overdose.* Saunders, 1983.

Olson KR et al: Physical assessment and differential diagnosis of the poisoned patient. Med Toxicol 1987;2:52.

Olson KR et al: *Poisoning & Drug Overdose.* Appleton & Lange, 1990.

Table 33–9. Common drugs screened for in blood and urine in the toxicology laboratory.[1]

Blood
  Acetaminophen, alcohols, barbiturates, benzodiazepines, cariosprodol, ethchlorvynol, glutethimide, meprobamate, methaqualone, phenytoin, salicylates.
Urine
  Acetaminophen, alcohols, barbiturates, chlorpheniramine, cocaine, codeine, dextromethorphan, diphenhydramine, ethchlorvynol, lidocaine, meperidine, meprobamate, methadone, methyprylon, morphine, pentazocine, phencyclidine, phenothiazines, propoxyphene, salicylates, tricyclic antidepressants.

[1] *Note:* The urine screen is generally more comprehensive, detecting drugs of abuse (opiates, stimulants), antihistamines, and, in many cases, drugs also found in serum.

Table 33–10. Specific quantitative levels and potential therapeutic interventions. [1]

Drug or Toxin	Treatment
Acetaminophen	Use of specific antidote (acetylcysteine) based on serum level.
Carbon monoxide	High carboxyhemoglobin level indicates need for 100% oxygen.
Digitalis	On basis of serum digitalis and potassium levels, treatment with Fab antibody fragments may be indicated.
Ethanol	Low serum level may suggest nonalcoholic cause for coma (eg, trauma, other drugs, other alcohols). May also be used in monitoring ethanol therapy for methanol or ethylene glycol poisoning.
Ethylene glycol	High level and acidosis indicate need for hemodialysis and ethanol therapy.
Iron	Level may indicate need for chelation with deferoxamine.
Lithium	Serum levels and calculated half-life can guide decision to hemodialyze.
Methanol	Acidosis, high methanol level indicate need for hemodialysis, ethanol therapy.
Methemoglobin	Methemoglobinemia can be treated with methylene blue intravenously.
Salicylates	High level may indicate need for hemodialysis, alkaline diuresis.
Theophylline	Immediate hemoperfusion may be indicated based on serum level.

[1] Some drugs or toxins may have profound and irreversible toxicity unless rapid and specific management is provided outside of routine supportive care. For these agents, laboratory testing may provide the serum level or other evidence required for administering a specific antidote or arranging for hemodialysis.

TREATMENT OF COMMON SPECIFIC POISONINGS (Alphabetical Order)

ACETAMINOPHEN

Acetaminophen is a common analgesic found in many nonprescription and prescription products. After absorption, it is metabolized mainly by glucuronidation and sulfation, with a small fraction metabolized via the P-450 mixed-function oxidase system to a highly toxic reactive intermediate. This toxic intermediate is normally detoxified by cellular glutathione. With acute acetaminophen overdose (> 140 mg/kg, or 7 g in an average adult), hepatocellular glutathione is rapidly depleted and the reactive intermediate attacks other cell proteins, causing necrosis.

Clinical Findings

Shortly after ingestion, patients may have nausea or vomiting, but there are no other signs of toxicity until 24–48 hours after ingestion, when hepatic transaminase levels increase. With severe poisoning, massive hepatic necrosis may occur, resulting in jaundice, hepatic encephalopathy, renal failure, and death.

The diagnosis of severe poisoning is based on measurement of the serum acetaminophen level. Plot the serum level versus the time since ingestion on the acetaminophen nomogram shown in Fig 33–1.

Treatment

A. Emergency and Supportive Measures: Empty the stomach by emesis or gastric lavage, and administer activated charcoal. If more than 3–4 hours have passed since ingestion, do not induce emesis, because it is ineffective and may delay oral administration of the antidote acetylcysteine. Although charcoal may bind the oral antidote acetylcysteine, this is not considered clinically significant.

Provide supportive care for hepatic injury. Some patients who progress to massive hepatic failure with encephalopathy may require emergency liver transplantation.

B. Specific Treatment: If the serum acetaminophen level is higher than the toxic line on the nomo-

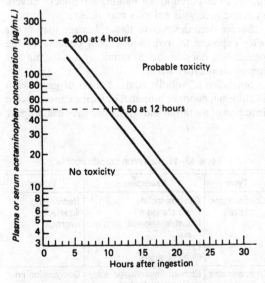

Figure 33–1. Nomogram for prediction of acetaminophen hepatotoxicity following acute overdosage. The upper line defines serum acetaminophen concentrations known to be associated with hepatotoxicity; the lower line defines serum levels 25% below those expected to cause hepatotoxicity. To give a margin for error, the lower line should be used as a guide to treatment. (Modified and reproduced, with permission, from Rumack BH, Matthew H: Acetaminophen poisoning and toxicity. Pediatrics 1975; 55:871.)

gram (Fig 33–1)), begin treatment with acetylcysteine, 140 mg/kg orally, followed by 70 mg/kg every 4 hours for 17 doses or until the serum acetaminophen level is zero. Treatment with acetylcysteine is most effective if started within 8 hours after ingestion; it is of little proved benefit if started after 16 hours.

Acetylcysteine may also be given intravenously; this is the preferred method in Europe and Canada, but there is no approved parenteral formulation or dosing schedule in the United States.

Ashbourne JF et al: Value of rapid screening for acetaminophen in all patients with intentional overdose. Ann Emerg Med 1989;18:1035.

Smilkstein MJ et al: Efficacy of oral N-acetylcysteine in the treatment of acetaminophen overdose. N Engl J Med 1988;319:1557.

ACIDS, CORROSIVE
(Table 33–11)

The strong mineral acids exert primarily a local corrosive effect on the skin and mucous membranes. In severe burns, circulatory collapse may result. Symptoms include severe pain in the throat and upper gastrointestinal tract, marked thirst, bloody vomitus; difficulty in swallowing, breathing, and speaking; discoloration and destruction of skin and mucous membranes in and around the mouth; and shock. Severe systemic metabolic acidosis may occur.

Severe deep destructive tissue damage may occur after exposure to hydrofluoric acid because of the penetrating fluoride ion. Systemic hypocalcemia and hyperkalemia may occur.

Inhalation of volatile acids, fumes, or gases such as chlorine, fluorine, bromine, or iodine causes severe irritation of the throat and larynx and may cause upper airway obstruction and noncardiogenic pulmonary edema.

Treatment

A. Ingestion: Do *not* induce emesis. Dilute immediately by giving a glass of milk or water to drink. Do *not* give bicarbonate or other neutralizing agents. Some experts recommend immediate gastric lavage.

Perform flexible endoscopic esophagoscopy promptly to determine the presence and extent of injury but do not attempt to pass beyond the injury. Perforation, peritonitis, and major bleeding are indications for surgery.

B. Skin Contact: Flood with water for 15 minutes. Use no chemical antidotes; the heat of the reaction may cause additional injury. For hydrofluoric acid burns, soak the affected area in magnesium sulfate solution or apply calcium gluconate gel; then arrange immediate consultation with a plastic surgeon or other specialist. Binding of the fluoride ion may be achieved by injecting 0.5 mL of 10% calcium gluconate per square centimeter under the burned area.

C. Eye Contact: Anesthetize the conjunctiva and corneal surfaces with topical local anesthetic drops. Flood with water for 15 minutes, holding the eyelids open. Check pH with pH 6.0–8.0 test paper, and repeat irrigation, using normal saline, until pH is 7.0. Check for corneal damage with fluorescein and slit-lamp examination; consult an ophthalmologist about further treatment.

D. Inhalation: Remove from further exposure to fumes or gas. Check skin and clothing. Treat pulmonary edema.

Caravati EM: Acute hydrofluoric acid exposure. J Emerg Med 1988;6:143.

Crain EF et al: Caustic ingestions: Symptoms as predictors of esophageal injury. Am J Dis Child 1984;138:863.

Schultz CH: Hydrofluoric acid burns of the hand. West J Med 1989;71.

ALKALIES
(Table 33–11)

The strong alkalies are common ingredients of household cleaning compounds and may be suspected by their ''soapy'' texture. Those with alkalinity above pH 12.0 are particularly corrosive. Clinitest tablets and disk batteries are also a source. Alkalies cause liquefactive necrosis, which is deeply penetrating. Symptoms include burning pain in the upper gastrointestinal tract, nausea, vomiting, and difficulty in swallowing and breathing. Examination reveals destruction and edema of the affected skin and mucous membranes and bloody vomitus and stools. X-ray may reveal the presence of disk batteries in the esophagus or lower gastrointestinal tract.

Table 33–11. Common caustic agents.[1]

Type	Examples	Injury
Concentrated alkalies	Clinitest tablets Drain cleaners Industrial-strength ammonia Lye Oven cleaners	Penetrating liquefaction necrosis
Concentrated acids	Etchers (hydrofluoric acid) Pool disinfectants Toilet bowl cleaners	Coagulation necrosis
Weaker cleaning agents	Cationic detergents (dishwasher detergents) Household ammonia Household bleach	Superficial burns and irritation; deep burns (rare)

[1] Reproduced, with permission, from Olson KR, Becker CE: Chapter 29 in: *Current Emergency Diagnosis & Treatment*, 3rd ed. Ho MT, Saunders CE (editors). Appleton & Lange, 1990.

Treatment

A. Ingested: Do *not* induce emesis. Dilute immediately with a glass of water. Some gastroenterologists recommend immediate gastric lavage after ingestion of liquid caustic substances to remove residual material.

Immediate endoscopy is recommended to evaluate the extent of damage. If x-ray reveals the location of ingested disk batteries in the esophagus, immediate endoscopic removal is mandatory.

The use of corticosteroids to prevent stricture formation is controversial and is definitely contraindicated if there is evidence of esophageal perforation.

B. Skin Contact: Wash with running water until the skin no longer feels soapy. Relieve pain and treat shock.

C. Eye Contact: Anesthetize the conjunctival and corneal surfaces with topical anesthetic. Irrigate with water or saline continuously for 20–30 minutes, holding the lids open. Check pH with pH test paper, and repeat irrigation, using normal saline, for additional 30-minute periods until the pH is 7.0. Check for corneal damage with fluorescein and slit-lamp examination; consult an ophthalmologist for further treatment.

Gaudreault P et al: Predictability of esophageal injury from signs and symptoms: A study of caustic ingestion in 378 children. Pediatrics 1983;71:767.
Kuhns DW et al: Button battery ingestions. Ann Emerg Med 1989;18:293.
Wasserman RL et al: Caustic substance injuries. J Ped 1985;107:169.

AMPHETAMINES & COCAINE

Amphetamines and cocaine are widely abused for their euphorigenic and stimulant properties. Both drugs may be smoked, snorted, ingested, or injected. The forms most commonly used for smoking are "ice" (amphetamine base) and "crack" or "freebase" (cocaine base). Amphetamines and cocaine produce central nervous system stimulation and a generalized increase in central and peripheral sympathetic activity. The toxic dose of each drug is highly variable and depends on the route of administration and individual tolerance. The onset of effects is most rapid after intravenous injection or smoking.

Clinical Findings

Patients may present with anxiety, tremulousness, tachycardia, hypertension, diaphoresis, dilated pupils, agitation, muscular hyperactivity, and psychosis. In severe intoxication, seizures and hyperthermia may occur. Sustained or severe hypertension may result in intracranial hemorrhage, aortic dissection, or myocardial infarction.

The diagnosis is supported by finding amphetamines, cocaine, or the cocaine metabolite benzoyl-ecgonine in the urine. Blood screening is not sensitive enough to detect these drugs.

Treatment

A. Emergency and Supportive Measures: Maintain a patent airway and assist ventilation, if necessary. Treat coma or seizures as described at the beginning of this chapter. Rapidly lower the body temperature in patients who are hyperthermic (40 °C). Treat agitation or psychosis with a benzodiazepine such as diazepam, 0.1–0.2 mg/kg intravenously, or midazolam, 0.1 mg/kg intramuscularly.

For poisoning by ingestion, perform gastric lavage and administer activated charcoal, or administer activated charcoal alone without prior gut emptying. Do *not* induce emesis, because of the risk of seizures.

B. Specific Treatment: Treat hypertension with a vasodilator drug such as phentolamine (1–5 mg intravenously) or nifedipine (10–20 mg orally) or a combined α- and β-adrenergic blocker such as labetalol (10–20 mg intravenously). Do *not* administer a pure beta-blocker such as propranolol alone, as this may result paradoxic worsening of the hypertension as a result of unopposed α-adrenergic effects.

Treat tachycardia or tachyarrhythmias with a short-acting beta-blocker such as esmolol (25–50 μg/kg/min by intravenous infusion).

Derlet RW et al: Emergency department presentation of cocaine intoxication. Ann Emerg Med 1989;18:182.
Ernst AA et al: Unexpected cocaine intoxication presenting as seizures in children. Ann Emerg Med 1989;18:774.
Olson KR et al: Life-threatening cocaine intoxication. Prob Crit Care 1987;1:95.

ANTICOAGULANTS

Warfarin and related compounds (including ingredients of many rodenticides) inhibit the clotting mechanism by blocking hepatic synthesis of vitamin K-dependent clotting factors.

Anticoagulants may cause hemoptysis, gross hematuria, bloody stools, hemorrhages into organs, widespread bruising, and bleeding into joint spaces. The prothrombin time is increased within 8–12 hours (peak 36–48 hours) after a single overdose. After ingestion of brodifacoum and indanedione rodenticides, inhibition of clotting factor synthesis may persist for several weeks after a single dose.

Treatment

Discontinue the drug at the first sign of gross bleeding, and determine the prothrombin time. If the patient has ingested an acute overdose, empty the stomach by emesis or lavage and administer activated charcoal. If the prothrombin time is elevated, give phytonadione (vitamin K), 5–10 mg subcutaneously and give fresh-frozen plasma if there is serious bleeding. If the patient is chronically anticoagulated and has strong medical indications for being maintained in that status (eg, prosthetic heart valve), give much smaller doses of vitamin K (1 mg) and fresh-frozen plasma (or both) to titrate to the desired prothrombin time.

If the patient has ingested brodifacoum or related super-rodenticides, prolonged observation (over weeks) and repeated administration of vitamin K may be required.

Katona B et al: Superwarfarin poisoning. J Emerg Med 1989;7:627.

Smolinske SC et al: Superwarfarin poisoning in children: A prospective study. Pediatrics 1989;84:490.

ARSENIC

Arsenic is found in pesticides and industrial chemicals. Symptoms of poisoning usually appear within 1 hour after ingestion but may be delayed as long as 12 hours. They include abdominal pain, vomiting, watery diarrhea, and skeletal muscle cramps. Profound dehydration and shock may occur. In chronic poisoning, symptoms can be vague but often include those of peripheral sensory neuropathy. Urinary arsenic levels may be misleading and are falsely elevated after certain meals (eg, seafood) that contain large quantities of relatively nontoxic organic arsenic.

Treatment
A. Emergency Measures: Induce vomiting or perform gastric lavage, and administer 60–100 g of activated charcoal.

B. Antidote: For symptomatic patients or those with massive overdose, give dimercaprol injection (BAL), 10% solution in oil, 2.5 mg/kg dimercaprol intramuscularly, then 2–3 mg/kg intramuscularly every 4 hours for 2 days. The side effects include nausea, vomiting, headache, and hypertension. An antihistamine such as diphenhydramine, 25–50 mg orally, will reduce the side effects if given 30 minutes before dimercaprol. Follow dimercaprol with oral penicillamine, 100 mg/kg/d in 4 divided doses (maximum 1 g/d) for 1 week. Consult a medical toxicologist or regional poison control center (Table 33–1) for advice regarding continued chelation.

DiNapoli J et al: Cyanide and arsenic poisoning by intravenous injection. Ann Emerg Med 1989;18:308.

Hutton JT: Source, symptoms and signs of arsenic poisoning. J Fam Pract 1983;17:423.

Peters HA et al: Seasonal arsenic exposure from burning chromium-copper-arsenate-treated wood. JAMA 1984; 251:2393.

ATROPINE & ANTICHOLINERGICS

Atropine, scopolamine, belladonna, Lomotil, *Datura stramonium, Hyoscyamus niger,* some mushrooms, tricyclic antidepressants, and antihistamines are antimuscarinic agents with variable central nervous system effects. The patient complains of dryness of the mouth, thirst, difficulty in swallowing, and blurring of vision. The physical signs include dilated pupils, flushed skin, tachycardia, fever (although hypothermia has been reported), delirium, myoclonus, ileus, and flushed appearance. Antidepressants and antihistamines may induce convulsions.

Treatment
Induce vomiting or perform gastric lavage, and administer activated charcoal. Do *not* induce emesis in patients who have ingested antidepressants, because seizures may occur abruptly.

Tepid sponge baths and sedation are indicated to control high temperatures. If symptoms are severe (eg, hyperthermia or excessively rapid tachycardia), give physostigmine salicylate, 1 mg slowly intravenously over 5 minutes, with electrocardiographic monitoring, until symptoms are controlled. Bradyarrhythmias and convulsions are a hazard with physostigmine administration, and it should not be used with antidepressant overdose.

Pentel PR, Benowitz NL: Tricyclic antidepressant poisoning: Management of arrhythmias. J Med Toxicol 1986;1:101.

BETA-ADRENERGIC BLOCKERS

There are a wide variety of β-adrenergic blocking drugs, with varying pharmacologic and pharmacokinetic properties. The most commonly used and most toxic beta-blocker is propranolol. Propranolol competitively blocks β_1 and β_2 adrenoceptors and also has direct membrane-depressant and central nervous system effects.

Clinical Findings
The most common findings with mild or moderate intoxication are hypotension and bradycardia. With more severe poisoning, cardiac depression may occur that is often unresponsive to conventional therapy with β-adrenergic stimulants such as dopamine and norepinephrine. In addition, with propranolol and other lipid-soluble drugs, seizures and coma may occur.

The diagnosis is based on typical clinical findings. Toxicology screening does not usually include beta-blockers.

Treatment
A. Emergency and Supportive Measures: Maintain a patent airway and assist ventilation, if necessary. Treat coma, hypotension, and seizures as described at the beginning of this chapter. Initially, treat bradycardia or heart block with atropine (0.5– 2 mg intravenously), isoproterenol (2–5 μg/min by

intravenous infusion), or an external transcutaneous cardiac pacemaker. Specific antidotal treatment may be necessary (see below).

For ingested drugs, empty the stomach by gastric lavage and administer activated charcoal. Do *not* induce emesis because of the risk of seizures.

B. Specific Treatment: If the above measures are not successful in reversing bradycardia and hypotension, give glucagon, 5 mg intravenously. Glucagon is an inotropic agent that acts at a different receptor site and is therefore not affected by beta-blockade.

CALCIUM ANTAGONISTS

Calcium antagonists used in the United States include verapamil, diltiazem, nifedipine, nicardipine and nimodipine. These drugs share the ability to cause arteriolar vasodilation and depression of cardiac contractility, especially after acute overdose. Patients may present with bradycardia, AV nodal block, hypotension, or a combination of these effects. With severe poisoning, cardiac arrest may occur. The diagnosis is made clinically; these drugs are not included in routine toxicology screening.

Treatment
A. Emergency and Supportive Measures: Maintain a patent airway and assist ventilation, if necessary. Treat coma, hypotension, and seizures as described at the beginning of this chapter. Treat bradycardia with atropine (0.5–2 mg intravenously), isoproterenol (2–5 μg/min by intravenous infusion), or a transcutaneous or internal cardiac pacemaker.

For ingested drugs, perform gastric lavage and administer activated charcoal. Do *not* induce emesis because of the risk of seizures.

B. Specific Treatment: If bradycardia and hypotension are not reversed with these measures, administer calcium chloride 10%, 5–10 mL intravenously, or calcium gluconate 10%, 10–15 mL intravenously. Calcium is most useful in reversing negative inotropic effects and is less effective for AV nodal blockade and bradycardia.

Horowitz BZ et al: Massive verapamil ingestion: A report of two cases and a review of the literature. Am J Emerg Med 1989;7:624.

Ferner RE et al: Pharmacokinetics and toxic effects of diltiazem in massive overdose. Human Toxicol 1989;8:497.

Weinstein RS: Recognition and management of poisoning with beta-adrenergic blocking agents. Ann Emerg Med 1984;13:1123.

CARBON MONOXIDE

Carbon monoxide is a colorless, odorless gas produced by the combustion of carbon-containing materials. Poisoning may occur as a result of suicidal or accidental exposure to automobile exhaust, smoke inhalation in a fire, or accidental exposure to an improperly vented gas heater or other appliance. Carbon monoxide avidly binds to hemoglobin, with an affinity approximately 250 times that of oxygen. This results in reduced oxygen-carrying capacity and altered delivery of oxygen to cells.

Clinical Findings
At low carbon monoxide levels (carboxyhemoglobin saturation 10–20%), victims have may headache, dizziness, abdominal pain, and nausea. With higher levels, confusion, dyspnea, and syncope may occur. Hypotension, coma, and seizures are common with levels greater than 50–60%. Survivors of acute severe poisoning may develop permanent neurologic deficits.

Carbon monoxide poisoning should be suspected in any person with severe headache or acutely altered mental status. Diagnosis depends on specific measurement of the arterial or venous carboxyhemoglobin saturation. Routine arterial blood gas testing and pulse oximetry are not useful because they give falsely normal calculated oxyhemoglobin saturation determinations.

Treatment
A. Emergency and Supportive Measures: Maintain a patent airway and assist ventilation, if necessary. Remove the victim from exposure. Treat patients with coma, hypotension, or seizures, as described at the beginning of this chapter.

B. Specific Treatment: The half-life of the carboxyhemoglobin complex is about 4–5 hours in room air but is reduced dramatically by high concentrations of oxygen. Administer 100% oxygen by tight-fitting high-flow reservoir face mask or endotracheal tube. Hyperbaric oxygen can provide 100% oxygen under higher than atmospheric pressures, further shortening the half-life; it may be useful if immediately available.

Caravati EM et al: Fetal toxicity associated with maternal carbon monoxide poisoning. Ann Emerg Med 1988; 17:714.

Olson KR: Carbon monoxide poisoning: Mechanisms, presentation, and controversies in management. J Emerg Med 1984;1:233.

Sloan EP et al: Complications and protocol considerations in carbon monoxide-poisoned patients who require hyperbaric oxygen therapy: Report from a ten-year experience. Ann Emerg Med 1989;18:629.

CHEMICAL WARFARE AGENTS

Agents used in chemical warfare work by cholinesterase inhibition and are most commonly organophosphates. Agents such as **tabun** (dimethylphosphoramidocyanidic acid ethyl ether) and **sarin** (methylphosphonofluoridic acid 1-methylethyl ester) are similar to insecticides such as malathion but are vastly more potent. They may be inhaled or absorbed through the skin. Systemic effects due to unopposed action of acetylcholine include miosis, salivation, abdominal cramps, diarrhea, and muscle flaccidity producing respiratory arrest. Inhalation also produces severe bronchoconstriction and copious nasal and tracheobronchial secretions.

Prevention involves use of masks and protective clothing. Physicians caring for such patients must be gloved, since cutaneous absorption may occur through normal skin.

Treatment with atropine in an initial dose of 2 mg intramuscularly is effective. United States military personnel are equipped with autoinjectable units containing this dose plus 600 mg of the cholinesterase-reactivating agent pralidoxime. Repeated doses of atropine are occasionally necessary. Some victims have required several hundred milligrams.

Therapy of exposure to vesicants such as mustard gas is similar to that of burns.

Jacob WH, Friedl KE: Drug delivery systems for chemical defense. Army Research Development and Acquisition Bulletin, Jan–Feb 1990, pp 14–16.

CHLORINATED INSECTICIDES
(Chlorophenothane [DDT], Lindane, Toxaphene, Chlordane, Aldrin, Endrin)

DDT and other chlorinated insecticides are central nervous system stimulants that can cause poisoning by ingestion, inhalation, or direct contact. The MLD is about 20 g for DDT, 3 g for lindane, 2 g for toxaphene, 1 g for chlordane, and less than 1 g for endrin and aldrin. The manifestations of poisoning are nervous irritability, muscle twitching, convulsions, and coma. Arrhythmias may occur. Hepatic and renal damage are reported.

Treatment

Do *not* induce emesis, since seizures may occur abruptly. Give activated charcoal at once, perform lavage, and give a cathartic. For convulsions, give diazepam, 0.1 mg/kg slowly intravenously, or other anticonvulsants.

Prendergast T et al: Endrin poisoning associated with taquito ingestion—California. MMWR 1989;38:345.
Telch J, Jarvis DA: Acute intoxication with lindane (gamma benzene hexachloride). Can Med Assoc J 1982;126:662.

CLONIDINE & OTHER SYMPATHOLYTIC ANTIHYPERTENSIVES
(Clonidine, Methyldopa, Prazosin)

Overdosage with these agents causes bradycardia, hypotension, miosis, respiratory depression, and coma. (Hypertension occasionally occurs after clonidine overdosage, a result of peripheral alpha effects of this drug in high doses.) Symptoms are usually resolved in less than 24 hours, and deaths are rare.

Treatment

Empty the stomach by emesis or lavage. Give activated charcoal and a cathartic. Maintain the airway and support respiration if necessary. Symptomatic treatment is usually sufficient even in massive overdose. Maintain blood pressure with intravenous fluids. Dopamine can also be used. Atropine is usually effective for bradycardia.

Wiley JF et al: Clonidine poisoning in young children. J Ped 1990;116:654.

CYANIDE

Cyanide is a highly toxic chemical used widely in research and commercial laboratories and many industries. Its gaseous form, hydrogen cyanide, is an important component of smoke in fires. Cyanide-generating glycosides are also found in the pits of apricots and other related plants. Cyanide is rapidly absorbed by inhalation, skin absorption, or ingestion. It disrupts cellular function by inhibiting cytochrome oxidase and preventing cellular oxygen utilization.

Clinical Findings

The onset of toxicity is nearly instantaneous after inhalation of hydrogen cyanide gas but may be delayed for minutes to hours after ingestion of cyanide salts or cyanogenic plants or chemicals. Symptoms of intoxication include headache, dizziness, nausea, abdominal pain, and anxiety, followed by confusion, syncope, shock, seizures, coma, and death. The odor of "bitter almonds" may be detected on the victim's breath or in vomitus, though this is not a reliable finding. The venous oxygen saturation may be elevated ($> 90\%$) in severe poisonings because tissues have failed to take up arterial oxygen. There are no reliable rapid bedside laboratory tests for cyanide.

Treatment

A. Emergency and Supportive Measures: Maintain a patent airway and assist ventilation, if necessary. Remove the victim from exposure, taking care to avoid exposure to rescuers. Treat coma, hypotension, and seizures as described at the beginning of this chapter.

For cyanide ingestion, empty the stomach by gastric lavage with charcoal, or immediate oral administration of charcoal, or immediate emesis (if lavage or charcoal is not available). Although charcoal has a low affinity for cyanide, it is adequate to bind typically ingested lethal doses (100—200 mg).

B. Specific Treatment: In the United States, the cyanide antidote kit (Table 33–12) contains nitrites

Table 33–12. Currently available (prepackaged) cyanide antidotes.[1,2]

Antidote	How Supplied	Dose
Amyl nitrite	0.3 mL (aspirol inhalant)	Break 1–2 aspirols under patient's nose.
Sodium nitrite	3 g/dL (300 mg in 10 mL [vials])	6 mg/kg intravenously (0.2 mL/kg)
Sodium thiosulfate	25 g/dL (12.5 g in 50 mL [vials])	250 mg/kg intravenously (1 mL/kg)

[1] Reproduced, with permission, from Olson KR, Becker CE: Chapter 29 in: *Current Emergency Diagnosis & Treatment,* 3rd ed. Ho MT, Saunders CE (editors). Appleton & Lange, 1990.
[2] In USA, manufactured by Eli Lilly & Co.

(to induce methemoglobinemia, which binds free cyanide) and thiosulfate (to promote conversion of cyanide to the less toxic thiocyanate). Administer amyl nitrite by crushing an ampule under the victim's nose or at the end of the endotracheal tube; and administer 3% sodium nitrite solution, 10 mL intravenously (300 mg; for children, 0.3 mg/kg to a maximum of 10 mL) over 3–5 minutes. *Caution:* Nitrites may induce hypotension and dangerous levels of methemoglobin, especially in children. Also administer 25% sodium thiosulfate solution, 50 mL intravenously (12.5 g; for children, 400 mg/kg, or 1.6 mL/kg up to maximum 50 mL).

Caravati EM et al: Pediatric cyanide intoxication and death from an acetonitrile-containing cosmetic. JAMA 1988; 260:3470.

Lambert RJ et al: The efficacy of superactivated charcoal in treating rats exposed to a lethal oral dose of potassium cyanide. Ann Emerg Med 1988;17:595.

DIGITALIS & OTHER CARDIAC GLYCOSIDES

Cardiac glycosides are derived from a variety of plants and are widely used to treat heart failure and supraventricular arrhythmias. These drugs have potent vagotonic effects and also paralyze the Na^+/K^+-AT Pase pump. Intracellular effects include enhancement of calcium-dependent contractility and shortening of the action potential duration. Digoxin and ouabain are highly tissue-bound, but digitoxin has a volume of distribution of just 0.6 L/kg, making it the only cardiac glycoside accessible to enhanced removal procedures such as hemoperfusion or repeated doses of activated charcoal.

Clinical Findings

Intoxication may result from acute single exposure or chronic accidental overmedication. After acute overdosage, patients frequently develop nausea and vomiting, bradycardia, hyperkalemia, and atrioventricular block. Patients who develop toxicity gradu-

ally during chronic therapy are often hypokalemic and hypomagnesemic owing to concurrent diuretic treatment and more commonly present with ventricular arrhythmias (eg, ectopy, bidirectional ventricular tachycardia, or ventricular fibrillation).

Treatment

A. Emergency and Supportive Measures: Maintain a patent airway and assist ventilation, if necessary. Treat ventricular arrhythmias initially with lidocaine or phenytoin, and treat bradycardia initially with atropine (0.5–2 mg intravenously), isoproterenol, or a transcutaneous external cardiac pacemaker. Consider the use of digoxin-specific antibodies (see below).

After acute ingestion, perform gastric lavage and administer activated charcoal. Emesis is not recommended because it may enhance vagotonic effects such as bradycardia and AV block.

B. Specific Treatment: For patients with severe intoxication (eg, marked bradycardia or AV block unresponsive to atropine, or ventricular arrhythmias unresponsive to lidocaine or phenytoin), administer digoxin-specific antibodies (digoxin immune Fab [ovine]; Digibind). Estimation of the Digibind dose is based on the body burden of digoxin calculated from the ingested dose or the steady-state serum digoxin concentration:

1. From the ingested dose–Number of vials = 1.7 × Ingested dose (in mg).

2. From the serum concentration–Number of vials = Serum digoxin (in ng/mL) × Body weight (in kg) × 0.0093.

Shumaik GM et al: Oleander poisoning: Treatment with digoxin-specific Fab antibody fragments. Ann Emerg Med 1988;17:732.

Springer M et al: Acute massive digoxin overdose: Survival without use of digitalis-specific antibodies. Am J Emerg Med 1986;4:364.

Stolshek BS et al: The role of digoxin-specific antibodies in the treatment of digitalis poisoning. Med Toxicol 1988;3:167.

ETHANOL, BARBITURATES, & OTHER SEDATIVE-HYPNOTIC AGENTS

The group of agents known as sedative-hypnotic drugs include a variety of products used for the treatment of anxiety, depression, insomnia, and epilepsy. Ethanol and other selected agents are also popular recreational drugs. All of these drugs depress the central nervous system reticular activating system, cerebral cortex, and cerebellum. Some agents (eg, glutethimide) also have anticholinergic properties.

Clinical Findings

Mild intoxication produces euphoria, slurred speech, and ataxia. Ethanol intoxication may produce hypoglycemia, even at relatively low concentrations. With more severe intoxication, stupor, coma, and respiratory arrest may occur. Death or serious morbidity is usually the result of pulmonary aspiration of gastric contents. Bradycardia, hypotension, and hypothermia are common. Patients with massive intoxication may appear to be dead, with no reflex responses and even absent electroencephalographic activity. Diagnosis and assessment of severity of intoxication is usually based on clinical findings. Ethanol serum levels greater than 300 mg/dL (0.3 g/dL; 65 mmol/L) usually produce coma in persons not chronically abusing the drug. Phenobarbital levels greater than 80–100 mg/L usually cause coma.

Treatment

A. Emergency and Supportive Measures: Maintain a patent airway, and assist ventilation if necessary. Treat coma, hypotension, and hypothermia as described at the beginning of this chapter.

Empty the stomach by emesis or gastric lavage and administer activated charcoal. Protect the airway with a cuffed endotracheal tube in deeply obtunded patients. Repeat-dose charcoal may enhance elimination of phenobarbital, and hemoperfusion may be necessary for patients with severe phenobarbital intoxication, but these procedures are not effective for most other drugs in this group.

B. Specific Treatment: There are as yet no specific antidotes available in the United States, but clinical studies are under way on a benzodiazepine antagonist already used in Europe (flumazenil).

Curry SC et al: Lack of correlation between plasma 4-hydroxyglutethimide and severity of coma in acute glutethimide poisoning: A case report and brief review of the literature. Med Toxicol 1987;2:309.
Eisen TF et al: Serum osmolality in alcohol ingestions: Differences in availability among laboratories of teaching hospital, nonteaching hospital, and commercial facilities. Am J Emerg Med 1989;7:256.
Hojer J et al: Benzodiazepine poisoning: Experience of 702 admissions to an intensive care unit during a 14-year period. J Int Med 1989;226:117.
Lopez GP et al: Survival of a child despite unusually high blood ethanol levels. Am J Emerg Med 1989;7:283.
Minion GE et al: Severe alcohol intoxication: A study of 204 consecutive patients. Clin Toxicol 1989;27:375.
Pond SM et al: Randomized study of the treatment of phenobarbital overdose with repeated doses of activated charcoal. JAMA 1984;251:3104.

IRON

Iron is widely used therapeutically for the treatment of anemia and as a daily supplement in multiple vitamin preparations. Most children's preparations contain about 12–15 mg of elemental iron (as sulfate, gluconate, or fumarate salt) per dose, compared with 60–90 mg in most adult-strength preparations. Severe iron intoxications occur most often in children who ingest adult-strength preparations. Iron is corrosive to the gastrointestinal tract and, once absorbed, has depressant effects on the myocardium and on peripheral vascular resistance. Intracellular toxic effects of iron include disruption of Krebs cycle enzymes.

Clinical Findings

Ingestion of less than 30 mg/kg of elemental iron usually produces only mild gastrointestinal upset. Ingestion of more than 40–60 mg/kg usually causes vomiting (sometimes with hematemesis), diarrhea, hypotension, and acidosis. Death may occur as a result of profound hypotension due to massive fluid losses and bleeding, metabolic acidosis, peritonitis from intestinal perforation, or sepsis. Survivors of the acute ingestion may suffer permanent gastrointestinal scarring.

Serum iron levels greater than 400–500 μg/dL are considered toxic, and levels over 1000 μg/dL are usually associated with severe poisoning. A plain abdominal x-ray may reveal radiopaque tablets.

Treatment

A. Emergency and Supportive Measures: Maintain a patent airway and assist ventilation if necessary. Treat hypotension aggressively with intravenous crystalloid solutions (normal saline or lactated Ringer's injection). Fluid losses may be massive owing to vomiting and diarrhea as well as third-spacing into injured intestine.

Empty the stomach by emesis or gastric lavage if more than 30 mg/kg of elemental iron has been ingested. Activated charcoal is not effective but may be used if other ingestants are suspected. If many tablets remain visible on abdominal x-ray, perform repeated lavage using a 2% bicarbonate solution—or perform whole bowel irrigation—and consider endoscopy or surgical removal.

B. Specific Treatment: Deferoxamine is a selective iron chelator. It may be given intramuscularly or intravenously but is not useful as an oral binding agent. For patients with established manifestations of toxicity—and particularly those with markedly elevated serum iron levels (eg, greater than 500–600 μg/dL)—administer 10–15 mg/kg/h by constant intravenous infusion. Continue the infusion until the iron level is less than 250 μg/dL. Deferoxamine is safe for use in pregnant women with acute iron overdose.

Proudfoot AT et al: Management of acute iron poisoning. Med Toxicol 1986;1:83.
Vernon DD et al: Hemodynamic effects of experimental iron poisoning. Ann Emerg Med 1989;18:863.

ISONIAZID

Isoniazid (INH) is an antibacterial drug used mainly in the treatment and prevention of tuberculosis. It may cause hepatitis in certain patients with chronic use. It produces acute toxic effects by competing with pyridoxal 5-phosphate, resulting in lowered brain γ-aminobutyric acid (GABA) levels. Acute ingestion of as little as 1.5–2 g of isoniazid can cause toxicity, and severe poisoning is likely to occur after ingestion of more than 100 mg/kg.

Clinical Findings

Confusion, slurred speech, and seizures may occur abruptly after acute overdose. Severe lactic acidosis—out of proportion to the severity of seizures—is probably due to inhibited metabolism of lactate.

Diagnosis is based on a history of ingestion and the presence of severe acidosis associated with seizures. Isoniazid is not usually included in routine toxicologic screening, and serum levels are not readily available.

Treatment

A. Emergency and Supportive Measures: Maintain a patent airway and assist ventilation if necessary. Treat coma, hypotension, and seizures as described at the beginning of this chapter. Seizures may require higher doses of diazepam (15–20 mg intravenously) or administration of pyridoxine as antidote (see below).

Empty the stomach by gastric lavage and administer activated charcoal. Do *not* induce emesis, because of the risk of abrupt onset of seizures.

B. Specific Treatment: Pyridoxine (vitamin B$_6$) is a specific antagonist of the acute toxic effects of isoniazid and is usually successful in controlling convulsions that do not respond to diazepam. Give 5 g intravenously or, if the amount is known, give a gram-for-gram equivalent amount of pyridoxine.

Hankins DG et al: Profound acidosis caused by isoniazid ingestion. Am J Emerg Med 1987;5:165.

Yarbrough BE et al: Isoniazid overdose treated with high-dose pyridoxine. Ann Emerg Med 1983;12:303.

LEAD

Lead is used in a variety of industrial and commercial products, such as storage batteries, solders, paints, pottery, plumbing, and gasoline. Children are susceptible to lead poisoning by repeatedly ingesting lead-containing paints or dusts. Lead toxicity is rare after a single exposure. Lead produces a variety of adverse effects on cellular function and primarily affects the nervous system, gastrointestinal tract, and hematopoietic system.

Clinical Findings

Lead poisoning often goes undiagnosed initially because presenting symptoms and signs are nonspecific and exposure is not suspected. Common symptoms include colicky abdominal pain, constipation, headache, and irritability. Severe poisoning may cause coma and convulsions. Chronic intoxication can cause learning disorders (in children) and motor neuropathy (eg, wrist drop).

Diagnosis is based on measurement of the blood lead level. Whole blood lead levels less than 25 μg/dL are usually considered nontoxic. Levels of 50–70 μg/dL are associated with moderate toxicity, and levels greater than 70–100 μg/dL are often associated with severe poisoning. Other laboratory findings of lead poisoning include microcytic anemia with basophilic stippling and elevated free erythrocyte protoporphyrin.

Treatment

A. Emergency and Supportive Measures: For patients with encephalopathy, maintain a patent airway and treat coma and convulsions as described at the beginning of this chapter.

For recent acute ingestion, give activated charcoal and a cathartic. If a large lead-containing object (eg, fishing weight) is still visible in the stomach on abdominal x-ray, repeated cathartics, whole bowel irrigation, endoscopy, or even surgical removal may be necessary to prevent subacute lead poisoning.

Conduct an investigation into the source of the lead exposure. Workers with lead levels greater than 60 μg/dL must by federal law be removed from the site of exposure.

B. Specific Treatment: Lead may be chelated parenterally with edetate calcium disodium (EDTA) or dimercaprol (BAL). The indications for chelation depend on the blood lead level and the patient's clinical state. A medical toxicologist or regional poison control center (Table 33–1) should be consulted for advice about selection and use of these antidotes.

1. Severe toxicity–Patients with severe intoxication (encephalopathy or levels greater than 70–100 μg/dL) should receive dimercaprol, 4–5 mg/kg intramuscularly every 4 hours for 5 days; and edetate calcium disodium, 30 mg/kg intramuscularly every 6 hours or as continuous intravenous infusion for 5 days.

2. Less severe toxicity–Patients with less severe symptoms and asymptomatic patients with blood lead levels between 55 and 69 μg/dL may be treated with edetate calcium disodium alone in dosages as above.

3. Challenge test–Edetate calcium disodium may also be used in patients with lower lead levels as a mobilization or "challenge" test to determine if there is a pool of chelatable lead. Administer 20–25 mg/kg (1 g maximum) in 100 mL of 5% dextrose intravenously over 1 hour, and then collect urine in a lead-free container over the next 24 hours. If the number of micrograms of lead excreted is greater than the number of milligrams of edetate calcium disodium given, the test is considered positive.

Rempel D: The lead-exposed worker. JAMA 1989;262:532.
Schneitzer L et al: Lead poisoning in adults from renovation of an older home. Ann Emerg Med 1990;19:415.

MERCURY

Acute mercury poisoning usually occurs by ingestion of inorganic mercuric salts or inhalation of metallic mercury vapor. Ingestion of the mercuric salts causes a metallic taste, salivation, thirst, a burning sensation in the throat, discoloration and edema of oral mucous membranes, abdominal pain, vomiting, bloody diarrhea, and shock. Direct nephrotoxicity causes acute renal failure. Inhalation of high concentrations of metallic mercury vapor may cause acute fulminant chemical pneumonia. Chronic mercury poisoning causes weakness, ataxia, intention tremors, irritability, and depression. Chronic intoxication in children may be a cause of acrodynia. Exposure to alkyl (organic) mercury derivatives from contaminated fish or fungicides used on seeds has caused ataxia, tremors, and convulsions and catastrophic birth defects.

Treatment
A. Acute Poisoning: There is no effective specific treatment for mercury vapor pneumonitis. Remove ingested mercuric salts by emesis and lavage, and administer activated charcoal and a cathartic. For acute ingestion of mercuric salts, given dimercaprol (BAL) at once, as for arsenic poisoning. Penicillamine, 100 mg/kg orally in divided doses (maximum 1 g/d), is also effective. Maintain urine output. Treat oliguria and anuria if they occur.

B. Chronic Poisoning: Remove from exposure. Neurologic toxicity is not considered reversible with chelation, although some authors recommend a trial of penicillamine.

Adams CR et al: Mercury intoxication simulating amyotrophic lateral sclerosis. JAMA 1983;250:642.
Aronow R et al: Mercury exposure from interior latex paint—Michigan. MMWR 1990;39:125.
Jaffe KM et al: Survival after acute mercury vapor poisoning. Am J Dis Child 1983;137:749.

METHANOL & ETHYLENE GLYCOL

Methanol (wood alcohol) is commonly found in a variety of products, including solvents, duplicating fluids, record cleaning solutions, and paint removers. It is sometimes ingested intentionally by alcoholics as a substitute for ethanol and may also be found as a contaminant in bootleg whiskey. Ethylene glycol is the most common constituent in antifreeze. The toxicity of both agents is caused by metabolism to highly toxic organic acids—methanol to formic acid; ethylene glycol to glycolic and oxalic acids.

Clinical Findings
Shortly after ingestion of either of these agents, patients usually appear "drunk." The serum osmolality is usually elevated, but acidosis is often absent early. After several hours, metabolism to toxic organic acids leads to a severe anion gap metabolic acidosis, tachypnea, confusion, convulsions, and coma. Methanol intoxication frequently causes visual disturbances, while ethylene glycol often produces oxalate crystalluria and renal failure.

Treatment
A. Emergency and Supportive Measures: Maintain a patent airway, and assist ventilation if necessary. Treat coma, hypotension, and seizures as described at the beginning of this chapter. Treat metabolic acidosis with sodium bicarbonate by intravenous infusion.

For patients presenting within 30–60 minutes after ingestion, empty the stomach by emesis or gastric lavage and administer activated charcoal. (*Note:* Charcoal is not very effective.)

Patients with significant toxicity (manifested by severe acidosis, altered mental status, serum methanol or ethylene glycol level > 50 mg/dL) should undergo hemodialysis as soon as possible to remove the parent compound and the toxic metabolites.

B. Specific Treatment: Ethanol blocks metabolism of the parent compounds by competing for the enzyme alcohol dehydrogenase. The desired serum ethanol concentration is 100 mg/dL. To achieve this, administer a loading dose of approximately 750 mg/kg orally or in a dilute intravenous solution (available from the pharmacy in 5% and 10% solution), and then provide a maintenance infusion of 100–150 mg/kg/h. The infusion will have to be increased to about 175–250 mg/kg/h during hemodialysis to replace dialysis elimination of ethanol.

Ekins BR et al: Standardized treatment of severe methanol poisoning with ethanol and hemodialysis. West J Med 1985;142:337.
Jacobsen D, McMartin KE: Methanol and ethylene glycol poisonings: Mechanisms of toxicity, clinical course, diagnosis and treatment. Med Toxicol 1986;1:309.

METHEMOGLOBINEMIA-INDUCING AGENTS

A large number of chemical agents are capable of oxidizing ferrous hemoglobin to its ferric state (methemoglobin), a form that cannot carry oxygen. Drugs and chemicals known to cause methemoglobinemia include benzocaine (a local anesthetic), aniline, nitrites, nitrogen oxide gases, nitrobenzene, dapsone, pyridium, and many others.

Clinical Findings

Methemoglobinemia reduces oxygen-carrying capacity and may cause dizziness, nausea, headache, dyspnea, confusion, seizures, and coma. The severity of symptoms depends on the percentage of hemoglobin oxidized to methemoglobin; severe poisoning is usually present with methemoglobin fractions of greater than 40–50%. Even at low levels (15–20%), victims appear cyanotic because of the "chocolate brown" color of methemoglobin. Hemolysis may occur, especially in patients susceptible to oxidant stress (ie, those with glucose-6-phosphate dehydrogenase deficiency).

Treatment

A. Emergency and Supportive Measures: Maintain a patent airway, and assist ventilation if necessary. Administer high-flow supplemental oxygen. Treat coma, hypotension, and seizures as described at the beginning of this chapter.

If the causative agent was recently ingested, empty the stomach by emesis or gastric lavage and administer activated charcoal. For dapsone ingestion, give repeat-dose activated charcoal to enhance dapsone elimination.

B. Specific Treatment: Methylene blue is a commonly used dye that enhances the conversion of methemoglobin to hemoglobin by increasing the activity of the enzyme methemoglobin reductase. For symptomatic patients, administer 1–2 mg/kg (0.1–0.2 mL/kg of 1% solution) intravenously. The dose may be repeated once in 15–20 minutes if necessary. Patients with hereditary methemoglobin reductase deficiency or glucose-6-phosphate dehydrogenase deficiency may not respond to methylene blue treatment.

Hall AH et al: Drug- and chemical-induced methaemoglobinemia: Clinical features and treatment. Med Toxicol 1986;1:253.

MONOAMINE OXIDASE INHIBITORS (Isocarboxazid, Phenelzine)

Overdoses cause ataxia, excitement, hypertension, and tachycardia, followed later by hypotension, convulsions, and hyperthermia.

Ingestion of tyramine-containing foods may cause a severe hypertensive reaction. These include aged cheese and red wines. Hypertensive reactions may also occur with any sympathomimetic drug. Fatal hyperthermia may occur if patients receiving monoamine oxidase inhibitors are given meperidine or fluoxetine.

Treatment

Remove ingested drug by gastric lavage, and administer activated charcoal and a cathartic. Treat severe hypertension with nitroprusside, phentolamine, or other rapid-acting vasodilator. Treat hypotension with fluids and positioning, but avoid use of pressor agents. Treat hyperthermia with aggressive cooling; neuromuscular paralysis may be required.

Kaplan RF et al: Phenelzine overdose treated with dantrolene sodium. JAMA 1986;255:642.

Mirchandani H et al: Fatal malignant hyperthermia as a result of ingestion of tranylcypromine (Parnate) combined with white wine and cheese. J Forensic Sci 1985; 30:217.

MUSHROOMS

There are thousands of mushroom species that cause a variety of toxic effects. The most dangerous species of mushrooms are *Amanita phalloides, Amanita verna, Amanita virosa, Gyromitra esculenta,* and the *Galerina* species, all of which contain amatoxin, a potent cytotoxin. Ingestion of part of one mushroom of a dangerous species may be sufficient to cause death.

The pathologic finding in fatalities from amatoxin-containing mushroom poisoning is acute necrosis of the liver, kidneys, heart, and skeletal muscles.

Clinical Findings
(Table 33–13)

A. Symptoms and Signs:

1. Amatoxin-type cyclopeptides (*Amanita phalloides, Amanita verna, Amanita virosa,* and *Galerina* species)—After a latent interval of 8–12 hours, severe abdominal cramps and vomiting begin and progress to profuse diarrhea, bloody vomitus and stools, followed by hepatic necrosis, hepatic encephalopathy, and frequently renal failure. The fatality rate is about 20%. Cooking the mushrooms does not prevent poisoning.

2. Gyromitrin type (*Gyromitra* and *Helvella* species)—Toxicity is more common following ingestion of uncooked mushrooms. Vomiting, diarrhea, hepatic necrosis, convulsions, coma, and hemolysis may occur after a latent period of 8–12 hours. The fatality rate is probably less than 10%.

3. Muscarinic type (*Inocybe* and *Clitocybe* species)—Vomiting, diarrhea, bradycardia, hypotension, salivation, miosis, bronchospasm, and lacrimation occur shortly after ingestion. Cardiac arrhythmias may occur. Fatalities are rare.

4. Anticholinergic type (eg, *Amanita muscaria, Amanita pantherina*)—This type causes a variety of symptoms that may be atropine-like, including excitement, delirium, flushed skin, dilated pupils, and muscular jerking tremors, beginning 1–2 hours after ingestion. Fatalities are rare.

**5. Gastrointestinal irritant type (eg, *Boletus*,

Table 33–13. Poisonous mushrooms.[1]

Toxin	Genus	Symptoms and Signs	Onset	Treatment
Amanitin	*Amanita* (*A phalloides, A verna, A virosa*)	Severe gastroenteritis, followed by delayed hepatic and renal failure after 48–72 hours.	6–24 hours.	Supportive. Correct dehydration. Thioctic acid is of unproved benefit.
Muscarine	*Inocybe, Clitocybe*	Muscarinic (salivation, miosis, bradycardia, diarrhea).	30 minutes to 1 hour	Supportive. Give atropine, 0.5–2 mg intravenously, for severe cholinergic symptoms and signs.
Ibotenic acid, muscimol	*Amanita muscaria* ("fly agaric")	Anticholinergic (mydriasis, tachycardia, hyperpyrexia, delirium).	30 minutes to 2 hours	Supportive. Give physostigmine, 0.5–2 mg intravenously, for severe anticholinergic symptoms and signs.
Coprine	*Coprinus*	Disulfiramlike effect occurs with ingestion of ethanol.	30 minutes to 2 days	Supportive. Abstain from ethanol for 3–4 days.
Monomethylhydrazine	*Gyromitra*	Gastroenteritis; occasionally hemolysis, hepatic and renal failure.	6–12 hours	Supportive. Correct dehydration. Pyridoxine, 2.5 mg/kg intravenously, may be helpful.
Psilocybin	*Psilocybe*	Hallucinations.	15–30 minutes	Supportive.
Gastrointestinal irritants	Many species	Nausea and vomiting, diarrhea.	30 minutes to 2 hours.	Supportive. Correct dehydration.

[1] Modified and reproduced, with permission, from Becker CE et al: *West J Med* 1976;**125**:100.

Cantharellus)–Nausea, vomiting, and diarrhea occur shortly after ingestion. Fatalities are rare.

6. Disulfiram type (*Coprinus* species)–Disulfiramlike sensitivity to alcohol may persist for several days. Toxicity is characterized by flushing, hypotension, and vomiting after coingestion of alcohol.

7. Hallucinogenic type (*Psilocybe* and *Panaeolus* species)–Mydriasis, nausea and vomiting, and intense visual hallucinations occur 1–2 hours after ingestion. Fatalities are rare.

B. Laboratory Findings: (Type 1 [amatoxin] or 2 [gyromitrin] mushrooms.) Creatinine and blood urea nitrogen may be elevated. Effects on the liver are revealed by increased transaminase and bilirubin levels and prothrombin time. The blood glucose should be monitored frequently when hepatotoxicity is present.

Treatment

A. Emergency Measures: After the onset of symptoms, efforts to remove the toxic agent are probably useless, especially in cases of type 1 (amatoxin) or type 2 (gyromitrin) poisoning, where there is a delay of 12 hours or more before symptoms occur. However, induction of vomiting is recommended for any recent ingestion of an unidentified or potentially toxic mushroom. Activated charcoal and a cathartic should also be given.

B. General Measures:

1. Amatoxin-type cyclopeptides–A variety of unproved antidotes (eg, thioctic acid, silibinin, penicillin, corticosteroids) have been suggested for amatoxin-type mushroom poisoning, but experimental re-

sults are equivocal. Aggressive fluid replacement for diarrhea and intensive supportive care for hepatic failure are the mainstays of treatment.

Interruption of enterohepatic circulation of the amatoxin by the administration of activated charcoal and laxatives may be of value. However, by the time this method is employed, most of the amatoxin has already caused cellular damage and has already been excreted.

Liver function has been known to begin to return 6–8 days after exposure, followed by eventual complete recovery. Liver transplant may be the only hope for survival in gravely ill patients (encephalopathy, severe coagulopathy).

2. Gyromitrin type–For gyromitrin poisoning, give pyridoxine, 25 mg/kg intravenously.

3. Muscarinic type–For mushrooms producing predominantly muscarinic-cholinergic symptoms, give atropine, 0.005–0.01 mg/kg intravenously, and repeat as needed.

4. Anticholinergic type–For anticholinergic type, physostigmine, 0.5–1 mg intravenously, may calm extremely agitated patients and reverse peripheral anticholinergic manifestations, but it may also cause bradycardia, asystole, and seizures.

5. Gastrointestinal irritant type–Treat with antiemetics and intravenous or oral fluids.

6. Disulfiram type–For *Coprinus* ingestion, avoid alcohol. Treat alcohol reaction with fluids and supine position.

7. Hallucinogenic type–Provide a quiet, supportive atmosphere. Diazepam or haloperidol may be used for sedation.

Klein AS et al: *Amanita* poisoning: Treatment and role of liver transplantation. Amer J Med 1989;86:187.

Pond SM et al: Amatoxin poisoning in Northern California, 1982–1983. West J Med 1986;145:204.

OPIOIDS
(Morphine, Heroin, Codeine, Propoxyphene, Etc)

Prescription and illicit opioids are popular drugs of abuse and the cause of frequent hospitalizations for overdose. These drugs have widely varying potencies and durations of action; for example, some of the illicit fentanyl derivatives are up to 2000 times more potent than morphine. All of these agents decrease central nervous system activity by acting on opiate receptors in the brain.

Clinical Findings
Mild intoxication is characterized by euphoria, drowsiness, and constricted pupils. More severe intoxication may cause hypotension, bradycardia, hypothermia, coma, and respiratory arrest. Pulmonary edema may occur. Death is usually due to apnea or pulmonary aspiration of gastric contents. While the duration of effect for heroin is usually 3–5 hours, methadone intoxication may last for 48–72 hours or longer. Most opioids, with the exception of illicit newer fentanyl derivatives, are detectable on urine toxicology screening.

Treatment
A. Emergency and Supportive Measures: Maintain a patent airway, and assist ventilation if necessary. Treat coma, hypothermia, and hypotension as described at the beginning of this chapter.

If the patient arrives for medical care shortly after ingestion, empty the stomach by emesis or gastric lavage and administer activated charcoal.

B. Specific Treatment: Naloxone is a specific opioid antagonist that can rapidly reverse signs of narcotic intoxication. Although it is structurally related to the opioids, it has no agonist effects of its own. Administer 0.4–2 mg intravenously, and repeat as needed to awaken the patient and maintain airway protective reflexes and spontaneous breathing. Very large doses (10–20 mg) may be required for patients intoxicated by some opioids (eg, propoxyphene, codeine, fentanyl derivatives). *Caution:* The duration of effect of naloxone is only about 2–3 hours; repeated doses may be necessary for patients intoxicated by long-acting drugs such as methadone. Continuous observation for at least 3 hours after the last naloxone dose is mandatory.

Goldfrank L et al: A dosing nomogram for continuous infusion of intravenous naloxone. Ann Emerg Med 1986; 15:566.

PARAQUAT

Paraquat is used as a herbicide. Concentrated solutions of paraquat are highly corrosive to the oropharynx, esophagus, and stomach. The fatal dose after absorption may be as small as 4 mg/kg. If not rapidly fatal because of its corrosive effects, paraquat causes pulmonary edema and fibrosis with respiratory insufficiency, and renal damage with anuria. Patients with plasma paraquat levels above 2 mg/L at 6 hours or 0.2 mg/L at 24 hours are likely to die.

Treatment
Remove ingested paraquat by immediate emesis, or by gastric lavage if the patient is already in a health care facility. Clay (bentonite or fuller's earth) and activated charcoal are effective adsorbents. Administer repeated doses of 60 g of activated charcoal by gastric tube every 2 hours for at least 3–4 doses. Charcoal hemoperfusion, 8 hours per day for 2–3 weeks, has been anecdotally reported to be lifesaving. Supplemental oxygen should be withheld unless the P_{O_2} is less than 70 mm Hg. For further information and for rapid determination of paraquat levels, call the nearest regional poison center or ICI America Inc ([800] 327–8633).

Bismuth C et al: Elimination of paraquat. Human Toxicol 1987;6:63.

Hampson EC et al: Failure of haemoperfusion and haemodialysis to prevent death in paraquat poisoning: A retrospective review of 42 patients. Med Toxicol 1988;3:64.

PESTICIDES: CHOLINESTERASE INHIBITORS
(Organophosphates: Parathion, TEPP, Malathion, Thimet, Phosdrin, Systox, HETP, EPN, OMPA, Etc; Carbamates: Carbaryl, Aldicarb, Benomyl)

Organophosphate and carbamate insecticides are widely used in commercial agriculture and home gardening and have largely replaced older, more environmentally persistent organochlorine compounds such as DDT and chlordane. The organophosphates and carbamates—also called anticholinesterases because they inhibit the enzyme acteylcholinesterase—cause an increase in acetylcholine activity at nicotinic and muscarinic receptors and in the central nervous system. There are a variety of chemical agents in this group, with widely varying potencies. Most of them are poorly water-soluble and are formulated with an aromatic hydrocarbon solvent such as xylene. Most of them are well absorbed through intact skin.

Clinical Findings
Inhibition of cholinesterase results in abdominal

cramps, diarrhea, vomiting, excessive salivation, sweating, lacrimation, miosis (constricted pupils), wheezing and bronchorrhea, seizures, and skeletal muscle weakness. Initial tachycardia is usually followed by bradycardia. Profound skeletal muscle weakness, aggravated by excessive bronchial secretions and wheezing, may result in respiratory arrest and death.

The diagnosis is suspected in patients who present with miosis, sweating, and hyperperistalsis. Serum and red blood cell cholinesterase activity can be measured in the laboratory and is usually depressed at least 50% below baseline in those victims who have severe intoxication.

Treatment

A. Emergency and Supportive Measures:
Maintain a patent airway, and assist ventilation if necessary. Administer supplemental oxygen. Suction excessive secretions from the airway.

If the agent was recently ingested, empty the stomach by emesis or gastric lavage and administer activated charcoal. Gastric lavage is preferred over emesis because of the risk of abrupt onset of seizures. If the agent is on the victim's skin or hair, wash repeatedly with soap or shampoo and water. Providers must take care to avoid skin exposure by wearing gloves and waterproof aprons.

B. Specific Treatment:
Atropine reverses excessive muscarinic stimulation and is effective for treatment of salivation, wheezing, abdominal cramping, and sweating. However, it does not interact with nicotinic receptors and has no effect on muscle weakness. Administer 2 mg intravenously, and give repeated doses as needed to dry bronchial secretions and decrease wheezing; as much as several hundred milligrams of atropine have been given to treat severe poisoning.

Pralidoxime (2-PAM, Protopam) is a specific antidote that reverses organophosphate binding to the cholinesterase enzyme; therefore, it is effective at all sites. Administer 1–2 g intravenously (20–40 mg/kg in children), and repeat every 3–4 hours as needed. A continuous infusion may be more effective because of the short duration of action of single doses. Pralidoxime is of questionable benefit for carbamate poisoning, because carbamates have only a transitory effect on the cholinesterase enzyme.

Clifford NJ et al: Organophosphate poisoning from wearing a laundered uniform previously contaminated with parathion. JAMA 1989;262:3035.

Zwiener RJ et al: Organophosphate and carbamate poisoning in infants and children. Ped 1988;81:121.

PETROLEUM DISTILLATES (Petroleum Ether, Charcoal Lighter Fluid, Kerosene, Paint Thinner, Benzine, Gasoline, Etc)

Petroleum distillate toxicity occurs almost entirely as a result of pulmonary aspiration during or after ingestion. Acute manifestations of aspiration pneumonitis are vomiting, coughing, and bronchopneumonia. Some hydrocarbons—ie, those with aromatic or halogenated subunits—can also cause severe systemic poisoning after oral ingestion. Most hydrocarbons can also cause systemic intoxication by inhalation, but only with very high concentrations of the vapors in an enclosed space. Vertigo, muscular incoordination, irregular pulse, myoclonus, and convulsions oc-

Table 33–14. Clinical features of hydrocarbon poisoning.[1]

Type	Examples	Risk of Pneumonia	Risk of Systemic Toxicity	Treatment
High-viscosity	Vaseline Motor oil	Low	Low	None.
Low-viscosity, nontoxic	Furniture polish Mineral seal oil Kerosene Lighter fluid	High	Low	Observe for pneumonia. *Do not* induce emesis.
Low-viscosity, unknown systemic toxicity	Turpentine Pine oil	High	Variable	Observe for pneumonia. *Do not* induce emesis if less than 1–2 mL/kg was ingested.
Low-viscosity, known systemic toxicity	Camphor Phenol Chlorinated insecticides Aromatic hydrocarbons (benzene, toluene, etc)	High	High	Induce emesis, or perform lavage. Give activated charcoal.

[1] Reproduced, with permission, from Olson KR, Becker CE: Chapter 29 in: *Current Emergency Diagnosis & Treatment,* 3rd ed. Ho MT, Saunders CE (editors). Appleton & Lange, 1990.

cur with serious poisoning and may be due to hypoxemia or the systemic effects of some agents (eg, camphor). Chlorinated and fluorinated hydrocarbons (trichloroethylene, freons, etc) can cause ventricular arrhythmias by a mechanism of myocardial sensitization after inhalation.

Treatment
(See Table 33–14.)

Remove the patient to fresh air. Since aspiration is the primary danger with many common products, use of lavage or emesis is controversial. Removal of ingested hydrocarbon is usually suggested only if the preparation contains toxic solutes (eg, an insecticide) or is an aromatic or halogenated product. If lavage is done in an obtunded or comatose patient, prophylactic insertion of a cuffed endotracheal tube is recommended to prevent aspiration. Watch the victim closely for 6–8 hours for signs of aspiration pneumonitis (cough, localized rales or rhonchi, tachypnea, and infiltrates on chest radiograph). The use of corticosteroids to treat pneumonitis is controversial. If fever occurs, give a specific antibiotic after identification of pathogens by laboratory studies. Because of the risk of arrhythmias, use bronchodilators only with caution in patients with chlorinated or fluorinated solvent intoxication.

Brook MP et al: Pine oil cleaner ingestion. Ann Emerg Med 1989;18:391.
Machado B et al: Accidental hydrocarbon ingestion cases telephoned to a regional poison center. Ann Emerg Med 1988;17:804.

PHENCYCLIDINE

Phencyclidine (PCP) was until recently one of the most commonly abused street drugs—second only to alcohol as a cause of emergency room visits for drug intoxication in many cities. It occurs under a variety of names or is misrepresented as other psychotomimetic agents. The drug has a wide range of toxic manifestations. Doses under 5 mg (adults) cause hyperactivity, horizontal and vertical nystagmus, incoordination, diaphoresis, flushing, rigidity, dissociative anesthesia, rhabdomyolysis with myoglobinuria, and wild movements. Doses over 10 mg cause, in addition, seizures, coma, hyperthermia, rhabdomyolysis, and myoglobinuria. Symptoms may persist for several days.

Treatment

A. General Measures: Maintain a quiet, calm atmosphere. Sedate the agitated patient with diazepam, 0.1 mg/kg intravenously, midazolam, 0.1 mg/kg intramuscularly, or haloperidol, 0.05–0.1 mg/kg intramuscularly. Endotracheal intubation and mechanical ventilation may be necessary. Restrict sensory input, prevent injuries, and monitor vital signs.

Control convulsions by giving diazepam, 0.1 mg/kg intravenously. Hyperthermia should be treated aggressively, with control of muscular rigidity or hyperactivity by paralysis with neuromuscular blockers and endotracheal intubation.

Lowering urine pH may slightly increase urinary elimination of phencyclidine by ion trapping but is hazardous and may promote myoglobinuric renal failure.

B. Gut Decontamination: If the patient is awake and cooperative, give activated charcoal orally. In obtunded patients, perform gastric lavage prior to charcoal administration. Repeated administration of activated charcoal may remove additional PCP secreted into the acidic stomach. However, repeated use of charcoal and cathartics may lead to dehydration and hypernatremia from massive fluid loss in stools.

Jackson JE: Phencyclidine pharmacokinetics after a massive overdose. Ann Intern Med 1989;111:613.
McCarron MM et al: Acute phencyclidine intoxication: Incidence of clinical findings in 1,000 cases. Ann Emerg Med 1981; 10:237.

PHENOTHIAZINE TRANQUILIZERS (Chlorpromazine, Promazine, Prochlorperazine, Etc)

Chlorpromazine and related drugs are synthetic chemicals derived in most instances from phenothiazine. They are used as antiemetics and psychic inhibitors and as potentiators of analgesic and hypnotic drugs.

Minimum doses induce drowsiness and mild orthostatic hypotension in as many as 50% of patients. Larger doses cause obtundation, miosis, severe hypotension, tachycardia, convulsions, and coma. Abnormal cardiac conduction may occur, resulting in prolongation of QRS or QT intervals (or both) and ventricular arrhythmias.

With therapeutic doses, some patients develop an acute extrapyramidal reaction similar to Parkinson's disease, with spasmodic contractions of the face and neck muscles, extensor rigidity of the back muscles, carpopedal spasm, and motor restlessness.

Treatment

Remove ingested overdoses by emesis or gastric lavage. Follow with activated charcoal and cathartic. For severe hypotension, treatment with fluids and pressor agents may be necessary. Control convulsions cautiously with diazepam, 0.1 mg/kg intravenously. Maintain cardiac monitoring. Hypotension and cardiac arrhythmias associated with widened QRS intervals on the ECG may respond to intravenous sodium bicarbonate as used for tricyclic antidepressants.

For extrapyramidal signs, give diphenhydramine, 0.5–1 mg/kg intravenously, or benztropine mesylate, 1–2 mg intramuscularly. Treatment with oral doses of these agents should be continued for 24–48 hours.

Kemper AJ et al: Thioridazine-induced torsade de pointes: Successful therapy with isoproterenol. JAMA 1983; 249:2931.

QUINIDINE & RELATED ANTIARRHYTHMICS

Quinidine, procainamide, and disopyramide are class Ia antiarrhythmic agents, and flecainide and encainide are class Ic agents. These drugs have membrane-depressant effects on the sodium-dependent channel responsible for cardiac cell depolarization. Manifestations of toxicity include diarrhea, arrhythmias, syncope, respiratory failure, and hypotension. The ECG may show widening of the QRS complex, a lengthened QT and PR interval, and atypical or polymorphous ventricular tachycardia (torsades de pointes). Associated toxicity due to digitalis may result from increased blood levels owing to concomitant quinidine administration.

Treatment

Remove ingested drug by gastric lavage followed by activated charcoal and catharsis. Treat cardiotoxicity (atrioventricular block, hypotension, QRS interval widening) with intravenous boluses of sodium bicarbonate, 50–100 meq. Ventricular tachycardia of the torsade de pointes variety may be treated with intravenous magnesium, isoproterenol, or overdrive pacing.

Swiryn S, Kim SS: Quinidine-induced syncope. Arch Intern Med 1983;143:314.

SALICYLATES

Salicylates (aspirin, methyl salicylate, etc) are found in a variety of over-the-counter and prescription medications. Salicylates uncouple cellular oxidative phosphorylation, resulting in anaerobic metabolism and excessive production of lactic acid and heat, and they also interfere with several Krebs cycle enzymes. A single ingestion of more than 200 mg/kg of salicylate is likely to produce significant acute intoxication. Poisoning may also occur as a result of chronic excessive dosing over several days. Although the half-life of salicylate is 2–3 hours after small doses, it may increase to 20 hours with intoxication.

Clinical Findings

Acute ingestion often causes nausea and vomiting, occasionally with gastritis. Mild to moderate intoxication is characterized by hyperpnea (deep and rapid breathing), tachycardia, tinnitus, and elevated anion

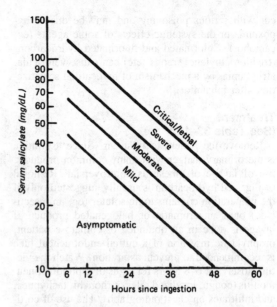

Figure 33–2. Nomogram for determining severity of salicylate intoxication. Absorption kinetics assume acute (one-time) ingestion of non-enteric-coated preparation. (Redrawn and reproduced, with permission, from Done AK: Salicylate intoxication: Significance of measurement of salicylate in blood in cases of acute ingestion. Pediatrics 1960;26:800.)

gap metabolic acidosis. Serious intoxication may result in agitation, confusion, coma, seizures, cardiovascular collapse, pulmonary edema, hyperthermia, and death.

Diagnosis is suspected in any patient with metabolic acidosis and is confirmed by measuring the serum salicylate level. Patients with levels greater than 100 mg/dL (1000 mg/L) after an acute overdose (see Fig 33–2) are more likely to have severe poisoning. On the other hand, patients with chronic intoxication may suffer severe symptoms with levels of only 60–70 mg/dL. The arterial blood gas typically reveals a respiratory alkalosis with an underlying metabolic acidosis.

Treatment

A. Emergency and Supportive Measures: Maintain a patent airway, and assist ventilation if necessary. Treat coma, hyperthermia, hypotension, and seizures as described at the beginning of this chapter. Treat metabolic acidosis with intravenous sodium bicarbonate.

After acute suicidal or accidental ingestion of more than 150–200 mg/kg salicylate, empty the stomach by emesis or gastric lavage and administer activated charcoal. Extra doses of activated charcoal may be needed in patients who ingest more than 10 g of aspirin.

B. Specific Treatment: Alkalinization of the urine enhances renal salicylate excretion by trapping the salicylate anion. Add 100 meq (2 ampules) of sodium bicarbonate to 1 L of 5% dextrose in 0.25-N saline, and infuse this solution intravenously at a rate of about 150–200 mL/h. Unless the patient is oliguric, add 20–30 meq of potassium to each liter of intravenous fluid.

Hemodialysis may be lifesaving and is indicated for patients with severe metabolic acidosis, markedly altered mental status, or significantly elevated salicylate levels (eg, > 100–120 mg/dL (1000–1200 mg/L) after acute overdose or > 60–70 mg/dL (600–700 mg/L) with chronic intoxication).

Dugandzic RM et al: Evaluation of the validity of the Done nomogram in the management of acute salicylate intoxication. Ann Emerg Med 1989;18:1186.
McGuigan MA: A two-year review of salicylate deaths in Ontario. Arch Intern Med 1987;147:510.

SNAKE BITES

The venom of poisonous snakes and lizards may be predominantly neurotoxic (coral snake) or predominantly cytolytic (pit viper). Neurotoxins cause respiratory paralysis; cytolytic venoms cause tissue destruction by digestion and hemorrhage due to hemolysis and destruction of the endothelial lining of the blood vessels. The manifestations of cytolytic envenomation (eg, rattlesnake venom) are local pain, redness, swelling, and extravasation of blood. Perioral tingling, metallic taste, nausea and vomiting, hypotension, and coagulopathy may also occur. Neurotoxic envenomation may cause ptosis, dysphagia, diplopia, and respiratory arrest.

Treatment

A. Emergency Measures: Immobilize the patient and the bitten part in a horizontal position. Avoid manipulation of the bitten area. Transport the patient to a medical facility for definitive treatment. Do *not* give alcoholic beverages or stimulants; do *not* apply ice; do *not* apply a tourniquet. The trauma to underlying structures resulting from incision and suction performed by unskilled people is probably not justified in view of the small amount of venom that can be recovered.

B. Specific Antidote and General Measures:
1. Pit viper (eg, rattlesnake) envenomation–With local signs such as swelling, pain, and ecchymosis but no systemic symptoms, give 4–5 vials of polyvalent crotalid antivenin by intravenous drip. (This should be preceded by skin testing for horse serum sensitivity with the kit supplied.) For more serious envenomation with marked local effects and systemic toxicity (eg, hypotension, coagulopathy), 10–20 vials may be required. Epinephrine should be available for immediate use in the event of an allergic reaction. Specific antiserum therapy is more effective if given

soon after the bite. Monitor vital signs and the blood coagulation profile. Type and cross-match blood. The adequacy of venom neutralization is indicated by improvement in signs and symptoms, and the rate of swelling slows. Serum sickness reactions are common after antivenin use, usually occur 5–10 days after antivenin administration, and may be treated with prednisone, 45–60 mg daily with tapering doses.

2. Elapid (coral snake) envenomation–Give 1–2 vials of specific antivenom as soon as possible.

To locate antisera for exotic snakes, call the Arizona Poison and Drug Information Center, Tucson ([602] 626–6016).

Nelson BK: Snake envenomation: Incidence, clinical presentation and management. Med Toxicol 1989;4:17.

SPIDER BITES & SCORPION STINGS

The toxin of most species of spiders causes only local pain, redness, and swelling. That of the more venomous black widow spiders *(Latrodectus mactans)* causes generalized muscular pains, muscle spasms, and rigidity. The brown recluse spider *(Loxosceles reclusa)* causes progressive local necrosis as well as hemolytic reactions (rare). Stings by most scorpions cause only local pain. Stings by the more toxic *Centruroides* species (found in the southwestern USA) may cause muscle cramps, twitching and jerking, and occasionally convulsions.

Treatment

A. Black Widow Spider Bites: Pain may be relieved with parenteral narcotics or muscle relaxants (eg, methocarbamol, 15 mg/kg). Calcium gluconate 10%, 0.1–0.2 mL/kg intravenously, may relieve muscle rigidity. Antivenin is rarely indicated, usually only for very young or elderly patients who do not respond to the above measures. Horse serum sensitivity testing is required.

B. Brown Recluse Spider Bites: Because bites occasionally progress to extensive local necrosis, some authorities recommend early excision of the bite site, whereas others use oral corticosteroids. Recently, interest has focused on the use of dapsone and colchicine and an antivenin is being developed. All of these treatments remain of unproved value.

C. Scorpion Stings: No specific treatment is available. For *Centruroides* stings, some toxicologists use a specific antivenom, but this is neither FDA-approved nor widely available.

Curry SC et al: Envenomation by the scorpion *Centruroides sculpturatus.* J Toxicol Clin Toxicol 1983–84;21:417.

THEOPHYLLINE

Theophylline is commonly used in the treatment of bronchospasm due to asthma, chronic lung disease, and congestive heart failure. Its toxicity may be caused by several of its pharmacologic effects, including inhibition of phosphodiesterase and adenosine and release of catecholamines. Theophylline may cause intoxication after an acute single overdose or as a result of chronic accidental repeated overmedication. The usual serum half-life of theophylline is 4–6 hours, but this may increase to more than 20 hours after overdose.

Clinical Findings

Mild intoxication causes nausea, vomiting, tachycardia, and tremulousness. Severe intoxication is characterized by ventricular and supraventricular tachyarrhythmias, hypotension, and seizures. Status epilepticus is common and often intractable to usual anticonvulsants. After acute overdose (but not chronic intoxication), hypokalemia, hyperglycemia, and metabolic acidosis are common. Seizures and other manifestations of toxicity may be delayed for several hours after acute ingestion, especially if a sustained-release preparation such as Theo-Dur was taken.

Diagnosis is based on measurement of the serum theophylline concentration. Acute overdose patients with serum levels greater than 100 mg/L are likely to develop seizures and hypotension. Patients with chronic intoxication may develop serious toxicity at lower levels (ie, 60 mg/L).

Treatment

A. Emergency and Supportive Measures: Maintain a patent airway, and assist ventilation if necessary. Administer supplemental oxygen. Treat seizures with diazepam and phenobarbital as described on p 1150.

After acute ingestion, empty the stomach by emesis or gastric lavage and administer activated charcoal and a cathartic. Repeated doses of activated charcoal may enhance theophylline elimination by "gut dialysis."

Hemoperfusion is effective in removing theophylline and is indicated for patients with status epilepticus or markedly elevated serum theophylline levels (eg, > 100 mg/L after acute overdose or > 60 mg/L with chronic intoxication).

B. Specific Treatment: There is no antidote for seizures, but hypotension and tachycardia—which are mediated through excessive β_2-adrenergic stimulation—may respond to beta-blocker therapy. Administer esmolol, 25–50 μg/kg/min by intravenous infusion, or propranolol, 0.5–1 mg intravenously.

Gaar GG et al: The effects of esmolol on the hemodynamics of acute theophylline toxicity. Ann Emerg Med 1987; 16:1334.

Gaudreault P et al: Theophylline poisoning: Pharmacological considerations and clinical management. Med Toxicol 1986;1:169.

TRICYCLIC ANTIDEPRESSANTS

Tricyclic antidepressants are among the most commonly implicated products in suicidal overdose. These drugs have anticholinergic and cardiac depressant properties. Tricyclic antidepressants produce more marked membrane-depressant cardiotoxic effects than the phenothiazines. All of these drugs are highly tissue-bound and are not effectively removed by hemodialysis procedures.

Clinical Findings

Signs of severe intoxication may occur abruptly and without warning within 30–60 minutes after acute overdose. Anticholinergic effects include dilated pupils, tachycardia, dry mouth, flushed skin, muscle twitching, and decreased peristalsis. Membrane-depressant cardiotoxic effects include QRS interval widening (> 0.12 s; see Fig 33–3), ventricular arrhythmias, atrioventricular block, and hypotension. Seizures and coma are common with severe intoxication. Life-threatening hyperthermia may result from status epilepticus and anticholinergic-induced impairment of sweating.

The diagnosis should be suspected in any overdose patient with anticholinergic side effects, especially

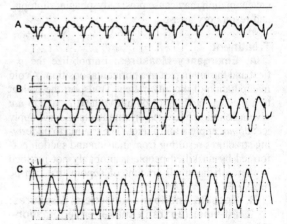

Figure 33–3. Cardiac arrhythmias resulting from tricyclic antidepressant overdose. **A:** Delayed intraventricular conduction results in prolonged QRS interval (0.18 s). **B and C:** Supraventricular tachycardia with progressive widening of QRS complexes mimics ventricular tachycardia. (Reproduced, with permission, from Benowitz NL, Goldschlager N: Cardiac disturbances in the toxicologic patient. Page 71 in: *Clinical Management of Poisoning and Drug Overdose.* Haddad LM, Winchester JF [editors]. Saunders, 1983.)

if there is widening of the QRS interval. For intoxication by most tricyclics, the QRS interval correlates with the severity of intoxication more reliably than the serum drug level. However, newer antidepressants such as amoxapine and fluoxetine may cause seizures without QRS interval prolongation.

Treatment

A. Emergency and Supportive Measures: Maintain a patent airway, and assist ventilation if necessary. Treat coma, hypotension, and seizures as described at the beginning of this chapter. Observe patients for at least 6 hours, and admit all patients with signs of cardiotoxicity.

Perform gastric lavage and administer activated charcoal. Do *not* induce emesis because of the risk of seizures.

B. Specific Treatment: Cardiotoxic membrane-depressant effects may respond to boluses of sodium bicarbonate (50–100 meq intravenously). Sodium bicarbonate provides a large sodium load that alleviates depression of the sodium-dependent channel. Reversal of acidosis may also have beneficial effects at this site. Maintain the pH between 7.45 and 7.5.

Boehnert MT, Lovejoy FH: Value of the QRS duration versus the serum drug level in predicting seizures and ventricular arrhythmias after an acute overdose of tricyclic antidepressants. N Engl J Med 1985;313:474.

Pentel PR, Benowitz NL: Tricyclic antidepressant poisoning: Management of arrhythmias. J Med Toxicol 1986; 1:101.

SOURCES OF INFORMATION ABOUT POISONS

Books

(1) Bryson P: *Critical Review in Toxicology.* Aspen Systems, 1988.

(2) Dreisbach RH, Robertson WO: *Handbook of Poisoning: Prevention, Diagnosis, & Treatment,* 12th ed. Appleton & Lange, 1987. (Lists 6000 poisons and trade-named mixtures.)

(3) Ellenhorn M, Barceloux D: *Medical Toxicology.* Elsevier, 1988.

(4) Goldfrank L et al: *Goldfrank's Toxicologic Emergencies.* Appleton & Lange, 1986.

(5) Gosselin RE et al: *Clinical Toxicology of Commercial Products,* 5th ed. Williams & Wilkins, 1985. (Lists ingredients of 17,500 products.)

(6) Haddad LM, Winchester JF (editors): *Clinical Management of Poisoning and Drug Overdose.* Saunders, 1983.

(7) *The Merck Index,* 11th ed. Merck, 1989.

(8) Olson KR et al: *Poisoning & Drug Overdose.* Appleton & Lange, 1990.

Microfiche Poison Information Systems

(1) Likes KE (editor): Toxifile. Chicago Micro Corporation, Chicago, IL 60625. A microfiche information system.

(2) Rumack BH (editor): Poisindex. National Center for Poison Information, Denver, CO 80204. A computerized and microfiche information system. Revised quarterly.

Other Sources of Information

(1) The manufacturer or the local representative. Another way to identify the contents of a substance is to telephone the manufacturer or the local distributor, who will be able to provide information concerning the type of toxic hazard to be expected from the material in question and what treatment should be given.

(2) Poisoning hotlines to manufacturers. Call the poison control center for the telephone number.

34

Medical Genetics

Reed E. Pyeritz, MD, PhD

The rapid and in some cases spectacular advances in human genetics during the past decade have had important implications for clinical medicine. Familiarity with the fundamental principles of both basic and clinical genetics is now necessary if the physician is to provide a high standard of care. Within the professional lifetimes of most physicians practicing today, all 3 billion nucleotides of the human genome will have been sequenced. The great hope, of course, is that with this exponential growth in information will come new insights into the causes and pathogenetic mechanisms of human disease, more accurate diagnosis, and effective treatment for many disorders now considered beyond the practitioner's therapeutic reach. Along with this optimistic prospect, however, have come some urgent concerns about (1) the ethical, legal, and sociologic implications of what is currently called "genetic engineering"; (2) the problem for medical educators of how best to transmit such an enormous body of information to their students and to physicians in practice; and (3) the seemingly esoteric nature of much of that information paired with the realization that any one of the obscure facts of medical genetics might achieve clinical relevance at any time.

This chapter is an attempt to introduce the medical reader to the field of knowledge encompassed by the term "medical genetics." The first section reviews basic genetic principles and emphasizes recent advances of clinical relevance. The second section focuses on the technology of medical genetics, the expanding scope of its clinical applications, and indications for use. For more detailed treatment of these topics, the following contemporary texts are recommended.

Gelehrter TD, Collins FS: *Principles of Medical Genetics.* Williams & Wilkins, 1990. (A comprehensive yet succinct text suitable for a medical school course in medical genetics.)

Holtzman NA: *Proceed With Caution.* Johns Hopkins Univ Press, 1989. (A critical assessment of the social, legal, and ethical implications of contemporary issues in medical genetics.)

Vogel F, Motulsky AG: *Human Genetics: Problems and Approaches,* 2nd ed. Springer, 1987. (The standard text in human genetics—the place to go for detailed answers to most questions of theory and some of practice.)

INTRODUCTION TO MEDICAL GENETICS

Physicians at one time concerned themselves only with what they could discover by bedside interrogation and inspection and laboratory investigation. In the parlance of genetics, the patient's appearance is called his or her **phenotype.** Now the means are at hand for defining a person's **genotype,** the actual information content inscribed in the 2 meters of coiled DNA present in each cell of the body—or half that amount in every mature ovum or sperm. Virtually all phenotypic characteristics—and this includes diseases as well as human traits such as personality, height, and intelligence—are to some extent determined by the genes. The importance of the genetic contribution varies widely among human phenotypes, and methods are not yet at hand for phenotypic description of complex traits or of most common diseases. Moreover, the importance of the environment and of interactions between environment and genotype in producing phenotypes cannot be overstated despite the obscurity of the actual mechanisms.

The billions of nucleotides in the nucleus of a cell are organized linearly along the DNA double helix in functional units called **genes,** and each of the 50,000–100,000 human genes is accompanied by various regulatory elements that control when it is active in producing **messenger RNA** by a process called **transcription.** In most situations, mRNA is transported from the nucleus to the cytoplasm, where its genetic information is **translated** into **proteins,** which perform the functions that ultimately determine phenotype. For example, proteins serve as enzymes that facilitate metabolism and cell synthesis; as DNA binding elements that regulate transcription of other genes; as structural elements of cells and the extracellular matrix; and as receptor molecules for intra- and intercellular communication.

Chromosomes are the vehicles in which the genes are carried from generation to generation. Each chromosome is a complex of protein and nucleic acid in which an unbroken double helix of DNA is coiled and supercoiled into a space many orders of magnitude less than the extended length of the DNA. Within the chromosome there occur highly complicated and integrated processes, including DNA replication, recombination, and transcription. Humans normally have 46 chromosomes, which are arranged in 23 pairs. One of these pairs, the **sex chromosomes** X and Y, determines the sex of the individual; females have the pair XX and males the pair XY. The remaining 22 pairs are called **autosomes** (Fig 34–1).

In all somatic cells, the 44 autosomes and one of the X chromosomes are transcriptionally active. In males, the active X is the only X; portions of the Y chromosome are also active. In females, the requirement for **dosage compensation** (to be equivalent to the situation in males) is satisfied by complete inactivation of one of the X chromosomes early in the cell cycle. This process of X chromosomal inactivation, while not understood biochemically, is known to be random, so that on average, in 50% of a female's cells, one of the X chromosomes will be active, and in the other 50% the **homologous** member of the pair will be active. The phenotype of the cell is determined by which genes on the chromosomes are active in producing mRNA at any given time.

GENES & CHROMOSOMES

Elucidation of the molecular organization of human genes has been one of the recent triumphs of biology. The traditional view of genes as "beads along a string" of the chromosome is too simplistic. In all genes, information is contained in parcels called **exons,** which are interspersed with stretches of DNA called **introns** that do not encode any information about the protein sequence. However, introns may contain regulatory sequences, and some introns are so large that they could encode an entirely distinct gene; indeed, some genes do overlap.

The exact location of a gene on a chromosome is its **locus,** and the array of loci constitutes the **human gene map.** Currently, the chromosomal site of about 2000 genes is known, often to a high degree of resolution. A variation of this map, identifying selected loci known to be involved in human disease, is shown in Fig 34–2. The difference in resolution of the ordering of genes achievable by molecular techniques (such as linkage analysis) compared to cytogenetic techniques (such as visualization of small defects) is enor-

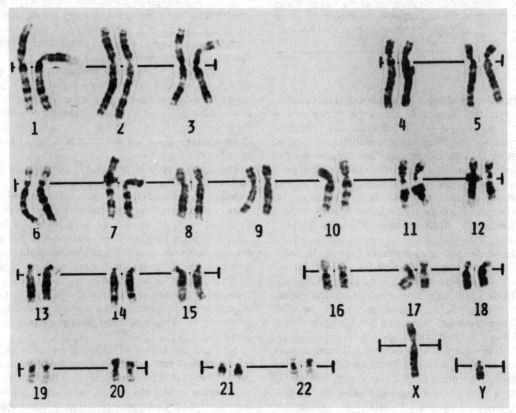

Figure 34–1. Normal karyotype of a human male. Prepared from cultured amniotic cells and stained with Giemsa's stain. About 400 bands are detectable per haploid set of chromosomes.

1176 / CHAPTER 34

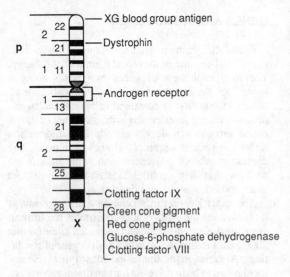

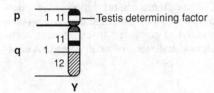

Figure 34–2. A partial "morbid map" of the human genome. Shown next to the ideogram of the human X and Y chromosomes are representative mendelian disorders caused by mutations at that locus. (Courtesy of McKusick and Strayer.)

mous, although the gap is narrowing. The chromosomes in the "standard" karyotype shown in Fig 34–1 have about 400 visible bands; under the best of cytologic and microscopic conditions, a total of about 1600 bands can be seen. But even in this extended configuration, each band contains dozens—sometimes hundreds—of individual genes. Thus, loss **(deletion)** of a small band, which is the smallest type of defect identifiable, will involve loss of many coding sequences and will have diverse effects on the phenotype.

The number and arrangement of genes on homologous chromosomes are identical even though the actual coding sequences of homologous genes may not be. Homologous copies of a gene are termed **alleles.** In comparing alleles, it must be specified at what level of analysis the comparison is being made. When alleles are truly identical—in that their coding sequences are invariant—the individual is **homozygous** at that locus. At a coarser level, the alleles may be functionally identical despite subtle variations in nucleotide sequence—with the result either that the proteins produced from the 2 alleles are identical or that whatever differences there may be in amino acid sequence will have no bearing on the function of

the protein. If the individual is being analyzed at the level of the protein phenotype, allelic homozygosity would again be an apt descriptor. However, if the analysis were at the level of the DNA—as occurs in restriction enzyme examination or nucleotide sequencing—then, despite functional identity, the alleles would be viewed as different and the individual would be **heterozygous** for that locus. Heterozygosity based on differences in the protein products of alleles has been detectable for decades and was the first hard evidence concerning the high degree of human biologic variability. In the past decade, analysis of DNA sequences has shown this variability to be much more remarkable—differences in nucleotide sequence between individuals occur about once every 400 nucleotides.

McKusick VA: Mapping and sequencing the human genome. N Engl J Med 1989;320:910. (Review of the methods of gene mapping and how the information is useful in clinical medicine.)
Watson JD et al: *Molecular Biology of the Gene*, 4th ed. Benjamin/Cummings, 1987.

MUTATION

Allelic heterozygosity most often results when different alleles are inherited from the egg and the sperm, but it also occurs as a consequence of spontaneous alteration in nucleotide sequence **(mutation).** Genetic change occurring during formation of an egg or a sperm is called a **germinal mutation.** When the change occurs after conception—from the earliest stages of embryogenesis to dividing cells in the body of the oldest adult—it is termed a **somatic mutation.** As is discussed below, the role of somatic mutation in the etiology of human disease is now increasingly recognized.

The coarsest type of mutation is alteration in the number or physical structure of chromosomes. For example, **nondisjunction** (failure of chromosome pairs to separate) during **meiosis**—the reduction division that leads to production of mature ova and sperms—causes the embryo to have too many or too few chromosomes, a situation called **aneuploidy.** Rearrangement of chromosome arms, such as occurs in **translocation** or **inversion,** is a mutation even if breakage and reunion does not disrupt any coding sequence. Thus, the phenotypic effect of gross chromosomal mutations can range from profound (as in aneuploidy) to nil.

A bit less coarse, but still detectable cytologically, are **deletions** of part of a chromosome. Such mutations almost always alter phenotype, because large numbers of genes are almost always lost; however, a deletion *may* involve only a single nucleotide, whereas about 1 million nucleotides (1 megabase) must be lost before the defect can be visualized by the most sensitive cytogenetic methods. Molecular biologic techniques are needed to detect smaller losses.

Mutations of one or a few nucleotides in exons have several potential consequences. Changes in one nucleotide can alter which amino acid is encoded; if the amino acid is in a critical region of the protein, function might in this way be severely deranged. On the other hand, some amino acid substitutions have no detectable effect on function, and the phenotype is therefore unaltered by the mutation. Similarly, because the genetic code is **degenerate** (2 or more different 3-nucleotide sequences called **codons** encode some amino acids), nucleotide substitution does not necessarily alter the amino acid sequence of the protein. Three specific codons signal termination of translation; thus, a nucleotide substitution in an exon that generates one of the stop-codons will result in a truncated protein, which is nearly always dysfunctional. Other nucleotide substitutions can disrupt the signals that direct splicing of the mRNA molecule and grossly alter the protein product. Finally, insertions and deletions of one or more nucleotides can have dramatic effects—any change that is not a multiple of 3 nucleotides disrupts the reading frame of the remainder of the exon—or potentially minimal effects (if the protein can tolerate the insertion or loss of an amino acid).

Mutations in introns may disrupt mRNA splicing signals or may be entirely silent with respect to the phenotype. A great deal of variation in nucleotide sequences among individuals (averaging one difference every few hundred nucleotides) resides within introns. Mutations in the DNA between adjacent genes may also be silent or may have a profound effect on phenotype if regulatory sequences are disrupted.

Mutations may occur spontaneously or may be induced by such environmental factors as radiation, medication, or viral infections. Both advanced maternal and paternal age favor mutation, but of different types. In women, nondisjunction of chromosomes becomes more common as ovulation occurs and the egg thereby completes meiosis, later in life. The risk that an aneuploid egg will result increases exponentially and becomes a major clinical worry for women in their early 30s. In men, mutations of a subtler sort—affecting nucleotide sequences—increase with age. Offspring of men over 40 are at an increased risk of having mendelian conditions, primarily autosomal dominant ones.

Antonarakis SE, Kazazian HH Jr: The molecular basis of hemophilia A in man. Trends Genet 1988;4:233. (Wide array of mutations as the cause of a single disease.)

GENES IN INDIVIDUALS

For some quantitative traits such as height or serum glucose concentration, it is impossible to distinguish the contributions of individual genes; this is because in general, phenotypes are the products of multiple genes acting in concert. However, if one of the genes in the system is aberrant, a major departure from the "normal" or expected phenotype might arise. Whether the aberrant phenotype is serious (ie, a disease) or even recognized will depend on the nature of the defective gene product and how resilient the system is to disruption. The latter point emphasizes the importance of homeostasis in both physiology and development—many mutations go unrecognized because the system can cope, even though tolerances for further perturbation might be narrowed.

In other words, virtually all human characteristics are **polygenic,** while many of the disordered phenotypes thought of as "genetic" are **monogenic** but still influenced by other loci in a person's genome.

Phenotypes due to alterations at a single gene are also characterized as **mendelian,** after the Austrian monk and part-time biologist who studied the reproducibility and recurrence of variation in garden peas. Gregor Mendel showed that some traits were **dominant** to others, which he called **recessive.** The dominant traits required only one copy of a "factor" to be expressed, regardless of what the other copy was, whereas the recessive traits required 2 copies before expression occurred. In modern terms, the mendelian factors are genes, and the alternative copies of the gene are alleles. Let A and a represent alleles at a locus: If the same phenotype is present no matter whether the genotype is A/a or A/A, it is dominant, whereas if the phenotype is present only when genotype is a/a, it is recessive.

In medicine, it is important to keep 2 considerations in mind: First, dominance and recessiveness are attributes of the phenotype, not the gene; and second, the concepts of dominance and recessiveness depend on how one defines the phenotype. To illustrate both points, consider sickle cell disease. This condition occurs when a person inherits 2 alleles for β^S globin, in which the normal glutamate at position 6 of the protein has been replaced by valine; the genotype for the β-globin locus is HbS/HbS, compared to the normal HbA/HbA. When the genotype is $HbS/HbA,$ the individual does not have sickle cell disease, so this condition satisfies the criteria for being a recessive phenotype. But now consider the phenotype of sickled erythrocytes. Red cells with the genotype HbS/HbS clearly sickle—but, if the oxygen tension is reduced, so do cells with the genotype HbS/HbA. Therefore, sickling is a dominant trait.

A mendelian phenotype is characterized not only in terms of dominance and recessiveness but also according to whether the determining gene is on the X chromosome or on one of the 22 pairs of autosomes. Traits or diseases are therefore called autosomal dominant, autosomal recessive, X-linked recessive, and X-linked dominant.

Pyeritz RE: Formal genetics in humans: Mendelian and

nonmendelian inheritance. In: *Genes, Brain and Behavior*. McHugh P (editor). Raven Press, 1990. (Review of behavior in families of phenotypes caused by autosomal, X-linked, and mitochondrial genes.)

GENES IN FAMILIES

Since the first decade of this century, the patterns of recurrence of specific human phenotypes have been explained in terms of principles first described by Mendel in the garden pea plant. Mendel's second principle—usually referred to as his first* —is called the **law of segregation** and states that a pair of factors (alleles) that determines some trait separates (segregates) during formation of gametes. In simple terms, a heterozygous (*A/a*) person will produce 2 types of gametes with respect to this locus—one containing only *A* and one containing only *a*, in equal proportions. Offspring of this person will have a 50–50 chance of inheriting the *A* allele and a similar chance of inheriting the *a* allele.

The concepts of genes in individuals and in families can be combined to specify how mendelian traits will be inherited.

Autosomal Dominant Inheritance

The characteristics of autosomal dominant inheritance in humans can be summarized as follows:

(1) There is a vertical pattern in the pedigree, with multiple generations affected (Fig 34–3).

(2) Heterozygotes for the mutant allele show an abnormal phenotype.

(3) Males and females are affected with equal frequency and severity.

(4) Only one parent must be affected for an offspring to be at risk for developing the phenotype.

(5) When an affected person mates with an unaffected one, each offspring has a 50% chance of inheriting the affected phenotype. This is true regardless of the sex of the affected parent—specifically, male-to-male transmission occurs.

(6) The frequency of sporadic cases is positively associated with the severity of the phenotype. More precisely, the greater the **reproductive fitness** of affected persons, the less likely it is that any given case resulted from a new mutation.

(7) The average age of fathers is advanced in the case of isolated (sporadic or new mutation) cases.

---

* Mendel's first law stated that—from the perspective of the phenotype—it mattered not from which parent a particular allele was inherited. For years this principle was thought to be too obvious to be codified as anybody's "law" and was therefore ignored. In fact, however, recent evidence from studies of human disorders suggests that certain genes are "processed" ("imprinted") as they move through the gonad and that processing in the testis is different from that in the ovary. Thus, not only is this first mendelian principle important, it was incorrect as originally formulated from observations in peas.

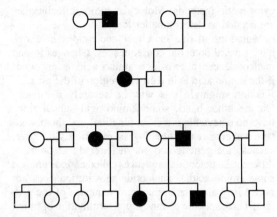

Figure 34–3. A pedigree illustrating autosomal dominant inheritance. Square symbols indicate males and circles females; open symbols indicate that the person is phenotypically unaffected, and filled symbols indicate that the phenotype is present to some extent.

Autosomal dominant phenotypes are often age-dependent, less severe than autosomal recessive ones, and associated with malformations or other physical features. They are **pleiotropic** in that multiple, even seemingly unrelated clinical manifestations derive from the same mutation; and **variable** in that expression of the same mutation among people will differ.

Penetrance is a concept often associated with mendelian conditions—especially dominant ones—and the term is often misused. It should be defined as an expression of the frequency of appearance of a phenotype (dominant or recessive) when one or more mutant alleles are present. For individuals, penetrance is an all-or-none phenomenon—the phenotype is either present (penetrant) or not (nonpenetrant). The term **variability**—not "incomplete penetrance"—should be used to denote differences in expression of an allele.

The most frequent cause of apparent nonpenetrance is insensitivity of the methods for detecting the phenotype. If an apparently normal parent of a child with a dominant condition were in fact heterozygous for the mutation, the parent would have a 50% chance at each subsequent conception of having another affected child. A common cause of nonpenetrance in adult-onset mendelian diseases is death of the affected person before the phenotype becomes evident but after transmission of the mutant allele to offspring. Thus, accurate genetic counseling demands careful attention to the family medical history and high-resolution scrutiny of both parents of a child with a condition known to be a mendelian dominant trait.

When both alleles are expressed in the heterozygote, as in blood group AB, in sickle trait (HbS/HbA), in the major histocompatibility antigens, or in sickle-C disease (HbS/HbC), the phenotype is called **codominant**.

In human dominant phenotypes, the homozygous state for the mutant allele is almost always more severe than in heterozygotes.

Autosomal Recessive Inheritance

The characteristics of autosomal recessive inheritance in humans can be summarized as follows:

(1) There is a horizontal pattern in the pedigree, with a single generation affected (Fig 34–4).

(2) Males and females are affected with equal frequency and severity.

(3) Inheritance is from both parents, each a heterozygote (carrier) and each usually clinically unaffected.

(4) Each offspring of 2 carriers has a 25% chance of being affected, a 50% chance of being a carrier, and a 25% chance of inheriting neither mutant allele. Thus, two-thirds of all clinically unaffected offspring are carriers.

(5) In matings between individuals, each with the same recessive phenotype, all offspring will be affected.

(6) Affected individuals who mate with unaffected individuals who are not carriers have only unaffected offspring.

(7) The rarer the recessive phenotype, the more likely it is that the parents are **consanguineous** (related).

Autosomal recessive phenotypes are often associated with deficient activity of enzymes and are thus termed **inborn errors of metabolism.** They are also more severe, less variable, and less age-dependent than dominant conditions.

When an autosomal recessive condition is quite rare, the chance that the parents of affected offspring are consanguineous is increased. As a result, the prevalence of rare recessive conditions is high among inbred groups such as the Old Order Amish. On the other hand, when the autosomal recessive condition is common, the chance of consanguinity between parents of cases is no higher than in the general population (about 0.5%).

Two different *mutant* alleles at the same locus, as in HbS/HbC, form a **genetic compound.** The phenotype usually lies between those produced by either allele present in the homozygous state. Because of the large number of mutations possible in a given gene, many autosomal recessive phenotypes are probably due to genetic compounds. Sickle cell disease is an exception. Consanguinity is strong presumptive evidence for true homozygosity of mutant alleles and against a genetic compound.

X-Linked Inheritance

The general characteristics of X-linked inheritance in humans can be summarized as follows:

(1) There is no male-to-male transmission of the phenotype (Fig 34–5).

(2) Unaffected males do not transmit the phenotype.

(3) All of the daughters of an affected male are heterozygous carriers.

(4) Males are usually more severely affected than females.

(5) Whether a heterozygous female is counted as affected—and whether the phenotype is called ''recessive'' or ''dominant''—depends often on the sensitivity of the assay or the examination.

(6) Some mothers of affected males will not themselves be heterozygotes (ie, they will be homozygous normal) but will have a germinal mutation. The proportion of heterozygous (carrier) mothers is negatively associated with the severity of the condition.

(7) Heterozygous women transmit the mutant gene to one-half of sons, who are affected, and to one-half of daughters, who are heterozygotes.

(8) If an affected male mates with a heterozygous female, half of the male offspring will be affected, giving the false impression of male-to-male transmis-

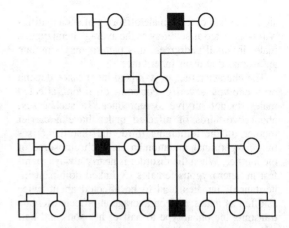

Figure 34–5. A pedigree illustrating X-linked recessive inheritance. (Symbols as in Fig 34–3.)

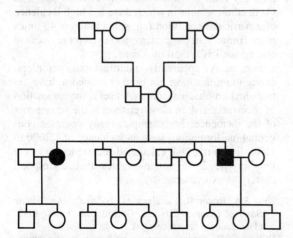

Figure 34–4. A pedigree illustrating autosomal recessive inheritance. (Symbols as in Fig 34–3.)

sion. One-half of the female offspring of such matings will be affected as severely as the average hemizygous male; in small pedigrees, this pattern may simulate autosomal dominant inheritance.

The characteristics of X-linked inheritance depend on phenotypic severity. For some disorders, affected males do not survive to reproduce. In such cases, about two-thirds of affected males have a carrier mother; in the remaining third, the disorder arises by new germinal mutation in an X chromosome of the mother. When the disorder is nearly always manifest in heterozygous females (X-linked dominant inheritance), females tend to be affected about twice as often as males; and on average an affected female transmits the phenotype to half of her sons and half of her daughters.

X-linked phenotypes are often clinically variable—particularly in heterozygous females—and suspected of being autosomal dominant with nonpenetrance.

Germinal mosaicism occurs in mothers of boys with X-linked conditions. The chance of such a mother having a second affected son or a heterozygous daughter depends on the fraction of her oocytes that carries the mutation. Currently, this fraction is impossible to determine. However, the presence of germinal mosaicism can be detected in a family by analysis of DNA, and this knowledge becomes crucial for genetic counseling.

About 5000 human genes have been identified through their phenotypes and inheritance patterns in families. This total represents 5–10% of all genes thought to be encoded by the 22 autosomes and 2 sex chromosomes. Victor McKusick coordinates an international effort to catalog human mendelian variation (see first reference, below).

McKusick VA: *Mendelian Inheritance in Man*, 9th ed. Johns Hopkins Univ Press, 1990. (A catalogue consisting, for each phenotype, of a 6-digit identification number—used extensively in the medical literature—for each phenotype, a summary statement, and a list of pertinent references. Editions are published biennially, but the catalogue is updated continuously and is computer-accessible as Online Mendelian Inheritance in Man [OMIM]. For information, contact OMIM User Support, Welch Medical Library, 1830 East Monument Street, Third Floor, Baltimore, MD 21205; [301] 955-7058.)

Wallace DC: Mitochondrial DNA mutations and neuromuscular disease. Trends Genet 1989;5:9. (Basic principles of "cytoplasmic" inheritance.)

DISORDERS OF MULTIFACTORIAL CAUSATION

Many disorders cluster in families but are not associated with evident chromosomal aberrations or mendelian inheritance patterns. Examples include congenital malformations such as cleft lip, pyloric stenosis, and spina bifida; coronary artery disease; adult-onset diabetes mellitus; and various forms of neoplasia. They are often characterized by varying frequencies in different racial or ethnic groups, disparity in sexual predilection, and greater frequency (but less than full concordance) in monozygotic than in dizygotic twins. This inheritance pattern is called "multifactorial" to signify that multiple genes interact with various environmental agents to produce the phenotype. The familial clustering is assumed to be due to sharing of both alleles and environment.

For most multifactorial conditions, there is little understanding of which particular genes are involved, how they and their products interact, and in what way different nongenetic factors contribute to the phenotype. For some disorders, biochemical and genetic studies have identified mendelian conditions within the coarse phenotype: Defects of the low-density lipoprotein receptor account for a small fraction of cases of ischemic heart disease (a larger fraction if only patients under age 50 are considered); familial polyposis of the colon predisposes to adenocarcinoma; and some patients with emphysema have inherited deficiency of α_1-proteinase inhibitor (α_1-antiproteinase, formerly called α_1-antitrypsin). Despite these notable examples, this reductionistic preoccupation with mendelian phenotypes is unlikely to explain the great majority of human disease; but even so, in the last analysis, much of human pathology will prove to be associated with genetic factors in cause, pathogenesis, or both.

Our profound ignorance about fundamental genetic mechanisms has not completely restricted practical approaches to the genetics of multifactorial disorders. For example, recurrence risks are based on empiric data derived from observation of many families. The risk of recurrence of multifactorial disorders is increased in several instances, as follows: (1) to close relatives (sibs, offspring, and parents) of an affected individual; (2) when 2 or more members of a family have the same condition; (3) when the first case in a family is in the less commonly affected sex; and (4) in ethnic groups in which there is a high incidence of a particular condition (eg, spina bifida is 40 times more common in Caucasians (and even more frequent among the Irish) than in Asians).

For many apparently multifactorial disorders, enough families have not been examined to have established empiric risk data. A useful approximation of recurrence risk in close relatives is the square root of the incidence. For example, many common congenital malformations have an incidence of 1:2000 to 1:500 live births; the calculated recurrence risks are thus in the 2–5% range—values that correspond closely to experience.

King RA, Rotter JI, Motulsky AG (editors): *The Genetic Basis of Common Disease*. Oxford Univ Press, 1990. (The standard reference work.)

Williams RR: Nature, nurture, and family predisposition. N Engl J Med 1988;318:769. (Prospects and pitfalls of understanding the causes and pathogenesis of disease.)

CHROMOSOMAL ABERRATIONS

Any deviation from the structure and number of chromosomes as displayed in Fig 34–1 is, technically, a chromosomal aberration. Not all aberrations cause problems in the affected individual, but some that do not may lead to problems in offspring. About 1:200 live-born infants have a chromosomal aberration that is detected because of some effect on phenotype. This frequency increases markedly the earlier in fetal life the chromosomes are examined. By the end of the first trimester of gestation, most fetuses with abnormal numbers of chromosomes have been lost through spontaneous abortion. For example, Turner's syndrome—due to absence of one sex chromosome and the presence of a single X chromosome—is a relatively common condition, but it is estimated that only 2% of fetuses with this form of aneuploidy survive to term. Even more striking in live-born children is the complete absence of most autosomal trisomies and monosomies despite their frequent occurrence in young fetuses.

Types of Chromosomal Abnormalities

Major structural changes occur in either **balanced** or **unbalanced** form. In the latter, there is a gain or loss of genetic material; in the former, there is no change in the amount of genetic material but only a rearrangement of it. At the sites of breaks and new attachments of chromosome fragments, there may be permanent structural or functional damage to one gene or to only a few genes. Despite no visible loss of material, the aberration may nonetheless be recognized as unbalanced through an abnormal phenotype and the chromosomal defect confirmed by molecular analysis of the DNA.

Aneuploidy results from nondisjunction—the failure of a chromatid pair to separate in a dividing cell. Nondisjunction in either the first or second division of meiosis results in gametes with abnormal chromosomal constitutions. In aneuploidy, more or fewer than 46 chromosomes are present (Table 34–1). The following are all forms of aneuploidy: (1) **monosomy,** in which only one member of a pair of chromosomes is present; (2) **trisomy,** in which 3 chromosomes are present instead of 2; and (3) **polysomy,** in which one chromosome is represented 4 or more times.

If nondisjunction occurs in mitosis, **mosaic** patterns occur in somatic tissue, with some cells having one karyotype and other cells of the same organism another karyotype. Patients with a mosaic genetic constitution often have manifestations of each of the genetic syndromes associated with the various abnormal karyotypes.

Translocation results from an exchange of parts of 2 chromosomes.

Deletion is loss of chromosomal material.

Duplication is the presence of 2 or more copies of the same region of a given chromosome. The redundancy may occur in the same chromosome or in a nonhomologous chromosome. In the latter case, a translocation will also have occurred.

An **isochromosome** is one in which the arms on either side of the centromere have the same genetic material in the same order—ie, the chromosome has at some time divided in such a way that it has a double dose of one arm and absence of the other.

In an **inversion,** a chromosomal region becomes reoriented 180 degrees out of ordinary phase. The same genetic material is present, but in a different order.

Bickmore WA, Sumner AT: Mammalian chromosome banding: An expression of genome organization. Trends Genet 1989;5:144. (Current knowledge and speculation about the association of chromosome bands and underlying genetic structure.)

deGrouchy J, Turleau C: Clinical Atlas of Human Chromosomes, 2nd ed. Wiley, 1984.

Gardner RJ, Sutherland GR: Chromosome Abnormalities and Genetic Counseling. Oxford Univ Press, 1989. (Mechanisms, clinical presentations, and recurrence risks.)

Hall JG: Somatic mosaicism: Observations related to clinical genetics. Am J Hum Genet 1988;43:355. (A review of the various mechanisms of somatic mosaicism at the single gene or chromosome level and their relevance to clinical diagnosis and counseling.)

Table 34–1. Clinical phenotypes resulting from aneuploidy.

Condition	Karyotype	Incidence at Birth
Trisomy 13	47,XX or XY,+13	1:15,000
Trisomy 18	47,XX or XY,+18	1:11,000
Trisomy 21 (Down's syndrome)	47,XX or XY,+21	1:900
Klinefelter's syndrome	47,XXY	1:1000 males
XYY	47,XYY	1:100 males
Turner's syndrome	45,X	1:7500 females
XXX syndrome	47,XXX	1:200 females

THE TECHNIQUES OF MEDICAL GENETICS

In the years leading to the creation of the American Board of Medical Genetics, which certifies clinical geneticists, genetic counselors, and clinical laboratory geneticists, some leading professionals argued against the need for a "subspecialty" designation on the grounds that medical genetics should only be viewed as the broadest of the medical specialties. Without a doubt, the diagnosis and management of hereditary disorders involves in the first instance the skills and knowledge of a general physician. The disorders affect multiple organ systems and people of all ages. Many disorders are chronic ones, but often there are acute crises. The concerns of patients and families span an enormous range of medical, psychologic, social, and economic issues. These characteristics emphasize the need for pediatricians, internists, obstetricians, and family practitioners to provide medical genetics services for their patients. Those physicians therefore need to know what laboratory and consultative services are available from clinical geneticists and the indications for their use. This section reviews these matters.

CYTOGENETICS

Cytogenetics is the study of chromosomes by light microscopy. The chromosomal constitution of a single cell or an entire individual is specified by a standardized notation. The total chromosome count is determined first, followed by the sex chromosome complement and then by any abnormalities. The autosomes are all designated by numbers from 1 to 22. A plus (+) or minus (–) sign indicates, respectively, a gain or loss of chromosomal material. For example, a normal male is 46,XY, while a girl with Down's syndrome caused by trisomy 21 is 47,XX,+21.

Chromosomal analyses are done by growing human cells in tissue culture, chemically inhibiting mitosis, and then staining, sorting, and counting the chromosomes. The display of all of the chromosomes is termed the **karyotype** (Fig 34–1) and is the end result of the technical aspect of cytogenetics. Interpretation of the karyotype is an additional step, as is communication of the interpretation to the referring physician.

Specimens for cytogenetic analysis can be obtained for routine analysis from the peripheral blood, in which case T lymphocytes are examined; from amniotic fluid for culture of amniocytes; from trophoblastic cells from the chorionic villus; from bone marrow; and from cultured fibroblasts, usually obtained from a skin biopsy. Enough cells must be examined so that the chance of missing a cytogenetically distinct cell line (a situation of mosaicism) is statistically low. For most clinical indications, 20 mitoses are examined and counted under direct microscopic visualization, and 2 are photographed and karyotypes prepared. Observation of aberrations usually prompts more extended scrutiny and in many cases further analysis of the original culture. Automated methods for cytogenetic analysis are being developed, but from the perspective of the patient and referring physicians, these will have little impact in the immediate future.

A variety of methods are available to reveal banding patterns—unique to each pair of chromosomes—that are invaluable in the analysis of aberrations. The number of bands that can be visualized is a function of how "extended" the chromosomes are, which in turn depends chiefly on how early in metaphase (or even in prophase for the most extensive banding) mitosis was arrested. The "standard" karyotype reveals about 400 bands per haploid set of chromosomes, whereas a prophase karyotype might reveal 4 times that number. As invaluable as extended karyotypes are in certain clinical circumstances, their interpretation is much more difficult—in terms both of the time and effort required and of ambiguity about what is abnormal, what is a normal variation, and what is a technical artifact. More recent techniques involve in situ hybridization of DNA probes for specific chromosomes. These probes can be labeled with radioactive isotopes or fluorescent dyes and can be used to identify chromosomes or fragments of chromosomes. The confluence of molecular biology and cytogenetics is rapidly becoming more imminent, so that some applications will find routine use before long.

Indications for Cytogenetic Analysis

The current indications are listed in Table 34–2. A wide array of clinical syndromes have been found to be associated with chromosomal aberrations, and analysis of the karyotype is useful any time a patient is discovered to have the manifestations of one of these syndromes. When a chromosomal aberration is revealed, not only does the patient's physician obtain valuable information about prognosis, but the parents gain insight into the cause of their child's problems and the family can be counseled accurately—and usually reassured—about the risks of recurrence.

Table 34–2. Indications for cytogenetic analysis.

1. Patients with malformations suggestive of one of the recognized syndromes associated with a specific chromosome aberration.
2. Patients of any age who are grossly retarded physically or mentally, especially if there are associated anomalies.
3. Any patient with ambiguous internal or external genitalia or suspected hermaphroditism.
4. Girls with primary amenorrhea and boys with delayed pubertal development. Up to 25% of patients with primary amenorrhea have a chromosomal abnormality.
5. Males with learning or behavioral disorders who are taller than expected (based on parental height).
6. Certain malignant and premalignant diseases (see Tables 34–9 and 34–10).
7. Parents of a patient with a chromosome translocation.
8. Parents of a patient with a suspected chromosomal syndrome if there is a family history of similarly affected children.
9. Couples with a history of multiple spontaneous abortions of unknown cause.
10. Couples who are infertile after more common obstetric and urologic causes have been excluded.
11. Prenatal diagnosis (see Table 34–8).

Mental retardation is a frequent component of congenital malformation syndromes because of coincident defective development of the central nervous system. However, one of the most frequent causes of mental retardation—especially in retarded males, in whom it is the second most common chromosomal aberration after Down's syndrome—is not associated with obvious systemic malformations. The fragile-X syndrome—so called because of the gap, or **fragile site,** evident at the end of the long arm of the X chromosome—occurs in one of every 2000 males. This aberration is inherited from mothers who are heterozygous for the fragile-X site; many carrier women have apparently normal intellect, but some are retarded. Thus, any person with unexplained mental retardation should be studied by chromosomal analysis, with particular attention paid to this aberration. Since special techniques are required, the laboratory request must clearly indicate that a search for fragile sites is needed.

Abnormalities of sexual differentiation can only be understood once the patient's **genetic sex** is clarified. Hormonal therapy and plastic surgery can to some extent determine **phenotypic sex** is, but genetic sex is dictated by the complement of sex chromosomes. The best-known example of dichotomy between the genetic sex and phenotypic sex is the testicular feminization syndrome, in which the chromosomal constitution is 46,XY but, because of a defect in the testosterone receptor protein (specified by a gene on the Y chromosome), the phenotype is completely female.

Failure or delay in developing secondary sexual characteristics occurs in Turner's syndrome (the most common cause being a form of aneuploidy, ie, monosomy for the X chromosome, 45,X), in Klinefelter's syndrome (the most common karyotype is 47,XXY), and in other much rarer chromosomal aberrations.

Tall stature is perhaps the only consistent phenotypic feature associated with having an extra Y chromosome (karyotype 47,XYY); most men with this chromosomal aberration lead normal lives, and thus tall stature in a male is itself no indication for chromosomal analysis. However, some evidence suggests that an increased prevalence of learning difficulties may be associated with this aberration. Furthermore, Klinefelter's syndrome often causes tall stature, albeit with a eunuchoid habitus, and learning and behavioral problems. Thus, the combination of learning or behavioral difficulties and unexpectedly increased height in a male should prompt consideration of cytogenetic analysis.

As discussed below, most tumors are associated with chromosomal aberrations, some of which are highly specific for certain malignancies. Cytogenetic analysis of tumor tissue may assist in diagnosis, prognosis, and management.

Whenever a person is shown to have a chromosome translocation—whether it be balanced and asymptomatic or unbalanced, causing a syndrome—the physician should consider the importance of identifying the source of the translocation. If the proband is a child and the parents are interested in having more children, both parents should be studied cytogenetically. How far the primary physician or consultant should go in tracking a translocation through a family is an unsettled question with legal and ethical as well as medical implications. Certainly the proband (if an adult) or the parents of the proband need to be counseled and the potential risks to relatives discussed. The physician should document, both in the medical record and by correspondence, that the burden of disclosing relevant data to the extended family has been assumed by specific named individuals.

Inability to produce offspring, either through failure to conceive or as a result of repeated miscarriages, is a frustrating and discouraging problem for affected couples and their physicians. Considerable progress in the urologic and gynecologic understanding of infertility has benefited many couples. However, chromosomal aberrations remain an important problem in reproductive medicine, and cytogenetic analysis should be utilized at some stage in extended evaluation. Infertility can be caused by Klinefelter's and Turner's syndromes; the external phenotype may be subtle, particularly if the chromosomal aberration is mosaic. Any early spontaneous abortion may be due to fetal aneuploidy. Recurrence may be due to parental translocation predisposing to an unbalanced fetal karyotype.

Hassold TJ: Chromosomal abnormalities in human reproductive wastage. Trends Genet 1986;2:105. (Summary of cytogenetic aberrations detected in spontaneously aborted fetuses at different stages of gestation.)

BIOCHEMICAL GENETICS

The field of biochemical genetics undertakes the study of **inborn errors of metabolism,** which can be defined more broadly than was done by Garrod at the turn of this century to include other than enzymatic defects. Today, biochemical genetics deals also with proteins of all functions, including cytoskeletal and extracellular structure, regulation, and receptors. The principal functions of the biochemical genetics laboratory are to determine the presence or absence of proteins, to assess the qualitative characteristics of proteins, and to verify the effectiveness of proteins in vitro. The key elements from the referring physician's perspective are (1) to indicate what the suspected clinical diagnoses are and (2) to make certain that the proper specimen is obtained and transported to the laboratory in a timely manner.

Indications for Biochemical Investigations

Some inborn errors are relatively common in the

Table 34–3. Representative inborn errors of metabolism.

General Class of Defect	Example	Biochemical Defect	Inheritance
Aminoacidopathy	Phenylketonuria	Phenylalanine hydroxylase	AR
Connective tissue	Osteogenesis imperfecta type II	α1(I) and α2(I) procollagen	AD
Gangliosidosis	Tay-Sachs disease	Hexosaminidase A	AR
Glycogen storage disease	Type I	Glucose-6-phosphatase	AR
Immune function	Chronic granulomatous disease	Cytochrome b, β chain	XL
Lipid metabolism	Familial hypercholesterolemia	LDL receptor	AD
Mucopolysaccharidosis	MPS II (Hunter's syndrome)	Iduronate sulfatase	XL
Porphyria	Acute intermittent	Porphobilinogen deaminase	AD
Transport	Cystic fibrosis	CF transmembrane conductance regulator	AR
Urea cycle	Citrullinemia	Arginosuccinate synthetase	AR

general population, eg, hemochromatosis, defects of the low-density lipoprotein receptor, and cystic fibrosis (Table 34–3). Others, while rare across the entire population, are common in certain ethnic groups, such as Tay-Sachs disease in Ashkenazic Jews, sickle cell disease in Afro-Americans, and thalassemias in populations from around the Mediterranean basin. Many of these disorders are autosomal recessive, and the frequency of heterozygotes is many times that of the diseases. Screening for carrier status can be effective if certain requirements are satisfied (Table 34–4). For example, all of the United States and the District of Columbia require screening of newborns for one or more metabolic diseases. Such programs are cost-effective even for rare conditions such as phenylketonuria, which occurs in only one of every 11,000 births. But economic concerns are only one issue to be considered in making decisions about establishing screening programs. Unfortunately, not all disorders that meet the requirements in Table 34–4 are screened for in every state. Furthermore, compliance is highly variable among programs, and follow-up diagnostic tests, management, and counseling are in some cases inadequate. Babies most likely to be missed are those born at home or in religious isolates. In some states, parents can refuse to have their infants studied.

Use of the biochemical genetics laboratory for other than screening purposes must be justified by the need for data on which to base a diagnosis of specific disorders or classes of related disorders. The possibilities are limited only by the extent of current knowledge (which changes daily), the enthusiasm of the primary physician or consultant, the willingness of the patient or family to pursue the diagnosis and specimens to be taken, and the availability of a laboratory to examine the specimens.

It is likely that inborn errors of metabolism underlie many disorders but that the defects are so subtle they have escaped detection. However, there are a number of clinical situations in which an inborn error should be part of the differential diagnosis; the urgency with which the investigation must be undertaken will vary depending on the severity of the disorder and the availability (or not) of treatment in case the diagnosis is made. Table 34–5 lists the various clinical presentations.

The possibility of acute metabolic disease of the neonate is the most important indication, because

Table 34–4. Requirements for effective screening for inborn errors of metabolism.

1. The disease should be clinically severe or have potentially severe consequences.
2. The natural history of the disease should be understood.
3. Effective treatment should be generally available and depend on early diagnosis for optimal results.
4. The disease incidence should be high enough to warrant screening.
5. The screening test should have favorable specificity (low false-positive rate) and sensitivity (low false-negative rate).
6. The screening test should be available for and used by the entire population at risk.
7. An adequate system for follow-up of positive results should be provided.
8. The economic cost-benefit analysis should favor screening and treatment.

Table 34–5. Manner of presentation of inborn errors of metabolism.

Presentation and Course	Examples
Acute metabolic disease of the neonate	Galactosemia, urea cycle disorders
Chronic disorders with little progression	Phenylketonuria, hypothyroidism
Chronic disorders with insidious, incessant progression	Tay-Sachs disease
Disorders causing abnormalities of structure	Skeletal dysplasias, Marfan's syndrome
Disorders of transport	Cystinuria, lactase deficiency
Disorders that determine susceptibilities	LDL receptor deficiency, agammaglobulinemia
Episodic disorders	Most porphyrias, glucose-6-phosphate deficiency
Disorders causing anemia	Pyruvate kinase deficiency, hereditary spherocytosis
Disorders interfering with hemostasis	Hemophilia A and B, von Willebrand disease
Congenital disorders with no possibility of reversal	Testicular feminization
Disorders with protean manifestations	Pseudohypoparathyroidism, hereditary amyloidoses
Inborn errors with no clinical effects	Pentosuria, histidinemia

prompt diagnosis and treatment can often make the difference between life and death. The clinical features, which may include diarrhea, vomiting, dehydration, acidosis, seizures, and coma, are nonspecific because the newborn has a limited repertoire of responses to severe metabolic insults. The physician must be both inclusive and systematic in evaluating such ill babies. Use of decision aids, one of which is illustrated in Table 34–6, can assist on both counts.

Brusilow SW, Valle DL, Arn P: Symptomatic inborn errors of metabolism. Pages 164–169 in: *Current Therapy in Neonatal-Perinatal Medicine.* Nelson NM (editor). BC Decker, 1990. (Summary of approaches to mendelian conditions that cause serious disease in early life.)

Scriver CR et al (editors): *The Metabolic Basis of Inherited Diseases,* 6th ed. McGraw-Hill, 1989. (The standard reference work and source of information about most hereditary disorders.)

Table 34–6. Systematic approach to the severely ill neonate with diarrhea.[1]

1. Administer oral glucose-electrolyte solution.
    If improvement occurs, go to 3.
    If no improvement, begin intravenous fluids to rehydrate.
        If diarrhea persists, go to 4 and 5.
        If diarrhea improves, go to 2.
2. Administer oral glucose-electrolyte solution.
    If improvement occurs, go to 3.
    If diarrhea recurs, administer an oral glucose load and follow blood glucose.
        If the blood glucose rises normally, go to 3.
        If the blood glucose does not rise, work up for glucose malabsorption.
3. Administer original formula.
    If diarrhea does not recur, workup ends (probably an infectious cause).
    If diarrhea recurs, go to 4 through 6.
4. Determine serum electrolytes and pH.
    If normal, go to 5.
    If acidotic, rehydrate intravenously, monitor serum bicarbonate, go to 5.
    If hypochloremic alkalosis, administer saline or KCl intravenously, go to 5.
5. Examine stool.
    5a. Culture and treat patients with positive results accordingly.
    5b. Check pH; if < 6.0, check for reducing substances. If positive for reducing substances, go to 7.
    5c. Check for steatorrhea; if present, go to 5d.
    5d. Check sweat chloride.
        If elevated, work up for cystic fibrosis.
        If normal, go to 5e.
    5e. Check plain radiograph of abdomen.
        If adrenals calcified, work up for Wolman's disease.
        If normal, go to 5f.
    5f. Check serum cholesterol and lipoproteins.
        If abnormal, work up for abetalipoproteinemia, etc.
        If normal, work up for other possible causes of malabsorption.
6. Examine urine for reducing substances.
    If positive, go to 7.
    If negative, go to 8.
7. Identify reducing substance (eg, galactose).
8. Check urine amino acids.
    If positive, identify which amino acids, consider transport defects.
    If negative, continue fluid and metabolic support and consider a metabolic or genetics consultation.

---

[1] Adapted from Holtzman NA: Rare diseases, common problems: Recognition and management. Pediatrics 1978;62:1056.

DNA ANALYSIS

Direct inspection of nucleic acids—often called "molecular genetics" or "DNA diagnosis"—is achieving an increasingly prominent role in a number of clinical areas, including oncology, infectious disease, forensic medicine, and the general study of pathophysiology. However, the greatest impact by far has been in the diagnosis of mendelian disorders. Once a particular gene is shown to be defective in a given condition, the nature of the mutation itself can be determined, often by sequencing the nucleotides and comparing the array with that of a normal allele. One of a variety of techniques can then be used to determine whether that same mutation is present in other patients with the same disorder. Genetic heterogeneity is so extensive that most mendelian conditions are associated with numerous mutations at one locus—or occasionally multiple loci—that produce the same phenotype. This fact complicates DNA diagnosis of patients and screening for carriers of defects in specific genes.

A few conditions are associated with relatively few mutations or with only one highly prevalent mutation. For example, all sickle cell disease is caused by exactly the same change of glutamate to valine at position 6 of β-globin, and that substitution in turn is due to a change of one nucleotide at the sixth codon in the β-globin gene. But such uniformity is the exception. In cystic fibrosis, about 70% of mutations are identical deletions of 3 nucleotides that cause loss of a phenylalanine residue from a chloride transport protein; however, the remaining 30% of mutations of that protein are diverse, so that a simple screening test that would detect all carriers of a cystic fibrosis mutation is not possible.

The actual methods of DNA diagnosis need not be described here; they are rapidly evolving, and some are being adapted in the form of kits for use in general clinical laboratories. Reviews of the current technical status of DNA analysis appear regularly in the medical journal literature. Polymerase chain reaction (PCR) studies have revolutionized many aspects of molecular biology, and DNA diagnosis has come to involve this technique in many instances.

Indications for DNA Diagnosis

The basic requirement for the use of nucleic acids in the diagnosis of hereditary conditions is that a **probe** be available for the gene in question. The probe may be a piece of the actual gene, a sequence close to the gene, or just a few nucleotides at the actual mutation. The closer the probe is to the actual mutation, the more accurate and the more useful will be the information derived. DNA diagnosis involves one of 2 general approaches: (1) direct detection of the mutation and (2) linkage analysis, whereby the presence of a mutation is inferred from the nature of a probe DNA sequence remote from the mutation.

In the latter approach, as the probe moves farther from the mutation, the chances increase that recombination will have separated the 2 sequences and confused the interpretation of the data.

The list of conditions for which direct detection of some mutations is possible continues to grow; some of the more common ones are listed in Table 34–7. Conditions that can be diagnosed only indirectly are also listed; while their number also is increasing, there is a gratifying shift of these disorders from diagnosis by indirect to diagnosis by direct detection as the molecular nature of mutations is defined.

DNA diagnosis is finding frequent application in presymptomatic detection of individuals with age-dependent disorders such as Huntington's disease and adult polycystic kidney disease, screening for carriers of autosomal recessive conditions such as cystic fibrosis and thalassemias, screening for female heterozygotes of X-linked conditions such as Duchenne's muscular dystrophy and hemophilia A and B, and prenatal diagnosis (see below). The full range of indications is undefined at this time.

Logistics of DNA Diagnosis

Lymphocytes are a ready source of DNA; 10 mL of whole blood yields up to 0.5 mg of DNA, enough for dozens of Southern hybridizations, each of which requires only 5 μg. If the analysis is quite narrowly focused on a specific mutation (such as in a family study, in which only one specific nucleotide change is addressed), polymerase chain reaction analysis can often be used and the amount of DNA needed is truly infinitesimal—a few hair bulbs or sperm can serve in a pinch. Once isolated, the DNA sample can be divided into aliquots and frozen. Alternatively, lymphocytes can be transformed with viruses into lymphoblasts; these cells are immortal, can be frozen, and—whenever DNA is required—can be thawed, propagated, and their DNA isolated. These stored specimens provide access to a person's genome long after the individual dies. This is such an important advantage that many clinical genetics centers and commercial laboratories "bank" DNA from patients and informative relatives even if the samples cannot be put to use immediately. The specimens may later prove invaluable to relatives or to other patients being evaluated. DNA in some instances has become more reliable than the medical record and even more readily retrievable!

Blood for DNA isolation should be drawn in EDTA anticoagulant (purple-top tubes); blood for lymphoblast culture should be drawn in heparin (green-top tubes). Neither should be frozen. Specimens for DNA isolation can be stored or shipped at room temperature over a period of a few days. Lymphoblast cultures should be established within 48 hours, so prompt shipment is essential.

Fetal DNA can be isolated from amniotic cells, from trophoblastic cells taken by chorionic villus sam-

Table 34–7. Selected DNA probes with current diagnostic applications.

Gene Probe	Disorder	Diagnostic Application
β-Globin	Sickle cell disease Beta thalassemia	Prenatal Prenatal
α-Globin	Alpha thalassemia Polycystic kidney disease	Prenatal Presymptomatic, prenatal screening
Factor VIII	Hemophilia A	Prenatal, carrier detection
Dystrophin	Duchenne's muscular dystrophy	Presymptomatic, prenatal, carrier detection
α_1-AT	α_1-Antiprotease deficiency	Prenatal, screening
Phe hydroxylase	Phenylketonuria	Prenatal
CFTR	Cystic fibrosis	Prenatal, presymptomatic, carrier screening
G8, other chromosome 4 markers	Huntington's disease	Presymptomatic, prenatal
Growth hormone	Growth hormone deficiency	Prenatal, carrier detection, early diagnosis
HLA	Hemochromatosis Congenital adrenal hyperplasia	Presymptomatic, prenatal Prenatal

pling, or from either cell type grown in culture. Samples need to be processed promptly but can be shipped by overnight mail and *must not be frozen.*

Antonarakis S: Diagnosis of genetic disorders at the DNA level. N Engl J Med 1989;320:153. (Current techniques and copious references.)

Brandt J et al: Presymptomatic diagnosis of delayed-onset disease with linked DNA markers. JAMA 1989; 261:3108. (A model program for diagnosis and counseling.)

Gusella JF: Recombinant DNA techniques in the diagnosis of inherited disorders. J Clin Invest 1986;77:1723. (State of the art up to the age of polymerase chain reactions.)

Kazazian HH Jr: Diagnosis by gene amplification. J Lab Clin Med 1989;114:95. (Utility of PCR in DNA diagnosis.)

Kerem B et al: Identification of the cystic fibrosis gene: Genetic analysis. Science 1989;245:1073. (One of 3 articles—with Riordan et al and Rommens et al; see below—describing the fundamental defect in this most common lethal hereditary disorder. A triumph of so-called reverse genetics.)

Landegren U, Kaiser R, Caskey CT, Hood L: DNA diagnostics: Molecular techniques and automation. Science 1988;242:229. (Current knowledge and projections for the near future.)

Riordan JR et al: Identification of the cystic fibrosis gene: Cloning and characterization of complementary DNA. Science 1989;245:1066. (See comment at Kerem B et al, above.)

Rommens JM et al: Identification of the cystic fibrosis gene: Chromosome walking and jumping. Science 1989;245:1059. (See comment at Kerem B et al, above.)

PRENATAL DIAGNOSIS

It is possible to diagnose in utero, before the middle of the second trimester, several hundred mendelian disorders, all chromosome aberrations, and a number of congenital malformations that are not mendelian. The first step toward prenatal diagnosis is taken when the expecting couple, the primary physician, or the obstetrician thinks of the need for it. Recent surveys suggest that even for the most common indication for such service—advanced maternal age—well under half of all women 35 years and older are offered prenatal testing.

Techniques Used in Prenatal Diagnosis

Prenatal diagnosis depends on the ability to assay the fetus directly (fetal blood sampling, fetoscopy), indirectly (analysis of amniotic fluid, amniocytes or trophoblastic cells, ultrasound), or remotely (analysis of maternal serum). Some of these approaches have been used for decades, while others are still being developed. Some satisfy the requirements for screening (Table 34–4) and should be offered to all pregnant women; others carry considerable risk and should be reserved for specific circumstances. The technical details can be found in standard texts.

Ultrasound scanning of the fetus is a safe, noninvasive procedure that can diagnose gross skeletal malformations as well as bony malformations known to be associated with specific diseases. Obstetricians often use ultrasound to gauge fetal age and developmental progress; repeated sonography of an apparently healthy fetus is an unwarranted expense. Level II ultrasound is reserved for the fetus with a suspected abnormality.

Other prenatal diagnostic procedures—fetoscopy, fetography, and amniography—are more invasive and a definite risk to the mother and fetus. They are indicated only if the risk of the suspected abnormality is high and the information cannot be obtained by other means.

All of the cytogenetic, biochemical, and DNA analytic techniques discussed above can be applied to specimens from the fetus. Aside from screening for alpha-fetoprotein in maternal serum, analysis of fetal chromosomes is the most frequently performed test. Chromosomal analysis can be performed on amniotic cells and on trophoblastic cells grown in culture and directly on any trophoblastic cells that happen to be undergoing mitosis. Amniotic fluid cells are derived chiefly from the fetal urinary system. Amniocentesis is best performed between gestational weeks 16 and 18 to permit unhurried sample analysis, transmission of results, and reproductive decisions. The time from obtaining the sample to a final reading of the karyotype has now been shortened to an average of 10 days, and automated methods may reduce the time a bit further. Sampling the chorionic villus for trophoblastic cells (derived embryologically from the same fertilized egg as the fetus) is usually done between gestational weeks 8 and 10. If the tissue can be analyzed directly, cytogenetic results can be obtained within a few hours; however, the quality of the karyotypes is inferior to that from cultured cells, and most laboratories routinely culture cells and reexamine any suspected abnormalities. The advantage of chorionic villus sampling is that the results are available early in pregnancy, so that if termination is elected the couple will have had less time to relate to the pregnancy and the obstetric complications of termination are fewer.

The risk of chorionic villus sampling is somewhat higher than that of amniocentesis, though both are relatively safe. Between 0.5% and 1% of pregnancies are lost after chorionic villus sampling—a few of which would have spontaneously aborted in any event—whereas less than one in 300 amniocenteses result in fetal loss.

Indications for Prenatal Diagnosis

The indications for prenatal diagnosis are listed in Table 34–8. A few deserve comment.

Most studies done for advanced maternal age will

Table 34–8. Indications for prenatal diagnosis.

Indications	Methods
Advanced maternal age, previous child with chromosome aberration, intrauterine growth delay	Cytogenetics (amniocentesis, chorionic villus sampling)
Biochemical disorder	Protein assay, DNA diagnosis
Congenital anomaly	Ultrasound, fetoscopy
Screening for neural tube defects and trisomy	Maternal serum α-fetoprotein

detect no chromosomal aberration, and the couple will be reassured by this news. However, it is always appropriate to emphasize that any pregnancy has about a 3% risk of producing a child with a defect evident at birth, such as a physical malformation or some inborn error of metabolism. Simply examining the chromosomes will do little to reduce this underlying risk. On the other hand, unless one of the other indications is present, it is simply not possible to "screen" a pregnancy for other birth defects (neural tube defects being an exception).

A history of cytogenetic aberrations includes a documented chromosomal defect in a parent, a family history of a chromosomal defect, or a previous child or conceptus with a defined or undefined chromosomal defect. The factors that render some couples susceptible to repeated episodes of aneuploidy are unclear, and routine prenatal testing is warranted once a defect has occurred.

Cytogenetic analysis of the fetus will of course give information about the sex chromosomes. Some couples do not desire advance knowledge of the sex of their child, and the person transmitting the results to the couple should always address this issue first. On the other hand, some couples *only* want to know the sex of the fetus and plan to terminate the pregnancy if the undesired sex is detected. Few centers in the United States consider sex selection to be an appropriate indication for prenatal diagnosis.

The level of α-fetoprotein in maternal serum changes with gestational age, with the mother's medical status, and with abnormalities of the fetus. If the first 2 factors can be well controlled, the assay can be used to provide information about the fetus. Levels are expressed as multiples of the median value for a particular gestational age. Higher than normal levels are associated with open neural tube defects (the conditions for which the test was developed), recent fetal demise, gastroschisis, and fetal renal disease. Extremely high levels are highly specific for fetal anomalies—a level 3 times the median increases 20-fold the risk of meningomyelocele or anencephaly. During the early days of using this test, it was found that low α-fetoprotein levels in maternal serum were associated with fetal trisomy, especially Down's syndrome. The reason for this association is unclear; however, both high and low levels should prompt further investigation using other prenatal diagnostic techniques.

Ledbetter DH et al: Cytogenetic results of chorionic villus sampling: High success rate and diagnostic accuracy in the United States collaborative study. Am J Obstet Gynecol 1990;162:495. (Part of a multicenter collaborative study of chorionic villus sampling that proved its utility and documented its risks. See also Rhoads et al, below.)

Palomaki GE, Haddow JE: Maternal serum alpha-fetoprotein, age, and Down syndrome risk. Am J Obstet Gynecol 1987;156:460. (Data for predicting risk of aneuploidy based on an indirect measure.)

Ramiro R et al: *Prenatal Diagnosis of Congenital Anomalies.* Appleton & Lange, 1988. (A comprehensive text by the people who developed the applications of many of the techniques.)

Rhoads GG et al: The safety and efficacy of chorionic villus sampling for early prenatal diagnosis of cytogenetic abnormalities. N Engl J Med 1989;320:609. (See comment at Ledbetter et al, above.)

NEOPLASIA: CHROMOSOMAL ANALYSIS

Studies of both chromosomes and nucleic acids support Boveri's 1914 hypothesis that cancer is caused by a change in genetic material at the cellular level. Two classes of genes have been discovered that function in neoplastic transformation.

Oncogenes arise from preexisting normal genes (proto-oncogenes) that have been altered by both viral and nonviral factors. As a result, the cells synthesize either normal proteins in inappropriate amounts or proteins that are aberrant in structure and function. Many of these proteins are cellular growth factors, controllers of messenger RNA, and initiators and regulators of RNA; others are receptors for growth factors. The result is unregulated cell division.

Tumor suppressor genes can be viewed as the antithesis of oncogenes. Their normal function is to suppress transformation; mutation of their sequence obliterates this important function.

It seems clear from numerous examples in both human and animal tumors that more than one step is involved in oncogenesis. Which oncogenes and tumor suppressor genes are involved—and in which tissue—probably have major roles in determining the type of tumor, the age at onset, and the aggressiveness of growth and metastasis. A large number of these genes have been identified, cloned, and sequenced. Although some were identified in—and are now even named by—specific tumors, none are yet known to be pertinent to a single cancer. In a few cases, however, it is possible to analyze a patient's DNA for the presence of a mutated gene and thereby assess that individual's risk for developing a tumor. Examples are retinoblastoma and certain forms of Wilms's

tumor associated with aniridia. As rapidly as this field is advancing, it may be possible to provide susceptibility counseling to members of kindreds that are especially prone to certain types of tumors—especially adenocarcinoma of the bowel and breast cancer.

This exciting work on the molecular nature of oncogenesis was preceded by years of study of the cytogenetics of tumors. Indeed, the retinoblastoma tumor suppression gene was ultimately isolated because a small number of patients with this tumor have a constitutive deletion of chromosome 13 where this gene maps. Other chromosomal aberrations have been found to be highly characteristic of—or even specific for—certain tumors (Table 34–9). Detection of one of these cytogenetic aberrations can thus aid in diagnosis.

Hematologic malignancies are especially amenable to study because of the relative ease of performing cytogenetic analysis. Such malignancies are associated with over 100 specific chromosomal rearrangements, chiefly translocations. Most of these rearrangements are restricted to a specific type of cancer (Table 34–10), and the remainder occur with many cancers.

In the leukemias, the chromosomal aberration is the basis of one of the subclassifications of the disease. When cytogenetic information is combined with the FAB classification, it is possible to define subsets of patients in which response to therapy, clinical course, and prognosis are predictable. If at the time of diagnosis there are no chromosomal changes in the bone marrow cells, the survival time is longer than if any or all of the bone marrow cells have abnormal cytogenetic characteristics. As secondary chromosomal changes occur, the leukemia becomes more aggressive, often associated with drug resistance and a reduced chance for complete or prolonged remission. The least significant of all chromosomal changes is numerical alteration without morphologic abnormality.

Less cytogenetic information is available for lym-

Table 34–9. Chromosome aberrations associated with representative solid tumors.

Tumor	Chromosome Aberration
Meningioma	del(22)(q11)[1]
Neuroblastoma	del(1)(p36)
Renal cell carcinoma	del(3)(p14.2–p25) or translocation of this region
Retinoblastoma, osteosarcoma	del(13)(q14.1) or translocation of this region
Small-cell lung carcinoma	del(3)(p14–p23)
Wilms's tumor	del(11)(p15)

[1] Nomenclature means, "a deletion at band q11 of chromosome 22."

Table 34–10. Chromosomal aberrations associated with representative hematologic malignancies.

Tumor	Chromosomal Aberration
Leukemias	
Acute myeloblastic	t(8;21)(q22;q22)[1]
Acute promyelocytic	t(15;17)(q22;q11–q12)
Acute monocytic	t(10;11)(p15–p11;q23)
Chronic myelogenous	t(9;22)(q34;q11)
Lymphomas	
Burkitt's	t(8;14)(q24.1;q32.3)
B cell	t(1;14)(q42;q43)
T cell	inv, del, and t of 1p13–p12
Premalignancy	
Polycythemia vera	del(20)(q11)

[1] Nomenclature means, "a translocation with the union at band q22 of chromosome 8 and q22 of chromosome 21."

phomas and premalignant hematologic disorders than for leukemia. In Hodgkin's disease, studies have been limited by the low yield of dividing cells and the low number of clear-cut aneuploid clones, so that complete chromosomal analyses with banding are available for far fewer patients with Hodgkin's disease than for any other type of lymphoma. In Hodgkin's disease, the modal chromosomal number tends to be triploid or tetraploid. About one-third of the samples have a 14q+ chromosome. In non-Hodgkin's lymphomas, high-resolution techniques of banding detect abnormalities in 95% of cases. With the new International Formulation and Rappaport Classification of these lymphomas, cytogenetic findings are now being correlated with the immunologic and histologic features and with prognosis. This is particularly true in the case of follicular lymphoma.

By far the most information is available about Bur-

kitt's lymphoma, a solid tumor of B cell origin. Ninety percent of patients with this disorder have a translocation between the long arm of chromosome 8 and the long arm of chromosome 14, with chromosomal breakage sites being at or near immunoglobulin and oncogene loci.

Instability of chromosomes also predisposes to the development of cancer. In certain autosomal recessive diseases such as ataxia-telangiectasia, Bloom's syndrome, and Fanconi's anemia, the cells have a tendency to **genetic instability,** ie, to chromosomal breakage and rearrangement in vitro. These diseases are associated with a fairly high incidence of neoplasia, particularly leukemia and lymphoma.

Some chromosomal aberrations, better known for their effect on phenotype, also predispose to tumors. For example, patients with Down's syndrome (trisomy 21) have a 20-fold increase in the risk of leukemia; 47,XXY males (Klinefelter's syndrome) have a 30-fold increase in the risk of breast cancer; and XY phenotypic females have a heightened risk of developing ovarian cancer, primarily gonadoblastoma.

Friend SH, Dryja TP, Weinberg RA: Oncogenes and tumor-suppressing genes. N Engl J Med 1988;318:619. (Basic science and potential clinical utility.)

Levine EG et al: Cytogenetic abnormalities predict clinical outcome in non-Hodgkin lymphoma. Ann Intern Med 1988;108:14. (Patients without chromosome aberrations at diagnosis were more likely to achieve remission and to survive longer.)

Stanbridge EJ: Identifying tumor suppressor genes in human colorectal cancer. Science 1990;247:13. (The multiple-step, multiple-gene pathway leading from normal epithelium to carcinoma.)

Appendix

I. SELECTED IMAGING PROCEDURES: DESCRIPTIONS, INDICATIONS, & COSTS

Susan D. Wall, MD

CT, US, MRI, & IVP

Selection of the proper radiographic examination is becoming increasingly difficult with the numerous new modalities available today. Complex and often overlapping examinations that have been developed in the past decade offer sophisticated diagnostic tools to today's clinicians. Physicians can best use this complex armamentarium of radiographic examinations by having a clear awareness of their indications and limitations. The "study of choice" for many presumptive diagnoses depends on many factors, some of which are discussed here. Indications for computerized tomography (CT), magnetic resonance imaging (MRI), ultrasound (US), intravenous pyelography (IVP), gastrointestinal radiography, and radionuclide imaging (nuclear mdicine) are summarized, along with a discussion of pertinent risks and contraindications for each examination. Patient preparation is included as well as approximate costs. The limitations of radiology often are overlooked or not recognized, and so they are listed in some detail. Alternative examinations are suggested, and the advantages of each modality are discussed.

It is important to recognize that local expertise and the availability of "state of the art" equipment are fundamental to the selection of imaging examination. Clear and direct communication with the radiologist allows him or her to modify each examination as needed in order to answer the specific question referable to each patient. No study is "routine." The radiologist should be consulted regarding which study to do, when, and in what order. The information below provides a guideline for the nonradiologist physician.

COMPUTED TOMOGRAPHY (CT)

Indications

A. Head: Acute cranial-facial trauma; acute neurologic dysfunction ($<$ 72 hours), such as stroke, suspected subarachnoid or intracranial hemorrhage; sinuses for evaluation of ostia and sinus drainage; orbit when disease can be isolated to orbital apex and anterior; temporal bone except for evaluation of asymmetric sensorineural hearing loss; also for further characterization of some intracranial lesions identified by MRI (eg, presence or absence of calcium, evaluation of bony extension).

B. Spine: Indicated for patients in whom MRI is contraindicated and for evaluation of a few specific limitations of MRI such as defining calcification of the posterior longitudinal ligament, tumoral calcification, osteophytic spurring, retropulsed bone fragments following trauma.

C. Chest: Mediastinal and hilar lymphadenopathy; staging of some lung cancers; interstitial lung disease with thin section images (1.5 mm); parenchymal versus pleural process, esophageal wall.

D. Abdomen and Pelvis: Morphologic evaluation of all abdominal and pelvic organs; differentiation of intraperitoneal versus retroperitoneal disorders; abscess; mesenteric and retroperitoneal lymphadenopathy; bowel wall thickening; site of gastrointestinal obstruction; aortoenteric fistula with perigraft abscess in patient with reconstructed aorta; abdominal aortic aneurysm; appendicitis and diverticulitis when diagnosis is unclear or when there is a question of extraluminal disease; staging of some carcinomas of the gastrointestinal tract; staging of hypernephroma; obstructive biliary disease; splenic infarction; course of ureters; trauma; spontaneous retroperitoneal hemorrhage; response to chemotherapy; pancreatitis and its complications; pancreatic cancer; liver metastasis with bolus of intravenous contrast and fast ("dynamic") imaging. *Note:* Increased sensitivity with delayed imaging (4–6 hours after intravenous contrast study) and especially with CT arterial portography (CTAP).

Risks & Contraindications

Intravenous contrast medium imposes a hazard of allergic reaction, resulting in death in 1:120,000–1:60,000 examinations; increasing data suggest reduced risk with nonionic contrast medium, which costs approximately $150.00 compared to $2.50 for the usual dose of 150 mL for ionic contrast medium. Serum urea nitrogen and serum creatinine may be increased in patients with diabetes mellitus and multiple myeloma. There is a risk of bleeding with percutaneous fine-needle aspiration, especially with abnormal clotting parameters.

Patient Preparation

Opacification of gastrointestinal tract; normal hydration; sedation in agitated patients. Limitations: Availability; generally limited to transaxial images; limited differentiation of cystic versus solid lesions; bowel opacification important; dense barium or Hypaque causes severe artifact that precludes a diagnostic study; patient must be able to hold still and to breath hold; surgical clips and metallic prostheses cause artifacts and degrade images; cachexia limits diagnostic quality of images. NB: Increasingly, patients are being asked to give written informed consent for intravenous contrast material.

Usual Billed Amount

$950.00–1250.00.

Alternatives

Ultrasound (often complementary) and sometimes MRI.

Advantages

Rapid; superb spatial resolution; not limited by overlying bowel, as in ultrasound; can guide percutaneous fine-needle aspiration of possible tumor or abscess; can evaluate success of prior drainage procedures and determine catheter course and tip position. Multiple organ systems can be evaluated simultaneously.

ULTRASOUND (US)

Indications

A. Abdomen and Pelvis: Intraperitoneal fluid; cystic versus solid lesions of liver and kidneys; intra- and extrahepatic biliary dilatation; hydronephrosis; pancreatic morphology; peripancreatic fluid collections and pseudocyst; aortic aneurysm; size of prostate and volume of residual urine; intraperitoneal abscess; primary and metastatic liver tumor; intrahepatic versus subhepatic lesion; cholelithiasis; gallbladder wall thickness; perigallbladder fluid; appendicitis; possible pregnancy; pelvic inflammatory disease.

B. Chest: Pleural fluid; supra- versus infradiaphragmatic fluid; paralyzed diaphragm.

C. Neck: Parathyroid adenoma; thyroid; lymphadenopathy versus vessels; patency of carotid arteries.

D. Vascular: Doppler flow of arteries and veins.

Risks & Contraindications

None.

Patient Preparation

Preferably NPO for 6 hours; full urinary bladder for pelvic studies.

Limitations

Abdominal and pelvic organs may be obscured by overlying bowel; somewhat operator-dependent (less so with newer equipment); presence of barium impairs sound waves.

Usual Billed Amount

$300.00–500.00.

Alternatives

Computed tomography (often complementary).

Advantages

No radiation; can be portable; imaging in all planes; endovaginal and endorectal probes enhance pelvic imaging; can guide percutaneous fine-needle aspiration of possible tumor or abscess.

MAGNETIC RESONANCE IMAGING (MRI)

Indications

A. Head: Essentially all intracranial pathologic processes except those listed above for CT.

B. Neck: Evaluation of the upper aerodigestive tract; staging of neck masses, including suspected vascular tumors; better than CT for evaluation of lymphadenopathy as well as supra- and infraglottic extension of laryngeal tumors.

C. Chest: Mediastinal lymphadenopathy; tumor staging with respect to invasion of vessels or pericardium; aortic dissection; aortic aneurysm; congenital anomalies of the heart (especially pulmonary atresia) when echocardiography is inconclusive.

D. Abdomen: Clarification of CT findings when surgical clip artifacts degrade images; retroperitoneal lymphadenopathy when CT cannot differentiate blood vessels or diaphragmatic crus; preoperative staging of large hypernephroma; some cases calling for differentiation of benign nonhyperfunctioning adrenal adenoma from malignant adrenal mass; complementary to CT in evaluation of liver lesions, especially regarding metastatic disease and possible tumor invasion of differentiation of cavernous hemangioma of the liver from cancer.

E. Pelvis: Staging of cancers of the uterus, cervix, and prostate; complementary to CT for staging of cancer of the urinary bladder and prostate; recurrent rectal cancer following abdominal-perineal resection.

F. Musculoskeletal System: Joints (except where a prosthesis is in place), especially knees and hips; shoulders for rotator cuff tear and instability; wrists for carpal tunnel syndrome; temporal mandibular joint; extent of primary or malignant tumor (bone and soft tissue); aseptic necrosis of the femoral head or elsewhere; infections of bone and soft tissue; marrow disorders and contusions; stress fractures.

G. Spine: MRI is the best examination to begin the workup of most abnormalities of the spine and cord especially disk disease; spinal stenosis; partial or complete block; metastatic or primary tumor syringohydromyelia; most arteriovenous malformations (AVM) (see limitations below); myelitis.

Risks & Contraindications

Cardiac pacemaker; intraocular metallic foreign body; intracranial aneurysm clips; cochlear implants; some artificial cardiac valves; life support devices.

Patient Preparation

Sedation for patients unable to lie still. Screening CT of orbits to rule out metallic foreign body in eye if history uncertain. For examination of the abdomen and pelvis, the patient should be NPO for 6 hours, followed by colon cleansing, glucagon during the study.

Limitations

Sensitivity to motion artifacts; need for intravenous contrast (such as gadolinium DTPA) for subarachnoid lesions and for small extra-axial masses; gastrointestinal opacification not yet readily available; claustrophobia; detection of calcification; dural-based or perimedullary AVMs are easily missed because of their small size (supine myelography better); detection of loose bodies; osseous encroachment of the spinal canal and neural foramina can be exaggerated by patient movement; cerebrospinal fluid pulsation artifacts may mimic flow void associated with AVM.

Usual Billed Amount

$900.00–1400.00.

Alternatives

CT scan.

Advantages

No beam-hardening artifacts; exquisite sensitivity to lesions; multiplanar capability; no ionizing radiation.

INTRAVENOUS PYELOGRAPHY (IVP)

Indications

Uroepithelial neoplasm, calculus, papillary necrosis and medullary sponge kidney, trauma.

Risks & Contraindications

Intravenous contrast media impose a hazard of allergic reactions, resulting in death in 1:40,000–1:30,000 examinations; increasing data suggest reduced risk with nonionic contrast medium, which costs approximately $100.00 for the usual dose of 100 mL compared to $1.67 for ionic contrast medium. Serum urea nitrogen and serum creatinine may be increased in patients with diabetes mellitus and multiple myeloma.

Patient Preparations

Adequate hydration; colon cleansing is not essential but is preferred.

Limitations

Optimal evaluation of the collecting system only; suboptimal evaluation of the renal parenchyma; does not adequately evaluate cause of ureteral deviation.

Usual Billed Amount

$300.00–350.00.

Alternatives

Ultrasound, CT, MRI.

Advantages

Better at evaluation of collecting system than alternative techniques listed above.

BARIUM RADIOLOGY

UPPER GASTROINTESTINAL STUDY

Indications

Double-contrast technique (air-contrast followed by thin barium) demonstrates esophageal, gastric, and duodenal mucosa for evaluation of inflammatory disease and early plaque lesions. Single-contrast technique is suitable for evaluation of possible outlet obstruction, peristaltic evaluation, gastroesophageal reflux and hiatal hernia, esophageal cancer, esophageal varices. Water-soluble contrast (Gastrografin) is suitable for evaluation of anastomotic leak or gastrointestinal perforation, but can be dangerous (see below).

Risks & Contraindications

Aspiration of water-soluble contrast material incites severe pulmonary edema and possibly death; perforation with barium can cause a granulomatous inflammatory reaction. Caution in pregnancy because of hazards of exposure of fetus to x-rays.

Patient Preparation

Patient *must* be NPO for 8 hours.

Limitations

Identification of a lesion does not prove it to be the site of blood loss in patients with gastrointestinal bleeding; endoscopy is required, and the presence of barium delays both endoscopy (because it will ruin the endoscope) and body CT examination (because it will cause severe artifact); retained gastric secretions prevent mucosal coating with barium; patient cooperation and ability to move about is required.

Usual Billed Amount

$320.00–400.00.

Alternatives

Endoscopy.

Advantages

Mucosal evaluation with double-contrast examination. No sedation required.

ENTEROCLYSIS

Indications

Evaluation of site of partial small bowel obstruction; extent of Crohn's disease; small bowel disease in patients with gastrointestinal bleeding who have normal upper gastrointestinal and colonic evaluations; metastatic disease to small bowel.

Risks & Contraindications

Because radiation exposure is substantial during the lengthy fluoroscopic examination required, this modality should be used sparingly in children and women of childbearing age. *Must not be used if the patient might be pregnant.*

Patient Preparation

Colonic cleansing and 24 hours of clear liquid diet. (The latter is the more important part of the preparation and is crucial in order to cleanse the small bowel of particulate matter.)

Limitations

Requires nasogastric or orogastric intubation and manipulation of tube to position it beyond the ligament of Treitz; "biphasic" examination is then performed with barium (for "single contrast") followed by methylcellulose (for "double contrast") introduced by means of a hemodialysis pump at a controlled rate; often cannot optimally evaluate the first loop of jejunum or terminal ileum.

Usual Billed Amount

$500.00–550.00.

Alternatives

Dedicated small bowel examination with oral inges-

tion of barium and frequent fluoroscopic imaging; CT of abdomen and pelvis.

Advantages

Clarification of possible lesions noted on more traditional barium examination of the small bowel; best means of establishing small bowel as normal; controlled high rate of flow of barium can elicit dilatation at site of intermittent partial obstruction.

PERORAL PNEUMOCOLON

Indications

The best means of evaluation of the terminal ileum by means of insufflation of air per rectum after orally ingested barium has reached the cecum.

Risks & Contraindications

Contraindicated in patients with toxic megacolon.

Patient Preparation

The patient should take a clear liquid diet for 24 hours as well as colon cleansing.

Limitations

Undigested food in the small bowel interferes with the evaluation.

Usual Billed Amount

Adds about $50.00 to the cost of upper gastrointestinal series.

Alternatives

CT for wall thickening.

Advantages

Best evaluation of terminal ileum; can be performed concurrently with upper gastrointestinal series.

BARIUM ENEMA

Indications

Double-contrast technique for evaluation of colonic mucosa in patients with suspected inflammatory or neoplastic disease; single-contrast technique for investigation of possible fistulous tracts or bowel obstruction, large or palpable masses in the abdomen, diverticulitis, and for debilitated patients.

Risks & Contraindications

Contraindicated in patients with toxic megacolon.

Patient Preparation

Colon cleansing with enemas, cathartic, and clear liquid diet (1 day in young patients; may take 2 days in older patients); possible use of intravenous glucagon for spasm versus mass lesion.

Limitations

Retained fecal material; requires patient cooperation and movement; marked diverticulosis precludes evaluation of possible neoplastic lesion in that area; evaluation of right colon occasionally incomplete or limited by reflux of barium across ileocecal valve as well as overlapping opacified small bowel; presence of barium delays colonoscopy and body CT.

Usual Billed Amount

Pneumocolon (air contrast) $450.00; single contrast $350.00.

Alternatives

Colonoscopy, abdominopelvic CT for possible wall thickening.

Advantages

Mucosal evaluation; no sedation required.

DIATRIZOATE SODIUM (HYPAQUE) ENEMA

Indications

Evaluation of sigmoid or cecal volvulus; anastomotic leak, or other type of perforation; differentiation of colonic versus small bowel obstruction; therapeutic for obstipation.

Risks & Contraindications

Contraindicated in patients with toxic megacolon.

Patient Preparation

Colonic cleansing is desirable but not always necessary.

Limitations

Demonstrates only colonic morphologic features and not mucosal changes.

Usual Billed Amount

About $350.00.

Alternatives

Colonoscopy.

Advantages

Water-soluble contrast medium is evacuated much faster than barium (because it does not adhere to the mucosa), so it can be followed immediately or within several hours by oral ingestion of barium for evaluation of possible distal small bowel obstruction.

DIAGNOSTIC NUCLEAR MEDICINE PROCEDURES

CENTRAL NERVOUS SYSTEM IMAGING

1. BRAIN SCAN

Radiopharmaceuticals

99m Tc pertechnetate (TcO_4)
99m Tc diethylenetriamine pentaacetic acid (DTPA)
99m Tc glucoheptonate
123 I iodoamphetamine (IMP)
99m Tc hexamethyl-propyleneamine oxime (HMPAO)

Indications

Establishment of brain death, suspected herpes simplex encephalitis, seizures, neuropsychiatric disorders.

Risks & Contraindications

Caution in pregnancy is advised because of the risk of ionizing radiation to the fetus.

Patient Preparation

Sedation in agitated patients. Premedication with potassium perchlorate when using TcO_4 in order to block choroid plexus uptake.

Limitations

Limited resolution. Delayed imaging (1–4 hours) often required. Limited availability of IMP and HMPAO. The latter 2 agents also require single photon emission computed tomography (SPECT) capabilities that may not be available at some institutions.

Usual Billed Amount

$350.00–750.00.

Alternatives

CT, MRI.

Advantages

Functional information. Portable capability of brain scan can be valuable in ICU for assessment of brain death.

2. CISTERNOGRAPHY

Radiopharmaceuticals

111 In DTPA.

Indications

Hydrocephalus (particularly normal pressure), shunt patency, CSF rhinorrhea or otorrhea.

Risks & Contraindications

Strict sterile precautions for intrathecal injection. Caution in pregnancy is advised because of the risk of ionizing radiation to the fetus.

Patient Preparation

For suspected cerebrospinal fluid leak, the patient's nose or ears should be packed with cotton pledgets prior to administration of dose. Sedation of agitated patients.

Limitations

Availability of 111 indium. Patients must be able to hold still. Requires multiple delayed imaging sessions up to 48–72 hours after injection.

Usual Billed Amount

$500.00–600.00.

Alternatives

CT often complementary.

Advantages

Functional information, particularly in distinguishing normal pressure hydrocephalus from senile atrophy in elderly patients. Very sensitive in detecting cerebrospinal fluid leaks.

ENDOCRINE

1. THYROID UPTAKE & SCAN

Radiopharmaceuticals

99m TcO_4
123 I sodium iodide
131 I sodium iodide

Indications

Uptake indicated for evaluation of hypothyroidism, hyperthyroidism, and thyroiditis and for calculation of therapeutic dosage. Thyroid scanning indicated for evaluation of palpable nodules, mediastinal mass, hyperthyroidism, and in patients with history of head and neck irradiation. Total body scanning used for evaluation of metastatic thyroid cancer.

Risks & Contraindications

Substances that interfere with thyroid uptake should be withheld for days to several weeks depending on substance (prior TcO_4 scan, iodides in vitamins and medicines, radiographic procedures using iodinated contrast, thyroid replacement medications, antithyroid drugs). Not advised in pregnancy because of the risk of ionizing radiation to the fetus (iodides cross placenta and concentrate in fetal thyroid). Because of significant radiation exposure in total body scanning with 131 I, patients should be instructed by nuclear medicine personnel regarding precautionary measures.

Patient Preparation

Administration of dose in the fasting state—nothing by mouth for 4–6 hours—aids absorption.

Limitations

Many common substances interfere with thyroid uptake and scanning. Small size of the thyroid gland requires use of a pinhole collimator. This technique does not distinguish solid from cystic masses. Poor resolution with 131 I limits use to uptake and total body scanning. Delayed imaging is required with iodides (123 I, 6 hours; 131 I total body, 72 hours).

Usual Billed Amount

$350.00–650.00.

Alternatives

Small parts ultrasound often complementary.

Advantages

Functional information. Identification of "cold" nodules that have a greater risk of malignancy. Identification of ectopic thyroid tissue. Imaging of total body with one dose (131 I).

2. PARATHYROID SCAN

Radiopharmaceuticals

201 thallium chloride
99m TcO_4 subtraction

Indications

Suspected parathyroid adenoma.

Risks & Contraindications

Patient must be able to hold still. Caution in pregnancy is advised because of the risk of ionizing radiation to the fetus. Use of agents that block thyroid uptake of TcO_4 (see above).

Patient Preparation

None required.

Limitations

Pinhole collimator recommended. Computer subtraction requires strict patient immobility between administration of radiopharmaceuticals. Small adenomas may not be detected (< 5–10 mm).

Usual Billed Amount

$400.00–500.00.

Alternatives
Ultrasound often complementary.

Advantages
Identification of hyperfunctioning tissue, particularly when planning surgery.

3. ADRENAL MEDULLARY IMAGING

Radiopharmaceuticals
131 I metaiodobenzylguanidine (MIBG)

Indications
Suspected pheochromocytoma.

Risks & Contraindications
Patient must be compliant (return for imaging on 1–3 consecutive days). Contraindicated in pregnancy because of the risk of ionizing radiation to the fetus. Because of the relatively high dose of 131 I, patients must be instructed regarding precautionary measures.

Patient Preparation
Administration of Lugol's iodine solution (to block thyroid uptake) prior to and following administration of dose.

Limitations
High radiation dose to adrenal gland. High cost and limited availability of radiopharmaceutical. Delayed imaging (1–3 days) necessitates return of patient.

Usual Billed Amount
$1000.00–1400.00.

Alternatives
CT, MRI.

Advantages
Test is useful for localization of pheochromocytomas—particularly those found in extra-adrenal tissue—and for multiple lesions.

CARDIOVASCULAR

1. MYOCARDIAL PERFUSION

Radiopharmaceuticals
201 thallium chloride.

Indications
Evaluation of chest pain. Detection of presence, location, and extent of myocardial ischemia.

Risks & Contraindications
Recent infarct. Risk of arrhythmia, ischemia, infarct, and, rarely, death. Patient must be able to exercise on a treadmill. In cases of peripheral vascular disease or of neurovascular or musculoskeletal disorders, pharmacologic stress with dipyridamole may be used. Dependence on aminophylline (inhibitor of dipyridamole) is a contraindication to the use of dipyridamole. Patient must be able to hold still for SPECT imaging. Caution in pregnancy because of the risk of ionizing radiation to the fetus.

Patient Preparation
Exercise and thallium administration should be performed in fasting state. Patients optimally should remain fasting between stress and redistribution. Dipyridamole may be administered orally or intravenously prior to thallium.

Limitations
The patient must be carefully monitored during stress on treadmill or pharmacologic stress—optimally, under the supervision of a cardiologist. Submaximal stress decreases sensitivity for ischemia. Imaging must begin immediately following stress to prevent early redistribution. Patients should not eat heavily or exercise between stress and redistribution images. Patients must return for redistribution images 4 hours following stress. SPECT, which increases sensitivity, may not be available at some institutions. Interpretation of study may be difficult in severe 3-vessel coronary artery disease.

Usual Billed Amount
$500.00–950.00.

Alternatives
Radionuclide ventriculography often complementary. Coronary angiography is "gold standard."

Advantages
Highly sensitive for detection of physiologically significant coronary stenosis. Noninvasive.

2. MYOCARDIAL INFARCT SCANNING

Radiopharmaceuticals
99m Tc pyrophosphate
201 thallium chloride

Indications
For determination of localization and extent of acute myocardial infarction.

Risks & Contraindications
Patient must be able to hold still. Caution in pregnancy because of the risk of ionizing radiation to the fetus.

Patient Preparation
Sedation of agitated patients.

Limitations

Pyrophosphate scan most sensitive at 24–72 hours. Sensitivity of thallium scan decreases after 24 hours. Sensitivity of both pyrophosphate and thallium scans lower for nontransmural infarcts. Location of infarct also affects sensitivity (highest for anterior wall). Patients with unstable angina may have falsely positive thallium scan. Pyrophosphate scan may be positive in patients who have undergone recent cardioversion. Pyrophosphate scan may be persistently positive in up to 20% of patients with remote histories of infarct.

Usual Billed Amount

$350.00–450.00.

Alternatives

Radionuclide ventriculography often complementary. Coronary angiography for identification of occluded vessels.

Advantages

Pyrophosphate imaging identifies acutely infarcted myocardium—in contrast to thallium and coronary angiography. Also helpful in the evaluation of perioperative infarcts in patients who have undergone recent cardiac surgery where CPK and electrocardiographic findings may be misleading.

3. RADIONUCLIDE VENTRICULOGRAPHY

Radiopharmaceuticals

99m Tc-labeled red blood cells.

Indications

Evaluation of patients with ischemic heart disease, other cardiomyopathies, response to pharmacologic therapy of heart disease, effects of cardiotoxic drugs.

Risks & Contraindications

Recent infarct is contraindication to exercise ventriculography. Arrhythmia, ischemia, infarct, and, rarely, death with exercise. Caution advised in pregnancy because of the risk of ionizing radiation to the fetus. Sterile technique required in handling of red cells.

Limitations

Requires labeling and reinjection of red cells. Gated data acquisition may be difficult in patients with severe arrhythmias. Limited to resting study in patients who are unable to exercise on a supine bicycle.

Usual Billed Amount

$500.00–1200.00.

Alternatives

Thallium perfusion scan often complementary. Cardiac echogram. Cardiac catheterization ventriculography. Gated magnetic resonance imaging.

Advantages

Noninvasive. Resting ejection fraction is a reproducible index that can be used to follow course of disease and response to therapy.

PULMONARY IMAGING

1. VENTILATION-PERFUSION SCAN

Radiopharmaceuticals

99m Tc macroaggregated albumin (MAA, perfusion)
133 xenon (ventilation)
99m Tc DTPA aerosol (ventilation)

Indications

Pulmonary embolism, preoperative evaluation of patients with COPD or those who are candidates for pneumonectomy, burn inhalation injury.

Risks & Contraindications

The number of particles injected should be reduced in patients with severe pulmonary artery hypertension. Patients must be able to cooperate for ventilation portion of examination. Caution advised in pregnancy because of the risk of ionizing radiation to the fetus.

Patient Preparation

None.

Limitations

Adequate means of trapping xenon. When ventilation with xenon is performed prior to perfusion scan, identification of ventilation-perfusion mismatch may be limited by single posterior ventilation image. Correlation with chest radiograph is mandatory for interpretation. High proportion of indeterminate studies in patients with underlying lung disease. Low probability scan still has an up to 10% possibility of pulmonary embolus.

Usual Billed Amount

$400.00–850.00.

Alternatives

Pulmonary angiography.

Advantages

Noninvasive. Functional information in preoperative assessment.

RETICULOENDOTHELIAL & BILIARY IMAGING

1. LIVER & SPLEEN SCAN

Radiopharmaceuticals
99m Tc sulfur colloid
99m Tc heat-damaged red blood cells (spleen)

Indications
Metastatic or primary tumor, inflammatory process, palpable mass, organomegaly, elevated hepatic enzymes, alcoholic liver disease, thrombocytopenia, search for accessory spleen, suspected subphrenic abscess.

Risks & Contraindications
Caution in pregnancy advised because of the risk of ionizing radiation to the fetus.

Patient Preparation
None.

Limitations
Diminished sensitivity for small (< 2 cm.), deep lesions. SPECT increases sensitivity; can detect 1–1.5 cm lesions. Nonspecific; unable to distinguish solid from cystic or inflammatory or neoplastic tissue. Lower sensitivity for diffuse hepatic tumor; may be difficult to distinguish from liver disease due to other causes. Artifacts can be caused by dense foreign body within gastrointestinal tract (eg, barium).

Usual Billed Amount
$400.00–750.00.

Alternatives
Ultrasound for evaluation of solid or cystic mass. CT more sensitive than scintigraphy and ultrasound, particularly for detection of deep lesions. MRI offers advantages of tissue specific diagnosis.

Advantages
Better sampling and more sensitive than ultrasound. May detect lesions missed by CT as a result of isodensity. Reproducible means of following response to chemotherapy.

2. HEPATOBILIARY SCAN

Radiopharmaceuticals
99m Tc N-substituted iminodiacetic acids (IDA).

Indications
Functional status of hepatocytes and biliary excretion. Hepatocellular dysfunction, obstruction from stone, tumor or infection, biliary atresia.

Risks & Contraindications
Caution in pregnancy because of the risk of ionizing radiation to the fetus.

Patient Preparation
Fasting 4–6 hours. Premedicate with CCK in some institutions.

Limitations
Does not demonstrate cause of obstruction (ie, tumor or gallstones). Sensitivity lower for acalculous cholecystitis (80%). May not be able to evaluate biliary excretion if hepatocellular function is severely impaired. May require delayed imaging (up to 24 hours) to distinguish acute from chronic cholecystitis. Visualization may be expedited by use of intravenous morphine sulfate. Nonvisualization can occur in hyperalimentation, nonfasting, prolonged fasting, acute pancreatitis, severe hepatocellular disease.

Usual Billed Amount
$400.00–500.00.

Alternatives
Oral cholecystogram, ultrasonography.

Advantages
Hepatobiliary functional information. Not dependent on intestinal absorption, as in oral cholecystography. Can be performed in patients with elevated bilirubin (up to 10–20 mg/dL). Does not expose patients to risk of iodinated contrast media.

GASTROINTESTINAL SYSTEM

1. GASTROINTESTINAL BLEEDING SCAN

Radiopharmaceuticals
99m Tc labeled red cells
99m Tc sulfur colloid

Indications
Evaluation of upper or lower gastrointestinal blood loss.

Risks & Contraindications
Caution advised in pregnancy because of the risk of ionizing radiation to the fetus. Sterile technique required in handling of red cells.

Patient Preparation
Nasogastric suction necessary for study with in vivo labeled red cells to eliminate free pertechnetate excreted by gastric mucosa.

Limitations
Bleeding must be active during time of imaging.

Sulfur colloid imaging time limited to approximately 1 hour, whereas red cells can be imaged for up to 24 hours. When sulfur colloid is used, upper gastrointestinal bleeding can be obscured by liver and spleen activity. Longer imaging time required for labeled red cells because of higher background activity. The presence of free pertechnetate (poor labeling efficiency) can lead to gastric, kidney, and bladder activity that can be misinterpreted as sites of bleeding. Penile activity is often present with both labeled red cells and sulfur colloid and may mimic rectal bleeding.

Usual Billed Amount
$500.00–700.00.

Alternatives
Angiography.

Advantages
Noninvasive compared to angiography. Longer period of imaging possible, which aids in detection of intermittent bleeding. Both labeled red cells and sulfur colloid can detect bleeding rates of as little as 0.05–0.10 mL/min. However, while there is greater potential for false-positive interpretation of labeled red cell scan, this method has been shown to be more sensitive than sulfur colloid for detection of gastrointestinal bleeding.

2. GASTRIC EMPTYING

Radiopharmaceuticals
99m Tc sulfur colloid in solid portion of meal.
111 In DTPA in liquid portion of meal.

Indications
Dumping syndrome, vagotomy, gastric outlet obstruction due to inflammatory or neoplastic disease, effects of drugs, diabetes mellitus, and other causes of gastroparesis.

Risks & Contraindications
Must be able to eat a 300-g meal consisting of liquids and solids. Not advisable in pregnancy due to risk of ionizing radiation to fetus.

Patient Preparation
Fasting for 4–6 hours.

Limitations
Meaningful data requires adherence to standard protocol and establishment of normal values.

Usual Billed Amount
$300.00–500.00.

Alternatives
Gastrointestinal endoscopy. Upper gastrointestinal series demonstrates peristalsis but cannot quantitate emptying.

Advantages
Gives functional information not available by other means of evaluations.

3. ESOPHAGEAL REFLUX

Radiopharmaceuticals
99m Tc sulfur colloid in 300 mL liquid.

Indications
Evaluation of heartburn and regurgitation.

Risks & Contraindications
Must be able to consume 300 mL of liquid. Not advisable in pregnancy because of the risk of ionizing radiation to the fetus.

Patient Preparation
Fasting for 4–6 hours.

Limitations
Incomplete emptying of esophagus may mimic reflux. Use of abdominal binder to increase lower-esophageal pressure may not be tolerated in patients who have undergone recent abdominal surgery.

Usual Billed Amount
$200.00–300.00.

Alternatives
Barium fluoroscopy, endoscopy, lower esophageal sphincter pressure measurements, acid reflux study.

Advantages
Noninvasive and well tolerated. More sensitive than fluoroscopy, endoscopy, and measurement of lower esophageal sphincter pressure. Similar to acid reflux test in sensitivity. Permits quantitation of reflux. Can also evaluate aspiration into lung fields.

GENITOURINARY SYSTEM

1. RENAL SCAN

Radiopharmaceuticals
99m Tc diethylenetriamine pentaacetic acid (DTPA, glomerular filtration rate agent)
131 I orthoiodohippurate (Hippuran, tubular agent)
99m Tc dimercaptosuccinic acid (DMSA, parenchymal agent)
99m Tc glucoheptonate (parenchymal agent)

Indications

Evaluation of renal blood flow and function in acute or chronic renal failure. Renal transplant evaluation. Estimation of glomerular filtration rate and effective renal plasma flow. Determination of relative function prior to nephrectomy. Parenchymal agents useful in assessment of obstruction. Captopril used in suspected renovascular hypertension.

Risks & Contraindications

Relatively high radiation dose with 131 I Hippuran. Good hydration and frequent bladder emptying advised. Caution in pregnancy because of the risk of ionizing radiation to the fetus.

Patient Preparation

None.

Limitations

Findings of poor renal blood flow and function are nonspecific. High background activity with extremely poor renal function limits usefulness in evaluation of other factors such as obstruction, relative function, cortical lesions. Estimation of GFR (glomerular filtration rate) and ERPF (effective renal plasma flow) based on anatomic presumptions that often introduce error. One- to 4-hour delayed images necessary with parenchymal agents. Parenchymal agents are nonspecific and do not give information about solid versus cystic nature of lesions.

Usual Billed Amount

$300.00–700.00.

Alternatives

Intravenous pyelography, ultrasound, CT.

Advantages

Functional information available without risk of iodinated contrast used in IVP. Quantitative information not available by other means.

MUSCULOSKELETAL SYSTEM

1. BONE SCAN

Radiopharmaceuticals

99m Tc phosphate compounds (methylene diphosphonate—MDP most widely used).

Indications

Primary or metastatic neoplasm, infection, arthritis, metabolic disorders, trauma, avascular necrosis, joint prosthesis.

Risks & Contraindications

Caution in pregnancy because of the risk of ionizing radiation to the fetus.

Patient Preparation

None.

Limitations

Nonspecific. Correlation with plain film radiographs often necessary. Two- to 3-hour delayed images necessary. In patients with poor renal function, image quality may be poor because of high background activity. Resolution often insufficient for localization of disease in distal extremities, head, and spine; in these instances, SPECT is often useful. In evaluation of infection, it may be difficult to distinguish osteomyelitis from cellulitis or septic joint. Dual imaging with gallium or with indium-labeled leukocytes can be helpful but not always definitive. Diagnosis of infection also limited by surgery or fracture. Bone scan may be hot, cold, or normal, depending on the stage of avascular necrosis. Bone scan may be negative within the first 24 hours after trauma.

Usual Billed Amount

$400.00–750.00.

Alternatives

Plain film radiography, MRI for tumor or infection. Leukocyte or gallium scan often complementary for infection.

Advantages

Entire body is surveyed. Highly sensitive compared to plain film radiography for detection of bone neoplasm. Bone scan may be positive much earlier in osteomyelitis (24 hours) compared to plain film (10–14 days).

INFLAMMATORY & NEOPLASTIC IMAGING

1. LEUKOCYTE SCAN

Radiopharmaceuticals

111 In oxine-labeled leukocytes.

Indications

Fever of unknown origin, postoperative patient, suspected abscess, pyelonephritis, osteomyelitis.

Risks & Contraindications

High radiation dose to spleen. Homologous donor leukocytes should be used in neutropenic patients. Sterile handling of leukocytes necessary. Contraindicated in pregnancy because of the hazard of ionizing radiation to the fetus. Patients must be able to hold still during relatively long acquisition times (5–10 minutes).

Patient Preparation

Venous blood drawn and leukocytes harvested and

labeled in vitro prior to reinjection. Process requires 1–2 hours. Leukocytes injected 24 hours prior to imaging.

Limitations

Twenty-four-hour delayed imaging may be contraindicated in critically ill patients. Imaging may be performed as early as 4 hours at the expense of lower sensitivity for detection of infection (30–50% of abscesses detected at 24 hours). False-negative scan possible in theory as a consequence of antibiotic administration or in chronic infection. Perihepatic or splenic infection foci can be missed as a result of normal leukocyte accumulation in these organs; liver and spleen scan is a necessary adjunct in this situation. Many causes of false-positive scans such as swallowed leukocytes, bleeding, indwelling tubes and catheters, surgical skin wound uptake, bowel activity due to inflammatory processes. Leukocytes may also accumulate in tumors in the absence of infection. Pulmonary uptake is nonspecific and has low predictive value for infection.

Usual Billed Amount

$700.00–800.00.

Alternatives

Ultrasound or CT for assessment of suspected abscess, particularly in critically ill patient, where 24-hour delayed imaging is undesirable. Bone scan and gallium scan often complementary in assessment of osteomyelitis.

Advantages

Although false-positive causes of uptake exist, the leukocyte scan is highly specific (98%) for infection—in contrast to gallium. Sensitivity for detection of abdominal source of infection is higher with indium, since leukocytes do not normally accumulate in abdominal organs other than liver and spleen. In patients with fever of unknown origin, total body imaging is advantageous compared to CT scan or ultrasound. Preliminary imaging as early as 4 hours is possible but less sensitive.

2. GALLIUM SCAN

Radiopharmaceuticals

67 Ga citrate.

Indications

Fever of unknown origin, infection (particularly chronic), inflammatory processes (most useful in lung), tumor (largely replaced by CT).

Risks & Contraindications

Not advisable in pregnancy because of the risk of ionizing radiation to the fetus. Patient must be reliable to return for imaging 72 hours after injection.

Patient Preparation

Gallium dose is injected 72 hours prior to imaging.

Limitations

Long time (2–3 days) necessary for clearance of background activity prior to imaging. Normal accumulation in bowel and reticuloendothelial system may obscure detection of abdominal abscess. Early accumulation of activity in kidneys (< 24 hours) may impair evaluation. Because of the poor imaging characteristics of gallium, resolution may be insufficient for detection of lesions less than 2 cm in lung, brain, and bone. Even larger lesions may be missed in the abdomen and pelvis, where background activity is high.

Usual Billed Amount

$700.00–800.00.

Alternatives

Leukocyte scan more specific for infection. Radionuclide bone scan often complementary in evaluation of osteomyelitis. CT has largely replaced gallium in evaluation of cancer. Plain chest radiograph or CT for evaluation of pulmonary disease.

Advantages

Gallium more sensitive than CT or chest x-ray in detection of pulmonary disease such as *Pneumocystis carinii* pneumonia, sarcoidosis, and other inflammatory processes. Gallium may be more helpful than leukocyte scan in assessment of chronic infection.

II. NORMAL LABORATORY VALUES (Blood [B], Plasma [P], Serum [S], Urine [U])

Marcus A. Krupp, MD

HEMATOLOGY

Bleeding time: Ivy method, 1–7 minutes (60–420 seconds). Template method, 3–9 minutes (180–540 seconds).

Cellular measurements of red cells: Average diameter = 7.3 μm (5.5–8.8 μm). Mean corpuscular volume (MCV): Men, 80–94 fL; women, 81–99 fL (by Coulter counter). Mean corpuscular hemoglobin (MCH): 27–32 pg. Mean corpuscular hemoglobin concentration (MCHC): 32–36 g/dL red blood cells (32–36%).

Clot retraction: Begins in 1–3 hours; complete in 6–24 hours. No clot lysis in 24 hours.

Fibrinogen split products: Negative > 1:4 dilution.

Fragility of red cells: Begins at 0.45–0.38% NaCl; complete at 0.36–0.3% NaCl.

Hematocrit (PCV): Men, 40–52% (0.4–0.52); women, 37–47% (0.37–0.47).

Hemoglobin: [B] Men, 14–18 g/dL (2.09–2.79 mmol/L as Hb tetramer); women, 12–16 g/dL (1.86–2.48 mmol/L). [S] 2–3 mg/dL.

Partial thromboplastin time: Activated, 25–37 seconds.

Platelets: 150,000–400,000/μL (0.15–0.4 × 10^{12}/L).

Prothrombin time: [P] Less than 2 seconds deviation from control.

Red blood count (RBC): Men, 4.5–6.2 million/μL (4.5–6.2 × 10^{12}/L); women, 4–5.5 million/μL (4–5.5 × 10^{12}/L).

Reticulocytes: 0.2–2% of red cells.

Sedimentation rate: Less than 20 mm/h (Westergren); 0–10 mm/h (Wintrobe).

White blood count (WBC) and differential: 5000–10,000/μL (5–10 × 10^9/L).

Myelocytes	0 %
Juvenile neutrophils	0 %
Band neutrophils	0–5 %
Segmented neutrophils	40–60%
Lymphocytes	20–40%
Eosinophils	1–3 %
Basophils	0–1 %
Monocytes	4–8 %
Lymphocytes: Total, 1500–4000/μL	
B cell	5–25%
T cell	60–88%
Suppressor	10–43%
Helper	32–66%
H:S	>1

BLOOD, PLASMA, OR SERUM CHEMICAL CONSTITUTENTS
(Values vary with method used.)

Acetone and acetoacetate: [S] 0.3–2 mg/dL (3–20 mg/L).

α-Amino acid nitrogen: [S, fasting] 3–5.5 mg/dL (2.2–3.9 mmol/L).

Aminotransferases:
Aspartate aminotransferase (AST; SGOT) (varies with method): 0–41 IU/L at 37 °C.
Alanine aminotransferase (ALT; SGPT) (varies with method): 0–45 IU/L at 37 °C.

Ammonia: [P] (as NH_3): 10–80 μg/dL (5–50 μmol/L).

Amylase: [S] 80–180 units/dL (Somogyi).

$α_1$–Antitrypsin: [S] > 180 mg/dL.

Ascorbic acid: [P] 0.4–1.5 mg/dL (23–85 μmol/L).

Base, total serum: [S] 145–160 meq/L (145–160 mmol/L).

Bicarbonate: [S] 24–28 meq/L (24–28 mmol/L).

Bilirubin: [S] Total, 0.2–1.2 mg/dL (2–20.5 μmol/L). Direct (conjugated), 0.1–0.4 mg/dL (< 7 μmol/L). Indirect, 0.2–0.7 mg/dL (< 12 μmol/L).

Calcium: [S] 8.5–10.3 mg/dL (2.1–2.6 mmol/L). Values vary with albumin concentration.

Calcium, ionized: [S] 4.25–5.25 mg/dL; 2.1–2.6 meq/L (1.05–1.3 mmol/L).

β-Carotene: [S, fasting] 50–300 μg/dL (0.9–5.58 μmol/L).

Ceruloplasmin: [S] 25–43 mg/dL (1.7–2.9 μmol/L).

Chloride: [S or P] 96–106 meq/L (96–106 mmol/L).

Cholesterol: [S or P] 150–220 mg/dL (3.9–5.72 mmol/L). (See Lipid fractions, below.)

Cholesteryl esters: [S] 65–75% of total cholesterol.

CO_2 content: [S or P] 24–29 meq/L (24–29 mmol/L).

Complement: [S] C3 ($β_{1C}$), 90–250 mg/dL. C4 ($β_{1E}$), 10–60 mg/dL. Total (CH_{50}), 75–160 mg/dL.

Copper: [S or P] 100–200 μg/dL (16–31 μmol/L).

Cortisol: [P] 8:00 AM, 5–25 μg/dL (138–690 nmol/L); 8:00 PM, < 10 μg/dL (275 nmol/L).

Creatine kinase (CK): [S] 10–50 IU/L at 30 °C.

Creatine kinase isoenzymes: BB, 0%; MB, 0–3%; MM, 97–100%.

Creatinine: [S or P] 0.6–1.2 mg/dL (50–110 μmol/L).

Cyanocobalamin: [S] 200 pg/mL (148 pmol/L).

Epinephrine: [P] Supine, < 100 pg/mL (< 550 pmol/L).

Ferritin: [S] Adult women, 20–120 ng/mL; men, 30–300 ng/mL. Children to 15 years, 7–140 ng/mL.

Folic acid: [S] 2–20 ng/mL (4.5–45 nmol/L). [RBC] > 140 ng/mL (> 318 nmol/L).

Glucose: [S or P] 65–110 mg/dL (3.6–6.1 mmol/L).

Glucose tolerance: See Chapter 21.

γ-Glutamyl transpeptidase: [S] < 30 units/L at 30°C.

Haptoglobin: [S] 40–170 mg of hemoglobin-binding capacity.

Hemoglobin A_{1c}: [B] See Chapter 21.

Iron: [S] 50–175 μg/dL (9–31 μmol/L).

Iron-binding capacity: [S] Total, 250–410 μg/dL (44.7–73.4 μmol/L). Percent saturation, 20–55%.

Lactate: [B, special handling] Venous, 4–16 mg/dL (0.44–1.8 mmol/L).

Lactatedehydrogenase (LDH): [S] 55–140 IU/L at 30 °C; SMA, 100–225 IU/L at 37 °C; SMAC, 60–200 IU/L at 37 °C. (Varies with method.)

Lipase: [S] < 150 units/L.

Lipid fractions: [S or P] Desirable levels: HDL cholesterol, > 50 mg/dL; LDL cholesterol, < 140 mg/dL; VLDL cholesterol, < 40 mg/dL. (To convert to mmol/L, multiply by 0.026.)

Lipids, total: [S] 450–1000 mg/dL (4.5–10 g/L).

Magnesium: [S or P] 1.8–3 mg/dL (0.75–1.25 mmol/L).

Norepinephrine: [P] Supine, < 500 pg/L (< 3 nmol/L).

Osmolality: [S] 280–296 mosm/kg water (280–296 mmol/kg water).

Oxygen:
Capacity: [B] 16–24 vol%. Values vary with hemoglobin concentration.
Arterial content: [B] 15–23 vol%. Values vary with hemoglobin concentration.
Arterial % saturation: 94–100% of capacity.
Arterial Po_2(Pao_2): 80–100 mm Hg (10.67–13.33 kPa (sea level). Values vary with age.

$PaCO_2$: [B, arterial] 35–45 mm Hg (4.7–6 kPa).

pH (reaction): [B, arterial] 7.35–7.45 ([H^+] 44.7–45.5 nmol/L).

Phosphatase, acid: [S] 1–5 units (King-Armstrong), 0.1–0.63 units (Bessey-Lowry).

Phosphatase, alkaline: [S] Adults, 5–13 units (King-Armstrong), 0.8–2.3 units (Bessey-Lowry); SMA, 30–85 IU/L at 37 °C; SMAC, 30–115 IU/L at 37 °C.

Phospholipid: [S] 145–200 mg/dL (1.45–2 g/L).

Phosphorus, inorganic: [S, fasting] 3–4.5 mg/dL (1–1.5 mmol/L).

Potassium: [S or P] 3.5–5 meq/L (3.5–5 mmol/L).

Protein:
Total: [S] 6–8 g/dL (60–80 g/L).
Albumin: [S] 3.5–5.5 g/dL (35–55 g/L).
Globulin: [S] 2–3.6 g/dL (20–36 g/L).
Fibrinogen: [P] 0.2–0.6 g/dL (2–6 g/L).
Separation by electrophoresis: Albumin, 52–68%; α_1-globulin, 2.4–4.4%; α_2-globulin, 6.1–10.1%; β-globulin, 8.5–14.5%; γ-globulin, 10–21%.

Pyruvate: [B] 0.6–1 mg/dL (70–114 μmol/L.

Serotonin: [B] 5–20 μg/dL (0.3–1.15 μmol/L).

Sodium: [S or P] 136–145 meq/L (136–145 mmol/L).

Specific gravity: [B] 1.056 (varies with hemoglobin and protein concentrations). [S] 1.0254–1.0288 (varies with protein concentration).

Sulfate: [S or P] As sulfur, 0.5–1.5 mg/dL (156–468 mmol/L).

Transferrin: [S] 200–400 mg/dL (23–45 μmol/L).

Triglycerides: [S] < 165 mg/dL (1.9 mmol/L). (See Lipid fractions, above.)

Urea nitrogen: [S or P] 8–20 mg/dL (2.9–7.1 mmol/L).

Uric acid: [S or P] Men, 3–9 mg/dL (0.18–0.54 mmol/L); women, 2.5–7.5 mg/dL (0.15–0.45 mmol/L).

Vitamin A: [S] 15–60 μg/dL (0.53–2.1 μmol/L).

Vitamin B$_{12}$: [S] > 200 pg/mL (> 148 pmol/L).

Vitamin D: [S]
  25-Hydroxycholecalciferol, 8–55 ng/mL (19.4–137 nmol/L)
  1,25-Dihydroxycholecalciferol, 26–65 pg/mL (62–155 pmol/L)
  24,25-Dihydroxycholecalciferol, 1–5 ng/mL (2.4–12 nmol/L)

Volume, blood (Evans blue dye method): Adults, 2990–6980 mL. Women, 46.3–85.5 mL/kg; men, 66.2–97.7 mL/kg.

Zinc: [S] 50–150 μg/dL (7.65–22.95 μmol/L).

HORMONES, SERUM OR PLASMA

Pituitary:
  Growth hormone (GH): [S] Adults, 1–10 ng/mL (46–465 pmol/L[by RIA).
  Thyroid-stimulating hormone (TSH): [S] < 10 μU/mL.
  Follicle-stimulating hormone (FSH): [S] Prepubertal, 2–12 mIU/mL; adult men, 1–15 mIU/mL; adult women, 1–30 mIU/mL; castrate or postmenopausal, 30–200 mIU/mL (by RIA).
  Luteinizing hormone (LH): [S] Prepubertal, 2–12 mIU/mL; adult men, 1–15 mIU/mL; adult women, < 30 mIU/mL; castrated or postmenopausal women, > 30 mIU/mL.
  Corticotropin (ACTH): [P] 8:00–10:00 AM, up to 20–100 pg/mL (4–22 pmol/L).
  Prolactin: [S] 1–25 ng/mL (0.4–10 nmol/L).
  Somatomedin C: [P] 0.4–2 U/mL.
  Antidiuretic hormone (ADH; vasopressin): [P] Serum osmolality 285 mosm/kg, 0–2 pg/mL; serum osmolality > 290 mosm/kg, 2–12 pg/mL or more.

Adrenal:
  Aldosterone: [P] Supine, normal salt intake, 2–9 ng/dL (56–250 pmol/L); increased when upright.
  Cortisol: [S] 8:00 AM, 5–25 μg/dL (14–69 μmol/L); 8:00 PM, < 10 μg/dL (28 μmol/L).

Deoxycortisol: [S] After metyrapone, > 7 μg/dL (> 20 μmol/L).
Dopamine: [P] < 135 pg/mL.
Epinephrine: [P] < 0.1 ng/mL (< 0.55 nmol/L).
Norepinephrine: [P] < 0.5 μg/L (< 3 nmol/L).
See also Miscellaneous Normal Values, below, for values in urine.

Thyroid:
  Thyroxine, free (FT$_4$): [S] 0.8–2.4 ng/dL (10–30 pmol/L).
  Thyroxine, total (TT$_4$): [S] 5–12 μg/dL (65–156 nmol/L) (by RIA).
  Thyroxine-binding globulin capacity: [S] 12–28 μg T$_4$/dL (150–360 nmol T$_4$/L).
  Triiodothyronine (T$_3$): [S] 80–220 ng/dL (1.2–3.3 nmol/L).
  Reverse triiodothyronine (rT$_3$): [S] 30–80 ng/dL (0.45–1.2 nmol/L).
  Triiodothyronine uptake (RT$_3$U): [S] 25–36%; as TBG assessment (RT$_3$U ratio), 0.85–1.15.
  Calcitonin: [S] < 100 pg/mL (< 100 ng/L).

Parathyroid: Parathyroid hormone levels vary with method and antibody. Correlate with serum calcium.

Islets:
  Insulin: [S] 4–25 μU/mL (29–181 pmol/L).
  C-peptide: [S] 0.9–4.2 ng/mL.
  Glucagon; [S, fasting] 20–100 pg/mL (20–100 μg/L).

Stomach:
  Gastrin: [S, special handling] Up to 100 pg/mL (47 pmol/L). Elevated, > 200 pg/mL (> 94 pmol/L).
  Pepsinogen I: [S] 25–100 ng/mL.

Kidney:
  Renin activity: [P, special handling] Normal sodium intake: Supine, 1–3 ng/mL/h; standing, 3–6 ng/mL/h. Sodium-depleted: Supine, 2–6 ng/mL/h; standing, 3–20 ng/mL/h (1 ng/mL/h = 2.778 ng/(L·s).

Gonad:
  Testosterone, free: [S] Men, 10–30 ng/dL; women, 0.3–2 ng/dL. (1 ng/dL = 0.035 nmol/L.)
  Testosterone, total: [S] Prepubertal, < 100 ng/dL; adult men, 300–1000 ng/dL; adult women, 20–80 ng/dL; luteal phase, up to 120 ng/dL.
  Estradiol (E$_2$): [S, special handling] Men, 12–34 pg/mL; women, menstrual cycle 1–10 days, 24–68 pg/mL; 11–20 days, 50–300 pg/mL; 21–30 days, 73–149 pg/mL (by RIA). (1 pg/mL = 3.6 pmol/L.)
  Progesterone: [S] Follicular phase, 0.2–1.5 mg/mL; luteal phase, 6–32 ng/mL; pregnancy, >

24 ng/mL; men, < 1 ng/mL. (1 ng/mL = 3.2 nmol/L.)

Placenta:

Estriol (E_3): [S] Men and nonpregnant women, < 0.2 μg/dL (< 7 nmol/L) (by RIA).

Chorionic gonadotropin: [S] Beta subunit: Men, < 9 mIU/mL; pregnant women after implantation, > 10 mIU/mL. (1 mIU/mL = 1 IU/L.)

NORMAL CEREBROSPINAL FLUID VALUES

Appearance: Clear and colorless.

Cells: Adults, 0–5 mononuclears/μL; infants, 0–20 mononuclears/μL.

Glucose: 50–85 mg/dL (2.8–4.7 mmol/L). (Draw serum glucose at same time.)

Pressure (reclining): Newborns, 30–90 mm water; children, 50–100 mm water; adults, 70–200 mm water (average = 125 mm water).

Proteins: Total, 20–45 mg/dL (0.2–0.45 g/L) in lumbar cerebrospinal fluid. IgG, 2–6 mg/dL (0.02–0.06 g/L).

Specific gravity: 1.003–1.008.

RENAL FUNCTION TESTS

p-Aminohippurate (PAH) clearance (RPF): Men, 560–830 mL/min; women, 490–700 mL/min.

Creatinine clearance, endogenous (GFR): Approximates inulin clearance (see below).

Filtration fraction (FF): Men, 17–21%; women, 17–23%. (FF = GFR/RPF.)

Inulin clearance (GFR): Men, 110–150 mL/min; women, 105–132 mL/min (corrected to 1.73 m^2 surface area). (Divide by 60 = mL/s.)

Maximal glucose reabsorptive capacity (Tm_G): Men, 300–450 mg/min; women, 250–350 mg/min.

Maximal PAH excretory capacity (Tm PAH): 80–90 mg/min.

Osmolality: On normal diet and fluid intake: Range 500–850 mosm/kg water. Achievable range, normal kidney: Dilution 40–80 mosm; concentration (dehydration) up to 1400 mosm/kg water (at least 3–4 times plasma osmolality).

Specific gravity of urine: 1.003–1.030.

MISCELLANEOUS NORMAL VALUES

Adrenal hormones and metabolites:

Aldosterone: [U] 2–26 μg/24 h (5.5–72 nmol/d). Values vary with sodium and potassium intake.

Catecholamines: [U] Total, < 100 μg/24 h. Epinephrine, < 10 μg/24 h (< 55 nmol/d); norepinephrine, < 100 μg/24 h (< 590 nmol/d). Values vary with method used.

Cortisol, free: [U] 20–100 μg/24 h (0.55–2.76 μmol).

11,17-Hydroxycorticoids: [U] Men, 4–12 mg/24 h; women, 4–8 mg/24 h. Values vary with method used.

17-Ketosteroids: [U] Under 8 years, 0–2 mg/24 h; adolescents, 2–20 mg/24 h. Men, 10–20 mg/24 h; women, 5–15 mg/24 h. Values vary with method used. (1 mg = 3.5 μmol.)

Metanephrine: [U] < 1.3 mg/24 h (< 6.6 μmol/d) or < 2.2 μg/mg creatinine. Values vary with method used.

Vanillylmandelic acid (VMA): [U] Up to 7 mg/24 h (< 35 μmol).

Fecal fat: Less than 30% dry weight.

Lead: [U] < 80 μg/24 h (< 0.4 μmol/d).

Porphyrins:

Delta-aminolevulinic acid: [U] 1.5–7.5 mg/24 h (11–57 μmol).

Coproporphyrin: [U] < 230 μg/24 h (< 350 nmol).

Uroporphyrin: [U] < 50 μg/24 h (< 60 nmol).

Porphobilinogen: [U] < 2 mg/24 h (< 8.8 μmol).

Urobilinogen: [U] 0–2.5 mg/24 h (< 4.2 μmol).

Urobilinogen, fecal: 40–280 mg/24 h (70–470 μmol).

Index

NOTE: Page numbers in bold face type indicate a major discussion. A *t* following a page number indicates tabular material and an *i* following a page number indicates an illustration. Drugs are listed under their generic names. When a drug trade name is listed, the reader is referred to the generic name.

biopsy of, 490
diseases of, **486–503**. *See also* Breast cancer
  nipple discharge in, differential diagnosis
    of, 502–503
  fat necrosis of, 503
  fibroadenoma of, 502
  fibrocystic disease of, 501–502
    breast cancer and, 486
  inspection of, 487–488
  male
    carcinoma of, **500–501**
    enlargement of, 790–791
  palpation of, 488
  physical examination of
    in cancer screening, 11*t*
    in elderly, 23
  reconstruction of, 496
  self-examination of, in cancer screening,
    11*t*, 491
Breast cancer, **486–501**
  adjuvant therapy in, 494–495
  advanced, **498–500**
  arm edema and, 495–496
  bilateral, 489
  biopsy in, 490
  chemotherapy in, 43*t*
    adjuvant, 494–495
    in advanced disease, 499
  clinical findings in, 487–491
  cytology in, 491
  differential diagnosis of, 491
  early detection of, 491
  follow-up care in, 495–496
  frequency of by anatomic site, 488*i*
  histologic types of, 492*t*
  and hormone receptor sites, 492
  hormone therapy in
    adjuvant, 494–495
    in advanced disease, 498–499
  imaging for metastasis in, 490
  incidence of, 37*t*
  inflammatory, 489
  laboratory findings in, 489–490
  during lactation, 489
  local recurrence of, 495
  malignant pleural effusion in, 499
  mammography in, 490
  mastectomy in
    radiation therapy and, 493–494
    radical, 493
    recommendations for, 494
    reconstructive surgery and, 496
    types of, 493–494
  in men, **500–501**
  Paget's, 489
    nipple erosion in, 488
  paraneoplastic syndromes associated with,
    38*t*
  pathologic types of, 491–492
  during pregnancy, 489, 549–550
  pregnancy risks and, 496
  prognosis for, 496
  radiation therapy in
    in advanced disease, 498
    and mastectomy, 493–494
  risk factors associated with, 486*t*
  screening programs for, 486–487, 491
    physical examination and, 11*t*, 491
  self-examination in detection of, 11*t*, 491
  signs of, 487–489
  staging of, 487
  symptoms of, 487, 488*t*
  treatment of
    curative, 492–493
    palliative, **498–500**
Breast feeding, **552–554**
  breast abscess and, 503

breast cancer during, 489
drug effects and, 552, 553*t*
oral contraceptive use and, 527
Breath sounds, 150
  in heart disease, 223
Breathing disorders, sleep-related, **209–210**
Brenner tumor, of ovary, 519*t*
Brethaire. *See* Terbutaline
Brethine. *See* Terbutaline
Bretylium, in arrhythmias, 278*t*
Brevibacterium, and tinea pedis, 87
Bricanyl. *See* Terbutaline
Brill's disease, 970, 971
Briquet's syndrome, 754
Brittle bones, **616–617**
Brodifacoum, poisoning with, 1157–1158
Bromocriptine
  for lactation suppression, 554
  nursing infant affected by, 553*t*
  ovulation induced by, 524
  in panhypopituitarism, 796
  in parkinsonism, 704–705
Brompheniramine, in allergic disorders, 574*t*
Bronchi
  foreign body in, 145–146
  obstruction of, 168
Bronchial adenomas, 187–188
Bronchial breath sounds, 150
Bronchial carcinoid tumors, **187–188**
Bronchial hygiene, in chronic obstructive pulmonary disease, 164
Bronchial provocation testing, in asthma, 157
Bronchiectasis, **168–169**
Bronchiolitis, **169–170**, 965
  obliterans, 169–170
    with organizing pneumonia, 170
    in silo-filler's disease, 206
  respiratory, 170
Bronchioloalveolar cell carcinoma, 182
Bronchitis
  antimicrobial therapy for, 1093*t*
  asthmatic, 156
  chronic, 162
    versus emphysema, 163*t*
  industrial, 206
Bronchoalveolar lavage
  in immunocompromised host, 176–177
  in interstitial lung disease, 190
Bronchocentric granulomatosis, **169**
Bronchodilators
  in asthma, 157, 158*t*
  in chronic obstructive pulmonary disease,
    158*t*, 164
Bronchogenic carcinoma, **182–185**. *See also*
  Lungs, cancer of
  paraneoplastic syndromes associated with,
    38*t*, 183
Bronchogenic cysts, **154–155**
  radiographic and clinical features of, 189*t*
Broncholithiasis, **170–171**
Bronchophony, 150
Bronchoprovocation testing, 573
Bronchopulmonary aspergillosis, allergic, **168**,
  1084
  treatment of, 575
Bronchopulmonary sequestration, **154**
Bronchoscopy, 153–154
  in pneumonia, 174
Bronchovesicular breath sounds, 150
Bronkometer. *See* Isoetharine
Bronkosol. *See* Isoetharine
Brown recluse spider bites, 93, 1171
Brown tumor of jaw, 822
Brown-Séquard syndrome, 715
Brucella
  abortus, 993
    bone infection caused by, 605

drugs for infections with, 1090*t*
  melitensis, 993
  suis, 993
Brucellosis, **993–994**
Bruch's membrane, degeneration of, 112–113
Brudzinski sign, in meningococcal meningitis,
  986
Brugia
  malayi, 1069
    drugs for infections with, 1054*t*
  timori, 1069
Bruits
  in cerebrovascular occlusive disease, 321
  in heart disease, 223
Brunsting-Perry variant, of cicatricial pemphi-
  goid, 68
Bruxism, earache and, 128
Bubo, in plague, 995
Buccal erythema, anticancer agents causing,
  49
Budd-Chiari syndrome, **470**
Buerger's disease, **324–325**
  Raynaud's disease/phenomenon differenti-
    ated from, 325, 327
Buffalo hump, in Cushing's syndrome, 788,
  833
Buffers, in hydrogen ion concentration regula-
  tion, 625
Bulbar palsy, progressive, 716
Bulimarexia, **908**
Bulimia, **908**
Bulk-forming laxatives, 398–399
Bullae
  drugs causing, 60
  in pemphigus, 67
  skin disorders characterized by, **68**
Bullous pemphigoid, 68
Bundle branch block, 287, 288
Bupropion, 741, 741*t*
  side effects of, 742
Burkitt's lymphoma, 374, 967
  chromosomal aberration and, 1190, 1190*t*
Burn team, 1137
Burns, **1132–1137**
  and body surface estimation, 1132
  classification of, 1132–1134
  electrical, 1133, 1137–1138
  fluid resuscitation in, 1135–1136
  initial management of, 1134–1135
  patient support in, 1137
  smoke inhalation and, 203
  wound care in, 1136
  and zones of tissue death, 1136*i*
Bursa of Fabricius, 558
Bursitis, **615**
Buruli ulcer, 1002
Buschke-Lowenstein giant condylomas, human
  papilloma virus and, 79
Buspar. *See* Buspirone
Buspirone, 743, 744*t*
Busulfan, 45*t*
  in chronic myeloid leukemia, 368
  dosage of, 45*t*
  toxicity of, 45*t*, 50
Butterfly rash
  in chronic discoid lupus erythematosus,
    76
  in polymyositis-dermatomyositis, 588
  in systemic lupus erythematosus, 584
Butyrophenones, 734–735, 734*t*
  movement disorders caused by, 708
Bypass grafting
  arterial
    in occlusive disease of aorta and iliac arte-
      ries, 317

Bypass grafting (*cont.*)
  arterial (*cont.*)
    in occlusive disease of femoral and popli-
      teal arteries, 317–318
    coronary artery, 263–264
Byssinosis, 206

C3
  in anti-glomerular basement membrane dis-
    ease, 641, 646
  in glomerulonephritis, 641
  in IgA nephropathy, 646
  in poststreptococcal glomerulonephritis, 642
  in rapidly progressive glomerulonephritis,
    647
c-myc gene, in non-Hodgkin's lymphoma, 374
C-peptide
  failure to suppress, in insulinoma, 882
  normal values of, 1205
CA19–9, in pancreatic cancer, 484
CABG. *See* Coronary artery bypass grafting
Cadmium, adverse effects and sources of, 202*t*
Café au lait spots, in neurofibromatosis, 702
"Café coronary," 204
Cafergot, in migraine, 678
Caffeine
  abuse of, 777
  in mammary dysplasia, 501
  nursing infant affected by, 553*t*
CAGE screening test for alcoholism, 11*t*
Caisson disease, **1142**
Calabar swellings, in loiasis, 1072
Calcareous tendinitis, scapulohumeral, 612
Calcifediol, in hypoparathyroidism, 821*t*
Calciferol, in renal osteodystrophy, 649
Calcimar. *See* Calcitonin
Calcitonin, 819
  normal values of, 1205
  in osteoporosis, 827
  in Paget's disease, 829
  in thyroid disorders, 805
Calcitriol
  in hypoparathyroidism, 821*t*
  in renal osteodystrophy, 649
Calcium, **630–631**
  characteristics of, 898*t*
  corticosteroid therapy and, 850
  defects of absorption of, 656
  deficit of, 631
  dietary recommendations for, 900*t*
  dietary supplementation of, 915
  excess of, 630–631
  intracellular, in hypertension, 245
  ionized, normal values of, 1203
  normal values of, 1203
  oral, for emergency treatment of hypopara-
    thyroid tetany, 821
  parathyroid gland secretion in homeostasis
    of, 819
  in pregnancy, 537
  RDA for, 895*t*
  in renal insufficiency, 647
  renal stone formation and, 665–666
Calcium antagonists. *See also* Calcium channel
    blockers
  overdose of, **1159**
Calcium bilirubinate, in gallstones, 473
Calcium carbonate, in peptic ulcers, 423
Calcium channel blockers. *See also* Calcium
    antagonists
  in angina pectoris, 262–263, 262*t*
  in hypertension, 249, 250*t*, 252
  in migraine, 678
  in psychiatric disorders, 745
  in unstable angina, 265

Calcium disodium edetate, in lead poisoning,
    1163
  challenge test and, 1163–1164
Calcium gluconate, for emergency treatment
    of hypoparathyroid tetany, 821
Calcium oxalate, renal stone formation and,
    666, 667
Calcium pyrophosphate dehydrate deposition
    disease, **598**
Calderol. *See* Calcifediol
Calendar method of contraception, 530
California encephalitis, 960*t*
Callosities (of feet or toes), **75–76**
  in diabetes mellitus or vascular disturbances,
    866
Calories
  dietary restriction of, 914*t*
  physical activities using, 896*t*
  in pregnancy, 537
Calymmatobacterium granulomatis, 998
Camalox. *See* Calcium carbonate
Camoquin. *See* Amodiaquine
Campylobacter
  diarrhea and gastroenteritis caused by, 932,
    933*t*, 934
  drugs for infections with, 1090*t*
  jejuni
    colitis caused by, 442
    diarrhea and gastroenteritis caused by,
      400, 932, 933*t*
    proctocolitis caused by, 451
    Reiter's syndrome following infection with,
      600
Cancer, **36–53**. *See also specific type*
  bacterial sepsis and, 40–41
  carcinoid syndrome and, 41
  chromosomal analysis and, 1189–1190
  chromosome instability and, 1190
  chronic effects of radiation and, 1140
  emergency complications of, management
    of, 37–41
  fever and hyperthermia caused by, 19
  fever of unknown origin and, 922–923
  human papilloma virus and, 79
  hypercalcemia and, 39–40, 823–824
  hyperuricemia and, 40
  incidence of most common types of, 37*t*
  malignant effusions and, 38–39
  neuropathy and, 720
  nonmetastatic neurologic complications of,
    700–701
  oral contraceptive use and, 526–527
  paraneoplastic syndromes and, 36–37
  prevention of, **10–11**
  primary treatment of, 41–42
  radiation therapy for, 41–42
  rheumatic manifestations of, 617
  risk factors for, 2*t*
  spinal cord compression and, 37–38
  surgery for, 41–42
  systemic therapy for, 42–52. *See also* Cancer
    chemotherapy
  thrombosis in, 392
  urate nephropathy and, 40
Cancer checkup, for screening, 11*t*
Cancer chemotherapy, **42–52**. *See also specific*
    agent and specific type of cancer
  adjuvant, 47–48
    in breast cancer, 494–495
      in men, 500
  in breast cancer
    in advanced disease, 499
    curative, 494–495
    in men, 500
    for postmenopausal women, 495*t*
    for premenopausal women, 494*t*
  cancers responsive to, 43–44*t*

  combination, in breast cancer, 494–495, 499
  eyes affected by, 120*t*
  in hydatidiform mole, 544
  and mechanisms of action of agents, 44–
    47
  nursing infant affected by, 553*t*
  renal stone formation and, 666
  single-agent dosage for, 45–46*t*
  and toxicity of agents, 45–46*t*, 48–51
  and tumor response evaluation, 51–52
Candida
  in acute leukemia, 370
  albicans, 1080
    keratitis caused by, 1087
    in sputum samples, 173
    vaginitis caused by
      clinical findings in, 508
      treatment of, 508
  dacryocystitis caused by, 106
  esophagitis caused by, 414
  neutropenia and, 363
  onychomycosis caused by, **89**, 90, 100
  oral infection with, 90, 409–410
  parapsilosis, 1080
  tropicalis, 1080
Candidiasis, **1080–1081**
  in AIDS, 148, 409, 944, 946, 947*t*, 1080
  hepatic, 471
  in hypoparathyroidism, 819, 849
  mucocutaneous, **90–91**, 409
  oral, 90, **409–410**
    in AIDS, 148, 409, 944, 1080
  in tetracycline therapy, 1106
Canker sore, **408**
Cannabinoids, in chemotherapy-induced nau-
    sea and vomiting, 49, 397
Cannabis. *See also* Cannabinoids; Tetrahydro-
    cannabinol
  abuse of, 776
  nursing infant affected by, 553*t*
Cantharellus mushrooms, poisoning caused
    by, 1166
Cantharidin, for warts, 80
Cantharone. *See* Cantharidin
Capillaria philippinensis, drugs for infections
    with, 1054*t*
Capillariasis, intestinal, drugs for treatment of,
    1054*t*
Capillary morphometry, in diabetes mellitus,
    857
Capillary wedge pressure, pulmonary, in
    shock, 341
Caplan's syndrome, 205
Capnocytophaga canimorsus, in bite wounds,
    929
Capsulitis, adhesive, of shoulder, **612–613**
Capsulotendinous cuff, inflammation of, 612
Captopril
  in heart failure, 296
  in hypertension, 250*t*, 252
  in hypertensive crises, 254*t*
  nutrient absorption and metabolism affected
    by, 899*t*
Carafate. *See* Sucralfate
Carbamates, poisoning with, 1167–1168
Carbamazepine
  and antipsychotic drug interactions, 735*t*
  overdose of, hemoperfusion in treatment of,
    1152*t*
  in psychiatric disorders, 745
  for seizures, 681*t*
Carbapenems, 1104
Carbaryl, poisoning with, 1167–1168
Carbenicillin, 1098–1099
  in patients with renal or hepatic failure, 1094*t*
Carbidopa, in parkinsonism, 704
Carbimazole, in hyperthyroidism, 812

keratitis caused by, 108
opportunistic infections caused by, 1087–1088
pulmonary alveolar proteinosis caused by, 193
skin infections caused by, **84–91**
in AIDS, 946
Funguria, candidal, 1080
FUO. *See* Fever of unknown origin
Furazolidone, in giardiasis, 1035
Furosemide
in hypertension, 249
in hypertensive crises, 254*t*
Furoxone. *See* Furazolidone
Furuncle (furunculosis), **82–83**, 979
antimicrobial therapy for, 1093*t*
Fusarium
keratitis caused by, 1087
opportunistic infections caused by, 1087
Fusobacterium nucleatum, and anaerobic pneumonia, 176

G6PD deficiency. *See* Glucose–6–phosphate dehydrogenase deficiency
⁶⁷Ga, nursing infant affected by, 553*t*
GABHS. *See* Pharyngitis, streptococcal
Gait
in parkinsonism, 703
unstable, in elderly, **29–30**
Galerina mushrooms, poisoning caused by, 1165
Gallbladder
carcinoma of, 479
diseases of, oral contraceptive use and, 527
gangrene of, 474
surgery of, during pregnancy, 550
Gallium scan, 1202
Gallops, 224
Gallstones, **473**
Gamete intra-fallopian tube transfer, 525
Gamma-chain disease, 558
Gamma-globulin
in alcoholic hepatitis, 462
in cirrhosis, 465
in hepatitis A, 458
in infantile X-linked agammaglobulinemia, 562
in infection in immunocompromised patient, 925
in rheumatoid arthritis, 595
in severe combined immunodeficiency, 563
Gamma-glutamyl transferase test, in alcoholism, 773
Gamma-glutamyl transpeptidase, normal values of, 1204
Gamma-interferon, 560*t*
Gammopathies, **557–558**. *See also specific type*
benign monoclonal, 557
neuropathy in, 719
Ganciclovir, in cytomegalovirus infection, 956, 1122
Gangliosidosis, 1184*t*
Gangrene
bacterial synergistic, 1000
gas, 981–982
drug treatment for, 1090*t*
of toes or feet, 319
in diabetics, 873
Ganja, abuse of, 776
Gardnerella, vaginosis caused by, 508
Gas gangrene, 981–982
drug treatment for, 1090*t*
Gases
gastrointestinal, **399–400**
inhalation of, 778

Gasoline, poisoning with, **1168–1169**
Gastrectomy
afferent (blind) loop syndrome after, 427–428
bile reflux after, 428
dumping syndrome after, 427
gastritis after, 420
hypoglycemia following, 883
miscellaneous complications of, 428
stomach cancer after, 428
Gastric acid
reduction of, in upper gastrointestinal hemorrhage, 403
reflux of, esophagitis caused by, 412–414
Gastric bypass, in obesity, 906
Gastric contents
acute aspiration of, 204
chronic aspiration of, 204
Gastric emptying, 1200
Gastric lavage, in poisoning and drug overdose, 1151–1152
Gastric resection, gastritis after, 420
Gastric ulcers, 426–427
gastritis and, 420
stomach cancer and, 428
in stressed noneating patient, 420
Gastrin
cells secreting, 841
in multiple endocrine neoplasia, 848
normal values of, 1205
in Zollinger-Ellison syndrome, 425
Gastrinoma, 425–426
and carcinoma of pancreas, 484
Gastritis, **419–421**
atrophic
in pernicious anemia, 351
stomach cancer and, 428
stomach cancer and, 428
Gastroenteritis
acute, **932**, 933*t*
antimicrobial therapy for, 1093*t*
appendicitis differentiated from, 440
Salmonella, 932, 933*t*, 934, 991–992
Gastrointestinal bleeding scan, 1199–1200
Gastrointestinal gas, **399–400**
Gastrointestinal system. *See also specific structure*
age-related changes in, 22*t*
anticancer drugs affecting, 49
barium radiology of
enema, **1194–1195**
upper, **1193–1194**
decontamination of, **1151–1153**
diseases of, **396–453**. *See also specific type*
in AIDS patients, 944–945
nuclear medicine studies in, 1199–1200
fever and hyperthermia caused by disorders of, 19
hemorrhage in
lower, **404–405**
nuclear medicine studies in, 1199–1200
peptic ulcer causing, 422
upper, **402–404**
late syphilitic lesions of, 1014
mushrooms irritating, 1165–1166, 1166*t*
stimulants of, in reflux esophagitis, 413
tetracyclines affecting, 1106
Gastrojejunostomy, afferent (blind) loop syndrome after, 427–428
Gastroparesis, in diabetes, 873
Gastropathy, in AIDS patients, 945
Gastroplasty, in obesity, 906
Gastrostomies, for tube feedings, 916–917
Gaze-evoked nystagmus, 104
GCSF. *See* Granulocyte colony-stimulating factor
Gellhorn pessary, in uterine prolapse, 517

Gemfibrozil, 890–891, 892*t*
Gender identity disorders, 757
treatment of, 758–759
Gene map, human, 1175, 1176*i*
Gene probe, 1186, 1187*t*
Genes, 1174, **1175–1176**
in familes, 1178–1180
immune response, 566
immunoglobulin, 556
in individuals, 1177–1178
tumor suppressor, 1189
Genetic code, 1177
Genetic compound, 1179
Genetic counseling, and sickle cell anemia, 357
Genetic disorders, prenatal diagnosis of, 1187–1189
indications for, 1188–1189
Genetic instability, 1190
Genetic sex, 1183
Genetics
biochemical, **1183–1185**
medical, **1174–1190**
introduction to, 1174–1181
techniques of, 1181–1190
molecular, 1186–1187
Genital warts
perianal, 452
vaginal, 508
treatment of, 508–509
Genitourinary tract
age-related changes in, 22*t*
anaerobic infection in in females, 1000
disorders of, **638–676**. *See also specific type*
and falls in elderly, 30
nonspecific manifestations of, 638–639
nuclear medicine studies in, 1200–1201
radiographic examination of, 640
tuberculosis of, **663–664**
tumors of, **671–675**
ultrasound examination of, 640
Genotype, 1174
Gentamicin, 1109
cost of, 1096*t*
dosage of, 1107, 1108*t*, 1109
Geriatric medicine, **21–35**. *See also* Aging; Elderly patients
five *I*'s of, **25–33**
Geriatric psychiatric disorders, **781–783**
German measles. *See* Rubella
Germinal mutation, 1176
Gerstmann's syndrome, in parietal lobe lesions, 697–698
Gestalt test, Bender, 733
Gestational diabetes, 546, 874
Gestational trophoblastic neoplasia, **543–544**
GFR. *See* Glomerular filtration rate
GH. *See* Growth hormone
Ghon focus, in tuberculosis, 178
Giant cell arteritis, **591–592**
headache and, 679
Giant cell thyroiditis, 817
Giant cell tumors of bone, 616
Giant condylomata, human papilloma virus and, 79
Giardia lamblia, 1034
diarrhea caused by, 400
Giardiasis, **1034–1035**
Gigantism, **796–798**
"cerebral," 788
Gilbert's syndrome, 463*t*
Gilles de la Tourette's syndrome, 708
Gingiva, abnormal pigmentation of, **411**
Gingivectomy, 407
Gingivitis, 407
in AIDS, 148, 407, 944
necrotizing ulcerating, **407**

Struma
  lymphomatosa (Hashimoto's thyroiditis), 817
    treatment of, 818
  ovarii, hyperthyroidism and, 810
Strychnine, seizures caused by, 1150*t*
Stupor, **711–713**. *See also* Coma
  metabolic disturbances causing, 712–713
  structural lesions causing, 712
Sturge-Weber syndrome, 702
Sty, 105
Subacute cerebellar degeneration, lung cancer and, 183*t*
Subacute combined degeneration of spinal cord, **711**
Subacute sclerosing panencephalitis, 969
  measles and, 954
  myoclonus in, 707
Subarachnoid hemorrhage, 692–693
  headache caused by, 680
Subareolar abscess, 503
Subclavian steal syndrome, 611
  transient vertebrobasilar ischemia caused by, 687
Subcortical arteriosclerotic encephalopathy, 26
Subcutaneous nodules
  in acute rheumatic fever, 230–231
  in rheumatoid arthritis, 579
Subdural hematoma
  and confusion in elderly, 27
  falls in elderly causing, 30
Subdural hemorrhage, 696, 714*t*
  chronic, 714
Suberosis, 206*t*
Subglottic hemangioma, 143
Subluxation, atlantoaxial, 608
Submandibular glands
  sialadenitis affecting, 141, 410
  tumors of, 142
Substance use and abuse, **771–778**. *See also specific agent and* Drug use and abuse
  and counseling patients 13–18 years of age, 3*t*
  and counseling patients 19–39 years of age, 4–5*t*
  and counseling patients 40–64 years of age, 6*t*
  and counseling patients 65 years and over, 7*t*
  prevention of, 11–12
Substitute homes, for psychiatric patients, 748
Subungual capillary pulsations, in aortic regurgitation, 240
Subungual fibromas, in tuberous sclerosis, 701
Subungual hemorrhages, in infective endocarditis, 242
Succinylcholine
  and lithium drug interactions, 739*t*
  and monoamine oxidase inhibitor interactions, 742*t*
Sucralfate, in peptic ulcers, 423
Sucrose hemolysis test, in paroxysmal nocturnal hemoglobinuria, 355
Sucrose-isomaltose intolerance, 438
Sudden death, **257**
  in myocardial infarction, 267
  survivors of, **289–290**
Sugar, dietary recommendations and, 900*t*
Suicide, 765–766
  in elderly, 22, 782
Sulbactam, penicillins combined with, 1099
Sulfacetamide solution, 1113
Sulfadiazine, 1113
Sulfamethoxazole, 1113
Sulfamylon. *See* Mafenide
Sulfasalazine, 1113
  in Crohn's disease, 431

nutrient absorption and metabolism affected by, 899*t*
  in ulcerative colitis, 445
Sulfate, normal values of, 1204
Sulfinpyrazone, in gout, 597
Sulfisoxazole, 1113
Sulfonamides, **1112–1114**
  eyes affected by, 20*t*
  nursing infant affected by, 553*t*
  nutrient absorption and metabolism affected by, 899*t*
  in recurrent rheumatic fever prevention, 231
Sulfones, in leprosy, **1114**
Sulfonylureas, 859–860, 859*t*
  and monoamine oxidase inhibitor interactions, 742*t*
  safety of, 861
  second-generation, 859*t*, 860
Sulfur dioxide, adverse effects and sources of, 202*t*
Sulindac, 18*t*
Summer grippe, 967–968
Sunburn, 61–62
"Sunday neuroses," 751
"Sundowning," 779
Sunlight (ultraviolet light)
  in acne vulgaris treatment, 74
  and cancer prevention, 10
  corneal burns caused by, 118
  drugs causing exaggerated response to, 60
  keratitis caused by, 118
  photodermatitis and, 61–62
  polymorphous sensitivity to, 61–62
  protection from
    and cancer prevention, 10
    and counseling patients 13–18 years of age, 4*t*
    and counseling patients 40–64 years of age, 6*t*
    and counseling patients 65 years and over, 8*t*
Sunscreens, 94
  in photodermatitis, 62
Superficial thrombophlebitis, 334–335
Superior vena cava
  dilatation of, radiographic and clinical features of, 189*t*
  obstruction of, **337**
Support hose
  in deep vein thrombophlebitis, 332
  varicose veins and, 330
Supportive psychotherapy, 747
Suppository
  contraceptive, 529
  glycerin, in constipation, 398
Suppressor T cells, 559
  in AIDS, 564
Suppressor-helper T cell ratio, 559
Suppressor-inducer T cells, 559
Supraclavicular nodes
  palpation of in breast cancer examination, 488
  pathology of, 660
Supraglottitis, 143
  differential diagnosis of, 143*t*
Suprapubic aspiration, for urine specimen collection, 660
Supratentorial arteriovenous malformation, 694
Supratentorial masses, stupor and coma caused by, 712
Supraventricular arrhythmias, **277–283**
Supraventricular beats
  aberrantly conducted, ventricular beats differentiated from, 282
  premature, in myocardial infarction, 271

Supraventricular tachyarrhythmias, in myocardial infarction, 271
Supraventricular tachycardia
  and accessory atrioventricular pathways, 283
  paroxysmal, 279–280
Suramin, in African trypanosomiasis, 1024
Surface antigens
  B cell, 559*t*, 560
  T cell, 559*t*
    receptors for, 560
Surgery
  anxiety disorders before and after, 784
    treatment of, 785
  in cancer treatment, 41–42
Surgery proneness, 784
  treatment of, 785
Surmontil. *See* Trimipramine
SVC. *See* Slow vital capacity
Swallowing, pain or difficulty in. *See* Dysphagia; Odynophagia
"Sweat test," in cystic fibrosis, 166–167
Swimmer's ear, 123–124
"Swimming pool granuloma," 1002
"Swinging light test," 104
Swyer-James syndrome, 170
Sycosis vulgaris, 81–82
Sydenham's chorea, in acute rheumatic fever, 231
Symmer's fibrosis, in schistosomiasis, 1052
Sympathectomy
  in Buerger's disease, 325
  in circulatory insufficiency in foot and toes, 320
  in frostbite, 1129
  in posttraumatic sympathetic dystrophy, 328–329
  in Raynaud's disease/phenomenon, 327
Sympathetic dystrophy
  posttraumatic, **328–329**
  reflex, **615**
Sympathetic nervous system, hyperactivity of, in hypertension, 244
Sympatholytic agents
  in hypertension, 250*t*, 252
  overdose of, 1160
Sympatholytic syndrome, in poisoning and drug overdose, 1153
Sympathomimetic agents
  in allergic disorders, 575
  in asthma, 157–159, 158*t*
  and monoamine oxidase inhibitor interactions, 742*t*
  and tricyclic and cyclic antidepressant drug interactions, 742*t*
Sympathomimetic syndrome, in poisoning and drug overdose, 1153
"Symptothermal" natural family planning, 530
Synarel. *See* Nafarelin
Synchronized intermittent mandatory ventilation, 212
  weaning and, 213
Syncope, **288–289**
  in aortic stenosis, 238
  cardiogenic, 222–223, 289
  falls in elderly caused by, 29
  heat causing, 1130–1131
  neurologic causes of, 686
  orthostatic, 686
    epilepsy differentiated from, 684
  vasomotor, 289
Syndrome of inappropriate antidiuretic hormone secretion, **801**
  cancer and, 38*t*
  confusion in elderly and, 27
  hyponatremia and, 624

REASON*
(Frequency of Symptoms and Signs)

	Percentage		Percentage
Prenatal examination	12.2	Depression	0.3
Abdominal pain, cramps, and spasms	2.3	Painful urination	0.29
Chest pain and related symptoms	2.2	Pain and related symptoms, generalized	0.29
Low back symptoms	1.8	Nasal congestion	0.29
Hypertension	1.78	Fever	0.28
Vaginal discharge and other vaginal		Irregular menses (interval)	0.28
symptoms	1.5	Stomach pain, cramps, and spasms	0.28
Headache, pain in head	1.35	Nausea	0.28
Cough	1.27	Diarrhea	0.27
Throat symptoms	1.18	Symptoms of infertility	0.27
Leg symptoms	1.18	Earache, or ear infection	0.26
Skin rash and other skin lesions	0.95	Menstrual symptoms, unspecified	0.25
Diabetes mellitus	0.94	Cervicitis, vaginitis	0.24
Tiredness, exhaustion	0.9	General ill feeling	0.2
Vertigo and dizziness	0.8	Infections	0.2
Lump or mass in breast	0.7	Labored breathing (dyspnea)	0.2
Pain, no specified reference	0.7	Other growths of skin	0.2
Head cold, upper respiratory infection	0.7	Diseases of the thyroid gland	0.2
Uterine and vaginal bleeding	0.66	Menopausal symptoms	0.19
Amenorrhea and irregular menses	0.66	Carbuncle, furuncle, boil, cellulitis,	
Shortness of breath	0.65	abscess	0.18
Neck symptoms	0.65	Hip symptoms	0.18
Knee symptoms	0.59	Disturbances of sensation	0.17
Anorectum symptoms	0.58	Hemorrhoids	0.17
Weight gain	0.56	Skin irritations, not elsewhere classified	0.15
Foot and toe symptoms	0.55	Ankle symptoms	0.14
Unspecified joint symptoms	0.55	Problems of pregnancy and postpartum	0.14
Shoulder symptoms	0.5	Swelling of skin	0.14
General weakness	0.5	Symptoms of skin moles	0.14
Hand and finger symptoms	0.5	Vulvar disorders	0.14
Ischemic heart disease	0.5	Warts, not otherwise specified	0.13
Hernia of abdominal cavity	0.47	Fractures and dislocations, upper extremity	0.13
Arthritis	0.45	Other diseases of skin	0.13
Abnormal pulsations and palpitations	0.4	Pain or soreness of breast	0.12
Pelvic symptoms (female)	0.4	Other diseases of female reproductive	
Anxiety and nervousness	0.4	system	0.1
Arm symptoms	0.36	Fibroids and other uterine neoplasms	0.1

*This chart and the one on the opposite page are based on the combined "Patterns of Ambulatory Care in Internal Medicine, General Surgery, and Obstetrics and Gynecology," published in the National Ambulatory Medical Care Survey, United States, January 1980– December 1981 (by Beulah K. Cypress), U.S. Department of Health and Human Services, Public Health Service, National Center for Health Statistics, Washington, DC. The study involved 314, 219,000 office visits.